Reproduced by permission of THE BETTMANN ARCHIVE, INC.

Compliments of: W. B. SAUNDERS CO.

EX LIBRIS: *John M. Arnold, M.D.*

PRINCIPLES OF NEUROLOGY

PRINCIPLES OF NEUROLOGY

SECOND EDITION

RAYMOND D. ADAMS, M.A., M.D.
Bullard Professor of Neuropathology, Emeritus, Harvard Medical School
Consultant Neurologist and Formerly Chief of Neurology Service,
Massachusetts General Hospital
Director, Eunice K. Shriver Research Center
Boston, Massachusetts
Médicin Adjoint, L'Hôpital Cantonale de Lausanne
Lausanne, Switzerland

MAURICE VICTOR, M.D.
Professor of Neurology, Case Western Reserve University School of Medicine
Chairman, Department of Neurology, Cleveland Metropolitan General Hospital
Cleveland, Ohio

McGraw-Hill Book Company

New York St. Louis San Francisco Auckland Bogotá Guatemala Hamburg
Johannesburg Lisbon London Madrid Mexico Montreal New Delhi Panama
Paris San Juan São Paulo Singapore Sydney Tokyo Toronto

PRINCIPLES OF NEUROLOGY

Copyright © 1981, 1977 by McGraw-Hill, Inc. All rights reserved.
Printed in the United States of America. No part of this publication may be reproduced, stored in a retrieval system, or transmitted, in any form or by any means, electronic, mechanical, photocopying, recording, or otherwise, without the prior written permission of the publisher.

1 2 3 4 5 6 7 8 9 0 VHVH 8 9 8 7 6 5 4 3 2 1

ISBN 0-07-000294-0

This book was set in Times Roman by Rocappi, Inc.
The editors were Richard S. Laufer and Timothy Armstrong; the designer was Anne Canevari Green; the production supervisor was Jeanne Skahan.
Von Hoffmann Press, Inc., was printer and binder.

Library of Congress Cataloging in Publication Data

Adams, Raymond Delacy, date
  Principles of neurology.

  Includes bibliographies and index.
  1. Nervous system—Diseases. I. Victor, Maurice,
date. II. Title. [DNLM: 1. Nervous system
diseases. WL 100 A216p]
RC346.A3 1981   616.8   81-549
ISBN 0-07-000294-0   AACR2

CONTENTS

PREFACE

In the first edition of this book it was remarked that the preface of a textbook is frequently considered to be a rather useless appendage, doing little more than adding to its weight or serving to distract critics from the study of its content. The value of a book is really to be judged by its substance and composition. Victor Hugo, in his foreword to *Cromwell,* expressed this sentiment more figuratively by pointing out that one seldom inspects the cellar of a house after visiting its salons or examines the roots of a tree after eating its fruit.

Yet there has to be a place where the authors can state the purpose of their work and the manner in which it was conceived, and the reasons for foisting yet another book on a medical public already overburdened with an immense literature. To continue our simile, although one seldom derives pleasure from inspecting the cellar of a house, one is not sorry sometimes to have examined its foundations, especially if one is to purchase it.

In the writing of this book the authors have adopted a method of exposition quite unlike that of the standard textbooks of neurology, in which the various diseases of the nervous system are described in endless succession. Instead, we have chosen to introduce the subject with a discussion of the phenomenology, or cardinal manifestations, of neurologic disease—a detailed exposition of the symptoms and signs of disordered nervous function, their anatomic and physiologic bases, and their clinical implications. This is followed by an account of the various syndromes of which these symptoms are a part and this, in turn, by a consideration of the diseases which express themselves by each syndrome. We believe this to be a logical approach to neu-

rologic disease, for in practice the patient presents with the symptoms of a disease, not with a disease already diagnosed. Furthermore, this sequence from symptoms to syndrome to disease recapitulates the rational process by which the neurologist makes a diagnosis. In teaching students and residents, we have found this method to be eminently successful, and it is to the student and resident that this work is primarily directed. In the strictest sense we believe this work to be an introduction to neurologic medicine.

The compass of our book differs in other ways from contemporary textbooks of neurology. A significant portion of it has been allotted to psychiatric syndromes and the major psychiatric diseases. This has been done in the belief that all physicians, including neurologists, should be knowledgeable about the diagnosis of the depressive states, neuroses, personality disorders, and schizophrenia and about the biologic facts that pertain to these disorders. Similarly, we have consigned a section of the book to a description of muscle diseases, which more and more are coming under the purview of neurologists. Also, pediatric neurology is emphasized, as it is in all neurology training programs in the United States. Finally, the effects of growth, maturation, and aging on the nervous system are elaborated in some detail, for the reason that all deviations from normal acquire significance only when viewed against the background of these natural, age-linked changes.

The warm reception accorded the first edition of this book has led us to believe that our plan of exposition has fulfilled a need and has emboldened us to carry this work forward. As often happens after the first writing, a number of glaring deficiencies came to our attention. We neglected to include a systematic account of hydrocephalus and related disorders of cerebrospinal fluid circulation, and we inadvertently omitted reference to a number of important topics such as episodic global amnesia and normal-pressure hydrocephalus. The writing of a second edition has given us the opportunity to correct these deficiencies and, at the same time, to amend each chapter thoroughly and update it with material that has been published since the first edition was issued. Also, in view of the increasing importance of computerized tomography in neurologic diagnosis, illustrations of all the common cerebral lesions have been inserted into the appropriate chapters.

We are indebted to many colleagues with whom we have repeatedly discussed much of the substantive material of the individual chapters. Robert Young, Bagwan Shihani, Keith Chiappa, and Robert Shields have kept us informed of important developments in clinical neurophysiology, and Miller Fisher, Jay Mohr, Philip Kistler, and Robert Ackerman, in cerebrovascular dis-

ease. Jean Rebeiz, Byron Kakulas, Betty Banker, and Maria Salam-Adams have shared their knowledge of muscle diseases, and Arthur Asbury, of peripheral nerve diseases. Henri Vander Eecken, Karl Åström, and Harry Webster had earlier collaborated with the authors in writing chapters on cerebral trauma and brain tumors, E. P. Richardson, on degenerative diseases, and Robert DeLong, on developmental disorders. Hugo Moser, Edwin Kolodny, and Ira Lott have helped in updating our ideas about hereditary metabolic diseases, and Thomas Hackett and Ross Baldessarini, about modern concepts of psychiatric disease. Other colleagues too numerous to mention have been sources of constant reference and constructive criticism.

Finally, we would like to express our gratitude to Mrs. Betty Wilson, who managed to collate, type, and retype the material of many chapters while at the same time attending to her other departmental duties. We must also thank Richard Laufer and Timothy Armstrong of McGraw-Hill, who have supervised the transcription of a difficult manuscript into the readable chapters of this book.

Raymond D. Adams
Maurice Victor

APPROACH TO THE PATIENT WITH NEUROLOGIC DISEASE

CHAPTER 1

THE CLINICAL METHOD OF NEUROLOGY

Neurology is often regarded as one of the most difficult and exacting specialties of medicine. Students coming to the neurology clinic for the first time are easily discouraged by what they see. Having had brief contact with neuroanatomy, neurophysiology, and neuropathology, they are already somewhat intimidated by the complexity of the nervous system. The ritual they then witness, of putting the patient through a series of maneuvers designed to evoke certain mysterious signs that are difficult to pronounce is hardly reassuring; in fact the procedure often appears to conceal the very intellectual processes by which neurologic diagnosis is attained. Moreover, the students have had no training in administering the many special tests which are used, such as the lumbar puncture and cerebrospinal fluid examination or the electroencephalographic, electromyographic, arteriographic, and scanning examinations, nor do they know how to interpret the results of such tests. Neurologic textbooks only confirm their fears as they read the myriad details of the countless rare diseases of the nervous system.

The authors believe that many of the students' difficulties with neurology can be overcome by adhering to the basic principles of clinical medicine. First and foremost it is necessary to know and acquire facility in use of the *clinical method*. Without a clear comprehension of this method the student is virtually as helpless with a new problem as a botanist or chemist who would attempt to do research without having an understanding of the steps in the scientific method.

The importance of the clinical method stands out more clearly in the study of neurologic diseases than in certain other fields of medicine, but the following remarks have universal application. The solution of any clinical problem is reached by a series of inferences and deductions—each an attempt to explain an item in the history of an illness or a physical finding. Diagnosis is the mental act of integrating all the interpretations and selecting the *one* explanation most compatible with all the facts of clinical observation.

It will be readily perceived that the logical processes involved in diagnosis are not the same in each and every case of neurologic disease and that in some cases the strict adherence to a particular sequence of reasoning is hardly necessary. The clinical picture of Parkinson's disease, for example, is so characteristic that the nature of the illness is at once apparent. Nevertheless, an analysis of the clinical method will show that in most cases it consists of an orderly series of steps, as follows:

1. The symptoms and signs are secured by history and physical examination.

2. The symptoms and physical signs which are considered relevant to the current problem are interpreted and translated in terms of disordered function of anatomical structures or systems of neurons. Often one recognizes a characteristic clustering of symptoms and signs, which constitute a syndrome, and the latter may be particularly helpful in ascertaining the locus and nature of the disease. This step may be called *syndrome diagnosis*.

3. These correlations permit the physician to localize the disease process, i.e., to name the part or parts of the nervous system involved. This step is called the *anatomic diagnosis*.

4. From the anatomic diagnosis and other medical data, particularly the mode of onset and course of the illness, the involvement of nonneurological organ systems, and the laboratory findings, one deduces the *pathologic diagnosis* and, when the mechanism and causation of the disease are determined, the *etiologic diagnosis*.

5. Finally the physician should assess the degree of disability and determine whether it is temporary or permanent. This *functional diagnosis* is important in management of the patient's illness and judging the potential for rehabilitation.

The accurate elicitation of symptoms and signs and their correct interpretation in terms of disordered function of the nervous system are the fundamental steps in diagnosis. When several physicians disagree on the diagnosis, it will frequently be discovered that the symptoms of disordered nervous function were incorrectly interpreted in the first place. Thus if a complaint of dizziness is identified as vertigo instead of lightheadedness or if partial continuous epilepsy is mistaken for an extrapyramidal movement disorder such as choreoathetosis, then surely the diagnosis will be erroneous. Repeated examinations may be necessary to establish these fundamental clinical data beyond doubt and, at times, to ascertain the course of the illness. This is why it is said that the second examination is the most helpful diagnostic test in a difficult neurologic case.

Different disease processes may cause identical symptoms, which is understandable from the fact that several diseases may involve the same parts of the nervous system. For example, a spastic paraplegia may result from spinal cord tumor, syphilitic meningomyelitis, or multiple sclerosis. Conversely, one disease may cause several different symptoms. However, despite the almost infinite number of possible combinations of symptoms and signs, a few occur with greater frequency than others in a given disease and can be recognized as the most characteristic clinical features of that disease. The experienced clinician acquires the habit of attempting to categorize every case in terms of one or another syndrome. Thus, the anatomic basis of the illness in question is more or less determined, and at the same time the range of possible etiologic factors is narrowed.

The final diagnosis must state the locality of the disease as well as its nature and, to be complete, should express the degree of functional impairment as well. Anatomic diagnosis takes precedence over etiologic diagnosis in neurology. To seek the cause of a disease of the nervous system without first ascertaining the parts or structures that are affected would be analogous in internal medicine to an attempt at etiologic diagnosis without knowledge of whether the disease involved the lungs, stomach, or kidneys.

The student must learn the identity and differential diagnosis of the common syndromes before the details of individual diseases. It should be kept clearly in mind, however, that syndromes are not diseases but rather abstractions set up by clinicians in order to facilitate the diagnosis of disease. The inherent danger in the method is that it may inculcate a rigidity of thinking and keep one from conceiving of diseases in new relationships.

TAKING THE HISTORY

The following three points about history taking in neurology deserve comment.

1. Special care must be exercised to avoid suggesting to the patient the symptoms that one seeks. The clinical interview is a bipersonal engagement, and the conduct of the examiner has a great influence on the patient. Repetition of this truism may seem tedious, but it is evident that many of the conflicting histories presented on ward rounds can be traced to leading questions that have suggested to the patient the symptoms that the examiner expects to find or to an unconscious distortion of the patient's story. Errors and inconsistency in recording the history are as often the fault of the physician as of the patient. Here the practice of making bedside notes is particularly to be recommended. The suggestible patient given to highly circumstantial accounts can be kept on the subject of the illness in question by discreet questions which draw out essential points. The immediate recording of the history assures greater reliability.

2. The mode of onset and the course of the illness are of paramount importance. Often the nature of the disease process can be decided by these facts alone. One must know how each symptom began and progressed. If such information cannot be supplied, it may be necessary to judge the course of the symptoms by what the patient was able to do at different times, i.e., how far he or she could walk, whether it was possible to carry on the usual work, etc., or by changes in the clinical findings between successive examinations, providing the clinician has quantitated the findings in some way.

3. Since neurologic diseases often derange the patient's mind, it is necessary in every case of cerebral disease to decide by an initial assessment of the mental status and the circumstances under which symptoms occurred whether or not the patient is competent to give the story of the illness. If not, the history must be obtained from a relative, friend, or employer. Certain illnesses, such as those characterized by convulsions or other forms of episodic confusion, obviously preclude the patient's knowledge of the details of those parts of the illness. In general, students (and some physicians as well) tend to be careless in estimating the mental capaci-

ties of their patients. Attempts are sometimes made to take histories from patients who are feebleminded or so confused that they have no idea why they are in a doctor's office or a hospital, or from one who could not possibly have been aware of the details of the illness.

THE NEUROLOGIC EXAMINATION

The neurologic examination always begins with the history. The manner in which patients tell the story of their illness may betray lack of coherence or confusion in thinking, impairment of memory or judgment, or difficulty in comprehending or expressing ideas. Observation of such matters is an essential part of the examination and provides information as to the adequacy of cerebral function. The physician should learn how to obtain this type of information without embarrassment to the patient. A common error is to pass over inconsistencies in history and inaccuracies about dates and symptoms as being unimportant, only to discover later that these are the major symptoms of the illness.

The remainder of the neurologic examination should be performed as the last part of the general physical examination, proceeding from the examination of the cranial nerves, the neck, and the trunk, to the testing of motor, sensory, and reflex function of the upper and the lower extremities, followed by an assessment of sphincteric and autonomic nervous system functions and suppleness of the neck and spine (meningeal irritation). Gait and station should be observed before or after the rest of the examination. The neurologic examination should always be carried out in an orderly, uniform manner, in order to avoid omissions and to facilitate the subsequent analysis of case records.

The thoroughness of the examination of the nervous system must of necessity depend on the type of clinical problem presented by the patient. To spend a half hour testing motor and sensory function in a patient seeking treatment for a sprained ankle is pointless and uneconomical. Furthermore, the procedure must be varied according to the condition of the patient. Obviously many tests cannot be done in a comatose patient; infants and small children and psychotic patients must be examined in special ways. The following comments about the examination procedure apply to these particular clinical circumstances.

THE MEDICAL OR SURGICAL PATIENT WITHOUT NEUROLOGIC SYMPTOMS

In this case, brevity is desirable, but any test that is undertaken should be done carefully and recorded accurately on the patient's chart. In examining the cranial nerves, the size of the pupils and their reaction to light, ocular movements, visual and auditory acuity (by question), and movements of face, jaw, palate, and tongue should be scrutinized. Observing the bare, outstretched arms for atrophy, weakness, tremor, or abnormal movements, inquiring about strength and subjective sensory disturbances, and eliciting the supinator, biceps, and triceps reflexes are usually sufficient for the upper extremities. Inspection of the legs as the feet, toes, and knees are actively flexed and extended, elicitation of the patellar, achilles, and plantar reflexes, and the testing of vibration and position sense in the fingers, ankles, and feet complete the essential parts of the neurologic examination. Coordination may be tested by having the patient place a finger on the tip of the nose and run the heel up and down the front of the leg. This entire procedure does not add more than 3 or 4 min to the physical examination. The routine performance of these few simple tests may offer clues to the presence of diseases of which the patient is not aware. For example, by finding Argyll Robertson pupils, absent tendon reflexes, and diminished vibratory and position sense in the legs, the physician is alerted to the possibility of tabes when there are no other symptoms of neurosyphilis.

Accurate recording of negative data may be useful in relation to some future illness.

PATIENTS WHO PRESENT SYMPTOMS OF A DISEASE OF THE NERVOUS SYSTEM

Numerous guides to the examination of the nervous system are available. For a full account of the methods the interested reader is referred to the monographs of Denny-Brown, DeJong, DeMyer, and the staff members of the Mayo Clinic, each of which approaches the subject from a special point of view. A large number of tests have been devised, and it is not proposed to review them here. Some are described in subsequent chapters dealing with disorders of mentation, cranial nerves, and motor, sensory, and autonomic functions. Many tests are of doubtful value and should not be taught to students of neurology. Merely to perform all of them on one patient would require several hours, and probably in many instances would not make the examiner any the wiser. The danger with all clinical tests is that the student and physician may regard them as indisputable symbols of disease rather than as ways of uncovering disordered functioning of the nervous system. The following few tests are relatively simple and provide the most useful information.

TESTING OF HIGHER CORTICAL FUNCTIONS

These functions are tested in detail if from the patient's history or behavior during the general examination there is reason to suspect some defect. Questions should then be directed toward determining orientation in time and place and insight into the current medical problem. Attention, speed of response, ability to give relevant answers to simple questions, and in general the capacity for sustained mental effort, all lend themselves to straightforward observation. Useful bedside tests of attention, memory, and clarity of thought are the immediate repetition of a series of digits in forward and reverse order, serial subtraction of 3s or 7s from 100, counting to 30 and back, the recall of the names of three objects or a short story after an interval of 3 min, and the names of the last six presidents or prime ministers. An account of the recent illness, medical consultations, and dates of hospitalizations, and the day-to-day recollection of medical procedures and incidents in the hospital are excellent tests of memory, and a narration of how they were done, of coherence of thinking. Other tests can be devised for the same purpose. Often the examiner can obtain a better idea of the clearness of the patient's sensorium and soundness of intellect by giving these few tests and noting the manner in which the patient deals with them than by relying on a score of a formal intelligence or achievement test.

If there is any suggestion of aphasia, a record of the patient's spontaneous speech should be made. In addition, accuracy in the naming of objects, execution of spoken commands, and repeating words and phrases of the examiner, and the ability to read and write should also be noted. Capacity to add, subtract, multiply, and divide and to solve simple arithmetical problems are ways of uncovering a dyscalculia. Drawing the floor plan of one's home or a map of one's country and copying figures are useful tests of visual-spatial perception and are indicated in cases of suspected cerebral disease (see Chap. 21).

TESTING THE CRANIAL NERVES

The function of the cranial nerves must be investigated more fully than in patients who have no neurologic symptoms. Tests of smell are carried out if one suspects

a lesion in the anterior fossa, and then it usually suffices to determine whether odors are perceived in each nostril. The visual fields should be outlined by confrontation testing; if any abnormality is suspected it should be checked on a perimeter and scotomas sought on the Bjerrum screen. Pupil size and reactivity to light and accommodation and the range of ocular movements should next be observed. Details of these test procedures and their indications are described in Chaps. 12 and 13.

Sensation over the face should be tested with a pin and wisp of cotton, and the presence or absence of the corneal reflexes should be determined. Facial movements should be observed as the patient speaks and smiles, for a slight weakness may be more evident in these circumstances than during voluntary movement. Audiograms and special tests of auditory and labyrinthine function are needed if there is any suspicion of disease of the eighth nerve (see Chap. 14). The vocal cords should be inspected in cases of suspected medullary disease, especially when there is hoarseness. Corneal and pharyngeal reflexes are usually of value only if there is a difference on the two sides; bilateral absence of these reflexes is seldom significant. Inspection of the protruded tongue is helpful; atrophy, fibrillation, and weakness may be seen. Slight deviation of the protruded tongue as a solitary finding may usually be disregarded. Articulation and the pronunciation of words should be noted. The jaw jerk and the buccal and sucking reflexes should be sought, particularly if there is suspicion of dysphagia or dysarthria.

TESTS OF MOTOR FUNCTION

In the assessment of motor function, students must remind themselves that observations of the speed and strength of movements and of muscle bulk, tone, and coordination are usually more informative than the tendon reflexes. It is essential to have the limbs fully exposed and to watch the patient maintain the arms outstretched in the prone and supine positions; to perform simple tasks, such as alternately touching the examiner's finger and the patient's own nose; to make rapid alternating movements that necessitate sudden acceleration and deceleration and changes in direction; and to do simple tasks such as buttoning clothes, opening a safety pin, or handling common tools. Estimates of the strength of leg muscles with the patient in bed are often unreliable; there may seem to be little or no weakness even though the patient cannot step up on a chair or arise from a squatting position. Running the heel down the front of the shin, alternately touching the examiner's finger with the toe and then the opposite knee with the heel, and rhythmically tapping the heel on the shin are the only tests of coordination that need be carried out in bed. The maintenance of both arms or both legs against gravity is a useful test; the weak one, tiring first, soon begins to sag. Also, abnormalities of movement and posture and tremors may appear (see Chaps. 4 and 5).

TESTS OF REFLEX FUNCTION

The testing of the biceps, triceps, supinator (radial-periosteal), knee, ankle, and the cutaneous abdominal and plantar reflexes permits an adequate sampling of reflex activity of the spinal cord. The plantar response offers special difficulty because several different reflex patterns can be evoked by stimulating the sole of the foot along its outer border from heel to toes. These are (1) the high-level, quick avoidance response, (2) the slower, spinal flexor nocifensor reflex (flexion of knee and hip and dorsiflexion of toes and foot), or Babinski sign, (3) grasp, and (4) support reactions.

TESTING OF SENSORY FUNCTION

This is undoubtedly the most difficult part of the neurologic examination. Usually sensory testing is reserved for the end of the examination, and if the findings are to be reliable, it should not be prolonged for more than a few minutes. An explanation of each test should be given; yet too much discussion of it with a meticulous, introspective patient may encourage the reporting of useless minor variations of stimulus intensity.

It is not necessary to examine all areas of the skin surface. A quick survey of the face, neck, arms, trunk, and legs with a pin takes only a few seconds. One is of course seeking differences between the two sides of the body (it is wise to ask whether stimuli on opposite sides of the body feel the same, not whether they feel different), a level below which sensation is lost, or a zone of relative or absolute anesthesia. Regions of sensory deficit can then be tested more carefully and mapped out. The finding of a zone of hyperesthesia may call attention in some patients to a disturbance of superficial sensation. Variations in the sensory findings from one examination to another reflect differences in technique of examination as well as inconsistency in the responses of the patient.

The details of sensory testing methods are described in Chap. 8.

TESTING OF GAIT AND STANCE

No examination is complete without watching the patient stand and walk. An ataxia of gait may be the only neurologic abnormality, as in certain cases of cerebellar degeneration. Stance, posture, and lack of highly automatic adaptive movements may provide the most definite clues in an early case of paralysis agitans (see Chap. 6).

THE COMATOSE PATIENT

Although subject to obvious limitations, examination of the stuporous or comatose patient may yield considerable information concerning the function of the nervous system. The special examination procedures are presented in Chap. 16. The demonstration of signs of focal cerebral or brainstem disease or of meningeal irritation is of aid in the differential diagnosis of the diseases which cause coma and which are the basis of the syndromes outlined in that chapter.

THE PSYCHIATRIC PATIENT

One is compelled in the examination of psychiatric patients to rely less on the cooperation of the patient and to be unusually critical of his statements and opinions. The depressed patient, for example, may claim to have impaired memory or weak or useless limbs when actually there is no amnesia or diminution in muscular power; or the psychopathic patient may feign paralysis. The opposite is sometimes true—psychotic patients may make accurate observations of their own symptoms, only to have them ignored because of their mental state.

If the patient will speak and cooperate even to a slight degree, much may be learned about the functional integrity of different parts of the nervous system. Aphasia can, in nearly every instance, be diagnosed by the manner in which the patient expresses ideas in phrases and sentences, or responds to spoken or written commands. Often it is possible to determine whether there are hallucinations, defective memory, or other symptoms of recognizable brain disease merely by watching and listening to the patient. The visual fields can be tested with fair accuracy by observing the patient's response to a moving stimulus or threat in all four quadrants of the fields. The tests of cranial nerve, motor, and reflex function in the legs, as outlined for the examination of the stuporous or comatose patient (Chap. 16), can be carried out even better if minimal cooperation is obtained from the patient. It must be remembered, however, that the neurologic examination is never complete unless the patient will speak and carry out the usual tests. On numerous occasions mute and resistive patients judged to be schizophrenic prove to have some widespread cerebral disease such as hypoxic or hypoglycemic encephalopathy, a brain tumor, a vascular lesion, or extensive demyelinative lesions.

INFANTS OR SMALL CHILDREN

The reader is referred to the methods of examination described by Gesell and Amatruda, André-Thomas, Paine and Opfré, and the staff members of the Mayo Clinic, summarized in Chap. 27.

IMPORTANCE OF A WORKING KNOWLEDGE OF NEUROANATOMY AND NEUROPHYSIOLOGY

Once the technique of obtaining reliable clinical data is mastered, students may find themselves handicapped in the interpretation of the findings by a lack of knowledge of neuroanatomy and neurophysiology. For this reason, each of the later chapters dealing with the motor system, sensation, special senses, etc., will be introduced by a review of the anatomic and physiologic facts that are necessary for an understanding of the clinical disorders.

A practical working knowledge of neuroanatomy should include the corticospinal tract, the motor unit of spinal cord, nerve, and muscle, basal ganglionic motor connections, cerebellar motor connections, the sensory pathways, cranial nerves, hypothalamus and pituitary connections, reticular formation of brainstem and thalamus, the limbic system, the areas of cerebral cortex and their connections, the visual system, the auditory system, the autonomic system, and the cerebrospinal fluid pathways. A working knowledge of neurophysiology should include the nerve impulse, neuromuscular transmission, and the contractile process of muscle; spinal reflex activity; central neurotransmission; the processes of neuronal excitation, inhibition, and release; and cortical activation and seizure production.

DIFFERENTIAL (ETIOLOGIC) DIAGNOSIS

The differential diagnosis of the cause of a clinical syndrome requires knowledge of an entirely different order.

One must be conversant with the clinical details and the course and natural history of the more common disease entities. Many of these facts are simple and well known and will be presented in later chapters of this textbook.

The findings in the general medical examination are of importance. To illustrate: low-grade fever, anemia, heart murmur, and splenomegaly in a case of unexplained apoplexy indicate that subacute bacterial endocarditis with embolic occlusion of a brain artery is the most likely cause. Pleocytosis in the cerebrospinal fluid with elevated protein and gamma globulin levels, and a positive serologic reaction establishes a syphilitic etiology in a patient with symptoms of apoplexy, a progressive dementia, or blindness.

The anatomic diagnosis may suggest the cause of a disease. Thus, when a unilateral Horner's syndrome, cerebellar ataxia, paralysis of a vocal cord, and analgesia of the face are combined with loss of pain and temperature sensation in the opposite arm, trunk, and leg, an occlusion of the vertebral artery is suggested, because all the involved structures lie within the territory of this artery. In a sense the anatomic diagnosis determines and limits the disease possibilities. If the signs point to disease of the peripheral nerves, it is usually not necessary to consider the causes of disease of the spinal cord. Some signs themselves are almost specific, e.g., Argyll Robertson pupils for neurosyphilis and oculogyric crises for postencephalitic parkinsonism or phenothiazine-induced dyskinesia.

If one adheres faithfully to the clinical method outlined here, neurologic diagnosis becomes relatively simple. In most patients one can reach an anatomic diagnosis. The cause of the disease may prove more elusive. It usually entails the intelligent and selective employment of a number of the laboratory procedures described in the next chapter. Even the most experienced neurologist is unable to ascertain the cause of many neurologic syndromes.

THE PURPOSE OF THE CLINICAL METHOD OF NEUROLOGY

Finally, a few words about the purpose of the clinical method of neurology. Actually, diagnosis accomplishes two main purposes: (1) it enables the physician to decide on the proper method of treating the patient, and (2) it serves as an essential method in the scientific study of clinical phenomena and disease. The medical profession is primarily concerned with the prevention and cure of illness, and all our knowledge is applied to this well-defined end. The practical physician attempts to diagnose diseases for which there is an effective treatment.

Each of the treatable causes of a given syndrome must be carefully considered and excluded by clinical and laboratory methods. For example, in the study of a case of disease of the spinal cord one must take special care to exclude the presence of a tumor, subacute combined degeneration, spinal syphilis, epidural abscess, ruptured disk, and cervical spondylosis, for these are treatable spinal cord diseases. Failure to recognize amyotrophic lateral sclerosis is a less serious error as far as the patient is concerned. Accurate diagnosis also permits prognosis, which is advantageous to both the physician and the patient.

Even when no therapy is possible, neurologic diagnosis is more than an intellectual pastime. There is no doubt that the first step in the scientific study of a disease process is the identification of it in the living patient. Until this is achieved it is impossible to apply adequately the "master method of controlled experiment." The clinical method of neurology thus serves both the physician, in the practical diagnosis and treatment of a patient's condition, and the clinical scientist, in the search for the ultimate cause of the disease.

LABORATORY DIAGNOSIS

From the foregoing description of the clinical method and its application, it is evident that the use of laboratory aids in the diagnosis of disease of the nervous system is always preceded by rigorous clinical examination. A plan of laboratory study can only be directed by clinical information. To reverse this process is unintelligent and wasteful of medical resources. However, in neurology the ultimate goal is prevention, for diseases that have destroyed the brain are irreversible. In the prevention of neurologic disease the clinical method is inadequate, and of necessity one resorts to two other methods, viz., the use of genetic information and laboratory screening. Genetic information enables the neurologist to identify patients at risk of developing a disease and it prompts him to look for biological markers before the advent of symptoms or signs. Biochemical screening tests are applicable to an entire population and permit the identification of neurologic disease in individuals who have yet to show their first symptom; in some of these diseases treatment can be instituted before the nervous system has suffered damage. In preventive neurology, therefore, laboratory methodology may take precedence over clinical methodology.

The laboratory methods that are available for neurologic diagnosis are discussed in the next chapter. The relevent principles of genetic and laboratory screening methods that are presently available for the prediction of disease will be presented in the discussion of the disease(s) to which they are applicable.

REFERENCES

ANDRÉ-THOMAS et al: *The Neurological Examination of the Infant.* London, National Spastics Society, 1960.

DEJONG RUSSELL N: *Neurologic Examination: Incorporating the Fundamentals of Neuroanatomy and Neurophysiology,* 4th ed. Hagerstown, Md, Harper & Row, 1979.

DEMYER W: *Technique of the Neurological Examination,* 2d ed. New York, McGraw-Hill, 1974.

DENNY-BROWN D: *Handbook of Neurological Examination and Case Recording,* rev ed. Cambridge, Mass, Harvard, 1957.

GESELL A, AMATRUDA CS: in Knoblock H, Pasamanick F (eds): *Gesell and Amatruda's Developmental Diagnosis,* 3d ed. Hagerstown, Md, Harper & Row, 1974.

HOLMES G: *Clinical Neurology.* Baltimore, Williams & Wilkins, 1952.

MAYO CLINIC AND MAYO FOUNDATION: *Clinical Examinations in Neurology,* 4th ed. Philadelphia, Saunders, 1976.

CHAPTER 2

SPECIAL TECHNIQUES FOR NEUROLOGIC DIAGNOSIS

The analysis and interpretation of the data elicited by a careful history and examination may prove to be adequate for diagnosis. Special laboratory examinations can then do no more than corroborate the initial impression. However, it happens more often that the conclusion as to the nature of the disease is not reached by simple "case study" alone; the diagnostic possibilities may be reduced to two or three, but the correct one is uncertain. Under these circumstances one resorts to the ancillary examinations outlined below. The aim of the neurologist is to arrive at a final diagnosis by artful analysis of the clinical data, aided by the *least* number of laboratory procedures. Similarly, the strategy of laboratory study of disease should be based purely on therapeutic and prognostic considerations, not on the physician's curiosity or presumed medicolegal exigencies.

A few decades ago the only laboratory procedures available to the neurologist were examination of a sample of CSF, radiology of the skull and spinal column, radiopaque myelography, pneumoencephalography, and electroencephalography. Now, through formidable advances in scientific technology, the physician's armamentarium has been expanded to include a multitude of laboratory methods. Some of these new methods are so impressive that there is a temptation to substitute them for a careful, detailed history and physical examination; this must be avoided. The neurologist should always keep in mind the primacy of the clinical method and that he or she is the final judge of the relevancy and significance of each laboratory datum. Hence the neurologist must be familiar with all the laboratory procedures and their reliability.

Below is a description of those laboratory procedures which have application to a diversity of neurologic diseases. Procedures that are pertinent to a single disease or category of disease will be presented in the chapter devoted to that disease.

LUMBAR PUNCTURE AND EXAMINATION OF CEREBROSPINAL FLUID

The information yielded by the examination of the cerebrospinal fluid (CSF) is often of crucial importance in the diagnosis of neurological disease.

INDICATIONS FOR LUMBAR PUNCTURE

1. To obtain pressure measurements and to procure a sample of CSF for cellular, chemical, and bacteriologic examination.

2. To aid in therapy by the administration of spinal anesthetics and occasionally antibiotics or antitumor agents.

3. To inject air, as in pneumoencephalography; a radiopaque substance (Pantopaque), a water-soluble contrast medium, or air, as in myelography; or a radioactive agent, ytterbium 169 bound to dimethyl triamine pentaacetic acid (DTPA), as in scintigraphic cisternography.

Lumbar puncture is risky if the CSF pressure is high (evidenced by headache and papilledema), for it increases the possibility of a fatal cerebellar or tentorial pressure cone. If, however, in a patient with suspected increased intracranial pressure, it is considered essential to have the information yielded by CSF examination, the lumbar puncture should be performed with a fine-bore (No. 22 or 24) needle as the last part of the clinical study. If the pressure proves to be very high—over 400

mmH_2O—one should obtain the necessary sample of fluid and then, according to the suspected disease and patient's condition, administer a unit of urea or mannitol and watch the manometer until the pressure falls. Dexamethasone (Decadron) should be started in a dose of 4 to 6 mg every 6 h.

Cisternal puncture and *cervical subarachnoid puncture*, although safe in the hands of the expert, are too hazardous to entrust to those without experience. The lumbar puncture is to be preferred except in obvious instances of spinal block requiring a sample of cisternal fluid or myelography above the lesion.

Experience teaches the importance of meticulous technique. Lumbar puncture should always be done under sterile conditions. If procaine is injected in and beneath the skin, the procedure should be painless. The puncture is easiest to perform at the L3-L4 interspace or in the space above or below; in infants and young children, in whom the spinal cord may extend to the level of the L3-L4 interspace, lower spaces should be used. Failure to enter the lumbar subarachnoid space after two or three trials can usually be corrected by doing the puncture with the patient in the sitting position and then assisting him to lie on one side for pressure measurements and fluid removal. The "dry tap" is more often due to an improperly placed needle than to an obliteration of the subarachnoid space by a compressive lesion of the spinal cord or chronic adhesive arachnoiditis.

EXAMINATION PROCEDURES

Once the subarachnoid space has been entered and a sample of CSF obtained, some or all of the following tests should be made: (1) pressure and "dynamics," (2) gross appearance of CSF, (3) number and type of cells and presence of microorganisms, (4) protein, glucose, and in special instances, analysis of pigments, (5) exfoliative cytology using millipore filters or other special apparatus, (6) protein immunoelectrophoresis for determination of gamma globulin and other protein fractions, and other special biochemical tests (for NH_3, pH, CO_2, enzymes, etc.), and (7) bacteriologic cultures and virus isolation.

Pressure and Dynamics When the CSF pressure is measured by a water manometer attached to a needle in either the lumbar subarachnoid space or the cisterna magna with the patient horizontal in the lateral decubitus position, the opening pressure varies from 80 to 200 mmH_2O. When measured with the needle in the lumbar region and the patient in a sitting position, the fluid in the manometer rises to the level of the cisterna magna

(about 280 mmH_2O). It fails to reach the level of the ventricles because the latter are in a closed system under slight negative pressure, whereas the fluid in the manometer is influenced by atmospheric pressure. Normally, with the needle properly placed in the subarachnoid space, the fluid in the manometer oscillates through a few millimeters in response to the pulse and to respiration, and rises promptly with coughing or straining or abdominal compression.

If a spinal subarachnoid block is suspected, jugular compression should be performed. The examiner stands behind the patient and slips a hand around the patient's neck, compressing first one side, then the other, and then both sides simultaneously and exerting enough pressure to compress the veins but not the carotid arteries (Queckenstedt's test). In the absence of a subarachnoid block, there should be a rapid rise in pressure of 100 to 200 mmH_2O, and the pressure should return to its original level within 10 s after release. A graded degree of jugular compression can be applied by wrapping a sphygmomanometer cuff around the neck, observing the pressure responses as the cuff is inflated rapidly to 20 mmHg for 10 s and then released, and repeating the procedure with inflation to 40 and then 60 mmHg. If there is no rise or only a slow rise and fall in CSF pressure with jugular compression, the effect of abdominal compression is checked to make certain that the needle is still in the subarachnoid space. A failure of rise in pressure with compression of one jugular vein but not the other (Tobey-Ayer test) may indicate lateral sinus thrombosis. Except for this circumstance, jugular compression should not be performed when intracranial disease is suspected.

Gross Appearance and Pigments Normally the CSF is clear and colorless, like water. Minor degrees of color change are best detected by comparing tubes of CSF and water against a white background or by looking down the tubes from above. A pleocytosis imparts a hazy or ground glass appearance; at least 200 cells per cubic millimeter must be present to detect this change. The presence of red cells (more than 1000 per cubic millimeter) imparts a pink to red color, depending on the amount of blood; centrifugation of the fluid or allowing it to stand causes a sedimentation of the red blood cells.

A traumatic tap may seriously confuse the diagnosis if it is falsely interpreted as indicating preexistent subarachnoid hemorrhage. To distinguish between the two types of "bloody tap," three samples of fluid should be taken at the time of the lumbar puncture. Usually, with a traumatic tap, there is a decreasing number of red cells in the second and third tubes. Also, the CSF pressure is usually normal, and if a large amount of blood is mixed with the fluid, it will clot or form fibrinous webs. These are not seen with preexistent hemorrhage because the blood is defibrinated in the spinal meninges. Finally, in subarachnoid hemorrhage the red cells undergo hemolysis, after a day or two, giving rise to a yellow discoloration (xanthochromia) in the supernatant fluid. Prompt centrifugation of bloody fluid from a traumatic tap will yield a colorless supernatant; only with large amounts of blood (RBC over 100,000 per cubic millimeter) will the supernatant fluid be faintly xanthochromic due to contamination with serum bilirubin and lipochromes.

The fluid from a traumatic tap should contain about 1 white blood cell per 700 red cells, assuming that the hemogram is normal, but this ratio varies widely and unpredictably. With subarachnoid hemorrhage, the proportion of white cells rises as red cells hemolyze, sometimes reaching a level of several hundred per cubic millimeter, but the vagaries of this reaction are such that it, too, cannot be relied upon to distinguish traumatic from preexistent bleeding. The same can be said for crenation of red cells, which occurs in both types of bleeding.

The reason that red blood corpuscles undergo rapid hemolysis in the CSF is not clear. It is surely not due to osmotic differences, for the osmolarity of plasma and CSF are essentially the same. Fishman suggests that the low protein content of CSF disequilibrates the red cell membrane in some way. The reason for the rapid phagocytosis of red cells in the CSF, which takes place within 48 h, is also obscure. Histiocytes engulf the red cells, forming macrophages, and hemosiderin appears in their cytoplasm within 5 to 6 days.

The pigments that discolor the CSF following subarachnoid hemorrhage are oxyhemoglobin, bilirubin and methemoglobin; in pure form, these pigments are colored red (orange to orange-yellow with dilution), canary yellow, and brown, respectively. Mixtures of these pigments produce combinations of these colors. Oxyhemoglobin appears first, within several hours of the hemorrhage, becomes maximal in the first few days, and, if no further bleeding occurs, diminishes over a 7- to 9-day period. Bilirubin appears in 2 to 3 days and increases in amount as the oxyhemoglobin decreases. Following a single, brisk bleed, bilirubin persists in the CSF for 2 to 3 weeks, the duration varying with the number of red cells that were present originally. Methemoglobin appears when hemorrhage is loculated in the meninges or in adjacent brain tissue.

If blood is added to spinal fluid in a test tube and allowed to stand for several days, oxyhemoglobin and then methemoglobin will form, but not bilirubin, suggesting that the action of living cells is necessary for the formation of the latter pigment. Barrows and his colleagues have devised three simple biochemical tests that reliably indicate the presence or absence of these pigments the benzidine reaction (for oxyhemoglobin), a modified Van den Bergh reaction (for bilirubin) and the potassium cyanide test for methemoglobin.

All xanthochromia of the CSF is not caused by hemolysis of red blood cells. With severe jaundice, bilirubin of both the direct and indirect reacting type will diffuse into the CSF. The quantity of bilirubin is from one-tenth to one-hundredth of that in the serum. Elevation of CSF protein from whatever cause results in xanthochromia, in this instance more or less in proportion to the albumin-bound fraction of bilirubin. Only at levels of more than 150 mg per 100 ml does the coloration due to protein become visible to the naked eye. Hypercarotinemia and hemoglobinemia (through its breakdown products, particularly oxyhemoglobin) also give a yellow tint to the CSF. Myoglobin does not enter the CSF, probably because of the low renal threshold which rapidly clears the blood.

Cellularity Normally the CSF contains no cells or at most up to five lymphocytes or other mononuclear cells per cubic millimeter. An elevation of white cells in CSF always signifies a reactive process to bacteria or other infectious agents, blood, chemical substances, or tumors. The white cells can be counted in an ordinary counting chamber, but their identification requires centrifugation of the fluid and a Gram stain of the sediment or the use of a millipore filter, cell fixation, and staining. One can then recognize and count differentially neutrophilic and eosinophilic leucocytes, lymphocytes, plasma cells, mononuclear cells, arachnoidal lining cells, macrophages, and tumor cells. Bacteria, fungi, fragments of echinococci and cysticerci can also be seen in cell-stained or Gram-stained preparations. An India-ink preparation is useful in distinguishing between lymphocytes and cryptococci or monilia. Dufresne's monograph is an excellent modern reference on CSF cytology. Special techniques applied to the cells of the CSF, such as electron microscopy, have demonstrated at a subcellular level such substances as phagocytosed fragments of myelin in multiple sclerosis. These and other types of reactive cell changes will be mentioned in the respective appropriate chapters.

Proteins In contrast to a blood protein level of approximately 7000 mg/ml, that of the lumbar spinal fluid is 50 mg per 100 ml or less. The protein content of fluid from the basal cisterns is 10 to 25 mg per 100 ml and that from the ventricles is 5 to 15 mg per 100 ml. This gradient of protein concentration probably depends upon the relatively greater permeability of the blood-CSF barrier to proteins in the basal meninges and the spinal subarachnoid space. Levels higher than these indicate a pathologic process in or near the ependyma or meninges, though the cause of modest elevations of the CSF protein frequently remains obscure.

As remarked above, bleeding into the ventricles or subarachnoid space results in the spillage not only of blood cells but of proteins. If the serum proteins are normal, the CSF protein should increase by 1 mg for every 700 RBC. The irritating effect of hemolyzed RBC increases the CSF protein to many times this amount.

The protein content of the CSF in bacterial meningitis, which increases capillary perfusion in choroidal and meningeal vessels, reaches several hundred milligrams per 100 ml. Viral infections induce a less intense and mainly lymphocytic inflammation and rarely elevate the total protein beyond 100 to 200 mg per 100 ml. Paraventricular tumors, by reducing the blood-CSF barrier, often raise the total protein to over 100 mg per 100 ml. Protein values of many hundreds of milligrams per 100 ml are found in an exceptional case of Landry-Guillain-Barré syndrome. Values of 1000 mg per 100 ml, or more, usually indicate loculation of the lumbar CSF (CSF block); the fluid is then deeply yellow and clots readily because of the presence of fibrinogen. This combination of CSF changes is called *Froin's syndrome.* Simpson and Cooper have reported mild elevations of protein after the prolonged administration of phenothiazines. Low CSF protein values sometimes are found in meningismus, in the condition known as meningeal hydrops (see Chap. 29), in hyperthyroidism, or after a recent lumbar puncture.

The quantitative partition of CSF proteins by electrophoretic and immunochemical methods demonstrates the presence of most of the serum proteins with a molecular weight of less than 150,000 to 200,000. The proteins that have been identified in this way fall within the following divisions: prealbumin and albumin, alpha$_1$, alpha$_2$, beta$_1$, beta$_2$, and gamma globulin fractions. Quantitative values of the different fractions are given in Table 2-1. These methods also demonstrate the presence of glycoproteins, haptoproteins, ceruloplasmin, transferrin and hemopexin. Large molecules, such as fibrinogen, IgM, and lipoproteins, are largely excluded from CSF.

There are other notable differences between the protein fractions of CSF and plasma. The CSF always contains a prealbumin fraction, and the plasma does

Table 2-1
Average values of constituents of normal CSF and serum

	Cerebrospinal fluid	Serum
Osmolarity	295 mosmol/liter	295 mosmol/liter
Sodium	138.0 meq/liter	138 meq/liter
Potassium	2.8 meq/liter	4.1 meq/liter
Calcium	2.4 meq/liter	5.2 meq/liter
Magnesium	2.7 meq/liter	1.9 meq/liter
Chloride	124.0 meq/liter	101.0 meq/liter
Bicarbonate	23.0 meq/liter	23.0 meq/liter
Carbon dioxide tension	48 mmHg	38 mmHg (arterial)
pH	7.31	7.41 (arterial)
Nonprotein nitrogen	19.0 mg/100 ml	27.0 mg/100 ml
Ammonia	30.0 μg/100 mg	70.0 μg/100 ml
Uric acid	0.24 mg/100 ml	4.0 mg/100 ml
Urea	4.7 mmol/liter	5.4 mmol/liter
Creatinine	1.1 mg/100 ml	1.6 mg/100 ml
Phosphorus	1.6 mg/100 ml	4.0 mg/100 ml
Total lipid	1.25 mg/100 ml	876.0 mg/100 ml
Total cholesterol	0.4 mg/100 ml	180.0 mg/100 ml
Cholesterol esters	0.3 mg/100 ml	126.0 mg/100 ml
Glucose	>45.0 mg/100 ml	90 mg/100 ml
Lactate	1.6 meq/liter	1.0 meq/liter
Total protein	15-50 mg/100 ml	6.5-8.4 g/100 ml
Prealbumin	1-7%	Trace
Albumin	49-73%	56%
Alpha$_1$ globulin	3-7%	4%
Alpha$_2$ globulin	6-13%	10%
Beta globulin (beta$_1$ plus tau)	9-19%	12%
Gamma globulin	3-12%	18%

Source: Fishman.

not. Although derived from plasma this fraction for an unknown reason concentrates in the CSF, and the level is greater in ventricular than in lumbar CSF (perhaps because of its concentration by choroidal cells). The CSF also has a beta$_2$ or tau fraction (transferrin) which is proportionately larger than that in the plasma and again higher in the ventricular than in the spinal fluid. The gamma globulin fraction in CSF is about 70 percent of that in plasma.

At present only a few of these proteins are known to be associated with specific diseases of the nervous system. The most important is IgG, which may exceed 12 percent of the total CSF protein in diseases such as multiple sclerosis, neurosyphilis, and subacute sclerosing encephalitis. The serum IgG is not correspondingly increased which means that this immune globulin must originate in the nervous system. However, an elevation of serum gamma globulin, as occurs in cirrhosis, sarcoidosis, myxedema, and multiple myeloma, will be accompanied by a rise in the CSF gamma globulins. To separate these two groups of conditions, the electrophoretic patterns of both the blood and CSF proteins should be determined. The albumin fraction in CSF increases in a wide variety of diseases of the CNS and craniospinal nerve roots which increase the permeability of the blood-CSF barrier, but no specific clinical correlations can be drawn. The use of precipitation tests (e.g., colloidal gold reaction) to demonstrate CSF proteins has been largely replaced by immunochemical and electrophoretic techniques, which measure the proteins directly.

Glucose Normally the range of CSF glucose is 45 to 80 mg per 100 ml, i.e., about two-thirds that in the blood. Higher levels parallel the blood glucose, but with marked hyperglycemia the ratio of CSF to blood glucose is less than 0.6. Values below 40 mg per 100 ml are abnormal. After the intravenous injection of glucose, approximately 2 h is required for equilibrium with the CSF to be reached; a similar delay follows the lowering of blood glucose. For these reasons, the proper evaluation of the CSF glucose requires that blood glucose be measured simultaneously, in the fasting state. Only decreased levels are of diagnostic significance. Low levels in the presence of pleocytosis usually indicate pyogenic, tubercular, or fungal meningitis, although the CSF glucose is sometimes reduced in sarcoidosis, in subarachnoid hemorrhage (most often between the fourth and eighth day), and in widespread neoplastic infiltration of the meninges.

The almost invariable rise of *CSF lactate* in meningitis informs us that some of the glucose is undergoing anaerobic glycolysis by the cells of the meninges and adjacent brain tissue. For a long time it was assumed that in meningitis the bacteria lowered the sugar content of CSF by their active metabolism and that the reactive inflammatory cells had only a slight effect on it, but the fact that the sugar remains at a subnormal level for 2 to 3 weeks after effective treatment of the meningitis indicates that another mechanism for the hypoglycorrhachia must be operative. Alterations of the membrane transport system must also be implicated. Interestingly, viral infections of the meninges and brain do not lower the CSF glucose nor raise the lactate levels, though Wilfert has reported low glucose values in a small proportion of patients with mumps meningoencephalitis and rarely in one or two other viral infections.

Serologic Tests for Syphilis The various serologic tests that are used on the blood (Wassermann complement-fixation test, Kahn flocculation or precipitation test, Kolmer complement-fixation test) can be performed on the CSF. When positive, they indicate neurosyphilis, but false-positive tests may occur when the CSF is contaminated with blood or with collagen diseases, malaria, and yaws. Tests which depend on the use of treponemal antigens, including the treponema immobilization test and the fluorescent treponemal antibody test are more specific and assist in the interpretation of false-positive reactions. The value of the CSF in the diagnosis and treatment of neurosyphilis is discussed in Chap. 31.

CHANGES IN SOLUTES AND OTHER COMPONENTS

The average osmolarity of the CSF (295 mosmol/liter) is identical to that of plasma. As the osmolarity of the plasma is increased by the injection of hypertonic intravenous solutions such as mannitol or urea, there is a delay of several hours in the rise of osmolarity of the CSF. It is during this period that the hyperosmolarity of the blood dehydrates the brain and decreases the volume of CSF.

The CSF and serum levels of sodium, potassium, calcium, and magnesium are listed in Table 2-1. Neurologic disease does not alter the CSF concentrations of these constituents in any characteristic way. The low CSF concentration of chloride that occurs in bacterial meningitis is not specific but a reflection of hypochloremia and elevated CSF protein.

Acid-base balance in the CSF is of considerable interest in relation to metabolic acidosis and alkalosis. Normally the pH of the CSF is about 7.31 and is lower than that of arterial blood, which is 7.41. The P_{CO_2} is higher in the CSF than in arterial blood, 48 to 38 mmHg. The bicarbonate levels of the two fluids are about the same, 23 meq/liter. There is a very precise regulation of CSF pH, and it tends to remain relatively unchanged even in the face of a subacute or chronic metabolic acidosis. However, when there are rapid changes in the blood pH, either in the direction of acidosis or alkalosis, the pH of CSF changes in parallel. Once it has changed, the return to normal levels, as the pH of the blood is regulated, is much slower. These phenomena are said to be explained by the rapid diffusion of CO_2 and the slower transport of bicarbonate and hydrogen ions. In metabolic acidosis or alkalosis, cerebral function is deranged only with relatively large changes in pH of the CSF, and it is likely to persist until the pH returns to normal. Cerebral and meningeal diseases and convulsive states contribute to the metabolic acidosis of the CSF by raising the lactic acid levels (anaerobic glycolysis).

The *ammonia content* of the CSF is approximately one-third to one-half that of the arterial blood; it rises in hepatic encephalopathy and in Reye's syndrome and the level correlates with the degree of encephalopathy. The *uric acid* content of CSF is about 5 percent of that in serum and varies with changes in the serum level (e.g., high in uremia and meningitis and low in Wilson's disease). The *urea* concentration in the CSF is slightly less than in the serum (see Table 2-1), and in uremia it rises in parallel with the blood level. An intravenous injection of urea raises the blood level immediately and the CSF level more slowly, during which interval it exerts its osmotic effect. All 24 of the *amino acids* have been isolated from the CSF. The concentration of the total amino acids is about one-third that of plasma. The CSF-to-plasma ratios of the individual amino acids varies from about 1.0 for glutamic acid to 0.1 for glutamate and even less for phenylalanine. Specific transport systems have been delineated for some of the acidic, basic, and neutral amino acids. Elevations of glutamine are found in hepatic coma and Reye's syndrome and of phenylalanine, histidine, valine, leucine, isoleucine, tyrosine, and homocystine in the corresponding aminoacidurias.

Many of the *enzymes* found in serum are known to rise in CSF under conditions of disease, usually in relation to a rise in CSF protein. None of the enzyme changes has proved to be a specific indicator of neurologic disease, with the possible exception of lactic dehydrogenase, especially isoenzymes 4 and 5, which are derived from granulocytes and are elevated in bacterial meningitis but not in aseptic or viral meningitis. As to *lipids* the quantities in CSF are small, and their mea-surement is difficult. In multiple sclerosis the proportions of the different types of lipid are said to change.

The catabolites of the *catecholamines* are now being measured in the CSF. Homovanillic acid (HVA), the major catabolite of dopamine, and 5-hydroxyindoleacetic acid (5-HIAA), the major catabolite of serotonin, are present in normal spinal fluid; both are five or six times higher in the ventricular than in the lumbar CSF. The levels of both catabolites are reduced in patients with idiopathic and drug-induced parkinsonism.

Finally, it may be said that with continued development of microchemical techniques for the analysis of the CSF, we can look forward to a better understanding of the metabolic mechanisms of the brain, particularly of the hereditary metabolic diseases. Ultrarefined methods such as gas-liquid chromatography will probably reveal many new catabolic products, the measurement of which will be of value in diagnosis and therapy.

RADIOGRAPHIC EXAMINATION OF SKULL AND SPINE

Although plain films of the cranium and vertebral column have for a long time been considered a "routine" part of the study of the neurologic patient, it has gradually become evident that the yield of useful information from this procedure is relatively small. Even in patients with head injury, where radiography of the skull would seem to be the optimal method of examination, a fracture is found in only one out of 25 cases, at an estimated cost of $2500 per fracture and an incalculable risk from radiation exposure.

Refinements of technique such as pneumoencephalography, carotid and vertebral arteriography, and serial autotomography greatly increase the yield of valuable information in special cases, but without question the most important advance since the discovery of the roentgen ray has been computerized tomography (CT scan). It has largely replaced pneumoencephalography and arteriography, except in a few diseases, and has greatly extended our ability to visualize living pathology. A new field of bioneuropathology has been created.

COMPUTERIZED TOMOGRAPHY (CT SCAN)

In this procedure the resistance offered by the skull, CSF, brain, and blood vessels to the passage of more than thirty thousand 2- to 4-mm beams of x-ray directed

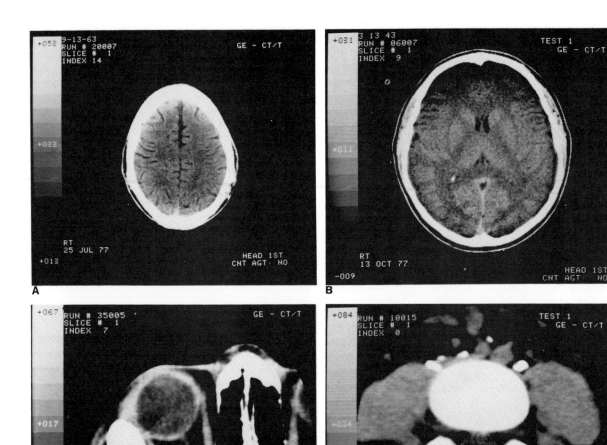

Figure 2-1

Computerized tomography (CT) scans of cerebrum, orbit, and cervical spine. Scale of densities, ranging from bone (+53) to water (+13) are shown on the left side of each figure. A. Cerebral hemispheres in the horizontal plane, at a level above the lateral ventricles. Note the differences in density between the skull, cerebral cortex, and white matter. Each of the major sulci are seen. B. Plane through the thalami and basal ganglia. The lower parts of the anterior horns are visible as two dark ovals. The lenticular nuclei and caudate nuclei are separated by the anterior limbs of the internal capsules. The thalami are separated from lenticular nuclei by the posterior limbs of the internal capsules. C. The eyeball and the optic nerve are seen in the orbit, as well as the lateral rectus and medial rectus muscles. D. The upper lumbar spine, including vertebral body, laminae, and spinous processes are white; the psoas muscles, on each side of the vertebral body, and the paravertebral muscles are gray. The spinal cord is visible within the spinal canal. (Courtesy of Medical Systems Division, General Electric Company.)

successively at several horizontal levels to the hemisphere of the cranium are computed and revisualized. The differing densities of bone, CSF, blood, gray and white matter are distinguishable in the resulting picture. One can see hemorrhage, softened and edematous brain, abscess, and tumor tissue and also the precise size and position of the ventricles. The radiation exposure is not significantly greater than that from plain skull films.

The results obtained by the first CT scanners were relatively crude, but new refinements now afford pictures of brain, spine, and orbit of truly remarkable clarity. As illustrated in Fig. 2-1, in transverse section of the brain one actually sees displayed the caudate and lenticular nuclei and the internal capsules and thalami. The position and width of all the main sulci can be measured, and the optic nerve and medial and lateral rectus muscles stand out clearly in the retroorbital space. The spinal cord is easily visible in the body scan.

The authors believe this new radiologic method to be so valuable that pictures of all the common lesions of the brain have been inserted in the appropriate chapters.

Other radiologic methods of value to neurology and neurosurgery are angiography, pneumoencephalography, and contrast myelography and ventriculography.

ANGIOGRAPHY

This technique has been developed over the last 30 years to the point where it is relatively safe and an extremely valuable method for the diagnosis of aneurysms, vascular malformations, occluded arteries and veins, and sometimes for mass lesions (hemorrhages, tumors, and abscesses). Following local anesthesia, a needle or cannula can be placed percutaneously into the lumen of any of the larger arteries of the neck; or, even better, a catheter can be used to cannulate any of the major cervical vessels in a retrograde fashion after being introduced into the brachial or femoral artery. In these ways radiopaque contrast media can be injected to visualize the arch of the aorta, the origins of the carotid and vertebral systems and their extent through the neck into the cranial cavity, occasionally the spinal cord arteries, cerebral arteries down to about 0.1 mm in lumen diameter (under optimal conditions), and small veins of comparable size. The procedure is not altogether without risk, and the indications should be clear. Approximately one percent of our patients have had a worsening of their condition or even a frank ischemic lesion in the territory of the catheterized artery. High concentrations of the injected media may induce vascular spasm and occlusion and clots may form on the catheter tip and embolize the artery.

PNEUMOENCEPHALOGRAPHY (PEG) AND VENTRICULOGRAPHY

The injection of air or oxygen into the lumbar subarachnoid space (PEG) with the patient in the sitting position permits visualization in considerable detail of the size and position of the ventricles, the subarachnoid space (upper spinal and cerebral), and, indirectly, the structures which lie between the ventricles and the meninges. Hydrocephalus, mass lesions which displace or deform the ventricles or cisterns, basal lesions which lie between the meninges and the sphenoid bone, sella turcica and clivus, and atrophic states of the cerebrum are revealed

by this technique. On rare occasions, in cases of greatly elevated intracranial pressure, air is injected directly into the ventricles (ventriculography) through burr holes placed in the skull. Air can also be used in the visualization of the spinal subarachnoid space for the demonstration of such abnormalities as spinal tumors and ruptured intervertebral disks.

RADIOOPAQUE MYELOGRAPHY (AND VENTRICULOGRAPHY)

By injecting 5 to 25 ml of Pantopaque through a lumbar puncture needle and then tipping the patient on a tilt table, the entire spinal subarachnoid space may be seen. The procedure is almost as harmless as the lumbar puncture, provided that the Pantopaque is afterward removed through the needle. Ruptured lumbar and cervical disks, cervical spondylotic bars and bony spurs encroaching on the spinal cord or roots, and spinal cord tumors can be diagnosed accurately. Occasionally, Pantopaque is injected into the lateral ventricles in order to visualize the third and fourth ventricles and the aqueduct of Sylvius (in tumors of the posterior fossa, for instance, when air does not enter from below). In some clinics air is preferred to Pantopaque in the demonstration of masses within the spinal canal because of the lesser risk of arachnoiditis (which results occasionally from the failure to remove all of the Pantopaque). It is of particular value when combined with polytomography in visualizing the size and position of the spinal cord and the relation to it of spondylotic bars and spurs. Water-soluble contrast media, such as metrizamide, are self-absorbing and are being used with increasing frequency.

RADIOACTIVE ISOTOPES

Radioactive isotopes of mercury, technetium, and arsenic are in regular use for the visualization of tumors, inflammatory masses, subdural hematomas, and some vascular lesions. Since this is a simple, noninvasive procedure, the only limitation in its use is the expense. The more vascular the lesion, the more consistent its demonstration by these methods. *Ultrasound* can also be used to show displacement of central structures of the brain by a mass lesion.

CRANIAL AND SPINAL BONE SCANS

These procedures are of inestimable value in visualizing tumors and inflammatory processes in cranial and spinal bones. Often the lesions can be visualized when plain films are negative. The bone scan can be combined with the gallium scan for the opacification of the soft tissues.

ELECTROENCEPHALOGRAPHY

The electroencephalographic examination is part of the clinical study of the patient suspected of having a cerebral disease; it is also used in the evaluation of the CNS effects of many medical diseases. It is described here in some detail, since it cannot suitably be assigned to any other single chapter.

The modern electroencephalograph has 8 to 16 or more separate amplifying units capable of recording from many areas of the scalp at the same time. The amplified brain rhythms are strong enough to move an ink-writing pen, which produces the waveform of the brain activity of frequency range 0.5 to 30 Hz (cycles per second) on paper moving at a standard speed of 3 cm/s. The resulting electroencephalogram (EEG), or *voltage-versus-time graph*, appears as a number of parallel, wavy lines, as many as there are amplifying units, or "channels." Electrodes, which usually are solder or silver–silver chloride disks 0.5 cm in diameter, are placed on the head by means of adhesive material such as bentonite or collodion, using ECG paste under the electrode to make contact with the scalp. Patients are usually examined with their eyes closed and while relaxed in a comfortable chair or bed. The procedure is entirely painless and takes ¾ to 1¼ h. The ordinary EEG, therefore, represents the electrocerebral activity recorded under restricted circumstances, usually during the waking state, from several parts of the cerebral convexities, during an almost infinitesimal segment of the person's life.

In addition to the resting record, a number of so-called activating procedures are usually carried out.

1. The patient is requested to breathe deeply twenty times a minute for 3 min. The resulting alkalosis and cerebral vasoconstriction may activate characteristic seizure patterns or other abnormalities.

2. A powerful light (stroboscope) is placed over the patient's face and flashed at frequencies from 1 to 20 per second with the patient's eyes opened and closed. The EEG leads may then show waves corresponding to each flash of light (photic driving) or abnormal discharges (Fig. 2-2C).

3. The EEG is recorded after the patient is allowed to fall asleep naturally or following sedative drugs

by mouth or by vein. Sleep is extremely helpful in bringing out abnormalities, especially where temporal lobe epilepsy and certain other seizures are concerned.

4. Special activating procedures, such as the parenteral administration of pentylenetetrazol (Metrazol) or insulin, are hazardous and rarely used now. Their purpose is to produce diagnostically useful abnormalities without actually inducing convulsions.

Through the medium of all-night EEG recordings, many abnormalities associated with sleep can be demonstrated (see Chap. 18). Some of these are important clinically, and the same may be said of EEGs recorded by telemetry from freely moving ambulatory patients.

The EEG consists of 150 to 300 or more pages, each representing 10 s in time. These are obtained by a technician who is primarily responsible for the entire procedure, including notation of movements or other events responsible for artifacts and successive modifications of technique based upon what the record shows. Certain preparations are necessary if electroencephalography is to be most useful. The patient should not be sedated (except as noted above) and should not have been without food for a long time, for both sedative drugs and relative hypoglycemia modify the normal EEG pattern. The same may be said of mental concentration and extreme nervousness or drowsiness, all of which tend to suppress the normal alpha rhythm and increase muscle and other artifacts. When dealing with patients who are suspected of having epilepsy and who are already being treated for it, most physicians prefer to record the first EEG while the patient continues to receive drugs. If it is normal, and if the referring physician and the electroencephalographer agree, the test can be repeated 24 h after withdrawal of anticonvulsants; it is well known that these drugs reduce the incidence of abnormal interictal records in patients with proved epilepsy. Though it is unusual for seizures to begin during this short interval, it may happen; longer periods without therapy are hazardous. It is helpful to indicate on the request form the suspected site of the lesion or the question to be answered.

TYPES OF NORMAL RECORDINGS

The normal record in adults usually shows somewhat asymmetric 8- to 13-per-second, 50-μV sinusoidal *alpha* waves in both occipital and parietal regions. These waves wax and wane spontaneously and disappear promptly when patients open their eyes or concentrate on something (Fig. 2-2A). Waves faster than 13 per second and of lower amplitude (10 to 20 μV), called *beta* waves, are also recorded from the frontal regions symmetrically. When the normal subject falls asleep, the

Figure 2-2

Abbreviations: R, right; L, left; a, anterior; m, mid; po, posterior; F, frontal; Fp, frontal poles; C, central (sensorimotor area); T, temporal; P, parietal; O, occipital; Ref, reference or inactive lead (such as to neck or ear). Calibrations are as noted.

A. Normal alpha (9 to 10 per second) activity is present posteriorly (bottom channel). The top channel contains a large blink artifact. Note the striking reduction of the alpha rhythm with eye opening.

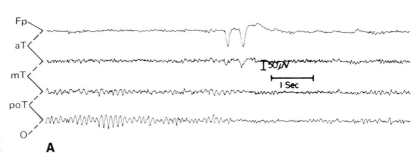

A

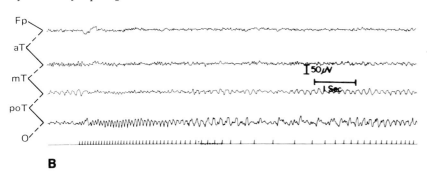

B

B. Photic driving. During stroboscopic stimulation of a normal subject a visually evoked response is seen posteriorly after each flash of light (signaled on the bottom channel).

C. Stroboscopic stimulation at 14 flashes per second (bottom channel) has produced a photoconvulsive response in this epileptic patient, evidenced by the abnormal spike and slow-wave activity toward the end of the period of stimulation.

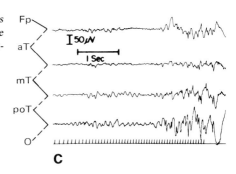

C

D. EEG from patient with focal motor seizures of the right side. Note focal spike discharge in left frontal region. The activity from the right hemisphere is relatively normal.

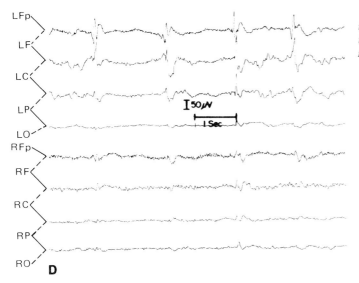

D

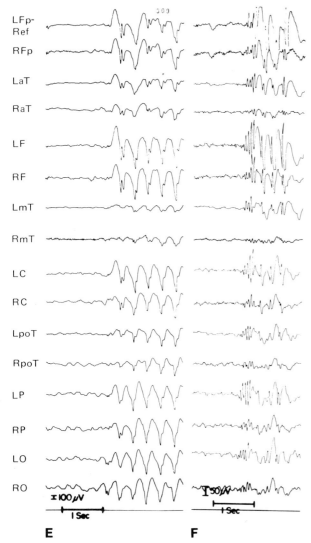

LFp-Ref
RFp
LaT
RaT
LF
RF
LmT
RmT
LC
RC
LpoT
RpoT
LP
RP
LO
RO

I 100 μV
1 Sec

E

I 50 μV
1 Sec

F

E. *Petit mal epilepsy, showing generalized 3-per-second spike and wave discharge. The abnormal activity arises abruptly from a normal background.*

F. *A spike-wave variant showing multiple spikes (polyspikes) and spike and slow-wave discharge at 4 per second in a patient with a mixed seizure pattern. Note that monopolar leads are used in E and F and that their calibrations differ.*

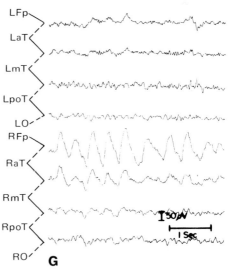

LFp
LaT
LmT
LpoT
LO
RFp
RaT
RmT
RpoT
RO

I 50 μV
1 Sec

G

G. *Large, slow, irregular delta waves are seen in the right frontal region (channels 5 and 6). In this case a glioblastoma was found in the left cerebral hemisphere, but the EEG picture does not differ basically from that produced by a stroke, abscess, or contusion.*

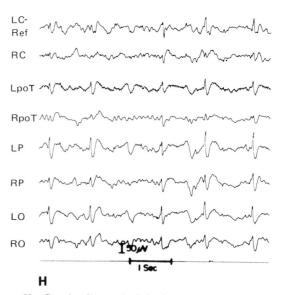

LC-Ref
RC
LpoT
RpoT
LP
RP
LO
RO

I 50 μV
1 Sec

H

H. *Grossly disorganized background activity interrupted by repetitive discharges consisting of large, sharp waves from all leads about once per second. This pattern is characteristic of Creutzfeldt-Jakob disease.*

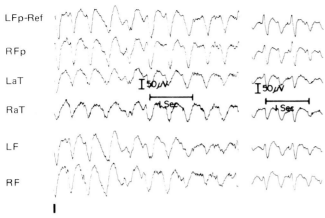

I. (Left) *Advanced hepatic coma. Bifrontal slow (about 2 per second) waves have replaced the normal activity in all leads. (Right) Hepatic coma. This record demonstrates the triphasic waves sometimes seen in this disorder (channels 1 and 2). The slowing is less marked than in the tracing on the left.*

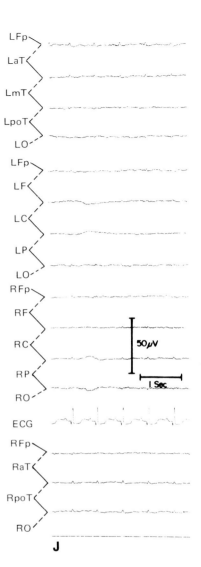

J. *Deep coma following cardiac arrest, showing electrocerebral silence. With the highest amplification, ECG and other artifacts may be seen, so that the record is not truly "flat" or isoelectric. However, no cerebral rhythms are visible. Note the ECG channel. (Illustrations courtesy of Dr. Susan Chester.)*

rhythm slows symmetrically, and characteristic waveforms (vertex sharp waves and sleep spindles) appear; if the sleep is induced by barbiturates, an increase in the fast frequencies is seen and is considered to be normal.

An occipital response to each flash may be seen in the normal EEG during stroboscopic stimulation and is called the *evoked response*, or, at faster repetition rates, photic "driving." The arrival of the visual response in the calcarine part of the occipital lobe occurs 20 to 30 ms after the flash of light. This evoked occipital response from flashes of light or a shifting pattern stimulus (see further on) has increased the scope of electroencephalography in several ways: (1) one can be sure that a person with such a response can at least perceive light, and a patient with such a response who claims to be totally blind is either hysterical or malingering; (2) when this evoked response is absent on one side of the head but present on the other, there is interruption of transmission between the thalamus and the occipital lobe on the one side; (3) when there is delay in the evoked response from one eye, there is usually disease in that optic nerve; (4) when the flashing light causes the occipital response to spread over the cortex with the production of abnormal waves, this provides evidence of abnormal excitability (Fig. 2-2B and C). Actual seizure patterns may be produced in the EEG if the activation procedure is continued and frank myoclonic jerks of face or arms, or major convulsions may be seen (photomyoclonus and photoconvulsions). This finding is to be differentiated from the purely muscular response, also myoclonic, produced normally in contracting scalp muscles and often visible in routine EEGs. Children and adolescents are more sensitive to all the activating procedures mentioned. It is customary for children to develop slow activity (3 to 4 per second) during the middle and latter part of a period of overbreathing. This disappears soon after the hyperventilation has stopped. The frequency of the dominant rhythms in infants is normally about 3 per second, and they are very irregular. There is a gradual increase in frequency and in rhythmicity of these occipital rhythms with maturation, and by the age of 12 to 14 years, normal 9- to 10-per-second alpha waves are the dominant pattern (see Chap. 27 for further discussion of maturation of brain as expressed in the EEG). Children's and infants' records are difficult to interpret because the wide range of normal values at each age makes rigid classification, using frequency criteria, impossible. Nevertheless, asymmetric records, or records with seizure patterns, are clearly abnormal in children of any age.

TYPES OF ABNORMAL RECORDINGS

The most pathologic finding of all is the disappearance of the EEG pattern and its replacement by "electrocerebral silence," which means that the electrical activity of the cortical mantle, measured at the scalp, is below 2 μV or absent. Artifacts of various types are seen as the gains are increased. Acute intoxication with anesthetic levels of drugs, such as barbiturates, can produce this sort of isoelectric EEG (Fig. 2-2J). However, in the absence of CNS depressants or hypothermia, a record which is "flat" (except for artifacts) all over the head is almost always a result of cerebral hypoxia or ischemia. Such a patient, without EEG activity, reflexes, spontaneous respiratory or muscular activity of any kind for 6 h or more, is said to be in "irreversible coma." The brain of such patients is largely necrotic, and there is no chance for neurologic recovery.

Localized regions of absence of brain waves may rarely be seen when there is a large area of softening or an extensive surface tumor or clot lying between the cerebral cortex and the electrodes. With such a finding, the localization of the abnormality is precise but of course the nature of the lesion is not disclosed. However, most such lesions are too small, relative to the recording arrangement, to be recognized, and the EEG may then record abnormal waves arising from functional though deranged brain at the borders of the lesion.

The abnormal waves are slower and of higher amplitude than normal. Those which are fewer than 4 per second with amplitude from 50 to 350 μV are called *delta* waves (Fig. 2-2G and I); those from 4 to 7 per second are called *theta* waves; and the higher-voltage, faster waves are known as *spikes* or *sharp* waves (Fig. 2-2F). These fast and slow waves may be combined, and when a series of them interrupts relatively normal EEG patterns in a paroxysmal fashion, they are highly suggestive of epilepsy. The ones associated with *petit mal* are 3-per-second spike-and-wave complexes that characteristically appear in all leads of the electroencephalogram at the same time and disappear almost as suddenly at the end of the seizure (Fig. 2-2E). This finding led to the theoretic localization of a pacemaker for petit mal discharges in the thalamus or other deep gray structures ("centrencephalon"), but such clinical and experimental evidence as exists has not verified this hypothesis.

NEUROLOGIC CONDITIONS WITH ABNORMAL EEG

Epilepsy (see also Chap. 15) All types of generalized epileptic seizures (grand mal and petit mal) are associated with some abnormality in the EEG, provided it is being recorded at the time. Also, the EEG is usually abnormal during the more restricted types of seizure activity (psychomotor, myoclonic, Jacksonian). One exception is certain deep temporal lobe foci where the discharge fails to reach the scalp in sufficient amplitude to be seen against the normal background activity of the EEG, particularly if there is a strong alpha rhythm. In these cases an anterior temporal electrode, which is most free of occipital alpha frequencies, or a nasopharyngeal lead may pick up the discharge, especially during sleep. In perhaps 2 to 5 percent of cases, the only way in which this deep activity can be sampled is by inserting an electrode into the substance of the brain, but this procedure is applicable only to the few who are having a craniotomy. Other exceptions in which, on occasion, no EEG abnormality may be recorded during a seizure include some of the patients with other types of focal seizure (sensory, Jacksonian, myoclonic, epilepsia partialis continua) and with polymyoclonus. This fact presumably means that the neuronal discharge is too deep, discrete, fast, or asynchronous to be transmitted by volume conduction through the skull and recorded via the EEG electrode, which is some 2 cm from the cortex. Much more frequently, a completely normal EEG during a seizure has been interpreted as indicating hysteria or a psychopathic reaction. Some of the different types of seizure patterns are shown in Fig. 2-2D to F. The petit mal, myoclonic jerk, and grand mal patterns correlate closely with the clinical seizure type and may be present in the interictal EEG.

A fact of importance is that between seizures as many as 20 percent of patients with petit mal and 40 percent with grand mal epilepsy show a normal pattern. Anticonvulsant therapy also tends to diminish the EEG abnormalities. The records of another 30 to 40 percent of epileptics, though abnormal between seizures, are nonspecifically so, and therefore the diagnosis of epilepsy can be made only by the correct interpretation of clinical data in relation to the EEG abnormality.

Brain Tumor, Abscess, and Subdural Hematoma Clinically significant intracranial mass lesions are associated with characteristic abnormalities in the EEG, depending on their type and location, in some 90 percent of patients. In addition to diffuse changes, described below, the classic abnormalities are focal or localized slow wave (usually delta, as in Fig. 2-2G) or, occasionally, seizure activity and decreased amplitude and synchronization of normal rhythms. As a rule, the more rapidly expanding lesions (abscess, some metastases, glioblastoma), especially those situated supratentorially, are associated with the greatest frequency of EEG abnormalities (90 to 95 percent of the latter two and virtually 100 percent of abscesses). More slowly growing tumors (astrocytomas) and particularly those outside the cerebral hemispheres (meningiomas, pituitary tumors) often produce no change in the EEG, though they may be very evident clinically. The EEG abnormality is found on the same side as the lesion in as many as 75 to 90 percent of patients with subdural hematomas and supratentorial tumors or abscesses. Therefore, when a patient in whom one of these conditions is suspected has a normal EEG, there are nine chances to one against its presence. Thus the EEG may be helpful in both a negative and positive way, particularly when integrated with the other laboratory and clinical findings. A normal EEG and brain scan together almost exclude the presence of a supratentorial brain tumor or abscess. The EEG is normal, however, in 20 to 25 percent of patients with infratentorial tumors.

Cerebrovascular Disease The EEG may be useful in the differential diagnosis of vascular hemiplegia. Both the diffuse and the localized EEG changes produced by vascular lesions such as cerebral infarcts and intracranial hemorrhages depend on the location and size of the disorder rather than its type. If the lesion responsible is in the distribution of the internal carotid or other major cerebral artery, an area of decreased normal activity and excessive slowing is practically always seen acutely in the appropriate region. If the hemiplegia is due to small-vessel disease, i.e., a lacunar infarction deep in the cerebrum or brainstem (see Chap. 33), the EEG is usually normal. Large hemispheral lesions associated acutely with depressed levels of consciousness produce widespread, diffuse, slow-wave activity, as is seen with stupor or coma from any cause; a few very large infarctions betray themselves acutely by ipsilaterally depressed EEG activity. Resolution begins after a few days, cerebral edema subsides, and focal abnormalities may then be seen (slow-wave activity or suppression of normal background rhythms). Smaller infarctions are associated with focal abnormalities acutely which lateralize the lesion well but do not localize it precisely. With further resolution after 3 to 6 months, roughly 50 percent of patients with cerebrovascular accidents have a normal EEG despite the persistence of clinical abnormalities. Once this occurs, the prognosis for further recovery is poor. Perhaps half these patients will have had normal EEGs even when recorded in the week or two following the ictus. Large lesions of diencephalon or midbrain produce bilaterally synchronous slow waves, but, interestingly, those of pons and medulla, i.e, below the mesencephalon, may be associated with a normal or near-normal wakeful type of EEG pattern, despite catastrophic clinical changes. The EEG may be of lateralizing value in acute subarachnoid hemorrhage, depending upon the extent to which the adjacent cerebrum is affected.

Brain Injury Cerebral concussion in animals is accompanied by a transitory disturbance in brain waves, but in humans this is usually over before a recording can be made. Cerebral contusion or laceration produces EEG changes similar to those described for cerebrovascular disease. Diffuse changes often give way to focal ones, especially if the lesions are on the lateral or superior surface of the brain, and these in turn usually disappear over a period of weeks or months. Sharp waves or spikes sometimes emerge as the focal slow-wave abnormality resolves and may precede the occurrence of posttraumatic epilepsy. Following head injury, therefore, serial EEGs may be of prognostic value as regards the prospect of epilepsy. They may also aid, as mentioned above, in evaluating patients for subdural hematoma.

Diseases That Cause Coma and States of Impaired Consciousness The EEG is abnormal in almost all conditions in which there is some impairment of consciousness. With hypothyroidism the brain waves are normal in configuration but are usually decreased in number. In general, the more profound the change in consciousness, the more abnormal the EEG recording. In these latter situations the slow (delta) waves are bilateral and of high amplitude, and tend to be more conspicuous over the frontal regions (Fig. 2-2*I*). This pertains to such differing conditions as acute meningitis or encephalitis, severe disorders of blood gases, glucose, electrolyte and water balance, uremia, diabetic coma, or impairment of consciousness accompanying the large cerebral lesions discussed above. In hepatic coma, the degree of abnormality in the EEG corresponds with the degree of confusion, stupor, or coma. Moreover, paroxysms of bilaterally synchronous large, sharp "triphasic waves" are characteristic (Fig. 2-2*I*), though they may also be seen with encephalopathies related to renal or pulmonary failure. Diffuse degenerative diseases (e.g., Alzheimer's disease) causing serious affection of the cerebral cortex are accompanied by relatively slight degrees of diffuse, slow-wave abnormality in the theta (4- to 7-Hz) range only late in their course. More rapidly progressive ones, such as subacute sclerosing panencephalitis (SSPE), Creutzfeldt-Jakob disease, and to a lesser extent the cerebral lipidoses have, in addition, very characteristic, almost pathognomonic, EEG changes, consisting of periodic bursts of high-amplitude, sharp waves, usually bisynchronous and symmetric (Fig. 2-2*H*). Even in situations where the EEG abnormality is not specific or diagnostic, it is useful in emphasizing the presence of physiologic, biochemical, and, sometimes, structural abnormalities of the brain. A normal EEG in a patient who is apathetic, slow, depressed, or forgetful is a point in favor of the diagnosis of an affective disorder or schizophrenia.

An EEG may also be of help in the diagnosis of coma when the pertinent history is unavailable. It may point to such otherwise unexpected causes as hepatic encephalopathy, intoxication with barbiturates or tranquilizers, clinically inapparent continuous epileptic discharges, or diffuse anoxia-ischemia.

Other Diseases of the Cerebrum Many disorders of nervous function cause little or no alteration in the EEG. Multiple sclerosis and other demyelinating diseases are examples, though as many as 50 percent of advanced cases will have an abnormal record of nonspecific type (slow wave frequencies in a focus or over a hemisphere). Delirium tremens and Wernicke-Korsakoff disease, despite the dramatic nature of the clinical picture, cause little or no change in the EEG. Some degree of slowing usually accompanies confusional states which have been designated elsewhere as hypokinetic delirium (see Chap. 19). Interestingly, neuroses and psychoses, such as manic-depressive disorders or schizophrenia, intoxication with hallucinogenic drugs such as LSD, and the majority of cases of mental retardation, are associated either with no important modification of the normal record or with minor nonspecific abnormalities.

CLINICAL SIGNIFICANCE OF MINOR EEG ABNORMALITIES

The gross EEG abnormalities discussed above are, by themselves, clearly abnormal and any formulation of the patient's clinical status should attempt to account for them. They include seizure discharge, generalized and extreme slowing, definite slow waves with a clear-cut asymmetry or a focus, and absence of normal rhythms. Certain other findings are of more doubtful significance and represent lesser degrees of abnormality which form a continuum between the undoubtedly abnormal and the completely normal. These records—which comprise such activity as 14- and 6-per-second positive spikes, small sharp waves, scattered 5- or 6-per-second slowing, voltage asymmetries, and moderate "breakdown" with hyperventilation—are termed *borderline* and are most difficult to interpret. The minor EEG abnormalities may be meaningful, but only if correlated with certain clinical phenomena. Whereas borderline deviations in an otherwise entirely normal person have no clinical significance, the same EEG findings, when associated with certain clinical signs and symptoms—even if they, too, are of minimal severity—become important. For example, a patient with tension headaches for 20 years is under neurologic study because of insomnia, weight loss, and an increase in the frequency of headaches. The neurologic examination, CSF, and skull films are all within normal limits. The EEG shows a reduction of voltage in the left occipitoparietal area and less alpha than the same area on the right side. The finding of such an asymmetry in the brain waves has no clinical significance in this case and may be disregarded. On the other hand, the same finding in someone who was rendered unconscious in an accident 9 days before and who shows slight awkwardness in the right hand and a continuous dull headache with a lack of usual alertness carries considerable diagnostic meaning. It points to the left hemisphere, which might show contusion or the presence of a subdural hematoma. The value of a normal or "negative" EEG in certain patients suspected of having a cerebral lesion has been discussed above.

In conclusion, the results of the EEG, like those of the EMG and ECG, are meaningful only in relation to the clinical status of the patient at the time they were recorded.

SPECIAL APPLICATIONS OF THE EEG

The EEG is useful in the operating room to monitor cerebral activity during the increasingly extensive procedures of modern cardiovascular surgery. EEG apparatus has long been available for indicating the level of anesthesia, and such simple equipment should be used by the anesthetist to monitor both the cardiac and cerebral status of *all* patients during surgical anesthesia.

In the neurosurgical operating room the EEG can be recorded from the exposed brain (electrocorticogram); seizure patterns can be localized more precisely than from the scalp, so that resection of such physiologically abnormal tissue may be undertaken.

The routine EEG can be of value in the diagnosis of hysterical blindness, as stated above. Similarly, a response evoked by noise during light sleep can be of help in confirming the presence of hearing in a patient who feigns total deafness. These responses may also be helpful in evaluating hearing and vision in infants. However, the visual and auditory evoked responses are usually too small to be visible in the melange of baseline noise and background activity of the routine EEG. Averaging techniques (computerized) may then be used to record them. This interesting field of electroencephalography is discussed below.

The EEG has been introduced into neonatal and infant neurology. The normal patterns from the seventh month of fetal life through infancy and childhood have been established. Full maturation, viz., the time when the stable adult pattern is achieved, varies considerably, making interpretation difficult. However, certain changes as described by Werner et al. are clearly indicative of a developmental disorder or disease.

COMPUTERIZED EVOKED POTENTIALS

The stimulation of sense organs or peripheral nerves evokes a response in the appropriate cortical receiving areas and affects a number of subcortical relay stations as well. However, one cannot place a recording electrode near the latter in the intact human organism; one can also not detect tiny potentials of only a few microvolts among the much larger background activity in the EEG or EMG. The use of the averaging method, introduced by Dawson, in 1954, and the more recent development of digital computers have provided the means of overcoming these problems. A series of waveforms, modified at each relay station and recorded by distant electrodes ("far-field recording") can be maximized by the com-

puter to a point where they can be easily measured in terms of their voltage and latency.

For many years it has been known that a light stimulus, flashing on the retina, initiated a discernible waveform over the occipital lobes. In 1969, it was observed by Regan and Heron that a visual evoked response could be produced by a sudden change of a viewed pattern. The responses produced in this way were easier to measure than flash responses and more consistent in waveform from one individual to another. It was found that this type of stimulus, applied first to one eye and then to the other, could demonstrate conductional delays in the visual pathways of patients who had formerly suffered a disease of the optic nerve—even though there were no residual signs of reduced visual

Figure 2-3

Pattern-shift visual evoked responses (PSVER). Upper two tracings, from right and left eye, are normal. Latency measured to first major positive peak (b); duration measured from beginning of positive peak (a) to return to baseline (c). Middle tracings: PSVER from the right eye is normal but the latency of the response from the left eye is prolonged and its duration is increased. Lower tracings: PSVER from both eyes show abnormally prolonged latencies, somewhat greater on the left than on the right. Calibration: 50 ms, 2.5 μV. (Redrawn from Shahrokhi et al.)

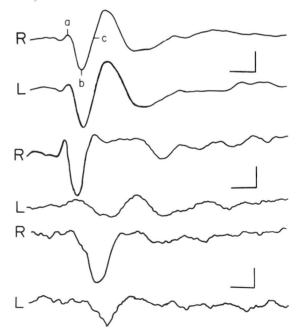

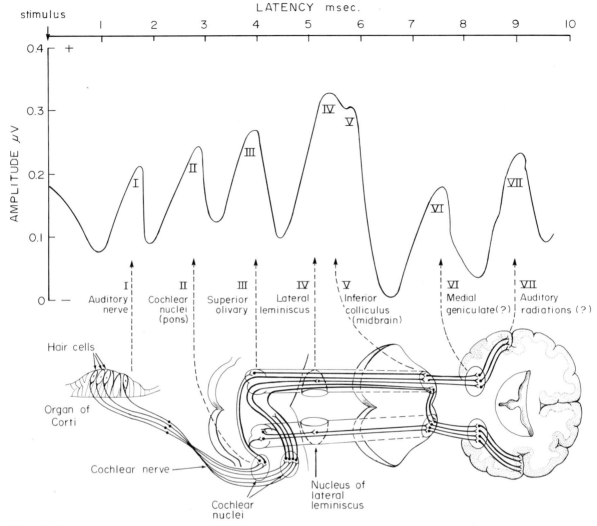

LATENCY msec.

Figure 2-4

Far-field brainstem auditory evoked responses (BAER). Diagram of the proposed electrophysiologic-anatomic correlations in human subjects.

acuity, visual field abnormality, alteration of the optic nerve head, or change in pupillary reflexes.

This procedure, which is called *pattern-shift visual evoked responses* (PSVER) has now become widely adopted as one of the most delicate tests of lesions in the visual system. Figure 2-3 illustrates the normal PSVER and two types of delayed responses. Examination of a large number of patients who were known to have had a retrobulbar neuritis showed a significantly prolonged latency from stimulus to cortical recording (from 102 ms in controls, with 1.3 ms difference between the two eyes,

to 132 ms); among 51 such patients only 4 had normal latencies (Shahrokhi, Chiappa, and Young). These authors found similar abnormalities of the PSVER in about one-third of multiple sclerosis patients who had no history or clinical evidence of optic nerve involvement. Usually, abnormalities of amplitudes and duration of PSVER accompany the abnormally prolonged latencies. A difference between responses from the two eyes signifies involvement of one optic nerve; bilateral prolongations could be due to lesions in both optic nerves or in the visual pathways posterior to the optic chiasm. Compressive lesions of an optic nerve will have the same effect as a demyelinative one. Glaucoma and other diseases anterior to the retinal ganglion cells may also produce increased latencies. Visual acuity has little effect on the latency but does correlate well with the amplitude of the PSVER.

The test of PSVER is especially valuable in proving the existence of active or residual disease of an optic nerve. The finding of abnormal PSVER in a patient with a clinically apparent lesion elsewhere in the central nervous system is presumptive evidence of multiple sclerosis (Chap. 36).

The cortical effects of auditory stimuli can be studied in the same way as visual ones, by a procedure called *far-field brainstem auditory evoked responses* (BAER). A large number of clicks, delivered first to one ear and then the other, are recorded through scalp electrodes and maximized by computer. A series of seven waves appear at the scalp within 10 ms after each stimulus. On the basis of depth recordings and the study of lesions produced in cats, it has been determined that each of the first five waves are generated by the brainstem structures indicated in Fig. 2-4. The generators of waves VI and VII are uncertain. A lesion which affects one of the relay stations or its immediate connections is said to be manifested by lower voltage of the wave or a delay in its appearance and an absence or reduction in amplitude of subsequent waves. These effects are more pronounced on the side of the stimulated ear than contralaterally, which is difficult to understand since the majority of the cochlear-superior olivary-lateral lemniscal-medial geniculate fibers cross to the opposite side. It

is also surprising that a severe lesion of one relay station would allow impulses to continue their ascent and be recordable in the cerebral cortex.

Short-latency somatosensory evoked potentials (SLSEP) are now being tested in several of the clinical neurophysiology laboratories in the United States. Here a series of electrical stimuli are delivered to the median nerve and recorded by electrodes over Erb's point (EP), in the supraclavicular region, over the C2 spine, over the cranial vertex (CZ) and over the midline of the forehead (FZ) after maximization by computer. Delay between stimulus and Erb's point indicates peripheral nerve disease (between arrow and EP in Fig. 2-5). Delay between Erb's point and waves A and B appears to occur with lesions in the cervical cord, medulla, and pons. Delay between B and P2 indicates a lesion in the thalamocortical radiations or primary sensory fields of the cortex, or both. Recordings with pathologically verified lesions at these levels are to be found in the article by Chiappa et al.

ELECTROMYOGRAPHY AND NERVE CONDUCTION STUDIES

These will be discussed in Chap. 44.

PSYCHOMETRY, PERIMETRY, AUDIOMETRY, AND TESTS OF LABYRINTHINE FUNCTION

These methods, drawn largely from the field of physiologic psychology, are used in quantitating and defining the nature of the psychic or sensory deficits produced by disease of the nervous system. The indications for doing these tests are (1) to obtain confirmation of a disorder of function in particular parts of the nervous system and to ascertain its nature or (2) to quantitate the disorder in order to determine, by subsequent examinations, the natural course of the underlying illness. A description of these methods and their clinical use will be found in the chapters dealing with developmental disorders of the cerebrum (Chap. 27), with dementia (Chap. 20), and with disorders of vision (Chap. 12) and of hearing and equilibrium (Chap. 14).

BIOCHEMICAL TESTS

With advances in the biochemistry of metabolic diseases a number of highly specific tests of serum, CSF, and

Figure 2-5

Short-latency somatosensory evoked potentials (SLSEP) from a normal subject. Stimulation of median nerve occurs at the arrow (1.28 ms before the start of the sweep). A positive potential is recorded by an upward deflection. For the upper three channels the calibration bar equals 2 μV; for the lowermost channel the bar equals 1.2 μV. EP, Erb's point; C2 and C4, second and fourth cervical spines; CZ, cranial vertex; FZ, midline of forehead; H, dorsum of hand opposite to that being stimulated. (Redrawn from Chiappa et al.)

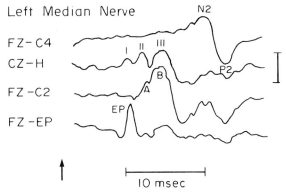

Left Median Nerve

circulating red and white blood cells have become available. These are too numerous and varied to describe here, and each one will be presented in relation to the metabolic diseases of which it is diagnostic.

The exact indications for the use of each of the above diagnostic procedures will be given in the following chapters, dealing with the cardinal manifestations of neurologic disease and the individual diseases of the nervous system.

REFERENCES

ALFIDI RJ et al: *Computed Tomography of the Human Body. An Atlas of Normal Anatomy.* St Louis, Mosby, 1977.

CHIAPPA KH, GLADSTONE KJ, YOUNG RR: Brainstem auditory evoked responses. *Arch Neurol* 36:81, 1979.

CHIAPPA KH, CHOI SK, YOUNG RR: Short latency somatosensory evoked potentials following median nerve stimulation in patients with neurological lesions, in Desmedt JE (ed): *Progress in Clinical Neurophysiology*, vol 7: *Somatosensory Evoked Potentials and Their Clinical Uses.* Basel, Karger, 1978.

DUFRESNE JJ: *Cytopathologie de CSF.* Basel, Ciba Foundation, 1973.

FISHMAN RA: *Cerebrospinal Fluid in Diseases of the Nervous System.* Philadelphia, Saunders, 1980.

HALLIDAY AM et al: The pattern-evoked potential in compression of the anterior visual pathways. *Brain* 99:357, 1976.

————, McDONALD WI, MUSHIN J: Visual evoked potentials in patients with demyelinating disease, in Desmedt JF (ed): *New Developments in Visual Evoked Potentials in the Human Brain.* London, Oxford University Press, 1976.

HARWOOD-NASH DC, FITZ CR: *Neuroradiology in Infants and Children,* vols 1-3. St Louis, Mosby, 1976.

KILOH LG, McCOMAS AJ, OSSELTON JW: *Clinical Electroencephalography,* 3d ed. London, Butterworth, 1972.

KLASS DW, DALY DD (eds): *Current Practice of Clinical EEG.* New York, Raven Press, 1979.

KOOI KA, TUCKER RP, MARSHALL RE: *Fundamentals of Electroencephalography,* 2d ed. Hagerstown, Md, Harper & Row, 1978.

NEWTON TH, POTTS DG (eds): *Radiology of the Skull and Brain,* vols 1-4. St Louis, Mosby, 1971-1978.

REGAN D, HERON JR: Clinical investigation of lesions of the visual pathway: A new objective technique. *J Neurol Neurosurg Psychiatry* 32:479, 1969.

SHAHROKHI F, CHIAPPA KH, YOUNG RR: Pattern shift visual evoked responses. *Arch Neurol* 35:65, 1978.

TAVERAS JM, WOOD EH: *Diagnostic Neuroradiology,* 2d ed. Baltimore, Williams & Wilkins, 1976.

WERNER SS, STOCKARD JE, BICKFORD RG: *Atlas of Neonatal Electroencephalography.* New York, Raven Press, 1977.

WESTMORELAND BF, KLASS DW, et al: Alpha-coma: Electroencephalographic, clinical, pathological and etiologic correlations. *Arch Neurol* 32:713, 1975.

WILFERT CM: Mumps meningoencephalitis with low cerebrospinal fluid glucose, prolonged pleocytosis and elevation of protein. *N Engl J Med* 280:855, 1969.

CARDINAL MANIFESTATIONS OF
NEUROLOGIC DISEASE

DISORDERS OF MOTILITY

Disturbances of motor function probably surpass all other neurologic symptoms in frequency and importance, for reasons that are not difficult to discern. The major portion of the human nervous system is designed for the purpose of moving the body in space and various parts of the body in relationship to one another. Damage to these parts of the nervous system or to the sensory pathways, which are intimately concerned with motor function, may result in a serious limitation of movement; and even injury of parts of the brain that are not concerned primarily with motor-sensory functions may affect motility, since much of the human nervous system is concerned with the planning of present and future action.

The following parts of the nervous system are known to be engaged primarily in the effectuation of movement, and in the course of disease, to yield a number of characteristic derangements of function:

1. The large motor nerve cells in the anterior horns of the spinal cord and the motor nuclei of the brainstem, the axons of which extend into the anterior spinal roots and spinal nerves and into the cranial nerves en route to the skeletal muscles, are called the primary, or lower, motor neurons. Complete lesions of them result in a loss of all movement—voluntary and reflex. In the strictest sense this is the "final common path" by which all nervous impulses are transmitted to muscle.

2. The motor cells in the cerebral cortex near Rolando's fissure are connected with the spinal motor neurons by a system of fibers known, because of their collective shape in transverse sections through the medulla, as the pyramidal tract. Since the motor neurons that run from the cerebral cortex to the spinal cord are not confined to the pyramidal tract, they are more accurately designated as the corticospinal tract, or, alternately, as the upper motor neuron, to distinguish them from the lower motor neuron.

3. Several nuclear masses deep in the brain, notably the caudate, lenticular, and subthalamic nuclei, the red nuclei, substantia nigra, and reticular formation in the brainstem, and also certain pontine nuclei and parts of the cerebellum, all of which subserve the neural mechanisms for posture and movement, are connected with one another and with the cerebral cortex and spinal cord by groups of neurons that are quite separate from the corticospinal ("pyramidal") tract. For this reason these structures are referred to as "extrapyramidal."

4. Many other parts of the cerebral cortex, viz., those concerned with tactile, visual, and auditory sensation as well as the more anterior parts of the frontal lobes, are connected by fiber tracts with the motor cortex. These association pathways provide for the sensory regulation of motor function and are also the means of coordinating thought and

action. They represent the highest level of motor function.

The impairment of motor function which results from lesions of these various parts of the nervous system may be somewhat arbitrarily divided into (1) paralysis due to affection of lower motor neurons, (2) paralysis due to affection of upper motor (corticospinal) neurons, (3) apraxic or nonparalytic disturbances of purposive movement due to involvement of the association pathways in the cerebrum, (4) abnormalities of movement and posture due to disease of the basal ganglia, and (5) abnormalities of coordination (ataxia) due to lesions in the cerebellum. The first two types of motor disorder and the apraxic disorders of movement will be discussed in Chap. 3; extrapyramidal motor abnormalities and disorders of coordination and gait will be considered in the chapters that follow. The impairment or loss of motor function which is due to primary disease of striated muscle or to a failure of neuromuscular transmission will be considered in a later section of this volume, in relation to diseases of striated muscle.

CHAPTER 3

MOTOR PARALYSIS

Definitions The term *paralysis* is derived from the Greek words *para*, "beside, off, amiss," and *lysis*, a "loosening" or "breaking up." In medicine it has come to refer to an abolition of function, either sensory or motor. When applied to motor function, *paralysis* means loss of voluntary movement due to interruption of one of the motor pathways from the cerebrum to the muscle fiber. A lesser degree of paralysis is sometimes spoken of as *paresis*, but in everyday medical parlance paralysis may stand for either partial or complete loss of function. The word *plegia* comes from a Greek word meaning "stroke," and the word *palsy*, from an old French word, has the same meaning as *paralysis*. All these words are used interchangeably in medical practice, though generally one uses *paresis* for slight and *paralysis* or *plegia* for severe loss of motor function.

AFFECTION OF THE LOWER MOTOR NEURON

ANATOMIC AND PHYSIOLOGIC CONSIDERATIONS

Each motor nerve cell, through the extensive arborization of the terminal part of its fiber, comes into contact with 100 to 200 or more muscle fibers; altogether they constitute "the motor unit." All the variations in force, range, rate, and type of movement are determined by differences in the number and size of motor units called into activity and the frequency of their action. Feeble movements involve only a few small motor units; powerful movements recruit many more units of increasing size. When a motor neuron becomes diseased, as in progressive muscular atrophy, it may manifest increased irritability, and all the muscle fibers that it controls may discharge sporadically, in isolation from other units. The result of the contraction of one or several such units is a

visible twitch, or *fasciculation*, which can be seen and recorded in the electromyogram as a large diphasic or multiphasic action potential. If the motor neuron is destroyed, all the muscle fibers which it innervates undergo a profound atrophy, viz., denervation atrophy. For some unknown reason the individual denervated muscle fibers become hypersensitive and contract spontaneously, though they can no longer do so in response to a nerve impulse as a part of the motor unit. This isolated activity of individual muscle fibers, called *fibrillation*, is so fine that it cannot be seen through the intact skin but can be recorded only as a small, repetitive, short-duration spike potential in the electromyogram (Chap. 44).

The motor nerve fibers of each ventral root intermingle as the roots join to form plexuses, and although the muscles are innervated roughly according to segments of the spinal cord, each large muscle comes to be supplied by two or more roots. In contrast, a single peripheral nerve usually provides the complete motor innervation of a muscle or group of muscles. For this reason the distribution of paralysis due to disease of the anterior horn cells or anterior roots differs from that which follows a lesion of a peripheral nerve.

All motor activity, even of the most elementary reflex type, requires the cooperation of many muscles. The analysis of a relatively simple movement, such as clenching the fist, affords some idea of the complexity of the underlying neural arrangements. In this act the primary movement is a contraction of the flexor muscles of the fingers, the flexor digitorum sublimis and profundus, the flexor pollicis longus and brevis, and the abductor pollicis brevis. In the terminology of Beevor, these muscles act as *agonists*, or *prime movers*. In order that flexion of these muscles may be smooth and forceful, the extensor muscles (*antagonists*) must provide a diminishing contraction, i.e., they must relax, at the same rate as the flexors contract. The muscles which flex the fingers also flex the wrist; and since it is desired that only the fingers flex, the muscles which extend the wrist must be brought into play to prevent its flexion. The action of the wrist extensors is synergic, and these muscles are called *synergists* in this particular act. Lastly, during this action of the hand, the wrist, elbow, and shoulder usually need to be stabilized by appropriate flexor and extensor muscles; the muscles which accomplish this serve as *fixators*. The coordination of agonists, antagonists, synergists, and fixators involves reciprocal innervation and is managed entirely by segmental spinal reflexes under the guidance of proprioceptive sensory stimuli. Only the agonist movement in a voluntary act is thought to be initiated at a cerebral level. In general, the more delicate the movement, the more precise must be the coordination between agonist and antagonist muscles.

In contrast to a slow so-called ramp movement, such as clenching the fist, in all fast ("ballistic") movements of either proximal or distal muscles there is first a burst of activity in the agonist muscles, then a burst in the antagonists, followed by a third burst in the agonists. The strength of the initial agonist burst determines the speed and distance of the movement, but always there is the same triad of agonist, antagonist, and agonist, according to Hallett and Khoshbin. Other muscles not selected in the movement sequence are inhibited. The basal ganglia and cerebellum prepare the pattern and set the timing of all the muscles involved in any projected motor performance. This will be discussed further in Chap. 4.

In addition, there are many basic motor activities which do not involve reciprocal innervation. In the support of the body in an upright posture, when the legs must act as rigid pillars, and in shivering, the agonists and antagonists contract simultaneously. The alternating coordinated movements of stepping are accomplished by multisegmental spinal reflexes.

PARALYSIS DUE TO DISEASE OF THE LOWER MOTOR NEURONS

If all or practically all peripheral motor fibers supplying a muscle are destroyed, all voluntary, postural, and reflex movements are abolished. The muscle becomes lax and soft, a condition known as *flaccidity*. Muscle tone—the slight resistance that normal relaxed muscle offers to passive movement—is reduced (*hypotonia* or *atonia*). The denervated muscle undergoes extreme atrophy,

being reduced to 20 or 30 percent of its original bulk within 3 months. The reaction of the muscle to sudden stretch, as by tapping its tendon, is lost. If only a portion of the motor fibers supplying the muscle is affected, partial paralysis or paresis will ensue. The atrophy will be less and the tendon reflexes will be reduced instead of lost. The electrodiagnosis of denervation depends upon the finding of certain abnormalities of nerve conduction and of fibrillations, fasciculations, and other abnormalities of needle electrode examination (see Chap. 44).

The tonus of muscle and the tendon reflexes are known to depend on the muscle spindles and the afferent fibers to which they give origin and on the small anterior horn cells whose axons terminate on the small muscle fibers within the spindles (intrafusal fibers). The specialized small motor neurons are called *gamma neurons*, in contrast to the large alpha neurons. Some of the gamma neurons are tonically active at rest, keeping the intrafusal muscle fibers taut and sensitive to external stretch. A tap on a tendon, by stretching the spindle muscle fibers, activates afferent nerve fibers which synapse with alpha motor neurons in the same and adjacent spinal segments, and they in turn send impulses to the skeletal muscle fibers, resulting in the familiar brief muscle contraction or stretch reflex (Fig. 3-1). Thus the setting of the spindle fibers and the state of excitability of the gamma neurons (normally inhibited by the corticospinal and other supranuclear fibers) determine the level of activity of the tendon reflexes and the responsiveness of muscle to stretch. Other mechanisms of an inhibitory nature, involving Golgi tendon organs, are brought into play in more powerful stretching of muscle. These receptors have mainly a protective function, preventing excessive muscle contraction, but they also play a role in naturally occurring limb movements, particularly in locomotion.

Lower motor neuron paralysis is the direct result of loss of function or destruction of anterior horn cells or their axons in anterior roots and nerves. The signs and symptoms vary according to the location of the lesion. Probably the most important question for clinical purposes is whether sensory changes coexist. The combination of flaccid, areflexic paralysis and sensory changes usually indicates involvement of mixed motor and sensory nerves or affection of both anterior and posterior roots. If sensory changes are absent, the lesion must be situated in the anterior gray matter of the spinal cord, in the anterior roots, in a purely motor branch of a peripheral nerve, or in motor axons alone. The distinction between nuclear (spinal) and anterior root (radicular) lesions may at times be impossible to make. Preserved tendon reflexes and spasticity in muscles weakened by a

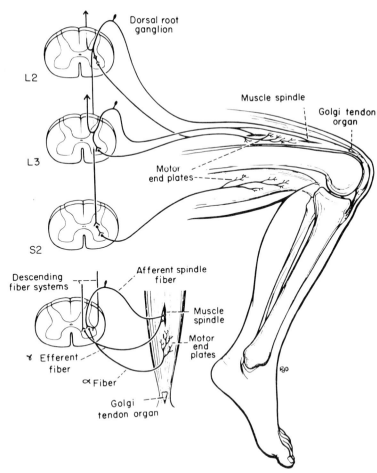

Figure 3-1

Patellar tendon reflex. Sensory fibers of the femoral nerve derived from spinal segments L2 and L3 mediate this myotatic reflex. The principal receptors are the muscle spindles, which respond to a brisk stretching of the muscle effected by tapping the patellar tendon. Afferent fibers from muscle spindles are shown entering only the L3 spinal segment, while afferent fibers from the Golgi tendon organ are shown entering only the L2 spinal segment. In this monosynaptic reflex, afferent fibers entering spinal segments L2 and L3 and efferent fibers issuing from the anterior horn cells of these and lower levels complete the reflex arc. Motor fibers shown leaving the S2 spinal segment and passing to the hamstring muscles demonstrate the disynaptic pathway by which inhibitory influences are exerted upon an antagonistic muscle group during the reflex.

The small diagram below illustrates the gamma loop. Gamma efferent fibers pass to the polar portions of the muscle spindle. Contractions of the intrafusal fibers in the polar parts of the spindle stretch the nuclear bag region and thus cause an afferent impulse to be conducted centrally. The afferent fibers from the spindle synapse with an alpha motor neuron, the peripheral processes of which pass to extrafusal muscle fibers, thus completing the loop. Both alpha and gamma motor neurons are influenced by descending fiber systems from supraspinal levels. (Redrawn from MB Carpenter, Human Neuroanatomy, 7th ed, Baltimore, Williams & Wilkins, 1976.)

corticospinal lesion point to the integrity of the segments below the level of the lesion.

AFFECTION OF THE CORTICOSPINAL (PYRAMIDAL), CORTICOBULBAR, AND OTHER UPPER MOTOR NEURONS

ANATOMIC AND PHYSIOLOGIC CONSIDERATIONS

The terms *pyramidal*, *corticospinal*, and *upper motor neuron* are often used interchangeably, but this is not altogether correct. The pyramidal tract, strictly speaking, refers only to those fibers which course longitudinally in the pyramid of the medulla oblongata. Of all the fiber bundles in the brain, the pyramidal tract has been known for the longest time, having been described by Türck in 1851. It descends from the cerebral cortex, tra-

verses the pons and the pyramid of the upper medulla, decussates in the lower medulla, and continues its caudal course in the lateral funiculus of the spinal cord; hence the alternate name, *corticospinal tract*. The corticospinal tract is the only *direct* long-fiber connection between the cerebral cortex and the spinal cord. There are, in addition, several *indirect* pathways, notably the corticorubrospinal and corticoreticulospinal, which do not run in the pyramid and by which the cortex influences the spinal motor neurons. All these pathways, direct and indirect, are embraced by the term *upper motor neuron*.

A major source of confusion about the pyramidal tract stems from the former belief that it originated entirely from the large motor cells of Betz in the fifth layer of the precentral convolution, or area 4 of Brodmann (Fig. 3-3). However, there are only 25,000 to 35,000 Betz cells, whereas the medullary pyramid contains about 1 million axons. The pyramidal tract, therefore, must con-

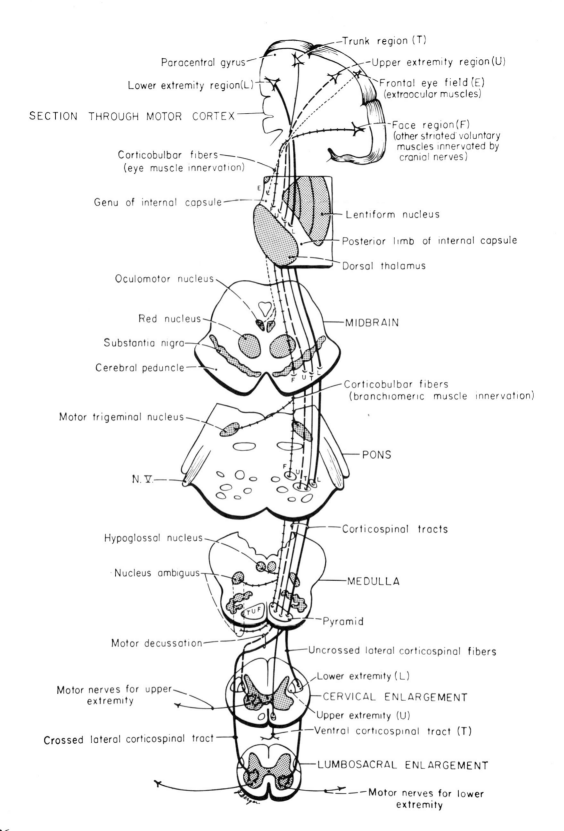

Trunk region (T)

Paracentral gyrus

Upper extremity region (U)

Lower extremity region (L)

Frontal eye field (E)
(extraocular muscles)

SECTION THROUGH MOTOR CORTEX

Face region (F)
(other striated voluntary
muscles innervated by
cranial nerves)

Corticobulbar fibers
(eye muscle innervation)

Genu of internal capsule

Lentiform nucleus

Posterior limb of internal capsule

Dorsal thalamus

Oculomotor nucleus

Red nucleus

MIDBRAIN

Substantia nigra

Cerebral peduncle

Corticobulbar fibers
(branchiomeric muscle innervation)

Motor trigeminal nucleus

N. V.

PONS

Corticospinal tracts

Hypoglossal nucleus

Nucleus ambiguus

MEDULLA

Pyramid

Motor decussation

Uncrossed lateral corticospinal fibers

Lower extremity (L)

Motor nerves for upper
extremity

CERVICAL ENLARGEMENT

Upper extremity (U)

Ventral corticospinal tract (T)

Crossed lateral corticospinal tract

LUMBOSACRAL ENLARGEMENT

Motor nerves for lower
extremity

36

tain many fibers that arise from other cortical neurons, particularly those in area 4 and area 6 (the frontal cortex immediately rostral to area 4, including the posterior portion of the superior frontal gyrus), in the primary somatosensory cortex (Brodmann's areas 3, 1, and 2), and in the superior parietal lobule (areas 5 and 7). The data concerning the origin of the pyramidal tract in humans are scanty, but in the monkey, counting the fibers remaining after cortical excisions and long survival periods, Russell and DeMyer found that 40 percent of descending pyramidal axons arise in the parietal lobe, 31 percent in area 4, and the remaining 29 percent in area 6.

The fibers from areas 4 and 6 and portions of the parietal lobe converge in the corona radiata and descend through the posterior limb of the internal capsule, crus cerebri, pons, and medulla. As the corticospinal tract descends in the brainstem, more or less distinct bundles of fibers separate successively as the corticomesencephalic, corticopontine, and corticobulbar tracts and cross the midline to the contralateral motor nuclei of the cranial nerves (Fig. 3-2). Insofar as the corticobulbar and corticospinal fibers have a similar origin and the motor nuclei of the brainstem are the homologues of the motor nuclei of the spinal cord, the term "upper motor neuron" may suitably be applied to both these systems of fibers.

The corticospinal tracts *decussate* at the lower end of the medulla, although some of their fibers may cross above this level. The proportion of crossed and uncrossed fibers varies greatly from one person to another. Most textbooks state that 75 percent of the fibers cross and that the remainder descend ipsilaterally, about equally divided between the lateral and ventral uncrossed corticospinal tracts. In exceptional cases, these tracts cross completely; rarely, none of the fibers cross. These variations are probably of functional significance in determining the amount of neurologic deficit that results from unilateral lesions such as capsular infarction. The presence of a large uncrossed segment of corticospinal fibers would account for a slight degree of paralysis of the affected extremities.

The corticospinal tracts and other upper motor neurons terminate mainly in relation to nerve cells in the intermediate zone of spinal gray matter (internuncial neurons), from which motor impulses are then transmitted to the anterior horn cells. Only a small proportion of corticospinal fibers (presumably the thick, rapidly conducting axons derived from Betz cells) establish direct synaptic connections with the large motor neurons of the anterior horns.

The *motor area of the cerebral cortex* is difficult to define precisely (Fig. 3-3). It includes that part of the precentral convolution which contains Betz cells (area 4), but, as already mentioned, it extends anteriorly into area 6 and posteriorly into the anterior parietal lobe

Figure 3-3

Lateral (A) and medial (B) surfaces of the human cerebral hemispheres, showing the areas of excitable cortex. (After Foerster.)

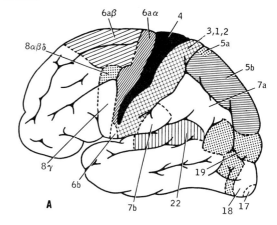

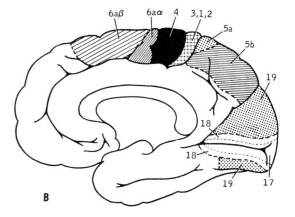

Figure 3-2

Corticospinal and corticobulbar tracts. The letters on the fiber tracts at various levels correspond to the letters which mark the origin of these fibers in the cortex. (From EC Crosby et al, Correlative Anatomy of the Nervous System, New York, Macmillan, 1962.)

where it overlaps the sensory areas. Physiologically it is defined as the region of electrically excitable cortex from which isolated movements can be evoked by stimuli of minimal intensity. The muscle groups of the contralateral face, arm, trunk, and leg are represented in the primary motor cortex (area 4), those of the face being at the lower end and those of the leg in the paracentral lobule on the medial surface of the cerebral hemisphere. The parts of the body capable of the most delicate movements have, in general, the largest cortical representation.

Area 6, the premotor area, is also electrically excitable, but requires more intense stimuli than area 4 to evoke movements. Stimulation of its caudal aspect (area 6a) produces responses that are similar to those elicited from area 4; these responses probably depend upon transmission of impulses to area 4 (since they cannot be obtained after ablation of this area) and discharge via the corticospinal tract. Stimulation of its most rostral portion (area 6aβ) elicits more general movement patterns, which discharge via pathways other than those derived from area 4 ("extrapyramidal"). Very strong stimuli elicit movement from a wide area of premotor frontal and parietal cortex, and the same movements may be obtained from several points. From this it may be assumed that one of the functions of the motor cortex is to synthesize agonist actions into an infinite variety of finely graded, highly differentiated patterns.

Stimulation of the supplementary motor area (the most anterior portion of area 6 on the medial surface of the cortex, rostral to the primary motor cortex) yields complex patterned movements and bilateral tonic contractions of the muscles of the trunk and legs. Presumably, much of the residual motor function following hemispherectomy depends on the ipsilateral innervation contributed by the supplementary motor area of the remaining hemisphere.

How the motor cortex controls movements is still a controversial matter. The long-entrenched view, based on the interpretations of Hughlings Jackson and of Sherrington, is that the motor cortex is organized in terms of movements, i.e., the coordinated contraction of groups of muscles, not of individual muscles. On the basis of observations that a patient could recover the use of a limb following destruction of a limb area that had been defined by cortical stimulation, Jackson visualized a widely overlapping representation of muscle groups in the cerebral cortex. This view was supported by Sherrington's experiments, in which stimulation of the corti-

cal surface activated not solitary muscles but a combination of muscles, and always in a reciprocal fashion, i.e., in a manner that maintained the expected relationship between agonists and antagonists. He noted also the inconstancy of stimulatory effects; a given cortical point may initiate flexion of a part at one time and extension at another.

These interpretations must be viewed with circumspection, as must all observations that are based on the electrical stimulation of the surface of the cortex. It has been shown that to stimulate motor cells from the surface, the electric current has to penetrate the cortex to a considerable depth, inevitably activating a large number of cortical neurons. The elegant experiments of Asanuma and his colleagues, who stimulated the depths of the cortex with a microelectrode, have demonstrated the existence of discrete zones of efferent neurons which control the contraction of individual muscles and have shown that stimulation of a given efferent zone often facilitates rather than inhibits the contraction of the antagonists. Furthermore, they noted that cells in the efferent zone receive afferent impulses from the particular muscle to which the efferent neurons project. These experimental findings must of necessity modify current views about the cortical control of movement, and the continued use of these techniques will undoubtedly serve to redefine the boundaries of the motor cortex.

The mode of termination of the corticospinal and other descending motor tracts has been studied in the monkey by interrupting these pathways in the medulla and more rostral parts of the brainstem and tracing the distribution of the degenerating elements in the spinal gray matter. On the basis of such experiments and a considerable body of physiologic data, Kuypers has suggested that the functional organization of the descending cortical and subcortical pathways is determined more by their patterns of termination and the motor capacities of the internuncial neurons upon which they terminate than by the location of their cells of origin. With reference to their differential terminal distribution, three groups of motor fibers can be distinguished: (1) A ventromedial pathway, which arises in the tectum, vestibular nuclei, and pontine and medullary reticular cells and terminates on the internuncial cells of the ventromedial part of the spinal gray matter. This system is mainly concerned with axial movements—the maintenance of posture, integrated movements of body and limbs, and total-limb movements. (2) A lateral pathway, which is derived mainly from the magnocellular part of the red nucleus and terminates in the dorsal and lateral parts of the internuncial zone. This pathway adds the capacity for independent use of the extremities, especially of the hands. (3) The corticospinal pathway, the major portion of which terminates diffusely throughout the nucleus proprius of the dorsal horn and the intermediate zone and greatly amplifies the control of hand movements. In addition, a small portion of the corticospinal tract synapses directly with the large motor neurons that innervate the distal parts of the extremities, face, and tongue; this system provides the capacity for a high degree of fractionation of movements, as exemplified by independent finger movements.

PARALYSIS DUE TO DISEASE OF THE UPPER MOTOR NEURONS

The corticospinal pathways may be interrupted by lesions at many levels, including the cerebral cortex, subcortical white matter, internal capsule, brainstem and spinal cord. Practically always, when paralysis is complete and permanent as a consequence of disease, much more is involved than the long, uninterrupted corticospinal pathway. In the cerebral white matter (corona radiata) and internal capsule the corticospinal fibers are intermingled with corticostriate, corticothalamic, corticorubral, corticopontine, corticoolivary, and corticoreticular fibers. It is noteworthy that thalamocortical fibers, which are a vital link in an ascending fiber system from the basal ganglia and cerebellum, also pass through the internal capsule and cerebral white matter. Thus lesions in these parts simultaneously affect both corticospinal and extrapyramidal systems. The terms *corticospinal* or *pyramidal* as designations for the spastic hemiplegia that results from a capsular lesion are misnomers, therefore. *Upper motor neuron paralysis* is a more suitable term, provided that it is used in a collective sense, indicating involvement of the several descending fiber systems that influence and modify the lower motor neuron.

The one place where corticospinal fibers are isolated as the pyramidal tract is in the medullary pyramids. In humans there are a few documented cases of a lesion more or less confined to this locality (see Ropper et al.). The result of such lesions has been a flaccid hemiplegia with sparing of the face, from which there is considerable recovery. Similarly, in monkeys, as shown by Tower, in 1940, and more recently by Lawrence and Kuypers, interruption of both pyramidal tracts results in a hypotonic paralysis; ultimately these animals recover control over a wide range of movements, though slowness of all movements and loss of individual finger movements remain as permanent deficits. These results inform us that spasticity cannot be interpreted as a manifestation of pure pyramidal tract disease. Also, the cerebral peduncle has been sectioned in human beings in an effort to abolish involuntary movements; in some of

these patients only a slight degree of weakness was produced and spasticity did not develop. These observations and the ones in monkeys indicate that control over a wide range of voluntary movements depends at least in part on nonpyramidal motor pathways. Animal experiments suggest that the corticorubrospinal and corticoreticulospinal pathways are important in this respect, since their fibers are arranged somatotopically and they are able to influence stretch reflexes. Further studies of human material are necessary to settle problems related to volitional movement and spasticity. The motor organization of the cat and even of the monkey is so different from that of humans and the range of volitional activity and motor skills so much less that direct comparisons are not justified.

The distribution of the paralysis due to upper motor neuron lesions varies with the locale of the lesion, but certain features are characteristic of all of them. A group of muscles is always involved, never individual muscles, and if any movement is possible, the proper relationships between agonists, antagonists, synergists, and fixators are preserved. The paralysis never involves all the muscles on one side of the body, even in the severest forms of hemiplegia. Movements that are invariably bilateral, such as those of the eyes, jaw, pharynx, larynx, neck, thorax, and abdomen, are little if at all affected. Upper motor neuron paralysis is rarely complete for any long period of time; in this respect it differs from the absolute paralysis due to a complete destruction of anterior horn cells or interruption of their axons.

Upper motor neuron lesions are characterized further by certain peculiarities of residual movement, known as *synkinesias*. The paralyzed arm may suddenly move during yawning and stretching. Attempts by the patient to move the hemiplegic limbs may result in a variety of associated movements. Thus, flexion of the arm may result in involuntary pronation; flexion of the leg may cause the foot to dorsiflex and evert automatically. Also, volitional movements of the normal limb may evoke imitative (mirror) movements in the paretic one or vice versa.

If the upper motor neurons are interrupted above the level of the facial colliculus in the pons, hand and arm muscles suffer most severely and the leg muscles next; of the cranial musculature only the muscles of the tongue and lower part of the face are involved to any significant degree. Broadbent was the first to call attention to this distribution of paralysis, sometimes referred to as "Broadbent's law." At lower levels, such as the cervical cord, acute lesions of the upper motor neuron may cause not only a paralysis of voluntary movement but also abolish temporarily the spinal reflexes subserved by segments below the lesion. This condition is referred to as *spinal shock*. After a few days to weeks the flaccidity and areflexia give way to a state of excessive muscular tonus (hypertonus) and heightened stretch reflexes, a phenomenon known as *spasticity* (see below). This sequence of changes is not as sharply defined with cerebral lesions as it is with spinal ones. With some acute lesions, spasticity and paralysis develop together; in others the limbs remain flaccid but reflexes are retained.

A predilection for involvement of certain muscle groups, a specific pattern of response to stretch, and manifestly exaggerated tendon reflexes are the identifying characteristics of spasticity. The antigravity muscles—flexors of the arms and the extensors of the legs—are predominantly affected. The arm tends to assume a flexed and pronated position and the leg an extended and adducted one, indicating that certain spinal neurons are reflexly more active than others. At rest in the shortened position to midposition, the muscles are flaccid to palpation and electromyographically silent. If the arm is extended or the leg flexed very slowly, there may be little or no change in muscle tone. In contrast, if these muscles are stretched more rapidly, the limb moves freely for a very short distance, beyond which there is an abrupt catch and then a rapidly increasing muscular resistance up to a point; thereafter, as the passive extension continues, the resistance melts away. This sequence constitutes the classical "clasp-knife" phenomenon. With the limb in the extended or flexed position, a new passive movement encounters the same sequence; this whole combination is the lengthening and shortening reaction. Thus the essential feature of spasticity is an increased reactivity to a stretch stimulus. The two-phased clasp-knife response is generally thought to result from the activation of the two varieties of stretch receptors, first the muscle spindles and then the Golgi tendon organs.

Not all hemiplegias of cerebral origin are associated with so pure a form of spasticity. In some cases, the arm flexors and leg extensors are spastic, while the antagonist muscles show an even resistance throughout the range of passive movement, i.e., rigidity (Chap. 4), or rigidity may be more prominent than spasticity in all muscles. In still other cases, severe weakness may be associated with only the mildest signs of spasticity, detectable as a catch in the pronators on passive supina-

tion of the forearm and in the flexors on extension of the wrist. Contrariwise, the most extreme degrees of spasticity, observed in certain cases of spinal cord disease, may so vastly exceed paresis of voluntary movement as to suggest that these two states depend on separate mechanisms. This notion is supported by the observation that anesthetic agents can selectively block small gamma neurons and abolish spasticity as well as hyperactive tendon jerks, leaving motor performance unimproved or worsened.

The hyperreflexic state that characterizes spasticity may take the form of *clonus*, a series of rhythmic involuntary muscular contractions, at a frequency of 5 to 7 Hz, in response to an abruptly and steadily applied stretch stimulus. It is usually designated in terms of the part of the limb to which pressure is applied (e.g., patella, ankle). The frequency is constant within 1 Hz and is not appreciably modified by altering peripheral or central nervous system activities. Clonus depends for its elicitation on the degree of voluntary relaxation of appropriate muscles, integrity of the spinal stretch reflex mechanisms, sustained hyperexcitability of alpha and gamma motor neurons (loss of suprasegmental effect), and synchronization of the contraction-relaxation cycle of muscle spindles (see Dimitrijevic et al.). The cutaneomuscular abdominal and cremasteric reflexes are usually abolished in these circumstances, and a Babinski sign is usually, but not invariably, present.

In addition to hyperactive *phasic myotatic reflexes*, lesions, particularly of the cervical segments of the spinal cord, may result in great enhancement of *tonic myotatic reflexes*. In standing or attempting voluntary movement, the entire limb becomes involved in intense muscular spasm that may last for several minutes. During this period the limb is quite useless. Presumably there is both an interruption of lower medullary inhibitory influences on the anterior horn cells and a release of the facilitatory effects needed in antigravity support (Henneman).

The *nociceptive spinal flexion reflexes*, of which the Babinski sign is a part, are not an essential component of spasticity. The most exaggerated forms of these release phenomena are observed in patients with severe paraparesis or paraplegia of spinal origin. Important characteristics of these responses are their capacity to be induced by weak superficial stimuli (such as a series of pinpricks) or by the patient's own efforts to move and their tendency to persist long after the stimulation or volitional effort ceases. Such hypertonus, based on tonic myotatic reflexes, retains few of the characteristics of the clasp-knife type of spasticity.

With bilateral cerebral lesions, exaggerated stretch reflexes can be elicited in cranial as well as in limb and trunk muscles, because of interruption of the corticobulbar pathways. In advanced cases this takes the form of spastic bulbar ("pseudobulbar") paralysis, characterized by dysarthria, dysphonia, dysphagia, and bifacial paralysis (see page 355).

Table 3-1 summarizes the main attributes of upper motor neuron lesions and contrasts them with those of the lower motor neurons.

Standing, all manner of postural adjustments, various positions of head and trunk, walking, and running all depend on integrations of proprioceptive, visual, and labyrinthine afferent impulses at the level of many spinal segments, medulla, pons, midbrain, and cerebellum. These will be discussed in Chap. 4 in connection with decerebrate rigidity.

APRAXIA AND OTHER NONPARALYTIC DISORDERS OF MOTOR FUNCTION

All that has been said about the cortical and spinal control of the effector apparatus gives one little idea of human motility. Viewed objectively, the conscious and sentient human organism is continuously active—fidgeting, adjusting posture and position, sitting, standing, walking, running, speaking, manipulating tools, or performing the intricate sequences of movements involved in

Table 3-1

Differences between paralysis of upper and lower motor neurons

Upper motor neuron or supranuclear paralysis	Lower motor neuron or nuclear-infranuclear paralysis
Muscles affected in groups, never individual muscles	Individual muscles may be affected
Atrophy slight and due to disuse	Atrophy pronounced up to 70 to 80% of total bulk
Spasticity with hyperactivity of the tendon reflexes and extensor plantar reflex (Babinski sign)	Flaccidity and hypotonia of affected muscles with loss of tendon reflexes
	Plantar reflex, if present, is of normal flexor type
Fascicular twitches absent	Fascicular twitches may be present
Normal nerve conduction studies; no denervation potentials in EMG	Abnormal nerve conduction studies; denervation potentials (fibrillations, fasciculations, positive waves) in EMG

athletic or musical activity. Some of these activities are relatively simple, automatic, and stereotyped. Others have been learned and mastered by great conscious effort and through practice have been reduced to an automatic level. Still others are complex and voluntary, parts of a carefully conceived conscious plan, and demand continuous attention and thought. What is more remarkable, human beings can indulge in several of these variably conscious and habitual activities simultaneously, as when driving through heavy traffic while lighting a cigarette and engaging in animated conversation. Moreover, when an obstacle prevents a sequence of movements from accomplishing its goal, a new sequence can be undertaken automatically for this purpose.

How is all this made possible? Neuropsychologists, studying patients with lesions of different parts of the cerebrum, tell us that the planning of complex activities, conceptualizing the final purpose, and continuous modification of the individual components of a motor sequence until the goal is achieved are under the control of the frontal lobes. Lesions in these parts of the brain have the opposite effect, i.e., they reduce the impulse to think, speak, and act ("cortical tone," to use Luria's expression, is reduced), and a complex activity will not be maintained for a long enough time for its completion. Some have called a defect at this level *ideational apraxia*, a term of which the authors do not approve because such disintegrations of complex motor sequences and the substitution of echopraxic and stereotyped pattern are virtually inseparable from the many nonmotor deficits of human mentation, as will be explained in several subsequent chapters (Sec. 5).

There is, however, another level of disordered motility for which the term apraxia is more appropriate. In this state, a patient who has no weakness, no ataxia or other extrapyramidal derangement, and no loss of the primary modes of sensation loses his ability to execute learned sequences of movement. This is the meaning given the term apraxia by Liepmann who first used it in the modern sense. In attempting to analyze this condition further, Luria points out that it is in the posterior part of the parietal lobe, where it joins the temporal lobe, that visual and somatic sensory (kinesthetic) information is integrated and from there projected to the motor areas; further, it is a lesion in this region, in the dominant hemisphere, that most consistently deranges learned motor sequences. Such sensory defects, although not detectable by the usual sensory tests, nevertheless remove some of the afferentation necessary for the successive facilitation and inhibition of the elements in a complex motor sequence. A particular deficit of this type, due mainly to a deficiency of proprioceptive afferentation, has been called *kinesthetic apraxia*. More specifically, the performing hand is not able to assume the proper positions for manipulating an object, and the perception of one's own movement—as part of the schema of the body—is not coordinated with the schema of objects in external space.

At a purely motor level one observes another type of apraxia in individuals who have a lesion that separates the left parietal lobe from the left motor cortex or a lesion of the anterior corpus callosum, separating the left from the right motor cortex (see below). The precise timing of each movement in a chain of consecutive movements is lost. Since each element requires its own impulse and then its suppression, the "kinetic melody" necessary for a given performance is broken. Patients no longer can perform simple acts such as eating with knife and fork, opening a door, or combing their hair either on command or in imitation. Moreover, their performances are often inconsistent. They may fail at one time, especially if the conditions for a given act are not habitual, and succeed later, when doing it alone.

In a practical sense the most frequent disorders of praxis involving both sides of the body are with lesions of the left parietal lobe, in the region of the supramarginal gyrus. This area is connected via long association pathways (probably the arcuate fasciculus) with the premotor cortex, and then by short association fibers with the motor cortex proper, for the control of the right limbs. The left premotor cortex is connected through the corpus callosum with the right premotor and motor cortex, for the control of the left side.

A failure to execute certain acts in the correct context while retaining the ability to carry out the individual movements upon which such acts depend is the main feature of apraxia. The most adequate clinical test of motor deficits of this type is to observe a series of self-initiated actions such as using a comb, a razor, a toothbrush, or a common tool, or gesturing, e.g., waving goodbye, saluting, shaking the fist as though angry, licking the lips or blowing a kiss. These actions may be called forth by verbal command or a request to imitate the examiner. Or, failing in these situations, the patient may perform certain acts appropriately in response to the usual stimuli for their production, e.g., being handed a hammer and nail or a match and cigarette. The patient may be unable to initiate the requested movement of

taking a pipe from a pocket and putting it in his mouth, or after the limb begins to move, it may do so in a hesitant uncertain manner. Yet if left alone, the patient may be seen to put the affected hand into the pocket or bring the pipe to his mouth "automatically," without obvious difficulty. Such a motor deficit, if it can be singled out, may be considered an amnesia for certain learned patterns of movement, analogous to the amnesia for words in aphasia. Of course, failure to follow a spoken or written request may be due to an aphasia that prevents understanding of what is asked, or to an agnosia, which prevents recognition of the tool or object to be used. And the presence of mental confusion tends often to obscure the disorder. Children with cerebral diseases that retard mental development are unable to learn the sequences of movement required in hopping, jumping over a barrier, hitting or kicking a ball, or dancing. They suffer a developmental motor apraxia. Certain tests quantitate failure in these age-linked motor skills (see Chap. 27).

In the authors' opinion, the time-honored division of apraxia into kinetic, ideokinetic or ideomotor, and ideational types is confusing and not useful clinically. It is more helpful to think of the various types in an anatomic sense, as disorders of association between different parts of the cerebral cortex. A lesion which interrupts the connections between the left supramarginal and premotor regions will cause an apraxia of both the right and left limbs. Such a lesion usually causes an aphasia as well, so it is important to determine that comprehension is intact by testing the patient's ability to imitate the examiner or to put a certain common tool to use automatically, without instructions.

A lesion of the callosal pathway, interrupting the connections between the left and right motor cortex, causes an apraxia of the left limbs only. As a rule, this pathway is involved at or near its origin, as part of a lesion that includes Broca's area and the left motor cortex; clinically there is a motor speech disorder, a right hemiplegia, and an apraxia of the nonparalyzed left hand, often referred to as a "sympathetic apraxia." Rarely this pathway is interrupted in the corpus callosum itself, thus separating the language areas from the right motor cortex. Patients with such a lesion carry out verbal commands correctly with the right hand but not with the left; they write correctly with the right hand if it is not paralyzed; but they write aphasically with the left.

Facial apraxia is probably the most common of all apraxias. It may occur with lesions that undercut the left supramarginal gyrus or the left motor association cortex and may be associated with apraxia of the limbs. Such patients will be unable to carry out facial movements to command (lick the lips, blow out a match, etc.), although they may do better when asked to imitate the examiner or when holding a lighted match. With lesions that are restricted to the facial area of the left motor cortex, the apraxia will be limited to the facial musculature, and usually will be associated with a motor speech disorder.

The disconnection syndromes will be discussed further in Chap. 21. So-called apraxia of gait will be considered in Chap. 6, "Disorders of Stance and Gait."

DIFFERENTIAL DIAGNOSIS OF PARALYSIS

The diagnostic considerations of paralysis may be simplified by the following subdivision, based on the location and distribution of weakness.

1. *Monoplegia* refers to weakness or paralysis of all the muscles in one limb, whether leg or arm. It should not be applied to paralysis of isolated muscles or groups of muscles supplied by a single nerve or motor root.

2. *Hemiplegia* is the commonest form of paralysis, involving arm, leg, and sometimes face on one side of the body.

3. *Paraplegia* indicates weakness or paralysis of both legs. It is most commonly found in spinal cord disease.

4. *Quadriplegia* or *tetraplegia* indicates weakness of all four extremities. It may result from lesions involving peripheral nerves, gray matter of the spinal cord, or the upper motor neuron bilaterally in the cervical cord, brainstem, or cerebrum. *Diplegia* is a special form of quadriplegia in which the legs are affected more than the arms.

5. Isolated paralysis of one or more muscle groups.

6. Nonparalytic disorders of movement.

7. Hysterical paralysis.

8. Muscular paralysis without visible changes in nerve and muscle.

MONOPLEGIA

The examination of patients who complain of weakness of one extremity often discloses an unnoticed weakness in another limb, and the condition is actually a hemiparesis or paraparesis. Or instead of weakness of all the muscles in a limb, only isolated groups are found to be affected. Ataxia, sensory disturbances, or pain in an extremity will often be interpreted by the patient as weak-

ness, as will the mechanical limitation resulting from arthritis and sometimes the rigidity of parkinsonism.

In general, the presence or absence of atrophy of muscles in a monoplegic limb can be of diagnostic help.

Monoplegia without Muscular Atrophy This is due most often to a lesion of the cerebral cortex. Only occasionally does it occur in diseases which interrupt the motor pathways at the level of the internal capsule, brainstem, or spinal cord. A vascular lesion (thrombosis or embolism) is the commonest cause, and of course, a circumscribed tumor or abscess may have the same effect. Multiple sclerosis and spinal cord tumor, early in their course, may cause weakness of one extremity, usually the leg. Weakness due to a lesion of the upper motor neuron is usually accompanied by spasticity, increased reflexes, and an extensor plantar reflex (Babinski sign), and nerve conduction studies are normal. However, acute diseases that destroy the motor tracts in the spinal cord may at first (for several days) reduce tendon reflexes and cause hypotonia (spinal shock). The latter does not occur in partial or slowly evolving lesions and only to a slight degree, if at all, with lesions of the brainstem and cerebrum. In acute diseases affecting the lower motor neurons the tendon reflexes are always reduced or abolished, but atrophy may not appear for several weeks. Hence before reaching an anatomic diagnosis one must take into account the mode of onset and the duration of the disease.

Monoplegia with Muscular Atrophy This is more frequent than monoplegia without muscular atrophy. Long-continued disuse of a limb may lead to atrophy, but it is usually of lesser degree than that which follows degeneration of the lower motor neurons. In disuse atrophy, the tendon reflexes are retained and nerve conduction studies are normal. In diseases that denervate muscles, in addition to the paralysis and reduced or abolished tendon reflexes, there may be visible fasciculations. If the limb is partially paralyzed, the electromyogram shows reduced numbers of motor unit potentials (often of large size), as well as fasciculations and fibrillations. The location of the lesion can usually be determined by the pattern of distribution of the palsied muscles (whether it is one of nerve, spinal root, or spinal cord involvement), by the associated neurologic symptoms and signs, and by special tests (cerebrospinal fluid examination, roentgenogram of spine, and myelogram).

Atrophic brachial monoplegia is relatively rare;

when present in an infant, it should suggest brachial plexus trauma; in a child, poliomyelitis or other viral infection; and in an adult, poliomyelitis, syringomyelia, amyotrophic lateral sclerosis, or brachial plexus lesions. Crural monoplegia is more frequent and may be caused by any lesion of the thoracic or lumbar cord, i.e., trauma, tumor, myelitis, multiple sclerosis, etc. Multiple sclerosis almost never causes severe atrophy, and ruptured intervertebral disk and the several varieties of mononeuropathy rarely paralyze all or most of the muscles of a limb. A unilateral retroperitoneal tumor may paralyze the leg by implicating the lumbosacral plexus.

HEMIPLEGIA

This is the most frequent form of paralysis in humans. With rare exceptions (a few unusual cases of poliomyelitis or motor system disease), this pattern of paralysis is due to involvement of the corticospinal pathways.

Location of Lesion Producing Hemiplegia The site or level of the lesion, i.e., cerebral, capsular, brainstem, or spinal cord, can usually be deduced from the associated neurologic findings. Diseases localized in the cerebral cortex, cerebral white matter (corona radiata), and internal capsule usually manifest themselves by weakness or paralysis of the face, arm, and leg on the opposite side. The occurrence of convulsive seizures or the presence of a language disorder (aphasia), a loss of discriminative sensation (astereognosis, impairment of tactile localization, etc.), anosognosia, or homonymous defects in the visual fields suggest a cortical or subcortical location.

Damage to the corticospinal and corticobrainstem tracts in the upper portion of the brainstem (see Fig. 3-2) also causes paralysis of the face, arm, and leg of the opposite side. The lesion in such cases is localized by the presence of a third nerve palsy on the same side as the lesion (Weber's syndrome) or other segmental abnormalities. Unilateral lesions of the upper part of the basis pontis have been shown by Fisher to cause a contralateral ataxic hemiplegia, i.e., cerebellar ataxia on the same side as the signs of corticospinal deficit. With low pontine lesions a unilateral abducens or facial palsy is combined with a contralateral weakness or paralysis of the arm and leg (Millard-Gubler syndrome). Lesions in the medulla affect the tongue and sometimes the pharynx and larynx on one side and the arm and leg on the other side. These "crossed paralyses," so common in brainstem diseases, are described further in Chap. 46.

Even lower in the medulla, a unilateral infarct in the pyramid causes a flaccid paralysis followed by slight spasticity of the contralateral arm and leg, sparing the face and tongue. Some motor function may be retained if any of the corticospinal fibers escape, as happened in the case of Ropper, Fisher, and Kleinman; interestingly, in their patient and in three others previously reported, there was considerable recovery of voluntary power even though the pyramid was almost completely destroyed.

Rarely, a homolateral hemiplegia may be caused by a lesion in the lateral column of the cervical spinal cord. At this level, however, the pathologic process more often induces bilateral signs, with resulting quadriparesis or quadriplegia. Homolateral paralysis, if combined with a loss of vibratory and position sense on the same side and a contralateral loss of pain and temperature, signifies disease of one side of the spinal cord (Brown-Séquard syndrome).

As indicated above, the muscle atrophy that follows upper motor neuron lesions never reaches the proportions seen in diseases of the lower motor neuron. The atrophy is due to disuse. When the motor cortex and adjacent parts of the parietal lobe are damaged in infancy or childhood, the normal development of the muscles and the skeletal system in the affected limbs is retarded. The palsied limbs and even the trunk on one side are small. This does not occur if the paralysis occurs after puberty, by which time the greater part of skeletal growth has been attained. In the hemiplegia due to spinal cord lesions, muscles at the level of the lesion may atrophy as a result of damage to anterior horn cells or ventral roots.

In the causation of hemiplegia, vascular diseases of the cerebrum and brainstem exceed all others in frequency. Trauma (brain contusion, epidural and subdural hemorrhage) ranks second. Other important causes, in order of frequency, are brain tumor, brain abscess and encephalitis, demyelinative diseases, and complications of meningitis. Most of these diseases can be recognized by their mode of evolution and the conjoined clinical and laboratory data, which are presented in the chapters on neurologic diseases. Alternating transitory hemiparesis may be due to a special type of migraine (see discussion in Chap. 9).

PARAPLEGIA

Paralysis of both lower extremities may occur with diseases of the spinal cord, spinal roots, or peripheral nerves. If the onset is acute, it may be difficult to distinguish spinal from neuritic paralysis because of the element of spinal shock which may result in abolition of reflexes and flaccidity. As a rule, in acute spinal cord diseases with involvement of corticospinal tracts, the paralysis affects all muscles below a given level; and often, if the white matter is extensively damaged, sensory loss below a particular level is conjoined (loss of pain and temperature sense due to spinothalamic tract damage, and loss of vibratory and position sense due to posterior column involvement). Also, in bilateral disease of the spinal cord, the bladder and bowel may be paralyzed. Alterations of cerebrospinal fluid (dynamic block, increase in protein or cells) are frequent. In peripheral nerve diseases, motor loss tends to involve the distal muscles of the legs more than the proximal ones (exceptions are certain varieties of acute idiopathic polyneuritis and diabetic neuropathy), and the sphincters are usually spared or impaired in function only transiently. Sensory loss, if present, is also more prominent in the distal segments of the limbs. The cerebrospinal fluid protein level may be normal or elevated.

For clinical purposes it is helpful to separate the acute paraplegias from the chronic ones and to divide the latter into two groups—those which occur in infancy and those which begin in adult life.

The most common cause of acute paraplegia (or quadriplegia, if the cervical cord is involved) is spinal cord trauma, usually combined with fracture-dislocation of the spine. Spontaneous hematomyelia due to a vascular malformation, thrombosis of a spinal artery, or dissecting aortic aneurysm or atherosclerotic occlusion of nutrient spinal arteries arising from the aorta with resulting infarction (myelomalacia) are less common causes. Paraplegia or quadriplegia due to postinfectious or postvaccinial myelitis, acute demyelinative myelopathy, necrotizing myelopathy, and epidural abscess or tumor with spinal cord compression tends to develop somewhat more slowly, over a period of hours or days, or longer. Epidural or subdural hemorrhage from bleeding diseases or coumadin has caused acute paraplegia in a number of our cases; in a few instances the bleeding followed a lumbar puncture. Paralytic poliomyelitis and acute idiopathic polyneuritis—the former a purely motor disorder with meningitis, the latter predominantly motor but often with minimal sensory disturbances—must be distinguished from the acute myelopathies and from each other.

In pediatric practice, delay in starting to walk and difficulty in walking are common problems. These conditions may indicate a systemic disease (such as rickets), mental deficiency, or, more commonly, some muscular or neurologic disease. Congenital cerebral disease accounts for a majority of cases of infantile diplegia (weakness predominantly of the legs, with minimal affection of the arms). Present at birth but becoming manifest in the

first months of life, it may appear to progress, but actually it is stationary and only becomes apparent as the motor system develops. Later there may seem to be slow improvement as a result of the normal maturation processes of childhood. Congenital malformation of the spinal cord or birth injury of the spinal cord are other possibilities. Friedreich's ataxia and familial paraplegia, progressive muscular dystrophy, and the chronic varieties of polyneuropathy tend to appear later during childhood and adolescence and are slowly progressive. Acute leukomyelopathy with total sensory and motor paralysis below a thoracic level is a rare condition of childhood. Normal CSF and normal myelography leave one without a tenable etiology, and few cases have been studied pathologically.

In adult life, multiple sclerosis, subacute combined degeneration (vitamin B_{12} deficiency), tumor, protruded cervical disk and cervical spondylosis, syphilitic meningomyelitis, chronic epidural infections (tuberculous, fungal, and other granulomatous diseases), motor system disease, syringomyelia, and degenerative disease of the lateral and posterior columns of unknown cause represent the most frequently encountered forms of spinal paraplegia. (See Chap. 35 for discussion of these spinal cord diseases.) Several varieties of polyneuropathy and polymyositis must be considered in the differential diagnosis, for they, too, may cause paraparesis.

QUADRIPLEGIA (TETRAPLEGIA)

All that has been said about the spinal causes of paraplegia applies to quadriplegia, the lesion being in the cervical rather than the thoracic or lumbar segments of the spinal cord. If the lesion is situated in the low cervical segments and involves the anterior half of the spinal cord, as in the anterior spinal artery syndrome and certain fracture-dislocations of the cervical spine, the paralysis of the arms may be flaccid and areflexic in type and the paralysis of the legs spastic. Dislocation of the odontoid process with compression of C1 and C2 spinal cord segments may occur with rheumatoid arthritis and Morquio's disease. In the latter there may also be pronounced pachymeningeal thickening. Bilateral infarction of the medullary pyramids from occlusion of the vertebral arteries or their anterior spinal branches is a rare cause of quadriplegia. In infants, aside from developmental abnormalities and anoxia of birth, certain cerebral diseases (Schilder's disease, metachromatic leukoencephalopathy, lipid storage disease) may be responsible for a quadriparesis or quadriplegia. Congenital forms of muscular dystrophy and also infantile muscular atrophy (Werdnig-Hoffmann disease) may be recognized soon after birth.

In adults, repeated cerebral vascular accidents may lead to bilateral hemiplegia, usually accompanied by pseudobulbar palsy.

PARALYSIS OF ISOLATED MUSCLE GROUPS

This condition usually indicates a lesion of one or more peripheral nerves, occasionally of several adjacent spinal roots. The diagnosis of an individual peripheral nerve lesion is made on the basis of weakness or paralysis of the muscle or group of muscles and impairment or loss of sensation in the distribution of the nerve in question. Complete transection or severe injury to a peripheral nerve is followed by atrophy of the muscles it innervates and by loss of their tendon reflexes. Paralysis of vasomotor and sudomotor functions and trophic changes in the skin, nails, and subcutaneous tissue may also occur.

Knowledge of the motor and sensory functions of the peripheral nerve in question is needed for a satisfactory diagnosis. Since lesions of individual nerves are relatively uncommon in civil life, it is not practical to memorize the precise motor-sensory distribution of each peripheral nerve; special manuals, such as the ones listed in the references, should be consulted. It is, however, of considerable importance to decide whether the lesion is a temporary one of conduction only or whether there has been a pathologic dissolution of continuity, requiring nerve regeneration or corrective surgery for recovery. Electromyography may be of value here.

If there is no evidence of upper or lower motor neuron disease, but certain acts are nonetheless imperfectly performed, one should look for a disorder of position sense or cerebellar coordination, or rigidity with abnormality of posture and movement due to disease of the basal ganglia (Chap. 4). In the absence of these disorders, the possibility of an apraxic disorder should be investigated by the methods outlined in the preceding part of this chapter.

HYSTERICAL PARALYSIS

In hysterical paralysis one arm or leg or all one side of the body may be affected. This is usually distinguishable from chronic lower motor neuron disease by absence of areflexia and of severe atrophy. Diagnostic difficulty arises only in certain acute cases of upper motor neuron disease that lack all the usual changes in reflexes and muscle tone. The hysterical gait is sometimes diagnostic (Chap. 6). Sometimes there is loss of sensation in the paralyzed parts and loss of sight, hearing, and smell on the paralyzed side—a group of sensory changes that is never seen in organic brain disease. When the patient is asked to move the affected limbs, the movement is seen to be slow and jerky, often with contraction of both agonist and antagonist muscles simultaneously or intermittently. Hoover's sign and the trunk-thigh sign of Babinski are helpful in distinguishing hysterical from organic hemiplegia. To elicit Hoover's sign the examiner places both hands under the heels of the recumbent patient, who is asked to press the heels down forcefully. With organic hemiplegia, pressure will be felt only from the nonparalyzed leg. The examiner then places a hand on top of the nonparalyzed foot and asks the patient to raise that leg. In true hemiplegia, no added pressure will be felt by the hand that remained beneath the heel of the paralyzed leg. In hysteria, the heel of the supposedly paralyzed leg will press down on the palm. To carry out Babinski's trunk-thigh test the recumbent patient is asked to sit up while keeping the arms crossed in front of the chest. In the patient with organic hemiplegia there is an involuntary flexion of the paretic limb; in paraplegia, both legs are raised as the trunk is flexed. In hysterical hemiplegia, only the normal leg may be elevated, while in hysterical paraplegia neither leg is raised.

MUSCULAR PARALYSIS AND SPASM UNATTENDED BY VISIBLE CHANGE IN NERVE OR MUSCLE

A discussion of motor paralysis would not be complete without some reference to a group of diseases in which there are no visible structural changes in motor nerve cells, nerve fibers, motor end plates, and muscle fibers. This group is comprised of myasthenia gravis, myotonia congenita (Thomsen's disease), familial periodic paralysis, disorders of potassium, sodium, calcium, and magnesium metabolism, tetany, tetanus, botulinus poisoning, black widow spider bite, and the thyroid myopathies. In these diseases, each of which possesses a fairly distinctive clinical picture, the abnormality is purely biochemical, and even if the patient survives for a long time, no light-microscopic changes develop. An understanding of these diseases requires knowledge of the processes involved in nerve and muscle excitation and in the contraction of muscle. They will be discussed in Chaps. 51 and 52.

REFERENCES

ASANUMA H: Cerebral cortical control of movement. *Physiologist* 16:143, 1973.

————, SAKATA H: Functional organization of a cortical efferent system examined with focal depth stimulation in cats. *J Neurophysiol* 30:35, 1967.

BRODAL A: Pathways mediating supraspinal influences on the spinal cord, in *Neurological Anatomy in Relation to Clinical Medicine*, 3d ed. New York, Oxford, 1981, chap 4.

BUCY PC et al: Destruction of the pyramidal tract in the monkey. *J Neurosurg* 25:1, 1966.

DIMITRIJEVIC MR, SHERWOOD AN, NATHAN PW: Clonus, peripheral and central mechanisms, in Desmedt JE (ed): *Physiological Tremor, Pathological Tremors and Clonus.* New York, Karger, 1978, pp 173–182.

FOERSTER O: Symptomatologie des Erkrankungen des Grosshirns. Motorische Felder und Bahnen, in Bumke O, Foerster O (eds): *Handbuch der Neurologie*, vol 6. Berlin, J Springer, 1936, pp 1–357.

GESCHWIND N: Disconnexion syndromes in animals and man. *Brain* 88:237, 1965.

HALLETT M, KHOSHBIN S: A physiological mechanism of bradykinesia. *Brain* 103:301, 1980.

HAYMAKER WE, WOODHALL B: *Peripheral Nerve Injuries: Principles of Diagnosis*, 2d ed. Philadelphia, Saunders, 1953.

HENNEMAN E: Motor functions of the brainstem and basal ganglia, in Mountcastle VB (ed): *Medical Physiology*, vol 1. St Louis, Mosby, 1974, pp 678–703.

KUYPERS HGJM: The anatomical organization of the descending pathways and their contributions to motor control especially in primates, in Desmedt JE (ed): *New Developments in EMG and Clinical Neurophysiology.* Basel, Karger, 1973, p 38.

LANDAU WM: Spasticity and rigidity, in Plum F (ed): *Contemporary Neurology Series*, vol 6: *Recent Advances in Neurology.* Philadelphia, Davis, 1970, chap 1.

LURIA AR: *The Working Brain: An Introduction to Neuropsychology.* New York, Basic Books, 1973.

LAWRENCE DG, KUYPERS HGJM: The functional organization of the motor system in the monkey. *Brain* 91:1, 15, 1968.

MEDICAL RESEARCH COUNCIL: *Aids to the Examination of the Peripheral Nervous System*, Memorandum no 45. London, HM Stationery Office, 1976.

NULSEN FE, KLINE DG: Acute injuries of peripheral nerves, in Youmans JR (ed): *Neurological Surgery*, vol 2. Philadelphia, Saunders, 1973, chap 61, pp 1089–1140.

NYBERG-HANSEN R, RINVIK E: Some comments on the pyramidal tract with special reference to its individual variations in man. *Acta Neurol Scand* 39:1, 1963.

ROPPER AH, FISHER CM, KLEINMAN GM: Pyramidal infarction in the medulla: A cause of pure motor hemiplegia sparing the face. *Neurology* 29:91, 1979.

RUSSELL JR, DEMYER W: The quantitative cortical origin of pyramidal axons of *Macaca rhesus*, with some remarks on the slow rate of axolysis. *Neurology* 11:96, 1961.

TOWER SS: Pyramidal lesion in the monkey. *Brain* 63:36, 1940.

CHAPTER 4

ABNORMALITIES OF MOVEMENT AND POSTURE DUE TO DISEASE OF THE EXTRAPYRAMIDAL MOTOR SYSTEM

In this chapter are discussed the automatic, static, postural, and other less modifiable motor activities of the human nervous system. They are believed, on good evidence, to be an expression of the older, or "extrapyramidal," motor system, meaning, according to S. A. K. Wilson, who introduced this term, the motor structures in the basal ganglia and certain related brainstem nuclei.

In health, the activities of the basal ganglia and the cerebellum are blended and modulate the corticospinal and cortical-brainstem-spinal systems. The static postural activities of the former are indispensable to the voluntary or willed movements of the latter. The close association of these two systems is also shown by human disease. Lesions that involve the corticospinal tracts predominantly result not only in paralysis of volitional movements of the contralateral half of the body but also in the appearance of a fixed posture or attitude in which the arm is maintained in flexion and the leg in extension (predilection type of Wernicke-Mann or hemiplegic dystonia of Denny-Brown). Similarly, interruption of the motor projection pathways by a lesion in the upper pons or midbrain releases another posture in which all four extremities are extended and the cervical and thoracolumbar portions of the spine are dorsiflexed. In these released action patterns one has evidence of postural and righting reflexes which are mediated through nonpyramidal bulbospinal and other brainstem systems. Observations such as these and the anatomic data presented in the preceding chapter have largely blurred the classical distinctions between pyramidal and extrapyramidal motor systems. Nevertheless, this division remains a useful if not an essential concept in clinical work, since it compels us to distinguish between two motor syndromes—one that is characterized by a loss of volitional movement and spasticity and another by akinesia without loss of voluntary movement, but with rigidity, involuntary movements, and tremor. The clinical differences between corticospinal and extrapyramidal disorders are summarized in Table 4-1.

Much of the criticism of the pyramidal-extrapyramidal concept derives from the terms themselves. The ambiguity related to the use of the term *pyramidal* has been discussed in the preceding chapter, where it was pointed out that pure pyramidal lesions do not cause total paralysis and when the latter exists there is always involvement of other descending corticospinal pathways. The term *extrapyramidal* is equally imprecise. Strictly interpreted, it refers to all the motor pathways except the pyramidal one, a term so all-embracing as to be practically meaningless. The concept of an extrapyramidal motor system becomes more meaningful if it is subdivided into two parts: (1) the striatopallidonigral and (2) the cerebellar. Disease in either of these parts will result in particular disturbances of movement and posture without significant paralysis. These two major systems and the symptoms that result when they are diseased are described on the following pages.

THE STRIATOPALLIDONIGRAL SYSTEM (BASAL GANGLIA)

ANATOMY AND PHARMACOLOGY

As an anatomic entity the basal ganglia have no precise definition. In addition to the caudate and lenticular nuclei, one usually includes the claustrum, the subthalamic nucleus (corpus Luysii), and the substantia nigra. The amygdaloid nuclear complex, because of its largely different connections and functions, is usually excluded. For reasons indicated below, some physiologists have expanded the list of basal ganglionic structures to include the red nucleus and the reticular formation of the brainstem. The latter structures receive direct cortical projections and give rise to rubrospinal and reticulospinal fibers; although these nonpyramidal linkages form indirect connections with the corpus striatum, they appear to be structurally independent of the latter structure.

The anatomic features of the extrapyramidal motor structures and the connections between them and other parts of the brain are too intricate to present in a textbook of neurology (cf. Brodal, *Neurological Anatomy;* also Carpenter, *Human Neuroanatomy*). Only a simplified version will be provided here. Knowledge of these anatomic data is essential to an understanding of normal motor function and provides a rational explanation for certain abnormalities of motor function as well, particularly for involuntary movements and tremor.

The main structures composing the basal ganglia are the caudate nucleus and the lentiform nucleus with its two subdivisions, the putamen and globus pallidus

Table 4-1

Clinical differences between corticospinal and extrapyramidal syndromes

	Corticospinal	Extrapyramidal
Character of the alteration of muscle tone	Clasp-knife effect (spasticity)	Plastic, equal throughout passive movement (rigidity), or intermittent (cogwheel rigidity); hypotonia in cerebellar disease
Distribution of hypertonus	Flexors of arms, extensors of legs	Flexors (predominantly) and extensors of all four limbs; flexors of trunk
Shortening and lengthening reaction	Present	Absent
Involuntary movements	Absent	Presence of tremor, chorea, athetosis, dystonia
Tendon reflexes	Increased	Normal or slightly increased
Babinski sign	Present	Absent
Paralysis of voluntary movement	Present	Absent or slight

(pallidum). Insofar as the caudate and putamen are really a single continuous structure, which is cytologically and functionally distinct from the pallidum, a more meaningful division of these nuclear masses is into the neostriatum (or striatum), comprising the caudate and putamen, and the paleostriatum or pallidum, with its medial (internal) and lateral (external) segments. The striatum and pallidum lie on the lateral aspect of the internal capsule, which separates them from the thalamus, subthalamic nucleus and substantia nigra on its medial side (Figs. 4-1 and 4-2).

The most important connections between these nuclei and with other structures are indicated in Figs. 4-1, 4-2, 4-3, and 4-6. The striatum receives topographically organized afferent fibers from all parts of the cerebral cortex (Fig. 4-3), particularly its anterior part, as well as from the substantia nigra and certain thalamic nuclei. The centromedian and parafascicular nuclei project mainly to the putamen, but also to portions of the body of the caudate; the rostral intralaminar nuclei project mainly to the head of the caudate. In turn, the caudate and putamen project topographically upon the lateral and medial segments of the pallidum and upon the substantia nigra, particularly on the cell-rich portion composed of large pigmented cells (pars compacta). Available evidence indicates that strionigral and nigrostriatal fibers are topographically and reciprocally organized. Terminals of the strionigral fibers in the pars reticulata contain glutamic acid decarboxylase (GAD), the enzyme utilized in the synthesis of γ-aminobutyric acid (GABA), suggesting that these fibers transport GABA. Nigrostriatal fibers convey dopamine to the striatum (see further on). In addition to the projections from the striatum, the pallidum receives fibers from the substantia nigra and has important reciprocal connections with the subthalamic nucleus.

All the impulses converging upon the pallidum are projected ultimately from its medial segment to the thalamus via well-developed fiber bundles known as the ansa and fasciculus lenticularis (Fig. 4-3). The ansa lenticularis sweeps around the internal capsule; the fasciculus lenticularis traverses the internal capsule in a number of small fascicles (Forel's field H_2) and then sweeps medially and caudally to join the ansa in the prerubral field (Forel's field H). Both these fiber bundles then join the *thalamic fasciculus* (Forel's field H_1), which contains not only pallidothalamic projections but also rubrothalamic and dentatothalamic ones. Together they project onto the ventrolateral nucleus of the thalamus and to a lesser

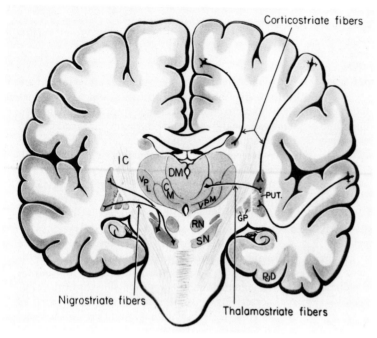

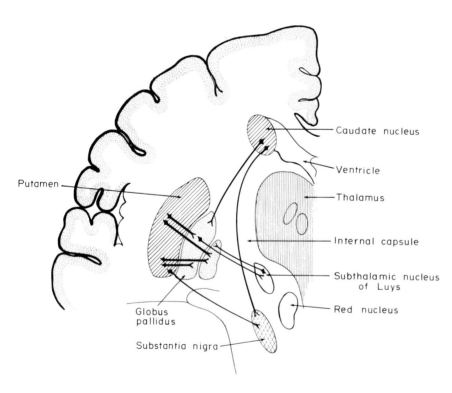

Figure 4-1
Diagram of the striatal afferent pathways. Cortico-striate fibers from broad cortical areas project to the putamen; fibers from the cortex on the medial surface project largely to the caudate nucleus. Nigrostriatal fibers arise from the pars compacta of the substantia nigra. Thalamostriate fibers arise from the centromedian-parafascicular complex of the thalamus. CM, centromedian nucleus; DM, dorsomedial nucleus; GP, globus pallidus; IC, internal capsule; Put., Putamen; RN, red nucleus; SN, substantia nigra; VPL, ventral posterolateral nucleus; VPM, ventral posterior medial nucleus. (From MB Carpenter, Human Neuroanatomy, 7th ed, Baltimore, Williams & Wilkins, 1976.)

Figure 4-2
Diagram of the basal ganglia in the coronal plane, illustrating the main striatal efferent pathways and pallidothalamic connections (details in text).

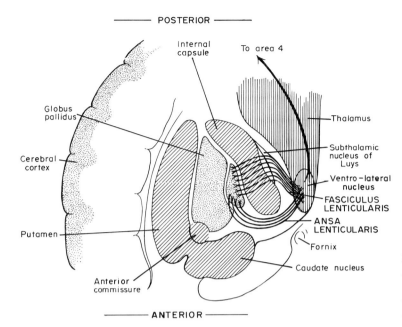

POSTERIOR

Internal capsule

To area 4

Globus pallidus

Thalamus

Subthalamic nucleus of Luys

Cerebral cortex

Ventro-lateral nucleus

FASCICULUS LENTICULARIS

ANSA LENTICULARIS

Putamen

Fornix

Caudate nucleus

Anterior commissure

ANTERIOR

Figure 4-3

Basal ganglia in the horizontal plane, illustrating the main efferent projections from the medial segment of the pallidum to the ventral nuclei of the thalamus (details in text).

extent onto the ventral anterior and intralaminar thalamic nuclei. The major projection of the ventrolateral nucleus of the thalamus is to the precentral motor cortex (area 4).

The principal anatomic datum to emerge from these observations is the central role of the ventrolateral (and anterior) nucleus of the thalamus. It is a vital link in an ascending fiber system from the basal ganglia and cerebellum to the motor cortex. Indeed, it would seem that most of the basal ganglionic and cerebellar influence on the motor system is funneled through the ventral tier of thalamic nuclei, which serve to integrate the extrapyramidal impulses and bring them to bear, via the thalamocortical fibers, on the corticospinal systems. Descending pathways from the cortex to the red nuclei and reticular formation of the brainstem are known. In addition there are cortical projections to the striatum. However, descending pathways from the basal ganglia to the spinal cord are disputed; a small group of efferent fibers projects from the pallidum to the tegmentum of the lower midbrain and probably from there, via polysynaptic pathways through the reticular formation of the pons and medulla, to the motor neurons of the spinal cord.

During the past two decades a series of exciting pharmacologic observations has considerably broadened our understanding of basal ganglionic function and has led to the discovery of a rational treatment of Parkinson's syndrome. Whereas physiologists had for years failed to discover the functions of the basal ganglia by

stimulation and ablation experiments, clinicians observed that the empirical use of certain drugs, such as reserpine and the phenothiazines, regularly produced extrapyramidal syndromes (parkinsonism, choreoathetosis, dystonia, etc.). This discovery greatly stimulated the study of transmitter substances in the central nervous system.

The most important neurotransmitter substances from the point of view of basal ganglionic function are acetylcholine, dopamine, and GABA. The basal ganglia contain several other biologically active substances, viz., norepinephrine and serotonin, but these are present in relatively low concentrations and their neurotransmitter functions in the basal ganglia, or in other parts of the brain, are less clearly defined than those of dopamine, acetylcholine, and GABA.

Acetylcholine, long established as the neurotransmitter at the neuromuscular junction as well as in the autonomic ganglia, is also physiologically active in the brain. The highest concentration of acetylcholine as well as of choline acetylase and acetylcholinesterase (the enzymes necessary for the synthesis and degradation of acetylcholine) is in the striatum. These facts suggest that acetylcholine is a physiologically potent substance and that the striatum is probably the major site of cholinergic activity. Acetylcholine appears to have an excitatory effect on the small (Golgi type 2) neostriatal neurons, and this effect is counteracted by dopamine. It is likely that the effectiveness of the belladonna alkaloids, which had been used empirically for many years in the treat-

51

ment of Parkinson's disease, also depends on their capacity to antagonize acetylcholine centrally.

Of the catecholamines—dopamine, epinephrine, and norepinephrine—the first has excited the greatest attention. The steps in the metabolic pathway for the biosynthesis of the catecholamines and the enzymes involved in each step are tabulated below:

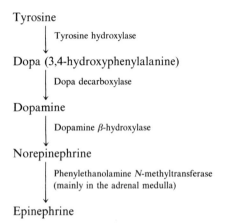

Tyrosine
↓ Tyrosine hydroxylase
Dopa (3,4-hydroxyphenylalanine)
↓ Dopa decarboxylase
Dopamine
↓ Dopamine β-hydroxylase
Norepinephrine
↓ Phenylethanolamine N-methyltransferase (mainly in the adrenal medulla)
Epinephrine

In the brain dopamine is metabolized by the enzymes monoamine oxidase and catechol-O-methyltransferase. The end products of dopamine metabolism are homovanillic acid (HVA) and dihydroxyphenylacetic acid (DOPAC). HVA is readily measured in the CSF and methods are now available for the measurement of both these metabolites in the plasma.

Dopamine has a specific function in the central nervous system, apart from being a precursor of norepinephrine. The areas richest in dopamine are the striatum, where it is contained almost exclusively in synaptic nerve endings from the substantia nigra, and the substantia nigra, where it is localized in the nerve cell bodies of the pars compacta. On the basis of experiments in rodents and monkeys, a dopamine-containing nigrostriatal pathway has been defined, originating in the pigmented cells of the substantia nigra and terminating diffusely in the striatum. Stimulation of the substantia nigra induces a specific response in the striatum, viz., a release of dopamine, which appears to have an inhibitory effect on neostriatal neurons.

In Parkinson's disease (both the idiopathic and postencephalitic varieties), the concentration of dopamine is greatly decreased in the striatum and substantia nigra, and the content of its major metabolite, homovanillic acid, is also decreased in these parts, as well as in

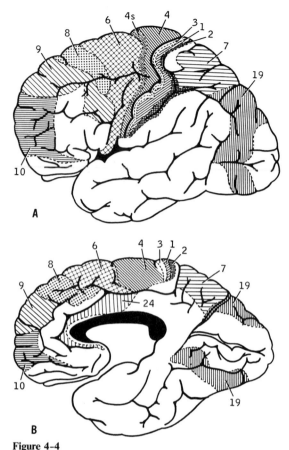

Figure 4-4

Lateral (A) and medial (B) surfaces of the brain, showing the areas of the cerebral cortex which send fibers into the extrapyramidal motor system. (From EL House et al, A Systematic Approach to Neuroscience, 3d ed, New York, McGraw-Hill, 1979.)

the globus pallidus and spinal fluid. The levels of norepinephrine and serotonin are also decreased, but to a much lesser degree. Furthermore, the degree of dopamine and homovanillic acid deficiency appears to correlate with the degree of cell loss in the substantia nigra, i.e., with the major pathologic change in Parkinson's disease.

Certain drugs, namely reserpine, the phenothiazines, and the butyrophenones, notably haloperidol, may induce parkinsonian syndromes in humans. Reserpine acts by depleting the striatum and other parts of the brain of dopamine; haloperidol and the phenothiazines produce parkinsonism by a different mechanism, probably by causing a blockade of dopamine receptors within the striatum.

Dopamine as such cannot pass the blood-brain

barrier and has no therapeutic effect. However, the immediate dopamine precursor, levodopa (L-dopa), does cross the barrier and is effective in decreasing the akinesia, rigidity, and to some extent the tremor of paralysis agitans (Parkinson's disease) and drug-induced parkinsonism. This effect is greatly enhanced by the inhibition of monoamine oxidase, an important enzyme in the catabolism of dopamine. The addition of a monoamine oxidase inhibitor to L-dopa results in a marked increase of dopamine levels in the brain, but only a slight increase of norepinephrine. These findings reinforce the generally held notion that dopamine depletion is responsible for the production of parkinsonian symptoms and that these symptoms are reversed by the replenishment of striatal dopamine, formed in the brain from the administered L-dopa.

Because of the aforementioned pharmacologic activities of acetylcholine and dopamine, it has been postulated that a functional equilibrium exists in the striatum between the excitatory cholinergic and the inhibitory dopaminergic mechanisms (Hornykiewicz). Thus, in Parkinson's disease, the deficiency of striatal dopamine results in a predominance of the cholinergic activity, a notion supported by the observation that parkinsonian symptoms are aggravated by centrally acting cholinergic drugs and improved by anticholinergic drugs. According to this theory, administration of anticholinergic drugs restores the ratio between dopamine and acetylcholine, but the new equilibrium would be set at a lower-than-normal level, because the striatal dopamine level is low to begin with. The repletion of striatal dopamine thus represents a more physiologic method of treatment of Parkinson's disease.

GABA is found in high concentrations in the spinal cord, dentate nucleus, and globus pallidus, where it probably acts as an inhibitory neurotransmitter. Specific neural pathways for this transmitter activity remain to be defined, however. GABA has been implicated in the pathogenesis of Huntington's chorea, vitamin B_6–dependent seizures, and many other neurologic disorders, as will be indicated at appropriate points in the text. Other central neurotransmitters such as serotonin and glycine will also be considered in relation to the disorders in which they play a part.

A more complete account of this subject than is possible here may be found in the writings of Klawans, of Hornykiewicz, and of others, referred to at the end of this chapter.

SYMPTOMS OF BASAL GANGLIA DISEASE

In broad terms, all motor disorders may be considered to consist of primary functional deficits (or *negative* symp-

toms) and secondary effects (or *positive* symptoms), the latter being ascribed to the release or disinhibition of the activity of undamaged parts of the motor nervous system. When various diseases of the basal ganglia are analyzed along these classic lines, then akinesia and loss of normal postural reflexes stand out as the principal deficits, or negative symptoms, and rigidity and involuntary movements (chorea, athetosis, and dystonia) as the positive symptoms. Disorders of phonation, articulation, and locomotion are more difficult to classify. In some cases they are clearly consequent upon rigidity and postural disorder; in others, where rigidity is slight or negligible, they seem to represent a primary deficiency. Difficulty in the performance of rapid alternating movements probably represents another negative effect in diseases of both the basal ganglia and the cerebellum. In fact, this latter symptom, presenting as clumsiness, may be the only fault manifest in certain maladroit children. Stress and nervous tension characteristically worsen both the motor deficiency and the abnormal movements in all extrapyramidal syndromes, just as relaxation helps the motor performance. All the movement disorders are abolished in sleep.

AKINESIA (BRADYKINESIA, HYPOKINESIA)

The term *akinesia* refers to the disinclination of the patient to use an affected part, to engage it freely in all the natural actions of the body. In contrast to what occurs in paralysis (the negative symptom of corticospinal lesions), strength is not significantly diminished in the part. Also, akinesia is unlike apraxia, where a lesion erases the memory of the pattern of movements necessary for the intended act. The parkinsonian patient manifests the phenomenon of akinesia most clearly in extreme underactivity (poverty of movement). The frequent automatic habitual movements observed in the normal state, such as putting the hand to the face, folding the arms, or crossing the legs, are absent or greatly reduced in parkinsonian patients. In looking to the side they move the eyes, not the head. In arising from a chair, they fail to make the little necessary adjustments such as putting feet back, hands on arms of chair, and so forth. Blinking is infrequent. Saliva is not swallowed as fast as it is produced, and sialorrhea results. The face lacks expressive mobility (hypomimia). They neglect the affected arm. Yet they can make all these movements by dint of will, so they are not weak (paretic) or apraxic. *Hypokinesia* refers to a similar phenomenon of lesser degree.

Bradykinesia connotes slowness rather than lack of movement. Not only is the parkinsonian patient "slow off the mark," but the transit time of various movements is longer than normal. Formerly, akinesia and bradykinesia were attributed to rigidity, which could reasonably hamper all movements, but the falsity of this explanation became apparent when it was discovered that an appropriately placed stereotactic lesion may abolish rigidity in a patient with paralysis agitans, but leave the akinesia unaltered. It would appear that apart from their contribution to the maintenance of postures, the basal ganglia must provide an essential element for the performance of the large variety of semiautomatic actions that make up the full repertoire of natural human motility. Hallett and Khoshbin have adduced evidence that the normal role of the basal ganglia is the selection and activation ("energizing") of specific sets of muscles to be used in a particular movement.

In some extrapyramidal diseases there are other disorders of voluntary movement. A persistent contraction of hand muscles, as in holding a pencil, may result in a tonic spasm that interferes with the next willed movement. Attempts to perform a sequence of movements may be blocked at one point, and a tremor then appears (digital impedence, see page 808). A simple projected movement may result in a spasm of several unneeded muscles, blocking the patient's intended action ("intention spasm").

DISORDERS OF POSTURAL FIXATION, EQUILIBRIUM, AND RIGHTING

These deficits are also demonstrated most clearly in the parkinsonian patient. They take the form of an involuntary flexion of the trunk and limbs and of the head, as in a person who falls asleep in an upright position. The incapacity of the patient to make appropriate postural adjustments to tilting or falling and to change from the reclining to the standing position are closely related phenomena. These postural abnormalities are not the result of weakness, nor are they related to obvious defects in proprioception or labyrinthine or visual function, the principal forces that control the normal posture of the head and trunk. They have been compared to the flexed postures of the head and neck and disorders of equilibrium and righting which have been produced in monkeys by the ablation of the globus pallidus bilaterally (Richter).

A point of interest is whether akinesia and disorders of postural fixation are invariable manifestations of all extrapyramidal diseases and whether without them there could be any secondary release effects such as dystonia, choreoathetosis, and rigidity. The question has no clear answer. Akinesia and abnormalities of posture are invariable features of Parkinson's and Wilson's disease; they seem to be present also in Huntington's and Sydenham's chorea and in double athetosis, but one cannot be sure of their existence in hemiballismus.

ALTERATIONS OF MUSCLE TONE

In the form of hypertonus known as *rigidity* the muscles are continuously or intermittently firm and tense. Although brief periods of electromyographic silence can be obtained in selected muscles by persistent attempts to relax the limb, there is obviously a low threshold for involuntary sustained muscle contraction, and this is present during most of the waking state, even when the patient appears quiet and relaxed. In contrast to spasticity, the increase in tone on passive movement that characterizes rigidity has no initial "free interval" and has an even or uniform quality throughout the range of movement of the limb, like that noted in bending a lead pipe or pulling a strand of toffee. When released, the limb does not spring back into its original position as may happen in spasticity.

Rigidity is present in all muscle groups, both flexor and extensor, but it tends to be more prominent in those which maintain a flexed posture, i.e., the flexor muscles of trunk and limbs. It appears to be somewhat greater in the large muscle groups, but this may be merely a question of muscle mass. Certainly the smaller muscles of the face and tongue and even those of the larynx are often affected. The tendon reflexes are not enhanced. Nevertheless, like spasticity, rigidity is said to be abolished by the extradural or subarachnoid injection of local anesthesia, and Foerster demonstrated long ago that it is eradicated by posterior root section, presumably by interrupting the afferent fibers of the gamma loop. In the electromyographic tracing, motor-unit activity is more continuous than in spasticity, persisting even after apparent relaxation.

A special type of rigidity, first noted by Negro in 1901, is the cogwheel phenomenon. When the hypertonic muscle is passively stretched, e.g., when the hand is dorsiflexed, one encounters a rhythmically interrupted, ratchet-like resistance. Wilson postulated that this phenomenon is a minor form of the lengthening-shortening reaction, but more likely it represents an associated static tremor which is masked by the rigidity during an attitude of repose but which emerges faintly during manipulation.

Rigidity is a prominent feature of many extrapyramidal diseases such as the advanced forms of paralysis agitans and the postencephalitic variety of Parkinson's disease, Wilson's disease, striatonigral degeneration, and dystonia musculorum deformans.

Except for the rare, rigid form of Huntington's chorea, the involuntary-movement disorders—chorea, athetosis, and ballism, which are described below—are not associated with a consistent abnormality of muscle tone. Usually in Sydenham's and Huntington's chorea a state of hypotonia prevails, sometimes striking in degree, such as one might find in acute cerebellar lesions, sensory polyneuropathies, and lower motor neuron paralyses. Some patients with choreoathetosis show an increased resistance to passive manipulation of the limbs, but this is variable from one moment to the next and paradoxic in that it may disappear when the limb is passively shaken. In still other cases, performance of a simple motor act (e.g., touching finger to nose) is rendered impossible by the simultaneous contraction of the muscles not only of the arm and hand but also of the neck, trunk, and even legs ("intention spasm"), or the limb may go in a direction opposite to the one intended as may happen at times in parietal lobe lesions.

A special type of variable resistance to passive movement is that in which the patient seems unable to relax a group of muscles on command. When the muscles are passively stretched, the patient's inability to cooperate interferes. This is sometimes called *gegenhalten* or *counterholding*. Actually, relaxation requires concentration on the part of the patient. If there is inattentiveness as happens with diseases of frontal lobes or senility or confusional states, the question of parkinsonian rigidity may arise. A similar difficulty in relaxing is observed in children.

INVOLUNTARY MOVEMENTS (CHOREA, BALLISM, ATHETOSIS, DYSTONIA)

In deference to usual practice, these symptoms will be described separately, as though each of them represents a discrete clinical phenomenon, readily distinguished one from the other. In fact, they usually occur together and have many points of similarity, and there are reasons to believe that they have a common anatomic and physiologic basis. One must also always be mindful that chorea, athetosis, and dystonia are only symptoms and are not to be equated with disease entities which happen to incorporate one of these terms (e.g., Huntington's chorea, dystonia musculorum deformans).

Chorea Derived from the Greek word meaning "dance," *chorea* refers to involuntary arrhythmic movements of a forcible, rapid, jerky type. These movements

may be simple or quite elaborate and of variable distribution. They may resemble a voluntary movement in their complexity, yet they are never combined into a coordinated act. The patient may, however, incorporate them into a deliberate movement, as if to make them less noticeable. When superimposed on voluntary movements, they may assume an exaggerated and grotesque character. Grimacing and peculiar respiratory sounds may be other expressions of the movement disorder. Usually the movements are discrete, but if very numerous, they become confluent and then resemble athetosis. If the involuntary movements can be held in abeyance, normal volitional movements are possible for there is no paralysis, but the latter tend also to be excessively quick and poorly sustained. The limbs are often slack or hypotonic, and because of this, the knee jerks tend to be pendular; with the patient sitting on the edge of the bed with the foot free of the floor, the leg swings back and forth four or five times in response to a tap on the patellar tendon, rather than once or twice, as it does normally. A choreic movement may be superimposed on the reflex movement, checking it in flight, so to speak, and giving rise to the "hung-up" reflex.

The hypotonia in chorea, as well as the pendular reflexes and some degree of interference with natural movements, are reminiscent of the syndrome that follows disease of the cerebellum. Lacking, however, are intention tremor and true incoordination or ataxia. Chorea differs from polymyoclonia only with respect to speed of the movements; the myoclonic jerk is much faster. Failure to recognize this difference accounts for inaccurate attribution of chorea to hypernatremia and other metabolic disorders.

Chorea appears in typical form in Sydenham's chorea and in the variety of that disease associated with pregnancy (chorea gravidarum). It is a feature also of Huntington's chorea (hereditary or chronic chorea), in which the movements tend more typically to be choreoathetotic. Phenothiazine drugs, haloperidol, and, rarely, hyperthyroidism may cause chorea.

Chorea may be limited to one side of the body (*hemichorea*), and the movements of the limbs may be unusually violent and flinging in nature, a disorder referred to as *hemiballismus*. The lesion in the latter cases is in or near the opposite subthalamic nucleus of Luys. As the severity of these hemiballismic movements subsides, they settle down to irregular flexions and extensions of the wrist and fingers, indistinguishable from chorea and athetosis of mild grades of severity.

Athetosis This term stems from a Greek word meaning "unfixed" or "changeable." The condition is characterized by inability to sustain the fingers and toes, tongue, or any other part of the body in one position. The maintained posture is interrupted by relatively slow, sinuous, purposeless movements which have a tendency to flow into one another. As a rule, the abnormal movements are most pronounced in the digits and hands, face, tongue, and throat, but no group of muscles is spared. One can detect as basic patterns of movement an alternation between extension-pronation and flexion-supination of the arm, and between flexion and extension of the fingers, the flexed and adducted thumb being trapped by the flexed fingers as the hand closes. Other characteristic movements are eversion-inversion of the foot, retraction and pursing of the lips, twisting of the neck and torso, and alternate wrinkling and relaxation of the forehead or opening and closing of the eyes. The movements appear to be slower than those of chorea, but all gradations between the two are seen, and in some cases it is impossible to distinguish between them (choreoathetosis). Attempts to perform discrete voluntary movements of the hand may result in a contraction of all the muscles in the limb ("intention spasm"). The overflow leading to excessive activation of inappropriate muscles is the opposite of bradykinesia.

Athetosis may affect all four limbs or may be unilateral, especially in children who have suffered a hemiplegia at some previous date (posthemiplegic athetosis). Many athetotic patients exhibit variable degrees of motor deficit, due to associated corticospinal tract disease, and variable degrees of rigidity, and these may account for the slower quality of athetosis, in contrast to chorea.

The combination of athetosis and chorea of all four limbs is a cardinal feature of Huntington's chorea and of a state known as double athetosis, which begins in childhood. Athetosis appearing in the first months of life is usually the result of a congenital or postnatal condition such as hypoxia or kernicterus. Postmortem examinations in some of the cases have disclosed a peculiar pathologic change of probable hypoxic etiology, a status marmoratus, in the striatum (Chap. 43); in others there has been a loss of medullated fibers, a status dysmyelinatus, in the same regions. In adults, athetosis may occur as an episodic or persistent disorder in hepatic encephalopathy, as a manifestation of chronic intoxication with phenothiazines or haloperidol, in a parkinsonian patient with overdosage of L-dopa, and in certain degenerative diseases, most notably Huntington's chorea (see Chap. 42).

Dystonia, or Torsion Spasm Dystonia is a persistent attitude in one or other of the extremes of athetoid movement. It may take the form of an overextended or overflexed posture of the hand, inversion of the foot, pulling of the head to one side, torsion of the lumbar portion of the spine, retraction of the head with arching and twisting of the back or closure of the eyes and a fixed grimace (Fig. 4-5). Defined in this way, dystonia is closely allied to athetosis, differing only in the duration or persistence of the postural abnormality and the disproportionate involvement of the larger axial muscles (those of the trunk and limb girdles). The term *dystonia* is generally used in this way, but it has also been given other meanings. S. A. K. Wilson designated any variability in muscle tone as dystonia. This term has also been applied to fixed abnormalities of posture which may be the end result of certain diseases of the motor system; thus Denny-Brown speaks of "hemiplegic dystonia" and the "flexion dystonia of parkinsonism." If the term is to be used in the latter sense, it would be better to speak of the persistent but reversible athetotic movements of the limbs and trunk as "torsion spasms" or "phasic dystonia," in contrast to "fixed dystonia." The former, like athetosis, may vary considerably in severity and may show remarkable fluctuations in individual patients. Torsion spasm may be limited to the facial, cervical, or trunk muscles or to those of one limb and may cease when the body is in repose. Severe dystonia results in grotesque movements and distorted positions of the body; sometimes the whole musculature of the body may be thrown into spasm by an effort to move an arm or to speak.

The term *dystonia* was introduced by Oppenheim and Vogt, in 1911, to describe the relatively slow, long-sustained, frequently forceful contorting movements of an uncommon heritable disease, dystonia musculorum deformans. Dystonia, or torsion spasm, is seen in its most pronounced form in this disease, but also occurs as a manifestation of many other diseases ("symptomatic dystonias"). These latter include double athetosis due to hypoxic damage to the brain, kernicterus, Hallervorden-Spatz disease, Huntington's chorea, Wilson's hepatolenticular degeneration, Parkinson's syndrome (both paralysis agitans and the postencephalitic type), lipid storage diseases, striatopallidodentatal calcification, and acute and chronic phenothiazine and haloperidol poisoning. Recently, Fahn has reported favorably on the treatment of the childhood form of dystonia with trihexyphenidyl (Artane) in high doses (6 to 30 mg/day).

Under the names of "paroxysmal choreoathetosis" and "periodic dystonia," among others, there has been described an uncommon familial disorder, characterized by paroxysmal attacks of dystonic spasms and choreoathetotic movements of the limbs and trunk. Chil-

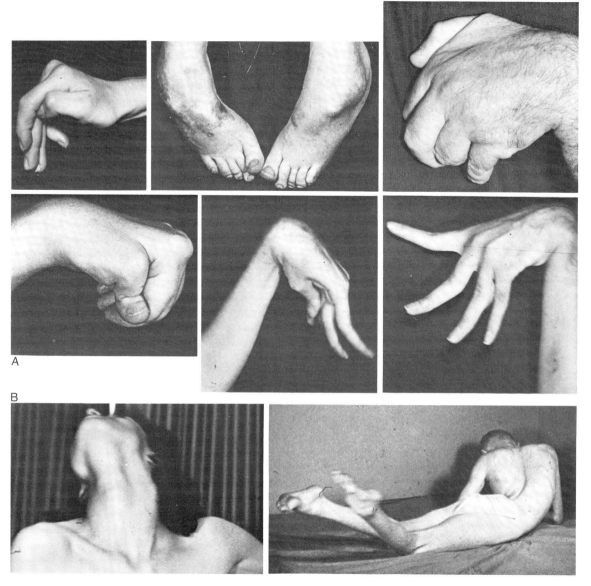

Figure 4-5

A. *Characteristic dystonic deformities of the hands and feet observed in parkinsonism.* B. *(Left) Severe dystonic retrocollis in a young woman. (Right) Incapacitating kyphoscoliotic postural deformity in a young man with dystonia. (A, from IS Cooper, Parkinsonism: Its Medical and Surgical Therapy, Springfield, Ill, Charles C Thomas, 1961; B, from IS Cooper, Involuntary Movement Disorders, Hagerstown, Md, Harper & Row, 1969.)*

dren and young adults are mainly affected. The electro-encephalogram is normal in these patients or shows only diffuse mild slowing, and consciousness is not lost during the attacks. In some families, such as those originally described by Mount and Reback and more recently by Lance, the attacks take the form predominantly of a persistent (5 min to 4 h) dystonic spasm. In others there are numerous brief attacks of choreoathetosis, often precipitated by sudden movement or startle, so that they probably represent an unusual "reflex" response questionably attributed to a seizure disorder originating in the basal ganglia. It should be recalled, however, that oculogyric crises and other spasms occur episodically in a pure basal ganglionic disease, such as postencephalitic parkinsonism. The usual mode of inheritance is autosomal recessive in the dystonic form and autosomal dominant in the paroxysmal, movement-induced choreoathetotic type (Lance). Also, sporadic instances of paroxysmal dystonia and choreoathetosis have been described in association with perinatal anoxia, basal ganglia disease, multiple sclerosis, hypoparathyroidism, and thyrotoxicosis. Rarely, the paroxysmal attacks take the form of cerebellar ataxia.

Restricted forms of athetosis and dystonia involve only the orbicularis oculi and face or mandibular muscles (blepharospasm-oromandibular dystonia), the tongue, the cervical muscles (spasmodic torticollis), the hand (writer's cramp) etc. These are described in the next chapter.

The Identity of Chorea, Athetosis, and Dystonia It must be evident, from the foregoing descriptions, that the distinctions between chorea and athetosis are probably not fundamental. Even their most prominent differences—the discreteness and rapidity of choreic movements and the slowness and confluence of athetotic ones—may be more apparent than real. As pointed out by Kinnier Wilson, involuntary movements may follow one another in such rapid succession that they become confluent and therefore appear to be slow. In practice, one finds that the patient with relatively slow, confluent movements also shows discrete, rapid ones, and vice versa, and that many patients with chorea and athetosis also show the persistent disorder of movement and posture that is generally designated as dystonia.

In a similar vein, no meaningful distinction, except one of degree, can be made between choreoathetosis and ballismus. Particularly forceful movements of large amplitude (ballismus) are observed in certain patients with Sydenham's and Huntington's chorea, who according to traditional teaching exemplify chorea and athetosis in their pure form. The intimate relationship between these involuntary movements is illustrated by the patient with hemiballismus, who, at the onset of illness exhibits wild flinging movements of the arm and, after a period of partial recovery, only choreoathetotic flexion-extension movements that are limited to the fingers. For this reason, the terms *hemiballismus* and *hemichorea* are often used interchangeably.

The Anatomic Basis of Choreoathetosis and Dystonia For many years it had been known that the abrupt onset of violent hemichorea or hemiballismus was associated

with a lesion in the contralateral subthalamic nucleus or its immediate connections. The implications of this relationship were not fully appreciated until relatively recently, however. In 1949, Whittier, Mettler, and Carpenter demonstrated that in monkeys a similar movement disorder, which they termed "choreoid dyskinesia," could be produced consistently in the limbs of one side of the body by a lesion localized to the opposite subthalamic nucleus. They showed also that for such a lesion to provoke dyskinesia, the adjacent pallidum and pallidofugal fibers had to be preserved; furthermore, a secondary lesion, placed in the pallidum, particularly its medial segment, or in the fasciculus lenticularis, or in the ventrolateral thalamic nuclear group, could abolish the dyskinesia. In a series of sequential studies, Carpenter and his colleagues also demonstrated convincingly that this form of experimental choreoid hyperkinesia could be abolished permanently by interruption of the lateral corticospinal tract, but not by interruption of the other motor or sensory pathways in the spinal cord. These observations have been interpreted to indicate that the subthalamic nucleus normally exerts an inhibitory or regulating influence on the globus pallidus and ventral thalamus. Removal of this influence, by selective destruction of the subthalamic nucleus, is expressed physiologically by bursts of irregular choreoid activity, which arise from the intact pallidum and are conveyed by pallidofugal fibers to the ventrolateral thalamic nuclei, thence by thalamocortical fibers to the motor cortex. Ultimately it expresses itself via the lateral corticospinal tract. In this instance a part of the "extrapyramidal" motor system functions not as an independent motor system but as a facilitating and inhibitory element in complex motor activities for which the corticospinal tract is the final executive pathway.

Conceivably, the abnormal movements that characterize Huntington's chorea or other disorders of the striatum have a similar explanation. Here there is a release of pallidal and thalamic activity by virtue of a loss of striatal neurons, which normally have a modulating effect upon the pallidum. Again, the upper motor neurons must be intact. In posthemiplegic choreoathetosis the corticospinal tract must have remained intact and recovered function (Dooling and Adams).

Some of these observations and interpretations can be corroborated in humans. It was appreciated for many years that if patients with involuntary movements suffered a stroke, the movement disorder would be abolished on the paralyzed side. Indeed it was this observation that led surgeons to interrupt the corticospinal tract—at its origin, in the precentral gyrus, in the cerebral peduncle, or in the dorsolateral funiculus of the spinal cord—in order to obtain the same effect. This operation was given up however, because of the attendant paresis and spasticity. The most important advance of recent years, credited largely to the pioneering efforts of neurosurgeons (Meyers; Cooper), has been the demonstration that tremor, rigidity, and involuntary movements of the limbs can be abolished by a surgical lesion in the medial segment of the globus pallidus or, preferably, in the ventrolateral nucleus of the thalamus (Fig. 4-6), without causing paralysis of voluntary movement. Again the effects are always contralateral. In the treatment of paralysis agitans, the oral administration of L-dopa has largely obviated the need for this surgical procedure, but it is still being used in certain cases of double athetosis and dystonia. Apart from these practical considerations, the salutary effects of ventrolateral thalamotomy indicate that the ventrolateral nucleus, probably through its connections with the motor cortex and the corticospinal pathway, is an essential link in the expression of the extrapyramidal syndromes, both of striatonigral and cerebellar types.

DIAGNOSIS OF DISEASES OF THE BASAL GANGLIA

The fully developed striatonigral syndromes can be recognized without difficulty once the physician has become familiar with their typical modes of clinical pre-

sentation. The picture of Parkinson's syndrome, with its slowness of movement, poverty of facial expression, flexed posture, immobility, and static tremor should be fixed in mind; it is the particular combination of these features that stamps the patient unmistakably as parkinsonian. Similarly, the torsion spasms and postural abnormalities of dystonia, whether widespread or involving only neck muscles, as in spasmodic torticollis, once seen, should thereafter be familiar. Choreoathetosis, with its instability of postures and ceaseless movements of fingers, hands, head, and facial muscles, and the shocklike movements of myoclonus that flit over the body, are other standard syndromes. Characteristic of all is the relatively mild defect in strength of volitional movement of the affected parts.

Early or mild forms of these conditions, like all medical diseases, may offer special difficulties in diagnosis. Cases of paralysis agitans, seen before the appearance of tremor, are often overlooked. The patient may complain of difficulty in performing a particular movement, of trembling, of being nervous and restless or may have experienced an indescribable stiffness and aching in certain parts of the body. Because of the absence of weakness and of reflex changes, the case may be considered psychogenic or rheumatic. It is well to remember

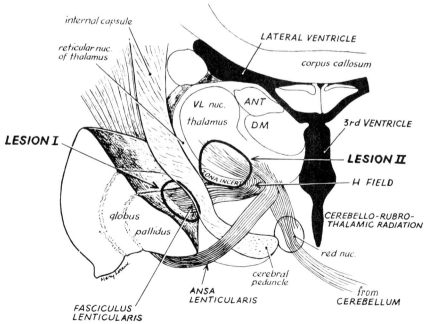

Figure 4-6
Basal ganglia and their connections, illustrating the location of lesions which abolish contralateral parkinsonian tremor. Lesion I involves the medial globus pallidus and fasciculus lenticularis; lesion II involves the ventrolateral nucleus of thalamus. (From TH Lin et al, Electroencephalogr Clin Neurophysiol 13:631, 1961.)

that the parkinsonian syndrome often begins in a hemiplegic distribution, and for this reason the illness may for a time be mistakenly attributed to cerebral thrombosis. A slight masking of the face, a suggestion of a limp, an inability to inhibit blinking when the bridge of the nose is tapped, a failure of an arm to swing naturally in walking, or loss of other automatic movements will help in diagnosis at this time. Every case presenting with Parkinson's syndrome or other abnormality of movement and posture in adolescence or early adult life should be investigated for hepatolenticular degeneration by tests of liver function, slit-lamp examination for corneal pigmentation (Kayser-Fleischer ring), and estimations of serum ceruloplasmin and urinary copper excretion. Dystonia in its early stages may be interpreted as an annoying mannerism or hysteria, and only later—in the face of persisting postural abnormality, the lack of the usual psychologic picture of hysteria, and the emerging character of the illness—is the correct diagnosis made.

INCOORDINATION OF MOVEMENT (ATAXIA) DUE TO DISEASE OF THE CEREBELLUM

Incoordination of movement may have more than one basis. It may be due to a lesion in the cerebellum or in the sensory pathways that control movement, i.e., cerebellar ataxia and sensory ataxia; there are also forms that are due to neither. This part of the chapter is devoted to cerebellar ataxia. Sensory and other types of ataxia will be considered in Chaps. 6, 8, and 14.

The cerebellum is concerned with the *regulation* or *control* of *muscular tone*, with the *coordination of movement,* especially skilled voluntary movement, and with the *control of posture and gait.* The mechanisms by which the cerebellum accomplishes these functions have been the subjects of intense interest and investigation in the last few decades. These investigations have yielded a mass of new data, testimony to the complexity of the organization of the cerebellum and its afferent and efferent connections. However, a coherent picture of cerebellar function has yet to emerge. Nor has it been possible, with a few notable exceptions, to relate the symptoms of cerebellar disease to discrete anatomic or functional units of the cerebellum. The following outline of cerebellar structure and function has of necessity been simplified; a full account can be found in the writings of Jan-

sen and Brodal, Dow and Moruzzi, and Gilman, listed at the end of this chapter.

ANATOMIC AND PHYSIOLOGIC CONSIDERATIONS

The classical studies of the comparative anatomy and the fiber connections of the cerebellum have led to the subdivision of the cerebellum into three parts (Fig. 4-7A and B): (1) The *flocculonodular lobe,* which is phylogenetically the oldest portion of the cerebellum (hence *archicerebellum*) and much the same in all animals, is separated from the main mass of the cerebellum, or corpus cerebelli, by the posterolateral fissure. (2) The *anterior lobe,* or *paleocerebellum,* which is the portion of the corpus cerebelli rostral to the primary fissure, constitutes most of the cerebellum in lower animals, but in humans it is relatively small, consisting of the anterior vermis and the contiguous paravermian cortex. (3) The *posterior lobe,* or *neocerebellum,* consists of the middle portions of the vermis and their large lateral extensions; practically all of the cerebellar hemispheres fall into this subdivision.

This anatomic subdivision corresponds roughly with a functional subdivision of the cerebellum, based on the arrangement of its afferent fiber connections. The flocculonodular lobe receives special proprioceptive impulses from the vestibular nuclei, and is therefore referred to as the "vestibulocerebellum"; it is concerned essentially with equilibrium. The anterior vermis and part of the posterior vermis are referred to as the "spinocerebellum," since the fibers to these parts are derived to a large extent from the proprioceptors of muscles and tendons in the limbs and are conveyed to the cerebellum by the dorsal spinocerebellar tract (from the lower limbs) and the ventral spinocerebellar tract (upper limbs). The main influence of the "spinocerebellum" appears to be on posture and muscle tone. The neocerebellum derives its afferent fibers from the cerebral cortex, via the pontine nuclei and brachium pontis, hence "pontocerebellum"; this portion of the cerebellum is concerned primarily with the coordination of skilled movements that are initiated at a cerebral cortical level.

On the basis of ablation experiments in animals, three rather characteristic clinical syndromes have been delineated, corresponding to these major divisions of the cerebellum. Lesions of the nodulus and flocculus have been found to cause a disturbance of equilibrium of the body and frequently a positional nystagmus as well; individual movements of the limbs are not affected, however. The main effects of anterior lobe ablation in primates are increased shortening and lengthening reactions, increased tendon reflexes, and an exaggeration

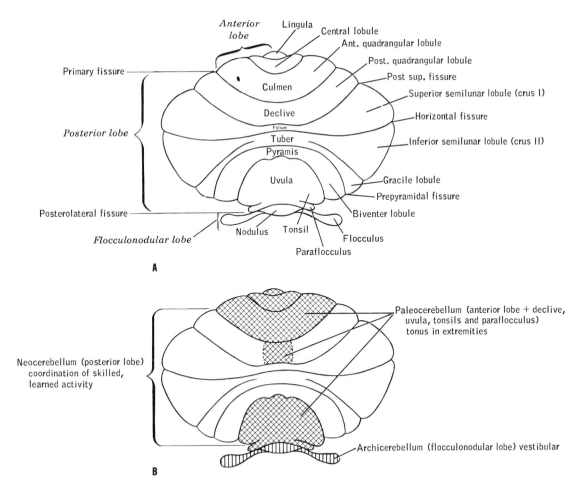

Figure 4-7
Cerebellum, illustrating (A) major fissures, lobes, and lobules, and (B) major divisions, on the basis of phylogenesis and function. (From EL House et al, A Systematic Approach to Neuroanatomy, 3d ed, New York, McGraw-Hill, 1979.)

of the postural reflexes, particularly of the "positive supporting reflex," which consists of an extension of the limb in response to light pressure on the foot pad. Ablation of the cerebellar hemisphere in cats and dogs yields inconsistent results, but in monkeys it causes hypotonia and clumsiness of the ipsilateral limbs; if the dentate nucleus is damaged in addition, these abnormalities are more enduring and the limbs also show an ataxic or "intention" tremor.

It should be emphasized that cerebellar function and structure are hardly as simple or precise as the foregoing outline indicates. The studies of Chambers and Sprague and of Jansen and Brodal indicate that in re-

spect to both afferent and efferent connections, the cerebellum is organized into longitudinal (sagittal) rather than transverse zones. There are three longitudinal zones—the vermian, paravermian or intermediate, and lateral, and there seems to be considerable overlapping between them. Chambers and Sprague, on the basis of their investigations in cats, concluded that the vermian zone controls the posture, tone, locomotion, and equilibrium of the entire body; the intermediate zone influences postural tone, but also individual movements of the ipsilateral limbs; the lateral zone is concerned mainly with the coordination of movements of the ipsilateral limbs, but is involved in other functions as well.

The efferent fibers of the cerebellar cortex, which consist essentially of the axons of Purkinje cells, project onto the deep cerebellar nuclei. According to the scheme of Jansen and Brodal, the vermis sends its fibers to the fastigial nucleus; the intermediate zone, to the globose

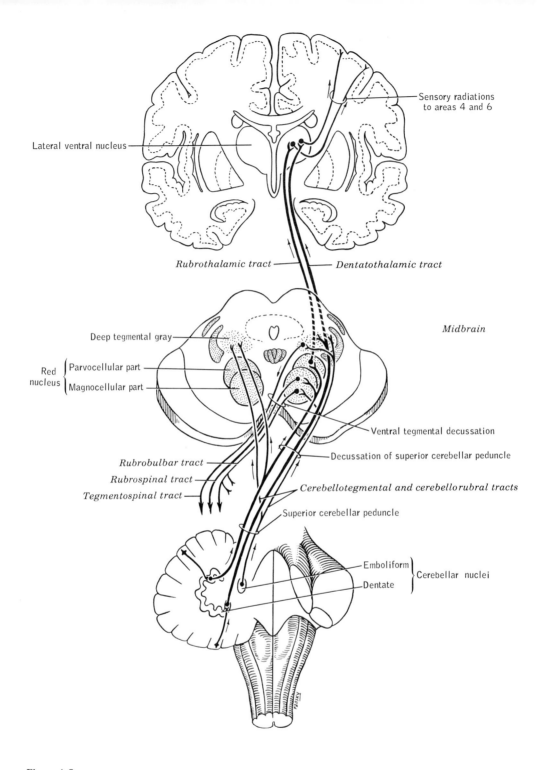

Figure 4-8
Cerebellar projections to the red nucleus, thalamus, and cerebral cortex. (After EL House et al, A Systematic Approach to Neuroanatomy, 3d ed, New York, McGraw-Hill, 1979.)

and emboliform nuclei (represented by the interpositus nucleus in animals); and the lateral zone, to the dentate nucleus. The deep cerebellar nuclei, in turn, project to the cerebral cortex and certain brainstem nuclei via two main pathways: (1) Fibers from the dentate, emboliform, and globose nuclei form the superior cerebellar peduncle, enter the upper pontine tegmentum as the brachium conjunctivum, decussate completely at the level of the inferior colliculus, and ascend to the ventrolateral nucleus of the thalamus and, to a lesser extent, to the intralaminar nuclei (Fig. 4-8). Some of these fibers, soon after their decussation, synapse in the red nucleus, but others traverse this nucleus without synapsing. The major projection from the ventral nuclei of the thalamus, it will be recalled, is to area 4 of the cerebral cortex. A small group of fibers of the superior cerebellar peduncle, following their decussation, descend in the ventromedial tegmentum of the brainstem and project to the reticulotegmental and paramedian reticular nuclei. These nuclei in turn project via the inferior cerebellar peduncle to the cerebellum, mainly the anterior lobe, thus completing a cerebelloreticular-cerebellar feedback system (Fig. 4-9). (2) The fastigial nucleus projects onto the vestibular nuclei of both sides, and to a lesser extent onto other nuclei

of the reticular formation of the pons and medulla. Thus, although the cerebellum has no direct pathways to the spinal cord comparable to the corticospinal tracts, it influences motor activity through its connections with the motor cortex and brainstem nuclei and their descending motor pathways.

The symptoms produced in animals by ablation of discrete anatomic or functional zones of the cerebellum bear only an imperfect relationship to the symptoms produced by cerebellar disease in humans. This is understandable for several reasons. Most of the lesions that occur in humans do not respect the boundaries established by experimental anatomists. However, even when the lesions are confined to discrete functional zones (e.g., flocculonodular lobe, anterior lobe), the clinical syndromes cannot be identified with those produced by the ablation of analogous zones in cats, dogs, and even in monkeys, indicating that the functions of these parts must have changed during phylogeny.

The evidence that flocculonodular lesions in humans cause a disturbance of equilibrium is quite flimsy. It rests entirely on the observation that with certain tumors of childhood, viz., medulloblastomas, there may be a gross ataxia of stance and gait, but no tremor or inco-

Figure 4-9
Dentatothalamic and dentatorubrothalamic pathways via the superior cerebellar peduncle. The "feedback" circuit via the reticular nuclei and reticulocerebellar fibers is also shown. (From EL House et al, A Systematic Approach to Neuroanatomy, 3d ed, New York, McGraw-Hill, 1979).

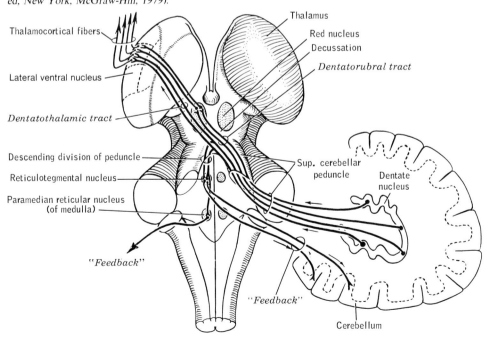

ordination of the limbs when the child is examined in the recumbent position. Insofar as these tumors are thought to originate from cell rests in the posterior medullary velum, at the base of the nodulus, it has been inferred that the disturbance of equilibrium results from involvement of this portion of the cerebellum. The validity of this deduction remains to be proved, however, because the tumors, by the time they are inspected at operation or autopsy, have spread beyond the confines of the nodulus, and no such strict clinicopathologic correlation is justified.

Cases in which accurate clinicoanatomic correlations can be made indicate that the syndrome of ataxia of stance and gait, with normality of movements of the limbs, corresponds more closely with lesions of the anterior vermis than with lesions of the flocculus and nodulus. This conclusion is based on the study of a highly stereotyped form of cerebellar degeneration in alcoholics (see Chap. 38). In such patients the cerebellar disturbance may be limited to one of stance and gait, and in these cases the pathologic changes are restricted to the anterior parts of the superior vermis. In more severely affected patients, there is also an incoordination of individual movements of the limbs, and in these cases the lesion will be found to extend laterally from the vermis, to involve the anterior portions of the anterior lobes (in cases with ataxia of the legs) and the more posterior portions of the anterior lobes (in patients whose arms are affected). Similar clinicopathologic relationships pertain in patients with familial cerebellar degeneration of the

"Holmes type." In either circumstance, despite a serious disturbance of equilibrium, the flocculonodular lobe may be spared completely.

These clinicopathologic observations suggest that the cerebellar cortex, and the anterior lobe in particular, is organized somatotopically, a view that has been amply confirmed experimentally. Originally, afferent projections to the cerebellum were thought to be entirely vestibular and proprioceptive, but now it is known that large portions of the hemispheres are involved in tactual, visual, auditory, and even visceral mechanisms. The mapping of evoked potentials from the cerebellar cortex, elicited by a variety of sensory stimuli, and an analysis of the motor effects produced by stimulation of specific parts of the cerebellar cortex, indicate that there is somatotopic localization of function in the cerebellum. The topographic representation of bodily parts, based on these experimental observations, is illustrated in Fig. 4-10. The similarities between this scheme and the one derived from the study of human disease are at once apparent.

Further experimental studies, utilizing the evoked potential technique (recording from the cerebral cortex while stimulating the cerebellar cortex, and then reversing the procedure), have demonstrated a close reciprocal connection between the anterior lobe of the cerebellum and the motor-sensory areas of the cerebral cortex, as well as between other functionally related parts of the two cortices (e.g., visual areas in the posterior vermis and the calcarine cortex). Furthermore, in these reciprocally connected areas there is considerable somatotopic organization. One can only deduce that the cerebellum must be concerned with the timing of the activity of various muscles utilized in a movement sequence and

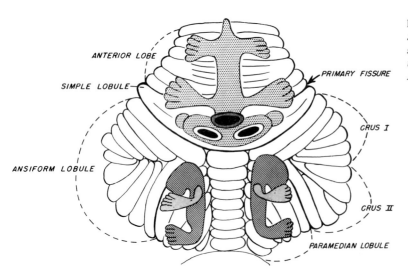

ANTERIOR LOBE

SIMPLE LOBULE

ANSIFORM LOBULE

PRIMARY FISSURE

CRUS I

CRUS II

PARAMEDIAN LOBULE

Figure 4-10
Somatotopic localization of motor and sensory function in the cerebellum. See text for explanation. (From M Victor et al, Arch Neurol 1:579, 1959.)

that the cerebellar and cerebral motor cortices and the basal ganglia must work closely together in effecting and controlling volitional movements.

CEREBELLAR SYMPTOMS

Lesions of the cerebellum in humans give rise to the following abnormalities: (1) loss of muscle tone, (2) incoordination (ataxia) of volitional movement, (3) minor degrees of muscle weakness, fatigability, and impairment of associated movements, and (4) disorders of equilibrium and gait. Extensive lesions of one cerebellar hemisphere, especially of the anterior lobe, cause hypotonia, postural abnormalities, ataxia, and mild weakness of the ipsilateral arm and leg. Lesions of the cerebellar peduncles have the same effects as extensive hemispheral lesions. If the lesion is limited to the cerebellar cortex and subcortical white matter, there may be surprisingly little disturbance of function, or the abnormality may be greatly attenuated with the passage of time. Lesions involving the superior cerebellar peduncle or the dentate nucleus cause the most severe and enduring cerebellar symptoms. Disorders of equilibrium and gait depend more upon vermian than upon hemispheral or peduncular involvement.

Clinically, *hypotonia* refers to the decrease in the normal resistance offered by the muscles to palpation or to passive manipulation (usually of a limb). Physiologically, it appears to be related to a depression of gamma motor neuron activity. In experimental animals (cats and monkeys), acute cerebellar lesions and hypotonia are associated with a depression of fusimotor efferent and spindle afferent activity; with the passage of time the fusimotor activity is restored as hypotonia disappears (Gilman, 1970). In the view of Gordon Holmes, hypotonia is the fundamental defect in cerebellar disease, accounting not only for the defects in postural fixation (see below) but also for the ataxia and tremor.

Hypotonia is much more apparent with acute than with chronic lesions and may be demonstrated in a number of ways. There may be undue flabbiness of the muscles on the affected side. Segments of the limbs may be displaced by the examiner through a wider range than normal. With recent, severe cerebellar lesions there may be gross asymmetries of posture, so that the shoulder slumps or the body tilts to the ipsilateral side. After flexing one arm against a resistance that is suddenly released, the patient may be unable to check the flexion movement to the point where the arm strikes the patient's own face; this is due to a delay in contraction of the triceps muscle, which ordinarily would arrest overflexion of the arm. This response, generally referred to as "Holmes" rebound phenomenon, is more appropriately

designated as an impairment of the check reflex. Stewart and Holmes, who first described this test, were careful to point out that when the resistance to flexion is suddenly removed, the normal limb moves only a short distance in flexion and then recoils or rebounds in the opposite direction. In this sense, rebound of the limb is actually deficient in cerebellar disease but exaggerated in spastic states.

A preferable method of testing for hypotonia is to tap the wrists of the outstretched arms, in which case the affected limb (or both limbs, in diffuse cerebellar disease) will be displaced through a wider range than normal, because of the failure of toneless muscles to fix the arm at the shoulder. When an affected limb is shaken, the flapping movements of the hands are of wider excursion than normal, although the abnormalities of postural fixation are usually less prominent in the distal than in the proximal segments of the limbs. Pendularity of the knee jerk, due to defective tonic contraction of the quadriceps and hamstring muscles, is another manifestation of cerebellar hypotonia. Patients with these abnormalities of tone may show little or no impairment of corticospinal function, indicating that the maintenance of posture involves more than the voluntary contraction of muscles.

The most prominent manifestations of cerebellar disease, those of *volitional movement*, are embraced under the general heading of cerebellar incoordination or ataxia. The terms dyssynergia, dysmetria, and dysdiadochokinesis, among others, are commonly used to describe cerebellar abnormalities of movement, but they have been used indiscriminately and have little precision. Gordon Holmes' characterization of these disturbances, as abnormalities in the rate, range, and force of movement, is at once less confusing and more accurate, as is apparent from an analysis of even a simple movement, e.g., the one elicited by finger-to-nose or toe-to-finger testing.

The speed of initiation of movement and its velocity are relatively little affected in cerebellar disease, but there is irregularity in both acceleration and deceleration of movement, these being sometimes slower and sometimes faster than intended. These abnormalities are particularly prominent as the finger or toe approaches its objective. Normally, deceleration of the movement is smooth and accurate, even if sharp changes in direction are demanded by moving the target. With cerebellar disease, the velocity and force of the movement are not checked in the normal manner. The excursion of the limb may be arrested prematurely, and the objective is then attained by a series of jerky movements. Or the limb overshoots the mark (hypermetria); then the error is corrected by a series of secondary movements, in which the finger or toe sways around the target before coming to rest, or moves from side to side a few times on the target itself. This side-to-side movement of the finger as it approaches its target may assume a rhythmic quality and is then referred to as "intention tremor." To some extent, as pointed out by Holmes, this defect is due to hypotonia, i.e., an instability of the arm at the shoulder and elbow (or at the hip and knee, in heel-to-shin testing), the result of defective postural fixation at these joints, and to the voluntary acts of deviation by which the patient attempts to correct the excessive swaying of the limb. Gilman has provided evidence that more than hypotonia is involved in the tremor of cerebellar disease. He found that deafferentation of the forelimbs of monkeys resulted in dysmetria and kinetic tremor; subsequent cerebellar ablation significantly increased both the dysmetria and tremor, indicating the presence of a mechanism, as yet unidentified, in addition to depression of the fusimotor efferent-spindle afferent circuit.

All the defects in volitional movement are more noticeable in acts that require alternation of movement, such as pronation-supination of the forearm or the successive touching of each finger to the thumb. The normal rhythm of these movements is interrupted by irregularities of force and speed, a disorder which Babinski named *adiadochokinesis*.

Another notable cerebellar disturbance is "decomposition" of a movement into its constituent parts. Electromyographic analysis has shown that decomposition of movement consists of abnormal duration and timing of bursts of contraction and relaxation of agonists and antagonists of a joint, usually a large one. This abnormality is most evident with compound movements, which involve a change in posture at two or more joints (e.g., in bringing finger to nose or heel to knee), but even a simpler movement may be fragmented, each component being effected with greater or lesser force than is required.

Cerebellar lesions commonly give rise to a disorder of *speech*, which may take one of two forms, either a simple slowing and slurring of repetitive movement resembling that which follows interruption of the corticobulbar tracts, or a *scanning dysarthria* with variable intonation, so called because words are broken up into syllables, much as a line of poetry is scanned for meter.

The latter disorder is uniquely cerebellar; in addition to its scanning quality, speech is slow, and each syllable, after an involuntary interruption, may be uttered with less force or more force ("explosive speech") than is natural.

A head tremor of moderate speed (3 to 4 per second) in the anterior-posterior direction often accompanies midline cerebellar lesions. This is called *titubation*. It is much faster than the nodding or bobbing of the head that accompanies lesions of the thalamus.

Ocular movement may be impaired as a result of cerebellar disease. Conjugate gaze is accomplished by a series of jerky movements, rather than by a smooth sweep of the eyes. On attempted fixation, the eyes may overshoot the target and then may oscillate through several cycles until precise fixation is attained. It will be recognized that these abnormalities, as well as those of speech, are of much the same nature as the ones which characterize volitional movements of the limbs. Other ocular abnormalities which may be related to cerebellar disease are skew deviation and ocular myoclonus; these are discussed in Chap. 13. Whether cerebellar lesions cause nystagmus is still not settled. Certainly large lesions of the cerebellar cortex and underlying white matter may be unaccompanied by nystagmus, but in at least one inferior cerebellar lesion, with no abnormality of the brainstem, there was sustained nystagmus (Duncan et al.). It is likely that the presence of nystagmus depends upon involvement of the fastigiovestibular connections.

A slight *loss of muscular power* and *excessive fatigability* of muscle may occur with acute cerebellar lesions. Also, in unilateral cerebellar disease, the ipsilateral arm may not swing normally in walking. Insofar as these symptoms cannot be explained by a loss of tone or other motor disorder, they must be regarded as primary manifestations of cerebellar disease, but they are never severe or persistent and are of little clinical importance.

Cerebellar disorders of equilibrium and gait are described in Chap. 6.

CLINICOPATHOLOGIC CORRELATIONS OF THE EXTRAPYRAMIDAL MOTOR DISORDERS

The extrapyramidal motor syndrome, as we know it today, was first delineated and so named by S. A. Kinnier Wilson, in 1912. The most striking abnormality in the nervous system of his patients was a degeneration of the putamens, to the extent of cavitation, and to these lesions Wilson attributed the characteristic symptoms of rigidity and tremor. Shortly thereafter, von Woerkom described a similar clinical syndrome in a patient with acquired liver disease (Wilson's cases were familial); in this case also the most prominent lesions consisted of foci of neuronal degeneration in the striatum. In 1920, Oskar and Cecile Vogt gave a detailed account of the neuropathologic changes in several patients who had been afflicted with choreoathetosis since early infancy; the changes, which they described as a status fibrosus or status dysmyelinatus, were confined to the caudate and lenticular nuclei. The studies of Huntington's chorea, beginning with those of Meynert (1871) and followed by those of Jelgersma (1908) and Alzheimer (1911), also had related the movement disorder to a loss of nerve cells in the striatum. Tretiakoff (1919) was the first to demonstrate the consistent affection of the substantia nigra in cases of paralysis agitans. A long series of observations, the most recent ones being those of J. Purdon Martin, have related hemiballismus to lesions in the subthalamic nucleus of Luys and its immediate connections.

Unfortunately, many of the classic cases leave much to be desired. We now know that in certain diseases, such as Wilson's disease, Huntington's chorea, and postencephalitic parkinsonism, parts of the brain other than the basal ganglia are involved. Also, lack of quantitative neuropathologic methods has hampered progress in this field. Even now the nature and topography of the pathologic findings in several of these diseases (e.g., dystonia musculorum deformans) have not been determined. The difficulties of clinicoanatomic correlations in cases of cerebellar disease have already been indicated. The lesions responsible for so-called palatal myoclonus have a specific localization, whereas the anatomic basis of diffuse myoclonus is quite vague (see Chap. 6).

Table 5-2 summarizes the clinicopathologic correlations accepted by most neurologists, but it must be reemphasized that there is still much uncertainty as to finer details.

Table 4-2
Clinicopathologic correlations of extrapyramidal motor disorders

Symptoms	Principal location of morbid anatomy
Unilateral plastic rigidity with static tremor (Parkinson's syndrome)	Contralateral substantia nigra plus (?) other structures
Unilateral hemiballismus and hemichorea	Contralateral subthalamic nucleus of Luys, prerubral area, and Forel's fields
Chronic chorea of Huntington type	Caudate nucleus and putamen
Athetosis and dystonia	Contralateral striatum and connections with the thalamus. The pathology of dystonia musculorum deformans (Oppenheim) is unknown.
Cerebellar incoordination, intention tremor, and hypotonia	Homolateral cerebellar hemisphere or middle and inferior cerebellar peduncles, superior brachium conjunctivum (ipsilateral if below the decussation, contralateral if above)
Decerebrate rigidity, i.e., opisthotonos, extension of arms and legs	Usually bilateral in tegmentum, involving upper brainstem, particularly red nucleus or structures between red and vestibular nuclei
Palatal and facial myoclonus (rhythmic)	Contralateral dentate nucleus or superior cerebellar peduncle or ipsilateral central tegmental tract (dentatoolivary pathway)
Diffuse myoclonus	Neuronal degeneration, usually diffuse or predominating in cerebral or cerebellar cortex and dentate nuclei

REFERENCES

CARPENTER MB: Brainstem and infratentorial neuraxis in experimental dyskinesia. *Arch Neurol* 5:504, 1961.

———: The basal ganglia, in *Human Neuroanatomy*, 7th ed. Baltimore, William & Wilkins, 1976, chap 17, pp 496–520.

———: Anatomy of the corpus striatum and brainstem integrating systems, in Brooks V (ed): *Handbook of Physiology*, sec 1: *The Nervous System*, vol 2: *Motor Control*. Bethesda, American Physiological Society (in press).

——— et al: Analysis of choreoid hyperkinesia in the rhesus monkey: Surgical and pharmacological analysis of hyperkinesia resulting from lesions of the subthalamic nucleus of Luys. *J Comp Neurol* 92:293, 1950.

CHAMBERS WW, SPRAGUE JM: Functional localization in the cerebellum. I. Organization in longitudinal cortico-nuclear zones and their contribution to the control of posture, both extrapyramidal and pyramidal. *J Comp Neurol* 103:104, 1955.

———, ———: Functional localization in the cerebellum. II. Somatotopic organization in cortex and nuclei. *Arch Neurol Psychiatry* 74:653, 1955.

COOPER IS: *Involuntary Movement Disorders.* New York, Hoeber-Harper, 1969.

COOPER JR, BLOOM FE, ROTH RH: *The Biochemical Basis of Neuropharmacology,* 3d ed. New York, Oxford, 1978.

DOOLING EC, ADAMS RD: The pathological anatomy of post-hemiplegic athetosis, Trans Am Neurol Assoc 99:33, 1974.

DOW RS, MORUZZI G: *The Physiology and Pathology of the Cerebellum.* Minneapolis, The University of Minnesota Press, 1958.

DUNCAN GW et al: Acute cerebellar infarction in the PICA territory. Arch Neurol 32:364, 1975.

FAHN S: Treatment of dystonia with high-dosage anticholinergic medication. *Neurology* 29:605, 1979.

——— et al: Monoamines in the human neostriatum; topographic distribution in normals and in Parkinson's disease and their role in akinesia, rigidity, chorea and tremor. *J Neurol Sci* 14:427, 1971.

GILMAN S: The nature of cerebellar dyssynergia, in Williams D (ed): *Modern Trends in Neurology—5.* London, Butterworth, 1970, chap 4, pp 60–79.

———, BLOEDEL J, LECHTENBERG R: *Disorders of the Cerebellum.* Philadelphia, Davis, 1980.

HALLETT M, KHOSHBIN S: A physiological mechanism of bradykinesia. *Brain* 103:301, 1980.

———, SHAHANI BT, YOUNG RR: EMG analysis of patients with cerebellar deficits. *J Neurol Neurosurg Psychiatry* 38:1163, 1975.

HOLMES G: The cerebellum of man. Hughlings Jackson lecture. *Brain* 62:1, 1939.

HORNYKIEWICZ O: Neurochemical pathology and pharmacology of brain dopamine and acetylcholine: Rational basis for the current drug treatment of parkinsonism, in Plum F (ed):

Contemporary Neurology Series, vol 6: *Recent Advances in Neurology.* Philadelphia, Davis, 1970, chap 2.

HUDGINS RL, CORBIN KB: An uncommon seizure disorder: Familial paroxysmal choreoathetosis. *Brain* 91:199, 1968.

JANSEN J, BRODAL A: *Aspects of Cerebellar Anatomy.* Oslo, Johan Grundt Tanum Forlag, 1954.

KLAWANS HL JR: *Monographs in Neural Sciences,* vol 2: *The Pharmacology of Extrapyramidal Movement Disorders.* Basel, Karger, 1973.

LANCE JW: Familial paroxysmal dystonic choreoathetosis and its differentiation from related syndromes. *Ann Neurol* 2:285, 1977.

MARTIN JP: *Papers on Hemiballismus and the Basal Ganglia.* London, National Hospital Centenary, 1960.

———: *The Basal Ganglia and Posture.* Philadelphia, Lippincott, 1967.

MEYERS R: The surgery of the hyperkinetic disorders, in Vinken PJ, Bruyn GW (eds): *Handbook of Clinical Neurology,* vol 6: *Basal Ganglia.* Amsterdam, North-Holland, 1968, chap 33, pp 844–878.

MOUNT LA, REBACK S: Familial paroxysmal choreoathetosis: Preliminary report on a hitherto undescribed clinical syndrome. *Arch Neurol Psychiatry* 44:841, 1940.

RICHTER R: Degeneration of the basal ganglia in monkeys from chronic carbon disulfide poisoning. *J Neuropathol Exp Neurol* 4:324, 1945.

SPRAGUE JM, CHAMBERS WW: Control of posture by reticular formation and cerebellum in the intact, anesthetized, unanesthetized and in the decerebrated cat. *Am J Physiol* 176:52, 1954.

WARD AA JR: The function of the basal ganglia, in Vinken PJ, Bruyn GW (eds): *Handbook of Clinical Neurology,* vol 6: *Basal Ganglia.* Amsterdam, North-Holland, 1968, chap 3, pp 90–115.

WHITTIER JR, METTLER FA: Studies on the subthalamus of the rhesus monkey. *J Comp Neurol* 90:281, 319, 1949.

WILSON SAK: Disorders of motility and of muscle tone, with special reference to the corpus striatum. The Croonian Lectures. *Lancet* 2:1, 53, 169, 215, 1925.

ZEMAN W: Pathology of the torsion dystonias (dystonia musculorum deformans). *Neurology* 20:79, 1970.

CHAPTER 5

TREMOR, MYOCLONUS, SPASMS, AND TICS

The subject of tremor may suitably be considered at this point because of its association with diseases of the basal ganglia and cerebellum. A miscellaneous group of other movement disorders—myoclonus, facial-cervical dyskinesias, occupational spasms, and tics—will also be described in this chapter. The latter disorders are largely involuntary in nature and can be quite disabling, but they have no known pathologic basis and no particular relationship to the extrapyramidal motor disorders or to other standard categories of neurologic disease. They are being brought together here mainly for convenience of exposition.

TREMOR

Tremor may be defined as a more or less regular, rhythmic oscillation of a part of the body around a fixed point or plane. This rhythmic quality distinguishes tremor from other involuntary movements. Two general categories are recognized: normal (or physiologic) and abnormal (or pathologic). The former, as the name implies, is a normal phenomenon; it is present in all muscle groups and persists throughout the waking state and sleep. It is so fine a movement that it cannot be seen by the naked eye and requires special instruments to be detected. It ranges in frequency between 8 and 13 Hz, the dominant rate being 10 Hz in adults and somewhat less in childhood and old age. Several hypotheses have been proposed to explain physiologic tremor, the most popular one being that it reflects the ballistocardiogram, i.e., the passive vibration of bodily tissues produced by mechanical activity of cardiac origin ("BCG tremor"). Assuredly, however, this is not the complete explanation of physiologic tremor. As Marsden points out, it is due to the complex interaction of several additional factors such as spindle input, the grouped firing rates of motor

neurons, and the natural resonating frequencies and inertia of the muscles and other structures. Certain abnormal tremors, namely the metabolic varieties of postural or action tremor and at least one type of familial tremor, seem to be variants or exaggerations of physiologic tremor; hence its clinical significance (see further on).

Abnormal or pathologic tremor, which is what one means when the term tremor is used clinically, preferentially affects certain muscle groups—the distal parts of the limbs (especially the fingers and hands), the head, tongue or jaw, and rarely the trunk—and is present only in the waking state. The rate in most forms of abnormal tremor is about half that of physiologic tremor, i.e., from 4 to 6 Hz. In any one individual the rate is fairly constant in all affected parts, regardless of the size of the muscles or the parts of the body involved. Abnormal tremors have been subdivided according to their rate and their relationship to posture of the limbs and volitional movement, the pattern of EMG activity in opposing muscle groups, and their response to certain drugs. The following types of tremor should be familiar to every physician.

REST (PARKINSONIAN) TREMOR

This is a coarse, rhythmic tremor with a frequency of 3 to 7 Hz. Electromyographically, it is characterized by bursts of activity which alternate between opposing muscle groups. The tremor is most often localized in one or both hands and less frequently in the feet, jaw, lips, or tongue. It occurs when the limb is in an *attitude of repose* and is suppressed or diminished by willed movement, at least temporarily, only to reassert itself once the limb assumes a new position. For this reason the parkinsonian tremor is often referred to as a "resting tremor" or "tremor at rest," but these terms need to be qualified. Maintaining the arm in an attitude of repose or keeping it still in other positions requires a certain degree of muscular contraction, albeit slight. If the tremulous hand is fully relaxed, as it is when the arm is fully supported at the wrist and elbow, the tremor usually disappears, but the patient rarely achieves this state. And under conditions of complete rest, i.e., in sleep, the tremor always disappears, as do all abnormal tremors.

Parkinsonian tremor takes the form of flexion-extension or abduction-adduction of the fingers or the hand; pronation-supination of the hand is also a common presentation. Flexion-extension of the fingers in combination with adduction-abduction of the thumb yields the classic "pill-rolling" tremor. When the legs are affected, the tremor takes the form of a flexion-extension movement of the foot, and in the jaw and lips an up-and-down and a pursing movement, respectively. The eyelids, if they are closed lightly, tend to flutter, and the tongue, when protruded, may move in and out of the mouth at about the same tempo as the tremor elsewhere. The rate of the tremor is surprisingly constant over long periods, but the amplitude is variable. Emotional stress, in particular, augments the amplitude, and increasing rigidity of the limbs may reduce it. The tremor interferes surprisingly little with voluntary movement; it is not uncommon, for example, to see a patient who has been trembling violently raise a full glass of water to his lips and drain its contents without spilling a drop. Parkinsonian tremor is suppressed most effectively by ethopropazine (Parsidol), by trihexphenydil (Artane), and somewhat less consistently by L-dopa. Stereotaxic lesions in the nucleus intermedius ventralis abolish tremor contralaterally.

Resting tremor is most often a manifestation of Parkinson's syndrome, whether it be the idiopathic variety described by James Parkinson (paralysis agitans) or the postencephalitic or the drug-induced type. In paralysis agitans the tremor is relatively gentle and more or less limited to the distal muscles, whereas the tremor of postencephalitic parkinsonism often has a greater amplitude and involves proximal muscles. A parkinsonian tremor may also be seen in elderly persons without akinesia, rigidity, or masklike facies. Unlike the tremor of paralysis agitans, it is unpredictably stationary or progressive. In some instances it is followed years later by paralysis agitans. Patients with Wilson's disease or the acquired form of hepatocerebral degeneration may also show a static tremor, but usually it is mixed with cerebellar ataxia and other extrapyramidal motor abnormalities.

INTENTION (ATAXIC) TREMOR

The word *intention* is ambiguous in this context because the tremor itself is not intentional and occurs not when the patient intends to make a movement, but only during the most demanding phases of active movement. In this sense it is a kinetic, or action, tremor, but the latter term has other connotations to neurologists, being used generally as a synonym for postural tremor. The term *ataxic* is a suitable substitute for "intention" because this tremor is always combined with and adds to cerebellar ataxia. The salient feature of this tremor is that it requires for its full expression the performance of an exacting, precise, projected movement. The tremor is absent when the limbs are inactive and during the first part of a voluntary movement, but as the action continues and fine adjustments of the movement are demanded (e.g., in touching a target such as the tip of the nose or the examiner's finger), a jerky, more or less rhythmic (4 to 6 Hz) interruption of forward progression, with side-to-side oscillation, appears, and may continue for a second or so after the act is completed. The tremor may seriously interfere with the patient's performance of skilled acts. Sometimes there is a rhythmic oscillation of the head on the trunk (titubation), or of the trunk itself, at approximately the same rate.

This type of tremor invariably indicates disease of the cerebellum or of its connections. It may be of such severity that every movement, even lifting the arm slightly from the side results in a wide-ranging tremor of sufficient violence to throw the patient off balance; in such cases, the lesion is usually in the midbrain, involving the upward projections of the dentatorubrothalamic fibers. This latter state is occasionally seen in multiple sclerosis, Wilson's disease, and vascular and other lesions of the tegmentum of the midbrain and subthalamus.

The mechanisms involved in the production of intention, or ataxic, tremor have been discussed in the preceding chapter (page 66).

POSTURAL AND ACTION TREMORS

These terms refer to a tremor that is present when the limbs and trunk are actively maintained in certain positions (such as holding the arms outstretched) and throughout active movement. More particularly, the tremor is absent when the limbs are relaxed but becomes evident when the muscles are activated; it is accentuated as greater precision of movement is demanded, but it never approaches the degree of augmentation seen in intention tremor. In contrast to static, or parkinsonian, tremor, which is characterized electromyographically by alternate activity in agonist and antagonist muscles, the rhythmicity of action tremor is accounted for by relatively rhythmic bursts of alpha motor neuron activity which occur *synchronously* and simultaneously in the opposing muscle groups. Presumably, inequalities in the strength and timing of contraction of opposing muscle groups account for the tremor.

Action tremors are of several different types, a feature which makes them more difficult to interpret than other tremors. Some action tremors seem to be mere exaggerations of normal or physiologic tremor; they have the same frequency as physiologic tremor but a greater amplitude. Such tremors, best elicited by holding the arms outstretched with fingers spread apart, are characteristic of hyperthyroidism and other toxic states (lithium), and of withdrawal from alcohol and other sedative-hypnotic drugs. A similar tremor is frequently observed in certain families (one type of familial tremor) and under conditions of intense muscular fatigue or anxiety. Also it is noteworthy that this type of action tremor can be reproduced by the intravenous injection of epinephrine or beta-adrenergic stimulating agents such as isoproterenol. All these clinical circumstances have in common an increased cardiac output, which may serve to increase the amplitude of physiologic or BCG tremor (see above). However, Young and his colleagues have adduced evidence that the enhancement of physiologic tremor that occurs in these various metabolic and toxic states is due to stimulation of peripheral tremorogenic beta-adrenergic receptors by increased levels of circulating catecholamines. Thus it appears that synchronization of motor units in physiologic tremor, though not primarily of neural origin, is nevertheless influenced by central and peripheral nervous activity.

A second group of action tremors is of a slower frequency (4 to 8 Hz) than physiologic tremor. Tremor of this slow-frequency type may occur as the only neurologic abnormality in several members of a family, in which case it is known as *familial tremor*. Such a tremor tends to be inherited as an autosomal dominant trait; it may begin in childhood, but usually comes on later in adult life and persists. If the inherited nature of the tremor is not evident, it is referred to as *essential tremor*, and if it becomes evident only in late adult life, as *senile tremor*. These tremors cannot be distinguished on the basis of their physiologic and pharmacologic properties, and should not therefore be considered as separate entities.

Familial, or *essential*, *tremor* most often makes its appearance in early adult life. The usual frequency is about 8 Hz, and it is of variable amplitude. Aging is associated with a decrease in the rate of the tremor, as is the case with physiologic tremor. The amplitude of the tremor may remain unchanged for long periods or may worsen slowly with advancing years. The tremor may be limited to the upper limbs, or a side-to-side or nodding movement of the head may be added. The tremor of the head may precede the tremor of the hand by several years, but more often it follows the hand tremor. The head tremor is also postural in nature and disappears when the head is supported. In advanced cases there is involvement of the jaw, lips, tongue, and larynx, the latter imparting a quaver to the voice. The lower limbs are practically always spared. In distinction to the rapid action tremors, which interfere little with voluntary movements, the slower, coarser types may increase in severity to a point where handwriting is altered and the patient can barely bring a cup or glass to the lips without spilling the contents. Eventually all tasks which require manual dexterity are difficult or impossible.

As indicated above, in most patients with essential tremor of fast frequency there is simultaneous activity in agonist and antagonist muscles. In about 10 percent of cases agonist and antagonist muscles are activated alternately. Some patients with the slow, "alternate beat" form of action tremor may later develop Parkinson's disease.

A curious fact about essential, or familial, tremor is that it can be suppressed by a few drinks of alcohol, but once the effects of the alcohol have worn off the tremor returns and may be even worse. It is also of interest that this type of tremor is often suppressed by the beta-adrenergic antagonist propranolol taken orally over a long period of time (average dose 40 mg tid), suggesting an autonomic basis for this tremor. Young et al. have shown that neither propranolol nor ethanol, when injected intraarterially into a limb, decrease the amplitude of essential tremor. These findings suggest that the therapeutic effects of alcohol and propranolol are due not to blockade of the peripheral beta-adrenergic tremorogenic receptors but to their action on structures within the central nervous system.

Action tremors are seen in a number of neurologic diseases in addition to those already mentioned. A coarse action tremor, sometimes combined with myoclonus, accompanies various types of meningoencephalitis (e.g., general paresis) and certain intoxications (methyl bromide and bismuth). Its anatomy and mechanism are obscure. Also it is important to note that an action tremor of either the fast-frequency or slower (essential) variety may accompany certain diseases of the basal ganglia, including parkinsonism, and may be combined with the more typical static tremor of the latter. An action tremor of varying severity is the most prominent feature of the alcohol withdrawal states. It may be of the fine fast-frequency variety, as indicated above, or it may take the form of a slower and coarser essential type of tremor. Alcoholic patients with the latter type often have a positive family history of tremor. Either type may occur as an isolated phenomenon following relatively short periods of intoxication and abstinence ("morning shakes"). The mechanisms involved in the genesis of alcohol withdrawal symptoms are discussed further in Chap. 40.

HYSTERICAL TREMOR

This is a relatively rare manifestation of hysteria, but it may simulate any of the better known types of organic tremor, thereby causing difficulty in diagnosis. Hysterical tremors are usually restricted to a single limb and are gross in nature. If the affected limb is restrained by the examiner, the tremor may move to another part of the body. Hysterical tremor is also less regular than static tremor. It persists in repose and during movement and is less subject than organic tremors to the modifying influences of posture and willed movement.

TREMORS OF MIXED TYPE

Not all tremors correspond exactly with the ones described above. There is frequently a variation in one or more particulars from the classic pattern, or one type of tremor may show a feature ordinarily considered characteristic of another. In some parkinsonian patients, for example, the tremor is accentuated rather than diminished by active movement; in others the tremor may be very mild or absent "at rest" and only become obvious with movement of the limbs. As mentioned above, a patient with classic parkinsonian tremor may have also a fine tremor of the outstretched hands, i.e., a postural or action tremor, and occasionally an element of ataxic tremor as well. In a similar vein, essential or familial tremor may, in its advanced stages, years after its onset, assume the aspects of a cerebellar, or intention, tremor. Gordon Holmes was careful to note that patients with acute cerebellar lesions sometimes showed a parkinsonian tremor in addition to the usual signs of ataxia and ataxic tremor.

The features of one type of tremor may be so mixed with those of another that satisfactory classification is impossible. In certain patients with essential or familial tremor or with cerebellar degeneration, one may observe a rhythmic tremor, characteristically parkinsonian in tempo, which is not apparent in repose but appears with certain sustained postures. It may take the form of an abduction-adduction or flexion-extension of the fingers when the patient's weight is partially supported by the hands, as in the writing position, or it may appear as a tremor of the thigh when the patient is seated or of the arms when they are outstretched. The term "rubral tremor" has been applied to this and to other types of mixed tremor, but there is no evidence that lesions of the red nucleus produce any motor disturbances other than those that accompany interruption of fibers of the brachium conjunctivum. The lesions are usually in the upper brainstem, involving both the dentatothalamic and dentatoolivary systems.

THE PATHOLOGIC ANATOMY OF TREMOR

The exact anatomic basis of parkinsonian tremor is not known. In paralysis agitans and postencephalitic Parkinson's syndrome, the visible lesions predominate in the substantia nigra. In animals, experimental lesions confined to the substantia nigra do not result in tremor, however; neither do lesions in the striatopallidal parts of the basal ganglia. Albe-Fessard and Narabayashi (see Desmedt) report rhythmic burst discharges of unitary cellular activity in the nucleus intermedius ventralis; these are synchronized with the beat of the tremor. Stereotaxic lesions here abolish parkinsonian tremor.

Ward and others have produced a Parkinson-like tremor in monkeys by placing lesions in the ventromedial tegmentum of the midbrain, just caudal to the red nucleus and dorsal to the substantia nigra. These lesions may interrupt ascending fibers from the substantia nigra and descending fibers from the red nucleus. Ward has postulated that interruption of the descending pathways permits a lower brainstem mechanism to oscillate, presumably involving the limb innervation via the reticulospinal pathway. Alternative possibilities are that the lesion in the ventromedial tegmentum interrupts the brachium conjunctivum destined for the contralateral thalamus, or the descending limb of the superior cerebellar peduncle, which functions as a link in a cerebellar-reticular-cerebellar feedback mechanism (Fig. 4-9).

Tremor has been consistently produced in monkeys by removal of the deep cerebellar nuclei or section of the superior cerebellar peduncle or brachium conjunctivum, below the decussation. The tremor is of the ataxic type, as one might expect, and is associated with other manifestations of cerebellar ataxia. In addition, however, the monkeys show a "simple tremor," which is the term that Carpenter has applied to a "resting" or parkinsonian tremor. The latter tremor is most prominent during the early postoperative period and is less enduring than ataxic tremor, but its presence suggests that ataxic and simple tremors have closely related neural mechanisms. Both forms of tremor, in humans as well as in animals, can be abolished by ablation of the ventrolateral thalamic nuclei, contralateral to the cerebellar lesion. The effectiveness of the thalamic lesion may be due to interruption of pallidothalamic and dentatothalamic projections or, what is more likely, to interruption of projections from the ventrolateral thalamus to the motor cortex, since the impulses responsible for cerebellar tremor, like those for choreoathetosis, are ultimately mediated by the lateral corticospinal tract. This concept explains why a lesion of the subthalamic nucleus causes *contralateral* dyskinesia, whereas a lesion of the brachium conjunctivum, below its decussation, gives rise to *ipsilateral* ataxia and tremor.

MYOCLONUS

Myoclonus is the name given to exceedingly abrupt, shocklike contractions of muscles which are irregular in rhythm and amplitude and, with few exceptions, asynchronous or asymmetric in distribution. In its brevity and arrhythmicity, the myoclonic movement resembles chorea, but it is much faster, being concluded in 10 to 30 ms. Variations in degree are noteworthy; the myoclonic jerk may consist of no more than a flick of a single muscle, but its true nature is always betrayed by larger movements that involve a group of muscles and may be of sufficient force to displace the affected limb or part of the limb, or even the trunk. Thus myoclonus can be distinguished from fasciculation.

Sensory relationships are another prominent attribute. In certain diseases that underlie myoclonus, flickering light, loud sounds, or abrupt contact with some part of the body may regularly initiate a jerk, either as a direct sensorimotor effect or through the mechanism of startle. Repeated stimuli may recruit a series of myoclonic jerks that crescendo to a full-blown seizure, as happens often in the familial myoclonic epilepsy syndrome of Unverricht-Lundborg. Another type of sensory myoclonus is the audiogenic form characteristic of Tay-Sachs disease. Each auditory stimulus results in abrupt blinking, elevation of the arms, and other movements. It does not fatigue with successive stimuli. This generalized myoclonic jerk also resembles the massive myoclonus (salaam spasm) of West's disease (see Chap. 15). Hence one may speak of stimulus-sensitive myoclonus or of auditory or visual myoclonus.

Intention (Action) Myoclonus One special variety of myoclonus is evoked by muscular activity, particularly by attempts to perform precise willed movements, hence the descriptive term *intention*, or *action*, *myoclonus*. It is often a sequela of anoxic encephalopathy, and may also be observed with cerebellar disease of other type and in patients with myoclonic epilepsy. Intention myoclonus can be suppressed by the benzodiazepine derivative, clonazepam (divided doses of 8 to 12 mg daily), and by 5-hydroxytryptophan (100 to 200 mg daily, increased slowly to 1 or 1.5 g daily) combined with carbidopa (150 to 400 mg daily).

Palatal Myoclonus Unfortunately the term *myoclonus* has also been assigned to a rather different motor phenomenon—that of persistent rhythmic movement of muscles derived from some part of the "branchial clefts" (i.e., craniocervical musculature). Palatal myoclonus or palatal nystagmus is the best-known form. The movement disorder affects not only the soft palate, but in some instances the pharynx, facial muscles, diaphragm, tongue, vocal cords, and even the shoulder muscles as well. The movement of the affected muscles is rhythmic, 60 to 100 per minute, and unlike all other forms of myoclonus, persists in sleep, unaltered in rhythm and rate. Its automatic rhythmicity, based on brainstem structures, is analogous to respiration.

The pathological change that has consistently been demonstrated in palatal myoclonus is a unique hypertrophic (presumably transsynaptic) degeneration of the inferior olive, associated with a primary lesion in the ipsilateral central tegmental tract or in the contralateral dentate nucleus. The pathway linking these structures originates in the dentate nucleus, enters the brainstem via the superior cerebellar peduncle, crosses the midline in the commissure of Wernekink, and turns caudally in the vicinity of the medial and dorsal part of the red nucleus to merge with the central tegmental tract (Lapresle and Ben Hamida). Thus palatal myoclonus, which we would prefer to designate as a form of continuous bulbar, facial, or diaphragmatic clonus, is a distinct clinicoanatomic entity that has little in common with other types of myoclonus.

Paramyoclonus Multiplex This is an outmoded term, first used by Friedreich, in 1881, to denote a nonfamilial type of myoclonus that began in adult life, involved all the muscles particularly those of the lower face and proximal segments of the limbs, and persisted, except during sleep, for many years, unassociated with other neurologic or systemic disease. The nature and pathologic basis of this disorder were never determined, and its status as a clinical entity was never secure. Over the years, the term paramyoclonus multiplex has been used to designate all variety of myoclonic disorders (and other motor phenomena as well) to the point where it no longer has a specific clinical connotation.

CLINICAL RELATIONSHIPS

Myoclonus is often observed in association with epilepsy, a relationship commonly designated as *myoclonic epilepsy.* Included under this title are several different seizure states, some quite benign and others associated with intellectual deterioration and a variety of abnormalities of the nervous system.

Patients with idiopathic epilepsy may complain of localized myoclonic jerks, usually confined to an arm or leg and occurring singly or in short bursts, often on awakening; or the myoclonic jerks may be more frequent and severe, particularly during the day or two preceding a major generalized seizure, after which they diminish in frequency. Relatively few patients with myoclonus and epilepsy of this type show progressive mental and physical deterioration. Myoclonus may also be associated with atypical petit mal and akinetic seizures in a variety of nonprogressive cerebral diseases. On the other hand, mental regression is a regular feature of a special variety of epilepsy in early childhood, in which the child collapses as a result of a massive myoclonic jerk of the trunk ("salaam" or "jack-knife" seizures).

The myoclonic epilepsy associated with dementia and other signs of progressive neurologic disease (the familial variety of Unverricht and Lundborg) has as its outstanding feature a remarkable sensitivity of the myoclonus to stimuli of all sorts. As indicated above, if a limb is passively displaced, the resulting myoclonic jerk may lead, by a series of progressively larger and more or less synchronous jerks, to a generalized convulsive seizure. In late childhood this type of myoclonus is usually a manifestation of the juvenile form of lipid storage disease and, in addition to myoclonus, is characterized by seizures, progressive dementia, rigidity, pseudobulbar paralysis, and, in the late stages, by quadriplegia in flexion. Another form of familial, stimulus-sensitive myoclonus beginning in late childhood or adolescence is that caused by the presence of neuronal inclusions (Lafora bodies) in the cerebral and cerebellar cortex and

in brainstem nuclei (see page 692). Under the title of "cherry-red spot–myoclonus syndrome," Rapin and her associates have drawn attention to a familial (autosomal recessive) form of diffuse incapacitating intention myoclonus associated with visual loss that develops insidiously in adolescence. The earliest sign is a cherry-red spot in the macula which may fade in the chronic stages of the illness. The intellect is relatively unimpaired. The specific enzyme defect appears to be a deficiency of lysosomal α-neuroaminidase (sialidase), resulting in the excretion of large amounts of sialylated oligosaccharides in the urine. Lowden and O'Brien, in a recent review, refer to this disorder as *type 1 sialidosis* and distinguish it from a second type in which patients have a short stature (due to chondrodystrophy) and often a deficiency of β-galactosidase in tissues and body fluids. In patients with sialidosis, a mucopolysaccharide-like material is stored in liver cells, but neurons show only a nonspecific accumulation of lipofuscin. A similar syndrome is seen in one form of Gaucher's disease and in a variant of neuroaxonal dystrophy.

In another group of myoclonic disorders, which may be loosely identified as the "myoclonic dementias," the most prominent associated abnormality is a progressive deterioration of intellect. Like the myoclonic epilepsies, the myoclonic dementias may be sporadic or familial and may affect both children and adults. An important childhood type is subacute sclerosing panencephalitis (SSPE), which is a subacute or chronic (occasionally remitting) disease, related in some way to infection with the measles virus (page 523). An analogous disorder, familial in nature, may occur in infants and young children (Ford); it has been called *progressive poliodystrophy.* On a background of normal birth and development over the first few months or years of life, there occurs a progressive psychomotor deterioration, with spastic quadriplegia, seizures, myoclonus, and blindness. In this condition, too, the fundamental pathologic alteration is a destruction of nerve cells in the cerebral and cerebellar cortices with replacement gliosis. The transmissible nature of this childhood form has not been established. In adults, there occurs a unique subacute illness characterized by dementia, disturbances of gait and coordination, all manner of mental aberrations, rigidity, and diffuse myoclonus. Originally the jerks are random in character, but late in the disease they may attain a certain rhythmicity and symmetry. In addition there is an exaggerated startle response. This disorder is commonly referred to as Creutzfeldt-Jakob disease. Pathologically it is characterized by a progressive destruction of the nerve cells, mainly but not exclusively of the cerebral and cerebellar cortices, and a striking degree of gliosis. In addition to the parenchymatous destruction, the cortical tissue may show a fine-meshed vacuolation, hence the preferable designation "subacute spongiform encephalopathy." Both the sporadic and rare familial forms of this disease are believed to be due to a transmissible agent (see page 525).

Myoclonus in association with signs of cerebellar incoordination, including opsoclonus (rapid, irregular, but predominantly conjugate movements of the eyes in all planes), is another syndrome that has been described both in children and adults under a variety of names. Most cases run a chronic course, waxing and waning in severity. Many of the childhood cases have been associated with occult neuroblastoma, and some have responded to the administration of corticosteroids. In adults a similar syndrome has been described in relation to bronchogenic carcinoma, but it also occurs at all ages as a manifestation of a benign postinfectious (possibly viral) illness (Baringer et al.). In some cases, myoclonus is associated only with cerebellar ataxia and tremor, opsoclonus being absent, and in others, myoclonus, seizures, cerebellar tremor, and ataxia have been combined (dyssynergia cerebellaris myoclonica of Ramsay Hunt). An acute onset of polymyoclonia with confusion may occur with methyl bromide and bismuth intoxication. Once ingestion is discontinued, there is improvement (over days to weeks) and the polymyoclonus is replaced by diffuse action tremors (see above) which themselves later subside.

Finally, it should be noted that myoclonus may occur as a transient or persistent phenomenon in viral encephalitis, suppurative meningitis, general paresis, advanced Alzheimer's disease, and with certain intoxications (strychnine, tetanus) and metabolic disorders (uremia, anoxic encephalopathy).

THE NATURE OF MYOCLONUS

The main difficulty with formulating a concept of myoclonus is that it embraces too many motor disorders. In addition to the several forms of myoclonus noted above, one must include the normal start or jerk of a limb as one falls asleep, and the motor components of a natural startle reaction. The obligatory Moro response also falls within the group, as well as the form of infantile epilepsy known as salaam spasms. Another problem arises in distinguishing diffuse myoclonus from other abrupt involuntary movements such as tremors, chorea, and restricted forms of epilepsy (epilepsia partialis continua). Speed of movement, lack of rhythmicity, and presence of special relationships to sensory stimulation prove to be the most reliable identifying features of myoclonus.

The pathophysiology of myoclonus remains to be clarified. It seems logical to assume that myoclonus is caused by abnormal discharges of aggregates of motor neurons or interneurons, due either to directly enhanced excitability of these cells or to removal of some inhibitory mechanism. Pathologic examinations have been of little help in determining the essential sites of this unstable neuronal discharge, because in most cases the neuronal disease is so diffuse. The most restricted lesions associated with myoclonus are seemingly located in the cerebellar cortex, dentate nuclei, and pretectal region. A lack of modulating influence of the cerebellum on the thalamocortical system of neurons has been postulated as a likely mechanism, but it is uncertain whether it is expressed through corticospinal or reticulospinal pathways. Metrazol injections evoke myoclonus of the limbs of animals, and the myoclonus persists after transection of corticospinal and other descending tracts until the lower brainstem (medullary reticular) structures are destroyed. In humans, also, evidence has been adduced that the mechanism of action myoclonus is hyperactivity of a reflex mediated in the reticular formation of the medulla (Halliday). In some such patients, however, the myoclonic jerks have a strict time relationship ("time-locked") to preceding spikes in the contralateral Rolandic area, indicating that the cerebral cortex may play an active and perhaps primary role in the elaboration of myoclonus (Sutton and Mayer, Chadwick et al.). Other clinical and experimental observations point to the spinal cord as the essential site in the genesis of myoclonus. Indeed, a sharply demarcated segmental myoclonus can be induced with Newcastle disease virus in purely "spinal" animals (i.e., after separation of spinal cord and brain), and examples of a purely spinal myoclonus have been observed in humans. Thus it may be concluded that all the necessary integrants for this type of movement exist at spinal levels.

SPASMODIC TORTICOLLIS AND OTHER FACIAL-CERVICAL SPASMS

These are intermittent and arrhythmic or continuous spasms of contraction of the facial, jaw, lingual, sternomastoid, trapezius, and other neck muscles. The involvement may be restricted to one muscle group: the orbicularis oculi may cause eye closure (blepharospasm); the muscles of the mouth and jaw may cause forceful opening or closure of the jaw and retraction or pursing of the mouth (oromandibular dystonia); the tongue may undergo prolonged involuntary protrusion; or the facial muscles may contract in a grimace. When the neck muscles are affected, the spasms may be more pronounced on one side, with rotation and partial extension of the head (torticollis). Occasionally the posterior or anterior neck muscles are involved predominantly, and the head is hyperextended (retrocollic spasm) or inclined forward (antero- or procollis). The movement disorder is involuntary and cannot be inhibited, thereby differing from habit spasm or tic. For many years this condition was thought to be a type of neurosis, but it should be considered a localized form of dystonia.

SPASMODIC TORTICOLLIS

This is the most frequent form of the syndrome, limited to the neck muscles. A condition of unknown cause, it usually begins in early to middle adult life and tends to worsen slowly. Pain in the contracting muscles is a common complaint. The quality of the torticollic movements varies; they may be deliberate and smooth, or jerky. Sometimes an irregular tremor accompanies deviation of the head, possibly representing an effort to overcome the contraction of the neck muscles. The spasms are worse when the patient stands or walks and are characteristically reduced or abolished by a contactual stimulus, such as occurs when the patient places a hand on the chin or neck on the side of the deviation, sometimes on the opposite side, or places the back of the head against a high chair or pillow. In chronic cases the affected muscles may undergo hypertrophy. Although the most prominently affected muscles are the sternomastoid and trapezius, electromyographic studies show sustained activity in all muscles on both sides of the neck. Rarely the muscle spasms spread beyond the neck, involving muscles of the shoulder girdle and back, or the limbs. No morphologic changes were found in the single case that has been studied post mortem (Tarlov).

Spasmodic torticollis is resistant to treatment with L-dopa and other antiparkinsonism agents, including bromocriptine, although occasionally they give slight relief. Psychiatric treatment has been ineffectual. Electrical feedback therapy has been proposed but has seldom resulted in sustained improvement. In severe cases, the sectioning of individual muscles (the sternomastoid) and spinal accessory nerves has helped slightly, but by far the most successful therapy has been bilateral cervical motor radiculotomy, which greatly reduces spasm without totally paralyzing the muscles. Bilateral thalamotomy has also been tried, but since it is less effective and

carries a considerable risk, it should be reserved for the most severely affected patients with more widespread dystonia.

BLEPHAROCLONUS AND BLEPHAROSPASM

A few patients in late adult life come to the clinic complaining of inability to keep their eyes open. Any attempt to look at a person or object is associated with a persistent tonic spasm or a series of clonic involuntary contractions of the eyelids. All customary activities are hampered. During conversation the patient struggles to overcome the spasm and is distracted by it. Reading and watching television are impossible at times, but surprisingly easy at others. There is fear even in crossing the street.

One's first inclination is to think of this disorder as photophobia, and indeed the patient may state that bright light is annoying. However, the spasms persist in dim light and even after anesthesia of the corneas. A psychological cause has been postulated, but psychiatric symptoms are lacking and psychotherapy has not proved of value. No neuropathologic lesion has been established. A similar closure of the eyes may be the initial symptom of dystonia musculorum deformans or of tardive dyskinesia.

A variety of antiparkinsonian and tranquilizing medications may be tried, but one should not be sanguine about the chances of success. Sometimes this disorder disappears spontaneously. In extremely persistent and disabling cases, crushing of part of the fibers in the branches of the facial nerves which innervate the orbicularis oculi muscles has weakened the spasms and rendered them tolerable.

SPASTIC DYSPHONIA

This is another unique movement disorder, in which the throat and neck muscles are thrown into spasm when the patient attempts to speak. It is described in Chap. 22, "Affections of Speech and Language."

FACIAL SPASM AND FACIAL MYOKYMIA

These conditions will be described in Chap. 52.

LINGUAL, FACIAL, AND OROMANDIBULAR SPASMS

These special varieties of involuntary movements appear in late adult life and the senium with a peak age of onset in the sixth decade. Women are affected more frequently than men. The most common type is characterized by forceful opening of the jaw, retraction of the lips, spasm of the platysma and protrusion of the tongue, or the jaw may be clamped shut and the lips may purse. Frequently blepharospasm and difficulty in speaking and swallowing are conjoined. Occasionally, patients with these disorders develop torticollis or dystonia of the trunk and limbs. All these prolonged forceful spasms of contraction of facial, tongue, and neck muscles have been provoked by administration of phenothiazine and butyrophenone drugs. Usually, however, the disorder induced by neuroleptics is of a different order, consisting of choreoathetotic chewing, lip smacking, and licking movements (orofacial dyskinesia; see page 777).

TICS AND HABIT SPASMS

Many persons throughout life are given to habitual movements such as sniffing, clearing the throat, protruding the chin, or blinking whenever they become tense. Stereotypy and irresistibility are their main identifying features. The patient admits to making the movements and feels compelled to do so in order to relieve tension. For a short time such movements can be inhibited by an effort of will, but they reappear as soon as attention is diverted. In certain cases they become so ingrained that the person is unaware of them and seems unable to control them. An interesting feature of many tics is that they correspond to purposive coordinated acts which normally serve the organism. It is only their incessant repetition when uncalled for that typifies the habit spasm or tic. It varies widely in its expression from a single isolated movement (e.g., blinking, sniffing, throat clearing or stretching the neck) to a complex of movements.

Children between the ages of 5 and 10 years are especially likely to develop habit spasms. Usually they consist of blinking, hitching up one shoulder, sniffing, throat clearing, etc. Seldom do they persist for longer than a few weeks if ignored; providing for more rest and a calmer environment are also helpful. In adults, relief of nervous tension by phenobarbital or other tranquilizing drugs and psychotherapy may be helpful, but the disposition to tic persists.

Adults often display, when idle, a wide variety of fidgeting types of movement and mannerisms which vary in degree from one patient to another. Special types of rocking, head bobbing, and other movements are features of motility unique to the mentally retarded. Apparently they represent a prolongation of some of the rhythmic, repetitive movements (head banging, etc.) of normal infants. If vision is impaired, and in some cases of photic epilepsy, eye rubbing or moving of the fingers rhythmically across the field of vision are commonly observed in children, especially in the mentally retarded.

These "rhythmias" have no known pathologic anatomy in the basal ganglia or elsewhere in the brain.

GILLES DE LA TOURETTE SYNDROME

Multiple tics, associated with sniffing, snorting, involuntary vocalization, and troublesome sexual and aggressive impulses constitute the rarest and most severe tic syndrome. It begins in childhood, usually as a simple tic, and may be precipitated by the administration of CNS stimulants such as methylphenidate and dextroamphetamine, prescribed for the control of hyperactivity. As the condition progresses, new tics are added to the repertoire. The compulsive utterance of obscenities (coprolalia) appears in 60 percent of cases, according to Shapiro et al., who have studied 250 patients. In one-third of their cases, tics have been observed in other members of the family. Several studies have reported a familial clustering of members with Tourette syndrome, but no consistent pattern of inheritance has emerged (Eldridge et al.). An ethnic bias (Ashkenazi Jews) has been reported, ranging from 19 to 62 percent in several series.

So-called soft neurologic signs are noted in half the patients. Hyperactivity and disorders of attention and perception are frequent. Evidence of "organic" impairment by psychological tests has been found in 40 to 60 percent of Shapiro's series. However, the intelligence does not deteriorate. Nonspecific abnormalities of the EEG are noted in more than half of the patients.

As to causation, little is known. The disease, if it is such, is unrelated to social class and to psychiatric illness; there is no consistent association with infection, trauma, or other disease. No neuropathologic lesion has been established.

The course of the illness is unpredictable. In some adolescents the illness subsides spontaneously and permanently or undergoes long remission, but in other patients it persists throughout life. Treatment with large doses of carbamazepine (1200 mg or more), chlorpromazine (25 to 50 mg tid), or haloperidol suppresses the tics in many cases. Others respond to pimozide, which has a more specific antidopaminergic activity than haloperidol.

WRITER'S CRAMP

This and other so-called craft or occupation cramps or spasms should be mentioned here, if only to indicate their unclassifiable status. The prevailing opinion is that they are restricted dystonias (Marsden). Men and women are equally affected, most often between the ages of 20 and 50 years. The patient observes, upon attempting to write, that all the muscles of thumb and fingers either go into spasm or are inhibited by a feeling of stiffness and pain or in some other inexplicable way. Usually it is the spasm that interferes, and if prolonged, it may be painful and spread into the forearm or even the shoulder. Sometimes the spasm fragments into a tremor that interferes with the execution of fluid, cursive movements. Immediately upon cessation of writing, the spasm disappears. Although the disturbance in writer's cramp is usually limited to the specific act of writing, it may involve other equally demanding motor acts. At all other times and in the execution of grosser movements the hand is normal, and there are no other neurologic abnormalities. Many patients learn to write in new ways or to use the other hand, though that, too, may become involved.

The performance of other highly skilled motor acts, such as piano playing or fingering the violin, may be similarly affected. The "loss of lip" in trombonists and other instrumentalists may represent an analogous phenomenon. In each case a delicate motor skill, perfected by years of practice and performed almost automatically, suddenly comes to require a conscious and labored effort for its execution.

The nature of these disorders is quite obscure. They have been classed traditionally as "occupational neuroses," and a psychiatric causation has been suggested repeatedly, but careful clinical analysis does not bear this out. Hypnosis and other forms of psychiatric treatment are usually without effect. Once developed, the disability persists in varying degrees of severity, even after long periods of inactivity of the affected part. It has been claimed that the patient can be helped by a deconditioning procedure that delivers an electric shock whenever the spasm occurs or by biofeedback, but these forms of treatment have not been rigorously tested.

REFERENCES

ALBE-FESSARD D et al: Activation of thalamocortical projections related to tremorogenic process, in Purpura D, Yahr MD (eds): *The Thalamus.* New York, Columbia, 1966, pp 237-254.

BARINGER JR et al: An acute syndrome of ocular oscillations and truncal myoclonus. *Brain* 91:473, 1968.

BRUMLIK J: On the nature of normal tremor. *Neurology* 12:159, 1962.

CARPENTER MB: Functional relationships between the red nucleus and the brachium conjunctivum. Physiologic study of lesions of the red nucleus in monkeys with degenerated superior cerebellar brachia. *Neurology* 7:427, 1957.

CHADWICK D et al: Clinical, biochemical, and physiological features distinguishing myoclonus responsive to 5-hydroxytryptophan, tryptophan with a monoamine oxidase inhibitor, and clonazepam. *Brain* 100:455, 1977.

DESMEDT JE (ed): *Progress in Clinical Neurophysiology,* vol 5: *Physiological Tremor, Pathological Tremors and Clonus.* New York, Karger, 1978.

ELDRIDGE R et al: Gilles de la Tourette's syndrome: Clinical, genetic, psychologic, and biochemical aspects in 21 selected families. *Neurology* 27:115, 1977.

FORD FR: Degeneration of the cerebral gray matter, in *Diseases of the Nervous System in Infancy, Childhood and Adolescence,* 6th ed. Springfield, Ill, Charles C Thomas, 1973, p 305.

HALLLIDAY AM: The neurophysiology of myoclonic jerking—a reappraisal, in Charlton MH (ed): *Myoclonic Seizures,* Roche Medical Monograph Series. Amsterdam, Excerpta Medica, 1975, pp 1-29.

HODSKINS MB, YAKOVLEV PI: Anatomico-clinical observations on myoclonus in epileptics and on related symptom complexes. *Am J Psychiatry* 86:827, 1930.

HUNT JR: Dyssynergia cerebellaris myoclonica—primary atrophy of the dentate system: A contribution to the pathology and symptomatology of the cerebellum. *Brain* 44:490, 1921.

LANCE JW, ADAMS RD: The syndrome of intention or action myoclonus as a sequel to hypoxic encephalopathy. *Brain* 87:111, 1963.

LAPRESLE J, BEN HAMIDA M: The dentato-olivary pathway. *Arch Neurology* 22:135, 1970.

LOWDEN JA, O'BRIEN JS: Sialidosis: A review of human neuroaminidase deficiency. *Am J Hum Genetics* 31:1, 1979.

MARSDEN CD: Blepharospasm-oromandibular dystonia syndrome (Brueghel's syndrome). *J Neurol Neurosurg Psychiatry* 39:1204, 1976.

————: The mechanisms of physiologic tremor and their significance for pathological tremors, in Desmedt JE (ed): *Physiological Tremor, Pathological Tremors and Clonus.* New York, Karger, 1978, pp 1-16.

MARSHALL J: Tremor, in Vinken PJ, Bruyn GW (eds): *Handbook of Clinical Neurology,* vol 6: *Basal Ganglia.* Amsterdam, North-Holland, 1968, chap 31, pp 809-825.

MOE PG, NELLHAUS G: Infantile polymyoclonia—opsoclonus syndrome and neural crest tumors. *Neurology* 20:7, 1970.

NARABAYASHI H, OHYE C: Parkinsonian tremor and nucleus ventralis intermedius of the human thalamus, in Desmedt JE (ed): *Physiological Tremor, Pathological Tremors and Clonus.* New York, Karger, 1978, pp 165-172.

RAPIN I et al: The cherry-red spot-myoclonus syndrome. *Ann Neurol* 3:234, 1978.

SHAHANI BT, YOUNG RR: Action tremors: A clinical neurophysiological review, in Desmedt JE (ed): *Progress in Clinical Neurophysiology,* vol 5. Basel, Karger, 1978, pp 129-137.

SHAPIRO AK et al: Gilles de la Tourette's syndrome: Summary of clinical experience with 250 patients and suggested nomenclature for tic syndromes, in Eldridge R, Fahn S (eds): *Advances in Neurology*, vol 14: *Dystonia*. New York, Raven Press, 1976, 277–283.

SUTTON GG, MAYER RF: Focal reflex myoclonus. *J Neurol Neurosurg Psychiatry* 37:207, 1974.

SWANSON PD et al: Myoclonus: A report of 67 cases and review of the literature. *Medicine* 41:339, 1962.

TARLOV E: On the problem of spasmodic torticollis in man. *J Neurol Neurosurg Psychiatry* 33:457, 1970.

WARD AA JR: The function of the basal ganglia, in Vinken PJ, Bruyn GW (eds): *Handbook of Clinical Neurology*, vol 6: *Basal Ganglia*. Amsterdam, North-Holland, 1968, chap 3, pp 90–115.

WATSON CW, DENNY-BROWN DE: Myoclonus epilepsy as a symptom of diffuse neuronal disease. *Arch Neurol Psychiatry* 70:151, 1953.

YOUNG RR, GROWDON JH, SHAHANI BT: Beta-adrenergic mechanisms in action tremor. *N Engl J Med* 293:950, 1975.

CHAPTER 6

DISORDERS OF STANCE AND GAIT

Certain disorders of motor function are manifested most clearly as an impairment of upright stance and locomotion, and their evaluation depends on a knowledge of the nervous mechanisms underlying these peculiarly human functions. Analysis of stance and gait is a particularly rewarding medical exercise; with some experience a neurologic diagnosis may be reached merely by noting the manner in which the patient walks.

NORMAL GAIT

The normal gait seldom attracts attention, but it should be observed with care, if slight deviations from normal are to be appreciated. The body is erect, the head straight, and the arms hang loosely and gracefully at the sides, each moving rhythmically forward with the opposite leg. The feet are slightly everted, and the steps are of moderate length and approximately equal, the internal malleoli of the tibias almost touching and each foot being placed almost in line with the other. With each step there is coordinated flexion of the hip and knee, dorsiflexion of the foot, and a barely perceptible elevation of the hip so that the foot clears the ground. The heel strikes the ground first, and inspection of the shoes will show that this part is most subject to wear. The muscles of greatest importance in maintaining the erect posture are the erector spinae and the extensors of the hips and knees.

When analyzed in greater detail, the requirements for locomotion in an upright, bipedal position may be reduced to the following elements: (1) antigravity support of the body, (2) stepping, (3) an adequate degree of equilibrium, and (4) a means of propulsion. The support of the body is provided by the antigravity reflexes which maintain firm extension of the knees, hips, and back, but which are modifiable by position of the head and neck.

These reflexes depend on the integrity of the spinal cord and brainstem (transection of the neuraxis between the red and vestibular nuclei leads to exaggeration of these antigravity reflexes—decerebrate rigidity). Stepping, the second element, is a basic movement pattern, present at birth and integrated at the midbrain level. Its appropriate stimuli are contact of the sole with a flat surface and inclination of the body forward and alternately from side to side. Equilibrium involves the maintenance of balance at right angles to the direction of movement. The center of gravity during the continuously unstable equilibrium which prevails in walking must shift from side to side within narrow limits as the weight is borne first on one foot, then on the other. Propulsion is provided by leaning forward and slightly to one side and permitting the body to fall a certain distance before being checked by the support of the leg. Here both forward and alternating lateral movements must occur. But in running, where at one moment both feet are off the ground, a forward drive or thrust by the hind leg is also needed. Locomotion may be impaired in the course of neurologic disease when one or more of these mechanical principles is prevented from operating, as we shall see.

There are many variations of gait from one person to another, and it is a commonplace observation that one may be identified by the sound of one's footsteps, notably the pace and lightness or heaviness of tread. The manner of walking and the carriage of the body may even provide clues to character, personality, and occupation. Furthermore, the gaits of men and women differ, the steps of women being quicker and shorter and the movement of their trunk and hips more graceful and delicate. Certain female characteristics of gait, if observed in the male, immediately impart an impression of femininity; or male characteristics in the female, one of masculinity. The changes in stance and gait which accompany aging—the slightly stooped posture and slow, stiff tread—are so familiar that they are regarded as variations of normal.

ABNORMAL GAIT

Since normal body posture and locomotion require intact labyrinthine function, proprioception, and vision (we see where we are going and pick our steps), the effect on normal function of deficits in these senses is worth noting.

A blind person or a normal one who is blindfolded may walk quite well, moving cautiously with arms slightly forward to avoid collision with objects, and on a smooth surface shortening the step slightly; with the shortening there is less rocking of the body, and the person seems unnaturally stiff.

A patient without labyrinthine function (as may happen after prolonged administration of streptomycin, kanamycin, or neomycin) shows a slight unsteadiness in walking and an inability to descend stairs without holding onto a banister. Running is more difficult. Such persons have great difficulty in visual focusing on a fixed target when they are moving or on a moving target when they are stationary. When the body is in motion, objects in the environment appear to jiggle up and down (oscillopsia; see page 186), so that they cannot drive a car or read on the train, and even when walking must stop in order to read a sign. These abnormalities indicate a loss of stabilization of ocular fixation by the vestibular system during body movements. Proof that the gait of such persons is dependent on visual cues comes from their performance blindfolded or in the dark when their unsteadiness and staggering increase, to the point of falling.

A loss of proprioception, as with a complete lesion in the posterior columns of the spinal cord at a high cervical level, abolishes the capacity for independent locomotion for a long time. After years of training such patients will still have difficulty in starting to walk and in forward propulsion. As Purdon Martin has illustrated, they hold their hands in front of the body, bend the body and head forward, walk with a wide base and irregular uneven steps, but still rock the body. If they are tilted to one side, they fail to compensate for their abnormal posture. If they fall, they cannot arise without help, and they cannot get up from a chair. They are unable to crawl or to get into an "all-fours" posture. When standing, if blindfolded, they immediately fall. Thus the postural reactions are primarily dependent on proprioceptive rather than on visual or labyrinthine information.

EXAMINATION OF THE PATIENT WITH
ABNORMAL GAIT

When confronted with a disorder of gait, the examiner must observe the patient's stance and the attitude and dominant positions of the legs, trunk, and arms. It is good practice to watch patients as they walk into the examining room, because they are apt to walk more naturally then than during special tests. They should be asked to stand with feet together, head erect, with eyes first open and then closed. Swaying due to nervousness may be overcome by asking the patient to touch the tip of the nose alternately with the forefinger of one hand and then the other. Next the patient should be asked to walk forward and backward, with eyes open and then closed. A tendency to veer to one side, as in cerebellar disease, can be checked by having the patient walk around a chair. When the affected side is toward the chair, the patient tends to walk into it; and when it is away from the chair, there is a veering outward in ever-widening circles. More delicate tests of gait are walking a straight line heel to toe, and having the patient arise quickly from a chair, walk briskly, stop or turn suddenly, and then sit down again. If all these tests are successfully executed, it may be assumed that any difficulty in locomotion is not due to impairment of proprioceptive or cerebellar mechanisms. Detailed neurologic examination is then necessary in order to determine which of the many other possible diseases is responsible for the patient's disorder of gait.

The following types of abnormal gait are so distinctive that with a little practice they can be recognized at a glance.

Cerebellar Gait The main features of this gait are a wide base (separation of legs), unsteadiness and irregularity of steps, and lateral veering. Steps are uncertain, some are shorter and others longer than intended, and the patient may stagger or lurch to one side or the other. The unsteadiness is more prominent on quickly arising from a chair, stopping suddenly while walking, or turning quickly. The irregular swaying of the trunk may be most evident when the patient has to stop walking abruptly and sit down, and it may be necessary for him or her to grasp the chair for support. Cerebellar ataxia may be so severe that the patient cannot stand without assistance. If it is less severe, standing with feet together and head erect may be difficult. In its mildest form the ataxia is best demonstrated by having the patient walk a line heel to toe; after a step or two, balance will be lost and it will be necessary to place one foot to the side to avoid falling. The patient with cerebellar ataxia who sways perceptibly when standing with feet together and eyes open will sway somewhat more with eyes closed, as will a normal person. Romberg's sign, i.e., marked swaying or falling with the eyes closed but not with the eyes open, indicates a loss of postural sense, not cerebellar disease (see Chap. 8). Compensation may be effected by shortening the step and shuffling, i.e., keeping both feet on the ground simultaneously. The defect in the cerebellar gait is not primarily in antigravity support, steppage, or propulsion but in the coordination of proprioceptive, labyrinthine, and visual information in reflex movements, particularly those which are required to make rapid adjustments to constant changes in posture. The abnormality of stance and gait is usually accompanied by other signs of cerebellar incoordination and intention tremor of the arms and legs, but it need not be. The presence of the latter signs depends on involvement of the cerebellar hemispheres, as distinct from the anterosuperior midline structures. If the lesion is unilateral, the signs of gait disorder are always on the same side.

Cerebellar gait is most commonly seen in multiple sclerosis, cerebellar tumors (particularly those which affect the vermis disproportionately—i.e., medulloblastoma), and the cerebellar degenerations. In certain forms of cerebellar degeneration (e.g., the type associated with chronic alcoholism), the disease process develops over days to weeks, reaches a plateau, and then remains stable for many years; the gait disorder, in these circumstances, becomes altered as compensations are acquired, and its designation as "drunken" or "reeling" is no longer appropriate. The base is wide, and the steps are still short, but more regular; the trunk is inclined slightly forward, the arms are held away from the sides, and the gait assumes a somewhat mechanical, rhythmic quality. In this way the patient can walk for long distances but lacks the capacity to make the necessary postural adjustments in response to sudden changes in position such as happen in walking on uneven ground. Many of these patients show pendularity of the patellar reflexes and other signs of hypotonia of the limbs when they are examined in the sitting and recumbent positions; paradoxically, walking without support brings out a certain stiffness of the legs and firmness of the muscles. Conceivably, the latter abnormality is analogous to the positive supporting reactions in cerebellectomized cats and dogs, which react to pressure on the foot pad with an extensor thrust of the leg.

Gait of Sensory Ataxia This disorder of gait is due to an impairment of joint-position sense resulting from interruption of afferent nerve fibers in the peripheral nerves, posterior roots, posterior columns of the spinal cords, or medial lemnisci; it may also be produced occasionally by a lesion of both parietal lobes. Whatever the location of the lesion, the effect is to deprive the patient of knowledge of the position of his or her limbs. The resulting disorder is characterized by varying degrees of difficulty in standing and walking, and in advanced cases there is a complete failure of locomotion, although muscular power is retained. The principal features of the gait disorder are the brusqueness of movement and the stamp of the feet. The legs are kept far apart to correct the instability, and patients carefully watch the ground and their legs. As they step out, the legs are flung abruptly forward and outward, often being lifted higher than necessary. The steps are of variable length, and many are attended by an audible stamp as the foot is brought down forcibly on the floor (possibly to enhance joint-position sense). The body is held in a slightly flexed position, and the weight is supported on the cane that the severely ataxic patient usually carries. Ramsay Hunt characterized this type of gait very well when he said that these patients are recognized by their "stamp and stick." The incoordination is greatly exaggerated when the patient is deprived of visual cues, as in walking in the dark. Most patients, when asked to stand with feet together and eyes closed, show greatly increased swaying or actual falling (Romberg's sign). It is said that the shoes are not worn in any one place in cases of sensory ataxia, because the entire sole strikes the ground at once. There is invariably a loss of sense of position in the feet and legs and usually a loss of vibratory sense as well.

A disordered gait of this type is observed in tabes dorsalis, Friedreich's ataxia and related forms of spinocerebellar degeneration, subacute combined degeneration (vitamin B_{12} deficiency), syphilitic meningomyelitis, chronic sensory polyneuropathy, and those cases of multiple sclerosis or compression of the spinal cord in which posterior column involvement predominates.

Hemiplegic and Paraplegic (Spastic) Gaits In hemiplegia, or hemiparesis, the leg is held stiffly and does not flex freely at the hip and knee. It tends to rotate outward and describes a semicircle, first away from and then toward the trunk (circumduction). The foot scrapes the floor, and the toe and outer side of the sole of the shoe are worn. One can recognize the spastic gait by the sound of the slow, rhythmic scuff of the foot along the floor. Other parts of the affected side are weak and stiff to a variable degree, particularly the arm, which is carried in a flexed position and does not swing naturally.

This type of gait disorder is most often a sequela of cerebral infarction or trauma but may result from a number of other conditions which damage the corticospinal pathway on one side.

The spastic paraplegic, or paraparetic, gait is in effect a bilateral hemiplegic gait affecting only the lower extremities. Each leg is advanced slowly and stiffly, with restricted motion at the hips and knees. The legs are extended or slightly bent at the knees and may be strongly adducted at the hips, tending almost to cross (scissors gait). The steps are regular and short, and the patient may be able to advance only with great effort, as though wading waist-deep in water. An easy way to remember the main features of the hemiplegic and paraplegic gaits is to recall the letter S, for slow, stiff, and scraping. The defect is in the stepping mechanism and in propulsion, not in support or equilibrium.

The spastic paraparetic gait is a major manifestation of cerebral diplegia, the result of anoxic or other forms of damage to the brain in the perinatal period. This disorder of gait is seen in a variety of chronic spinal cord diseases in which the dorsolateral and ventral funiculi are involved, including multiple sclerosis, syringomyelia, syphilitic meningomyelitis, combined system disease of both the pernicious anemia (PA) and non-PA types, chronic spinal cord compression, and familial forms of spinal cord degeneration. Frequently the effects of posterior column disease are added, giving rise to a mixed gait disturbance—a spinal spastic ataxia.

Festinating Gait   The term *festinating* is derived from the Latin *festinare*, "to hasten," and appropriately describes the involuntary acceleration or hastening of the gait that characterizes both paralysis agitans and postencephalitic Parkinson's syndrome. Rigidity and shuffling, in addition to festination, are the cardinal features of this gait. When they are joined to the typical tremor, the unblinking and masklike facial expression, the general attitude of flexion, immobility, and poverty of movement, there can be little doubt as to the diagnosis.

In walking, the trunk is bent forward. The arms are carried slightly flexed and ahead of the body and do not swing. The legs are stiff and bent at the knees and hips. The steps are short, and the feet barely clear the ground as the patient shuffles along. Once forward or backward locomotion is started, the upper part of the body advances ahead of the lower part, as though the patient were chasing his or her center of gravity. The steps become more and more rapid, and the patient may fall if not assisted. This is the festination, and it may occur when the patient is walking forward or backward, taking the form of either propulsion or retropulsion. The defects are in rocking the body from side to side so that

the feet may clear the floor and in moving the legs quickly enough to catch the center of gravity.

Other unusual gaits are sometimes observed in postencephalitic patients. For example, such a patient may be unable to take the first step forward because of being unable to lift one foot, or the patient may be unable to step forward until a few hops or one or two steps are taken backward. Walking may be initiated by a series of short steps or a series of steps of increasing size. Occasionally such a patient may run better than he or she walks or walk backward better than forward.

Choreoathetotic and Dystonic Gaits   Diseases that are characterized by involuntary movements and abnormal postures seriously affect gait. In fact, a disturbance of gait may be the initial and dominant manifestation of these diseases, and the testing of gait often brings out abnormalities of movement and posture that are otherwise not conspicuous.

As the patient with congenital athetosis or Huntington's chorea stands or walks there is a continuous play of irregular movements affecting the face, neck, hands, and, in the advanced stages, the large proximal joints and trunk. The positions of the trunk and upper parts of the body vary with each step. There are jerks of the head, grimacing, squirming, twisting movements of the trunk and limbs, and peculiar respiratory noises. One arm may be held aloft and the other one behind the body, with wrist and fingers alternately undergoing flexion and extension, supination and pronation. The head may be inclined in one direction, the lips alternately retract and then purse, and the tongue intermittently protrudes from the mouth. The legs advance slowly and awkwardly, the result of superimposed involuntary movements and postures. Sometimes the foot is plantar-flexed at the ankle, and the weight is carried on the toes; or it may be dorsiflexed or inverted. A superimposed involuntary movement may cause the leg to be suspended in the air momentarily, imparting a lilting or waltzing character to the gait, or it may twist the trunk so violently that the patient may fall.

In dystonia musculorum deformans the first symptom may be a limp due to inversion or plantar flexion of the foot or a distortion of the pelvis. The patient stands with one leg rigidly extended or one shoulder elevated, and the trunk may be in a position of exaggerated lordosis or scoliosis or both. Because of the muscle spasms that deform the body in this manner, the patient may have to walk with knees flexed. The gait may seem normal as the first steps are taken, but as the patient walks, the buttocks become prominent, owing to the lumbar lordosis, and one leg or both legs become flexed at the hip, giving rise to the "dromedary gait" of Oppenheim. In the more advanced stages walking becomes impossible, owing to torsion of the trunk or the continuous flexion of the legs. Gilman and Romanul have observed a special form of dystonic paraplegia with amyotrophy.

The general features of choreoathetosis and dystonia have been described more fully in Chap. 4.

Steppage, or Equine, Gait This is caused by paralysis of the pretibial and peroneal muscles, with resultant inability to dorsiflex and evert the foot. The steps are regular and even, but the advancing foot hangs with the toes pointing toward the ground (foot drop). Walking is accomplished mainly by flexion at the hip, and the leg must be lifted abnormally high in order for the feet to clear the ground. There is a slapping noise as the foot strikes the floor. The anterior and lateral borders of the sole of the shoe become worn. Foot drop may be unilateral or bilateral and occurs in diseases that affect the peripheral nerves of the legs or motor neurons in the spinal cord, such as poliomyelitis, progressive spinal muscular atrophy, and Charcot-Marie-Tooth disease (peroneal muscular atrophy). It may also be observed in certain types of muscular dystrophy in which the distal musculature of the limbs is involved. The most common cause of unilateral foot drop is compression of the common peroneal nerve, where it crosses the head of the fibula.

A particular disorder of gait, also of peripheral origin, may be observed in patients with painful dysesthesias of the soles of the feet. Peripheral neuropathy (most often of the alcoholic-nutritional type), causalgia, and erythromelalgia are the usual causes. Because of the exquisite pain evoked by weight bearing, the patient treads gingerly, as though walking barefoot on hot sand or pavement, with the feet rotated in such a position as to avoid pressure on their most painful portions.

Waddling Gait This gait is characteristic of progressive muscular dystrophy, but may occur also in chronic forms of spinal muscular atrophy (Wohlfart-Kugelberg-Welander syndrome) and in congenital dislocation of the hips.

In normal walking, as weight is placed alternately on each leg, the hip is fixated by the gluteal muscles, particularly the gluteus medius, allowing for a slight rise of the opposite hip and tilt of the trunk to the weight-bearing side. With weakness of these muscles, there is a failure to stabilize the weight-bearing hip, causing the opposite side of the pelvis to drop and the trunk to incline to that side. The alteration in lateral trunk movements results in the roll or waddle.

In progressive muscular dystrophy, an accentuation of the lumbar lordosis is often associated. Also, childhood cases may be complicated by muscular contractures leading to an equinovarus position of the foot, so that the waddle is combined with circumduction of the legs and "walking on the toes."

Staggering, or Drunken, Gait This is characteristic of alcoholic and barbiturate intoxication. The drunken patient totters, reels, tips forward and then backward, appearing each moment to be about to lose balance and fall. Control over trunk and legs is greatly impaired. The steps are irregular and uncertain. Such patients appear stupefied and indifferent to the quality of their performance, but under certain circumstances they can momentarily correct the defect.

The adjectives *drunken* and *reeling* are used frequently to describe the gait of cerebellar disease, but the similarities between a drunken and a cerebellar gait are only superficial. The severely intoxicated patient reels or sways in many different directions, and no effort is made to correct the staggering by watching the legs or the ground, as in cerebellar or sensory ataxia. Despite the wide excursions of the body and deviation from the line of march, the drunken patient may walk on a narrow base, and balance may be exquisitely maintained. Cerebellar stance and gait are characterized, in contrast, by a wide base, and patients have great difficulty in maintaining their balance if they sway or lurch too far to one side. Milder degrees of the drunken gait more closely resemble the gait disorder that follows loss of labyrinthine function (see above).

Toppling Gait Toppling, meaning tottering and falling, may occur with brainstem lesions, especially in the older person who has recently had a stroke. It is a feature of the lateral medullary syndrome. In patients with progressive supranuclear palsy (see page 813), where dystonia of the neck is combined with paralysis of vertical gaze and parkinsonian features, sudden lurches and frequent falls may be an early and prominent feature. The gait, in addition, is uncertain and hesitant, features that are enhanced no doubt by the hazard of falling unpredictably. The exact cause of the toppling phenomenon is not known; it does not have its basis in weakness, ataxia, or loss of deep sensation. It simply appears to be a disorder of balance occasioned momentarily by the wrong placement of a foot.

Hysterical Gait This may take one of several forms: monoplegic, hemiplegic, or paraplegic. Monoplegic or hemiplegic patients do not lift the foot from the floor while walking; instead, they drag the leg as a useless member or push it ahead of them as though it were on a skate. The characteristic circumduction is absent in hysterical hemiplegia, and the typical hemiplegic posture, hyperactive tendon reflexes, and Babinski sign are missing. The hysterical paraplegic cannot very well drag both legs, and usually depends on canes or crutches or remains helpless in bed; the muscles may be rigid, with contractures, or flaccid. The hysterical gait may take other dramatic forms. Some patients look as though they were walking on stilts, and others lurch wildly in all directions, actually demonstrating by their gyrations a remarkable ability to make rapid and appropriate postural adjustments.

Astasia-abasia, in which patients, though unable to either stand or walk, retain normal use of their legs while in bed, is nearly always a hysterical condition. When such patients are placed on their feet, they may take a few steps and then become unable to advance their feet; they lurch wildly and crumple to the floor if not assisted. On the other hand, one should not assume that a patient who manifests a disorder of gait but no other neurologic abnormality is necessarily suffering from hysteria. Lesions that are restricted to the anterosuperior cerebellar vermis may cause an ataxia which becomes manifest only when the patient attempts to stand and walk; this is true of frontal lobe disease as well (see below).

Frontal Lobe Disorder of Gait The capacity to stand and walk may be severely disturbed by diseases that affect the frontal lobes, particularly their medial parts. This disorder of gait is sometimes spoken of as a frontal lobe ataxia or as an apraxia, since the difficulty in walking cannot be accounted for by weakness or loss of sensation. Neither designation is entirely accurate, for reasons indicated below. Most likely the disorder represents a loss of integration at the cortical and basal ganglionic level of the essential elements of stance and locomotion which were acquired in infancy and are often lost in senility.

Patients assume a posture of slight flexion, with the feet placed farther apart than normal. They advance slowly, with small, shuffling, hesitant steps. At times they halt, unable to advance without great effort, although they do much better with a little assistance or with exhortation to march in step with the examiner.

Turning is accomplished by a series of tiny, uncertain steps that are made with one foot, the other being planted on the floor as a pivot. The initiation of walking becomes progressively more difficult, and in advanced cases patients may be unable to take a step, as though their feet were glued to the floor. Finally they become unable to stand or even to sit, and without support they fall backward or to one side. In normal pressure hydrocephalus one observes this progression of difficulties, as the patient's gait and stance deteriorate from an inability to walk, to stand, to sit, and to lie, and the reverse, following treatment.

Some patients are able to make complex movements with their legs, such as drawing imaginary figures, at a time when their gait is seriously impaired. Eventually, however, all movements of the legs become slow and awkward, and the limbs, when passively moved, offer variable resistance (*gegenhalten*). Difficulty in turning over in bed is highly characteristic, and may eventually become complete. These motor disabilities are usually associated with dementia, but the two disorders need not evolve in parallel. Thus, some patients with Alzheimer's disease may show a serious degree of dementia for several years before the gait disorder becomes apparent; in other conditions, such as normal pressure hydrocephalus, the opposite may pertain. Or both disorders may evolve together, in a subacute manner. Grasping, groping, hyperactive tendon reflexes, and Babinski signs may or may not be present. The end result in some cases is a "cerebral paraplegia in flexion" (Yakovlev), in which the patient lies curled up in bed, immobile and mute, the limbs fixed by contractures in an attitude of flexion (Fig. 6-1).

Senile Gait Elderly persons often complain of difficulty in walking. Examination discloses a slightly flexed posture and short, uncertain steps (*marche à petit pas*); lost are the speed, balance, and many of the graceful, adaptive movements that one associates with normal gait. The nature of this gait disorder is not understood. The uncertainty of balance and short-stepped gait in the elderly are often incorrectly attributed to loss of confidence and fear of falling. More likely, they represent a relatively mild degree of the frontal lobe disorder of gait, described above. It should be noted, however, that a short-stepped, cautious gait lacks specificity, being a general defensive reaction to all forms of defective locomotion. Senile gaits are more fully discussed in Chap. 28, on aging.

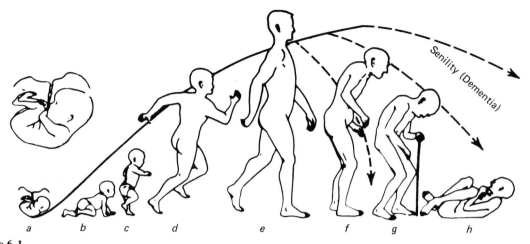

Figure 6-1

The evolution of erect stance and gait and of paraplegia in flexion of cerebral origin according to Yakovlev. The ripening forebrain of the fetus (a) drives the head and body up and moves the individual onward (b through e). When the "driving brain" (frontal lobe, striatum, and pallidum) degenerates, the individual "curls up" again (e through h). (From Yakovlev.)

Gaits of the Mentally Retarded There are, in addition to the disorders of locomotion described above, peculiarities of gait that defy analysis. One has only to observe the assortment of gait abnormalities in an institution for the mentally handicapped to appreciate this fact. Ungainly stance with the head too far forward or the neck extended, wide-based gait with awkward lurches or feet stomping the floor, arms held in odd positions, and each patient with his or her own ungraceful style—these are but a few of the peculiarities that meet the eye. In vain does one try to relate them to a disorder of proprioception, cerebellar deficit, or extrapyramidal disease.

The only plausible explanation that comes to mind is that these are pathologic variants of human locomotion based on a retardation of the natural developmental sequences of locomotion. The acquisition of the refinements of locomotion, such as hopping, jumping, running, dancing, twirling, balancing on one foot, kicking a ball, etc., are age-linked; i.e., each has its average age of acquisition. There are wide individual variations, but the most striking extremes are found in the mentally handicapped, who may be retarded in these ways as well as in scholastic pursuits. Rhythmic rocking movements, waving of the arms, tremors, and the like make their performances even more eccentric. The Lincoln-Oseretsky scale is an attempt to quantitate maturational delays in the locomotory sphere.

REFERENCES

GILMAN S, ROMANUL FCA: Hereditary dystonic paraplegia with amyotrophy and mental deficiency: Clinical and neuropathological characteristics, in Vinken PJ, Bruyn GW (eds): *Handbook of Clinical Neurology,* vol 22: *System Disorders and Atrophies,* pt II. Amsterdam, North-Holland, 1975, chap 120, pp 445–465.

MARTIN JP: The basal ganglia and locomotion. *Ann R Coll Surg Engl* 32:219, 1963.

YAKOVLEV PI: Paraplegia in flexion of cerebral origin. *J Neuropathol Exp Neurol* 13:267, 1954.

SECTION II

PAIN AND OTHER DISORDERS OF SOMATIC SENSATION, HEADACHE, AND BACKACHE

CHAPTER 7
PAIN

Pain, it has been said, is one of "nature's earliest signs of morbidity," and it stands preeminent among all the sensory experiences by which humans judge the existence of disease within themselves. Only a few maladies do not have painful phases, and in many of them pain is a characteristic without which diagnosis must always be in doubt.

The painful experiences of the sick pose manifold problems for physicians, and students must learn something of these problems in order to prepare themselves for the task ahead. They must be prepared to diagnose disease in patients who have felt only the first rumblings of discomfort, before other symptoms and signs have appeared. Even more problematical are patients who seek treatment for pain that appears to have no structural basis, and further inquiry may disclose that fear, worry, and other troubling emotional states have aggrandized some relatively minor ache and pain. They must also cope with the "difficult" pain cases in which no amount of investigation brings to light either medical or psychiatric illness. Finally, the physician must be prepared to manage patients with intractable pain caused by established and incurable disease, who demand relief either by the use of drugs or the "less moderate means of surgery." To deal intelligently with such pain problems requires a familiarity with the anatomy of sensory pathways and the sensory supply of body segments, an insight into the psychological factors that influence behavior, and a knowledge of medical and psychiatric disease.

The dual nature of pain is responsible for some of our difficulty in understanding it. Easiest to understand is its evocation by particular stimuli and the transmission of pain impulses along certain pathways. Far more abstruse is its quality as a mental state which defies definition, description, and quantification—"a passion of the mind," in the words of Aristotle. This duality is of practical importance, for certain drugs or surgical proce-dures, such as frontal leukotomy, may reduce the patient's reaction to pain, leaving much of the sensation intact. In contrast, interruption of certain neural pathways may abolish all sensation in an affected part, but the symptom of pain may persist (viz., denervation dysesthesia or anesthesia dolorosa). Unlike most sensations, which are aroused by a specific (adequate) stimulus such as pressure, heat, or cold, pain may be invoked by *all* these forms of stimuli, if they are intense enough.

The authors have noted that even in highly specialized medical centers few, if any, physicians are capable of handling unusual pain problems. In fact, it is to the neurologist that other physicians turn for help with these problems. Although much has been learned recently about the anatomy of pain pathways, their physiologic mechanisms, and which structures to ablate in order to produce analgesia, little is known about which patients should be subjected to these destructive operations or how to manage them by medical means. Here is a subspecialty that should challenge every thoughtful physician, for it demands the highest skill in medicine, neurology, and psychiatry.

END ORGANS, AFFERENT PATHWAYS, AND THALAMIC AND CORTICAL TERMINATIONS

PAIN RECEPTORS AND PERIPHERAL AFFERENT PATHWAYS

The traditional teaching, since the time of Von Frey (1894), has been that the free nerve endings in the skin and other organs are the receptors for pain and that such endings have their private pathway into the brain. These free endings are fine, profusely branched nerve fibers that are covered by Schwann cells and contain little or none of the laminated structure called "myelin." Actu-

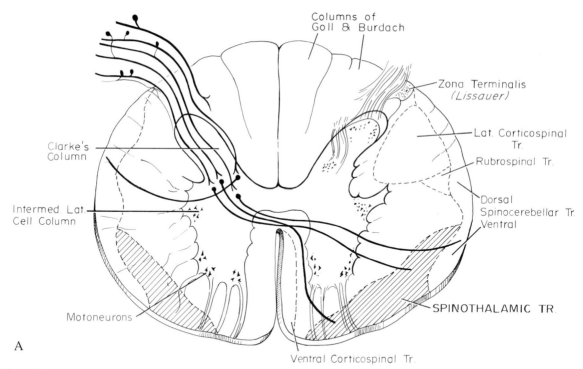

Columns of
Goll & Burdach

Zona Terminalis
(Lissauer)

Lat. Corticospinal
Tr.

Rubrospinal Tr.

Dorsal
Spinocerebellar Tr.
Ventral

SPINOTHALAMIC TR.

Ventral Corticospinal Tr.

Motoneurons

Intermed Lat.
Cell Column

Clarke's
Column

A

Figure 7-1

*A. Spinal cord in transverse section, illustrating the course of
the afferent fibers and the major ascending pathways. B. Transverse section through the sixth cervical segment of the spinal
cord of the cat, illustrating the subdivision of the gray matter
into laminas according to Rexed. LM and VM, lateromedial
and ventromedial groups of motor neurons. (After A Brodal,
Neurological Anatomy, 3d ed, New York, Oxford, 1981.)*

ally they are the terminations of the distal axons of sensory neurons, some of which are of the unmyelinated
type known as C fibers (0.3 to 1.5 μm in diameter) and
others that are thinly myelinated, designated the A-delta
(A-δ) fibers (1.0 to 5.0 μm in diameter). Although there
is no doubt that many such endings transduce only the
painful effects of noxious stimuli, their specificity has
been called into question by the observation that other
modes of sensation can be evoked from structures such
as the cornea, which is innervated solely by free nerve
endings.

The peripheral afferent fibers have their cell bodies in the dorsal root ganglia; central extensions of these
nerve cells project, via the dorsal root, to the dorsal horn
of the spinal cord. The fine myelinated and unmyelinated fibers occupy mainly the lateral part of the root
entry zone; and within the spinal cord many of the thin-
nest fibers form a discrete bundle, the tract of Lissauer
(Fig. 7-1A). That Lissauer's tract is predominantly a
pain pathway is shown (in animals) by the ipsilateral

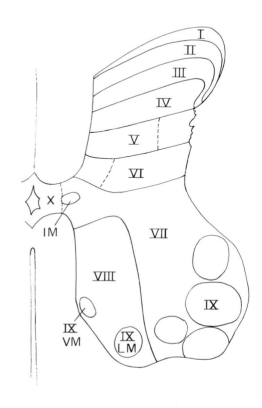

B

segmental analgesia that results from its transection, but it contains propriospinal fibers as well. Although it is customary to speak of lateral and medial divisions of the posterior root (the former contain the small pain fibers and the latter the large myelinated fibers), the separation into discrete functional bundles is not complete, and these two groups of fibers cannot be differentially interrupted by selective rhizotomy. The termination of these fibers is in the dorsal horn of the same and adjacent segments, rostral and caudal.

DERMATOMIC DISTRIBUTION OF PAIN FIBERS

Before considering the central terminations of pain fibers, brief reference should be made to their segmental distribution. This subject will be elaborated in the next chapter, which includes maps of the sensory dermatomes, but as a means of quick orientation to the topography of peripheral pain pathways, it should be remembered that the facial structures and anterior cranium lie in the field of the trigeminal nerves; the back of the head, second cervical; the neck, third cervical; the epaulet area, fourth cervical; the deltoid area, fifth cervical; the radial forearm and thumb, sixth cervical; the index and middle fingers, seventh cervical; the little finger and ulnar border of hand and forearm, first thoracic; the nipple, fifth thoracic; the umbilicus, tenth thoracic; the groin, first lumbar; medial side of knee, third lumbar; the great toe, fifth lumbar; the little toe, first sacral; back of thigh, second sacral; and the genitoanal zones, the third, fourth, and fifth sacral. The segmental distribution of pain fibers from deep structures, though not fully corresponding to those from the skin, also follows a segmental pattern. The first to fourth thoracic nerve roots are the important sensory pathways for the intrathoracic viscera; the sixth to eighth thoracic, for the upper abdominal organs.

THE DORSAL HORN

The afferent pain fibers, after traversing Lissauer's tract, terminate in the posterior gray matter or dorsal horn. Most of the fibers terminate within the segment of their entry into the cord, but some extend rostrally and caudally to several adjacent segments. The cytoarchitectonic studies of Rexed in the cat (the same organization pertains in primates and probably in humans) have shown that neurons in the dorsal horn are arranged in a series of six layers or laminae (Fig. 7-1B). Pain fibers terminate principally in lamina I of Rexed (also known as the marginal cell layer of Waldeyer and the substantia gelatinosa) and in lamina V. Cells in lamina I are directly activated by stimulation of A-δ nerve fibers,

whereas cells in lamina V are activated either directly or indirectly by both A-δ and C fibers. Secondary neurons from these cells of termination connect with ventral and lateral horn cells in the same and adjacent spinal segments, and subserve both somatic and autonomic reflexes. Cells of lamina I project ipsilaterally and contralaterally to higher levels, some to the thalamus. Part of the axons of cells of lamina V cross in the anterior commissure and ascend in the contralateral spinothalamic system (Fig. 7-2).

AFFERENT TRACTS FOR PAIN

Immediately upon entering the dorsal horn, nociceptive afferents synapse with secondary neurons, the axons of which decussate in the anterior spinal commissure, and ascend in the anterolateral fasciculus to other brainstem and thalamic structures (Fig. 7-2). The axons from each

Figure 7-2

The main somatosensory pathways. Offsets from the ascending anterolateral fasciculus (spinothalamic tract) to nuclei in the medulla, pons, and mesencephalon, and precise nuclear terminations of the tract are not indicated in the diagram (see text). (After A Brodal, Neurological Anatomy, 3d ed, New York, Oxford, 1981.)

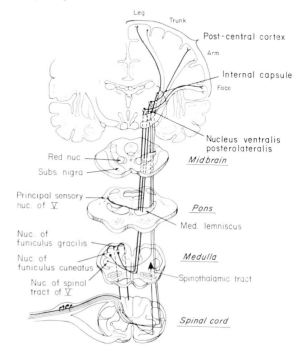

dermatome decussate one to three segments higher than the level of root entry; in this way the dorsal horns and anterior spinal commissure form a continuous pain pathway the full length of the spinal cord. Crossing fibers are added to the inner side of the spinothalamic tract (the principal afferent pathway of the anterolateral fasciculus), so that the longest fibers from the sacral segments come to lie most superficially, and fibers from successively more rostral levels occupy a progressively deeper position (Fig. 7-3). This somatotopic arrangement is of practical importance to the neurosurgeon; the depth to which the funiculus is cut will govern the level of analgesia that is achieved. It should be noted that in addition to the spinothalamic tract, the anterolateral fasciculus contains several other pain-transmitting pathways, of which the spinoreticular projection is the most important.

The afferent fibers in the anterolateral fasciculus ascend to the medulla where part of them terminate in the nucleus lateralis medullae oblongatae, which in turn projects somatotopically to the cerebellum. A second offset of fibers, somewhat more rostral, is in the region of the paramedian reticular nuclei. Another group terminates in the mesencephalon, in the nucleus subcoeruleus or the "paralemniscal nucleus" of the mesencephalic tectum and in the region of the periaqueductal gray matter. The remaining fibers of the lateral spinothalamic tract end in the magnocellular part of the medial geniculate body, in the nucleus ventralis posterolateralis (VPL), and in the intralaminar nuclei, in the region of the nucleus centralis lateralis.

The aforementioned medullary-pontine nuclei give rise to brainstem segmental connections and to a bundle of tertiary afferent fibers that lie just ventrolateral to the medial longitudinal fasciculus. This pathway deviates laterally and is incorporated for a portion of its ascending course in the central tegmental tract; within the diencephalon it bifurcates into a thalamic portion (which terminates in the intralaminar nuclei) and a subthalamic component. Other projections, derived from the mesencephalic offset of ascending spinothalamic pathways, terminate in limbic regions.

There is, in animals at least, a spinal afferent pathway that arises from cells in laminae I, IV, and V of the dorsal horn of the spinal cord and continues *ipsilaterally* in the dorsolateral column as *the spinocervical tract*, terminating in an aggregate of neurons in the cervical cord (C1 to C3 levels)—the *lateral cervical nucleus*. The latter, in turn, projects via the contralateral medial lemniscus to the nucleus ventralis posterolateralis and then to the cortical somatosensory areas I and II (see further on). Electrophysiologic studies indicate that this pathway is the most rapidly conducting afferent tract in the feline spinal cord and suggest that it may have a function in the transmission of pain. However, behavioral studies do not confirm such a function, so that the exact significance of this tract has yet to be settled. There is no evidence for an analogous tract in humans, even though a lateral cervical nucleus can be identified.

It should be emphasized that *all* the foregoing data, concerning the cells of termination of cutaneous nociceptive stimuli and the cells of origin of ascending spinal afferent pathways, have been derived from studies in *animals*. In humans, the cells of origin of the long anterospinal tract fibers have not been identified. Information about this pathway in humans has been derived

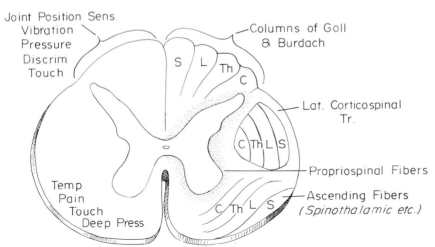

Joint Position Sens.
Vibration
Pressure
Discrim
Touch

Columns of Goll & Burdach

S L Th C

Lat. Corticospinal Tr.

C Th L S

Propriospinal Fibers

Temp.
Pain
Touch
Deep Press

C Th L S

Ascending Fibers
(Spinothalamic etc.)

Figure 7-3

Spinal cord showing the segmental arrangement of nerve fibers within major tracts. On the left side are indicated the "sensory modalities" which appear to be mediated by the two main ascending pathways. Note the broad zone close to the gray matter occupied by propriospinal fibers. C, cervical; L, lumbar; S, sacral; Th, thoracic. (After A Brodal, Neurological Anatomy, 3d ed, New York, Oxford, 1981.)

from the study of postmortem material, and mainly from the examination of patients subjected to anterolateral chordotomy for intractable pain. Unilateral section of the anterolateral funiculus produces a relatively complete loss of pain and thermal sense on the opposite side of the body, extending to a level one to three segments below the lesion. After a variable period of time sensation of pain often returns perhaps because of the presence of uncrossed spinothalamic fibers.

THALAMIC TERMINUS

Thalamic zones where neurons can be activated by stimulation of A-δ and C fibers have been less well established than the zones activated by other types of sensory fibers. Evidently, the posterior thalamic complex, the nuclei ventralis posterolateralis (VPL) and posteromedialis, and the ventrobasal (VB) complex all receive spinothalamic projections. Some afferent connections are also made with hypothalamic nuclei. However, few if any units within these nuclei respond exclusively to noxious stimuli. Thalamic regions outside VPL which receive spinothalamic projections are referred to collectively by neurophysiologists as the "posterior group of nuclei" and are considered to be important in the transmission of pain impulses to the cortex.

There are also descending fibers from brainstem structures to the posterior horns of spinal segments. One such pathway emanates from nuclei in the periaqueductal region of the midbrain; presumably it descends in the anterolateral columns of the spinal cord. The importance of this pathway in the inhibition of pain is discussed further on.

The practical conclusion to be reached from current anatomic and physiologic studies is that at thalamic levels, fibers and cell stations transmitting the sensation of pain are not organized into discrete loci that might provide a site or sites for surgical intervention for relief of pain. In general, current neurophysiologic evidence indicates that as one ascends from peripheral nerve to spinal, medullary, mesencephalic, thalamic, and limbic levels, the predictability of neuron responsivity to noxious stimuli diminishes. Thus it comes as no surprise that neurosurgical procedures for interrupting afferent pathways become less and less successful in the brainstem and thalamus.

THALAMOCORTICAL PROJECTIONS

The nuclei of the posterior thalamic complex send their axons to three main cortical areas: the postcentral cortex (a small number terminate in the precentral cortex), the parasylvian region in the inferior parietal lobe, and the superior parietal lobe. These are described more fully in Chap. 8, "Disorders of Somatic Sensation." Here it can be stated that these cortical areas are concerned mainly with the reception of tactile and proprioceptive stimuli and with discriminative sensory function. That any of them is activated by thermal and painful stimuli is unlikely. As a corollary, stimulation of these (or any other) cortical areas in an alert human being does not produce pain. As indicated above, some pain afferents, derived from the mesencephalic offset of the ascending fibers of the anterolateral funiculus, project to the amygdaloid nuclei, areas related to affect and emotion.

PHYSIOLOGY AND PSYCHOLOGY OF PAIN

Stimuli that activate pain receptors vary from one tissue to another. An adequate stimulus for skin is one that injures tissue, i.e., pricking, cutting, crushing, burning, and freezing. Interestingly these stimuli are ineffective when applied to the stomach and intestine. Pain in the gastrointestinal tract is produced instead by the local effects of an engorged or inflamed mucosa, distention or spasm of smooth muscle, and traction on the mesenteric attachment. In skeletal muscle, pain is caused by ischemia (the basis of the condition known as intermittent claudication), as well as by injuries of connective tissue sheaths, necrosis, hemorrhage, and the injection of irritating solutions. Prolonged contraction of skeletal muscle evokes an aching type of pain. Ischemia is also the most important cause of pain in cardiac muscle. Joints are insensitive to pricking, cutting, and cautery, but pain is induced in the synovial membrane by inflammation and by exposure to hypertonic saline. Arteries are a source of pain when pierced by a needle or involved in an inflammatory process. Excessive arterial pulsation is believed to be the basis of migraine; other mechanisms of headache relate to traction and displacement of arteries and the meningeal structures by which they are supported (see Chap. 9).

In the painful lesions due to tissue damage, proteolytic enzymes are released which act on gamma globulins to liberate substances that are irritating to free nerve endings. Bradykinins, histamine, prostaglandins and similar polypeptides, as well as acid metabolites which are known to appear in such lesions, elicit pain when injected intraarterially or applied to the base of a blister. Such substances are viewed as the mediators of the pain stimulus.

THE GATE-CONTROL THEORY OF PAIN

A theory of pain mechanisms has been propounded by Melzack and Wall. They observed, in decerebrate and spinal cats, that the stimulation of large myelinated fibers produced a negative dorsal root potential and that the stimulation of small C fibers (pain) caused a positive dorsal root potential. Since dorsal root potentials are concerned with presynaptic effects (negative potentials with inhibition and positive potentials with activation), they reasoned that a presynaptic control of inhibition and facilitation by nonpain and by pain fibers might determine the activity of secondary, transmitting neurons (T cells) in the dorsal horn. They postulated that small neurons in the substantia gelatinosa, also activated by sensory input, participate in the presynaptic "gate control" of the afferent fiber activity in the dorsal roots. It was suggested that descending fibers from such areas as the brainstem, thalamus, or limbic system also exert effects on this gate mechanism. The balance of presynaptic activity at the "gate" would determine, then, the effect of any cutaneous input. Postsynaptic activity was also of importance. According to this theory, the large, myelinated, "fast-fiber" input inhibits the central transmission of the overall effects of small myelinated and unmyelinated fiber input. A diminution in large fiber inhibition would leave the T cells continuously active, whereas stimulation of these fibers would suppress T-cell activity and control pain.

The gate-control mechanism offered a hypothetical explanation of the pain of ruptured disk and of other chronic neuropathies (large fiber outfall). Further, on the basis of this hypothesis attempts have been made to relieve pathologic pain by subjecting the peripheral nerves and dorsal columns (presumably their large myelinated fibers) to sustained electrical stimulation. Such stimulation would theoretically "close" the gate. These procedures have reportedly given some relief from pain, although this may not be due to stimulation of large myelinated fibers alone. Taub and Campbell have presented evidence that analgesia from electrical stimulation may be due to peripheral blockade of the A-δ fibers. In any event, these procedures must be considered as still in the experimental stage.

Several other observations are not in keeping with the gate-control hypothesis. In certain forms of peripheral neuropathy which are characterized by a selective loss of large myelinated fibers (resulting in a pathologic predominance of small C fibers), pain is not a feature; in fact, some neuropathies characterized by a predominant loss of small fibers may be quite painful. There are serious experimental difficulties with this theory as well, the most important being that several investigators have failed to substantiate the fundamental observation upon which it is based, viz., that with bipolar dorsal root recording, volleys from small myelinated and unmyelinated fibers induce a prolonged positive dorsal root potential. These and other aspects of the gate-control theory of pain have been thoroughly reviewed by P. W. Nathan.

Regardless of the inadequacies of the gate-control theory of pain, it has set neurologists to thinking along new lines. There is no doubt as to the existence of pain receptors in at least two portions (A-δ and C) of the primary afferent spectrum of fibers. Some nociceptive fibers are multimodal, and certain cells in the dorsal horn are able to respond to nonpainful and painful stimuli. These are points in favor of the "pattern theory" of Weddell and Sinclair (see Chap. 8). There are interactions between the effects of the several afferent fiber systems converging upon the dorsal horns of the spinal cord and upon the nuclei of the trigeminal nerves, but there are also many other levels of convergence in the central nervous system. One suspects that the secret of the long-persisting, nonadaptive quality of some pain, the ready conversion of nonnoxious stimuli to painful ones, the maintenance of states of hyperpathia and tissue sensitivity, and the obvious influences of emotion will all ultimately be clarified by new knowledge of the detailed physiology of afferent system convergence in the spinal cord and higher structures.

PERCEPTION OF PAIN

The *threshold for the perception of pain*, i.e., the lowest intensity of stimulus recognized as pain, is approximately the same in all persons. It is lowered by inflammation and raised by local anesthetics (e.g., procaine), lesions of the nervous system, and certain centrally acting analgesic drugs. Distraction and suggestion, by turning attention away from the painful part, reduce the awareness of and the response to pain. Strong emotion (fear or rage) suppresses pain. Neurotic patients in general have the same pain threshold as normal subjects, but their reaction may be excessive or abnormal. The pain thresholds of frontal lobotomized subjects are also unchanged, but they react briefly if at all to pain. The degree of emotional reaction and the verbalization (complaint) also vary with the personality and character of the patient.

The conscious awareness of perception of pain occurs only upon the arrival of pain impulses at the thalamocortical level. The precise roles of the thalamus and cortical sensory areas in this mental process are not fully understood, however. It is often said that impulses reaching the thalamus create awareness of the attributes of sensation and that the parietal cortex is necessary for the appreciation of the intensity and localization of the sensation. This seems to be an oversimplification. Probably a close and harmonious relationship between thalamus and cortex must exist in order for a sensory experience to be complete. The traditional separation of sensation (in this instance awareness of pain) and perception (awareness of the nature of the painful stimulus) has been abandoned in favor of the view that sensation, perception, and the various conscious and unconscious responses to a pain stimulus comprise an indivisible process.

That the cerebral cortex governs the patient's reaction to pain cannot be doubted, as will be indicated further on. It is also likely that the cortex can suppress or otherwise modify the perception of pain in the same way that corticofugal projections from the sensory cortex modify the rostral transmission of impulses from thalamic and dorsal column nuclei. It has been shown that central transmission in the spinothalamic tract can be inhibited by stimulation of the sensorimotor areas of the cerebral cortex, and descending fiber systems have been traced to the dorsal horn laminae from which this tract presumably originates.

ENDOGENOUS PAIN CONTROL MECHANISMS

The most important advance in recent years in our understanding of pain has been the discovery of an endogenous neuronal system for analgesia, which can be activated by the administration of opiates or by naturally occurring brain substances with the pharmacological properties of opiates.

Evidence for an endogenous analgesia system was first presented by Reynolds (1969), who found that stimulation of the ventrolateral periaqueductal gray matter in the rat produced a profound analgesia without altering behavior or motor activity. Stimulation of other discrete sites, particularly the diencephalic periventricular region and the raphe nuclei were later shown to have the same effect. Under the influence of such electrical stimulation, the animal could be operated upon without anesthesia and move around in an undisturbed manner despite the administration of noxious stimuli. More recent observations indicate that in humans the stimulation of analogous brainstem and diencephalic loci also produces a state of analgesia, which is even longer lasting than that produced in rats and subhuman primates. Further investigation has disclosed that stimulation-pro-

duced analgesia (now commonly referred to as SPA) produces its effects by inhibiting the neurons of laminae I and V of the dorsal horn, i.e., the neurons that are activated by noxious stimuli.

Morphine, it has been shown, also acts on the neurons of laminae I and V, suppressing the input from the nonmyelinated (C) fibers and lightly myelinated (A-δ) fibers of the posterior roots. Furthermore, these effects can be reversed by the narcotic antagonist, naloxone. Interestingly, naloxone also reverses SPA. It has been known for many years that morphine acts at several loci in the brainstem, and now it appears that the sites of action of morphine correspond with the sites that produce analgesia when they are stimulated electrically.

The aforementioned observations, summarized here in their briefest form, stimulated the search for morphine binding sites in the central nervous system. High densities of specific opiate receptors have been found in the spinal cord, in the dorsal horn where A-δ and C fibers dominate, and in the trigeminal nuclei, the medial thalamus, and the amygdaloid nuclei. What is more, it has been shown that the analgesic potency of an opiate is directly proportional to its affinity for the receptors.

The discovery of specific opiate receptors in the CNS led to the search for and ultimately the identification of several naturally occurring peptides, which proved to have a potent analgesic effect and to bind opiate receptors (Hughes et al.). These endogenous, morphine-like compounds are called *enkephalins*, or *endorphins*, meaning "the morphine within." The most widely studied of these compounds, β-endorphin, is a fragment of the pituitary hormone β-lipotropin, and has been shown to have powerful analgesic effects when given intraventricularly or systemically. C. H. Li had earlier found large amounts of this substance in the pituitary glands of camels, an animal known to be peculiarly insensitive to pain.

Thus it would appear that the central effects of a painful condition might be determined by the brain's level of endorphins. A deficiency at a particular level would explain persistent or excessive pain experience. Opiate addiction could be accounted for in this way and also the discomfort that follows withdrawal of the drug. Indeed, it has recently been shown that β-endorphins not only relieve pain but suppress withdrawal symptoms. In the limbic regions disturbances of endorphin formation and other neurotransmitters could be the basis of unpleasant and distressing emotional states (e.g., depression). Levine and his colleagues have demonstrated that the narcotic antagonist naloxone not only enhances clinical pain but that it interferes with the pain relief produced by placebos. These observations suggest that the heretofore mysterious beneficial effects of placebos (and perhaps of acupuncture) are due to activation of a neurological system that shuts off pain through the release of endorphins.

A peptide called substance P (substance preparation) has been strongly endorsed in recent years as a transmitter in the pain fiber systems. The most convincing evidence for this role is its concentration in the region of free nerve endings where it also has a vasoactive effect, and in the posterior horn of spinal cord. Its combined excitatory pain and vasoactive effects makes it a candidate for the causation of migraine. Capsaicin, a derivative of homovanillic acid found in Hungarian red peppers which causes first intense pain and then renders animals analgesic for months, suppresses substance P; and in newborn animals it causes a selective degeneration of chemosensitive primary pain afferents (see review by Nicoll et al.).

A theoretical construct of the roles of enkephalins and substance P at the point of entry of pain fibers into the spinal cord is illustrated in Fig. 7-4.

SOME CLINICAL ASPECTS OF PAIN

As indicated above, the nerve endings in each tissue are activated by different mechanisms, and the pain that results is characterized by its quality, locale, and temporal attributes. *Skin pain* is of two types: a pricking pain, evoked immediately by the penetration of the skin by a needle point, and a stinging or burning pain, which follows in 1 to 2 s. Together they constitute the "double response" of Lewis. Ischemia of nerve by the application of a tourniquet to a limb abolishes pricking pain before burning pain. The first pain is thought to be transmitted by the larger (A-δ) fibers and the second (slow) pain, which is somewhat more diffuse and longer lasting, by the thinner, unmyelinated C fibers. Both types of dermal pain are localized with precision, made possible by the overlap of sensory neurons.

Deep pain, from visceral and skeletomuscular structures, basically has the quality of aching, but if intense, it may be sharp and penetrating (knifelike). Occasionally there is a burning type of pain, as in the heartburn of esophageal irritation and rarely in angina pectoris. The pain is felt as being deep to the body surface. The double response is absent, localization is poor (no closer than two or three segments), and the margins of the pain are not well delineated, presumably because of the paucity of nerve endings in viscera.

The matter of localization raises a number of problems. Although deep pain has indefinite boundaries, its location always bears a fixed relationship to the skel-

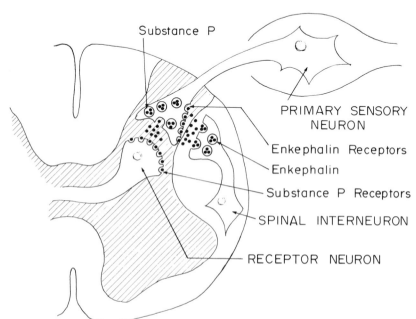

Figure 7-4
Theoretical mechanism of action of enkephalin (endorphin) and morphine on the transmission of pain impulses from the periphery to the CNS. Spinal interneurons containing enkephalin synapse with the terminals of pain fibers and inhibit the release of the transmitter, substance P. As a result, the receptor neuron in the dorsal horn receives less excitatory (pain) impulses and transmits fewer pain impulses to the brain. Morphine binds to unoccupied enkephalin receptors, mimicking the pain-suppressing effects of enkephalin (endorphin).

Substance P

PRIMARY SENSORY NEURON

Enkephalin Receptors

Enkephalin

Substance P Receptors

SPINAL INTERNEURON

RECEPTOR NEURON

etal or visceral structure that is involved. It tends to be referred not to the skin overlying the viscera of origin, but to skin innervated by the same spinal segments. This pain, projected to some fixed site away from the source, is called *referred pain*. The fact that nerves subserving pain are more numerous in the skin than in the viscera or skeletal structures is the reason usually given for this projection to the body surface. But since the nerves of any given dermatome may be distributed through several adjacent spinal or brainstem segments, the pain may be fairly widely distributed. For example, cardiac pain arising within the T1 to T4 dermatomes may be projected superficially to the inner side of the arm and the ulnar border of the hand (T1 and T2) and the precordium (T3 and T4), more often to the left, from which side most of the stimuli arise. Once this pool of sensory neurons in the dorsal horns of the spinal cord is activated, additional noxious stimuli may heighten the activity in the whole sensory field.

Another peculiarity of localization is *aberrant reference*, explained by an alteration of the physiologic status of the pools of neurons in adjacent segments of the spinal cord. For example, cervical arthritis or gallbladder disease causing low-grade discomfort by constantly activating segmental neurons may induce a shift of cardiac pain cephalad or caudad from its usual locale. And any pain, once it becomes chronic, may spread quite widely in a vertical direction on one side of the body.

The terms *hyperesthesia* and *hyperalgesia* refer to an increased sensitivity and a lowering of the threshold to tactile and painful stimuli. The term *hyperpathia* is used to designate an excessive reaction to pain, but usually with a raised threshold to stimulation. Distinctions between hyperalgesia and hyperpathia are somewhat pedantic. Seldom is it possible in any painful state except inflammation and burns of the skin to demonstrate a distinct hypersensitivity. Instead, in most cases of chronic pain, especially with diseases of the nervous system, there is usually a demonstrable defect in pain perception in the affected part, associated with an unusual sensitivity to all stimuli, even those which normally do not evoke pain; and the elicited pain may have unusual features, being unnatural, diffuse, modifiable by fatigue, emotion, etc., and often mixed with other sensations. In addition, central structures, e.g., the thalamus, if chronically stimulated, may become autonomously overactive, i.e., "kindled," and remain so after peripheral pathways are interrupted; painful states such as *causalgia, spinal cord pain*, and *phantom pain* are not, therefore, abolished by cutting spinal nerves or spinal tracts.

One of the most remarkable characteristics of pain is the strong tone or affect with which it is endowed, nearly always one of unpleasantness. Furthermore, pain does not appear to be subject to negative adaptation. Somatic stimuli, if applied continuously, soon cease to be effective, whereas pain may persist as long as the stimulus is operative. Moreover, it would seem that once a central excitatory state of some kind has been set up, pain may then be evoked by an inappropriate stimulus such as touch or movement, and the sensory experience may outlast the stimulus.

Since pain has this affective element, psychological conditions assume great importance in all persistent painful states. Furthermore, the patient's tolerance of pain and capacity to experience it without verbalization are also influenced by race, culture, and religion. It is a matter of common knowledge that some individuals, by virtue of training, habit, and phlegmatic temperament, remain stoic in the face of pain and that others react in an opposite fashion. Pain may be a presenting symptom in a depressive psychosis (Chap. 54). Then, too, there are rare individuals who seem totally incapable of feeling pain at any time in life, either from a lack of sensory endings in their skin and other peripheral parts or from some peculiarity of the central receptive apparatus (see Chap. 8).

Finally, a comment should be made about the devastating effects of chronic pain on a patient's behavior. As Ambroise Paré remarked, "There is nothing that abateth so much the strength as paine." Continuous pain increases irritability and fatigue, troubles sleep, and impairs appetite. Persons capable of great courage can be reduced to a whimpering, pitiable state that may arouse the scorn of healthy observers. Persons in pain may seem irrational about their illness and make unreasonable demands of family and physician. This condition, sometimes spoken of as "pain shock," if once established, requires delicate but firm management. Depression (reactive?) is a common sequel. Of course, demand for and dependency on narcotic drugs often complicate the clinical problem.

CLINICAL APPROACH TO THE PATIENT WITH PAIN AS THE PREDOMINANT SYMPTOM

One learns quickly in dealing with such patients that not all pain is the consequence of serious disease. Everyday, healthy persons of all ages have pains which must be taken as part of normal sensory experiences. To mention a few, there is the momentary hard pain over an eye, temporal region, occiput, or jaw which strikes with such alarming suddenness as to raise suspicion of a ruptured intracranial aneurysm; the more persistent ache in the fleshy part of the shoulder, hip, or extremity, relieved quickly by change in position; the fleeting but fluctuant precordial discomfort of gastrointestinal origin, which conjures up fear of cardiac disease; the breath-taking "stitch in the side" due to intercostal or diaphragmatic cramp. These normal pains, as they should be called, tend to be brief and to depart as obscurely as they came. Such pains come to notice only when elicited by an inquiring physician, or when experienced by a patient given to worry and introspection. They must always be distinguished from abnormal pains.

Whenever pain, by its intensity, duration, and the circumstances of its occurrence, appears to be abnormal, or when it constitutes one of the principal symptoms of disease, the physician must attempt to reach a tentative decision as to the mechanism of its production and cause. This is accomplished by a thorough interrogation of the patient, carefully seeking out the main characteristics of the pain in terms of its *location, provoking and relieving factors, quality and time-intensity attributes, mode of onset, duration, severity,* and *time of occurrence.* These diagnostic features are discussed in detail in *Principles of Internal Medicine* and are not appropriate for a textbook of neurology. Needless to say, they are put to use everyday in the practice of internal medicine. In conjunction with practical tests designed to reproduce or relieve pain, they enable the physician to identify many diseases.

INTRACTABLE PAIN

Once the pains due to the more common visceral diseases are eliminated, there remains a significant number of chronic pains which fall into one of four categories: intractable pain of inobvious medical disease which may turn out to be carcinomatosis, aneurysm, etc.; pain in association with psychiatric illness; pain with neurologic diseases; and pain of unknown cause.

PAIN DUE TO MEDICAL DISEASES

Carcinomatosis may be presented as the most frequent example. Osseous metastases, peritoneal implants, invasion of retroperitoneal tissues, and implication of nerves of the brachial or lumbosacral plexuses may be ex-

tremely painful, and the origin of the pain may be obscure for a long time. Sometimes it is necessary to repeat all diagnostic procedures after an interval of a few months, even though at first they were negative. Once the diagnosis has been established, therapy must include some type of pain control. Radiation therapy and other medical and surgical measures often fail to relieve the pain. Then comes the delicate decision of whether to administer opiates with the certainty of producing drug addiction, or to resort to one of several neurosurgical procedures for the destruction of pain-sensitive or pain-conducting structures.

One is influenced in reaching this decision by a number of factors, such as prospects of long survival, attitudes of the patient and the patient's family, location of the pain, and whether the locus is amenable to a surgical procedure. If the patient is ridden with disease and will not live more than a few weeks or months, or is opposed to surgery, or has widespread pain, then surgical measures are out of the question. With pain from widespread osseous metastases, radiation therapy, chemical hypophysectomy from the instillation of alcohol into the sella turcica, or radiation hypophysectomy by proton beam bombardment may give relief, even with hormone-insensitive tumors. Pain confined to a restricted area of the jaw or face may be relieved by section or alcohol injection or radio-frequency destruction of nerve, root, or ganglion. Usually section of nerve(s) has not been a satisfactory way of relieving restricted pain of trunk and limbs, because the overlap of adjacent nerves prevents complete denervation. Section of appropriate sensory roots may be considered in this situation. Bedfast patients with paralysis of the legs and painful flexor spasms have in some cases benefited from crushing of the obturator nerves or intrathecal phenol injections which partially interrupt spinal roots.

Spinothalamic tractotomy, in which the anterior half of the spinal cord on one side is sectioned at an upper thoracic level to relieve pain in the opposite leg and lower trunk, is effective in many instances. This may be done as an open operation or as a transcutaneous procedure in which a radio-frequency lesion is produced by an electrode. The analgesia and thermoanesthesia may last a year or longer, but with a tendency for the level to descend and the pain to return to some extent. Bilateral chordotomy is also feasible, but with greater risk of loss of voluntary control of sphincters and, at higher levels, of respiratory failure. Motor power is nearly always spared because of the position of the corticospinal tract in the posterior part of the lateral funiculus.

Pain in the arm, shoulder, and neck is more difficult to relieve. High cervical transcutaneous chordotomy has been used successfully, with achievement of analgesia up to the chin. Commissural myelotomy by longitudinal incision of the anterior commissure of the spinal cord over many segments has also been performed, with variable success. Lateral medullary tractotomy is another possibility, but must be carried almost to the midline to relieve cervical pain. The risks of this latter procedure and also of lateral mesencephalic tractotomy (which may actually produce pain) are so large that neurosurgeons have abandoned these operations.

Stereotactic surgery on the thalamus for one-sided chronic pain is still used in a few clinics, and the results have been instructive. Lesions placed squarely in the nucleus ventralis posterolateralis are said to abolish pain and temperature sensation over the contralateral side of the body, while leaving the patient with all the misery or affect of pain; lesions in the intralaminar or parafascicular-centrum medianum nuclei relieve the painful state without altering sensation (Mark). Thus, at this level there must also be a balance of inhibitory and facilitatory sensory systems, for one cannot explain intractable pain simply in terms of continuous stimulation of chains of pain neurons. Since these procedures have not yielded predictable benefits to the patient, they are now seldom practiced. The same unpredictability of result pertains to cortical ablations. Patients in whom a severe depression of mood is associated with a chronic pain syndrome have been subjected to bilateral stereotactic cingulotomy; the lesions are placed in the white matter above and just lateral to the corpus callosum. A considerable degree of success has been claimed for this operation, but the results are difficult to evaluate. The orbitofrontal leukotomy has been largely discarded because of the personality change which it produces (see Chap. 21).

PAIN IN ASSOCIATION WITH PSYCHIATRIC DISEASES

It is not unusual for patients with endogenous depression to have pain as the predominant symptom. And most patients with chronic pain of all types are depressed. In such cases one is faced with an extremely difficult clinical problem—that of determining whether a depressive state is primary or secondary. In some instances the diagnostic criteria cited in Chap. 54 give the answer, but in others it is impossible to differentiate between the two. Empirical treatment with antidepressant medication or electroconvulsive therapy is one way out of the dilemma. If the pain disappears or recedes to a minor arthritic ache or some similar trivial disorder, one can conclude that depression was the primary problem. If the depression lifts as the pain is brought under medical control, one may assume it was secondary.

Chronic hysterical neurosis and compensation neurosis may both be associated with intractable pain. Every experienced physician is familiar with the "battle-scarred abdomen" of the woman who has demanded and yielded to one surgical procedure after another, losing appendix, ovaries, fallopian tubes, uterus, gallbladder, etc., in the process. The recognition and management of this type of patient are discussed in Chap. 53.

Compensation neurosis is often colored by persistent headaches, neck pain (whiplash injuries), low-back pain, etc. Questions of ruptured disk are often raised, and not infrequently laminectomy is performed on the basis of dubious myelographic findings. Fatigue, depression, anxiety, insomnia, nervousness, irritability, palpitations, etc., are woven into the clinical syndrome, attesting to the prominence of psychiatric disorder. Long delay in settlement of litigation, in order allegedly to determine the seriousness of the injury, only enhances symptoms and prolongs the disability. The medical and legal professions have no certain approach to such problems and are often found to be working at cross-purposes. We have found that a frank objective appraisal of the injury, an assessment of the psychiatric problem, and encouragement to settle the legal claims as quickly as possible, work usually in the best interest of the patient. While hypersuggestibility (relief of pain by placebos, etc.) may reinforce the physician's belief that there is a prominent factor of hysteria or malingering (see Chap. 53), such data are difficult to interpret and are not acceptable in court.

CHRONIC PAIN WITH NEUROLOGIC DISEASES

Comprising this category are certain chronic mono- and multiple neuropathies, particularly those due to herpes zoster, diabetes, and trauma, including causalgias, and polyneuropathies, radiculopathies, spinal arachnoiditis, spinal cord injuries, and the thalamic pain syndrome of Déjerine-Roussy. It is noteworthy that lesions of the cerebral cortex and white matter are not usually associated with pain, but with contralateral hypalgesia. Parenthetically it should be mentioned that pain sensation is not entirely abolished by such lesions, even if they include the hemisphere and thalamus on one side.

In most of these diseases or syndromes, for some of the latter are due to multiple diseases, the painful phases of the illness may not come at the onset of the disease. For example, the posterolateral thalamic lesion that gives rise to the Déjerine-Roussy syndrome (which may also occur with lesions of white matter of the parietal lobe) is at first characterized by hemianesthesia; as weeks and months pass and sensory function begins to return, the pain syndrome commences. Should recovery continue, which it rarely does in thalamic infarcts and hemorrhages, the pains may cease. In other instances, however, pain with little sensory loss is the mode of presentation, and if confined to face or arm is difficult to recognize as neurologic. This sequence of events informs us that persistent pain, like the paresthesias and dysesthesias described in Chap. 8, is based on some mysterious imbalance of afferent sensory impulses, and it may be abolished by more severe and less severe lesions. The same applies to postherpetic neuralgia and causalgia (Chap. 10) and the painful diabetic neuropathies (Chap. 45). In each of these disorders natural stimuli play on a disequilibrated sensory system.

Uniquely, the patient's description of pain in these several neurologic diseases, particularly in the Déjerine-Roussy syndrome, is more varied and bizarre than in other pain syndromes, probably because the pain is really a dysesthesia combined with sensations of pressure, hotness, coldness, etc. Such expressions as "knifelike," "stabbing," "crushing," "burning" (less often, "freezing"), "a constricting band," "a storm," "a shock," "as if the flesh is being torn away," "indescribable" are metaphoric attempts to describe a complex of totally unfamiliar sensory experiences that cause suffering. Another interesting feature of these neurologic pains is the way in which various activities and external agencies affect the patient's unpleasant sensations. Changes in ambient temperature and barometric pressure, increase in static electricity, abrupt contact, certain musical scores and sounds, the use of the painful part or area, a fright or argument, all are reported to aggravate the condition. Continuously aware of the affected part, the patient may talk about it incessantly in hypochondriacal fashion. The painful part becomes virtually a separate entity, to be watched, shielded, and comforted.

Medical assistance would, in theory, follow several designs: to increase tolerance by impairing the receptive and reporting apparatus of the brain, i.e., the sensitivity and responsivity of the patient (use of tranquilizing and antidepressant medication); to worsen the sensory disorder by reducing the number of functioning elements (interrupting more fibers in the damaged nerve pathway, thus reverting the patient to the original state of anesthesia or analgesia without pain); or to reduce both the sensory input and response by a combination of analgesic and tranquilizing medications. The use of amitriptyline or imipramine and thioridazine or fluphenazine in combination may be more successful as a therapy than neurosurgical procedures which increase the sensory deficit.

CHRONIC PAIN OF INDETERMINATE CAUSE

This is the most difficult group of all—pain in the thorax, abdomen, face, or other part which cannot be traced to any visceral abnormality. Supposedly all neurologic sources such as a spinal cord tumor have been excluded by myelography and other tests. The patient's symptoms and behavior are not consonant with any known psychiatric disease or state. Yet the patient continuously complains of pain, is disabled, and spends large sums of money seeking medical aid.

When faced with such a circumstance, sympathetic physicians or surgeons may be persuaded to resort to extreme measures such as exploratory thoracotomy, laparotomy, and laminectomy. Or they may attempt to alleviate the pain and avoid drug addiction by severing roots and spinal tracts, often with the result that the pain moves to an adjacent segment or the other side of the body.

We are inclined to the view that this type of patient should be observed for a time in the hospital and should be seen frequently by the physician. All the medical facts should be reviewed and the clinical and laboratory examinations repeated, if some time has elapsed since they were last done. Tumors in the hilum of the lung or mediastinum, retropharyngeal region, retroperitoneal and paravertebral spaces, cervix uteri and prostate are known to offer special difficulty in diagnosis, often not being detected for many months. Neurologic pain is almost invariably accompanied by alterations in cutaneous sensation and other neurologic signs, the finding of which facilitates diagnosis. The possibility of drug addiction as a motivation should be eliminated. It is impossible to assess pain in the addicted individual, for the patient's complaints are woven into the need for medication. Temperament and mood should be evaluated carefully from day to day; the physician must remember that the depressed patient often denies being depressed and may occasionally smile. When no medical, neurologic, or psychiatric disease can be established, we are convinced that it is usually better to let the patient suffer than to prescribe opiates or subject the patient to ablative surgery.

PHARMACOLOGIC MANAGEMENT OF PAIN

The new information about endogenous pain control mechanisms (summarized on pages 95 and 96), in addition to providing an explanation for a number of clinical observations, also provides a theoretical basis for the management of intractable pain by pharmacologic means. In some instances the therapeutic agent may block pain transmission directly by preventing the activation of nociceptors in the periphery; in others, the transmission of pain impulses may be blocked in the central nervous system. In still others, pain may be modulated by the physiological activation of an intrinsic analgesic system.

Concerning the first of these mechanisms, aspirin and other nonsteroidal anti-inflammatory analgesics are believed to prevent the activation of nociceptors by blocking the release of prostaglandins in skin, joints, viscera, etc. Morphine and meperidine given orally, parenterally, or intrathecally produce analgesia by acting as "false" neurotransmitters at receptor sites in the posterior horns of the spinal cord—sites that are normally activated by endogenous opioid peptides (see Fig. 7-4). Yet another mechanism consists of the physiologic activation of the intrinsic analgesic system (descending pathways from brain to spinal cord?) by electrical stimulation, by administration of placebo, and possibly by acupuncture; transcutaneous stimulation may suppress pain in this way. Not only do opioids act directly on the pain-conducting sensory system, but they also exert a powerful action on the affective component of pain. Serotoninergic neurons are also thought to play a role in pain modulation. Tricyclic antidepressants, especially the methylated forms (imipramine, amitriptyline, and doxepin), block serotonin reuptake and thus enhance the action of this neurotransmitter at synapses and facilitate the action of opioid agonists.

RARE AND UNUSUAL DISTURBANCES OF PAIN PERCEPTION

Lesions of the parietooccipital regions of one cerebral hemisphere sometimes have had peculiar effects on the patient's capacity to feel and react to pain. One interesting syndrome, described by Marie and Fauré-Beaulieu, goes under the term *pain hemiagnosia*. In the reported cases the left arm and leg have been paralyzed from a right parietal lesion and at the same time rendered hypersensitive to noxious stimuli. When pinched on the affected side, after a delay the patient becomes agitated, moans, and seems distressed but makes no effort to fend

off the painful stimulus with the other hand or to retreat from it. In contrast, if the good side is pinched the patient reacts normally and moves the normal hand at once to the site of the stimulus to remove it. If asked what is being felt when the paralyzed side is hurt, the patient reports unbearable discomfort and cannot identify the source. A hemiagnosia for painful stimuli seems to be present, but the usual autonomic and emotional reactions appear, even in excess. The motor responses are no longer guided by sensory information from one side of the body.

The phenomenon of *asymbolia for pain* is another unusual state, wherein the patient, although capable of distinguishing the different types of pain stimuli from one another and from touch, makes none of the usual emotional, motor, or verbal responses to pain. This patient seems totally unaware of the painful or hurtful nature of stimuli delivered to any part of the body, whether on one side or the other. As pointed out by Schilder and Stengel, who first described the condition, not only are the patient's reactions to noxious stimuli judged to be insufficient and incomplete, but the same is true of responses to all signals of danger. In the few reported cases, pain asymboly has been a part of a larger syndrome, including various combinations of sensory aphasia, impairment of body schema and spatial disorientation, right-left confusion, and dyscalculia (i.e., Gerstmann's syndrome—see Chap. 21). There is also fluctuation of attention to stimuli and extinction of stimuli on one side of the body, when both sides are simultaneously stimulated, but these abnormalities are thought to be insufficient to explain the asymboly.

The currently accepted interpretation of asymbolia for pain is interruption of transcortical integration. Piéron sees it as a particular type of agnosia (analgoagnosia) or apractoagnosia (cf. Chap. 21) in which the organism loses its ability to adapt its emotional, motor, and verbal actions to the consciousness of a nociceptive impression. *"Le sujet a perdu la comprehension de la signification de la douleur."* A few verified lesions have involved the supramarginal convolution as well as other parts of the dominant parietal lobe, according to Hécaen and Ajuriaguerra.

REFERENCES

Burgess PR, Perl ER: Cutaneous mechanoreceptors and nociceptors, in Iggo A (ed): *Handbook of Sensory Physiology*, vol

II: *Somatosensory System*. Berlin, Springer-Verlag, 1973, pp 29–78.

DYKES RW: Nociception. *Brain Res* 99:229, 1975.

FIELDS H: Mechanisms and management of pain, in Isselbacher KJ et al (eds): *Update II: Harrison's Principles of Internal Medicine*, 9/e. New York, McGraw-Hill (in press).

———, BASBAUM AI: Brainstem control of spinal pain-transmission neurons. *Annu Rev Physiol* 40:217, 1978.

HÉCAEN H, DE AJURIAGUERRA J: Asymbolie à la douleur, étude anatomoclinique. *Rev Neurol* 83:300, 1950.

HUGHES J et al: Identification of two related pentapeptides from the brain with potent opiate agonist activity. *Nature* 258:577, 1975.

LELE PP, WEDDELL G: The relationship between neurohistology and corneal sensibility. *Brain* 79:119, 1956.

LEVINE JD, GORDON NC, FIELDS HL: The mechanism of placebo analgesia. *Lancet* 2:654, 1978.

MARK VH: Stereotactic surgery for the relief of pain, in White JC, Sweet WH (eds): *Pain and the Neurosurgeon*. Springfield, Ill, Charles C Thomas, 1969, chap 18, pp 843–887.

MELZACK R, WALL PD: Pain mechanisms: a new theory. *Science* 150:971, 1965.

MOUNTCASTLE VB: Central nervous mechanisms in sensation, in Mountcastle VB (ed): *Medical Physiology*, 13th ed. St Louis, Mosby, 1974, vol 1, chaps 9–11.

NATHAN PW: The gate-control theory of pain. A critical review. *Brain* 99:123, 1976.

———: Pain. *Br Med Bull* 33:149, 1977.

NICOLL RA, SCHENKER C, LEEMAN SE: Substance P as a transmitter candidate. *Annu Rev Neurosci* 3:227, 1980.

PIERON H: *La Sensation*. Paris, Presses Universitaires de France, 1953.

REXED B: A cytotectonic atlas of the spinal cord in the cat. *J Comp Neurol* 100:297, 1954.

SCHILDER P, STENGEL E: Asymbolia for pain. *Arch Neurol Psychiatry* 25:598, 1931.

SINCLAIR D: *Cutaneous Sensation*. London, Oxford, 1967.

SNYDER SH: Opiate receptors in the brain. *N Engl J Med* 296:266, 1977.

TAUB A: The use of psychotropic drugs alone and adjunctively in the treatment of otherwise intractable pain: postherpetic neuralgia; disseminated visceral neoplasm, in Voris HC, Whisler WW (eds): *Treatment of Pain*. Springfield, Ill, Charles C Thomas, 1975, chap 3, pp 32–42.

———, CAMPBELL JN: Percutaneous local electrical analgesia; peripheral mechanisms, in *Advances in Neurology*, vol 4: *Pain*. New York, Raven Press, 1974, pp 727–732.

———, COLLINS WF: Physiological anatomy of pain, in Youmans JR (ed): *Neurological Surgery*. Philadelphia, Saunders, 1972, chap 85, pp 1587–1614.

WALL PD: The gate-control theory of pain mechanisms. *Brain* 101:1, 1978.

WEDDELL G: The multiple innervation of sensory spots in the skin. *J Anat* 75:441, 1941.

WHITE JC, SWEET WH: *Pain and the Neurosurgeon: A Forty Year Experience*. Springfield, Ill, Charles C Thomas, 1969.

WOOLSEY CN, MARSHALL WH, BARD P: Note on the organization of the tactile sensory area of the cerebral cortex of the chimpanzee. *J Neurophysiol* 6:287, 1943.

CHAPTER 8
OTHER DISORDERS OF SOMATIC SENSATION

Under normal conditions, sensory and motor functions are interdependent, as was dramatically illustrated by the early animal experiments of Claude Bernard and Sherrington, in which practically all movements of a limb were abolished by sectioning only its posterior roots. Interruption of other sensory pathways and destruction of the parietal cortex also have a profound effect upon motility. Sensory and motor neurons are intimately connected at all levels of the nervous system from the spinal cord to the cerebrum. To a large extent, human activity depends upon a constant influx of sensory impulses (most of them not consciously perceived) which are integral to motor adaptations. Truly, in a physiologic sense, "movement is sensation."

However, under conditions of disease, motor and sensory functions may be affected independently. Loss or impairment of sensory function may occur, and these may represent the principal manifestations of neurologic disease. The logic of this is clear enough, since the major anatomic pathways of the sensory system are distinct from those of the motor system and may be selectively disturbed by disease. The analysis of sensory symptoms involves the use of special tests, designed to indicate the nature of the sensory disorder and its locality, and it is from this point of view that disorders of sensory function are considered here.

Only *general somatic sensation*, i.e., afferent impulses which arise from the skin, muscles, or joints and which reach the level of consciousness, will be discussed in this chapter. One form of somatic sensation—pain—has been presented in detail in the preceding chapter. The *special* senses—vision, hearing, taste, and smell—are considered in the next section (Chaps. 11 and 12), and visceral (interoceptive) sensation, most of which does not reach consciousness, is considered with the disorders of the autonomic nervous system (Chap. 26).

ANATOMIC AND PHYSIOLOGIC CONSIDERATIONS

An understanding of the sensory disorders depends upon a knowledge of applied anatomy. Ideally, one should be familiar with the sensory receptors in the skin and deeper structures, the distribution of the peripheral nerves and roots, and the pathways by which sensory impulses are conveyed through the spinal cord and brainstem to the thalamus and cortex of the parietal lobe. These aspects of the anatomy of the sensory system and its physiology have already been touched upon in Chap. 7 and will be summarized here briefly. Charts showing the cutaneous distribution of the peripheral nerves (Fig. 8-1) are included in this section, and little more will be said about this aspect of the subject.

Every sensation depends on impulses excited by the adequate stimulation of receptors and conveyed to the central nervous system by afferent, or sensory, fibers. Sensory receptors are of two main types: those in the skin (exteroceptors) and those in the deeper somatic structures (proprioceptors). The skin receptors are particularly numerous and transduce four types of sensory experience: warmth, cold, touch, and pain. The proprioceptors inform us of the position of our body in space, of the force, direction, and range of movement of the joints (kinesthetic sense), and of pressure, both painful and painless. Histologically, a wide variety of sense organs has been described, varying from simple, free axon terminals to highly branched and encapsulated structures, many of the latter bearing the names of the anatomists who first described them.

For many years it was taught that each of the primary modalities of cutaneous sensation is subserved by a morphologically distinct end organ, each with its separate peripheral nerve fibers. According to this hy-

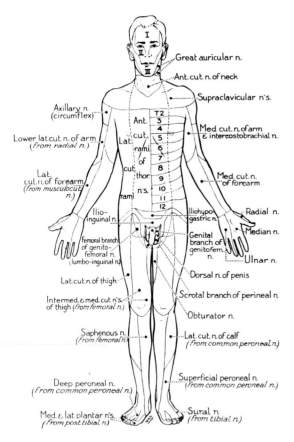
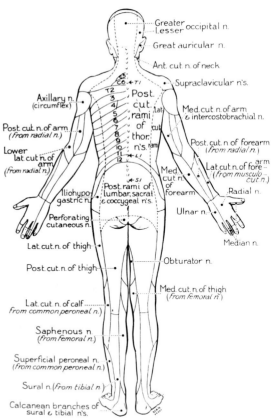

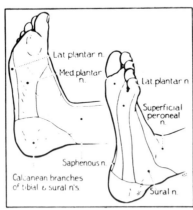

Figure 8-1
The cutaneous fields of peripheral nerves. (From W Haymaker, B Woodhall, Peripheral Nerve Injuries, 2d ed, Philadelphia, Saunders, 1953.)

pothesis, usually associated with the names of Müller and Volkmann and later of von Frey and Goldscheider, each type of end organ responds only to a particular sensory stimulus and gives rise to a specific modality of sensation. This hypothesis holds up reasonably well in respect to the perception of pain (see Chap. 7) and of temperature and perhaps to the perception of mechanical disturbances. Particularly instructive in this regard

are the observations of Kibler and Nathan, who studied the responses of warm and cold spots to different stimuli. (Warm and cold spots are those small areas of skin which most consistently respond to thermal stimuli with a sensation of warmth or cold.) They found that a cold stimulus applied to a warm spot gave rise to a sensation of cold and vice versa, that a pain stimulus applied to a warm or cold spot gave rise only to a painful sensation, and that mechanical stimulation of these spots gave rise to a sensation of touch or pressure. Observations such as these emphasize the specific quality of the different primary sensations and the importance of stimulus specificity in somatic sensibility.

The specialization of cutaneous afferent fibers is not absolute, however. The so-called pain (A-δ and C) fibers, for example, may be activated to some extent by nonnoxious stimuli. The concept of specificity of sensory endings has had to be modified as well. With a few exceptions (e.g., the pacinian corpuscle, which responds to compression and deformation), it has not been possible to ascribe a discrete function to each of the many varieties of receptors. Thus, Merkel's disks, Meissner's corpuscles, the nerve plexuses around the hair follicles, and free nerve endings can all be activated by a tactile stimulus. Conversely, a single type of receptor may mediate more than one sensory modality. Weddell and his colleagues found that with appropriate stimulation of the cornea each of the four primary modalities of somatic sensibility (touch, warmth, cold, pain) can be recognized, even though the cornea contains only fine, freely ending nerve filaments. In the ear, which is also sensitive to these four modalities, only two types of receptors—freely ending and perifollicular—are present. The lack of organized receptors, e.g., the end bulbs of Krause and Ruffini, in the cornea and ear make it evident that these types of receptors are not essential for the recognition of cold and warmth, respectively, as had been thought.

An alternate hypothesis of cutaneous sensibility, based on the foregoing observations, proposes that *any* given nerve fiber and its ending may convey impulses, that different stimuli set up different spatial and temporal "patterns" of impulses, and that the recognition of the nature of the stimulus (the psychical state called *sensation*) depends on the particular pattern of impulses reaching the brain. These observations, however, cannot be taken to mean that there is *no* specificity among the receptors and that sensory perception depends *only* on spatial and temporal "patterns" of impulses. The two concepts are not mutually exclusive, as has been pointed out in the discussion of pain perception (Chap. 7). There is still uncertainty about the mysterious step by which a particular mechanical stimulus is translated into a sensory experience, but it is fair to say that certain types of endings in certain localities facilitate the transductive process.

Proprioceptive fibers run mainly in the motor nerves; cutaneous fibers are carried in sensory or in mixed sensory and motor nerves. All the sensory neurons have their cell bodies in the dorsal root ganglia; the central projections of these cells enter the spinal cord via the dorsal or posterior roots. Each dorsal root contains all the fibers from skin, muscles, connective tissue, ligaments, tendons, joints, bones, and viscera which lie within the distribution of a single body segment, or somite. This segmental innervation has been amply demonstrated in humans and animals by observing the effects of diseases that involve one or two spinal nerves, such as herpes zoster, which also causes visible vesicles in the corresponding areas of skin, or ruptured disks, which cause hypalgesia in single root zones, or surgical section of several roots, leaving one intact (method of residual sensitivity). Maps of the dermatomes derived from these several types of data are shown in Fig. 8-2. It should be

noted that there is considerable overlapping from one segment to the other and that this is more so for touch than for pain (Fig. 8-3). The zone of pain loss is more dense and proves to be the most reliable means of testing for radicular disease. When such tests were done in leg and arm in patients with single root lesions, bands of hypalgesia were shown by Keegan and Garrett to be continuous longitudinally from foot or hand to the spine (Fig. 8-4). The segmental distribution of pain fibers from deep structures, though not fully corresponding to that of pain fibers from the skin, also follows a segmental pattern.

In the dorsal roots, the sensory fibers are first rearranged according to function. Large and heavily myelinated fibers enter the cord just medial to the dorsal horn and divide into an ascending and descending branch. The descending fibers and some of the ascending ones enter the gray matter of the dorsal horn within a few

Figure 8-2

Distribution of the sensory spinal roots on the surface of the body. (From G Holmes, Introduction to Clinical Neurology, 2d ed, Baltimore, Williams & Wilkins, 1952.)

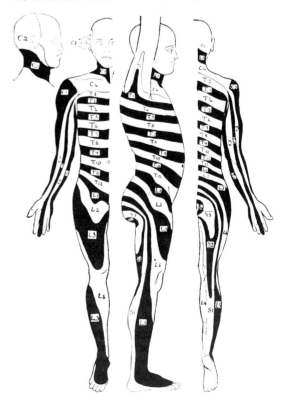

segments of their entrance and synapse with nerve cells in the gray matter of posterior and anterior horns, including large ventral horn cells, subserving segmental reflexes. Some of the ascending fibers run uninterruptedly in the dorsal columns of the same side of the spinal cord, terminating in the gracile and cuneate nuclei. In this column are contained the fibers mediating the senses of pressure, vibration, direction of movement, and position of joints and a portion of those for touch (see Fig. 7-3); it is unlikely, however, that the fiber pathways in the posterior columns are the sole mediators of proprioception in the spinal cord (see further on, under "posterior column syndrome"). The nerve cells of the nucleus gracilis and cuneatus give rise to a secondary afferent path, which crosses the midline in the medulla and ascends in the brainstem to the thalamus as the medial lemniscus (Fig. 7-2).

Thinly myelinated or unmyelinated fibers enter the cord on the lateral aspect of the dorsal horn and synapse with the dorsal horn cells within a segment or two of their point of entry into the cord. The dorsal horn cells in turn give rise to secondary sensory fibers, some of which may ascend ipsilaterally but most of which decussate and ascend in the anterolateral fasciculus of the

cord. These anatomic arrangements have already been considered in Chap. 7. Observations based on the surgical interruption of the anterolateral funiculus indicate that fibers mediating pain and temperature occupy the dorsolateral part of the anterolateral funiculus, and those for touch and deep pressure, the ventromedial part.

The pathways mediating cutaneous sensation from the face and head, especially touch, pain, and temperature, are conveyed to the brainstem mainly by the trigeminal nerve; after entering the pons, the pain and temperature fibers run caudally as the descending tri-

Figure 8-4
Dermatomes of the upper and lower extremities, outlined by the pattern of sensory loss following lesions of single nerve roots. (From Keegan and Garrett.)

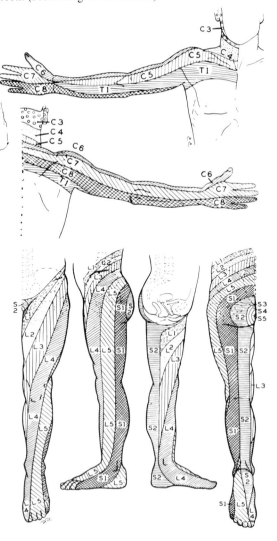

Figure 8-3
Radicular (A) and peripheral nerve innervation (B) of cutaneous areas showing overlapping of nerve fibers in the dermatomes. (From MB Carpenter, Human Neuroanatomy, 7th ed, Baltimore, Williams & Wilkins, 1976.)

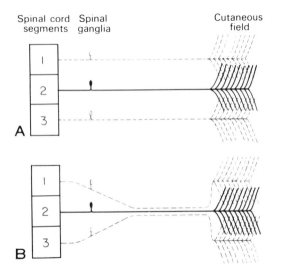

geminal root and terminate in a long vertically oriented nucleus which lies beside it and extends to the upper cervical segments of the cord. Axons from the neurons of this nucleus then cross the midline and join the most medial portion of the ascending spinothalamic tract (Fig. 7-2). Ascending fibers from the reticular nuclei, medial lemniscus, and spinothalamic pathways merge in the midbrain and terminate in the posterior complex of thalamic nuclei, particularly in the nucleus ventralis posterolateralis (VPL).

The posterior thalamic complex projects mainly to three cortical areas: (1) The postcentral cortex, or first somatic sensory area (S1), which corresponds to Brodmann's areas 3, 1, and 2. Afferents to S1 are derived primarily from VPL and the nucleus ventralis posteromedialis (VPM) and are distributed somatotopically, with the leg represented uppermost and the face lowermost. Electrical stimulation of this area yields sensations of tingling, numbness, and warmth in specific regions on the *opposite* side of the body. The information transmitted to S1 is tactile and proprioceptive, derived mainly from the dorsal column–medial lemniscus system, and is concerned with sensory discrimination. (2) The second somatosensory area (S2) which lies on the upper bank of the sylvian fissure, adjacent to the insula. Localization of function is less discrete in S2 than in S1, but S2 is also organized somatotopically, with the face rostrally and hind leg or leg caudally. The feelings evoked by electrical stimulation of S2 are much the same as those of S1 but may be bilateral in distinction to the latter. (3) The superior parietal lobule (areas 5 and 7 of Brodmann), electrical stimulation of which gives rise to feelings of warmth, tingling, and numbness over the entire contralateral side of the body and frequently over both sides. This area is not organized somatotopically and is of particular importance in regard to discriminative function.

Undoubtedly, the perception of sensory stimuli involves more of the cerebral cortex than the discrete areas described above. Furthermore, these areas are not purely sensory in function; motor effects can be obtained from all of them by electrical stimulation. It has been shown that sensory neurons in VPL, cuneate and gracile nuclei, and sensory neurons in the dorsal horn of the spinal cord all receive descending cortical projections. This reciprocal arrangement probably influences movement and the transmission and interpretation of pain.

Provided that the subcortical structures, especially the thalamus, are intact, certain sensations such as pain, touch, pressure, and extremes of temperature can reach consciousness. Their accurate localization, however, as well as the patient's ability to make fine sensory discriminations, depends on the integrity of the sensory cor-

tex. This is a fundamental clinical distinction and will be elaborated in discussions of the individual sensory syndromes.

Brief reference should be made to the concept of *protopathic and epicritic sensibility*. These terms were coined by Head and his coworkers, on the basis of observations of the sensory changes which followed the division of the cutaneous branch of the radial nerve in Head's own forearm. They described an area in which superficial sensation was completely abolished, surrounded by a narrower ("intermediate") zone, in which pain sensation was preserved and extreme degrees of temperature were recognized, but where perception of touch, lesser differences of temperature, and two-point discrimination were abolished. Pain from this latter zone was particularly unpleasant and diffuse and could not be localized accurately. These findings were explained by postulating the existence of two distinct systems of receptive end organs and conducting neurons: (1) a protopathic system, subserving pain and extreme differences in temperature and yielding ungraded, diffuse impressions of an all-or-none type, and (2) an epicritic system, which mediated touch, two-point discrimination, and lesser differences in temperature.

That an intermediate zone is regularly found between normal and anesthetic areas of skin is generally agreed upon. However, the nature of the changes in this intermediate zone has been much debated. The experiment of Head et al. was repeated by Trotter and Davies, who failed to substantiate the original observations. The latter investigators found that the intermediate zone was not anesthetic, only hypoesthetic, and attributed the other intermediate-zone changes—involving pain, temperature and two-point discrimination—to a hypoesthesia of these modalities. The particular structures postulated by Head to underlie each of his functional systems were not established. Actually, the fringe of hypoesthetic and altered sensation was later shown by Wedell to be due to collateral regeneration of surrounding nerve fibers. The concept of protopathic and epicritic sensibility has been criticized on theoretical as well as factual grounds (see review by Walshe), but it still has its proponents.

EXAMINATION OF THE PATIENT

Most neurologists would agree that sensory testing is the most difficult part of the neurologic examination. For one thing, test procedures are relatively crude and inadequate, unlike natural modes of stimulation with which the patient is familiar. Embarrassingly often, no objective sensory loss can be demonstrated despite symptoms that indicate the presence of such a deficit. Further, the response to sensory stimuli may be difficult to evaluate, since it depends on the patient's interpretation of sensory experiences. This in turn will depend on the patient's general awareness and responsiveness, desire to cooperate, as well as intelligence, education, and suggestibility. At times, children and relatively uneducated persons, by virtue of their simple and direct responses, are better witnesses than more sophisticated individuals who are likely to analyze their feelings minutely and report small inconsequential differences in stimulus intensity.

Before proceeding to sensory testing, the physician should question patients about their symptoms, and this too may pose special problems. Patients are confronted with derangements of sensation that may be unlike anything they have previously experienced, and they have few words in their vocabulary to describe what they feel. They may say that a limb feels "numb" and "dead" when in fact they mean that it is weak. Observant individuals may occasionally discover a loss of sensation, e.g., inability to feel discomfort on touching an object hot enough to blister the skin or unawareness of articles of clothing and other objects in contact with the skin. But more often disease induces new and unnatural sensory experiences. If nerves, sensory roots, or spinal tracts are partially interrupted, the patient may complain of tingling or prickling ("like Novocain," "pins and needles") feelings, that occur either spontaneously or in response to tactile stimulation; presumably some of the remaining touch and pain fibers are conducting impulses but the peripheral sensory mechanism is not functioning normally. Similarly, sensations of burning, coldness, and pain may represent overactivity or disinhibition of preserved thermal and pain fibers. Feelings of tightness, drawing and pulling, or of a band or girdle around the limb or trunk are common with partial involvement of proprioceptive fibers. All these abnormal sensations are called *paresthesias* or *dysesthesias*, and their character and distribution inform us of the anatomy of the lesions involving the sensory system.

Paresthesias should always raise suspicion of a lesion of the sensory pathways in nerves, spinal cord, or higher structures. However, they may, if evanescent, be of no significance. Every person has had the experience of resting on the ulnar, sciatic, or peroneal nerve and having the limb "fall asleep." Anxiety with hyperventila-

tion may cause paresthesias of the lips and hands (sometimes unilateral) from diminution of CO_2 and of ionized calcium. Tetany has the same effects with added carpopedal spasms.

The detail with which sensation is tested is determined by the clinical situation. If the patient has no sensory complaints, it is sufficient to test vibration and position sense in the fingers and toes and the perception of pinprick over the face, trunk, and extremities, and to determine whether the findings are the same in symmetric parts of the body. A rough survey of this sort may detect sensory defects of which the patient is unaware. On the other hand, more thorough testing is in order if the patient has complaints referable to the sensory system, or if one finds localized atrophy or weakness, ataxia, trophic changes of joints, or painless ulcers.

A few other general principles should be mentioned. One should not press the sensory examination in the presence of fatigue, for an inattentive patient is a poor witness. The examiner must also avoid suggesting symptoms to the patient. After having explained in the simplest terms what is required, the examiner should interpose as few questions and remarks as possible. Consequently, patients must not be asked, "Do you feel that?" each time they are touched; they should simply be told to say "yes" or "sharp" every time they have been touched or feel pain. Patients should not be permitted to see the part under examination. For short tests it is sufficient that they close the eyes; during more detailed testing it is preferable to screen the eyes from the part being examined. Finally, the findings of the sensory examination should be accurately recorded on a chart.

Somatic sensation is frequently classified as superficial (cutaneous, exteroceptive) and deep (proprioceptive); the former comprises the modalities of light touch, pain, and temperature; the latter includes the sense of position, passive motion, vibration, and deep pressure-pain.

SENSE OF TOUCH

This is usually tested with a wisp of cotton. Patients are first acquainted with the nature of the stimulus by applying it to a normal part of the body. Then they are asked to say "yes" each time various other parts are touched. A patient simulating sensory loss may say "no" in response to a tactile stimulus. Cornified areas of skin, such as the soles and palms, will require a heavier stimulus than elsewhere, and the hair-clad parts a lighter one, because of the numerous nerve endings around the follicles. The patient is more sensitive to a moving contactual stimulus of any kind than to a stationary one. The deft application of the examiner's or preferably the patient's fingertips is a useful method of mapping out an area of tactile loss, as Trotter originally showed.

More precise testing is possible by using a von Frey hair. By this method, a stimulus of constant strength can be applied and the threshold for tactile sensation determined by measuring the weight required to bend a hair of known length.

SENSE OF PAIN

This is most efficiently estimated by pinprick, although it may be evoked by a great diversity of noxious stimuli. Patients must understand that they are to report the degree of sharpness of the pin or the degree of penetration of the skin, not simply the feeling of contact or pressure of the point. If the pinpricks are applied rapidly in one area, their effect may be summated and excessive pain may result; therefore, they should be delivered about one per second, and not over the same spot.

It is almost impossible, using an ordinary pin or needle, to apply each stimulus with equal intensity. This difficulty can be largely overcome by the use of an algesimeter, which enables one not only to deliver stimuli of constant intensity but also to grade the intensity and determine threshold values. Even with this instrument an isolated stimulus may be reported as being excessively sharp, apparently because of direct contact with a pain spot.

If an area of diminished or absent touch or pain sensation is encountered, its boundaries should be demarcated to determine whether it has a segmental or peripheral nerve distribution or whether sensation is lost below a certain level. Such areas are best delineated by proceeding from the region of impaired sensation toward the normal, and the changes may be confirmed by dragging a pin lightly over the parts in question.

DEEP PRESSURE-PAIN

One can estimate this modality simply by pinching firmly or pressing deeply on the tendons and muscles; no special virtue is attached to the traditional and somewhat sadistic use of the testicle for this test. Pain can often be elicited by heavy pressure even when superficial sensation is diminished; conversely, in some diseases, such as tabetic neurosyphilis, loss of deep pressure-pain may be more prominent than loss of superficial pain.

THERMAL SENSE

The proper evaluation of this form of sensation requires attention to certain details of procedure. One may fail consistently to evoke a sensation of hot or cold if small test objects are used. The perception of thermal stimuli is relatively delayed, especially if the test objects are applied only lightly and momentarily against the skin. If the temperature of the test object is below 10°C or above 50°C, sensations of cold or warmth become confused with pain. As the temperature of the test object approaches that of the skin, the patient's response will be modified by the temperature of the skin itself.

The following procedure for testing thermal sensation is therefore suggested. The areas of skin to be tested should be exposed for some time before the examination. The test objects should be large, preferably Erlenmeyer flasks containing hot or cold water. Thermometers, which extend into the water through the flask stoppers, indicate the temperature of the water at the moment of testing. At first, extreme degrees of heat and cold (e.g., 10 and 45°C) are employed to delineate roughly an area of thermal sensory disturbance; the patient should be asked to report whether the flask feels "less hot" or "less cold" over such an area in comparison to a normal part. If areas of impaired sensation are found, the borders can be accurately determined by moving the flask along the skin from the insensitive to the normal region. The qualitative change should then be quantitated as far as possible by estimating the differences in temperature which the patient is able to recognize. The patient is asked to state whether one stimulus feels warmer or colder than another, not whether a given stimulus is warm or cold, since the cooler of the two may be interpreted as warm. The difference in temperature between the two flasks is gradually reduced by mixing their contents. Normally, one can detect a difference of 1°C or less when the temperature of the flasks is in the range of 28 to 32°C. In the warm range, a normal person readily recognizes differences between 35 and 40°C, and in the cold range, between 10 and 20°C. In some normal older persons and in others with poor peripheral circulation (especially in cold weather), the responses may not meet these standards.

The sensation of heat or cold depends not only on the temperature of the test object but also on the duration of the stimulus and the area over which it is applied. This principle may be employed to detect slight degrees of sensory impairment; the patient may be able to distinguish small differences in temperature when the bottom of the flask is applied for 3 s but be unable to do so if only the side of the flask is applied for 1 s. Throughout the test procedure, especially when small temperature differences are involved, the area of sensory disturbance should be continually checked against perception in normal parts.

POSTURAL SENSE AND THE PERCEPTION OF PASSIVE MOVEMENT

These modalities are usually lost together, although cases do occur in which the perception of the position of a limb in space is lost while that of passive movement of the toes or fingers is retained. The opposite has also been said to occur, but must be very rare.

Abnormalities of postural sensation may be revealed in several ways. With the arms outstretched and eyes closed, the affected arm will wander from its original position; if the fingers are spread apart, they may undergo a series of changing postures ("piano-playing" movements, or pseudoathetosis); in attempting to touch the tip of the nose with the index finger, the patient may miss the target repeatedly.

The lack of position sense in the legs may be demonstrated by displacing the limb from its original position and asking the patient to point to the large toe with eyes closed. If postural sensation is defective in both legs, the patient will be unable to maintain balance with feet together and eyes closed (Romberg's sign). This sign should be interpreted with caution. Even a normal person in the Romberg position will sway slightly with the eyes closed. A patient with lack of balance due to cerebellar ataxia or other motor disorder will also sway more if visual cues are removed. Only if there is a marked discrepancy between the state of balance with eyes open and closed can one confidently state that the patient shows Romberg's sign. Mild degrees of unsteadiness in nervous or suggestible patients may be overcome by diverting their attention, e.g., by having them touch the index finger of each hand alternately to the nose while standing with eyes closed.

Perception of passive movement is first tested in the fingers and toes, since the defect, when present, is reflected maximally in these parts. It is important to grasp the digit firmly at the sides opposite the plane of movement; otherwise the pressure applied by the examiner in displacing the digit may allow the patient to identify the direction of movement. This applies also to the testing of the more proximal segments of the limb. The patient should be instructed to report each movement as "up" or "down" from the previous position. It is useful to demonstrate the test with a large and easily identified movement, but once the idea is clear to the patient, the

smallest detectable changes in position should be determined. The part being tested should be moved rapidly. The range of a quick movement that is normally appreciated in the digits is said to be as little as 1°. In practice, defective perception of passive movement is judged by comparison with a normal limb or, if perception is bilaterally defective, on the basis of what the examiner has learned through experience to be normal. Slight impairment may be disclosed by a slow response or, if the digit is displaced very slowly, by an unawareness or uncertainty that movement has occurred; or, after the digit has been displaced in the same direction several times, the patient may misjudge the first movement in the opposite direction; or, after the examiner has moved the toe, the patient may make a number of small voluntary movements of the toe, in an apparent attempt to determine its position or the direction of the movement. Inattentiveness will cause some of these errors.

THE SENSE OF VIBRATION

This is a composite sensation comprising touch and rapid alterations of deep-pressure sense. Its conduction depends on both cutaneous and deep afferent fibers which ascend in the dorsal columns of the cord. It is therefore rarely affected by lesions of single nerves but will be disturbed in cases of polyneuritis and disease of the dorsal columns, medial lemniscus, and thalamus. Vibration and position sense are usually lost together, although one of them (most often vibration sense) may be affected disproportionately. With advancing age, vibration sense may be diminished at the toes and ankles.

Vibration sense is tested by placing a tuning fork with a low rate and long duration of vibration (128 dv) over the bony prominences. The examiner must make sure that the patient responds to the vibration, not simply to the pressure of the fork, and that the patient is not trying to listen to it. There are mechanical devices to quantitate vibration sense, but it is sufficient for clinical purposes to compare the point tested with a normal part of the patient or the examiner. Thus, the vibrating fork is allowed to run down until the moment that vibration is no longer perceived, and the fork is then transferred quickly to the corresponding point on the opposite limb; if vibration is then perceived and if this finding is consistent, one can be certain of an impairment of vibration sense. The perception of vibration at the tibial tuberosity after it has disappeared at the ankle, or at the anterior iliac spine after it has disappeared at the tibial tuberosity, is an indication of a peripheral nerve lesion. The level of vibration sense loss due to spinal cord lesions may be estimated by placing the fork over successive vertebral spines.

Damage to the sensory cortex or to the thalamocortical projections results in a special type of disturbance that affects mainly the patient's ability to make sensory discriminations. Lesions in these structures usually disturb postural sense but leave the so-called primary modalities (touch, pain, temperature, and vibration sense) relatively little affected. In such a situation, or if a cerebral lesion is suspected on other grounds, discriminative function should be tested further by the following tests.

Two-Point Discrimination The ability to distinguish two points from one is tested by using a compass, the points of which should be blunt and applied simultaneously and painlessly. The distance at which such stimuli can be recognized as double varies but is roughly 1 mm at the tip of the tongue, 2 to 3 mm on the lips, 3 to 5 mm at the fingertips, 8 to 15 mm on the palm, 20 to 30 mm on the dorsa of the hands and feet, and 4 to 7 cm on the body surface. It is characteristic of the patient with a lesion of the sensory cortex to mistake two points for one, although occasionally the opposite occurs.

Cutaneous Localization and Figure Writing The ability to localize cutaneous stimuli is tested by touching various parts of the body and asking the patient to point to the part touched or to the corresponding part on the examiner's limb. Recognition of numbers or letters (these should be larger than 4 cm) or the direction of lines drawn on the skin also depends on localization of tactile stimuli. According to Wall and Noordenbos, figure writing and detection of the direction of movement on the skin are the most useful and simplest tests of posterior column function.

Appreciation of Texture, Size, and Shape Appreciation of texture depends mainly on cutaneous impressions, but the recognition of the shape and size of objects is based on impressions from deeper receptors as well. The lack of recognition of shape and form, therefore, though frequently a manifestation of cortical disease, may occur also with lesions of the spinal cord and brainstem because of interruption of tracts transmitting postural and tactile sensation. The latter type of sensory defect, called *stereoanesthesia*, should be distinguished from *astereognosis*, which connotes an inability to identify an object by palpation, the primary sense data (touch, pain, temperature, and vibration) being intact. In practice, a pure astereognosis is rarely encountered, and the term is employed where the impairment of superficial and vibratory sensation in the hands seems to be of insufficient severity to account for the defect. Defined in this way,

astereognosis is either right- or left-sided, and, with the qualifications mentioned below, is the product of a lesion in the opposite hemisphere, involving the postcentral gyrus or the thalamoparietal projections.

The traditional teaching that somatic sensation is represented only in the contralateral parietal lobe is probably not strictly correct. Beginning with Oppenheim, in 1906, there have been sporadic reports of patients who showed bilateral astereognosis, or loss of tactile sensation, with an apparently unilateral cerebral lesion. The validity of these observations was established by Semmes et al., who carefully tested a large series of patients with traumatic lesions involving either the right or left cerebral hemisphere. These authors found that a substantial number of these patients showed an ipsilateral or bilateral impairment of "cortical" or discriminative sensation (pressure, two-point discrimination, point localization, and passive movement) as a result of unilateral cerebral disease, right or left. These observations, with minor qualifications, have been confirmed by Carmon and also by Corkin et al., who investigated the sensory effects of cortical excisions in patients with focal epilepsy.

Thus it appears that certain somatic sensory functions are mediated not only by the contralateral hemisphere, but also by the ipsilateral one, although the contribution of the former is undoubtedly the more significant.

Finally, astereognosis needs to be distinguished from *tactile agnosia*, in which a lesion of one hemisphere lying posterior to the postcentral gyrus of the *dominant* parietal lobe results in an inability to recognize an object by touch in *both* hands. Tactile agnosia is a disorder of perception of symbols and concepts akin to the defect in naming parts of the body, or visualizing a plan or a route, or understanding the meaning of the printed or spoken word (visual or auditory verbal agnosia). Again, recent observations have called into question the traditional concept of left hemispheric dominance in respect to tactile perception. The findings of Carmon and Benton, that the right hemisphere is particularly important in the tactile perception of direction, and of Corkin, that patients with right-hemisphere lesions show a consistently greater failure of tactile-maze learning than those with left-sided lesions, point to a relative dominance of the right hemisphere in the mediation of tactile performance involving a spatial component. This matter is considered further in Chap. 21.

A few other terms require definition, since they may be encountered in reading about sensation. Many of them lack precision and others are pedantic. It is recommended that the simplest possible terms be used. *Dysesthesia* refers to any unpleasant or painful sensory experience induced by a stimulus that is ordinarily painless, such as the pressure of bedclothes. *Paresthesias* refer to crawling, burning, tingling, or "pins-and-needles" feelings that arise spontaneously. *Anesthesia* refers to a complete loss of all forms of sensation, and *hypesthesia* to a diminution of sensation. Loss or impairment of specific cutaneous sensations may be indicated by an appropriate prefix or suffix, e.g., thermoanesthesia or thermohypesthesia, analgesia (loss of pain) or hypalgesia, tactile anesthesia and pallanesthesia (loss of vibratory sense). The term *hyperesthesia* refers to an abnormally increased sensitivity to various stimuli, and is usually used with respect to cutaneous sensation. The term implies a heightened activity of the sensory apparatus. Under certain conditions (e.g., sunburn) there does appear to be an enhanced sensitivity of cutaneous receptors, but usually the presence of hyperesthesia betrays an underlying sensory defect; careful testing will demonstrate an elevated threshold to tactile, painful, or thermal stimuli, but once the stimulus is perceived it may have a severely painful or unpleasant quality (*hyperpathia*). Some clinicians use the latter term to denote an exaggerated response to a painful stimulus.

SENSORY SYNDROMES

SENSORY CHANGES DUE TO INTERRUPTION OF A SINGLE PERIPHERAL NERVE

These changes will vary with the composition of the nerve involved, depending on whether it is predominantly muscular, cutaneous, or mixed. In lesions of cutaneous nerves, the area of tactile anesthesia is more extensive than the one for pain, because of greater overlapping of pain fibers. Also, because of overlap from adjacent nerves, the area of sensory loss following division of a cutaneous nerve is always less than its anatomic distribution. If a large area of skin is involved, the sensory defect characteristically consists of a central portion, in which all forms of cutaneous sensation are lost, surrounded by a zone of partial loss, which becomes less marked as one proceeds from the center to the periphery. The perception of deep pressure and passive movement are intact because these modalities are mediated by nerve fibers from subcutaneous structures and joints. Along the margin of the hypesthetic zone the skin becomes excessively sensitive. A light contact may be felt as smarting and mildly painful. According to Weddell, this is because of collateral regeneration from surrounding healthy nerves into the denervated region.

Particular types of lesions differentially affect the fibers in a sensory nerve. Compression may paralyze large touch and pressure fibers and leave the small pain, thermal, and autonomic fibers intact; procaine and cocaine have the opposite effect.

In lesions involving the brachial and lumbosacral plexuses, the sensory disturbance is no longer confined to the territory of a single nerve and is accompanied by muscle weakness and reflex changes.

SENSORY CHANGES DUE TO MULTIPLE NERVE INVOLVEMENT (POLYNEUROPATHY)

In most instances of polyneuropathy the sensory changes are accompanied by varying degrees of motor and reflex loss. Usually the sensory impairment is symmetric, with notable exceptions in some instances of diabetic and periarteritic neuropathy. Since the longest and largest fibers tend to be the most affected, the sensory loss is most severe over the feet and legs and less severe over the hands and arms. The abdomen, thorax, and face are spared except in the most severe cases. The sensory loss usually involves all the modalities, and although it is manifestly difficult to equate the impairment of pain, touch, temperature, vibration, and position senses, one of these may seemingly be impaired out of proportion to the others (exceptions are discussed in Chaps. 40 and 45). One cannot accurately predict, from the patient's symptoms, which mode of sensation will be disproportionately affected. The term *glove-and-stocking anesthesia,* frequently employed to describe the sensory loss of polyneuropathy, draws attention to the predominantly distal pattern of involvement. The term is inaccurate insofar as the change from normal to impaired sensation is not sharp but gradual. In hysteria, by contrast, the border between normal and absent sensation is usually sharp.

SENSORY CHANGES DUE TO INVOLVEMENT OF MULTIPLE SPINAL NERVE ROOTS

Because of considerable overlap from adjacent roots, division of a single sensory root does not produce complete loss of sensation in any area of skin. Compression of a single sensory cervical or lumbar root (e.g., in herniated intervertebral disks) causes varying degrees of impairment of cutaneous sensation in a segmental pattern, however. When two or more roots have been completely divided, a zone of sensory loss can be found, greater for pain than for touch. Surrounding the area of complete loss is a narrow zone of partial loss, in which a raised threshold accompanied by overreaction (hyperpathia) may or may not be demonstrated. Tendon and cutaneomuscular reflexes may be lost. The presence of muscle weakness and atrophy indicates involvement of ventral roots as well.

THE TABETIC SYNDROME (See Fig. 8-5)

This results from damage to the large proprioceptive and other fibers of the posterior lumbosacral (and sometimes the cervical) roots. It is typically caused by neurosyphilis, but also by diabetes mellitus and other diseases that involve the posterior roots. Numbness or paresthesias and lightning or lancinating pains are frequent complaints; areflexia, atonicity of the bladder, abnormalities of gait (Chap. 6), and hypotonia without muscle weakness are found on examination. The sensory loss may consist only of loss of vibration and position senses in the lower extremities, but in severe cases, loss or impairment of superficial or deep pain sense or of touch may

Figure 8-5
Some of the sites of lesions that produce characteristic spinal cord syndromes (shaded areas indicate lesions).

be added. The feet and legs are most affected, much less often the arms and trunk. Atonicity of the bladder with retention of urine is often associated.

COMPLETE SPINAL SENSORY SYNDROMES
(See Fig. 8-5)

In a complete transverse lesion of the spinal cord, all forms of sensation are abolished below a level that corresponds to the lesion. However, there may be a narrow zone of hyperesthesia at the upper margin of the anesthetic zone. Loss of pain, temperature, and touch begins one or two segments below the level of the lesion; of course vibratory and position senses have a less discrete level. It is important to remember that during the evolution of such a lesion there may be a greater discrepancy between the level of the lesion and that of the sensory loss, the latter ascending as the lesion progresses. This can be understood if one conceives of a lesion evolving from the periphery to the center of the cord, affecting first the outermost fibers carrying pain and temperature sensation from the legs. Conversely, a lesion advancing from the center of the cord may affect these modalities in the reverse order.

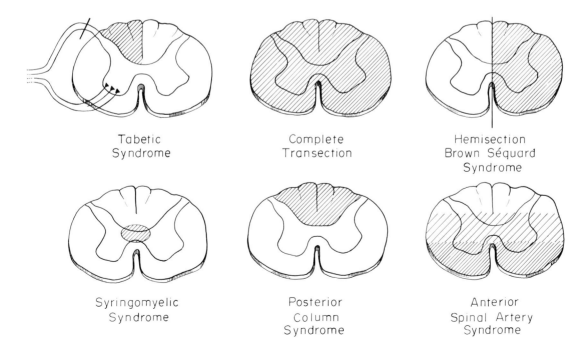

Tabetic
Syndrome

Complete
Transection

Hemisection
Brown Séquard
Syndrome

Syringomyelic
Syndrome

Posterior
Column
Syndrome

Anterior
Spinal Artery
Syndrome

PARTIAL SPINAL SENSORY SYNDROME (HEMISECTION OF THE SPINAL CORD, BROWN-SÉQUARD SYNDROME)

In rare instances disease is confined to one side of the spinal cord; pain and thermal sensation are affected on the opposite side of the body, and proprioceptive sensation is affected on the same side as the lesion. The loss of pain and temperature sensation begins one or two segments below the lesion. An associated motor paralysis on the side of the lesion completes the syndrome (Fig. 8-5). Tactile sensation is not involved, since the fibers from one side of the body are distributed in tracts (posterior columns and anterior spinothalamic) on both sides of the cord.

LESIONS OF THE CENTRAL GRAY MATTER (SYRINGOMYELIC SYNDROME)

Since fibers conducting pain and temperature cross the cord in the anterior commissure, a lesion in this location of considerable vertical extent will characteristically abolish these modalities on one or both sides over several segments (dermatomes) but will spare tactile sensation (Fig. 8-5). The most common cause of such a lesion is syringomyelia; less common causes are tumor and hemorrhage. This type of dissociated sensory loss usually occurs in a segmental distribution, and since the lesion frequently involves other parts of the gray matter, varying degrees of segmental amyotrophy and reflex loss are usually present as well. If the lesion has spread to the white matter, corticospinal, spinothalamic, and posterior column signs may be conjoined.

POSTERIOR COLUMN SYNDROME (See Fig. 8-5)

Loss of vibratory and position senses occur below the lesion, but the perception of pain, temperature, and touch are affected relatively little or not at all. Since this condition is due to the interruption of central projections of the dorsal root ganglia cells, it may be difficult to distinguish from an affection of large fibers in sensory roots (tabetic syndrome). In some diseases that involve the dorsal columns, vibratory sensation may be involved predominantly, whereas in others position sense is more affected. An interruption of proprioceptive fibers may also impair discriminative ("cortical") sensory functions such as two-point discrimination, figure writing, and the ability to detect the direction of a moving stimulus on the skin. Paresthesias in the form of tingling and pins-and-needles sensations or girdle- and bandlike sensations are common complaints with posterior column disease, and pinprick may produce a diffuse, burning, unpleasant sensation.

In several cases on record, interruption of the posterior columns by surgical incision or other type of injury did not cause a permanent loss of the sensory modalities thought to be subserved by these pathways (Cook and Browder, Wall and Noordenbos). Since post-mortem studies of these cases were not carried out, it is possible that some of the posterior column fibers had been spared, or following injury to the posterior columns, some proprioceptive function may have been assumed by other spinal sensory pathways. Also, it should be realized that all the posterior column fibers do not ascend to the nuclei of Goll; some synapse with secondary neurons at a lower level. The proposition of Wall and Noordenbos, which is debatable, is that such patients lose not the classical modalities of posterior column sensation but the ability to perform tasks that demand simultaneous analysis of spatial and temporal characteristics of the stimulus.

ANTERIOR MYELOPATHY (ANTERIOR SPINAL ARTERY SYNDROME)

With infarction of the spinal cord in the distribution of the anterior spinal artery or other destructive lesions that predominantly affect the ventral portion of the cord, one finds a loss of pain and temperature sensation below the level of the lesion and a relative or absolute sparing of proprioceptive sensation. Since the corticospinal tracts and the ventral gray matter also lie within the area of distribution of the anterior spinal artery, paralysis of motor function forms a prominent part of this syndrome (Fig. 8-5).

DISTURBANCES OF SENSATION DUE TO LESIONS OF THE BRAINSTEM

A chacteristic feature of lesions of the medulla is that in many instances the sensory disturbance is crossed, i.e., there is loss of pain and temperature sensation of one side of the face and the opposite side of the body. This is accounted for by involvement of the trigeminal tract or nucleus and the lateral spinothalamic tract on one side of the brainstem. This is nearly always caused by a lateral medullary infarction (Wallenberg's syndrome). In the upper medulla, pons, and midbrain, the crossed trigeminothalamic and lateral spinothalamic tracts run together and a lesion causes loss of pain and temperature sense on the opposite half of the body. In the upper brainstem the spinothalamic tract and the medial lemniscus become confluent, so that an appropriately placed lesion may cause a loss of all superficial and deep sensation over the contralateral side of the body. Cranial nerve palsies, cerebellar ataxia, or motor paralysis are often associated, as indicated in Chap. 33.

SENSORY LOSS DUE TO A LESION OF THE THALAMUS (SYNDROME OF DÉJERINE-ROUSSY)

Involvement of the nucleus ventralis posterolateralis of the thalamus, usually due to a vascular lesion, less often to a tumor, causes loss or diminution of all forms of sensation on the opposite side of the body. Position sense is affected more frequently than any other sensory function, and deep sensory loss is usually but not always more profound than cutaneous loss. There may be spontaneous pain or discomfort (*thalamic pain*), sometimes of the most distressing type, on the affected side of the body (see page 100), and any form of stimulus may then have a diffuse, unpleasant, lingering quality. Emotional disturbance also aggravates the painful state. In spite of this overresponse to pinprick or other stimuli, the patient usually shows an elevated pain threshold, i.e., a stronger stimulus than normal is necessary to produce a sensation of pain. The "thalamic" pain syndrome may occasionally accompany lesions of the white matter of the parietal lobe (see Chap. 33) or the medial lemniscus or even the posterior columns of the spinal cord.

SENSORY LOSS DUE TO A LESION OF THE PARIETAL LOBE

This results in a disturbance mainly of discriminative sensory functions on the opposite side of the body, particularly the face, arm, and leg. Loss of position sense, impaired ability to localize touch and pain stimuli, elevation of two-point threshold, astereognosis, and tactile agnosia (if the lesion is in the dominant hemisphere) are the most prominent findings. Another characteristic manifestation of parietal lobe lesions is sensory extinction or inattention. In response to bilateral simultaneous testing of symmetric parts, patients may acknowledge only the stimulus on the sound side, or they may improperly localize the stimulus on the affected side, whereas stimuli applied to each side separately are properly appreciated. This phenomenon and other features of parietal lobe lesions are considered further in Chap. 21.

It is generally taught that the primary modalities of sensation (pain and temperature, touch and vibratory sense) are not affected by lesions that involve the parietal cortex or underlying white matter, but this statement needs to be modified in several ways. In acute parietal cortical lesions, and occasionally in chronic ones, the primary modalities may be impaired, although not to the extent that one observes with deep lesions involving the thalamus. Frequently the impairment takes a form different from that due to thalamic lesions. With cortical lesions, the patient's reports are variable; one examination may disclose no sensory abnormalities, whereas another does. This type of response is often attributed to hysteria. In other circumstances, a lesion confined to the parietal cortex (the best examples have been due to glancing bullet wounds of the skull) has resulted in a circumscribed loss of superficial sensation in an opposite limb, mimicking a root or peripheral nerve lesion.

SENSORY LOSS DUE TO SUGGESTION AND HYSTERIA

The possibility of suggesting sensory loss to a patient is a very real one, as has already been indicated. Hysterical patients rarely complain spontaneously of cutaneous sensory loss, although they may use the term "numbness" to indicate a paralysis of a limb. Examination, on the other hand, may suggest to the patient a complete hemianesthesia, often with reduced hearing, sight, smell, and taste, as well as impaired vibration sense over only half the skull, which persists thereafter. Anesthesia of one entire limb or a sharply defined sensory loss over part of a limb, not conforming to the distribution of root or cutaneous nerve, may also be observed. Postural sensation is rarely affected. The diagnosis of hysterical hemianesthesia is best made by eliciting the other relevant symptoms of hysteria or, if this is not possible, by noting the discrepancies between this type of sensory loss and that which occurs as part of the usual sensory syndromes. Sometimes in a patient with no other neurologic abnormality or in one with a definite neurologic syndrome, one is dismayed by sensory findings which are completely unexplainable and discordant. In such cases one must try to reason through to the diagnosis by disregarding the sensory findings.

REFERENCES

BRODAL A: The somatic afferent pathways, in *Neurological Anatomy*, 3d ed. New York, Oxford, 1981, pp 46-147.
CARMON A: Disturbances of tactile sensitivity in patients with unilateral cerebral lesions. *Cortex* 7:83, 1971.

————, BENTON AL: Tactile perception of direction and number in patients with unilateral cerebral disease. *Neurology* 19:525, 1969.

COOK AW, BROWDER ES: Function of posterior columns in man. *Arch Neurol* 12:72, 1965.

CORKIN S: Tactually guided maze learning in man: Effects of unilateral cortical excision and bilateral hippocampal lesions. *Neuropsychologia* 3:339, 1965.

———— et al: Effects of different cortical excisions on sensory thresholds in man. *Trans Am Neurol Assoc* 89:112, 1964.

HEAD H, RIVERS WHR, SHERREN J: The afferent nervous system from a new aspect. *Brain* 28:99, 1905.

HOLMES GM: *Introduction to Clinical Neurology*, 2d ed. Baltimore, Williams & Wilkins, 1952, chaps 8, 9.

KEEGAN JJ, GARRETT, FD: The segmental distribution of the cutaneous nerves in the limbs of man. *Anat Rec* 102:409, 1948.

KIBLER RF, NATHAN PW: A note on warm and cold spots. *Neurology* 10:874, 1960.

MAYO CLINIC: *Clinical Examinations in Neurology*, 4th ed. Philadelphia, Saunders, 1976.

MOUNTCASTLE VG: Central nervous mechanisms in sensation, in Mountcastle VB (ed): *Medical Physiology*, 13th ed. St Louis, Mosby, 1974, vol 1, chaps 9-11.

SEMMES J et al: *Somatosensory Changes after Penetrating Brain Wounds in Man*. Cambridge, Mass, Harvard, 1960.

TROTTER W, DAVIES HM: Experimental studies in the innervation of the skin. *J Physiol* 38:134, 1909.

WALL PD, NOORDENBOS W: Sensory functions which remain in man after complete transection of dorsal columns. *Brain* 100:641, 1977.

WALSHE FMR: The anatomy and physiology of cutaneous sensibility: A critical review. *Brain* 65:48, 1942.

CHAPTER 9

HEADACHE AND OTHER CRANIOFACIAL PAINS

Of all the painful states to which humans are prey, headache is undoubtedly the most frequent. In fact, there are so many vexatious cases of headache in every medical center that it has become necessary to have special headache clinics where physicians with extensive experience in this problem may direct diagnostic study and therapy. Of course, many headaches are due to medical rather than neurologic diseases; hence the subject is the legitimate concern of the general physician. Yet always there is a question of intracranial disease. Therefore, it is difficult to approach the subject without a knowledge of neurologic medicine.

Why so many pains are centered in the head is a matter of some interest. Several explanations come to mind. For one thing the face and scalp are more richly supplied with pain receptors than many other parts of the body, perhaps in order to protect the precious contents of the skull. Then, too, the nasal and oral passages, the eye, and the ear, all delicate and highly sensitive structures, reside here and need to be protected; when afflicted by disease, each is capable of inducing pain in its own way. Finally, for the intelligent person there is greater concern about what happens to the head than to other parts of the body, since the former carries the risk of cerebral injury. A body without an adequately functioning brain is not of much use.

The term *headache* should encompass all aches and pains located in the head, but in practice its application is restricted to discomfort in the region of the cranial vault. Facial, lingual, and pharyngeal pains are put aside as something different, and are discussed separately in the latter part of this chapter.

GENERAL CONSIDERATIONS

In the introductory chapter on pain, reference was made to the necessity, when dealing with any painful state, of determining its quality, severity, location, duration and time course, and the conditions which produce, exacerbate, or relieve it. When headache is considered in these terms, a certain amount of useful information is obtained, but often less than one might expect. Unfortunately, physical examination of the head itself is seldom useful.

As to the quality of cephalic pain, the patient's description is rarely helpful. In fact, persistent questioning on this point may occasion surprise, for the patient often assumes that the word *headache* should have conveyed enough information to the examiner about the nature of the discomfort. Most headaches, regardless of type, tend to be dull, aching, and not sharply localized, as is usually the case with disease of structures deep to the skin. Seldom does the patient describe the pricking or stinging type of pain that is localized to the skin. When asked to compare the pain to some other sensory experience, the patient may allude to tightness, pressure, bursting, sharpness, or stabbing. The most important datum to be obtained is whether the headache has a throbbing or pulsatile quality, indicating a vascular origin.

Similarly, statements about the intensity of the pain must be accepted with caution, since they reflect as much the patient's attitudes and customary ways of describing symptoms as the true severity of the symptoms. As usual, the bluff, hearty person tends to minimize the discomfort, and the neurotic is more inclined to dramatize it. The degree of incapacity is a better index, especially if the patient is not prone to illness. A severe migraine attack seldom allows performance of the day's work. The pain which awakens the patient from sleep or prevents sleep is also likely to have a demonstrable organic basis. As a rule the most intense cranial pains are those which accompany meningitis and subarachnoid hemorrhage, which have grave implications, or migraine and cluster headaches, which are benign.

Data regarding location of the headache are apt to be more informative. Inflammation of an extracranial artery causes pain localized to the site of the vessel. Lesions of paranasal sinuses, teeth, eyes, and upper cervical vertebrae induce less sharply localized pain but one that is still referred to a certain region. Intracranial lesions in the posterior fossa cause pain in the occipitonuchal region, homolateral if the lesion is one-sided. Supratentorial lesions induce frontotemporal pain, again homolateral to the lesion. Localization, however, may also be deceiving. Pain in the frontal regions may be due to such diverse lesions and mechanisms as sinusitis, thrombosis of the basilar artery, pressure on the tentorium, or increased intracranial pressure. Similarly, although ear pain may signify disease of the ear itself, more often it is referred from other regions, such as cervical muscles, cervical spine, or structures in the posterior fossa.

The *mode of onset, time-intensity curve,* and *duration* of the headache, with respect both to a single attack and to the natural behavior of the headache over a period of years, are also useful data. The headache of bacterial meningitis and that of subarachnoid hemorrhage occurs in a single attack and attains its maximal severity in a matter of minutes (in the case of a ruptured aneurysm) or more gradually, over several hours or days in the case of bacterial meningitis. Single, brief (1- to 2-s) pains in the cranium are presently uninterpretable and are significant only for reason of their benignity. Migraine of the classic type has its onset in the early morning hours or daytime, reaches its peak of severity in a half hour or so, and lasts, unless treated, for a period varying from several hours up to 1 to 2 days, often terminated by sleep. In the life history, a frequency of more than a single attack every few weeks is exceptional. A migrainous patient having several attacks per week usually proves to have a combination of migraine and tension headaches. In contrast, the nightly occurrence of unilateral temporoorbital pain 2 to 3 h after falling asleep, over a period of several weeks to months, is typical of cluster headache. Usually it dissipates within 30 to 60 min. The headache of intracranial tumor may come

at any time of day or night, may interrupt sleep, vary in intensity, and last a few minutes to hours. Tension headaches may persist, with varying intensity, for weeks to months or even longer.

The more or less constant relationship of headache to certain biologic events and also to environmental changes must always be noted. Headaches that occur regularly in the premenstrual period in relation to oliguria and edema are usually generalized and mild in degree ("premenstrual tension"), but attacks of migraine may occur at this time. The headaches of cervical arthritis are most typically intense after a period of inactivity, and the first movements of the neck are stiff and painful. Hypertensive headaches, like those of cerebral tumor, tend to occur early in the morning; as with all vascular headaches, excitement and tension may provoke them. Headache from infection of nasal sinuses may appear, with clocklike regularity, upon awakening or in midmorning, and is characteristically worsened by stooping and changes in atmospheric pressure. Eyestrain headaches naturally follow prolonged use of the eyes, as in reading, peering for a long time against glaring headlights, or watching a cinema. Alcohol, intense exercise or coughing, and sexual intercourse are known to initiate a special type of bursting headache lasting a few seconds to minutes in certain individuals. Atmospheric cold may evoke pain in the so-called "fibrositic" or "nodular" form of headache or when the underlying condition is arthritic or neuralgic. Anger, excitement, or worry may initiate common migraine in certain disposed persons; this is more typical of common migraine than of the classic type. In other patients migraine occurs several hours after or on the day following a period of intense activity and stress ("weekend migraine").

PAIN-SENSITIVE STRUCTURES AND MECHANISMS OF HEADACHE

Understanding of headache has been greatly augmented by the observations of surgeons during operations on the brain. These observations inform us that the following cranial structures are sensitive to mechanical stimulation: (1) skin, subcutaneous tissue, muscles, arteries, and periosteum of the skull; (2) delicate structures of the eye, the ear, and the nasal cavity; (3) intracranial venous sinuses and their tributary veins; (4) parts of the dura at the base of the brain and the arteries within the dura mater and pia-arachnoid; and (5) the trigeminal, glossopharyngeal, vagus, and first three cervical nerves. The bony skull, much of the pia-arachnoid and dura, and the parenchyma of the brain lack sensitivity. Interestingly, pain is practically the only sensation produced by stimulation of the listed structures.

The pathways whereby sensory stimuli, whatever their source, are conveyed to the central nervous system are the trigeminal nerves for supratentorial structures in the anterior and middle fossae of the skull, and the first three cervical nerves for posterior fossa and infratentorial structures. The ninth and tenth cranial nerves supply part of the posterior fossa and refer the pain to the ear and throat. The tentorium is the border zone between the trigeminal and cervical innervation. The central connections through spinal cord and brainstem to thalamus have been described in the preceding chapter.

The pain of intracranial disease is referred, by a mechanism already discussed, to some part of the cranium lying within the areas supplied by the fifth, ninth, and tenth cranial nerves and the first three cervicals. There may be local tenderness of the scalp at the site of the referred pain. Dental or jaw pain may also have cranial reference. The pain of disease in other parts of the body is not referred to the head, although it may initiate headache by other means.

By analysis of several types of headache, Wolff and his colleagues have demonstrated that most "spontaneous" cranial pains can be traced to the operation of one or more of the following mechanisms:

1. Distention, traction, and dilatation of the intracranial or extracranial arteries

2. Traction or displacement of large intracranial veins or the dural envelopes in which they lie

3. Compression, traction, or inflammation of sensory cranial and spinal nerves

4. Voluntary or involuntary spasm and possibly interstitial inflammation of cranial and cervical muscles

5. Meningeal irritation and raised intracranial pressure

More specifically, intracranial mass lesions cause headache only if in a position to deform, displace, or exert traction on vessels and dural structures at the base of the brain, and this may happen long before intracranial pressure rises. In fact the artificial induction of high intraspinal and intracranial pressure by the subarachnoid or intraventricular injection of sterile saline solution does not result in headache. Some have interpreted this to mean that raised intracranial pressure does not cause headache, a conclusion which is called into question by the demonstrable relief of headache by lumbar puncture and lowering the cerebrospinal fluid (CSF) pressure in some patients. Actually, most patients with high intracranial pressure complain of bioccipital and bifrontal headache that fluctuates in severity, probably

because of traction on vessels or dura. As to localization, the pain follows the patterns mentioned above; lesions deflecting the falx or pressing on the superior longitudinal or straight sinuses induce pain behind or above the eye; if the lateral part of the lateral sinus is involved, the pain is felt in the ear. Displacement of the tentorium elicits pain in the supraorbital region.

Dilatation of the temporal arteries in the scalp with stretching of surrounding sensitive structures is believed to be the mechanism of most of the pain of migraine. Extracranial temporal and occipital arteries, when involved in giant-cell arteritis (cranial or "temporal" arteritis), give rise to severe, persistent headache, at first localized and then more diffuse. Evolving atherosclerotic thrombosis of internal carotid, anterior, and middle cerebral arteries is sometimes accompanied by pain in the forehead or temple; with vertebral artery thrombosis, the pain is postauricular, and basilar artery thrombosis causes pain to be projected to the occiput and sometimes to the forehead.

Infection or *blockage of paranasal sinuses* is accompanied by pain, usually over the maxillary sinuses or in the forehead. Pain from the ethmoid and sphenoid sinuses is localized around the eyes on one or both sides, or in the vertex (especially in disease of the sphenoid sinus) or other part of the cranium. The mechanism in these cases involves changes in pressure and irritation of pain-sensitive sinus walls. Usually it is associated with tenderness of the skin in the same distribution. Sinus pain may have two remarkable properties: (1) when throbbing, it may be abolished by compressing the carotid artery on the same side, and (2) it recurs and subsides periodically, depending on the drainage. With frontal and ethmoidal sinusitis, the pain is worse on awakening and gradually subsides when the person is upright; the opposite pertains with maxillary and sphenoidal sinusitis. These relationships are believed to disclose their mechanism; pain is ascribed to filling of the sinuses and its relief to their emptying, induced by the dependent position of the ostia. Stooping intensifies the pain by causing changes in pressure, as does blowing the nose, sometimes; during air flights both earache and sinus headache tend to occur on descent, when the relative pressure in the blocked viscus falls. Sympathomimetic drugs such as phenylephrine hydrochloride, which reduce swelling and congestion, tend to relieve the pain. However, the pain may persist after all purulent secretions have disappeared, probably because of blockage of the orifice by boggy membranes and a vacuum or suction effect on the sensitive sinus wall (*vacuum sinus headaches*). The condition is relieved when aeration is restored.

Headache of ocular origin, located as a rule in the orbit, forehead, or temple, is of steady, aching type and tends to follow prolonged use of the eyes in close work. The main faults are hypermetropia and astigmatism (rarely myopia), which result in sustained contraction of extraocular as well as frontal, temporal, and even occipital muscles. Correction of the refractive error abolishes the headache. Traction on the extraocular muscles and on the iris during eye surgery will evoke pain. Another mechanism is involved in iridocyclitis or in acute glaucoma, in which raised intraocular pressure causes steady, aching pain in the region of the eye. When intense, it may radiate throughout the distribution of the ophthalmic division of the trigeminal nerve. As for ocular pain in general, it is important that the eyes be refracted, but eyestrain is probably not as frequent a cause as one would expect from the wholesale dispensing of spectacles for its relief.

The headaches accompanying disease of ligaments, muscles, and apophyseal joints in the upper part of the spine, which are referred to the occiput and nape of the neck on the same side, can be reproduced in part by the injection of hypertonic saline solution into these structures. Such pains are especially frequent in late life, because of rheumatoid and hypertrophic arthritis, and tend also to occur after whiplash injuries or other forms of sudden flexion, extension, or torsion of the head on the neck. If the pain is arthritic in origin, the first movements after being still for some hours are both stiff and painful. The headache of myofibrositis, evidenced by tender nodules near the cranial insertion of cervical and other muscles, is a questionable entity. There are no pathologic data as to the nature of these vaguely palpable lesions, and it is uncertain whether the pain actually arises in them. They may represent only the deep tenderness felt in the region of referred pain or the involuntary secondary protective spasm of muscles. Characteristically, the pain is steady (nonthrobbing) and spreads from one to both sides of the head. Exposure to cold or draft may precipitate it. Though severe at times, it seldom prevents sleep. Massage of muscles, heat, and injection of the tender spots with local anesthetic have unpredictable effects but relieve the pain in some cases.

The *headache of meningeal irritation* (infection or hemorrhage) is of acute onset, severe, generalized, deepseated, constant, and associated with stiffness of the neck on bending forward. It has been ascribed by some authorities to increased intracranial pressure. Indeed the withdrawal of CSF may afford some relief. But dilatation and congestion of inflamed meningeal vessels and the chemical irritation of nerve endings in the meninges must also be factors in the production of pain.

Lumbar puncture headache, which is characterized by a steady occipital-nuchal pain but also by frontal pain coming on a few minutes after arising from a recumbent position and relieved within a few minutes by lying down, has as its cause a persistent leakage of CSF into the lumbar tissues through the needle tract. The CSF pressure is low (often zero in the lateral decubitus position), and the injection of sterile isotonic saline solution intrathecally relieves the headache. Usually this type of headache is increased by compression of the jugular veins and unaffected by digital obliteration of one carotid artery. It seems probable that in the upright position a low intraspinal and negative intracranial pressure exert traction on dural attachments and dural sinuses by caudal displacement of the brain. Understandably, then, headache following cisternal puncture is rare. As soon as the leakage of CSF stops and CSF pressure is restored (usually from a few days to a week), the headache disappears. "Spontaneous" low-pressure headache may follow a sneeze or strain, presumably because of rupture of the spinal arachnoid along a nerve root (see Chap. 29).

Headaches that are aggravated by lying down occur with chronic subdural hematoma and tumors, especially in the posterior fossa of the skull.

The throbbing or steady headache which accompanies febrile illnesses, is probably vascular in origin. It may be generalized or predominate in the frontal or occipital regions and is much like histamine headache in being relieved on one side by carotid artery compression and on both sides by jugular vein compression or the subarachnoid injection of saline solution. It is increased by shaking the head. It seems probable that the increased pulsation of meningeal vessels stretches painsensitive structures around the base of the brain. In certain cases the pain may be lessened by compression of temporal arteries, and in these cases a component of the headache seems to be derived from the walls of extracranial arteries, as in migraine.

PRINCIPAL VARIETIES OF HEADACHE

There is little difficulty in recognizing the headache of glaucoma, purulent sinusitis, bacterial meningitis, and brain tumor; a fuller account of these types of headache will be found where the underlying diseases are described in later sections of the book. It is when headache is chronic, recurrent, and unattended by other important signs of disease that the physician faces one of his most difficult medical problems.

The following types of headaches should then be considered.

MIGRAINE

Migraine is a familial disorder characterized by periodic, commonly unilateral, throbbing headaches which begin in childhood, adolescence, or early adult life and recur with diminishing frequency during advancing years.

Two closely related clinical syndromes have been identified. The first is called "classic," "neurologic," or "typical" migraine; the second "common," or "atypical." The typical syndrome is ushered in by a disturbance of neurologic function (photopsia, teichopsia, hemianopia or central blindness, hemiparesthetic disturbance, slight speech abnormality or aphasia, or hemiparesis), followed in a few minutes by hemicranial or, occasionally, bilateral headache, nausea, and vomiting, all of which last for hours or as long as a day or two. The other syndrome is characterized by an unheralded onset of hemicranial or generalized headache with or without nausea and vomiting but following the same temporal pattern. Both headache syndromes usually respond to ergotamine, if administered early in the attack. The genetic nature of typical migraine is evidenced by occurrence in several members of the family of the same and successive generations in 60 to 80 percent of cases; a family history is less frequently elicited in atypical migraine, perhaps because diagnosis is less certain.

Neurologic migraine frequently has its onset soon after awakening, but may occur at any time of day. The patient may have a vague premonition of an attack. Then abruptly there is a disturbance of vision consisting usually of unformed flashes of light (photopsia) or dazzling zigzag lines (fortification spectra or teichopsia), which give way within minutes to scotomatous defects; usually they are bilateral and often homonymous (involving corresponding parts of the field of vision of each eye). Soon thereafter, numbness and tingling of lips, face, hand (on one or both sides), slight confusion of thinking, weakness of an arm or leg, mild aphasia, dizziness and uncertainty of gait, or drowsiness (rarely coma) are added to the clinical picture. Only one or a few of these neurologic phenomena are present in any given patient, and they tend to occur in the same combination in each attack. If the weakness or numbness spreads from one part of the body to another or one symptom follows another, it does so *slowly* in a period of minutes (not in seconds, as in a seizure). These symptoms last 5

to 15 min, and as they begin to recede they are followed by a unilateral throbbing headache (usually on the side of the cerebral disturbance), which slowly increases in intensity. At its peak, in an hour or so, the patient is forced to lie down and to shun light and noise, and nausea and vomiting may occur. The headache lasts hours or a day or two and is always the most unpleasant feature of the illness.

Much variation occurs. The headache may accompany rather than follow the neurologic abnormalities. Though typically hemicranial (the word *migraine* is said to be derived from *megrim,* meaning hemicrania), the pain may be frontal, temporal, or generalized. Milder forms of migraine, especially if partially controlled by medication, do not force withdrawal from accustomed activities. Any one of the three principal components—neurologic abnormality, headache, or vomiting—may be absent. With advancing age, there is a tendency for the headache and vomiting to become less severe, finally leaving only the neurologic abnormality that recurs with decreasing frequency. The latter is also subject to variation. Although visual disturbances are by far the most common manifestation, they differ in detail from patient to patient; numbness and tingling of the lips and the fingers of one hand are probably next in frequency, followed by transient aphasia or a thickness of speech and hemiparesis.

A relatively uncommon variant of the migraine syndrome has been described by Bickerstaff. The patients, usually young women with a family history of migraine, first develop visual phenomena, like those of typical migraine, except that they occupy the whole of both visual fields. This stage is rapidly followed by vertigo, staggering, dysarthria, and tingling in both hands and feet and sometimes around both sides of the mouth. Exceptionally there is quadriplegia. These symptoms last 10 to 30 min and are followed by headache, which is usually occipital. In some patients, at the stage when the headache is likely to begin, there is a transient disturbance of consciousness. In all respects but their transience, the symptoms closely resemble those due to lesions in the territory of the basilar-posterior cerebral arteries—hence the name *basilar-artery migraine.*

Recurrent unilateral headaches associated with extraocular muscle palsies have been called *ophthalmoplegic migraine.* A transient third nerve palsy with ptosis is the usual picture; rarely, the sixth nerve is affected. Mental disturbances may appear: irritability or depression, or an episode of mental confusion, which is the

Table 9-1
Common types of headache

Type	Site	Age and sex	Clinical characteristics	Diurnal pattern	Life profile	Provoking factors	Associated features	Treatment
Common migraine	Frontotemporal Uni- or bilateral	Children, young to middle-aged adults, more common in women	Throbbing; worse behind one eye or ear Becomes dull ache and generalized Sensitive scalp	Upon awakening or later in day Duration: hours to 1–2 days	Irregular intervals, weeks to months Tends to decrease in middle age and during pregnancy	Bright light, noise, tension, alcohol Relieved by darkness and sleep	Nausea and vomiting in some cases	Ergotamine and phenergan at onset Propranolol or methysergide for prevention
"Neurologic" migraine	Same as above	Same as above	Same as above Family history frequent	Same as above	Same as above	Same as above	Scintillating lights, blindness and scotomas Unilateral numbness and weakness Disturbed speech Vertigo Confusion	Same as above
Cluster (histamine headache, migrainous neuralgia)	Orbital- temporal Unilateral	Adolescent and adult males (80–90%)	Intense, nonthrobbing pain, unilateral	Usually nocturnal, one or more hours after falling asleep Occasionally diurnal	Nightly for several weeks to months Recurrence after many months or years	Alcohol in some	Lacrimation Stuffed nostril Rhinorrhea Injected conjunctivum	Ergotamine at bedtime Amitriptyline Methysergide and corticosteroids in recalcitrant cases

Table 9-1 (continued)
Common types of headache

Type	Site	Age and sex	Clinical characteristics	Diurnal pattern	Life profile	Provoking factors	Associated features	Treatment
Tension headaches	Generalized	Mainly adults, both sexes	Pressure (nonthrobbing), tightness, aching	Continuous, variable intensity, for days, weeks, or months	One or more periods of months to years	Fatigue and nervous strain Fear of brain tumor	Depression, worry, anxiety, insomnia	Antianxiety and antidepressant drugs
Meningeal irritation (meningitis, subarachnoid hemorrhage)	Generalized, or bioccipital or bifrontal	Any age, both sexes	Intense, steady deep pain, may be worse in neck	Duration: days to a week or more	Single episode	None	Neck stiff on forward bending Kernig and Brudzinski signs	For meningitis or bleeding (see text)
Brain tumor	Unilateral or generalized	Any age, both sexes	Variable intensity May awaken patient Steady pain	Lasts minutes to hours; increasing severity	Once in a lifetime: weeks to months	None Sometimes position	Papilledema Vomiting Impaired mentation Seizures Focal signs	Corticosteroids Mannitol Treatment of tumor
Temporal arteritis	Unilateral, temporal, or occipital	Over 50 years, either sex	Throbbing, then persistent aching and burning, arteries thickened and tender	Intermittent, then continuous	Persists for weeks to a few months	None	Loss of vision Polymyalgia rheumatica Fever, weight loss, increased sedimentation rate	Corticosteroids

more common. A particularly vexing variant occurs in a child or adolescent who, after a trivial head injury, may lose sight, suffer severe headache, or be plunged into a state of confusion with belligerent and irrational behavior that lasts for hours or several days before clearing. Another migraine variant in the child is episodic vertigo and staggering ("paroxysmal dysequilibrium") followed by headache (Watson and Steele).

There is also a state known as *hemiplegic migraine* where an infant, child or adult has episodes of unilateral paralysis that may long outlast the headache. Several families have been described in which this condition was inherited as an autosomal dominant trait (familial hemiplegic migraine). Instances of this disorder may account for some of the inexplicable strokes in young women. We have seen several infants and children from 6 months to a few years of age who have had attacks of hemiplegia, first on one side then the other, every few weeks. Recovery was complete, and four-vessel arteriography in one child, after more than 70 attacks, was normal. The mode of onset and lack of seizures stamped the illness as vascular, but its relationship to neurologic migraine remains an open question.

The attacks, instead of beginning in childhood and recurring in the usual fashion every few weeks or months with diminishing frequency in middle and late adult years, may have their onset in the latter periods or suddenly increase in frequency during the menopause or when hypertension and vascular disease develop. Some of the transient hemianesthetic or hemiplegic strokes of late life may be of migrainous origin; Fisher has provided some documentation of this hypothesis. In some individuals the migraine, for unaccountable reasons, may increase in frequency for several months. As many as three or four attacks may occur each week, leaving the scalp continuously tender. Rarely, the focal neurologic symptoms may be prolonged or constantly recurrent for days or weeks on end. This has been referred to as "status migrainosus," but again, the relationship of this disorder to migraine is uncertain.

Rarely, neurologic symptoms, instead of being transitory, may leave a permanent deficit (e.g., a homonymous visual field defect) like an ischemic stroke. Couch and Hassanein have found an increase in platelet aggregability in migraine patients, especially during an attack of headache, and they suggest that this abnormality may be responsible for the strokes that complicate migraine. The use of hormones to prevent pregnancy has increased the frequency and severity of migraine and in

several reported instances has resulted in a permanent neurologic deficit. The recent report by Dorfman et al., in which cerebral infarction was revealed by CT scan in four young adults (16 to 32 years) with migraine, suggests that this complication may be more prevalent than is generally appreciated.

Between attacks the migrainous patient is normal. For a time, when psychosomatic medicine was much in vogue, there was insistence on a migrainous personality, characterized by tenseness, rigidity in thinking, meticulousness, and perfectionism. The migrainous attack was said to occur often during the "let-down period," after many days of hard work or stress. Further analyses, however, have not established a particular personality type in migrainous patients. Moreover, the fact that the headaches may begin in early childhood, when the personality is relatively amorphous, would argue against this idea. Further, the temporal relations between headache and the day's or week's activities have not proved to be consistent.

Migraine is prevalent, found in an estimated 3 to 5 percent of the general population; the incidence in females is about twice that in males, and the headaches tend to occur during the period of premenstrual tension and fluid retention. The attacks usually cease during pregnancy, and estrogens and progesterone may increase their frequency. A considerable number of patients link their attacks to certain articles of diet, particularly chocolate, fatty foods, oranges, tomatoes, and onions. Alcohol regularly provokes an attack in some persons. There is no clear relationship, despite many statements to the contrary, between migraine and psychoneurosis. The relationship to epilepsy is also unclear; the incidence of seizures is slightly higher in migrainous patients and their relatives than in the general population.

During an attack, the electroencephalogram reveals a nonspecific decrease of wave frequency in one-third to one-half of all patients. Cerebral circulation has been found by blood-flow studies to be slowed early in the attack. Vasodilatation and excessive pulsation of branches of the *external carotid artery* have been observed during the headache. Further, as the pulsation decreases, either spontaneously or after the administration of ergotamine, the headache disappears. Vasoconstriction of cerebral arteries was early postulated as the basis of the neurologic symptoms; decreased filling of the internal carotid artery branches has been confirmed in at least one chance carotid arteriogram and has been inferred from prompt abolition, in some patients, of the visual or neurologic disorder upon the inhalation of amyl nitrite or 10% carbon dioxide, both of which dilate intracranial arteries. Thus the vascular theory of migraine has come to be accepted, supported further by surgical observations that the extracranial arteries can be a source of pain. However, the theory does not explain why the intracranial and extracranial arteries should periodically undergo spasm and dilatation in the migrainous individual, nor does it account for the nausea and vomiting (infrequent in all other headaches except those due to tumor) or the tenderness and swelling of the temporal vessels and surrounding tissues.

A hypothesis has been put forth that the constriction of certain vessels and subsequent hyperemic pulsations are induced by a release of amines such as norepinephrine and epinephrine and of serotonin in individuals whose vessels are peculiarly sensitive. These substances are known to be powerful vasoconstrictors. Some migraine patients during their attack excrete increased amounts of the terminal metabolites of the catecholamines, particularly 5-hydroxyindoleacetic acid (5-HIAA), derived from serotonin, and of vanillylmandelic acid (VMA), a product of norepinephrine and epinephrine. A corresponding reduction in platelet serotonin levels at the onset of migraine and in platelet monoamine oxidase activity has also been detected. Other observations in line with this are that (1) reserpine, which reduces the level of serotonin in platelets, brain, and other tissues, may provoke migraine in susceptible persons but not in normal individuals, (2) the injection of serotonin relieves both spontaneous and induced migraine attacks, and (3) serotonin antagonists such as cyproheptadine, pizotifen, and methysergide may prevent attacks. These agents, it is postulated, protect against the cephalalgia induced by serotonin that is released from the brain and sequestered in blood vessel walls. However, the catecholamine-serotonin hypothesis does not explain the paroxysmal nature of the headache or its unilaterality. It is also difficult to reconcile the aforementioned data with the finding that during a migraine headache a polypeptide with some of the properties of bradykinin (one of the plasma kinins) not only can be aspirated from the tissue around the dilated scalp arteries but if reinjected at another site will cause increased capillary permeability, pain, and lowered pain threshold in the overlying skin. Its algogenic action is potentiated by serotonin. Whether this substance, which was called *neurokinin* by Wolff and his colleagues and which may be related to the peptide substance P, escapes secondarily during the phase of vasodilatation or initiates the vasodilatation is not known. Of interest is a recent hypothesis which links the mechanism of migraine to the accumulation of substance P in the walls of extracranial and intracranial arteries. Substance P has been shown to be vasoactive and to excite pain receptors (Chap. 7). Though these data are incomplete and several of the findings need ver-

ification, they do promise to clarify the migraine syndrome and possibly other forms of vascular headache.

Diagnosis Neurologic migraine should occasion no difficulty in diagnosis if the above facts are kept in mind and if a good history is obtained. The difficulties come from a lack of awareness that (1) a progressively unfolding neurologic syndrome may be migrainous in origin, (2) the neurologic disorder may occur without headache, and (3) recurrent headaches, which may be an isolated phenomenon, may take many forms, some of which may prove difficult to distinguish from the other common types of headache.

Some of these problems merit elaboration because of their practical importance.

The neurologic part of the migraine syndrome may resemble focal epilepsy, the clinical effects of an arteriovenous malformation or aneurysm, a transient ischemic attack, or a thrombotic or embolic stroke. It is the pace of the neurologic symptoms of migraine, more than their character, that reliably distinguishes the condition from epilepsy. The evolution of an epileptic aura and spread of focal seizure activity are measured in seconds, for they depend on spreading neural excitation, in contrast to the much slower progression of neurologic migraine, which has been attributed by neurophysiologists to "spreading depression"—a phenomenon in which waves of inhibition move across the cerebral cortex at a rate of about 3 mm/min, and which, in migraine, is presumably triggered by vasoconstriction.

Ophthalmoplegic migraine will always suggest a carotid aneurysm, but in very few cases has carotid arteriography revealed such an abnormality. There have been many claims that the habitual occurrence of migraine on the same side of the head increases the likelihood of an underlying vascular malformation, but studies of numerous cases, both of migraine and of vascular malformations, indicate that the association between these two disorders is only slightly greater than could be accounted for by chance. Nevertheless, arteriovenous malformation is an acknowledged cause of recurrent headache, and the latter may be frequent and troublesome for years before the malformation is discovered. In more than 200 such patients seen by the authors, the headaches, though often of throbbing type, usually do not have the other features of either migraine or cluster headache.

A special problem relates to paroxysms of throbbing headache, not hemicranial in distribution, not preceded by a neurologic aura, and not accounted for by other known cause. Are they examples of common (non-neurologic) migraine or of some other cephalalgia? Unfortunately, since diagnosis depends on the interpretation of the patient's symptoms and since there is as yet no valid confirmatory laboratory test, the controversy as to where migraine begins and ends is of the armchair type. Favoring the diagnosis of migraine are lifelong history, childhood onset, positive family history, and response of the headache to ergotamine.

A variety of episodic attacks have been described as migraine equivalents: attacks of abdominal pain with nausea, vomiting, and diarrhea; pain localized in the thorax, pelvis, and extremities; bouts of fever; transient disturbances in mood (psychic equivalents); or recurrent nocturnal orbital (cluster) headache. The only advantage of considering such attacks as migrainous is that this view protects some patients from unnecessary diagnostic procedures and surgical intervention, but it may also prevent necessary surgery.

CLUSTER HEADACHE

This type of headache is also called *paroxysmal nocturnal cephalgia, migrainous neuralgia,* and *(Horton's) histamine cephalgia.* It occurs predominantly in young adult men and is characterized by a constant, unilateral orbital localization with onset usually 2 or 3 h after falling asleep; it is less frequent during the waking hours. The pain is felt deep in and around the eye, is intense and nonthrobbing as a rule, and often radiates into the forehead, temple, and cheek. Associated phenomena are a blocked nostril followed by rhinorrhea, nausea, injected conjunctivum, and occasionally miosis, ptosis, flush and edema of the cheek, all lasting for 10 min to 2 h. The homolateral temporal artery may become prominent and tender during an attack, and the skin over the scalp and face may be hyperalgesic. The pain of a given attack may leave as rapidly as it began or fade away gradually. It tends to recur nightly or several times during the night and day for a period of 2 to 8 weeks, sometimes much longer, followed by complete freedom for many months or even years (hence the term *cluster*). Almost always the same orbit is involved during a bout of headaches as well as in recurring bouts. A similar type of headache may occasionally occur in the postauricular or occipital areas. During the period of freedom, alcohol, which commonly precipitates cluster headaches, no longer has the capacity to do so.

The picture of cluster headache is usually so characteristic that it cannot be confused with any other disease, though to those unfamiliar with it a diagnosis of migraine, trigeminal neuralgia, carotid aneurysm, brain tumor, or sinusitis may be entertained. Appropriate investigations (CT scan with contrast, carotid arteriography) will always exclude the latter conditions, but are rarely necessary. To be distinguished also is the *paratrigeminal syndrome of Raeder,* which consists of pain in the distribution of the ophthalmic and maxillary divisions of the fifth nerve, in association with ocular sympathetic paralysis (ptosis and miosis) but with preservation of sweating. An unpleasant disturbance of taste has been noted in some patients. Many of the cases of paroxysmal pain behind the eye or nose or in the upper jaw or temple, associated with blocking of the nostril or lacrimation and described under the titles of sphenopalatine (Sluder's), petrosal, vidian, and ciliary (Charlin's or Harris') neuralgia, probably represent instances of cluster headache or variants thereof. There is no evidence to support the separation of these neuralgias as distinct entities.

The relationship of the cluster headache to migraine remains conjectural. No doubt certain headaches have some of the characteristics of both migraine and cluster headaches (hence the term migrainous neuralgia). Lance and others, however, have pointed out important differences: flushing of the face on the side of a cluster headache and pallor in migraine; increased intraocular pressure in cluster headache, normal in migraine; and increased skin temperature over the forehead, temple, and cheek in cluster headache, decreased in migraine.

The fact that cluster headache could be reproduced by the intravenous injection of 0.1 mg histamine (an early experimental device for studying the mechanism of headache) led to the notion, popular for many years, that this form of headache was caused by the spontaneous release of histamine, and to a form of treatment which consisted of "desensitizing" the patient by slow intravenous injections of this drug, given daily for several weeks. Experience has shown that this form of treatment accomplishes nothing more than temporization; and it can be pointed out that the intravenous injection of histamine induces or worsens many forms of focal or generalized headache (due to fever, trauma, brain tumor) that are dependent upon stretching of pain-sensitive tissue around the vessels derived from the internal carotid artery.

Chronic paroxysmal hemicrania is the name given by Sjaastad and Dale to a unilateral headache syndrome that resembles cluster headache in some respects but has several distinctive features. The headaches are paroxysmal and of short duration (20 to 30 min), invariably affect the temporoorbital region of one side, and are accompanied by conjunctival hyperemia, rhinorrhea and a partial Horner's syndrome. Unlike cluster headache, however, the paroxysms occur many times each day, recur daily for years on end (the patient of Price and Posner had an average of 16 attacks daily for more than 40 years) and, most importantly, respond dramatically to the administration of indomethacin.

TENSION HEADACHES

This headache is usually bilateral, often with occipital-nuchal, temporal, or frontal localization, or with diffuse extension over the top of the cranium. The pain is described as dull and aching, but close questioning may uncover other sensations, such as fullness, tightness, or pressure (as if the head is surrounded by a band or a vise), on which waves of aching pain are engrafted. The onset of a given attack is more gradual than in migraine, and the headache, once established, may persist unremittingly for weeks, months, or even years. In fact, this is the only type of headache that exhibits the peculiarity of being absolutely continuous day and night for long periods of time. Although sleep is usually undisturbed, the headache is present when the patient awakens or develops soon afterward, and the common analgesic remedies have no beneficial effect unless the pain is intense.

Tension headaches are more common in women than in men. Unlike migraine, they infrequently begin in childhood or adolescence but are more likely to occur in middle age and coincide with anxiety and depression in the trying times of life. Many premenstrual headaches are of this type and there is an increased incidence of tension headache at the menopause. Migraine and traumatic headaches may be complicated by tension headache, which, because of its persistence, often arouses fears of a brain tumor. However, as Patten points out, not more than one or two patients out of every thousand with tension headaches will be found to harbor an intracranial tumor.

As to mechanism, the ascription of tension headache to sustained muscle contraction is only a partial explanation. Many persons persistently frown or clench their teeth but do not develop tension headaches. The continuous pressing quality of tension headache, at times when the patient is relaxed, hardly seems attributable to continuous muscle activity. Moreover, it must be remembered that all types of headache in their advanced stages may give rise to muscle tension and that this is of an aching rather than a pressure type.

HEADACHE AND OTHER CRANIOFACIAL PAIN WITH PSYCHIATRIC DISEASE

When psychiatric symptoms are searched for in patients with headache, it is evident that the majority of those with anxiety neurosis, hysteria, obsessive-compulsive neurosis, and various forms of depressive illness will complain of headache of the tension type. As a corollary, psychological studies of groups of patients with tension headache have revealed prominent symptoms of anxiety, hypochondriasis, and depression. In our outpatient clinics, the most common cause of generalized intractable headache, both in adolescents and adults, is depression or anxiety in one of its several forms.

The authors have noted that among seriously ill psychiatric patients many have frequent headaches that are not of the tension type. These patients report unilateral or generalized throbbing cephalic pain lasting for hours every day or two. The nature of these headaches, which in some instances resemble common migraine, is unsettled. As the psychiatric symptoms subside, the headaches usually disappear.

Odd cephalic pains, e.g., boring pain, a sensation of having a nail driven into the head ("clavus hystericus"), may occur in hysteria and raise perplexing problems in diagnosis. The bizarre character of these pains, their persistence in the face of every known therapy, the absence of other signs of disease, and the presence of other manifestations of hysteria provide the basis for correct diagnosis (see Chap. 53).

TRAUMATIC HEADACHE

Severe, chronic, continuous or intermittent headaches appear as the cardinal symptom of several posttraumatic syndromes, separable in each instance from the headache that immediately follows head injury (i.e., that of scalp laceration and cerebral contusion with blood in the CSF and increased intracranial pressure) and that lasts several days or a week or two.

The headache of chronic subdural hematoma is deep-seated, steady, unilateral or generalized, and is accompanied by drowsiness, confusion, stupor, coma, and hemiparesis. The head injury may have been minor and forgotten by the patient and family. Typically the headache and other symptoms increase in frequency and severity over several weeks or months. Diagnosis is established by arteriography or CT scan.

Headache is a prominent feature of a complex

syndrome comprised of giddiness, fatigability, insomnia, nervousness, trembling, irritability, inability to concentrate, and tearfulness (*posttraumatic nervous instability*). This type of headache and associated symptoms are described fully in Chap. 34, "Craniocerebral Trauma."

Tenderness and aching pain sharply localized to the scar of the scalp laceration represent in all probability a different problem, raising the question of a *traumatic neuralgia*. With *whiplash injuries* to the neck, unilateral or bilateral retroauricular or occipital pain occurs, due usually to stretching or tearing of muscles at the occipitonuchal junction. Much less frequently, cervical intervertebral disks and roots are involved.

Under the heading of *posttraumatic dysautonomic cephalalgia*, Vijayan and Dreyfus have described severe, episodic, throbbing, unilateral headaches, accompanied by ipsilateral mydriasis and excessive sweating of the face. Between bouts of headache, the patients showed partial ptosis and miosis, as well as pharmacologic evidence of partial sympathetic denervation. The condition followed injury to the soft tissues of the neck in the region of the carotid artery sheath. The headaches did not respond to treatment with ergotamine, but prompt relief was obtained in each case with propranolol, a beta-adrenergic blocking agent.

HEADACHES OF BRAIN TUMOR

Headache is a significant symptom in about two-thirds of all patients with brain tumor (Rooke). Unfortunately the quality of the pain has no specific feature. It tends to be deep-seated, nonthrobbing (or throbbing), and aching or bursting. Attacks last a few minutes to an hour or more and occur once or many times during the day. Activity and frequent change in the position of the head may provoke pain, whereas rest diminishes its frequency. Nocturnal awakening because of pain, although typical, is by no means diagnostic. Unexpected forceful (projectile) vomiting may punctuate the illness in its later stages. As the tumor grows, the pain becomes more frequent and severe and eventually continuous, but there are exceptions. Some headaches are mild and tolerable; others are as agonizing as those of bacterial meningitis and subarachnoid hemorrhage. If unilateral, the headache is nearly always on the same side as the tumor. Pain from supratentorial tumors is felt anterior to the interauricular circumference of the skull; from posterior fossa tumors, behind this line. Bifrontal and bioccipital

headaches, coming on after unilateral headaches, signify the development of increased intracranial pressure.

CRANIAL ARTERITIS (TEMPORAL ARTERITIS, GIANT-CELL ARTERITIS)

This particular type of inflammatory disease of cranial arteries is an important cause of headache in elderly persons. All of our patients have been over 50 years of age and most of them over 60 years. From a state of normal health they develop an increasingly intense throbbing or nonthrobbing pain over the affected arteries, which persists throughout the day and is particularly severe at night. It lasts for several months if untreated. The superficial temporal and other scalp arteries are frequently thickened and tender and without pulsation. Many of the patients feel generally unwell and have lost weight, and some have a low-grade fever. The sedimentation rate is nearly always elevated, and a few patients have a neutrophilic leukocytosis. As many as 15 to 20 percent have generalized aching of muscles, a condition that proves to be *polymyalgia rheumatica*.

The importance of early diagnosis relates to the threat of blindness from thrombosis of the ophthalmic arteries. This may be preceded by several episodes of amaurosis fugax. Ophthalmoplegia may also occur but is less frequent. The intracranial vessels have rarely been affected. Once vision is lost, it is seldom recoverable. For this reason the earliest suspicion of cranial arteritis should lead to hospital admission and cranial artery biopsy; microscopic examination of the offending artery discloses an intense granulomatous or "giant-cell" arteritis. Treatment consists of the administration of prednisone, 45 to 60 mg/day in divided doses over a period of several weeks, with gradual reduction to 10 to 20 mg/day and maintenance at this dosage for several months.

UNUSUAL VARIETIES OF HEADACHE

COUGH AND EXERTIONAL HEADACHE

A patient may complain of transient, severe cranial pain on coughing, sneezing, laughing, heavy lifting, stooping, and straining at stool. Pain is most severe in the front of the head but is also felt in the occipital region and may be unilateral or bilateral. As a rule it follows the initiating action within a few seconds, and lasts a few seconds to a few minutes. Its character is that of a bursting pain and may be of such severity as to cause certain patients to cradle their head in their hands.

This syndrome most often occurs as a benign idiopathic state that may last months to a year or two and then may subside. In a report of 103 patients followed for 3 years or longer, Rooke found that additional symptoms of neurologic disease developed in only ten, and Symonds also attested to the usually benign nature of the condition. Its cause and mechanism have not been determined. During the attack the CSF pressure is normal. Bilateral jugular compression may induce an attack, possibly because of traction on the walls of veins and dural sinuses. In a few instances we have observed this type of headache after lumbar puncture.

As indicated above, patients with cough or strain headache may occasionally be found to have serious intracranial disease; interestingly, this is most often of the posterior fossa and foramen magnum—Arnold-Chiari malformation, platybasia, basilar impression, or tumor. It may be necessary, therefore, to supplement the neurologic examination by CT scan, EEG, radioisotopic scanning, and exceptionally, pneumoencephalography.

We have tried a variety of medications but can report no consistent therapeutic success with any of them.

HEADACHES RELATED TO SEXUAL ACTIVITY

Lance has recently described 21 cases of this type of headache. Two groups were recognized, one in which headache of the tension type developed with sexual excitement, and another in which a severe, throbbing, "explosive" headache occurred at the time of orgasm. The latter headaches were of such abruptness and severity as to suggest a ruptured aneurysm, but the neurological examination was negative in every instance, as was arteriography in seven patients who were subjected to this procedure. In 18 patients who were followed for a period of 2 to 7 years no other neurological symptoms developed. Of course, a hypertensive hemorrhage or rupture of an aneurysm or vascular malformation may occur during the exertion and excitement of sexual intercourse.

ERYTHROCYANOTIC HEADACHE

On rare occasions, an intense, generalized, throbbing headache may occur in conjunction with flushing of the face and hands and numbness of the fingers (erythromelalgia or erythermalgia). Episodes tend to be present on awakening from sound sleep. This condition has been reported in a number of unusual settings: (1) in mastocytosis (infiltration of tissues by mast cells which elaborate histamine, heparin, and serotonin), (2) in carcinoid, (3) with serotonin secreting tumors, (4) with some tumors of pancreatic islets, and (5) with pheochromocytoma.

HEADACHE RELATED TO MEDICAL DISEASES

About 50 percent of patients with *hypertension* complain of headache, but the relationship of the one to the other is not entirely clear. Minor elevations of blood pressure may be a result rather than the cause of tension headaches. Severe hypertension, with diastolic pressure of more than 120 mmHg, is regularly associated with headache, and measures that reduce the blood pressure relieve the headache. However, it is the moderately severe hypertensive individual with frequent severe headaches who gives the most concern. In many of these patients there is undoubtedly an underlying anxiety or tension state or a common migraine syndrome, but in some the headaches defy explanation. According to Wolff, the mechanism of the hypertensive headache is similar to that of migraine, i.e., increased vascular pulsations. The headaches, however, bear no clear relation to peaks in blood pressure. Nevertheless, vasoconstricting drugs such as ergotamine are said to be as effective in the common hypertensive headache as in migraine. Curiously, headaches that occur toward the end of renal dialysis or soon after its completion are associated with a fall in blood pressure as well as a decrease in blood sodium levels and osmolarity. The mechanism of occipital pain that may awaken the hypertensive patient and wear off during the day is not understood.

Experienced physicians are aware of many other conditions in which headache may be a dominant symptom. These include: fevers of any cause, carbon monoxide exposure, chronic lung disease with hypercapnia (headaches often nocturnal), hypothyroidism, Cushing's disease, withdrawal from corticosteroid medication, chronic ingestion of ergotamine, chronic exposure to nitrites, occasionally adrenal insufficiency, aldosterone-producing adrenal tumors, use of the "pill," pheochromocytoma with acute rises in blood pressure, and acute anemia with hemoglobin below 10 g.

TREATMENT

TREATMENT OF MIGRAINE

The time to initiate treatment of an acute attack is during the neurologic disorder or, if the latter is absent, at the beginning of the headache. If the headaches are mild, the patient may already have learned that 0.6 g acetylsalicylic acid repeated once or twice at short intervals or small doses of codeine will suffice to control the pain. For more severe attacks ergotamine tartrate is the most effective form of treatment. This drug can be administered subcutaneously or intramuscularly in a dose of 0.25 to 0.5 mg and repeated in 30 min if necessary, but the parenteral route is rarely practical. The use of uncoated 2-mg tablets of ergotamine tartrate, held under the tongue until dissolved and repeated every half hour until the headache is relieved or until a total of 8 mg is taken, is almost as effective. A single dose of promethazine (Phenergan) 50 mg by mouth should be given with the ergotamine. It relaxes the patient and allays nausea and vomiting. Caffeine, 100 mg, combined with 1 mg of ergotamine (Cafergot) can be taken in tablet form (two at onset of headache and a third in half an hour), or as a rectal suppository (2 mg of ergotamine and 100 mg of caffeine) if vomiting prevents oral administration. When ergotamine is administered early in the attack, the headache will be abolished or reduced in severity and duration in some 90 percent of patients. Once the headache has become intense, ergotamine is of little help, and one must resort to codeine sulfate, 30 mg, or meperidine (Demerol), 50 mg, to control the pain.

Because of the danger of prolonged arterial spasm in patients who have vascular disease or who are pregnant, ergotamine must be used cautiously, if at all. Even in healthy individuals, more than 10 to 15 mg of ergotamine per week is risky. Obviously the use of reserpine and "the pill" should be interdicted, because of the propensity of these agents to induce migraine.

In individuals with frequent migrainous attacks, efforts at prevention are worthwhile. Some success has been obtained with propranolol (Inderal), 20 to 40 mg thrice daily, clonidine, 0.05 mg thrice daily, or indomethacin 150 to 200 mg daily. Also Bellergal, a preparation of ergotamine tartrate, 0.3 mg, phenobarbital, 20 mg, and belladonna alkaloids, 0.1 mg, two or three times a day for a few weeks has been helpful in some patients during periods of frequent migrainous attacks. ACTH (40 units/day) or prednisone (45 mg/day for 3 to 4 weeks) has also been helpful in some difficult refractory cases. Methysergide (Sansert), in doses of 2 to 6 mg daily given for several weeks or months, is probably the most effective agent in the prevention of migraine. Retroperitoneal fibrosis, which is the most serious complication of methysergide administration can be avoided by discontinuing the medication for 3 to 4 weeks after every 5-month course of treatment. In patients who cannot toler-

ate methysergide, pizotifen (Sandomigran) or cyproheptadine (Periactin) may be tried.

Some patients know, or allege to know, that certain items of food induce attacks, and it is obvious enough that they should avoid these foods, if possible. In certain cases it has been claimed that the correction of a refractive error, an elimination diet, or psychotherapy for some personality disorder has relieved migraine. However, this is so exceptional that a cause-and-effect relationship must be doubted, in view of the variability of the disease itself. All experienced physicians appreciate the importance of helping patients rearrange their schedules with a view to controlling tensions and hard-driving ways of living. There is no one way of accomplishing this. In general, long and costly psychotherapy has not been helpful; or at least one can say that there are no substantial data as to its value.

TREATMENT OF NONMIGRAINOUS HEADACHES

The most important measures in the treatment of these headaches are those which uncover and remove the underlying disease or functional disturbance.

For common headaches due to fatigue, stuffy atmosphere, or excessive use of alcohol and tobacco, it is simple enough to advise avoidance of the offending activity or agent, and symptomatic therapy in the form of acetylsalicylic acid, 0.6 g (aspirin or Anacin) will suffice. Some patients who invariably have headache when constipated and hypochondriacs who suffer incapacitating headache, fatigue, and depression whenever bowel elimination does not meet their expectation, are not easily helped. Certainly, simple explanation, an anticonstipation regimen, and drugs which counteract depression (see Chap. 54) are preferable to the continuous use of analgesics. Premenstrual headache, if troublesome, can usually be helped by the use of a diuretic compound for the week preceding the menstrual period and mild analgesic and tranquilizing medications (acetylsalicylic acid, 0.6 g, and diazepam, 5 mg).

Hypertensive headaches respond to agents which lower blood pressure and relieve muscle tension. Chlorothiazide (Diuril), 25 to 50 mg/day, and methyldopa (Aldomet), 500 to 1500 mg/day, when combined with diazepam, 5 mg bid, have given the best results. Meprobamate, 200 mg tid, or chlordiazepoxide (Librium), 5 mg tid, may be administered in place of diazepam. For the morning occipital ache, a capsule containing sodium nitrite, 30 mg, caffeine sodium benzoate, 0.5 g, and acetophenetidin, 0.6 g, has been useful. A simplified method of treating this kind of headache is to supply the caffeine in a cup of strong black coffee and to give acetylsalicylic acid with it. Blocks under the head of the bed may be helpful.

Muscle contraction and other types of tension headaches respond best to massage, relaxation, and the use of one of several drugs which relieve anxiety (phenobarbital, meprobamate, diazepam, or chlordiazepoxide). Simple analgesics such as aspirin may be helpful, but with severe tension headaches, stronger analgesic medication may be needed (codeine or meperidine). Psychotherapy is usually not beneficial in this group of patients.

Nocturnal attacks of cluster headache should be treated with a single dose of ergotamine at bedtime (3 mg orally or 1 mg by injection). In other patients, ergotamine has to be given once or twice during the day, at times when an attack of pain is expected. Some patients have responded to high doses (200 to 300 mg/day) of amitriptyline (Elavil), the larger dose being given at bedtime. For the exceptional cluster, in which headache recurs daily for many months on end, indomethacin, corticosteroids, and methysergide have been used, with variable success. Several recent reports suggest that lithium carbonate (600 mg daily for 1 week and 900 mg daily for 2 weeks more) may be useful in the treatment of the protracted attack.

The patient with posttraumatic nervous instability requires supportive psychotherapy in the form of reassurance and frequent explanation of the benign and transient nature of the symptoms, a program of increasing physical activity, and the use of drugs which allay anxiety and depression. Tender scars from scalp laceration may be treated by the repeated subcutaneous injection of 5 ml of 1% procaine. Settlement of litigation as soon as possible works to the patient's advantage.

Heat, massage, salicylates, and indomethacin (Indocin), or phenylbutazone (Butazolidin) usually effect some improvement in arthritic diseases of the cervical spine which are associated with cervicocranial pain.

Corticosteroids are highly effective in the treatment of cranial arteritis, as has been indicated. The headaches of cranial tumor often respond surprisingly well to large doses of prednisone and similar compounds.

In conclusion, it is well to mention the importance of general hygienic measures. Young physicians in particular are apt to seek a specific therapy for each headache syndrome and to give little thought to the general health of the patient. We have observed that most of the recurrent and chronic headaches are likely to be more severe and disabling whenever the patient becomes nervous, sick, and tired. A well-rounded diet, adequate rest, a reasonable amount of physical exercise, and a balanced view of the sources of daily anxieties and how to

cope with them should be the goal of all therapeutic programs.

OTHER CRANIOFACIAL PAINS

TRIGEMINAL NEURALGIA (TIC DOULOUREUX)

This is a disorder of middle age and later life and consists of excruciating paroxysms of pain in the distribution of the mandibular and maxillary divisions (rarely in the ophthalmic division) of the fifth cranial nerve. The pain seldom lasts more than a few seconds or a minute or two but may be so intense that the patient winces; hence the term *tic*. The paroxysms recur frequently, both day and night, for several weeks at a time. Another characteristic feature is the initiation of pain by obvious stimuli applied to certain areas of the face, lips, or tongue, or by movement of these parts in chewing, talking, or yawning—the so-called trigger zones. Sensory or motor loss in the distribution of the fifth nerve cannot be demonstrated in these cases though there are minor exceptions to this rule. In addition to the paroxysms some of the patients complain of a more or less continuous pain and sensitivity of face, features always regarded as atypical even though not infrequent.

In studying the relationship between stimuli applied to the trigger zone and the paroxysms of pain, it is found that the paroxysms are induced by touch and possibly tickle, rather than by pain or a thermal stimulus. Usually a spatial and temporal summation of impulses is necessary to trigger an attack, which is followed by a refractory period of up to 2 or 3 min. This suggests that the mechanism for the paroxysmal pain involves the nucleus of the spinal tract of the fifth nerve.

The diagnosis of tic douloureux must rest upon the strict clinical criteria enumerated above, and the condition must be distinguished from other forms of facial and cephalic neuralgia and pain arising from diseases of the jaw, teeth, or sinuses. This form of trigeminal neuralgia is usually without assignable cause (*idiopathic*), in contrast to *symptomatic trigeminal neuralgia*, in which paroxysmal facial pain is a manifestation of other neurologic disease. Thus, tic douloureux is occasionally a manifestation of multiple sclerosis (may be bilateral) and rarely of an aneurysm of the basilar artery or of a tumor (acoustic or trigeminal neuroma, meningioma, epidermoid) in the cerebellopontine angle. Each of these disorders may give rise only to pain in the distribution of the fifth nerve, but usually they produce a loss of sensation as well.

The conventional treatment for tic douloureux is alcohol or phenol injection of the affected nerve at the foramen ovale and rotundum or section of the root of the trigeminal nerve between the ganglion and the brainstem. Stereotaxic coagulative lesions of the roots have also been made. Antiepileptic drugs such as phenytoin (Dilantin), and particularly carbamazepine (Tegretol) have been found to suppress or shorten the duration of the attacks. Temporizing and using these drugs may permit a spontaneous remission to occur. Most of the patients with severe pain come to surgery.

GLOSSOPHARYNGEAL NEURALGIA

This syndrome is much less common than trigeminal neuralgia, but resembles the latter in many respects. The pain is intense and paroxysmal; it originates in the throat, approximately in the tonsillar fossa. In some cases the pain is localized in the ear or may radiate from the throat to the ear, implicating the auricular branch of the vagus nerve. For this reason White and Sweet have suggested the term *vagoglossopharyngeal neuralgia*. This is the only craniofacial neuralgia which may be accompanied by bradycardia and even by syncope, presumably because of the triggering of cardiovascular regulatory fibers by afferent pain impulses. Spasms of pain are initiated most commonly by swallowing, but also by talking, chewing, yawning, laughing, etc. There is no demonstrable sensory or motor deficit. Rarely, carcinoma or epithelioma of the oropharyngeal-infracranial region or peritonsillar abscess may give rise to pain clinically indistinguishable from glossopharyngeal neuralgia. A trial of phenytoin or carbamazepine or cocainization of the throat may be useful, but if these are unsuccessful, the glossopharyngeal nerve and upper rootlets of the vagus near the medulla need to be interrupted surgically.

POSTHERPETIC NEURALGIA

Neuralgia associated with a vesicular eruption, due to infection with the virus of herpes zoster, may affect cranial as well as peripheral nerves. In the region of the cranial nerves, two syndromes are frequent: so-called *geniculate herpes* and *ophthalmic herpes*. Both are exceedingly painful in the acute phase of the infection. In the former, herpes of the external auditory meatus and pinna and sometimes of the palate and occipital region, with or without deafness, tinnitus, and vertigo, is com-

bined with facial paralysis. This syndrome, since its original description by Ramsay Hunt, has been generally known as *geniculate herpes,* despite the lack, to this day, of pathologic proof that it depends upon a herpetic lesion of the geniculate ganglion (see Chap. 46). Pain and herpetic eruption due to herpes zoster infection of the gasserian ganglion and the peripheral and central pathways of the trigeminal nerve are practically always limited to the first division (herpes zoster ophthalmicus). We do not recognize a form of zoster infection with facial or other painful states but no cutaneous eruption. The latter will invariably appear within 4 to 5 days after the onset of the pain.

The acute discomfort associated with the herpetic eruption usually subsides after several weeks, or it may linger on for several months. Infrequently, and in the elderly as a rule, the pain becomes chronic and intractable. It is described as a constant burning, with superimposed waves of stabbing pain, and the skin in the territory of the preceding eruption is exquisitely sensitive to the slightest stimuli. This unremitting postherpetic neuralgia of long duration represents one of the most difficult pain problems with which the physician has to deal. Some relief of pain may be provided by massage of the affected areas, infiltration with local anesthesia, and application of a mechanical vibrator or by the administration of phenytoin and carbamazepine. In some patients the pain gradually subsides; others can be managed by administration of antidepressants and tranquilizing agents (amitriptyline, 75 mg at bedtime, and fluphenazine, 1 mg tid, is a particularly useful combination) and strong psychological support. Extensive trigeminal rhizotomy and nucleotomy or other destructive procedures should be avoided, since these surgical measures are not universally successful and may superimpose a diffuse refractory dysesthetic component upon the radicular neuralgia.

OCCIPITAL NEURALGIA

Paroxysmal pain may occasionally occur in the distribution of the greater occipital nerve (suboccipital, occipital, and posterior parietal areas). Pain can be provoked from "trigger zones" in this general territory. Procaine blocks of the occipital nerve, repeated as necessary, usually relieve this disorder. Sectioning of the second and third cervical dorsal roots may be necessary in particularly difficult cases.

CAROTIDYNIA

This term was coined by Temple Fay, in 1927, to designate a special type of cervicofacial pain that could be elicited by pressure on the common carotid arteries of

Table 9-2
Types of facial pain

Type	Site	Clinical characteristics	Aggravating-relieving factors	Associated diseases	Treatment
Trigeminal neuralgia (tic douloureux)	Second and third divisions of trigeminal nerve, unilateral	Men/women = 1:3 Over 50 years Paroxysms (10–30 s) of stabbing, burning pain; persistent for weeks or longer Trigger points No sensory or motor paralysis	Touching trigger points, chewing, smiling, talking, blowing nose, yawning	Idiopathic If in young adults, multiple sclerosis Vascular anomaly Tumor of fifth cranial nerve	Carbamazepine Phenytoin Alcohol injection, coagulation, or surgical section of nerve
Atypical facial neuralgia	Unilateral or bilateral; cheek or angle of cheek and nose; deep in nose	Predominantly female 30–50 years Continuous intolerable pain Mainly maxillary areas	None	Depressive and anxiety states Hysteria Idiopathic	Antidepressant and antianxiety medication
Postzoster neuralgia	Unilateral Usually ophthalmic division of fifth nerve	History of zoster Aching, burning pain; jabs of pain Paresthesiae, slight sensory loss Dermal scars	Contact, movement	Herpes zoster	Carbamazepine, phenytoin, and antidepressants
Costen's syndrome	Unilateral, behind or front of ear, temple, face	Severe aching pain, intensified by chewing Tenderness over temporo-mandibular joints Malocclusion, missing molars	Chewing, pressure over temporo-mandibular joint	Loss of teeth, rheumatoid arthritis	Correction of bite Surgery in some
Tolosa-Hunt syndrome	Unilateral, mainly orbital	Intense sharp, aching pain, associated ophthalmoplegias Pupil inequality, sensory loss over forehead	None	Lesion of cavernous sinus or superior orbital fissure	Surgery; cortico-steroids for granulomatous lesions
Raeder's paratrigeminal syndrome	Unilateral, frontotemporal and maxilla	Intense sharp or aching pain, ptosis, miosis, preserved sweating	None	Tumors, granulomatous lesions, injuries in parasellar region	Depends on type of lesion
"Migrainous neuralgia"	Orbitofrontal, temple, upper jaw, angle of nose and cheek	See cluster headache, Table 9-1	Alcohol in some		Ergotamine
Carotidynia, lower-half headache, sphenopalatine neuralgia, etc.	Unilateral face, ear, jaws, teeth, upper neck	Both sexes, constant dull ache 2–4 h	Compression of common carotid below bi-furcation reproduces pain in some	Occasionally with cranial arteritis, carotid tumor, and cluster headache	Ergotamine acutely; methysergide for prevention

patients with "atypical facial neuralgia," or the so-called lower-half headache of Sluder. Compression of the artery in these patients, at a point just below the bifurcation, produced a dull ache which was referred to the ipsilateral face, ear, jaws, and teeth, or down the neck. Later (1932), Fay showed that pain of this type and distribution could be reproduced by mild faradic stimulation of the carotid artery at and near its bifurcation.

Fay's observations were followed by a number of reports describing the occurrence of spontaneous pain of similar type and radiation, associated with tenderness of the carotid artery at its bifurcation and swelling of the overlying tissues. This syndrome occurs rarely as part of cranial (giant-cell) arteritis and displacement of the carotid artery by tumor and during attacks of cluster headache. Carotidynia is frequently associated with a throbbing headache, indistinguishable from common migraine. In other patients migraine and carotidynia occur separately. Another variant of carotidynia, with a predilection for young adults, has been described by Roseman. This latter syndrome takes the form of recurrent, self-limited attacks, lasting a week or two. During the attack, aggravation of the pain by head movement, chewing, and swallowing is characteristic.

Many patients with carotidynia respond favorably to the administration of ergotamine, methysergide, and other drugs that are effective in the treatment of migraine.

COSTEN'S SYNDROME

This refers to a form of craniofacial pain consequent upon dysfunction of one temporomandibular joint. Malocclusion due to ill-fitting dentures or loss of molar teeth on one side, with loss of the normal masticatory movements, may lead to distortion of and ultimately degenerative changes in the joint and to pain behind or in front of the ear with radiation to the temple and over the face. Management depends upon careful adjustment of the bite by a dental surgeon.

"ATYPICAL" FACIAL PAIN

There remains, after all the classic pain syndromes and all the possible intracranial and local sources of pain from throat, mouth, sinuses, orbit, and carotid vessels have been excluded, a small number of patients with pain in the face for which no cause can be found. These patients are most often young women, who describe the pain as constant and unbearably severe, deep in the face or at the angle of cheek and nose and unresponsive to all varieties of analgesic medication. Because of the failure to identify an organic basis for the pain, one is tempted to attribute it to psychological or emotional factors or to abnormal personality traits; these can rarely be defined, however, and only a small proportion of the patients satisfy the diagnostic criteria for hysteria or depression. Facial pain of this type, like other chronic pain of indeterminate cause, should be managed by the methods outlined in the preceding chapter, and not by thalamotomy, leukotomy, or other forms of destructive cerebral surgery.

OTHER FACIAL PAINS

A number of other types of facial pain syndromes include ciliary, nasociliary, supraorbital, and Sluder's neuralgia. These are vague entities at best, and some are merely different descriptive terms given to pains localized around the eye and nose (see "Cluster Headache" above; also Table 9-2). The Tolosa-Hunt syndrome of pain behind the eye and granulomatous involvement of the ocular nerves is discussed in Chap. 46.

Trigeminal neuritis following dental extractions or oral surgery is another vexing problem. There may be sensory loss in the tongue or lower lip and weakness of the masseter or pterygoid muscle. Eventually the patients recover.

REFERENCES

BICKERSTAFF, ER: Basilar artery migraine. *Lancet* 1:15, 1961.

CLOVER V et al: Transitory decrease in platelet monoamine oxidase activity during migraine attacks. *Lancet* 1:391, 1977.

COUCH JR, HASSANEIN, RS: Platelet aggregability in migraine. *Neurology* 27:843, 1977.

DORFMAN LS, MARSHALL WH, ENZMANN DR: Cerebral infarction and migraine: Clinical and radiologic correlations. *Neurology* 29:317, 1979.

FISHER CM: Late-life migraine accompaniments as a cause of unexplained transient ischemic attacks. *Can J Neurol Sci,* 7:9, 1980.

FRIEDMAN A (ed): *Research and Clinical Studies of Headache.* Baltimore, Williams & Wilkins, 1967.

FROMANTIN M et al: La forme céphalalgique pure du pheochromocytome. *Ann Med Interne* 124:587, 1973.

GURALNICK W, KABAN, LB, MERRILL, RG: Temporomandibular-joint afflictions. *N Engl J Med* 299:123, 1978.

LANCE JW: Headaches related to sexual activity. *J Neurol Neurosurg Psychiatry* 39:1126, 1976.

LANCE JW: *The Mechanism and Management of Headache,* 3d ed. London, Butterworth, 1978.

PATTEN J: *Neurological Differential Diagnosis.* London, Harold Starke, 1977.

PRICE, RW, POSNER JB: Chronic paroxysmal hemicrania: A disabling headache syndrome responding to indomethacin. *Ann Neurol* 3:183, 1978.

RASKIN NH, APPENZELLER O: *Headache*, vol 19: *Major Problems in Internal Medicine.* Philadelphia, Saunders, 1980.

ROOKE, ED: Benign exertional headache. *Med Clin North Am* 52:801, 1968.

ROSEMAN DM: Carotidynia. *Arch Otolaryngol* 85:103, 1967.

SJAASTAD O, DALE I: A new (?) clinical headache entity "chronic paroxysmal hemicrania." *Acta Neurol Scand* 54:140, 1976.

VIJAYAN N, DREYFUS PM: Posttraumatic dysautonomic cephalalgia. *Arch Neurol* 32:649, 1975.

VINKEN PJ, BRUYN GW (eds): *Handbook of Clinical Neurology,* vol. 5: *Headaches and Cranial Neuralgias.* Amsterdam, North-Holland, 1968.

WATSON P, STEELE JC: Paroxysmal dysequilibrium in the migraine syndrome of childhood. *Arch Otolaryngol* 99:177, 1974.

WHITE JC, SWEET WH: *Pain and the Neurosurgeon.* Springfield, Ill, Charles C Thomas, 1969.

WOLFF HG: *Headache and Other Head Pain,* 2d ed. New York, Oxford, 1963.

CHAPTER 10

PAIN IN THE BACK, NECK, AND EXTREMITIES

The diagnosis of pain in these parts of the body often requires the assistance of a neurologist. The task is to determine whether a disease of the spine, intervertebral disks, or articulations has implicated roots and spinal nerves. The primary disease often falls within the province of the orthopedist, rheumatologist, or internist, and a proper study of such cases requires a knowledge of diseases outside the specialty of neurology.

The purpose of including a chapter on this subject in a textbook of neurology is to help the student appreciate the neurologic implications of back and neck pain and to develop a systematic mode of inquiry and method of examination.

Since pains in the lower part of the spine and legs are caused by rather different types of disease than those in the neck, shoulder, and arms, we shall consider them separately.

PAIN IN THE LOWER BACK AND EXTREMITIES

The lower parts of the spine and pelvis, with their massive muscular attachments, are relatively inaccessible to palpation and inspection. Although some physical signs and radiographs are helpful, it is often necessary to depend on the patient's description of the pain (which may not be altogether accurate) and on the patient's behavior during the execution of certain maneuvers, to assess fully the nature of the problem. Seasoned clinicians, for these reasons, have come to appreciate the need of a systematic clinical approach, the description of which will be one of the main purposes of this chapter.

ANATOMY AND PHYSIOLOGY OF THE LOWER PART OF THE BACK

The bony spine is a complex structure, roughly divisible into an anterior and a posterior part. The former consists of a series of cylindric vertebral bodies, articulated by the intervertebral disks and held together by the anterior and posterior longitudinal ligaments. The posterior elements are more delicate and extend from the bodies as pedicles and laminas which form, with the posterior aspects of the bodies, the vertebral canal. Stout transverse and spinous processes project laterally and posteriorly, respectively, and serve as the origins and insertions of the muscles which support and protect the spinal column. The bony processes are also held together by sturdy ligaments, the most important being the ligamentum flavum.

The stability of the spine depends on two types of supporting structures, the ligamentous (passive) and muscular (active). Although the ligamentous structures are quite strong, neither they nor the vertebral body-disk complexes have sufficient integral strength to resist the enormous forces that act on the column, and most of the stability is dependent on the voluntary and reflex contractions of the sacrospinalis, abdominal, glutei maximi, and hamstring muscles.

The vertebral and paravertebral structures derive their innervation from the meningeal branches (also known as recurrent meningeal or sinuvertebral nerves) of the spinal nerves. Pain endings and fibers have been demonstrated in the ligaments, muscles, periosteum of bone, outer layers of the annulus fibrosus, and synovium of the articular facets. The sensory fibers from these structures and sacroiliac and lumbosacral joints join to form the sinuvertebral nerves. These filaments number two to four on each side and are present at every vertebral level. They join the spinal nerves just beyond the point where the latter emerge from the intervertebral foramens. Sensory fibers reenter the vertebral canal via the dorsal root and synapse in the gray matter of the spinal cord; efferent fibers emerge from corresponding segments and extend to the paravertebral muscles through the same nerves. Each of the sinuvertebral nerves receives fibers from a neighboring gray ramus or directly from a thoracic sympathetic ganglion; the sympathetic nerves contribute only to the innervation of blood vessels and appear to play no part in voluntary and reflex movement. However, they do contain sensory fibers.

The parts of the back that possess the greatest freedom of movement, and hence are most frequently subject to injury, are the lumbar and cervical. In addition to the voluntary motions required for bending, twisting, and other movements, many actions of the spine are reflex in nature and are the basis of posture.

GENERAL CLINICAL CONSIDERATIONS

Types of Low-Back Pain Of the several symptoms of disease of the spine (pain, stiffness or limitation of movement, and deformity), pain is of foremost importance by virtue of its frequency and its disabling effects. Four types of pain may be differentiated: local, referred, radicular, and that arising from secondary (protective) muscular spasm. One may identify these several types of pain by the patient's description; reliance is placed mainly on the character of the pain, its location, and the modifying conditions.

Local pain is caused by any pathologic process which impinges upon or irritates sensory endings. Involvement of structures which contain no sensory endings is painless. The substance of the vertebral body may be destroyed by tumor, for example, without evocation of pain, whereas lesions of periosteum, synovial membranes, muscles, annulus fibrosus, and ligaments are often exquisitely painful. Although painful states are often accompanied by swelling of the affected tissues, this is not apparent if a deep structure of the back is the site of disease. Local pain is often described as steady but may be intermittent and subject to variation in position or activity. The pain may be sharp or dull and, although often diffuse, is always felt in or near the affected part of the spine. Often there is involuntary splinting of the corresponding spine segments by paravertebral muscles, and certain movements or postures that alter the position of the injured tissues aggravate or relieve the pain.

Firm pressure or percussion upon superficial structures in the region involved usually evokes tenderness which is of aid in identifying the site of the abnormality.

Referred pain is of two types, that projected from the spine into viscera and other structures lying within the area of the lumbar and upper sacral dermatomes and that projected from the pelvic and abdominal viscera to the spine. Pain due to diseases of the upper part of the lumbar spine is usually referred to the anterior aspects of the thighs and legs. On the other hand, disease in the upper lumbar vertebrae, such as fracture or postmenopausal osteoporosis, will often cause pain across the lower part of the back. This has been attributed to irritation of the superior cluneal nerves, which are derived from the posterior divisions of the first three lumbar spinal nerves and which innervate the superior portions of the buttocks. Pain from the lower part of the lumbar spine is usually referred to the lower buttocks, and is due to irritation of lower spinal nerves which activate the same pool of neurons as posterior thighs and calves. Pain of this type, although of deep, aching quality and rather diffuse, tends at times to be more superficially projected. In general the referred pain parallels in intensity the local pain in the back. In other words, maneuvers which alter local pain have a similar effect on referred pain, though not with such precision and immediacy as in "root pain." Pain from visceral disease usually is felt within the abdomen, flanks, or lumbar region, and may be modified by the state of activity of the viscera. Its character and temporal relationships are those of the particular visceral structure involved, and posture and movement of the back have relatively little effect, either on the local pain or on that referred to the back.

Radicular, or "root," pain has some of the characteristics of referred pain but differs in its greater intensity, distal radiation, circumscription to the territory of a root, and the factors which excite it. The mechanism is distortion, stretching, irritation, or compression of a spinal root, central to the intervertebral foramen. The pain is sharp and often quite intense; it nearly always radiates from a central position near the spine to some part of the lower extremity. It is usually superimposed on the dull ache of referred pain. Cough, sneeze, and strain characteristically evoke this sharp radiating pain, although these maneuvers may also jar or move the spine and enhance local pain. In fact, any action which stretches the nerve, e.g., forward bending with the knees extended or "straight-leg raising" excites radicular pain; and jugular vein compression, which raises intraspinal pressure and may cause a shift in the position of the root, may have a similar effect. Involvement of the fourth and fifth lumbar and first sacral roots, which form the sciatic nerve, causes pain which extends down the posterior aspects of thigh and the postero- and anterolateral aspects of the leg and into the foot in the distribution of this nerve—so-called sciatica. Paresthesias or superficial sensory loss, soreness of the skin, and tenderness in certain regions along the nerve usually accompany radicular pain. Also reflex loss, weakness, atrophy, fascicular twitching, and stasis edema may occur if anterior roots are involved.

Pain resulting from muscular spasm usually occurs in relation to local pain. The spasm is reflexive, to guard the diseased parts against injurious motion. Muscle spasm is associated with many disorders of the low back and can produce distortions of the normal posture. Chronic tension in muscles may give rise to a dull, sometimes cramping ache. One can feel the tautness of the sacrospinalis and gluteal muscles and demonstrate by palpation that the pain is localized to them.

Other pains, often of undetermined origin, are sometimes described by patients with chronic disease of the lower part of the back. Drawing and pulling in the legs, cramping sensation (without involuntary muscle spasm), tearing, throbbing, or jabbing pains, feelings of burning or coldness—like paresthesias and numbness, they should always suggest the possibility of nerve or root disease.

Since it is often difficult to obtain physical or laboratory confirmation of painful disease of the low back, the importance of an accurate history cannot be overemphasized. In addition to assessing the character and location of the pain, one should determine the factors which aggravate and relieve it, its constancy, and its relationship to recumbency and to forward bending, cough, sneeze, and strain. Frequently the most important lead comes from knowledge of the mode of onset and circumstances which initiated the pain. Inasmuch as many painful affections of the back are the result of injury incurred during work or in an accident, the possibility of exaggeration or prolongation of pain for personal reasons, or even of hysteria or malingering, must always be kept in mind.

Much information may be gained by *inspection* of the back, buttocks, and lower extremities in various positions. The normal spine shows a dorsal kyphosis and

lumbar lordosis in the sagittal plane, which in some individuals may be somewhat exaggerated (swayback). In the coronal plane, the spine is normally straight or shows a slight curvature, particularly in females. One should observe the spine closely for excessive curvature, list, flattening of the normal lumbar lordosis, presence of a gibbus (a short, sharp, kyphotic angulation usually indicative of a fracture), pelvic tilt or obliquity, or asymmetry of the paravertebral or gluteal musculature. In severe sciatica one may observe abnormalities of posture of the affected leg, presumably to reduce tension on the irritated nerve.

The next step in the examination is observation of the spine, hips, and legs during certain motions. It is well to remember that no advantage accrues from finding out how much pain the patient can tolerate. It is more important to determine when and under what conditions the pain commences. One looks for limitation of the natural motions of the patient during disrobing and while standing, sitting, and reclining. When standing, the motion of forward bending normally produces flattening and reversal of the lumbar lordotic curve and exaggeration of the dorsal curve. With lesions of the lumbosacral region which involve the posterior ligaments, articular facets, or sacrospinalis muscles, and with ruptured lumbar disks, protective reflexes prevent stretching of these structures. As a consequence, the sacrospinalis muscles remain taut and prevent motion in the lumbar part of the spine. Forward bending then occurs at the hips and at the thoracolumbar junction; also, the patient bends in such a way as to avoid tensing the hamstring muscles and putting undue leverage on the pelvis.

Lateral bending is usually less instructive than forward bending. In unilateral ligamentous or muscular strain, bending to the opposite side aggravates the pain by stretching the damaged tissues. With unilateral *sciatica,* the patient lists to one side and strongly resists bending to the opposite side. When the herniated disk lies lateral to the nerve root and compresses it medially, tension on the root is reduced by bending the trunk away from the lesion; with herniation medial to the root, the patient inclines the trunk to the side of the lesion.

In the sitting position, flexion of the spine can be performed more easily, even to the point of bringing the knees in contact with the chest. The reason for this is that knee flexion relaxes the often tightened hamstring muscles or relieves stretch of the sciatic nerve.

The study of motions in the reclining position yields the same information as study of motions in the standing and sitting positions. With lumbosacral lesions and sciatica, passive lumbar flexion causes little pain and is not limited as long as the hamstrings are relaxed and there is no stretching of the sciatic nerve. With disease of the spine (e.g., arthritis), passive flexion of the hips is free, whereas flexion of the lumbar spine may be impeded and painful. Passive straight-leg raising (possible in normal individuals up to 90° except in those who have unusually tight hamstrings), like forward bending in the standing posture with the legs straight, places the sciatic nerve and its roots under tension, thereby producing pain. It may also cause an anterior rotation of the pelvis around a transverse axis, increasing stress on the lumbosacral joint and thus causing pain if this joint is arthritic or otherwise impaired. Consequently, in diseases of the lumbosacral joints and of the lumbosacral roots, this movement is limited on the affected side and, to a lesser extent, on the opposite side. Lasègue's sign (pain and limitation of movement during elevation of the leg with knee extended) is a useful test of these conditions. Straight raising of the opposite leg may also cause some pain on the affected side, believed by some to be an even more reliable sign of a ruptured disk. There is some evidence that this sign is indicative of a more extensive lesion, such as an extruded disk fragment, rather than a prolapse or protrusion. It is important to remember, however, that the evoked pain is always referred to the diseased side, no matter which leg is elevated.

Hyperextension may be performed with the patient standing or lying prone. If the condition causing back pain is acute, it may be difficult to extend the spine in the standing position. A patient with lumbosacral strain or disk disease (except in the acute phase) can usually extend or hyperextend the spine without aggravation of pain. If there is an active inflammatory process or fracture of the vertebral body or posterior elements, hyperextension may be markedly limited. In some cases of disk disease with thickening of the ligamentum flavum this movement gives rise to pain; and in narrowing of the spinal canal (spondylosis, spondylolisthesis), upright stance and extension produce neurologic symptoms (see below).

Gentle palpation and percussion of the spine are the last steps in the examination. It is preferable to palpate first those regions which are the least likely to evoke pain. At all times the examiner should know what structures are being palpated (see Fig. 10-1). Localized tenderness is seldom pronounced in disease of the spine, because the involved structures are so deep. Nevertheless, tenderness of a spinous process (or jarring by gentle percussion) may indicate the presence of inflammation (as in disk space infection), pathologic fracture, or a disk lesion at the site deep to it.

Tenderness over the costovertebral angle often indicates genitourinary disease, adrenal disease, or an in-

jury to the transverse process of the first or second lumbar vertebra [Fig. 10-1, (1)]. Tenderness on palpation of the paraspinal muscles may signify a strain of muscle attachments or injury to the underlying transverse processes of the lumbar vertebrae.

Upon palpation of the spinous processes it is important to note any deviation in the lateral plane (this may be indicative of fracture or arthritis) or in the anteroposterior plane. A "step-off" forward displacement of the spinous process may be an important clue to the presence of spondylolisthesis. Tenderness of the interspi-

Figure 10-1

(1) Costovertebral angle. (2) Spinous process and interspinous ligament. (3) Region of articular facet (fifth lumbar to first sacral). (4) Dorsum of sacrum. (5) Region of iliac crest. (6) Iliolumbar angle. (7) Spinous processes of fifth lumbar to first sacral vertebrae (tenderness = faulty posture or occasionally spina bifida occulta). (8) Region between posterior superior and posterior inferior spines. Sacroiliac ligaments (tenderness = sacroiliac sprain, often tender with fifth lumbar to first sacral disk). (9) Sacrococcygeal junction (tenderness = sacrococcygeal injury, i.e., sprain or fracture). (10) Region of sacrosciatic notch (tenderness = fourth to fifth lumbar disk rupture and sacroiliac sprain). (11) Sciatic nerve trunk (tenderness = ruptured lumbar disk or sciatic nerve lesion).

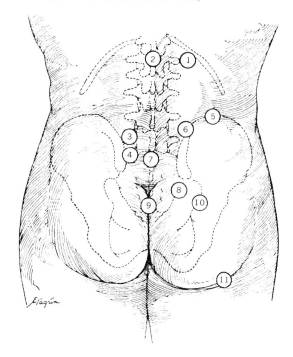

nous ligaments is indicative of disk lesions [Fig. 10-1, (2)].

Tenderness in the region of the articular facets between the fifth lumbar and first sacral vertebrae is consistent with lumbosacral disk disease [Fig. 10-1, (3)]. Tenderness in this region and in the sacroiliac joints is also a frequent manifestation of ankylosing spondylitis.

Abdominal, rectal, and pelvic examination, in addition to assessment of the integrity of the peripheral vascular systems, is essential in the study of the patient with complaints in the lower part of the back. Examination of these regions may disclose evidence of neoplastic, inflammatory, or degenerative disorders which may produce symptoms referred to the lower part of the spine.

Upon completion of the examination of the back, a search for motor, reflex, and sensory changes, particularly in the lower extremities, should be made (see "Protrusion of Lumbar Intervertebral Disks," further on in this chapter).

SPECIAL LABORATORY PROCEDURES

Laboratory tests often aid in the diagnosis of disorders of the lower part of the spine. Depending on the circumstances, these may include a complete blood count, erythrocyte sedimentation rate (especially helpful in screening for infection or myeloma), measurement of the serum proteins, calcium, phosphorus, uric acid, alkaline phosphatase, acid phosphatase (if one suspects metastatic carcinoma of the prostate), serum protein electrophoresis (myeloma proteins), tuberculin test, agglutination test for *Brucella*, and rheumatoid factor. Radiographs should be taken in every case of low-back pain and sciatica, preferably with the patient standing, in the anteroposterior, lateral, and oblique planes of the lumbar part of the spine. Special spot views or stereoscopic or laminographic films may provide further information in certain cases. Examination of the spinal canal with a contrast medium (myelogram) may be necessary, especially if a spinal cord tumor is suspected or if a patient thought to have a prolapsed disk fails to improve with conservative measures. This study can be combined with tests of dynamics of the cerebrospinal fluid, and a sample of the fluid should always be removed for cytologic and chemical examination prior to the installation of the contrast medium (Pantopaque, Myodil, air, or some of the newer contrast media such as metrizamide, which are resorbed). Injection and removal of Pantopaque require special skill and should not be attempted

without previous experience with the procedure. If done properly, the procedure has a very low incidence of significant complications. Injection of contrast medium directly into the intervertebral disk (diskogram) is a popular procedure in some institutions but is more difficult to interpret than myelography and carries the risk of damage to nerve roots or the introduction of infection. In the authors' opinion, diskography is indicated only in special circumstances and should be undertaken only by those who are specialized in its performance. Isotope bone scans are useful in demonstrating tumors and inflammatory processes. Computerized tomography of the spine is now being developed. It should accurately visualize protruded disks, tumors, etc., and eventually replace contrast myelography.

PRINCIPAL CONDITIONS THAT GIVE RISE TO PAIN IN THE LOWER BACK

Congenital Anomalies of the Lumbar Spine Anatomic variations of the spine are frequent, and although rarely of themselves the source of pain and functional derangement, they may predispose an individual to diskogenic and spondylotic complications, because of altered mechanics and alignment of the vertebrae or size of the spinal canal.

There may be a lack of fusion of the laminas of the neural arch of one or several of the lumbar vertebrae, or of the sacrum (spina bifida). Occasionally hypertrichosis or hyperpigmentation in the sacral area betrays the condition, but in most patients it remains occult until disclosed by x-ray. The anomaly may be accompanied by malformation of vertebral joints and usually induces pain only when aggravated by injury. The neurologic aspects of defective fusion of the spine (dysraphism) will be discussed in Chap. 43.

Many congenital anomalies affect the lower lumbar vertebrae: asymmetric facetal joints, abnormalities of the transverse processes, "sacralization" of the fifth lumbar vertebra (in which L5 appears to be fixed to the sacrum), or lumbarization of the first sacral (in which S1 looks like a sixth lumbar vertebra), are all seen occasionally in patients with low-back symptoms, but with apparently equal frequency in asymptomatic individuals. Their role in the genesis of low-back derangement is unclear, but in the authors' opinion, they are rarely the cause of specific symptoms.

Spondylolysis consists of a bony defect in the pars interarticularis (a segment near the junction of the pedicle with the lamina) of the lower lumbar areas, probably based on some genetic abnormality. The defect is best visualized on oblique projections. In some individuals it is unilateral; under these circumstances it usually relates to single or multiple injuries. In the usual bilateral form, the vertebral body, pedicle, and superior articular facet may move anteriorly, leaving the posterior elements behind. This latter disorder, known as *spondylolisthesis*, may cause little difficulty at first, but eventually becomes symptomatic. The patient complains of pain in the low back radiating into the thighs, and limitation of motion. Examination discloses tenderness near the segment which has "slipped" (most often L5 or occasionally L4), a palpable "step" of the spinous process forward from the segment below, hamstring spasm, and, in severe cases, shortening of the trunk and protrusion of the lower abdomen (both of which result from the abnormal forward shift of L5 on S1), and signs of involvement of spinal roots—paresthesias and sensory loss, muscle weakness, and reflex impairment. The fourth or fifth lumbar vertebra may sometimes slip forward, narrowing the spinal canal, without there being a defect in the pars interarticularis.

Traumatic Disorders of the Low Back   Traumatic disorders constitute the most frequent cause of low back pain; these will be touched upon only briefly, for they are mainly the concern of the orthopedist. In severe acute injuries, the examining physician must be careful to avoid further damage. All movements must be kept to a minimum until an approximate diagnosis has been made and adequate measures have been instituted for the proper care of the patient. If the patient complains of pain in the back and cannot move the legs, the spine may have been fractured and the cord compressed. The neck should not be flexed, and the patient should not be allowed to sit up. (See Chap. 35 for further discussion of spinal cord injury.)

   Sprains and strains   The terms *lumbosacral strain*, *sprain*, and *derangement* are used loosely by most physicians, and it is probably not possible to differentiate among them. What formerly was regarded as sacroiliac strain or sprain is now known to be due, in most instances, to disk disease. The authors prefer the term "low-back strain" for minor, self-limited injuries usually associated with lifting a heavy object, a fall, or sudden deceleration, as may occur in an auto accident. A common cause is lifting heavy objects with the spine in a position of imperfect mechanical balance, as when lifting and turning at the same time. Sudden unexpected motion is particularly likely to cause this type of injury. Sometimes these syndromes are more chronic in nature, being regularly exacerbated by a modicum of bending or lifting and suggesting that postural, muscular, or arthritic factors may play a role.

   The discomfort of low-back strain is often severe,

and the patient may assume unusual postures related to spasm of the sacrospinalis muscles. The pain is usually confined to the lower part of the back and is almost always relieved by rest. The diagnosis of lumbosacral strain depends upon the description of the injury or activity that precipitated the pain, the localization of the pain by the patient, the finding of localized tenderness, and the augmentation of pain when tension is exerted on the involved structures by the appropriate maneuvers. Alleviation of the pain by rest and relaxation indicates the existence of a strain. The pain may be relieved by local infiltration of an anesthetic agent, a finding which is also helpful in diagnosis.

   Vertebral fractures   Fractures of the lumbar vertebral body are usually the result of flexion injuries. Such trauma may occur in a fall or jump from a height (and if the patient lands on the feet, the calcanei may also be fractured) or as a result of auto accidents or other violence. When fractures occur with minimal trauma (or spontaneously), the bone has presumably been weakened by some pathologic process. Most of the time, particularly in older individuals, osteoporosis is the cause of such an event, but there are many other causes, including osteomalacia, hyperparathyroidism, hyperthyroidism, myeloma, metastatic carcinoma, and a large number of local conditions. Spasm of the lower lumbar muscles, limitation of movements of the lumbar section of the spine, and the radiographic appearance of the damaged lumbar portion (with or without neurologic abnormalities) are the basis of clinical diagnosis. The pain is usually immediate, though occasionally it may be delayed for days.

   Fractured transverse processes, which are almost always associated with tearing of the paravertebral muscles, cause deep tenderness at the site of the injury, local muscle spasm on one side, and limitation of all movements which stretch the lumbar muscles. The radiologic findings confirm the diagnosis. In some circumstances, tears of the paravertebral musculature may be associated with extensive bleeding in the retroperitoneal space and profound shock.

Protrusion of Lumbar Intervertebral Disk   This condition is now recognized as the major cause of severe and chronic or recurrent low-back and leg pain. It is most likely to occur between the fifth lumbar and first sacral vertebrae, and, with lessening frequency, between the fourth and fifth, third and fourth, second and third, and first and second lumbar vertebrae. Rare in the thoracic portion of the spine, disk disease is again frequent at the sixth and seventh and fifth and sixth cervical vertebrae (see further on).

The cause of protruded lumbar disk is usually a flexion injury, but in a considerable proportion of patients no trauma is recalled. Degeneration of the posterior longitudinal ligaments and the annulus fibrosus, which occurs in most adults of middle and advanced years, may have taken place silently or have been manifested by mild, recurrent lumbar ache. A sneeze, lurch, or other trivial movement may then cause the nucleus pulposus to prolapse, pushing the frayed and weakened annulus posteriorly. In more severe cases of disk disease, the nucleus may protrude through the annulus or become extruded and lie as a free fragment in the vertebral canal. Fragments of the nucleus pulposus protrude through rents in the annulus, usually to one side or the other (occasionally central), where they impinge upon a root or roots. The latter are compressed against the articular apophysis or the ligament between the articular processes (ligamentum flavum). This hernia may reduce itself spontaneously or be reabsorbed, but more often it persists, causing chronic irritation of the root or a discarthrosis with posterior osteophyte formation.

The fully developed syndrome of prolapsed intervertebral lumbar disk consists of (1) stiff, deformed spine, (2) pain radiating into the thigh, calf, and foot, and (3) some combination of paresthesias, weakness, and reflex impairment.

The pain of protruded intervertebral disk is of several types. First there are the spontaneous pains that range from a mild discomfort to the most severe knifelike stabs, radiating the length of the leg and superimposed on a constant intense ache. In the most acute cases patients must stay in bed, avoiding the slightest movement; cough, sneeze, or strain is intolerable. They are usually most comfortable lying on the back with legs flexed at the knees and hips (dorsal decubitus position) and with the shoulders raised on pillows to obliterate the lumbar lordosis. A particular lateral decubitus position may be more comfortable. When the condition is less severe, walking is possible, though fatigue sets in quickly, with the appearance of heaviness and pulling pains. Sitting may be particularly painful. The pain is usually located deep in the buttock, just lateral to and below the sacroiliac joint, and in the posterolateral region of the thigh, with radiations to the calf, heel, and other parts of the foot.

Pain may be characteristically provoked by pressure over the L5 and S1 vertebral spines and along the course of the sciatic nerve at the classic points of Valleix (sciatic notch, retrotrochanteric gutter, posterior surface of thigh, head of fibula). Pressure at one point may cause pain and tingling to radiate down the leg. Elongation of the nerve by straight-leg raising or extending the knee when the leg is flexed at the hip (Lasègue's maneuver) is the most consistent of all signs in provoking pain. When the sciatica is severe, the straight-leg raising is restricted to 20 to 30°; when it is less severe, or with improvement, the angle formed by leg and bed widens to 50 to 60° and finally to 90°. The same maneuver with the healthy leg evokes a lesser degree of pain, but always on the side of the spontaneous pain (Fajerstagn's sign). The presence of the crossed straight-leg-raising sign is strongly indicative of a ruptured disk as a cause of sciatica (in 56 of 58 cases in the series of Hudgkins). With the patient standing, forward bending of the trunk will cause flexion of the knee on the affected side (Neri's sign). Forced flexion of the head and neck may provoke the sciatica, as does pressure on both jugular veins, a maneuver which increases the intraspinal pressure (Naffziger's sign).

In the upright position the posture of the body is altered by the pain. The patient stands with the affected leg slightly flexed at the knee and hip, so that only the ball of the foot rests on the floor. The trunk tends to tilt forward and to one side or the other, depending on the relationship of the protruded disk material to the root (see above). This posture is referred to as "sciatic scoliosis." These antalgic postures of defence are maintained by reflex contraction of the paraspinal muscles which can be both seen and palpated. In walking, the knee is slightly flexed, and weight bearing on the painful leg is brief and cautious, giving a limp. Ascending and descending stairs is particularly painful.

The signs of spinal root involvement are hypotonia, loss or impairment of sensation and tendon reflexes, and muscle weakness. The hypotonia is evident on palpation of the buttock and calf, and the Achilles tendon tends to be less salient. Paresthesias (rarely hyperesthesia or hypoesthesia) are a frequent complaint; they are felt in the foot or leg usually. Less often there is a loss of pain perception over the appropriate dermatome(s). Muscle weakness is exceptional. The ankle or knee jerk is usually diminished or lost on the side of the lesion. Bilaterality of symptoms and signs is rare, as is sphincteric paralysis, but they may occur with large central protrusions. The CSF protein is often elevated (50 to 100 mg per 100 ml).

Since herniations of the intervertebral lumbar disks most often occur between the fifth lumbar and first sacral vertebrae and between the fourth and fifth lumbar vertebrae, respectively, it is important to recognize the clinical characteristics of root compression at these two sites. *Lesions of the fifth lumbar root* produce pain in the region of the hip, groin, posterolateral thigh, lateral calf to the external malleolus, dorsal surface of the foot, and the first or second and third toes. Paresthesias may be felt in the entire territory or only in its distal parts. The tenderness is in the lateral gluteal region and near the head of the femur. Weakness, if present, involves the extensors of the big toe and of the foot. A definite diminution of the knee and ankle jerks is seldom observed. Walking on the heels may be more difficult and uncomfortable than walking on the toes, because of weakness of dorsiflexion.

With *lesions of the first sacral root* the pain is felt in the midgluteal region, posterior part of the thigh, posterior region of the calf to the heel, and the outer plantar surface of the foot and fourth and fifth toes. Tenderness is most pronounced over the midgluteal region (in the region of the sacroiliac joint), posterior thigh areas, and calf. Paresthesias and sensory loss are mainly in the lower part of the leg and outer toes, and weakness, if present, involves the flexor muscles of the foot and toes, abductors of the toes, and hamstring muscles. The ankle reflex is diminished or absent in the majority of cases. Walking on the toes is more difficult and uncomfortable

than walking on the heels, because of weakness of plantar flexors. With lesions of either root there may be limitation of straight-leg raising during the acute painful stages.

The *rarer lesions of the third and fourth lumbar roots* give rise to pain in the anterior part of the thigh and knee and medial part of the leg (fourth lumbar) with corresponding sensory loss. The knee jerk is diminished or abolished.

Rarer still are protrusions of intervertebral disks in the thoracic region (0.5 percent of all surgically verified disk protrusions, according to Love and Schorn). The lowermost four thoracic interspaces are most frequently involved. Trauma, particularly hard falls on the heels or buttocks, appears to be an important causative factor. Paresthesias below the level of the lesion, loss of sensation, both deep and superficial, and paraparesis or paraplegia are the usual clinical manifestations. Careful myelography is the most important diagnostic maneuver.

Frequently, the herniated disk at one interspace involves more than one root (Fig. 10-2), and it follows

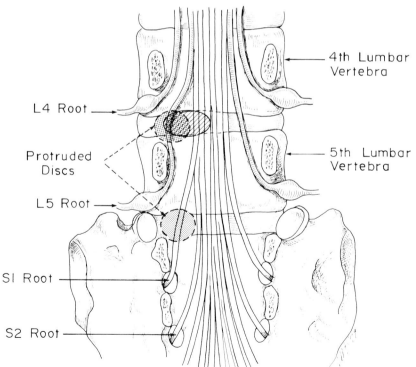

Figure 10-2

Mechanisms of compression of the fifth lumbar and first sacral roots. A lateral disk protrusion at the L4–L5 level usually involves the fifth lumbar root and spares the fourth; a protrusion at L5-S1 involves the first sacral root and spares the fifth lumbar root. Note that a more medially placed disk protrusion at the L4–L5 level may involve the fifth lumbar root as well as the first (or second and third) sacral root.

that the symptoms will then reflect involvement of two roots. The combined rupture of two or more disks occurs occasionally and further complicates the clinical picture.

Low back pain may also be caused by degeneration of the intervertebral disk, without frank extrusion of disk tissue. Or the herniation may occur into the adjacent vertebral body, giving rise to a so-called Schmorl's nodule. In such cases there are no signs of nerve root involvement, although back pain may be present, which sometimes is referred to the thigh and leg.

All or part of the above syndromes may be present. Back pain may be present with little or no leg pain; sometimes the back pain will disappear and only limb pain and neurologic loss persist; rarely will only leg pain be experienced from the beginning.

When all components of the syndrome are present the diagnosis is easy, but most neurologists prefer to corroborate their clinical impression by contrast myelography. Usually this will demonstrate the protruding disk at the suspected site and also will rule out protrusions at other sites or an unsuspected tumor. At the lumbosacral junction there may be a wide gap between the posterior margins of the vertebrae and the dural sac, so that a centrally protruded L5-S1 disk may fail to indent the Pantopaque column. Diskography may demonstrate a rent in the annulus fibrosus. In this situation (and in others where myelography presents technical difficulties) the EMG may be useful. Loss or marked asymmetry of the H reflex is a useful index of S1 radiculopathy. The finding of denervation potentials in the paraspinal muscles and in other muscles in a root distribution is also helpful, provided that at least 3 weeks have elapsed from the onset of root pain.

Far more vexing is the problem of patients who have had a disk removed but still have back and leg pain. Residual symptoms from the previous rupture or from operative damage to a nerve root may still be present. First one must exclude by myelography the possibility of a further rupture of more disk material at the same site or at another level. Tomograms may show spondylotic encroachment on an intervertebral foramen. All too often, however, nothing can be found, and further exploration reveals only a slight thickening of the arachnoid and adhesions around the roots ("arachnoiditis" with radiculopathy). Freeing the roots from adhesions and fusion of the spine has benefited less than 50 percent of such patients, and often both donor and recipient sites of the bone graft have become additional sources of pain. Further surgery in patients with no de-

monstrable disk protrusion should be avoided. It is far better to settle litigation if any is pending, to use nonaddicting pain medication, and to encourage resumption of activities. Many such patients will eventually recover. Drug addiction and depression must not be overlooked as sources of continued disability and pain.

Radiculitis and lumbosacral neuritis or plexitis (analogous to brachial neuritis); arachnoiditis; tumors of bone, cauda equina, and meninges; and acute sciatic neuropathy in the diabetic may produce a syndrome similar to that of ruptured disk (see Chaps. 35 and 45).

Arthritis and Arthropathy   Arthritis of the spine is a major cause of backache, cervical pain, and occipital headache.

Osteoarthritis, or osteoarthropathy, the more frequent type, occurs usually in later life and may involve all or any part of the spine. It is most prevalent in the cervical and lumbar regions, however. The pain is centered in the affected part of the spine, is increased by movement, and is associated almost invariably with stiffness and limitation of motion. There is a notable absence of systemic symptoms such as fatigue, malaise, and fever, and the pain usually can be relieved by rest. The severity of the symptoms often bears little relation to the radiologic findings; pain may be present when there are minimal findings on x-ray, and conversely, marked osteophytic overgrowth with spur formation, ridging, and bridging of vertebrae can be seen in asymptomatic patients in middle and late life. Osteoarthritic changes in the cervical region of the spine and to a lesser extent in the lumbar region may by their location compress roots or spinal cord, giving rise to the spondylotic form of radiculopathy or myelopathy.

In the lumbar region, osteoarthritic changes, superimposed on a smaller-than-normal spinal canal, may lead to compression of the caudal roots—so-called spondylotic caudal radiculopathy (SCR). The roots are actually caught between the posterior surface of the vertebral body and the ligamentum flavum posterolaterally. Tiredness, weakness, and paresthesias of the legs and buttocks are produced by standing, walking, or heavy exertion and are relieved by sitting or lying down. The clinical picture, with its intermittency, corresponds to the so-called intermittent claudication of the cauda equina described in 1911, by Déjerine. It has been shown by Verbiest to be due not to ischemia, but to encroachment on the cauda by apophyseal joints, thickened ligaments, and small protrusions of disks, engrafted upon a canal that is developmentally shallow in the anteroposterior diameter. It has been shown also that the canal in these cases is narrow from side to side (reduced interpedicular distance on x-ray). Decompression of the spinal canal relieves the symptoms in a considerable proportion of the cases. SCR is the lumbar equivalent of spondylotic cervical myelopathy and radiculopathy. SCR is a cauda equina syndrome, and its differential diagnosis will be discussed in Chap. 35, Diseases of the Spinal Cord.

Rheumatoid Arthritis and Ankylosing Spondylitis Arthritic disease of the spine takes two distinct forms—ankylosing spondylitis (the more common) and rheumatoid arthritis.

Ankylosing spondylitis (also called Marie-Strümpell arthritis) affects young males predominantly. The main complaint is pain, usually centered in the low region of the back, at least in the initial stages of the disease. Often it radiates to the back of the thighs and groin. At first the symptoms are vague (tired back, "catches" up and down the back, sore back), and the diagnosis may be overlooked for many years. Although the pain is recurrent, limitation of movement is constant and progressive and over time tends to dominate the picture. Early in the course, this is experienced as "morning stiffness" or increasing stiffness after periods of inactivity; these findings may be present long before radiologic changes are manifest. Rarely, a cauda equina syndrome may complicate ankylosing spondylitis, the result apparently of an inflammatory reaction and later a proliferation of connective tissue in the caudal canal (Mathews). Limitation of chest expansion, tenderness over the sternum, and decreased motion and tendency to flexion of the hips may be present early in the course of the disease. The radiologic hallmarks are at first destruction and subsequently obliteration of the sacroiliac joints, followed by bridging of the vertebral bodies by bone to produce the characteristic "bamboo spine." When this occurs, the entire spine is immobilized and usually the pain subsides, but the patient has little motion of the back and neck. Patterns indistinguishable from that of ankylosing spondylitis may also accompany Reiter's syndrome, psoriasis, and inflammatory diseases of the intestine (see also Chap. 35).

Occasionally ankylosing spondylitis is complicated by destructive vertebral lesions. This complication should be suspected whenever the pain returns, after a period of quiescence, or becomes localized. The cause of these lesions is not known, but they may represent a response to nonunion of fractures with an excessive production of fibrous inflammatory tissue. Rarely they may result in collapse of a vertebral segment and compression of the spinal cord. Ankylosing spondylitis of a very severe nature may involve both hips, greatly accentuating the back deformity and disability.

Spinal rheumatoid arthritis tends to be localized to the cervical apophyseal joints and atlantoaxial articulation; the pain, stiffness, and limitation of motion are then in the neck and back of the head. In contrast to ankylosing spondylitis, rheumatoid arthritis is rarely confined to the spine. Because of major affection of other joints, the diagnosis is relatively easy to make, but significant involvement of the neck may be overlooked in patients with diffuse disease. In advanced stages of the disease, one or several of the vertebrae may be displaced anteriorly; or a synovitis of the atlantoaxial joint may damage the transverse ligament of the atlas, resulting in forward displacement of the atlas on the axis, i.e., atlantoaxial subluxation. In either instance, serious and even life-threatening compression of the spinal cord, gradual or sudden, may occur (see Chap. 35). Cautiously taken lateral roentgenograms in flexion and extension are useful in visualizing atlantoaxial dislocation or subluxation of the lower segments.

Destructive Diseases of the Spine *Infections, neoplastic and metabolic diseases* Metastatic carcinoma (breast, bronchus, prostate, thyroid, kidney, stomach, uterus), multiple myeloma, and reticulum-cell sarcoma are the common malignant tumors which involve the spine. Since the primary lesion may be small and asymptomatic the presenting complaint caused by these or other tumors may be pain in the back due to metastatic deposits. The pain is described as constant and dull; it is often unrelieved by rest and may be worse at night. At the time of onset of the back pain there may be no radiographic changes, but when they appear they usually take the form of destructive lesions in one or several vertebral bodies with only limited involvement of the disk space, even in the face of a compression fracture. Before such destructive changes become evident, an isotope scan may be helpful in detecting areas of osteoblastic activity due to neoplastic or inflammatory disease.

Infection of the vertebral column is usually the result of pyogenic organisms (staphylococci or coliform bacilli) or tuberculosis, and these are often difficult to distinguish on the basis of clinical findings. Both groups of patients complain of pain in the back, of subacute or chronic nature, which is exacerbated by motion but not materially relieved by rest. Motion becomes limited, and there is tenderness over the spine in the involved segments and pain with jarring of the spine, such as occurs with walking on the heels. Usually, these patients are afebrile and do not have a leukocytosis. The erythrocyte sedimentation rate is usually elevated. Radiographs may demonstrate narrowing of a disk space with erosion and destruction of the two adjacent vertebrae. A soft tissue mass may be present, indicating an abscess, which may in the case of tuberculosis drain spontaneously, at sites quite remote from the vertebral column.

Special mention should be made of *spinal epidural abscess*, which necessitates urgent surgical treatment. This is usually due to staphylococci, sometimes to *Pseudomonas*, which may be introduced by a contaminated lumbar puncture needle or drug injection. The main symptom is localized pain, occurring spontaneously and intensified by percussion and pressure upon the vertebral spines; the pain may have a radicular radiation. A rapidly developing flaccid paraplegia appearing in a febrile patient should suggest compression of the spinal cord by epidural abscess. A noninflammatory form of acute epidural compression may be caused by rheumatoid arthritis or by hemorrhage (as in anticoagulant therapy and vascular malformations).

In so-called metabolic bone disease (osteoporosis of either the postmenopausal or senile type, or osteomalacia), a considerable degree of loss of bone substance may occur without any symptoms whatsoever. Many patients with such conditions do, however, complain of aching in the lumbar or thoracic area and a few have brief paroxysms of pain accompanied by flexor spasms of the legs and lower back. This is most likely to occur following an injury, sometimes of trivial degree, which leads to collapse or wedging of a vertebra. Certain movements greatly enhance the pain, and certain positions relieve it. One or more spinal roots may be involved. *Paget's disease of the spine* may be associated with aching in the lumbar or thoracic areas; or it may be painless. Occasionally, it may lead to compression of the spinal cord or nerve roots. In general, the condition of patients thought to have neoplastic, infectious, or metabolic disease of the spine should be thoroughly evaluated by means of radiographs, bone scans, and myelography where indicated. Laboratory studies such as a complete blood count, sedimentation rate, calcium, phosphorus, alkaline and acid phosphatase, protein electrophoresis, immunoelectrophoresis, tuberculin test, febrile agglutinins, and blood cultures may be helpful in establishing the diagnosis.

Referred Pain from Visceral Disease   The pain of disease of the pelvic, abdominal, or thoracic viscera is often felt in the region of the spine, i.e., it is referred to the

more posterior parts of the spinal segment which innervates the diseased organ. Occasionally back pain may be the first and only sign. The general rule is that the pain of pelvic disease is referred to the sacral region, lower abdominal disease to the lumbar region (centering around the second to fourth lumbar vertebrae), and upper abdominal disease to the lower thoracic portion of the spine (eighth thoracic to the first and second lumbar vertebrae). Characteristically there are no local signs, no stiffness of the back, and motion is of full range without augmentation of the pain. However, some positions, e.g., flexion of the lumbar areas of the spine in the lateral recumbent positions, may be more comfortable than others.

Low thoracic–upper lumbar back pain in abdominal disease   Peptic ulceration or tumor of the stomach and duodenum most typically induces pain in the epigastrium; but if the posterior wall is involved, particularly if there is retroperitoneal extension, the pain may be felt in the dorsal spine, centrally or to one side or in both locations. If very intense, it may seem to encircle the body. It tends to retain the characteristics of pain from the affected organ; e.g., if due to peptic ulceration, it appears about 2 h after a meal and is relieved by food and antacids.

Diseases of the pancreas are apt to cause pain in the back, being more to the right of the spine if the head of the pancreas is involved and to the left if the body and tail are implicated.

Diseases of retroperitoneal structures, e.g., lymphomas, sarcomas, and carcinomas, may evoke pain in the dorsal or lumbar spine with some tendency toward radiation to the lower part of the abdomen, groins, and anterior thighs. A tumor in the iliopsoas region often produces a unilateral lumbar ache with radiation toward the groin and labia or testicle; there may also be signs of involvement of the upper lumbar spinal roots. An aneurysm of the abdominal aorta may induce a pain which is localized to an analogous region of the spine.

The sudden appearance of lumbar pain in a patient receiving anticoagulants should arouse the suspicion of retroperitoneal bleeding.

Inflammatory diseases or tumor of the colon causes pain which may be felt in the lower abdomen or in the midlumbar region, or in both places. If very intense, the pain may have a beltlike distribution. Pain from a lesion in the transverse colon or first part of the descending colon may be central or left-sided, and its level of reference is to the second and third lumbar vertebrae. If the sigmoid colon is implicated, the pain is lower, in the upper sacral spine and anteriorly in the midline suprapubic region or left lower quadrant of the abdomen.

Sacral pain in pelvic (urologic and gynecologic) diseases Gynecologic disorders often manifest themselves by back pain, but their diagnosis is seldom difficult. Thorough abdominal palpation, vaginal and rectal examination, supplemented by certain laboratory procedures (sigmoidoscopy, barium enema, pyelography, and culdoscopy) usually disclose the source of pain.

The most important source of chronic back pain from the pelvic organs is the uterosacral ligaments. Endometriosis or carcinoma of the uterus (body or cervix) may invade these structures, causing pain which is localized in the sacrum below the lumbosacral joint either centrally or more on one side. In endometriosis the pain begins during the premenstrual phase and often continues until it merges with menstrual pain. Malposition of the uterus (retroversion, descensus, and prolapse) characteristically leads to sacral pain, especially after the patient has been standing for several hours. Postural adjustments may also evoke pain here when a fibroma of the uterus pulls on the uterosacral ligaments.

Carcinomatous pain due to implication of nerve plexuses is continuous and becomes progressively more severe; it tends to be more intense at night. The primary lesion may be inconspicuous, being overlooked on pelvic examination. Papanicolaou smears and a pyelogram are the most useful diagnostic procedures. X-ray therapy of these tumors may produce sacral pain consequent to swelling and necrosis of tissue, the so-called radiation phlegmon of the pelvis.

Low-back pain with radiation into one or both thighs is a common phenomenon during the last weeks of pregnancy. Menstrual pain may be felt in the sacral region. It is rather poorly localized, tends to radiate down the thighs and is of a crampy nature.

Carcinoma of the prostate with metastases to the lower part of the spine is a common cause of sacral or lumbar pain. It may present without urinary symptoms. Spinal nerves may be infiltrated by tumor cells, or the spinal cord itself may be compressed if the epidural space is invaded. The diagnosis is established by rectal examination, roentgenograms of the spine, and measurement of acid phosphatase (particularly the prostatic phosphatase fraction). Chronic prostatitis, evidenced by prostatic discharge, burning and frequency of urination, and slight reduction in sexual potency, may be attended by a nagging sacral ache; it may be mainly on one side, with radiation into one leg if the seminal vesicle is involved on that side. Lesions of the bladder and testes are usually not accompanied by back pain. When the kidney is the site of disease, the pain is ipsilateral, being felt in the flank or lumbar region.

Obscure Types of Low-Back Pain and the Question of Psychiatric Disease A safe rule is to assume that all patients who complain of low-back pain of obscure origin have some type of primary or secondary disease of the spine and its supporting structures or of the abdominal or pelvic viscera. However, even after exhaustive study there remains a group of patients in whom no pathologic basis can be found for the back pain. Two categories can be recognized: those with postural back pain and those with psychiatric illness, but there are others in whom the diagnosis remains obscure.

Postural back pain Many slender, asthenic individuals and some fat, middle-aged ones have discomfort in the back. Their backs ache much of the time, and the pain interferes with effective work. The physical examination is negative except for slack musculature and poor posture. The pain is diffuse in the mid or low region of the back; characteristically it is relieved by bed rest and induced by the maintenance of a particular posture over a period of time. Pain in the neck and between the shoulder blades is a common complaint among thin, tense, active women and seems to be related to taut trapezius muscles.

Adolescent girls and boys are subject to an obscure form of epiphyseal disease of the spine (Scheuermann's disease) which, over a period of 2 to 3 years, may cause low-back pain upon exercise.

Psychiatric illness Low-back pain may be encountered in hysteria, malingering, anxiety neurosis, depression, hypochondriasis, and in many nervous persons whose symptoms do not conform to any of these psychiatric illnesses.

Again it is good practice to assume that pain in the back in such patients may signify disease of the spine or adjacent structures, and this should always be carefully sought. However, even when some organic factors are found, the pain may be exaggerated, prolonged, or woven into a pattern of invalidism or disability because of coexistent or secondary psychologic factors. This is especially true when there is the possibility of secondary gain (notably compensation). Patients seeking compensation for protracted low-back pain without obvious structural disease tend, after a time, to become suspicious, uncooperative, and hostile toward their physicians or anyone who might question the authenticity of their illness. One notes in them a tendency to describe their pain poorly and a preference, instead, to discuss the degree of their disability and their mistreatment at the hands of the medical profession. These features and a negative examination of the back should lead one to suspect a psychological factor. A few patients, usually frank malingerers, adopt the most bizarre attitudes, such as walking with the trunk flexed at almost a right angle (camptocormia) and being unable to straighten up.

The depressed and anxious patient represents a troublesome problem. A common error is to minimize the importance of anxiety and depression or to ascribe them to worry over the illness and its social effects. In these circumstances common and minor back ailments, e.g., those due to osteoarthritis and postural ache, are enhanced and rendered intolerable. Such patients are often subjected to surgical procedures, which prove ineffective. The disability seems excessive for the degree of spinal malfunction, and misery, irritability, and despair are the prevailing features of the syndrome. One of the most reliable diagnostic measures is the response to drugs that alleviate the depression (see Chap. 54).

PAIN IN THE NECK AND SHOULDER

In this connection, it is useful to distinguish *three major categories of painful disease*—that of the *spine, brachial plexus* (*thoracic outlet*), and *shoulder*. Although the pain from each of the sources may overlap, the patient usually can indicate its site of origin.

Pain arising from the *cervical part of the spine* is felt in the neck and back of the head (although it may be projected to the shoulder and arm), is evoked or enhanced by certain movements or positions of the neck, and is accompanied by tenderness and limitation of motions of the neck.

Pain of brachial plexus origin is experienced in and around the shoulder and in the supraclavicular region, is induced by the performance of certain tasks with the arm and by certain positions, and is associated with tenderness of structures above the clavicle. There may be a palpable abnormality above the clavicle (aneurysm of the subclavian artery, tumor, cervical rib). The combination of circulatory symptoms and signs referable to the medial cord of the brachial plexus are characteristic of the thoracic outlet syndrome. These are manifested in the hand by obliteration of the pulse when the patient

takes and holds a full breath with the head tilted back or turned (Adson's test) and swelling, venous distension and cyanosis of the dependent hand when the subclavian vein is compressed. Unilateral Raynaud's phenomenon, trophic changes in the fingers, and sensory loss over the ulnar side of the hand with or without interosseous atrophy, complete the clinical picture.

Pain localized to the shoulder region, influenced by motion, and associated with tenderness and limitation of motion (especially internal rotation) points to a calcific tendonitis, or to a tear of the rotator cuff, which is made up of the tendons of the muscles surrounding the shoulder joint. The term *bursitis* is often used loosely to designate this tendonitis, capsulitis, or muscular tear. Shoulder pain, like spine and plexus pain, may radiate into the arm or hand, but sensory, motor, and reflex changes, which always indicate disease of nerve roots, plexus, or nerves, are absent. However, trophic changes may develop in the hand (see further on, under Sudeck's atrophy).

Osteoarthritis of the cervical spine may cause pain which radiates into the back of the head, shoulders, and arms on one or both sides. Coincident involvement of nerve roots is manifested by paresthesias, sensory loss, weakness and atrophy and tendon reflex changes in the arms and hands. Should bony ridges form in the spinal canal (spondylosis), the spinal cord may be compressed, with resulting spastic weakness, ataxia, and loss of vibratory and position sense in the legs. A cervical myelogram reveals the encroachment on the spinal canal (narrowing to 10 to 11 mm or less in the anteroposterior diameter) and the level at which the spinal cord is affected. There may be great difficulty in distinguishing spondylosis with root and spinal cord compression from primary neurologic diseases (syringomyelia, amyotrophic lateral sclerosis, or tumor) with an unrelated osteoarthritis of the cervical portion of the spine, particularly at the C5-C6 and C6-C7 levels, where the disk spaces are often narrowed in the adult. Here the myelogram is of particular importance (see Chap. 35 for differential diagnosis). A combination of osteoarthritis of the cervical spine with nervous tension or with injury to ligaments and muscles in which the neck is forcibly extended and flexed (e.g., whiplash injury to spine) raises vexatious clinical problems. If the pain is persistent and limited to the neck, the problem will sometimes prove to be due to disruption of a disk, but more often it is complicated by psychologic factors, and disk disease is absent.

CERVICAL DISK PROTRUSION

One of the most common causes of neck, shoulder, and arm pain is disk herniation in the lower cervical region

(Fig. 10-3*A* and *B*). It may develop after trauma, which may be major or minor (from sudden hyperextension of the neck, diving, forceful manipulations, chiropractic treatment, etc.). The roots most commonly involved in cervical disk protrusion are the seventh (in 70 percent of cases) and the sixth (20 percent); fifth and eighth root involvement make up the remaining 10 percent (Yoss et al.).

With laterally situated disk lesions between the fifth and sixth cervical vertebrae, the symptoms and signs are referred to the sixth cervical roots. The full syndrome is characterized by pain at the trapezius ridge and tip of the shoulder, with radiation into the anterior-upper part of the arm, radial forearm, and often into the thumb; paresthesias and sensory impairment in the same regions; tenderness in the area above the spine of the scapula and in the supraclavicular and biceps regions; weakness in flexion of the forearm; diminished to absent biceps and supinator reflexes (triceps retained or exaggerated).

When the protruded disk lies between the sixth and seventh vertebrae, there is involvement of the seventh cervical root and the pain is in the region of the shoulder blade, pectoral region and medial axilla, posterolateral upper arm, dorsal forearm and elbow, index and middle fingers, or all the fingers; tenderness is most pronounced over the medial aspect of the shoulder blade opposite the third to fourth thoracic spinous processes, in the supraclavicular area and triceps region; paresthesias and sensory loss are most pronounced in the second and third fingers or tips of all the fingers; weakness is seen in extension of the forearm (occasionally wrist drop is present) and in the hand grip; the triceps reflex is diminished to absent, and the biceps and supinator reflexes are preserved.

Either of these syndromes may be incomplete in that only one or several of the typical findings are present. The article by Friis et al., listed in the references, describes in detail the distribution of pain in 250 cases of herniated disk or spondylotic nerve root compression in the cervical region. Virtually every patient, irrespective of the particular root(s) involved, shows a limitation in the range of motion of the neck and aggravation of pain with movement (particularly hyperextension). Usually the patient states that cough, sneeze, and downward pressure on the head in the hyperextension position exacerbate pain, and traction (even manual) tends to relieve it.

Unlike lumbar disks, the cervical ones, if large and centrally situated, may result in compression of the spinal cord (central disk, all of the cord; paracentral disk, part of the cord) (Fig. 10-3*B*). The centrally situated disk may be painless, and the cord syndrome may simulate a degenerative disease (amyotrophic lateral sclerosis, combined system disease). A common error is to fail to think of a protruded cervical disk in patients with obscure symptoms in the legs. The diagnosis should be confirmed by myelography.

THORACIC OUTLET SYNDROMES

A variety of anatomical anomalies occur in the lateral cervical region, which may, under certain circumstances, compress the brachial plexus, the subclavian artery, and the subclavian vein, causing pain in the neck, shoulder, arm, and hand. The most frequent of these abnormali-

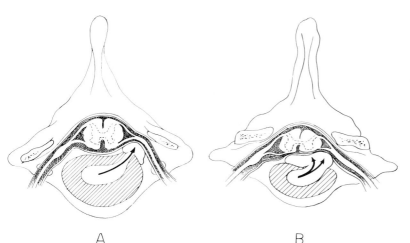

Figure 10-3
A. *Mechanism of root compression in lateral herniation of nucleus pulposus.* B. *Mechanism of root and cord compression from central herniation of nucleus pulposus. (After Kristoff and Odom.)*

A　　　　　B

ties are complete cervical ribs, which articulate with the first rib; incomplete cervical ribs, with a sharp fascial band passing from their tips to the first rib; sharp fibrous bands passing from the transverse process of C7 to the first rib; and anomalies of the position and insertion of the anterior and medial scalene muscles. Depending on the postulated abnormality and mechanism of symptom production, the terms *cervical rib, anterior scalene, costoclavicular, neurovascular compression,* and *hyperabduction* have been applied to this syndrome. The international anatomical term is "superior thoracic aperture syndrome."

Variations in regional anatomy could explain these several postulated mechanisms, but it must be conceded that to this day there is not full agreement about them. An anomalous cervical rib, which arises from the seventh cervical vertebra and extends laterally between the anterior and medial scalene muscles, then under the brachial plexus and subclavian artery to attach to the first rib, obviously disturbs anatomic relationships and may compress these structures. The other anomalies may have similar effects on the brachial plexus and the subclavian artery and vein at a number of points (Fig. 10-4). These are understandable when it is remembered

that the subclavian artery leaves the thorax and passes over the first rib, at which point it lies between the anterior scalene muscle anteriorly and the brachial plexus and medial scalene posteriorly; as it courses laterally under the clavicle and subclavian muscle, it encounters another potential narrowing and then a third one as it passes under the pectoralis minor to enter the axilla. The subclavian vein follows the same course except that it lies in front of the anterior scalene muscle. The brachial plexus issues from the paravertebral region, passes between the anterior and medial scalene muscles, and runs parallel to the subclavian artery and vein to the axilla. Thus it is that the lower part of the brachial plexus and the subclavian artery and vein tend to be compressed together, and this may happen at any one of the several potential narrowings which are modified by posture of the shoulders and arms, sleeping position, carrying of objects in the arm or over the shoulder, and the position of the head.

Since an estimated 0.5 percent of the population has cervical ribs on one or both sides and only about 10 percent of these persons have symptoms, other factors must be operative in most instances. The majority of the patients are women of early or midadult years in whom sagging of the shoulders and poor muscular tone may be of importance. Occupational activities may also play a part.

In 138 cases of thoracic outlet syndrome reported

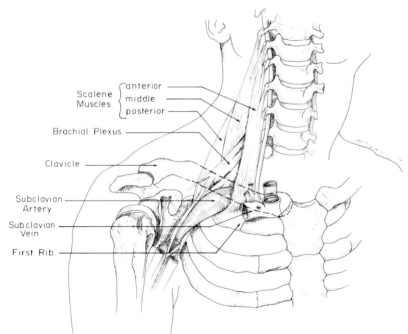

Figure 10-4

Course of the brachial plexus and subclavian artery between the anterior scalene and middle scalene muscles. Dilatation of the subclavian artery just distal to the anterior scalene muscle is illustrated. Immediately distal to the anterior and middle scalene muscles is another potential area of constriction, between the clavicle and the first rib. With extension of the neck and turning of the chin to the affected side (Adson's maneuver), the tension on the anterior scalene muscle is increased and the subclavian artery compressed, resulting in a supraclavicular bruit and obliteration of the radial pulse.

Scalene Muscles
{ anterior
  middle
  posterior }

Brachial Plexus

Clavicle

Subclavian Artery

Subclavian Vein

First Rib

by Urschel et al., all but 6 had symptoms of nerve compression, manifested by pain and paresthesia. The pain is usually of insidious onset and involves the neck, shoulder, arm, and hand. Paresthesias in a specific nerve distribution occurred in 102 of their patients usually in the distribution of the ulnar nerve, occasionally the median. In contrast, compression of the subclavian artery was present in about 25 percent of their series, and of the subclavian vein in only 10 percent. Objective sensory findings are demonstrable in only 38 percent of patients, and motor deficit, mainly weakness and wasting of hand muscles, in 58 percent (Lascelles et al.). In about one-half of these patients there will be one or more of the findings associated with vascular compression—loss of radial pulse during Adson's maneuver, in bracing and pushing down on shoulders, or abducting arm over head; tenderness and bruit over the subclavian artery above the clavicle with easy obliteration of pulse and pain with pressure above the clavicle; unilateral Raynaud's phenomenon; pallor on elevating arm; brittle nails; and ulceration of fingers. Compression of the subclavian vein causes a dusky discoloration of the arm, venous distension, and edema, and the vein may become thrombosed after prolonged exercise, the so-called effort thrombotic syndrome of Paget and Schroetter. Occasionally a narrowed or atherosclerotic artery is the source of brachial embolism. Rarely, the artery may become thrombosed.

Diagnosis is difficult unless there is evidence of compression of both vascular structures and brachial plexus and easy reproduction of symptoms by the aforementioned maneuvers. Nerve conduction studies are usually normal. EMG frequently shows a decrease in sensory amplitudes and signs of denervation in the abductor pollicis brevis. Arteriography, with the arm in abduction, can be used to corroborate arterial compression. Sensitivity of the hand to cold with production of Raynaud's phenomenon is another useful finding, attributed by Telford and Mottershead to a compression of a small branch of postganglionic sympathetic fibers which courses separately from the brachial plexus in this region.

In the authors' experience, neck and arm pain, especially in slender, neurotic women, presents especially difficult problems in diagnosis; often the physician assumes it to be due to a thoracic outlet syndrome, only to discover that operation affords little or no relief. One should be skeptical of the diagnosis unless there is evidence of both circulatory difficulty and sensory changes along the ulnar side of hand and forearm. Nerve conduction studies and arteriography are helpful, but we have had patients who were immediately relieved by operation, even though the results of these tests were completely normal. Common mistakes are to confuse this syndrome with cervical arthritis or disk disease, postural muscular aches, carpal tunnel syndrome, and ulnar nerve compression at the elbow. EMG is helpful in ruling out the latter two disorders.

OTHER CONDITIONS

Metastases to the cervical region of the spine are less common than to other parts of the vertebral column. They are frequently painful and may cause root compression. Extension of a tumor posteriorly or compression fractures may lead to the rapid development of quadriplegia.

The Pancoast tumor, usually a squamous cell carcinoma in the superior sulcus of the lung, may implicate the lower cervical and upper thoracic (T1 and T2) spinal nerves as they exit from the spine. Horner's syndrome, numbness of the inner side of arm and hand, weakness of all muscles of the hand and of the triceps muscle are combined with pain beneath the upper scapula and in the arm. The neurological abnormalities may occur long before the tumor becomes visible radiographically.

Shoulder injuries (rotator cuff), subacromial or subdeltoid bursitis, and "frozen shoulder" (periarthritis or capsulitis), tendonitis, and arthritis may develop in patients who are otherwise well, but these conditions also occur occasionally as a complication of hemiplegia. The pain is often severe and extends toward the neck and down the arm into the hand. The dorsum of the hand may tingle without other signs of nerve involvement. Immobility of an arm following myocardial infarction may be associated with pain in the shoulder and arm and with vasomotor changes in the hand (shoulder-hand syndrome); after a time, osteoporosis and atrophy of cutaneous and subcutaneous structures occur (Sudeck's atrophy or Sudeck-Leriche syndrome). These conditions fall within the province of the orthopedist and cardiologist and will not be discussed in detail. The neurologist, however, must know that they can be prevented by proper exercises.

Medial and lateral epicondylitis (tennis elbow) are readily diagnosed by demonstrating tenderness over the affected parts and an aggravation of pain on certain movements of the wrist. We have observed entrapment of the ulnar nerve in some cases of medial epicondylitis.

The pain of the carpal tunnel syndrome (Chap. 45) often extends into the forearm and sometimes higher, and may be mistaken for disease of the shoulder or neck. Similarly, involvement of the ulnar, radial, or median nerves may be mistaken for brachial plexus or root lesions. Electromyography and nerve conduction studies are helpful in these circumstances. Tenosynovitis may be associated with the carpal tunnel syndrome or occur separately.

OTHER PAINFUL DISORDERS OF THE UPPER AND LOWER EXTREMITIES

PAINFUL ARTHRITIS OF EXTREMITIES

The principal symptom of *osteoarthritis* is pain which is brought on by use and relieved by rest. Stiffness after sitting and immediately upon rising in the morning is common but seldom persists for more than a few minutes. The more common locations are the terminal phalanges, carpal-metacarpal joint of the thumb, knees, hips, and spine. *Rheumatoid arthritis* most commonly involves the proximal interphalangeal and metacarpophalangeal joints, toes, wrists, ankle, knee, elbow, hip, and shoulder. Other types of arthritis are numerous—infectious, posttraumatic, and that associated with connective tissue, gastrointestinal, pulmonary, and psoriatic disease. The synovial membranes and periarticular structures are primarily involved in early rheumatoid disease, infectious arthritis, and gout, whereas the cartilage and bone are mainly affected in osteoarthritis and in the later stages of rheumatoid arthritis.

POLYMYALGIA RHEUMATICA

This syndrome is observed in middle-aged and elderly persons and is characterized by severe pain, aching, and stiffness in the proximal muscles of the limbs and a markedly elevated erythrocyte sedimentation rate. In many patients it is a manifestation of giant-cell (temporal) arteritis and may be the only symptomatic expression of that disease (page 583). This disorder is self-limited, lasting 6 months to 2 years, and responds dramatically to corticosteroid therapy.

ARTERIOSCLEROSIS OBLITERANS

Atherosclerosis of large and medium-sized arteries, the most common vascular disease of humans, often leads to symptoms which are induced by exercise (intermittent claudication) but may occur also at rest (ischemic rest pain). The diabetic patient is especially susceptible. The muscle pain that is brought on by exercise and promptly relieved by rest most frequently involves the calf and thigh muscles. If the atherosclerotic narrowing or occlusion involves the aortic and iliac arteries, it may also cause hip and buttock claudication and impotence in the male (Leriche syndrome). Ischemic rest pain, and sometimes attendant ulceration and gangrene, is usually localized to the foot and toes and the consequence of multiple sites of vascular occlusion. Pain at rest is characteristically worse at night and totally or partially relieved by dependency.

The examination of such patients will reveal a loss of one or more peripheral pulses, trophic changes in skin and nails (in advanced cases), and the presence of bruits or thrills over or distal to sites of narrowing. A search should always be made in such patients for an abdominal aortic aneurysm, since it is prone to rupture and can be corrected by operation. Arteriography is necessary only for confirmation of the location and extent of the vascular narrowing in planning surgical therapy. The upper extremities are rarely involved. Aneurysms of the peripheral arteries do not usually produce pain unless they compress adjacent nerves; they are of importance primarily because they become the source of distal arterial embolization or undergo thrombosis.

PAINFUL CIRCULATORY DISORDERS

In evaluating patients with cold sensitivity it is important to distinguish Raynaud's disease from Raynaud's phenomenon. *Raynaud's disease* is a benign, symmetric disorder of unknown cause which usually has its onset in the late teens or early twenties. Females are more commonly affected than males, and cold and emotional stimuli are the factors which trigger the response in the digits. The fingers become white, then blue, and finally red (the triphasic color response). Pain and paresthesias are common during the ischemic phase. Ulcerations are rarely observed.

Raynaud's phenomenon is always a symptom (sometimes it is the initial manifestation) of some underlying disease. It may occur at any period of life and may be asymmetric. When severe it is accompanied by tender, painful fingertip ulcers. It is associated most often with one of the collagen-vascular diseases, but also with rheumatoid arthritis, thromboangiitis obliterans, the dysproteinemias, occupational trauma (e.g., working with pneumatic drill, sculling on a cold day), and the thoracic outlet syndromes.

Reflex Sympathetic Dystrophy   This is an excessive or abnormal response of the sympathetic nervous system to injury of the shoulder and arm, rarely the leg. It consists of protracted pain in association with cyanosis or pallor, swelling, coldness, pain on passive motion, and osteoporosis. The condition is variously described under such terms as Sudeck's atrophy, posttraumatic osteoporosis, and shoulder-hand syndrome. According to Carlson et al., bone scans are positive. Pharmacologic or surgical sympathectomy hastens recovery.

Erythromelalgia   This rare disorder of the microvasculature produces a burning pain, usually in the toes and forefoot, in association with changes in ambient temperature. Since it was first carefully described by Weir Mitchell in 1878, many articles have been written about it, but the cause of the primary form is still obscure. Each patient has a temperature threshold above which symptoms appear and the feet become bright red and warm. Those afflicted rarely wear stockings or regular shoes, since these tend to bring out the symptoms. Patients characteristically relieve the pain by walking on a cold surface or soaking their feet in ice water. The peripheral pulses are intact and there are no motor, sensory, or reflex changes. There are secondary forms of the disease associated in rare cases with myeloproliferative disorders, particularly polycythemia vera, and occlusive vascular diseases; in some instances it is a manifestation of a painful neuropathy (Chap. 45). According to Abbott and Mitts, aspirin is useful in the treatment of paroxysms of primary erythromelalgia; others recommend methysergide maleate (Pepper).

MANAGEMENT OF BACK AND LIMB PAIN

Muscular and ligamentous strains and minor disk prolapses are usually self-limited, responding to simple measures in a relatively short period of time. The basic principle of therapy in both is rest, in a recumbent position, for several days to weeks. Usually lying on the side with knees and hips flexed is the favored position. With strains of the sacrospinalis muscles and sacroiliac ligaments, the optimal position is hyperextension. This position is best maintained by having the patient lie with a small pillow or blanket under the lumbar portion of the spine or lie face down. Physical measures, such as application of cold in the acute phase and heat after the third or fourth day, diathermy, or massage, are of limited value. Analgesic medication should be given liberally during the first few days [codeine, 30 mg, and aspirin, 0.6 g; pentazocine (Talwin), 50 mg; or meperidine (Demerol), 50 mg]. Muscle relaxants are often useful [diazepam (Valium), 8 to 40 mg in divided doses; carisoprodol (Soma), 350 mg twice daily] if only to make bed rest more tolerable. If an inflammatory component is suspected, indomethacin (Indocin), 75 mg/day (in di-

vided doses), or ibuprofen (Motrin), 400 mg three or four times daily, may be helpful. When weight bearing is resumed, a light lumbosacral support should be worn until the pain has subsided. Thereafter, corrective exercises are prescribed, designed to strengthen trunk muscles, especially the abdominal, overcome faulty posture, and increase the mobility of the spinal joints.

In the treatment of an *acute or chronic rupture of a lumbar or cervical disk,* complete bed rest is essential, and strong analgesic medication may be required. Traction is of little value in lumbar disk disease, and it is best to permit the patient to find the most comfortable position. In the case of a cervical disk syndrome, traction with a halter may be of considerable benefit. Treatment can be administered with the patient in recumbency, or if the patient improves sufficiently to be ambulatory, it can be performed intermittently in the sitting position using special equipment. During the recumbent phase of treatment of lumbar disk disease, muscle relaxants and antiinflammatory agents as described above may be of considerable value. After 2 or 3 weeks in bed, the patient can be allowed to resume activities gradually, usually with the protection of a brace or light spinal support (or a soft collar, in the case of cervical disk disease). In lumbar disk disease exercise programs designed to increase the strength of the abdominal and gluteal muscles are helpful at this point. The patient may suffer some minor recurrence of the pain but will be able to continue his or her usual activities and eventually will recover. If the pain and neurologic findings do not disappear on prolonged conservative management or the patient suffers frequent recurrent acute episodes, surgical treatment may be indicated. This should always be preceded by a myelogram to localize the lesion (and rule out the presence of intra- or extradural tumors). The surgical procedure most often indicated is a hemilaminectomy, with excision of the disk involved. Arthrodesis of the involved segments is indicated only in cases in which there is extraordinary instability, usually related to anatomic abnormality (such as spondylolysis) or, in the cervical region, when an extensive laminectomy has rendered the spine unstable.

For a time, chemonucleolysis was used for the management of lumbar disk lesions which did not respond to conservative measures. Chymopapain, a polysaccharide-splitting enzyme of plant origin, is introduced into the damaged nucleus pulposus by a laterally placed needle under radiographic control. The enzyme, by its lytic action, causes a decrease in intradiskal pressure. We have discontinued its use because of poor results, but it is still in vogue in some clinics. The choice and performance of such procedures as laminectomy, chemonucleolysis, and spinal arthrodesis should be weighed carefully in the light of the patient's occupation, emotional response, compensation status, etc.

Spondylosis of the cervical part of the spine, if painful, is helped by bed rest and traction; if signs of spinal cord and root involvement are present, a collar to limit movement may halt the progression and even lead to improvement. Decompressive laminectomy or anterior excision of single spondylotic spurs and fusion is reserved for severe instances of the disease with advancing neurologic symptoms (see Chap. 35).

In the management of the thoracic outlet syndromes, treatment is indicated when pain with or without paresthesias is the only symptom. Exercises to build up the shoulder muscles, sleeping with shoulders braced by pillows in an anteroflexed position, and not carrying heavy objects with the arm and hand at the side of the body have often relieved the symptoms. If not, and especially if there are symptoms of vascular insufficiency, surgery should be advised. The procedure favored by some thoracic surgeons is excision through the axilla of a segment of the first rib; others decompress the thoracic outlet by scalenectomy through a supraclavicular approach. Symptoms have been relieved immediately in over 95 percent of cases when there had been signs of neural and vascular compression. Pain may recur if nerves become entrapped in scar, and it is relieved by surgical freeing of the nerve. Atherosclerosis with thrombosis and embolism of the subclavian artery and thrombosis of the vein require decompression and arterioplasty and venous thrombectomy, respectively. Brachial sympathectomy is indicated in exceptional patients with persistent Raynaud's phenomenon. (For further details, see Imparato and Spencer.)

It is important to note that vasomotor, sudomotor, and trophic changes in the skin, with atrophy of the soft tissues and decalcification of bone, may follow the prolonged immobilization and disuse of an arm or leg for whatever reason. The patient may be reluctant to move the limb because of pain, lack of motivation to get well, or reasons of monetary gain. Surgery in this group of patients is ill-advised, and the physician's efforts should be directed to mobilization of the affected part through an intensive physical therapy program and settlement of litigation, if this is a factor.

PREVENTIVE ASPECTS OF BACK PAIN

Without doubt these are important. There would be many fewer back problems if adults kept their trunk muscles in optimal condition by regular exercise such as swimming, walking briskly, running, and calisthenic programs of the Canadian Air Force type. Morning is the ideal time for exercising, since the back of the older adult tends to be stiffest following a night of inactivity. This happens regardless of whether a bed board or a stiff mattress is used. Sleeping with back hyperextended and sitting for long times in an overstuffed chair or a badly designed car seat are particularly likely to aggravate backache. It is estimated that intradiskal pressures are increased 200 percent by changing from a recumbent to a standing position and 400 percent when slumped in an easy chair. Correct sitting posture lessens this pressure. Long trips in a car or plane without change in position put maximal strain on disk and ligamentous structures in the spine. Lifting from a position of flexed trunk, as in removing a suitcase from the trunk of a car, is risky (always lift with object close to body). Also, sudden strenuous activity without conditioning and warm-up are likely to injure disks and their ligamentous envelopes, and certain families seem disposed to injury to these structures.

POSTTRAUMATIC PAIN SYNDROMES

Included under this heading are a variety of painful conditions of the extremities caused by trauma or disease of individual peripheral nerves.

Persistent and often incapacitating pain and dysesthesias may follow any type of injury that leads to *neuroma formation or intraneural scarring*—fracture, contusion of the limbs, compression from lying on the arm in a drunken stupor, severing of sensory nerves in the course of surgical operations, or incomplete regeneration after nerve suture. It is stated that the nerves in these cases contain a preponderance of unmyelinated C fibers and a reduced number of A-δ fibers, and this imbalance is presumably related to the genesis of painful dysesthesias. These cases are best managed by complete excision of the neuromas with end-to-end suture of healthy nerve, but not all cases lend themselves to this procedure.

Another special type of neuroma is the one that forms at the end of a nerve severed at amputation (stump neuroma). Pain from this source is occasionally abolished by relatively simple procedures such as resection of the end bulbs, proximal neurotomy, or resection of the regional sympathetic ganglia. Anterolateral tractotomy with achievement of complete analgesia is the surest way to abolish pain from stump neuroma (as well as pain from a phantom limb), but is of limited value because of the failure to maintain full analgesia for a protracted time; with some return of sensation (6 months in the case of the lower extremities and earlier in the arms), pain usually returns as well.

NEUROGENIC LIMB PAIN (NONTRAUMATIC)

Many diseases may affect the peripheral nerves and cause pain in the limbs. The nerves may be affected singly (e.g., meralgia paresthetica), or multiple nerves may be affected, in a symmetric or asymmetric fashion. Painful neuropathies are associated most often with alcoholic-nutritional disease (beriberi), polyarteritis, and diabetes mellitus. Idiopathic polyneuritis (Guillain-Barré) may occasionally be painful. These disorders are considered in Chap. 45.

REFERENCES

ABBOTT KH, MITTS MG: Reflex neurovascular syndromes, in Vinken PJ, Bruyn GW (eds): *Handbook of Clinical Neurology*, vol 8. Amsterdam, North-Holland, 1970, chap 20, pp 321-356.

ARMSTRONG JR: *Lumbar Disc Lesions: Pathogenesis and Treatment of Low Back Pain and Sciatica*, 3d ed. Baltimore, Williams & Wilkins, 1965.

BALLANTINE HT JR: Extradural spinal cord and nerve root compression from benign lesions of the cervical areas, in Youmans J (ed): *Neurological Surgery*. Philadelphia, Saunders, 1973, chap 65, pp 1194-1212.

CARLSON DH, SIMON H, WEGNER W: Bone scanning and the diagnosis of reflex sympathetic dystrophy. *Neurology* 27:791, 1977.

DEPALMA AF, ROTHMAN RH: *The Intervertebral Disc*. Philadelphia, Saunders, 1970.

FRIIS ML, GULLIKSEN GC, RASMUSSEN P: Distribution of pain with nerve root compression. *Acta Neurosurgica* 39:241, 1977.

HUDGKINS WR: The crossed straight leg raising sign (of Fajerstagn). *N Engl J Med* 297:1127, 1977.

IMPARATO AM, SPENCER FC: Peripheral arterial disease, in Schwartz SI et al (eds): *Principles of Surgery*, 3d ed. New York, McGraw-Hill, 1979, chap 21, pp 946-951.

KRISTOFF FV, ODOM GL: Ruptured intervertebral disc in the cervical region. *Arch Surg* 54:287, 1947.

LASCELLES RG et al: The thoracic outlet syndrome. *Brain* 100:601, 1977.

LOVE JG, SCHORN VG: Thoracic-disc protrusions. *JAMA* 191:627, 1965.

MATHEWS WB: The neurological complications of ankylosing spondylitis. *J Neurol Sci* 6:561, 1968.

PEPPER H: Primary erythromelalgia. Report of a case treated with methysergide maleate. *JAMA* 203:1066, 1967.

Primer on the Rheumatic Diseases, 7th ed. *JAMA*, vol 224, no 5, suppl, April 30, 1973.

TELFORD ED, MOTTERSHEAD S: Pressure at the cervicobrachial junction: An operative and anatomical study. *J Bone Joint Surg* 30B:249, 1948.

URSCHEL HD, PAULSON DL, MCNAMARA JJ: Thoracic outlet syndrome. *Ann Thorac Surg* 6:1, 1968.

VERBIEST H: Further experiences on the pathological influence of a developmental narrowness of the bony lumbar vertebral canal. *J Bone Joint Surg* 37B:576, 1955.

WEINSTEIN PR, EHNI G, WILSON CB: *Lumbar Spondylosis. Diagnosis, Management and Surgical Treatment*. Chicago, Year Book, 1977.

WHITE JC, SWEET WH: *Pain and the Neurosurgeon*. Springfield, Ill, Charles C Thomas, 1969.

YOSS RE et al: Significance of symptoms and signs in localization of involved root in cervical disc protrusion. *Neurology* 7:673, 1957.

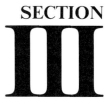

SECTION

III

DISORDERS OF THE SPECIAL SENSES

The four chapters in this section are concerned with the highly specialized functions of taste and smell, vision and ocular movement, hearing, and the sense of balance. These special senses and the cranial nerves that subserve them represent the most finely developed parts of the sensory nervous system. The sensory dysfunctions of the eye and ear are, of course, the proprietary interest of the ophthalmologist and otologist, but they are of interest to the clinical neurologist as well. Some of them reflect the presence of serious systemic disease, and others represent the initial or leading manifestation of neurologic disease. It is from both these points of view that they will be considered here. In keeping with the general approach being used in this volume, the disorders of the special senses and of ocular movement will be considered in a particular sequence: first, their cardinal clinical manifestations, along with the certain facts of anatomic and physiologic importance, followed by a consideration of the syndromes of which these manifestations are a part. Because of their specialized nature, some of the diseases which produce these syndromes will be discussed here rather than in other parts of the book.

CHAPTER 11

DISORDERS OF SMELL AND TASTE

The sensations of smell (olfaction) and taste (gustation) are suitably considered together. Physiologically, these modalities share the singular attribute of responding primarily to chemical stimuli, i.e., the end organs that mediate olfaction and gustation are chemoreceptors. Clinically, taste and smell are also interdependent. The appreciation of the flavor of food and drink depends to a large extent on their aroma, and an abnormality of one of these senses is frequently associated with an abnormality of the other. In contrast to vision and other special senses, taste and smell play a relatively unimportant role in the life of the individual, and only rarely is the loss of either of these latter modalities a serious handicap. Nevertheless, a loss of taste and smell may serve to identify a number of intracranial and systemic disorders, and they assume clinical importance from this point of view.

OLFACTORY SENSE

ANATOMIC AND PHYSIOLOGIC CONSIDERATIONS

Nerve fibers subserving the sense of smell have their cells of origin in the mucous membrane of the upper and posterior part of the nasal cavity. The entire olfactory mucosa covers an area of 2.5 cm and contains two vertically oriented cell types, the receptor cells and the sustenacular, or supporting, cells. The receptor cells are actually bipolar neurons. Each cell has a peripheral process (the olfactory rod), from which project 6 to 12 fine hairs, or cilia. The central processes of these cells, or *olfactory fila*, are very fine (0.2 μm in diameter) unmyelinated fibers which converge to form small fascicles and pass through openings in the cribriform plate of the ethmoid bone into the olfactory bulb (Fig. 11-1). Collec-

tively, the central processes of the olfactory receptor cells constitute the *first cranial*, or *olfactory, nerve*.

In the olfactory bulb, the receptor cell axons synapse with mitral cells (triangular in shape, like a bishop's mitre), the dendrites of which form brushlike terminals or olfactory glomeruli (Fig. 11-1). Smaller, so-called tufted cells in the olfactory bulb also contribute dendrites to the glomerulus. Several thousand olfactory-cell axons converge on a single glomerulus.

The axons of the mitral and tufted cells enter the olfactory tract, which courses along the olfactory groove of the frontal bones to the cerebrum. Caudal to the olfactory bulbs are scattered groups of cells which constitute the anterior olfactory nucleus (Fig. 11-1). Dendrites of these cells synapse with fibers of the olfactory tract, while their axons project to the olfactory nucleus and bulb of the opposite side; these neurons are thought to function as a reinforcing mechanism for olfactory impulses.

Posteriorly the olfactory tract divides into medial and lateral olfactory striae. The medial stria contains fibers from the anterior olfactory nucleus which pass to the opposite side, via the anterior commissure. Fibers in the lateral stria originate in the olfactory bulb, give off collaterals to the anterior perforated substance, and terminate in the medial and cortical nuclei of the amygdaloid complex and the prepiriform area (also referred to as the lateral olfactory gyrus). The latter represents the *primary olfactory cortex*, which in humans occupies a restricted area on the anterior end of the hippocampal gyrus and uncus (area 34 of Brodmann; see Figs. 21-1 and 2). Thus olfactory impulses reach the cerebral cortex without relay through the thalamus; in this respect olfaction is unique among sensory systems. From the prepiriform cortex, fibers project to the neighboring entorhinal cortex (area 28 of Brodmann), the medial dorsal nucleus of the thalamus, and the hypothalamus, but the role of these latter structures in olfaction is not well understood.

In quiet breathing, little of the air entering the nostril reaches the olfactory mucosa; sniffing carries the air into the olfactory crypt. To be perceived as an odor, an inhaled substance must be volatile, i.e., spread in the air as very small particles, and soluble in water or lipids. When a jet of scented vapor is directed to the sensory epithelium, a slow negative potential shift, called the electroolfactogram (EOG) can be recorded from an electrode placed on the mucosa. The conductance changes that underlie the potential of the receptor are induced by molecules of odorous material dissolved in the mucus overlying the receptor. This olfactory potential can be

eliminated by destroying the olfactory receptor surface or the olfactory filaments. The loss of EOG occurs 8 to 16 days after severance of the nerve; the receptor cells disappear, but the sustenacular cells are not altered.

CLINICAL MANIFESTATIONS

Disturbances of olfaction may be subdivided into three groups, as follows:

1. Quantitative abnormalities: loss or reduction of smell (anosmia, hyposmia) or increased olfactory acuity (hyperosmia)

2. Qualitative abnormalities: distortion of smell or dysosmia

3. Illusions and hallucinations of smell caused by local diseases of the nose, central neurologic diseases, or psychiatric diseases

Figure 11-1

Diagram illustrating the relationships between the olfactory receptors in the nasal mucosa and neurons in the olfactory bulb and tract. Cells of the anterior olfactory nucleus are found in scattered groups, caudal to the olfactory bulb. Fibers from the anterior olfactory nucleus project centrally (A). A fiber from the contralateral anterior olfactory nucleus is labeled B. Inset. Diagram of the olfactory structures on the inferior surface of the brain (see text for details).

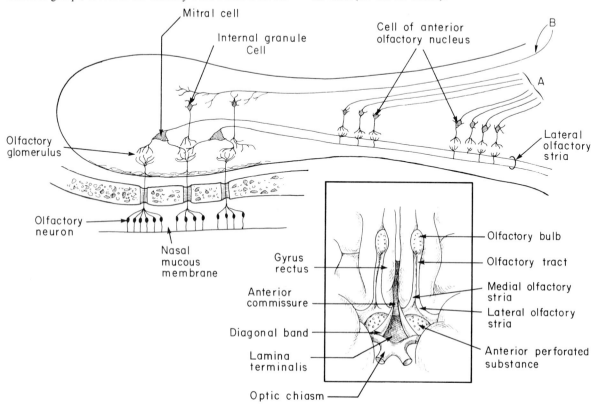

Anosmia (loss of sense of smell) is the most frequent clinical abnormality, and if unilateral it will not be recognized by the patient. Unilateral anosmia is sometimes demonstrated in the hysterical patient on the side of anesthesia, blindness, and deafness. Bilateral anosmia, on the other hand, is not an uncommon complaint, and the patient is usually convinced that the sense of taste has been lost as well (*ageusia*). This calls attention to the fact that taste depends largely on the volatile substances in foods and beverages, and the sensation of flavor is a combination of smell and taste. This can be proved by demonstrating that such patients are able to distinguish the elementary taste sensations (sweet, sour, bitter, and salty). The olfactory defect can be verified readily enough by presenting a series of nonirritating olfactory stimuli (vanilla, lemon, cigarette, coffee, etc.), first in one nostril, then in the other, and asking the patient to sniff and identify them. If the odors can be detected in each nostril, even if they cannot be identified, it may be assumed that the olfactory nerves are relatively intact.[1] Ammonia and similar pungent substances should not be used because they stimulate the trigeminal nerves.

Regarding the nasal diseases responsible for bilateral hyposmia or anosmia, the most frequent are those in which hypertrophy and hyperemia of the nasal mucosa prevent olfactory stimuli from reaching the receptor cells. Heavy smoking, it is said, is the most frequent cause of hyposmia. Chronic rhinitis of allergic, vasomotor, or infective types are common causes, though hormones and metabolic disorders may also cause congestion and swelling of the nasal mucosa. In biopsies of the olfactory mucosa in allergic rhinitis the sensory epithelial cells are still present but their cilia are deformed and shortened and are buried under other mucosal cells. Influenza may be followed by hyposmia or anosmia. This may be permanent since the receptor cells are destroyed by the virus (Douek). There is also a group of diseases in which the primary receptor neurons are congenitally absent or are hypoplastic and lack cilia. One type is Kallman's syndrome of congenital anosmia and hypogonadotropic hypogonadism. Also, congenital anosmia occurs in albinos, because of the absence of "olfactory pigment" or other congenital structural defect.

Head injury causes anosmia by severing the delicate filaments of the receptor cells as they pass through the cribriform plate, especially if the injury is severe enough to cause fracture. The damage may be unilateral or bilateral and is usually permanent. Cranial surgery (especially if much cerebrospinal fluid escapes while the patient is sitting and inclined backward so that the olfactory bulbs retract from the ethmoid bones), subarachnoid hemorrhage, and chronic meningeal inflammation may have a similar effect.

The gradual development of anosmia should prompt an investigation of the anterior base of the skull. Meningiomas of the olfactory region may implicate the olfactory bulbs and tracts and may extend posteriorly to involve the optic nerves. With meningiomas on one side, the anosmia may be strictly unilateral. Upward extension of the tumor into the frontal lobes causes also a lack of initiative (abulia) and personality changes such as apathy, silliness, carefree joking (witzelsucht), and forgetfulness (see Chap. 21). Large aneurysms of the anterior cerebral and anterior communicating arteries may produce a similar syndrome. Children with anterior meningoencephaloceles are usually anosmic and, in addition, may exhibit CSF rhinorrhea when the head is held in certain positions (demonstrated by chemical examination of the fluid, which contains more sugar than mucous secretions, and by watching, under ultraviolet light, fluorescein issue from the nostrils after it has been instilled in the spinal subarachnoid space). Nasal injury and hydrocephalus are other causes of CSF rhinorrhea. These defects in the sense of smell are all attributable to lesions of receptor cells and their axons or the olfactory bulbs. It is not known whether olfactory symptoms may be produced by lesions of the anterior perforated space or medial and lateral olfactory striae. In some cases of increased intracranial pressure, the olfactory sense has been impaired without evidence of lesions in the olfactory bulbs.

Whether a true *hyperosmia* exists is a matter of conjecture. Neurotic individuals may complain of being unduly sensitive to odors, but there is no proof of a lowered threshold of the sense organ.

Dysosmia or parosmia (perversion of the sense of smell) may occur with local nasal conditions such as empyema of the nasal sinuses and ozena. Partial injuries of olfactory bulbs may have a similar effect. Parosmia may also be a troublesome symptom in middle-aged and elderly persons who have symptoms of depression. Every article of food is said to have an extremely unpleasant odor (cacosmia). Sensations of disagreeable taste are of-

---

[1] The analysis of olfactory disorders in humans was put on a quantitative basis by Elsberg, who attempted to detect partial olfactory deficits by measuring the quantity of a scent needed to elicit a minimal identifiable odor (MIO). The continuous stimulation by a stream of odors was used to determine "fatigue" or "adaptation." Though an interesting approach, it has not been widely accepted or used by neurologists.

ten associated (cacogeusia). Nothing is known of the basis of this state; there is usually no loss of discriminative sensation. Minor degrees of parosmia are not necessarily abnormal, for unpleasant odors have a way of lingering for several hours and of being reawakened by other olfactory stimuli, as every pathologist knows (phantosmia).

Olfactory hallucinations are always of central origin. Here the patient claims to smell an odor that no one else can detect. If the patient is convinced of its presence and personal reference, despite all evidence to the contrary, the symptom assumes the status of a *delusion*. Aside from uncal seizures, in which the olfactory experience is brief and accompanied by an alteration of consciousness and other epileptic components (see page 217), olfactory hallucinations and delusions usually signify a psychiatric illness. Zilstorff has written informatively on this subject. There is complaint of a large array of odors, most of them foul. In some, the smell seems to emanate from the patient (intrinsic hallucinations); in others they seem to come from an external source (extrinsic hallucinations). Both types vary in intensity and are remarkable with respect to their persistence. According to Pryse-Phillips, who took note of the psychiatric illness in a series of 137 patients with olfactory hallucinations, most were associated with endogenous depression and schizophrenia. In schizophrenia the olfactory stimulus is usually interpreted as arising externally and as being induced by someone for the purpose of harming the patient. In depression, the stimulus is usually intrinsic and is more overwhelming. All manner of ways are used to get rid of the stench, the usual ones being excessive washing, use of deodorants, and social withdrawal.

Olfactory hallucinations and delusions also occur in conjunction with senile dementia, but when this happens one should consider the possibility of an associated involutional depression. Occasionally an alcoholic withdrawal syndrome with prominent auditory and visual hallucinations is accompanied by olfactory hallucinations. Peculiar reactions to smell characterize certain sexual psychopathies. Usually the stimuli appear to be extrinsic, but in this regard it should be noted that odors imagined by normal individuals are also perceived as coming from outside the person through inspired air, and unpleasant ones are more clearly represented than pleasant ones. In interpreting these phenomena, Bromberg and Schilder suggest that smell is an important orienting sense, has value as a "social indicator," and

serves to initiate attraction behavior (if pleasant or sexual) or avoidance behavior if disagreeable.

GUSTATORY SENSE

ANATOMIC CONSIDERATIONS

The sensory receptors for taste (taste buds) are distributed over the surface of the tongue and, in smaller numbers, over the palate, pharynx, and larynx. Mainly they are located in the epithelium along the lateral surfaces of the circumvallate papillae and to a lesser extent in the epithelium of the fungiform papillae. The taste buds are round or oval structures, each composed of about 20 vertically oriented receptor cells, arranged like the staves of a barrel. The ends of these cells surround a small opening, the taste pore, which opens onto the mucosal surface. The tips of the sensory cells project through the pore as a number of filiform microvilli ("taste hairs"). Fine unmyelinated nerve fibers penetrate the base of the taste bud to innervate the sensory cells. Each receptor is capable of being activated by chemical substances in solution and transmits its activity along the sensory nerves to the brainstem. Any one taste bud is capable of responding to a number of sapid substances, but always it is more sensitive to one type of stimulus than another. In other words, the receptor for each primary taste is only relatively specific. The sensitivity of these receptors is remarkable: as little as 0.05 mg per 100 ml of quinine sulfate will arouse a bitter taste when applied to the base of the tongue.

As stated above, the four primary taste sensations are salty, sweet, bitter, and sour; more complex flavors are combinations of olfactory and gustatory sensations. All four submodalities are perceived at the tip of the tongue, though this part is more sensitive to sweet and salt. The sides of the tongue are more sensitive to sour and the base to bitter.

The number of taste buds is not large and diminishes with age. In each taste bud the receptor cells have a brief life cycle being replaced constantly by mitotic division of adjacent epithelial cells. Therefore gustatory acuity is highly variable. It is tested by withdrawing the tongue with a gauze sponge and using a moistened applicator to place a few crystals of salt or sugar on small discrete parts of the tongue; the tongue is then wiped clean, and the subjects are asked to report what they have sensed. A useful stimulus for sour sensation is a low-voltage direct current, the electrodes of which can be accurately placed on the tongue surface. Special procedures have been devised for the measurement of taste intensity and for determining the detection and recognition thresholds of taste and olfactory stimuli (Henkin et al.), but these are beyond the scope of the usual clinical examination.

From the anterior two-thirds of the tongue, taste fibers first run in the lingual nerve (a major branch of the mandibular nerve). After coursing within it for a short distance the taste fibers diverge to enter the chorda tympani (a branch of the seventh nerve); thence they pass through the pars intermedia and geniculate ganglion of the seventh nerve to the rostral part of the nucleus of the tractus solitarius in the medulla. Fibers from the palatal taste buds pass through the pterygopalatine ganglion and greater superficial petrosal nerve, join the facial nerve at the level of the geniculate ganglion, and proceed to the nucleus of the solitary tract (see Fig. 46-2). Possibly, also, taste fibers from the tongue may reach the brainstem via the mandibular division of the trigeminal nerve. The presence of these alternate pathways probably accounts for instances of unilateral taste loss that have followed section of the root of the trigeminal nerve and instances in which no loss of taste has occurred with section of the chorda tympani. From the posterior third of the tongue, soft palate, and palatal arches, the sensory impulses for taste are conveyed through the glossopharyngeal nerve and ganglion nodosum to the nucleus of the tractus solitarius. Taste fibers from the extreme dorsal part of the tongue and the few that arise on taste buds on the pharynx and larynx are carried by the vagus nerve. Rostral and lateral parts of the nucleus solitarius, which receive the special afferent (taste) fibers from the facial and glossopharyngeal nerves, constitute the "gustatory nucleus." Probably both sides of the tongue are represented in this nucleus.

The second sensory neuron for taste has been difficult to track. The neurons of the nucleus solitarius send axons to adjacent nuclei (e.g., dorsal motor nuclei of vagus, ambiguus, salivatorius superior and inferior, trigeminal, and facial) which serve in viscerovisceral and viscerosomatic reflex functions, but those concerned with the conscious recognition of taste are believed to form a gustatory (solitariothalamic) lemniscus, the fibers of which ascend in association with the medial lemniscus on the same and opposite sides and synapse in the ventral posteromedial (VPM) nucleus. Some secondary fibers end in the hypothalamus and probably influence autonomic function. Experiments in animals indicate that taste impulses from the thalamus project to the tongue-face area of the postrolandic sensory cortex, and in humans, also to the region of the second somatic sensory cortex.

Richter has explored the biological role of taste in normal nutrition. Animals made deficient in sodium, calcium, certain vitamins, proteins, etc., will automati-

cally select the correct foods, on the basis of their taste, to compensate for their deficiency.

CLINICAL MANIFESTATIONS

Heavy smoking, particularly pipe smoking, is probably the commonest cause of impairment of taste sensation. Extreme drying of the tongue with desquamation and damage to the taste buds may lead to temporary loss or reduction of the sense of taste (*ageusia* or *hypogeusia*). Dryness of the mouth (xerostomia) from inadequate saliva, as occurs in Sjögren's syndrome, x-ray irradiation of head and neck, and pandysautonomia, also interferes with taste because taste stimuli, like olfactory ones, are effective only in a fluid medium. If unilateral, ageusia is seldom the source of complaint. Taste is frequently lost over one-half of the tongue (except posteriorly) in cases of Bell's palsy, providing the lesion extends far enough centrally to involve the nerve after it is joined by the chorda tympani. The loss is always homolateral.

A permanent decrease in acuity of taste and smell (hypogeusia and hyposmia), sometimes associated with perversions of these sensory functions (dysgeusia and dysosmia) may follow influenza-like illnesses. These abnormalities have been shown to be associated with pathological changes in the taste buds, as well as in the nasal mucous membranes. In a group of 143 patients who presented with hypogeusia and hyposmia, 87 (59 percent) were of this postinfluenzal type (Henkin et al.). The remaining patients in this series developed their symptoms in association with a wide variety of disorders, including scleroderma, acute hepatitis, viral encephalitis, myxedema and other hormonal disorders, occult and overt malignancies, deficiency of vitamins B_{12} and A, and the administration of a wide variety of drugs (see below).

An interesting syndrome, called *idiopathic hypogeusia*, in which a decreased taste acuity is associated with dysgeusia, hyposmia, and dysosmia, has been described by Henkin et al. The taste and aroma of food is unpleasant to the point of being revolting (cacogeusia and cacosmia), and the persistence of these symptoms may lead to a loss of weight, anxiety, and depression. Patients with this disorder have been shown to have a decreased concentration of zinc in their parotid saliva and their symptoms have responded to small oral doses of zinc sulfate.

Persistent misinterpretations of taste and distortions (dysgeusia) tend to occur with certain medications, e.g., with griseofulvin, amitriptyline, antithyroid drugs, chlorambucil, and colestyramine; with penicillamine, in the course of treatment of Wilson's disease and rheumatoid arthritis; and with procarbazine, vincristine, and vinblastine, used in the treatment of carcinoma and lymphoma.

Unilateral lesions of the medulla oblongata have not been reported to cause ageusia, perhaps because the nucleus of the tractus solitarius is usually outside the zone of infarction. Unilateral thalamic and parietal lobe lesions have both been associated with contralateral impairment of taste sensation, and stimulation of the anterior part of the second sensorimotor cortex (where it approaches the insula) has given rise to sensations of taste. A gustatory aura occasionally marks the beginning of a convulsive attack originating in this part of the cortex. A gustatory aura may be part of an uncinate seizure, and if conjoined with auditory or visual hallucinations and "dreamy" states, the seizure activity has probably spread laterally and rostrally from the uncus. Gustatory hallucinations are much less frequent than olfactory ones but may occur both with structural lesions of the temporoparietal regions (e.g., encephalitis) and in the functional psychoses.

REFERENCES

BRODAL A: *Neurological Anatomy in Relation to Clinical Medicine*, 3d ed. Fair Lawn, NJ, Oxford, 1981.

BROMBERG W, SCHILDER P: Olfactory imagination and hallucinations. *Arch Neurol Psychiatry* 32:467, 1934.

DOUEK E: *The Sense of Smell and its Abnormalities*. London, Churchill-Livingstone, 1973.

ELSBERG CA: A new and simple method of quantitative olfactometry. *Bull Neurol Inst* 4:1, 1935.

HENKIN RI, GILL JR JR, BARTTER FC: Studies on taste thresholds in normal man and in patients with adrenal cortical insufficiency: The effect of adrenocorticosteroids. *J Clin Invest* 42:727, 1963.

———, LARSON AL, POWELL RD: Hypogeusia, dysgeusia, hyposmia and dysosmia following influenza-like infection. *Ann Otol* 84:672, 1975.

———, SCHECHTER PJ, HOYE R, MATTERN CFT: Idiopathic hypogeusia with dysgeusia, hyposmia, and dysosmia. A new syndrome. *JAMA* 217:434, 1971.

PRYSE-PHILLIPS W: Disturbances in the sense of smell in psychiatric patients. *Proc Roy Soc Med* 68:26, 1975.

ZILSTORFF W: Parosmia. *J Laryngol Otol* 80:1102, 1966.

CHAPTER 12

COMMON DISTURBANCES OF VISION

The eye, with its diverse composition of epithelial, vascular, collagenous, neural, and pigmentary tissue, is a medical microcosm, susceptible to manifold diseases. Moreover, its transparency makes it accessible to direct inspection by the ophthalmoscope and affords an opportunity to observe during life many of the specific lesions of medical diseases.

Since the eye is the organ of vision, it is obvious that impairment of visual acuity of various degrees should stand as the most frequent and important symptom of eye disease. Irritation, redness and photophobia, pain, diplopia and strabismus, and drooping or closure of the eyelids are the other major symptoms. The impairment of eyesight may be unilateral or bilateral, sudden or gradual, episodic or enduring. The common causes of impairment of vision vary with age. In late childhood and adolescence nearsightedness, or *myopia*, is the usual cause though a retinal, optic nerve, or suprasellar tumor must not be overlooked. In middle-age, farsightedness (hyperopia) is almost invariable. Still later in life, *cataracts, glaucoma, retinal hemorrhages, detachments, and degenerations* are the most frequent causes of visual disturbance.

Episodic blindness in early life is usually due to migraine; later, transient blindness, or *amaurosis fugax*, is related to stenosis of the carotid artery or embolism of retinal arterioles, or there may be no discernible cause. Cerebrovascular disease deranges vision with increasing frequency in later life. The term *amaurosis* refers to blindness from any cause, whereas *amblyopia* refers to an impairment or loss of vision which is not due to an error of refraction or to other disease of the eye itself. *Nyctalopia* means poor twilight or night vision and is associated with vitamin A deficiency, retinitis pigmentosa, and, often, color blindness.

In approaching the problem of disturbance of vision one always begins by inquiring as to precisely what patients mean when they say that they cannot see properly, for they may be referring to symptoms as varied as near- or far-sightedness, excessive tearing, diplopia, partial syncope, or even giddiness or dizziness. Fortunately their statements can be checked by the measurement of visual acuity, which is the single most important part of the ocular examination. Inspection of the fundi and plotting of the visual fields complete the examination of the second cranial nerves.

NONNEUROLOGIC CAUSES OF REDUCED VISION

In the measurement of visual acuity the *Snellen Chart*, which contains rows of letters of diminishing size (the height of each letter subtends 5 min of an arc when held at various distances from the eye), is utilized. The letter at the top of the chart subtends 5 min of an arc at a distance of 200 ft (or roughly 60 m); then follow rows of letters which should be read at lesser distances. Thus if the patient can read only the top letter at 20 rather than 200 ft, the acuteness of vision is expressed as 20/200 (V = 20/200, or 6/60 if distances are measured in meters rather than feet). If the patient's eyesight is normal, the visual acuity will equal 20/20, or 6/6, using the metric scale. Many persons, especially during youth, can read at 20 ft the line which should be read at 15 ft from the chart (V = 20/15). Patients with a corrected refractive error should wear their eyeglasses for the test. For bedside testing, a "near card" can be used. In young children, acuity can be estimated by having them mimic the examiner's finger movements.

If the visual acuity (with glasses) is less than 20/20, either the refractive error has not been properly corrected or there is some other reason for the diminished acuity. The former possibility can be ruled out if the patient can read the 20/20 line through a pinhole in a cardboard held in front of the eye; the pinhole permits a narrow shaft of light to fall on the macular fovea (the area of greatest visual acuity).

Light entering the eye is focused on the outer layer of the retina, which contains two types of photoreceptor cells, the slender *rods* and flask-shaped *cones.* Consequently the tissue and fluid through which the light passes must be transparent. These media are the cornea, the aqueous humor of the anterior chamber, the lens, the vitreous humor of the vitreous cavity, and the retina itself. The clarity of these media can be determined ophthalmoscopically, and this examination usually requires that the pupil be dilated, to at least 6 mm in diameter. This is best accomplished by instilling a few drops of 10% phenylephrine (Neo-Synephrine) in each eye after the visual acuity has been measured, the pupillary responses recorded, and the intraocular pressure estimated. The mydriatic action of phenylephrine lasts only a few hours. Rarely, an *attack of angle-closure glaucoma with ocular pain, nausea, and vomiting may be precipitated by pupillary dilation;* this can be prevented by instilling 2% pilocarpine immediately after the ocular examination. Usually the pupils will have returned to normal size by the time the physical examination is completed.

By looking through a high-plus lens of the ophthalmoscope, from a distance of 6 to 12 in, the examiner can visualize opacities in the refractive media; by adjusting the lenses from a high-plus to a zero or minus setting, it is possible to "depth-focus" from the cornea to the retina. Depending upon the refractive error of the examiner, lenticular opacities are best seen within a $+20$ to $+12$ range; vitreous opacities in the $+10$ to $+2$ range; and the retina comes into focus with $+1$ to -1 lenses. The pupil appears as a red circular structure (red reflex), the color being provided by the oxyhemoglobin of the capillaries of the choroid layer. Clarity of all the refractile media means that reduced vision uncorrected by glasses is due to a defect in the macula, the optic nerve, or the parts of the brain with which they are connected.

It is not feasible to mention all the causes of opacification of the refractive media; only those with important medical or neurologic implications are listed below. In the *cornea,* the most common cause is scarring due to trauma and infection. Hypercalcemia secondary to sarcoid, hyperparathyroidism, and vitamin D intoxication may give rise to precipitates of calcium phosphate and carbonate, beneath the corneal epithelium and primarily in a plane corresponding to the interpalpebral tissue, so-called *band keratopathy.* The latter disorder also occurs with multiple myeloma, juvenile rheumatoid arthritis and dry eyes. Diffuse deposition of calcium in the cornea and conjunctivum may occur in the milk alkali syndrome. Cystine crystals are deposited in cystinosis, chloroquine crystals in cases of discoid lupus treated by this drug, polysaccharides in Hurler's disease, and copper in hepatolenticular degeneration (Kayser-Fleischer ring, page 687). Crystal deposits may also be observed in multiple myeloma and cryoglobulinemia. The occurrence of an arcus senilis at an early age is commonly associated with familial hypercholesterolemia. Ulceration and subsequent opacification of the cornea may also occur with herpes simplex and herpes zoster infections or may complicate the conjunctivitis and uveitis of Behcet's disease and other mucocutaneous-ocular syndromes (Stevens-Johnson, Reiter's). Keratitis may be a manifestation also of congenital syphilis, tuberculosis, malignant exophthalmos, and of more innocent states such as drying and injury of the corneas during coma. Corneas are diffusely cloudy in certain lysosomal storage diseases (see Chap. 37).

In relation to the *anterior chamber,* the common problem is one of impediment to the outflow of the aqueous fluid, excavation of the optic disk, and visual loss, or *glaucoma.* In more than 90 percent of cases (of the wide-angle type) the cause of this syndrome is unknown; in about 5 percent the angle between pupil and lateral cornea is narrow and blocked when the pupil is dilated; and in the remaining cases the condition is secondary to some disease process that blocks outflow channels [inflammatory debris of uveitis, red blood cells from hemorrhage in the anterior chamber (hyphema), or new formation of vessels and connective tissue on the surface of the iris (rubeosis iridis), a rare complication of diabetes mellitus]. Some degree of increased intraocular pressure is said to occur in 2 percent of all persons over the age of 40; in most of these cases it is asymptomatic and goes unrecognized for years, but in some it may progress to rapid loss of vision. Therefore the intraocular pressure should be measured routinely, using a Schiotz tonometer. This is a simple procedure which should be practiced by every physician. With the patient supine, a drop of local anesthetic is put into each eye and the tonometer is then placed on the cornea so that the instrument is perfectly vertical. When the tonometer is pressed against the eye, the scale is read and the units are converted into millimeters of mercury from the chart in the tonometer case. The normal pressure is about 15 mmHg. Pressures of 20 to 30 mmHg may damage the optic nerve. The damage is manifest first as a quadrantic defect in the nasal field and may lead to blindness; with the ophthalmoscope one can see also that the optic disk is excavated and the margins of the optic cup are broadened.

In the *lens,* cataract formation is the common abnormality. The "sugar cataract" of diabetes mellitus is the result of sustained high levels of blood glucose, which is changed in the lens to sorbitol, the accumulation of which leads to a high osmotic gradient with swelling and disruption of the lens fibers. Galactosemia is a much rarer disease, but the mechanism of cataract formation is similar, i.e., the accumulation of dulcitol in the lens. In hypoparathyroidism, lowering of the concentration of calcium in the aqueous humor is in some way responsible for the opacification of newly forming lens fibers. Prolonged high doses of chlorpromazine and corticosteroids and radiation therapy are believed to induce lenticular opacities. Down's syndrome and oculocerebrorenal syndrome (Chap. 43), spinocerebellar ataxia with oligophrenia (Chap. 42), and certain dermatologic syndromes (atopic dermatitis, congenital ichthyosis, incontinentia pigmenti) are other causes of lenticular opacities. Myotonic dystrophy (Chap. 49) and, rarely, Wilson's disease (Chap. 37) are associated with special types of cataract. Subluxation of the lens, the result of weakening of its zonular ligaments, occurs in syphilis, Marfan's syndrome, and homocystinuria.

In the *vitreous humor,* hemorrhage may occur from rupture of a ciliary or retinal vessel. On ophthalmoscopic examination, the hemorrhage appears as a diffuse haziness of part or all of the vitreous or as a sharply defined mass, if the blood displaces rather than mixes with the vitreous gel. The common causes are trauma, rupture of newly formed vessels of proliferative retinopathy in patients with diabetes mellitus, and retinal tears, in which the hemorrhage breaks through the internal limiting membrane. The deep portions of the vitreous humor may also be affected by deposition of calcium soaps, which are seen as small white opacities with the ophthalmoscope; these are referred to as *asteroid hyalitis,* and are observed in older patients, particularly those with amyloidosis. Occasionally crystals of fatty acids or cholesterol appear as small glistening opacities which fall in a shower when the eyeball is moved. These are known as *synchisis scintillans.* The commonest vitreous opacities are the benign "floaters" or "spots before the eyes" which appear as gray dots when the individual changes the position of the eyes; they may be annoying or even alarming until the patient stops looking for them.

NEUROLOGIC CAUSES OF REDUCED VISION

The search begins with an ophthalmoscopic examination of the retina. This thin (100- to 350-μm) sheet of transparent tissue and the nerve head (*optic disk*) into which the visual information is channeled are the only parts of the central nervous system that can be inspected directly during life.

ANATOMIC AND PHYSIOLOGIC CONSIDERATIONS

Light entering the eye passes through the full thickness of the retina to reach the first neuronal elements in the visual pathway—the receptor layer of rods and cones. The cones are responsible for color discrimination and sharp vision, and they alone are present in the fovea, the portion of the retina upon which objects are focused under photopic conditions. The rods, which are more sensitive to low intensities of light, predominate in the rest of the retina. Impulses arising in these photoreceptors are transmitted by means of a second system of neurons, the bipolar cells, to the innermost ganglion-cell layer. The third system of visual neurons consists of the ganglion cells and their axons, which run uninterruptedly through the optic nerve, chiasm, and optic tracts, synapsing with cells in the lateral geniculate body. From these cells arises the fourth system of neurons, the final visual pathway, consisting of the geniculocalcarine tract. The visual pathway is discussed further on in relation to the visual fields.

The axons of the retinal ganglion cells penetrate the lamina cribrosa, a sievelike structure which consists of elements of sclera and fibrous tissue of the optic nerve. It appears ophthalmoscopically within the optic cup, in the central or nasal part of the optic disk. The absence of visual end organs at this point accounts for the blind spot in the field of vision. Normally, the ganglion cell axons acquire a myelin sheath only after they penetrate the lamina cribrosa and form the optic nerve. But sometimes the retinal nerve fibers adjacent to the disk acquire a myelin sheath. This variant of the normal state appears as white patches with fine linear streaks near the disk and must not be confused with exudates. The optic nerve, unlike other cranial and spinal nerves, is truly a part of the central nervous system, with glial cells rather than Schwann cells between its fibers.

The vascular supply of the retina comes from the ophthalmic branch of the internal carotid artery, which gives origin first to the posterior ciliary arteries (which supply the optic disk and adjacent portion of the optic nerve and the choroid and ciliary body) and then to the central retinal artery. The latter issues from the optic disk, divides into four branches, which, after a short distance, lose their internal elastic membrane and continuous muscular coat, and are properly classed as arterioles. Each branch supplies a quadrant of the retina. The ganglion and bipolar cells receive their blood supply from these arterioles and their capillaries, whereas the photoreceptor elements receive their nourishment from the underlying choroidal vascular bed, by diffusion through the semipermeable Bruch's membrane.

LESIONS OF THE RETINA

In disease, the retinal vessels react like vessels of corresponding size in the brain. Atheromatous deposits with subsequent *occlusion* may occur in the posterior ciliary arteries and in the *central retinal artery* and its branches close to the disk, since these are true arteries. Pallor of the retina, narrowing of the arterioles, and a cherry-red appearance of the fovea are the important ophthalmoscopic findings in thrombosis of the central retinal artery. Ultimately, optic atrophy of the consecutive type develops. Thrombosis of the posterior ciliary arteries may cause sudden blindness due to ischemic optic neuropathy with no visible change in the retinal circulation or retina itself (Hayreh), though in some of our cases we have observed edema of the optic disk and swelling of the optic nerve in the CT scan. Later there may develop cupping of the optic disk, resembling that of glaucoma, except for more severe pallor. Occasionally, *atheromatous and other emboli* from the carotid arteries and aorta may reach the smaller retinal vessels. Since the central retinal vein and artery share a common adventitial sheath, atheromatous plaques in the artery may be associated with thrombosis of the vein. *Venous engorgement* and *tortuosity, segmentation* of columns of venous blood, and *retinal hemorrhages* are often associated with *occlusion of the central retinal vein;* these changes are most frequently observed in patients with diabetes mellitus or hypertension, or both, less frequently with sickle-cell disease, and rarely with multiple myeloma and macroglobulinemia.

Since the walls of the retinal arterioles are transparent, what is seen with the ophthalmoscope is a column of blood. The central light streak of many normal arterioles is thought to represent the reflection of light

from the ophthalmoscope as it strikes the interface of the column of blood and the concave vascular wall. In *arteriolosclerosis* (usually coexistent with hypertension), the lumina of the vessels appear irregularly narrowed because of fibrous tissue replacement of the media and thickening of the basement membrane. *Tortuosity of arterioles, arteriolar-venular compressions,* and *narrowed segments* are other signs of hypertension and arteriolosclerosis. It is generally believed that the vein is compressed by the thickened arteriole within the adventitial envelope shared by both vessels at the site of crossing. Progressive vascular disease, to the point of occlusion of the lumen, results in a narrow, white ("silver-wire") vessel with no visible blood column. This change is associated most often with severe hypertension, but may follow other types of occlusion of the central retinal artery or its branches. Sheathing of the arterioles is observed in some patients with leukemia, malignant hypertension, sarcoid, Behcet's disease, or other forms of vasculitis.

In malignant hypertension there are, in addition to the arteriolar changes noted above, a number of extravascular lesions: the so-called *soft exudates or cotton-wool patches, sharply marginated, glistening "hard" exudates, retinal hemorrhages,* and *papilledema;* in many patients who show these retinal changes, analogous lesions are to be found in the brain (necrotizing arteriolitis and microinfarcts).

The ophthalmoscopic appearance of retinal hemorrhages is determined by the structural arrangements of the particular zones in which they occur. In the superficial layer of the retina they are linear or flame-shaped, because of their confinement by the horizontally coursing nerve fibers in that layer. These hemorrhages usually overlie and obscure the retinal vessels. Round or oval ("dot and blot") hemorrhages lie behind the vessels, in the outer plexiform layer (synaptic layer between bipolar cells and nuclei of rods and cones); in this layer, blood accumulates in the form of a cylinder between vertically oriented nerve fibers, and appears round when viewed end-on with the ophthalmoscope. Rupture of arterioles on the inner surface of the retina, such as occurs with ruptured intracranial saccular aneurysms, arteriovenous malformations and other conditions causing sudden severe elevation of intracranial pressure, permits the accumulation of a sharply outlined lake of blood between the internal limiting membrane of the retina and the coalescing vitreous fibers (hyaloid membrane); this is the subhyaloid or preretinal hemorrhage. Either the superficial or the deep retinal hemorrhage may show a central or eccentric pale (Roth) spot, which is caused by an accumulation of white blood cells, fibrin, or amorphous material. This lesion is characteristic of bacterial endocarditis, but may be observed in leukemia and multiple myeloma.

Cotton-wool patches, like splinter hemorrhages, overlie and tend to obscure the retinal blood vessels. Large patches, or small ones involving the macula, cause serious disturbances of vision. The soft exudates are in reality infarcts of the nerve fiber layer, due to occlusion of arterioles and capillaries; they are composed of clusters of ovoid structures called *cytoid bodies*, representing the terminal swellings of interrupted axons. *"Hard exudates"* appear as punctate, white or yellow bodies; they lie in the outer plexiform layer, behind the retinal vessels, as do punctate hemorrhages. If present in the macular region, they are arranged in lines radiating toward the fovea (*macular star*). Hard exudates consist of fibrin strands, neutral fat, and fatty acids, and their pathogenesis is not understood. They are observed most often in cases of diabetes mellitus and accelerated hypertension. *Drusen* (*colloid*) *bodies*, which are benign excrescences of Bruch's membrane, are difficult to distinguish ophthalmoscopically from hard exudates, except when they occur alone; as a rule, hard exudates are accompanied by other funduscopic abnormalities. Drusen that are located near the optic disk may simulate papilledema.

Aneurysms of retinal vessels appear as small, discrete red dots and are located, in the largest number, in the paracentral region. They occur with or without other vascular lesions of the retina and are most often a sign of diabetes mellitus, sometimes appearing before the usual clinical manifestations of that disease have become obvious. Microscopically, the aneurysms take the form of small (20- to 90-μm) saccular outpouchings from the walls of capillaries, venules, or arterioles. The vessels of origin of the aneurysms are invariably abnormal, being either acellular branches of occluded vessels or themselves occluded by fat or fibrin.

Aside from vascular lesions, other more specific alterations of the retina, namely, tears and detachments, may impair vision acutely. The rods and cones may be separated from the pigment layer of the retina, or in cases of proliferative retinopathy, the contraction of fibrous tissue may pull the entire retina away from the choroid.

Minimal changes in the retina or retinal pigment epithelium, not readily detectable by ophthalmoscopy, may nevertheless impair visual acuity. The diminished visual acuity in these circumstances is characterized by a prolonged recovery time following light stimulation. This attribute forms the basis of the "light-stress test," in which a strong light is shone through the pupil of the affected eye for 10 s; the time necessary for the acuity to return to its previously determined level is recorded and compared to the recovery time in the normal eye (50 s or

less). Lesions of the optic nerve do not alter the recovery time, so that the test is useful in distinguishing the loss of vision due to retinal disease from that due to optic nerve disease.

In summary, sudden painless loss of vision should always raise the question of *disease of the optic nerve* (retrobulbar neuropathy, see further on) *or of the retina*, more specifically of occlusion of the central retinal artery or vein or of the posterior ciliary artery with ischemic optic neuropathy, detachment of the retina, macular hemorrhage, vitreous hemorrhage, or acute glaucoma.

Degenerations of the retina are an important cause of chronic visual loss and are of several varieties: (1) Degeneration of the outer receptor layer and subjacent pigment epithelium occurs as a hereditary trait in retinitis pigmentosa and also in the Laurence-Moon-Biedl syndrome; in Bassen-Kornzweig disease, Refsum's disease, Kearns-Sayre syndrome, and Batten-Mayou juvenile lipid storage disease (Chap. 37); and in idiopathic senile macular degeneration. (2) Degeneration of Bruch's membrane (which supports the layer of pigment epithelium next to the rods and cones) and its repair by fibrosis give rise to angioid streaks typical of pseudoxanthoma elasticum, Paget's disease, hyperphosphatemia, sickle cell anemia, and acromegaly. (3) Phenothiazine derivatives may conjugate with the melanin of the pigment layer, with resulting degeneration of the outer retinal layers. When these drugs are used, the doses should be kept low and the patient tested frequently for defects in visual fields and color vision. Other degenerative disorders involving the retina are described in Chap. 42 (see pages 827 to 828). In still other disorders, such as toxoplasmosis, histoplasmosis, syphilis, tuberculosis, and sarcoidosis, both the retina and the choroid may be involved. The choroid is also a frequent site of viral and noninfective inflammatory reactions, often in association with iridocyclitis.

THE OPTIC DISK

The optic nerves, chiasm, and tracts, which constitute the third visual neuron, can be inspected only in part, from the foveal or macular region to the optic disk. Changes in the optic disk are of particular importance, since they reflect the presence of raised intracranial pressure (papilledema or choked disk), disease of the optic nerve affecting its ophthalmoscopically visible portion (papillitis), atrophy of the optic nerve, and glaucoma.

Illustrations of these and other abnormalities of the disk can be found in the ninth edition of *Harrison's Principles of Internal Medicine*.

Of the various abnormalities of the optic disk, *papilledema* is of the greatest significance, neurologically speaking, for it provides evidence of increased intracranial pressure. In its mildest form the papilledema may present only as a blurring and slight elevation of the disk margins. Since many normal individuals, especially those with hypermetropia, have ill-defined nasal disk margins, this early stage of papilledema is difficult to detect. Pulsations of retinal veins will have disappeared by the time intracranial pressure is raised, but since 10 to 15 percent of normal individuals have no pulsations, this criterion is not absolute. On the other hand, the presence of spontaneous venous pulsations is a reliable indicator of an intracranial pressure below 180 to 190 mmH$_2$O and thus usually excludes early papilledema. The more advanced degrees of papilledema appear as a "mushrooming" of the entire disk and surrounding retina with edema and obscuration of marginal vessels, congested veins, and peripapillary hemorrhages. When advanced, papilledema is always bilateral but may be more pronounced on the side of an intracranial tumor. A purely unilateral edema of the optic disk, usually with impaired vision, is caused by perioptic meningiomas and other tumors and lesions of the optic nerve. As papilledema becomes chronic, the elevation of the disk margin is less restricted, and pallor of the optic nerve head appears. As the papilledema subsides, it leaves a secondary optic atrophy.

Papilledema from increased intracranial pressure must be distinguished from a combined edema of the optic nerve and retina which may occur in malignant hypertension and in iridocyclitis with retinitis. These two conditions are usually divulged by changes in the periphery of the retinae and other data. As remarked earlier, visual function is usually retained with papilledema, except for enlargement of the blind spots and constriction of the visual fields.

The pathogenesis of papilledema has recently been restudied in terms of orthograde axoplasmic transport (Minckler and others). It appears that with increased intracranial pressure the initial changes consist of intraaxonal swelling and blockage of axoplasmic transport, followed by obstruction of the fine prelaminar venous channels and extravasation of fluid. Since the optic nerve head is nourished by the posterior ciliary arteries and not by the central retinal artery, the former

vessels and associated veins assume greater importance in the mechanism of papilledema. While interesting, this is only a refinement of the hypothesis advanced many years ago by Holmes and Patton, viz., that an increased pressure in the perioptic subarachnoid spaces blocks both the central retinal and posterior ciliary veins, leading to vascular engorgement and accumulation of intercellular fluid. The newer techniques of fluorescein angiography, infrared ophthalmoscopy (which shows the increasing separation and prominence of retinal nerve fibers), and stereoscopic fundus photography are ways of verifying early edema of optic disks.

Other abnormalities of the optic disk and their significance will be discussed in relation to the particular syndromes and diseases of which they are a part.

NEUROLOGY OF THE CENTRAL VISUAL PATHWAY

From the retina, there is a point-to-point projection to the lateral geniculate ganglion, and from the latter a point-to-point projection to the calcarine cortex of the occipital lobe. Thus the visual cortex receives a spatial pattern of stimulation that corresponds with the retinal image of the visual field. For purposes of description, each retina and macula (the central portion of the retina for acute vision) is divided into a temporal and nasal half by a vertical line passing through the fovea centralis. A horizontal line, also through the fovea, divides each half of the retina and macula into upper and lower quadrants (Fig. 12-1).

The anatomic features of the central projections of the retinas are illustrated in their simplest form in Fig. 12-1: (1) Fibers from the *right half of each retina* project exclusively to the right geniculate ganglion and in turn to the right occipital cortex; the converse, of course, applies to fibers from the left halves of the retinas. (2) Fibers from the upper retinal quadrants (peripheral to the maculae) project to the medial portion of the lateral geniculate ganglion, and, in turn, to the anterior two-thirds of the visual cortex, *above* the calcarine sulcus. (3) From the lower peripheral retinal quadrants, the projection is to the lateral portion of the geniculate ganglion and the anterior two-thirds of the visual cortex, *below* the calcarine sulcus. (4) Macular fibers project to a relatively large posterior area of the lateral geniculate ganglion with a relay to the visual cortex of the occipital pole; the upper portion of the macula is represented above and the lower portion below the calcarine fissure. Nearly 90 percent of the primary visual cortex (area 17) is activated by the macular regions of the retina and only 10 percent by the rest of the retina. In addition, there are other geniculocalcarine projections to the occipital and parietal cortex, concerned with visual alerting reactions and perception.

ABNORMALITIES OF THE VISUAL FIELDS

Visual defects caused by lesions in the retina, optic nerves and tracts, lateral geniculate bodies, geniculocalcarine path, and striate cortex of occipital lobes are manifested by changes in the *visual fields*. In the alert, cooperative patient, the visual fields can be plotted accurately at the bedside. With one of the patient's eyes covered and the other looking directly into the corresponding eye of the examiner (patient's right eye and examiner's left), a target, such as a moving finger, or a cotton pledget or white disk mounted on a stick is brought from the outside toward the center of the visual field. With the target at an equal distance between the

Figure 12-1

Projection of the retina on the lateral geniculate nucleus and the visual cortex. (From ML Barr, The Human Nervous System, 3d ed, Hagerstown, Md, Harper & Row, 1979.)

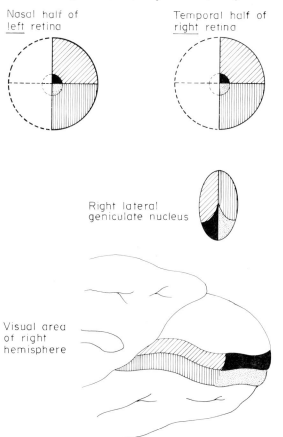

Nasal half of left retina

Temporal half of right retina

Right lateral geniculate nucleus

Visual area of right hemisphere

examiner's and patient's eyes, the patient's fields are compared with those of the examiner.

The patient's blind spot should be aligned with the examiner's and its size determined by moving the target outward from the blind spot until it is seen. Central and paracentral defects in the field can be outlined the same way.

Glaser uses a simple and effective method for the detection of subtle hemianopic defects. The examiner's hands are presented simultaneously to either side of the vertical meridian separating the temporal from the nasal hemifield; the hand in the hemianopic depression appears blurred or darker than the other. Similarly, a scotoma may be defined by asking the patient to report changes in color or brightness of a test object as it is moved toward or away from the point of fixation. Alternately, two test objects can be used, one placed centrally and the other eccentrically, and the patient is asked to describe differences in color intensity.

If any defect is found or suspected by confrontation testing, *the fields should be charted on a perimeter and scotomas outlined on a Bjerrum screen.* In testing the visual fields, the sense of movement represents the coarsest stimulus, so that a perception of motion may be preserved while a stationary target of the same size may not be seen. Similarly, there may be impairment of perception of color, but not of form. Inability to recognize color may depend on the size of the target; the smaller the target, the less likely the patient is to recognize it. Careful perimetry and scotometry should take each of these features into account.

The method of double simultaneous stimulation may elicit visual field defects that are undetected by conventional perimetry. Movement of one finger in all parts of each temporal field may disclose no abnormality, but if movement is simultaneous in analogous parts of both temporal fields, the patient may see only the one in the normal half. In young children or uncooperative patients the integrity of the fields may be roughly estimated by observing whether the patient is attracted to objects in the peripheral field or blinks in response to sudden threatening gestures in one-half the visual field.

A common abnormality disclosed by visual field examination is *concentric constriction*. This may be due to papilledema, in which case it is usually accompanied by an enlargement of the blind spot. A concentric constriction of the visual field, at first unilateral and later bilateral, associated with pallor of the optic disk (optic atrophy), should suggest chronic syphilitic optic neuritis.

Glaucoma is another cause of this type of field defect. *Tubular* ("gun-barrel," "tunnel") *vision*, i.e., constriction of the visual field to the same degree regardless of the distance of the visual test stimulus from the eye, is a sign of hypersuggestibility or hysteria. In organic disease, e.g., syphilitic optic neuritis, the area of the constricted visual field naturally enlarges as the distance between the patient and the test object increases.

The types of visual field defect resulting from lesions in different parts of the visual pathways are shown in Fig. 12-2. *These defects are always described in terms of the visual field, rather than the retina.* The retinal image of an object in the visual field is inverted and reversed from right to left (like the image on the film of a camera). The rules which govern the representation of regions in the visual field in the geniculate ganglion and cerebral cortex are, therefore, the reverse of those which apply to the retinal representation (see above): (1) The left visual field of each eye is represented in the right geniculate nucleus and the visual cortex of the right occipital lobe. (2) The upper half of the visual field is represented in the lateral part of the geniculate ganglion and below the calcarine fissure in the visual cortex; the opposite holds for the lower half of the visual field.

Figure 12-2

Diagram showing the effects on the fields of vision produced by lesions at various points along the optic pathway: A, complete blindness in left eye; B, bitemporal hemianopia; C, nasal hemianopia of left eye; D, right homonymous hemianopia; E and F, right upper and lower quadrant hemianopias; and G, right homonymous hemianopia with preservation of central vision. (From J Homans, A Textbook of Surgery, Springfield, Ill, Charles C Thomas, 1945.)

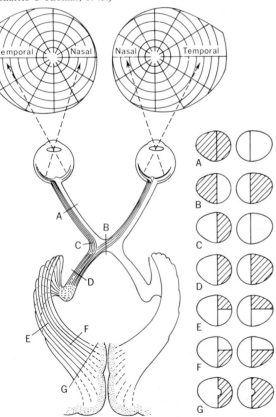

PRECHIASMAL LESIONS

These cause either a scotoma (an island of impaired vision within the visual field) or a cut in the peripheral part of one visual field. A small scotoma in the macular part of the visual field may seriously impair visual acuity. Demyelinative, toxic (methyl alcohol, quinine, and chloroquine, and certain of the phenothiazine tranquilizing drugs), nutritional (so-called tobacco-alcohol amblyopia), and vascular diseases (ischemic optic neuropathy) are the usual causes of scotomas. The toxic states are characterized by symmetric bilateral scotomas, and the nutritional disorders by more or less symmetric bilateral central scotomas (involving the fixation point) or centrocecal ones (involving both the fixation point and the blind spot). The centrocecal scotoma represents a lesion that is predominantly in the distribution of the papillomacular bundle and is more sensitive to red than to white test objects. However, the finding of this visual field abnormality does not establish whether the primary defect is in the cells of origin of the bundle, i.e., the retinal ganglion cells, or their fibers. Demyelinative disease (retrobulbar neuritis and multiple sclerosis) is characterized by unilateral or asymmetric bilateral scotomas. Vascular lesions which take the form of retinal hemorrhages and infarctions of the nerve-cell layer (cotton-wool patches) give rise to unilateral scotomas; occlusion of the central retinal artery or its branches causes infarction of the retina and gives rise, as a rule, to cuts of varying size in the visual field. Vascular lesions (ischemic optic neuropathy) may also occur in the optic nerve, causing sudden blindness or a scotoma without visible change in the retina.

Since the optic nerve also contains the afferent fibers for the pupillary light reflex, lesions of the nerve will cause alterations of the pupil. These are described in the next chapter (see page 188).

With most diseases of the optic nerve the optic disk will eventually become pale (*optic atrophy*). This usually requires 4 to 6 weeks to occur. If the optic nerve degenerates (e.g., in multiple sclerosis, Leber's hereditary optic atrophy, traumatic transection, tumor of nerve, or syphilitic optic atrophy), the disk becomes chalk white, with sharp, clean margins. If the atrophy is secondary (consecutive) to papillitis or papilledema, the margins are obscure and irregular and the adjacent retina is altered.

SYNDROME OF RETROBULBAR NEUROPATHY

Acute impairment of vision in one eye or both eyes (in the latter case the eyes may be affected either simultaneously or successively) develops in a number of clinical settings. The most frequent is one in which a child, adolescent, or young adult notes a rapid diminution of vision in one eye (as though a veil or haze had covered the eye), sometimes progressing to complete blindness. The optic disk and retina may appear normal, but if the lesion is near the nerve head, there may be swelling of the optic disk, i.e., papillitis, and the disk margins are elevated and blurred, and rarely surrounded by hemorrhages. Papillitis is distinguished from the papilledema of increased intracranial pressure by the marked impairment of vision and the scotomas it produces. Less consistent symptoms of retrobulbar neuropathy (neuritis) are pain on movement of the eye, tenderness on pressure of the globe, a subjective difference in light brightness and an increase in blurring of vision with exertion or following a hot bath. Examination, in addition to papillitis, may disclose an impairment of color vision and the presence of fine opacities in the vitreous. After some few days or weeks the other eye may be similarly involved; the blindness may then be complete or nearly complete, and the pupillary light reflex impaired. In a large proportion of such patients, no cause of the retrobulbar neuropathy can be found, and after several more weeks there is spontaneous recovery. Vision returns to normal in more than two-thirds of all instances; occasionally a scotoma is left, or even blindness. The optic disk, particularly its temporal portion, later becomes slightly pale in many of the patients. The CSF may be normal or may contain from 10 to 200 lymphocytes, and the levels of total protein and of gamma globulin may be elevated.

Nearly half such patients will develop other symptoms and signs of multiple sclerosis within 10 to 15 years, and probably even more will do so if the patients are observed for longer periods. Less is known about children with retrobulbar neuropathy, but the prognosis for them is probably better than that for adults. Formerly the syndrome was blamed on sinusitis and treated as such, but Cushing long ago proved the error of this assumption. Sinus disease rarely affects vision, except for

an occasional mucocele which presses on an ocular or optic nerve. Demyelinative disease is the only common cause of a unilateral retrobulbar neuritis, but the nature of those forms which do not progress to multiple sclerosis remains obscure. Regression of symptoms may occur spontaneously or may be hastened by the administration of ACTH or corticosteroids (see page 657).

Simultaneous impairment of vision in the two eyes, with central or centrocecal scotomas, usually is caused not by a demyelinative process but rather by a toxic or nutritional disorder. The latter condition is observed most commonly in the chronically alcoholic patient. Impairment of visual acuity evolves over several days or weeks, and examination discloses bilateral, roughly symmetric central or centrocecal scotomas, the peripheral fields being intact. With appropriate treatment (nutritious diet and B vitamins) instituted soon after the onset of amblyopia, complete recovery is possible; if treatment is delayed, patients are left with varying degrees of permanent defect in central vision and pallor of the temporal portions of the optic disks. This disorder is commonly referred to as "tobacco-alcohol amblyopia," the implication being that it is due to the toxic effects of tobacco or alcohol, or both. In fact the disorder is caused by nutritional deficiency and is properly designated as *nutritional amblyopia* or *nutritional optic neuropathy* (Chap. 38). The same disorder may be seen in nonalcoholic patients, under conditions of severe nutritional deprivation, and in patients with vitamin B_{12} deficiency (pernicious anemia).

Impairment of vision due to *methyl alcohol intoxication* is abupt in onset and is characterized by large symmetric central scotomas, as well as by symptoms of systemic disease and acidosis. Treatment is directed mainly to correction of the acidosis. The subacute development of central field defects has been attributed to several other toxins and the chronic administration of certain therapeutic agents: halogenated hydroxyquinolines (Enterovioform, Clioquinol), chloramphenicol, ethambutol, isoniazid, streptomycin, chlorpropamide (Diabinese), and ergot. Rarely, the optic nerves may be involved as part of exophthalmic ophthalmoplegia.

Rarely, the syndrome of retrobulbar neuropathy is caused by cranial arteritis, systemic lupus erythematosis, thyrotoxicosis, or diabetes. Congenital and hereditary forms of optic atrophy are known (Chaps. 37 and 43; see also Table 14-1). Chiasmal and optic nerve compression by tumors may also cause scotomas and optic atrophy (Chap. 30).

LESIONS OF THE CHIASM, OPTIC TRACT, AND GENICULOCALCARINE PATHWAY

Hemianopia (hemianopsia) means blindness in one-half the visual field. *Bitemporal hemianopia* indicates a lesion of the decussating fibers of the optic chiasm and is usually caused by tumor of the pituitary gland (showing as a ballooned sella in films of the skull). However, it may also be caused by craniopharyngiomas, saccular aneurysms of the circle of Willis, meningiomas of the tuberculum sellae, and rarely sarcoidosis, metastatic carcinoma, and Hand-Schüller-Christian disease. The lesion is always in the chiasm, involving the decussating nasal fibers from each retina, although in some instances the tumor pushing upward presses the medial parts of the optic nerves against the anterior cerebral arteries. Heteronymous field defects, i.e., scotomas or field defects that differ in the two eyes, are also a sign of involvement of the optic chiasm or adjoining optic nerves; they are caused by craniopharyngioma or other tumors or to opticochiasmic arachnoiditis.

Homonymous hemianopia (a loss of vision in corresponding halves of the visual fields) signifies a lesion of the visual pathway behind the chiasm and, if complete, gives no more information than that. *Incomplete homonymous hemianopia* has more localizing value; as a general rule, if the field defects in the two eyes are identical (congruous), the lesion is likely to be in the calcarine cortex; if *incongruous*, the visual fibers in the parietal or temporal lobe are more likely to be implicated.

Actually, absolute congruity of the field defects is rare, even with occipital lesions. Further, lesions of the optic tract may produce fairly congruent defects, and are difficult to distinguish from those of the occipital lobe on the basis of visual field testing alone.

Lower fibers of the geniculocalcarine pathway (from the inferior retina) swing in a wide arc over the temporal horn of the ventricle into the temporal lobe, before joining the upper fibers of the pathway on their way to the calcarine cortex (Fig. 12-3). This arc of fibers is known as Flechsig's or Meyer's loop, and a lesion that interrupts them will produce an opposite-sided defect involving the upper quadrants of the visual fields (Fig. 12-2), i.e., an *upper homonymous quadrantanopia*. This clinical effect was first described by Harvey Cushing, so that his name also has been applied to the loop of temporal visual fibers. Parietal lobe lesions may affect the lower quadrants of the visual fields more than the upper ones.

Finally, it should be mentioned that defects in visual perception due to cerebral lesions are practically always associated with impairment of color perception, either a loss (achromatopsia) or alteration of perception (metachromatopsia). When all images are tinged one color, the disorder is referred to as *monochromatopsia*. This latter disorder may affect both eyes, as in digitalis intoxication, in which patients complain that everything appears yellow (xanthopsia), or one eye, as in cases of macular hemorrhage, which imparts a reddish hue to all images (erythropsia).

If the entire optic tract or calcarine cortex on one side is destroyed, the homonymous hemianopia is complete, including that part of the field subserved by the

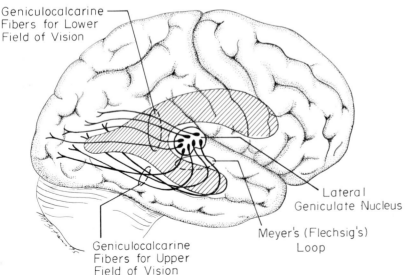

Figure 12–3
The geniculocalcarine projection. (Redrawn from ML Barr, The Human Nervous System, 3d ed, Hagerstown, Md, Harper & Row, 1979.)

Geniculocalcarine Fibers for Lower Field of Vision

Lateral Geniculate Nucleus

Geniculocalcarine Fibers for Upper Field of Vision

Meyer's (Flechsig's) Loop

macula. Incomplete lesions of the optic tract and radiation usually spare central (macular) vision. Apparent macular sparing is frequently due to imperfect fixation of gaze. A lesion of the tip of one occipital lobe produces central homonymous hemianopic scotomata because half the macular fibers of both eyes terminate there. Lesions of both occipital poles (as in embolization of the posterior cerebral arteries) result in bilateral central scotomas; and if all the calcarine cortex on both sides is completely destroyed, there is "cortical" blindness. *Homonymous altitudinal or horizontal hemianopia* is due more often to lesions of both occipital lobes below or above the calcarine cortex than to a lesion of the optic chiasm. The most common cause is infarction due to occlusion of the posterior cerebral arteries.

In addition to blindness, i.e., "visual anesthesia," there is another category of visual impairment in which patients cannot understand the meaning of what they see, i.e., *visual agnosia.* Primary visual perception is intact, and patients may describe accurately the shape, color, and size of objects that are presented. Despite this, they cannot identify the objects unless they hear, smell, taste, or palpate them. The failure of visual recognition of words alone is called *alexia.* The ability to recognize visually presented objects and words depends upon the integrity not only of the visual pathways and primary visual area of the cerebral cortex (area 17 of Brodmann), but also of those cortical areas which lie just anterior to area 17 (areas 18 and 19 of the occipital lobe and the angular gyrus of the dominant hemisphere). Visual-object agnosia and alexia result from lesions of these latter areas or from a lesion of the left calcarine cortex combined with one which interrupts the fibers crossing from the right occipital lobe (see also page 320). Failure to understand the meaning of an entire picture even though some of its parts are recognized (simultagnosia) and failure to recognize familiar faces (prosopagnosia) are variants of visual agnosia. Patients with these forms of visual agnosia practically always show some impairment of other visual or mental function or various degrees of aphasia, so that certain authorities have questioned the existence of a pure visual agnosia (see Chap. 21).

Other disturbances of vision include various types of distortion in which images seem to recede into the distance (teleopsia), or appear too small (micropsia), or, less frequently, too large (macropsia). If such a disturbance is in one eye only, a local retinal lesion should be suspected. Micropsia and teleopsia have also been described in patients with lesions of the chiasm, occurring in the defective temporal half-fields of vision (Bender and Savitsky). When these phenomena are bilateral, however, they usually signify disease of the temporal lobes, in which case the visual disturbances tend to occur in attacks and are accompanied by other manifesta-

tions of temporal lobe seizures (Chap. 15). With parietal lobe lesions, objects may appear to be askew. Lesions of the vestibular nucleus or its immediate connections may produce the illusion that objects are tilted or that straight lines are curved.

Visual hallucinations may be simple or unformed (e.g., flashes of light, colored spots, or scintillating zigzag lines), or they may be complex or formed (consisting of people, animals, landscapes, etc.). The former are related to lesions in the occipital lobes, and are observed characteristically in migraine (Chap. 9). Formed hallucinations are observed in a variety of conditions, notably in the withdrawal state following chronic intoxication with alcohol and other sedative-hypnotic drugs (Chaps. 40 and 41), in Alzheimer's disease (Chap. 42), and in disease of the temporal or parietal lobes or the diencephalon (peduncular hallucinosis; see Chap. 19).

Occasionally, patients with an attention hemianopia may displace an image to the nonaffected half of the field of vision (*visual allesthesia*), or a visual image may persist for minutes to hours after the exciting stimulus has been removed (*palinopsia*); the latter disorder also occurs in defective, but not blind, homonymous fields of vision. *Oscillopsia*, or illusory movement of the environment occurs with lesions of the labyrinthine-vestibular apparatus, and is described with disorders of ocular movement (see page 186).

The clinical effects and syndromes that result from occipital lobe lesions are discussed further in Chap. 21.

REFERENCES[1]

GLASER JS: *Neuro-ophthalmology.* Hagerstown, Md, Harper & Row, 1978.

HAYREH SS: Pathogenesis of oedema of the optic disc (papilloedema). *Br J Ophthalmol* 48:522, 1964.

———: Blood supply of the optic nerve head and its role in optic atrophy, glaucoma, and oedema of the optic disc. *Br J Ophthalmol* 53:721, 1969.

LEVIN BE: The clinical significance of spontaneous pulsations of the retinal vein. *Arch Neurol* 35:37, 1978.

MINCKLER DS, TSO MOM, ZIMMERMAN LE: A light microscopic autoradiographic study of axoplasmic transport in the optic nerve head during ocular hypotony, increased intraocular pressure, and papilledema. *Am J Ophthalmol* 82:741, 1976.

[1] See also references at end of Chap. 13.

CHAPTER 13

DISORDERS OF OCULAR MOVEMENT AND PUPILLARY FUNCTION

Abnormalities of ocular movement are of two basic types. In one, the disorder of motility can be traced to a lesion of the extraocular muscles themselves or to the cranial nerves that supply them (*nuclear or infranuclear palsy*). In the other, the derangement is in the highly specialized neural mechanisms that enable the eyes to move simultaneously in the same direction, i.e., conjugately (*supranuclear palsy*). Such a distinction, in keeping with the general concept of upper and lower motor neuron paralysis, hardly conveys the complexity of the neural mechanisms that govern ocular motility; nevertheless it is a useful, if not an essential first step in the approach to the patient with defective eye movements. In both cases, it must be recognized, a knowledge of the anatomy of normal movement is essential to an undertanding of abnormal movement.

SUPRANUCLEAR DISORDERS OF EYE MOVEMENT

ANATOMIC AND PHYSIOLOGIC CONSIDERATIONS

Accurate binocular vision is achieved by the associated action of the ocular muscles, which allows a visual stimulus to fall on exactly corresponding parts of the two retinas. The symmetrical and synchronous movement of the eyes in the same direction is termed conjugate (yoked or joined together) movement, or conjugate gaze, and is controlled by centers in the cerebral cortex and brainstem.

Area 8 in the frontal lobe is the region which initiates *voluntary conjugate movements* of the eyes to the opposite side, referred to also as movements on command, since they can be elicited by instructing the patient to look to the right or left. These movements are characteristically rapid and jerky or *saccadic* and their purpose is to quickly change ocular fixation, i.e., to bring new images of objects of interest onto the fovea. Saccadic movements (or saccades) may also be elicited *reflexly*, as when a sudden sound or appearance of an object in the peripheral field of vision causes the eyes to move in the direction of the stimulus.

Saccades are to be distinguished from the slower and smoother, largely involuntary *pursuit, or following, movements*, for which the major stimulus is a moving target upon which the eyes are fixated. The function of pursuit movements is to stabilize the image of a moving object on the fovea as the head is turned or as a fixated object is tracked by the eyes ("smooth tracking"). Pursuit movements to each side appear to be generated in the ipsilateral parietooccipital cortex, but also in ipsilateral brainstem structures (as in the vestibuloocular reflex) and ipsilateral cerebellum, particularly the flocculus (Zee et al.).

Knowledge about the corticofugal pathways for conjugate gaze is fragmentary. Using the Marchi technique, Brucher has traced the efferent fibers from the ablated frontal eye fields of 12 monkeys. The fibers descend in the anterior limb of the internal capsule and then separate into two bundles: (1) a noncrossed pathway which runs through the diencephalon and terminates diffusely in the periaqueductal gray matter, pretectum, superior colliculus, and above all in the homolateral mesencephalic reticular formation; and (2) the so-called aberrant pyramidal system of Déjerine, which descends in the median third of the basis pedunculi, crosses the midline just caudal to the substantia nigra and descends in the pontine reticular formation to the level of the abducens nucleus (Fig. 13-1). The reticular formation in this particular area is sometimes designated as the pontine paramedian reticular formation

(PPRF) and constitutes the pontine center for horizontal gaze (see below).

One pathway for pursuit movements probably originates in the parietooccipital cortex and descends in the internal sagittal stratum, through the pulvinar, to the midbrain. Its further course in the brainstem has not been identified.

Ultimately, all the pathways mediating saccadic, pursuit, and vestibuloocular movements converge onto the pontine centers for horizontal gaze. The center for right lateral gaze is situated in the right paramedian tegmentum, ventral to the medial longitudinal fasciculus, and lateral to the abducens nucleus (Fig. 13-1). Since the precise location of the center is unclear, the alternate designation, *paraabducens center*, is sometimes used.

The center for left lateral gaze is near the left abducens nucleus. The pontine center accomplishes conjugate lateral gaze by the simultaneous innervation of the ipsilateral external rectus and the contralateral internal rectus, the latter through fibers that run in the medial portion of the medial longitudinal fasciculus. It is the interruption of these latter fibers that accounts for the discrete impairment or loss of adduction of the ipsilateral eye, a phenomenon referred to as *unilateral internuclear ophthalmoplegia*. These connections are illustrated in Figs. 13-1 and 13-2.

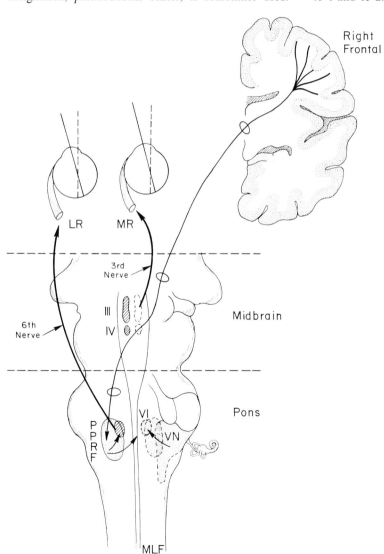

Right
Frontal

Figure 13-1

The supranuclear pathways subserving conjugate horizontal gaze to the left. Pathway originates in the right frontal cortex, descends in the internal capsule, decussates at the level of the lower midbrain and descends to synapse in the left pontine paramedian reticular formation (PPRF). Further connections with the third and sixth nerve nuclei are illustrated in Fig. 13-2. Cranial nerve nuclei III and IV are labeled on left; nucleus of VI and vestibular nuclei (VN) are labeled on right. LR, lateral rectus; MR, medial rectus; MLF, medial longitudinal fasciculus. (Redrawn from JS Glaser, Neuro-ophthalmology, Hagerstown, Md, Harper & Row, 1978.)

The arrangements of nerve cells and fibers for vertical upward gaze are situated in the pretectal areas of the midbrain tegmentum and the region of the posterior commissure. An autopsied case with upward-gaze paralysis revealed lesions in the interstitial nuclei of Cajal and the nuclei of Darkschewitsch (Sachsenweger). The "centers" for downward gaze are in the same vicinity. In several carefully studied patients who showed an isolated palsy of downward gaze, autopsy has disclosed bilateral lesions (infarction) of the rostral midbrain, situated in the ventral portion of the pretectal tegmentum, on either side of the aqueduct, just medial and dorsal to the red nuclei (Jacobs et al., Halmagyi et al.). In monkeys, a defect in downward gaze has been produced by the placement of bilateral lesions, 1.7 mm in diameter, centered in the same regions (Kömpf et al.). The so-called rostral interstitial nucleus of the medial longitudi-

nal fasciculus and the nucleus campi Foreli, which receive fibers from the PPRF and project onto the oculomotor nucleus, appear to be destroyed in this lesion.

The course of the cortical-mesencephalic fibers that govern vertical gaze has not been established. Fibers from the frontal "eye areas" are thought to connect with the ipsilateral third and fourth nerve nuclei via the diencephalic-mesencephalic pathway of Brucher, described above. Fibers from the occipital areas probably reach both oculomotor nuclei via the pretectal and posterior commissural nuclei.

PARALYSIS OF CONJUGATE MOVEMENT (GAZE)

An acute lesion, such as an infarct in one frontal lobe, usually causes paralysis of contralateral gaze, and the eyes will turn toward the side of the cerebral lesion. This rule is not absolute, however; occasionally a deep cerebral lesion, particularly a thalamic hemorrhage extending into the midbrain, will cause the eyes to deviate conjugately to the side opposite the lesion.

In the case of cerebral infarction, the gaze palsy is temporary, lasting only for a day or two, rarely longer. Almost invariably, it is accompanied by hemiparesis. In this circumstance, forced closure of the eyelids frequently causes the eyes to move conjugately to the side of the hemiparesis, and not upward. During sleep, a similar phenomenon may occur; the eyes deviate conjugately from the side of the lesion to the side of the paralysis. In bilateral frontal lesions the patient may be unable to turn the eyes voluntarily in any direction, but retains fixation and following movements, which are believed to be initiated in the parietooccipital cortex. Gaze paralysis of central origin is not attended by strabismus or diplopia. The usual causes are vascular occlusion with infarction, hemorrhage, and abscess or tumor of the frontal lobe. With certain extrapyramidal disorders (e.g., postencephalitic parkinsonism, Huntington's chorea) ocular movements may be limited in all directions, especially upward. In the disorder known as progressive supranuclear palsy there may be an early selective paralysis of downward gaze, combined with nuchal dystonia and other extrapyramidal symptoms (Chap. 42).

Midbrain lesions affecting the pretectum on both sides of the midline and lesions in the region of the posterior commissure interfere with conjugate movements in the vertical plane. Paralysis of gaze in the vertical plane is frequently referred to as *Parinaud's syndrome* or the *syndrome of the sylvian aqueduct*. Upward gaze is affected far more frequently than downward gaze and is often associated with mydriasis, loss of convergence movements and of pupillary light reflexes, and occasionally with convergence or retractory nystagmus (see page

Figure 13-2

Dorsal surface of the brainstem, showing the connection of the pontine centers for conjugate lateral gaze with the abducens nuclei and with the oculomotor nuclei by way of the medial longitudinal fasciculus. Internuclear ophthalmoplegia, characterized by paralysis of the medial recti on attempted conjugate lateral gaze, is due to lesions of the medial longitudinal fasciculus. The internuclear ophthalmoplegia is accompanied by paresis of convergence with anterior lesions (1) and by weakness of conjugate gaze and nystagmus with posterior lesions (3), while there may be normal convergence and normal excursions of the abducting eye with midzone lesions (2). (From DG Cogan, Neurology of the Ocular Muscles, 2d ed, Springfield, Ill., Charles C Thomas, 1956.)

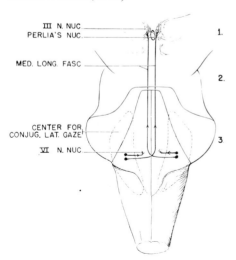

186), and blepharospasm, or fluttering of the eyelids. Vestibular or optically induced nystagmus in the vertical plane is usually lost in association with these abnormalities. The range of upward gaze is frequently restricted by a number of extraneous factors, such as aging, drowsiness, and increased intracranial pressure. In patients who cannot elevate their eyes voluntarily, reflex upward deviation of the eyes in response to forced flexion of the head (doll's head maneuver) or to forced closure of the eyelids (*Bell's phenomenon*) indicates that the nuclear and infranuclear mechanisms for upward gaze are intact and that the defect is supranuclear. It must be remembered that about 15 percent of normal adults do not show a Bell's phenomenon. Lesions confined to one cerebral hemisphere do not cause abnormalities of vertical gaze.

A lesion in the rostral midbrain tegmentum, by interrupting the cerebral pathways for conjugate gaze before their decussation, will cause a horizontal gaze palsy to the opposite side. A lesion in the pontine horizontal gaze complex, in the vicinity of each abducens nucleus, causes *ipsilateral* gaze palsy, with the eyes tending to turn to the opposite side. As a rule, the horizontal gaze palsies of cerebral and pontine origin are readily distinguished. The former are usually accompanied by a hemiparesis, and the paralysis of gaze is on the same side as the hemiparesis. Palsies of pontine origin are associated with other signs of pontine disease, particularly peripheral facial and external rectus palsies which occur on the same side as the paralysis of gaze, whereas the hemiparesis is on the side opposite to the gaze palsy. Gaze palsies due to cerebral lesions tend not to be as long-lasting as those due to pontine lesions. Also, in the case of a cerebral lesion (but not with a pontine lesion), the eyes can be turned to the paralyzed side if a target is fixated and the head is rotated passively to the opposite side.

Skew deviation is a poorly understood disorder of gaze in which there is a maintained vertical deviation of one eye above the other. The deviation may be the same (comitant) in all fields of gaze, or it may be variable for different directions of gaze. The patient complains of vertical diplopia. Skew deviation does not have precise localizing value, but occurs with a variety of lesions of the brainstem and cerebellum. With brainstem disease, the eye on the side of the lesion is lower than the other eye.

Another unusual disturbance of gaze is the *oculogyric crisis or spasm*, which consists of conjugate spasmodic movements of the eyes, usually upward and less frequently laterally or downward. Recurrent attacks, sometimes associated with spasms of the neck, mouth, and tongue muscles and lasting from a few seconds to an hour or two, are pathognomonic of postencephalitic parkinsonism (pages 521 and 809). This phenomenon is also observed as an acute reaction in patients who have been given phenothiazine drugs (see page 777). The pathogenesis of these ocular spasms is not known.

NUCLEAR AND INFRANUCLEAR DISORDERS OF EYE MOVEMENT

ANATOMIC CONSIDERATIONS

The third (oculomotor), fourth (trochlear), and sixth (abducens) cranial nerves innervate the extrinsic musculature of the eye. Their actions are closely integrated, and many diseases involve all of them at once, so that they are suitably considered together.

The oculomotor nuclei consist of several paired groups of nerve cells, adjacent to the midline and ventral to the aqueduct of Sylvius, at the level of the superior colliculi. A centrally located group of nerve cells that innervate the pupillary sphincters and ciliary bodies (muscles of accommodation) is situated dorsally in the so-called Edinger-Westphal nucleus; this is the parasympathetic portion of the oculomotor nucleus. Ventral to this nuclear group are the cells which mediate the action of the levator of the lid, superior and inferior recti, inferior oblique, and medial rectus, in this dorsal-ventral order. This functional arrangement has been determined in cats and monkeys by extirpating individual extrinsic ocular muscles and observing the retrograde cellular changes (Warwick). These experiments have also indicated that the medial and inferior recti and the inferior oblique have a strictly homolateral representation in the oculomotor nuclei, whereas the superior rectus receives only crossed fibers, and the levator palpebrae superioris has a bilateral innervation. For many years it has been taught that convergence is under the control of an unpaired medial group of large motor cells, not clearly separate from the rest of the third nerve complex, called Perlia's nucleus. However, the critical studies of Warwick and others have cast serious doubt on the existence of such a center.

It is important to note that the efferent fibers of the oculomotor and abducens nuclei have a considerable intramedullary extent (Fig. 13-3*A* and *B*). The fibers of the third nerve nucleus course ventrally in the brainstem, traversing the medial longitudinal fasciculus, the red nucleus, substantia nigra, and the medial part of the cerebral peduncle, and may therefore be interrupted by lesions involving these latter structures. The sixth nerve arises at a considerably lower level, from a paired group of cells in the floor of the fourth ventricle, adjacent to the midline, at the level of the lower pons. The intrapontine portion of the facial nerve loops around the sixth nerve nucleus before it turns anterolaterally to make its exit; a lesion in this locality, therefore, may cause a homolateral paralysis of the lateral rectus and facial muscles. The cells of origin of the trochlear nerves are just caudal to those of the oculomotor nerves. Unlike the third and sixth nerves, the fourth nerve decussates before emerging, a short distance from its origin, from the dorsal surface of the brainstem, just caudal to the inferior colliculi.

The oculomotor nerve, soon after it emerges from the brainstem, comes into close relationship with the posterior cerebral artery. Both these structures may be compressed at this point by herniation of the uncus through the tentorium. More anteriorly, the oculomotor nerve crosses the internal carotid artery at its junction with the posterior communicating artery. An aneurysm at the latter site frequently damages the third nerve and serves to localize the site of the compression or bleeding. The sixth cranial nerve sweeps upward, after leaving the brainstem, and joins the third and fourth cranial nerves; together, the ocular motor nerves course anteriorly, pierce the dura, and enter the cavernous sinus, where they are closely applied to the various divisions of the fifth nerve. In the posterior part of the cavernous sinus, compressive lesions, notably infraclinoid extradural aneurysms and tumors, tend to involve all three trigeminal divisions, together with the nerves to the extraocular muscles; in the middle portion of the sinus, the first and second trigeminal divisions are involved; and in the anterior portion, only the ophthalmic division. Together with the latter division, the third, fourth, and sixth nerves enter the orbit through the superior orbital fissure. The oculomotor nerve supplies all the extrinsic ocular muscles except two—the superior oblique and the external rectus—which are innervated by the trochlear and abducens nerves, respectively. The voluntary part of the levator palpebrae muscle is also supplied by the oculomotor nerve, the autonomic part being under the control of sympathetic fibers.

Although all the extraocular muscles probably participate in every movement of the eyes, a movement in a specific direction should clinically be thought of as requiring the action of one particular muscle, e.g., the lateral rectus rotates the eye outward; the medial rectus, inward. The action of the superior and inferior recti and the oblique muscles varies according to the position of the eye. When the eye is turned outward, the elevator is the superior rectus, and the depressor is the inferior rec-

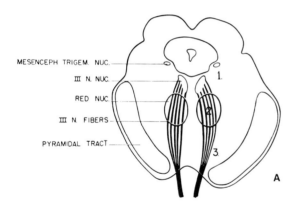

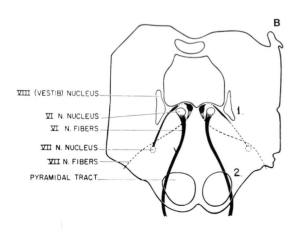

Figure 13-3

A. Brainstem in horizontal section, at level of third nerve nucleus, indicating structures involved by lesions at different loci in the midbrain. Lesions at 1 result in homolateral third nerve paralysis and homolateral anesthesia of the cornea. Lesions at 2 result in homolateral third nerve paralysis and contralateral tremor (Benedikt's syndrome). Lesions at 3 result in homolateral third nerve paralysis and crossed corticospinal tract signs (Weber's syndrome).

B. Brainstem at the level of the sixth nerve nuclei, indicating structures involved by lesions at different loci. Lesions at 1 result in homolateral sixth and seventh nerve paralyses with varying degrees of nystagmus and weakness of conjugate gaze to the homolateral side. Lesions at 2 result in homolateral sixth nerve paralysis and crossed hemiplegia (Millard-Gubler syndrome). (From DG Cogan, Neurology of the Ocular Muscles, 2d ed, Springfield, Ill, Charles C Thomas, 1956.)

tus. When the eye is turned inward, the elevator and depressor are the inferior and superior oblique muscles, respectively. The actions of the ocular muscles in different positions of gaze are illustrated in Fig. 13-4.

STRABISMUS

Strabismus (*squint*) refers to a muscle imbalance that results in improper alignment of the visual axes of the two eyes. It may be caused by weakness of an individual eye muscle (*paralytic strabismus*) or to an unexplained imbalance of muscular tone due to a faulty "central" mechanism which normally maintains a proper angle between the two visual axes (*nonparalytic strabismus*). Almost everyone has a slight tendency to the latter, i.e., to misalign the visual axes (*phoria*), but normally this tendency is overcome by the fusion mechanisms. In persons with strabismus the misalignment becomes manifest and can no longer be overcome (*tropia*). Paralytic strabismus is primarily a neurologic problem; nonparalytic strabismus (referred to as *concomitant strabismus* if the angle between the visual axes is the same in all fields of gaze) is more strictly an ophthalmologic problem.

Once binocular fusion is established, usually by 6 months of age, any type of ocular muscle imbalance causes diplopia, since images then fall on disparate or noncorresponding parts of the two functionally active retinas. After a time, however, the young patient learns to eliminate the diplopia by suppressing the image in one eye. After a variable period the suppression becomes permanent, and the individual grows up with a diminished visual acuity in that eye, the result of prolonged disuse (*amblyopia ex anopsia*). With proper early treatment, the amblyopia can be reversed, but if it persists beyond the age of 5 or 6 years, recovery of vision does not occur. Occasionally, when the eyes are used alternately for fixation (*alternating strabismus*), visual acuity remains good in each eye.

PARALYSIS OF INDIVIDUAL OCULAR MUSCLES

Characteristic clinical disturbances result from lesions of the third, fourth, and sixth cranial nerves. A complete third nerve lesion causes ptosis or drooping of the upper eyelid (since the levator palpebrae is supplied mainly by the third nerve) and an inability to rotate the eye upward, downward, or inward. When the lid is passively elevated, the eye is found to be deviated outward and slightly downward because of unopposed intact actions of the lateral rectus and superior oblique muscles; in addition, one finds a dilated nonreactive pupil (iridoplegia) and paralysis of accommodation (cycloplegia), due to interruption of the parasympathetic fibers in the third nerve.

Fourth nerve lesions result in extorsion and weakness of downward movement of the affected eye, most marked when the eye is turned inward, so that the patient commonly complains of special difficulty in reading or going downstairs. This defect may be overlooked in the presence of a third nerve palsy if the examiner fails to note the absence of intorsion as the patient tries to move the paretic eye downward. Head tilting to the opposite shoulder (Bielschowsky's sign) is especially characteristic of fourth nerve lesions; this maneuver causes a compensatory intorsion of the unaffected eye, and ameliorates the double vision. Lesions of the *sixth nerve* result in a paralysis of lateral or outward movement and a crossing of the visual axes. With incomplete sixth nerve palsies, turning the head toward the side of the paretic muscle may overcome diplopia.

Diplopia and the Red-Glass Test The foregoing signs may occur with various degrees of completeness. When the ocular paresis is slight, there may be no obvious squint or defect in ocular movement; yet the patient ex-

Figure 13-4

Muscles chiefly responsible for vertical movements of the eyes in different positions of gaze. (From DG Cogan, Neurology of the Ocular Muscles, 2d ed, Charles C Thomas, Springfield, Ill, 1956.)

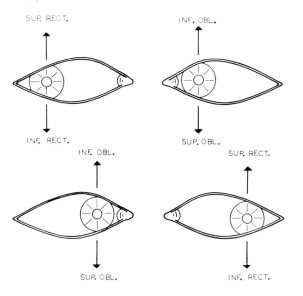

periences diplopia. Study of the relative positions of the images of the two eyes then becomes a useful way of determining which muscle might be involved. The image seen by the affected eye is usually less distinct, but a more reliable way of distinguishing the weak muscle is by the *red-glass test*. A red glass is placed in front of the patient's right eye (the choice of the right eye is arbitrary, but if the test is always done in the same way, interpretation is simplified). The patient is then asked to look at a flashlight (held at a distance of 1 m), to turn both eyes to various points in the visual fields, and to

state or indicate with the two index fingers the position of the red and white images and the relative distances between them. The positions of the two images are plotted as indicated in Fig. 13-5.

Three rules aid in the analysis of ocular movements by the red-glass test. (1) The direction in which the distance between the images is at a maximum is the direction of action of the paretic muscle. For example, if the greatest horizontal separation is in looking to the right, either the right abductor or the left adductor muscle is weak. (2) If the separation is mainly horizontal, the paresis will be found in one of the horizontal recti (a small vertical disparity should be disregarded); if the separation is mainly vertical, the paresis will be found in the vertically acting muscles, and a small horizontal deviation should be disregarded. (3) The image projected farther from the center belongs to the paretic eye. If the patient looks to the right and the red image is farther to the right, then the right lateral rectus muscle is weak. If the white image is to the right of the red, then the left internal rectus muscle is weak. In testing vertical movements, again the image seen with the eye with the paretic muscle is the one projected most peripherally. It must be remembered that *one* of *two* muscles responsible for the movement in the direction of maximal separation of images is distinguished by the red-glass test. For example, if the maximum vertical separation of images occurs on looking downward and to the *left*, and

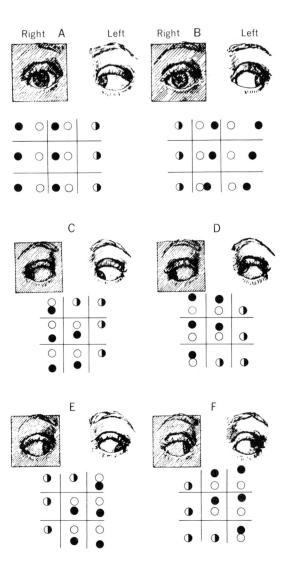

Figure 13-5

Diplopia fields with individual muscle paralysis. The dark glass is in front of the right eye, and the fields are projected as the patient sees the images. A. Paralysis of right external rectus. Characteristic: right eye does not move to the right. Field: horizontal homonymous diplopia increasing on looking to the right. B. Paralysis of right internal rectus. Characteristic: right eye does not move to the left. Field: horizontal crossed diplopia increasing on looking to the left. C. Paralysis of right inferior rectus. Characteristic: right eye does not move downward when eyes are turned to the right. Field: vertical diplopia (image of right eye lowermost) increasing on looking to the right and down. D. Paralysis of right superior rectus. Characteristic: right eye does not move upward when eyes are turned to the right. Field: vertical diplopia (image of right eye uppermost) increasing on looking to the right and up. E. Paralysis of right superior oblique. Characteristic: right eye does not move downward when eyes are turned to the left. Field: vertical diplopia (image of right eye lowermost) increasing on looking to left and down. F. Paralysis of right inferior oblique. Characteristic: right eye does not move upward when eyes are turned to the left. Field: vertical diplopia (image of right eye uppermost) increasing on looking to left and up. (From DG Cogan, Neurology of the Ocular Muscles, 2d ed, Springfield, Ill, Charles C Thomas, 1956.)

the white image is projected farther down than the red, the paretic muscle is the left inferior rectus. If the maximum separation occurs on looking down and to the left and the red image is lower than the white, the paretic muscle is the right superior oblique. Separation of images on looking up and to the right or left will similarly distinguish paresis of the inferior oblique and superior rectus muscles.

Monocular diplopia may occur occasionally in relation to diseases of the retina or lens; usually the images are overlapping or superimposed rather than discrete. In most cases, no disease can be found to explain monocular diplopia. Occasionally patients with homonymous scotomas due to a lesion of the occipital lobe will see multiple images (polyopsia) in the defective field of vision, particularly when the target is moving.

Rarely, the acute onset of convergence paralysis may give rise to diplopia and blurred vision at all near points; most cases are due to head injury, some to encephalitis or multiple sclerosis. Many cases of convergence paralysis do not have an organic basis. The acute onset of divergence paralysis causes diplopia at a distance because of crossing of the visual axes; in patients with divergent paralysis, images fuse at near distance. This disorder, the pathological basis of which is unknown, is difficult to distinguish from mild bilateral sixth nerve palsies and from convergence spasm, which is common in malingerers and hysterics.

The Causes of Third, Fourth, and Sixth Nerve Palsies
Ocular palsies may be central, i.e., due to a lesion of the nucleus or of the intramedullary portion of the cranial nerve, or they may be peripheral. Weakness of ocular muscles due to a lesion in the brainstem is usually accompanied by involvement of other cranial nerves or long tracts. Peripheral lesions, which may or may not be solitary, have a great variety of causes. Rucker (1958, 1966), who analyzed 2000 cases of paralysis of the ocular motor nerves, found that the most common causes were tumors of the base of the brain (primary, metastatic, meningeal carcinomatosis), trauma to the head, ischemic infarction of a nerve, and aneurysms of the circle of Willis, in that order. Much less common causes included herpes zoster, subdural hematoma, giant-cell arteritis, ophthalmoplegic migraine, sarcoid, and tuberculous, syphilitic, and other chronic forms of meningitis. Myasthenia gravis must always be considered in cases of acute ocular muscle palsy. Actually, in the single largest group of patients (20 to 30 percent) no cause could be assigned. Fortunately, in most of the cases of undetermined cause, the palsy disappears in a few weeks to months.

The acute development of a sixth, third, or fourth

nerve palsy on one side is a relatively common occurrence in the adult. In Rucker's series, the sixth nerve was affected in about one-half the cases; third nerve palsies were about one-half as common as those of the sixth nerve; and the fourth nerve was involved in less than 10 percent of cases.

An isolated sixth nerve palsy frequently proves to be caused by neoplasm. In children, the most common tumor that involves the sixth nerve is a pontine glioma; in adults, it is metastatic tumor from the nasopharynx. Thus it is essential that the nasopharynx be examined carefully in every case of unexplained sixth nerve palsy, particularly if it is accompanied by sensory symptoms on the side of the face.

The fourth nerve is particularly vulnerable to head trauma and is practically never involved by aneurysm. The sixth nerve also is rarely damaged by aneurysm. This reflects the relative infrequency of carotid artery aneurysms in the infraclinoid portion of the cavernous sinus, where they can impinge on the sixth nerve. In contrast, supraclinoid aneurysms commonly involve the third nerve.

In third nerve lesions due to compression by aneurysm, tumor, or temporal lobe herniation, enlargement of the pupil is an early sign, because of the peripheral location in the nerve of the pupilloconstrictor fibers. In cases of infarction of the third nerve, as occurs in patients with diabetes, the pupil is spared, since the infarction characteristically involves the central portion of the nerve. The oculomotor palsy that occurs with diabetes is of acute onset, developing over a few hours, and is accompanied by pain around the eye and forehead. The prognosis for recovery in cases of diabetic third nerve palsy (as in other nonprogressive lesions of the ocular motor nerves) is usually good, because of the potentiality of nerve regeneration.

Rarely, children or young adults may have one or more attacks of ocular palsy in conjunction with an otherwise typical migraine (ophthalmoplegic migraine). The muscles (both extrinsic and intrinsic) innervated by the oculomotor or, very rarely, the abducens nerve are affected. Presumably, intense spasm of the vessels supplying these nerves causes a transitory ischemic paralysis. Arteriograms done after the onset of the palsy usually disclose no abnormality. The patient with oculomotor palsy tends to recover, but after repeated attacks there may be some permanent residual paresis.

The slow development of a *complete ophthalmoplegia* is most often traced to an aneurysm, tumor, ocular myopathy (progressive external ophthalmoplegia; see Chap. 49), or an inflammatory process in the anterior portion of the cavernous sinus or at the superior orbital fissure (syndrome of Tolosa-Hunt; see Table 46-1). The various intramedullary and extramedullary syndromes involving the ocular and other cranial nerves are summarized in Tables 46-1 and 46-2. See also the diagrams of the angioanatomic syndromes in Chap. 33.

Several causes of *pseudoparalysis of ocular muscles* need to be distinguished. In thyroid disease a tight inferior rectus muscle limits upward gaze (most frequent) or a tight medial rectus muscle limits abduction (both are demonstrable by forced ductions). Duane's retraction syndrome, due to congenital fibrosis of the lateral rectus, causes retraction of the globe on adduction and limitation of abduction. Convergence spasm, in which both eyes converge on attempted fixation straight ahead or to the side, is usually hysterical and can be arrested by mydriatics (atropine). An old squint or tropia with secondary fibrosis of an ocular muscle should also be considered.

MIXED GAZE AND OCULAR MUSCLE PARALYSIS

We have already considered two types of paralysis of the extraocular muscles: paralysis of conjugate movements (gaze) and paralysis of individual ocular muscles. Now we must consider a third, viz., mixed gaze and ocular muscle paralysis. The latter is always a sign of an intrapontine or mesencephalic lesion, due usually to vascular, demyelinative, or neoplastic disease. A lesion of the lower pons in or near the sixth nerve nucleus causes a homolateral paralysis of the lateral rectus muscle and a failure of adduction of the opposite eye, i.e., a combined paralysis of the sixth nerve and of conjugate lateral gaze.

Lesions of the medial longitudinal fasciculi interfere with lateral conjugate gaze in another way. As already indicated, the pontine or paraabducens center accomplishes horizontal conjugate gaze by simultaneously innervating the ipsilateral abducens nucleus and the contralateral oculomotor nucleus, the latter through fibers conveyed in the medial longitudinal fasciculus (MLF). With a lesion of the left MLF, the left eye fails to adduct when the patient looks to the right; this condition is referred to as *left internuclear ophthalmoplegia*. With a lesion of the right MLF, the right eye fails to adduct when the patient looks to the left *(right internuclear ophthalmoplegia)*. Nystagmus is more prominent in or is limited to the abducting eye. Since the MLF also

contains axons that originate in the vestibular nuclei and that govern vertical eye and head position, a lesion of the MLF causes vertical nystagmus and impairment of vertical fixation and pursuit. Since the two medial longitudinal fasciculi lie close together, each being situated adjacent to the midline, they are frequently affected together, yielding a bilateral internuclear ophthalmoplegia; this condition should always be suspected when only adduction of the eyes is affected. Lesions involving the medial longitudinal fasciculi in the high midbrain may result in a loss of convergence in conjunction with paralysis of the medial recti on attempted lateral gaze ("anterior" internuclear ophthalmoplegia); if the MLF is involved by a lesion in the pons, convergence is normal, but there may be some degree of associated limitation of conjugate lateral gaze or sixth nerve palsy ("posterior" internuclear ophthalmoplegia, Figs. 13-1 and 13-2).

NYSTAGMUS AND RELATED DISORDERS OF OCULAR MOVEMENT

Nystagmus refers to involuntary rhythmic movements of the eyes and is of two general types. In so-called *jerk nystagmus*, the movements alternate between a slow component and a fast corrective component, or jerk, in the opposite direction. In *pendular nystagmus*, the oscillations are roughly equal in rate for the two directions, although on far lateral gaze the pendular type is converted to the jerk type, with the fast component to the side of the gaze.

In testing for nystagmus, the eyes should be examined first in the central position and then during upward, downward, and lateral movements. Nystagmus of labyrinthine origin, e.g., the type induced by irrigation of the external auditory canal with hot or cold water, is most obvious when visual fixation is prevented by shielding the patient's eyes or by fitting the patient with Frenzel's spectacles, which also magnify the eyes and aid the detection of nystagmus. On the other hand, nystagmus of brainstem and cerebellar origin is brought out best by having the patient fixate upon and follow a moving target. Labyrinthine nystagmus may vary with the position of the head. In particular, the postural nystagmus of Barany is evoked by hyperextension and rotation of the neck, with the patient in the supine position. Optokinetic nystagmus, the type of nystagmus induced in normal persons by looking at a moving object, should be tested by asking the patient to look at a striped rotating cylinder or at a striped cloth that is moved across the field of vision.

In some normal individuals a few irregular jerks are observed as they turn their eyes to one side ("nystagmoid" jerks), but no sustained rhythmic movements occur once fixation is attained. Occasionally a fine rhythmic nystagmus may occur in extreme lateral gaze, beyond the range of binocular vision, but if it is bilateral and disappears as the eyes move a few degrees toward the midline it usually has no clinical significance. These movements are probably analogous to the tremulousness of skeletal muscles that are contracted maximally.

Pendular nystagmus is found in a variety of conditions in which central vision is lost early in life, such as albinism and various other diseases of the retina and refractive media (congenital ocular nystagmus). Occasionally it is observed in patients with multiple sclerosis, and it occurs as a congenital abnormality, even without poor vision. The syndrome of miner's nystagmus, formerly a common cause of industrial disability, occurs in patients who have worked for many years in comparative darkness. The oscillations of the eyes, in pendular nystagmus, are usually very rapid, increase on upward gaze, and may be associated with compensatory oscillations of the head and intolerance of light. *Spasmus nutans*, a specific type of pendular nystagmus of infancy, is accompanied by head nodding and occasionally by wry positions of the neck. It begins between the fourth and twelfth months of life, never after the third year. The nystagmus may be horizontal, vertical, or rotatory, is usually more pronounced in one eye than the other (or limited to one eye) and can be intensified by immobilizing or straightening the head. The prognosis is good, and most infants recover within a few months or years.

Jerk nystagmus is the more common type. It may be horizontal or vertical, particularly on ocular movement in these planes, or it may be rotatory and rarely retractory or vergent. By custom, in the English-speaking world, the direction of the nystagmus is named according to the direction of the fast component. There are several varieties of jerk nystagmus. Some occur spontaneously, others are readily induced in normal persons by drugs, or by labyrinthine or visual stimulation. Deviations from the patterns of normally induced nystagmus may provide important clues to the locus of disease.

When one is watching a moving object (e.g., the passing landscape from a train window or a rotating drum with vertical stripes), a rhythmic jerk nystagmus, *optokinetic nystagmus (OKN)*, normally appears. The usual explanation of this phenomenon is that the slow component of the nystagmus represents an involuntary pursuit movement to the limit of comfortable conjugate gaze; the eyes then make a quick corrective movement in the opposite direction and fixate another object. With unilateral cerebral lesions, specifically of the parietal region (and transiently with acute frontal lobe lesions), OKN may be lost or diminished when a moving stimu-

lus, e.g., the striped OKN drum is rotated *toward* the side of the lesion, whereas rotation of the drum to the opposite side elicits a normal response. It should be noted that patients with hemianopia may show a normal optokinetic response. On the other hand, patients with a parietal lobe lesion and hemianopia consistently show an abnormal optokinetic response. These observations suggest that an abnormal response does not depend upon a lesion of the geniculocalcarine tract. Presumably it is due to the interruption of the efferent pathways from the parietal region to the lower centers for conjugate gaze.

Perhaps the most important fact about OKN is that its demonstration proves that the patient is not blind. Thus it is of particular value in the examination of hysterical patients and malingerers who claim that they cannot see and of neonates and infants (OKN is established within minutes or hours after birth).

Labyrinthine stimulation, e.g., irrigation of the external auditory canal with hot or cold water, produces nystagmus; in addition, cold water induces a slow tonic deviation of the eyes in a direction opposite to that of the nystagmus. The slow component reflects the effect of impulses derived from the semicircular canals, and the fast component is a corrective movement. The production of nystagmus by labyrinthine stimulation and other features of vestibular nystagmus are discussed further in Chap. 14.

Drug intoxication, particularly with barbiturates, is the most frequent cause of induced nystagmus. Alcohol, other sedative-hypnotic drugs, and phenytoin are other common offenders. This form of nystagmus is most prominent on deviation of the eyes in the horizontal plane, but occasionally it may appear in the vertical plane as well, and rarely in the vertical plane alone, suggesting a tegmental brainstem lesion.

Nystagmus occurring spontaneously in patients may signify the presence of labyrinthine-vestibular, brainstem, or cerebellar disease. Vestibular-labyrinthine nystagmus may be horizontal, vertical, or oblique and characteristically has a rotatory component. Tinnitus and hearing loss are associated with disease of the peripheral labyrinthine mechanism; vertigo, nausea, vomiting, and staggering are the usual accompaniments of peripheral or central lesions (see Chap. 14). Brainstem lesions often cause a coarse, unidirectional, gaze-dependent nystagmus, which may be horizontal or vertical; the latter is brought out usually on upward gaze, less often on downward gaze. The presence of vertical nystagmus is pathognomonic of disease in the tegmentum of the brainstem, usually the pons. Vertigo is inconstant, and signs of disease of other nuclear structures and tracts in the brainstem are frequent. Vertical nystagmus of this type is observed frequently in patients with demyelinative or vascular disease, tumors, Wernicke's disease, syringobulbia, and Arnold-Chiari malformation. Vertical nystagmus in a downward direction is said to be characteristic of the last disorder and of other lesions near the foramen magnum. Cerebellopontine-angle tumors may cause a coarse bilateral horizontal nystagmus, coarser to the side of the lesion. Nystagmus of several types, including downbeat nystagmus and "rebound nystagmus" (gaze-evoked nystagmus which changes direction with fatigue or refixation to the primary position), occurs with cerebellar disease, but the specific structures involved in the genesis of these symptoms have not been defined. Characteristic also of cerebellar disease are the closely related disorders of saccadic movement (opsoclonus, flutter, dysmetria) described below. The nystagmus that occurs only in the abducting eye (dissociated nystagmus) and is a common sign of multiple sclerosis probably represents an incompletely developed form of internuclear ophthalmoplegia; on attempted lateral gaze, the adducting eye (which does not show nystagmus) will lag behind the abducting one.

Convergence nystagmus is a rhythmic oscillation in which a slow abduction of the eyes in respect to each other is followed by a quick movement of adduction. It is usually accompanied by other types of nystagmus and by one or more features of Parinaud's syndrome. There may also be quick rhythmic retraction movements of the eyes *(nystagmus retractorius)* and movements of the eyelids, or a maintained spasm of convergence, best brought out on attempted elevation of the eyes to command or downward rotation of an OKN drum. These unusual phenomena all point to a lesion of the upper midbrain tegmentum and are usually manifestations of vascular disease or of tumor, notably pinealoma. *Seesaw nystagmus* is a torsional-vertical oscillation in which the intorting eye moves up and the opposite (extorting) eye moves down, and then both move in the reverse direction. It is occasionally observed in conjunction with bitemporal hemianopia due to sellar or parasellar masses. Rhythmic "palatal nystagmus," due to a lesion of the central tegmental tract, may be accompanied by a pendular nystagmus or a convergence-retraction nystagmus that has the same beat as the palatal and pharyngeal muscles.

Oscillopsia refers to illusory movement of the environment in which stationary objects seem to move back and forth—either up or down or from side to side. It may be associated with severe nystagmus of any type due to lesions of the brainstem, involving the vestibular nucleus on one or both sides. With lesions of the labyrinths (as in streptomycin toxicity), oscillopsia is characteristically provoked by motion, e.g., riding in an automobile, and indicates a loss of stabilization of ocular fixation by the vestibular system during body movement. Examination of the eyes in these latter circumstances discloses no abnormalities.

Similar subjective phenomena may be produced by parietal-occipital lesions. These take the form of visual hallucinations or illusions in the contralateral homonymous fields. It may seem to the patient, for example, that a venetian blind is continually being opened and closed, or that objects are moving or waving or shimmering in that field.

Ocular bobbing is a term coined by C. M. Fisher to describe a distinctive spontaneous fast jerk of the eyes in a downward direction, followed by a slow drift to the midposition. It occurs usually with large destructive lesions of the pons in comatose patients in whom horizontal eye movements are absent. The phenomenon itself and the clinical setting in which it occurs are variable, however (Susac et al.), and its pathophysiology is obscure.

Opsoclonus is the term applied to rapid, conjugate oscillations of the eyes in a horizontal, rotatory, and vertical direction, which are made worse by voluntary movement or the need to fixate the eyes. These eye movements are usually associated with widespread myoclonus of diverse causes, as indicated in Chap. 5. Similar movements have been produced in monkeys by creating bilateral lesions in the pretectum. A fine oscillation of the eyes can be induced by volition in some persons. *Ocular dysmetria* consists of an overshoot of the eyes on attempted fixation, followed by several cycles of oscillations of diminishing amplitude until precise fixation is attained. The overshoot may occur on eccentric fixation or on refixation in the primary position of gaze. This abnormality is a sign of disease of the cerebellum or its pathways and is analogous to cerebellar dysmetria of the limbs. *Ocular flutter* refers to quick, multiphasic, usually horizontal oscillations around the point of fixation; this abnormality is also associated with cerebellar disease. Opsoclonus, ocular dysmetria, and flutter-like oscillations are closely related disorders. A patient may show only one of these ocular abnormalities or more than one, either simultaneously or in sequence. Evidence has been presented that these ocular dyskinesias represent abnormal saccadic movements (Ellenberger et al.).

THE PUPILS

The testing of pupillary size and reactivity, which can be accomplished by the use of a flashlight, yields important, often vital, clinical information. Essential, of course, is the proper interpretation of the pupillary reactions, and this requires some knowledge of their underlying neural mechanisms.

The diameter of the pupil is determined by the balance of innervation between the autonomically innervated sphincter and radially arranged dilator muscles of the iris, the sphincter muscle playing the major role. *The pupilloconstrictor (parasympathetic) fibers arise in the Edinger-Westphal nucleus in the high midbrain, join the third cranial (oculomotor) nerve, and synapse in the ciliary ganglion with the postganglionic neurons which innervate the sphincter pupillae and the ciliary body. The pupillodilator (sympathetic) fibers arise in the posterolateral part of the hypothalamus and descend uncrossed, in the lateral tegmentum of the midbrain, pons, medulla, and cervical spinal cord to the eighth cervical and first and second thoracic segments, where they synapse with the lateral horn cells.* These cells give rise to preganglionic fibers, most of which leave the cord by the first

ventral thoracic root and proceed through the stellate ganglion to synapse in the superior cervical ganglion; the postganglionic fibers course along the internal carotid artery and traverse the cavernous sinus, where they join the first division of the trigeminal nerve, finally reaching the eyes as the two long ciliary nerves.

The Pupillary Light Reflex The commonest stimulus for pupillary constriction is exposure of the retina to light. Reflex pupillary constriction is also part of the act of convergence and accommodation for near objects (near synkinesis).

The pathway for the pupillary light reflex consists of three parts (Fig. 13-6): (1) An afferent limb, which has its origin in the retinal receptor cell, passes through the bipolar cell, and synapses with the retinal ganglion cell, the axon of which runs in the optic nerve and tract. The light reflex fibers leave the optic tract just rostral to the lateral geniculate body and enter the high midbrain, where they synapse in the pretectal nucleus. (2) Interca-

Figure 13-6
Diagram of the pupillary light reflex. (Redrawn from FB Walsh, WF Hoyt, Clinical Neuro-Ophthalmology, 3d ed, Baltimore, Williams & Wilkins, 1969.)

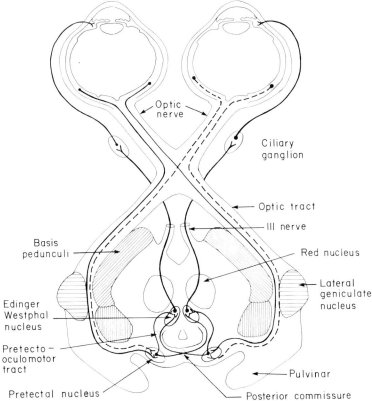

lated neurons, by which the pupillomotor fibers pass ventrally to the ipsilateral Edinger-Westphal nucleus, and, via fibers that cross in the posterior commissure, to the contralateral Edinger-Westphal nucleus. (3) An efferent two-neuron pathway from the Edinger-Westphal nucleus by which all motor impulses reach the pupillary sphincter, as described above.

Alterations of the Pupils Normally the pupil constricts under a bright light (direct reflex) and the other unexposed pupil also constricts (consensual reflex). With complete or nearly complete interruption of the optic nerve the pupil will fail to react to direct light stimulation; however, the pupil of the blind eye will show a consensual reflex, i.e., it will constrict when light is shone in the healthy eye. The lack of a direct reflex in the blind eye together with a lack of a consensual reflex in the sound one means that the afferent limb of the reflex arc (optic nerve) is the site of the lesion. A lack of direct light reflex with retention of the consensual reflex places the lesion in the efferent limb of the reflex arc, i.e., in the homolateral oculomotor nerve or its nucleus. It is evident that a lesion of the afferent limb of the light reflex pathway will not affect the near responses of the pupil and that lesions of the visual pathway caudal to the point where the light reflex fibers leave the optic tract will not alter the pupillary light reflex.

Following initial constriction, the pupil may dilate slightly in spite of a light shining steadily in one or both eyes. This failure to sustain pupillary constriction, or "pupillary escape," is sometimes referred to as the Gunn pupil sign; a mild degree of it may be observed in normal persons, but it is far more prominent in cases of damage to the retina or optic nerve. A variant of this abnormal pupillary response may be used to expose mild degrees of retrobulbar neuropathy. If a light is shifted immediately from the normal to the impaired eye, the direct light stimulus is no longer sufficient to maintain the previously evoked pupillary constriction, and both pupils dilate. These abnormal pupillary responses form the basis of "the swinging-flashlight test," in which each pupil is alternately exposed to light at 5-s intervals.

The Gunn pupil sign is not to be confused with the Marcus Gunn or "jaw-winking" phenomenon, a congenital and sometimes hereditary anomaly, in which a ptotic eyelid retracts momentarily when the mouth is opened or the jaw is moved to one side. In other cases, inhibition of the levator muscle and ptosis occurs with opening of the mouth ("inverse Marcus Gunn phenomenon"). These associated movements of lid and jaw have been referred to as a trigeminooculomotor synkinesis and attributed to abnormal connections between the central mechanisms innervating the pterygoid and levator muscles.

Interruption of the sympathetic fibers either centrally, between the hypothalamus and their point of exit from the spinal cord (first thoracic segment), or peripherally (cervical sympathetic chain, superior cervical ganglion or along the carotid artery) results in miosis and ptosis (because of paralysis of the pupillary dilator muscle and of Müller's muscle, respectively), enophthalmos, loss of sweating of the same side of the face and neck, and redness of the conjunctiva. The entire complex is called the *Horner-Bernard*, or *Horner's, syndrome*. Stimulation or irritation of the sympathetic fibers has the opposite effect, i.e., lid retraction, slight proptosis, and dilatation of the pupil. The ciliospinal pupillary reflex, evoked by pinching the neck (afferent, C2, C3), is effected through these efferent sympathetic fibers. Extreme constriction of the pupils (miosis) is commonly observed with pontine lesions, presumably because of bilateral interruption of the pupillodilator fibers. Interruption of the parasympathetic fibers yields an abnormal dilatation of the pupils (mydriasis), often with loss of pupillary light reflexes; this is frequently the result of midbrain lesions and is a common finding in cases of deep coma.

The functional integrity of the sympathetic and parasympathetic nerve endings in the iris may also be determined by the use of certain drugs. Atropine and homatropine dilate the pupils by paralyzing the parasympathetic nerve endings; physostigmine and pilocarpine constrict them, the former by inhibiting cholinesterase activity at the neuromuscular junction, and the latter by direct stimulation of the sphincter muscle of the iris. Epinephrine and phenylephrine dilate the pupil by direct stimulation of the dilator muscle. Cocaine dilates the pupils by preventing the reabsorption of norepinephrine into the nerve endings. Morphine acts centrally to constrict the pupils.

In chronic syphilitic meningitis and other forms of late syphilis, particularly tabes dorsalis, the pupils are usually small, irregular, and unequal; they do not dilate properly in response to mydriatic drugs and fail to react to light, although they do constrict on accommodation. In some cases atrophy of the iris is also associated. This is known as the *Argyll Robertson pupil*. The exact locality of the lesion is not certain; it is generally believed to be in the tectum of the midbrain proximal to the oculomotor nuclei, where the descending pupillodilator fibers are in close proximity to the light reflex fibers (Fig. 13-6). The possibility of a partial third nerve lesion or a lesion of the ciliary ganglion seems more plausible to the authors. A dissociation of the light reflex from the accommodation-convergence reaction is sometimes observed with other midbrain lesions, e.g., pinealoma, multiple sclerosis, and occasionally in patients with diabetes mellitus; in these diseases, miosis, irregularity of pupils, and failure to respond to a mydriatic are not constantly present. S. A. K. Wilson referred to this condition as the Argyll Robertson pupillary phenomenon and contrasted it to the Argyll Robertson pupil.

Another interesting pupillary abnormality is the tonic reaction sometimes referred to as *Adie's pupil*. This syndrome is due to an affection of the postganglionic parasympathetic fibers which normally constrict the pupil and cause accommodation. The patient may complain of blurring of vision or may have suddenly noticed that one pupil is larger than the other. The reaction to light and sometimes to accommodation are absent if tested in the customary manner, although the size of the pupil will change slowly on prolonged maximal stimulation. Once contracted or dilated, the pupil remains in this state for some minutes. The affected pupil reacts promptly to the common mydriatic and miotic drugs and is usually sensitive to a 0.125% solution of pilocarpine, a strength that will not affect a normal pupil. The myotonic pupil usually appears during the third or fourth decade of life; it may be associated with absence of knee or ankle jerks and hence be mistaken for tabes dorsalis. From all available data it represents a mild polyneuropathy.

Ocular movement, pupillary reaction, and visual acuity may be affected by diseases which alter the contents of the orbit. Usually this is accompanied by bilateral exophthalmos, as in thyroid or pituitary disease, or unilateral exophthalmos with thyroid disease, orbital tumors (dermoids, hemangiomas, adenoma of lacrimal gland, optic nerve glioma, neurofibroma, metastatic carcinoma, meningioma), granuloma, orbital cellulitis or abscess, or cavernous sinus thrombosis. Progressive paralysis of the eyelids, which may obstruct vision, occurs separately or as part of an external ophthalmoplegia, as in the ocular dystrophy of Kiloh and Nevin or in oculopharyngeal dystrophy.

REFERENCES

BENDER MB, SAVITSKY N: Micropsia and teleopsia limited to the temporal fields of vision. *Arch Ophthalmol* 29:904, 1943.

BRUCHER JM: The frontal eye fields of the monkey. *Int J Neurol* 5:262, 1966.

CHESTER EM: *The Ocular Fundus in Systemic Disease*. Chicago, Year Book, 1973.

COGAN DG: *Neurology of the Ocular Muscles*, 2d ed. Springfield, Ill, Charles C Thomas, 1956.

———: *Neurology of the Visual System*. Springfield, Ill, Charles C Thomas, 1966.

DAROFF RB: Ocular oscillations. *Ann Otol Rhinol Laryngol* 86:102, 1977.

ELLENBERGER C JR et al: Ocular dyskinesia in cerebellar disease. *Brain* 95:685, 1972.

GLASER JS: *Neuro-ophthalmology*. Hagerstown, Md, Harper & Row, 1978.

HALMAGYI AM, EVANS WA, HALLINAN JM: Failure of downward gaze. The site and nature of the lesion. *Arch Neurol* 35:22, 1978.

JACOBS L, ANDERSON PJ, BENDER MG: The lesions producing paralysis of downward but not upward gaze. *Arch Neurol* 28:319, 1973.

KÖMPF D et al: Downward gaze in monkeys. Stimulation and lesion studies. *Brain* 102:527, 1979.

RUCKER CW: Paralysis of the third, fourth, and sixth cranial nerves. *Am J Ophthalmol* 46:787, 1958.

———: The causes of paralysis of the third, fourth and sixth cranial nerves. *Am J Ophthalmol* 61:1293, 1966.

SACHSENWEGER R: Clinical localization of oculomotor disturbances, in Vinken PJ, Bruyn GW, (eds): *Handbook of Clinical Neurology*, vol 2. Amsterdam, North-Holland, 1969, chap 13, pp 286-357.

SUSAC JO et al: Clinical spectrum of ocular bobbing. *J Neurol Neurosurg Psychiatry* 33:771, 1970.

THOMAS JE, REAGEN TJ: Nonhemorrhagic complications of intracranial aneurysms of the internal carotid artery. *Neurology* 20:1043, 1970.

WALSH FB, HOYT WF: *Clinical Neuro-ophthalmology*, 3d ed. Baltimore, Williams & Wilkins, 1969.

WARWICK R: Representation of the extraocular muscles in the oculomotor nuclei of the monkey. *J Comp Neurol* 98:449, 1953.

———: The so-called nucleus of convergence. *Brain* 78:92, 1955.

ZEE DS et al: Ocular motor abnormalities in hereditary cerebellar ataxia. *Brain* 99:207, 1976.

CHAPTER 14

DEAFNESS, DIZZINESS, AND DISORDERS OF EQUILIBRIUM

ANATOMIC CONSIDERATIONS

The vestibulocochlear or eighth cranial nerve has two components: the cochlear nerve, which subserves hearing or acoustic function, and the vestibular nerve, which is concerned with equilibrium and orientation of the body in space. The acoustic division has its cell bodies in the spiral ganglion of the cochlea. This ganglion is composed of bipolar cells, the peripheral processes of which convey auditory impulses from the specialized neuroepithelium of the inner ear, the spiral organ of Corti. This is the end organ of hearing, and consists of numerous hair cells, aligned in rows along the entire $2\frac{1}{2}$ turns of the cochlea. The vestibular division arises from cells in the vestibular or Scarpa's ganglion, which is situated in the internal auditory meatus. This ganglion also is composed of bipolar cells, the peripheral processes of which terminate in hair cells of the specialized sensory epithelium of the labyrinth (semicircular canals, saccule, and utricle). The sensory epithelium is distributed in patches in the dilated openings or ampullae of the semicircular canals, where they are called the *cristae ampullaris* and in the utricle and saccule, where they are called *maculae acusticae*. The hair cells of the maculae are covered by a mucilaginous material which contains small calcareous formations, or *otoliths*.

The central fibers from the spiral and vestibular ganglia are united in a common trunk, which enters the cranial cavity through the internal auditory meatus (accompanied by the facial and intermediate nerves), traverses the cerebellopontine angle, and enters the brainstem at the junction of the pons and medulla. Here the cochlear and vestibular fibers become separated. The cochlear fibers bifurcate and terminate almost at once in the dorsal and ventral cochlear nuclei. Secondary acous-

tic fibers project via the trapezoid body and lateral lemniscus to the inferior colliculi and medial geniculate bodies, which in turn project via the auditory radiations (situated in the most posterior part of the internal capsule) to the primary receptive areas for hearing in the transverse temporal gyri of Heschl (Fig. 14-1). Since each cochlear nucleus is connected with the cortex of both temporal lobes, hearing is unaffected by unilateral cerebral lesions.

The vestibular fibers of the eighth nerve terminate in the four vestibular nuclei: superior (Bechterev's), lateral (Deiter's), medial (principal or Schwalbe's), and inferior (spinal or descending). In addition, some of the fibers from the semicircular canals project directly to the cerebellum, via the juxtarestiform body, to terminate in the flocculonodular lobe and adjacent vermian cortex. Efferent fibers from this portion of the cerebellar cortex project to all four vestibular nuclei of the ipsilateral side. Other fibers from one side of the "vestibulocerebellum" project to the ipsilateral fastigial nucleus (see Chap. 4); fibers from this nucleus project in turn to the contralateral vestibular nuclei, again via the juxtarestiform body. Thus the cerebellum of each side exerts an influence on the vestibular nuclei of both sides (Fig. 14-2).

The lateral and medial vestibular nuclei also have important connections with the spinal cord, mainly via the uncrossed lateral vestibulospinal and the crossed and uncrossed medial vestibulospinal tracts (Fig. 14-3). The nuclei of the third, fourth, and sixth cranial nerves come under the influence of the vestibular nuclei, mainly the superior and medial nuclei, through the projection fibers that course up and down in both medial longitudinal fasciculi. In addition, all the vestibular nuclei have afferent and efferent connections with the pontine reticular formation (Fig. 14-3). Finally, there are projections from the vestibular nuclei to the cerebral cortex, although the exact anatomic pathways are not known. In the monkey the projections are almost exclusively contralateral, terminating near the "face area" of the first somatosensory cortex (area 2 of Brodmann).

These brief remarks convey some notion of the complexity of the anatomic and functional organization of the vestibular system (for a full discussion, see Brodal's *Neurological Anatomy*). It is apparent that acoustic and vestibular function (as well as other cranial nerve function) may be affected together in the course of disease, or that each may be affected separately.

Figure 14-1

The ascending auditory pathways. The lower part of the diagram is a horizontal section through the upper medulla. (From CR Noback, The Human Nervous System, 3d ed, New York, McGraw-Hill, 1981.)

DEAFNESS AND TINNITUS

TINNITUS

Tinnitus aurium literally means "ringing of the ears" (Latin *tinnire*, "to ring or jingle") and is a common symptom in adults. Although the term always refers to sounds originating in the ear, they need not be ringing in character. Buzzing, humming, whistling, roaring, hissing, clicking, or pulselike sounds are also reported. Some otologists use the term *tinnitus cerebri* to distinguish other head noises from those that arise in the ear, but most often the term *tinnitus* is used without qualification and refers to *tinnitus aurium*.

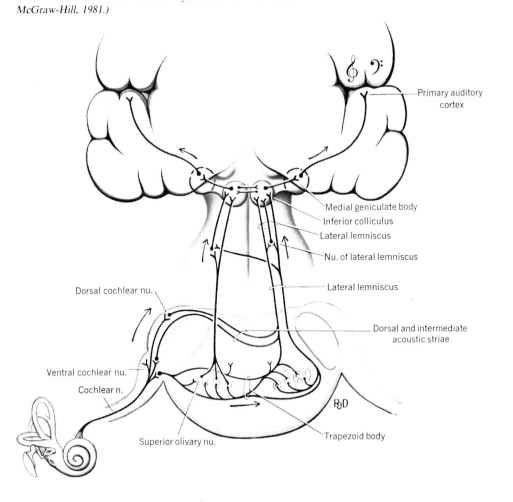

Primary auditory cortex

Medial geniculate body

Inferior colliculus

Lateral lemniscus

Nu. of lateral lemniscus

Lateral lemniscus

Dorsal and intermediate acoustic striae

Dorsal cochlear nu.

Ventral cochlear nu.

Cochlear n.

Superior olivary nu.

Trapezoid body

Tinnitus may be defined more precisely as any sensation of sound for which there is no source outside the individual. Fowler divides it into two basic types: vibratory and nonvibratory. The latter, and by far the more common form, is also called *subjective tinnitus*, because it can be heard only by the patient. The vibratory form is referred to as *objective tinnitus*, because under certain conditions, it can be heard by the examiner as well as by the patient. In either case, whether tinnitus is produced in the ear or in some other part of the head and neck, sensory auditory neurons must be stimulated, for only the auditory neural pathways can transmit an impulse that will be perceived as sound.

Vibratory head noises are mechanical in origin and conducted to the inner ear through the various hard or soft, fluid or gaseous media of the body. They are not due to a primary dysfunction of the auditory neural mechanism but have their origin in the contraction of muscles of the eustachian tube, middle ear (stapedius, tensor tympani), the palate (palatal myoclonus), or the muscles of deglutition. One type of vibratory tinnitus is caused by opening and closing of the eustachian tubes.

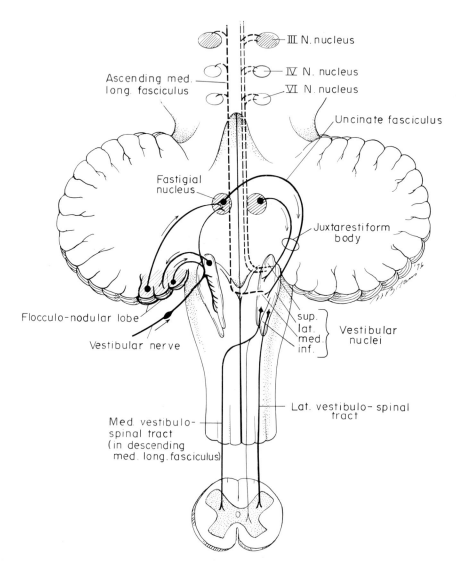

Figure 14-2

A simplified diagram of the vestibulocerebellar and vestibulospinal pathways and connections between vestibular and ocular motor nuclei. (See text and also Fig. 13-1.)

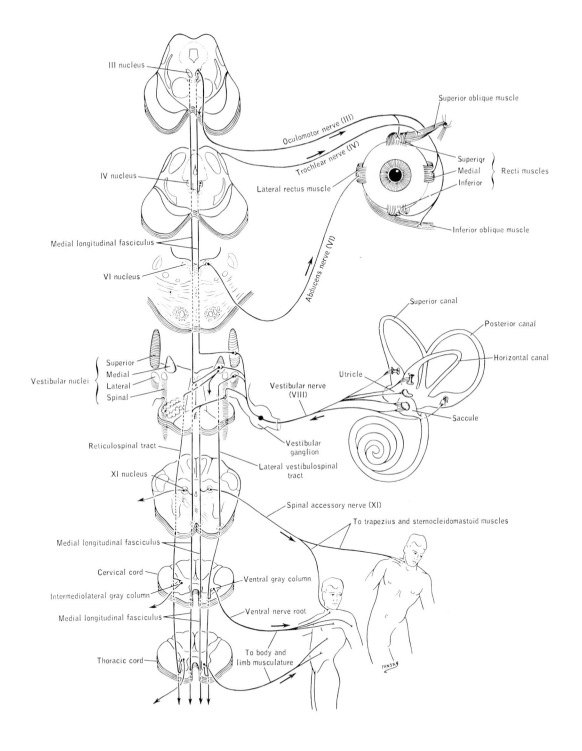

Figure 14-3
The vestibular reflex pathways. (From EL House et al, A Systematic Approach to Neuroscience, New York, McGraw-Hill, 1979.)

The most common form of objective tinnitus is a vascular bruit from the large vessels of the neck or arteriovenous malformations of the brain. In these latter cases, the tinnitus corresponds to the pulse (pulsatile tinnitus), and the examiner may hear a bruit over the mastoid process. One must be cautious in interpreting this symptom because normal persons can hear their pulse when lying with one ear on a pillow, and introspective individuals may worry about it.

Nonvibratory tinnitus arises in the middle or inner ear. Under ideal acoustical circumstances (in a sound-proof room, having an ambient noise level of 18 dB or less), it is present in 80 to 90 percent of adults ("physiologic tinnitus"). The ambient noise level in ordinary living conditions usually exceeds 35 dB and is of sufficient intensity to mask physiologic tinnitus, which remains inaudible. However, tinnitus due to disease of the middle ear and auditory neural mechanism may also be masked by environmental noise and hence becomes troublesome only in quiet surroundings—at night, in the country, etc.

Most often, tinnitus signifies a disorder of the inner ear, ossicles of the middle ear, tympanic membrane, or eighth nerve. The large majority of patients who complain of persistent tinnitus also have some degree of deafness as well. Tinnitus that is localized to one ear and is described as having a tonal character (such as a ringing or bell-like or high, steady musical tone) is usually associated with an impairment of cochlear or neural function. Tinnitus due to middle ear disease (e.g., otosclerosis, etc.) tends to be more constant than the tinnitus of sensorineural disorders, and is of variable intensity and lower pitch. All clicks, pops, rushing sounds, etc., are believed to be due to middle ear disease.

As was remarked, the pitch of tinnitus associated with a conductive hearing loss is of low-frequency (median frequency of 490 Hz, with a range of 90 to 1450 Hz). That which accompanies sensorineural loss is higher (median frequency of 3900 Hz, with a range of 545 to 7500 Hz). This rule does not apply to Ménière's disease, in which the tinnitus usually has a low-pitched buzzing or roaring sound (median frequency of 320 Hz, with a range of 90 to 900 Hz), thus resembling the tinnitus that accompanies a conductive rather than a sensorineural hearing loss (Nodar and Graham).

For most forms of tinnitus there is little effective treatment. Patients reconcile themselves to its presence as a rule, once the nature of the disorder is explained to them. If tinnitus is the basis of repeated complaints, one usually discovers that the patient is anxious or depressed, and a careful medical history will reveal the other symptoms of these psychiatric illnesses.

DEAFNESS

This is a problem of immense proportions. In 1969, Konigsmark estimated that there were in the United States at least 6 million persons with hearing loss of sufficient severity to impair the understanding of speech; there are probably three times this many with some impairment of hearing. He estimated that in about one-half the affected children and about one-third the affected adults, the deafness was on a hereditary basis.

Deafness is of two general types: (1) *conductive deafness*, which is a defect in the mechanism by which sound is conducted to the cochlea and is due to conditions such as otosclerosis, chronic otitis, cholesteatoma, or occlusion of the external auditory canal or eustachian tube, and (2) *sensorineural deafness* (also called perceptive or nerve deafness), which is due to disease of the cochlea or of the cochlear division of the eighth cranial nerve or its central connections. It is important to distinguish these two types, since important remediable measures are available for conductive deafness. Also, potentially serious causes of both types of deafness, e.g., cholesteatoma, acoustic neuroma, etc., must be recognized.

In differentiating conductive from nerve deafness, the tuning-fork tests are often of value. When a vibrating fork of 512-Hz frequency is held about an inch from the ear (the test for air conduction), sound waves can be appreciated only as they are transmitted through the middle ear and will be reduced with disease in this location. When the vibrating fork is applied to the skull (test for bone conduction), the sound waves are conveyed directly to the cochlea, without the intervention of the sound-transmission apparatus of the middle ear, and will therefore not be reduced or lost. Normally air conduction is better than bone conduction. These principles form the basis for several simple tests of auditory function.

In *Weber's test*, the vibrating fork is applied to the forehead in the midline. In nerve deafness, the sound is localized in the normal ear; in conductive deafness the sound is localized in the affected ear. In *Rinne's test* the fork is applied to the mastoid process. At the moment the sound ceases the fork is held at the auditory meatus. In middle ear deafness the sound cannot be heard by air conduction after bone conduction has ceased (abnormal or negative Rinne test). In nerve deafness the reverse is true (normal or positive Rinne test), although both air and bone conduction may be quantitatively decreased.

In *Schwabach's test*, the patient's bone conduction is compared with that of a normal observer.

In general, sensorineural deafness is characterized by a partial loss of perception of high-pitched sounds and conductive deafness by a partial loss of perception of low-pitched sounds. This can be ascertained with the use of tuning forks of different frequencies, but the most accurate results are obtained by the use of an electric audiometer and the construction of an audiogram which reveals the entire range of hearing at a glance. The audiogram represents the nucleus of any diagnostic evaluation of loss of hearing and the point of departure for subsequent diagnostic evaluation.

SPECIAL AUDIOLOGIC PROCEDURES

A number of special tests have proved to be helpful in distinguishing cochlear from retrocochlear (nerve) lesions. Although an absolute distinction cannot be made on the basis of any one test, the results of the tests when taken together make it possible to predict the site of the lesion with considerable accuracy. These tests, usually carried out by an otologist or audiologist, include the following:

1. *Loudness recruitment.* This phenomenon is thought to depend upon selective destruction of low-intensity elements subserved by the external hair cells of the organ of Corti. The high-intensity elements are preserved, so that loudness is appreciated at high intensities. In testing for loudness recruitment, the difference in hearing between the two ears is estimated, and the loudness of the stimulus of a given frequency delivered to each ear is then increased by regular increments. In nonrecruiting deafness (characteristic of nerve trunk lesion), the original difference in hearing persists in all comparisons of loudness above threshold, since both high- and low-intensity fibers are affected. In recruiting deafness (which occurs with a lesion in the organ of Corti, i.e., Ménière's disease), the more affected ear gains in loudness and may finally be equal to the better one.

2. *Speech discrimination.* This consists of presenting the patient with a list of 50 phonetically balanced monosyllabic words (e.g., thin, sin) at suprathreshold levels. Speech-discrimination score is the percentage of the 50 words correctly repeated by the patient. Marked reduction (less than 30 percent) in the speech-discrimination test scores with respect to threshold sensitivity is characteristic of eighth nerve lesions.

3. *Short-increment sensitivity index (SiSi).* The patient is asked to respond to a series of twenty 1-dB increments in amplitude superimposed on a steady tone

of the same frequency presented at a sensation level of 20 dB. In normal persons and in those with retrocochlear lesions, most of these small 1-dB pips of sound are not heard; with cochlear lesions most of them are heard.

4. *Threshold "tone decay."* This test requires only a conventional pure-tone audiometer. With lesions of the cochlear nerve, e.g., acoustic neuroma, a continuous tone presented at threshold intensity gradually seems to decrease in loudness, in contrast to what happens with cochlear lesions.

5. *Békésy audiometry.* Continuous and interrupted tones are presented at various frequencies. Tracings are made which measure the increments by which the patient must increase the volume in order to continue to hear the continuous and interrupted tones just above threshold. Analysis of many tracings has shown that there are four basic configurations, referred to as types I to IV Békésy audiograms. Types III or IV usually indicate the presence of retrocochlear lesions, the type II response points to a lesion of the cochlea itself, and type I is considered normal.

6. *Computerized auditory evoked potentials.* This is the newest method and provides information as to the integrity of primary and secondary neural pathways from the cochlea to the temporal lobe cortex.

MIDDLE EAR DEAFNESS

The common causes are otosclerosis, otitis media, and trauma. Of the various types of progressive conductive deafness, *otosclerosis* is the most frequent, being the cause of about half the cases of deafness that have their onset in adult life (usually in the second or third decade). It is transmitted as an autosomal dominant trait with variable penetrance. Pathologically this disorder is characterized by an overgrowth of labyrinthine capsular bone around the oval window, leading to progressive fixation of the stapes. The remarkable advances in microotologic surgery, designed to mobilize or replace the stapes, have greatly altered the prognosis in this disease; significant improvement in hearing can now be achieved in the majority of patients.

The use of antibiotic drugs has greatly reduced the incidence of suppurative otitis media, both the acute and chronic forms, which in former years were a common cause of conductive hearing loss. Chronic serous otitis media is still an important cause of this type of deafness.

Fractures of the temporal bone, particularly those in the long axis of the petrous pyramid, may damage middle ear structures, and frequently there is bleeding into the middle ear as well, from a ruptured tympanic membrane. Transverse fractures through the petrous pyramid are more likely to damage the cochlear-labyrinthine structures and the facial nerve.

SENSORINEURAL DEAFNESS

This has many causes. The cochlea may be aplastic from birth (hereditary deaf-mutism). This is the most common form of hereditary deafness and is characterized by an autosomal dominant transmission and normality of vestibular function (caloric responses are normal). Less frequently, hereditary deafness that is unassociated with vestibular or other congenital abnormalities may be unilateral or have its onset in childhood and run a progressive course; these forms of hereditary deafness are characterized by autosomal dominant, recessive, or sex-linked transmission, in that order of frequency. The cochlea may be damaged by rubella in the pregnant mother. Mumps, acute purulent meningitis, or chronic infection spreading from the middle to the inner ear may cause nerve deafness in childhood.

Little is known about the syndrome of sudden unilateral deafness without vertigo. Presumably it is of cochlear origin. A vascular causation has been postulated, on uncertain grounds. A few cases have complicated herpes zoster and mumps parotitis, but there is no proven relationship with the usual viral respiratory infections. In a prospective study of 88 such cases, Mattox and Simmons found that two-thirds of them recovered their hearing completely within a few days or a week or two, and that none of the currently popular treatments, such as histamine and steroids, had any effect on the outcome. In the remaining patients, recovery was much slower and often incomplete; in this latter group, the hearing loss was predominantly for high tones and was associated with varying degrees of vertigo and hypoactive caloric responses.

Explosions or intense, sustained noise in certain industrial settings or from gun blasts or even from rock music may result in a high-tone sensorineural hearing loss. Certain antimicrobial drugs (viz., streptomycin, kanamycin, neomycin, and gentamicin) may damage cochlear hair cells. Quinine and acetylsalicylic acid may impair sensorineural function transiently. The most

common type of hearing loss in the aged (presbycusis) is a high-frequency sensorineural type, which is probably due to progressive atrophic changes in the cochlea. Otologists have described a progressive sensorineural type of hearing loss as a late manifestation of congenital syphilis, and it may occur despite prior treatment of the latter disorder with adequate doses of penicillin. It has been claimed that the long-term administration of steroids may be useful in these circumstances. The pathologic basis of the hearing loss in such cases has not been determined, and the causal relationship to congenital syphilis remains to be established.

The *auditory nerve* may be involved by tumors of the cerebellopontine angle or by syphilitic meningitis. Deafness may also result from a demyelinative plaque, infarction, or tumor involving the cochlear nerve fibers or nuclei in the *brainstem*.

A large series of *genetically determined syndromes* which feature a neural or conductive type of deafness, some congenital and others having their onset in childhood or early adult life, have recently come to light (see articles by Konigsmark and by Proctor and Proctor). Most of them are inherited as an autosomal dominant trait, but some are characterized by a recessive or sex-linked transmission. Konigsmark has classified these forms of hereditary deafness on the basis of associated defects caused by the same gene: malformations of the external ear; integumentary abnormalities such as hyperkeratosis, hyperplasia or scantiness of eyebrows, albinism, large hyperpigmented or hypopigmented areas, brittle twisted hairs, and coniform and missing teeth; ocular abnormalities such as hypertelorism, severe myopia, optic atrophy, congenital and juvenile cataracts, and retinitis pigmentosa; neurologic abnormalities such as polyneuropathy and sensory ataxia (Refsum's syndrome), polyneuropathy, progressive ophthalmoplegia and cerebellar ataxia, bilateral acoustic neuromas, photomyoclonic seizures, and mental deficiency; skeletal abnormalities; and renal, thyroid, or cardiac abnormalities (see Table 14-1). The associations of neurosensory deafness with degenerative neurologic diseases are discussed further in Chap. 43.

HYSTERICAL DEAFNESS

It is possible to distinguish hysterical deafness from organic disease in several ways. In the case of bilateral deafness, the distinction can be made by observing a blink (cochleoorbicular reflex) or an alteration in skin sweating (psychogalvanic skin reflex) in response to loud sound. Unilateral hysterical deafness may be detected by

(continued on page 200)

Table 14-1
Hereditary cochleovestibular atrophies

Mode of inheritance	Age of onset	Type of hearing loss	Associated abnormalities	Eponymic disease or syndrome
Type I: Progressive hearing loss with involvement of kidneys, skin, or bones				
Autosomal dominant	Childhood	Onset with loss of low, mid, or high frequencies, variably progressive	None	
Recessive	Congenital	Neural; rapidly progressive with failure of speech development	None	
Sex-linked recessive	Early childhood	Neural, rapidly progressive, with speech impairment	None	
Autosomal dominant or recessive	Early adulthood	Neural, with tinnitus; progressive, with unilateral or bilateral vestibular paresis	Episodic paroxysmal vertigo ("hereditary Ménière's")	
Autosomal dominant	Congenital or first decade	Sensorineural; variable severity and progression	Progressive nephritis with uremia	Alport
Autosomal recessive	Childhood	Neural; progressive	Renal tubular acidosis	
Autosomal dominant	Childhood or adolescence	Sensorineural; slowly progressive	Nephrotic syndrome with amyloidosis; recurrent urticaria and fever	Muckle-Wells
Autosomal dominant (probable)	Childhood	Neural; progressive	Ichthyosis of extremities; prolinuria; glomerulosclerosis and uremia in some cases	Goyer
Autosomal dominant	Early adulthood	Neural; progressive	Congenital anhidrosis with absence of sweat and sebacious glands	Helweg-Larsen
Autosomal dominant	Middle age	Conductive loss at onset, then sensorineural; progressive	Osteitis deformans	Paget
Dominant	Childhood	Conductive or neural or mixed; usually progressive	Craniometaphyseal dysplasia with sclerosis of base of skull and narrowing of foramina; sometimes optic atrophy and facial palsy	Pyle
Recessive	Childhood or adolescence	Neural or mixed; progressive	Osteosclerosis of skull and mandible with narrowing of foramina; facial paresis	Van Buchem
Autosomal dominant	Second or third decade	Conductive; sometimes neural or mixed	Osteogenesis imperfecta tarda	Ekman-Lobstein or Van der Hoeve

197

Table 14-1 *(continued)*
Hereditary cochleovestibular atrophies

Mode of inheritance	Age of onset	Type of hearing loss	Associated abnormalities	Eponymic disease or syndrome
Type II: Hereditary hearing loss with retinal disease				
Recessive	Congenital	Sensorineural, with vestibular hypofunction	Progressive retinitis pigmentosa and ataxia beginning in late childhood or adolescence. Sometimes mental defect, cataracts and glaucoma	Usher
Recessive	Early in second decade	Sensorineural; progressive	Retinitis pigmentosa, polyneuropathy, ataxia, mental deterioration	Refsum
Recessive	Infancy	Sensorineural; progressive	Retinal pigmentary degeneration, cataracts, diabetes mellitus	Alström
Recessive	Childhood	Sensorineural; variable progression	Dwarfism, senile appearance, variable mental retardation	Cockayne
Autosomal dominant	Childhood	Neural; variably progressive	Optic atrophy, ataxia, muscle wasting of shoulder girdle and hands, mental dullness, degeneration of optic nerves, posterior columns, spinocerebellar and corticospinal tracts	Sylvester
Recessive	Infancy	Neural; progressive with failure of speech development	Optic atrophy, polyneuropathy	Rosenberg-Chutorian
Autosomal recessive	First decade	Neural; progressive	Optic atrophy, juvenile diabetes mellitus	Tunbridge-Paley
Autosomal recessive	Infancy	Neural; progressive	Opticocochleodentate degeneration, progressive quadriparesis and mental deterioration	Nyssen-Van Bogaert
Sex-linked recessive	Congenital (ocular signs)	Onset of neural deafness in second and third decade; progressive	Retinal vascular and glial proliferation, progressive microphthalmia and mental retardation	Norrie
Recessive	Congenital	Neural	Tortuosity of retinal vessels and exudative retinitis, muscle wasting, immobile facies	Small

Table 14-1 *(continued)*
Hereditary cochleovestibular atrophies

Mode of inheritance	Age of onset	Type of hearing loss	Associated abnormalities	Eponymic disease or syndrome
Type III: Hereditary hearing loss with nervous system disease				
Dominant	Third decade	Neural; progressive	Nephropathy, photomyoclonic seizures, mental deterioration, diabetes mellitus. Diffuse cerebral and cerebellar cortical neuronal loss	Hermann
Dominant	Childhood	Neural, slowly progressive	Myoclonus, progressive ataxia and dysarthria	May-White
Recessive	Congenital	Neural; with failure of speech development	Mild chronic myoclonic epilepsy	Latham-Munro
Dominant	Congenital	Neural, varying severity	Piebald trait and variable absence of pigmentation of skin; ataxia and mental retardation frequent	Telfer
Dominant	Second or third decade	Sensorineural	Hyperuricemia, decreased renal function, progressive ataxia and dysarthria, proximal muscle weakness and wasting	Rosenberg-Bergstrom
Recessive	Childhood	Progressive, severe	Progressive ataxia, hypotonia and dysarthria, mild mental retardation	Lichtenstein-Knorr
Autosomal recessive	Infancy or early childhood	Neural, slowly progressive	Progressive ataxia of gait, hypogonadism, mental deficiency, wasting and weakness of distal limb muscles	Richards-Rundle
Recessive	Childhood	Neural; rapidly progressive	Progressive cerebellar ataxia, mental deficiency, extensor plantar signs, pigmented spots on face and limbs; heart block	Jeune-Tommasi
Autosomal dominant	Second or third decade	Neural; progressive with tinnitus and loss of vestibular function	Bilateral acoustic neuromas	Gardner
Dominant	Childhood	Neural deafness, not in all cases	Progressive sensory radicular neuropathy	Denny-Brown

Table 14-1 *(continued)*
Hereditary cochleovestibular atrophies

Mode of inheritance	Age of onset	Type of hearing loss	Associated abnormalities	Eponymic disease or syndrome
		Type III: Hereditary hearing loss with nervous system disease (continued)		
Dominant	First or second decade	Neural; progressive	Myopia, cataracts and retinitis pigmentosa; sensorimotor peripheral neuropathy; skin atrophy with ulceration; dental caries; kyphoscoliosis, cystic bone changes	Flynn-Aird
Autosomal recessive	Childhood	Neural, progressive	Proteinutria, progressive distal muscle wasting and weakness with claw hand and foot	Lemieux-Neemeh
? Dominant with incomplete penetrance	Congenital	Auditory imperception with failure of speech development	Indifference to pain	Osuntokun
Autosomal recessive	Childhood or adolescence	Progressive; neural with loss of vestibular function	Slowly progressive bulbar palsy	

Source: Konigsmark.

(continued from page 196)

an audiometer, with both ears connected, or by whispering into the bell of a stethoscope attached to the patient's ears, closing first one and then the other tube without the patient's knowledge. The elicitation of brainstem auditory evoked potentials provides indisputable evidence that the patient can hear.

DIZZINESS AND VERTIGO

Dizziness and other sensations of unbalance are among the commonest symptoms confronting the neurologist. The significance of these complaints varies greatly. For the most part they are benign, but always there is the possibility that they signal the presence of an important neurologic disorder. The diagnosis of such disorders demands that the complaint of dizziness be analyzed correctly—with the exact nature of the disturbance of function determined first, and then its anatomic localization. This classic approach to neurologic diagnosis is nowhere more valuable than in the patient whose main complaint is dizziness.

The term *dizziness* is applied by the patient to a number of different sensory experiences—a feeling of rotation or whirling, as well as nonrotatory swaying, weakness, faintness, light-headedness, or unsteadiness. Blurring of vision, feelings of unreality, syncope, and even petit mal, or other seizure phenomena may be called "dizzy spells." Hence a close questioning as to how the patient is using the term becomes a necessary first step in clinical study. Essentially, the physician must determine whether the symptoms have the specific quality of *vertigo*—which in this chapter will refer to all subjective and objective illusions of motion or position—or whether they are more properly categorized as nonrotatory *giddiness* or *pseudovertigo*. The distinction between these two groups of symptoms will be elaborated presently, following a brief discussion of the factors that are involved in the maintenance of equilibrium.

PHYSIOLOGIC CONSIDERATIONS

Several mechanisms are responsible for the maintenance of a balanced posture and for the awareness of the position of the body in relation to its surroundings.

Continuous afferent impulses from the eyes, labyrinths, muscles, and joints inform us of the position of the body. In response to these impulses the adaptive movements necessary to maintain equilibrium are carried out. Normally we are unaware of these many fine adjustments, since they operate for the most part at a reflex level. The most important of these afferent impulses are:

1. Visual impulses from the retinas of both eyes and possibly impulses derived from proprioceptors of the ocular muscles which enable us to judge the distance of objects from the body. These impulses are coordinated by ocular motor mechanisms and supply information about the position and movement of the body and its surroundings.

2. Impulses from the labyrinths, which function as highly specialized spatial proprioceptors and register changes in direction of motion (either acceleration or deceleration) and position of the body. The semicircular canals respond primarily to movement and angular acceleration, while the otoliths, which are the sense organs of the utricle and saccule, are mainly concerned with static head position and linear acceleration. In each of these locations displacement of the sensory hair cells is the effective stimulus. In the semicircular canals this is accomplished by movement of the endolymphatic fluid, which in turn is induced by rotation of the head in relation to the vertical axis. In the utricle and saccule the hairs are displaced in response to the force of gravity on the otoliths.

3. Impulses from the proprioceptors of the joints and muscles, which are essential to all reflex, postural, and volitional movements. Those from the neck are of special importance in relating the position of the head to the rest of the body.

These sense organs are connected with the cerebellum and certain ganglionic centers in the brainstem (particularly the oculomotor, red, and vestibular nuclei) and the medial longitudinal fasciculi. These are the important coordinators of the sensory data and provide for postural adjustments and the maintenance of equilibrium. Conversely, any disease that disrupts these neural mechanisms may give rise to vertigo and dysequilibrium.

Important psychophysiologic mechanisms are involved in the maintenance of equilibrium and the proper relationship of our bodies to the external world. Early in life we come to coordinate parts of our body in relation to one another and to perceive that portion of space occupied by our bodies. We construct from these integrated sensory data a general concept that has been designated by Russell Brain as the *body schema*. The space around our body is represented by another set of data, the *environmental schema*. These two schemata are neither static nor independent; they are constantly being modified and adapted to one another; their interdependence is ascribed to the fact that the various sense or-

gans which supply the information on which the two schemata are based are usually simultaneously activated by any movement of our bodies. By a process of learning we come to see objects as stationary while we are moving, and moving objects as having motion when we are either moving or stationary. Motion of an individual in space is always relative. At times, especially when our own sensory information is incomplete, we mistake movement of our surroundings for movements of our own body. A well-known example of this is the feeling of movement which one experiences while seated in a stationary train, when actually a neighboring train is moving. Hence, in this frame of reference, orientation of the body in space is made possible only by the maintenance of an orderly relationship between the bodily schema and the schema of the external world; as a corollary, disorientation in space, or disequilibrium, occurs when this relationship is upset.

CLINICAL CHARACTERISTICS OF VERTIGO AND GIDDINESS

A careful history and physical examination usually afford the basis for separating true vertigo from the dizziness of the anxious patient and from the other types of pseudovertigo. The recognition of vertigo is relatively easy when the patient states that objects in the environment spun around or moved in one direction or that there was a sensation of the head and body whirling. (A distinction is sometimes drawn between subjective vertigo, meaning a sense of turning of one's body, and objective vertigo, an illusion of movement of the environment, but its validity is doubtful.) Often, however, the patient is not so explicit. The feeling may be described as a to-and-fro or up-and-down movement of the body, usually of the head. Or the floor or walls may seem to tilt or to sink or rise up. In walking, the patient may have felt unsteady and veered to one side. Or there may have been a sensation of being pulled to the ground or to one side or another, as though being drawn by a strong magnet. This feeling of *impulsion* is particularly characteristic of vertigo.

Some patients may be able to identify their symptoms only when they are asked to compare them with the feeling of movement experienced when coming to a halt after rapid rotation. If the patient is unobservant or imprecise in his or her descriptions, a helpful tactic is to provoke a number of dissimilar sensations by rotating the patient rapidly, irrigating the ears with warm and cold water, asking the patient to stoop for a minute and straighten up, to stand relaxed for 3 min and check blood pressure for orthostatic effect, and to hyperventilate for 3 min. Should the patient be unable to distinguish among these several types of induced dizziness or to ascertain the similarity of one of the types to his or her own condition, the history is probably too inaccurate for purposes of diagnosis.

When the patient's symptoms are mild or poorly described, small items of the patient's history, such as disinclination to walk during an attack, tendency to list to one side, aggravation by riding in a vehicle, and preference for one position help to identify them as vertigo.

In some patients an attack of vertigo is so abrupt and violent that they are virtually flung to the ground, sometimes injuring themselves. This attack has been given the quaint term, the "otolithic catastrophe of Tumarkin," and attributed, with little evidence, to involvement of the utricle or saccule. The diagnosis is usually substantiated by the presence of vertigo, nausea, and vomiting while the patient is on the ground, distinguishing it from a seizure or faint. Probably it differs from other forms of labyrinthine vertigo only in its severity.

All but the mildest forms of vertigo are accompanied by varying degrees of nausea, vomiting, pallor, and perspiration. As a rule, patients have some difficulty with walking, and cannot walk at all if the vertigo is intense. Forced to lie down, they realize that one position, usually on one side with eyes closed, reduces the vertigo and nausea and that the slightest motion of the head aggravates them. One form of vertigo, the *benign positional vertigo of Bárány*, occurs only for a few seconds after lying down, sitting up, or turning. If the vertigo is less severe, the patient can walk unsteadily but may veer to one side. The source of the ataxia that is associated with vertigo (vertiginous ataxia) is recognized as being "in the head," not as being related to control of the legs and trunk. It is noteworthy that in these circumstances the coordination of the individual movements of the limbs is not impaired—a point of difference from most instances of cerebellar disease. There may be headache, generalized or in the region of the offending ear. Loss of consciousness as part of a vertiginous attack nearly always signifies another type of disorder (seizure or faint).

Giddiness and other types of pseudovertigo are usually described as feelings of swaying, light-headedness, a swimming sensation, or, more rarely, of uncertainty, of walking on air, of being "queer in the head,"

or being about to fall or "pass out." These sensory experiences are particularly common in illnesses featured by anxiety attacks, viz., anxiety neurosis, hysteria, and depression. They are in part reproduced by hyperventilation; and then it is appreciated that apprehensiveness, panic, palpitation, breathlessness, trembling, and sweating are concurrent.

Other pseudovertiginous symptoms are less definite. In severe anemic states weakness and languor may be attended by a light-headedness related to postural change and exertion, the basis of which must be a mild hypoxia. In the emphysematous patient physical effort may be associated with weakness and peculiar cephalic sensations, and coughing may lead to giddiness and even fainting (tussive syncope) because of impaired return of venous blood to the heart. The dizziness that so often accompanies hypertension is difficult to evaluate; sometimes it is an expression of anxiety, or it may conceivably be due to an unstable adjustment of cerebral blood flow. *Postural dizziness* is another example of unstable vasomotor reflexes which prevent a constancy of cerebral circulation; it is notably frequent in persons with primary orthostatic hypotension and polyneuropathy, in those recently bedfast, in the weak and ill, and maybe in the elderly. Abrupt arising from a recumbent or sitting position may be followed immediately by a swaying type of dizziness, dimming of vision, and spots before the eyes which last a few seconds. Patients are forced to stand still and steady themselves by holding onto a nearby object. Occasionally, a syncopal attack may occur at this time (see page 250).

In practice it is usually not difficult to separate these types of pseudovertigo from true vertigo, for there is none of the feeling of impulsion or rotation or other disturbance of motion so characteristic of the latter. Lacking also are the ancillary symptoms of true vertigo, viz., nausea, vomiting, tinnitus and deafness, staggering, and the need to remain immobile during an attack.

THE NEUROLOGIC AND OTOLOGIC CAUSES OF VERTIGO

The fact that vertigo may constitute the aura of an epileptic seizure, the origin of which is in the temporal cortex, supports the view that a cerebral cortical lesion can produce vertigo. Electrical stimulation of the cerebral cortex, either of the posterolateral aspects of the temporal lobe or the inferior parietal lobule, near the sylvian fissure may evoke intense vertigo (see page 217). The occurrence of vertigo as the initial symptom in a seizure is infrequent. In such a case, a sensation of movement—either of the body away from the side of the lesion or of the environment in the opposite direction—lasts for a few seconds before being submerged in other seizure activity. Vertiginous epilepsy of this type should be differentiated from vestibulogenic seizures, in which an excessive vestibular discharge serves as the stimulus for a seizure. In this latter form of reflex epilepsy, tests which induce vertigo may provoke the seizure.

Oculomotor disorders, such as recent ophthalmoplegia with diplopia, are a source of spatial disorientation, and may give rise to brief sensations of vertigo, accompanied by mild nausea and staggering. This is maximal when the patient looks in the direction of action of the paralyzed muscle; it is attributable to the receipt of two conflicting visual images. In fact some normal people even experience dizziness for a brief time when adjusting to bifocal glasses or when looking down from a height.

Whether lesions of the cerebellum produce vertigo seems to depend on which part of the cerebellum is involved. Large destructive processes in the cerebellar hemispheres and vermis may cause no vertigo. However, lesions involving the cerebellum in the territory of the posterior inferior cerebellar artery (distal to the branches to the medulla oblongata) may cause an intense vertigo, indistinguishable from that due to labyrinthine disorder (Duncan et al.). In two such cases that were studied pathologically, the lesion (ischemic infarction) extended to the midline and involved the flocculonodular lobe. Falling, in these cases, was to the side of the lesion; nystagmus was present on gaze to each side but was more prominent on gaze to the side of the infarct. Labyrinthine disease, on the other hand, usually causes unidirectional nystagmus away from the side of the lesion and swaying or falling toward the side of the lesion—i.e., the nystagmus is in the opposite direction of the falling.

The observations of Biemond and DeJong document a kind of nystagmus and vertigo induced by disturbances of upper cervical roots and the cervical muscles and ligaments which they innervate (so-called cervical vertigo). Spasm of the cervical muscles, trauma to the neck, and irritation of the upper cervical sensory roots are said to produce asymmetric spinovestibular stimulation and thus evoke nystagmus and prolonged vertigo and disequilibrium. The existence of this type of vertigo and nystagmus, or at least this interpretation of it, is still open to question.

Although lesions of the cerebral cortex, eyes, cerebellum, and perhaps the cervical muscles may give rise to vertigo, they are not common sources of vertigo, and vertigo is not the dominant manifestation of disease in these parts. For all practical purposes, vertigo indicates a disorder of the vestibular end organs, the vestibular division of the eighth nerve, or the vestibular nuclei in the brainstem and their immediate connections. The clinical problem usually resolves itself into deciding which portion of the labyrinthine-vestibular apparatus is primarily involved. This decision is usually made on the basis of the form of the vertiginous attack and, particularly, the associated symptoms. The common labyrinthine-vestibular syndromes are described below.

LABYRINTHINE VERTIGO AND MÉNIÈRE'S DISEASE

Labyrinthine disease is the most common cause of true vertigo. The classical variety, *Ménière's disease,* is characterized by recurrent attacks of vertigo associated with tinnitus and deafness. One or the other of the latter symptoms—rarely both—may be absent during the initial attacks of vertigo, but they invariably assert themselves as the disease progresses and are increased in severity during an acute attack.

The attacks of vertigo are characteristically abrupt and last for minutes to an hour or longer. The vertigo is clearly of the whirling or rotational type and usually so severe that the patient cannot stand or walk. Varying degrees of nausea and vomiting, tinnitus, and a feeling of fullness in the ear are practically always associated. Nystagmus is present during the acute attack. It is horizontal in type, usually with a rotary component and with the slow phase toward the affected ear. The patient preferentially lies with the faulty ear uppermost and is disinclined to look toward the normal side because of exaggeration of the nystagmus and dizziness.

The attacks vary considerably in frequency and severity. They may recur several times weekly for many weeks on end, or there may be remissions of several years' duration. Frequently recurring attacks may give rise to mild chronic states of disequilibrium. With milder forms of the disease the patient may complain more of head discomfort and of difficulty in concentration than of vertigo and may be considered neurotic. Symptoms of anxiety are common in patients with Ménière's disease, particularly in those who suffer frequent, severe attacks.

Irrigation of the ear canal with cold and warm water (*caloric testing*) usually discloses an impairment or loss of thermally induced nystagmus on the involved side. In caloric testing, the patient's head is tilted forward 30° from the horizontal (bringing the horizontal semicircular canal into a vertical plane, which is the position of maximal sensitivity of this canal to thermal stimuli). The external auditory meati are irrigated in turn for 30 s with water at 30°C and 44°C (7°C below and above body temperature), with a pause of at least 5 min between each irrigation. In normal persons, cold water induces a slight tonic deviation of the eyes to the side being irrigated, followed, after a latent period of about 20 s, by nystagmus to the opposite side (direction of the fast phase). Warm water induces nystagmus to the irrigated side. The nystagmus usually persists for 90 to 120 s, but the spread of values in normal subjects is much larger.

Simultaneous irrigation of both canals with cold water causes a tonic downward deviation of the eyes, with nystagmus (quick component) upward. Bilateral irrigation with warm water yields movement and nystagmus in the opposite direction.

Caloric tests will reliably answer whether or not the vestibular end organs react, and comparison of the responses from the two ears will indicate which one is paretic. The presence of "directional preponderance" can be determined (if the two stimuli that induce nystagmus to one side provoke a stronger reaction than the two stimuli that provoke nystagmus to the other side). It is questionable whether the measurement of directional preponderance provides diagnostic information that cannot be gained from irrigating each ear with either cold or warm water.

Vestibular (labyrinthine) stimulation can also be produced by rotating the patient in a Bárány chair or any type of swivel chair. The patient's eyes should be kept closed or blindfolded during rotation to avoid the effects of optokinetic nystagmus. Electronystagmography represents a more refined method of detecting disordered labyrinthine function, since it obviates completely the effects of visual fixation (which may suppress nystagmus even in patients wearing Frenzel's glasses).

The hearing loss in Ménière's disease usually begins before the first attack of vertigo, but may appear later. Frequently there is a decrement in hearing with each attack, i.e., a saltatory progressive unilateral hearing loss (in only 10 percent of cases are both ears involved). Early in the disease, deafness occurs mainly in the low tones and fluctuates in severity; later the fluctuations cease and high tones are affected. The attacks of vertigo usually cease when the hearing loss is complete. Audiometry reveals a sensorineural type of deafness, with air and bone conduction equally depressed. Provided that deafness is not complete, loudness recruitment can be demonstrated in the involved ear (see above). In general, the association of vertigo and deafness signifies a disease process of the end organ or eighth nerve. The precise locus of the disease is determined by tests of labyrinthine and auditory function and by finding neurologic and radiologic signs of affection of structures adjacent to the eighth cranial nerve.

Ménière's disease affects the sexes about equally and has its onset most frequently in the fifth decade of life, although it may occur in younger adults and the elderly. Cases of Ménière's disease are usually sporadic, but rare hereditary forms (both autosomal dominant and recessive) have been described (see reviews by Konigsmark). The pathologic changes consist of distension of the endolymphatic system, which leads to a degeneration of the delicate cochlear hair cells. It has been speculated that the paroxysmal attacks of vertigo are related to ruptures of the membranous labyrinth, leading to disruption of sensory receptors and a dumping of potassium into the perilymph, which has a paralyzing effect on vestibular nerve fibers (Friedmann).

During an acute attack of Ménière's disease, rest in bed is the most effective treatment, since the patient can usually find a position in which vertigo is minimal. The antihistaminic agents dimenhydrinate (Dramamine), cyclizine (Marezine), or meclizine (Bonine, Antivert), in doses of 25 to 50 mg every 4 h, are useful in the more protracted cases. For many years a low-salt diet, ammonium chloride, and diuretics have been used in the treatment of Ménière's disease, but their value has never been established. Mild sedative drugs may help the anxious patient between attacks. If the attacks are continuous and disabling, permanent relief can be obtained by surgical means. Destruction of the labyrinth is the measure employed in patients with strictly unilateral disease and complete or nearly complete loss of hearing. In patients with bilateral disease or significant retention of hearing, the vestibular portion of the eighth nerve can be sectioned intracranially; an endolymphatic-subarachnoid shunt is the operation favored by some surgeons, and selective destruction of the vestibule by a cryogenic probe by others.

PAROXYSMAL POSITIONAL VERTIGO

Another disorder of labyrinthine function is characterized by the occurrence of paroxysmal vertigo and nystagmus with the assumption of certain critical positions of the head, particularly lying down in bed or tilting the head backward. The symptoms may recur periodically for several days or for many months and examination usually discloses no abnormalities of hearing or evidence of vestibular paresis. This is the *positional vertigo of Bárány,* of the so-called benign paroxysmal type. The diagnosis of this disorder is settled at the bedside by moving the patient from the sitting position to recumbency with the head straight or preferably tilted 30° over the end of the table and 30° to one side. This maneuver produces, after a latency of a few seconds, a paroxysm of vertigo, and the patient may become frightened and grasp the examiner or the table or struggle to sit up. The vertigo is accompanied by nystagmus which may be rotatory, horizontal, or mixed in type, with the slow phase directed toward the dependent ear; both the vertigo and nystagmus last for less than 15 s, as a rule. Changing from a recumbent to a sitting position reverses the direction of vertigo and nystagmus. With repetition of the maneuver, the vertigo and nystagmus are less apparent and are absent after three or four trials; they can then be reproduced in their original severity only after a protracted period of rest. There are, in addition, variants of benign positional vertigo in which turning suddenly will induce vertigo for a few seconds. It may come and go for years, particularly in the elderly, and requires no treatment.

It should be pointed out that changes in position may induce vertigo and nystagmus or cause a worsening of these symptoms in patients with all types of vestibular-labyrinthine disease, including that of posterior fossa tumors. Only if the paroxysm has the special characteristics noted above, viz., latency of onset, reversal of direction on lying down and sitting, fatigability with repetition of the test, the presence of distressing subjective symptoms of vertigo or its persistence for months or years without other symptoms, can it be regarded as "benign positional" in type. This latter disorder is presumably labyrinthine in origin, but its pathologic basis has not been established.

VESTIBULAR NEURONITIS

This is the term applied originally by Dix and Hallpike to a distinctive disturbance of vestibular function, characterized clinically by a paroxysmal and usually a single attack of vertigo and by a conspicuous absence of tinnitus and deafness.

This disorder occurs mainly in young adults (children and older individuals may be affected), without preference for either sex. The patient frequently gives a history of an antecedent upper respiratory infection of nonspecific viral type. Usually the onset of vertigo is abrupt, although some patients describe a prodromal period of several hours or days in which they felt "lightheaded" or "off balance." The vertigo is severe as a rule, and is associated with nausea, vomiting, and the need to remain immobile. Examination discloses vestibular paresis on one side (absent response to caloric stimulation),

nystagmus with the quick component to the opposite side, and, notably, normality of auditory function. In some patients the caloric responses are abnormal bilaterally, and in some the vertigo may recur.

Vestibular neuronitis is a benign disorder. The severe vertigo and associated symptoms subside in a matter of several days, but lesser degrees of these symptoms, made worse by rapid movements of the head, may persist for several weeks. The caloric responses are gradually restored to normal as well.

The portion of the vestibular pathway that is primarily affected in this disease, and the nature of the affection are not known; hence the general designation *vestibular neuronitis*. Dix and Hallpike reasoned that the lesion was located central to the labyrinth, since hearing is spared and vestibular function usually returns to normal. It is likely that many of the conditions described under the terms *epidemic vertigo, epidemic labyrinthitis*, and *acute labyrinthitis* are examples of the same syndrome.

OTHER FORMS OF PAROXYSMAL VERTIGO

The term *labyrinthine apoplexy* has been applied to a clinical syndrome consisting of a single abrupt attack of severe vertigo, nausea, and vomiting, without tinnitus or hearing loss, but with *permanent ablation of labyrinthine function* on one side. It has been suggested that this syndrome is due to occlusion of the labyrinthine division of the internal auditory artery, but so far anatomic confirmation of this idea has not been obtained.

A particular form of paroxysmal vertigo occurs in childhood. The attacks occur in a setting of good health and are of sudden onset and brief duration. Pallor, sweating, and immobility are prominent manifestations, and occasionally vomiting and nystagmus occur. No relation to posture or movement has been observed. The attacks are recurrent but tend to cease spontaneously after a period of several months or years. The outstanding abnormal finding is demonstrated by caloric testing, which shows impairment or loss of vestibular function, bilateral or unilateral, frequently persisting after the attacks have ceased. Cochlear function is unimpaired. The pathologic basis of this disorder has not been determined.

Cogan has described an infrequent syndrome in young adults, in which a *nonsyphilitic interstitial keratitis is associated with vertigo*, tinnitus, nystagmus, and rapidly progressive deafness. The prognosis for life and vision is good, but the deafness is usually permanent. The cause of Cogan's syndrome is unknown although many patients later develop aortitis or a systemic vasculitis that resembles polyarteritis nodosa. Also, a viral origin has been suggested but remains unproved.

There are many other causes of aural vertigo, such as purulent labyrinthitis complicating meningitis, serous labyrinthitis due to infection of the middle ear, "toxic labyrinthitis" due to intoxication with alcohol, quinine, or salicylates, motion sickness, and hemorrhage into the internal ear. In these instances the attacks of vertigo tend to last longer than in the recurrent form, but in other respects the symptoms are similar. Vertigo with varying degrees of spontaneous or positional nystagmus and reduced vestibular responses is a frequent complication of head trauma, both of the type called "whiplash" injury and of concussion. The vertigo, though sometimes long-lasting, invariably improves in these circumstances and rarely is it accompanied by impairment of hearing, in distinction to the vertigo that follows fractures of the temporal bones (as described earlier in this chapter under deafness). Streptomycin and gentamicin may damage the fine hair cells of the vestibular end organs and cause a permanent disorder of equilibrium (as well as of hearing).

VERTIGO OF VESTIBULAR NERVE ORIGIN

This may occur with diseases that involve the nerve in the petrous bone or the cerebellopontine angle. Except that it is less severe and is less frequently paroxysmal, it has many of the characteristics of labyrinthine vertigo. The adjacent auditory division of the eighth cranial nerve may also be affected, which explains the frequent coincidence of tinnitus and deafness. The function of the seventh and fifth cranial nerves may be disturbed by tumors of the lateral recess (especially acoustic neuroma), as well as by meningeal inflammation in this region, or, rarely, by compression from an abnormal vessel.

The most common cause of vertigo of eighth nerve origin is an *acoustic neuroma*. Vertigo is rarely observed as the initial symptom; the usual sequence is deafness affecting the high-frequency tones initially, followed some months or years later by chronic vertigo and impaired caloric responses, then additional cranial nerve palsies (involving the seventh, fifth, and tenth nerves), ipsilateral ataxia of limbs, and headache (see page 462).

Variations of this sequence of development of symptoms are frequent, however. In the diagnosis of acoustic neuroma, certain ancillary examinations are important. These include the special audiologic tests which serve to separate lesions of the eighth nerve from those of the cochlea (absence of loudness recruitment, low SiSi scores, poor speech discrimination, pronounced tone decay, and type III or IV Békésy audiograms); CT scans with contrast medium; tests of the spinal fluid, which show an elevation of protein content in most cases; roentgenograms of the skull, including polytomography of the temporal bones, or metrizamide cisternography, which may show erosion of the internal auditory meatus.

VERTIGO OF BRAINSTEM ORIGIN

In these cases, vestibular nuclei and their connections are implicated. Auditory function is nearly always spared, since the vestibular and cochlear fibers separate upon entering the medulla and pons. As a general rule, the vertigo and the accompanying nausea, vomiting, nystagmus, and disequilibrium are more protracted with brainstem than with labyrinthine lesions. The nystagmus which accompanies such central lesions tends also to be more persistent than that from peripheral lesions. The nystagmus may be uni- or bidirectional, purely horizontal, vertical or rotary, and is characteristically worsened by attempted visual fixation. In contrast, nystagmus of labyrinthine origin is unidirectional, and the direction of past-pointing and falling is toward the slow phase. A purely vertical nystagmus does not occur, and a purely horizontal nystagmus without a rotary component is unusual. Furthermore, the nystagmus is inhibited by visual fixation.

The central localization is evidenced further by the attendant signs of involvement of other structures within the brainstem (cranial nerves, sensory and motor tracts, etc.). Mode of onset, duration, and other features of the clinical picture depend upon the nature of the causative disease, which is usually vascular, demyelinative, or neoplastic.

Vertigo is a prominent symptom of ischemic attacks and of brainstem infarction occurring in the territory of the vertebral-basilar arteries. On the other hand, pure vertigo as a manifestation of disease of the brainstem is rare, and the rule we have found trustworthy is that unless other symptoms and signs of brainstem disorder appear within 1 or 2 weeks, one can nearly always postulate an aural origin and exclude vascular disease of the brainstem. The same is true of multiple sclerosis, which may be the explanation of a persistent vertigo in some adolescents or young adults.

Attacks of vertigo followed by an intense unilateral and often suboccipital headache and vomiting have been described under the title of *basilar artery migraine* (see page 121). Test results of cochlear and vestibular function in these patients are normal, and the visual symptoms of classic migraine are usually absent, although they are said to be present frequently among family members of such patients. The relationship of this "migraine equivalent" to disease of the vertebral and basilar arteries is obscure.

REFERENCES

BIEMOND A, DEJONG JMBV: On cervical nystagmus and related disorders. *Brain* 92:437, 1969.

BRODAL A: The cranial nerves, in *Neurological Anatomy*, 3d ed. New York, Oxford, 1981, pp 448-577.

COATS AC: Vestibular neuronitis. *Acta Otolaryngol*, suppl 251, 1969.

DIX MR: Modern tests of vestibular function, with special reference to their value in clinical practice. *Br Med J* 3:317, 1969.

DUNCAN GW et al: Acute cerebellar infarction in the PICA territory. *Arch Neurol* 32:364, 1975.

FOWLER EP: Head noises in normal and in disordered ears. *Arch Otolaryngol* 39:498, 1944.

FRIEDMANN I: Ultrastructure of ear in normal and diseased states, in Hinchcliffe R, Harrison D (eds): *Scientific Foundations of Otolaryngology*. London, Heinemann, 1976, pp 202-211.

GRAHAM JT: Tinnitus aurium. *Acta Otolaryngol*, suppl 202, 1965.

———, NEWBY HA: Acoustical characteristics of tinnitus. *Arch Otolaryngol* 75:162, 1962.

HELLER MF, BERGMAN M: Tinnitus aurium in normally hearing persons. *Ann Otol Rhinol Laryngol* 62:73, 1953.

KONIGSMARK BW: Hereditary deafness in man. *N Engl J Med* 281:713, 774, 827, 1969.

———: Hereditary progressive cochleovestibular atrophies, in Vinken PJ, Bruyn GW (eds): *Handbook of Clinical Neurology*, vol 22. Amsterdam, North-Holland, 1975, chap 22, pp 481-497.

———: Hereditary diseases of the nervous system with hearing loss, in Vinken PJ, Bruyn GW (eds): *Handbook of Clinical Neurology*, vol 22. Amsterdam, North-Holland, 1975, chap 23, pp 499-526.

MATTOX DE, SIMMONS FB: Natural history of sudden sensorineural hearing loss. *Ann Otol* 86:463, 1977.

NODAR RH, GRAHAM JT: An investigation of frequency characteristics of tinnitus associated with Ménière's disease. *Arch Otolaryngol* 82:28, 1965.

PAGE J: Audiologic tests in the differential diagnosis of vertigo. *Otolaryngol Clin North Am* 6(1):53, 1973.

PROCTOR CA, PROCTOR B: Understanding hereditary nerve deafness. *Arch Otolaryngol* 85:23, 1967.

TILLMAN TW: Special hearing tests in otoneurologic diagnosis. *Arch Otolaryngol* 89:51, 1968.

EPILEPSY AND DISORDERS OF CONSCIOUSNESS

CHAPTER 15

EPILEPSY AND OTHER CONVULSIVE STATES

In contemporary society the frequency and importance of epilepsy can hardly be overstated. From the statistical studies of Hauser and Kurland, who determined the prevalence in a small urban community, it can be estimated conservatively that more than 1 million individuals in the United States are subject to recurring seizures, exclusive of those in whom convulsions complicate intercurrent illnesses. The chronicity of many seizure states adds to their statistical importance. Indeed, epilepsy follows apoplexy in being the second major neurologic disorder. Therefore it is desirable for every physician, if he or she is to achieve some degree of competency in the diagnosis and treatment of seizure states, to know something of the nature of these disorders.

Epilepsy may be described basically as an intermittent derangement of the nervous system due presumably to a sudden, excessive, disorderly discharge of cerebral neurons. This was the postulation of Hughlings Jackson, the eminent British neurologist of the nineteenth century, and modern electrophysiology offers no evidence to the contrary. The discharge results in an almost instantaneous disturbance of sensation, loss of consciousness or psychic function, convulsive movements, or some combination thereof. A terminologic difficulty arises from the diversity of the clinical manifestations. It seems improper to call a condition a *convulsion* when only an alteration of sensation or consciousness takes place. The word *seizure* is preferable as a generic term, and also for the reason that it lends itself to qualification. The term *motor* or *convulsive seizure* is therefore not tautologic, and one may likewise speak of a *sensory seizure*. The word *epilepsy* is derived from Greek words meaning "to seize upon" and "to lay hold of." Our fore-

fathers referred to it as the *falling sickness* or the *falling evil*. Although a useful medical term, the word *epilepsy* still has unpleasant connotations, and is probably best avoided in dealing with patients, until such time as the general public becomes more enlightened.

Viewed in its many clinical contexts, the first solitary seizure or brief outburst of seizures may occur during the course of many medical illnesses. It indicates always that the nervous system has been affected by disease, either primarily or secondarily. By their very nature, if repeated every few minutes as in status epilepticus, seizures may threaten life. Even more important, a seizure or a series of them may be the manifestation of an ongoing primary neurologic disease that demands the full employment of special diagnostic and therapeutic facilities, as in the case of a brain tumor.

A more common and less grave circumstance is for a seizure to be but one in an extensive series occurring over long periods of life, with most of the attacks being more or less similar in type. In this instance they may represent a burned-out lesion that originated in the past and remains as a scar. The original disease may have passed unnoticed; or perhaps it occurred in utero, at birth, or in infancy in parts of the brain too immature to manifest signs. Again, it may have affected a silent area in a mature brain. Patients with such old lesions probably make up the majority of those with recurrent seizures, but are necessarily classified as having "idiopathic epilepsy," because it is impossible to ascertain the nature of the original disease; and the seizure may be the only sign of the brain abnormality. In this sense, all epilepsy is "symptomatic," or "secondary," although the latter terms generally indicate that the seizures have an identifiable and usually acquired structural cause. There are other types of epilepsy for which no pathologic basis has ever been established. Included in this category are hereditary types, such as photogenic epilepsy and certain types of grand mal and petit mal. Some authors (Lennox and Lennox, Forster) apply the term idiopathic only to seizures of these types; in the International Classification (see below) they are classified as primary generalized epilepsies.

COMMON TYPES OF SEIZURE

Seizures have been classified in many ways: according to their supposed etiology and site of origin, on the basis of physiological (EEG) correlates, and even in terms of their response to therapy. The International Classification, mentioned above, divides all seizures into two groups, generalized and partial (focal). The generalized epilepsies are divided in turn into primary and secondary types. In the *primary generalized epilepsies* (also referred to as *essential, idiopathic,* and *centrencephalic*) there is no apparent underlying cause except perhaps a genetic one. In the *secondary generalized epilepsies,* as well as the partial or focal ones, the seizures can be related more directly to acquired cerebral or systemic disease—hence the alternate designations "acquired" or "symptomatic." The following classification, abstracted from Gastaut, is based mainly on the clinical form of the seizure, but conforms in all essential details with the International Classification.

I. Generalized seizures (bilaterally symmetric and without local onset)
    A. Tonic-clonic seizures (grand mal)
    B. Absence (petit mal)
    C. Bilateral myoclonus
    D. Infantile spasms } Infants
    E. Atonic seizures } and
    F. Tonic seizures } children
II. Partial seizures (seizures beginning locally)
    A. Simple (generally without loss of consciousness)
        1. Motor (includes Jacksonian)
        2. Sensory (somatic sensory, visual, auditory, olfactory, vertiginous)
        3. Affective
    B. Complex (usually with loss of consciousness): temporal lobe or psychomotor seizures
III. Partial (focal) seizures with secondary generalization

GENERALIZED SEIZURES

THE GENERALIZED CONVULSIVE SEIZURE (GRAND MAL)

The term *convulsion* is most applicable to this form of seizure. The patient may sense its possible approach by any one of several subjective phenomena (the prodrome). For some hours the patient may feel apathetic, depressed, irritable, or, very rarely, just the opposite—ecstatic. One or more myoclonic jerks of the trunk or limbs, on awakening, may herald the occurrence of a seizure later in the day. Abdominal pains or cramps, pallor or redness of the face, throbbing headache, constipation or diarrhea have also been given prodromal status, but we have not found them frequent enough to be helpful. In approximately half the cases there is some type of movement (usually turning of the head and eyes or whole body), palpitation, a sinking, rising, or gripping feeling in the epigastrium, or an unnatural sensation in another part of the body, before consciousness is lost. Such an experience is called the *aura,* which the patient regards as a sign of an impending seizure, but which is actually the initial event of the seizure itself. The aura is important, for it may provide a clue as to the location of the "discharging focus" or lesion.

Equally often, however, the seizure strikes "out of the blue," i.e., without warning, beginning with a sudden loss of consciousness and fall to the ground. The initial motor signs are an opening of the mouth and eyes associated with abduction of the arms, flexion at the elbows and pronation of the hands ("hands-up" position), and extension of the legs. These are followed by snapping shut of the jaws, often biting of the tongue, and there may be a piercing cry as the whole musculature is seized in a spasm and air is forcibly emitted through the closed vocal cords. Since the respiratory muscles are caught in the tonic spasm, breathing is impossible, and after some seconds the skin and mucous membranes become cyanotic. The bladder may empty at this stage or later, during the postictal stupor. The pupils are dilated and unreactive to light. This is the so-called *tonic phase* of the seizure, and lasts for 10 to 15 s.

There then occurs a gradual transition from the tonic to the *clonic phase* of the convulsion. At first there is a mild generalized trembling, which rapidly gives way to violent muscular contractions which come in rhythmic salvos and agitate the entire body. The eyes roll, and the violaceous face is contorted in a series of grimaces. The pulse is rapid. There is a bloody froth on the lips from the bitten tongue and excessive salivation, and, rarely, periorbital hemorrhages appear. Sweating is now abundant. The clonic jerks decrease in amplitude and frequency over a period of about 30 s, the entire clonic phase lasting 1 to 2 min, as a rule. The patient remains apneic until the end of the clonic phase, which is marked by a large inspiration.

Next comes the terminal phase of the seizure. All movements have now ended, and the patient lies still and limp in a deep coma. The pupils, equal or unequal, now begin to contract to light. Breathing has become quiet, and the skeletal muscles have relaxed. This state persists for about 5 min, after which the patient opens the eyes, begins to look about, and is obviously disoriented and confused. The patient may speak and later not remember anything that was said. If undisturbed, the patient often falls into an exhausted sleep for several hours and then awakens with a pulsatile headache. When fully recovered, such a patient has no memory of any part of the spell except possibly the aura, and he or she knows that something has happened only because of the strange surroundings (in ambulance or hospital), the obvious concern of others, and a sore, bitten tongue and aching muscles from violent contractions. The contractions may even have crushed or fractured a vertebral body, or a serious injury (fracture or burn) may have been sustained in the fall.

Convulsions of this type ordinarily come singly or in groups of two or three and may occur when the patient is awake and active or during sleep. About 5 to 8 percent of such patients will at some time have a series of such seizures without completely regaining consciousness between them. This so-called status epilepticus demands urgent treatment. Conversely, instead of the whole dramatic sequence described above, only a part of the seizure may occur. For example, there may be only the aura without loss of consciousness, or only a brief tonic spasm followed by a few moments of confusion. Seizures may be abbreviated by anticonvulsive medications, and the partial motor activity may then point to the site of the discharging lesion.

"ABSENCE" (MINOR EPILEPSY, PETIT MAL)

In contrast to major generalized seizures, these are notable for their brevity and the paucity of motor activity. Indeed, they are so brief that sometimes the patients themselves are not aware of them, and to an onlooker they resemble a moment of absentmindedness.

The attack, coming without warning, consists of a sudden interruption of consciousness. Usually such patients are motionless; they stare and briefly stop the conversation or cease to respond. During the attack, clonic movements of the eyelids, facial muscles, or fingers or

synchronous movements of both arms may occur, usually bilaterally and symmetrically at the 3-per-second rate that characterizes the EEG abnormality. Automatisms, taking the form of lip smacking, chewing, and fumbling movements of the fingers, are common during an absence attack. Lip smacking is especially prominent in seizures induced by hyperventilation. Postural tone may be slightly decreased or increased, and occasionally there is a mild vasomotor disorder. As a rule such patients do not fall, and they may even continue such complex acts as walking or riding a bicycle. After 2 to 10 s, occasionally longer, the patient reestablishes contact with the environment and resumes all preseizure activity. Only the loss of the thread of the conversation or of the place in reading matter signals the occurrence of a momentary "blank" period (an absence). Voluntary hyperventilation for 2 to 3 min is an effective way of inducing these petit mal attacks.

Closely related to the typical absence are varieties in which the loss of consciousness is less complete and the EEG abnormalities are less regularly of a 3-per-second spike-and-wave type (they may be 2 to 2.5 per second, or take the form of multiple sharp waves, or there may be no EEG abnormalities). In about 30 percent of children with absence attacks, symmetric or asymmetric myoclonic jerks (without loss of consciousness) occur. About 50 percent of such children will also at some time have tonic-clonic convulsions. Photic or some other type of sensory stimulation may reproduce these atypical seizures more reliably than hyperventilation. Rarely is postural tone sufficiently diminished in an absence attack to cause the patient to fall. However, akinetic seizures (atonic or astatic, "drop attacks") occur in infants and young children, and these may be succeeded by tonic seizures and mental retardation. This is the so-called Lennox-Gastaut syndrome, which is associated with slow spike-and-wave complexes in the EEG. The notion that absences, myoclonic seizures, and akinetic seizures constitute a triad typical of petit mal, as originally proposed by Lennox, should be abandoned. The typical absence should be considered a separate entity, because of its benignity. Its association with tonic-clonic, myoclonic, and akinetic seizures always has grave implications, because of their frequent association with serious neurologic disease and their relative refractoriness to treatment. In the International Classification they are placed in the category of secondary epilepsies. Many have followed an infectious febrile encephalopathy of childhood, and are misinterpreted as benign febrile seizures (see further on, under "Febrile Seizures").

Typical petit mal absences are most characteristic of the epilepsy of childhood; rarely do they begin before 4 years of age or following puberty. Another attribute is their great frequency. As many as several hundred may occur in a single day, sometimes in bursts at certain times of the day. Most often they relate to periods of inattention and may occur in the classroom when the child is sitting quietly rather than participating actively in his lessons. If frequent, they may disturb attention and derange thinking so that the patient does poorly in school. Such attacks may last for hours with no interval of normal mental activity between them—so-called petit mal or absence status. The majority of such cases has been described in adults; they are very rare in children. *Pyknolepsy* is an obsolete term for the frequent, brief attacks of unawareness of childhood that terminate by puberty. Petit mal may be the only type of seizure during childhood. The attacks tend to diminish in frequency in adolescence and may disappear; often petit mal gives way to grand mal. In contrast, atypical petit mal and the Lennox-Gastaut syndrome may persist into adult life and are the most difficult to treat of all forms of epilepsy.

FOCAL SEIZURES

All forms of seizure, possibly even the primary generalized types, are believed to originate in a discharging focus or lesion in some part of the cerebrum, and in this sense all epilepsy is focal in nature. But in the generalized seizure without aura and in the petit mal absence, as will be pointed out further on in this chapter, the location of the focus of origin is unknown, and there is no reason to think—if it exists at all—that it resides in the cerebral cortex. In contrast, what we are referring to here as a focal seizure is clearly the product of a demonstrable lesion in some part of the cerebral cortex. The specific type and pattern of the seizure vary with the locale of the lesion. Psychomotor seizures usually have their focus in the temporal lobe on one side or the other; seizures characterized by somatic motor or sensory symptoms originate in the contralateral sensorimotor cortex; attacks characterized by auditory and vertiginous sensations emanate from the superior temporal cortex, etc. *The seizure types and patterns that are tabulated below are so helpful in the localization of the offending lesion that their relationships should be memorized by every student of medicine (Table 15-1).

COMPLEX PARTIAL SEIZURES (PSYCHOMOTOR EPILEPSY, TEMPORAL LOBE EPILEPSY)

These differ from the major generalized and petit mal seizures discussed above in that ① the aura is often a complex hallucination or perceptual illusion, indicating a temporal lobe origin, and ② instead of completely losing control of thought and action, patients behave in a confused manner, for which they are later found to be amnesic.

Though it is difficult to enumerate all the psychic experiences which may occur during complex partial seizures, they may be categorized into a somewhat arbitrary hierarchy of hallucinations, illusions, dyscognitive states, and affective experiences. Hallucinations are most often visual and auditory (consisting of formed or un-

Table 15-1
Common seizure patterns

Clinical type	Localization
Somatic motor	
Jacksonian (local motor)	Prerolandic gyrus
Masticatory	Amygdaloid nuclei
Simple contraversive	Frontal
Somatic and special sensory (auras)	
Somatosensory	Postrolandic
Visual	Occipital or temporal
Auditory	Temporal
Vertiginous	Temporal
Olfactory	Mesial temporal
Gustatory	Insula
Visceral: autonomic	Insuloorbital-frontal cortex
Complex partial seizures	
Formed hallucinations	Temporal
Illusions	Temporal
Dyscognitive experiences (déjà vu, dreamy states, depersonalization)	Temporal
Affective states (fear, depression, or elation)	Temporal
Automatism (ictal and postictal)	Temporal and frontal
Absence	"Reticulocortical"
Bilateral epileptic myoclonus	
	"Reticulocortical"

Source: Modified from Penfield and Jasper.

formed visual images, sounds, and voices), less frequently olfactory (usually unpleasant, unidentifiable sensations of smell), gustatory, or vertiginous. Illusions, or distortions of ongoing perceptions, are even more common. Objects or persons in the environment may shrink or recede into the distance, or, less frequently, they may enlarge. The dyscognitive states involve feelings of increased reality or familiarity (déjà vu) or of strangeness or unfamiliarity (jamais vu) or depersonalization. A certain old memory or scene may insert itself into the patient's mind and recur with striking clarity, or there may be an abrupt interruption of memory. Epigastric and abdominal sensations are frequent; usually they are difficult to describe but are recognized as not being part of normal experience. Fear and anxiety are the most common affective experiences. Relatively rarely does the patient describe feelings of rage or intense anger as part of a psychomotor seizure.

These subjective experiences may constitute the entire seizure, or they may be followed by a period of unresponsiveness. The motor components of the psychomotor seizure occur during this latter phase. Patients may smack their lips and make sucking, chewing, or swallowing movements. Such a patient may walk about in a daze or perform acts inappropriate to the occasion (undressing in public, speaking incoherently, etc.). Habitual acts, such as driving a car or turning the pages in a book, may continue. However, if asked a specific question or given a command, it becomes evident that the patient is out of contact. He or she may not respond at all, or may look toward the examiner in a confused way or utter a few stereotyped phrases. Usually such a patient can be led gently but may resist and strike out at the examiner. The violence and aggression that are said to characterize patients with temporal lobe seizures usually take this form of nondirected resistance in response to restraint, during the period of *automatic behavior* (so called because the patient presumably acts like an automaton). Unprovoked assault is distinctly unusual. Rarely, laughter or running may be the most striking feature of an automatism (*gelastic epilepsy* and *epilepsia procursiva*, respectively), or wandering may occur, either as an ictal or postictal phenomenon (*poriomania*).

Seizures of this type may proceed to tonic spasms or other forms of secondarily generalized seizures. This tendency to generalization is true of all forms of focal epilepsy.

Any patient with this form of epilepsy may exhibit only one of these types of seizure or various combinations of them. In a series of 414 patients studied by Lennox, 43 percent displayed some of the motor changes; 32 percent, the automatic state; and 25 percent, the alterations in psychic function. Because of the frequent con-

currence of these three symptom complexes, he referred to them as the *psychomotor triad.* Probably their clinical pattern varies with the locality and the direction and extent of spread of electrical discharge in the temporal lobe cortex. Because of their common focal origin and complex symptomatology, all these types of seizures are best subsumed under the inclusive title of *complex partial seizures.* This term is preferable to *temporal lobe seizures,* since typical *psychomotor* seizures can apparently arise from a focus in the frontal lobe, and the seizure discharge in such cases can be limited to the frontal lobe.

Such seizures are not peculiar to any period of life but show an increased incidence in adolescence and adult years, as though recurrent generalized (grand mal) seizures had led to secondary damage to the temporal lobe. In Ounsted's series, there was a high incidence of seizures beginning during a febrile illness (see further on); it is noteworthy that 5 percent of patients with febrile seizures continued to have seizures during adolescence and adult life, and in the latter group there were many in whom the seizures were of temporal lobe type. Also, in Falconer's series of temporal lobectomies for intractable epilepsy, there were many that had had this special type of febrile epilepsy. Two-thirds of patients with psychomotor seizures also have generalized seizures or have had them at some earlier time. Psychomotor seizures are notably variable in duration. Behavioral automatisms rarely last longer than 4 or 5 min, although postictal confusion and amnesia may persist for a considerably longer time. Some psychomotor seizures consist only of a momentary change in facial expression and a blank spell, resembling an absence seizure. EEG recording during natural sleep or following hyperventilation, especially if carried out for more than 3 min, is useful in disclosing the temporal lobe focus.

FOCAL AND JACKSONIAN MOTOR SEIZURES

Focal, or partial, motor seizures are attributable to a discharging lesion of the opposite frontal lobe. Their most common manifestation is a turning movement of the head and eyes to the side opposite the irritative focus, often associated with tonic contractions of the trunk and extremities. These movements may constitute the entire motor component of the seizure or may be followed by generalized clonic movements, and they may occur before or simultaneously with loss of consciousness. On the other hand, a lesion in one or other frontal lobe may give rise to a major generalized convulsion without an introductory turning of the head and eyes. It has been postulated that in both types of seizure, the one with and the one without versive movements, there is an immediate spread of the discharge from the frontal lobe into an integrating center in the thalamic or midbrain reticular formations, accounting for the loss of consciousness.

Adversive is the term usually applied to seizures that begin with turning of head and eyes to the side opposite the irritative focus, but *contraversive* would be more correct, or ipsiversive, in the rare cases of turning toward the focus. Contraversive movements of the head and eyes can be induced most consistently by electrical stimulation of the intermediate frontal region (area 8), just anterior to the precentral gyrus. However, the same movements can be obtained by stimulation of more anterior portions of the frontal cortex, the posterior part of the superior frontal gyrus (the supplementary motor area), and the temporal or occipital cortex, so that contraversive movements, as such, cannot be equated with a focus in the frontal cortex.

Do most cases of generalized motor seizure (grand mal) of idiopathic type have a frontal lobe focus? Unfortunately this question cannot be answered unequivocally. Actually an epileptogenic frontal lobe focus, determined by EEG recording or pathologic examination, has been found in only a small number of such cases, and these may not be representative of the whole group.

The *Jacksonian motor seizure* begins with a tonic contraction of the fingers of one hand, the face on one side, or one foot. This transforms into clonic movements in these parts, in a fashion analogous to that in a generalized tonic-clonic convulsion. These seizures may occur in bursts or paroxysms. The disorder then spreads ("marches") from the part first affected to other muscles on the same side of the body. In the classical form, which is a clinical rarity, the seizure spreads from the hand, up the arm, to the face, and down the leg; or if the first movement is in the foot, the seizure marches up the leg, down the arm, and to the face, usually in a matter of 20 to 30 s. Consciousness is not lost if the motor-sensory symptoms are confined to one side (a small proportion of cases of focal motor epilepsy are associated with sensory symptoms). The first muscular contraction may (rarely) be in the abdomen, thorax, or neck. In some cases the one-sided motor signs are followed by turning of the head and eyes to the convulsing side, occasionally

the opposite, and by a generalized seizure with loss of consciousness.

The high incidence of onset of focal motor epilepsy in the lips, fingers, and toes probably is related to the greater cortical representation of these parts of the body. The disease process or focus of excitation is usually in the rolandic cortex, i.e., area 4 (Fig. 3-3) on the opposite side; in a few cases it has been found in the postrolandic convolution. Lesions confined to the premotor cortex (area 6) are said to induce tonic contractions of the contralateral arm, face, neck, or all of one side of the body. Perspiration and piloerection, sometimes of the parts of the body involved in a focal motor seizure, suggest that these autonomic functions have a cortical representation in the rolandic area. Some neurologists distinguish *focal motor* and *Jacksonian motor seizures* by the absence of a characteristic march in the former, but both have essentially the same localizing significance.

Epilepsia Partialis Continua This is a special type of focal motor epilepsy, characterized by clonic twitching of one group of muscles, usually in the face, arm, or leg, which is repeated at fairly regular intervals of a few seconds and persists for hours, days, or months without spreading to other parts of the body. Thus epilepsia partialis continua is in effect a focal motor status epilepticus. The distal muscles of the leg and arm, especially the flexors of the hand and fingers, are affected more frequently than the proximal ones. In the face, seizures involve either the corner of the mouth or one eyelid, or both. Occasionally, isolated muscles of the neck or trunk are affected on one side. The clonic spasms may be accentuated by active or passive movement of the involved muscles and may be reduced in severity, but not abolished during sleep.

Described first by Kozhevnikov, in patients with Russian spring and summer encephalitis, these partial seizures may be induced by a variety of acute or chronic cerebral lesions. In some cases the underlying disease is not apparent, and the twitchings are mistaken for some types of tremor or extrapyramidal movement disorder. Most patients with epilepsia partialis continua show focal EEG abnormalities, either slow-wave abnormalities or sharp waves or spikes over the central areas of the contralateral hemisphere. And in some cases, the spike activity can be related precisely in location and time to the motor activity (Thomas et al.). As a rule, this form of epilepsy responds poorly or not at all to anticonvulsant medications.

An unresolved controversy surrounds the question whether cortical or subcortical mechanisms are responsible for the continuous seizure activity. The electrophysiologic evidence adduced by Thomas and his colleagues favors a cortical origin of epilepsia partialis continua. The pathologic evidence is less definite. In each of eight cases in which the brain was examined postmortem, they found some degree of involvement of the motor cortex or adjacent cortical area, contralateral to the affected limbs. However, all but one of these patients also had some involvement of deeper structures on the same side as the cortical lesion or on the opposite side, or on both sides.

Seizure discharges arising from the cortical areas concerned with language function may give rise to a brief aphasic disturbance (*ictal aphasia*) or, more frequently, to vocal arrest. Ictal aphasia is usually succeeded by other focal or generalized motor manifestations, but may occur in isolation, without loss of consciousness, and can be described later by the patient. Postictal aphasia is more common and has much the same localizing value. Vocalization at the outset of a seizure has no such significance. These disturbances should be distinguished from the stereotyped repetition of words or phrases or garbled speech that characterize the postictal confusional state.

SOMATOSENSORY, VISUAL, AND OTHER TYPES OF SENSORY SEIZURE

Somatic-sensory seizures, either focal or "marching" to other parts of the body on one side, are nearly always indicative of a focus in or near the postrolandic convolution of the opposite cerebral hemisphere. In the series of Penfield and Kristiansen, the seizure focus was found in the postcentral or precentral convolution in 49 out of 55 cases. The usual sensory disorder is described as a numbness, tingling, or "pins-and-needles" feeling, occasionally as a sensation of crawling (formication), electricity, or a sense of movement of the part. Pain and thermal sensations are infrequent. The onset is in the lips, fingers, and toes in the majority of cases, and the spread to adjacent parts of the body follows a pattern determined by sensory arrangements in the postcentral (postrolandic) convolution of the parietal lobe. If the sensory symptoms are localized to the head, the focus is in the lowest part of the convolution, near the sylvian fissure; and if they are in the leg or foot, the upper part near the superior sagittal sinus or medial surface of the hemisphere is involved.

Visual seizures are also of localizing significance. Lesions in or near the striate cortex of the occipital lobe usually produce elemental visual sensations of darkness or of spots or lights, which may be stationary or moving and colorless or colored. According to Gowers, red is the most frequent color, followed by blue, green, and yellow.

These images may be referred to the visual field on the side opposite the lesion, or may appear to be straight ahead of the patient. Often, if they occur on one side of the visual field, patients believe that only one eye is affected, the one opposite the lesion, probably because the average person is aware only of the temporal half of a homonymous field defect. It is curious that a lesion arising in one occipital lobe may cause momentary blindness in both eyes. It has been noted that lesions on the lateral surface of the occipital lobes (Brodmann's areas 18 and 19) are likely to cause twinkling or pulsating lights. Complex or formed visual hallucinations are usually due to a focus in the posterior part of the temporal lobe, near its junction with the parietal, and may be associated with auditory hallucinations. Often the visual images, either those of the hallucination or of objects seen, are distorted, being too small (micropsia) or too large (macropsia) or unnaturally arranged.

Auditory hallucinations are infrequent as an initial manifestation of a seizure. Occasionally a patient with a focus in one superior temporal convolution will report a buzzing or a roaring in the ears. A human voice sometimes repeating unrecognizable words has been noted a few times with lesions in the more posterior part of one temporal lobe.

Vertiginous sensations of a type suggesting vestibular stimulation may be the first symptom of a seizure. The lesion is usually localized in the superior-posterior temporal region or at the junction between parietal and temporal lobes. In one of the cases reported by Penfield and Jasper, a sensation of vertigo was evoked by stimulating the cortex at the junction of the parietal and occipital lobes. Occasionally with a temporal focus the vertigo is followed by an auditory sensation. Giddiness is also a frequent prelude to a seizure, but this has so many different meanings that it is of little diagnostic import.

Olfactory hallucinations are often associated with disease of the inferior and medial part of the temporal lobe, usually in the region of the hippocampal convolution or the uncus (hence the term *uncinate seizures*, after Jackson). Usually the smell is exteriorized, i.e., projected to some place in the environment, and is described as disagreeable or foul, though otherwise unidentifiable. Gustatory hallucinations have also been recorded in proven cases of temporal lobe disease. Sensations of thirst and salivation may be associated. Electrical stimulation in the depths of the sylvian fissure, extending into the insular region, has reproduced peculiar sensations of taste.

Vague and often indefinable visceral sensations arising in the thorax, epigastrium, and abdomen are among the most frequent of auras, as already indicated. In several such cases the seizure discharge has been localized to the upper bank of the sylvian fissure, but in a few cases the focus was located in the upper or middle frontal gyrus, or in the medial frontal area near the cingulate gyrus. Palpitation and acceleration of the pulse at the beginning of the attack have also been related to a temporal lobe focus.

MYOCLONUS AND OTHER MOTOR SEIZURES

The phenomenon of myoclonus has already been discussed in Chap. 5, where the relationship to seizures was also indicated. Characterized by a brusque, brief, muscular contraction, some myoclonic jerks are so small as to involve only one muscle or part of a muscle, and others so large as to implicate whole limbs on one or both sides of the body or the entire trunk musculature. They may occur intermittently every few seconds or present as a single jerk or a brief salvo.

Single myoclonic jerks occur occasionally in patients with absence seizures and frequently in patients with generalized tonic-clonic seizures. Disseminated myoclonus, having its onset in childhood, raises the suspicion of an acute viral encephalitis or, if lasting a few weeks, of a progressive subacute sclerosing encephalitis juvenile lipidosis, Lafora type of familial myoclonic epilepsy, or other chronic familial degenerative diseases of undefined type (Friedreich's paramyoclonus multiplex, Ramsay Hunt's dyssynergia cerebellaris myoclonica). In middle and late adult years, disseminated myoclonus, when joined with dementia, usually indicates the presence of so-called Creutzfeldt-Jakob disease. At any age diffuse myoclonus may be a sequel of hypoxic injury to the brain. An interesting feature of all forms of disseminated myoclonus is the tendency for sensory stimulation or movement to elicit the myoclonus. When numerous and generalized, notably in the familial types, they may be recruited under certain stimulus conditions into a generalized seizure with loss of consciousness. In a sense, such random, arrhythmic myoclonus might be designated as *epilepsia partialis discontinua* and *disseminata*. The causative diseases will be discussed in Chaps. 32, 37, and 39.

Massive myoclonus (West's disease) is the term applied to a particular form of epilepsy of infancy and early childhood. West described the condition in his own son in the middle of the nineteenth century. The seizure disorder, which in most cases appears during the first year of life, is characterized by recurrent, gross flexion and less frequently by extension movements of the trunk and limbs (hence the alternative terms, *infantile, salaam,* or *jackknife spasms*). Most but not all patients with this disorder show severe EEG abnormalities, consisting of continuous multifocal spikes and slow waves of large amplitude; this pattern, referred to as *hypsarrhythmia* ("mountainous" dysrhythmia) by Gibbs and Gibbs, is not specific for infantile spasms, however. These seizures are frequently associated with developmental or acquired abnormalities of the brain. Of the latter the most common type is an unknown, presumably metabolic disease. The seizures tend to diminish as the child matures (usually they disappear by the fourth to fifth year), and both seizures and EEG abnormalities may respond dramatically to treatment with ACTH or adrenal corticosteroids. However, most patients, even those who were apparently normal when the seizures appeared, are left mentally impaired.

Paroxysmal attacks of *choreoathetotic and dystonic movements,* usually without loss of consciousness, are thought by some to be epileptic in nature, perhaps originating in the basal ganglia. We are skeptical of this interpretation (see page 58). Occasionally the movements are in the form of pronounced trembling, torsions of the trunk, or ballistic or ataxic motions of the limbs (see Chap. 4).

REFLEX EPILEPSY

For a long time it has been known that seizures could be evoked in certain epileptic individuals by a physiologic or psychologic stimulus. Forster has classified the evoking stimuli into five types: (1) *visual*—flashing light (by far the commonest type of stimulus-induced epilepsy), visual patterns, closure of eyes in bright light, and specific colors (especially red); (2) *auditory*—sudden unexpected noise, specific sounds, specific musical themes, and specific types of voices; (3) *somatosensory*—either a brisk unexpected tap or prolonged tactile stimulus to a certain part of the body; (4) *reading* of words or numbers; and (5) *eating.*

The evoked seizure may be focal (beginning often in the part of the body which has been stimulated) or generalized, and may take the form of one or a series of myoclonic jerks, petit mal, or grand mal. Seizures induced by music, voice, reading, and eating are usually of temporal lobe type. In a few instances such reflex epilepsy, as it is called, has been due to a focal cerebral disease, such as tumor, but more often its cause cannot be ascertained.

Anticonvulsant medication is generally ineffective in controlling reflex epilepsy. Some patients learn to avert the seizure by undertaking some mental task, e.g., thinking about some distracting subject, counting, etc., or by initiating some physical activity. [Similarly, spontaneously occurring focal motor seizures, e.g., those beginning in the toes or fingers, may be arrested (inhibited) by applying a ligature above the affected part or, in the case of focal sensory seizures, by applying a vigorous sensory stimulus ahead of the advancing sensory aura.] Forster has demonstrated that in certain types of reflex epilepsy the repeated and carefully controlled presentation of the noxious stimulus may eventually render the stimulus innocuous. This technique requires a great deal of time and assiduous reinforcement, which limits its therapeutic value.

THE NATURE OF THE DISCHARGING LESION

Physiologically, the epileptic seizure has been defined as a sudden alteration of central nervous system function, resulting from a paroxysmal high-frequency or synchronous low-frequency, high-voltage electrical discharge (Schmidt and Wilder). This discharge may arise from an assemblage of neurons in any part of the cerebrum, cortical or subcortical, and perhaps in the brainstem and spinal cord as well, but it is the visible focal lesion in the cerebral cortex that has been the most thoroughly investigated. There need not be a visible lesion, for under the proper circumstances, a seizure discharge can be initiated in an entirely normal cerebral cortex, as when the cortex is activated by a drug or stimulated repeatedly by subconvulsive electrical stimuli ("kindling phenomenon").

Just why the neurons in or near a focal lesion discharge is not fully understood. Some of the electrical properties of a cortical epileptogenic focus suggest that its neurons have been deafferented. Such neurons are known to be hypersensitive, and they may remain chronically in a state of partial depolarization, able to fire irregularly at rates of 700 to 1000 per second. The cytoplasmic membranes of such cells appear to have an increased permeability which renders them susceptible to activation by hyperthermia, hypoxia, hypoglycemia, hypocalcemia, and hyponatremia, as well as by repeated sensory (e.g., photic) stimulation and during certain phases of sleep (where hypersynchrony of neurons is known to occur). Another hypothesis is that the groups of cortical neurons exhibiting giant excitatory postsynaptic potentials are no longer being acted upon by inhibitory cortical or thalamic neurons.

Biochemical studies of the involved clone of neurons of a seizure focus have not clarified the problem. Epileptic foci are known to be sensitive to acetylcholine and to be slower in binding and removing it than normal cerebral cortex. A deficiency of the inhibitory neurotransmitter, γ-aminobutyric acid (GABA), a disturbance of cytochrome oxidase with decrease in ATP production, a reduction in the Krebs cycle function with a shift to a GABA-succinate shunt, or a disturbance in local regulation of extracellular K, Na, Ca, or Mg are other plausible hypotheses that have been proposed to explain the heightened excitability of epileptic neurons. Calcium is of particular interest in this regard, for it is known to stabilize cell membranes and to be essential for transmitter release at presynaptic terminals. Heinemann et al. recorded a decrease in Ca in experimental epileptic foci preceding both the onset of ictal activity and associated changes in K. (See Pedley for a review of the subject.)

Concurrent EEG recordings from an epileptogenic cortical focus and subcortical, thalamic, and brainstem centers have enabled investigators to construct a sequence of electrical and clinical events that characterize an evolving focal seizure. The firing of the involved neurons in the cortical focus is reflected in the EEG as a series of periodic spike discharges, which increase progressively in amplitude and frequency. Once the intensity of the seizure discharge exceeds a certain point, it spreads to normal neurons in the immediate neighborhood, via short corticocortical synaptic connections. Probably, if the abnormal discharge remains confined to the cortical focus and immediately surrounding cortex, there are no clinical symptoms or signs of seizure. Presumably, the EEG abnormality that persists during the interseizure period reflects this type of confined abnormal cortical activity. The mechanism of this restriction of electrical spread is unknown.

If unchecked, cortical excitation spreads to the contralateral cortex across interhemispheric pathways and across anatomically and functionally related pathways to subcortical (particularly basal ganglionic, thalamic, and brainstem reticular) nuclei. Then it is that the first clinical manifestations of the convulsion begin, the particular signs and symptoms depending upon the portion of the brain from which the seizure originates. The excitatory activity from the subcortical nuclei is fed back to the original focus and to the other parts of the forebrain, a mechanism which serves to amplify the excitatory activity and gives rise to the characteristic high-voltage polyspike discharge in the EEG. There is propagation downward to spinal neurons as well, via corticospinal and reticulospinal pathways.

The spread of excitation to the subcortical, thalamic, and brainstem centers corresponds with the tonic phase of the seizure and loss of consciousness, as well as with the signs of autonomic nervous system overactivity (salivation, mydriasis, tachycardia, increase in blood pressure, etc.). Vital functions may be arrested but usually for only a few seconds. In rare instances, however, death may occur owing to a cessation of respiration, derangement of cardiac action, or some unknown cause.

Shortly thereafter a diencephalocortical inhibition begins and intermittently interrupts the seizure discharge, changing it from the persistent discharge of the tonic phase to the intermittent bursts of the clonic phase. Electrically, a transition occurs from a continuous polyspike to a spike-and-wave pattern. The intermittent clonic bursts become less and less frequent and finally cease altogether, leaving in their wake an "exhaustion" of the neurons of the epileptic focus. The latter is thought to be the basis of *Todd's postepileptic paralysis* (and of postictal aphasia and hemianopia) and the diffuse slow waves in the EEG. The basis of this phenomenon is not known. Plum and his associates have observed a two- to threefold increase in glucose utilization during seizure discharges, and the following paralysis might be due to depletion of glucose or some other substrate. However, inhibition of epileptogenic neurons may occur in the absence of neuronal exhaustion and undoubtedly is important in the termination of seizures. One must conclude that the exact roles played by inhibition and metabolic exhaustion of neurons in producing postictal paralysis of function is not entirely settled.

The development of unconsciousness and the generalized tonic contraction of muscles is reflected in the EEG by a high-voltage discharge which appears simultaneously over the entire cortex. The generalization of the clinical and electrical manifestations depends upon activation of a deep, centrally located physiologic mechanism which, for reasons outlined in Chap. 16, includes the midbrain reticular formation and its diencephalic extension, the intralaminar and nonspecific thalamic projection systems (originally referred to by Penfield as the centrencephalon, now as the reticulocortical activating system). Apparently, the same central mechanism is operative whether the generalized seizure is triggered by spread from a cortical focus or whether loss of consciousness and generalized seizure activity are the initial manifestations.

The characteristic 3-per-second, high-voltage, spike-and-wave discharge and seizures resembling absence attacks have been produced in animals by the topical application of epileptogenic substances in both prefrontal regions. The EEG discharges persist after thalamectomy, but are interrupted by callosal section. The spike-and-wave complex, which represents brief excitation followed by slow-wave inhibition, is the type of EEG pattern which characterizes the clonic (inhibitory) phase of the focal motor or grand mal seizure. In contrast to what occurs in grand mal seizures, this strong element of inhibition is present from the beginning of a petit mal attack, a feature perhaps that accounts for the failure of excitation to spread to lower brainstem and spinal structures (viz., tonic-clonic movements do not occur).

Temporal lobe seizures are known to arise in foci in the medial temporal lobe, amygdaloid nuclei, and hippocampus. They may arise also in the convexity of the temporal lobe and propagate to the amygdaloid nuclei and hippocampus. Electrical stimulation in these areas reproduces feelings of depersonalization and automatic behavior. The latter, so characteristic of psychomotor epilepsy, appears in some instances to be a direct effect of the temporal lobe discharge and in others is a postexcitatory, inhibitory, or paralytic effect. Loss of consciousness following electrical stimulation does not occur unless it excites an afterdischarge which spreads to the opposite hemisphere.

A discovery of no little importance is that a seizure focus—if active for a time—may establish, via commissural connections, a persistent secondary focus in the corresponding area of cortex in the opposite hemisphere (mirror focus). The nature of this development is not fully understood. It may be similar to the "kindling" phenomenon, mentioned above. No morphologic change is visible in the mirror focus by light microscopy. Possibly Golgi studies, like those performed by the Scheibels on the epileptic temporal lobe, would show the same irregularity and tortuosity of dendrites and loss of dendritic spines which they consider significant (see below). The mirror focus becomes a source of confusion in trying to identify electrographically the side of the primary lesion.

Severe seizures may secondarily disturb the chemistry of the brain by causing hypoxia, acidosis with rise in Pco_2, and an accumulation of lactic acid. Some of these effects are secondary to respiratory spasm, blockage of airway, and excessive muscular activity. In paralyzed and artificially ventilated subjects receiving electroconvulsive therapy, these changes are minimal, and oxygen tension in cerebral venous blood may actually rise. According to Plum and his associates, the brisk rise in blood pressure evoked by the seizure causes a sufficient increase in cerebral blood flow to meet the increased metabolic needs of the brain.

THE ELECTROENCEPHALOGRAM IN EPILEPSY

The electroencephalogram (EEG) provides a delicate confirmation of J. Hughlings Jackson's theory of epilepsy—that it is an excessive disorderly discharge of cortical neurons. The EEG is undoubtedly the most sensitive, indeed the indispensable, tool for the diagnosis of epilepsy, but like other laboratory tests it must be used in conjunction with clinical data. Many epileptic patients have a perfectly normal interictal EEG; occasionally, using standard methods of scalp recording, the EEG may even be normal during a partial or psychomotor seizure. Conversely, a small segment of the normal population shows paroxysmal EEG abnormalities. Some of these patients have a family history of epilepsy and may themselves later develop seizures.

The EEG abnormalities that characterize an evolving epileptogenic focus and generalization of seizure activity, both the grand mal and petit mal types, have been described in the preceding section. At first there was thought to be a characteristic EEG picture for psychomotor epilepsy, but further studies have not confirmed this. The postseizure state, or *postconvulsive paralysis of cerebral function,* also has its EEG correlate, taking the form of random generalized slow waves. With recovery of normal mentation, the EEG returns to normal or to the preseizure state. The EEG tracing obtained during the interval between seizures is abnormal to some degree in approximately 40 percent of fully conscious and 75 percent of sleeping patients.

The EEG changes in epilepsy are discussed further in Chap. 2.

PATHOLOGY OF THE SEIZURE STATE

In some cases of idiopathic (primary) epilepsy of grand mal and petit mal type the brain has been grossly and microscopically normal, though it is unlikely that the entire brain has been subjected to serial sectioning in any single case. Certainly the convulsive states attending drug withdrawal, intoxication, etc., must represent derangements at the subcellular level.

Many of the so-called secondary types of epilepsy have definable pathologies. These include zones of neuronal loss and gliosis (scars), hamartomas, vascular malformations, and tumors. The latter are rare in early life. The frequency of these lesions is not fully known. Certainly the focal epilepsies have the highest incidence of a structural substratum, although in certain cases no morphological change is visible. In many series of cases of temporal lobe excisions, such as that of Falconer, incisural sclerosis in the hippocampal and amygdaloid regions and neuronal loss with gliosis were found in the majority of cases; vascular malformations, hamartomas, and astrocytomas were infrequent, and in a small number no abnormalities could be found.

The widespread use of computerized tomography offers another approach to the pathologic study of epilepsy. Gastaut and Gastaut have reported that in primary grand mal and petit mal epilepsies a CT abnormality was found in approximately 10 percent of cases, whereas in the Lennox-Gastaut syndrome, the West syndrome, and partial complex epilepsies it was found in 52, 77, and 63 percent, respectively. Atrophy, calcification, and malformations were the most frequent abnormalities.

With reference to the focal epilepsies it has not been possible to determine which component of the lesion is responsible for the seizures. In other words, one cannot say from microscopic examination whether or not any given lesion was epileptogenic. Gliosis, fibrosis, vascularization, and meningocerebral cicatrix have all been incriminated, but they occur in nonepileptic foci as well. The Scheibels' Golgi studies of neurons from epileptic foci in the temporal lobe reveal distortions of dendrites, loss of dendritic spines, and disorientation of residual neurons near the scars, but similar nonepileptic lesions were not compared. Golgi or electron microscopic studies of Goddard's "kindled cortex" have shown no morphologic abnormality. Partial disconnection of groups of cortical neurons from those of the neighboring cortex, of the other cerebral hemisphere, and of the thalamus seems likely to have occurred. Certain systems of inhibiting neurons may have been destroyed. In the highly epileptogenic experimental lesions produced by application of aluminum cream and penicillin to the cortex, one can see that some neurons are surely destroyed, especially in the superficial layers, and the synaptic connections of the remaining ones are reduced in number. Probably a disorganization of these cortical interneural relationships is more important than the nature of the lesion since diseases as different as hemorrhage, infarction, and neoplastic invasion, for example, are all epileptogenic at times. Once a gliotic focus of whatever cause, bordered by groups of discharging neurons, becomes epileptogenic, it may remain so throughout the lifetime of the patient.

Another aspect of the pathology of the epileptic

brain relates to effects (traumatic, hypoxic) secondary to the seizures themselves, an epileptic encephalopathy, so to speak. Cortical contusions are seen in some cases in which the original seizure disorder was on a nontraumatic basis. Norman and his colleagues have called attention to recent lesions in the cerebellum and hippocampus of hypoxic-hypotensive origin in longstanding severe epileptics. According to Salcman et al. degeneration of Purkinje cells may occur in chronic epileptics who had never experienced a generalized convulsion; the pathogenesis of these neuropathologic changes is unclear but is probably not hypoxic.

CLINICAL APPROACH TO THE EPILEPSIES

Medical Diseases in Which Seizures Are a Prominent Clinical Manifestation Among the medical diseases which may be complicated by a seizure or a burst of seizures, the following are the most frequent.

1. Generalized convulsions of the "tonic-clonic" type appear prominently during the *abstinence or withdrawal period in patients addicted to alcohol, barbiturates, or other sedative-hypnotic drugs.* Suspicion of this mechanism is raised by the telltale marks of alcohol abuse or the history of prolonged nervousness requiring sedation. Also disturbances of sleep, tremulousness, disorientation, illusions, and hallucinations often precede and follow the convulsive phase of the illness. Seizures in this setting may occur singly, more often in brief flurries, the entire convulsive period lasting for several hours, rarely for a day or longer, during which time the patient is unduly sensitive to photic stimulation (see Chaps. 40 and 41).

2. *Bacterial meningitis* is another type of illness with a strong convulsive tendency, more in children than in adults. Fever and stiff neck usually provide the clue, and lumbar puncture yields the salient diagnostic data. Seizure(s) may be the initial manifestation of syphilitic meningitis.

3. *Uremia* is another condition with a prominent convulsive tendency. Of interest is the relation of seizures to the sequence of events in complete anuria. This condition is tolerated for 2 or 3 days without neurologic signs, and then there is a rapid onset of twitching, trembling, myoclonic jerks, and generalized motor seizures. Tetany may be added. The motor display, one of the most dramatic in medicine, lasts several days until the patient sinks into terminal coma or recovers. When this

syndrome accompanies lupus erythematosus, idiopathic epilepsy, or generalized neoplasia, one can nearly always be sure that it has its basis in renal failure.

4. Cardiac arrest, suffocation or respiratory failure, NO_2 anesthesia, CO poisoning—the common causes of *hypoxic encephalopathy*—induce a diffuse myoclonic jerking of all the musculature and generalized seizures as soon as cardiac function is resumed. The convulsive phase of this condition may last only a few days, in association with coma, stupor, or confusion; or it may persist indefinitely as an intention myoclonus-convulsive state.

5. Other acute illnesses complicated by generalized and multifocal motor seizures are hyponatremia and water intoxication, thyrotoxic storm, hypertensive encephalopathy, porphyria, hypoglycemia, hyperglycemia, pyridoxine deficiency, argininosuccinic aciduria, and phenylketonuria. Picrotoxin and Metrazol are two highly convulsant drugs but are now used very little. Lead (in children) and mercury (in children and adults) are the most frequent convulsive metallic intoxicants.

Generalized seizures, with or without twitching, may occur in the terminal phase of many other illnesses, such as gram-negative septicemia with shock, liver coma, and intractable congestive heart failure.

6. Several primary diseases of the brain are also announced by an acute convulsive state. Myoclonic jerking and seizures appear early in acute herpes simplex encephalitis and other forms of viral, treponemal, and parasitic encephalitides, in subacute sclerosing panencephalitis, as well as in lipid storage diseases, subacute spongiform encephalopathy (Creutzfeldt-Jakob disease), and diffuse gliomatosis of the brain.

Convulsive seizures are a relatively uncommon occurrence in patients with stroke. Only exceptionally will an acute cerebral embolus cause a focal fit, though old embolic infarcts become epileptogenic in about 25 percent of cases. Similarly, thrombotic occlusions of cerebral arteries are almost never convulsive in the evolving phases of the stroke, but ischemic infarcts that involve the cortex may later become so. The rupture of an aneurysm is occasionally marked by one or two generalized convulsions. Subcortical hypertensive hemorrhages occasionally become sources of recurrent focal epilepsy. The rare cortical phlebothrombosis or thrombophlebitis with cortical ischemia and infarction is probably the most highly convulsive vascular lesion.

Febrile and Other Seizures of Infancy and Childhood The well-known *febrile seizure*, peculiar to infants and children between 6 months and 6 years of age (peak incidence 9 to 20 months) and tending to be familial, is generally regarded as a benign condition that does not progress to epilepsy in later years. Usually it takes the form of a single, generalized motor seizure, occurring as the temperature rises or reaches its peak. Seldom does the seizure last longer than 10 min, and by the time an EEG can be obtained there is usually no abnormality. Recovery is complete. Since such a seizure may recur with the next febrile episode, phenobarbital is recommended at the first hint of any subsequent infection or in the interval between infections.

This benign type of febrile seizure should not be confused with a second type of illness in which the outlook is more serious. In some instances an acute encephalitic or encephalopathic state will present as a febrile illness with severe and prolonged seizures, generalized or focal EEG abnormalities, and other neurologic signs. Status epilepticus may be the first seizure disorder and the illness may end fatally, or the child may survive and be left with mental impairment, hemiparesis, or other neurologic abnormalities. The seizures may continue, not only with infections, but at other times. Lennox and others have failed to separate these two types of febrile convulsions and a third one in which an antecedent birth injury of the brain or other disease is exposed by an episode of fever with convulsions. When cases of all three types are lumped together under the rubric of febrile convulsions, it is not surprising that a high percentage are complicated by atypical petit mal and atonic and astatic spells followed by tonic seizures, mental retardation (Lennox-Gastaut syndrome), and psychomotor epilepsy. Ormerod and Falconer, who have studied psychomotor seizures in adult life, note retrospectively a high incidence of "febrile seizures" during infancy and childhood. The authors believe that they are referring to the second and third types described above, which we prefer not to label as febrile convulsions.

Other types of epilepsy are also notable with reference to certain diseases of childhood and certain stages in the development of the nervous system. In the young child, a focal vascular or encephalitic lesion may cause hemiparesis or other focal or lateralizing signs. Unilateral seizures follow, and some of these are of the inhibitory type with a sudden hemiplegia representing the seizure; or the seizure may be followed by a Todd's paralysis lasting hours to several days. Some of these patients improve within a few years and have no further seizures. Tumor is rarely the cause of unilateral seizures in the child. A unilateral form of epilepsy in childhood, characterized by sensory and motor seizure activity (especially of the face), associated with anarthria and a midtemporal spike focus, has been described by Lombroso. Both the EEG seizure focus and the seizures disappear within a few years.

Infantile spasms, as noted above, are of primary and secondary types. The former is probably of metabolic origin, but the specific abnormality is unknown. The latter may be caused by tuberous sclerosis, phenylketonuria or other amino acid abnormality, Sturge-Weber disease, birth injury, or developmental anomaly of the brain (see Chap. 43 for further discussion and therapy).

Neonatal seizures are of special type and have significance with reference to birth injury, hypoxic-ischemic encephalopathy of parturition, and certain infectious and inherited diseases. They also are discussed in Chap. 43.

Generalized and Recurrent Focal Seizures Beginning in Adult Life The usual causes are traumatic scars, cerebral tumors, old cerebrovascular foci such as embolic or thrombotic infarcts that involve the cortex and small subcortical hemorrhages, suppurative diseases, especially thrombophlebitis and abscesses, and neurosyphilis. Each of these groups of disease will be discussed in its appropriate chapter. Obviously their clinical analysis must be backed up by the most refined diagnostic procedures available to neurologists, such as localizing EEG, cytology and chemical tests of CSF, arteriography, and CT scanning.

Recurrent Seizures of Unknown Cause (Idiopathic Epilepsy) Some physicians may find it curious that neurologists are so concerned with the treatment of an entity, the cause of which is unknown. The plain fact is that we are defeated by the imprecise relation of epilepsy to disease. As pointed out in the introduction to this chapter, seizures have a way of appearing long after the inception of a disease that has left in its wake a discharging focus. The latter may attract attention only when it happens to evoke a seizure. Even if tardive epilepsy were fatal—which it rarely is—pathologic study is so remote from the active phase of the causative disease that one is left with only an uninterpretable neuronal loss and glial scarring or with a lesion that cannot be discerned even after microscopic study of the brain.

The clinical approach to recurrent seizures in childhood and adolescence is much influenced by these facts. Rarely can the cause be determined. Usually one must conclude that the underlying disease is burned out and further pursuit of the cause will be unsuccessful or that the epilepsy is of primary type and the morphological basis has never been determined. In either instance the reality of the seizure problem is equally serious and equally challenging to control. If one surveys the entire population of epileptic patients, the majority will fall into this "idiopathic" category, not into the group with acute medical disease or with an advancing focal lesion.

When analyzed in greater detail, patients with idiopathic epilepsy tend to fall into three groups: (1) those whose seizures begin in infancy and early childhood and who are abnormal in other ways (some neurologists would exclude these cases from the category of idiopathic epilepsy because of the signs of cerebral disease, even though the cause is unknown); (2) those who are thought to be normal or only slightly abnormal until the first seizure at the age of 5 to 10 years; and (3) those who appear entirely normal until about puberty or adolescence, when they have their first generalized convulsion. The first two groups are much larger than the third, because with every passing year after the occurrence of a brain lesion the chances of its becoming an epileptic focus lessen. In the mature brain the usual interval between receipt of the lesion and first seizure is 9 to 15 months, but it may be as brief as a few months or as long as several years. In the immature brain the interval may be longer, but in either instance, once the epilepsy begins there is a tendency for it to lessen in frequency with each passing year as the static lesion becomes more remote. Children are said to outgrow their epilepsy, but the same trend has been noted in soldiers whose brain injury and subsequent epilepsy were acquired in adult life.

Patients in whom seizures begin in infancy and early childhood show a higher incidence of parturitional difficulties than is found in the population of normal children. Developmental anomalies of the cerebral cortex are also frequent. Seizures may have occurred in the neonatal period, and of this group approximately half turn out to be developmentally retarded. The infantile twitches and brief tonic spasms tend to be replaced after a few months by infantile myoclonic flexor spasms (salaam spasms), which may persist for 4 to 5 years, in diminishing severity, before giving way to atypical petit mal and generalized seizures. The specific seizure pattern is a function, then, not only of the topography of the discharging foci but of the level of maturation of the nervous system. Also there are changes in pattern consequent upon the occurrence of a series of convulsions. For example, anoxic damage to the temporal lobes during seizures may cause an increasing incidence of psychomotor seizures.

The clinical investigation of seizures beginning early in life involves differentiation of many diseases. The most frequent ones are developmental defects of many types, hypoxic-hypotensive perfusion failures of the brain, intrauterine and infantile infections, metabolic diseases and tuberous sclerosis. In this group the control of seizures is only one of many problems relating to such factors as training, discipline, schooling, and correction of specific disabilities.

Seizures beginning in the 4- to 8-year period may be typical petit mal, with grand mal appearing some time later, or the initial seizure may be grand mal in type. The neurologic history may disclose no antecedent illness or other disturbance of nervous function. Films of the skull, CSF examination, and brain scans may disclose no abnormalities, or at most some minor one such as a slight enlargement of the temporal horn of a ventricle. If the seizures are infrequent and responsive to anticonvulsant medication, the child's progress in scholastic, emotional, and social adjustment is unimpaired. Fully 80 percent of cases fall into this favorable group. If the seizures are frequent and not easily suppressed by medication and if they show other unusual features (several different types of seizure such as atypical petit mal, psychomotor, or one-sided seizures), the child's life may be seriously deranged. Such a child may fail in school, spend much time in hospitals, and be derailed from the normal developmental track. Poor motivation, parental dependence, immature reactions, difficulty in learning, muddled thinking, bizarre ideation, and religiosity sometimes pose problems as difficult as the seizures themselves. In adult life the seizures may continue to interfere with work, marriage, etc. The most disabled members of this group usually have associated cerebral deficits.

Patients with temporal lobe seizures, during the interictal period, may exhibit a number of behavioral abnormalities. Often they are slow and rigid in their thinking, subject to outbursts of bad temper and aggressivity, and show a tendency to be circumstantial and tedious in conversation and preoccupied with rather naive religious and philosophical ideas. Altered sexual interest (more in the direction of loss of libido and hyposexualism than the opposite), obsessionalism, humorless sobriety, emotionality (mood swings, anger, and sadness), and a tendency to paranoia are other frequently described traits.

That such personality traits are more common in patients with temporal lobe epilepsy than in nonepileptics has been shown convincingly by Bear and Fedio. Moreover, these authors have suggested that certain of these traits (obsessionalism, elation, sadness, and emotionality) are more common with *right* temporal lesions and that anger, paranoia, and cosmologic or religious conceptualizing are more characteristic of *left* temporal lesions. Whether such behavioral changes actually distinguish patients with temporal lobe epilepsy from other groups of epileptics remains to be determined. Despite the widespread belief that temporal lobe epileptics are more prone to develop interictal psychosis than patients with other forms of epilepsy, this question also has not been settled with finality (see reviews of Stevens and of Pincus and Tucker).

The group with the best outlook are adolescents or young adults who have their first generalized seizure while performing adequately in high school or college. All laboratory tests, including the interictal EEG, may be normal. In the authors' experience, such patients, if treated intelligently, have no more trouble in continuing their education and social adjustment than they would have if the seizures had never occurred.

The common causes of recurrent seizures according to the age of onset are summarized in Table 15-2.

Other Problems in Differential Diagnosis The clinical differences between a seizure and a syncopal attack will be considered in detail in Chap. 17. It must be emphasized that there is no single criterion that will distinguish them unequivocally. The authors have erred in calling akinetic seizures simple faints and in mistaking cardiac or carotid sinus faints for seizures. Petit mal may be difficult to identify because of the brevity of attacks.

Table 15-2
Causes of recurrent seizures in different age groups*

Age of onset, years	Probable cause
Infancy, 0-2	Congenital maldevelopment, birth injury, metabolic disorders (hypocalcemia, hypoglycemia), vitamin B_6 deficiency, phenylketonuria, and others
Childhood, 2-10	Perinatal anoxia, injury at birth or later, infections, thrombosis of cerebral arteries or veins, or indeterminate cause ("idiopathic" epilepsy)
Adolescence, 10-18	Idiopathic epilepsy, trauma, congenital defects
Early adulthood, 18-25	Idiopathic epilepsy, trauma, neoplasm, withdrawal from alcohol or other sedative-hypnotic drugs
Middle age, 35-60	Trauma, neoplasm, vascular disease, alcohol or drug withdrawal
Late life, over 60	Vascular disease, tumor, degenerative disease

*Meningitis may be a cause of seizures at any age.

Helpful maneuvers are to have the patient hyperventilate or to count aloud for 5 to 10 min. Patients who have frequent petit mal attacks will pause in counting or skip one or two numbers. Psychomotor seizures are the most difficult of all to diagnose. These attacks are so variable in character and so likely to induce minor disturbances in conduct—rather than obvious interruptions of consciousness—that they may be misdiagnosed as temper tantrums, hysteria, psychopathic behavior, or acute psychosis. Careful questioning of witnesses of an attack is essential. Verbalizations that cannot be remembered or walking aimlessly into another room are characteristic.

Epilepsy complicated by states of mental dullness and confusion poses a special problem in diagnosis. Most epileptic patients seen in hospital and office practice show no mental deterioration, regardless of the type of seizure. Therefore, the appearance of dementia, confusion, or some other derangement of mental functions should suggest the possibility of frequently recurrent subclinical seizures not controlled by medication, drug intoxication, postseizure psychosis, or a brain disease that has caused both dementia and seizures.

TREATMENT

The treatment of epilepsy of all types can be divided into three parts: the removal of causative and precipitating factors, the regulation of physical and mental hygiene, and the use of antiepileptic drugs.

REMOVAL OF CAUSATIVE AND PRECIPITATING FACTORS

Central nervous system infections, such as the meningitides and syphilis, which may give rise to convulsive seizures, should be treated by appropriate measures. The same may be said of hyponatremia, hypocalcemia, and similar conditions. Disturbances of the endocrine system resulting from islet-cell adenomas or hypoparathyroidism require surgery and appropriate replacement therapy, respectively. The logic of this approach is self-evident and does not need to be elaborated.

When convulsive seizures are associated with cerebral tumor or abscess, surgical management is usually indicated. It must be remembered, however, that the surgical removal of a meningioma of the brain will relieve seizures in only about 50 percent of cases and that in cases of glioma or abscess of the brain, the percentage is much smaller. In such cases, further treatment with drugs is necessary.

Surgery has also been advocated for the removal of cortical scars secondary to cerebral trauma, vascular lesions, and birth injuries, on the assumption that such scars are surrounded by irritable foci which act as a trigger mechanism for the seizures. A number of neurosurgeons have reported a reduction in the frequency of seizures as a sequel to these operations. This form of treatment should be limited to patients with frequent and severe focal attacks which cannot be controlled by medical means. In addition, such lesions should be excised only by neurosurgeons who have facilities for the adequate localization of the discharging focus. Practically all these patients will still require medical treatment after operation.

The anterior tip of the temporal lobe and the amygdaloid nuclei have been removed or destroyed by stereotaxis in patients with psychomotor seizures who have failed to respond to medical therapy and in whom it was possible to demonstrate a temporal lobe focus by electroencephalography. Favorable results have been reported for this procedure by some neurosurgeons. The effect of such operations upon the interseizure disorders of personality and behavior, which are thought to have a disproportionately high incidence in patients with temporal lobe seizures, remains to be determined.

PHYSICAL AND MENTAL HYGIENE

The most important factors in seizure breakthrough, next to the abandonment of medication, are loss of sleep and alcoholic excess. The need for moderation in the use of alcohol must be stressed, as well as the need to maintain regular hours of sleep.

The epileptic patient should have a wholesome, regular diet consisting of simple foods with an abundance of vegetables and fresh fruits. Constipation can be a troublesome symptom and should be avoided by the establishment of regular bowel habits, proper diet, and the use of mild laxatives when necessary.

A moderate amount of physical exercise is desirable. With proper safeguards, even the more dangerous sports, such as swimming, may be permitted. However, a person with incompletely controlled epilepsy should not be allowed to drive an automobile, operate unguarded machinery, climb ladders, swim alone, or take tub baths behind locked doors.

Simple psychotherapy will frequently prevent or

help overcome the feelings of inferiority and self-consciousness of many epileptic patients. Patients and their families will benefit from such therapy, and proper family attitudes should be cultivated. Oversolicitude and overprotection should be discouraged. It is important to emphasize that the patient should be allowed to live as normal a life as possible. Every effort should be made to keep children in school, and adults should be encouraged to work. Once seizures are under medical control, the driving of an automobile is allowed in most western countries. Many communities have vocational rehabilitation centers and special social agencies for epileptics, and advantage should be taken of such facilities. Patients should be encouraged to participate in available recreational activities as well.

THE USE OF ANTIEPILEPTIC DRUGS— GENERAL PRINCIPLES

Approximately 75 percent of patients with convulsive seizures can have their attacks controlled completely or reduced in frequency by the use of antiepileptic drugs. Although these drugs are not a cure for epilepsy, their use is the most important facet of treatment of convulsive disorders. The most commonly used drugs are listed in Table 15-3, along with their dosages, effective blood levels, and serum half-life. It should be noted that because of the long half-life of phenytoin, phenobarbital, and ethosuximide, these drugs need be taken only once daily, preferably at bedtime.

Certain drugs are more effective in one type of seizure than in another, and it is necessary to use the proper drugs in the optimum dosages for the different types of seizures. If satisfactory results are not obtained with one drug, then another should be tried, but frequent shifting of drugs is not advisable. Each should be given an adequate trial before another is substituted. In some patients a combination of two drugs will produce better results than one alone. Rarely are more than two drugs necessary, and the physician should make an effort to succeed with no more than two drugs, given in adequate dosage.

Initially, only one drug should be used and the dosage increased until therapeutic levels have been assured. If seizures are still not controlled, a second drug can then be added. Changes in medication should be made only if such a program is inadequate. In changing medication, the dosage of the new drug should be gradually increased to an optimum level at the same time that the dosage of the old drug is gradually decreased. The sudden withdrawal of a drug may lead to status epilepticus, even though a new drug is substituted. Once an anticonvulsant or a combination of anticonvulsants is found to be effective, its use should be maintained for a period of years.

The therapeutic dose for any patient must be determined, to some extent, by trial and error. Not uncommonly a drug is discarded as being ineffective, whereas a slightly increased dosage would have led to a complete disappearance of all the attacks. It is, however, a common error to administer a drug to the point where the patient is so dull and stupefied that the toxic effects of the drug are more incapacitating than the seizures. It is highly doubtful whether the prolonged administration of anticonvulsant medication is a factor in the development of the mental deterioration that occurs in a small percentage of the patients with convulsive seizures. In fact, improvement in mental faculties sometimes occurs following control of the seizures by the use of anticonvulsant drugs. We believe the same to be true of psychoses which are said by some psychiatrists to be more likely to occur when seizures are suppressed.

The management of seizures with drugs is greatly facilitated by having the patient chart daily medication and the number, time, and circumstances of seizures. Ideally such a baseline should be established before medication is begun, since each patient tends to have an individual pattern of seizures, but this is impractical.

Some patients find it helpful to use a dispenser that would be filled on Sunday, for example, for the week. This indicates to the patient whether a dose was missed and whether the supply of medications is running low. The efficacy of anticonvulsant drugs is increased also by frequent measurements of their serum levels. The levels of phenytoin, barbiturate, primidone, ethosuximide, and carbamazepine can all be measured on a single specimen by gas-liquid chromatography. These measurements are helpful in regulating dosage, revealing irregular drug intake, identifying the responsible agent in intoxicated patients who are taking more than one drug, and assuring compliance on the part of the patient.

USE OF SPECIFIC DRUGS IN TREATMENT OF SEIZURES (See Table 15-3)

Tonic-Clonic Seizures (Grand Mal) In children, or in adults with infrequent seizures (from one to four per year), phenobarbital (0.1 to 0.3 g daily in adults) can be tried first, because it is relatively nontoxic and inexpen-

Table 15-3
Common antiepileptic drugs

Generic name	Trade name	Usual daily dosage		Principal therapeutic indications	Serum half-life, h	Effective blood level, $\mu g/ml$
		Children	Adults, mg			
Phenobarbital	Luminal	3–5 mg/kg (8 mg/kg infants)	60–200	Tonic-clonic seizures; simple and complex partial seizures; absence	96 ± 12	15–30
Phenytoin	Dilantin	4–7 mg/kg	300–400	Tonic-clonic seizures; simple and complex partial seizures	24 ± 12	10–20
Carbamazepine	Tegretol	20–30 mg/kg	600–1200	Tonic-clonic seizures; complex partial seizures	12 ± 3	6–8
Primidone	Mysoline	10–25 mg/kg	750–1500	Tonic-clonic seizures; simple and complex partial seizures	12 ± 6	6–12
Ethosuximide	Zarontin	20–30 mg/kg	750–1500	Absence	30 ± 6	40–100
Methsuximide	Celontin	10–20 mg/kg	500–1000	Absence	30 ± 6	40–100
Diazepam	Valium	0.15–2 mg/kg (intravenously)	10–150	Status epilepticus		
ACTH		40–60 units/day		Infantile spasms		
Valproic acid	Depakene	30–60 mg/kg	1000–3000	Absence; simple and complex partial seizures	8 ± 2	25–100
Clonazepam	Clonopin	0.01–0.2 mg/kg	1.5–20	Absence; myoclonus	18–50	0.01–0.07

sive; in some cases this drug alone will control the seizures. Usually another drug has to be added, in which case phenytoin (0.3 to 0.4 g/day) or carbamazepine (0.6 to 1.2 g/day) may be used. When either of these drugs is used in combination with phenobarbital, a full therapeutic dose of each drug must be given. Where such a regimen fails to control the seizures, a combination of primidone and phenytoin or primidone and carbamazepine is often successful. Primidone should be *added* to full therapeutic doses of phenytoin or carbamazepine in increments of 50 mg every few days, to a maximum of 750 to 1500 mg daily.

The *toxic effects* of *phenobarbital,* which are drowsiness and mental dullness, nystagmus, and staggering, should be used as indications of excessive dosage. Rash, fever, lymphadenopathy, eosinophilia and other blood dyscrasias, and polyarteritis are manifestations of phenytoin hypersensitivity, and their occurrence calls for discontinuation of the medication. The prolonged use of *phenytoin* often leads to hirsutism (mainly in young girls) and hypertrophy of gums; these can be largely prevented by reduction in dose and careful oral hygiene. Chronic phenytoin intoxication may rarely be associated with peripheral neuropathy, but there is no conclusive evidence, in animals or in humans, that the administration of this drug can lead to cerebellar degeneration (Dam). An antifolate effect on blood and a reduction of protein-bound iodine (without lowering of the basal metabolism rate) have been reported. The claim of occurrence of pulmonary fibrosis seems to be unfounded. Congenital abnormalities, including mental deficiency, may rarely occur in children whose mothers have taken phenytoin during pregnancy. Overdose with phenytoin leads to ataxia, stupor, and coma. The adverse effects of *primidone* and *carbamazepine* are much like those of phenobarbital and phenytoin, respectively. In general, carbamazepine is better tolerated than phenytoin.

Complex Partial Seizures   Drugs effective in the treatment of grand mal seizures are also effective in the treatment of complex partial seizures. Phenytoin, 300 to 400 mg/day, carbamazepine, 0.6 to 1.2 g/day, and primidone, 750 to 1000 mg/day, have given the best results in adults. Most neurologists use carbamazepine initially in preference to phenytoin. On the whole, the results of anticonvulsant treatment are not as good as in tonic-clonic seizures.

Petit Mal Attacks   Drugs effective in the treatment of grand mal and psychomotor seizures are relatively ineffective in the treatment of patients with petit mal attacks. In the latter, ethosuximide (Zarontin), 750 to 1500 mg/day, has been the most successful and has replaced trimethadione (Tridione) and paramethadione (Paradione). It is good practice to begin with a single dose of 250 mg of ethosuximide per day and increase it every week until the optimum therapeutic effect is achieved. Phensuximide (Milontin), methsuximide (Celontin), valproic acid and acetazolamide (Diamox) are somewhat less effective but may be useful in individual cases where ethosuximide has failed.

Minor Seizures and Focal Attacks   The drugs that are effective in the treatment of grand mal and psychomotor seizures are also effective against focal attacks and minor seizures. The latter, which appear in patients whose grand mal attacks have been controlled, can occasionally be checked by simply increasing the dose of the drug(s) that the patient is already taking. If the minor attacks are very infrequent and not incapacitating, no great effort need be made to treat them.

Atypical Petit Mal plus Other Types   Patients who are subject to petit mal as well as grand mal or psychomotor seizures should be given ethosuximide plus phenytoin, carbamazepine, phenobarbital, or primidone. The treatment of the special types of convulsions in the neonatal period and in infancy and childhood is discussed further in Chap. 43.

Probably the form of epilepsy that is most difficult to treat is the atypical petit mal syndrome of Lennox-Gastaut (see above). Some of these patients have as many as 50 or more seizures per day, and every combination of anticonvulsant medications has no effect. Recently valproic acid (900 to 2400 mg/day) has been tried, and in approximately half the cases the frequency of spells has been reduced. Clonazepam also has had limited success.

In patients who obtain no therapeutic benefit from medication one may in desperation resort to surgical methods of therapy. In patients with massive destruction of one cerebral hemisphere, associated with neurologic deficits and intractable seizures, hemispherectomy was tried at one time with some success in a small number of cases. More recently, Cooper et al. have implanted a cerebellar stimulator, taking advantage of the inhibitory effects of Purkinje cells on motor activity. They have reported some success, but the authors have not confirmed this in three personally studied cases. Section of the corpus callosum, designed to prevent the transcallosal spread of seizures, is another procedure that has not been fully evaluated.

Myoclonus   Ethosuximide is often effective in the treatment of myoclonus associated with absence seizures. Phenobarbital, by itself, is less effective in this type of seizure but may be used in conjunction with ethosuximide. In the treatment of massive myoclonus in infants, ACTH or adrenal corticosteroids have been the most effective. Postanoxic intention myoclonus (see page 73) can be suppressed by clonazepam (8 to 12 mg/day) and by 5-hydroxytryptophan (1 to 1.5 g/day) combined with carbidopa (150 to 400 mg/day).

Status Epilepticus   Recurrent generalized convulsions at a frequency which does not allow consciousness to be regained in the interval between seizures (grand mal status) probably constitute the most serious therapeutic problem. Most patients who die of epilepsy do so because of uncontrolled seizures of this type or an injury sustained as a result of seizure. Rising temperature, circulatory collapse, and lower-nephron nephrosis is a sequence of events which may be encountered in fatal cases of status epilepticus.

It must be conceded that at present no known drug will safely control all recurrent convulsions. This is not surprising, for there are many causes of convulsions, and not all cases are alike. Clinical experience teaches that in some patients the convulsive tendency is so overwhelming that no amount of anticonvulsant medication, even ether anesthesia, will prevent recurrence of seizures. In others the liability to recurrent convulsions lasts only a few hours or at most a few days, regardless of whether anticonvulsant medication is given. The real hazard in treating resistant recurrent convulsions is that consciousness and vital functions may be suppressed to a degree incompatible with life. The risk of deep coma without convulsions is greater than semicoma or stupor with an occasional convulsion.

The following medications have been recommended for recurrent convulsions with brain disease and for status epilepticus:

1. *Sodium phenobarbital* in a dose of 0.2 to 0.4 g intramuscularly and a repeated dose of 0.1 to 0.2 g every 30 min until a maximum of 0.8 to 1 g per 24 h is reached.

2. *Thiopental* (Pentothal sodium) in doses of 0.3 to 0.6 g intravenously or intramuscularly.

3. *Phenytoin* (Dilantin) in a dose of 0.5 to 1 g/day orally (through stomach tube) or intravenously. This drug is not consistently effective in terminating seizures abruptly.

4. *Diazepam* (Valium) in intravenous doses of 5 to 10 mg repeated every 30 min (to a maximum of 100 to 150 mg per 24 h). If the patient is intubated, the total dosage may be doubled. In general it is better to depend on maintenance doses of phenobarbital and phenytoin, using diazepam for only an occasional uncontrolled outburst of seizures.

5. *Ether* by inhalation.

6. *Paraldehyde*, in a dose of 5 to 10 ml intramuscularly (avoiding injection near nerves, which may be damaged by it), is a rapidly acting anticonvulsant. The slow (over 2 min) intravenous administration of 1 to 4 ml is sometimes highly effective, but carries the danger of respiratory arrest.

These many treatments attest to the fact that no one of them is altogether satisfactory. The authors have had the most success with the following program. When the patient is first seen, 10 mg diazepam (adult) is administered intravenously over a period of 2 to 10 min. At the same time the 24-h maintenance doses of phenytoin and phenobarbital are started. An intravenous injection of 0.3 g sodium phenobarbital is first given. Phenytoin, 0.5 g, is then administered through a stomach tube, and this should constitute the daily dose. If seizures continue, either diazepam or sodium phenobarbital are given intravenously, according to the regimen outlined above. If after 24 h the seizures continue, all medication except phenytoin should be discontinued, and either a light ether anesthesia or Pentothal anesthesia, up to 0.5 g intravenously, should be tried. Should the seizures continue despite all these medications, one is justified in the assumption that the convulsive tendency is so strong that it cannot be checked by reasonable quantities of anticonvulsants. One then depends entirely on phenytoin, 0.5 g, and sodium phenobarbital, 0.4 g/day (smaller doses in infants and children, as shown in Table 15-3), and on safeguarding the patient's vital functions. For recurrent seizures such as those associated with brain abscess, subdural empyema, or thrombophlebitis, paraldehyde may be effective where phenytoin and other drugs have failed. The dose is 5 to 10 ml injected intramuscularly, with care taken to avoid nerves, and it may be repeated once or twice at 4-h intervals.

REFERENCES

BEAR DM, FEDIO P: Quantitative analysis of interictal behavior in temporal lobe epilepsy. *Arch Neurol* 34:454, 1977.

COOPER IS, AMIN I, GILMAN S: The effect of chronic cerebellar stimulation upon epilepsy in man. *Trans Am Neurol Assoc* 98:192, 1973.

DAM M: The density and ultrastructure of the Purkinje cells following diphenylhydantoin treatment in animals and man. *Acta Neurol Scand Suppl* 49:3, 1972.

Drugs for epilepsy. *Med Lett* 21:25, 1979.

EADIE MJ, TYRER JH: *Anticonvulsant Therapy: Pharmacological Basis and Practice,* 2d ed. London, Churchill Livingstone, 1980.

FALCONER MA: Genetic and related aetiological factors in temporal lobe epilepsy. A review. *Epilepsia* 12:13, 1971-1972.

FORSTER FM: *Reflex Epilepsy, Behavioral Therapy and Conditional Reflexes.* Springfield, Ill, Charles C Thomas, 1977.

GASTAUT H: Clinical and electroencephalographical classifications of epileptic seizures. *Epilepsia* 11:102, 1970.

———, GASTAUT JL: Computerized transverse axial tomography in epilepsy. *Epilepsia* 17(3):325, 1976.

GODDARD GV, MCINTYRE DC, LEECH CK: A permanent change in brain function resulting from daily electrical stimulation. *Exp Neurol* 25:295, 1969.

GOWERS WR: *Epilepsy and Other Chronic Convulsive Diseases: Their Causes, Symptoms and Treatment.* New York, Dover, 1964. (Originally published in 1885; reprinted as Amer Acad Neurol Reprint Series, vol 1.)

HAUSER WA, KURLAND LT: The epidemiology of epilepsy in Rochester, Minnesota. *Epilepsia* 16:1, 1975.

HEINEMANN U, LUX HD, GUTNICK MJ: Extracellular free calcium and potassium during paroxysmal activity in the cerebral cortex of the cat. *Exp Brain Res* 27:237, 1977.

JASPER HH et al: *Basic Mechanisms of the Epilepsies.* Boston, Little, Brown, 1969.

KUTT H, PENRY JK: Usefulness of blood levels of antiepileptic drugs. *Arch Neurol* 31:283, 1974.

LENNOX MA: Febrile convulsions in childhood. *Am J Dis Child* 78:868, 1949.

LENNOX W, LENNOX MA: *Epilepsy and Related Disorders.* Boston, Little, Brown, 1960.

LOMBROSO CT: Sylvian seizures and midtemporal spike foci in children. *Arch Neurol* 17:52, 1967.

NORMAN RN, SANDRY S, CORSELLIS JAN: The nature and origin of patho-anatomical change in the epileptic brain, in Vinken PJ, Bruyn GW (eds): Amsterdam, North-Holland, 1974, vol 15, pp 611-620.

OUNSTED C, LINDSAY J, NORMAN RA: *Biological Factors in Temporal Lobe Epilepsy, Clinics in Developmental Medicine,* vol 22. London, Heineman/Spastic Society, 1966.

PEDLEY TA: The pathophysiology of focal epilepsy: neurophysiological considerations. *Ann Neurol* 3:2, 1978.

PENFIELD W, JASPER HH: *Epilepsy and Functional Anatomy of the Human Brain.* Boston, Little, Brown, 1954.

———, KRISTIANSEN K: *Epileptic Seizure Patterns.* Springfield, Ill, Charles C Thomas, 1951.

PENRY JK, DALY DD (eds): *Complex Partial Seizures and Their Treatment.* New York, Raven Press, 1975.

——— et al: Simultaneous recording of absence seizures with video tape and electroencephalography. *Brain* 98:427, 1975.

PINCUS JH, TUCKER GJ: *Behavioral Neurology.* London, Oxford University Press, 1974, pp 29-36.

PLUM F, HOWSE DC, DUFFY TE: Metabolic effects of seizures. *Res Publ Assoc Res Nerv Ment Dis* 53:141, 1974.

SALCMAN M et al: Neuropathological changes in cerebellar biopsies in epileptic patients. *Ann Neurol* 3:10, 1978.

SCHEIBEL ME, SCHEIBEL AB: Hippocampal pathology in temporal lobe epilepsy: A Golgi survey, in Brazier MAB (ed): *Epilepsy: Its Phenomena in Man.* New York, Academic, 1973, pp 315-357.

SCHMIDT RP, WILDER BJ: *Epilepsy.* Philadelphia, Davis, 1968.

STEVENS JR: Psychiatric implications of psychomotor epilepsy. *Arch Gen Psychiatry* 14:461, 1966.

SUTHERLAND JM, EADIE MJ: *The Epilepsies.* London, Churchill Livingstone, 1980.

THOMAS JE, REGAN TJ, CLASS DW: Epilepsia partialis continua. A review of 32 cases. *Arch Neurol* 34:266, 1977.

WOODBURY DM et al: *Anti-epileptic Drugs.* New York, Raven, 1972.

CHAPTER 16

COMA AND RELATED DISORDERS OF CONSCIOUSNESS

In the hospital practice of neurology the clinical analysis of unresponsive and comatose patients becomes a practical necessity. There is always an urgency about such medical problems and a need to determine the underlying disease process and the direction in which it is evolving and to protect the brain against more serious or irreversible damage. The attending physician must therefore have an immediately accessible and systematic approach to the problems of coma; the need for prompt therapeutic and diagnostic action allows no time for leisurely, scholarly investigation.

Some idea of the dimensions of these types of disorders is obtained from published statistics. In two large municipal hospitals it was estimated that as many as 3 percent of total admissions to an emergency ward were due to diseases that had caused coma (Table 16-1). Although this figure seems high, it serves to emphasize the importance of this class of neurologic diseases and the necessity for every student of medicine to acquire a theoretic as well as a practical knowledge of them.

The terms *consciousness, confusion, stupor, unconsciousness,* and *coma* have been endowed with so many different meanings that it is almost impossible to avoid ambiguity in their usage. They are not strictly medical terms, but literary, philosophic, and psychological ones as well. The word *consciousness* is the most difficult of all. William James once remarked that one knows what consciousness is until one attempts to define it. To the psychologist, consciousness denotes a state of awareness of one's self and one's environment. Knowledge of one's self includes all "feelings, attitudes and emotions, impulses, volitions, and the active or striving aspects of conduct" (English)—in short, an awareness of all one's own mental functioning, particularly of the cognitive processes. These can be judged only by the patients' verbal accounts of their introspections and, in-

directly, by their actions. Physicians, being practical for the most part, have learned to place greater confidence in their observations of the patient's behavior and reactions to overt stimuli than in what the patient says. For this reason when they employ the term *consciousness,* they usually give it its commonest and simplest meaning, viz., the state of the patient's awareness of self and environment. This narrow definition has another advantage in that the word *unconsciousness* is its exact opposite—a state of unawareness of self and environment or a suspension of those mental activities by which people are made aware of themselves and their environment. To add to the ambiguity, psychoanalysts have given the word *unconscious* a still different meaning; for them it stands for a repository of impulses and memories of previous experiences that cannot immediately be recalled to the conscious mind.

Much more could be said about the history of our ideas concerning consciousness, and the theoretic problems with regard to its definition, but this would serve no practical purpose. The reader is better referred to the discussion of consciousness by Frederiks, in the *Handbook of Clinical Neurology* (see References at end of chapter).

DESCRIPTION OF STATES OF NORMAL AND IMPAIRED CONSCIOUSNESS

The following definitions, though probably unacceptable to most psychologists, are of service to medicine, and they will provide the student with a convenient terminology for describing the states of awareness and responsiveness of patients.

Normal Consciousness This is the condition of the normal person when awake. In this state the individual is fully responsive to stimuli and indicates by behavior and speech the same awareness of self and environment as we have ourselves. This normal state may fluctuate during the course of the day from keen alertness or deep concentration with a marked constriction of the field of attention, to general inattentiveness and drowsiness.

Inattention, Confusion, and Clouding of Consciousness
In these conditions patients do not take into account all elements of their immediate environment. These states always imply, as does delirium, an element of sensorial clouding or imperceptiveness and distractibility of attention. The term *confusion* lacks precision, but in a general way it denotes an inability to think with customary speed and clarity. Here the difficulty is in defining *thinking*, a term which variably refers to problem solving and coherence of ideas about a subject. The patient may fail in either way for several different reasons, viz., inattentiveness, disorder of language, forgetfulness, or abulia (see Chap. 19).

Severely confused and inattentive persons are usually unable to do more than carry out the simplest commands. Few if any thought processes are in operation. Their speech may be limited to a few words or phrases, or they may be voluble. They are unaware of much that goes on around them and do not grasp their immediate situation. Moderately confused persons can carry on a simple conversation for short periods of time, but their thinking is slow and incoherent, and they are unable to stay on one topic. They are distractible and at the mercy of every stimulus. Periods of irritability and excitability alternate with drowsiness. Often they are disoriented in time and place. In mild degrees of confusion the disorder may be so slight that it is overlooked unless the examiner is searching particularly for alterations in the patient's behavior and conversation. The patient may even be roughly oriented as to time and place, with only occasional irrelevant remarks betraying an incoherence of thinking. Patients with mild or moderately severe confusion may be subjected to psychological testing. The degree of confusion often varies from one time of day to another. It tends to be least pronounced in the early morning and most pronounced in the evening or night, when environmental cues are less clear-cut and the patient is fatigued. Many events that happen to confuse patients leave no trace in their memory; in fact, capacity to recall events that transpired in any given period is one of the most delicate tests of mental clarity. However, careful analysis will show the defect to be one of inadequate registration and fixation of items, rather than a fault in retentive memory.

Some neurologists regard *delirium* as a state of confusion with excitement and hyperactivity, and in some medical writings the terms *delirium* and *confused-cloudy states* are used interchangeably. However, the vivid hallucinations which characterize delirious states, the relative inaccessibility of patients to events other than those to which they are reacting at any one moment, their extreme agitation, their tendency to tremble, to startle easily, and to convulse, and the overactivity of the autonomic nervous system suggest a cerebral disorder of distinctive type. The clearest evidence of the relationship of inattention, confusion, stupor, and coma is that patients may pass through all these states as they become comatose or emerge from coma. The authors have not observed such a relationship between coma and delirium, with the possible exception of hepatic stupor and coma, which may be *preceded* by a brief period of delirium. No doubt in certain acute mental syndromes the distinction between delirium and other confusional states is difficult to make, since some of the attributes of delirium are lacking. These problems are elaborated in Chap. 19.

At times a patient with certain types of aphasia, especially jargon aphasia, may create the impression of confusion, but close observation will reveal that the disorder is confined to the sphere of language and that behavior is otherwise natural and appropriate to the situation.

Stupor In stupor, mental and physical activity are reduced to a minimum. Patients can be aroused only by vigorous and repeated stimuli, at which time they open their eyes, look at the examiner, and do not appear to be unconscious; response to spoken commands is either absent or slow and inadequate. Tremulousness of movement, coarse twitching of muscles, restless or stereotyped motor activity, and grasping and sucking reflexes are not infrequent, and tendon and plantar reflexes may or may not be altered, depending on the way in which the underlying disease has affected the nervous system. In psychiatry, *stupor* refers to a state in which impressions of the external world are normally received but activity is suspended or marked by negativism, e.g., catatonic schizophrenia.

Coma The patient who appears to be asleep and is at the same time incapable of sensing or responding either to external stimuli or to inner needs is in a state of coma. Coma may vary in degree, and in its deepest stages no reaction of any kind is obtainable; corneal, pupillary, pharyngeal, tendon, and plantar reflexes are all absent. With lesser degrees of coma, pupillary reflexes and ocular movements and other brainstem reflexes are preserved, and there may or may not be extensor rigidity of the limbs and opisthotonos—signs which, as Sherrington showed, indicate decerebration. Respirations are often slow or rapid and may be periodic (Cheyne-Stokes breathing) or deranged in other ways (see below). In still lighter stages, referred to as *semicoma,* most of the above reflexes can be elicited, and the plantar reflexes may be either flexor or extensor (Babinski sign). Moreover, pricking or pinching the skin, shaking and shouting at the patient, or distention of the bladder may cause a stirring or moaning and a quickening of respirations.

These physical signs vary somewhat, depending on the cause of coma. For example, patients with alcoholic intoxication may be unresponsive to noxious stimuli and arreflexic, even when respirations and other vital signs are not threatened. Drug overdose rarely produces decerebrate rigidity, no matter what the degree of coma. The signs of depth of coma and stupor, when compared in serial examinations, are most useful in assessing the direction in which the disease is evolving.

RELATIONSHIP OF SLEEP TO COMA

Persons in sleep give little evidence of being aware of themselves or their environment; in this respect they are unconscious. Sleep shares a number of other features with the pathologic states of drowsiness, stupor, and coma. These include yawning, closure of the eyelids, cessation of blinking and swallowing, upward deviation or divergence or roving movements of the eyes, loss of muscular tone, decrease or loss of tendon reflexes and even Babinski signs, irregular respirations, sometimes Cheyne-Stokes in type, and occasionally incontinence of urine. Nevertheless, sleeping persons may still respond to unaccustomed stimuli and at times are capable of some mental activity in the form of dreams which leave their traces in memory, thus differing from persons in stupor or coma. The most important difference, of course, is that persons in sleep, when stimulated, can be recalled from their physical and mental inactivity to normal consciousness. There are important physiologic differences as well. Cerebral oxygen uptake does not decrease during sleep as it does in coma, and the EEG, which may be similar in sleep and in coma, is much more often different, as will be indicated later in this chapter and in Chap. 18. The anatomic basis for these differences is not clear.

THE PERSISTENT VEGETATIVE STATE, PSEUDOCOMA, AND AKINETIC MUTISM

With increasing refinements in the treatment of severe cerebral injury, more and more patients who formerly would have died have survived for indefinite periods, without regaining any recognizable mental function. For the first week or two after the cerebral injury these patients are in a state of deep coma. Then they begin to open their eyes, at first in response to painful stimuli and later spontaneously and for increasingly prolonged periods. The patient may blink in response to threat. Intermittently the eyes move from side to side, seemingly following objects or fixating on the physician or a family member, and giving the erroneous impression of cognition. However, the patient remains inattentive, never speaks, and shows no signs of awareness of the environment or inner need; responsiveness is limited to primitive postural and reflex movements of the limbs. In brief, there is arousal or wakefulness, without awareness or responsiveness. The EEG, which originally may have been isoelectric, approaches normality, even showing alpha rhythm and sleep patterns. This syndrome is most appropriately referred to as the *persistent vegetative state* (Jennett and Plum).

The foregoing states of coma and persistent vegetative state must be clearly distinguished from a clinical state in which there is little or no disturbance of awareness (consciousness), but only an inability of the patient to respond adequately. The latter state—referred to variously as *pseudocoma,* the *locked-in* syndrome, or the *deefferented* state—is due most often to a lesion of the basis pontis. Such a lesion spares the pathways for somatic sensation and the nonspecific ascending system of neurons and fibers responsible for arousal and wakefulness but interrupts the corticobulbar and corticospinal pathways, depriving the patient of speech or the capacity to respond in any other way. Severe degrees of motor neuropathy may have a similar effect. One could logically refer to this state as *akinetic mutism* (*coma vigile* of the French), insofar as the patient is akinetic and mute, but this term was originally used by Cairns in another sense—to describe a patient who appeared to be awake but was unresponsive (actually Cairns' patient was able to answer in whispered monosyllables). Cairns' patient, following repeated evacuation of a third ventricular cyst, would regain consciousness but was unable to remember any of the events that had occurred when she was in the akinetic-mute state. Unfortunately this term has been applied to patients who are silent and immobile as a result of bilateral frontal lobe lesions, despite the integrity of motor and sensory pathways; lacking in these latter patients is the psychic drive or impulse to action (abulia).

It is apparent from these remarks that considerable imprecision surrounds the terms which are used to describe the states of consciousness. The student would be better advised to avoid the use of arbitrary designations such as *coma* and *akinetic mutism,* which are open to differing interpretations and to use simple descriptive language instead, indicating whether the patient appears awake or asleep, drowsy or alert, the degree of awareness of surroundings, and the nature of responses to a variety of designated stimuli.

BRAIN DEATH

In the late 1950s European neurologists called attention to a state of coma in which the brain was irreversibly damaged and had ceased to function but in which pulmonary and cardiac function could still be maintained by artificial means. Mollaret and Goulon referred to this condition as *coma dépassé* (a state beyond coma). It has also been called *irreversible coma, brain death,* and *cerebral death,* terms that are now used interchangeably. The concept that a person is dead if the brain is dead and that death of the brain may precede the cessation of cardiac function posed a number of important ethical, legal, and social problems as well as medical ones. The various aspects of brain death have been the subject of close study by several professional committees, which have provided rather clear and generally accepted guidelines for determining that the brain is dead.

The central considerations in the diagnosis of brain death are (1) the absence of cerebral functions, (2) the absence of brainstem functions, including spontaneous respirations, and (3) the irreversibility of the state.

The absence of cerebral function is judged by the lack of spontaneous movement and lack of motor and vocal response to all visual, auditory, and cutaneous stimulation. Spinal reflexes may be present, however. The EEG is a valuable indicator of cerebral death and most institutions require proof of electrocerebral silence (ECS), also called a flat or isoelectric EEG, which is considered to be present if there is no change in electrical potentials over 2 μV during two 30-min recordings taken 6 h apart. It needs to be emphasized that cerebral unresponsivity and a flat EEG do not always signify

brain death but that both may occur, and be completely reversible, in states of profound hypothermia and intoxication with sedative-hypnotic drugs.

Brainstem functions are considered to be absent if there are no pupillary reactions to light, no corneal, oculocephalic, vestibuloocular, oropharyngeal, or tracheal reflexes, no decerebrate or decorticate responses to noxious stimuli, and no spontaneous respirations. For practical purposes, absolute apnea is present if the patient makes no effort to override the respirator for at least 15 min. As a final test, the patient can be disconnected from the respirator long enough (a few minutes) to ensure that arterial Pco_2 rises above the threshold for stimulation of respiration.

When examination has disclosed that all brain functions are absent, it should be repeated in 6 h, for confirmation that the state is irreversible. If an appropriate history and comprehensive screening procedures for drugs are not available, an observation period of 72 h may be required to assess reversibility. Although they are rarely practical, cerebral perfusion studies, demonstrating complete cessation of intracranial circulation, provide absolute evidence of brain death.

Finally it should be mentioned that the clinical and EEG criteria for brain death in infants and young children are not well established.

THE ELECTROENCEPHALOGRAM AND DISTURBANCES OF CONSCIOUSNESS

One of the most delicate confirmations of the fact that the states of impaired consciousness are expressions of neurophysiologic changes is the altered electroencephalogram (EEG). In the normal waking state the electrical potentials of the cortical neurons are integrated into regular waves of two frequency ranges, from 8 to 13 per second (alpha rhythm) and from 16 to 25 per second (beta rhythm). These waveforms are established by adolescence, but certain individual differences in general pattern and dominance of alpha waves are maintained throughout adult life. With sleep there is a decrease in the frequency of these cortical potentials and increased synchrony of the EEG tracing. At one stage in light sleep characteristic bursts of 14 to 16 waves per second appear (the so-called sleep spindles), and in deep sleep all the waves of normal frequency and amplitude are replaced by $1\frac{1}{2}$ - to 3-per-second waves of high voltage. In rapid-eye-movement (REM) sleep the EEG becomes desynchronized (see Chap. 18). Similarly, some alteration in brain waves occurs in all disturbances of consciousness except the milder degrees of confusion. This alteration usually consists of a disorganization of the EEG pattern, which shows random, slow waves of high voltage in stages of confusion; more regular, slow, 2- to 3-per-second waves of high voltage in stupor and semi-coma; and slow waves or even suppression of all organized electrical activity (isoelectric state) in the deep coma of hypoxia and ischemia—the so-called brain-death syndrome. The EEGs of deep sleep and of light coma resemble each other. However, not all diseases that cause confusion and coma have the same effect on the EEG. Some, such as barbiturate intoxication, may cause an increase in frequency and amplitude of the brain waves. In epilepsy the disturbance of consciousness is usually attended by paroxysms of sharp waves or "spikes" (fast waves of high amplitude) or by the characteristic alternating slow waves and spikes of petit mal. Other diseases, such as hepatic coma, characteristically cause a decrease in frequency and an increase in amplitude of brain waves and the appearance of bilaterally synchronous triphasic waves. Whether all metabolic diseases of the brain induce similar changes in the EEG has not been determined. Probably there are differences among them, some of which may be significant (see Chap. 2).

MORBID ANATOMY AND PHYSIOLOGY OF COMA

In recent times there has been some clarification and amplification of earlier neuropathologic observations that the smallest lesions associated with protracted coma are always to be found in the midbrain and thalamus. The essence of more recent neurophysiologic studies is that an ascending series of destructive lesions of spinal cord, medulla, cerebellum, and lower pons has no effect on the state of consciousness, until the level of the upper pons is reached. Destruction of the high brainstem reticular formation invariably induces states of prolonged unresponsiveness, accompanied by a slow, synchronized EEG, whereas stimulation by an electrode placed in the substance of the reticular formation causes a drowsy or sleeping animal to become suddenly alert and its EEG to change correspondingly (desynchronization). Furthermore, the state of unresponsiveness induced by destruction of the reticular formation cannot be reversed by strong sensory stimulation, even if the primary sensory pathways from the periphery via the thalamus to the cortex are preserved. Similarly, as anesthetic agents abolish consciousness, they are found to suppress the activity of the upper reticular activating system, without interfering, at least at certain levels, with the transmission of specific sensory impulses to the cerebral cortex.

The anatomic boundaries of the reticular activating system of the upper brainstem are indistinct. It is interspersed throughout the paramedian regions of the upper pontine and midbrain tegmentum, the septal re-

gion, and the hypothalamus, and includes the functionally related medial, intralaminar, and reticular nuclei of the thalamus. In the brainstem it receives collaterals from the specific sensory pathways and projects not just to the sensory cortex of the parietal lobe, as do the thalamic relay nuclei for somatic sensation, but to the whole of the cerebral cortex. Sensory stimulation, it would seem, then, has the double effect of conveying to the brain information about the outside world and also of activating those parts of the nervous system on which consciousness depends. The cerebral cortex not only receives impulses from the ascending reticular activating system but also modulates this incoming information via corticofugal connections which feed back nerve impulses to the reticular formation.

These new data are in line with the older ideas of Herbert Spencer and Hughlings Jackson—that the diencephalon and cerebral cortex always function together as a unit and represent the highest level of integrative nervous activity, called by Penfield *centrencephalic.* Though the anatomic details of the reticular activating system have yet to be worked out and the physiology is more complicated than this simple formulation would suggest, it nevertheless, as a working idea, makes some of the following neuropathologic observations more comprehensible.

The study of a large series of human cases in which coma has preceded death by several days discloses two major types of lesion. (1) In one group, a readily discernible lesion such as a tumor, abscess, intracerebral, subarachnoid, subdural, or epidural hemorrhage, massive infarct, or meningitis is demonstrable. Usually the lesion involves only a portion of the cortex and white matter, leaving much of the cerebrum intact. Rarely, it is located in the thalamus or midbrain, which would make the coma understandable, but in the other instances the coma will be related to a temporal lobe-tentorial herniation with compression, ischemia, and secondary hemorrhage in the midbrain and lower thalamus, or with distortion or displacement of these parts (see Chap. 30). A detailed clinical record will show the coma to have coincided with these secondary displacements and herniations. Exceptionally, widespread bilateral damage to the cortex and subcortical white matter will be found—the result of bilateral infarcts or hemorrhages, viral encephalitis, hypoxia, or ischemia—without visible thalamic or midbrain lesions. Presumably, the coma in these cases is the result of complete interruption of the corticofugal impulses that normally sustain diencephalic and midbrain reticular activity. (2) In the second group (larger than the first) no lesion is visible to the naked eye. In some instances the grossly normal brain will reveal a microscopic change that may be characteristic, e.g., hepatic coma. Usually the microscopic lesions are too diffuse for clinicoanatomic correlation. Often no abnormality is divulged by any technique of pathology; the lesion, caused by a metabolic or toxic state, is subcellular or molecular.

Thus pathologic changes are compatible with physiologic deductions—that the state of prolonged coma correlates with lesions of all parts of the cortical-diencephalic system of neurons, but it is only in the upper brainstem that the lesions may be small and discrete.

MECHANISMS WHEREBY CONSCIOUSNESS IS DISTURBED IN DISEASE

Knowledge of diseases of the nervous system is so limited that it is not possible to identify all the different mechanisms by which consciousness is disturbed. Already several ways in which the mesencephalic-diencephalic-cortical systems are deranged have been identified; there are many others.

In a number of disease processes there is direct interference with the metabolic activities of the nerve cells in the cerebral cortex and the central nuclear masses of the brain. Hypoxia, hypoglycemia, hyper- and hypoosmolar states, acidosis, alkalosis, hypokalemia, hyperammonemia, and deficiencies of thiamine, nicotinic acid, vitamin B_{12}, pantothenic acid, and pyridoxine are well-known examples (see Chap. 39 and Table 39-1). The relevant point for our discussion is that cerebral metabolism or blood flow is reduced in all metabolic disorders leading to coma. Oxygen values below 2 ml/min per 100 g brain tissue are incompatible with an alert state. In hypoglycemia the cerebral blood flow is normal or above normal, whereas the cerebral metabolic rate is diminished, owing to deficiency of substrate. In thiamine and vitamin B_{12} deficiency the cerebral blood flow is normal or slightly diminished, and the cerebral metabolic rate is diminished, presumably because of insufficiency of coenzymes. Extremes of body temperature [over 41°C (106°F) or below 36°C (97°F)] probably induce coma by exerting a nonspecific effect on the metabolic activity of neurons. Diabetic acidosis, uremia, hepatic coma, and the coma of systemic infections are examples of endogenous intoxications. The identity of the toxic agents is not entirely known. In diabetes, acetone bodies (acetoacetic acid, β-hydroxybutyric acid,

and acetone) are present in high concentration, and in uremia there is probably accumulation of dialyzable toxins, perhaps phenolic derivatives of the aromatic amino acids. In both conditions "dehydration" and serum acidosis may also play an important role. In many cases of hepatic coma, elevation of blood NH_3 to levels five to six times normal has been found. Lactic acidosis may affect the brain by lowering arterial blood pH to less than 7.0. The impairment of consciousness that accompanies pulmonary insufficiency is related to both hypoxia and hypercapnia, the elevated carbon dioxide tension probably being the main factor (see Table 39-1). The mode of action of bacterial toxins is unknown. In all these conditions the cerebral metabolic rate tends to be reduced, whereas cerebral blood flow remains normal. In water intoxication the membrane excitability of nerve cells is altered by hyponatremia and changes in intracellular levels of potassium.

Drugs such as barbiturates, bromides, phenytoin, alcohol, glutethimide, and phenothiazines induce coma by their direct depressant effects on the neurons of the cerebrum and diencephalon. Others such as methyl alcohol, ethylene glycol, and paraldehyde produce a metabolic acidosis. Many additional pharmacologic agents have no direct action on the nervous system but lead to coma through the mechanism of circulatory collapse and inadequate cerebral blood flow. In toxic and metabolic diseases, although the patient usually approaches coma through a state of drowsiness, confusion, and stupor, and the reverse sequence occurs during emergence, each disease has its special effects, manifesting itself by a characteristic clinical picture. Probably this means that the mechanism in each case and topography of the lesions are different.

A critical decline in blood pressure, usually to a systolic level below 70 mmHg, affects neural structures by causing a decrease in cerebral blood flow and, secondarily, in cerebral metabolic rate. If decline in blood pressure is episodic, the corresponding clinical picture is syncope (see Chap. 17). Here the clinical picture is one of physical weakness preceding and following the loss of consciousness, the whole process being acute and promptly reversible.

The sudden, violent, and excessive neuronal discharge that characterizes *epilepsy* is another common mechanism. Usually focal seizure activity has little effect on consciousness until it spreads from one side of the body to the other. Coma then ensues, presumably because the spreading of the seizure discharge to central neuronal structures paralyzes their function. Other types of seizure in which consciousness is interrupted from the very beginning are believed to originate in the diencephalon.

Concussion exemplifies still another special pathophysiologic mechanism of coma. In "blunt" head injury it has been shown that there is an enormous increase in intracranial pressure, of the order of 200 to 700 lb/in^2, lasting a few thousandths of a second. Either the vibration set up in the skull and transmitted to the brain or sudden high intracranial pressure is believed to be the basis of the abrupt paralysis of nervous function that follows head injury. That the increased pressure itself may be the main factor has been suggested by experiments in which raising the intraventricular pressure to a level approaching diastolic blood pressure has abolished all vital functions. A swirling motion of the brain with torque of the upper brainstem imparted by a blow to the head is another factor involved in concussion and is the mechanism favored by most neurologists.

As was pointed out above, large, destructive, and space-consuming lesions of the brain, such as hemorrhage, tumor, or abscess, interfere with consciousness in two ways. One is by direct destruction of the midbrain and diencephalon. The other, far more frequent, is by producing herniation of the medial part of the temporal lobe(s) through the opening of the tentorium and crushing the upper midbrain against the opposite free edge of the tentorium (see Chap. 30). Whether a distinction can and should be drawn between central and lateral herniations, as has been suggested by Plum and Posner, has not been settled. There is also a less frequent upward herniation of the cerebellum and displacement of the brainstem with masses in the posterior fossa (usually in the cerebellum).

CLINICAL APPROACH TO THE COMATOSE PATIENT

Coma is not an independent disease entity but is always a symptomatic expression of disease. Sometimes the underlying disease is perfectly obvious, as when a healthy individual is struck on the head and rendered unconscious. All too often, however, the patient is brought to the hospital in a state of coma, and little or no information is immediately available. The clinical problem must then be scrutinized from many directions. To do this efficiently, the physician must have a broad knowledge of disease and a methodical approach that leaves none of the common and treatable causes of coma unexplored.

When the comatose patient is seen for the first time, one must quickly see if the patient's airway is clear. It is equally important to ascertain that the patient is not in shock (circulatory collapse) or, if trauma has occurred, that there is no bleeding from a wound or ruptured organ (e.g., spleen or liver). In these circumstances, simple therapeutic measures (insertion of an endotracheal tube, administration of pressor agents, oxygen, blood, or glucose solutions, *after* drawing blood for glucose determinations) take precedence over diagnostic procedures. In the patient who has suffered a head injury there may be a fracture of the cervical vertebrae, in which case one must be cautious about moving the head and neck lest the spinal cord be inadvertently crushed. There must be an immediate inquiry as to the previous health of the patient, whether there had been a head injury or a convulsion, and the circumstances in which the person was found. The persons who accompany the comatose patient to the hospital should not be permitted to leave until they have been questioned.

From an initial survey many of the common types of disease causing coma, such as severe head injuries, alcoholic or other forms of drug intoxication, and hypertensive brain hemorrhage, are readily recognized. As can be seen in Table 16-1, which summarizes data from the emergency wards of the Boston City and the Cook County Hospitals, they comprise about two-thirds of all cases of coma seen in such emergency wards. In large university hospitals, which tend to attract the more obscure and difficult cases, the statistics are quite different. For example, in the series of Plum and Posner (Table 16-2), which resembles more that of the Massachusetts and Cleveland Metropolitan General Hospitals, only 113 of 500 patients proved to have cerebrovascular disease (60 of the 113 were cerebral, brainstem, and cerebellar hemorrhage), and in 31 the coma was the consequence of trauma (epidural and subdural hemorrhages). Indeed, all "mass lesions," such as tumors, abscesses, hemorrhages, and infarcts, made up less than one-third of all coma-producing diseases. Instead, the majority were the result of exogenous and endogenous intoxications and hypoxia, with subarachnoid hemorrhage, meningitis, and encephalitis adding up to another 5 percent of the total. Thus the order is reversed, but still intoxication, stroke, and cranial trauma stand as the "big three" of coma-producing conditions.

DIAGNOSIS

Alterations in vital signs—temperature, pulse, respiratory rate, and blood pressure—are important aids in diagnosis. Fever suggests a systemic infection such as pneumonia, bacterial meningitis, or a brain lesion that has disturbed the temperature-regulating centers. An excessively high body temperature [42 or 43°C (107 to 110°F)] associated with dry skin, should arouse the suspicion of heat stroke. Hypothermia, on the other hand, is frequently observed in alcoholic or barbiturate intoxication, extracellular fluid deficit, peripheral circulatory failure, and myxedema. Slow breathing points to morphine or barbiturate intoxication, or hypothyroidism, whereas deep, rapid breathing suggests pneumonia but may occur in diabetic or uremic acidosis (Kussmaul respiration) or with intracranial diseases that cause central neurogenic hyperventilation. The rapid breathing of pneumonia is often accompanied by an expiratory grunt, cyanosis, and fever. Diseases that elevate the intracranial pressure or damage the brain, especially the brain-

stem, often cause slow, irregular, or periodic (Cheyne-Stokes) breathing. The pulse rate is less helpful, but if exceptionally slow, it should suggest heart block, or if combined with periodic breathing and hypertension, an increase in intracranial pressure. A tachycardia of 140 beats per minute or more calls attention to the possibility of an ectopic cardiac rhythm with insufficiency of cerebral circulation. Marked hypertension occurs in patients with cerebral hemorrhage and hypertensive encephalopathy and, at times, in those with increased in-

Table 16-1

Relative incidence of diseases which cause coma*

Disease	Boston City Hospital series (clinical cases)†			Cook County series‡ (autopsied cases)	
	No.	Percent	Mortality, percent	No.	Percent
Alcoholism	690	59.1	2.0	16	4.6
Trauma	152	13.0	31.5	94	27.5
Cerebral vascular disease	118	10.0	77.0	120	35.0
Poisoning	33	3.0	9.0		
Epilepsy	28	2.4	0		
Diabetes	20	1.7	55.0	8	2.3
Bacterial meningitis*	20	1.7	100.0	29	8.5
Pneumonia	20	1.7	90.0	18	5.4
Cardiac decompensation	17	1.4	70.0		
Neurosyphilis	7	0.6	0	4	1.2
Uremia	7	0.6	100.0	37	10.9
Eclampsia	7	0.6	68.4		
Miscellaneous	48	1.1	75.0	16	4.6
Total	1167	100.0		342	100.0

* These figures were collected in 1933 before the introduction of most of the sulfonamide drugs or antibiotics.

† Reported by P Solomon, CD Aring, *Am J Med Sci* 188:805, 1934.

‡ Reported by B Holcomb, *JAMA* 77:2112, 1921.

Table 16-2

Final diagnosis in 500 patients admitted to hospital with "coma of unknown etiology"*

Supratentorial mass lesions	101
Intracerebral hematoma	44
Subdural hematoma	26
Epidural hematoma	4
Cerebral infarct	9
Thalamic infarct	2
Brain tumor	7
Pituitary apoplexy	2
Brain abscess	6
Closed-head injury	1
Subtentorial lesions	65
Brainstem infarct	40
Pontine hemorrhage	11
Brainstem demyelination	1
Cerebellar hemorrhage	5
Cerebellar tumor	3
Cerebellar infarct	2
Cerebellar abscess	1
Posterior fossa subdural hemorrhage	1
Basilar migraine	1
Metabolic and other diffuse disorders	326
Anoxia or ischemia	87
Hepatic encephalopathy	17
Uremic encephalopathy	8
Pulmonary disease	3
Endocrine disorders (including diabetes)	12
Acid-base disorders	12
Temperature regulation	9
Nutritional	1
Nonspecific metabolic coma	1
Encephalomyelitis and encephalitis	14
Subarachnoid hemorrhage	13
Drug poisoning	149
Psychiatric disorders	8

*Listed here are only those patients in whom the initial diagnosis was uncertain and a final diagnosis was established. Thus, obvious poisonings and closed-head injuries are underrepresented.

Source: F Plum, JB Posner, *Diagnosis of Stupor and Coma,* 3d ed, Philadelphia, Davis, 1980.

tracranial pressure; whereas hypotension is the usual finding in the states of depressed consciousness that are due to diabetes, alcohol or barbiturate intoxication, internal hemorrhage, myocardial infarction, dissecting aortic aneurysm, gram-negative bacillary septicemia, and Addison's disease.

Inspection of the skin may also yield valuable information. Cyanosis of the lips and nail beds means inadequate oxygenation. Cherry-red coloration indicates carbon monoxide poisoning. Multiple bruises, and in particular a bruise or boggy area in the scalp, bleeding from an ear or the nose, or orbital hemorrhage always raise the possibility of cranial fracture and intracranial trauma. Telangiectases, puffiness of the face, and hyperemia of the face and conjunctivae are the usual stigmata of alcoholism; myxedema also imparts a characteristic puffiness of the face. Marked pallor suggests internal hemorrhage. In pituitary hypoadrenalism the skin is sallow. The presence of a maculohemorrhagic rash indicates the possibility of meningococcal infection, staphylococcal endocarditis, typhus, or Rocky Mountain spotted fever. Pellagra may be recognized by the typical skin lesions on face, arms, and legs. Excessive sweating suggests hypoglycemia or shock, and dry skin suggests diabetic acidosis or uremia. Skin turgor is reduced in dehydration. Blisters, sometimes hemorrhagic, will have formed over pressure points if the patient has been motionless for a time; these blisters are particularly characteristic of acute barbiturate poisoning, and their presence in a comatose patient should always raise this diagnostic possibility.

The odor of the breath may provide a clue to the nature of a disease causing coma. The odor of alcohol is easily recognized (except for vodka, which is odorless). The spoiled-fruit odor of diabetic coma, the uriniferous odor of uremia, and the musty fetor of hepatic coma are distinctive enough to be identified by physicians who possess a keen sense of smell.

Neurologic examination of the stuporous or comatose patient, although limited in many ways, is of crucial importance. Careful observation of what the patient does may yield considerable data concerning the functions of different parts of the nervous system. The predominant postures of the body, the presence or absence of spontaneous movements, the position of the head and eyes, the rate, depth, and rhythm of respiration, and the pulse should be noted. The state of responsiveness should then be estimated by noting the patient's reaction to calling his or her name or a request to execute a simple command, or to painful stimuli such as supraorbital or sternal pressure, or to pinching of the side of the neck or inner parts of the upper arms or thighs. By grading these stimuli, one may evaluate both the degree of unresponsiveness and changes from hour to hour in the course of the disease. Vocalization may persist in stupor and light coma and is the first response to be lost as coma deepens. Grimacing and deft avoidance movements of parts stimulated are preserved in light coma; their presence substantiates the integrity of corticobulbar and corticospinal tracts.

It is usually possible to determine whether or not coma is accompanied by meningeal irritation or focal disease in the cerebrum or brainstem. In all but the deepest forms of coma, meningeal irritation, from either bacterial meningitis or subarachnoid hemorrhage, will cause resistance to passive flexion of the neck but not to extension, turning, or tipping the head. (It should be noted that in some patients the signs of meningeal irritation do not develop for 12 to 24 h after the occurrence of subarachnoid hemorrhage, during which time lumbar puncture is the most reliable diagnostic measure.) Resistance to movement of the neck in all directions indicates disease of the cervical spine or is part of generalized rigidity. In the infant, bulging of the anterior fontanel is at times a more reliable sign of meningitis than stiff neck. A temporal lobe or cerebellar pressure cone or decerebrate rigidity may also limit passive flexion of the neck and may be confused with meningeal irritation.

Evidence of a lesion in a cerebral hemisphere, or in the diencephalon, midbrain, pons, or medulla can be obtained even though the patient is comatose, by noting the residual movements, prevailing postures of the body, rhythm and frequency of respiration, and status of the cranial nerves. This is of more than passing importance, because severe and persistent derangements of these functions are frequent with mass lesions of the brain and are rare in metabolic disorders (except in the terminal stages). A hemiplegia is revealed by lack of restless movements of the arm and leg and of avoidance movements in response to painful stimuli. The paralyzed limbs are slack; if placed in uncomfortable positions, they tend to remain there, and if lifted from the bed, they "fall flail." The hemiplegic leg lies in a position of external rotation (this may also be due to a fractured femur), and the thigh may appear wider and flatter than the nonhemiplegic one. The cheek puffs out in expiration on the paralyzed side, and the eyes are often turned away from the paralysis (toward the lesion). In most cases a hemiplegia reflects a contralateral hemispheral lesion, but with temporal lobe herniation and compression of the cerebral peduncle against the opposite tentorium, the hemiparetic signs may be ipsilateral to the lesion (false localizing sign).

A moan or grimace may be provoked by painful stimuli on one side but not on the other, reflecting a hemianesthesia. A homonymous hemianopia in a stuporous patient may be disclosed by noting whether the patient is attracted to visual stimuli presented on one side and not the other, or fails to blink in reaction to a threatening movement on one side.

Of the various indicators of brainstem function, the most useful are the pattern of breathing, pupillary size and reactivity, ocular movement, and oculovestibular reflexes. These functions, like consciousness itself, are to a large extent dependent upon the integrity of structures in the midbrain and subthalamus.

A massive supratentorial lesion, bilateral deep-seated cerebral lesions, or metabolic disturbances of the brain give rise to a characteristic pattern of breathing, in which a period of waxing-and-waning hyperpnea regularly alternates with a shorter period of apnea (Cheyne-Stokes respiration, or CSR). This means that the respiratory centers in the brainstem, now isolated from the cerebrum, are rendered more sensitive than usual to CO_2 (hyperventilation drive). As a result of overbreathing, the blood CO_2 drops below the level where it stimulates the centers, and breathing stops. CO_2 then reaccumulates until it exceeds the respiratory threshold, and the cycle repeats itself.

Clinically, the presence of CSR signifies bilateral dysfunction of cerebral structures, usually those deep in the hemispheres or diencephalon. In itself, CSR is not a grave sign. Only when it gives way to other abnormal respiratory patterns, which implicate the brainstem more directly, is the patient in imminent danger. Lesions of the lower midbrain-upper pontine tegmentum, either primary or secondary to a tentorial herniation, may give rise to central neurogenic hyperventilation (CNH). Here respirations are increased in rate and in depth, to the extent that respiratory alkalosis may result. The reflex mechanisms for respiratory control in the lower brainstem have in this instance been released, and the threshold of respiratory activation is low. This respiratory drive continues despite low arterial CO_2 tensions and elevated pH. The administration of oxygen does not modify the pattern (unlike its effect in certain cases of pneumonia and pulmonary congestion, in which the drive to hyperventilation is hypoxia).

Low pontine lesions, usually due to basilar artery occlusion, sometimes cause apneustic breathing (a pause

of 2 to 3 s after full inspiration) or other varieties of periodic breathing (short-cycle Cheyne-Stokes respiration) in which the breathing and apneic cycles are very short—there may be three or four rapid, deep breaths, the waxing and waning phases of which consist of only one or two breaths; or seven to ten breaths may alternate with periods of apnea without waxing and waning; or occasional small breaths are interposed between full breaths; or a few breaths are omitted from time to time (respiration alternans). With lesions of the dorsomedial part of the medulla the rhythm of breathing is chaotic, being irregularly interrupted, each breath varying in rate and depth (Biot's breathing). This has also been called "ataxia of breathing," not a very appropriate term. The latter progresses to infrequent, prolonged inspiratory gasps and finally to apnea, as may also CSR or CNH; in fact, respiratory arrest is the mode of death of most patients with serious central nervous system disease. As Fisher and Plum and Posner point out, when certain supratentorial lesions progress to the point where the temporal lobe and cerebellum herniate, one may observe a succession of respiratory patterns (CSR-CNH-Biot's breathing), indicating extension of the functional disorder from upper to lower brainstem. Rapidly evolving lesions of the posterior fossa may cause acute respiratory failure, without intervention of any of the aforementioned abnormalities of breathing. Also it should be noted that in patients with acute head injuries and other forms of diffuse brain damage, the patterns of abnormal breathing may overlap and it is difficult to relate particular breathing patterns with discrete sites of brain damage.

With midbrain lesions the pupils dilate to 4 or 5 mm and become unreactive to light; thus, the preservation of pupillary light reflexes indicates integrity of the pupillary dilation and constriction mechanisms in the midbrain (see Fig. 13-6). Pontine tegmental lesions cause miotic pupils with only slight reaction to strong light. This is characteristic of pontine hemorrhage. Ciliospinal pupillary dilation is also lost in brainstem lesions (see page 188). Horner's syndrome (miosis, ptosis, enophthalmos, and reduced sweating) may be observed homolateral to a lesion of one side of the brainstem, thalamus, or hypothalamus or to a dissecting aneurysm of the internal carotid artery. The pupillary reactions are of great importance, because drug intoxications and metabolic disorders which cause coma usually leave the pupils unaffected. Exceptions are glutethimide (Doriden) and deep ether anesthesia, which cause the pupils to be of medium size or slightly enlarged and unreactive for several hours; opiates (heroin and morphine), which cause pinpoint pupils with so slight a constriction to light that it can be seen only with a magnifying glass; and atropine poisoning, in which the pupils are widely dilated and fixed.

Ocular movements are altered in a variety of ways. In light coma of metabolic origin the eyes rove from side to side in random fashion. These movements disappear as brainstem function becomes depressed. Oculocephalic reflexes (doll's-eye movements), elicited by briskly turning or tilting the head, with eyes moving conjugately in the opposite direction, are not present in the normal person, and if they are elicitable in the comatose patient provide evidence of the integrity of the tegmental structures of the midbrain and pons, which integrate ocular movements, and of the third, fourth, and sixth cranial nerves. Irrigation of each ear with 30 to 100 ml ice water (or just cold water if the patient is not comatose) will normally cause nystagmus (fast component) away from the stimulated side (see page 200). In comatose patients in whom the fast "corrective" phase of nystagmus is lost, the eyes are deflected to the side irrigated with cold water or away from the side irrigated with hot water. The position is held for 2 to 3 min. These vestibuloocular reflexes are also lost with brainstem lesions. If while one is eliciting lateral conjugate movements, only one eye abducts and the other fails to adduct, there is indication of interruption of the medial longitudinal fasciculus (on the side of adductor paralysis). Irrigating both ears simultaneously with ice water with the head flexed 30° from horizontal will induce vertical conjugate movements. An abducens (sixth nerve) palsy is reflected by medial deviation of the eye because of unopposed action of the medial rectus muscle, and oculomotor (third nerve) palsy results in an outward and slight downward position of the eye, from the unopposed action of the lateral rectus and superior oblique muscles. The eyes may be held conjugately to one side at all times—away from the side of the paralysis with large cerebral lesions (looking toward the lesion) and toward the side of the paralysis with unilateral pontine lesions (looking away from the lesion). "Wrong-way" conjugate deviation may occur with thalamic lesions (see page 178). And during a one-sided seizure the eyes turn toward the convulsing side (opposite to the irritative focus). The eyes may be turned down and inward (looking at the nose) in thalamic and upper midbrain lesions (Parinaud's syndrome; see page 178). Retraction and convergence nystagmus and ocular bobbing (see page 186) occur with lesions in the tegmentum of the midbrain and lower pons, respectively. The major brainstem structural lesions, including temporal lobe herniation, abolish most if not all conjugate ocular movements when producing coma, whereas metabolic disorders do not. Of the intoxicants, barbiturates and phenytoin (Di-

lantin) are the only common drugs which abolish ocular movements, but they leave pupillary reactions intact.

Restless movements of the arm(s) and of the leg(s) and grasping and picking movements signify that the corticospinal tract(s) is probably intact. Variable resistance to passive movement (paratonic rigidity) and complex avoidance movements have the same meaning, and if they are bilateral, the coma usually is not profound. Also, the occurrence of focal motor epilepsy usually indicates intactness of the corticospinal motor system. With massive destruction of a cerebral hemisphere, such as occurs in hypertensive hemorrhage, focal seizures are seldom seen on the paralyzed side; seizure activity may occur in the ipsilateral limbs alone, with the paralysis probably preventing the contralateral limbs from participating. Often elaborate forms of semivoluntary movement are present on the "good side" in patients with extensive disease in one hemisphere; they probably represent some type of disequilibrium of cortical and subcortical movement patterns. Definite choreic, athetotic, or hemiballistic movements indicate disorder of the basal ganglionic and subthalamic structures, just as they do in the alert patient.

Postural changes are often instructive in the comatose patient. *Decerebrate rigidity*—jaw clenched, neck retracted, arms and legs stiffly extended and internally rotated—appears with temporal lobe herniation and midbrain compression, with certain metabolic disorders such as hypoglycemia and hypoxia, and rarely with hepatic coma. Occasionally the mechanism of the decerebrate posture is unclear, as with certain bilateral subacute inflammatory, demyelinative, and infarctive cerebral lesions. In some instances the lesions are clearly in the cerebral white matter or basal ganglia, but, of course, functional disorder of structures in the midbrain and upper pons (due to brain swelling, distortion, etc.) cannot be excluded.

Decorticate rigidity, with arm or arms in flexion and adduction and leg(s) extended, signifies higher lesions in cerebral white matter, internal capsules, and thalamus. *Diagonal postures*, e.g., flexion of one arm and extension of the opposite arm and leg, probably mean supratentorial lesions; extended arms and flexed legs are probably fragments of decerebrate postures and point to midpontine lesions. *Abolition of all postures and movements* usually indicates acute interruption of corticospinal function bilaterally and low pontine-medullary lesions involving reticular facilitatory (extrapyramidal) mechanisms. The coma is usually profound.

Lower brainstem reflexes are seldom helpful in the analysis of coma. Only in the most profound metabolic comas and intoxications and in the hypoxic necrosis of the entire brain are coughing, swallowing, and spontaneous respirations all abolished. Further, the tendon and plantar reflexes may give little indication of what is happening. Tendon reflexes are sometimes preserved until the late stages of coma due to metabolic disturbances and intoxications. In coma due to a large cerebral infarction or hemorrhage, the tendon reflexes may be normal or only slightly reduced on the hemiplegic side, and the plantar reflexes may be absent or extensor. Flaccidity and lack of motion in the arm and leg are reliable indicators of a cerebral hemiplegia in an unresponsive patient, except in states of deep coma and decerebrate rigidity.

A history of headache before or at the onset of coma, recurrent vomiting, and papilledema are the best clues to increased intracranial pressure. Papilledema may develop within 12 to 24 h in brain trauma and brain hemorrhage, but, if pronounced, it usually signifies brain tumor or abscess, i.e., a lesion of longer duration. Multiple retinal or large subhyaloid hemorrhages are usually associated with ruptured saccular aneurysm or hemorrhage from an arteriovenous malformation. Papilledema, with widespread retinal exudates, hemorrhages, and arteriolar changes, is an almost invariable accompaniment of malignant hypertension. In patients with evidence of increased intracranial pressure a CT scan should be obtained. Lumbar puncture, although carrying a certain danger because it may promote further herniation, is nevertheless necessary in some instances (to rule out suppurative meningitis, encephalitis, and primary subarachnoid hemorrhage).

LABORATORY PROCEDURES

Unless the diagnosis is established at once by history and physical examination, it is necessary to carry out a number of laboratory procedures. If poisoning is suspected, the gastric contents must be aspirated and saved for chemical analysis. A specimen of urine is obtained by catheter for determination of specific gravity, glucose, acetone, and albumin content. Urine of low specific gravity and high protein content is found in uremia, but proteinuria may also occur for 2 or 3 days after a subarachnoid hemorrhage or with fever. Urine of high specific gravity, glycosuria, and acetonuria are almost invariable in cases of diabetic coma; but glycosuria and

hyperglycemia may result from a massive cerebral lesion. Accurate means are available for measuring the blood levels of phenytoin, bromide, barbiturates, and other substances if drug intoxication is suspected. A blood count is made, and in malarial districts a blood smear is examined for malarial parasites. Neutrophilic leucocytosis occurs in bacterial infections and also with brain hemorrhage and softening. Venous blood should be examined for glucose, nonprotein nitrogen, CO, sodium bicarbonate, pH, NH_3, sodium, potassium, chlorides, Ca, P, and SGOT (serum glutamic oxaloacetic transaminase). The CSF should be examined, as indicated in Chap. 2. Bloody CSF occurs in cerebral contusion, subarachnoid hemorrhage, brain hemorrhage, anthrax meningitis, and occasionally with infarcts due to thrombophlebitis or arterial embolism. If meningitis is suspected, a stained smear of the sediment should be searched for bacteria, and the nature of the cells verified. The standard cerebrospinal fluid formula in bacterial meningitis is elevated pressure, high white blood cell count (5000/20,000), elevated protein level, and subnormal glucose values. The fluid should be submitted for quantitative tests for glucose and protein, bacterial and fungus cultures, and serologic tests for syphilis. If the pressure is greatly elevated (>400 mmH$_2$O), urea, mannitol, or other hypertonic solutions should be given intravenously. Then, using a No. 22 needle, 6 to 10 ml of spinal fluid should be withdrawn over a period of 15 to 20 min. Also, a corticosteroid may be given to reduce brain swelling over a longer period of time. Jugular compression is obviously contraindicated. In appropriate cases, skull films should be obtained as soon as possible after these procedures, preferably between the emergency ward and the hospital room.

CLASSIFICATION OF COMA AND DIFFERENTIAL DIAGNOSIS

The demonstration of focal brain disease or of meningeal irritation with abnormalities of cerebrospinal fluid is of particular help in the differential diagnosis of coma, and serves to divide the diseases that cause coma into three classes, as follows:

I. Diseases that cause no focal or lateralizing neurologic signs or alteration of the cellular content of the cerebrospinal fluid (CSF)
   A. *Intoxications:* alcohol, barbiturates, opiates, etc. (Chaps. 40 and 41)
   B. *Metabolic disturbances:* anoxia, diabetic acidosis, uremia, hepatic coma, hypoglycemia, Addisonian crises (Chap. 39)
   C. *Severe systemic infections:* pneumonia, typhoid fever, malaria, Waterhouse-Friderichsen syndrome

D. Circulatory collapse (shock) from any cause, and cardiac decompensation in the aged

E. Epilepsy (Chap. 15)

F. Hypertensive encephalopathy and eclampsia (Chap. 33)

G. Hyperthermia or hypothermia

H. Concussion (Chap. 34)

II. Diseases that cause meningeal irritation with blood or an excess of white cells in the CSF, usually without focal or lateralizing signs

A. Subarachnoid hemorrhage from ruptured aneurysm, occasionally trauma (Chaps. 33 and 34)

B. Acute bacterial meningitis (Chap. 31)

C. Some forms of viral encephalitis (Chap. 32)

III. Diseases that cause focal or lateralizing neurologic signs, with or without changes in the CSF

A. Brain hemorrhage (Chap. 33)

B. Cerebral infarction due to thrombosis or embolism (Chap. 33)

C. Brain abscess, subdural empyema (Chap. 31)

D. Epidural and subdural hemorrhage and brain contusion (Chap. 34)

E. Brain tumor (Chap. 30)

F. Miscellaneous: e.g., thrombophlebitis, some forms of viral encephalitis, focal embolic encephalomalacia due to bacterial endocarditis, acute hemorrhagic leukoencephalitis, disseminated (postinfectious) encephalomyelitis

Using the clinical criteria outlined above, one can usually ascertain whether a given case of coma falls into one of these three categories. Concerning the group without focal, lateralizing, or meningeal signs [which includes most of the acquired metabolic diseases of the brain, intoxications (both exogenous and endogenous), concussion, and postseizure states], it should be pointed out that residues from a previous neurologic disease may confuse the clinical picture. Thus, an earlier hemiparesis, from vascular disease or trauma, may reassert itself in the course of uremic or hepatic coma, or with hypotension, hypoglycemia, diabetic acidosis, or following a seizure. In hypertensive encephalopathy, focal signs may also be present, and occasionally, for no understandable reason, one leg may seem to move less, or one plantar reflex may be extensor, or seizures may be predominantly or entirely unilateral in a metabolic coma. In actuality, the diagnosis of concussion or of postepileptic coma depends on observation of the precipitating event or indirect evidence thereof. Usually the diagnosis in the latter case is not long obscure, for another seizure or burst of seizures may occur, and recovery of consciousness, once the seizures cease, is usually prompt. The final determination of the exact toxic or metabolic disorder requires the synthesis of a variety of clinical and laboratory data (see Table 16-3).

With respect to the second group in the above outline, the signs of meningeal irritation (head retraction, stiffness of neck on forward bending, Kernig's and Brudzinski's leg-flexion signs) can usually be elicited in both bacterial meningitis and subarachnoid hemorrhage. However, if the coma is profound, stiff neck may be absent. In such cases the spinal fluid has to be examined in order to establish the diagnosis. In bacterial meningitis, unless it is associated with brain swelling and cerebellar herniation, the CSF pressure is not exceptionally high (usually less than 400 mmH$_2$O); if the pressure is high, as death approaches, the pupils become fixed and dilated and there are signs of compression of the medulla, with fall in arterial blood pressure and arrest of respiration. Patients in coma from ruptured aneurysms also have high CSF pressure and often a massive hemispheral and ventricular extension of the hemorrhage.

In patients with the group III type of coma, it is the focality of sensorimotor signs, the aforementioned changes in respiratory pattern, pupillary and ocular reflexes, and the remaining postural states that provide the clues to serious structural lesions in the cerebral hemispheres and their effects upon segmental brainstem functions. As the latter become prominent, they may obscure earlier signs of cerebral disease. It is noteworthy that the comatose state due to bilateral cerebral infarction or traumatic necrosis of and hemorrhage into the cerebral hemispheres may resemble the coma of metabolic and toxic diseases, since brainstem mechanisms may be preserved; contrariwise, hepatic, hypoglycemic, and hypoxic coma will sometimes resemble coma due to brainstem lesions, by causing decerebrate postures. Usually, however, the CSF is bloody and under increased pressure in massive cerebral hemorrhage. Unilateral infarction due to anterior, middle, or posterior cerebral artery occlusion seldom produces more than a stupor or light coma; however, with massive unilateral infarction due to carotid artery occlusion or with bilateral infarction, coma may be profound. Evidence of temporal lobe herniation and brainstem displacement is manifested by increased or altered ventilation (CSR, CNH), bilateral Babinski signs, dilated pupil and ptosis on the side of the lesion, decerebrate postures, and later by dilated pupils and loss of full ocular movements. The coma itself gives no clue as to the nature of the underlying mass lesion. The terminal pattern of a descending gradient of diencephalic, mesencephalic, and pontomedullary paralysis of nervous function is identical in all. Differential diagnosis must depend on the other data.

Table 16-3
Important points in the differential diagnosis of the common causes of coma

General group	Specific disorder	Important clinical findings	Important laboratory findings	Remarks
Coma with focal or lateralizing signs of brain disease	Brain tumor	Stertorous breathing, neurologic signs dependent on location, papilledema	CSF pressure elevated; protein often > 100 mg	Steady progression of signs and symptoms
	Cerebral hemorrhage	Stertorous breathing, hypertension, flushed skin, hemiplegia	CSF grossly bloody and under increased pressure	Sudden onset, elderly patients
	Cerebral thrombosis	Unilateral and bilateral paralysis of abrupt onset	CSF normal or protein modestly elevated	Stupor or coma
	Cerebral embolism	Sudden onset of paralysis	Same as above; occasionally up to 5000 RBC/mm^3	Evidence of heart disease
	Fracture or concussion	Signs of skin trauma	Skull fracture by x-ray; CSF bloody and under increased pressure	Bleeding from nose or ears; history of trauma
	Subdural hematoma	Slow respiration, rising blood pressure, hemiparesis, dilated pupil	Normal or increased CSF pressure; xanthochromia with relatively low protein	History of trauma; progressively severe headache and confusion
	Brain abscess	Neurologic signs depending on location; symptoms and signs of increased intracranial pressure	Fever, leucocytosis; increased pressure, protein and white cells, but normal glucose in CSF	Subacute evolution of headache and neurologic signs on background of sinus, ear, or lung infection or septicemia
	Hypertensive encephalopathy	Headache, severe hypertension, hypertensive retinopathy, convulsions	CSF pressure normal or increased; protein 50-200 mg	Confusion, stupor or coma; rapid evolution; duration, several days
Coma without focal or lateralizing signs but with evidence of meningeal irritation	Meningitis	Stiff neck, positive Kernig's sign, fever, headache	Changes in CSF	Subacute or acute onset
	Subarachnoid hemorrhage	Stertorous breathing, hypertension, stiff neck, positive Kernig's sign	Bloody or xanthochromic CSF under increased pressure	Sudden onset with headache
Coma without focal neurologic signs or evidence of meningeal irritation	Alcohol intoxication	Hypothermia, hypotension, flushed skin, alcohol breath	Elevated blood alcohol	
	Barbiturate intoxication	Hypothermia, hypotension	Barbiturate in urine	History of intake of intoxicating substance
	Opium intoxication	Slow respiration, cyanosis, constricted pupils		Administration of naloxone causes withdrawal signs
	Bromide intoxication	Hyperthermia, delirium	Blood bromides + +	

General group	Specific disorder	Important clinical findings	Important laboratory findings	Remarks
Coma without focal neurologic signs or evidence of meningeal irritation (*continued*)	Carbon monoxide intoxication	Cherry-red skin	Carboxyhemoglobin	
	Anoxia	Rigidity, decerebrate postures, fever, seizures, involuntary movements	CSF normal; EEG may be isoelectric, or show high voltage delta	Abrupt onset following cardiopulmonary failure; damage permanent if anoxia exceeds 3-5 min
	Diabetic coma	Signs of extracellular fluid deficit, hyperventilation with Kussmaul respiration, "fruity" breath	Glycosuria, hyperglycemia, acidosis; reduced serum bicarbonate; ketonemia and ketonuria	History of polyuria, polydipsia, weight loss, or diabetes
	Hypoglycemia	Same as for anoxia	Low blood glucose; coeliac angiography may disclose insulinoma	Characteristic slow evolution through stages of nervousness, hunger, sweating, flushed face; then pallor, shallow respirations and seizures
	Uremia	Hypertension, sallow, dry skin, uriniferous breath, twitch-convulsive syndrome	Protein and casts in urine; elevated BUN and serum creatinine; acidosis, hypocalcemia, etc.; anemia	Progressive apathy, confusion, and asterixis precede coma
	Hepatic coma	Jaundice, ascites and other signs of portal hypertension	Elevated blood NH_3 levels CSF yellow with normal protein	Onset over a few days or after hemorrhage from varices or paracentesis; confusion, stupor, asterixis and characteristic EEG changes precede coma
	Hypercapnia	Papilledema, diffuse myoclonus, asterixis	Increased CSF pressure; P_{CO_2} may exceed 75 mmHg; EEG theta and delta activity	Advanced pulmonary disease; profound coma and brain damage uncommon
	Severe infections; heat stroke	Extreme hyperthermia, rapid respiration	Vary according to cause	Evidence of a specific infection or exposure to extreme heat
	Idiopathic epilepsy	Episodic disturbance of behavior or convulsive movements	Characteristic EEG changes	History of previous attacks

An error which must be cautioned against is the diagnosis of brain-death syndrome on the basis of complete abolition of all brainstem and cerebral activity and isoelectric (flat) EEG, in patients with hypothermia or evidence of intoxication. Only in those with hypoxia and cerebral ischemia can this diagnosis be made securely.

Finally, it should be stated that diagnosis has as its prime purpose the direction of therapy, and it matters little to the patient whether or not we diagnose a disease for which we have no treatment. The treatable causes of coma are drug intoxications, shock due to infection or exsanguination, epidural and subdural hematoma, brain abscess, bacterial, fungal and tuberculous meningitis, diabetic acidosis, hypoglycemia, and hypertensive encephalopathy.

CARE OF THE COMATOSE PATIENT

Impaired states of consciousness, regardless of their cause, are often fatal because they not only represent an advanced stage of many diseases but also add their own characteristic burden to the primary disease. The physician's main objective, of course, is to find the cause of the coma, according to the procedures already outlined, and to treat it appropriately. It often happens, however, that the disease process is one for which there is no specific therapy; or, as in hypoxia or hypoglycemia, the disease process may already have expended itself before the patient comes to the attention of the physician. Again, the problem may be infinitely complex, for the disturbance may be attributable not to a single cause but rather to several possible factors acting in unison, no one of which could account for the total clinical picture. In lieu of direct therapy, supportive measures must be used, and, indeed, it may be said that the patient's chances of surviving the original disease often depend in large measure on their effectiveness.

The successful management of the insensate patient requires the services of a well-coordinated team of nurses under the constant guidance of a physician. The necessary treatment must be instituted immediately, even if all the diagnostic needs have not been fulfilled; diagnosis and treatment have to proceed concurrently, not seriatim. The following is a brief outline of the principles involved in the treatment of such patients. The details of management of shock, fluid and electrolyte imbalance, and other complications that threaten the comatose patient (pneumonia, urinary tract infections,

phlebothrombosis, etc.) are found in *Harrison's Principles of Internal Medicine.*

1. The management of shock, if it is present, takes precedence over all other diagnostic and therapeutic measures.

2. Shallow and irregular respirations, stertorous breathing (indicating obstruction to inspiration), and cyanosis require the establishment of a clear airway and delivery of oxygen. The patient should be placed in a lateral position so that secretions and vomitus do not enter the tracheobronchial tree. Pharyngeal reflexes are usually suppressed, and therefore an endotracheal tube can be inserted without difficulty. Stagnant secretions should be removed by suctioning as soon as they accumulate, since they will lead to atelectasis and bronchopneumonia. Oxygen can be administered by mask in a 100% concentration for 6 to 12 h, alternating with 50% concentration for 5 h. The depth of respiration can be increased by the use of 5 to 10% carbon dioxide for periods of 3 to 5 min every hour. Atropine should not be given; edema of the lungs and fluid in the tracheobronchial passages are not glandular secretions. Furthermore, atropine thickens this fluid and also may disturb temperature regulation. Aminophylline is helpful in controlling Cheyne-Stokes breathing. Respiratory paralysis dictates the use of endotracheal intubation and a positive-pressure respirator, but in the authors' experience neither has been effective in comatose states in which there is disorganization of the respiratory centers.

3. Concomitantly, an intravenous line should be established and blood samples drawn for the measurement of the blood elements as well as glucose, toxins, and electrolytes and for tests of liver and kidney function. Arterial blood gases should also be measured. Naloxone, 0.5 mg, should be given intravenously if a narcotic overdose is suspected.

4. A lumbar puncture should be performed if meningitis or subarachnoid hemorrhage is suspected. If there are signs of increased intracranial pressure, mannitol, 50 g, in a 20% solution, should be given intravenously over 10 to 20 min. Corticosteroids help to maintain the reduction in intracranial pressure. CT scan may disclose subarachnoid hemorrhage (no lumbar puncture necessary).

5. Convulsions should be controlled by measures outlined in Chap. 15.

6. If coma is due to drug ingestion, gastric aspiration and lavage with normal saline may be useful. Salicylates, opiates, and anticholinergic drugs (tricyclic antidepressants, phenothiazines, scopolamine), all of which induce gastric atony, may be recovered many hours after ingestion. Caustic materials should not be lavaged be-

cause of the danger of perforation. Lavage of strychnine and other analeptic drugs carries the danger of precipitating seizures and cardiac arrhythmias. Emesis induced by ipecac or apomorphine should be reserved for alert patients.

7. The temperature-regulating mechanisms may be disturbed, and extreme hypothermia, hyperthermia, or poikilothermia may occur. In hyperthermia, removal of blankets and use of alcohol sponges and a cooling mattress are indicated.

8. The bladder should not be permitted to become distended; if the patient does not void, a retention catheter should be inserted. If the bladder is found to be greatly distended, decompression should be carried out slowly, over a period of hours. Urine excretion should be kept between 500 and 1000 ml/day. The patient should not be permitted to lie in a wet or soiled bed.

9. Diseases of the central nervous system may upset the control of water, glucose, and salt. The unconscious patient can no longer adjust the intake of food and fluids by hunger and thirst. Salt-losing and salt-retaining syndromes have both been described with brain disease. Water intoxication and severe hyponatremia may of themselves prove fatal. If coma is prolonged, the insertion of a stomach tube will ease the problems of feeding the patient and maintaining fluid and electrolyte balance.

10. Aspiration pneumonia should be avoided by prevention of vomiting (stomach tube), position, and restriction of oral fluids. Should it occur, corticosteroid therapy is beneficial. The legs should be examined each day for signs of phlebothrombosis.

11. If the patient is capable of moving, suitable restraints should be used to prevent falling out of bed.

REFERENCES

BENNETT DR et al: *Atlas of Electroencephalography in Coma and Cerebral Death.* New York, Raven, 1976.

CARONNA JJ, SIMON RP: The comatose patient: A diagnostic approach and treatment. *Int Anesthesiol Clin* 17(2/3):3, 1979.

FISHER CM: The neurological examination of the comatose patient. *Acta Neurol Scand Suppl* 36, 1969.

FREDERIKS JAM: Consciousness, in Vinken PJ, Bruyn GW (eds): *Disorders of Higher Nervous Function, Handbook of Clinical Neurology,* vol 4. Amsterdam, North-Holland, 1969, chap 4, p 48.

JENNETT B, PLUM F: Persistent vegetative state after brain damage. *Lancet* 1:734, 1972.

MOLLARET P, GOULON M: Le coma dépassé. *Rev Neurol* 101:3, 1959.

PLUM F, POSNER JB: *Diagnosis of Stupor and Coma,* 3d ed. Philadelphia, Davis, 1980.

POSNER JB: The comatose patient. *JAMA* 232:1313, 1975.

CHAPTER 17

FAINTNESS AND SYNCOPE

The term *syncope* (Greek, *synkope*) literally means a "cessation, a cutting short, or pause." Medically, it refers to an episodic interruption of consciousness and is synonymous in everyday language with *faint*. The terms faint and faintness are also commonly used to describe the sudden loss of strength and other symptoms that characterize the impending or incomplete fainting spell. This latter state is referred to as *presyncope*, whereas syncope comprises the more advanced or complete state with generalized loss of postural tone, inability to stand, and loss of consciousness. Relatively abrupt onset, brief duration, and complete recovery are other distinguishing features.

Faintness and syncope are among the most common nervous symptoms. Practically every adult has experienced some presyncopal symptoms, if not a fully developed syncopal attack, or has observed such an attack in others. Description of these symptoms, as with other purely subjective states, is often ambiguous. The patient, usually untrained in introspection, may refer to them as light-headedness, giddiness, dizziness, "drunk feeling," weak spells, or if consciousness was lost, as "blackouts." Careful questioning may be necessary to ascertain that these words refer to sudden weakness and an impaired alertness. In many instances the condition is clarified by the fact that these symptoms have proceeded to a sensation of faintness and then a momentary loss of consciousness, which is easily recognized as a faint, or syncope. This sequence also informs us that under certain conditions any difference between faintness and syncope appears to be only quantitative. These symptoms must be clearly set apart from disorders such as cataplexy, transient ischemic attacks, "drop attacks," or vertigo, which are also characterized by episodic attacks of generalized weakness or inability to stand upright, without

loss of consciousness, and from epilepsy, the other major cause of episodic unconsciousness.

CLINICAL FEATURES OF SYNCOPE

Faints may vary somewhat, according to their mechanisms, but all of them conform roughly to the following pattern.

Though the syncopal attack may develop rapidly, it is doubtful if consciousness is ever abolished as abruptly as with a seizure. Even with an arrest of cardiac function, i.e., cardiac syncope, the onset requires several seconds. With few exceptions, e.g., the Stokes-Adams syndrome, the patient is usually in the upright position at the beginning of the attack, either sitting or standing. A number of subjective symptoms, known as the prodrome, mark the onset of the faint. The person feels uneasy and queasy, is assailed by giddiness, a sense of swaying, and a severe headache. What is most noticeable, even at the beginning of the attack, is a pallor or ashen-gray color of the face, and often the face and body become bathed in a cold perspiration. Nausea and sometimes vomiting may accompany these symptoms; patients try to protect themselves by yawning, sighing, or breathing deeply. Vision may dim and the ears ring, and it may be impossible to think clearly. If the person can lie down promptly, the attack may be averted without complete loss of consciousness; otherwise, consciousness is lost and the patient falls to the ground. As a rule, the deliberate onset enables patients to lie down or at least to protect themselves as they slump. A hurtful fall is exceptional.

The depth and duration of the unconsciousness vary. Sometimes the person is not completely oblivious of the surroundings. It may still be possible to hear voices or see the blurred outlines of people or there may be a complete lack of awareness and responsiveness. The patient may remain in this state for seconds to minutes, rarely longer, unless for some reason kept in the upright position.

If unconsciousness persists for 15 to 20 s, convulsive movements may occur. These usually take the form of tonic extension of the trunk and clenching of the jaw, or brief, mild, clonic jerks of the limbs and trunk and twitchings of the face. Occasionally the extensor rigidity and jerking flexor movements are severe, lasting for 2 to 3 min. Very rarely is there a generalized tonic-clonic convulsion. Usually the person who has fainted lies motionless, with skeletal muscles fully relaxed. Sphincteric control is maintained in nearly all cases. The pulse is thin and slow or cannot be felt; the systolic blood pressure is reduced (to 60 mmHg or less, as a rule), and breathing is almost imperceptible. The depressed vital functions, the striking pallor, and unconsciousness simulate death.

Once the patient is horizontal from having fallen or deliberately lain down, gravitation no longer hinders the flow of blood to the brain. The strength of the pulse soon improves, and color begins to return to the face. Breathing becomes quicker and deeper. Then the eyelids flutter, and consciousness is quickly regained. There is from this moment onward a correct perception of the environment. Confusion, headache, and drowsiness, the common sequelae of a convulsive seizure, do not follow a syncopal attack. The patient is nevertheless keenly aware of physical weakness, and by arising too soon, may precipitate another faint.

CAUSES OF EPISODIC FAINTNESS AND SYNCOPE

The following classification is based on established or assumed physiologic mechanisms.

I. Circulatory (deficient quantity of blood to the brain)
  A. Inadequate vasoconstrictor mechanisms
    1. Vasodepressor (vasovagal)
    2. Postural hypotension
    3. Primary autonomic insufficiency
    4. Sympathectomy (pharmacologic or surgical)
    5. Peripheral and central nervous system diseases
    6. Carotid sinus irritability
  B. Hypovolemia
  C. Mechanical reduction in venous return to heart
    1. Valsalva maneuver
    2. Cough
    3. Micturition
    4. Atrial myxoma (ball-valve thrombus)
  D. Reduced cardiac output
    1. Obstruction to left ventricular outflow: aortic stenosis, hypertrophic subaortic stenosis

    2. Obstruction to pulmonary flow: pulmonic stenosis, tetralogy of Fallot, primary pulmonary hypertension, pulmonary embolism
    3. Myocardial: massive myocardial infarction with "pump" failure
    4. Pericardial: cardiac tamponade
  E. Cardiac arrhythmias
    1. Bradyarrhythmias
      a. Atrioventricular (AV) block (second- and third-degree) with Stokes-Adams attacks
      b. Ventricular asystole
      c. Sinus bradycardia, sinoatrial block, sinus arrest
      d. Carotid sinus syncope (see also "Inadequate Vasoconstrictor Mechanism")
      e. Vagoglossopharyngeal neuralgias (and other painful states)
    2. Tachyarrhythmias
      a. Episodic ventricular fibrillation with or without associated bradyarrhythmias
      b. Ventricular tachycardia
      c. Supraventricular tachycardia without AV block
II. Other causes of episodic faintness and syncope
  A. Altered state of blood to the brain
    1. Hypoxia
    2. Anemia
    3. Diminished CO_2 due to hyperventilation (faintness common, syncope rare)
    4. Hypoglycemia (faintness frequent, syncope rare)
  B. Emotional disturbances
    1. Hysterical fainting
    2. Anxiety attacks (weakness common, syncope rare)

This list of conditions which cause faintness and syncope is deceptively long and involved. It will be recognized that the usual types are reducible to a few simple mechanisms, viz., a temporary reduction in the flow of blood to the brain (which in turn is due to a decrease in peripheral resistance, as in vasovagal syncope, or to a diminished cardiac output, as in the Stokes-Adams attack), or an altered state of the blood itself, so that an essential component, such as O_2, CO_2, or glucose, is not delivered to the brain in adequate amount. In order not to obscure the central problem of fainting by too many details, only the varieties of fainting commonly encountered in clinical practice will be discussed below.

COMMON TYPES OF SYNCOPE

Vasodepressor (Vasovagal) Syncope This is the common faint. It always occurs when the patient is in the erect position, and may be averted or relieved by lying down. There is a short premonitory phase of pallor, nausea, epigastric distress, perspiration, yawning, tachypnea, and weakness, with pupillary dilatation and bradycardia. The period of unconsciousness lasts only a few seconds or minutes. Jaw clenching, extensor rigidity or clonic movements may occur 15 to 20 s after the loss of consciousness. Sudden vasodilatation, particularly of intramuscular arterioles, caused by strong emotion or physical injury, is thought to be the initial event. Peripheral vascular resistance decreases due to active vasodilatation of "resistance vessels" and blood pressure falls. Cardiac output fails to exhibit the expected rise which normally occurs in hypotension. Vagal stimulation may then occur (hence the term *vasovagal*), causing bradycardia, possibly leading to a further drop in blood pressure and perspiration, increased peristaltic activity, nausea, and salivation. The loss of consciousness and pallor are caused by inadequate flow of blood to the brain and extracranial structures.

Although bradycardia does appear in the course of the common fainting spell, it probably contributes little to the loss of consciousness. The term vasovagal is therefore not entirely apt and should be avoided as a synonym for vasodepressor syncope.

The common, or vasodepressor, faint occurs (1) in normal health under the influence of strong emotion (sight of blood or an accident) or in conditions which favor peripheral vasodilatation, e.g., hot, crowded rooms ("heat syncope"), especially if the person is hungry or tired or has had a few drinks, or (2) during a painful illness or after bodily injury as a consequence of fright, pain, and other factors. Where pain is involved, the vasovagal element is more prominent in the genesis of the faint.

Postural (Orthostatic) Hypotension with Syncope This type affects persons whose vasomotor reflexes are variably unstable or defective. Although the character of the faint differs little from the vasodepressor type, the effect of posture in its initiation is its most typical attribute. Sudden arising from a recumbent position or prolonged periods of standing are the circumstances under which it is most likely to happen.

Postural syncope tends to occur under the following conditions: (1) in individuals who for an unknown reason have defective pressor-receptor reflexes (pressor-receptors are sensory receptors in blood vessels that are sensitive to changes in pressure); (2) as part of a syndrome known as chronic orthostatic hypotension or pri-

mary autonomic insufficiency (see below); (3) after prolonged illness with recumbency, especially in elderly individuals with flabby muscles; (4) in association with diseases of the peripheral nerves, including autonomic nerves (diabetic neuropathy, tabes dorsalis, amyloid and other polyneuropathies, which interrupt vasomotor reflexes and also cause the muscles to be weak and flabby; (5) after sympathectomy; (6) in persons with large varicose veins of the legs which facilitate the pooling of blood; (7) in patients receiving L-dopa, antihypertensive drugs (particularly ganglionic blocking agents such as guanethidine), and certain sedative and antidepressant drugs; and (8) in patients who are hypovolemic from diuretics, excessive sweating, or acute hemorrhage (as occurs with a bleeding peptic ulcer).

These conditions are easily understood if one keeps in mind that the pooling of blood in the lower parts of the body is normally prevented by (1) reflex arteriolar and arterial constriction, (2) reflex acceleration of the heart by means of aortic and carotid reflexes, and (3) muscular activity which improves venous return. A normal individual placed on a table to relax the muscles and tilted with head upward has some accumulation of venous blood in the legs and a slightly diminished cardiac output. This is followed by a transitory fall in blood pressure and then a compensatory rise. However, in about 20 percent of normal persons, after the blood pressure has fallen slightly and stabilized at a lower level, the compensatory reflexes suddenly fail, with a precipitant drop in pressure. A strong autonomic reaction then occurs, with pallor, sweating, nausea, etc., and sometimes a brief faint.

Primary Autonomic Insufficiency (Idiopathic Orthostatic Hypotension) When the autonomic nervous system is defective for any reason, the patient, on assuming an upright position, shows a steady fall in blood pressure to a level at which cerebral circulation cannot be supported. Compensatory tachycardia does not occur, however, and contrary to what occurs in vasopressor syncope, there are no autonomic responses such as pallor, sweating, or nausea, and there is no release of norepinephrine. Clouding of the sensorium may precede unconsciousness or be the only evidence of cerebral disorder.

Primary autonomic insufficiency, also called *idiopathic orthostatic hypotension*, presents in two forms. In one there is probably a selective degeneration of neurons in the sympathetic ganglia with denervation of smooth muscle and glands (pathology not fully delineated); in the other there is a degeneration of preganglionic neurons in the lateral columns of gray matter in the spinal cord, leaving postganglionic neurons isolated from spinal control. The latter lesion is often associated with degeneration of other systems of neurons in the central nervous system. Three pathologic syndromes have been identified: (1) degeneration of the substantia nigra and locus ceruleus (described by Shy and Drager), (2) striatonigral degeneration, and (3) cerebellar and spinocerebellar degenerations. In the first two syndromes, Parkinson's syndrome is combined with orthostatic hypotension; in the third, with cerebellar ataxia.

All these forms of autonomic degeneration have their onset in adult life, and hypotension and syncope are usually part of a more widespread paralysis of autonomic function that includes loss of sweating in the lower parts of the body, atonicity of the bladder, and impotence in the male. These conditions are discussed more fully in Chap. 26.

Micturition syncope is a condition usually seen in men, often in young adults as well as in the elderly, who arise from bed at night to urinate. The syncope occurs at the end of micturition or soon thereafter, and the loss of consciousness is abrupt, with rapid and complete recovery. The mechanism is not fully understood. A full bladder tends to cause vasoconstriction; as the bladder empties it gives way to vasodilatation which, in the erect posture, might be sufficient to cause fainting in some individuals. Vagally mediated bradycardia may also be a factor, and alcohol ingestion, hunger, fatigue, and upper respiratory infection are common predisposing factors. In some instances, especially in the elderly, the nocturnal collapse has led to serious head injury.

Syncope may occur occasionally in the course of prostatic examination, but only if the patient is standing (*prostatic syncope*). The Valsalva maneuver and reflex vagal stimulation may be contributing factors.

Hyperbradykininism is the term applied to a syndrome of orthostatic hypotension, characterized by postural faintness and syncope, a rise in heart rate, facial erythema, and purple discoloration of the legs after standing. Most of the patients have been young females. The syndrome is familial and associated with abnormally high plasma concentrations of the polypeptide bradykinin, which presumably causes dilatation of cutaneous venules and capillaries in the legs and reduction in venous return. Improvement has attended the use of propranolol, fludrocortisone and cyproheptadine.

Syncope of Cardiac Origin   This is due to a sudden reduction in cardiac output, usually because of a dysrhythmia. Normally, a pulse as low as 35 to 40 beats per minute or as high as 150 beats per minute is well tolerated, especially if the patient is recumbent. Changes in pulse rate beyond these extremes impair cerebral circulation and lead to syncope. Upright posture, anemia,

coronary and myocardial lesions, and valvular disease all render the individual more susceptible to these alterations.

Syncope of cardiac origin occurs most frequently in patients with complete atrioventricular block and a pulse rate of 40 or less per minute (Adams-Stokes-Morgagni syndrome). The causation of heart block need not concern us here. The block may be persistent or intermittent; it is often preceded by disturbed conduction in two or three fascicles of the conduction system or by a second-degree heart block. When the block is complete and the pacemaker below the block fails to function, ventricular contraction ceases altogether. Ventricular arrest of 4 to 8 s, if the patient is upright, is enough to cause coma; when the patient is supine the asystole must last 12 to 15 s. At 12 s, according to Engel, the patient turns pale and is momentarily weak or may lose consciousness without warning. This may occur at any time of day or night and regardless of the position of the body. If the duration of cerebral ischemia exceeds 15 to 20 s there may be a few tonic spasms or clonic jerks, and if it persists up to 5 min, the ashen-gray pallor gives way to cyanosis, stertorous breathing, incontinence, fixed pupils, and bilateral Babinski signs. As heart action is resumed, the face and neck become flushed. In cases of prolonged asystole there may be cerebral injury, caused by a combination of hypoxia and ischemia. Coma may persist or may be replaced by confusion, and other neurologic signs and focal ischemic changes, often irreversible, may then be traced to the field of occluded atherosclerotic cerebral arteries. Cardiac faints of the Stokes-Adams type may recur several times a day. Occasionally the heart block is transitory, and between attacks the electrocardiogram may show only evidence of myocardial disease. A continuous taped electrocardiogram or monitor is then needed to demonstrate the intermittent AV block.

Less often there is a decreased rate of discharge of the sinoatrial node (from sinoatrial block or sinus pauses). The lesion in the node is usually due to ischemia, inflammatory disease (myocarditis), augmented vagal activity, or cardiodepressant drugs (quinidine), but it may immediately follow tachycardia. A bout of ventricular fibrillation or some other tachyrhythmia such as atrial flutter and paroxysmal atrial and ventricular tachycardia with normal AV conduction may also reduce cardiac output to a degree sufficient to cause syncope.

In other types of cardioinhibitory syncope, the

heart block is purely reflexive, because of irritation of the vagus nerves (from esophageal diverticula, mediastinal tumors, gallbladder stones, carotid sinus disease, vagoglossopharyngeal neuralgia, bronchoscopy and needling of body cavities). Here the reflex bradycardia is more often of sinoatrial than atrioventricular type. Weiss and Ferris called such faints "vagovagal."

Cardiac syncope may also result from acute massive myocardial infarction, particularly when associated with cardiogenic shock; fright, pain, or arrhythmias may also be involved. Aortic stenosis often sets the stage for exertional syncope, because cardiac output is inadequate to meet the demands of exercise. This may result in myocardial and cerebral ischemia and arrhythmias. Idiopathic hypertrophic subaortic stenosis may also lead to exertional syncope by the same mechanism. In primary pulmonary hypertension bouts of right-sided heart failure may be associated with syncope. However, vagal overactivity may be responsible for the syncope in this condition, as well as for the syncope that accompanies pulmonary embolism. Ball-valve thrombus in the left atrium, left atrial myxoma, malfunction of a prosthetic valve, or cardiac tamponade from rupture of a dissecting aortic aneurysm may produce sudden mechanical obstruction of the circulation and syncope. Tetralogy of Fallot is the congenital cardiac malformation that most often leads to syncope. Here systemic vasodilatation, possibly associated with infundibular spasm, greatly increases right-left cardiac shunting, thereby producing hypoxia.

Carotid Sinus Syncope The carotid sinus is normally sensitive to stretch and gives rise to sensory impulses carried via the nerve of Hering, a branch of the glossopharyngeal nerve, to the medulla oblongata. Massage of one of the carotid sinuses or of both of them alternately, particularly in elderly persons, causes (1) a reflex cardiac slowing (sinus bradycardia, sinus arrest, or even atrioventricular block), the so-called vagal type of response, or (2) a fall of arterial pressure without cardiac slowing, the *depressor type* of response, or (3) possibly an interference with the circulation of the ipsilateral cerebral hemisphere, the *central type*.

Faintness or syncope due to carotid sinus sensitivity has reportedly been initiated by turning of the head to one side while wearing a tight collar, or even by shaving over the region of the sinus. But the absence of such stimuli is of no aid in diagnosis, since spontaneous attacks may occur. The attack nearly always begins when the patient is upright, usually standing. The onset is sudden, often with falling. Convulsive movements occur quite frequently in the vagal and depressor types of carotid sinus syncope. A central type was described by Weiss et al., but the authors find it difficult to distinguish from carotid stenosis due to atherosclerosis. The latter condition is characterized by homolateral blindness or contralateral sensory or motor deficits. The period of unconsciousness in carotid sinus syncope seldom lasts longer than a few minutes. The sensorium is immediately clear when consciousness is regained. The majority of the reported cases have been in males.

In a patient displaying faintness on massage of one carotid sinus, it is important to distinguish between the benign disorder (hypersensitivity of one carotid sinus) and a much more serious condition—atheromatous narrowing of the opposite carotid or of the basilar artery (see Chap. 33). In testing for carotid sinus sensitivity in the latter circumstances, it is important to avoid compression of the carotid artery, which may represent the major vascular supply to both hemispheres.

Vagoglossopharyngeal Neuralgia This is known occasionally to induce a reflex type of fainting. Again the sequence is always pain, then syncope; in this instance the pain is localized to the base of the tongue, pharynx or larynx, tonsillar areas, and an ear. It may be triggered by pressure at these sites or simply by chewing or swallowing. Section of the appropriate branches of the ninth and tenth cranial nerve relieves the condition (see page 130). It has been suggested that the cardiovascular effects are attributable to excitation of the dorsal motor nucleus of the vagus via collateral fibers from the nucleus of the tractus solitarius. Other examples of fainting due to reflex vagal stimulation have been mentioned above, in the discussion of cardiac syncope.

Tussive Syncope ("Laryngeal Vertigo") This is a rare condition that results from a severe paroxysm of coughing, first described by Charcot, in 1876. Patients with this type of syncope are usually heavy-set males who smoke and have chronic bronchitis. Occasionally it occurs in children, particularly following paroxysmal coughing spells of pertussis and laryngitis. After hard coughing, the patient suddenly becomes weak and may lose consciousness momentarily. The intrathoracic pressure becomes elevated and interferes with the venous return to the heart. The Valsalva maneuver of trying to exhale against a closed glottis produces the same effect. The unconsciousness that results from breath holding in infants is probably based on this mechanism as well. The loss of consciousness that occurs during competitive weight lifting ("weight-lifters' blackout") also is due to the Valsalva maneuver, compounded by the effects of vascular dilatation, produced by squatting and hyperventilation. Lesser degrees of this phenomenon (faintness and light-headedness) not infrequently follow other kinds of strenuous activity such as laughing, straining at stool, or lifting.

Syncope Associated with Cerebrovascular Disease This is infrequent and has usually been caused by partial or complete occlusion of the large arteries in the neck. The best examples are found in the "aortic-arch syndrome" (pulseless disease), in which the brachiocephalic and common carotid and vertebral arteries have become narrowed. Physical activity may then critically reduce blood flow to the upper part of the brainstem, causing abrupt loss of consciousness; stenosis or occlusion of vertebral arteries and the "vertebral steal syndrome" are other examples (see Chap. 33). Fainting is said also to occur occasionally in patients with congenital anomalies of the upper cervical part of the spine (Klippel-Feil syndrome) or cervical spondylosis, in which the vertebral circulation is compromised. Head turning may then cause vertigo, nausea and vomiting, visual scotomas, and finally unconsciousness.

Hysterical Fainting Hysterical fainting is rather frequent and usually occurs under dramatic circumstances (Chap. 53). The attack is unattended by any outward display of anxiety. The evident lack of change in pulse and blood pressure or color of the skin distinguishes it from the vasodepressor faint. The diagnosis is based on these negative findings in a person who exhibits the general personality and behavioral characteristics of hysteria. Several interesting instances of mass faintness and syncope of hysterical type have been described in school marching bands (Levine).

PATHOPHYSIOLOGY OF SYNCOPE

In the final analysis the loss of consciousness in these different types of syncope must be caused by a change in the neural elements in those parts of the brain which subserve consciousness (high brainstem reticular activating system). In this respect syncope and epilepsy have a common ground; yet there is an important difference. In epilepsy, whether major or minor, the arrest in mental function is almost instantaneous, and, as revealed by the EEG, it is accompanied by a paroxysm of activity occurring simultaneously in all of the cerebral cortex. Syncope, on the other hand, is not so sudden. The difference relates to the essential pathophysiology—a sudden spread of an electric discharge in epilepsy, and the more gradual failure of the cerebral circulation in syncope.

During syncopal attacks, there are demonstrable reductions in cerebral blood flow, cerebral oxygen utilization, and cerebral vascular resistance. It has been estimated that the critical level of blood flow necessary to maintain consciousness is about 30 ml per 100 g brain per minute (normal 50 to 55 ml). If the ischemia lasts only a few minutes, there are no lasting effects on the brain. If it persists for a longer time, it may result in necrosis of the border zones between the major cerebral or cerebellar arteries.

The EEG changes during syncope have been investigated by Gastaut and Fischer-Williams. Attacks of cardiac arrest and syncope were produced by compression of the eyeballs (oculovagal reflex) in 20 of 100 patients who had a history of syncopal attacks—mainly of the vasopressor type. These investigators found that after a 7- to 13-s period of cardiac arrest there was a loss of consciousness, pallor, and muscle relaxation. Toward the end of this period, runs of bilaterally synchronous theta and delta waves appeared, predominantly in the frontal lobes, and in some patients one or more myoclonic jerks occurred in time with the slow waves. If the cardiac arrest persisted beyond 14 or 15 s, the EEG became flat. This period of electrical silence lasted for 10 to 20 s and was sometimes accompanied by a generalized tonic spasm with incontinence. Following the spasm, heartbeats and large-amplitude delta waves reappeared, and after another 20 to 30 s the EEG reverted to normal. It is noteworthy that rhythmic clonic seizures or epileptiform EEG activity was not observed at any time during the periods of cardiac arrest, syncope, and tonic spasm.

DIFFERENTIAL DIAGNOSIS

OF CONDITIONS ASSOCIATED WITH EPISODIC WEAKNESS AND FAINTNESS BUT RARELY WITH SYNCOPE

Anxiety Attacks and the Hyperventilation Syndrome These are discussed in detail in Chaps. 24 and 53. The giddiness of anxiety and hyperventilation is frequently described as a feeling of faintness, but consciousness is not lost. Such symptoms are not accompanied by facial pallor and not relieved by recumbency. The diagnosis is made on the basis of the associated symptoms, and part of the attack can be reproduced by having the patient hyperventilate. Two of the mechanisms known to be involved in the attacks are reduction in carbon dioxide as the result of hyperventilation, and the release of epinephrine. Hyperventilation results in hypocapnia, alkalosis, increased cerebrovascular resistance, and decreased cerebral blood flow.

Hypoglycemia Another cause of obscure episodic weakness is hypoglycemia. When severe, hypoglycemia is usually traceable to a serious disease, such as a tumor of the islets of Langerhans or advanced adrenal, pituitary, or hepatic disease. The clinical picture is one of trembling, flushed facies, and sweating, progressing to confusion or even seizures and coma. When mild, hypoglycemia is usually of the reactive type, occurring 2 to 5 h after eating, and is not associated with a disturbance of consciousness. The diagnosis depends largely upon the history, documentation of reduced blood glucose during an attack, and the reproduction by an injection of insulin or an oral dose of tolbutamide (or ingestion of a high-carbohydrate meal, in the case of reactive hypoglycemia) of a symptom complex exactly the same as that occurring in the spontaneous attacks.

Acute Hemorrhage Acute blood loss, usually within the gastrointestinal tract, is a cause of weakness, faintness, or even unconsciousness. In the absence of pain and hematemesis, the cause (peptic ulcer is the most common) may remain obscure until the passage of a black stool.

Transient Cerebral Ischemic Attacks These occur in some patients with arteriosclerotic narrowing or occlusion of the major arteries of the brain. The main symptoms, varying from patient to patient, include dim vision, hemiparesis, numbness of one side of the body, dizziness, and thick speech; to these may be added an impairment of consciousness. In any one patient the attacks are usually of one type and indicate a temporary deficit of function in a certain region of the brain due to inadequate circulation. The mechanism of the deficit has not been fully elucidated; recurrent embolism is the probable explanation in some cases (see Chap. 33).

Drop attacks is another condition that has been attributed to vascular disease of the brainstem but the evidence is far from convincing. The patient, usually elderly and more often female, while walking suddenly falls down. The knees inexplicably buckle. There is no dizziness or loss of consciousness and the fall is forward with scuffing of knees and sometimes the nose. Immediately the patient arises, unless obese, and goes her way quite embarrassed. There may be several attacks during

a period of a few weeks and none thereafter. EEGs are normal. There is no treatment. Drop attacks occur in hydrocephalics, and the patient, though conscious, may not be able to arise for several hours. Seizures of akinetic type also cause drop attacks, but nearly always with brief loss of consciousness.

OF SEIZURE AND SYNCOPE

Fully developed syncope must be distinguished from other cerebral disturbances causing loss of consciousness, the most frequent of which is akinetic or some other form of epilepsy (see Chap. 15). The epileptic attack may occur day or night, regardless of the position of the patient; syncope rarely appears when the patient is recumbent, the only common exception being the Stokes-Adams attack. The patient's color does not usually change at the onset of an epileptic attack; pallor is an early and invariable finding in all types of syncope, except chronic orthostatic hypotension and hysteria, and it precedes unconsciousness. Epilepsy is more sudden in onset; if an aura is present, it rarely lasts longer than a few seconds before consciousness is abolished. The onset of syncope is usually more deliberate, and the prodromal symptoms are quite distinctive and different from those of seizures. Injury from falling is frequent in epilepsy and rare in syncope, for the reason that only in the former are protective reflexes instantaneously abolished. Tonic spasm of muscles with upturning eyes is a prominent and often an initial feature of epilepsy but occurs only rarely and late in the course of a faint; however, several clonic contractions of the limbs may occur several seconds after the patient has fainted (see above). The period of unconsciousness and subsequent confusion tends to be longer in epilepsy than in syncope. Urinary incontinence is frequent in epilepsy and rare in syncope, but it may not occur during an epileptic attack, in which case it cannot be used as a means of excluding the latter disorder. The return of consciousness is slow in epilepsy, prompt in syncope; mental confusion, headache, and drowsiness are common sequelae in the former state, and physical weakness with clear sensorium characterizes the latter. Repeated spells of unconsciousness in a young person at a rate of several per day or month are much more suggestive of epilepsy than of syncope. No one of these points will absolutely differentiate epilepsy from syncope, but taken as a group and supplemented by electroencephalograms, they usually enable one to distinguish the two conditions.

OF DIFFERENT TYPES OF SYNCOPE

When faintness is related to reduced cerebral blood flow resulting directly from a disorder of cardiac function, there may be a combination of pallor and cyanosis, with pronounced dyspnea, and often the jugular veins are distended. When, on the other hand, the peripheral circulation is at fault, pallor is not accompanied by cyanosis or respiratory disturbances, and the veins are collapsed. During the attack a heart rate faster than 150 beats per minute indicates an ectopic cardiac rhythm, while a rate of less than 40 suggests complete heart block. In a patient with faintness or syncope attended by bradycardia, one has to distinguish between the neurogenic reflex and the cardiogenic (Stokes-Adams) types. The electrocardiogram is decisive, but even without it, Stokes-Adams attacks can be recognized clinically by their longer duration, the greater constancy of the slow heart rate, the presence of audible sounds synchronous with atrial contraction, and the marked variation in intensity of the first sound, despite the regular rhythm. The clinical diagnosis may at times be difficult or impossible, however.

The color of the skin, character of the breathing, appearance of the veins, and rate of the heart are therefore valuable data in diagnosis if the patient is seen during the attack. Unfortunately, the physician rarely has the opportunity to witness the syncopal attack and must obtain the proper clues from the patient's relatives and nearby observers. It is of primary importance that the physician be familiar with the circumstances and the precipitating and alleviating factors in a given episode of weakness or fainting. The following points are also helpful in the differential diagnosis of syncope.

Type of Onset When the attack begins with relative suddenness, i.e., over the period of a few seconds, carotid sinus syncope, postural hypotension, or sudden atrioventricular block is likely. When the symptoms develop gradually during a period of several minutes, hyperventilation or hypoglycemia should be considered. Onset of syncope during or immediately after exertion is seen occasionally in persons with aortic stenosis or aortic insufficiency and with severe occlusive disease of cerebral arteries.

Position at Onset of Attack Attacks due to hypoglycemia, hyperventilation, or heart block are not dependent upon posture. Faintness associated with a decline in blood pressure (including carotid sinus attacks) and with ectopic tachycardia usually occurs only in the sitting or standing position, whereas faintness resulting from orthostatic hypotension is apt to set in shortly after change from the recumbent to the standing position.

Associated Symptoms The associated symptoms during an attack are important; palpitation is likely to be present when the attack is due to anxiety or hyperventilation, to ectopic tachycardia, or to hypoglycemia. Numbness and tingling in the hands and face are frequent accompaniments of hyperventilation. Irregular jerking movements and generalized spasms without loss of consciousness or change in the EEG are typical of the hysterical faint.

Duration and Frequency of Attacks When the duration is very brief, i.e., a few seconds to a few minutes, carotid sinus syncope or one of the several forms of vasodepressor syncope or postural hypotension is most likely. A duration of more than a few minutes but less than an hour suggests hypoglycemia or hyperventilation.

When an otherwise healthy adult has many fainting attacks over a period of days one must consider myocardial disease with dysrhythmia, action of antihypertensive and psychotropic drugs, and hysteria.

SPECIAL METHODS OF EXAMINATION

In many patients who complain of recurrent weakness or syncope but do not have a spontaneous attack while under observation of the physician, an attempt to reproduce attacks is of great assistance in diagnosis.

When hyperventilation is accompanied by faintness, the pattern of symptoms can be reproduced readily by having the subject breathe rapidly and deeply for 2 to 3 min. This test is often of therapeutic value also, because the underlying anxiety tends to be lessened when the patient learns that symptoms can be produced and alleviated at will simply by controlling breathing.

Other conditions in which the diagnosis is clarified by reproducing the attacks are carotid sinus hypersensitivity (massage of one or the other carotid sinus) and orthostatic hypotension (observations of pulse rate, blood pressure, and symptoms in the recumbent and standing positions). Most patients with tussive syncope cannot reproduce an attack by the Valsalva maneuver, but can sometimes do so by voluntary coughing, if severe enough. In each of these instances the crucial point is not whether symptoms are produced (the procedures mentioned frequently induce symptoms in healthy persons), but whether the exact pattern of symptoms that occurs in the spontaneous attacks is reproduced in all the artificial ones. Careful continuous monitoring of the ECG in the hospital or recording the ECG over many hours using a portable lightweight tape recorder may identify an arrhythmia responsible for the syncopal episode. Monitoring may show that the syncopal episode is characterized by a bout of cardiac standstill, extreme bradycardia, or severe tachyarrhythmia.

The EEG may be helpful in differentiating syncope from epilepsy. In the interval between epileptic seizures it may show some degree of abnormality in 40 to 75 percent of cases, whereas it should be normal between syncopal attacks.

TREATMENT

Fainting in most instances is relatively benign. In dealing with patients who have fainted, the physician should think first of those causes of fainting that constitute a therapeutic emergency. Among them are massive internal hemorrhage and myocardial infarction, which may be painless, and cardiac arrhythmias. In an elderly person a sudden faint, without obvious cause, should arouse the suspicion of complete heart block, even though all findings are negative when the physician sees the patient.

Patients seen during the preliminary stages of fainting or after they have lost consciousness should be placed in a position which permits maximal cerebral blood flow, i.e., with head lowered between the knees, if sitting, or in the supine position with legs elevated. All tight clothing and other constrictions should be loosened and the head turned so that the tongue does not fall back into the throat, blocking the airway. Peripheral stimulation, such as sprinkling or dashing cold water on the face and neck or the application of cold towels, is helpful. If the temperature is subnormal, the body should be covered with a warm blanket. If available, aromatic spirit of ammonia may be given cautiously by inhalation. Since emesis is frequent, one should be prepared for a possible aspiration of vomitus. Nothing should be given by mouth until the patient has regained consciousness. The patient should not be permitted to rise until the sense of physical weakness has passed, and should be watched carefully for a few minutes after rising.

As a rule, the physician sees the patient after recovery from the faint, and is asked to explain why it happened and how it can be prevented in the future. The prevention of fainting depends on the mechanisms involved. In the usual vasodepressor faint of adolescents, which tends to occur in circumstances favoring vasodilatation and periods of emotional excitement, fatigue,

hunger, etc., it is enough to advise the patient to avoid such circumstances. In postural hypotension, patients should be cautioned against arising suddenly from bed. Instead, they should first exercise the legs for a few seconds, then sit on the edge of the bed and make sure they are not light-headed or dizzy before starting to walk. They should sleep with the headposts of the bed elevated on wooden blocks 8 to 12 in high. A snug elastic abdominal binder and elastic stockings are often helpful. Drugs of the ephedrine group (ephedrine sulfate, 40 to 50 mg) may be useful if they do not cause insomnia.

In the syndrome of chronic orthostatic hypotension, special corticosteroid preparations [fludrocortisone acetate (Florinef), 0.01 to 0.02 mg/day in divided doses] and increased salt intake to expand blood volume are helpful. Binding of the legs (i.e., wearing a G suit) and sleeping with head and shoulders elevated are other useful measures. Tyramine and monoamine oxidase inhibitor have given relief in some cases of Shy-Drager syndrome.

The treatment of carotid sinus syncope involves first of all instructing the patient in measures that minimize the hazards of a fall (see below). Loose collars should be worn, and the patient should learn to turn the whole body, rather than the head alone, when looking to one side. Atropine or one of the ephedrine group of drugs should be used, respectively, in patients with pronounced bradycardia or hypotension during attacks. If atropine is not successful and the syncopal attacks are incapacitating, the insertion of a demand pacemaker into the right ventricle should be considered. Radiation or surgical denervation of the carotid sinus has apparently yielded favorable results in some patients, but it is rarely necessary. Once it has been concluded that the attacks are due to a narrowing of major cerebral arteries, some of the surgical measures discussed in Chap. 33 must be considered. Vagovagal attacks usually respond well to anticholinergic drugs (propantheline, 15 mg tid).

Treatment of the hyperventilation syndrome and of hysteria are considered in Chap. 53. For a discussion of the treatment of the various cardiac arrhythmias which may induce syncope and of hypoglycemia, the reader is referred to *Harrison's Principles of Internal Medicine*.

The chief hazard of a faint in elderly persons is not the underlying disease but rather fracture or other trauma due to the fall. Therefore, patients subject to recurrent syncope should cover the bathroom floor and bathtub with rubber mats, and should have as much of their home carpeted as is feasible. Especially important is the floor space between the bed and the bathroom, because faints are common in elderly persons when walking from bed to toilet. Outdoor walking should be on soft ground rather than hard surfaces, and the patient should avoid standing still for prolonged periods, which is more likely to induce an attack than walking.

REFERENCES

COMPTON D et al: Weight-lifters' blackout. *Lancet* 2:1234, 1973.

ENGEL GL: *Fainting*, 2d ed. Springfield, Ill, Charles C Thomas, 1962.

FRIEDBERG CK: Syncope: Pathological physiology: Differential diagnosis and treatment. *Mod Concepts Cardiovasc Dis* 40:55, 1971.

GASTAUT H, FISCHER-WILLIAMS M: Electro-encephalographic study of syncope: Its differentiation from epilepsy. *Lancet* 2:1018, 1957.

JOHNSON RH, SPALDING JMK: *Disorders of the Autonomic Nervous System*. Philadelphia, Davis, 1974.

KONTOS HA, RICHARDSON DW, NORVELL JE: Norepinephrine depletion in idiopathic orthostatic hypotension. *Ann Int Med* 82:336, 1975.

LEE JE et al: Episodic unconsciousness, in Barondess JA (ed): *Diagnostic Approaches to Presenting Syndromes*. Baltimore, Williams & Wilkins, 1971, pp 133–167.

LEVINE B, POSNER JB: Swallow syncope. Report of a case and review of the literature. *Neurology* 22:1086, 1972.

LEVINE RJ: Epidemic faintness and syncope in a school marching band. *JAMA* 238:2373, 1977.

SCHOENBERG BS, KUGLITSCH JF, KARNES WE: Micturition syncope—not a single entity. *JAMA* 229:1631, 1974.

SHY GM, DRAGER GA: A neurological syndrome associated with orthostatic hypotension: A clinical-pathologic study. *Arch Neurol* 2:511, 1960.

STREETEN DHP et al: Hyperbradykininism: A new orthostatic syndrome. *Lancet* 2:1048, 1972.

WEISS S et al: Syncope and convulsions due to a hyperactive carotid sinus reflex: Diagnosis and treatment. *Arch Int Med* 58:407, 1936.

———, FERRIS EB JR: Adams-Stokes syndrome with transient complete heart block of vagovagal reflex origin: Mechanism and treatment. *Arch Int Med* 54:931, 1934.

WRIGHT KE JR, MCINTOSH MD: Syncope: Review of pathophysiological mechanisms. *Prog Cardiovasc Dis* 13:580, 1971.

ZIEGLER DK, LIN J, BAYER WL: Convulsive syncope: Relationship to cerebral ischemia. *Trans Am Neurol Assoc* 103:150, 1978.

ZIEGLER MG, LAKE CR, KOPIN IJ: The sympathetic nervous system defect in primary orthostatic hypotension. *N Engl J Med* 296:293, 1977.

CHAPTER 18
SLEEP AND ITS ABNORMALITIES

Sleep, that familiar yet inexplicable condition of repose in which consciousness is in abeyance, is obviously not abnormal, yet it is not illogical to consider it in connection with abnormal phenomena. There are no doubt irregularities of sleep which approach serious extremes, just as there are unnatural forms of waking consciousness.

Everyone has had a great deal of personal experience with sleep, or lack of it, and has observed people in sleep, so it requires no special knowledge of neurology to know something about this condition or to appreciate its importance to health and well-being. The psychological and physiologic benefits of sleep have seldom been so eloquently expressed as in the words of Tristram Shandy:

> *Tis the refuge of the unfortunate—the enfranchisement of the prisoner, the downy lap of the hopeless, the weary, the broken-hearted; of all the soft delicious functions of nature this is the chiefest; what a happiness it is to man, when the anxieties and passions of the day are over.*

Physicians are often consulted by patients who suffer some derangement of sleep. Most often the problem is one of sleeplessness, but sometimes it concerns excessive sleep or other peculiar phenomena occurring in connection with sleep. Certain points concerning the physiology of normal sleep and of the sleep-waking mechanisms will first be reviewed, since familiarity with these concepts is necessary for an understanding of sleep disorders and their treatment.

NORMAL SLEEP

Sleep, as everyone knows, is an elemental phenomenon of life and an indispensable phase of human existence. It represents one of the basic 24-h cyclic changes in the nervous system, traceable through all mammalian, avian, and reptilian species.

Observations of the human sleep-waking cycle show it to be age-linked. The newborn baby sleeps from 16 to 20 h a day, the child, 10 to 12 h, and the adult, approximately 7 h, but wide individual differences, due apparently to genetic factors, early-life conditioning, and the physical and psychological state, are to be noted in the amount of sleep that occurs.

The pattern of sleeping, which in terrestrial life is adjusted to the 24-h day, also varies in the different epochs of life. A nocturnal predominance begins to appear only after the first few weeks of postnatal life of the full-term infant; as the child matures, the morning nap is omitted, then by the fourth or fifth year the afternoon nap, and the night's sleep becomes consolidated into a single long period. Actually, half the world's population, or more, continues to have an afternoon nap (siesta, etc.) as a lifelong sleep-wake pattern. This alternating pattern of sleeping and waking persists throughout adolescence and adult years, unless altered by emotional or physical disease, and not until old age does fragmentation of the sleep pattern occur. Night awakenings then increase in frequency, and the daytime waking period becomes interrupted frequently by paroxysmal bursts of sleep lasting seconds to minutes (microsleep), as well as by longer naps. From about 35 years of age onward, the female tends to sleep slightly more than the male.

Loomis and his associates and Dement and Kleitman have made important contributions to our understanding of sleep through electroencephalographic (EEG) and polygraphic analysis. Five stages of sleep, representative of two alternating physiologic mechanisms, have been defined. Relaxed wakefulness is accompanied by sinusoidal alpha waves of 9 to 11 Hz (cycles per second) and low-voltage fast activity of mixed frequency in the EEG; there are the usual artifacts due to blinking and movements of the eyes and limbs; the electromyogram is silent when the patient is sitting or lying quietly in bed, except for the facial (mimetic) muscles. As a person falls asleep and the muscles relax further, the eyelids droop and the EEG pattern changes to one of progressively lower voltage and mixed frequency, with loss of alpha waves; this is associated with slow rolling eye movements. This is called stage 1 sleep. As sleep changes into stage 2, $\frac{1}{2}$ - to 2-s bursts of 12- to 16-Hz waves (sleep spindles) and high-amplitude, sharp slow-wave (K) complexes appear. The deep sleep of stages 3 and 4, also referred to as slow-wave sleep, is composed of an increasing proportion of high-amplitude (>100 μV), slow-wave (1 to 2 Hz) activity in the EEG. In the next stage of sleep, bursts of rapid eye movements (REMs) occur, and the mentalis and other facial muscles lose their tonic activity, but are activated by brief phasic discharges which also involve the distal muscles of the extremities. The EEG becomes desynchronized, i.e., it has a lower-voltage and higher-frequency discharge pattern, but 10-Hz alpha bursts are rare. The first four stages of sleep are called nonrapid eye movement (NREM) sleep or quiet or synchronized sleep; the last stage is variously designated as rapid eye movement (REM), paradoxical, active, or desynchronized sleep (see Fig. 18-1).

In the first portion of a typical night's sleep the normal young and middle-aged adult passes successively through stages 1, 2, 3, and 4 of NREM sleep. After about 70 to 100 min, a high proportion of which is spent in stages 3 and 4, the first REM period occurs, usually heralded by a transient increase in body movements and a shift in the EEG pattern from stage 4 to 2. This NREM-REM cycle (activity-rest cycle of Kleitman) is repeated at about the same interval four to six times during the night, depending on the length of sleep. The first REM period may be brief, and the later cycles have much less stage 4 NREM sleep (in most cases, actually none). In the latter portion of a night's sleep, the cycles consist essentially of two alternating stages—REM sleep and stage 2 (spindle-K-complex) sleep. The newborn full-term infant spends about 50 percent of sleep in the REM stage (although having different EEG and eye movement characteristics from the adult). The newborn sleep cycle lasts about 60 min (50 percent REM, 50 percent NREM, generally alternating through a 3- to 4-h interfeeding period), but with age the sleep cycle lengthens to 90 to 100 min. About 20 to 25 percent of total sleep time in young adults is spent in REM sleep, 3 to 5 percent in stage 1, 50 to 60 percent in stage 2, and 10 to 20 percent in stages 3 and 4 combined. The amount of sleep in stages 3 and 4 decreases with age, and the el-

derly (over 70 years) have virtually no stage 4 sleep and only small amounts of stage 3 sleep (Fig. 18-2). The 90- to 100-min cycle is fairly stable in any one person and is believed to continue to operate in a less perceptible degree during wakefulness in relation to cyclic gastric motility, hunger, degrees of alertness, and capacity for cognitive activity.

PHYSIOLOGIC CHANGES IN SLEEP

A comparison of the physiologic changes in NREM and REM sleep has been instructive. The change in the EEG pattern has already been indicated. Cortical neurons tend to discharge in synchronized bursts during NREM sleep and in nonsynchronous bursts in the wakeful states; in REM sleep the unit activity rate is quite high and generally asynchronous. Most complex, visual dreaming occurs in the REM period and is recalled most consistently if the subject is awakened at this time. However, it has been shown that similar mental activity occurs in non-REM sleep as well.

During REM sleep, tonic muscle activity is minimal, but there are small twitching, trembling movements in facial and distal extremity (hands and feet) muscles. Gross body movements occur in all stages of sleep, but their frequency is maximal in the transition between REM and NREM sleep. Eye movements of REM sleep are conjugate and occur in all directions (horizontal more than vertical), like those of the waking state.

It has long been known that the body temperature falls during sleep; however, if sleep does not occur, there still is a drop in body temperature, as part of the circadian (24-h) temperature curve. This fall is also independent of the 24-h lying-ambulatory cycle. During sleep, the fall in temperature occurs mainly during the NREM period, and the same is true of the heart beat and respiration, both of which become slow and more regular in this period. Oxygen consumption in muscle diminishes during NREM sleep and increases markedly in brain during REM sleep. Urine excretion decreases during sleep, and the absolute quantity of sodium and potassium that is eliminated also decreases; however, the specific gravity and osmolality increase, presumably because of increased antidiuretic hormone excretion and reabsorption of water. The autonomic nervous functions tend to be activated in REM sleep. Breathing is more irregular; heart rate and blood pressure fluctuate, and cerebral blood flow and metabolic rate increase. Penile erections appear about every 90 min, usually in REM

Figure 18-1

EEG recordings from a 29-year-old woman in the awake state and various stages of sleep.

Awake state *(uppermost tracing).*

1. Stage 1 sleep: *EEG decreases in amplitude and increases in frequency, giving a "flat" appearance.*

2. Stage 2 sleep: *bursts of 13- to 16-Hz waves (sleep spindles) as well as high-amplitude, single-complex (K) waves appear, against a background of low frequency.*

3. Stage 3 sleep: *appearance of high-voltage slow waves (delta activity) with some spindling.*

4. Stage 4 sleep: *predominant delta slow-wave activity.*

REM sleep: *concomitant appearance of relatively low-voltage mixed-frequency EEG (stage 1) and REM (rapid-eye-movement) episodes.*

Technical note: *Four recording sites from the same montage are illustrated in each tracing: F_1-F_7, left frontal; C_3-A_2, left central to right ear; O_3-O_zP_z (between O_z and P_z), left parietooccipital; LE-A_2, left eye to right ear. Recordings were made at conventional sleep-laboratory speed of 15 mm/s (i.e., half the paper speed of standard clinical EEG recordings). (Adapted from Williams et al.)*

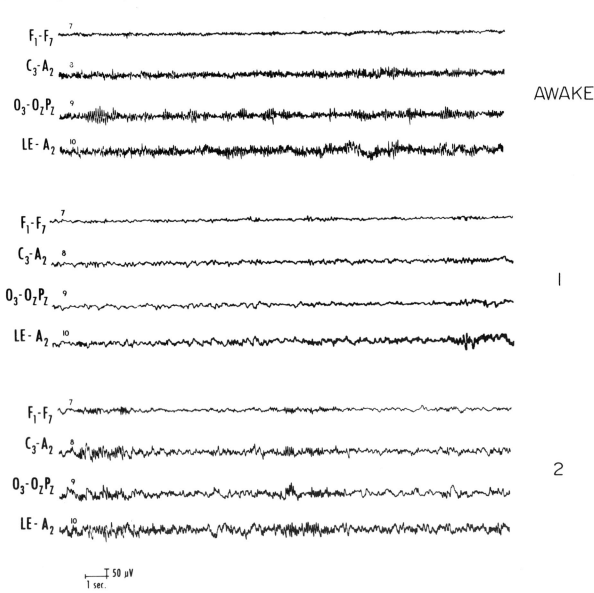

AWAKE

1

2

⊥ 50 µV
1 sec.

periods. Three or four episodic bursts of cortisol and ACTH secretion occur in the latter half of the night's sleep period. Sleep-related secretion of growth hormone (during the first 2 h of sleep) and of prolactin and luteinizing hormones in pubertal children have also been shown to occur. The sleep-wake hormonal relationships are quite complex and are only beginning to be understood (see review by Weitzman et al.).

On closer study, REM sleep has been found to have phasic and tonic components. During the phasic period the eyes move rapidly in all directions, the pupils alternately dilate and constrict, the blood pressure, pulse, and respiration increase and become more irregular, and small twitches or myoclonic jerks appear in the limbs and face. The phasic activities are related to bursts of neuronal activity in the vestibular nuclei and are me-

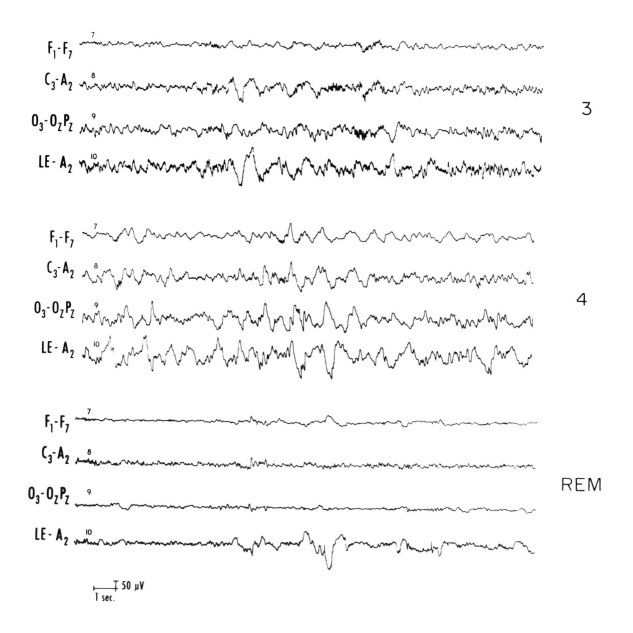

diated through the medial longitudinal fasciculi and ocular nuclei, the median raphe nuclei, and the corticospinal tracts. In the nonphasic periods of REM sleep, alpha and gamma spinal neurons are inhibited and both postural and flexor reflexes diminish or are abolished.

Evidence derived from studies in animals shows that the physiologic mechanisms that govern NREM and REM sleep lie in the brainstem and are influenced by acetylcholine and the monoamine neurotransmitters, 5-hydroxytryptamine (serotonin) and norepinephrine. Serotoninergic neurons are located in and near the midline or raphe regions of the pons; the lower groups of cells project to the medulla and spinal cord; the medial raphe nuclei project to the medial temporal (limbic) cor-

Figure 18-2
Normal sleep cycles. REM sleep (darkened areas) occurs cyclically throughout the night at intervals of approximately 90 min in all age groups. REM sleep shows little variation in the different age groups, whereas stage 4 sleep decreases with age. (From Kales and Kales.)

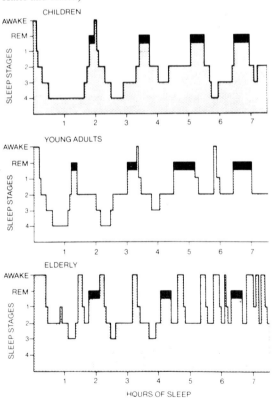

tex and the dorsal raphe nuclei to the neostriatum, cerebral and cerebellar cortices, and thalamus. Norepinephrine-rich neurons are concentrated in the locus coeruleus and related nuclei in the central tegmentum of the caudal pons as well as in other lateral-ventral tegmental regions. These neurons project downward to the lateral horn cells of the spinal cord and upward via centrally located tegmental tracts to specific thalamic and subthalamic nuclei and all of the cerebral cortex, and via the superior cerebellar peduncle to the cerebellar cortex. Acetylcholine also appears to function as a neurotransmitter in the brainstem reticular activating system, but the cells of origin of this neurotransmitter and its projection system have not been defined.

Serotonin is probably the most important of the neurotransmitters, as far as sleep mechanisms are concerned. Activation of the serotoninergic neurons [by "factor S"(?), see below] or injection of 5-hydroxytryptophan, the precursor of serotonin, may induce and maintain NREM sleep, presumably by inhibiting neuronal systems of the reticular activating system; serotonin also may trigger and facilitate REM sleep. Contrariwise, inhibition of serotonin synthesis causes decreased sleep, with disappearance of both NREM and REM sleep. Local microapplications of cholinergic drugs in several brainstem sites can produce striking motor-inhibitory effects and other REM sleep characteristics in the intact animal. The detailed studies of Pompeiano and his colleagues have shown that fibers from the rostral medullary reticular formation exert a tonic postsynaptic inhibition on spinal motor neurons during REM sleep. It is also known that this portion of the bulbar reticular formation receives fibers from the locus coeruleus, and that lesions in the latter structure abolish the muscle atonia of REM sleep. These findings indicate that the noradrenergic neurons of the locus coeruleus and its projection system are somehow involved in the motor inhibition of REM sleep. Monoamine oxidase inhibitors have been shown selectively to diminish or abolish REM sleep, probably by influencing the monoamine neurotransmitters.

The details of the neuropharmacology of sleep are not yet fully known, nor do we know how these neuronal systems are normally activated at both 24-h and short-term regular intervals to produce sleep and sleep-stage cycling. The systems involved in REM sleep are suppressed for a time during NREM sleep but periodically become active and interrupt it. The plasma of drowsy or sleeping animals has been shown by Monnier and Hosli to contain a substance with properties that induce somnolence and increase NREM sleep in alert animals. Pappenheimer and his associates have isolated an "S factor" from the CSF and brain of animals deprived of sleep.

When injected into rats and rabbits it induces slow-wave sleep lasting 4 to 6 h. Its molecular weight is about 350, and it is destroyed by pronase, indicating the presence of peptides. Its origin and specific nature are as yet unknown.

THE EFFECTS OF TOTAL AND PARTIAL SLEEP LOSS

Deprived of sleep, experimental animals will die within a few days, no matter how well they are fed, watered, and housed, and under similar circumstances human beings suffer a variety of unpleasant symptoms that must be separated from the usual types of insomnia.

Despite many studies of the deleterious emotional and cognitive effects of sleeplessness, we still know too little about them. Human beings deprived of sleep (NREM and REM) for periods of 60 to 200 h experience increasing fatigue and irritability and find it difficult to concentrate, to perceive accurately, and to maintain their orientation. Illusions and hallucinations, mainly visual and tactile ones, may intrude in consciousness and become more intense as the period of sleeplessness is prolonged. Performance of skilled motor activities deteriorates. If the tasks are of short duration and of slow pace, the subject can keep up, but if speed and perseverance are demanded, he cannot. Incentive to work weakens, and sustained thought and action are interrupted by lapses of attention. Neurologic signs to be noted include a mild and fleeting nystagmus, a slight tremor of the hands, ptosis of eyelids, expressionless face, and thickness of speech, with mispronunciation and incorrect choice of words. A decrement of alpha waves appears in the EEG, and closing of the eyes no longer generates alpha activity. The concentration of 17-hydroxycorticosteroids increases in the blood, and catecholamine output rises.

Occasionally, probably only in predisposed persons, loss of sleep provokes psychotic episodes. Rarely, the subject may go berserk, with screaming, sobbing, and incoherent muttering about seeing things. Fragmentary delusions and paranoid thoughts are more frequent.

During recovery from prolonged sleep deprivation, the amount of sleep obtained is never equal to the amount lost. This is probably due to the intrusive nature of sleep in the waking period (it is virtually impossible to deprive a human being or animal totally of sleep) and the microsleep periods which occur and which represent a sizable amount of time, if summated. When falling asleep after a long period of deprivation, the subject rapidly enters stage 4 of NREM sleep, which continues for several hours at the expense of stage 2 and REM sleep. But by the second recovery night, REM sleep rebounds and exceeds that of the predeprivation period. Stage 4

NREM sleep seems to be the most important sleep stage in restoring the altered functions of the nervous system which result from prolonged sleep deprivation.

The effects of partial and differential deprivation are somewhat different. If subjects are prevented from having REM sleep night after night, they show an increasing tendency to become hyperactive, emotionally labile, and less able to control their impulses, a state which corresponds to the heightened activity, excessive appetite, and oversexuality of REM sleep-deprived animals. Differential deprivation of NREM sleep (stages 3 and 4) leads, instead, to hyporesponsiveness and excessive sleepiness.

Since the need for sleep varies considerably from person to person, it is difficult to decide what is partial sleep deprivation. Certain rare individuals apparently function well on 4 h or less of sleep per 24-h period, and others, who sleep long hours, claim not to obtain the maximum benefit from it.

SLEEP DISORDERS

INSOMNIA

This word signifies an inability to sleep at the time of day when sleep is expected normally to occur, and is used popularly to indicate any impairment in its duration, depth, or restorative properties. Insomnia may consist of difficulty in falling asleep or in remaining asleep, or a too early final awakening; or there may be a combination of these abnormalities. Precision as to what constitutes insomnia is impossible at the present time because of our uncertainty as to the exact amounts of sleep that are required and also its role in the economy of the human body.

Two general classes of insomniac disturbance may be defined—one in which there appears to be a primary abnormality of the normal sleep mechanism, another in which sleep impairment is secondary to a medical or psychological disorder. Polygraphic studies have defined another subgroup of insomniacs—"pseudoinsomniacs"—who actually sleep quite well but who perceive their sleep time to be shortened.

The term *primary insomnia* should be reserved for the condition in which nocturnal sleep is disturbed for prolonged periods and in which none of the recognized symptoms of neurosis, depression, or other psychiatric or medical diseases can be elicited to explain the sleep disturbance. Unlike the rare individuals who seem to be satisfied with 3 to 4 h of sleep a night, insomniacs suffer the effects of partial sleep deprivation and resort to all manner of drugs and various techniques to induce or maintain sleep. Their life comes to revolve around sleep to such an extent that they have been called "sleep pedants" or "sleep hypochondriacs." Although statements of insomniacs are often not to be trusted, Rechtschaffen and Monroe have confirmed that they do indeed sleep poorly. They sleep for shorter periods, move and awaken more often, spend less time in stage 4 sleep than normal persons, and show a heightened physiologic arousal. Personality inventories have revealed a high incidence of psychological disturbances in this group of patients, but whether these are a cause or effect is not known. Although victims of insomnia, regardless of the cause, tend to exaggerate the amount of sleep lost, primary insomnia should be recognized as an entity and not passed off as a quirk of the neurotic.

Secondary insomnia can often be ascribed to pain or some other discomfort, or to anxiety, worry, or depression. This latter type, also called *situational insomnia,* is usually transient and clearly related to a specific anxiety-provoking condition. Of the sensory disorders conducive to abnormal wakefulness, pain in the spine with or without nerve root involvement stands out, and also abdominal discomfort from peptic ulcer and carcinoma. Aching, restless legs, an obscure and usually benign state known as the "restless legs syndrome" (anxietas tibiarum), may regularly delay the onset of sleep. Excessive fatigue may give rise to abnormal muscular sensations of similar nature. Another syndrome, *nocturnal myoclonus,* has been shown to be a cause of insomnia. In this condition, prolonged periods of repetitive flexor or extensor movements of the legs, occurring every 20 to 30 s, produce frequent microarousals or, if severe, periodic full arousals. The patient, usually unaware of these sleep-related movements, is often told of them by a bedmate. Acroparesthesias, a predominantly nocturnal tingling and numbness of the fingers and palms due to tight carpal ligaments (carpal-tunnel syndrome), may awaken the patient at night, as does also cluster headache. The headaches tend to occur in the REM sleep period.

More frequently, insomnia is secondary to some type of psychological disturbance. Domestic or business worries may keep the patient's mind in a turmoil (situational insomnia). Also, vigorous mental activity late at night, or excitement, which leaves the muscles tense, may counteract drowsiness and sleep. A strange bed or

surroundings may do likewise. Under these circumstances there is mainly a difficulty in falling asleep, with a tendency to sleep late in the morning. These facts emphasize that a certain degree of conditioning is involved in readying the mind and body for sleep.

Illnesses in which anxiety and fear are prominent symptoms also result in difficulty in falling asleep and in light, fitful, or intermittent sleep. Also, disturbing dreams are frequent and may awaken the patient. Some patients even try to stay awake in order to avoid them, but this is the exception. In contrast, the depressive illnesses characteristically produce early-morning waking and inability to return to sleep; quantity of sleep is reduced, and nocturnal motility is increased; REM sleep, although not always reduced, comes earlier in the night—this is termed the "increased pressure of REM sleep." If anxiety is combined with depression there is a tendency for both the above patterns to be observed. Yet another pattern of disturbed sleep can be discerned in individuals who are under great tension and worry or are overworked and exhausted. These people sink into bed and sleep through sheer exhaustion, but around 4 or 5 A.M. they awaken with their worries and are unable to get back to sleep.

In states of mania and acute agitation, sleep diminishes and REM sleep may be abolished. Chronic intoxication with barbiturates and certain nonbarbiturate sedative-hypnotic drugs markedly reduces REM sleep, as well as stages 3 and 4 of NREM sleep. Following withdrawal of these drugs there is a rapid and marked increase of REM sleep and of dreaming. The patient has difficulty in falling asleep, and once asleep, arousals are frequent. Thus insomnia may be produced by the drugs that were intended to cure the disorder ("drug-withdrawal insomnia"; see Kales et al.). Furthermore, a form of drug-withdrawal insomnia may actually occur during the night in which the drug is administered. The drug produces its hypnotic effect in the first half of the night and the withdrawal symptoms during the latter half of the night, and the patient and the physician may be misled into thinking that these insomniac symptoms require more of the hypnotic drug or a different one.

The sleep rhythm may be totally deranged in acute confusional states and delirium, and the patient may doze for only short periods, both day and night, the total amount and depth of sleep in a 24-h period being reduced. Frightening hallucinations may prevent sleep. The senile patient tends to catnap during the day and to remain alert for progressively longer periods during the night, until sleep is obtained in a series of short naps throughout the 24 h; the total amount of sleep may be increased or decreased. Disturbed and decreased total sleep also occurs when the normal circadian rhythm of the sleep-wake cycle is altered, as occurs in shift workers who periodically change their work schedule from day to night, or in transmeridional jet flights (jet-lag syndrome).

Treatment of Insomnia In general, sedative-hypnotic drugs for the management of insomnia should be prescribed only as a short-term adjuvant during illness or some unusual circumstance. For patients who have difficulty in falling asleep or staying asleep, or both, a quick-acting, fairly rapidly destroyed hypnotic is useful; e.g., secobarbital (Seconal), 0.1 g given 15 to 20 min before going to bed; flurazepam (Dalmane), 30 mg; chloral hydrate (Noctec), 1 to 2 g; or glutethimide (Doriden), 0.5 g. These drugs are more or less equally effective in inducing and maintaining sleep; however, they affect sleep stages differently. Flurazepam reduces stage 4 but not REM sleep, whereas the barbiturates and glutethimide reduce REM sleep as well. If these drugs have to be given for longer than a week or two, all of them, with the possible exception of flurazepam, begin to lose their effectiveness, and larger doses are required to regain the initial effect. Patients who awaken too early in the morning may be given a longer-acting barbiturate, such as barbital, 0.3 g at bedtime. For debilitated patients tablets should be crushed to ensure proper absorption, or an injectable form should be used. Chloral hydrate may be substituted if barbital is undesirable.

When pain is a factor in insomnia, acetylsalicylic acid, 0.3 to 0.6 g, may be given with the sedative or codeine phosphate, 30 mg, when the pain is severe. For cardiac patients with moderate orthopnea or Cheyne-Stokes respiration, a rectal suppository of aminophylline, 0.5 g at bedtime, will frequently relieve the respiratory distress and promote sleep. The use of drugs in patients with delirium and manic-depressive disease is discussed in Chaps. 40 and 54.

A word of caution about oversedation is appropriate in any discussion of sedative drugs. All too frequently they are given when not needed, the dosage is too great, or the wrong preparation is chosen. These drugs are a common source of constipation, lead to fatigue and lack of strength, and may interfere with the patient's recovery from the illness.

When large dosages of fast-acting barbiturates, 0.4 to 0.6 g daily, are given for more than a few weeks, there is a real danger of addiction, which once developed, is pernicious in character. Withdrawal, unless accomplished skillfully, may cause serious mental disturbance or precipitate convulsions (see Chap. 41).

The chronic insomniac who has no other symptoms should not be permitted to use sedative drugs as a crutch on which to limp through life. The solution of this problem is rarely to be found in medication. One should search out and correct, if possible, any underlying situational or psychological difficulty, using medication only as a temporary measure. A helpful approach is to lessen the patient's concern about the sleeplessness by pointing out that the human organism will always get as much sleep as needed, and that there is pleasure to be derived from staying awake and reading a good book.

DISTURBANCES IN THE TRANSITIONAL PERIOD BETWEEN WAKING AND SLEEP (SOMNOLESCENT STARTS, SENSORY PAROXYSMS, AND SLEEP PARALYSIS)

As sleep comes on, certain motor centers may be excited to a burst of insubordinate activity. The result is a sudden "start" or bodily jerk that rouses the incipient sleeper. It may involve one or both legs or the trunk (less often, the arms) and be associated with a frightening dream or sensory experience. If the "start" occurs repeatedly during the process of falling asleep and is a nightly event, it may become a matter of great concern to the patient. These "starts" are more apt to occur in individuals in whom the sleep process develops slowly, and are especially frequent under conditions of tension and anxiety. Polygraphic recordings have shown that these bodily jerks occur only during light sleep. Sometimes they appear as part of an arousal response to a faint external stimulus. It is probable that some relationship exists between these nocturnal starts and the sudden isolated jerk of a leg, or arm and leg, which occurs occasionally in healthy, fully conscious persons.

The brusque bodily jerks that occur at the moment of falling asleep are not a variant of epilepsy. Oswald, who first studied this phenomenon by means of polygraph recordings, considers the jerks to be physiologic events, exaggerations of the common "somnolescent starts." EEG recordings in relation to the jerks do not disclose any epileptic discharges, and association with other manifestations of epilepsy is exceptional. Nor should these "starts" be referred to as *nocturnal myoclonus*, a term now used to designate the twitches that occur *during* sleep, mainly in stages 3 and 4 (see above, under "Insomnia").

Sensory centers may be disturbed in a similar way, either as an isolated phenomenon or in association with motor phenomena. The patient, dropping off to sleep, may be roused by a sensation that darts through the body, a sudden clang or crashing sound, or a sudden flash of light. Sometimes there is a sensation of being lifted and dashed to the earth or turned; conceivably these are sensory paroxysms involving the labyrinthine mechanism.

Curious paralytic phenomena, referred to as pre- and postdormital paralyses, may occur in the transition from the sleeping to the waking state. Sometimes, in otherwise healthy individuals, a state supervenes in the morning, less frequently when falling asleep, in which, although awake, conscious, and fully oriented, they are unable to innervate their muscles (respiratory and diaphragmatic function is not affected, however). They lie as though still asleep, with eyes closed and may become quite frightened while engaged in a struggle for movement. They have the impression that if they could move one muscle, the paralysis would be dispelled instantly and they would regain full power. It has been stated that the slightest cutaneous stimulus, such as the touch of a hand, or calling the patient's name, will abolish the paralysis. Such attacks may be related to narcolepsy (see later in this chapter). Usually they are transient, and if they occur in isolation and only on rare occasions are of no special significance.

NIGHT TERRORS AND NIGHTMARES

The night terror (*pavor nocturnus*) is more frequent in children than in adults. It usually occurs soon after falling asleep, often within 30 min, during stage 3 or 4 sleep. The child awakens abruptly in a state of intense fright, screaming or moaning, with marked tachycardia (150 to 170 beats per minute) and deep, rapid respirations. Children with night terrors are often sleepwalkers as well, and both kinds of attacks may occur simultaneously. The entire episode lasts only a minute or two, and in the morning the child recalls nothing of it or only a vague unpleasant dream. It has been suggested that night terrors, somnambulism, and confusion represent impaired or partial arousal out of deep sleep, since EEGs taken during such episodes show a waking type of mixed frequency and alpha pattern. Children with night terrors and somnambulism do not show an increased incidence of psychological abnormalities and tend to outgrow these disorders. In adults, however, recurring night-terror attacks are often associated with psychological disturbances. There is evidence that diazepam, which reduces the duration of stage 4 sleep, will prevent night terrors, and this drug should be tried in persistent cases.

Frightening dreams or nightmares are far more frequent than night terrors and affect children and adults alike. They occur during periods of normal REM sleep and are particularly prominent during periods of increased REM sleep (REM rebound), following the withdrawal of alcohol or other sedative-hypnotic drugs that had suppressed REM sleep chronically. Autonomic changes are slight or absent, and the content of the dreams can usually be recalled in considerable detail. Some of these dreams (e.g., the ones occurring in the alcohol-withdrawal period) are so vivid that the patient may have difficulty in separating them from reality.

Nightmares are of little significance as isolated events. Fevers dispose one to them, as may conditions such as indigestion, or the reading of bloodcurdling stories, or seeing such stories enacted on television before bedtime. Persistent nightmares may be a pressing medical complaint, and are said to be accompanied frequently by other behavioral disturbances or neuroses. In adults they should always arouse the suspicion of chronic alcohol or barbiturate intoxication and withdrawal.

SOMNAMBULISM AND SLEEP AUTOMATISM

Examples of sleepwalking come to the attention of the practicing physician not infrequently. This condition likewise occurs more often in children than in adults, and is associated with an increased incidence of enuresis and of night terrors, as has been indicated. The motor performance and responsiveness during the sleepwalking incident vary considerably. The most common behavioral abnormality is for patients to sit up in bed or on the edge of the bed without actually walking. When walking about the house, they may turn on a light or perform some other familiar act. There may be no outward signs of emotion, or the patient may be frightened (night terror). Usually the eyes are open, and such sleepwalkers are guided by vision, thus avoiding familiar objects; the sight of an unfamiliar object may awaken them. Sometimes these patients make no attempt to avoid obstacles and may injure themselves. If spoken to, they make no response; if told to return to bed, they may do so but more often must be led back to it. Sometimes they mutter strange phrases or sentences over and over or perform certain repetitive acts such as pushing against a wall or turning a doorknob back and forth. The episode lasts for only a few minutes, and the following morning they usually have no memory of it.

Half-waking somnambulism, or sleep automatism, is a closely related disorder. This is a state in which an adult, half-roused from sleep, goes through a fairly complex routine such as going to a window, opening it, and looking out, but afterward recalls only a part of the episode.

A popular belief is that the sleepwalker is acting out a dream. Sleep-laboratory observations are at variance with this view, since somnambulism has been found to arise almost exclusively from stages 3 and 4 of NREM sleep, when dreaming is least likely to occur. And the entire nocturnal sleep pattern of such individuals does not differ from normal. Similarly, there is no evidence that somnambulism is a form of epilepsy. It is probably allied to talking in one's sleep, although the two conditions seldom occur together.

Some psychiatrists hold that somnambulism represents a dissociated mental state, similar to the hysterical trance of fugue, except that it begins during sleep. To them sleepwalking is evidence of a nervous disorder, probably of psychoneurotic variety. This interpretation is probably incorrect, at least in children and adolescents, since they usually do not show any other signs of psychopathology. Adult somnambulists, on the other hand, are said to show a high incidence of psychoneurosis and schizophrenia.

The major consideration in the treatment of somnambulism is to guard patients against injury by locking doors and windows, removing dangerous objects from their usual routes of march, having them sleep on the ground floor, etc. Children usually outgrow this disorder, and parents should be reassured on this score and disabused of the notion that somnambulism is a sign of psychiatric disease.

NOCTURNAL EPILEPSY

It has long been known that convulsive seizures often occur during sleep. This is such a frequent occurrence that the practice of inducing sleep in order to obtain confirmation of epilepsy has been adopted as an activating procedure in most EEG laboratories. Seizures may occur soon after the onset of sleep or at any time during the night, but mainly in stage 4 of NREM sleep or in REM sleep.

Sleeping epileptic patients attract attention to their seizure by a cry, violent motor activity, or labored breathing. As in the diurnal seizure, after the tonic-clonic phase, they become quiet and fall into a state resembling sleep but from which they cannot be roused. Their appearance depends on the phase of the seizure they happen to be in when first observed. If the nocturnal seizure is unobserved, the only indication of it may be disheveled bedclothes, a few drops of blood on the pillow, wet bed linen from urinary incontinence, a bitten tongue, or sore muscles. In some, the occurrence of a seizure is betrayed only by inappropriate behavior or a

headache, the common aftermaths of convulsive disorder. Rarely, a patient may die in an epileptic seizure during sleep, presumably from smothering in the bedclothes or aspirating vomitus, or for some more obscure reason. These accidents, and similar ones in awake epileptics, account for the higher mortality rate in epileptics than in nonepileptics.

Rarely, epilepsy may occur in conjunction with night terrors and somnambulism, and the question then arises whether the latter disorders are in the nature of postepileptic automatisms. Usually no such relationship is established. EEG studies during a nocturnal period of sleep are most helpful in such cases.

EXCESSIVE SLEEP (HYPERSOMNIA) AND REVERSAL OF SLEEP-WAKING RHYTHM

Encephalitis lethargica, or "epidemic encephalitis," that remarkable illness which appeared on the medical horizon as a pandemic following World War I, has provided some of the most dramatic instances of prolonged somnolence. In fact, protracted sleep lasting from days to weeks was such a prominent symptom of this disease that it was called *sleeping sickness*. The patient appeared to be in a state of continuous sleep, or *somnosis*, and could be kept awake only while stimulated. Although the infective agent was never isolated, the pathologic anatomy was fully divulged by many excellent studies, all of which demonstrated a destruction of neurons in the midbrain, subthalamus, and hypothalamus. Patients who survived the acute phase of the illness often had difficulty in reestablishing their normal sleep-waking rhythm. As the somnolence disappeared, some patients exhibited a reversal of the sleep-wake rhythm, tending to sleep by day and stay awake at night; many of them also developed Parkinson's syndrome, months or years later.

Hypersomnia also occurs in trypanosomiasis, the common cause of "sleeping sickness" in Africa, and with a variety of diseases localized to the mesencephalon and the floor and walls of the third ventricle. Small tumors in this area have been associated with arterial hypotension, diabetes insipidus, and somnolence lasting many weeks. Such patients can be aroused, but if left alone, they immediately fall asleep. Tumors of the brain, in general, have a tendency to cause drowsiness and excessive sleep, but this effect occurs more with diencephalic tumors than with any other. Traumatic lesions and other diseases affecting the mesencephalon and diencephalon produce similar clinical pictures. Severe myxedema causes hypersomnia, as does hypercapnia, the latter with nocturnal headache and confusion.

Periodic hypersomnia is a manifestation of the *Kleine-Levin syndrome*. Three or four times a year, for periods lasting a few days to several weeks, these patients (most often adolescent boys) may have daily attacks of prolonged diurnal sleep lasting many hours, or the duration of nocturnal sleep may be greatly prolonged, or they may sleep for days on end. The food intake during the period of hypersomnia may exceed three times the normal (bulimia), and to a variable extent there are other behavioral changes such as social withdrawal, negativism, slowness of thinking, incoherence, inattentiveness, and disturbances of memory. The basis of this condition has never been elucidated. A psychogenic mechanism has been proposed but is without foundation.

SLEEP APNEA SYNDROMES

As mentioned above, REM sleep is characterized by irregular breathing, and this may include several brief periods of apnea, up to 15 s in duration. Such apneas, occurring during REM sleep or at the onset of sleep, are not considered to be pathologic. During the past decade it has come to be recognized that in some individuals sleep-induced apneic periods are particularly frequent and prolonged (15 to 120 s) and that such a condition may be responsible for a variety of clinical disturbances in children and adults. This pathologic form of sleep apnea may be due to a cessation of respiratory drive (so-called central apnea) or to an obstruction of the upper airway, or to a combination of these two mechanisms. The central form of sleep apnea has been observed in patients with bulbar poliomyelitis, brainstem infarction, spinal (high cervical) surgery, and with a disorder referred to as the primary, or idiopathic, hypoventilation syndrome. Obesity and adenotonsillar hypertrophy, and less frequently acromegaly, myxedema, micrognathia and myotonic dystrophy have been associated with apnea of the obstructive type.

The occurrence of a prolonged period of sleep apnea, from whatever cause, is accompanied by progressive hypercapnia and hypoxemia, a transient increase in systemic and pulmonary arterial pressures, and sinus bradycardia or other arrhythmias. The blood gas changes, or perhaps other stimuli, induce an arousal response, either a lightening of sleep or a very brief awak-

ening, which is followed by an immediate resumption of breathing. The patient quickly falls asleep again and the sequence is repeated, several hundred times a night in severe cases. Noisy snoring and excessive body movement throughout the night are characteristic features of the obstructive type of sleep apnea; snoring ceases briefly with apnea and returns when breathing is resumed. Paradoxically these patients are very difficult to rouse at all times during the night.

Sleep apnea syndromes occur in persons of all ages. In adults, obstructive sleep apnea is predominantly a disorder of overweight, middle-aged men, and usually presents as *excessive daytime sleepiness*, a complaint that is often mistaken for narcolepsy (see below). Other patients, usually those with the central form of apnea complain mainly of a disturbance of sleep at night, or insomnia, which may be incorrectly attributed to anxiety or depression. Morning headache, inattentiveness, and decline in school or work performance are other symptoms attributable to sleep apnea. Ultimately, systemic and pulmonary arterial hypertension, cor pulmonale, polycythemia, and heart failure may develop. These symptoms, if combined with obesity, are frequently referred to as the Pickwickian syndrome, so named by Burwell et al. (1956), who identified this clinical syndrome with that of the extraordinarily sleepy, red-faced fat boy described by Dickens, in *The Pickwick Papers*. The term is no longer apt, since it fails to indicate the central role of sleep apnea in the genesis of the syndrome. Furthermore, obesity is found in only a minority of patients with sleep apnea; conversely, apnea occurs in only a small proportion of obese persons. Severe and life-threatening sleep apnea may occur with lateral medullary infarction and other brainstem lesions.

In infants with delayed maturation of the respiratory centers, sleep apnea is a not infrequent and dangerous condition. It accounts for a certain number of crib deaths. In approximately half of the observed infants with this latter condition, the apnea represents a respiratory arrest during a seizure. This can be demonstrated by EEG.

Cheyne-Stokes respiration (CSR) may occur only at night in certain individuals, especially in the elderly and during illness or postoperatively. It does not have the same serious significance as diurnal CSR.

The full-blown syndrome of sleep apnea is readily recognized. In patients who complain only of excessive daytime sleepiness or insomnia, the diagnosis may be elusive and requires special respiratory tests in addition to all-night polygraphic sleep monitoring. Treatment is governed by the severity of symptoms and the predominant type of apnea, central or obstructive. In the former, medications such as medroxyprogesterone and theophylline may be helpful. The apneas of infants are often caused by seizures and respond to anticonvulsant drugs. In apnea caused by upper-airway obstruction, weight loss and surgical correction of an anatomic defect, when present, are often effective. Tracheostomy in severe cases has been found to reverse dramatically the hypersomnia, cardiopulmonary signs, and systemic hypertension. Severe sleep apnea may require a respirator or a rocking bed.

NARCOLEPSY AND CATAPLEXY

This clinical entity has long been known to the medical profession. Gelineau gave it the name *narcolepsy* in 1880, although several authors had described the recurring attacks of irresistible sleep even before that time (see historical review of Passouant). Loewenfeld (1902) was probably the first to recognize the common association between the sleep attacks and the temporary paralysis of the somatic musculature during bouts of laughter, anger, and other emotional states; this was referred to as *cataplectic inhibition* by Henneberg (1916) and later as *cataplexy* by Adie (1926). The term *sleep paralysis*, to designate the brief, episodic loss of voluntary movement that occurs during the period of falling asleep (hypnagogic or predormital) or of awakening (hypnopompic or postdormital), was introduced by Kinnier Wilson in 1928. Actually, Weir Mitchell had described this disorder in 1876, under the title of *night palsy*. Sometimes sleep paralysis is accompanied or just preceded by vivid and terrifying hallucinations (*hypnagogic hallucinations*). The hallucinations may be visual, auditory, vestibular (a sense of motion), or somatic (a feeling that a limb or finger or other part of the body is enlarged or otherwise transformed). These four conditions constitute a clinical tetrad. The association of hypnagogic hallucinations with narcolepsy was first described by Lhermitte and Tournay, in 1927.

Clinical Features This syndrome is not infrequent, as shown by the fact that about 100 new cases a year appear at the Mayo Clinic (Daly and Yoss). Males are affected more often than females. As a rule the condition begins in late childhood, adolescence, or early adult life; narcolepsy is usually the presenting symptom, less often cataplexy, and rarely sleep paralysis. The essential disorder is one of irresistible attacks of sleepiness. Several times a day, usually after meals, or while sitting in class or being in other states of physical inactivity, these subjects are assailed by an uncontrollable desire to sleep. Their eyes close, their muscles relax, their breathing deepens slightly and they have all the appearances of dozing. A noise, a touch, or even the cessation of the lecturer's voice are enough to awaken them. The periods of sleep rarely last longer than 15 min, unless the patient is reclining, when they may continue for an hour or longer. What distinguishes the narcoleptic sleep attacks from the commonplace postprandial drowsiness is the frequent occurrence of the former (two to six attacks every day, as a rule) and their occurrence in unusual situations, as while standing, eating, or carrying on a conversation. Blurring of vision, diplopia, and ptosis may attend drowsiness and may bring the patient to an ophthalmologist.

It is not generally appreciated that in addition to episodes of outright sleep, narcoleptics frequently experience episodic lapses in consciousness, characterized by automatic behavior and amnesia. These latter phenomena, which may last for a few seconds or as long as an hour or more, occur more often in the afternoon and evening than in the morning, usually when the patient is alone and performing some monotonous task, such as driving. Initially the patient feels drowsy and may recall attempts to fight off the drowsiness, but gradually he or she loses track of what is going on. The patient may continue to perform routine tasks but cannot respond appropriately to a new demand or answer complex questions. Often there is a sudden burst of words, without meaning or relevance to what was just said. Such an outburst may terminate the attack, for which there is complete or nearly complete amnesia. In many respects the attacks resemble episodes of nocturnal sleepwalking. Such attacks of automatic behavior and amnesia are common, occurring in more than half of a large series of patients with narcolepsy-cataplexy (Dement).

Approximately 70 percent of these patients, if questioned carefully, will admit having some form of cataplexy, and if the narcoleptic attacks can be shown by polygraph recordings to represent episodes of REM sleep (see below), then almost all such patients will give a history of cataplectic attacks. Cataplexy refers to the curious circumstances in which hearty laughter, more rarely excitement, sadness, or anger will cause the patient's head to fall forward, the jaw to drop, the knees to buckle, even with falling to the ground, all with perfect preservation of consciousness. The attacks last only a few seconds or a minute or two. Rarely, cataplexy precedes the onset of sleep attacks, but usually it follows them, sometimes by many years. Sleep paralysis and hypnagogic hallucinations (see above) occur in about one-quarter of the patients, and the full tetrad occurs in about 10 percent.

Once the condition begins, it usually continues for the remainder of the patient's life, perhaps becoming less severe with age. No other abnormality is associated with it, and none develops later.

Cause and Pathogenesis The cause of narcolepsy is unknown. It bears no relation to epilepsy or migraine. A psychogenesis has been proposed, but the relevance of the psychological observations remains open to question. Furthermore, Mitler has described the occurrence of narcolepsy and cataplexy, as well as unambiguous sleep-onset REM periods, in animals (the miniature poodle)—a finding that certainly challenges the psychiatric view of this condition. No autopsies in which the brain was thoroughly examined have been reported.

Rarely, the narcolepsy-cataplexy syndrome follows cerebral trauma or accompanies multiple sclerosis, craniopharyngioma, or diabetes insipidus (*secondary or symptomatic narcolepsy*). Narcolepsy was said to be a frequent sequela of encephalitis lethargica, but now only a handful of such cases still exist.

The most important development in our understanding of narcolepsy has been the demonstration, by Dement and his group, that this disorder is associated with an inversion of the two states of sleep, with REM rather than NREM sleep occurring at the onset of the sleep attacks. Not all the diurnal sleep episodes of the narcoleptic begin with REM sleep, but almost always such an onset can be identified in narcoleptic-cataplectic patients in the course of a polygraphic sleep study. The hypnagogic hallucinations (which in this formulation are viewed as dream phenomena), cataplexy, and sleep-onset paralysis (inhibition of anterior horn cells) are all identified as events that characterize the REM period. Rechtschaffen and Dement have shown also that the night sleep pattern of the narcoleptic characteristically begins with a REM period. This, too, almost never occurs in normal subjects or in patients with other types of hypersomnia. Furthermore, the nocturnal sleep pattern is altered in narcoleptics, with frequent body movements and transient awakenings and decrease in sleep stages 3 and 4 and in total sleep. In addition, Passouant and his colleagues, on the basis of continuous 24-h polygraphic monitoring, have presented evidence that in some patients there is a 90- to 120-min periodicity of the narcolepsy REM sleep attacks all during the day. Recently evidence has been presented that *sleep latency* (the time between the point when an individual tries to sleep and the point of onset of EEG sleep patterns), measured re-

peatedly in diurnal nap situations, is greatly reduced in narcoleptics (Richardson et al.). Thus narcolepsy is not simply a matter of excessive diurnal sleepiness or even a disorder of REM sleep, but a generalized disorganization of sleep-waking functions.

Diagnosis The greatest difficulty in the diagnosis of narcolepsy relates to the problem of separating it from the normal sleep pattern. Many sedentary, obese adults, if unoccupied, doze readily after meals, or during a game of bridge, or in the theater, but characteristic of narcolepsy is the insistent sleeping under unusual circumstances (such as standing up) and the tendency of the sleep attacks to recur many times a day. When cataplexy is conjoined, diagnosis becomes virtually certain. The brief attacks of automatic behavior and amnesia of the narcoleptic need to be distinguished from hysterical fugues and partial complex seizures. Excessive somnolence, easily mistaken for idiopathic narcolepsy, may attend obesity, heart failure, hypothyroidism, excessive use of barbiturates and alcohol, cerebral trauma, certain brain tumors (e.g., craniopharyngioma) and the sleep-apnea syndromes. Where polygraphic sleep recording facilities are available, the finding of short latency (less than 5 min) REM sleep during normal waking hours or just after nocturnal sleep begins will confirm the diagnosis of narcolepsy.

Treatment No single therapy will control all the symptoms. The narcolepsy responds best to ① strategically placed 15-min naps (during lunch hour, before or after dinner, etc.) and ② the use of analeptic drugs [dextroamphetamine sulfate (Dexedrine) or methylphenidate hydrochloride (Ritalin)] or tricyclic antidepressants (imipramine or clomipramine). Monoamine oxidase inhibitors (phenelzine, pargyline) are also effective in controlling narcoleptic symptoms, but their severe side effects make them impractical for long-time use. All these drugs presumably produce their effects by inhibiting REM sleep.

The ideal frequency of the naps has to be determined for each individual, and similarly the time of medication should be adjusted to the study or work habits of the patient. The usual dose of amphetamine is 5 to 10 mg given three to five times a day. This is ordinarily well tolerated and does not cause wakefulness at night. The dose of methylphenidate is 10 to 20 mg thrice daily. These have rather little effect on cataplexy but are partially effective in the Kleine-Levine syndrome. Imipramine (Tofranil) and clomipramine are given in doses of 25 mg three to four times a day. Since amphetamines are particularly effective in reducing the sleep attacks and imipramine or clomipramine in reducing cataplexy and sleep paralysis, the combined use of these drugs is often useful.

A problem with all these drugs is the development of tolerance over a 6- to 12-month period, which requires the switching of drugs and periods of drug cessation in the clinical management.

PATHOLOGIC WAKEFULNESS

This state has been induced in animals by lesions in the tegmentum (median raphe nuclei) of the pons. Comparable states are known to occur in humans, but must be rare. The commonest causes of asomnia in hospital practice are delirium tremens and drug-withdrawal psychoses. Drug-induced psychoses and hypomania may also cause hyposomnia.

SLEEP PALSIES AND ACROPARESTHESIAS

Curious and at times distressing paresthetic disturbances develop during sleep. Everyone is familiar with the phenomenon of an arm or leg "falling asleep." The immobility of the limbs and the maintenance of uncomfortable postures without being aware of them permits undue pressure to be applied to exposed nerves. The ulnar, radial, and peroneal nerves are quite superficial in places, and pressure of the nerve against the underlying bone may interfere with intraneural circulation of blood in the compressed segment. If such pressure is continued for half an hour or longer, a sensory and motor paralysis—sometimes referred to as *sleep* or *pressure palsy*—may develop. This condition usually lasts only a few hours or days, but if the compression is prolonged, the nerve may be severely damaged so that functional recovery awaits regeneration. Unusually deep sleep or stupor, as in alcoholic intoxication or anesthesia, renders patients especially liable to pressure palsies, merely because they do not heed the discomfort of an unnatural posture.

Acroparesthesias are frequent in adult women and are not unknown to men. The patient, after being asleep for a few hours, is awakened by a numbness, tingling, prickling, "pins and needles" feeling in the fingers and hands. There are also aching, burning pains or tightness and other unpleasant sensations. At first there is a suspicion of having slept on an arm, but the frequent bilaterality of the symptoms and their occurrence regardless of the position of the arms, dispels this notion. Usually the paresthesias are in the distribution of the median nerves. With vigorous rubbing or shaking of the hands the paresthesias subside within a few minutes, only to return later, upon first awakening in the morning. The condition tends not to occur during the daytime unless the patient is lying down or sitting with the arms and hands in one position. In severe cases, the hands at all times feel swollen, stiff, clumsy, slightly numb, and sometimes distressingly painful. Examination may disclose little or no objective sensory loss, though in some cases touch and pain sensation are diminished in parts supplied by the median nerves. Atrophy and weakness of the abductor pollicis brevis and opponens pollicis muscles have also been noted, and in a few cases have been marked in degree (carpal tunnel syndrome; see also pages 151 and 921). The use of the hands for heavy work during the day seems to aggravate the condition, and a holiday or a period of hospitalization may relieve it. It often occurs in young housewives with a new baby or in factory workers who perform a routine skill. The disorder is particularly common in rheumatoid arthritis, myxedema, acromegaly, primary amyloidosis, mucopolysaccharidoses and multiple myeloma (due to amyloid deposits); common to all of these is a thickening of the transverse carpal ligaments or the synovia of the flexor tendons, with compression of the median nerve. The injection of 50 mg hydrocortisone beneath the carpal ligaments and the use of chlorothiazide (Diuril) or one of its analogues has given relief in a respectable number of cases, particularly those with a tenosynovitis. The section of the transverse carpal ligament and palmar aponeurosis nearly always cures recalcitrant cases.

NOCTURNAL ENURESIS

Nocturnal bedwetting with daytime continence is a frequent disorder of sleep during childhood but may persist into adult life. Approximately one of ten children 4 to 14 years of age is affected, boys more frequently than girls, and even among adults (military recruits) the incidence is 1 to 3 percent. Though the condition was formerly thought to be functional, i.e., psychogenic, the studies of Gastaut and Broughton have revealed a peculiarity of bladder physiology. Intravesicular pressures periodically rise to much higher levels in enuretic patients than in normal persons, and their arousal time under such conditions is delayed. Also, the bladders of enuretic patients tend to be smaller. This suggests a maturational failure of certain modulating nervous influences. The urinary incontinence has been found to occur usually during the first third of the night, especially during stage 4 of NREM sleep, and is preceded by a burst of rhythmic delta waves associated with a general body movement. If the patient is awakened at this point, he does not report any dreams. Imipramine (Tofranil) has proved to be an effective agent in reducing the frequency of enuresis. Diseases of the urinary tract, diabetes mellitus or diabetes insipidus, epilepsy, sickle-cell anemia, and spinal cord or cauda equina disease must be differentiated as causes of symptomatic enuresis.

RELATION OF SLEEP TO OTHER MEDICAL ILLNESSES

Patients with duodenal ulcer secrete more HCl during sleep (peaks coincide with REM sleep) than normal subjects. Patients with coronary arteriosclerosis show ECG changes during REM sleep, and nocturnal angina has been recorded at this time. Asthmatics frequently have their attacks at night, but not concomitantly with any specific stage of sleep; they do have a decreased amount of stage 4 NREM sleep and frequent awakenings, however. Patients with hypothyroidism have shown a decrease of stages 3 and 4 NREM sleep, and a return to a normal pattern when they become euthyroid.

The senile dement exhibits reduced amounts of REM sleep and stage 4 NREM sleep, as do mongolian idiots, phenylketonurics, and brain-damaged children. A correlation has been demonstrated between the level of intelligence and the amount of REM sleep in all these conditions, and in normal persons as well. Alcohol, barbiturates, and other sedative-hypnotic drugs, which suppress REM sleep, permit extraordinary excesses of it to appear during withdrawal periods, which may in part account for the hyperactivity and confusion seen in these states.

REFERENCES

BURWELL CS et al: Extreme obesity associated with alveolar hypoventilation. A Pickwickian syndrome. *Am J Med* 21:811, 1956.

DANIELS L: Narcolepsy. *Medicine* 13:1, 1935.

DALY D, YOSS R: Narcolepsy, in Vinken PJ, Bruyn GW (eds): *Handbook of Clinical Neurology, The Epilepsies.* Amsterdam, North-Holland, 1974, chap 43, pp 836–852.

DEMENT WC, KLEITMAN N: Cyclic variations in EEG during sleep and their relation to eye movements, bodily motility and dreaming. *EEG Clin Neurophysiol* 9:673, 1957.

GUILLEMINAULT C, DEMENT WC: 235 cases of excessive daytime sleepiness. Diagnosis and tentative classification. *J Neurol Sci* 31:13, 1977.

————, ————, PASSOUANT P (eds): Narcolepsy, in *Advances in Sleep Research,* vol 3. New York, Spectrum, 1976.

———— et al: Sleep-related periodic myoclonus in patients complaining of insomnia. *Trans Am Neurol Assoc* 100:19, 1975.

KALES A, KALES JD: Sleep disorders: Recent findings in the diagnosis and treatment of disturbed sleep. *N Engl J Med* 290:487, 1974.

————: Chronic hypnotic use: Ineffectiveness, drug withdrawal insomnia and hypnotic drug dependence. *JAMA* 27:513, 1974.

MITLER MM: Toward an animal model of narcolepsy-cataplexy, in Guilleminault C, Dement WC, Passouant P (eds): *Narcolepsy.* New York, Spectrum, 1976, pp 387–409.

MONNIER M, HOSLI L: Humoral regulation of sleep and wakefulness by hypnogenic and activating dialysable factors. *Prog Brain Res* 18:118, 1965.

OSWALD I: Sudden bodily jerks on falling asleep. *Brain* 82:92, 1959.

PAPPENHEIMER JR et al: Sleep-promoting effects of cerebrospinal fluid from sleep-deprived goats. *Proc Natl Acad Sci USA* 58:513, 1967.

PASSOUANT P: The history of narcolepsy, in Guilleminault C, Dement WC, Passouant P (eds): *Narcolepsy.* New York, Spectrum, 1976, pp 3–13.

PHILLIPSON EA: Breathing disorders during sleep. *Basics RD* 7 (3):1, Jan 1979.

POMPEIANO O: Vestibular influences during sleep, in Kornhuber HH (ed) *Handbook of Sensory Physiology,* vol VI/1: *Vestibular System,* pt 1: *Basic Mechanisms.* Berlin, Springer-Verlag, 1974, pp 583–622.

RECHTSCHAFFEN A, KALES A (eds): *A Manual of Standardized Terminology, Techniques, and Scoring System for Sleep Stages of Human Subjects.* Washington, Public Health Service, 1968.

————, MONROE LJ: Laboratory studies of insomnia, in Kales A (ed): *Sleep: Physiology and Pathology, A Symposium.* Philadelphia, Lippincott, 1969, p 158.

RICHARDSON GS: Excessive daytime sleepiness in man: Multiple sleep latency measurement in narcoleptic and control subjects. *EEG Clin Neurophysiol* 45:621, 1978.

WEITZMAN ED et al: The relationship of sleep and sleep stages to neuroendocrine secretion and biological rhythms in man. *Recent Prog Horm Res* 31:399, 1975.

WILLIAMS RL et al: *Electroencephalography (EEG) of Human Sleep: Clinical Applications.* New York, Wiley, 1974.

ZARCONE V: Narcolepsy. *N Engl J Med* 288:1156, 1973.

DERANGEMENTS OF INTELLECT, BEHAVIOR, AND LANGUAGE DUE TO DIFFUSE AND FOCAL CEREBRAL DISEASE

Physicians sooner or later discover through clinical experience the need for special competence in assessing the mental faculties of their patients. They must be able to observe with detachment and complete objectivity the patient's character, intelligence, mood, memory, judgment, and other attributes of personality, in much the same fashion as they observe the nutritional state and the color of the mucous membranes. The systematic examination of these affective and intellectual functions permits the physician to reach certain conclusions regarding mental status, and it is also of value in helping the physician understand the patient and his or her illness. Without such data, errors will be made in evaluating the reliability of the history in the diagnosis of the patient's neurologic or psychiatric disease and in conducting an appropriate therapeutic program.

Perhaps the content of this section will be more clearly understood if we anticipate a few of the introductory remarks to the section on psychiatric diseases. The main thesis of the neurologist is that mental and physical functions of the nervous system are simply two aspects of the same neural process. Mind and behavior both have their roots in the self-regulating, goal-seeking activities of the organism, the same ones that provide impulse to all forms of mammalian life. The prodigious complexity of the human brain permits, to an extraordinary degree, the solving of difficult problems, the capacity for remembering past experiences and phrasing them in a symbolic language that can be written and read, and the planning of events that have not taken place. Somehow there emerges in the course of these complex cerebral functions a more complete and continuous awareness of one's self and of the operation of one's own psychic processes than is found in any other species. It is this continuous inner consciousness of past experiences and ongoing cognitive activities that is called mind. Any separation of the mental from the observable behavioral aspects of nervous functioning is illusory. Biologists and psychologists have reached the modern monistic view by placing all protoplasmic activities of the nervous system (growth, development, behavior, and mental function) in a continuum and noting the inherent purposiveness and creativity common to all of them. The physician is persuaded of the truth of this view through daily clinical experience, in which every known aberration of behavior and intellect appears as an expression of cerebral disease. Further, in many brain diseases the physician witnesses parallel disorders of the patient's behavior and introspective awareness of functional capacities.

Chapters 19 and 20 will be concerned with common disturbances of the sensorium and of intellection which have not been discussed previously and which stand as cardinal manifestations of certain cerebral diseases. The most frequent of these are the acute confusional states, delirium, and disorders of learning, memory, and other intellectual functions. A consideration of these abnormalities, indicative as a rule of a diffuse disturbance of cerebral function, leads naturally to an examination of the symptoms consequent upon focal cerebral lesions (Chap. 21), and of language mechanisms (Chap. 22), which fall between the readily localizable functions of the cerebrum and those which cannot be localized.

CHAPTER 19

DELIRIUM AND OTHER ACUTE CONFUSIONAL STATES

The singular event in which a patient with previously intact mentality becomes acutely psychotic is observed almost daily on the medical and surgical wards of a general hospital. Occurring as it often does during an infective fever, in the course of another illness (such as renal or hepatic failure), or as an effect of medication or abuse of alcohol, it never fails to create grave problems for the physician, nursing personnel, and family. The physician has to cope with the problem of diagnosis often without the advantage of a lucid history, and any program of therapy to be initiated is constantly threatened by the patient's agitation, sleeplessness, and inability to cooperate. The nursing personnel is often sorely taxed by the necessity of providing satisfactory care for the patient and, at the same time, maintaining a tranquil atmosphere for other patients. The family must be supported as it faces the appalling spectre of insanity and all it signifies.

These problems are greatly magnified when the patient arrives in the emergency ward, having behaved in some irrational way, and the physician must begin the clinical analysis without knowledge of the patient's background and underlying medical problems. Under such circumstances it is tempting to rid oneself of the clinical problem by transferring the patient to a psychiatric hospital. This is unwise in the authors' opinion, for there may not be adequate facilities for the management of the great variety of medical diseases with which the psychosis may be associated. It is far better to study such patients initially on a general medical or neurologic ward and to transfer them to a psychiatric service only if the behavioral disorder proves impossible to manage in a general hospital, or, if warranted, when the underlying medical problems have been brought under control.

DEFINITION OF TERMS

The definition of normal and abnormal states of mind is difficult, because the terms used to describe these states have been given so many different meanings in both medical and nonmedical writings. Compounding the difficulty is the fact that the pathophysiology of the confusional states, delirium, and dementia is not fully understood, and the definitions depend on their clinical relationships, with all the lack of precision which this entails. The following nomenclature, though tentative, has proved useful to us and will be employed throughout this textbook.

Confusion is a general term denoting an incapacity of the patient to think with customary speed, clarity, and coherence. Disorientation, impaired attention and concentration, inability to register properly immediate happenings and to recall them later, reduced perceptiveness with visual and auditory illusions (sometimes hallucinations), and a general diminution of all mental activity are other features. These psychological disturbances may be due to any one of several factors. A confusional state is an essential element in delirium, in which case it depends mainly on a disorder of perception. It appears at a certain stage in the evolution and devolution of a series of diseases which lead to stupor and coma, as was pointed out in Chap. 16, in which instance it must be aligned with disorders of consciousness. It may occur in association with a chronic syndrome such as dementia where already there has been a failure of memory and other intellectual impairments. Finally, intense emotional disturbances may interfere with coherence of thinking.

Delirium will be used to denote a special type of confusional state. In addition to all the negative elements described above, delirium is marked by a prominent disorder of perception, terrifying hallucinations and vivid dreams, a kaleidoscopic array of strange and absurd fantasies, inability to sleep, tendency to convulse, and intense emotional disturbances. All these positive aspects of disordered consciousness, after the classic studies of the French authors, are designated by the term *oneirism* or *oneiric consciousness* (from the Greek *oneiros*, "dream"). The *twilight states* are closely related disorders, but the clinical descriptions have been so divergent that the term now has little useful meaning. We would add that delirium is distinguished also by heightened alertness, i.e., an increased readiness to respond to stimuli, and by marked overactivity of psychomotor and autonomic nervous system functions. Implicit in the term *delirium* are its nonmedical connotations—intense agitation, frenzied excitement, and trembling.

It should be noted that this distinction between delirium and other acute confusional states is not universally accepted. Some authors attach no particular significance to the autonomic and psychomotor overactivity and oneiric or dreamlike features of delirium, or to the underactivity and somnolence that characterize other confusional states. All such states are lumped together under the heading of toxic psychosis, infective-exhaustive psychosis, febrile delirium, exogenous reaction type of psychosis, or acute organic reaction or symptomatic psychosis, with the implication that they are induced by toxic or metabolic disturbances of the brain. We believe that delirium should be set apart from other confusional states, for the reason that the two conditions are descriptively different and occur in different clinical contexts, as will be indicated further on. Nevertheless, implicit in both is the idea of an acute, transient, completely reversible disorder.

The term *amnesia* means loss of the ability to form memories despite an alert state of mind. It presupposes an ability to grasp the problem, to use language normally, and to maintain adequate motivation. The failure is mainly one of retention, recall, and reproduction, and it should be distinguished from states of drowsiness and acute confusion, in which information and events seem never to have been adequately perceived and registered in the first place.

Dementia literally means an undoing of the mind or, more particularly, a deterioration of all intellectual or cognitive functions, without disturbances of consciousness or perception. Implied in the word is the idea

of a gradual enfeeblement of mental powers in a person who formerly possessed a normal mind. *Amentia*, by contrast, indicates a congenital feeblemindedness. Dementia and amnesia are defined further in the next chapter.

OBSERVABLE ASPECTS OF BEHAVIOR AND THEIR RELATION TO CONFUSION, DELIRIUM, AMNESIA, AND DEMENTIA

The intellectual, emotional, volitional, and behavioral activities of the human organism are so complex and varied that one may question the feasibility of using derangements of them as reliable indicators of cerebral disease. Certainly they have not the same reliability and ease of anatomic and physiologic interpretation as sensory and motor paralysis or aphasia. Yet one observes particular disturbances of these higher cerebral functions recurring with such regularity in certain diseases as to be useful in clinical medicine; and some of them gain in specificity because they are often combined in certain ways to form syndromes, which are essentially what states of confusion, delirium, amnesia, and dementia are.

The components of mentation and behavior that lend themselves to bedside examination are (1) the processes of sensation and perception; (2) the capacity of memorizing; (3) the ability to think and reason; (4) temperament, mood, and emotion; (5) initiative, impulse, and drive; and (6) insight. Of these (1) is sensorial, (2) and (3) are cognitive, (4) is affective, and (5) is conative or volitional. Insight includes the introspective observations made by patients concerning their own normal or disordered functioning. Each component of behavior and intellection has its objective side, expressed in the behavioral responses that are produced by certain stimuli and its subjective side, expressed in the thinking and feeling described by the patient in relation to the stimuli.

DISTURBANCES OF PERCEPTION

Perception, i.e., the process involved in acquiring through the senses a knowledge of the "world about" or of one's own body, involves much more than the simple sensory process of being aware of the attributes of a stimulus. It includes the maintenance of attention, the selective focusing on a stimulus, elimination of all extraneous stimuli, and identification of the stimulus by recognizing its relationship to personal remembered experiences. The perception of a stimulus undergoes predictable types of derangement in disease. Most often there is a reduction in the number of perceptions in a given unit of time and failure to synthesize them properly and relate them to the ongoing activities of the mind. Or there may be apparent inattentiveness or fluctuations of attention, distractibility (pertinent and irrelevant stimuli now having equal value), and inability to persist in an assigned task. Qualitative changes also appear, mainly in the form of sensory distortions, causing misinterpretation and misidentification of objects and persons (illusions); and these, at least in part, form the basis of hallucinatory experience in which the patient reports and reacts to stimuli not present in the environment. There is an inability to perceive simultaneously all elements of a large complex of stimuli, which is sometimes explained as a "failure of subjective organization." These major disturbances in the perceptual sphere, often referred to as "clouding of the sensorium," occur most often in deliria and other acute confusional states, but quantitative deficiency may also become evident in the advanced stages of amentia and dementia.

DISTURBANCES OF MEMORY

Memory, i.e., the retention of learned experiences, is involved in all mental activities. It may be arbitrarily subdivided into several parts, viz., (1) registration, which includes all that was mentioned under perception; (2) mnemonic integration and retention; (3) recall; and (4) reproduction. As stated above, in disturbances of perception and attention there may be a complete failure of learning and memory for the reason that the material to be learned was never registered and assimilated. In Korsakoff's amnesic syndrome (Korsakoff's psychosis), newly presented material appears to be temporarily registered but cannot be retained for more than a few minutes, and there is always an associated defect in the recall and reproduction of memories that had been formed several days, or weeks, or even years before the onset of the illness (retrograde amnesia). The fabrication of stories, called *confabulation*, constitutes a third feature of the syndrome, but not a specific or invariable one. Sound retention with failure of recall is at times a normal state; when it is severe and extends to all events of past life it is usually due to hysteria or malingering. Proof that the processes of registration and recall are intact under these circumstances comes from hypnosis and suggestion, by means of which the lost items are fully recalled and reproduced. Patients with Korsakoff's psychosis fail on all tests of learning and recent memory, and their behavior accords with their deficiencies of information. Hypnosis does not facilitate recall. Since memory is involved to some extent in all mental processes, it becomes the most testable component of mentation and behavior.

DISTURBANCES OF THINKING

Thinking, the highest order of intellectual activity, remains one of the most elusive of all mental operations. If by thinking we mean selective ordering of symbols for problem solving and capacity to reason and form sound judgments (the usual definition), obviously the working units of most mental activity of this type are words and numbers. The substitution of words and numbers for the objects for which they stand (symbolization) is a fundamental part of the process. These symbols are formed into ideas or concepts, and the arrangement of new and remembered ideas into certain orders or relationships, according to the rules of logic, constitutes another intricate part of thought, presently beyond the scope of analysis. On page 303, reference is made to Luria's analysis of the steps involved in problem solving in connection with frontal lobe function, but actually the whole cerebrum is implicated. In a general way one may examine thinking for speed and efficiency, ideational content, coherence and logical relationships of ideas, quantity and quality of associations to a given idea, and the propriety of the feeling and behavior engendered by an idea.

Information concerning the thought processes and associative functions is best obtained by analyzing the patient's spontaneous verbal productions and by engaging him or her in conversation. If the patient is taciturn or mute, one may have to depend on responses to direct questions or upon written material, i.e., letters, etc. One notes the prevailing trends of the patient's thoughts; whether the ideas are reasonable, precise, and coherent or vague, circumstantial, tangential, and irrelevant; and whether the thought processes are shallow and fragmented.

Disorders of thinking are frequent in deliria and other confusional states, in dementia, and in schizophrenia. The organization of thought may be disrupted, with fragmentation, repetition, and perseveration. This is spoken of as an "incoherence of thinking" and marks confusional states of all types. The patient may be excessively critical, rationalizing, and hairsplitting; this is a type of thinking often manifest in depressive psychoses. Derangements of thinking may also take the form of a flight of ideas; patients move nimbly from one idea to another, and their associations are numerous and loosely linked. This is a common feature in hypomanic and manic states. The opposite condition, poverty of ideas, is characteristic both of depression, where it is combined with gloomy thoughts, and of dementing diseases, where it is part of a reduction of all intellectual activity. Thinking may be distorted in such a way that ideas are not checked against reality. When a false belief is maintained in spite of normally convincing contradictory evidence, the patient is said to have a delusion. Delusions are common to many illnesses, particularly manic-depressive and schizophrenic states. Patients may declare that ideas have been implanted in their minds by some outside agencies, such as radio, television, or atomic energy. These reflect the "passivity feelings" characteristic of schizophrenia. Other distortions of logical thought, such as gaps in sequential thinking and condensation of associations, are typical of schizophrenia, of which they constitute diagnostic features.

DISTURBANCES OF EMOTION, MOOD, AND AFFECT

The emotional life of the patient is expressed in a variety of ways. In the first place, rather marked individual differences in basic temperament are to be observed in the normal population; some persons are throughout their life cheerful, gregarious, optimistic, and free from worry, whereas others are just the opposite. The usually volatile, cyclothymic person is said to be liable to manic-depressive psychosis, and the suspicious, withdrawn, introverted person to schizophrenia and paranoia, but there are frequent exceptions to this statement. Strong, persistent emotional states, such as fear and anxiety, may occur as reactions to life situations and may be accompanied by derangements of visceral function. If excessive and disproportionate to the stimulus, they are usually manifestations of an anxiety neurosis or depression. Variations in the degree of responsiveness to emotional stimuli are also frequent, and when extreme and persistent, assume importance. In depression, all stimuli tend to enhance the somber mood of unhappiness. Emotional responses that are excessively labile and poorly controlled or uninhibited are a common manifestation of many diseases of the cerebrum, particularly those involving the corticopontine and corticobulbar pathways. This disorder constitutes a part of the syndrome of spastic bulbar (pseudobulbar) palsy. All emotional expression may be lacking, as in apathetic states or severe depressions, or the patient may be a victim of every trivial problem in daily life, i.e., unable to control worry. Finally, the emotional response may be inappropriate to the stimulus, e.g., a depressing or morbid thought may seem amusing and be attended by a smile, as in schizophrenia.

Temperament, mood, and other emotional experiences described above are evaluated by the appearance of patients and by verbalized accounts of their feelings. For these purposes it is convenient to divide emotionality into mood and feeling (or affect). By *mood* is meant the prevailing emotional state of individuals without reference to the stimuli immediately impinging upon them. It may be pleasant and cheerful or melancholic. The language (e.g., the adjectives used) and the facial expression, attitude, posture, and speed of movement most reliably betray the patient's mood. By contrast, *feelings* (or *affect*) are said to be emotional experiences evoked by environmental stimuli. According to some psychiatrists, feeling is the subjective component, and affect, the overt manifestation. Others apply either word to the subjective state. The difference between mood as a prevailing emotional state and feeling, or affect, as an emotional reaction to stimuli may seem rather tenuous, but these distinctions are considered valuable by psychiatrists. The significance of various types of emotional disturbance is discussed more fully in Chap. 25.

DISTURBANCES OF IMPULSE

Impulse, that basic biologic urge, driving force, or purpose, by which every organism is directed to reach its full potentialities, appears to be another observable and extremely important, though somewhat neglected, dimension of behavior. Again, one notes wide normal variations from one person to another in strength of impulse, and these individual differences are present throughout life. One of the most conspicuous pathologic deviations is an apparent constitutional weakness of impulse in certain neurotic persons. Moreover, with many types of cerebral disease (particularly those which involve the posterior orbital parts of the frontal lobes), a reduction in impulse is coupled with an indifference or lack of concern about the consequences of actions. In such cases all other measurable aspects of psychic function may be normal. The lack of impulse, or *abulia*, may be extreme in degree, to the point of mutism and immobility (*akinetic mutism;* see pages 233 and 302). Psychomotor retardation is a lesser degree of the same state and is a feature of cerebral disease or of depression. In the latter instance, alteration of mood and extreme fatigability are added.

LOSS OF INSIGHT

Insight, the state of being fully aware of the nature and degree of one's deficits, becomes manifestly impaired or abolished in relation to all types of cerebral disease that cause complex disorders of behavior. Rarely do patients with any of the aforementioned states seek advice or help for their illness. Instead, the family usually brings the patient to the physician. Thus, it appears that the diseases which produce all these abnormalities not only evoke observable changes in behavior but also alter or reduce the capacity of patients to make accurate introspections concerning their own psychic function. This fact stands as proof that the cerebrum is the organ both of behavior and of all inner psychic experiences; i.e., behavior and mind are but two inseparable aspects of the function of the nervous system.

COMMON SYNDROMES

The entire group of acute confusional and delirious states is characterized principally by an impairment of consciousness with prominent disorders of attention and perception that interfere with the speed and clarity of thinking and the formation of memories. Three major clinical syndromes can be recognized. One is a *confusional state* in which there is manifest reduction in alertness and psychomotor activity. The second syndrome, here called *delirium,* is characterized by overactivity, sleeplessness, tremulousness, and hallucinations, with convulsions often preceding or associated with the delirium. A third syndrome consists of a confusional state occurring in persons with some other cerebral disease. The latter disposes the patient to the acute psychosis which we have chosen to designate as a *beclouded dementia.* These illnesses tend to develop acutely, to have multiple causes, and to terminate within a relatively short period of time (days to weeks), leaving the patient without residual damage or with whatever defects were present before their onset.

ACUTE CONFUSIONAL STATES ASSOCIATED WITH REDUCED ALERTNESS AND PSYCHOMOTOR ACTIVITY

Clinical Features Some features of this syndrome have already been described in Chap. 16, "Coma and Related Disorders of Consciousness." In the most typical example, all mental functions are reduced to some degree; but alertness, attentiveness, and the ability to grasp all elements of the immediate situation suffer most. In its mildest form, the patient may pass for normal, and only failure to recollect and reproduce happenings of the past few hours or days reveals the inadequacy of mental function. The more obviously confused patients spend much of their time in idleness, and what they do may be inappropriate and annoying to others. Only the more automatic acts and verbal responses are performed properly, but these may permit the examiner to obtain from the patient a number of relevant and accurate replies to questions about age, occupation, and residence. Reactions are slow and indecisive. Such patients may repeat every question that is put to them, before answering, and their responses tend to be brief and mechanical. It is difficult or impossible for them to sustain a conversation. Their attention wanders and they have constantly to be brought back to the subject at hand. They may even fall asleep during the interview, and, if left alone, they are observed to sleep more hours each day than is natural, or the usual number at irregular intervals. Frequently there are perceptual disturbances in which voices, common objects, and the actions of other persons are misinterpreted. Often one cannot discern whether these patients hear voices and see things that do not exist, i.e., whether they are hallucinating, or are merely misinterpreting stimuli in the environment. Inadequate perception and forgetfulness result in a constant state of bewilderment. Failing to recognize their surroundings fully and having lost all sense of time, they repeat the same question and make the same remarks over and over again. Irritability may or may not be present. Some patients are extremely suspicious; in fact, a paranoid trend may be the most pronounced and troublesome feature of the illness.

As the confusion deepens, conversation becomes more difficult, and at a certain stage these patients no longer notice or respond to much of what is going on around them. Replies to questions may be a single word or a short phrase spoken in a soft tremulous voice or whisper. The patient may be mute. In its most advanced stages confusion gives way to stupor and finally to coma. As these patients improve, they may pass again through the stage of stupor and confusion in the reverse order. All this informs us that at least one category of confusion is but a manifestation of the same disease processes that in their severest form cause coma.

In the most typical case, this type of confusional state is readily distinguished from delirium; in others with more than the usual degree of irritability and restlessness, one cannot fail to notice their resemblance to each other. Further, when a delirium is complicated by an illness that superimposes stupor (e.g., delirium tremens with pneumonia, meningitis, or hepatic encephalopathy), it may be difficult to distinguish from other acute confusional states. Difficulty in distinguishing these two states explains why some psychiatrists (Engel and Romano, Lipowski) insist that there is only one disorder, which they call *delirium*. The present writers would disagree, for they believe that several pathogenetic mechanisms of different types and involving different parts of the brain are included in this category of acute, reversible cerebral disease.

Morbid Anatomy and Pathophysiology All that has been said on this subject in Chap. 16, "Coma and Related Disorders of Consciousness," is applicable to at least one subgroup of the confusional states. In the others no consistent pathologic change has been found. The EEG is of interest, because it is almost invariably abnormal in more severe forms of this syndrome, in contrast to delirium, where the changes are relatively minor. High-voltage slow waves in the 2- to 4-per-second (delta) range or the 5- to 7-per-second (theta) range are the usual findings.

DELIRIUM

Clinical Features These are most perfectly depicted in the alcoholic patient. The symptoms usually develop over a period of 2 or 3 days. The first indications of the approaching attack are difficulty in concentration, restless irritability, tremulousness, insomnia, and poor appetite. One or several generalized convulsions are the initial major symptom in almost 30 percent of the cases. The patient's rest is troubled by unpleasant or terrifying dreams. There may be momentary disorientation, an occasional inappropriate remark, or transient illusions or hallucinations.

These initial symptoms rapidly give way to a clinical picture that, in severe cases, is one of the most colorful in medicine. The "sensorium is clouded" in that the patients are inattentive and unable to perceive all elements of their situation. They may talk incessantly and incoherently and look distressed and perplexed; their expression is in keeping with their vague notions of being annoyed or threatened by someone who seeks to injure them. From their manner and the content of their speech it is evident that they misinterpret the meaning of ordinary objects and sounds, misidentify the people around them, and have vivid visual, auditory, and tactile hallucinations, often of a most unpleasant type. At first they can be brought momentarily into touch with reality and may in fact identify the examiner and answer other questions correctly; but almost at once they relapse into their preoccupied, confused state, giving wrong answers and being unable to think coherently. Before long they

are unable to shake off their hallucinations even for a second and do not recognize their physician or even their family. They are unable to make meaningful responses to even the simplest questions and are profoundly disoriented, as a rule.

Tremor and restless movements are usually present and may be violent. Sleep is impossible or occurs only in brief naps. The countenance is flushed, the pupils are dilated, and the conjunctivas are injected; the pulse is rapid and soft, and the temperature may be raised. There is much sweating, and the urine is scanty and of high specific gravity. The signs of overactivity of the autonomic nervous system, more than any other, distinguish delirium from all other confusional states.

The symptoms abate, either suddenly or gradually, after 2 or 3 days, although in exceptional cases they may persist for several weeks. The most certain indication of the end of the attack is the occurrence of sound sleep and of lucid intervals of increasing length. Recovery is usually complete.

Delirium is subject to all degrees of variability, not only from patient to patient but in the same patient from day to day and hour to hour. The entire syndrome may be observed in one patient, and only one or two symptoms in another. In its mildest form, as so often occurs in febrile diseases, it consists of an occasional wandering of the mind and incoherence of verbal expression. This form, lacking motor and autonomic overactivity, is sometimes referred to as a *quiet delirium* (or *hypokinetic delirium*) and is difficult to distinguish from other confusional states. The more severe form of delirium, best exemplified by delirium tremens, ends fatally in 5 to 15 percent of patients (see Chap. 40).

Morbid Anatomy and Pathophysiology The brains of patients who have died in delirium tremens usually show no pathologic changes of significance. A number of diseases, however, may cause delirium and also give rise to focal lesions in the brain, such as viral encephalitis, Wernicke's disease, trauma, or focal embolic encephalomalacia. The topography of these lesions is of particular interest. They tend to be localized in the midbrain and subthalamus and in the temporal lobes, where they involve the reticular activating and limbic systems. Electrical stimulation studies of the human cerebral cortex during surgical exploration have clearly indicated the importance of the temporal lobe in the genesis of visual, auditory, and olfactory hallucinations. With subthalamic and midbrain lesions, visual hallucinations may occur that are not unpleasant and may be accompanied by good insight (the "peduncular hallucinosis" of Lhermitte).

The EEG in delirium usually shows nonfocal slow

activity in the 5- to 7-per-second range, a state that rapidly returns to normal as the delirium clears. However, in other cases only activity in the fast beta frequency range is seen, and in milder degrees of delirium there is usually no abnormality at all.

An analysis of the several conditions conducive to delirium suggests at least three different physiologic mechanisms. The withdrawal of alcohol, barbiturates, or other sedative-hypnotic drugs, following a period of chronic intoxication, is the most common one (see Chaps. 40 and 41). These drugs are known to have a strong depressant effect on certain areas of the central nervous system; presumably, the disinhibition and overactivity of these parts, after withdrawal of the drug, are the basis of delirium. In this respect it is interesting to note that the symptoms of delirium tremens are the antithesis of those of alcoholic intoxication. In the case of bacterial infections and poisoning by certain drugs, such as atropine and scopolamine, the delirious state probably results from the direct action of the toxin or chemical agent on these same parts of the brain. Thirdly, destructive lesions, such as those of the temporal lobes in herpes simplex encephalitis, may cause delirium by disturbing the function of these particular areas.

Psychophysiologic mechanisms have also been postulated. It has long been suggested that some persons are much more liable to delirium than others. There is much reason to doubt this hypothesis, for it has been shown that all of a group of randomly selected persons develop delirium if the causative mechanisms are strongly operative (Wolff and Curran). This is not surprising, for any healthy person under certain circumstances may experience phenomena akin to those found in delirium. After repeated auditory and visual stimulation, the same impressions may continue to be perceived even though the stimuli are no longer present. A soldier, for example, may continue to hear the whine of artillery shells long after the bombardment has ceased. Also, a healthy person can be induced to hallucinate by being placed for several days in an environment as free as possible of sensory stimulation. A relation between delirium and dream states has been postulated because both are characterized by a loss of appreciation of time, a richness of visual imagery, indifference to inconsistencies, and "defective reality testing." Moreover, patients may refer to some of these delirious symptoms as a "bad dream," and normal persons may experience so-called hypnagogic hallucinations in the period between sleeping and waking. In general, however, formulations in the field of dynamic psychology seem more reasonably to account for the topical content of delirium than to explain its occurrence. Wolff and Curran, having observed the same content in repeated attacks of delirium due to different causes, concluded that the content depends more on age, sex, intellectual endowment, occupation, personality traits, and past experiences of the patient than on the cause or mechanism of the delirium.

The main difficulty in understanding delirium arises from the fact that it has not been possible to ascertain which of the many symptoms have physiologic significance. What is the basis of this altered consciousness, this sensorial disturbance, this lack of harmony between actual sensory impressions of the present and memory of those in the past? Obviously, something has been removed from the perceptive process, something that leaves the patient at the mercy of certain sensory stimuli and unable to attend to others, yet at the same time incapable of discriminating between sense impression and fantasy. The lack of inhibition of sensory processes may also be the basis of the sleep disturbance (insomnia).

SENILE AND OTHER DEMENTING BRAIN DISEASES COMPLICATED BY MEDICAL OR SURGICAL ILLNESS (BECLOUDED DEMENTIA)

Many elderly patients who enter the hospital with a medical or surgical illness are mentally confused. Presumably the liability to this state is determined by preexisting brain disease, most often senile dementia, which may or may not have been obvious to the family before the onset of the complicating illness. Other cerebral diseases (vascular, neoplastic, demyelinative) may have the same effect.

All the clinical features that one observes in the acute confusional states may be present. The severity may vary greatly. The confusion may be reflected only in the patient's inability to relate sequentially the history of the illness, or it may be so severe that the patient is virtually non compos mentis.

Although almost any complicating illness may bring out the confusion in such a person, the most common are infectious diseases, especially in those cases which resist the effects of antibiotic medication; posttraumatic states, notably concussive brain injuries; operations, particularly the removal of cataracts (in which case the confusion is probably related to temporary deprivation of vision); and with congestive heart failure, chronic respiratory disease, and severe anemia, especially pernicious anemia. Often it is difficult to determine which of several possible factors is responsible for the confusion, and there may be more than one. In a cardiac patient with a confusional psychosis for example, there may be fever, a marginally reduced cerebral blood flow, intoxication with one or more drugs, and electrolyte imbalance. The same may be true of a patient in a postoperative confusional state, in which a number of factors such as fever, infection, dehydration, and drug intoxication may be incriminated. Alcoholism may further complicate the problem.

When such patients recover from the medical or surgical illness, they usually return to their premorbid state, though their shortcomings, now drawn to the attention of the family and physician, may be more obvious than before.

COINCIDENTAL DEVELOPMENT OF SCHIZOPHRENIC OR MANIC-DEPRESSIVE PSYCHOSIS DURING A MEDICAL OR SURGICAL ILLNESS

A certain proportion of psychoses of the schizophrenic or manic-depressive type first become manifest during an acute medical illness or following an operation or parturition and need to be distinguished from an acute confusional state. A causal relationship between the psychosis and medical illness is sought but cannot be established. The psychosis may have preceded the medical illness but was not recognized, or it emerges during the convalescent period. The diagnostic studies of the psychiatric illness must proceed along the lines suggested in Chaps. 54 and 56. Close observation will usually reveal a clear sensorium and relatively intact memory, which permits differentiation from the acute confusional states.

CLASSIFICATION AND DIAGNOSIS OF DELIRIUM AND OTHER ACUTE CONFUSIONAL STATES

The syndromes themselves and their main clinical relationships are the only satisfactory basis for classification until such time as the actual cause and pathophysiology are discovered (Table 19-1). The practice of classifying the syndromes according to their most prominent symptom or degree of severity, e.g., "picking delirium," "microptic delirium," "acute delirious mania," and "muttering delirium," has no fundamental value.

The first step in *diagnosis* is to recognize that the patient is confused. This is obvious in most cases, but, as pointed out above, the mildest forms of confusion, par-

Table 19-1

Classification of delirium and acute confusional states

I. Delirium
  A. In a medical or surgical illness (no focal or lateralizing neurologic signs; CSF usually clear)
    1. Typhoid fever
    2. Pneumonia
    3. Septicemia, particularly erysipelas and other streptococcal infections
    4. Rheumatic fever
    5. Thyrotoxicosis and ACTH intoxication (rare)
    6. Postoperative and postconcussive states
  B. In neurologic disease that causes focal or lateralizing signs or changes in the CSF
    1. Vascular, neoplastic, or other diseases, particularly those involving the temporal lobes and upper part of the brainstem
    2. Cerebral contusion and laceration (traumatic delirium)
    3. Acute purulent and tuberculous meningitis
    4. Subarachnoid hemorrhage
    5. Encephalitis due to viral causes (e.g., infectious mononucleosis) and to unknown causes
  C. The abstinence states, exogenous intoxications, and postconvulsive states; signs of other medical, surgical, and neurologic illnesses absent or coincidental
    1. Withdrawal of alcohol (delirium tremens), barbiturates, and nonbarbiturate sedative drugs, following chronic intoxication (Chaps. 40 and 41)
    2. Drug intoxications: camphor, caffeine, ergot, bromides, scopolamine, atropine, amphetamine, etc.
    3. Postconvulsive delirium
II. Acute confusional states associated with psychomotor underactivity
  A. Associated with a medical or surgical disease (no focal or lateralizing neurologic signs; CSF clear)
    1. Metabolic disorders; hepatic stupor, uremia, hypoxia, hypercapnea, hypoglycemia, porphyria
    2. Infective fevers, especially typhoid
    3. Congestive heart failure
    4. Postoperative, posttraumatic, and puerperal psychoses
  B. Associated with drug intoxication (no focal or lateralizing signs; CSF clear): opiates, barbiturates, bromides, Artane, etc.
  C. Associated with diseases of the nervous system (with focal or lateralizing neurologic signs and/or CSF changes)
    1. Cerebral vascular disease, tumor, abscess
    2. Subdural hematoma
    3. Meningitis
    4. Encephalitis
  D. Beclouded dementia, i.e., senile or other brain disease in combination with infective fevers, drug reactions, heart failure, or other medical or surgical diseases

ticularly when some other acute alteration of personality is prominent, may be overlooked. In these mild forms a careful analysis of the patient's thinking as the history of the illness and the details of personal life are given will usually reveal an incoherence. Digit span and serial subtraction of 3s and 7s from 100 are useful bedside tests of the patient's capacity for sustained mental activity. Memory of recent events is one of the most delicate tests of adequate mental function and may be accomplished by having the patient relate all the details of entry to the hospital, laboratory tests, the names of the last six presidents, etc.

Once it is established that the patient is confused, the differential diagnosis must be made between delirium, an acute confusional state associated with psychomotor underactivity, and a beclouded dementia. This can usually be done by taking into account the degree of the patient's alertness, wakefulness, psychomotor and hallucinatory activity, and the presence or absence of signs of autonomic nervous system overactivity. The distinction between the acute confusional states and dementia may be difficult at times. The patient with acute confusional psychosis is said to have a "clouded sensorium," i.e., is inattentive, sometimes drowsy, and inclined to inaccurate perceptions and sometimes to hallucinations and delusions, whereas the patient with dementia usually has a clear sensorium. However, some demented patients are as beclouded as those with confusional psychosis, and the two conditions are at times indistinguishable, except for their different time courses. All this suggests that the parts of the nervous system affected may be the same in both conditions. When the physician is faced with this problem, the history of the mode of onset is of prime importance. The confusional psychosis usually has an acute onset and is reversible, whereas dementia has an insidious onset and chronic course and is more or less irreversible, as will be elaborated in the following chapter. Schizophrenia and manic-depressive psychosis can usually be separated from the confusional states by the presence of a clear sensorium and relatively good memory.

Once a case has been classified as either type of acute confusional state or as a beclouded dementia it is important to determine its clinical associations. A thorough medical and neurologic examination and lumbar puncture should be performed. The medical and neurologic findings are of great value in indicating the underlying disease to be treated, and they also give information concerning prognosis. In the neurologic examination, particular attention should be given to language functions, visual fields and visual-spatial discriminations, cortical sensory functions, calculations, and other test performances that require normal functioning

of the temporal, parietal, and occipital lobes. Confusional states are frequent with diseases of these parts of the brain. Contrariwise, some of the signs of the latter are often mistaken for a confusional psychosis.

CARE OF THE DELIRIOUS AND CONFUSED PATIENT

▷ The primary therapeutic effort is directed to the control of the underlying medical disease. Other important objectives are to quiet these patients and protect them against injury. A private nurse, an attendant, or a member of the family should be with such patients at all times if this can be arranged. Depending on how active and vigorous they are, a locked room, screened windows that cannot be opened by the patient, and a low bed should be arranged. It is often better to let patients walk about the room than to tie them into bed, which may excite or frighten them so that they struggle to the point of complete exhaustion and collapse. If they are less active, they can usually be kept in bed by side rails, wrist restraints, or a restraining sheet or net. Unless it is contraindicated by the primary disease, the patient should be permitted to sit up or walk about the room part of the day.

▷ All drugs that could possibly be responsible for the acute confusional state or delirium should be discontinued (unless withdrawal effects are believed to underlie the illness). Paraldehyde and chloral hydrate are trustworthy sedatives under these circumstances. Chlorpromazine, chlordiazepoxide, and diazepam are equally effective if given in full doses, and should be continued until natural sleep is restored. One must be cautious in attempting to suppress agitation completely. To accomplish this may require very large doses of drugs, and vital functions may then be dangerously impaired. The purpose of sedation is to assure rest and sleep so that patients do not exhaust themselves, and to facilitate nursing care. Continuous warm baths are also effective in quieting the delirious patient, but very few general hospitals have proper facilities for this valuable method of treatment.

A fluid intake and output chart should be kept, and any fluid and electrolyte deficit should be corrected. The pulse and blood pressure should be recorded at frequent intervals in anticipation of circulatory collapse. Transfusions of whole blood and vasopressor drugs may be lifesaving.

Finally, the physician should be aware of many small therapeutic measures that may allay fear and suspicion and reduce the tendency to hallucinations. The room should be kept dimly lighted at night, and if possible, the patient should not be moved from one room to another. Every procedure should be explained in detail, even such simple ones as the taking of blood pressure or temperature. The presence of a member of the family may enable the patient to maintain contact with reality.

It may be some consolation and also a source of professional satisfaction to remember that most delirious patients recover if they receive competent medical and nursing care. The family should be reassured on this point. They must also understand that the patient's abnormal behavior is not willful but rather symptomatic of a brain disease.

See also Chaps. 40 and 41 for specific aspects of management of delirium due to withdrawal of alcohol, barbiturates, and other sedative-hypnotic drugs.

REFERENCES

ENGEL GL, ROMANO J: Delirium, a syndrome of cerebral insufficiency. *J Chronic Dis* 9:260, 1959.

EY H: Disorders of consciousness in psychiatry, in Vinken PJ, Bruyn GW (eds): *Handbook of Clinical Neurology, Disorders of Higher Nervous Activity.* Amsterdam, North-Holland, 1969, chap 7, pp 112-136.

LIPOWSKI ZJ: Delirium, clouding of consciousness and confusion. *J Nerv Ment Dis* 145:227, 1967.

————: *Delirium: Acute Brain Failure in Man.* Springfield, Ill, Charles C Thomas, 1980.

LISHMAN WA: *Organic Psychiatry. The Psychological Consequences of Cerebral Disorder.* Oxford, Blackwell, 1978.

WOLFF HG, CURRAN D: Nature of delirium and allied states. *Arch Neurol Psychiatry* 33:1175, 1935.

CHAPTER 20

THE DEMENTIAS AND KORSAKOFF'S PSYCHOSIS

Increasingly, as the number of elderly adults in our population rises, the neurologist is consulted because an otherwise healthy person begins to lose his or her capacity to function effectively as a worker or head of a family. This may indicate the beginning of a brain tumor, the formation of a chronic subdural hematoma, or the development of chronic drug intoxication, chronic meningoencephalitis (syphilis), degenerative cerebral disease, chronic low-pressure hydrocephalus, or depressive psychosis. In former times, when there was little that could be done about these clinical states, no great premium was attached to diagnosis. But modern medicine offers the means of treating several of these conditions and in some instances of restoring the patient to normal health and effectiveness. Moreover, a number of new diagnostic technologies now allow earlier recognition of the underlying pathologic process, improving the chances of recovery.

DEFINITIONS

In current neurologic parlance the term *dementia* usually denotes a clinical syndrome composed of failing memory and loss of other intellectual functions due to chronic progressive degenerative disease of the brain. Such a definition is too narrow. Actually the term covers a number of closely related syndromes that are characterized not only by intellectual deterioration but also by certain nonintellectual behavioral abnormalities and changes in personality. Moreover it is illogical to set apart any one constellation of cerebral symptoms on the basis of their speed of onset, rate of evolution, or duration. Alternatively, we would propose that there are several states of dementia of multiple causation and mechanism and that a diffuse degeneration of neurons (usually

chronic) is only one of the many causes. Therefore it is more nearly correct to speak of *the dementias* or the dementing diseases.

To understand the phenomenon of intellectual deterioration, it is helpful to have some idea of how intellectual activity is normally organized and sustained by the brain, and the manner in which deficits in intelligence relate to diffuse and focal cerebral disease.

THE NEUROLOGY OF INTELLIGENCE

As every educated person knows, intelligence has something to do with normal cerebral function. Further, humans obviously differ in intelligence, and the members of certain families are exceptionally bright and intellectually accomplished while others are just the opposite. Intelligent children, if properly motivated, excel in school and score high on intelligence tests, which are themselves predictive of scholastic success. Indeed the first intelligence tests devised by Binet and Simon in 1905 were for this purpose. The term *intelligence quotient*, or *IQ*, was introduced by Terman in 1916 to denote a figure obtained by dividing mental age (as determined by the Binet-Simon scale) by chronologic age and multiplying the result by 100. The IQ correlates with achievement in school and eventual success in professional work. The IQ calls attention to other qualities of intelligence—that it increases with age up to the sixteenth to eighteenth year and that at any given age a large sample of normal children attain test scores that distribute in conformity with the normal, or Gaussian, curve. Older individuals are known to do less well on certain parts of intelligence tests.

The original studies of pedigrees of highly intelligent and mentally inferior families, which revealed a striking concordance between parent and child, lent support to the idea that intelligence is largely inherited. However, it soon became evident that the tests being used depended on the verbal skills and other scholastic attainments which educated parents offered their children, and were less reliable in selecting others who were talented but never had similar opportunities for schooling. In recent times this has led to the widespread belief that intelligence tests are only achievement tests and that environmental factors that foster high performance are the only important ones in determining intelligence. Neither of these views is entirely correct. The studies of monozygotic and dizygotic twins raised in the same or different families has put the matter in a clearer light. Identical twins reared together or apart are more alike in intelligence than nonidentical twins brought up in the same home (see reviews of Shields and of Slater and Cowie). There can be no doubt, therefore, that genetic endowment is the more important factor; Piercy has estimated the ratio of the hereditary and environmental components of intelligence to be from 6:4 to 8:2. However, such estimates can never be absolute. There is convincing evidence that early learning may greatly modify the level of ability that is finally obtained. The latter should not be looked upon as the sum of genetic and environmental factors, but as the product of the two.

As to psychological theories of intelligence, two have held sway. One is known as the two-factor theory of Spearman, who noted that all tests of cognitive ability correlated positively, suggesting a general (g) factor which enters into all performance. Since none of the correlations approached unity, he postulated that every test measures not only this general ability (commonly identified with intelligence), but also a smaller subsidiary factor, specific to the individual test. The latter he designated as the s factor. The other theory, the multifactorial theory of Thurstone, proposes that intelligence consists of a number of primary mental abilities, such as memory, verbal skill, numerical ability, visual-spatial perception, all of approximately equal magnitude. These primary abilities, although correlated, are not subordinate to a more general ability.

Concerning the way in which adult intelligence develops, the most widely known theory is that of Piaget, who traced the process through several stages—sensorimotor, from 0 to 2 years; preconceptual thought, from 2 to 4 years; intuitive thought, from 4 to 7 years; concrete "operations" (conceptualization), from 7 to 11 years; and finally the period of "formal operations"

(logical or abstract thought), from 11 years on. Surely one can perceive these stages in the child, but Piaget's theory has been criticized as being too anecdotal and lacking the quantitative validation that could be derived only from studies of a large normal population. Another theory is that of Hebb, based on his observations that cerebral injury caused a more diffuse disturbance of intellect in children than in adults. The latter tended to suffer more focal impairment, or else showed little intellectual change, even with large frontal lesions. On the basis of these observations Hebb postulated two forms of intelligence. One is an innate capacity to form concepts (intelligence A), which determines the speed and level of intellectual development and which is delayed or impaired in a nonspecific way by lesions of many parts of the brain. Intelligence B is the level of intellectual efficiency actually attained, which, once developed, is relatively little affected by cerebral lesions. Hebb suggested further that those cognitive abilities which are seriously impaired by cerebral lesions require an unimpaired brain for their optimal performance, i.e., they involve intelligence A. This subject is discussed further in Chap. 27.

One would suppose that in neurology, where we are confronted with many diseases affecting the cerebrum, it might be possible to verify one of the several theories of intelligence. Diffuse lesions might be expected to impair the g factor of intelligence in proportion to the mass of brain involved ("mass-action" principle of Lashley). Chapman and Wolff believe that there is a correlation between the volume of tissue lost and a general deficit of cerebral function. Others have disagreed, claiming that no universal psychological deficit can be recognized with lesions affecting various parts of the cerebrum. Probably the truth lies between these two extreme points of view. With lesions above a certain size (50 ml of tissue, according to Tomlinson et al.) there is some general reduction in performance, especially in speed, and an impairment of reasoning. It is noted also that levels of g do not decline consistently with age. On the other hand, in a closely reasoned analysis of specific intellectual deficits, Piercy has found positive correlations between losses of particular functions and lesions of particular parts of the left and right hemispheres. These are discussed in detail in Chap. 21. Each of these special abilities, although to some extent under genetic control, is influenced by early learning. Thus, neurologic studies provide evidence that is more consistent with a concept of intelligence as a gestalt of multiple primary abilities, each with a certain degree of anatomic localization, than as a unitary function. However, they do not eliminate the possibility of a g factor (perhaps equivalent to thinking or abstract reasoning ability that is only operative if the connections of the frontal lobes with other parts of the brain are intact).

THE NEUROLOGY OF DEMENTIA

The study of dementia also shows it to consist of a loss of several seemingly separable but overlapping abilities. This type of intellectual impairment occurs as the preeminent clinical abnormality in several cerebral diseases, and sometimes as the only abnormality. The most common types of dementing diseases and their relative frequency are listed in Table 20-1. These figures, which are in accord with our experience, have been compiled by Wells, and are based on the findings in three neurological centers as well as his own.

What is noteworthy about these figures is the apparently high level of accuracy of diagnosis. This is somewhat misleading, however. In the atrophic-degenerative group, for example, there is surely an incalculable number of cases of Pick's disease and other degenerative

Table 20-1

The common types of dementing diseases and their relative frequency

Dementing disease	Relative frequency, %
Cerebral atrophy, mainly Alzheimer–senile dementia (ASD)	50
Multiinfarct dementia	10
Alcoholic dementia*	5–10
Intracranial tumors	5
Normal pressure hydrocephalus	6
Huntington's chorea	3
Chronic drug intoxications	3
Miscellaneous diseases (hepatic failure; pernicious anemia; hypo- or hyperthyroidism; dementias with Parkinson's disease, amyotrophic lateral sclerosis, cerebellar atrophy; neurosyphilis; Cushing's disease; Creutzfeld-Jakob disease; multiple sclerosis; epilepsy)	7–10
Undiagnosed types	3
Pseudodementias (depression, hypomania, schizophrenia, hysteria, undiagnosed)	7

*Frequency varies with incidence of alcoholism in the population studied.

Source: C Wells (ed), *Dementia*, New York, Davis, 1977.

diseases that cannot be diagnosed clinically, but in our experience they probably do not make up more than 5 or 10 percent of the entire group. These data also do not indicate the frequency of combined types, particularly of Alzheimer's disease and vascular disease(s). Impressive also is the fact that approximately one in twenty patients seen in a neurologic center with a question of dementia proved to have a potentially reversible psychiatric illness simulating dementia (pseudodementia).

In the following pages we shall consider the prototype syndromes. The special features of individual dementing diseases will be presented in the appropriate chapters.

The earliest signs of *dementia due to degenerative disease* may be so subtle as to escape the notice of the most discerning physician. Often an observant relative of the patient or an employer is the first to become aware of a certain lack of initiative, a lack of interest in work, a neglect of routine tasks, or an abandonment of pleasurable pursuits. Initially, these changes may be attributed to fatigue or boredom. The gradual development of forgetfulness is another prominent early symptom. Common names are no longer remembered, the purpose of an errand is forgotten, appointments are not kept, a recent conversation or social event is forgotten. The patient may repeatedly ask the same question, the answers that were previously given not being retained. Sometimes the mental failure is brought to light more dramatically by a severe confusional state that attends a febrile illness or the taking of some new medicine. Later it becomes evident that the patient is easily distracted by every passing incident. No longer is it possible to think about or discuss a problem with the usual clarity, and there is a failure to comprehend all aspects of complex situations. One feature may become a source of unreasonable concern or worry. Tasks that require several steps cannot be accomplished, and all but the simplest directions cannot be followed. The patient may get lost, even along habitual routes of travel. Day-to-day events are not recalled, and perseveration in speech, action, and thought is noted. There may be sudden outbursts of emotion, taking the form of anger, tears, or aggressiveness. Frequently a change in mood becomes apparent, deviating more toward depression than elation. Some patients are grumpy and bad-tempered. A few are cheerful and facetious. The direction of the mood change is said to depend on the previous personality of the patient, rather than on the character of the disease, but one can recall glaring exceptions. Excessive lability of mood may also be observed, i.e., easy fluctuation from laughter to tears on slight provocation. Loss of social graces and indifference to social customs occur but usually later in the course of illness. Judgment becomes impaired, early in some, late in others. At certain phases of the illness, suspiciousness or frank paranoia may develop. Visual and auditory hallucinations, sometimes quite vivid in nature, may be added. As a rule these patients have little or no realization of such changes within themselves. They lack insight, so to speak.

As the condition progresses, all intellectual faculties are impaired, but memory most of all. Patients may fail to recognize their relatives or to recall their names. Apractagnosias may be prominent, and the defects may alter the performance of the simplest tasks, such as preparing a meal or setting the table, or even using the telephone or a knife and fork, or dressing, or walking. The disordered gait which tends to occur in the late stages of disease has been described fully in Chap. 6.

Language functions suffer almost from the beginning of the disease. Lost early are the suppleness and spontaneity of verbal expression. Vocabulary becomes restricted; conversation, rambling and repetitious. Patients forget or misuse proper names and no longer formulate ideas with well-constructed phrases or sentences. There is a tendency to resort instead to clichés, stereotyped phrases, and exclamations, which may hide the underlying defect during social intercourse. More severe degrees of aphasia and dysarthria are added to the clinical picture, but only in the later stages. As pointed out by Chapman and Wolff, there is loss also of the capacity to express feelings and impulses, to tolerate frustration and restrictions, and to modulate defence reactions. Disagreeable behavior—petulance, agitation, shouting and whining if restrained, palilalia, and echolalia—may occur.

There is also a physical deterioration. Food intake, which may be increased in the beginning of the illness, is in the end reduced, with resulting emaciation. Any febrile illness, drug intoxication, or metabolic upset is poorly tolerated, leading to severe confusion, stupor, or coma, an indication of the precarious state of cerebral compensation (see "Beclouded Dementia," Chap. 19). Finally, these patients remain in bed most of the time, oblivious of their surroundings, and succumb to pneumonia or to some other intercurrent infection.

Should intercurrent illness not carry them off, some patients become virtually decorticate. They are totally unaware of their environment, no longer speak or respond to others, and lie with eyes open but do not look about. Food and drink are no longer requested but are swallowed if placed in the mouth. Grasping and sucking reflexes are easily elicited. The limbs may exhibit a combination of spasticity and rigidity, the tendon reflexes are hyperactive, and occasionally diffuse choreoathetotic movements or random myoclonic jerking can be observed. The sphincters are incontinent. Pain or an uncomfortable posture goes unheeded. The course of the disease extends over 5 to 10 years or more.

It would be an error to think that the abnormalities in degenerative diseases are confined to the intellectual sphere. The appearance of the patient and the physical examination alone yield highly informative data. The first impression is helpful; patients may be unkempt, sloppy in dress, and unbathed. They may look bewildered, as though lost, or their expression is vacant, and they do not maintain a lively interest or participate in the interview. Deference to other members of the family when unable to answer the examiner's questions is characteristic. The posture appears to be stiff and inflexible. All movements are slow, and gait is altered in a characteristic manner (Chap. 6). Attempts to move the limbs passively encounter a fluctuating resistance (gegenhalten). Grasp and sucking reflexes, lip puckering, mouthing movements, uninhibited blink on tapping the glabella, snout reflex (lip pursing when lips are lightly tapped), biting or jaw clamping (bulldog) reflex, corneomandibular reflex (jaw clenching when cornea is touched), and palmomental reflex (retraction of one side of mouth and chin when the thenar eminence of the palm is stroked), all occur with increasing frequency in the more advanced stages of the dementia. Many of these will be recognized as mild motor disinhibitions which appear only when the premotor areas of the brain are involved.

Naturally every case does not follow the exact sequence outlined above. Not infrequently patients are brought to a physician because of a loss of facility in language. In other patients impairment of retentive memory with relatively intact reasoning power may be the dominant clinical feature in the first months or even years of the disease, or low impulsivity (abulia) may be the dominant feature of the dementing syndrome, resulting in an apparent loss in all the more specialized higher cerebral functions. Gait disorder, though usually a late development, may occur early, particularly in cases where the dementia is superimposed on Parkinson's disease, cerebellar ataxia, or amyotrophic lateral sclerosis, which sometimes happens. These variations and others will be described in Chap. 42.

Many of these alterations of behavior are the direct consequence of neuronal loss in the cerebrum. Expressed in another way, the symptoms are the primary manifestations of neurologic disease. However, other symptoms are secondary, i.e., they are the patient's reactions to the catastrophe of losing his or her mind. For example, demented persons may seek solitude to hide their affliction and may thus appear asocial or apathetic. Again, excessive orderliness may be an attempt to compensate for failing memory; apprehension, gloom, irritability may reflect a general dissatisfaction with a necessarily restricted life. According to Kurt Goldstein, who has written about these "catastrophic reactions," as he calls them, patients even in a state of fairly advanced deterioration are still capable of reacting to their illness and to persons who care for them.

Special psychological tests aid in the quantitation of some of these abnormalities. The Wechsler Adult Intelligence Scale (WAIS) reveals scores well below the patient's norm, with a disproportionate failure on the nonverbal parts of the test. The Wechsler Memory Scale is highly sensitive to the amnesic feature of the illness. The Rorschach test is said to disclose a paucity of associations, as well as a tendency to fixate on small details rather than to see the whole figure. The Reitan battery, popular in certain circles, permits wide testing of many functions, including topographic memory, visual perception, and personality traits, and it includes parts of the above tests.

This syndrome is presented in rough outline, divested of a number of special features which characterize particular so-called degenerative diseases, such as Alzheimer's disease, senile dementia, Pick's disease, Huntington's chorea, etc. The details of the Alzheimer-senile dementia complex and other degenerative diseases will be considered in Chap. 42.

Arteriosclerotic dementia represents a special problem and merits a few words. Often the term *arteriosclerotic* is incorrectly applied to the dementia of Alzheimer's disease or other degenerative diseases. Undoubtedly, the compounded effect of recurrent strokes impairs intellect, but then the stroke-by-stroke advance of the disease is usually apparent. Of course, having senile dementia does not indemnify the patient against cerebrovascular disease; in fact, this combination is very frequent, in which case the clinical picture may be a composite of the two diseases. Then, too, special cerebrovascular lesions may cause unusual and at times highly characteristic syndromes—that of pseudobulbar palsy or pathologic emotionality, due usually to multiple small lacunar infarcts in the corticobulbar motor pathways; the combination of Korsakoff's psychosis with visual field alterations, caused by bilateral posterior cerebral artery occlusion; and the frontal lobe–sympathetic apraxia syndrome, with anterior cerebral artery oc-

clusion (see Chap. 21, under "Disconnection Syndromes").

The dementia of *normal-pressure hydrocephalus* often simulates that of the degenerative diseases, although the former tends to evolve more rapidly. Normal-pressure hydrocephalus, usually distinguished by the triad of gait disorder, psychomotor slowing, and sphincter incontinence, is discussed further in Chap. 29. Since it is correctible by ventriculoatrial shunting, one must now look closely at the whole population of dementing patients and subject them to appropriate clinical and diagnostic tests.

Cerebral tumors, particularly those involving the corpus callosum, right temporal, and frontal lobes, may alter mental function for some time before headaches, seizures, and focal signs of cerebral disease appear, and the latter may be inconspicuous. The same is true of *chronic subdural hematoma.*

MORBID ANATOMY AND PATHOPHYSIOLOGY OF DEMENTIA

Attempts to relate the impairment of particular intellectual functions to lesions in certain parts of the brain have been eminently unsuccessful. Two types of difficulty have obstructed progress in this field. (1) There is the problem of defining, analyzing, and determining the significance of the so-called intellectual functions. (2) The morbid anatomy of the dementing diseases is often so diffuse and complex that it cannot be fully localized and quantitated. The memory impairment, which is a constant feature, may occur with extensive disease in any part of the cerebrum. Yet it is important to note that the functions of certain parts of the diencephalon and temporal lobes are more fundamental to retentive memory than the rest of the cortex, as will be pointed out below. Failure in tests of verbal function (the most advanced degree of which is aphasia) is closely associated with disease of the dominant cerebral hemisphere, particularly the perisylvian parts of the frontal, temporal, and parietal lobes. Loss of capacity for reading and numerical calculation is related to lesions in the posterior part of the left (dominant) cerebral hemisphere. Impairment in drawing or constructing simple and complex figures with blocks, sticks, picture arrangements, etc., as shown by tests of visual construction, is observed most often in right (nondominant) parietal lobe lesions. Thus, the clinical picture resulting from cerebral disease depends in part on the extent of the lesion, i.e., the amount of cerebral tissue destroyed, and on the specific locality of the lesion.

Dementia is related usually to obvious structural disease of the cerebrum and the diencephalon. In some diseases, such as Alzheimer's and Pick's, the main process appears to be a degeneration and loss of nerve cells in the association areas, with secondary changes in the cerebral white matter. In others, such as Huntington's chorea and other cerebral-basal ganglionic degenerations, loss of neurons in the cerebral cortex is accompanied by a similar degeneration of neurons in the putamen and caudate nuclei and other parts of the basal ganglia and cerebellum. Finally, purely thalamic degenerations may be the basis of a dementia, because of the integral relationship of the thalamus to the cerebral cortex.

Arteriosclerotic vascular disease (Chap. 33), which pursues a different course than the degenerative diseases results in multiple foci of infarction throughout the thalami, basal ganglia, brainstem, and cerebrum and, in the latter, in the motor, sensory, or visual projection areas as well as in the association areas. Severe trauma may cause contusions of cerebral convolutions and, rarely, degeneration of the central white matter (page 598), which may result in protracted stupor, coma, or dementia. Most diseases that produce dementia are quite extensive, and the frontal and temporal lobes tend to be affected more often than other parts of the cerebrum.

Mechanisms other than the destruction of brain tissue may operate in some cases. *Chronic increased intracranial pressure* or *chronic hydrocephalus* (with large ventricles the pressure may not exceed 180 mmHg), regardless of cause, is often associated with a general impairment of mental function. Compression of cerebral white matter is the main factor. The compression of one or both of the cerebral hemispheres by chronic subdural hematomas may have the same effect. *A diffuse inflammatory process* is at least in part the basis of dementia in syphilis, cryptococcosis, and virus infections such as herpes simplex ("inclusion-body") encephalitis; presumably there are loss of some neurons and also inflammatory derangement of the function of other neurons. Lastly, several of the *metabolic* and *toxic* disorders discussed in Chaps. 37 and 41 may interfere with nervous function over a period of time and create a clinical picture similar to, if not identical with, that of dementia. One must suppose that the altered biochemical environment has affected neuronal function.

BEDSIDE CLASSIFICATION OF DEMENTING DISEASES OF THE BRAIN

The conventional classification of dementing diseases of the brain is usually according to cause, if known, or to the pathologic changes. Another more practical approach, which follows logically from the method by which the whole subject has been presented in this book, is to subdivide the diseases into three categories on the basis of the associated clinical and laboratory signs of medical disease and the accompanying neurologic signs. Once it has been determined that the patient suffers a dementing illness, it must then be decided, from the medical, neurologic, and laboratory data, into which category the case fits. This classification may at first seem somewhat artificial. However, it is likely to be more useful to the student or physician not conversant with the many diseases that cause dementia than a classification based on pathology.

I. Diseases in which dementia is associated with clinical and laboratory signs of other medical disease
  A. Hypothyroidism
  B. Cushing's syndrome
  C. Nutritional deficiency states such as pellagra, the Wernicke-Korsakoff syndrome, and subacute combined degeneration of spinal cord and brain (vitamin B_{12} deficiency)
  D. Chronic meningoencephalitis: general paresis, meningovascular syphilis, cryptococcosis
  E. Hepatolenticular degeneration, familial and acquired
  F. Bromidism; chronic barbiturate intoxication

II. Diseases in which dementia is associated with other neurologic signs but not with other obvious medical disease
  A. Invariably associated with other neurologic signs
    1. Huntington's chorea (choreoathetosis)
    2. Schilder's disease and related demyelinative diseases (spastic weakness, pseudobulbar palsy, blindness, deafness)
    3. Amaurotic familial idiocy and other lipid-storage diseases (myoclonic seizures, blindness, spasticity, cerebellar ataxia)
    4. Myoclonic epilepsy (diffuse myoclonus, generalized seizures, cerebellar ataxia)
    5. Subacute spongiform encephalopathy or one type of Creutzfeldt-Jakob disease
    6. Cerebrocerebellar degeneration (cerebellar ataxia)
    7. Cerebral-basal ganglionic degenerations (apraxia-rigidity)
    8. Dementia with spastic paraplegia (spastic legs)
  B. Often associated with other neurologic signs
    1. Thrombotic or embolic cerebral infarction
    2. Brain tumor (primary or metastatic) or abscess
    3. Brain trauma, such as cerebral contusion, midbrain hemorrhage, chronic subdural hematoma
    4. Marchiafava-Bignami disease (often with apraxia and other frontal lobe signs)

5. Communicating (low-pressure) or obstructive hydrocephalus (often with ataxia of gait)

III. Diseases in which dementia is usually the only evidence of neurologic or medical disease

A. Alzheimer's disease
B. Pick's disease
C. Kraepelin's disease

These diseases are discussed fully in other sections of this book. The special clinical features and morbid anatomy of the dementias that accompany arteriosclerotic, syphilitic, traumatic, nutritional, and degenerative diseases are discussed in the appropriate chapters.

DIFFERENTIAL DIAGNOSIS

Although the form of confusion or dementia does not indicate a particular disease, certain combinations of symptoms and neurologic signs are more or less characteristic and may aid in diagnosis. The mode of onset, the clinical course, the associated neurologic signs, and the accessory laboratory data constitute the basis of differential diagnosis. It must be admitted, however, that some of the rarer types of "degenerative" brain disease are at present recognized only by pathologic examination. The correct diagnosis of treatable forms of dementia—neurosyphilis, cryptococcosis, subdural hematoma, brain tumor, bromide or other chronic drug intoxication, normal-pressure hydrocephalus, pellagra and other deficiency states, hypothyroidism and other metabolic and endocrine disorders—is of course of greater practical importance than the diagnosis of the untreatable ones.

The first task in dealing with this class of patients is to verify the presence of intellectual deterioration and personality change. It may be necessary to examine the patient several times before one is confident of the clinical findings.

There is always a tendency to assume that mental function is normal if a patient complains only of nervousness, fatigue, insomnia, or vague somatic symptoms, and to label the patient psychoneurotic. *This will be avoided if one keeps in mind that psychoneurosis rarely begins in middle or late adult life.* A practical rule is to assume that all mental illnesses beginning during this period are due either to structural disease of the brain or to depressive psychosis.

A mild dysphasia must not be mistaken for dementia. Aphasic patients appear uncertain of themselves, and their speech may be incoherent. Furthermore, they may be anxious and depressed over their ineptitude. Careful attention to the patient's language performance will lead to the correct diagnosis in most instances. Further observation will disclose that the patient's behavior, except that which is related to the language disorder, is not abnormal.

Depressed patients present another type of problem. They may remark that their mental function is poor or that they are forgetful and cannot concentrate. Scrutiny of their remarks will show, however, that they usually can remember the details of their illness and that no qualitative change in mental ability has taken place. Their difficulty is either lack of energy and interest, or preoccupation and anxiety that prevent the focusing of attention on anything except their own problems. Even during mental tests their performance may be impaired by their emotions, in much the same way as that of the worried student during examinations. This condition of emotional blocking is called *experiential confusion*. When such patients are calmed by reassurance, their mental function improves, indicating that intellectual deterioration has not occurred. Hypomanic patients fail in tests of intellectual function because of their restlessness and distractibility. It is helpful to remember that demented patients rarely have sufficient insight to complain of mental deterioration, and if they admit to poor memory, they do so without conviction or full appreciation of the degree of their disability. The physician must never rely on the patient's statements as to the efficiency of mental function and must always evaluate a poor performance on tests in the light of the emotional state and motivation at the time the test is given.

The neurologic syndrome associated with metabolic or endocrine disorders (i.e., ACTH or corticosteroid therapy, hypothyroidism, Cushing's syndrome, hypercalcemia, Addison's disease, hepatic encephalopathy, hypoglycemia, uremia, chronic barbiturate intoxication, and bromidism) may present difficulties in diagnosis because of the wide variety of clinical pictures by which they manifest themselves. Some patients appear to be suffering from a dementia, others from an acute confusional psychosis, or if mood change, negativism, hallucinations, and delusions predominate, a manic-depressive psychosis or schizophrenia is suggested. In these conditions some degree of clouding of sensorium and impairment of intellectual function can usually be recognized, and these findings alone should be enough to exclude schizophrenia and manic-depressive psychosis. It is well to remember that the abrupt onset of mental symptoms always suggests a confusional psychosis or delirium; inattention, clouding of the sensorium, perceptual disturbances, and often drowsiness are conjoined

(Chap. 19). Inasmuch as these latter conditions are practically always reversible, they must be distinguished from dementia.

Once it is decided that the patient suffers from a dementing disease, the next step is to determine by careful physical examination whether there are other neurologic signs or indications of a particular medical disease. This enables the physician to place the case in one of the three categories in the bedside classification (see above). Ancillary examinations, such as skull films, EEG, lumbar puncture, and CT scan or (if not available) pneumoencephalography should be carried out in most cases. Usually these procedures necessitate admission to a hospital. The final step is to determine, from the total clinical picture, the particular disease within any one category.

KORSAKOFF'S PSYCHOSIS (Amnesic or Amnestic-Confabulatory Psychosis)

These terms are used interchangeably to designate a unique but common disorder of cognitive function, in which memory is deranged out of all proportion to all other components of mentation and behavior. It possesses two salient features which may vary in severity but are always conjoined: (1) an impaired ability to recall events and other information that had been well established before the onset of the illness (retrograde amnesia) and (2) an impaired ability to acquire new information, i.e., to learn or to form new memories (anterograde amnesia). Other cognitive functions (particularly the capacity for concentration, spatial organization, visual and verbal abstraction), which depend little or not at all on memory, may also be impaired, but to a relatively minor degree. The patient is usually lacking in initiative and spontaneity. Confabulation, an ill-defined symptom that refers to fabrication of stories or false accounts of recent events, is variably present.

The definition of Korsakoff's psychosis is predicated also upon the integrity of certain aspects of behavior and mental function. The patient must be awake and attentive, responsive, and capable of understanding the written and spoken word, of making appropriate deductions from given premises, and of solving such problems as can be concluded within the patient's forward memory span. These "negative" features are of particular importance, because they help to distinguish Korsakoff's psychosis from a number of other disorders in which the basic defect is not in retentive memory, but in some other psychologic mechanism, e.g., in attention and perception (as in the delirious, confused, or stuporous patient), in recall (as in the hysterical patient), or in volition, i.e., the will to learn (as in the abulia of the patient with frontal lobe disease).

The anatomic structures of particular importance in memory function are the diencephalon (specifically the medial portions of the dorsomedial nuclei of the thalamus) and the hippocampal formations (gyrus dentatus, hippocampus, and parahippocampal gyrus). Bilaterally placed lesions in either of these regions derange memory and learning out of all proportion to other cognitive functions, and unilateral lesions of the dominant hemisphere can probably produce a lesser degree of the same effect. Horel, who has critically reviewed the neuroanatomy of learning and memory, points out that the critical structure which is damaged in lesions of the inferomedial temporal lobe is not the hippocampus itself, but the underlying white matter, the so-called temporal stem; the latter structure contains fiber tracts that connect the middle and inferior temporal convolutions with the medial (magnocellular) part of the dorsomedial nucleus of the thalamus.

The physiologic basis of Korsakoff's psychosis is obscure. An acceptable hypothesis, which is still to be conceived, would have to explain how a single pathologic process, acting over a circumscribed period of time, impairs not only all future learning but also the ability to recall information that had been acquired before the illness began, and why the most recently acquired information is the most vulnerable. Such a hypothesis would also have to explain why the anterograde and retrograde amnesias, in patients who recover, always recover together and why certain types of memory function (immediate recall, long-standing social habits and motor skills, memory for words, etc.) are not damaged at all. Detailed discussions of these subjects will be found in the references at the end of this chapter.

CLASSIFICATION OF DISEASES CHARACTERIZED BY AN AMNESIC SYNDROME

The amnesic (Korsakoff's) syndrome, as defined above, may be a manifestation of several neurologic disorders that are identified by their mode of onset and clinical course, the associated neurologic signs, and ancillary findings.

I. Amnesic syndrome of sudden onset—usually with gradual but incomplete recovery
   A. Bilateral hippocampal infarction due to atheroscle-

rotic-thrombotic or embolic occlusion of the posterior cerebral arteries or their inferior temporal branches

B. Trauma to the diencephalic or inferomedial temporal regions

C. Spontaneous subarachnoid hemorrhage (mechanism of amnesia not understood)

D. Carbon monoxide poisoning and other hypoxic states (rare)

II. Amnesia of sudden onset and short duration

A. Temporal lobe seizures

B. Postconcussive states

C. "Transient global amnesia"

III. Amnesic syndrome of subacute onset with varying degrees of recovery, usually leaving permanent residua

A. Wernicke-Korsakoff disease

B. Herpes simplex encephalitis

C. Tuberculous and other forms of meningitis characterized by a granulomatous exudate at the base of the brain

IV. Slowly progressive amnesic states

A. Tumors involving the floor and walls of the third ventricle

B. Alzheimer's disease and other degenerative disorders with disproportionate affection of the temporal lobes

The foregoing amnesic states, and the disorders of which they are a part, are discussed in the appropriate chapters. The only exception is so-called *transient global amnesia,* the nature of which is uncertain. It cannot with assurance be included with the epilepsies, or with the cerebrovascular diseases, or with any other category of disease and is therefore being considered here.

"TRANSIENT GLOBAL AMNESIA"

This is the name applied by Fisher and Adams to a particular type of memory disorder which occurs not infrequently in middle-aged and elderly persons and which is characterized by an episode of confusion and bewilderment that lasts for several hours. The patient's symptoms have their basis in a defect in memory for events of the present and the recent past. During the attack there is no impairment in the state of consciousness and no overt sign of seizure activity, and personal identification is intact, as are motor, sensory, and reflex functions. Unlike psychomotor epilepsy the patient is capable of high-level intellectual activity during the attacks. As soon as the attack has ended, no abnormality of mental function can be detected.

Recurrence of such attacks is uncommon, being noted in only 6 of 33 patients who were followed for periods of 1 to 17 years (Shuping et al.). In one of the authors' cases there were more than 50 attacks, but in all the rest (more than 100 cases) 5 was the maximum. Two patients in the series of Shuping et al. were exceptional in that they had multiple attacks of transient global am-

nesia which ceased after treatment of an associated medical condition (polycythemia vera in one and myxomatous degeneration of the mitral valve in the other). Shuttleworth and Wise have also reported transient global amnesia consequent upon embolism, and, of course, embolism in the posterior artery territories is known to cause strokes with permanent loss of memory (see Chap. 33).

The pathogenesis of transient global amnesia has not been settled. Possibly it represents an unusual form of temporal lobe epilepsy, or, more likely, a transient ischemic attack involving these areas; rarely does this disorder progress to stroke, however. By electroencephalography with nasopharyngeal leads, Rowan and Protass found independent mesial temporal spike discharges in five of seven patients. They attributed the discharges to ischemic lesions. In some reported cases such spike discharges disappeared after a few months, an unlikely happening if the attacks were due to hippocampal epilepsy.

The benignity and infrequency of episodic global amnesia in most patients is noteworthy. No treatment is required.

THE CLINICAL APPROACH TO THE PROBLEM OF DEMENTIA AND THE AMNESIC STATE

The physician presented with a patient suffering from dementia and amnesia must adopt an examination technique designed to expose fully the intellectual defect. Abnormalities of posture, movement, sensation, and reflexes cannot be relied upon to disclose the disease process, since the association areas of the brain may be severely damaged without demonstrable neurologic signs of this type. Suspicion of a dementing disease is aroused when the patient presents multiple complaints that seem totally unrelated to one another and to any known syndrome, when irritability, nervousness, and anxiety are vaguely described by a patient and the symptoms do not fit exactly into one of the major psychiatric syndromes, and when the patient is incoherent in describing the illness and the reasons for consulting a physician.

Three categories of data are required for the recognition and differential diagnosis of dementing brain disease:

1. A reliable history of the illness

2. Findings on mental examination, i.e., so-called "mental status," as well as on the rest of the neurologic examination

3. Special laboratory procedures: CT scan, lumbar puncture, radiographs of the skull, EEG, radionuclide scanning of the brain, and sometimes pneumoencephalogram

The history should always be supplemented by information obtained from a person other than the patient, because, through lack of insight, patients are often unaware of their illness; indeed, they may be ignorant even of their chief complaint. Special inquiry should be made about the patient's general behavior, capacity for work, personality changes, language, mood, special preoccupations and concerns, delusional ideas, hallucinatory experiences, personal habits, and such faculties as memory and judgment.

The performance of an examination of the mental status must be systematic. At a minimum it should include the following:

1. *Insight* (patient's replies to questions about the chief symptoms): What is your difficulty? Are you ill? When did your illness begin?

2. *Orientation* (knowledge of personal identity and present situation): What is your name? What is your occupation? Where do you live? Are you married?

Place: What is the name of the place where you are now? How did you get here? What floor is it on? Where is the bathroom?

Time: What is the date today? What day of the week is it? What time of the day is it? What meals have you had? When was the last holiday?

3. *Memory.*

Remote: Tell me the names of your children and their birth dates. When were you married? What was your mother's maiden name? What was the name of your first school teacher? What jobs have you held?

Recent past: Tell me about your recent illness (compare with previous statements). What did you have for breakfast today? What is my name (or the nurse's name)? When did you see me for the first time? What tests were done yesterday? What were the headlines of the newspaper today? Give the patient a simple story, oral or written, and ask him to retell it after 3 to 5 min.

Immediate recall ("short-term memory"): Repeat these numbers after me (give series of 3, 4, 5, 6, 7, 8 digits at speed of one per second). Now when I give a series of numbers, repeat them in reverse order.

Memorization (learning): The patient is given three simple data (examiner's name, date, time of day) and asked to repeat them until he or she can do so without prompting. The capacity to reproduce them at intervals after committing them to memory is a test of *retentive memory span.*

Visual span: Show the patient a picture of several objects; then ask him or her to name the objects and note any inaccuracies.

4. *General information:* Ask about names of presidents, well-known historic dates, the names of large rivers, of large cities, etc.

5. *Capacity for sustained mental activity.*

Calculation: Test ability to add, subtract, multiply, and divide. Subtraction of serial 7s from 100 is a good test of calculation as well as of concentration.

Abstract thinking: See if the patient can detect similarities and differences between classes of objects, or explain a proverb or a fable.

6. *General behavior:* Attitudes, general bearing, stream of thought, attentiveness, mood, manner of dress, etc.

7. *Special tests of localized cerebral functions:* Grasping, sucking, aphasia battery, praxis with both hands, cortical sensory function, drawing of clock face, map of United States or Europe, floor plan of house, etc.

In order to enlist the full cooperation of patients, the physician must prepare them for questions of this type. Otherwise, the first reaction will be one of embarrassment or anger because of the implication of unsound mind. It should be pointed out to the patient that some individuals are rather forgetful and that it is necessary to ask specific questions in order to form some impression about their degree of nervousness when being examined. Reassurance that these are not tests of intelligence or of sanity is helpful. If the patient is extremely agitated, suspicious, or belligerent, intellectual functions must be inferred from his or her remarks.

Whether or not to resort to formal psychological tests is certain to arise. Such tests yield quantitative data of comparative value but cannot of themselves be used for diagnostic purposes. Pfeiffer's test and Roth's dementia index rely essentially on the points mentioned above. All the clinical and psychological tests are measuring the same aspects of behavior and intellectual function. Probably the Wechsler Adult Intelligence Scale (WAIS) is the most widely used. The Wechsler Memory Scale is useful in estimating the degree of memory failure. Using the WAIS, the discrepancy between the vocabulary, picture-completion, and object-assembly tests as a group (these correlate well with premorbid intelligence and are relatively insensitive to dementing brain disease) and arithmetic, block-design, digit-span, and digit-symbol tests provide an index of deterioration. The Mini-Mental Status of Folstein et al. is a useful bedside method of scoring cognitive impairment and following its progress.

MANAGEMENT OF THE DEMENTED PATIENT

Dementia is a clinical state of the most serious nature, and usually it is worthwhile to admit patients to the hospital for a period of observation. The physician then has an opportunity to see them on different occasions in a new and fairly constant hospital environment, where the laboratory procedures mentioned above can be carried out (blood counts, vitamin B_{12} and drug levels, evaluation of thyroid, adrenal, renal, and liver function and cardiac and vascular status, examination of CSF for syphilis, and the special tests of CNS function such as EEG, CT scan, etc.). The management of demented patients in the hospital may be relatively simple if they are quiet and cooperative. If the disorder of mental function is severe, it is helpful if a nurse, attendant, or member of the family can stay with the patient at all times. Provision must be made for adequate food and fluid intake and control of infection, using the same measures outlined for the delirious patient.

The primary responsibility of the physician is to diagnose the treatable forms of dementia and to institute appropriate methods of therapy. Once it is established that the patient has an untreatable dementing brain disease, a responsible member of the family should be apprised of the medical facts and prognosis, if the diagnosis is sufficiently certain for this to be done. Patients themselves need only be told that they have a nervous condition for which they are to be given rest and treatment. Nothing is accomplished by telling them more. If the dementia is slight and circumstances are suitable, patients should remain at home, continuing activities of which they are capable. They should be spared responsibility and guarded against injury that might result from imprudent action. If they are still at work, plans for occupational retirement should be carried out. In more advanced stages of the disease, when mental and physical enfeeblement become pronounced, institutional care should be advised. Seizures should be treated symptomatically. Nerve tonics, vitamins, vasodilators, and hormones are of no value in checking the course of the

illness or in regenerating decayed tissue. They may, however, offer some support to the patient and family. Sometimes stimulants in the form of dextroamphetamine, caffeine, and nicotinic acid cause transitory improvement in mental function. Undesirable restlessness, nocturnal wandering, belligerency, or anxiety may be reduced by administration of one of the tranquilizing drugs (see Chap. 41).

REFERENCES

FISHER CM, ADAMS RD: Transient global amnesia. *Acta Neurol Scand*, vol 40, suppl 9, 1964.

FOLSTEIN M, FOLSTEIN S, McHUGH PR: "Mini-mental status." A practical method for grading the cognitive state of patients for the clinician. *J Psychiatr Res* 12:189, 1975.

GOLDSTEIN K: *The Organism. A Holistic Approach to Biology.* New York, American Book, 1939, pp 35-61.

HEBB DO: Intelligence, brain function and the theory of mind. *Brain* 82:260, 1959.

HOREL JA: The neuroanatomy of amnesia. A critique of the hippocampal memory hypothesis. *Brain* 101:403, 1978.

LASHLEY KS: *Brain Mechanisms and Intelligence.* Chicago, University of Chicago, 1929.

PIAGET J: *The Psychology of Intelligence.* London, Routledge and Kegan Paul, 1950.

PIERCY M: Neurological aspects of intelligence, in Vinken PJ, Bruyn GW (eds): *Handbook of Clinical Neurology*, vol 3: *Disorders of Higher Nervous Activity.* Amsterdam, North-Holland, 1969, chap 18, pp 296-315.

ROWAN AJ, PROTASS LM: Transient global amnesia: Clinical and electroencephalographic findings in 10 cases. *Neurology* 29:869, 1979.

SHIELDS J: *Monozygotic Twins Brought Up Apart and Brought Up Together. An Investigation Into the Genetic and Environmental Causes of Variation in Personality.* London, Oxford University Press, 1962.

———: Heredity and psychological abnormality, in Eysenck HJ (ed): *Handbook of Abnormal Psychology*, 2d ed. London, Pitman, 1973.

SHUPING JR, ROLLINSON RD, TOOLE JF: Transient global amnesia. *Ann Neurol* 6:159, 1979.

SHUTTLEWORTH EC, WISE GR: Transient global amnesia due to arterial embolism. *Arch Neurol* 29:340, 1973.

SLATER E, COWIE V: *The Genetics of Mental Disorders.* London, Oxford University Press, 1971, pp 196-200.

TOMLINSON BE, BLESSED G, ROTH M: Observations on the brains of demented old people. *J Neurol Sci* 11:205, 1970.

WELLS C (ed): *Dementia.* Philadelphia, Davis, 1977, p 250.

CHAPTER 21

NEUROLOGIC DISORDERS CAUSED BY LESIONS IN PARTICULAR PARTS OF THE CEREBRUM

The age-old controversy about cerebral functions—whether they are diffusely represented in the cerebrum, with all parts equivalent, or localized to certain lobes or regions—has long ago been resolved. Clinicians and physiologists have demonstrated beyond doubt that particular cortical regions are related to certain functions. For example, the pre- and postrolandic zones are motor, the striate-parastriate occipital zones are visual, the superior temporal and Heschl's transverse gyri are auditory, etc. Along strictly histologic lines Brodmann was able to divide the cerebral cortex into 47 different areas (Figs. 21-1 and 21-2), each showing cytologic differences (based on cytoarchitechtonics), and von Economo identified more than twice this number. From the anatomic point of view, the six-layered neocortex [also called isocortex (Vogt) and homogenetic cortex (Brodmann) because of its uniform embryogenesis and morphology] has been shown not to be homogeneous but to differ in its various parts by virtue of particular connections with other areas of the cortex in the same and opposite cerebral hemispheres and with the thalamus and other lower centers. Hence, one must regard the neocortex or neopallium as a heterogeneous array of many anatomic systems, each with a rather complex intercortical and central (thalamic) arrangement, but what still remains unresolved is whether any particular region acts as a single unit by a kind of mass action or is organized according to a complex preordained plan. If vision is to be taken as an example, the latter seems more likely. Recent anatomic and physiologic evidence shows the relations between the visual receptive and associational zones to be quite intricately patterned, even though the degree of functional deficit occurring in disease states seems to be roughly in proportion to the volume of tissue destroyed.

As was emphasized in the preceding chapter on dementia and Korsakoff's amnesic state, one must not assume that each of the neocortical systems exists in isolation unrelated to the rest of the cerebrum and thalamus. It will be evident in the discussions which follow that each part bears certain fixed relations to others. Deterioration of intellect has already been presented, not simply as a failure of a unitary function of intelligence that is diffusely represented in the cerebrum, but as a failure of a constellation of functions, some more strictly localized than others. Inescapably there will be some overlap between the previous chapter and this one since the anatomy of each element of dementia will have to be discussed again, in a different context.

Another aspect of cerebral localization has been emphasized by the Soviet school of physiologists and psychologists. The Soviets do not view function as the direct property of a particular, highly specialized group of cells but as the product of complex reflex activity by which sensory stimuli are analyzed and integrated at various levels of the nervous system and are united, through a system of temporary connections, into a working mosaic, adapted to accomplish a particular task. Within such a functional system, the initial and final links (the task and the effect) remain unchanged but the intermediate links (the means of performance of a given task) may be modified within wide limits, and will never be exactly the same on two consecutive occasions. Thus, when a certain act is called for by a spoken command, the dominant temporal lobe must receive the message and transmit it to the motor areas; and the latter are always under the dynamic control of the proprioceptive, visual, and vestibular systems. These are some of the recognizable elements in the motor performance, and the symptom, which is a loss of the skilled act, may be

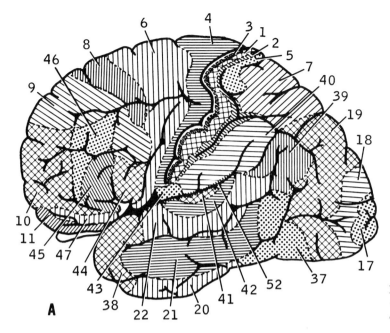

Figure 21-1
Cytoarchitectural zones of the human cerebral cortex. A. Lateral surface. B. Medial surface.

Figure 21-2
Cytoarchitectural zones of the cerebral cortex, basal surface, adapted from Brodmann.

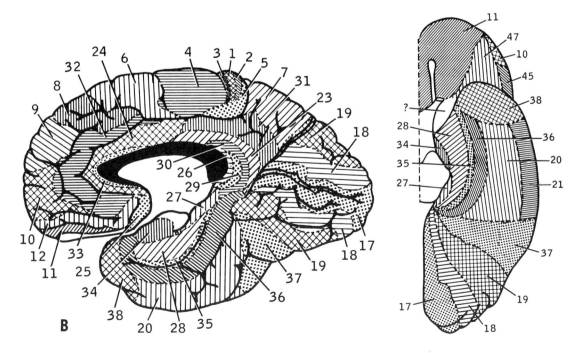

caused by a lesion which affects any one of several elements in the act, either the motor centers or its connections with the other elements. All parts comprise a recognizable functional system, and the purpose of neuropsychology is to localize defects in different parts of the system.

This conception of cerebral function and localization, which applies to all mental activities, differs from that which postulates equivalence of all cerebral function and also from that which assumes strict localization of any given activity within one part of the brain. It is open to precise neuropsychological analysis, which has been the approach of the Vigotskii-Anokhin-Bernshtein-Luria school (see Luria).

From these remarks it follows that subdivision of the cerebrum into frontal, temporal, parietal, and occipital lobes has no real validity. It was made long before the first glimmer of knowledge about the function of the cerebrum. Even when the neurohistologists began parcelling the neocortex, they found that their areas did not fall within zones bounded by sulci and fissures. Therefore, when the words *frontal, parietal, temporal,* and *occipital* are used in the text below, it is only to provide the reader with a familiar anatomic reference.

SYNDROMES CAUSED BY LESIONS OF THE FRONTAL LOBES

ANATOMIC AND PHYSIOLOGIC CONSIDERATIONS

In Fig. 21-3 it is seen that the frontal lobes lie anterior to the central, or Rolando's, sulcus and superior to the sylvian fissure. Several different systems of neurons are located here, and they subserve different functions. Areas 4, 6, and 8 and the lateral parts of the prefrontal cortex relate specifically to motor activities but are integrated with somatic sensory neurons of the anterior part of the postcentral gyrus (Chap. 3), as well as with other parietal areas, thalamic nuclei, and reticular formation of the upper brainstem. As was pointed out in earlier chapters, all motor activity needs sensory guidance, and this comes from the somesthetic, visual, and auditory cortices (which are connected with the ventroposterolateral thalamic nuclei, lateral geniculate bodies, and medial geniculate bodies, respectively) and from the cerebellum, through the ventrolateral, ventromedial, and ventro-

Figure 21-3
Photograph of lateral surface of the human brain. (From MB Carpenter, Human Neuroanatomy, 7th ed, Baltimore, Williams & Wilkins, 1976.)

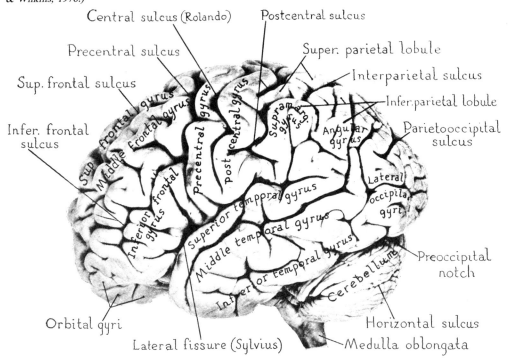

anterior thalamic nuclei. In turn the frontal motor areas exert a controlling influence on the afferent parts of the brain.

Area 8 is concerned with the turning of eyes and head contralaterally. Area 44 of the dominant hemisphere (Broca's area) and the contiguous part of area 4 are "centers" of motor speech and related functions of the lips, tongue, etc., and if these areas are affected bilaterally, there is paralysis of articulation, phonation, and deglutition. The limbic and piriform cortex (allocortex of Vogt) are bilaterally organized and concerned with control of certain of the respiratory, circulatory, and other vegetative functions. These areas of the cortex receive input from the somatic sensory and olfactory afferents and in turn are connected with other parts of the limbic brain. The most anterior parts of the frontal lobes (areas 9 to 12 and 45 to 47), sometimes referred to as the *prefrontal areas*, are particularly well developed in human beings but have no clearly assigned functions. For a long time intelligence was believed to be seated here, and it came as a surprise that limited ablation of these regions caused no significant reduction in scores on intelligence tests. These parts do not belong to the motor areas, in the sense that electrical stimulation evokes no direct movement; the prefrontal cortex is said to be inexcitable.

Concerning the detailed histology of the motor and premotor cortices, it should be pointed out that six

layers can be distinguished, from the pial surface to the underlying white matter (molecular or plexiform, external granular, external pyramidal, internal granular, ganglionic or internal pyramidal, and multiform or fusiform). The precentral cortex is dominated by pyramidal rather than granular cells; hence the term *agranular* (Fig. 21-4). This type of cortex characterizes areas 4 and 6, as well as the anterior parts of the insula and gyrus cinguli. The frontal agranular cortex, especially areas 4 and 6, provides most of the cerebral efferent system known as the *pyramidal,* or *corticospinal, tract* (Figs. 3-2 and 3-3). In contrast, the primary sensory cortex (anterior wall of the postcentral gyrus, banks of the calcarine sulcus, and the transverse gyri of Heschl), where layers II and IV are strongly developed for the receipt of afferent impulses, has been termed *granular,* or *koniocortex* (Greek *konia,* "dust"), because of the marked predominance of granular cells (Fig. 21-4).

In the frontal cortex, rostral to areas 4 and 6, and in the prefrontal cortex the granular layers are more distinct than in the motor cortex. Further, the transverse fiber systems (external and internal bands of Baillarger) are less well developed than in the strongly agranular cortex (Fig. 21-5). In these respects the frontal and pre-

Figure 21-4
The five fundamental types of cerebral cortex, according to von Economo: 1, agranular; 2, frontal; 3, parietal; 4, polar; and 5, granulous.

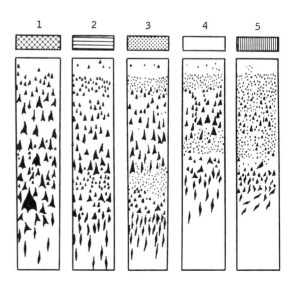

frontal cortices (types 2 and 3 of von Economo) resemble the associative cortex of parietal and temporal lobes (Fig. 21-4).

The intrinsic organization of the isocortex follows the pattern elucidated by Lorente de Nó. Figure 21-4 illustrates the fundamental vertical (columnar) organization of these neuronal systems. Afferent fibers terminate in layers IV, III, and II (Fig. 21-6). Internuncial neurons transmit impulses to adjacent superficial and deep layers through horizontal and vertical fiber systems. Neuronal connections are mainly through axonal-dendritic synapses. In the macaque brain, each pyramidal neuron in layer IV has about 60,000 synapses, and one afferent axon may encompass an area that contains up to 5000 neurons. These figures convey some idea of the wealth of cortical connections.

The so-called secondary motor unit (area 6) has connections with area 4 and is itself under the influence of afferent systems, and the same may be said of the prefrontal or tertiary unit. However, unlike the sensory areas, where the hierarchical organization is from primary projection to associational cortex, the organization is reversed in the motor areas—from tertiary to secondary to primary projection cortex.

Of the human efferent fiber systems, the largest is the corticospinal, which arises from the agranular cortex, mainly from the pyramidal cells of layer V of the pre- and postcentral convolutions (see Figs. 3-2 and 3-3). Another massive projection is the frontopontocerebellar tract. In addition there are other fiber systems which pass from frontal cortex to caudatum, putamen, subtha-

Figure 21-5

The basic cytoarchitecture of the cerebral cortex, adapted from Brodmann.

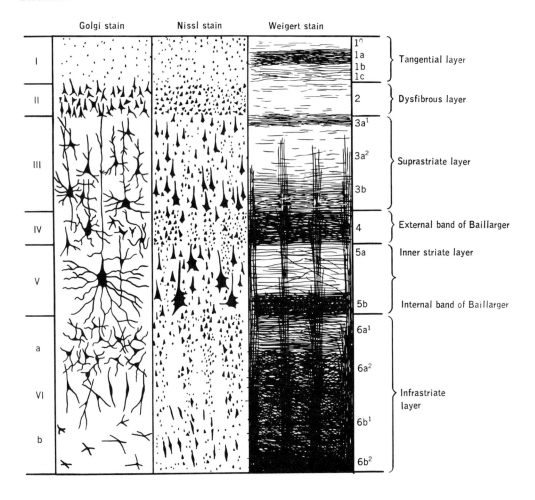

lamic nucleus, red nucleus, brainstem reticular formation, substantia nigra, inferior olive, as well as to the ventrolateral, medial dorsal, and dorsolateral nuclei of the thalamus. Areas 8 and 6 are connected with the sensorimotor cortex, and also with the oculomotor, abducens, and other brainstem motor nuclei, and with identical areas of the other cerebral hemisphere through the corpus callosum. Area 44 also has transcortical connections. A massive bundle connects the frontal with the occipital lobes. An uncinate bundle connects the orbital part of the frontal lobe with the temporal lobe.

The granular frontal cortex has a rich system of connections both with lower levels of the brain (medial and ventral nuclei and pulvinar of the thalamus) and with virtually all other parts of the cerebral cortex.

CLINICAL EFFECTS AND SYNDROMES

Lesions of the motor areas of the frontoparietal cortex and subcortical white matter produce a spastic paralysis of the contralateral face, arm, and leg. Lesions of the

more anterior part of the motor cortex cause spasticity, with less paresis, and a release of sucking and grasping reflexes, the mechanisms of which reside in the parietal lobe, according to Denny-Brown, and which presumably are normally inhibited by these parts of the frontal cortex. Electrical stimulation of the motor cortex elicits contraction of the corresponding muscle groups, and focal seizure activity has a similar effect. Temporary paralysis of contralateral head and eye turning follows a destructive lesion in area 8 (seizure activity in this area has the opposite effect). Destruction of Broca's and adjacent insular areas in the dominant hemisphere results in motor aphasia, agraphia, and apraxia of face, lips, and tongue. All these effects are discussed in Chaps. 3 and 22.

When one speaks in general terms of the frontal lobes, reference is usually made to the nonmotor, nonlin-

Figure 21-6

The organization of neuronal systems in the granular cortex, following the plan of Lorente de Nó. The black spheres represent points of synapse. A. Connections of efferent cortical neurons. B. Connections of intracortical neurons. C. Connections of afferent (thalamocortical) neurons. D. Mode of termination of afferent cortical fibers. P, pyramidal cell; M, Martinotti cell; S, spindle cell; 1, projection efferent; 2, association efferent; 3, specific afferent; 4, association afferent.

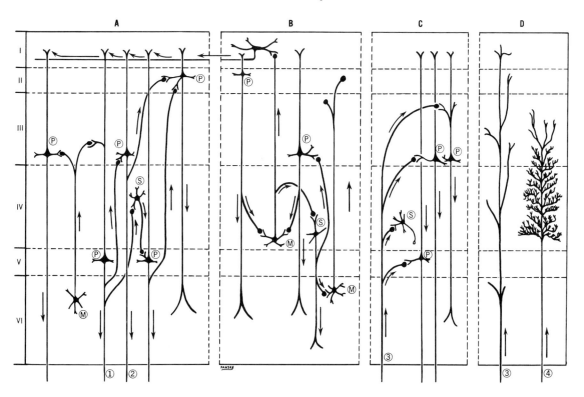

guistic parts. Here one faces a paradox. On one hand the frontal lobes are considered the "organ of civilization," the "part that is uniquely human"; on the other, the negligible effects that follow extensive lesions and surgical ablations of one frontal lobe have led some to believe that they have no assignable function.

Our knowledge of the effects of lesions in the prefrontal areas has been derived mainly from experiments on chimpanzees. Jacobsen and his collaborators observed that removal of these parts of the frontal lobes led to social indifference, tameness, and placidity, and also to forgetfulness and a diminished capacity to solve problems. It was these effects in chimpanzees that encouraged Egaz Moniz to undertake prefrontal leukotomy for the treatment of chronic schizophrenia and obsessive and depressive states. Bilateral excision of the lateral orbital region (area 47 and parts just medial to it) of chimpanzees resulted in an extreme degree of hyperactivity which continued for months, as long as the animals were awake.

The effects of frontal lobe lesions in humans have been the subject of endless controversy. Some workers, such as Hebb and Penfield, claim that there are no discernible effects, even of bilateral lesions. Others, such as Chapman and Wolff, Halstead, Reitan, and Hécaen, insist that there are predictable and diagnostic changes in behavior. The arguments pro and con and the inadequacies of many of the studies, both in clinical testing and anatomical verification of the lesions, are well summarized by Walsh.

The following abnormalities have been observed in humans with prefrontal leukotomy and lesions of whatever cause:

1. *Change of personality,* usually expressed as lack of concern over the consequences of any action, social indifference, placidity, lack of aggression, loss of anxiety and of depressive mood, sometimes childish excitement (moria of Jastrowitz), an inappropriate joking and punning (witzelsucht of Oppenheim), or an instability and superficiality of emotion

2. *Slight impairment of intelligence,* usually described as lack of concentration, vacillation of attention, inability to carry out planned activity, difficulty in changing from one task to another, and slight loss of memory (see below)

3. *Lack of initiative,* impulsivity, and spontaneity (abulia), and reduction in amount and rate of activity with *slowing of all mental processes,* extreme degrees of which verge on *akinetic mutism* (see page 233)

4. *Motor abnormalities,* such as decomposition of gait and upright stance ("Bruns' ataxia"), paratonic rigidity or gegenhalten (counterholding), reflex grasping and sucking, and sphincteric incontinence

The most pronounced changes have been observed in cases with bilateral disease of the frontal lobes, and there has been much doubt as to whether a lesion involving only one frontal lobe has any effect. Rylander, by careful psychological testing, has shown that patients with lesions of either frontal lobe manifest a slight elevation of mood with increased talkativeness and tendency to joke, lack of tact, inability to adapt to a new situation, instability of mood, and loss of initiative.

Studies of leukotomized patients are difficult to interpret because very few of the subjects were normal before the operation. However, this operation has been performed for severe neurosis or intractable pain in some patients of normal intellect. When tested later, they were said to have shown little or no impairment of performance on intelligence tests, depending on the extent of the procedure, and if worry, fears, compulsions, and suffering from pain were incapacitating, the loss of these symptoms resulted in test scores actually higher than before the operation. Interestingly, the obsessions, delusions, or depression with chronic pain, for which the frontal leukotomy was performed, usually persisted, but the patient was less troubled by them. Careful examination of the patient's behavior in everyday tasks usually disclosed diminished drive or psychic energy, slowness of all types of performance, lack of concentration, and a change of personality in the form of shallow emotional life, loosening of ethical standards, lack of tact, and inability to direct and sustain activity toward future goals. There was also a diminution of traits related to neuroticism, such as suggestibility, rigidity of character, self-criticism, and introversion.

Although it is generally believed that frontal lesions cause no impairment of orientation and memory, Hécaen noted an incidence of amnesia in 20 percent of his series of 131 frontal tumors. Luria believes that so-called frontal amnesia is a manifestation of the patient's pathologic distractibility and inertia, an inability to create a "stable intention to remember."

Apart from the Broca types of aphasia in which the dominant inferofrontal convolution is implicated (Chap. 22), other verbal defects are associated with frontal lobe disease of either side. Laconic speech, lack of spontaneity of speech, loss of word fluency, and an inability to resist the habit of using words according to their conventional meanings have all been commented upon. Characteristically these abnormalities are most prominent when the patient is expected to carry on an unprompted narrative; the same information, obtained in the course of a dialogue or prompted conversation, may disclose little or no abnormality of speech. The exact location of lesions that cause this reduction in rate and complexity of speech are not known, but the defect is common in patients with hydrocephalus, frontal tumors, and other forms of disease deep in the anterior frontal regions.

Luria has offered an interesting analysis of the role of the frontal lobes in intellectual activity, based on his general premise that meaningful correlations of disturbed behavior and brain lesions must be preceded by a qualitative analysis of the structure of the symptom. He postulates that problem solving of whatever type (perceptive-motor, constructive, arithmetic, psycholinguistic, mnemic, or logical—definable also as goal-related behavior) proceeds in four steps: (1) the specification of a problem and the conditions in which it has arisen (in other words, a goal is perceived and the conditions associated with it are set); (2) a plan of action (strategy) for the solution of the problem is formulated, requiring that certain necessary activities expressible linguistically be initiated in orderly sequence; (3) the execution, including implementation and control of the plan; and (4) a checking or comparison of the results against the original idea of the problem. Obviously such a complex psychological activity must involve many parts of the cerebrum and will suffer as a result of destruction of any part which contributes to the functional system. Luria observes that when the frontal lobes are impaired by disease, in addition to a certain inertia or psychomotor slowing there is an erroneous analysis of the conditions of the problem: "The plan of action that is selected quickly loses its regulating influence on behavior as a whole and is replaced by perseveration of one particular link of the motor act or by the influence of some connection established during the patient's past experience." Furthermore, there is a failure to distinguish the essential links in the analysis and to compare the final solution with the original conception of the problem. Expressed otherwise, there is difficulty in initiating and sustaining the activities required in the solution of the problem, a kind of incoherence of the reasoning process, with easy distraction by irrelevant data, a lack of inhibition and control, and perseveration.

Plausible as this scheme appears, such psychophysiologic analyses of mental processes impress the authors as being somewhat artificial. Such a dissection of intellectual activity is entirely theoretical, and the factors

to which it refers correspond to no known physiologic functions. One cannot discern in it definable and easily measurable basic processes. Such schemes are likely to suffer the fate of Goldstein's concept of intellectual activity, which predicted a deterioration from abstract to concrete thinking, as disease develops. It fell into obsolescence because it was not a complete explanation of intellectual activity.

Our experience with syndromes of the prefrontal cortex impresses us with their subtle and elusive character. We agree that an abulic-hypokinetic disorder and a slowing of mental processes impairs the patient's performance on all tests of cerebral function. This is usually revealed by inattentiveness and lack of persistence in all assigned activity and sometimes by drowsiness. Luria refers to this as an impairment of "cortical tone," a failure of the frontal lobes to regulate the "activation processes lying at the basis of voluntary attention." The depression of alpha activity is an expression of this diminution or absence of "expectancy waves." Such a state cannot be ascribed specifically to the prefrontal regions since it may be a reflection of a more general cerebral disorder [thalamic-limbic(?), upper reticular formation(?)]. The problem is to distinguish this syndrome in cases of frontal lobe disease from any other disorder in which there is a failure to synthesize all elements of a problem in its solution. Unfortunately, in any given patient one seldom sees all the so-called frontal lobe defects or any one of them in their fully developed forms. Only some finding such as unilateral anosmia, optic atrophy, or unilateral grasping may then provide the clue to an orbital frontal lesion, such as an olfactory groove meningioma. Harlow's (1868) famous patient, Phineas Gage, a capable, God-fearing foreman, who became irreverent, irresponsible, and vacillating following an injury in which a crowbar was driven by an explosive through his left frontal lobe, and Dandy's patient with bilateral frontal lobectomy for meningioma, studied by Brickner, are notable examples in the medical literature which illustrate most clearly the entire syndrome of severe frontal lobe defect.

In some diseases, such as Pick's form of frontal lobe atrophy, the lesions may extend into the anterior motor areas, causing instinctual and reflex grasping, hyperreflexia, and impairment of motor speech and writing. Gait disturbances, taking the form of short, hesitant steps, slight imbalance, and impaired capacity to make postural adjustments may later become prominent (see "Apraxia of Gait," page 85). *Cerebral paraplegia in flexion* is the most severe form of deterioration of upright stance and locomotion, wherein the individual lies curled up in bed, incapable of even a slight change in position, unable to turn over or to sit (Fig. 6-1). This condition is usually due to advanced bifrontal lesions with involvement also of the basal ganglia, particularly the globus pallidus (the morbid anatomy has not been carefully studied).

Right- or left-sided lesions involving the posterior part of the superior frontal gyrus and anterior cingulate gyrus, and the intervening white matter, cause loss of control of micturition and defecation (Andrew and Nathan). The awareness of fullness of the bladder and imminence of micturition are impaired, and the patient is surprised to find that he or she has been incontinent of urine. Less complete forms of the syndrome are associated with frequency and urgency when the patient is awake. With large lesions that invade the anterior half of the frontal lobes an element of indifference to the incontinence, so-called frontal lobe incontinence, may be added.

Frontal gliomas, abscesses, etc., may also extend posteriorly into motor and speech areas. Impaired use of the limbs on one side, especially if the movements are slow and poorly coordinated, may raise the suspicion of cerebellar ataxia. Described first by Bruns, the disorder is sometimes called *Bruns' frontal lobe ataxia*. The most severe forms of nonparalytic *akinetic mutism* are associated with lesions in the posterior orbitofrontal region, adjacent to the diencephalon. Although ascribed to the diencephalon by Cairns, who first described the syndrome in a patient with a neoplastic cyst in the third ventricle, we have the impression that low frontothalamic connections are usually involved. A pure hyperactivity syndrome, the "organic drivenness" of von Economo and Kahn, when it has occurred in our clinical material, has been associated with frontal and temporal lobe lesions, usually encephalitic, but exact clinicoanatomic correlations have not been possible.

In diffuse diseases of the brain one may assume that the frontal lobes are involved when any one or a combination of the aforementioned symptoms become manifest. However, it must be remembered that involvement of the so-called association areas, especially if both cerebral hemispheres are involved, may compound clinical effects in ways that have never been fully analyzed.

Finally it should be emphasized that the function of the frontal lobes or other discrete parts of the brain cannot be determined simply by the study of human beings who have suffered injury or disease of that part. *Symptoms from lesions of a part of the nervous system are not to be equated with the function of that part.* The symptoms of frontal lobe deficit are the product of both a loss of certain structures and the functional activity (sometimes overactivity) of the portions of the nervous system that remain intact. To date, a unified concept of frontal lobe function has not emerged. There is no doubt that the mind is changed by disease of the frontal lobes, but it is difficult to say exactly how it is changed. Perhaps at present it is best to regard the frontal lobes as that part of the brain which quickly and effectively orients and drives the individual, with all percepts and concepts formed from past life experiences, toward action that is projected into the future.

Effects of frontal lobe diseases may be summarized as follows:

  I. Effects of unilateral frontal disease, either left or right
    A. Contralateral spastic hemiplegia
    B. Slight elevation of mood, increased talkativeness, tendency to joke, lack of tact, difficulty in adaptation, loss of initiative
    C. If entirely prefrontal, no hemiplegia; grasp and suck reflexes may be released.
    D. Anosmia with involvement of orbital parts
 II. Effects of right frontal disease
    A. Left hemiplegia
    B. Changes as in I*B, C,* and *D.*
III. Effects of left frontal disease
    A. Right hemiplegia
    B. Motor speech disorder with agraphia, with or without apraxia of the lips and tongue (see Chap. 22)
    C. Loss of verbal associative fluency
    D. Sympathetic apraxia of left hand
    E. Changes as in I*B, C,* and *D*
 IV. Effects of bifrontal disease
    A. Bilateral hemiplegia
    B. Spastic bulbar (pseudobulbar) palsy
    C. If prefrontal, abulia or akinetic mutism, lack of ability to sustain attention and solve complex problems, rigidity of thinking, bland affect and labile mood, and varying combinations of grasping, sucking, decomposition of gait, and sphincteric incontinence

SYNDROMES CAUSED BY LESIONS OF THE TEMPORAL LOBES

ANATOMIC AND PHYSIOLOGIC CONSIDERATIONS

The boundaries of the temporal lobes are indicated in Fig. 21-3. The sylvian fissure separates the superior surface of each temporal lobe from the frontal and anterior parts of the parietal lobes. There is no definite anatomic boundary between the temporal lobe and the occipital or posterior part of the parietal lobe. The temporal lobe includes the superior, middle, and inferior temporal, fusiform, and hippocampal convolutions and the transverse gyri of Heschl, which are the primary auditory receptive area on the superior surface, within the sylvian fissure. The cortical receptive zone has a somatotopic arrangement; fibers carrying high tones terminate in the medial portion of the gyrus and those carrying low tones, in the lateral portion. The cortical receptive zone for labyrinthine impulses is not as well demarcated as that for hearing, but probably is situated on the banks of the sylvian fissure, just posterior to the auditory receptive area. The superior part of the dominant temporal lobe is concerned with the acoustic aspects of language (see page 324) and the middle and inferior convolutions with learning and memory (see page 292). The hippocampal convolution was formerly thought to be related to the olfactory system, but now it is known that lesions here do not alter the sense of smell.

Most of the temporal lobe cortex, including Heschl's gyri, has fairly equally developed pyramidal and granular layers. In this respect it resembles more the granular cortex of the frontal and prefrontal regions and inferior parts of the parietal lobes (types 2 and 3 of von Economo; see Fig. 21-4). Unlike the neocortex (isocortex, neopallium), or "homogenetic," six-layered cortex, the hippocampus and gyrus dentatus are typical of the three-layered allocortex, or "heterogenetic," cortex, the phylogenetically older portions of the cerebral cortex (archipallium).

A massive fiber system connects the striate and parastriate zones of the occipital lobes to the inferior and medial parts of the temporal lobes. The temporal lobes are connected to one another through the anterior commissure and middle of the corpus callosum, and the inferior, or uncinate, fasciculus passes between the anterior temporal and orbital frontal regions. The arcuate fasciculus connects the posterosuperior temporal lobe to the motor cortex and Broca's area (see page 324).

The planum temporale, i.e., isthmus of the temporal lobe, has been shown by Geschwind and Levitsky to be larger in the left (dominant) hemisphere than the right.

CLINICAL EFFECTS AND SYNDROMES

Visual Field Defects Lesions of the temporal lobe characteristically produce a contralateral upper homonymous quadrantanopia, due to involvement of the lower arching fibers of the geniculocalcarine pathway (as described on page 174).

Cortical Deafness Bilateral lesions of the transverse gyri of Heschl are known to cause deafness. Henschen, in his famous review of all reported cases of aphasia, found nine in which these parts were destroyed by restricted vascular lesions, with resulting deafness. There are now some 20 cases of this type in the medical literature; lesions in other parts of the temporal lobes had no effect on hearing. From these data it has been adduced that the primary auditory receptive area is located in the cortex of the transverse gyri (chiefly the first). Subcortical lesions which interrupt the fibers from both medial geniculate bodies to the transverse gyri have the same effect. Usually there is an aphasia as well because of the proximity of the transverse gyri to the left superior temporal gyrus. Hécaen has remarked that cortically deaf persons may seem to be unaware of their deafness, a state similar to blind persons who act as though they can see (Anton's syndrome; see further on, under "Visual Anosognosia").

Unilateral lesions of Heschl's gyri were for a long time believed to have no effect on hearing, but it has been found that if very brief auditory stimuli are delivered, the threshold of sensation in the opposite ear is elevated. The receptive zone appears to prolong and stabilize the effects of stimulation. Also, while unilateral lesions do not diminish the perception of pure tones or clearly spoken words, the ear contralateral to a temporal lesion is less efficient if the conditions of hearing are rendered more difficult. For example, if words are slightly distorted (electronically filtered to alter consonants), they are heard less well in that ear; also the patient has more difficulty in equalizing sounds that are presented to both ears and in perceiving rapidly spoken numbers or different words presented to the two ears.

Auditory Agnosias Lesions of the secondary zones of the auditory cortex—area 22 and part of area 21 of Brodmann—have no effect on the perception of sounds and pure tones. However, the perception of complex combinations of sounds is severely impaired. This of course makes it impossible to differentiate the sounds of speech. A patient with such a lesion of the dominant temporal lobe has difficulty memorizing a series of *spoken* words; such a patient will succeed in reproducing only a small fraction of them, even though no difficulty is encountered in memorizing a *written* series (acoustic-amnestic defect). Comparable lesions of the nondominant temporal lobe disturb the hearing of rhythm and music, a so-called sensory amusia. These several forms of auditory agnosia have been divided by Kleist into three groups—inability to recognize sounds, music (amusia), and words—and presumably each has a slightly different anatomic basis.

In agnosia for sounds, all noises are indistinguishable. Such varied sounds as the tinkling of a bell, the rustling of paper, running water, or a siren all sound alike. The condition is usually associated with auditory verbal agnosia or with amusia. Hécaen states that an agnosia for sounds alone has been reported in only two cases; one patient could identify only half of 26 familiar sounds, and the other could recognize no sound other than the ticking of a watch. Yet in both patients the audiogram was normal, and neither had trouble understanding spoken words. In both, the lesion involved the right temporal lobe, and the corpus callosum was intact.

Amusia proves to be more complicated, for the appreciation of music has several aspects: the recognition of a familiar melody and the ability to name it, the perception of pitch and timbre, and the ability to read and write music. There are many reports of musicians who became word-deaf with lesions of the dominant temporal lobe and retained their recognition of music and their skill in producing it. Others became agnosic for music but not for words, and still others were agnosic for both words and music. According to Segarra and Quadfasel, impaired recognition of music depends on lesions in the middle temporal gyrus and not on lesions at the pole of the temporal lobe, as formerly postulated by Henschen.

That the appreciation of music is impaired by lesions of the nondominant temporal lobe finds support in Milner's studies of patients who had undergone temporal lobectomy. She found a statistically significant lowering of the patient's appreciation of the duration of notes, timbre, intensity of sounds, and memory of melodies following right temporal lobectomy; these abilities were preserved in patients with left temporal lobectomies, regardless of whether Heschl's gyri were included. Similar observations were made by Shankweiler, but in addition he found that patients had difficulty in the denomination of a note or the naming of a melody following left temporal lobectomies.

These data suggest that the nondominant hemisphere is important for the perception of musical notes and melodies but that the naming of musical scores and all the semantic aspects of music require the integrity of the dominant temporal lobe.

Word Deafness (Auditory Verbal Agnosia) This important element in Wernicke's aphasia will be discussed in Chap. 22. While often combined with agnosia for sounds and music, there is no doubt that it can occur separately.

Auditory Illusions Temporal lobe lesions that leave hearing intact may cause paracusia; i.e., sounds may be heard more loudly or less loudly than normally. There may also be modifications of timbre or tonality. Sounds or words may seem strange or disagreeable, or they may seem to be repeated, a kind of perseveration. If auditory hallucinations are also present, they may undergo similar alterations. Such paracusias may last indefinitely and alter musical appreciation as well.

Auditory Hallucinations These may be elementary (murmurs, blowing, sound of running water or motors, whistles, clangs, sirens, etc.) and either steady or rhythmical, or they may be complex (musical themes, choruses, voices). Usually sounds and musical themes are heard more clearly than voices. Patients may recognize the illusions and hallucinations for what they are (i.e., abnormalities of hearing), or they may be convinced that the voices are real, in which case they respond to them with intense feeling and emotion. Hearing may fade before or during the hallucination.

In temporal lobe epilepsy the auditory hallucinations may occur alone or in combination with visual or gustatory hallucinations, dizziness, aphasia, and visual distortions. There may be hallucinations based on remembered experiences (experiential hallucinations, in the terminology of Penfield and Rasmussen).

The anatomy of the lesions underlying auditory illusions and hallucinations has been incompletely studied. In some instances these sensory phenomena have been combined with auditory verbal (or nonverbal) agnosia and inability to draw a named object (while still able to copy it); the superior and posterior parts of one or both temporal lobes are then involved. Clinicoanatomic correlation is difficult in cases of tumors that distort the brain without completely destroying it and also cause edema of the surrounding tissue. Moreover, it is often uncertain whether some of the symptoms have been produced by destruction of cerebral tissue or the excitation of it, i.e., by way of seizures, which act in a fashion similar to electrical stimulation of the audiopsychic zones during surgical operations. Elementary hallucinations and dreamy states have been reported with lesions of either temporal lobe, whereas the more complex auditory hallucinations and particularly polymodal ones (visual plus auditory) occur more often with left-sided lesions. Also it should be noted that elementary (unformed) auditory hallucinations (e.g., the sound of an orchestra tuning up) occur with lesions that appear to be restricted to the pons ("pontine auditory hallucinosis").

It is tempting to relate complex auditory hallucinations to disorders in the auditory association areas surrounding Heschl's gyri, but the data do not fully justify such an assumption. The most one can say is that the superolateral part of the temporal lobe usually is affected, and if the hallucinations are polymodal, the lesions lie more posteriorly, usually in the dominant hemisphere.

Vestibular Disturbances In the superior and posterior part of the temporal lobe (posterior to auditory cortex, first and second temporal convolution) there is an area which responds to vestibular stimulation. If destroyed on one side, the only clinical effect is a change in the pattern of eye movements on optokinetic stimulation. Epileptic activation of this area occurs and may then induce vertigo or a sense of disequilibrium. As was pointed out on page 199, pure vertiginous epilepsy is a rarity, and if vertigo does precede a fit, it is usually momentary and is quickly submerged in the other components of the seizure.

Disturbances of Time Perception These may occur with lesions of either temporal lobe. In a temporal lobe seizure, time may seem to stand still or pass with great speed, or it cannot be estimated. On recovery from such a seizure the patient may repeatedly look at the clock, having lost all sense of time. Serious cerebral diseases (amentias and dementias) may prevent or abolish the capacity to reckon personal events in terms of a time scale. The patient with Korsakoff's psychosis, presumably because of failure of retentive memory, is unable to correlate experiences in their proper time relationships. Other than these clinical instances the authors have not been impressed with derangements of the sense of time as having any importance in clinical neurology.

Other (Nonauditory) Syndromes Between the hippocampal formation (on the inferomedial surface of the temporal lobe) and the primary and secondary auditory areas (Heschl's transverse gyri and superior temporal convolution, respectively) there is a large expanse of temporal lobe that has no assignable function. Patients with tumors and vascular lesions in this region have been examined on numerous occasions, but usually the full extent of the disease has not been determined, even by arteriography or scanning procedures. Cases of partial or complete temporal lobectomy for tumor have been more valuable, but again it has seldom been possible to be certain that other parts of the brain were not involved. With lesions in these parts of the dominant temporal lobe, a defect in the retrieval of words (amnesic dysnomia) has been the most frequently observed abnormality.

Careful psychological studies have disclosed a difference between patients with loss of the dominant temporal lobes and those with loss of the nondominant temporal lobes. With the former there is impairment in the learning of material presented through the auditory sense; with the latter there is failure in the learning of visually presented material. In addition, about 20 percent of patients who had undergone lobectomy, left or right, showed a syndrome similar to that described for the prefrontal regions, but perhaps more significant is the fact that in the remainder of the cases, little or no defect in personality or behavior was observed. The study of cases of uncinate epilepsy, with the characteristic dreamy state, olfactory or gustatory hallucinations, and masticatory movements, suggests that all these functions are organized through the temporal lobes. Similarly, stimulation of the posterior parts of the first and second temporal convolutions of fully conscious epileptic patients can arouse complex memories and visual and auditory images, some with strong emotional content. Penfield and Roberts, who reported these observations, call this part of the temporal lobe the "interpretive cortex."

Studies of the effect of stimulation of the amygdaloid complex of nuclei, which is in the anterior and medial part of the temporal lobe, have shown that olfactory sensations were evoked. In addition, symptoms not unlike some of those of schizophrenic patients have been elicited. Complex emotional experiences that have occurred previously may be revived. There are remarkable autonomic effects: blood pressure rises, pulse rate increases, respirations increase in depth and frequency, and the patient looks frightened. Sexual aberrations (excessive arousal, overactivity, reduced capacity) have also been reported in some patients, and MacLean has reproduced some of these and other visceral effects in monkeys by stimulation of the medial periamygdaloid regions, i.e., the part that he has labeled the "visceral brain." Some seizures arising from foci in this region are manifested by a complex of disordered thought, hallucinations, and strange, detached, and at times violent, uncontrollable behavior. This complex of symptoms resembles schizophrenia and hypomania. Aggressive behavior in some sociopaths has been associated with discharging foci in one or both temporal lobes. There are cases on record in which ablation of the amygdaloid nuclei has eliminated uncontrollable rage reactions in psychotic patients. Temporal lobe epileptics with psychosis, on the other hand, while improved with respect to seizures, persist in their psychotic behavior. Hippocampal and adjacent convolutions have been excised bilaterally, for a distance of 7 cm from the temporal pole, with a disastrous loss of ability to learn or to establish new memories (Korsakoff's psychosis). All this indicates an important role of the temporal lobes in auditory and visual perception and imagery, in learning and memory, and in the emotional life of the individual.

Bilateral removal of the temporal lobes in the macaque monkey produces a behavioral state in which the animal reacts to every visual stimulus without seeming to recognize it (psychic blindness, or visual agnosia). The animal sees small objects but in order to recognize them must examine them by oral and manual contact. Placidity, i.e., lack of the usual emotional response to stimuli, and increase in sexual activity are other prominent features. This is the Klüver-Bucy syndrome, and the full form, as produced in monkeys, has so far not been observed in humans. In a person with a stable personality, unilateral temporal lobectomy has had little recognizable effect on emotion and temperament (see page 307). If the lesions are bilateral, a syndrome resembling that of Klüver and Bucy has been described. (See Chap. 25 for discussion of emotional aspects.)

To summarize, human temporal lobe syndromes include the following:

   I. Effects of unilateral disease of the dominant temporal lobe
      A. Homonymous quadrantanopia
      B. Wernicke's aphasia
      C. Amusia (some types)
      D. Impairment in tests of verbal material presented through the auditory sense
      E. Dysnomia or amnesic aphasia
  II. Effects of unilateral disease of nondominant temporal lobe
      A. Homonymous quadrantanopia
      B. Inability to judge spatial relation in some cases
      C. Impairment in tests of visually presented nonverbal material
      D. Agnosia for sounds and some qualities of music
 III. Effects of disease of either hemisphere
      A. Auditory illusions and hallucinations
      B. Psychotic behavior (aggressivity)
  IV. Effects of bilateral disease
      A. Korsakoff's amnesic defect (hippocampal formations)
      B. Apathy and placidity   ⎫ Klüver-Bucy
      C. Disturbance of sexual functions ⎬ syndrome
      D. Loss of other of the unilateral functions

SYNDROMES CAUSED BY LESIONS OF THE PARIETAL LOBES

ANATOMIC AND PHYSIOLOGIC CONSIDERATIONS

This part of the cerebrum is least well demarcated from the rest (Fig. 21-3). Lying behind Rolando's sulcus and above the sylvian fissure, it has no sharp boundaries inferiorly and posteriorly, where it merges with the temporal and occipital lobes. On its medial side the parietooccipital sulcus marks the posterior border which is completed by extending the line of the sulcus downward to the preoccipital notch on the inferolateral border of the hemisphere. Within the parietal lobe there are two important sulci: the postcentral sulcus, which forms the posterior boundary of the somesthetic cortex, and the interparietal sulcus, which runs anteroposteriorly from the middle of the posterior central sulcus and separates the mass of the parietal lobe into superior and inferior parietal lobules (Fig. 21-3). The posterior extremity of the sylvian fissure curves upward to terminate in the inferior parietal lobule where it is surrounded by the supramarginal gyrus (Brodmann's area 40). The superior temporal sulcus also turns up, into the more posterior part of the inferior parietal lobule, and is surrounded by the angular gyrus (area 39). The supramarginal and angular gyri are sometimes referred to as Ecker's inferior parietal lobule. These two gyri and the posterior third of the first temporal gyrus make up what continental neuroanatomists call Wernicke's speech area.

The architecture of the postcentral convolution is typical of all primary receptive areas (koniocortex or special granular cortex) and that of the rest of the parietal lobe resembles the associational cortex of the frontal and temporal lobes. The superior and inferior parietal lobules and adjacent parts of the temporal and occipital lobes are more extensive in humans than any of the other primates and are relatively slow in development, not being fully functional until the seventh year of age. This area has large fiber connections with the frontal, occipital and temporal lobes of the same hemisphere and, through the middle part of the corpus callosum, with corresponding parts of the opposite hemisphere.

Electrical stimulation of the cortex of the superior and inferior parietal lobules evokes no specific motor or sensory effects. Overlapping here, however, are the tertiary zones for vision, hearing, and somatic sensation, the supramodal integration of which is essential to our awareness of space and person and certain aspects of language and calculation, as will be described below.

The reader is referred to Critchley's monograph for a more complete account of the anatomy and physiology of this uniquely human "middle third" of the cerebrum.

Within the brain no other territory surpasses the parietal lobes in the rich variety of clinical phenomena that are exposed under conditions of disease. This state of neurological affairs contrasts sharply with that of the late nineteenth century, when the parietal lobes, in the classic textbooks of Oppenheim and Gowers, were considered to be "silent areas." However, the clinical manifestations may be subtle, requiring special techniques for their elicitation, and even more difficult are the interpretations of these abnormalities of function in terms of a coherent and plausible physiology.

Despite Critchley's pessimistic prediction that to establish a formula of normal parietal function will prove to be a "vain and meaningless pursuit," the activities of this part of the brain are beginning to assume some degree of order. There is now little reason to doubt that the anterior parietal cortex contains the mechanisms for tactile percepts. Here, discriminative tactile functions are organized and integrated with visual and auditory information in the building up of an awareness of the body (body schema) and of its relation to extrapersonal space. Proprioception and vision are combined for the manipulation of the body and of objects and for certain constructional activities, and impairment of these functions implicates the parietal lobes, especially the right. The understanding of the grammatical and syntactical aspects of language is a function of the dominant parietal lobe, as will be elaborated in Chap. 22. The recognition and utilization of numbers, arithmetic, principles and acts of calculation, which have important spatial attributes, stand as other functions that are integrated principally through the dominant parietal lobe.

CLINICAL EFFECTS AND SYNDROMES

Cortical Sensory Syndromes The effects of a parietal lobe lesion on somatic sensation were first described by Verger and then more completely by Déjerine, in his monograph *L'agnosie corticale*, and by Head and Holmes. In the French medical literature these effects are sometimes referred to as the Verger-Déjerine syndrome. As was pointed out in Chap. 8 the sensory defect is essentially one of sensory discrimination, i.e., an impairment or loss of the sense of position and of passive movement, of the ability to localize tactile, thermal, and noxious stimuli applied to the body surface, to judge the size, shape, and texture of objects (astereognosis), to recognize figures written on the skin, and to distinguish between single and double contacts (two-point discrimination). In contrast, the perception of pain, touch, pressure, vibratory, and thermal stimuli is relatively intact. This type of sensory defect is sometimes referred to

as "cortical," although these effects can be produced just as well by lesions in the thalamocortical connections that traverse the cerebral white matter. Clinicoanatomical studies implicate the postcentral gyrus, particularly the hand area on the opposite side of the body; parietal-cortical lesions that do not involve the postcentral gyrus produce only transient somatosensory changes or none at all (Corkin et al.; Carmon and Benton).

The question of unilateral versus bilateral sensory deficits with lesions in only one postcentral convolution was raised by the studies of Semmes et al. and of Corkin et al. In tests of pressure sensitivity, two-point discrimination, point localization, position sense, and tactual object recognition, they found bilateral disturbances in nearly half of their cases, but the deficits were always most severe contralaterally and mainly in the hand.

These disturbances of disciminative sensation and the subject of tactile agnosia are discussed more fully in Chap. 8.

Déjerine and Mouzon have described another parietal lobe sensory syndrome in which touch, pressure, pain, thermal, vibratory, and position sense are lost on the opposite side of the body or in a limb. This type of hemisensory syndrome usually occurs with large, acute lesions in the cerebral white matter (infarcts, hemorrhages) and recedes in time, leaving more subtle defects in sensory discrimination. As indicated in Chap. 8, lesser lesions, particularly ones that result from a glancing blow to the parietal region, may cause a defect in cutaneous-kinesthetic perception in a discrete part of a limb, e.g., the ulnar half of the hand and forearm, in which case it mimics to some extent a peripheral nerve or root lesion.

Head and Holmes drew attention to a number of interesting points about subjects with parietal sensory defects—the easy fatigability of the patient's sensory perceptions, the inconsistency of feedback about such perceptions, the difficulty in distinguishing more than one contact at a time, the tendency of superficial pain sensations to outlast the stimulus and to be hyperpathic, and the occurrence of hallucinations of touch.

The Asomatognosias The idea that visual and tactile sensory information is normally synthesized during development into a body schema or image (perception of one's body and of the relations of bodily parts to one another) was first clearly conceptualized by Pick and was extensively elaborated by Brain. Long before their time, however, it was suggested that such information was the basis of our emerging awareness of ourselves as persons, and philosophers had assumed that there must be a constant interplay between percepts of ourselves and those of the surrounding world.

The formation of the body schema is believed to be based on the constant influx of sensations from our bodies as we move about; hence, motor activity is important in its development. Always, however, this involves a sense of extrapersonal space as well, which depends upon visual and labyrinthine impulses. The mechanisms upon which these perceptions depend are best appreciated by studying their derangements in the course of neurologic disease.

Unilateral asomatognosia (Anton-Babinski syndrome) The observation that a patient with a dense left hemiplegia may be indifferent to, or unaware of, the paralysis was first made by Anton. Babinski gave it the name *anosognosia*.

This disorder may express itself in several ways: The patient may act as if nothing is the matter. If asked to lift the paralyzed arm, the patient may lift the intact one or do nothing at all. If asked whether the paralyzed arm has been moved, the patient may say "yes." If the failure to do so is pointed out, the patient may admit that the arm is slightly weak. If told it is paralyzed, the patient may deny that this is so or offer an excuse: "My shoulder hurts." If asked why the paralysis went unnoticed, the response may be, "I'm not a doctor." Some patients report that they feel as though their left side has disappeared, and when shown their paralyzed arm, they may deny it is theirs and assert that it belongs to someone else, or even take hold of it and fling it aside. This mental derangement, which Hughlings Jackson referred to as a kind of "imbecility," obviously includes a somatic sensory defect as well as a conceptual negation of paralysis, a neglect and even a disturbed visual perception of that half of the body, and a blunted emotionality.

Anosognosia is usually associated with other abnormalities. The patient looks dull, is inattentive and apathetic, and shows varying degrees of general confusion. There may be an indifference to failure, a feeling of something missing, visual and tactile illusions when sensing the paralyzed part, hallucinations of movement, and allocheiria (one-sided stimuli are felt on the other side).

A particularly common group of parietal symptoms consists of neglect of one side of the body in dressing and grooming ("dressing apraxia"), recognition only on the intact side of bilaterally and simultaneously presented stimuli ("sensory extinction"), deviation of head and eyes to the side of the lesion, and torsion of the body in the same direction. Homonymous hemianopia, visual inattention, and varying degrees of hemiparesis may or may not be present, and there may be grasping and groping with the nonparalyzed hand.

According to Denny-Brown et al., the basic disturbance in cases such as these is an inability to summate a series of "spatial impressions"—tactile, kinesthetic, visual, or auditory—a defect they refer to as *amorphosynthesis*. In their view, imperception or neglect of one side of the body and of extrapersonal space represents the full extent of the disturbance, which in lesser degree consists only of tactile and visual extinction. They make the additional points that the disorder of spatial summation is strictly contralateral to the damaged parietal lobe, right or left, and has to be distinguished from a true agnosia, which is a disorder of perception of symbols and concepts and applies to both sides of space as a result of damage to one (the dominant) hemisphere (see below).

The lesion responsible for the various forms of unilateral asomatognosia lies in the cortex and white matter of the superior parietal lobule but extends variably into the postcentral gyrus, frontal motor areas, and temporal and occipital lobes, which accounts for some of the associated abnormalities. The right (nondominant) parietal lobe is affected seven times more frequently than the left, according to Hécaen's statistics. Nevertheless, symptoms identical to those which follow a right parietal lesion may occur with a left parietal lesion. The apparent infrequency of right-sided symptoms is attributable, at least in part, to their obscuration by an associated aphasia.

From the above descriptions it is evident that the left and right parietal lobes function differently. The most obvious difference, of course, is that language functions are centered in the left hemisphere. It is hardly surprising therefore that verbally mediated or verbally associated spatial functions are more affected with left-sided than right-sided lesions. It must also be realized that speech involves cross-modal connections and is central to all cognitive functions. Hence cross-modal matching tasks (auditory-visual, visual-auditory, visual-tactile, tactile-visual, auditory-tactile, etc.) are most clearly impaired with dominant hemisphere lesions. Indeed this is what Butters and Brody have found. Similarly, faults in what Luria has called logicogrammatical and syntactic aspects of language (which he considers to be quasispatial) occur with left parietal lesions. Such patients can read and understand spoken words but cannot grasp the meaning of a sentence if it contains elements of relationship (e.g., the mother's daughter versus the daughter's mother; the father's brother's son; Jane's complexion is lighter than Marjorie's but darker than her sister's). In calculation there are similar effects; the patient may be able to read numbers and describe the rules of a required computation but not be able to carry it out with pencil and paper. It should be noted that addition, subtraction, multiplication, and division all require the placing of numbers in specific spatial relationships. The recognition and naming of parts of the body and the distinction of right from left and up from down are other learned, verbally mediated spatial percepts which are disturbed by lesions in the dominant parietal lobe.

The symptoms comprised by *Gerstmann's syndrome* provide the most striking examples of bilateral asomatognosia due to a left, or dominant, parietal lesion. The characteristic features are: confusion of the right and left sides of the body; inability to designate or name the different fingers of the two hands; and inability to calculate and to write. Each of these deficits depends on learned spatial relationships conditioned by verbal clues. These patients cannot put words, numbers, and parts of the body into proper relationships. They may try to add a column of figures transversely or obliquely and start the subtraction or multiplication of a column of figures from the wrong side. Although they do better calculating mentally, they still make errors, supporting Ehrenfeld's idea that there is also a fault in recognition of numbers and in ordination.

There has been a dispute as to whether the four main elements of Gerstmann's syndrome (agraphia, right-left confusion, digital agnosia, and acalculia) have a common basis or only a chance association. Benton states that they occur together in a parietal lesion no more often than do constructional apraxia, alexia, and loss of visual memory and that every combination of these symptoms and those of Gerstmann's syndrome occurs with equal frequency in parietal lobe disease. Others disagree and believe that digital agnosia, agraphia, and acalculia have special significance, being linked through a unitary defect in spatial orientation.

Disturbances of the perception of space, other than language-related ones, are most evident in patients with lesions in the right, nondominant parietal lobe. These include disorders of topographic (extrapersonal) orientation, topographic and geographic memory with resulting difficulties in route finding, and an inability to reproduce geometric figures ("constructional apraxia"). A number of tests have been designed to elicit these disturbances, such as indicating the time by placing of hands on the figure of a clock, spontaneous (free) drawing, copying a complex figure, reproducing stick-pattern constructions and block designs (constructional apraxia), three-dimensional constructions, and reconstruction of puzzles. In the majority of cases, as remarked above, the lesions responsible for these deficits prove to be in the right hemisphere, though the dominance is not as striking as that of language and language-associated functions.

A great variety of other more general examination techniques are used to elicit these left and right parietal defects: optokinetic nystagmus; reading; all the main operations of calculation; indicating right and left sides of the body; naming and indicating to command the different digits of the two hands; writing dictated sentences and copying; drawing figures of multiple parts on command and copying from memory; reconstructing patterns with blocks or match sticks; drawing maps and floor plans of rooms and home; drawing the route from home to work; putting on a dressing gown, one sleeve of which has been turned inside out; naming all the objects in the room (to note unilateral spatial neglect); and holding both arms outstretched (to show postural arm drift).

Consciousness of Self and Depersonalization   There are many other circumstances in which the patient's appreciation of self in relation to environment is disturbed in a more general sense. Some of these, such as diplopia and labyrinthine vertigo (discussed in Chaps. 13 and 14), are readily understandable, for they present to the sensorium conflicting data about the external world, e.g., double images or unnaturally moving images. In other clinical conditions, however, there is no evidence of sensory deficit. Rather, some disorder occurs in the state of continuous self-consciousness, which depends on the influx of sensations and their association with past memories, the stream of life experiences and feelings that keep us continuously aware of ourselves as entities. Patients with depression of mood may say that they do not feel natural, as they move about in the world; it is as though they were frozen in their reactions, as though something has altered their way of feeling and experiencing. The schizophrenic may feel unreal, or *depersonalized*. Extreme degrees of this are observed in the delusions of negativism (*délire de negativisme*), in which such patients deny their own existence. In a manic attack every experience may be more vivid, enjoyable, and personalized than ever before. Also delusions of transformation, of being someone else (a royal figure, God, or Jesus) occur in schizophrenia, manic states, and general paresis (delusions of grandeur). It is tempting to view all these clinical phenomena as manifestations of more general disturbances of the body-environmental schemata, but the evidence is inconclusive. Ideomotor apraxia, another symptom complex due to left parietal lesions, has been discussed in Chap. 3.

The effects of disease of the parietal lobes may be summarized as follows:

I. Effects of unilateral disease of the parietal lobe, right or left
   A. Cortical sensory syndrome and sensory extinction (or total hemianesthesia with large acute lesions of white matter)
   B. Mild hemiparesis, unilateral muscular atrophy in children
   C. Homonymous hemianopia (incongruent or inferior quadrantic) or visual inattention, and sometimes anosognosia, neglect of one-half of the body and of extrapersonal space (observed more frequently with right than with left parietal lesions)
   D. Abolition of optokinetic nystagmus to one side
II. Effects of unilateral disease of the dominant parietal lobe (left hemisphere in right-handed patients); additional phenomena include:
   A. Disorders of language (especially alexia)
   B. Gerstmann's syndrome
   C. Tactile agnosia (bimanual astereognosis; see page 111)
   D. Bilateral apraxia of the ideomotor type
III. Effects of unilateral disease of the nondominant (right) parietal lobe
   A. Topographic memory loss
   B. Anosognosia and dressing apraxia. These disorders may occur with lesions of either hemisphere but have been observed more frequently with lesions of the nondominant one.

In all these lesions, if the disease is sufficiently extensive, there may be a reduction in the capacity to think clearly, inattentiveness, and impaired memory.

It is impossible at this time to present an all-embracing formula of parietal lobe function. It does seem reasonably certain that in addition to the perception of somatosensory impulses (postcentral gyrus) the parietal lobe participates in the integration of all sensory data, especially those which provide consciousness of one's surroundings, of the relation of objects in the environment to one another, and of the position of the body in space. In this respect, the parietal lobe may be regarded as a special, high-order sensory organ, the locus of transmodal (intersensory) integrations, particularly tactile and visual ones, which are the basis of our concepts of spatial relations.

SYNDROMES CAUSED BY LESIONS OF THE OCCIPITAL LOBES

ANATOMIC AND PHYSIOLOGIC CONSIDERATIONS

The occipital lobes are the terminus of the geniculocalcarine pathways and are essential for visual perception and recognition. This part of the brain has a large medial surface and somewhat smaller lateral and inferior surfaces. The parietooccipital fissure is its obvious medial boundary with the parietal lobe, but laterally it merges with the parietal and the temporal lobes. The large calcarine fissure courses in an anteroposterior direction from the pole of the occipital lobe to the splenium of the corpus callosum, and area 17, the primary visual receptive cortex, lies in its banks (Fig. 21-1). It is typical koniocortex but is unique in that its fourth layer is divided into two granular cell layers by a greatly thickened outer band of myelinated fibers, the band of Baillarger. The grossly visible stripe in area 17 is also called the band of Gennari and has given this area the name *striate* cortex. The largest part of area 17 is the terminus of the macular fibers (see Fig. 12-1). The parastriate cortex (areas 18 and 19) lacks the line of Gennari and resembles the granular association cortex of the rest of the cerebrum. Area 17 contains cells that are activated by the homolateral geniculocalcarine pathway and sends fibers to areas 18 and 19. The latter are connected with one another and with the angular gyri, medial temporal and parietal gyri, frontal motor areas, and with corresponding areas of the opposite hemisphere through the posterior third (splenium) of the corpus callosum.

The connections between these several areas in the occipital lobe are complicated, and the old idea that area 17 is activated by the lateral geniculate neurons and that their activity is then transferred and elaborated in areas 18 and 19 is surely not the complete story. Actually there are four or five occipital receptive fields, activated by the lateral geniculate neurons, and as Hubel and Wiesel have shown, the response patterns of neurons in both occipital lobes to edges and moving visual stimuli and to on-and-off effects of light are much different than was originally supposed. The monographs of Polyak and of Walsh and Hoyt contain detailed information about the anatomy and physiology of this part of the brain.

CLINICAL EFFECTS AND SYNDROMES

Visual Field Defects The most familiar clinical disorder resulting from a lesion of one occipital lobe, homonymous hemianopia, has already been discussed in

Chap. 12. Extensive destruction abolishes all vision in the corresponding half of each visual field. With a neoplastic lesion that eventually involves the entire striate region, the field defect may extend from the periphery toward the center, and loss of color vision (hemiachromatopsia) precedes loss of black and white. Lesions that destroy only part of the striate cortex on one side yield characteristic field defects that accurately indicate the loci of the lesions. A lesion confined to the pole of the occipital lobe results in a central hemianopic defect which splits the maculas and leaves the peripheral fields intact. This observation indicates that half of each macula is unilaterally represented and settles once and for all the old debate as to whether they may be spared in hemianopia. Bilateral lesions of the occipital poles, as in embolism of the posterior cerebral arteries, result in bilateral central hemianopias often of different sizes. Quadrant defects and altitudinal field defects due to striate lesions indicate that the cortex on one side of the calcarine fissure is damaged. The cortex below the fissure is the terminus of fibers from the lower half of the retina, and the resulting field defect is in the upper quadrant, and vice versa. Most bilateral altitudinal defects are traceable to incomplete occipital lesions (cortex or terminal parts of geniculocalcarine pathways). Head and Holmes described several such cases due to gunshot wounds; embolic or thrombotic infarction has been the usual cause in our material.

Cortical Blindness With bilateral lesions of the occipital lobes (destruction of area 17 of both hemispheres), there is a loss of sight. The degree of blindness may be equivalent to that which follows enucleation of the eyes or severance of the optic nerves. Since the pupillary light reflexes depend upon visual fibers that do not pass through the lateral geniculate bodies but terminate in the midbrain, they are preserved (see Fig. 13-6). Usually no changes are detectable in the retinas, though van Buren has described slight optic atrophy in monkeys long after occipital ablations. The eyes are still able to move through a full range, but optokinetic nystagmus cannot be elicited. Visual imagination and visual imagery in dreams are preserved. No cortical potentials can be evoked in occipital lobes by light flashes, and the alpha rhythm is lost in the EEG.

Less complete lesions may leave some degree of perception of light. There may also be visual hallucinations of either elementary or complex types, as described on page 175. The mode of recovery from cortical blindness has been studied carefully by Pötzl, who describes three stages: (1) obscurity with hallucinations, (2) gray vision with vague outlines, (3) recovery of color (red first, blue last). Even with recovery the patient may complain of visual fatigue (asthenopia) and difficulties in fixation and fusion.

The usual cause of cortical blindness is occlusion of the posterior cerebral arteries (embolic or thrombotic). The infarction may also involve the medial temporal regions and thalami with resulting Korsakoff's psychosis, alexia with loss of ability to name colors, and Déjerine-Roussy syndrome (see pages 100 and 541). Hypoxic encephalopathy, the leukodystrophies, and bilateral gliomas are other causes of cortical blindness. A transitory form of cortical blindness may occur with head injury.

Visual Anosognosia (Anton's Syndrome) The main characteristic is denial of blindness in patients who obviously cannot see. The patients act as though they can see, and when attempting to walk, they collide with objects, even to the point of injury. Excuses may be offered for their difficulties: "I lost my glasses," "The light is dim," etc., or there may be only an indifference to the loss of sight. The lesions in cases of negation of blindness extend beyond the striate cortex to involve the visual association areas.

The opposite condition may also arise: a patient can see small objects, but claims to be blind. This individual walks about avoiding obstacles, picks up crumbs or pills from the table, and catches a small ball thrown from a distance. The anatomy of this disorder is not known.

Visual Illusions and Hallucinations While these may occur in relation to lesions in any part of the visual system, they are particularly frequent with occipital lobe lesions. Electrical stimulation of the occipital cortex elicits visual phenomena of this type, and it seems likely, therefore, that seizures reproduce them by activating the visual system directly. In these instances the hallucinations are *positive phenomena*. Certain lesions disturb the equilibrium of the visual system in other ways, possibly by disinhibiting other parts, thereby liberating the hallucinations (*negative* phenomena). Difficulties in distinguishing between positive and negative hallucinatory phenomena also arise in the interpretation of the effects of drugs and the process of withdrawal, if the patient had been habituated. Although illusions and hallucinations are considered separately here, they may be difficult to separate, especially in epilepsy and delirium.

Visual Illusions (Metamorphopsias) These may present as distortions of form, size, movement, or color; also visual images may fail to arouse visual memories and their associated affect, resulting in a sense of strangeness or inexplicable familiarity, as occurs in the "dreamy state" of temporal lobe epilepsy. Some of these have already been mentioned in Chaps. 12 and 15.

Visual illusions take the form of objects seeming too small (micropsia) and distant or too large (megalopsia or macropsia) and moving toward the patient. In other cases, objects may appear elongated, swollen, or run together, or the vertical and horizontal orientation of the image may shift. Inverted vision, irradiation of contour, disappearance of color (achromatopsia), illusional coloring (erythropsia), polyopia (one object appearing as two or more objects) or monocular diplopia (vertical, concentric, especially triplopia), illusions of movement of stationary objects, too rapid displacement of moving objects, or imperception of movement are other forms of illusory visual experience. There may be also a loss of stereoscopic vision, perseveration of visual images (palinopsia), a false orientation of objects in space (optic alloesthesia), or metamorphosis of objects. In a group of 83 patients with visual perceptual abnormalities Hécaen found that 71 fell under one of four headings: deformation of the image, change in size, illusions of movement, or a combination of all three.

Illusions of these types have been reported with lesions of the occipital, occipitoparietal, or occipitotemporal regions, and the right hemisphere appears to be involved somewhat more often than the left. Illusions of movement occur more frequently with posterior temporal lesions, polyopsia more frequently with occipital lesions, and palinopsia with both parietal and occipital lesions. Visual field defects are present in many of the cases.

Hoff and Pötzl have insisted that an element of vestibular disorder underlies the metamorphopsias of parietooccipital lesions (the vestibular system is represented in the parietal lobe; see page 199). Polyopia, ascribed to faulty ocular fixation, has usually proved to be a manifestation of occipital lesions, although it may occur in hysteria.

Pharmacologic agents also alter vision, and one may surmise that occipital or temporooccipital regions are involved. Lysergic acid and mescaline cause many of these illusory phenomena. Atropine may make objects appear smaller than normal as such patients look from a distance toward themselves and larger if they look from

nearby to a distance. Disintegration of sensory information due to parietal lesions may explain some of the failures to synthesize ocular movement and vestibular function.

Visual Hallucinations These phenomena may be elementary or complex, and both have sensory as well as cognitive aspects. Elementary (or unformed) hallucinations include flashes of light, colors, luminous points, stars, multiple lights (like candles), and geometric forms (circles, squares, and hexagons). They may be stationary or moving (zigzag, oscillations, vibrations, or pulsations). Complex, or formed, hallucinations include objects, persons, or animals. They may be of natural size, lilliputian, or grossly enlarged. With hemianopia they may appear in the defective field or move from the intact field toward the hemianopic one. The patient may realize that the hallucinations are false experiences or may be convinced of their reality. Since the patient's feeling or emotion is usually in accord with the character of the hallucination, the patient may react with fear to a threatening vision or contemplate the hallucinations with amusement if their content is benign.

The clinical setting for the occurrence of visual hallucinations varies. Often they are associated with a homonymous hemianopia, as indicated above. Frequently the background is one of confusion and clouding of consciousness, as in the syndrome of delirium (Chap. 19). In the "peduncular hallucinosis" of Lhermitte, the hallucinations are objectified, have a natural spatial orientation, move about as in an animated cartoon, and are usually considered to be unreal, abnormal phenomena (preserved insight). Similar phenomena occur as part of hypnagogic hallucinations in the narcolepsy-cataplexy syndrome (see page 269).

A special syndrome of ophthalmopathic hallucinations occurs in the blind or partially blind person (syndrome of Bonnet). The visual images may be of elementary or complex type, usually of people or animals. Polychromic (unusually vivid colors), animated scenes appear in all parts of the visual field bilaterally, in corresponding fields in homonymous hemianopia, or in one eye if that eye is blinded. Moving the eyes or closing the affected eye has variable effects, sometimes abolishing the hallucinations.

In patients with visual hallucinations, the lesions, if they can be identified, are usually situated in the occipital lobe or posterior part of the temporal lobe. According to Penfield and Rasmussen, elementary hallucinations have their origin in lesions of the occipital cortex, and complex ones, in the temporal cortex. Another peculiarity of posterior temporal lesions is that the hallucinations often fill both visual fields whereas occipital ones appear to be seen only by the opposite eye.

In our material, so-called peduncular hallucinosis has been associated mainly with diencephalic lesions and not strictly with mesencephalic ones. The hallucinations in this disorder are purely visual. If hallucinations are polymodal, the lesion is always in the cerebrum.

The hallucinatory phenomena of delirium are nonlocalizable, as was pointed out in Chap. 19, but sometimes the evidence points to an origin in the temporal lobe. In ophthalmopathic hallucinations there is a visual loss from ocular, optic nerve or tract, or occipital lobe lesions, and also a slight impairment of mental function.

The Visual Agnosias These rare conditions consist of failure to name or indicate the use of a seen object by spoken or written word or by gesture. Vision is intact, the mind is clear, and the patient is not aphasic—conditions requisite for the diagnosis of agnosia. If the object is palpated, it is recognized at once, and it can also be identified by smell or sound if it has an odor or makes a noise. Movement of the object or placing it in its customary surroundings facilitates recognition.

Object agnosia In most reported instances of this condition, first described by Lissauer in 1880, the patient retains normal visual acuity but cannot identify, match, or name objects presented in any part of the visual fields. The underlying lesions are usually extensive in the basal and lateral parts of the occipital lobes and are often bilateral. In Kleist's case there was a lesion in area 19, on the left side. A lesion of the left occipital lobe causes a right homonymous hemianopia (a frequent accompaniment of visual object agnosia) and, by its deep extent into the white matter or the splenium of the corpus callosum, interrupts the fibers that project from the right occipital lobe to the speech areas of the left hemisphere.

The latter lesion accounts for a dyslexia and an inability to name objects and colors (see below under "Corpus Callosum and the Disconnection Syndromes").

Simultagnosia Wolpert originally described a patient in which there was a failure to read and to perceive simultaneously all the elements of a scene and to properly interpret the scene. In the framework of Gestalt psychology the patient could see the parts but not the whole. A cognitive defect of synthesis of the visual impressions was thought to be the basis of this condition, which Wolpert called *simultagnosia*. Some of the patients have a right homonymous hemianopia; in others the visual fields are "full." Components of Balint's syndrome (see below) have been observed in other cases of this kind, suggesting that a fault in ocular scanning might underlie the failure of synthesis. Through tachistoscopic testing, Kinsbourne and Warrington have noted that, by reducing the time of stimulus exposure, single objects are perceived in an instant, but not two objects. Levine and Calvanio, whose review of this subject is recommended, find the basis of simultagnosia to be a quantitative defect in "the capacity for perceptual analysis and form synthesis, resulting in a decrease in the span of visual form apprehension." Nielsen has attributed this disorder to a lesion of the inferolateral part of the dominant occipital lobe (area 18), but more often bilateral occipital lesions have been present. The anatomy has not been studied carefully.

Prosopagnosia In this form of visual agnosia patients cannot identify a familiar face either by looking at the person or a picture, even though they know that it is a face and can point to the features. Such patients may also have trouble in interpreting the meaning of facial expressions (observed in one-half of Hécaen's cases). In identifying persons, the patient depends on other data such as the presence and type of spectacles or moustache, the type of gait, or the sound of a voice. As a rule, other agnosias are present in such cases (color agnosia, simultagnosia), and there may be topographical disorientation, disturbances of body schema, and constructional or dressing apraxia. Visual field defects are nearly always present, a left upper quadrantanopsia being the most frequent. Impairment of highly discriminative visual skills, such as recognition of species of birds or types of fruit, have been described. Some neurologists have interpreted this condition as a simultagnosia involving facial features. Another interpretation is that the face, though satisfactorily perceived, cannot be matched to a memory store of faces. In the small number of cases that have been studied anatomically there was evidence of bilateral disease predominantly of the inferior occipitotemporal lobes. Clinically, this disorder has been attributed to unilateral occipitotemporal lesions, more frequently on the right than left side, in keeping with Milner's observations that visual memory for faces is impaired in patients with right temporal lobectomies.

Visual agnosia for words See Chap. 22 and below in the present chapter, under "Corpus Callosum and the Disconnection Syndromes."

Visual disorientation and disorders of spatial (topographic) localization Spatial orientation, which depends upon visual, tactile, and kinesthetic perception, has already been discussed under "Parietal Lobes." There are instances, however, where the defect in visual perception predominates. Patients cannot draw the floor plan of their house or a map of their town or the United States and cannot describe a familiar route, say, from their home to their place of work or find their way in familiar surroundings. In brief, they have lost topographic memory. Furthermore, they may have difficulty visualizing and describing the shapes of common objects and also in localizing objects seen in their own visual field. Yet, there is no agnosia for the objects themselves or of the word symbols that represent them. Holmes' patients had occipital lesions, and the right side has been involved more often than the left. Presumably when the visual aspects of space are disturbed, the lesion lies more posteriorly in the occipital lobe, rather than in the parietal lobe.

Color agnosia Here one must distinguish several different aspects of the identification of colors such as the correct perception of color (the loss of which is called *color blindness*) or the naming of a color. In the latter instance the patient has no difficulty in matching a series of skeins of wool of the same hue (test of Holmgren) but refers to them by incorrect names. Usually the patient can state the color of an object named by the examiner. If color perception is altered, the patient may, in painting, choose an incorrect color for the sky, a lawn, or a tomato.

Lhermitte and colleagues have described three types of defects in chromatic vision: (1) loss of perception of all the chromatic aspects of objects, due to bilateral occipital lesions; (2) difficulty in matching colors and sorting colored objects on the basis of hue; and (3) difficulty in designating a color by name while still being able to match colors. The latter two disorders are associated with a lesion of the left occipital area, though in many cases the lesions are bilateral, and, as in other agnosias, performance is erratic, chromatic perception undergoes rapid fatigue (asthenopia for colors), and there may be a failure in associating the proper color with an object. In the third disorder, the lesion always is located in the left parietooccipital region, and the splenium of the corpus callosum is often involved as well.

As with other agnosias, the one for color rarely occurs in isolation. In all forms, visual field defects are common, and there may be other agnosias as well as signs of parietal lobe dysfunction.

Balint's Syndrome This consists of (1) an inability to turn the eyes to a point in the visual field, despite the fact that eye movements are full (psychic paralysis of gaze); (2) a failure to precisely grasp or touch an object under visual guidance, as though hand and eye were not coordinated (optic ataxia); and (3) visual inattention, with intactness of attention to other sensory stimuli.

The psychic paralysis of gaze is apparent when the patient attempts to turn his or her eyes to fixate an object in the right or left visual field and to follow a moving object into all four quadrants of the field once the eyes are fixed on it. Optic ataxia is detected when the patient reaches for an object, either spontaneously or in response to verbal command. To reach the object, the patient engages in tactile search with the palm and fingers, presumably using somatosensory cues to compensate for a lack of visual information. This may give the erroneous impression that the patient is blind. In contrast, movements which do not require visual guidance, such as those directed to the body, or movements of the body itself, are performed naturally. This disorder may involve one or both hands. The presence of visual inattention is tested by asking the patient to carry out tasks such as looking at a series of objects or connecting a series of dots by lines; often only one of a series of objects can be found even though the visual fields seem to be full.

The essential feature in Balint's syndrome appears to be a failure to properly direct oculomotor function in the exploration of space. Thus it is closely related to simultagnosia and to a disorder of spatial summation (amorphosynthesis). In all the reported cases of Balint's syndrome the lesions have been bilateral in the parietooccipital regions, although instances of optic ataxia alone have been described within a single visual field, contralateral to a right or left parietooccipital lesion.

The effects of disease of the occipital lobes may be summarized as follows:

I. Effects of unilateral disease, either right or left
   A. Contralateral (congruent) homonymous hemianopia, which may be central (splitting the macula) or peripheral; also homonymous hemiachromatopsia
   B. Irritative lesions—elementary (unformed) hallucinations
II. Effects of left occipital disease
   A. Right homonymous hemianopia
   B. If deep white matter or splenium of corpus callosum is involved, alexia and color-naming defect
   C. Object agnosia

III. Effects of right occipital disease
   A. Left homonymous hemianopia
   B. With more extensive lesions, visual illusions (metamorphopsias) and hallucinations; more frequent with right-sided than left-sided lesions
   C. Loss of topographic memory and visual orientation
IV. Bilateral occipital disease
   A. Cortical blindness (pupils reactive)
   B. Loss of perception of color
   C. Prosopagnosia, simultagnosia
   D. Balint's syndrome
   E. Bonnet's syndrome

THE THEORETICAL PROBLEM OF VISUAL AND OTHER AGNOSIAS

From the foregoing discussion it is apparent that the term *optic agnosia* applies to a series of visual perceptive disorders which include, in varying combinations, faults of discrimination, identification, and recognition of faces, objects, pictures, colors, spatial arrangements, and words. The diagnosis of these states is predicated on the assumption that the failure in perception occurs in spite of intact visual acuity and adequate mental function, and an essentially normal language mechanism. When examined carefully, agnosic patients usually do not satisfy all these criteria and instead have a number of derangements that may at least in part explain their perceptual incompetence. Often there is a unisensory or polysensory disturbance, or an inadequacy of memory or of naming, or an impairment of visuooculomotor control. Anatomic studies have established that disturbances of recognition of complex forms, human faces, and spatial arrangements accompany right (nondominant) parietooccipital lesions more often than left-sided ones. Disturbances of perception of graphic symbols of objects, of color discrimination and naming—in short all of the lexical aspects of recognition—are virtually always associated with left parietooccipital lesions. Variations in the clinical effects of such lesions are dependent to a large extent on the tests used to elicit them and whether they involve learning, recognition, and recall.

There have been many critics of the concept of agnosia as a higher-order perceptual disturbance that can be clearly separated from loss of elementary sensation. Such a division is said to perpetuate an archaic view of sensory reception in the brain as consisting of two separable functional attributes, elementary sensation and perception. Bay, for example, claims that careful testing of patients with visual agnosia always brings to light some degree of diminished vision, in combination with general defects such as confusion and mental deterioration. Others (Geschwind; Sperry, Gazzaniga, and Bogen) emphasize that the visual agnosias depend

upon disconnections of the visual receptive zones of the brain and the language areas of the left hemisphere, the learning and memory zones of the temporal lobes, the suprasensory zones of the parietal lobes, and the motor regions. Hécaen and Gassel have presented the evidence for and against these points of view.

The reported cases of visual agnosia emphasize the complexity of the perceptive process and the inadequacy of our knowledge of the physiology of the several receptive zones of the occipital lobes. The fact that in some cases there are impairments of primary sensation that can be elicited by careful testing of visual function—using visual adaptation, perception of pattern, flicker-fusion, etc., as Bay recommends—cannot be disputed. However, even when present, such abnormalities would not fully explain the loss of discrimination and the inability to visualize or imagine the form and color of objects, their spatial arrangements, and their names. Failure of a sensation to activate these visual memories must involve a higher-order disturbance of cerebral function in the association areas. To reduce the agnosias to a series of disconnections between the striate and parastriate cortex and other parts of the brain, although an interesting approach, leads to an overly simplified mechanistic view of cerebral activity which probably will not be sustained as more knowledge of cerebral physiology is acquired. There is still a great need of cases in which sensation and perception have been tested in detail and in which the anatomy of the lesion, in its stable end stage, has been studied by serial microscopic sections of the whole brain.

SPECIAL PSYCHOLOGICAL TESTS

In the study of focal cerebral disease there are two approaches—the clinical-neurological and the psychometric. The first consists of the observation and recording of qualitative changes in behavior and performance and the identification of syndromes from which there may be deductions as to the locus and nature of certain diseases. The second consists of recording a patient's level of performance on a variety of psychological tests that have been standardized in a large population of age-matched normal individuals. These tests provide data that can be graded and treated statistically. An example is the *deterioration index* deduced from the difference in performance on subtest items of the Wechsler Adult Intelligence Scale which hold up well in cerebral diseases (vocabulary, information, picture completion, and object assembly) and those which undergo impairment (digit span, similarities, digit symbol, and block design). The main criticism of this and other scatter patterns, such as the Halstead-Reitan impairment index, is the implicit assumption that cerebral activity is a unitary function, the defects of which are quantitative and related to the volume of the lesion rather than its location. The neurological arguments against this notion were given in the introduction to this chapter.

Nonetheless it cannot be denied that there are certain psychometric scales which reveal disease in certain parts of the cerebrum more than in others and provide data that allow comparison of the patient's deficits from one point in the course of an illness to another. Walsh has listed those that he finds most valuable in his recent text on neuropsychology. In addition to the Wechsler Adult Intelligence Scale, Wechsler Memory Scale, and an aphasia screening test he recommends the following for quantitation of:

I. *Frontal lobe disorders*
   A. Milan sorting test, Halstead category test, and Wisconsin card-sorting test, as tests of ability to abstract
   B. The Porteus Maze Test, Reitan Trail Making Test, the recognition of figures in the Figure of Rey as tests of planning, regulating and checking programs of action
   C. Benton's Verbal Fluency Test for estimating verbal skill and verbal regulation of behavior.

II. *Temporal lobe disorders*
   A. Figure of Rey, Benton Visual Retention Test, Illinois Nonverbal Sequential Memory Test, Recurring Nonsense Figures of Kimura, and Facial Recognition Test as modality specific memory tests
   B. Milner's Maze Learning Task and Lhermitte-Signoret amnesic syndrome tests for general retentive memory
   C. Seashore Rhythm Test, Speech-Sound Perception Test from the Halstead-Reitan battery, Environmental Sounds Test, and Austin Meaningless Sounds Test, as measures of auditory perception.

III. *Parietal lobe disorders*
   A. Figure of Rey, Wechsler Block Design and Object Assembly, Benton Figure Copying Test, Halstead-Reitan Tactual Performance Test, and Fairfield Block Substitution Test as tests of constructional praxis
   B. Several mathematical and logicogrammatical tests as tests of spatial synthesis
   C. Cross-modal association tests as tests of suprasensory integration
   D. Benson-Barton Stick Test, Cattell's Pool Reflection Test, and Money's Road Map Test, as tests of spatial perception and memory

IV. *Occipital lobe disorders*
   A. Color naming, color form association, visual irreminiscence, as tests of visual perception

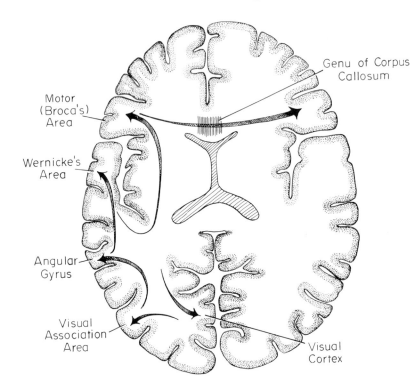

Figure 21-7
Intrahemispheric connections involved in naming a seen object, according to Wernicke's model. The visual pattern is transferred from the visual cortex and association areas to the angular gyrus, which contains the memories for arousing the auditory pattern in Wernicke's (auditory association) area. The auditory form, in turn, is transmitted, via the arcuate fasciculus, to the motor (Broca's) association area. There the articulatory form is aroused and transferred to the face area of the motor cortex, and the word is spoken.

Interruption of the association fibers in the anterior part of the corpus callosum, connecting left and right motor areas, causes a failure of the left hand to obey spoken commands (left-sided apraxia). (Redrawn, with permission, from N Geschwind, Sci Am 226:76, 1972.)

It is the authors' opinion that the data obtained from the above tests should supplement clinical observations. Taken alone, they cannot be depended upon for the localization of cerebral lesions.

DISCONNECTION SYNDROMES

Several clinical syndromes result from interruption of the connections between the two cerebral hemispheres in the corpus callosum or adjacent white matter (commissural syndromes) or between different parts of one hemisphere (intrahemispheric dissociation syndromes). Some of these are illustrated in Figs. 21-7 and 21-8.

When the entire corpus callosum is missing from birth because of a congenital defect or has been destroyed (anterior four-fifths) by an occlusion of the anterior cerebral artery, the language and perception areas of the left hemisphere are isolated from the right hemisphere. These patients, if blindfolded, are unable to match an object held in one hand with that in the other. Furthermore, they cannot match an object seen in the right half of the visual field with one in the left half. If

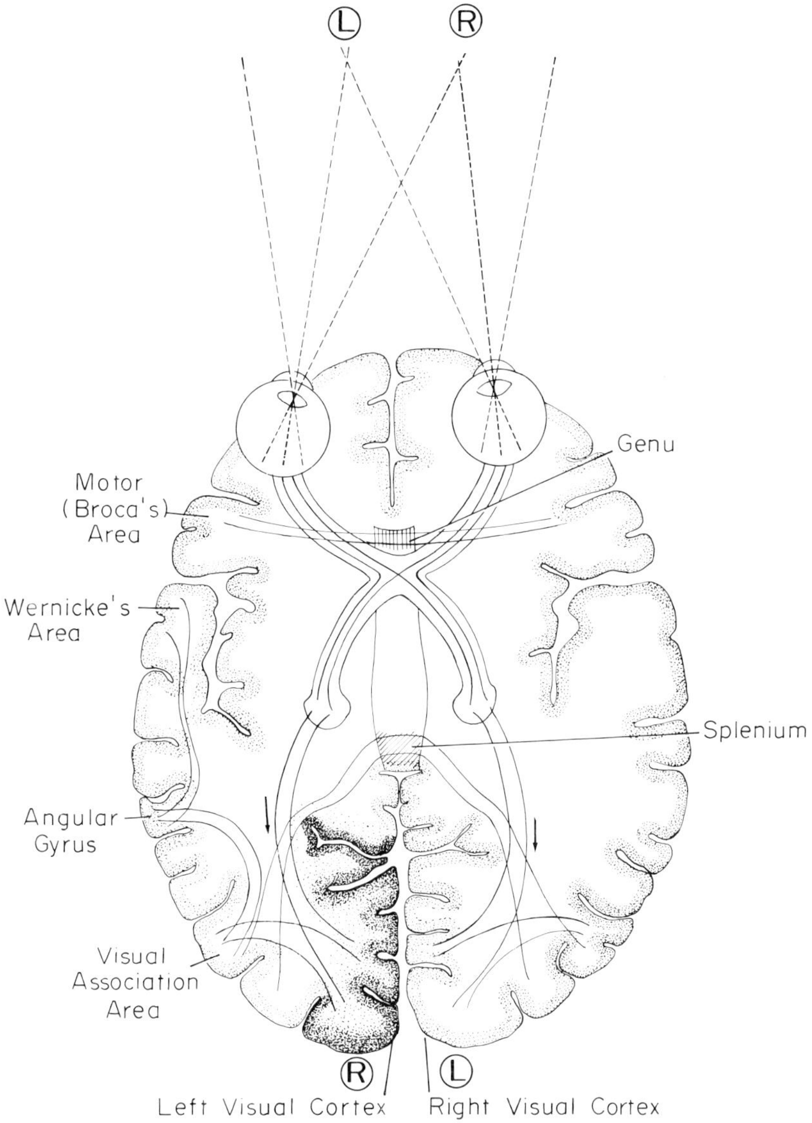

Figure 21-8
The visual part of the disconnection syndrome, based on the classical case study of J. J. Déjerine (1892). The left visual cortex and splenium were destroyed as a result of a left posterior cerebral artery occlusion. The patient was blind in his right visual field (R), and words from the left (L), perceived in the right visual cortex, could not cross over to the language areas because of destruction of the splenium. The patient was unable to read, despite normal visual acuity and the capacity to copy written words. (Redrawn from N Geschwind, Sci Am 226:76, 1972.)

given a verbal command, they execute it correctly with the right hand, but not with the left. For example, if asked to write from dictation with the left hand, they make only an illegible scrawl. Without vision, objects placed in the right hand are named correctly, but not those in the left.

In lesions confined to the posterior fifth of the corpus callosum (splenium), only the visual part of the disconnection syndrome occurs. Occlusion of the left posterior cerebral artery provides the best examples of the latter. Since infarction of the left occipital lobe causes a right homonymous hemianopia, all visual information needed for activating the speech areas of the left hemisphere must thereafter come from the right occipital lobe and cross the splenium of the corpus callosum. Patients with such a lesion cannot read or name colors because the visual information cannot reach the left angular gyrus. There is no difficulty in copying words (though they cannot read what they have written); presumably the visual information for activating the left motor area crosses the corpus callosum more anteriorly. Matching of colors without naming them is done without error.

A disconnection in the anterior third of the corpus callosum, where fiber systems pass between left and right motor areas, results in failure of only the left hand to obey spoken commands, the right one performing normally (left-sided apraxia); the patient may still be able to imitate the examiner's movements with the left hand.

Of intrahemispheric disconnections, the following are the most important. They are mentioned here only briefly and are considered in detail in the following chapter.

1. *Conduction* (also called "central") *aphasia.* The patient has fluent, but paraphasic, speech and writing, impaired repetition, and relatively intact comprehension of spoken and written language. Wernicke's area in the temporal lobe is separated from Broca's area by a lesion in the arcuate fasciculus.

2. *Sympathetic apraxia in Broca's aphasia.* By destroying the origin of the fibers that connect the left and right motor association cortices, a lesion in the subcortical white matter underlying Broca's area and contiguous cortex causes an apraxia of command movements of the left hand. This condition may also result from a lesion in the anterior corpus callosum.

3. *Pure word deafness.* Although the patient is able to hear and to identify nonverbal sounds, there is loss of ability to comprehend spoken language. The patient's speech remains normal. This defect has been attributed to a subcortical lesion of the left temporal lobe, spanning Wernicke's area, interrupting also those fibers that cross from one Wernicke's area to another in the corpus callosum, and preventing them from activating the right auditory region. Bilateral temporal lesions have the same effect.

OTHER BEHAVIORAL DISORDERS ASSOCIATED WITH CEREBRAL DISEASE

When one attempts to categorize all the patients with relatively acute or subacute disorders of mentation and behavior discussed above, a considerable number still remain that are difficult to classify. They present as an almost infinite variety of syndromes in which the following abnormalities of function may occur: reduced or increased levels of speech, thought, and action; disorientation as to time and place; idleness and lack of interest; loss of sense of humor, or inappropriate jocularity; resistiveness and negativism; lack of observance of social custom, use of abusive and vulgar language; inexplicable euphoria and lack of proper concern; complaint of excess sensitivity to sounds; distortions of smell and taste; inability to find the names of objects, to follow a conversation, to think coherently; sexual indiscretion, lack of modesty, and other signs of disinhibition; and disturbances of sleep. Obviously not all these many symptoms have the same basic significance, and the majority possess only relative localizing value. They may be associated with definite hemiparesis, hemihypesthesia, aphasia, or homonymous hemianopia; but even without these lateralizing signs they point to the existence of cerebral disease.

Syndromes comprising these elements may be observed in subacute inclusion body encephalitis, Behçet's meningoencephalitis, adult toxoplasmosis, infectious mononucleosis, acute or subacute demyelinative diseases (acute or subacute recurrent multiple sclerosis), granulomatous and other forms of angiitis, gliomatosis cerebri, carcinomatous meningitis, endothelial angiomatosis, multiple tumor metastases, acute and subacute bacterial endocarditis, widespread atheromatous or myxomatous embolization, Whipple's disease, and thrombopenia with small vessel thrombosis. A fuller account of some of these cerebral symptoms will be found in the chapters dealing with these diseases.

REFERENCES

ANDREW J, NATHAN PW: Lesions of the anterior frontal lobes and disturbances of micturition and defecation. *Brain* 87:233, 1964.

BAY E: Disturbances of visual perception and their examination. *Brain* 76:515, 1953.

BENTON AL: The fiction of Gerstmann's syndrome. *J Neurol Neurosurg Psychiatry* 24:176, 1961.

BRAIN R: Visual disorientation with special reference to lesions of the right hemisphere. *Brain* 64:244, 1941.

BRICKNER RM: *The Intellectual Functions of the Frontal Lobes*. New York, Macmillan, 1936.

BUTTERS N, BRODY BA: The role of the left parietal lobe in the mediation of intra- and cross-modal associations. *Cortex* 4:328, 1968.

CARMON A: Sequenced motor performance in patients with unilateral cerebral lesions. *Neuropsychologia* 9:445, 1971.

————, BENTON AL: Tactile perception of direction and number in patients with unilateral cerebral disease. *Neurology* 19:525, 1969.

CHAPMAN LF, WOLFF HF: The cerebral hemispheres and the highest integrative functions of man. *Arch Neurol* 1:357, 1959.

CORKIN S, MILNER B, RASMUSSEN T: Effects of different cortical excisions on sensory thresholds in man. *Trans Am Neurol Assoc* 89:112, 1964.

CRITCHLEY M: *The Parietal Lobes*. London, Arnold, 1953.

DAMASIO AR, BENTON AL: Impairment of hand movements under visual guidance. *Neurology* 29:170, 1979.

DÉJERINE J, MOUZON J: Un nouveau type de syndrome sensitif corticale observé dans un cas de monoplégie corticale dissociée. *Rev Neurol* 28:1265, 1914-1915.

DENNY-BROWN D: The frontal lobes and their functions, in Feiling A (ed): *Modern Trends in Neurology*. New York, Hoeber-Harper, 1951, p 13.

————, BANKER B: Amorphosynthesis from left parietal lesion. *Arch Neurol Psychiatry* 71:302, 1954.

————, MEYER JS, HORENSTEIN S: Significance of perceptual rivalry resulting from parietal lesions. *Brain* 75:433, 1952.

GASSEL MM: Occipital lobe syndromes (excluding hemianopia), in Vinken PJ, Bruyn GW (eds): *Handbook of Clinical Neurology*, vol 2. New York, American Elsevier, 1969, chap 19, pp 640-679.

GASTAUT H, MORIN G, LEFEVRE N: Étude de comportement des épileptiques psychomoteurs dans l'intervalle de leurs crises. *Ann Med Psychol* 1:1, 1955.

GESCHWIND N: The clinical syndromes of cortical disconnections, in Williams D (ed): *Modern Trends in Neurology*, vol 5. London, Butterworth, 1970, p 29.

————, LEVITSKY W: Human brain: Left-right asymmetries in temporal speech region. *Science,* 161:186, 1968.

GOLDSTEIN K: The significance of the frontal lobes for mental performance. *J Neurol Psychopathol* 17:27, 1936.

HALSTEAD WC: *The Brain and Intelligence*. Chicago, University of Chicago Press, 1947.

HARLOW JM: Quoted in Denny-Brown D: The frontal lobes and their functions, in Feiling A (ed): *Modern Trends in Neurology*. New York, Hoeber, 1951, p 65.

HEAD H, HOLMES G: Sensory disturbances from cerebral lesions. *Brain* 34:102, 1911.

HEBB DO, PENFIELD W: Human behavior after extensive bilateral removal of the frontal lobes. *Arch Neurol Psychiatry* 44:421, 1940.

HÉCAEN H: Clinical symptomatology in right and left hemispheric lesions, in Mountcastle VB (ed): *Interhemispheric Relations and Cerebral Dominance*. Baltimore, Johns Hopkins, 1962.

HENSCHEN SE: Clinical and anatomical contributions on brain pathology (abstracts and comments by Walter F. Schaller); Fifth part: Aphasia, amusia, akalkulia. *Arch Neurol Psychiatry* 13:226, 1925.

HOFF H, PÖTZL O: Zur diagnostischen Bedeutung der Polyopie bei Tumoren des Occipitalhirnes. *Z Gesamte Neurol Psychiatr* 152:433, 1935.

HUBEL DH, WIESEL TN: Receptive fields, binocular interaction and functional architecture in the cat's visual cortex. *J Physiol* 160:106, 1962.

JACOBSEN CF: Functions of frontal association in primates. *Arch Neurol Psychiatry* 33:558, 1935.

JOYNT RJ, GOLDSTEIN MN: Minor cerebral hemisphere, in Friedlander WJ (ed): *Advances in Neurology*, vol 7. New York, Raven, 1975, p 147.

KINSBOURNE M, WARRINGTON EK: A disorder of simultaneous form perception. *Brain* 85:461, 1962.

KLÜVER H, BUCY PC: An analysis of certain effects of bilateral temporal lobectomy in the rhesus monkey with special reference to psychic blindness. *J Psychol* 5:33, 1938.

LEVINE DN, CALVANIO R: A study of the visual defect in verbal alexia-simultanagnosia. *Brain* 101:65, 1978.

LURIA AR: *Higher Cerebral Function in Man*. New York, Basic Books, 1966.

————: Frontal lobe syndromes, in Vinken PJ, Bruyn GW (eds): *Handbook of Clinical Neurology*, vol 2. Amsterdam, North-Holland, 1969, chap 22, p 725.

————: *The Working Brain*. London, Allen Lane, 1973.

MEADOWS JC: The anatomical basis of prosopagnosia. *J Neurol Neurosurg Psychiatry* 37:489, 1974.

MILNER B: Interhemispheric differences in the localization of psychological processes in man. *Br Med Bull* 27:272, 1971.

NIELSEN JM: *Agnosia, Apraxia, Aphasia: Their Value in Cerebral Localization*, 2d ed, New York, Hoeber, 1946.

OBRADOR S: Temporal lobotomy. *J Neuropathol Exp Neurol* 6:185, 1947.

PENFIELD W, RASMUSSEN P: *The Cerebral Cortex of Man*. New York, Macmillan, 1950.

————, ROBERTS L: *Speech and Brain Mechanisms*. Princeton, Princeton University Press, 1956.

POLYAK SL: *The Vertebrate Visual System*, Chicago, University of Chicago Press, 1957.

REITAN RW: Psychological deficits resulting from cerebral deficits in man, in Warren JM, Akert K (eds): *The Frontal Granular Cortex and Behavior.* New York, McGraw-Hill, 1964, chap 14.

RYLANDER G: Personality changes after operations on the frontal lobes. *Acta Psychiatr Scand Suppl* 20: 1939.

SEGARRA JM, QUADFASEL FA: Destroyed temporal lobe tips; preserved ability to sing. *Proc VII Internat Cong Neurol* 2:377, 1961.

SEMMES J, WEINSTEIN S, GHENT L, TEUBER HL: *Somatosensory Changes After Penetrating Brain Wounds in Man.* Cambridge, Harvard University Press, 1960.

SHANKWEILER DP: Performance of brain-damaged patients on two tests of sound localization. *J Comp Physiol Psychol* 54:375, 1961.

SPERRY RW, GAZZANIGA MS, BOGEN JE: The neocortical commissures; syndrome of hemisphere disconnection, in Vinken PJ, Bruyn GW (eds): *Handbook of Clinical Neurology,* vol 4. Amsterdam, North-Holland, 1969, chap 14, pp 273-290.

VAN BUREN JM: Trans-synaptic retrograde degeneration in the visual system of primates. *J Neurol Neurosurg Psychiatry* 26:402, 1963.

WALSH FB, HOYT WF: The visual sensory system: Anatomy, physiology and topographic diagnosis, in Vinken PJ, Bruyn GW (eds): *Handbook of Clinical Neurology,* vol 2. Amsterdam, North-Holland, 1969, chap 18, pp 506-639.

WALSH KW: *Neuropsychology. A Clinical Approach.* Edinburgh, Churchill-Livingstone, 1978.

WOLPERT I: Die Simultanagnosie-Störung der Gesamtauffassung. *Z Gesamte Neurol Psychiatr* 93:397, 1924.

CHAPTER 22
AFFECTIONS OF SPEECH AND LANGUAGE

Speech and language functions are of fundamental human significance, both in social intercourse and in private intellectual life. When these functions are disturbed as a consequence of brain disease, the resultant physiologic loss exceeds all others in gravity—even blindness, deafness, and paralysis.

The neurologist must be concerned with all derangements of speech and language, including those of reading and writing, because they are the source of great disability and are almost invariably manifestations of disease of the brain. In a broader context, however, language is the means whereby patients communicate their complaints and their feelings to the physician and at the same time the medium for that interpersonal transaction between physician and patient that we call psychotherapy. Therefore any disease process that interferes with speech or the understanding of spoken words touches the very core of the physician-patient relationship. Finally, the clinical study of language disorders serves to illuminate the abstruse relation between psychological functions and the anatomy and physiology of the brain. Language mechanisms fall somewhere between the well-localized sensorimotor functions and the more complex mental functions such as imagination and thinking, which cannot be localized.

GENERAL CONSIDERATIONS

It has been remarked that, as human beings, our commanding position in the animal world rests on the possession of two faculties: (1) the ability to develop and employ verbal symbols as a background for our own ideation and as a means of transmitting thoughts, by spoken and written word, to others of our kind; and (2) the remarkable facility in the use of our hands. One curious and provocative fact is that the evolution of both language and manual dexterity occurs in relation to neurophysiologic pathways in one (the dominant) cerebral hemisphere. This is a departure from most other localized neurophysiologic activities, which are organized according to a contralateral or bilateral and symmetrical plan. The dominance of one hemisphere, usually the left, emerges with speech and the preference for the right hand, especially for writing; and a lack of development or loss of cerebral dominance as a result of disease entails a disturbance of both these traits.

There is abundant evidence that higher animals are able to communicate with one another by vocalization and gestures. However, the content of their communication is their feeling tone of the moment. This emotional language, as it is called, was studied by Charles Darwin, who noted that it undergoes increasing differentiation in the animal kingdom. Only in the chimpanzee are the first semblances of propositional speech recognizable.

Similar instinctive patterns of emotional expression are observed in human beings. In fact they are the earliest forms of speech to appear (in infancy) and may have been the first to develop in primitive human beings. Moreover, the language we use to express joy, anger, and fear is retained even after destruction of all the language areas in the dominant cerebral hemisphere. The neural arrangements which subserve emotional expression are bilateral and symmetrical and do not depend on the cerebrum. The experiments of Cannon and Bard have amply demonstrated that emotional expression is possible in animals after removal of both cerebral hemispheres, provided the diencephalon and particularly the hypothalamic part of it remain intact. In the human infant, emotional expression is well developed at a time when much of the cerebrum is still immature.

Propositional or symbolic speech differs from

emotional speech in several ways. Instead of communicating feeling it is the means of transferring ideas from one person to another, and it requires in its development the substitution of a series of sounds or marks for objects, persons, and concepts. As was stated, this type of speech is not found in animals or in the human infant. It is not instinctive but learned and is therefore subject to all the modifying influences of social environment and culture. However, the learning process becomes possible only after the nervous system has reached a certain degree of development. Facility in symbolic language, which is acquired over a period of 15 to 20 years, depends then on both the maturation of the nervous system and education.

Although speech and language are closely interwoven functions, they are not strictly synonymous. A derangement of language function always is a reflection of an abnormality of the brain and, more specifically, of the dominant cerebral hemisphere. A disorder of speech may have a similar origin, but not necessarily; it may be due to abnormalities in different parts of the brain, or to extracerebral mechanisms. Whereas language function involves the comprehension and transmission of ideas and feelings by the use of conventionalized signs, marks, sounds, and gestures and the sequential ordering of them according to accepted rules of grammar, speech refers more to the articulatory and mechanical aspects of verbal expression.

The profound importance of language in contemporary society may be overlooked unless one reflects on the proportion of our time devoted to purely verbal pursuits. *External speech,* or *exophasy,* by which is meant the expression of thought by spoken or written words and the comprehension of the spoken or written words of others, is an almost continuous activity when human beings are gathered together; and *inner speech,* or *endophasy,* i.e., the silent processes of thought and the formulation in our minds of unuttered words on which thought depends, is "the coin of mental commerce." The latter is almost incessant during our preoccupations, since we think always with words, and we may, in doing so, subconsciously mutter.

ANATOMY OF THE LANGUAGE FUNCTIONS

The conventional teaching is that there are three main language areas, situated, in most persons, in the left cerebral hemisphere (Fig. 22-1). Two are receptive and one is executive. The two receptive areas are closely related and embrace what may be referred to as the central language zone. One, subserving the perception of spoken language, occupies a crescentic zone in the posterior one-third of the first temporal convolution (areas 41 and 42, or Wernicke's area), just lateral to the primary auditory receptive area in Heschl's gyri; the other, subserving the perception of written language, occupies the angular convolution (area 39) in the inferior parietal lobule, anterior to the visual receptive areas. The supramarginal gyrus, which lies between these auditory and visual language "centers," and the inferior temporal region (area 37), just anterior to the visual association cortex, are probably part of this central language zone as well. Here are centered cross-modal visual and auditory functions. The area situated at the posterior end of the third (inferior) frontal convolution is referred to as Broca's area or Brodmann's area 44 and is concerned with motor aspects of speech.

These sensory and motor areas are connected by a large bundle of nerve fibers, the arcuate fasciculus, which passes through the isthmus of the temporal lobe and around the sylvian fissure; other connections may traverse the external capsule of the lenticular nucleus (subcortical white matter of the insula). There are many corticocortical connections as well. From Broca's area there are fiber connections with the lower rolandic cortex, which in turn innervates the speech apparatus. These language areas are also connected with the thalamus and to corresponding areas in the minor cerebral hemisphere through the corpus callosum and anterior commissure (Figs. 21-9 and 21-10).

Figure 22-1

Diagram of the brain showing the classical language areas, numbered according to the scheme of Brodmann. The elaboration of speech and language probably depends on a much larger area of cerebrum, indicated roughly by the entire shaded zone (see text).

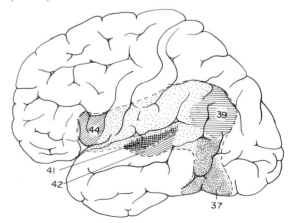

There has been much difference of opinion concerning these cortical areas, and objection has been made to calling them centers, for they do not represent histologically circumscribed structures of constant function. Actually there is relatively little information concerning their anatomy and physiology. A competent neuroanatomist could not distinguish these cortical language areas microscopically from the cerebral cortex that surrounds them. Electrical stimulation of the parts of the cortex concerned with language while the patient is alert and talking (during craniotomy under local anesthesia)—except for a simple vocalization, usually a single-vowel monotone—causes only an arrest of speech. Knowledge of the location of language functions has come almost exclusively from the postmortem study of humans with focal brain diseases. From the available information it seems almost certain that the whole language mechanism is not divisible into discrete parts, each specifiable language function depending on a certain fixed group of neurons. Instead, language must be regarded as an integrated sensorimotor process, roughly localized in the opercular, or perisylvian, region of the left cerebral hemisphere; the more complex elaborations of speech and language depend on other parts of the cerebrum as well. Undeniably there is, within the language area, a kind of localization, as discussed below, but there is also a presently undifferentiable *mass effect,* viz., a degree of deficit that is influenced by the size of the lesion.

Carl Wernicke, of Breslau, more than any other person, must be credited with the anatomic-psychological scheme upon which contemporary ideas of aphasia rest. Earlier, Paul Broca, of Paris, had made the fundamental observations that a lesion of the insula and the overlying operculum deprived a person of speech, and that such lesions were always in the left hemisphere. Wernicke's thesis was that only the most elementary visual, olfactory, tactile, and auditory perceptions can be assigned to defined areas of cortex; the higher mental functions depend on the association of different regions, achieved by fiber tracts which connect these regions. He pointed out that there were two major anatomic loci for language: (1) an anterior locus, in the posterior part of the inferior frontal lobe (Broca's area), which functioned as the center for the "memory images" of speech movements, and (2) the insular region, or adjoining parts of the perisylvian cortex, which was the center for the images of sounds (Meynert had already shown that aphasia could occur with lesions in the temporal lobe, Broca's area being intact). Wernicke believed that the fibers between these regions ran in the insula and mediated the psychic reflex arc between the heard and spoken word. Later, Wernicke came to accept von Monakow's view

that the connecting fibers ran around the posterior end of the sylvian fissure, in the arcuate fasciculus.

Wernicke gave a comprehensive description of the receptive aphasia that now bears his name. The four main features, he pointed out, were a disturbance of comprehension of spoken language, agraphia, alexia, and fluent paraphasic speech. In Broca's aphasia, by contrast, comprehension was intact, but the patient was mute or employed only a few simple words. Wernicke theorized that lesions which interrupted the fibers connecting the two cortical speech areas would give rise to a disturbance in which the patient's comprehension would be undisturbed, but the intact sound images would be unable to exert an influence on the choice of words. Wernicke proposed that this variety of aphasia be called *Leitungsaphasie,* or conduction aphasia; later it was given the name "central aphasia" by Kurt Goldstein.

This anatomic scheme was the basis of **Wernicke's** classification of aphasia, and although it was much criticized by Pierre Marie, Henry Head, von Monakow, Arnold Pick, and Goldstein, the anatomic plans which they offered differed little from that of Wernicke. Careful case analysis since the time of Broca and Wernicke has repeatedly documented an association between the receptive type of aphasia (Wernicke's aphasia) and lesions in the posterior perisylvian region and between a predominantly motor aphasia (Broca's aphasia) and lesions in the posterior part of the inferior frontal convolution and the adjacent motor, insular, and opercular regions of the cortex. The concept of a conduction aphasia, based upon an interruption of pathways between Wernicke's and Broca's zones, has been the most difficult to accept, because it presupposes a neat separation of sensory and motor functions, which is not in line with contemporary views of sensorimotor physiology of the rest of the body. Nevertheless, there are in the medical literature excellent descriptions that conform to Wernicke's model of conduction aphasia; the lesion in these cases most often lies in the parietal operculum, involving the white matter deep to the supramarginal gyrus, where it presumably interrupts the arcuate fasciculus.

Thus it appears that human language function depends upon the integrity of an anatomic region situated between the primary input zones of the temporal and occipital lobes and their association areas in the parietal and temporal lobes, and the output zones in the inferior frontal lobe of the dominant hemisphere. This places the language area in close connection with the cortical sensory association and cross-modal elaboration areas of the superior temporal and inferior parietal lobes, with the corresponding parts of the opposite cerebral hemisphere through the corpus callosum, and with the medial parts of the temporal lobes and diencephalon (learning-memory mechanism). The acquisition of language appears to involve, in part, the establishment of specific, item-by-item, cross-modal, verbally mediated associations. But how these regions of the brain are organized, how they can be activated (controlled) by a variety of visual and auditory stimuli, resulting in the complex behavior of which we make casual daily use in interpersonal communication, remain to a large extent unknown.

Although localization of the lesion that produces aphasia is in most instances roughly predictable from the clinical deficit, there are wide variations in the degree of deficit that follows focal brain disease. Inconsistency of anatomic findings in certain types of aphasia has been explained in several ways. The most popular explanation has been that the net effect of any lesion depends not only on the locus and extent of the lesion but also on the degree of cerebral dominance, i.e., on the degree to which the minor hemisphere assumes language function after damage to the major one. If cerebral dominance is poorly established, a left-sided lesion has less effect on language function than if dominance is strong. Unfortunately, handedness and cerebral dominance are not recorded in many of the 1500 cases collected by Henschen from the world's medical literature. Another factor which imparts an element of unpredictability to the anatomy of language is the poorly understood concept that individuals differ in the way they acquire language as children. This is believed to play a role in making available alternative means for accomplishing language tasks when the method initially learned has been impaired through brain disease. The extent to which improvement of aphasia represents "recovery" of function or generation of new response methods has not been settled to the present day.

CEREBRAL DOMINANCE AND ITS RELATION TO SPEECH AND HANDEDNESS

The functional supremacy of one cerebral hemisphere is crucial to language function. There are three ways of determining that the left side of the brain is dominant: (1) the loss of speech when disease occurs in certain parts of the left hemisphere and its preservation with lesions involving corresponding parts of the right hemi-

sphere; (2) the greater facility in the use of the right hand, foot, and eye; and (3) the arrest of speech immediately after the injection of amobarbital or some other drug in the left internal carotid artery. Only (2) and (3) are of use in deciding the cerebral dominance of a living, healthy person. Unfortunately the injection of amobarbital (Wada test) does not reproduce the syndrome of major hemisphere inactivation; there is only mutism and contraversive turning of the head and eyes, followed by a groping for names. The entire abnormality lasts for about 30 s. Presumably this test gives information about the localization of language-output areas rather than of sensory ones.

Approximately 90 to 95 percent of the general population is right-handed; the remainder prefers the left hand. A person who is said to be right-handed chooses the right hand for intricate, complex acts and is more skillful with it. The preference is more complete in some persons than in others. Most individuals are neither completely right-handed nor completely left-handed but favor one hand for more complicated tasks.

The reason for hand preference is still controversial. There is strong evidence of a hereditary factor, but the mode of inheritance is uncertain. Learning is also a factor; many children are shifted at an early age from left to right (shifted sinistrals), because it is a handicap to be left-handed in a right-handed world. Many right-handed persons sight with the right eye, and it has been said that eye preference determines hand preference. Even if true, this still does not account for eye dominance. It is noteworthy that handedness develops simultaneously with language, and the most that can be said at present is that localization of language and preference for one eye, one hand, and one foot are all manifestations of some fundamental, inherited tendency not yet defined. Anatomic differences between the dominant and the nondominant cerebral hemispheres cannot be demonstrated, with one exception—the planum temporale, the region on the superior surface of the temporal lobe between Heschl's gyri and Wernicke's language zone, is slightly larger in the left than in the right hemisphere, in a ratio of about 6:1.

Left-handedness may result from disease of the left cerebral hemisphere in early life, and this probably accounts for its higher incidence among the feeble-minded and brain-injured. Presumably the neural mechanisms for language then become centered in the right cerebral hemisphere. Handedness and cerebral dominance may fail to develop in some individuals, and this is particularly true in certain families. Developmental defects in speech and reading, stuttering, mirror writing, and general clumsiness are much more frequent in these individuals.

Differences in degree of cerebral dominance unquestionably account for some of the inconsistency in the cerebral localization of language in different persons. In studies of groups of left-handed individuals with aphasia it has been noted that approximately 75 percent of them have had lesions in the left cerebral hemisphere. Further, in the rare cases of aphasia due to right cerebral lesions, the patient is nearly always left-handed, and the speech disorder tends to be less severe and enduring. Rarer still, but well documented, is the occurrence of aphasia in a right-handed individual as a result of a lesion confined to the right cerebral hemisphere.

The language capacities of the minor hemisphere are not fully documented by careful anatomic studies. As mentioned above, there is always some uncertainty whether any residual function after lesions of the major hemisphere can be traced to recovery of parts of its language zones or to activity of the minor hemisphere. The observations of Levine and Mohr suggest that the nondominant hemisphere has only a limited capacity to produce oral speech after extensive damage of the dominant hemisphere; stated in another way, the extent of recovery from motor speech disorders depends mainly upon the degree of preservation of the frontoparietal opercular areas of the dominant hemisphere. The observation by Kinsbourne of the effect of intraarterial amytal in the right hemisphere of patients aphasic from left-sided lesions shows the contribution of the right hemisphere to residual language functions.

SPEECH AND LANGUAGE DISORDERS DUE TO DISEASE

These may be divided into four categories:

1. Disturbances of speech and language that occur with diseases affecting the higher nervous integrations, i.e., with diseases causing delirium and dementia. Speech is seldom lost in these conditions but is deranged as part of a general impairment of perceptual and intellectual functions. In Alzheimer's disease, a gradual impairment of all elements of language constitutes an important part of the clinical picture (Chap. 20). *Echolalia* and *palilalia* are special abnormalities observed in states of profound dementia with bilateral cerebral lesions. In echolalia the patient repeats, parrot-like, words and phrases that he or she hears. In palilalia, the patient repeats the last word or two of a statement with decreasing volume and increasing rapidity, finally making only silent articulatory movements of the lips (*aphonic palilalia*).

2. A cerebral disturbance in which there is a loss more or less exclusively of the production or of compre-

hension of spoken or written language, or both. This condition is called *aphasia* or *dysphasia*.

3. A defect in articulation, with intact mental functions and normal comprehension and memory of words. This is a pure motor disorder of the muscles of articulation and may be due to flaccid or spastic paralysis, rigidity, repetitive spasms (stuttering), or ataxia. The terms *dysarthria* and *anarthria* have been applied to some of these conditions.

4. Loss of voice due to a disease of the larynx or its innervation—*aphonia* or *dysphonia*. Articulation and inner language are unaffected.

CLINICAL VARIETIES OF APHASIA

Systematic examination will usually enable one to decide whether a patient has a *motor*, or *Broca's*, *aphasia*, sometimes called expressive or executive aphasia; a *receptive*, or *Wernicke's*, *aphasia*, with impairment in all language-dependent behavior; a *total*, or *global*, *aphasia*, with loss of all or nearly all speech and language functions; or one of the *dissociative speech syndromes*, such as conduction aphasia, word deafness (auditory verbal agnosia), word blindness (visual verbal agnosia or alexia), anomic (nominal or amnestic) aphasia, and several types of mutism. Impaired ability to communicate by writing (agraphia) is found to some degree in practically all types of aphasia; rarely does it exist alone.

MOTOR, OR BROCA'S, APHASIA

Although the precise nature of Broca's aphasia remains somewhat in doubt, we have chosen to apply the term, as have others, to a primary deficit in language output or speech production. In our experience there is a wide range of variation in the motor deficit from the mildest cortical type of dysarthria, with intact inner language and ability to write, to a complete loss of all means of communication through lingual, phonetic, and manual action. Since the muscles that can no longer be used in speech still function in other learned acts, i.e., they are not paralyzed, the term *apraxia* seems applicable to certain elements of the deficit.

In the most advanced form of the syndrome patients will have lost all power of speaking aloud. No longer can a word be uttered in conversation, in reading aloud, or in trying to repeat words that are heard. Occasionally, the words *yes* or *no* or expletives can be uttered, usually in the correct context. One might suspect that the lingual and phonatory apparatus are paralyzed, until patients are observed to have no difficulty chewing, swallowing, clearing the throat, and even vocalizing without words. Often the lower part of the face and arm are weak on the opposite (right) side, and occasionally the leg as well. The tongue may deviate away from the lesion, i.e., to the right, and be slow and awkward in rapid movements. For a time, despite the relative preservation of auditory comprehension and ability to read, commands to purse or lick the lips, to blow, smack, and make other purposeful movements are poorly executed, which means that the apraxia has extended to certain other learned oropharyngeal acts. In these circumstances, imitation of the examiner's actions is better performed than execution of acts on command. Self-initiated actions, by contrast, may be normal. Patients may repeat a few stereotyped utterances over and over again, as if compelled to do so, a disorder referred to as *monophasia* (Critchley), *recurring utterance* (Hughlings Jackson), or *verbal stereotypy* or *automatism*. If speech is possible at all, certain habitual expressions, such as "Hi," "Fine, thank you," or "Good morning," seem to be the easiest, and the words of well-known songs may be sung. When angered or excited, patients may explode with an expletive, thus emphasizing that they are *speechless,* but not *wordless.* Patients recognize their ineptitudes and mistakes. Repeated failures in speech may cause exasperation or despair.

In the milder form of Broca's aphasia and in the recovery phase of the severe form, patients are able to speak aloud to some degree. Words are uttered slowly and laboriously. Enunciation (articulation) and the melody of language (prosody) are disordered. This dysfluency takes the form of improper accent or stress on certain syllables and incorrect intonation and phrasing of words in a series and pacing of word utterances. Speech is sparse (10 to 15 words per minute compared to the normal 100 to 115 words per minute) and consists mainly of nouns, transitive verbs, or important adjective modifiers; many of the small words (articles, prepositions, conjunctions) are omitted, giving the speech an agrammatical and telegraphic character. The substantive content allows the patient to communicate ideas to some extent, despite the gross expressive difficulties.

Most patients with Broca's aphasia have a correspondingly severe impairment in writing. Should the right hand be paralyzed, the patient cannot print with the left one, and if the right hand is spared, the patient fails as miserably in writing requests or replies to questions as in speaking them. Writing to dictation is impossible, though letters and words can still be copied.

The comprehension of spoken and written language, though normal under many conditions of testing, is usually defective in Broca's aphasia and will break down under stringent testing, especially when novel or complicated material is introduced. This is the most variable and controversial aspect of Broca's aphasia. In some patients who suffer a loss of motor speech and agraphia as a result of cerebral infarction, the understanding of spoken and written language may be virtually normal. Mohr has shown that in such patients the mutism is replaced by a rapidly improving dyspraxic and effortful articulation, usually leading to complete recovery; the lesion in these cases is restricted to a zone in and immediately around the posterior part of the inferior frontal convolution (Broca's area). Mohr has stressed the distinctions between this relatively mild and restricted form of motor speech disorder and the more complex syndrome that is traditionally referred to as Broca's aphasia. The latter is characterized by more difficulty in understanding spoken and written language and by protracted mutism; verbal stereotypes, agrammatism and dysprosody are prominent during the recovery phase. Pathologically, there is in the latter condition a lesion that involves the operculum, insula, and adjacent cerebrum. In other words, the lesion in typical Broca's aphasia extends far beyond Broca's area.

It is noteworthy that in one of Broca's original patients, in whom speech had been limited to a few verbal stereotypes for 10 years before death, inspection of the surface of the brain (the brain was never cut) disclosed an extensive lesion, encompassing the left insula, the frontal, central, and parietal operculum, and even part of the inferior parietal lobe, posterior to the sylvian fissure. Curiously, Broca attributed the aphasic disorder in his patient to the lesion of the frontal operculum alone and deliberately ignored the rest of the lesion which he considered to be a later spreading effect of the stroke. Perhaps Broca was influenced by the prevailing opinion of that time (1861), that articulation was a function of the inferior frontal lobes. The fact that Broca's name later became attached to a discrete part of the inferior frontal cortex (Brodmann's area 44) helped to entrench the idea that Broca's aphasia could be equated with a lesion in Broca's area. However, as pointed out above, a lesion confined to Broca's area gives rise to a relatively modest and transient motor speech disorder (Mohr et al.) or to no disorder of speech at all (Goldstein).

Motor speech disorders, both Broca's aphasia and

the more restricted and transient types, are most often due to a vascular lesion. An embolus in the upper main (rolandic) division of the middle cerebral artery is probably the most frequent type of vascular lesion and results in the most abrupt onset and sometimes the most rapid regression (occurring in hours or days), depending on whether the ischemic paralysis proceeds to tissue necrosis. Even with the latter, however, transient ischemia around the zone of infarction causes a more extensive syndrome than that of the infarct alone. In other words, the physiologic impairment of function exceeds the pathologic. Because of the distribution of this artery, there are frequently an associated *right*-sided faciobrachial paresis and a *left*-sided brachial apraxia (due probably to interruption of the corpus callosal fibers that connect left and right motor cortices). Atherosclerotic thrombosis, tumor, subcortical hypertensive hemorrhage, traumatic hemorrhage, etc., should they involve the appropriate parts of the motor cortex, may also declare themselves as Broca's aphasia.

A closely related syndrome, *pure word mutism*, also causes the patient to be wordless but leaves inner speech intact and writing undisturbed. Anatomically, this is believed to be in the nature of a dissociation of the motor cortex for speech from lower centers and will be described with the dissociative speech syndromes further on in this chapter.

WERNICKE'S APHASIA

This syndrome comprises two main elements: (1) an impairment in the comprehension of word elements (discriminative or phonemic hearing), which reflects involvement of auditory association areas or their separation from the angular gyrus and the primary auditory cortex of Heschl's transverse gyri; and (2) a general impairment of language-dependent behavior, which reveals the major role the auditory region plays in the regulation of language. The defect in auditory language functions is manifested further by a varying inability to repeat spoken words.

The patient talks volubly, gestures freely, and appears strangely unaware of the deficit. Speech is produced without effort; the phrases and sentences appear to be of normal length and are properly intonated and articulated. Despite the fluency and normal prosody, the patient's speech is remarkably devoid of meaning. In contrast to Broca's aphasia, the patient with Wernicke's aphasia produces words that are nonsubstantive. Also, the words themselves are often malformed or inappropriate, a disorder referred to as *paraphasia*. A phoneme (the minimum unit of sound that permits the differentiation of the meaning of a word) or a syllable may be

substituted within a word (e.g., "The grass is greel"); this is called *literal paraphasia*. The substitution of one word for another ("The grass is blue") is called *verbal paraphasia* or *semantic substitution*. Neologisms, i.e., phonemes, syllables, or words that are not part of the language, may also appear ("The grass is grumps"). Fluent paraphasic speech may be entirely incomprehensible (*gibberish* or *jargon aphasia*). Fluency is not an invariable feature of Wernicke's aphasia. Speech may be hesitant, in which case it tends to occur in that part of a phrase which contains the central communicative (predicative) item, such as a key noun, verb, or descriptive phrase. The patient with such a disorder conveys the impression of constantly searching for the correct word and of having difficulty in finding it.

Although the motor apparatus required for the activation and expression of language behavior may be quite intact, patients with Wernicke's aphasia are unable to function as social organisms because they are deprived of all means of communication. They cannot understand what is said to them; a few simple commands may still be executed, but there is failure to carry out complex ones. They cannot read aloud or silently with comprehension, tell others what they want or think, or write to them. When trying to designate an object that they see or feel, they cannot find the name, even though they may be able to repeat it from dictation; nor can they write from dictation the very words that they can copy from sight or touch. The copying performance is notably slow and laborious and conforms to the contours of the model, including the examiner's handwriting style. These patients cannot match words that they hear with those that they see. All these defects, of course, may be present in varying degrees of severity. In general, the defects in reading, writing, naming, and repetition parallel in severity the defect in comprehension.

Wernicke's aphasia that is due to stroke usually improves in time, sometimes to the point where the deficits can be detected only by asking the patient to repeat unfamiliar words from dictation, to name unusual objects or parts of objects, to spell difficult words, or to write complex self-generated sentences. A more favorable prognosis attends those forms of Wernicke's aphasia in which some of the elements, e.g., visual comprehension, are only slightly impaired.

As a rule, the lesion lies in the posterior perisylvian region (comprising posterosuperior temporal, opercular supramarginal and posterior insular gyri) and usually it is due to embolic (less often thrombotic) occlusion of the lower division of the left middle cerebral artery. A "slit hemorrhage" in the subcortex of the temporoparietal region or involvement of this area by tumor, abscess, or extension of a small putaminal or thalamic hemorrhage may have similar effects.

The posterior perisylvian region appears to encompass a variety of language functions, since seemingly minor changes in size and locale of the lesion are associated with important variations in the elements of Wernicke's aphasia or lead to *conduction aphasia* or to *pure word deafness* (see below). The interesting theoretical problem is whether all the deficits observed are indicative of a unitary language function that resides in the posterior perisylvian region or, instead, of a series of separate sensorimotor activities whose anatomic pathways happen to be crowded together in a small region of the brain. In view of the multiple ways in which language deteriorates in disease, the latter hypothesis seems more likely.

TOTAL, OR GLOBAL, APHASIA

This syndrome is due to a lesion that destroys a large part of the language area of the major cerebral hemisphere; usually it is due to occlusion of the left internal carotid or middle cerebral artery, but it may be caused by hemorrhage, tumor, or other lesions, and it may occur as a postictal effect. The middle cerebral artery nourishes all of the language area, and nearly all the aphasic disorders due to vascular occlusion are caused by involvement of this artery or its branches.

All aspects of speech and language are affected in global aphasia, as the term implies. At the most, the patients can say only a few words, usually some cliché or habitual phrase. They may understand a few words and phrases of the speech of others, but they characteristically fail to carry out a series of simple commands or to name objects because of verbal and motor perseveration (the obligate repetitive evocation of a word or motor act just after it has been employed in another context). They cannot read or write or repeat what is said to them. Related signs include right hemiplegia, hemianesthesia, and homonymous hemianopia. The state of consciousness may vary from full alertness to semicoma; in the latter condition the lack of verbal response is obviously difficult to interpret, for the diagnosis of aphasia presupposes a relatively alert state of mind and integrity of other cerebral functions. The patient may participate in common gestures of greeting, show modesty and avoid-

ance reactions, and engage in self-help activities. With the passage of time some degree of understanding of speech may return, and what then emerges is the clinical picture of Broca's aphasia. Rapid improvement frequently occurs when the main cause is cerebral edema, postconvulsive paralysis, or transient metabolic derangements such as hypoglycemia, hyponatremia, etc., which worsen old lesions that had involved language areas. Although speech loss from a disintegrating embolus of the left middle cerebral artery may be transient, some part of the deficit may persist, being easily demonstrated by presenting the patient with complex words or double negatives in sentences.

DISSOCIATIVE SPEECH SYNDROMES

These are characterized by an impairment in the access of nervous impulses to and from the language areas, due to an interruption of one of the major afferent or efferent pathways. Included also in this category are aphasias due to lesions that separate the more strictly receptive parts of the language mechanism from the purely motor ones ("conduction aphasia") and to lesions that isolate the perisylvian speech areas from the other parts of the cerebral cortex ("transcortical aphasias").

The anatomic basis for most of these so-called conduction or transcortical aphasias is poorly defined. The concept, however, is an interesting one and emphasizes the importance of afferent, intercortical, and efferent connections of the language mechanism. Its weakness is that it leads to premature acceptance of anatomic and physiologic arrangements that are overly simplistic.

Conduction Aphasia As indicated earlier, it was Carl Wernicke, in his monograph of 1874, who pointed out that there were two major centers for language, one in the frontal and the other in the temporal region. He theorized that certain clinical symptoms would follow a lesion that effectively separated these centers, without damaging either of them. Since then, many cases of aphasia have been described that conform to Wernicke's proposed model of conduction aphasia, which is the name he gave to it.

In many respects the features of conduction aphasia resemble those of Wernicke's aphasia. There is a similar fluency and paraphasia in self-initiated speech, in repeating what is heard, and in reading aloud, and writing is invariably impaired. Also, dysarthria and dysprosody are lacking. In contrast to Wernicke's aphasia, patients have little or no difficulty in understanding words that are heard or seen, and are aware of their deficit. Characteristically, repetition is severely affected, and the contrast between defective repetition and relatively normal comprehension is said to be an essential feature of the syndrome. One of the best ways of eliciting the defect is to have the patient repeat nonsense syllables. The mistakes are then of the literal paraphasic type, i.e., substitution of a closely but detectably different letter or syllable. The disorder in repeating from dictation becomes more apparent when the rate of presentation of material is increased and the words become more polysyllabic. Since nouns are the longest words in a sentence, one may gain an impression that they are specifically affected.

The lesion in autopsied cases is located in the cortex and subcortical white matter in the upper bank of the sylvian fissure, involving the supramarginal gyrus of the inferior parietal lobule and occasionally the most posterior part of the superior temporal region. It appears that the critical structure involved is the arcuate fasciculus. This is a fiber tract that streams out of the temporal lobe, proceeding deep and somewhat posteriorly, around the posterior end of the sylvian fissure; there it joins the superior longitudinal fasciculus, deep in the anteroinferior parietal region, and proceeds forward through the suprasylvian opercular region to the motor association cortex, including Broca's area (Figs. 21-9 and 21-10). The usual cause of conduction aphasia is an embolic occlusion of the ascending parietal or posterior temporal branch of the middle cerebral artery, but other forms of vascular disease, neoplasm, or trauma in this region may produce the same syndrome.

Pure Word Deafness (Auditory Verbal Agnosia) This uncommon disorder is characterized by impaired auditory comprehension and inability to repeat what is said or to write to dictation, being similar in these respects to Wernicke's aphasia. By contrast, self-initiated utterances are correctly phrased and the patient's writing and ability to comprehend written language are normal or near normal. Such patients may declare that they cannot hear, but shouting does not help, sometimes to their surprise. By audiometric testing no hearing defect is found. Nonverbal sounds can be distinguished. The patient is forced to depend heavily on visual cues and frequently uses these cues well enough to understand most of what is said. However, tests which prevent the use of visual cues readily uncover the deficit. If able to describe the auditory experience, the patient says that words sound like a jumble of noises. Often the syndrome is not pure, particularly at the onset, and elements of paraphasia enter, which also help the examiner to distinguish the condition from true deafness.

In most recorded autopsy studies the lesion has been bilateral, in the middle thirds of the superior temporal gyri, in position to damage the connections between the primary auditory cortex in the transverse gyri of Heschl and the association areas of the superoposterior part of the temporal lobe. The few unilateral lesions have been localized in this part of the dominant temporal lobe. Requirements of small size and superficiality of the lesion in the cortex and subcortical white matter are best fulfilled by an embolic occlusion of a small branch of the lower division of the middle cerebral artery.

Pure Word Blindness This also is a rare syndrome, in which a literate person loses the ability to read and, often, to name colors. Such a person can no longer name or point on command to letters or to the words of which they are composed, although often able to read and name numbers. Understanding spoken language, repetition of what is heard, writing to dictation, and conversation are all intact. The striking feature of this syndrome is the retained capacity to write fluently, after which the patient cannot read what has been written (*alexia without agraphia*). Often no complaint about the difficulty is registered; it is discovered almost by accident. In lesser degrees of the affection, reading aloud is possible, but the patient manages only a single letter at a time.

Autopsies of such cases have usually demonstrated a lesion that destroys the left visual cortex and underlying white matter, particularly the geniculocalcarine tract, as well as the connections of the right visual cortex with the intact language areas of the dominant hemisphere. This latter "disconnection" usually occurs in the posterior part (splenium) of the corpus callosum, wherein lie the connections between the visual association areas of the two hemispheres (Fig. 21-10). Since the patient is blind in the right half of each visual field by virtue of the left occipital lesion, visual information reaches only the right occipital lobe and must be transferred across the corpus callosum to the angular gyrus of the left (dominant) hemisphere.

In other cases, the lesion is confined to the deep central white matter of the left parietooccipital region, in a position to interrupt the connections between the angular gyrus and both occipital lobes. In such cases, a right homonymous hemianopia may be absent, and the *alexia may be combined with agraphia*, with anomic aphasia (see below) and the other elements of Gerstmann's syndrome, i.e., right-left confusion, acalculia, and difficulty in naming of fingers and other parts of the body (see page 311). The entire constellation of symptoms is sometimes referred to as the *syndrome of the angular gyrus*.

Pure Word Mutism (Subcortical or Peripheral Motor Aphasia of Goldstein, Anarthria of Marie) Occasionally, as a result of a vascular lesion or other type of localized injury, the patient loses all capacity to speak, while retaining perfectly the ability to write, to understand spoken words, and to read silently with comprehension. Faciobrachial palsy may be associated. With improvement, it is possible to distinguish between two types of expressive disorder, as Bastian first pointed out. In one, a few words, such as yes or no or a few phrases return, which are understandable but are used inappropriately. In a second type, it is evident, from the time speech becomes audible, that language is syntactically complete, showing neither loss of vocabulary nor agrammatism and normal language function when allowed to write. This Bastian called *aphemia*, a term that Broca had used originally as a substitute for aphasia. The essential point is that this second type of speech disorder is nearly always transitory. Within a few weeks or months language is restored to normal. This syndrome should be distinguished from what is described above under Broca's aphasia.

The anatomic basis of pure word mutism has not been determined precisely, although reference is made in a few postmortem cases to a lesion in Broca's area. Bastian speculated that there was a separation of Broca's convolution from subcortical motor centers; hence the complete escape of intellectual function, even in the stage of mutism. A particularly well-studied case has recently been reported by Roch-LeCours and Lhermitte. Their patient uttered only a few sounds for 4 weeks, after which he recovered rapidly and completely. From the onset of the stroke the patient showed no disturbance of comprehension of language or of writing. Autopsy, 10 years later, disclosed an infarct that was confined to the cortex and subjacent white matter of the lowermost part of the precentral gyrus. Broca's area, one gyrus forward, was completely spared.

Anomic (Amnestic, Nominal) Aphasia This may be a relatively early or an isolated manifestation of disease of the nervous system. The patient loses only the ability to name objects. There are typical pauses in speech, groping for words, circumlocution, and substitution of another word or phrase that conveys the meaning. When shown a series of common objects, the patient may tell of their use instead of giving their names. The difficulty applies not only to objects seen but to the names of things heard or felt, but this is more difficult to demonstrate. Recall of the names for letters, digits, and other printed verbal material is almost invariably preserved, and immediate repetition of a spoken name is intact. That the deficit is principally one of naming is shown by the patient's correct use of the object and, usually, by an ability to point to the correct object on hearing or seeing the name. There is a tendency for patients to attribute their failure to forgetfulness or to give some other lame excuse for the disability, suggesting that they are not completely aware of the nature of their difficulty.

Anomic aphasia has been associated with lesions in different parts of the language area. In some cases the lesion has been deep in the basal portion of the posterior temporal lobe, in position probably to interrupt connections between sensory language areas and the hippocampal regions concerned with learning and memory. Mass lesions, such as a tumor or an otogenic abscess, are the most frequent causes, and as they enlarge a contralateral upper quadrantic visual field defect or a Wernicke's aphasia is added. Occasionally, anomia appears with lesions due to occlusion of the temporal branches of the posterior cerebral artery. Anomia may be a prominent manifestation of transcortical motor aphasia or be associated with Gerstmann's syndrome, in which case the lesions are found in the frontal lobe and angular gyrus respectively. Alzheimer's disease may begin with an anomic type of aphasia. This deficit may also be discovered in testing patients with a confusional state caused by metabolic or infectious disease, but then it has no localizing value. By the time the patient's difficulty is fully recognized, other disorders of speech and indifference, apathy, and abulia are conjoined.

Isolation of the Speech Areas (Transcortical Aphasias) Destruction of the border zones between anterior, middle, and posterior cerebral arteries, usually as a result of prolonged hypotension, carbon monoxide poisoning, or other forms of anoxia, may effectively isolate the intact motor and sensory speech areas from the rest of the cortex of the same hemisphere. In so-called transcortical sensory aphasia (Goldstein) the patient suffers a deficit of auditory and visual word comprehension, and writing and reading are impossible. Presumably information from the nonlanguage areas of the cerebrum cannot be transferred to Wernicke's area for conversion into verbal form. Speech remains fluent, with marked paraphasia, anomia, and empty circumlocution. There may be a remarkable facility in echoing, parrotlike, word phrases and songs that are heard (echolalia), unlike the deficit in Wernicke's aphasia, in which the ability to repeat the spoken word is lost or severely impaired. In transcortical motor aphasia ("anterior isolation syndrome," "dynamic aphasia" of Luria) the patient is unable to initiate con-

versational speech, producing only a few grunts or syllables. Comprehension is relatively preserved and repetition is strikingly intact.

These syndromes are of great theoretical interest
and may be more common than is currently appreciated.

THE AGRAPHIAS

Writing is of course an integral part of language function but a less essential and universal component, for a
considerable segment of the world's population talks but
does not read or write. Interestingly, this defect in the
illiterate illustrates the importance of visual perception
of form and space in the act of writing and explains why
writing is acquired in close association with reading during the developmental phases of language.

It might be supposed that all the rules of language
derived from the study of motor aphasia would be applicable to agraphia. In part this is true. One must be able
to formulate ideas into words and phrases in order to
have something to say as well as to write; hence disorders of writing like disorders of speaking reflect all the
basic defects of language. But there is an obvious difference between these two expressive activities. In speech
only one final motor pathway coordinating the movements of lips, tongue, larynx, and respiratory muscles is
available, whereas if the right hand is paralyzed, one can
still write with the left one, or with a foot, and even with
the mouth by holding a pencil between the teeth.

Pure agraphia as the initial and sole disturbance
of language function is a great rarity, but such cases
have been described (see Rosati and de Bastiani for a
recent review). Pathologically verified cases are virtually
nonexistent, but CT examination of the case of Rosati
and de Bastiani disclosed a lesion of the posterior perisylvian area. This is in keeping with the observation that
a lesion in or near the angular gyrus will occasionally
cause a disproportionate disorder of writing, with relative intactness of reading. The notion of a specific center
for writing in the posterior part of the second frontal
convolution ("Exner's writing area") has been generally
abandoned (Leischner).

Quite apart from the *aphasic agraphias* where
spelling and grammatical errors abound, there are special forms of agraphia caused by abnormalities of spatial
perception and praxis. Spatial agnosia appears to underlie *constructional agraphia*. In this circumstance letters
and words are formed clearly enough but wrongly arranged on the page. Words may be superimposed, written diagonally, in haphazard arrangement, from right to
left, or reversed, and with right parietal lesions and left-
sided spatial agnosia only the right half of the page is
used. Usually other constructional difficulties such as in-

ability to copy geometric figures or to make drawings of
clocks, flowers, and maps, etc., will be found as well.

A third group may be called the *apraxic agraphias*. Here language formulation is correct and the spatial
arrangements of words respected, but the hand has lost
its skill in forming letters and words. Handwriting becomes a scrawl, losing all personal character. There may
be an uncertainty as to how the pen should be held and
applied to paper. As a rule, other learned manual skills
are simultaneously disordered. Speculations as to the basic fault here are similar to those discussed in Chap. 3,
under "Nonparalytic (Apraxic) Motor Disorders," and
in Chap. 21, in relation to functions of the frontal and
parietal lobes.

OTHER CEREBRAL DISORDERS OF LANGUAGE

It would be incorrect to conclude that the syndromes
described above, all related to perisylvian lesions of the
dominant cerebral hemisphere, represent all the ways in
which cerebral lesions disturb language. The effects on
speech and language of diffuse cerebral disorders, such
as delirium tremens and Alzheimer's disease have already been mentioned (see page 327). Pathologic
changes in parts of the cerebrum other than the perisylvian regions may secondarily affect language function.
The lesions that occur in the border zones between major cerebral arteries and effectively isolate perisylvian
areas from other parts of the cerebrum fall into this category (see above). Another example is the lesion in the
medial and orbital parts of the frontal lobes, which impair all motor activities, to the point of abulia or akinetic
mutism (see page 233). If there is any emitted speech in
this latter circumstance, it tends to be laconic with long
pauses and an inability to sustain a monologue. Extensive occipital lesions impair reading and reduce the utilization of all visual and lexical stimuli. Deep cerebral
lesions, by causing fluctuant states of inattention and
disorientation, induce fragmentation of words and
phrases and protracted uncontrollable talking (logorrhea). Strong stimulation, which momentarily stabilizes
behavior and speech, proves the essential integrity of
language mechanisms.

Thalamic lesions, usually vascular, may cause an
aphasia that is characterized by mutism to begin with,
then paraphasic, hypophonic speech. Characteristically
also, the patient's comprehension of spoken language
and ability to name objects and to repeat dictated words
and phrases are unimpaired. Reading and writing may

or may not be affected. Complete recovery, in a matter of weeks, is the rule.

DISORDERS OF ARTICULATION AND PHONATION

The act of speaking is a highly coordinated sequence of contractions of the larynx, pharynx, palate, tongue, lips, and respiratory musculature. These are innervated by the vagal, hypoglossal, facial, and phrenic nerves. The nuclei of these nerves are controlled by both motor cortices through the corticobulbar tracts. As with all movements, there are also extrapyramidal influences from the cerebellum and basal ganglions. For speaking, air has to be expired in regulated bursts, and each expiration must be maintained long enough (by pressure mainly from the intercostal muscles) to permit utterance of phrases and sentences. The current of expired air is then finely regulated by the activity of the various muscles engaged in speech.

Phonation, or the production of vocal sounds, is a function of the larynx. The pitch of the voice depends upon the tension of the vocal cords, and this is adjusted by means of the intrinsic laryngeal muscles before any audible sound emerges. The controlled intratracheal pressure forces air past the glottis and separates the margins of the cords, setting up a series of vibrations and recoils. Sounds thus formed are modified as they pass through the nasopharynx and mouth, which act as resonators. *Articulation* consists of contractions of the pharynx, palate, tongue, and lips, which interrupt or alter the vocal sounds. Vowels are of laryngeal origin, as are some consonants, but the latter are formed for the most part during articulation; the consonants *m, b,* and *p* are labial, *l* and *t* are lingual, and *nk* and *ng* are guttural (throat and soft palate).

Defective articulation and phonation are recognized at once by listening to the patient speaking during ordinary conversation or reading aloud from a newspaper or a book. Test phrases or attempts at rapid repetition of lingual, labial, and guttural consonants (e.g., *la-la-la-la, me-me-me-me,* or *k-k-k-k*) bring out the particular abnormality. Disorders of phonation call for a precise analysis of the voice and its apparatus. The movements of the vocal cords should be inspected with a laryngoscope, and those of the tongue, palate, and pharynx by direct observation.

DYSARTHRIA AND ANARTHRIA

Dysarthria and anarthria comprise a third group of speech abnormalities. In pure dysarthria or anarthria there is no abnormality of the cortical language areas. The dysarthric patient is able to understand perfectly what is heard, and, if literate, has no difficulty in reading and writing, although unable to utter a single intelligible word. This is the strict meaning of being inarticulate.

Defects in articulation may be subdivided into several types: paretic (lower motor neuron) dysarthria, spastic and rigid dysarthria, and ataxic dysarthria.

Paretic Dysarthria (Lower Motor Neuron Paralysis, Atrophic Bulbar Paralysis) This is due to weakness or paralysis of the articulatory muscles. the result of disease of the motor nuclei of the medulla and lower pons or their peripheral extensions, the cranial nerves (*lower motor neuron paralysis*). In advanced forms of this disorder, the shriveled tongue lies inert and fasciculating on the floor of the mouth, and the lips are relaxed and tremulous. Saliva constantly collects in the mouth because of dysphagia, and drooling is troublesome. Speech becomes slurred and progressively less distinct. There is special difficulty in the distinct enunciation of vibratives, such as *r,* and as the paralysis becomes more complete, lingual and labial consonants are finally not pronounced at all. Bilateral paralysis of the palate may occur with diphtheria, poliomyelitis, and progressive bulbar palsy. Bilateral paralysis of the lips, as in the facial diplegia of idiopathic polyneuritis, interferes with enunciation of labial consonants; *p* and *b* are slurred and sound more like *f* and *v.* Degrees of this abnormality are also observed in myasthenia gravis.

Spastic and Rigid Dysarthrias These are more frequent than the lower motor neuron variety. Diseases that involve the corticobulbar tracts, usually vascular disease or motor system disease, result in the syndrome of spastic bulbar (pseudobulbar) palsy. The patient may have had a clinically inevident vascular lesion at some time in the past, affecting the corticobulbar fibers on one side. Since the bulbar muscles are probably innervated by both motor cortices, there may be no impairment in speech or swallowing from a unilateral lesion. Should another stroke then occur, involving the other corticobulbar tract at the pontine, midbrain, or capsular level, the patient immediately becomes dysphagic and anarthric or dysarthric, often with paresis of the facial muscles. This condition, unlike bulbar paralysis due to lower motor neuron involvement, entails no atrophy or fasciculation of the paralyzed muscles; the jaw jerk and other facial reflexes soon become exaggerated, the palatal reflexes are retained or increased, emotional control is impaired (pathologic laughter and crying), and sometimes breathing becomes periodic (Cheyne-Stokes). When the frontal operculum alone is involved, the speech may be dysarthric (cortical dysarthria), usually without the impairment in emotional control. In the beginning, the patient may be totally anarthric and aphonic, but as improvement progresses or in mild degrees of the same condition, speech is notably slow, thick, and indistinct, much like that of partial bulbar paralysis. In many cases of partially recovered Broca's aphasia the patient is left with a dysarthria that may be difficult to distinguish from a pure articulatory defect. Careful testing of other language functions, especially writing, will reveal the aphasic quality.

In paralysis agitans, or in postencephalitic Parkinson's syndrome, one observes an extrapyramidal disturbance of articulation, characterized by slurring of words and syllables and trailing off the end of sentences. The voice is low-pitched, monotonous, and lacks both volume and inflection. The words are pronounced hastily. In advanced cases speech is almost unintelligible; only whispering is possible. It may happen that the patient finds it impossible to talk while walking but can speak if sitting or lying down.

With chorea and myoclonus, speech may also be affected in a highly characteristic way. Unlike the defect of pseudobulbar palsy or paralysis agitans, chorea and myoclonus cause abrupt interruptions of the words by superimposition of the abnormal movements. The idea is best conveyed by the phrase "hiccup speech," in that the breaks are unexpected, as in singultus. Grimacing and other characteristic motor signs must be depended upon for diagnosis.

Corticobulbar and extrapyramidal disturbances of speech may be combined in double athetosis (see page 854) and Hallervorden-Spatz disease (see page 688) and in generalized cerebral diseases such as general paresis, in which slurred speech is one of the cardinal signs.

Ataxic Dysarthria This is characteristic of acute and chronic cerebellar lesions. It may be observed in multiple sclerosis, Friedreich's ataxia, cerebellar atrophy, and heatstroke. The principal speech abnormality is slowness; imprecise enunciation, monotony, and unnatural separation of the syllables of words (scanning) are other features. Coordination of speech and of respiration is disordered. There may not be enough breath to utter certain words or syllables, and others are uttered with greater force than intended (explosive speech). *Scanning dysarthria* (see page 66) is distinctive and is due most often to mesencephalic lesions involving the brachium conjunctivum. However, in some cases of cerebellar disease, especially if there is a possibility of spastic weakness of the tongue from corticobulbar tract involvement, there may be only a slurring dysarthria, and it is not possible to predict the anatomy of disease from analysis of speech alone. Myoclonic jerks involving the speech musculature may be superimposed on cerebellar ataxia in a number of diseases.

APHONIA AND DYSPHONIA

Finally, a few points should be made concerning the fourth group of speech disorders, i.e., disturbances of voice. In adolescence there may be a persistence of the unstable "change of voice" normally seen in boys during puberty. As though by habit, the patient speaks part of the time in falsetto. This condition may persist into adult life. Its basis is unknown. Voice training has been helpful in the majority of patients.

Paresis of respiratory movements, as in poliomyelitis and acute infectious polyneuritis, may affect the voice because insufficient air is provided for phonation and articulation. Also, disturbances in the rhythm of respiration may interfere with the fluency of speech. This is particularly noticeable in so-called extrapyramidal diseases, where one may observe that the patient tries to talk during part of inspiration. In the latter conditions, another common feature is reduced volume of the voice due to limited excursion of the breathing muscles; the patient is unable to shout or to speak above a whisper. Whispering speech is also a feature of stupor, but strong stimulation may make the voice audible.

With paresis of both vocal cords, the patient can speak only in whispers. Since the vocal cords normally separate during inspiration, their failure to do so when paralyzed may result in an inspiratory stridor. If one vocal cord is paralyzed, as a result of involvement of the tenth cranial nerve by tumor, for example, the voice becomes hoarse, low-pitched, rasping, and somewhat nasal in quality because the posterior nares do not close during phonation. The pronunciation of certain consonants such as b, p, n, and k are followed by escape of air into the nasal passages. The abnormality is sometimes less pronounced in recumbency and increased when the head is thrown forward. Hoarseness may also be due to structural changes in the vocal cords caused by cigarette smoking, chronic inflammation, polyps, etc.

Another curious condition about which little is known is *spastic dysphonia*. Spasmodic dysphonia would be a better term; the adjective *spastic* suggests corticospinal involvement, whereas the disorder is probably of extrapyramidal origin. The authors have seen many patients, middle-aged or elderly men and women, otherwise healthy, who gradually lost the ability to speak quietly and fluently. Any attempt to speak results in contraction of all the speech musculature so that the patient's voice is strained and speaking is a great effort. The patient sounds as though he or she were trying to speak while being strangled. Shouting is easier than quiet speech, and whispering is unaltered. Other actions utilizing approximately the same muscles (swallowing and singing) are usually unimpeded.

Spastic dysphonia is usually nonprogressive and occurs as an isolated phenomenon, but we have observed exceptions in which it is combined with blepharoclonus or spasmodic torticollis, or both.

The nature of spastic dysphonia is unclear. As a neurologic disorder it is apparently similar to writer's cramp (see page 77). Speech therapists watching such a patient strain to achieve vocalization often assume that the patient can be relieved by making him or her relax; and psychotherapists believe at first that a search of the patient's personal life around the time when the dysphonia began will enable the patient to understand the problem and regain a normal mode of speaking. But both these methods have failed without exception. Drugs useful in extrapyramidal diseases such as paralysis agitans have only exceptionally proved beneficial. Crushing of one recurrent laryngeal nerve is said to be beneficial (Dedo). No pathologic studies have been made, and since the condition is restricted and nonprogressive, it is doubtful if present methods of neuropathologic study would demonstrate an anatomic abnormality.

CLINICAL APPROACH TO THE PATIENT WITH SPEECH AND LANGUAGE DISORDERS

APHASIA

In investigating a case of aphasia it is first necessary to inquire into the patient's native language, handedness, and previous education. For many years it has been taught that following the onset of aphasia, individuals who had been fluent in more than one language (polyglots) improved more quickly in their native tongue than in a subsequently acquired language. There are many exceptions to this rule. In our experience, when adequate testing is possible, the first language is invariably affected as part of an aphasic disorder, and more or less to the same extent as the more recently acquired one. Many naturally left-handed children are trained to use their right hand for writing; therefore, in determining this point we must ask which hand is used for throwing a ball, threading a needle, sewing, or using a spoon or common tools such as a hammer, saw, or bread knife. It is important before the beginning of the examination to determine whether the patient is alert and can be made to participate reliably in testing, as accurate assessment of language depends on these factors.

One should quickly ascertain whether the patient has other signs of a gross cerebral lesion such as hemiplegia, facial weakness, homonymous hemianopia, or cortical sensory loss. When such a constellation of major neurologic signs is present, the aphasic disorder is usually of the total (global) type. Dyspraxia of limbs and speech musculature, in response to spoken commands or to visual mimicry, is generally associated with Broca's aphasia and sometimes with Wernicke's aphasia. Bilateral or unilateral homonymous hemianopia without motor weakness tends often to be linked to pure word blindness or to alexia with agraphia, and to anomic aphasia.

The special types of aphasia—Broca's, Wernicke's, conduction, pure word deafness or blindness—are sometimes associated with evidence of embolism to the nondominant cerebral hemisphere or to other organs.

Conversational testing permits quick assessment of the motor aspects of speech (praxis and prosody), fluency, language formulation, and auditory comprehension. If the disability consists mainly of sparse, laborious speech, it suggests, of course, Broca's aphasia, and this possibility can be pursued further by tests of repeating from dictation and by special tests of praxis of the oropharyngeal muscles. Fluent, empty, paraphasic speech with impaired comprehension is indicative of Wernicke's aphasia. Impaired comprehension but perfectly normal formulated speech and intact ability to read suggest the rare syndrome of pure word deafness. Disorders confined to naming, generally without paraphasias, when other language functions (reading, writing, spelling, etc.) are found adequate, are diagnostic of amnesic or anomic aphasia.

When conversation discloses virtually no abnormalities, other tests may still be revealing. The most important of these are reading, writing, repetition, and naming. Reading aloud single letters, words, and text may reveal the dissociative syndrome of pure word blindness. Except for this syndrome and for Bastian's aphemia (see above), writing is disturbed in all forms of aphasia. Literal and verbal paraphasic errors may appear in milder cases of Wernicke's aphasia as the patient reads aloud from text or from words in the examiner's handwriting. Similar errors appear even more frequently when the patient is asked to explain the text, read aloud, or give an explanation in writing.

Testing the patient's ability to repeat spoken language is a simple and important maneuver in the evaluation of aphasic disorders. As with other tests of aphasia, it may be necessary to increase the complexity of the test, from digits and simple words to complex words, phrases, and sentences, in order to disclose the full disability. Defective repetition occurs in all forms of aphasia (Broca's, Wernicke's, and total) due to lesions in the perisylvian language areas. The patient may be unable to repeat despite adequate comprehension—the hallmark of conduction aphasia. Contrariwise, normal repetition in an aphasiac indicates that the perisylvian area is intact. Thus the capacity for repetition may be preserved despite grossly disordered comprehension, as in transcortical sensory aphasia. In fact, in the latter circumstance, the tendency to repeat may be excessive (echolalia). Preserved ability to repeat is also characteristic of anomic aphasia and of the aphasia that occasionally occurs with putaminal and thalamic lesions.

Quantitation of these deficits can be obtained by the use of any one of several examination procedures. A recent one is that of Goodglass and Kaplan.

ARTICULATION-PHONATION DISORDERS

Disturbances of articulation point to involvement of a different set of neural structures, such as the motor cortices, the corticobulbar pathways, the nuclei of the fifth, seventh, ninth, tenth, and twelfth cranial nerves, and extrapyramidal nuclei and tracts. Often is is necessary to use other neurologic findings to decide which of these structures are implicated. The fundamental distinction between the atrophic bulbar (nuclear or infranuclear) and the spastic bulbar (pseudobulbar or supranuclear) palsies is grasped only with difficulty by most students. The information obtained by localizing these two major types of dysarthria is extremely helpful in differential diagnosis.

Dysphonia should lead to an investigation of laryngeal disease, either primary or secondary to an abnormality of innervation. Inspection of vocal cords is a necessary step in the clinical study.

TREATMENT

The sudden onset of aphasia would be expected to cause great apprehension, but except for pure or almost pure motor defects, most patients show remarkably little concern. It appears that the very lesion that deprives them of speech also causes at least a partial loss of insight into their own disability. This reaches almost a ludicrous extreme in some cases of Wernicke's aphasia, in which patients become indignant when others cannot understand their jargon. Nonetheless, as improvement occurs, many patients do become discouraged. Reassurance and a positive program of speech rehabilitation are the best ways of helping the patient at this stage.

The contemporary methods of training and reeducation in overcoming an aphasic defect have never been critically evaluated. Most aphasic difficulty is due to vascular disease of the brain, and nearly always this is accompanied by some degree of spontaneous improvement in the days, weeks, and months that follow the stroke. Sometimes recovery is complete within hours or days; at times not more than a few words are regained after a year or two of assiduous speech training. Nevertheless, it is the opinion of many experts in the field that speech training is worthwhile (see review by Benson).

One must decide for each patient whether speech training is needed and when it should be started. As a rule, therapy is not advisable in the first few days of an aphasic illness, because one does not know how lasting it will be. Also, if the patient suffers a severe global aphasia and can neither speak nor understand spoken and written words, the speech therapist is helpless. Under such circumstances, one does well to wait a few weeks until one of the language functions has begun to return. Then the physician may begin to encourage and help the patient to use the function to a maximum degree. In milder aphasic disorders the patient may be sent to the speech therapist as soon as the illness has stabilized.

The methods of speech training are specialized, and it is advisable to call in a person who has been trained in this field. However, inasmuch as the benefit is largely psychological, an interested member of the family or a schoolteacher can be of help if a speech therapist is not available in the community.

The language problems of children pose special problems and demand skillful diagnosis and treatment. These are considered fully in Chap. 27.

REFERENCES

BENSON DF: Aphasia rehabilitation. *Arch Neurol* 36:187, 1979.

———: *Aphasia, Alexia and Agraphia*. New York, Churchill Livingstone, 1979.

———, GESCHWIND N: The aphasias and related disturbances, in Baker AB, Baker LH (eds): *Clinical Neurology*. New York, Harper & Row, 1976, chap 8.

CRITCHLEY M: Aphasiological nomenclature and definitions, *Cortex* 3:3, 1967.

DEDO HH: Recurrent laryngeal nerve section for spastic dysphonia. *Ann Otol* 85:451, 1976.

GESCHWIND N: Disconnection syndromes in animals and man. *Brain* 88:237, 585, 1965.

———: Wernicke's contribution to the study of aphasia. *Cortex* 3:449, 1967.

GOLDSTEIN K: *Language and Language Disturbances*. New York, Grune & Stratton, 1948, pp 190–216.

GOODGLASS H, KAPLAN E: *The Assessment of Aphasia and Related Disorders*. Philadelphia, Lea & Febiger, 1972.

HALLGREN B: Specific dyslexia. *Acta Psychiatr Neurol Scand Suppl* 65, 1950.

HENSCHEN SE: Clinical and anatomical contributions on brain pathology. *Arch Neurol Psychiatry* 13:226, 1925.

KINSBOURNE M: *Hemispheric Disconnection and Cerebral Function*. Springfield, Ill, Charles C Thomas, 1974.

LEISCHNER A: The agraphias, in Vinken PJ, Bruyn GW (eds): *Handbook of Clinical Neurology*, vol 4. Amsterdam, North-Holland, 1969, pp 141–180.

LEVINE DN, MOHR JP: Language after bilateral cerebral infarctions: Role of the minor hemisphere in speech. *Neurology* 29:927, 1979.

MOHR JP: Broca's area and Broca's aphasia, in Whitaker H, Whitaker H (eds): *Studies in Neurolinguistics*. New York, Academic, 1976, vol 1, pp 201–235.

——— et al: Broca aphasia: Pathologic and clinical. *Neurology* 28:311, 1978.

NIELSEN JM: *Agnosia, Apraxia, Aphasia: Their Value in Cerebral Localization*, 2d ed. New York, Hafner, 1962.

ROCH-LE COURS H, LHERMITTE F: The pure form of the phonetic disintegration syndrome (pure anarthria). *Brain and Language* 3:88, 1976.

ROSATI G, DE BASTIANI P: Pure agraphia: A discrete form of aphasia. *J Neurol Neurosurg Psychiatry* 42:266, 1979.

SYMONDS C: Aphasia. *J Neurol Neurosurg Psychiatry* 16:1, 1953.

ANXIETY AND DISORDERS OF ENERGY, MOOD, EMOTION, AND AUTONOMIC FUNCTIONS

CHAPTER 23

LASSITUDE AND FATIGUE

In this chapter and the next we will consider the clinical phenomena of lassitude, fatigue, anxiety, and depression. These cardinal manifestations of disease, though more abstruse than paralysis, sensory loss, seizures, or aphasia, are no less important, if for no other reason than their frequency. They may provide clear indication of the existence of a psychiatric illness, as will be pointed out later, but are often observed as reactive states in association with all manner of medical and neurologic diseases, in which case it may be difficult to separate their effects from those of the underlying diseases.

The terms *weakness* and *tiredness,* among many others, are used by patients to describe a variety of subjective complaints which vary in their diagnostic and prognostic significance. The complaints can usually be fitted into one of the following categories:

I. *Lassitude, fatigue, lack of energy, listlessness, and languor.* (These terms, though not synonymous, shade into one another; all refer to a weariness and a loss of that sense of well-being typically found in persons who are healthy of body and mind.)

II. *Weakness, loss of strength, paresis, paralysis.* These may be persistent or episodic.

A. *Persistent weakness.* This may be (1) restricted to certain muscles or groups of muscles (see Chap. 3), or (2) more or less generalized, i.e., involving the entire musculature (see Chaps. 48 and 49).

B. *Episodic.* Attacks of weakness may occur in myasthenia and the periodic paralyses. Many patients confuse "attacks of weakness" with a diminished sense of alertness, lightheadedness, or feeling of faintness. These usually turn out to be episodes of partial or threatening syncope, attacks of anxiety or vertigo, or seizures (see Chaps. 17, 14, and 15, respectively).

Of all the symptoms in this group lassitude and fatigue are the most frequent and often the most vague.

More than half of all patients entering a general hospital register a direct complaint of fatigability or admit to it when questioned. During the Second World War, fatigue was so prominent in combat personnel as to be given a separate place in medical nosology, viz., "combat fatigue," which referred to all acute psychiatric illnesses that happened on the battlefield. The common clinical antecedents and accompaniments of fatigue, its significance, and its physiologic and psychological bases should, therefore, be matters of interest to all physicians.

Patients who complain of lassitude and fatigue have a more or less characteristic way of describing their symptoms. They say that they are "all in," "tired all the time," "weary," "turned off," or "fed up," or that they have "no pep," "no ambition," or "no interest." They manifest their condition by showing an indifference to the tasks at hand, by talking much about how hard they are working; they are inclined to sit around or lie down, occupying themselves with trivial tasks. On closer analysis one observes that they have a difficulty in initiating activity and also in sustaining it.

This condition is the familiar aftermath of prolonged labor or great physical exertion, and under such circumstances it is accepted as a normal, physiologic reaction. When, however, the same symptoms or similar ones appear in no relation to such antecedents, they are suspected of being the manifestations of disease.

The physician's task begins, then, with an attempt to determine whether the patient is merely suffering from the physical and mental effects of overwork without realizing it. Overworked, overwrought people are everywhere observable in our society. Their actions are both instructive and pathetic. They seem to be impelled by notions of duty and refuse to think of themselves. Or, as is often the case, some personal inadequacy seems to prevent them from deriving pleasure from any activity except their work, in which they indulge themselves as a kind of defense mechanism. Such persons show their fatigue by other symptoms, such as irritability, restlessness, and sleeplessness. Their symptoms and behavior may be better understood by considering certain psychological studies of the effects of fatigue on the normal individual.

EFFECTS OF FATIGUE ON THE NORMAL PERSON

According to several authoritative sources, fatigue has both explicit and implicit effects, grouped under (1) a series of biochemical and physiologic changes in many organs of the body, (2) an overt disorder in behavior taking the form of a reduced output of work (*work decrement*), and (3) an expressed dissatisfaction and a subjective feeling of tiredness.

As to the biochemical and physiologic changes, continuous muscular work leads to depletion of muscle glycogen and an accumulation of lactic acid and other metabolites, which in themselves reduce the power of muscular contraction and delay recovery. Extreme degrees of muscular effort, in which activity exceeds provision of substrate, results in necrosis of fibers and rise in serum levels of creatine phosphokinase and aldolase in normal persons (and much more so in individuals with one of the hereditary metabolic diseases of muscle described in Chap. 49). The muscles are slightly swollen and sore for several days. It is said that the injection of blood from a fatigued animal into a rested one will produce overt manifestations of fatigue in the latter, but the authors are skeptical of such reports. With repeated contraction of muscles, their action is observed to become tremulous, movements are less adept, and the coordination of agonist, antagonist, and synergic muscles is less precise. The rate of breathing increases, the pulse quickens, the blood pressure rises and pulse pressure widens, and the white blood cell count and metabolic rate are increased. These alterations bear out the hypothesis that fatigue is in part a manifestation of altered metabolism.

The decreased capacity for work or productivity which is a direct consequence of fatigue has been investigated by industrial psychologists. Their findings show clearly the importance of the motivational factor on work output, whether it be in manual or mental tasks. Also, individual differences in energy potential appear to

be important, as are differences in physique, intelligence, and temperament.

The subjective aspects of fatigue have been carefully recorded. Aside from feeling weary and tired, the fatigued person is unable to deal effectively with complex problems and tends to be unreasonable, often about trivialities. The number and quality of his associations in psychological tests are reduced. The ability to deliberate and to reach judgments is impaired; decisions made late at night may appear unsound the next day. The worker, after a long, hard day, is unable to perform adequately the demanding duties of head of the household; the tired business executive who becomes the tyrant of the family is proverbial. A disinclination to try and the appearance of ideas of inferiority are other characteristics of the fatigued mind.

Instances of fatigue and lassitude resulting from overwork are not difficult to recognize. A description of the patient's daily routine and a talk with family members and associates will usually suffice. Moreover, if the person can be persuaded to live at a more reasonable pace and allow time for outside pleasurable activities, the symptoms will promptly subside. A common error in diagnosis, however, is the ascription of fatigue to overwork when actually it is a manifestation of a psychoneurosis or depression.

FATIGUE AS A MANIFESTATION OF PSYCHIATRIC DISORDER

The great majority of patients who enter a hospital because of unexplained chronic fatigue and lassitude are found to have some type of psychiatric illness. Formerly this state was called "neurasthenia," but since fatigue rarely exists as an isolated phenomenon, the current practice is to label such cases according to the total clinical picture. The usual associated symptoms are nervousness, irritability, anxiety, depression, insomnia, headaches, difficulty in concentrating, reduced sexual impulse, and loss of appetite. In one series in a general hospital 75 percent of persons admitted because of a chief complaint of chronic fatigue were diagnosed, finally, as having *anxiety neurosis* and *tension states*. Depression accounted for another 10 percent, and the remainder of the patients had a miscellanea of medical and psychiatric illnesses.

Several features are common to the psychiatric group. The fatigue may be worse in the morning. There is an inclination to lie down and rest, but sleep does not come. The fatigue relates more to some activities than to others. Inquiry may disclose that the fatigue was first experienced in temporal relation to a grief reaction, a surgical operation, a medical illness, or some other unpleasant event. The feeling of fatigue interferes with mental as well as physical activities; the patient is worried easily, is mentally inactive, and finds it difficult to concentrate during the attempted solution of a problem or in carrying on a conversation.

Depression, as will be elaborated in the following chapter, has a characteristic effect on impulse and energy. Also, sleep is disturbed, with a tendency to early-morning waking, so that such persons are at their worst in the morning, both in spirit and in energy output. Their tendency is to improve as the day wears on, and they may even feel fairly normal by evening. It is difficult to decide whether the fatigue is a primary manifestation of disease or is secondary to a lack of interest.

Not all chronically fatigued individuals deviate enough from normal to justify the diagnosis of psychoneurosis or depression. Many people in society, because of circumstances beyond their control, have no purpose in life and much idle time. They are bored with the monotony of their routine. Such circumstances are conducive to fatigue, just as the opposite, a new enterprise that excites optimism and enthusiasm, will dispel fatigue. Other persons seem normal until some adversity is encountered, arousing worry or fear, and then it becomes apparent that their adjustment was unstable. Such reactions are understandable to anyone who has ever had stage fright and who remembers the sense of physical weakness, the utter incapacity to act, the intellectual chaos that overwhelms the previously well-ordered mind, and the exhaustion that follows.

PSYCHOLOGICAL THEORIES

The enervating effect of a strong emotion such as anxiety is well known, and it might be supposed that the simple prolongation of the emotional experience would provide a rational explanation for the chronic fatigue of anxiety neurosis. Even if true, however, this explanation does not account for the occurrence of fatigue at a time when there is no apparent emotional disorder.

The dynamic schools of psychiatry, particularly the psychoanalytic, have postulated that chronic fatigue, in the broadest sense, is like the anxiety from which it derives; it is a danger signal that something is wrong—that some attitude or activity has been too intense or too persistent. The fatigue is self-preservative, serving not merely as a protection against physical injury but also as a protection of the person's self-esteem and self-confidence. As to mechanism, it is claimed that the fatigue is

the result of exhaustion of the store of psychic energy required to maintain repression of unacceptable ideas. Another psychoanalytic theory holds that fatigue is not a negative symptom, a lack or depletion of energy, but an unconscious desire for inactivity. A reciprocal relation is said to exist between fatigue and anxiety. Both are protective, but anxiety is the more imperative. It calls for taking some positive action to get out of a predicament, whereas fatigue calls for inactivity. Both operate blindly, however, for the person cannot perceive what it is that must be done or stopped. All this allegedly happens at the subconscious level.

Some persons are low in impulse and energy throughout life, being more so at times of stress; some psychiatrists believe that they have a constitutional inadequacy. Kahn classifies such persons as "psychopaths weak in impulse" and points out in his description their inability throughout life to play games vigorously, to compete successfully, to work hard without exhaustion, to withstand or recover quickly from illness, or to assume a dominant role in a social group.

It is obvious that these several psychologic hypotheses could not all be correct, nor could they be applicable to all situations in which chronic fatigue is the complaint. Undoubtedly there are persons who, because of genetic factors or early life experiences, are underactive, and are lacking in stamina and the capacity to sustain physical or mental activity, or both. It is equally clear that psychic and physical energy are closely linked to mood. The more chronic varieties of acquired fatigue, without associated medical disease, have in nearly all instances a psychological basis.

LASSITUDE AND FATIGUE WITH CHRONIC INFECTION AND WITH ENDOCRINE AND OTHER MEDICAL DISEASES

Infection is another cause of chronic fatigue, though a much less frequent one. All of us have at some time or other sensed the abrupt onset of extreme exhaustion, a tired ache in the muscles or an inexplicable listlessness, only to discover later that we were "coming down with the flu." In chronic infections such as hepatitis, tuberculosis, brucellosis, and infectious mononucleosis, the infection may not be at once evident, but it should always be suspected when the fatigue is acute in onset and out of proportion to other symptoms such as mood change, nervousness, and anxiety. More often the fatigue begins with an obvious infection but persists for several weeks after the signs of the infection have subsided, and it may then be difficult to decide whether there is still a lingering infection or the infection has been complicated by psychological symptoms during convalescence. In discases such as those just mentioned and a host of other systemic viral infections, it may appear that longstanding neurotic symptoms have been uncovered. Nevertheless it is not possible to dismiss an obscure secondary metabolic disorder consequent to the infection.

Metabolic and endocrine diseases (Chaps. 26 and 39) of various types may cause inordinate degrees of lassitude and fatigue. Sometimes there is in addition a true muscular weakness. In Addison's disease and Simmonds' disease, fatigue may dominate the clinical picture. Aldosterone deficiency is another established cause of fatigue. In persons with hypothyroidism, with or without frank myxedema, lassitude and sluggishness are frequent complaints, and also muscle aching and joint pains. Fatigue may also be present in patients with hyperthyroidism but is usually less troublesome than nervousness. Uncontrolled diabetes mellitus may be accompanied by excessive fatigability, as are hyperparathyroidism, hypogonadism, and Cushing's disease.

Anemia, when moderate or severe, should be considered as a possible cause of unexplained lassitude. Mild grades of anemia are usually asymptomatic; lassitude is far too often ascribed to it.

Any type of nutritional deficiency may, when severe, cause lassitude, and in its earlier stages this may be the chief complaint. Weight loss and the history of dietary inadequacy may provide the only other clues to the nature of the illness.

For several weeks or months following myocardial infarction, most patients complain of fatigue out of all proportion to effort. In many of these patients there is an accompanying anxiety or depression. Much more difficult to understand is the complaint of fatigue that may precede myocardial infarction.

Among neurologic diseases in which fatigability is a prominent symptom one should mention the syndrome of posttraumatic nervous instability, Parkinson's disease, and multiple sclerosis. The fatigue of Parkinson's disease may precede the recognition of neurologic signs by months or even years. It is probably a reaction to the subjective awareness of increasing disability occasioned by the akinesia. The majority of patients who recover from a stroke complain of being weak and tired. The fatigue that accompanies multiple sclerosis may be greatly worsened by exposure to high temperatures, e.g., a hot bath.

DIFFERENTIAL DIAGNOSIS

If one looks critically at the patients who enter a hospital because of lassitude and fatigability (sometimes incorrectly called "weakness"), it is evident that the most commonly overlooked diagnoses are psychoneurosis and depression. The correct conclusion can usually be reached by keeping these illnesses in mind as one elicits the symptoms of the illness from patient and family. Difficulty arises when symptoms of the psychiatric illness are so inconspicuous as not to be appreciated; one comes then to suspect the diagnosis only by having eliminated the common medical causes. Observation in the hospital may bear out the existence of an anxiety state or gloomy mood, as the patient resists rehabilitation. Strong reassurance in combination with a therapeutic trial of tranquilizing and antidepressant drugs may suppress symptoms of which the patient was barely aware and may clarify the diagnosis. The possibility of mistaking a depression for a neurosis has already been mentioned above. Of course the asthenic psychopath is recognized by the characteristic lifelong behavioral pattern revealed in the biography.

Infections such as pulmonary tuberculosis, brucellosis, subclinical hepatitis, subacute bacterial endocarditis, malaria, hookworm, and other parasitic infections should always be included in the differential diagnosis and a search made for their characteristic symptoms and signs and laboratory findings. There should be a search for occult tumor. An endocrine survey is also in order in all obscure cases. The measurement of serum T_4, cortisol, and electrolytes may prove helpful in identifying an endocrine cause of a patient's fatigue syndrome.

It should be remembered that chronic intoxications with barbiturates, alcohol, or bromides, some of which are given to suppress nervousness, may contribute to fatigability. Finally, when onset of fatigue is rapid and recent, the cause is likely to be an infection, a disturbance in fluid balance, or rapidly developing circulatory failure of either peripheral or cardiac origin.

GENERALIZED WEAKNESS

As can be judged from the foregoing remarks, weakness must be distinguished from lassitude and fatigue. The demonstration of reduced muscular power sets the case analysis along different lines, bringing up for particular consideration diseases of the peripheral nervous system or of the musculature.

True neural or myopathic weakness is probably never caused by psychological factors, though the hysteric or malingerer may claim weakness. Usually this can be detected by the criteria outlined in Chap. 53. In anemia, chronic infection, malignancy, and nutritional depletion (except when polyneuropathy is present), the thin muscles are always stronger during tests of peak contraction than one would expect, though strength falls short of that of a healthy individual (see Chap. 44 for description of tests of peak power and endurance of muscles).

The presence of muscular weakness is ascertained by (1) obtaining a history of reduced strength and (2) demonstrating a failure to contract the muscles forcefully one or more times. By testing each of the major groups of muscles from head to foot, one may ascertain whether all or certain groups fall below standard. Quantitative and qualitative changes (myasthenia, inverse myasthenia, myotonia, paramyotonia, pathologic cramping) may also be detected by the methods to be outlined in Chaps. 51 and 52. The topography of weakness and associated neurologic findings permit distinction between the various types of spinal, peripheral nerve, and myopathic pareses. Rare diseases, difficult to diagnose, that cause inexplicable muscle weakness are masked hyperthyroidism, hyperparathyroidism, ossifying hemangiomas with hypophosphatemia, some of the kalemic periodic paralyses, and hyperinsulinism.

REFERENCES

ADAMS RD: Thayer lectures: I. Principles of myopathology. II. Principles of clinical myology. *Johns Hopkins Med J* 131:24, 1972.

KAHN E: *Psychopathic Personalities.* New Haven, Yale University Press, 1931.

MAYER-GROSS W et al: *Clinical Psychiatry,* 3d ed. Baltimore, Williams & Wilkins, 1969.

WALTON JN (ed): *Diseases of Voluntary Muscle,* 4th ed. Boston, Little, Brown, 1981.

CHAPTER 24

NERVOUSNESS, ANXIETY, AND DEPRESSION

Nervousness, anxiety, and depression, like lassitude and fatigue, are among the most frequent disorders encountered in office and hospital practice. It might be supposed that the stresses of contemporary urban life or the prospect of real or imaginary illness are enough to induce these reactions. If they stand in clear temporal relation to a stressful event or situation such as worry over economic reverses or grief over the death of a loved one, such symptoms can be accepted as normal. Only when excessively intense, uncontrollable, or prolonged, or when the visceral derangements which accompany them are prominent do they become a matter of medical concern.

The symptoms of anxiety and depression become more difficult to understand when they occur in persons who are not being subjected to immediately stressful or unhappy experiences. One assumption has been that such experiences, if they exist at all, lie buried in the subconscious mind of the patient and that they have either been suppressed from consciousness or are part of an elaborate subjective transformation of which the patient is unaware. The relation between social stimulus and prevailing anxiety or nervousness can then be discovered only through the probings of a psychologically sophisticated physician. But once the connection is established and the problem dealt with realistically, the symptoms become understandable and either disappear or are better tolerated. This is what analytical psychiatrists speak of as the *catharsis* of a *psychoneurotic reaction*. The line of separation between psychoneurotic and normal emotional reactions is admittedly ambiguous. (These matters will be dealt with more fully in Chap. 53.)

There is still another category of nervousness, anxiety, and depression wherein the emotional states are intense and prolonged but without obvious explanation.

Such states may be overwhelming and derange these patients in all their activities. One recognizes here a more complete, pervasive *psychotic reaction*. In many such instances a genetic factor appears to operate, and the features of the illness are so stereotyped as to indicate a disease of the parts of the nervous system which control the affective, emotional life. Yet a consistent biochemical change in the blood or brain tissue has not been found, and no lesion has been discerned.

The problem confronting the physician is to recognize all the nuances of these psychological reactions and diseases which obviously shade into one another, and to determine to what extent they dominate the medical condition of the patient. Some type of therapeutic maneuver must then be initiated, varying from simple reassurance and realistic management of existing personal difficulties to suppression of symptoms by drugs. Often referral to a psychiatrist is necessary for more expert management, including electroconvulsive therapy.

In this chapter the cardinal manifestations of these emotional states will be considered, together with currently accepted views of their origins. The major diseases of which they are part are discussed in Chaps. 53 and 54.

NERVOUSNESS

By this vague term the lay person usually refers to a state of restlessness, tension, uneasy apprehension, irritability, or hyperexcitability, but it may connote other states, such as thoughts of suicide, fear of killing one's child or spouse, a distressing hallucination, a paranoid idea, or a frankly hysterical outburst. Careful inquiry as to what the patient means when complaining of nervousness is always a necessary first step.

Most often nervousness represents no more than a psychic and behavioral state in which the person is maximally challenged by difficult personal problems, and there are times in life when this is more likely to happen. For example, adolescence rarely passes without its period of turmoil as persons attempt to emancipate themselves from parental dominance or to adjust to scholastic demands or to the opposite sex. The menses are regularly accompanied by increased tension and moodiness, and the menopause may be another critical period. Some persons, because of early patterning or character formation, claim to have been nervous in all their social relationships throughout life; one should then suspect a psychoneurosis, depression, or schizophrenia, even though performance within the family unit, at school, and at work were adequate. Others complain of a recent development of nervousness, and one must consider such possibilities as an upheaval in personal affairs, the first attack or exacerbation of a psychoneurosis, an endogenous depression, an endocrine disease (hyperthyroidism, adrenal cortical disease, or corticosteroid therapy), or withdrawal from a sedative drug (alcohol, barbiturate). Some patients complain of a nervousness that attends the onset of a medical or neurologic disease; it would then appear to be secondary, occasioned by fear of disability, dependency, or death.

Nervousness, even in its simplest form, is reflected in many important activities of the human organism. There are often a mild somberness of mood, an increased tendency to tears and anger (irritability), fatigue that bears no proper relation to activity and rest, and disturbed sleep, eating, and drinking habits. Headaches may increase in number and intensity. There is a tendency to sweat, tremble, be aware of heart action, feel a bit "queer in the head" or giddy, have an upset stomach, and urinate more often, though these autonomic accompaniments are seldom as conspicuous as in anxiety neurosis. Thus, it would appear that what is being described here as nervousness and anxiety constitute a graded series of reactions and that the latter in many instances is only a more intense and protracted form of the former (see Chap. 53).

THE ANXIETY STATE

Anxiety is "the fundamental phenomenon and central problem of the neuroses . . . a nodal point, linking up all kinds of most important questions, a riddle of which the solution must cast a flood of light upon our whole mental life" (Freud). From the viewpoint of the social historian, anxiety is thought to be the most prominent mental characteristic of Occidental civilization. These com-

ments should convey some notion of the broad implications of this reaction.

The more strictly medical meaning of the term *anxiety*, and the one used in this chapter, is a state characterized by a subjective feeling of fear and uneasy anticipation (apprehension), usually with a definite topical content and associated with the physiologic accompaniments of strong emotion, i.e., breathlessness, choking sensation, palpitation, restlessness, increased muscular tension, tightness in the chest, giddiness, trembling, sweating, and flushing. By topical content is meant the idea, person, or object about which the person is anxious. The several vasomotor and visceral alterations that underlie the symptoms are mediated through the autonomic nervous system, particularly the sympathetic part of it, and involve also the thyroid and adrenal glands.

FORMS OF ANXIETY

Anxiety is manifested in acute episodes, each lasting several minutes, or as a protracted state that may last for weeks, months, or years. In the *acute attacks*, or *panics* as they are called, patients are plunged into an inexplicable mental state in which they fear they will die, lose their reason or self-control, become insane, or commit some horrible crime. They are breathless, choke, sweat, tremble, and have intense palpitation, gastric distress, and anorexia. As a persistent protracted state they experience fluctuating degrees of nervousness, restlessness, irritability, fatigue, insomnia, intolerance of physical exertion, and tension headaches. Discrete anxiety attacks and chronic states of anxiety merge into one another.

Episodic anxiety without disorder of mood (i.e., depression) is usually classified as *anxiety neurosis*. The chronic form with prominent exercise intolerance is called *neurocirculatory asthenia*. Anxiety may, however, be combined with other somatic symptoms in hysteria and may be the restraining factor in *phobic neurosis*. Persistent anxiety with insomnia, lassitude, and fatigue, regardless of mood, should always raise the suspicion of a *depressive psychosis*, especially when it begins in middle adult life or beyond. Panic attacks may also occur at the beginning of a schizophrenic illness. Both anxiety and depression are prominent features of the syndrome of posttraumatic nervous instability (see pages 126 and 610).

Thus, the differential diagnosis of an anxiety state includes all the major syndromes in psychiatry. Often it is but one component of a far more serious condition, one which may result in suicide or some other antisocial act. Also when the psychic counterparts of fear and apprehension are absent, the visceral symptoms alone should arouse suspicion of thyrotoxicosis, corticosteroid overdosage, pheochromocytoma, hypoglycemia, and menopause.

PHYSIOLOGIC AND PSYCHOLOGICAL BASIS

The cause, mechanism, and biologic meaning of anxiety have been the subjects of much speculation, and completely satisfactory explanations are not available. The psychologist regards anxiety as anticipatory behavior, i.e., a state of uneasiness about something which may happen in the future. William McDougall spoke of it as "an emotional state arising when a continuing strong desire seems likely to miss its goal." The primary emotion, somewhat muted perhaps, is that of fear, and its arousal under conditions not overtly threatening may be explained as a conditioned response to some recondite component of a formerly threatening stimulus.

The psychoanalytic school looks upon anxiety as a response to a situation that in some manner undermines the security of the individual. The topical content or cause of potential danger lies in the unconscious mind. The postulated danger is internal rather than external; a primitive drive has been aroused that is not compatible with current social practices, and it can be satisfied only at risk of harm to the person.

Physicians have searched for evidence of impairments of visceral function without success. The asthenic patient with a neurocirculatory disorder is in poor physical condition and has an elevated blood lactate level in the resting state and after exercise, and infusions of lactic acid are said to make the symptoms worse. The patient will not tolerate the work or exercise needed to build up stamina. The urinary excretion of epinephrine has been found elevated in some patients; in others, there is an increased urinary excretion of norepinephrine and its metabolites. Aldosterone excretion is raised to two or three times the normal level during intense anxiety. Medical students experiencing fear and anxiety while preparing for an examination also excrete increased amounts of aldosterone. The interpretation of these data (whether primary or secondary) is not certain, but it is becoming increasingly evident that prolonged and diffuse anxiety is a pattern of behavior related to certain biochemical abnormalities of blood, and probably of the brain.

DEPRESSION

There are few persons who do not experience periods of discouragement and despair. As with nervousness and anxiety, depression of mood that is appropriate to a given situation in life is a natural reaction and seldom is the basis of medical concern. Patients in these situations tend to seek help only when they cannot control their grief or unhappiness, but there are numerous instances in which these symptoms assert themselves for reasons that are not apparent. Often the symptoms are interpreted as a medical illness, bringing the patient first to the internist. Sometimes another disease is found (such as chronic hepatitis, brucellosis or other infection, or postinfluenzal asthenia) in which chronic fatigue is confused with depression, but often the opposite pertains, i.e., an endogenous depression is itself the essential problem even when there has been evidence earlier of a viral or bacterial infection. Since the risk of suicide is not inconsiderable in depression, an error in diagnosis may be life-threatening.

Information about depression, like that of all psychiatric syndromes, is gained from three sources: the history obtained from the patient, the history obtained from the family or a close friend, and the findings on examination.

From the patient and the family it is learned that the patient has been "feeling unwell," "low in spirits," "blue," "glum," "unhappy," or "morbid." There has been a change in emotional reactions of which the patient may not be fully aware. Activities that were formerly pleasurable are no longer so. Often, however, change in mood is less conspicuous than reduction in psychic and physical energy, and it is this type of case that is so often misdiagnosed by internists and neurologists. Fatigue is almost invariable; not uncommonly, it is worse in the morning after a night of restless sleep. The words "loss of pep," "weak," "tired," "no energy to work," "my job seems more trying and difficult" appear in the language of the patient. The outlook is pessimistic. The patient is preoccupied with uncontrollable worry over trivialities. With excessive worry the ability to think with accustomed efficiency is reduced; there is complaint that the mind does not function properly, of being forgetful and unable to concentrate. If the patient is naturally of suspicious nature, paranoid tendencies may assert themselves.

Particularly troublesome in medical diagnosis is the patient's tendency to hypochondriasis. Indeed, most cases formerly diagnosed as hypochondriasis are now regarded as depression. Pain from whatever cause—a stiff joint, a toothache, fleeting abdominal pains, or other troubles such as constipation, frequency of urination, insomnia, pruritus, burning tongue, weight loss—may become an obsessive focus of complaint. The patient passes from doctor to doctor seeking relief from symptoms that would not trouble the average person, and no amount of reassurance relieves his or her state of mind. The anxiety and depressed mood of these persons may be obscured by their preoccupation with visceral functions.

When examined, the patient's facial expression is often plaintive, troubled, pained, or anguished. The attitude and manner of the patient betray a prevailing mood of depression, discouragement, and despondency. In other words, the affective response, which is the outward expression of feeling, is consistent with the depressed mood. During the interview the patient's eyes may be tearful. Occasionally, such patients cry openly. In some there is a kind of immobility of the face that mimics parkinsonism, though others are restless and agitated (pacing, wringing their hands, etc.). Occasionally the patient will smile, but the smile impresses one as more a social gesture than an expression of feeling.

The stream of speech, from which the ideational content is determined, is slow. At times the patient is mute and speaks neither spontaneously nor in response to questions. Again there may be a long pause between questions and answers. The latter are brief and may be monosyllabic. There is a paucity of ideas. The retardation extends to all topics of conversation and affects movement of limbs as well. The most extreme forms of decreased motor activity, rarely seen in the medical clinic, border on stupor.

Content of speech is found to be abnormal if examined carefully. Conversation is replete with pessimistic thoughts, fears, expressions of unworthiness, inadequacy, inferiority, and sometimes guilt. In severe depressions, bizarre ideas, delusions about the body ("blood drying up," "bowels are blocked with cement," "I am half dead") may be expressed.

ETIOLOGY OR MECHANISM

Three theories have emerged concerning the cause of the pathologic depressive state: (1) the endogenous form is hereditary; (2) a biochemical abnormality results in a periodic depletion in the brain of serotonin and norepinephrine; (3) a basic fault in character development exists. These theories will be elaborated in Chap. 54.

It is the authors' belief that depression is one of the most commonly overlooked diagnoses in clinical medicine. Part of the trouble is with the word itself, which implies being unhappy about something. The persistent or recurrent endogenous depression should be suspected in all chronic states of ill health, hypochondriasis, disability that exceeds manifest signs of a medical disease, neurasthenia, chronic pain syndromes, and suicide attempts. Inasmuch as recovery is the rule, suicide is a tragedy for which the medical profession must often share responsibility.

REFERENCES

CASSIDY WL et al: Clinical observations in manic depressive disease. *JAMA* 164:1535, 1953.

FREUD S: On the grounds for detaching a particular syndrome from neurasthenia under the description "anxiety neurosis," in *Standard Edition of the Complete Psychological Works of Sigmund Freud.* London, Hogarth Press, 1962, vol 3, p 90.

KLERMAN GL: Overview of affective disorders, in Kaplan HI, Freedman AM, Sadock BJ (eds): *Comprehensive Textbook of Psychiatry,* 3d ed. Baltimore, Williams & Wilkins, 1980, Chap 18.1, pp 1305-1319.

WHEELER EO et al: Neurocirculatory asthenia (anxiety neurosis, effort syndrome, neurasthenia). *JAMA* 142:878, 1950.

CHAPTER 25

THE LIMBIC LOBES AND THE NEUROLOGY OF EMOTION

The medical literature is replete with references to illnesses believed to be based on emotional disorders. Careful examination of clinical records reveals that a diversity of phenomena are being so classified: anxiety states, cycles of depression and mania, nervous reactions to distressing life situations, so-called psychosomatic diseases, and illnesses of obscure nature. Obviously great license is being taken with the term *emotional,* referring no doubt to its indiscriminate nonmedical usage. Such ambiguity discourages neurologic analysis. Nevertheless, in certain clinical states patients appear to be hyperemotional under conditions that normally are not conducive to emotionality, and apathetic under conditions that are exciting. It is with these disturbances that the following remarks are mainly concerned. First, however, one must be clear as to what is meant by emotion.

According to the *Dictionary of Psychology* (Drever) emotion is a complex state of the organism involving certain types of bodily changes (mainly visceral and under the control of the autonomic nervous system) in association with a mental state of excitement or perturbation, and leading usually to an impulse to action or to a certain type of behavior. If the emotion is intense, there may ensue some disturbance of intellectual functions, viz., a measure of dissociation of normal sequences of ideas and actions, and a tendency toward a more automatic behavior of ungraded, stereotyped character.

In its most easily recognized human form, emotion is initiated by a stimulus (real or imagined), the perception of which involves recognition, memory, and specific associations. The emotional state that is engendered is mirrored in a psychic experience, i.e., a feeling, or affect, that is known only to the patient and possibly to others through the patient's communication or by judgment of his or her behavioral manifestations. The

latter, which are in part hormonal-visceral and in part motor, may show themselves in facial expression, attitude of the body, vocalizations, or directed voluntary activity. Subdivided, the components of emotion appear to consist of (1) the stimulus, (2) the affect or feeling, (3) the autonomic-visceral changes, and (4) the impulse to a certain type of activity. In many cases of neurologic disease, however, it is not possible to separate these components from one another, and to emphasize one of them does no more than indicate the particular bias of the examiner.

ANATOMIC RELATIONSHIPS

The occurrence of emotional reactions in the course of disease has been regularly attended by lesions in certain parts of the nervous system. These have been grouped under the term *limbic* and are among the most complex and least understood parts of the nervous system. The Latin word *limbus* means a border or margin. Credit for introducing the term limbic to neurology is usually given to Broca (of aphasia fame) who used it to describe the ring of gray matter (formed primarily by the cingulate and parahippocampal gyri) that encircles the upper brainstem. Actually Thomas Willis had pictured this region of the brain and referred to it as the limbus in 1664. Broca preferred his term *le grand lobe limbique* to *rhinencephalon,* which refers more specifically to structures related to the olfactory sense. Neuroanatomists of more recent times have affirmed his position and have extended the boundaries of the *limbic lobe* to include the subcallosal gyrus as well as the cingulate and parahippocampal gyri, and the underlying hippocampal formation and dentate gyrus. The term *limbic system* has an even wider designation; in addition to all parts of the limbic lobe, it includes a number of associated subcortical nuclei, such as those of the amygdaloid complex, septal region, hypothalamus, anterior thalamus, and upper midbrain.

To visualize the relationship of the limbic structures, it is useful to imagine two adjacent rings of tissue molded around the neck of the outpouching cerebral vesicle as it forms during embryonic life. The simple anatomical relationship is distorted to some extent by

the growth of the thalamus, the expansion of the temporal lobe and the development of the corpus callosum which penetrates and divides the two rings.

If one looks at Fig. 25-1 and begins at the caudal part of the orbital surface of the frontal lobe, near the midline, the next structures posteriorly are the uncus,

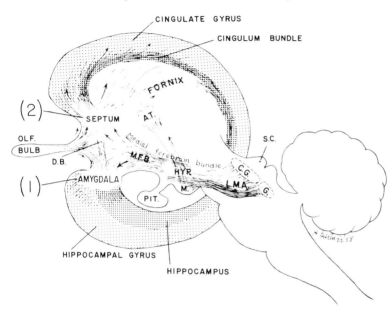

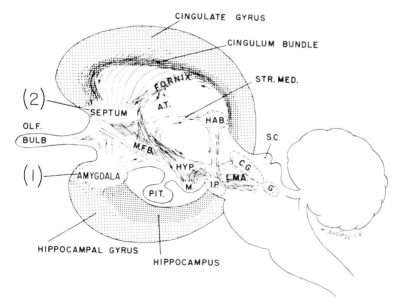

Figure 25-1

The limbic lobe and its major connections with the hypothalamus and midbrain, with emphasis on the origin and destination of the medial forebrain bundle. Concentric areas of archicortex and mesocortex are portrayed in dark and light stipple, respectively. Upper. Afferent pathways to rostral limbic structures. Lower. Efferent pathways from these structures. AT, anterior thalamic nuclei; CG, central gray of midbrain; DB, diagonal band of Broca; G, dorsal and ventral tegmental nuclei of Gudden; hab., habenular nuclei; IP, interpeduncular nucleus; LMA, limbic midbrain area (of Nauta); M, mamillary body; pit., pituitary gland; SC, superior colliculus; str. med., stria medullaris thalami. (From MacLean.)

which overlies the amygdaloid nuclei, and then the hippocampal formation, which can be followed backward and upward over the splenium of the corpus callosum. The hippocampal formation can be traced forward into the subcallosal and septal areas thus completing the inner or more rhinencephalic circle of gray matter. The outer ring of limbic structures is more complex. Beginning again at the base of the frontal lobe, but more laterally, is a region that can be followed posteriorly to the insula, and then to the hippocampal and parahippocampal gyri. These structures curve upward into the cingulate gyrus, which is continuous anteriorly with the paraolfactory gyrus. These gyri merge laterally with the medial parts of the temporal, parietal, and frontal lobes.

The cytologic arrangements of the two rings of limbic cortex clearly distinguish them from the neocortex (isocortex) and from one another. The neocortex, as stated in Chap. 21, differentiates into a characteristic six-layered structure. In contrast, the outer ring of the limbic cortex, or *mesocortex*, is less elaborately structured; the inner ring, or *allocortex*, differs even more, being composed of irregularly arranged aggregates of nerve cells that tend to be trilaminate. The hippocampal formation has a highly specialized architecture, consisting of two interlocking convolutions, the dentate gyrus and hippocampus proper; the latter extends via the subiculum (gateway) to the hippocampal gyrus. The main component of the hippocampal formation is a band of pyramidal neurons, one segment of which (Sommer's sector) is known to be especially susceptible to hypoxia. The amygdaloid complex, a nuclear component of the rhinencephalic part of the limbic system, also has a unique composition, consisting of several separable nuclei each with special connections to other limbic structures.

The connections between neocortex and the limbic lobes, between the individual components of the limbic lobes, and between the limbic lobes and the hypothalamus and midbrain reveal some of the potential functional relationships. The medial forebrain bundle is of particular importance. It is a complex system of ascending and descending fibers that connect the orbital parts of the frontal lobes (preoptic), the septal nuclei, the hypothalamus, and certain nuclei in the midbrain and pons. Another important tract consists of ascending fibers from the lateral hypothalamus which diverge into two mainstreams, one that turns laterally into the region of the amygdaloid nuclei and another that continues rostrally and medially into the septal area of the inner ring. The septal nuclei, in turn, project by a system of fibers to the hippocampal formation via the fimbria of the fornix. Efferent fibers from the hypothalamus descend in the medial forebrain bundle through the ventral tegmentum of the midbrain to the dorsal and ventral tegmental nuclei. This system, of which the hypothalamus is the central part, has been designated by Nauta as the *septohypothalamomesencephalic continuum*. Through this system flow the principal pathways connecting the hippocampus and amygdala with the thalamic nuclei and brainstem reticular formation.

There are many other interrelationships between the various parts of the limbic system, only a few of which can be indicated here. The preoptic (medial orbital-frontal) cortex projects onto the amygdala, which in turn projects by way of the stria terminalis to the nuclei of the stria terminalis and anterior hypothalamus. The amygdaloid nuclei send fibers to the hippocampal formation; and other fibers enter the latter structure via the fornix from the septal nuclei. The amygdala also projects to the dorsomedial nucleus of the thalamus via the inferior thalamic peduncle, and to specific cortical regions.

The main efferent pathway from the hippocampus is the fornix, which terminates in the mammillary body and septal and preoptic regions. The bundle of Vicq d'Azyr connects these latter parts with the anterior nuclei of the thalamus, which in turn project to the cingulate gyrus; from the latter structure, impulses can reach the hippocampus via the cingulum, thus forming another circuit. The main efferent pathway from the outer mesocortical limbic ring is the cingulum, which loops around the interior of the ring, concentric to the curvature of the corpus callosum; it connects various parts of the limbic lobe to one another and projects also to the striatum and to certain brainstem nuclei.

PHYSIOLOGY OF THE LIMBIC SYSTEM

The functional properties of the limbic structures first became known during the third and fourth decades of this century. From ablation and stimulation studies, Cannon, Bard, and others established the fact that the hypothalamus contained the suprasegmental integrations of the autonomic nervous system, both the sympathetic and parasympathetic parts (see Chap. 26). Soon after, anatomists found efferent pathways from the hypothalamus to the neural structures subserving the segmental parasympathetic and sympathetic reflexes. Bard localized the central regulatory apparatus for emotional reactions as well as that for respiration, wakefulness, and sexual activity in the hypothalamus. The hypothalamus was also found to contain neurosecretory cells, which controlled the secretion of the pituitary hormones, and special sensory devices for the control of hunger, thirst, body temperature and levels of circulating electrolytes. Gradually there has emerged the idea of a hypothalamic-pituitary-autonomic nervous system that is essential to both the basic homeostatic and emergency reactions of the organism.

The impressions of the great psychologists of the nineteenth century that autonomic reactions were an essential motor part of the instinctual emotions were corroborated. In fact, for a time, it was proposed that emotional experience was merely the awareness of these visceral activities (the James-Lange theory of emotion). The fallacy of this theory became evident when it was demonstrated by Sherrington that the capacity to manifest emotional changes remained after all visceral afferent fibers had been interrupted.

Although emotion involves the same perceptive-cognitive activities as does any nonemotional sensorimotor experience, it was realized that the important difference relates to its prominent visceral effects, and the particular behavioral reactions that are evoked. Clearly, specific parts of the nervous system must be utilized.

As mentioned above, Bard, in 1928, first produced "sham rage" in cats by removal of the cerebral hemispheres, leaving the hypothalamus and brainstem intact. This is a state in which the animal reacts to all stimuli with an expression of intense anger and the signs of autonomic overactivity. In subsequent studies, Bard and Mountcastle found that only if the ablations involved the amygdaloid nuclei on both sides would sham rage be produced; removal of all the neocortex, but sparing the limbic lobe, resulted in a placid animal. Interestingly, in the macaque monkey, a normally aggressive and recalcitrant animal, removal of the amygdaloid nuclei bilaterally greatly reduced the reactions of fear and anger.

On the basis of the physiologic observations of Cannon and Bard and his knowledge of neuroanatomy, Papez postulated that the limbic parts of the brain "elaborate the functions of central emotion as well as participate in emotional expression." Their intermediate position permits them to establish rich to-and-fro connections with the hypothalamus on its inner side and to transmit neocortical effects coming from its outer side.

The experimental observations of MacLean indicated that the functions of the limbic system are much more complex than was first believed; in reality it consists of two circuits or systems (see above, under "Anatomic Relationships"), the outer subserving mainly parasympathetic functions and the inner, sympathetic

functions, both capable of being activated by ascending fiber systems and modifiable by neocortical-brainstem fiber systems. The physiologic effects of stimulating these regions and of ablating them have established their role as the *visceral brain*, to use the terminology of MacLean.

The discovery that the hippocampal formation and underlying white matter is also important in memory emerged more recently through the observations of Scoville and Milner and others who observed the effects of medial temporal lobectomies or infarction of these parts (see page 308). Why this part of the brain should be essential to memory function is indeed perplexing. The only explanation that comes to mind is that in animals at least, the memory of olfactory experiences is vital to survival and the propagation of the species.

Another aspect of limbic function has come to light as information is being acquired about neurotransmitters, and more particularly, about the distribution of amines in the central nervous system. The level of norepinephrine is highest in the hypothalamus and next in the medial parts of the limbic system, and at least 70 percent of it is concentrated in axon terminals of neurons which lie in the medulla and pons (see Chap. 18). The axons of other ascending fibers, especially those coming from the reticular formation of the midbrain and terminating in the amygdala and septal nuclei as well as in lateral parts of the limbic lobe, are rich in serotonin. The axons of neurons in the ventral tegmental parts of the midbrain which ascend in the medial forebrain bundle and the nigrostriatal pathway contain much of the brain dopamine. Also notable is the fact that the zinc content of the limbic system is the highest of any part of the nervous system.

EMOTIONAL DISTURBANCES DUE TO DISEASES INVOLVING THE LIMBIC SYSTEM

Nearly all the foregoing ideas about the role of the limbic system have come from experimentation in laboratory animals. Only in relatively recent years have neurologists, primed by knowledge of these studies, begun to observe in their patients emotional disturbances in association with disease of limbic structures. These clinical observations, summarized in the following pages, begin to form an interesting chapter in neurology. The authors have listed the most readily recognized derangements of emotion in Table 25-1. The list is tentative, and our understanding of many of these states is incomplete. As knowledge of emotional disorders increases, it will undoubtedly bring together large segments of psychiatry and neurology.

EMOTIONAL DISTURBANCES IN HALLUCINATING AND DELUDED PATIENTS

These are best portrayed by the patient with a florid delirium. Threatened by imaginary figures and hearing their admonitions, which seem real and inescapable, the patient trembles, cringes, cowers, asks for protection, and displays the full picture of terror. Assuming the reality of the hallucinations, the patient's affect, emotional reaction, and vegetative and somatic motor responses are altogether appropriate. We have seen a patient slash his wrists and another try to drown himself in response to hallucinatory voices that told them of their worthlessness and the shame they would bring upon their families.

The abnormality under these circumstances is in the field of disordered perception, and we have no reason to believe that there is a derangement of the mechanism for emotional expression. That the latter may be more readily activated in such an individual than in a normal one cannot be discounted, however, for the degree of sweating, palpitation, trembling, insomnia, tachycardia, and hyperpyrexia are so excessive and prolonged.

An emotional outburst, seemingly inappropriate or excessive in the patient's environmental setting, is a common occurrence in a psychotic person. Here the patient is deluded but experiences intense emotion and reacts appropriately. Believing that somebody is threatening him or her, the patient may in a state of fury injure or kill the imagined tormentor. Again the emotional state becomes comprehensible once the content of the delusion has been divulged.

However, many psychotic patients whose hallucinations and delusions persist for months or years appear to become inured to them. No longer does the natural emotional reaction and impulse follow. Either the patient denies having the hallucinations or appears to disregard them. Perhaps we observe here the emergence of the bland affect and less appropriate emotional reaction of the schizophrenic. We have had occasion, in patients with alcoholic auditory hallucinosis, to trace this state from the early terrifying hallucinosis with appropriate emotional response to a state indistinguishable from paranoid schizophrenia with inappropriate reaction (see Chap. 40).

In these aforementioned conditions the experienced clinician appreciates that although the emotional outburst is the overt manifestation of abnormal nervous functioning, the basic abnormality is in the sphere of perception and cognition. The emotional state is secondary.

DISINHIBITION OF EMOTIONAL EXPRESSION

Emotional Lability It is a commonplace clinical experience that cerebral diseases of many types, and seemingly without respect to location, weaken the mechanism of control of emotional expression that has been acquired over years of maturation. To be grown up means that one can inhibit one's emotions; not that one has less feeling with aging, but rather that it can be hidden from others. The degree to which this pertains varies with sex and ethnicity. In certain cultures, women are permitted to cry in public, but men are not. Men and women of Mediterranean races exhibit their feelings more openly than Anglo-Saxons.

A patient whose cerebrum has been damaged by a single vascular lesion may suffer the humiliation of crying in public upon meeting an old friend or hearing the national anthem. Less often a mildly amusing remark or an attempt to tell a funny story may cause excessively prolonged and loud laughter. There may also be easy vacillation from one state to another; this is called *emo-*

Table 25-1
Neurology of emotional disturbances

I. Disturbances of emotionality due to:
   A. Perceptual abnormalities (illusions and hallucinations)
   B. Cognitive derangements (delusions)
II. Disinhibition of emotional expression
   A. Emotional lability
   B. Pathologic laughter and crying
III. Rage reactions and aggressivity
IV. Apathy and placidity
   A. Klüver-Bucy syndrome
   B. Other syndromes
V. Hypersexuality
VI. "Diencephalic" epilepsy
VII. Endogenous fear, anxiety, depression, and euphoria

tional lability and has for more than a century been accepted as a sign of "organic brain disease." Perhaps lesions of the frontal lobes more than those of other parts of the brain are conducive to this state, but the authors are unaware of a critical clinicoanatomic study that substantiates this impression. It is certainly a frequent accompaniment of diffuse cerebral diseases such as the Alzheimer-senile-dementia complex, but of course these diseases also involve the limbic cortex.

Pathologic (Forced, Spasmodic) Laughter and Crying
This form of disordered emotional expression, whether in the guise of uncontrollable laughter or of crying, has been well recognized since the late nineteenth century. Numerous references to these conditions (the *Zwangslachen* and *Zwangsweinen* of German neurologists and the *rire et pleurer spasmodiques* of the French) are to be found in the writings of Oppenheim, von Monakow, and Wilson.

The terms in the heading of this section specify a state in which involuntary, irresistible laughing or crying, or both, have entered the foreground of a clinical syndrome. The depression of spirits with tearfulness and irritability that so often follows chronic diseases of the nervous system and also the facile moods and outbursts of the neurotic are not included. Forced laughing and crying always signify a pathologic substratum in the brain, either diffuse or focal; hence it stands as a syndrome of multiple causes. It may occur with degenerative and vascular diseases of the brain and no doubt is the direct result of them, but often their diffuse nature precludes useful topographic analysis and clinicoanatomic correlation. More instructive in this regard are those cases in which a vascular, degenerative or demyelinative process is discretely localized, but unfortunately few well-documented clinical cases of these types have been studied by proper anatomic methods.

The best examples of pathologic laughing and crying are provided by lacunar vascular disease and less often by amyotrophic lateral sclerosis and multiple sclerosis. It may also be part of the residue of the diffuse or more widespread lesions of hypoxic-hypotensive encephalopathy, cerebral trauma, or encephalitis. Most often by far, a sudden hemiplegia or double hemiplegia sets the stage for the pathologic emotionality which emerges as part of the syndrome of pseudobulbar palsy (see page 41). In the latter there is a striking incongruity between the loss of voluntary movements of muscles innervated by the motor nuclei of the lower pons and medulla (inability to forcefully close the eyes, elevate and retract the corners of the mouth, open and close the mouth, chew, swallow, phonate, articulate, and move

the tongue) and the preservation of movement of the same muscles in yawning, coughing, throat clearing, and spasmodic laughing or crying (reflexive pontomedullary activities). In some such cases, on the slightest provocation or sometimes for no apparent reason, the patient is thrown into hilarious laughter that may last for many minutes to the point of exhaustion, or, far more often, the opposite happens—the patient, at the mere mention of family or the sight of the doctor begins to cry uncontrollably. The severity of the emotional incontinence or the ease with which it is provoked does not correspond precisely with the severity of the faciobulbar paralysis. There are, however, patients with forced crying and laughing in whom voluntary control of the facial and bulbar muscles remains virtually intact or at most there is but a slight unilateral facial weakness. Therefore the pathologic emotional state cannot be equated with pseudobulbar palsy even though there is a strong tendency in that direction.

Much interest has centered on the patient's affect, or feeling, while in the throes of involuntary laughter and crying. Are these states actuated by appropriate stimuli, and once initiated do they then induce the appropriate emotion? There are no simple answers to these questions. One problem, of course, is to determine what constitutes an appropriate stimulus. Virtually always the emotional response is set off by some stimulus but in most cases it is trifling, or at least it appears so to the physician; merely addressing the patient or making some casual remark in the presence of the patient may suffice. Certainly in such cases the emotional response is out of all proportion to the stimulus. As to the affect, Oppenheim and others stated that these patients need not feel sad when crying or mirthful when laughing, and at least in some cases this is in agreement with our experience. Other patients, however, report a congruence of affect and expression.

Noteworthy also are the invariability of the initial motor response and the relative dedifferentiation of the emotional reaction. Laughter and crying, as they proceed, may merge with one another. Poeck puts great emphasis on the latter point, but it does not seem surprising when one considers how close are the two forms of emotional expression. Some normal persons cry when happy and smile when sad. More impressive to us is the fact that in some patients with pseudobulbar palsy, laughing and crying are the only available forms of emotional expression; intermediate phenomena, such as smiling and frowning, are lost. Impressive also are the patients with complete loss of motor function, in whom spasmodic laughing or crying, or a caricature thereof, is the only available form of expression, emotional or voluntary.

Wilson, in his discussion of the anatomic basis and mechanism of this state, points out that laughter and crying involve the same facial, vocal, and respiratory musculature and have similar visceral accompaniments (dilatation of facial vessels, secretion of tears, etc.). Two major supranuclear pathways are involved in the control of the pontomedullary mechanisms of facial and other movements required in laughter and crying. One is the familiar corticobulbar pahway, from motor cortex through the posterior limb of the internal capsule, for the control of volitional movements; the other is a more anterior frontopontomedullary connection, for emotional expression. The latter is believed to descend near the knee of the internal capsule and to contain facilitatory and inhibitory fibers, but it has not been accurately traced to the lower pons. Unilateral involvement of this latter tract leaves the opposite side of the face under volitional control but paretic during laughter and crying (emotional facial paralysis) and the opposite is observed with a unilateral corticobulbar lesion. Wilson's argument, based to some extent on clinicopathologic evidence, assumed that the descending motor pathways which naturally inhibit the expression of the emotions were interrupted, but he could not decide where. Almost 40 years later, Poeck and Pillieri, after reviewing all the published pathologic anatomy in 30 verified cases, were able to do no more than conclude that supranuclear motor pathways are always involved with loss of some control mechanism lying in the brainstem between thalamus and medulla. However, this clinical state is observed in amyotrophic lateral sclerosis where the corticobulbar tracts may be involved at a cortical and subcortical level. The lesions are bilateral in most instances (see references under Poeck).

A rare but probably closely related syndrome is *le fou rire prodromique* (prodromal laughing madness) of Féré, in which uncontrollable laughter begins abruptly and is followed after hours or a longer time by hemiplegia. Martin cites examples where patients laughed themselves to death. Again the pathologic anatomy is unsettled. Laughing and (less often) crying may occur also as a manifestation of epileptic seizures, usually of psychomotor type. Daly and Mulder have referred to these as "gelastic" seizures.

AGGRESSIVE BEHAVIOR, RAGE REACTIONS, VIOLENCE

Viewed ethnologically, aggressivity is an integral part of social behavior. During early life the emergence of aggressive action enables the individual to secure a position in the family and later in an ever-widening social circle. Individual differences are noteworthy from infancy on, and males are generally more aggressive than females.

The degree to which excessively aggressive behavior is tolerated varies in different cultures. In most civilized societies, tantrum behavior, rage reactions, and destructiveness are not condoned, and one of the principal objectives of training and education is the suppression and sublimation of such behavior. The rate at which this developmental process proceeds varies from one individual to another. In some, especially males, it is not complete until 25 to 30 years of age (see Chap. 27).

That groundless outbreaks of unbridled rage may present as the main manifestation of disease is an idea not fully appreciated by the medical profession. Such patients with little provocation may change from an entirely reasonable state to one of the wildest rage, with a blindly furious impulse to violence and destruction. They charge at those around them, strike, kick, bite, and throttle whomever they can reach; they smash every object which they can lay hands on, tear their clothes, shout, and curse; their eyes flash and roll; their faces are suffused with blood, and their hearts beat violently. Every incoming sensation excites them to the point of frenzy. On attempting to subdue such a person, one finds that he or she has the strength of five people. In such states patients appear out of contact with reality and are impervious to all argument or pleading. As well as one can tell, they are experiencing anger appropriate to their actions. What is abnormal is the provocation of the attack by some trifling event and violence out of all proportion to the stimulus, but there are examples also of dissociation of affect and behavior, in which the patient may spit, cry out, attack, or bite without seeming to be angry. This is especially true of the mentally retarded.

Rage reactions of the intensity described above may be encountered in the following medical settings: (1) as part of a psychomotor seizure, (2) as an episodic reaction without recognizable seizures or other neurologic abnormality, or (3) in the course of some recognizable acute or chronic neurologic disease. With reference to the last, several of our patients have had evidence of disease of the left cerebral hemisphere, and Fisher has remarked upon anger associated with dysphasia of the Wernicke type. Placidity is more frequent with lesions of the right (nondominant) hemisphere. However, the crucial structure in the genesis of these reactions appears to be the amygdaloid nuclear complex. Bilateral ablation of these nuclei causes "sham rage" in cats, as was remarked earlier; in human beings these and related limbic structures are also of special importance (see below).

Rage in Psychomotor Seizures   According to Gastaut et al., a directed attack of uncontrollable rage may occur both as part of a seizure and as an interictal phenomenon. Some patients describe a gradual heightening of emotional excitability for 2 to 3 days, either before or after a seizure, before bursting into a rage. Certainly such attacks have been observed, but they are not common, as pointed out by Gloor and Feindel. When aggressive behavior occurs as part of a temporal lobe seizure, it is usually in the late stages of the attack and is part of the behavioral automatism, brief in duration, and poorly directed (see page 215). Usually the lesion is in the temporal lobe of the dominant hemisphere. Similarly, a feeling of rage or severe anger is rare as an ictal emotion—much less common than feelings of fear, sadness, or pleasure (only 17 cases of anger among 165 patients with ictal emotion were reported by Williams). Geschwind emphasizes the frequency of a profound deepening of the patient's emotional experiences in temporal lobe epilepsy.

Rage Attacks without Visible Seizure   In some instances of this type the patient has always been hotheaded, intolerant of frustration, and impulsive, exhibiting behavior that would be classed as sociopathic (Chap. 55). There are others, however, who, at certain periods of life, usually adolescence or early adulthood, begin to have episodes of wild, aggressive behavior. A small amount of alcohol or some other drug may set them off. One suspects epilepsy but cannot elicit a history of recognizable seizure, and the EEG is either normal or nonspecifically abnormal. In a few such patients where the aggressive action has caused serious injury to others (or homicide), depth electrodes have been placed in the amygdaloid nuclear complex and seizure discharges recorded. Attacks of excitement and various autonomic accompaniments have been aroused by stimulation of the same regions, and the abnormal behavior has in some instances been relieved by electrocoagulation. Mark and Ervin have documented a number of impressive examples of this type of "discontrol syndrome."

Violent Behavior in Acute or Chronic Neurologic Disease From time to time one encounters patients in whom intense excitement, rage, and aggressivity begin abruptly in association with an acute neurologic disease. One of our patients, who was brought to the hospital in coma and with bloody cerebrospinal fluid after an occipital

injury, became exceedingly violent as he regained consciousness and could only be controlled by the use of restraints and heavy sedation. When he died several days later, the medial portions of the orbital and temporal lobes were found to be reduced to a hemorrhagic pulp. Hemorrhagic leukoencephalitis and herpes simplex encephalitis rarely have had the same effect. Akert and Hess and Poeck and Pillieri have described cases of this type with a ruptured aneurysm of the circle of Willis and a hypophyseal adenoma (see Poeck for references).

Of interest also in this connection are the effects of slow-growing tumors of the temporal lobe. Of 18 such cases with mental disorder reported by Malamud, several had fits of rage; all the latter were cases of temporal lobe glioma. Other patients harboring such tumors were without rage reactions but exhibited a clinical picture resembling schizophrenia. It is noteworthy that eight of his nine patients with temporal lobe glioma also had seizures. Zeman and King, Poeck and Pillieri, Cushing, Dott, Alpers, MacLean and Bingley have reported other examples (see Poeck for references). The anteromedial part of the left temporal lobe has been the site of the tumor in the majority of cases, but the hypothalamus and fornices were involved in a few. Falconer and Serafetinides have described temporal lobe cases with rage reactions in which there was a hamartoma or sclerotic focus in this region. However, the precise anatomy has not been demarcated.

PLACIDITY AND APATHY

In our experience the most frequent of all psychobehavioral alterations in patients with cerebral disease is a quantitative reduction in all activity. There are fewer thoughts, fewer words uttered, fewer movements per unit of time. That this is not a purely motor phenomenon is disclosed in conversation wherein the patient seems to think more slowly, to make fewer associations with a given idea, and to exhibit less inquisitiveness and interest. This reduction in psychomotor activity is recognized as a personality change by the family.

Depending upon how this state is viewed, it may be interpreted as a heightened threshold to stimulation, inattentiveness and inability to maintain an attentive attitude, impaired thinking, apathy, or lack of impulse (abulia). All are correct in a sense, for each represents a different aspect of the reduced mental activity. Clinicoanatomic correlates are inexact, but bilateral interruption of the medial inferior frontal connections are sometimes observed to result in a striking lack of impulse, spontaneity, and conation, out of proportion to thinking, e.g., akinetic mutism. In this state we would assume the apathy and placidity to be secondary to reduced impulse.

Quite apart from this abulic syndrome, which has already been discussed in relation to lesions of the frontal lobes (Chap. 21), there is another clinical state where a lively, sometimes volatile, person has been rendered placid by a disease of the nervous system. The most consistent changes of this type follow bilateral frontal leukotomy. If the lesions interrupt the anteromedial frontothalamic connections, anxiety, depression, and agitation immediately are eliminated but always at the expense of certain personality alterations such as indifference, lack of concern, and superficiality of thinking. These effects, too, have been discussed in relation to the frontal lobes. Barris and Schuman have documented states of extreme placidity in lesions of the anterior cingulate gyri.

This alteration in emotional behavior was also found by Klüver and Bucy to be part of a syndrome resulting from total bilateral temporal lobectomy in adult rhesus monkeys. In addition, their animals lost the ability to recognize objects visually (they could not distinguish edible from inedible objects), had a striking tendency to examine orally everything seen, were unusually alert and responsive to visual stimuli (they touched or mouthed every object in their visual fields), became hypersexual, and increased their food intake.

This constellation of behavioral changes has been sought in human beings, but the complete syndrome has been described only infrequently (Marlowe et al). Pillieri and Poeck have listed other cases that come the closest to reproducing the syndrome (Fig. 25-2A and B). Unfortunately many human examples have occurred in conjunction with diffuse diseases (Alzheimer's and Pick's cerebral atrophies, meningoencephalitis of toxoplasmic or herpes simplex type) and hence of little use for anatomic analysis. With bitemporal surgical ablations it is to be noted that placidity and enhanced oral behavior were the most frequent consequences and altered sexual behavior and visual agnosia less so. In all patients who showed placidity and the amnesic state the hippocampi had been destroyed, but not the amygdaloid nuclei. It is also of interest that the cingulate gyri, where lesions are sometimes made to reduce anxiety and depression, were involved in only one of five cases with placidity.

The full range of placidity reactions in neurology

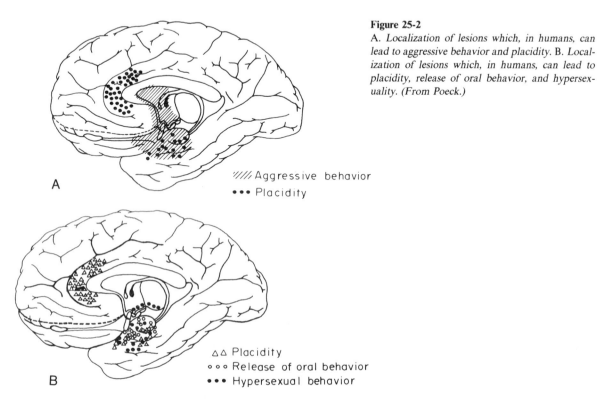

A. ///// Aggressive behavior
••• Placidity

B. △△ Placidity
∘∘∘ Release of oral behavior
••• Hypersexual behavior

Figure 25-2

A. Localization of lesions which, in humans, can lead to aggressive behavior and placidity. B. Localization of lesions which, in humans, can lead to placidity, release of oral behavior, and hypersexuality. (From Poeck.)

has not been cataloged. Unfortunately neurologists and psychiatrists have tended to neglect this aspect of behavior.

ALTERED SEXUALITY

The normal pattern of sexual behavior in both male and female may be altered by cerebral disease quite apart from impairment due to obvious physical disability or to diseases which destroy or isolate the segmental reflex mechanisms (see Chap. 26).

Hypersexuality in either sex is a rare but well-documented complication of neurologic disease. Kleist pointed out that lesions of the orbital parts of the frontal lobes remove moral-ethical restraints and may lead to indiscriminate sexual behavior, and that superior frontal lesions may be associated with a general loss of initiative which reduces all impulsivity, including sexual. In rare cases, extreme hypersexuality begins with an attack of encephalitis or develops gradually with tumors of the temporal region. Presumably the limbic parts of the brain are affected, the ones from which MacLean could evoke penile erection and orgasm by electrical stimulation (medial dorsal thalamus, medial forebrain bundle, and septal preoptic region). Persistence of this behavior suggests disinhibition rather than stimulation as the mechanism. We know of no case where a stable lesion has been studied carefully by serial sections of the whole brain.

In our clinical work we find that hyposexuality, meaning loss of libido, is usually due to a depressive illness, but a variety of cerebral diseases often have this effect. Lesions which involve the tuberoinfundibular region of the hypothalamus are also known to cause disturbances in sexual function. If acquired early in life, pubertal changes are prevented from occurring; hamartomas of the hypothalamus, as in von Recklinghausen's neurofibromatosis and tuberous sclerosis, may cause sexual precocity.

Blumer and Walker have reviewed the literature on epilepsy and abnormal sexual behavior. They note that sexual arousal is apt to occur only in relation to temporal lobe seizures, particularly when the discharging focus is in the medial temporal region. Temporal lobectomy for such lesions has sometimes been followed by a period of hypersexuality. These have been called *sexual seizures*. They also cite numerous references to global hyposexuality with temporal lobe epilepsy.

Panautonomic neuropathy and lesions in the sacral parts of the parasympathetic system also abolish normal sexual performance.

"DIENCEPHALIC" AUTONOMIC EPILEPSY

Penfield, in 1929, recorded a clinical illness characterized by episodes of flushing, lacrimation, salivation, shivering, hiccups, decrease in respiratory rate, tachycardia, hypertension, sweating, and dilatation or contraction of the pupils. Consciousness was altered so that it was impossible to ascertain the patient's emotional state. Such attacks occurred several times a day and lasted for 1 or 2 to 15 min. The cause was a tumor wedged into the foramina of Monro and compressing the dorsomedial (or anterior) nuclei of the thalamus on either side.

Most neurologists have found it impossible to evaluate this case. The nature of the lesion and its location leave open the possibility of intermittent hydrocephalus. Although certain autonomic changes commonly appear in the course of seizures (dilatation of one or both pupils, sweating, hyperpnea, etc.; see page 212), we have never observed a seizure of precisely the type described by Penfield nor have any convincing examples been reported by others. However, attacks of autonomic overactivity without loss of consciousness may occur with basal ganglionic disease and with pheochromocytomas.

ANXIETY, FEAR, AND DEPRESSION

The phenomenon of acute fear and anxiety occurring as a prelude to, or part of, a seizure is familiar to every physician. Williams' study, already alluded to, is of particular interest; in a series of about 2000 epileptics, he was able to cull 100 patients who felt an emotion as part of the epileptic experience. Of these latter cases, 61 experienced feelings of fear and anxiety and 21 experienced depression. Daly has made similar observations. These clinical data call to mind the effects of stimulating the upper, anterior and inferior parts of the temporal lobe during surgical procedures (Penfield and Jasper). Sometimes by altering the intensity of stimulation, anxiety was changed to rage. Usually the patient described feelings of strangeness, uneasiness, and fear. Consciousness was variably impaired at the same time in most instances, and some patients had hallucinatory experiences as well.

Less frequent as an ictal emotion is depression, though this state may occur as an interictal phenomenon, but odd mixtures of depression and anxiety are often associated with temporal lobe tumors. Similar alterations have been observed with tumors of the hypothalamus and third ventricle (see review by Alpers).

Elation and euphoria are less well documented as limbic phenomena, nor has the elevation in mood in some patients with multiple sclerosis ever been adequately explained. Feelings of pleasure, satisfaction, and "stirring sensations" are unusual but well-described emotional experiences in patients with temporal lobe seizures, and this type of affective response has been elicited by Penfield and Jasper in stimulating certain parts of the temporal lobe.

DIFFERENTIAL DIAGNOSIS

Aside from clinical observation there are no reliable means of evaluating the above-described emotional disorders, and while neurologic medicine has done little more than describe and classify some of the clinical states dominated by emotional derangement, an activity considered by some to be the lowest level of science, knowledge of this type is nonetheless of both theoretical and practical importance. In theory it prepares one for the next step, of passing from a superficial to a deeper order of inquiry, where questions of genesis can be broached. Practically, it provides certain clues which are useful in the differential diagnosis of disease, as the following clinical problems indicate.

Uninhibited Laughter and Crying and Emotional Lability As indicated earlier, one may confidently assume that the syndrome of forced laughter and crying signifies cerebral disease and more specifically bilateral disease of the corticobulbar tracts. Usually the motor and reflex changes of pseudobulbar palsy are associated, especially heightened facial and mandibular reflexes, but occasionally these are minimal or absent altogether. Also extreme emotional lability always suggests bilateral cerebral disease, although here, too, only the signs of unilateral disease may be apparent clinically. The most common pathologic states are lacunar infarction, other cerebrovascular diseases, diffuse hypoxic-hypotensive encephalopathy, amyotrophic lateral sclerosis, and multiple sclerosis. Abrupt onset, of course, indicates vascular disease.

Placidity and Apathy These may be the earliest and most important signs of cerebral disease. Clinically, placidity and apathy must be distinguished from the retardation of Parkinson's disease and depressive illness. Their pathologic associations are usually Alzheimer's disease, low-pressure hydrocephalus and frontal-corpus

callosal tumors, but they may occur in conjunction with a variety of other frontal and temporal lesions.

An Outburst of Violent Anger and Aggressive Action Most often such an outburst is but another episode in a lifelong sequence of sociopathy (see Chap. 55). More significance attaches to its abrupt appearance as a sudden departure from normal character. If there are seizures, and if rage accompanies the seizures, the outburst of rage should be viewed as the consequence of the seizure activity on temporal lobe function or of its causative lesion. Usual causes are birth injury, cranial trauma, encephalitis, and earlier seizures. Amygdaloid seizures as a cause of blind rage are suggested by (1) abruptness of onset, (2) easy provocation, (3) evocation by alcohol or small amounts of other drugs, (4) other signs (clinical or EEG) of temporal lobe disease. Rarely, rage and aggressivity are expressive of an acute neurologic disease of medial temporoorbital frontal regions. We have several times observed such states transiently in a stable individual as an expression of an obscure encephalopathy.

An Acute Panic Attack, Extreme Fright and Agitation Here the central problem must be clarified by determining whether the patient is delirious (clouding of consciousness, psychomotor overactivity, and hallucinations), deluded (schizophrenia), in an anxiety attack (anxiety neurosis, anxious depression), or hypomanic (overactive, flight of ideas). Rarely does panic prove to be an expression of temporal lobe epilepsy.

Depression, Anxiety, Bizarre Ideation Developing over Weeks, Months, or a Few Years While these symptoms are usually due to a psychosis (schizophrenia or manic-depressive disease), one should consider a tumor or other lesion of the temporal lobe when there are psychomotor seizures, aphasic difficulty, rotatory vertigo (rare), and quadrantic visual field defect. Such states have been described in hypothalamic disease, suggested by somnolence, diabetes insipidus, visual field defects, and hydrocephalus.

REFERENCES

AKERT K, HESS WR: Über die neurobiologischen Grundlagen akuter affektiver Erregungszustände. *Schweiz Med Wochenschr* 92:1524, 1962.

ALPERS BJ: Personality and emotional disorders associated with hypothalamic lesions. *Res Publ Assoc Nerv Ment Dis* 20:725, 1939.

BARD P: A diencephalic mechanism for the expression of rage with special reference to the sympathetic nervous system. *Am J Physiol* 84:490, 1928.

————, MOUNTCASTLE VB: Some forebrain mechanisms involved in the expression of rage with special reference to suppression of angry behavior. *Assoc Res Nerv Ment Dis Proc* 27:362, 1947.

BARRIS RW, SCHUMAN HR: Bilateral anterior cingulate gyrus lesions: Syndrome of the anterior cingulate gyri. *Neurology* 3:44, 1953.

BINGLEY T: Mental symptoms in temporal lobe epilepsy and temporal lobe gliomas. *Acta Psychiatr Scand* 33 (suppl 120):1958.

BLUMER D, WALKER AE: The neural basis of sexual behavior, in Benson F, Blumer D (eds): *Psychiatric Aspects of Neurologic Disease.* New York, Grune & Stratton, 1975, chap 11, p 199.

CANNON WB: *Bodily Changes in Pain, Hunger and Fear,* 2d ed. New York, Appleton-Century, 1929.

CUSHING H: *Pituitary Body, Hypothalamus and Parasympathetic Nervous System.* Springfield, Ill, Charles C Thomas, 1932.

DALY DD: Ictal affect. *Am J Psychiatry* 115:97, 1958.

————, MULDER DW: Gelastic epilepsy. *Neurology* 7:189, 1957.

DOTT NM: Surgical aspects of the hypothalamus, in WE Clark et al (eds), *The Hypothalamus: Morphological, Functional, Clinical and Surgical Aspects.* Edinburgh, Oliver & Boyd, 1938.

FALCONER MA, SERAFETINIDES EA: A follow-up study of surgery in temporal lobe epilepsy. *J Neurol Neurosurg Psychiatry* 26:154, 1963.

FERE MC: Le fou rire prodromique. *Rev Neurol* 11:353, 1903.

FISHER CM: Anger associated with dysphasia. *Trans Am Neurol Assoc* 95:240, 1970.

GASTAUT H, MORIN G, LEFEVRE N: Etude de comportement des épileptiques psychomoteurs dans l'intervalle de leurs crises. *Ann Med Psychol* 1:1, 1955.

GESCHWIND N: The clinical setting of aggression in temporal lobe epilepsy, in Field WS, Sweet WH (eds). *The Neurobiology of Violence.* St. Louis, Warren H Green, 1975.

GLOOR P, FEINDEL W: Affective behavior and the temporal lobe, in *Physiologie und Pathophysiologie des Vegetativen Nervensystems,* vol 2: *Pathophysiologie.* Stuttgart, Hippokrates-Verlag, 1963, pp 685–716.

ISAACSON RL: *The Limbic System.* New York, Plenum, 1974.

KLEIST K: Gehirnpathologie und lokalisatorische Ergebnisse; die Störungen der Ichleistungen und ihre Lokalisation im Orbital-, Innen- und Zwischenhirn. *Monatsschr Psychiatr Neurol* 79:338, 1931.

KLÜVER H, BUCY PC: An analysis of certain effects of bilateral temporal lobectomy in the rhesus monkey with special reference to psychic blindness. *J Psychol* 5:33, 1938.

MACLEAN PD: Contrasting functions of limbic and neocortical systems of the brain and their relevance to psychophysiological aspects of medicine. *Am J Med* 25:611, 1958.

MALAMUD N: Psychiatric disorder with intracranial tumors of limbic system. *Arch Neurol* 17:113, 1967.

MARK VH, ERVIN FR: *Violence and the Brain.* New York, Harper & Row, 1970.

MARLOWE WB, MANCALL EL, THOMAS JJ: Complete Klüver-Bucy syndrome in man. *Cortex* 11:53, 1975.

MARTIN JP: Fits of laughter (sham mirth) in organic cerebral disease. *Brain* 70:453, 1950.

NARABAYASHI H, NACAO Y, YOSHIDA M, NAGAHATA M: Stereotaxic amygdalectomy for behavior disorders. *Arch Neurol* 9:1, 1963.

NAUTA WJH: The central visceromotor system: A general survey, in Hockman CH (ed): *Limbic System Mechanisms and Autonomic Function.* Springfield, Ill, Charles C Thomas, 1972, chap 2, pp 21–33.

PAPEZ JW: A proposed mechanism of emotion. *Arch Neurol Psychiatry* 38:725, 1937.

PENFIELD W, JASPER H: *Epilepsy and the Functional Anatomy of the Human Brain.* Boston, Little, Brown, 1954, pp 413–416.

PILLIERI G: The Klüver-Bucy syndrome in man. *Psychiatr Neurol* 152:65, 1967.

POECK K: Pathophysiology of emotional disorders associated with brain damage, in Vinken PJ, Bruyn GW (eds): *Handbook of Clinical Neurology,* vol 3. Amsterdam, North-Holland, 1969, chap 20, pp 343–367.

————, PILLIERI G: Pathologisches Lachen und Weinen. *Schweiz Arch Neurol Psychiatr* 92:323, 1963.

SCOVILLE WB, MILNER B: Loss of recent memory after bilateral hippocampal lesions. *J Neurol Neurosurg Psychiatry* 20:11, 1957.

WILLIAMS D: The structure of emotions reflected in epileptic experiences. *Brain* 79:29, 1956.

WILSON SAK: Some problems in neurology: II. Pathological laughing and crying. *J Neurol Psychopathol* 16:299, 1924.

ZEMAN W, KING FA: Tumors of the septum pellucidum and adjacent structures with abnormal affective behavior: An anterior or midline structure syndrome. *J Nerv Ment Dis* 127:490, 1958.

CHAPTER 26

DISORDERS OF THE AUTONOMIC NERVOUS SYSTEM AND NEUROENDOCRINE FUNCTION

The human internal environment is regulated in large measure by the autonomic nervous system and endocrine glands and by the integrated activity of these two systems. The visceral and homeostatic functions, essential to life and the survival of our species, are involuntary. Why nature has divorced them from volition is an interesting question. One would like to think that the mind, being preoccupied with discriminative, moral, and esthetic matters, should not have to be troubled with such mundane activities as breathing, regulation of heart rate, lactating, hunger, and sleep. Claude Bernard expressed this idea in more sardonic terms when he wrote that "nature thought it prudent to remove these important phenomena from the caprice of an ignorant will."

Diseases that exert their morbid effects exclusively on the neuroendocrine axis are not numerous and would deserve only limited consideration in a textbook on neurology. On the other hand, there are many medical diseases whose symptoms are to some extent expressed by a derangement of autonomic or neuroendocrine function (e.g., hypertension, syncope, asthma). Also there is a wide variety of pharmacologic agents that influence these disorders and are of concern to neurologists. What is more, these parts of the neuraxis represent the effector apparatus utilized in all emotional and affective experience.

Before discussing the many clinical derangements of autonomic and neuroendocrine function, it is necessary to review some facts about the anatomy and physiology of the autonomic nervous system and the modes of interaction between this system and the endocrine glands.

ANATOMIC CONSIDERATIONS

Probably the most remarkable feature of the autonomic nervous system (also called the visceral or vegetative nervous system) is the location of a major part of it outside the cerebrospinal axis in proximity to the structures which it innervates. This position alone seems to symbolize its relative independence from the cerebrospinal system. Also, in distinction to the somatic neuromuscular system, where a single motor neuron bridges the gap between the central nervous system and the effector organ, in the autonomic nervous system there are always two motor neurons (Fig. 26-1).

From the strictly anatomic viewpoint the autonomic nervous system is divided into the thoracolumbar (sympathetic) and the craniosacral (parasympathetic) divisions (see Figs. 26-2 and 26-3). The *parasympathetic division* consists of the special visceral nuclei in the brainstem, viz., the anteromedian and dorsal visceral cell columns of the oculomotor nuclei, the superior and inferior salivatory nuclei, and the dorsal motor nucleus of the vagus. The axons (preganglionic fibers) of the anteromedian nucleus and dorsal visceral cell columns (only the latter constitute the Edinger-Westphal nucleus) course through the oculomotor nerve and synapse in the ciliary ganglion in the orbit; the axons of the latter innervate the ciliary muscle and sphincter pupillae (Fig. 13-6). The preganglionic fibers of the superior salivatory nucleus enter the facial nerve, and at a point near the geniculate ganglion they form the greater superficial petrosal nerve, by which they reach the sphenopalatine ganglion; the cells of this ganglion innervate the lacrimal gland (see also Fig. 46-1). Other fibers of the facial nerve traverse the tympanic cavity as the chorda tympani and eventually join with the submandibular ganglion; the cells of this ganglion innervate the submandibular and sublingual glands. The axons of the nerve cells of the inferior salivatory nucleus enter the glossopharyngeal nerve and reach the otic ganglion through the tympanic plexus and lesser superficial petrosal nerve; cells of the otic ganglion send fibers to the parotid gland. The preganglionic neurons of the dorsal motor nucleus of the vagus enter the vagus nerve and terminate in ganglia situated in the walls of the many thoracic and abdominal viscera which it supplies. Their postganglionic fibers activate smooth muscle and glands of the pharynx, esophagus, and remainder of the gastrointestinal tract, as well as the heart, pancreas, liver, and gallbladder. In addition to parasympathetic fibers, the plexuses to the aforementioned organs contain sympathetic fibers as well.

The sacral part of the parasympathetic system is largely made up of preganglionic neurons originating in the lateral horns of the second, third, and fourth sacral segments. Their axons traverse the sacral nerves and synapse in ganglia which lie within the walls of the colon, bladder, and other pelvic organs. These sacral autonomic neurons, like the cranial ones, have long preganglionic and short postganglionic fibers, which would be expected from the peripheral location of the ganglion cells.

Figure 26-1

The principles of the sympathetic outflow from the spinal cord and the course and distribution of sympathetic fibers. The preganglionic fibers are in heavy lines; postganglionic fibers are in thin lines. (From Pick.)

The *sympathetic division* consists essentially of aggregates of motor neurons whose cell bodies are collected into two large ganglionated chains, or cords, one on each side of the vertebral column, and into isolated ganglions elsewhere. The axons of the sympathetic ganglion cells (*the postganglionic neurons*) pass via the gray communicating rami to the spinal nerves and supply the blood vessels, sweat glands, and pilomotor structures in the various segments of the body; they also form plexuses of fibers which are distributed to the viscera. The autonomic ganglia are under the influence of the motor nerve cells of the lateral horns of the spinal cord and of the special visceral nuclei in the brainstem. The axons of these craniospinal nuclei traverse the anterior roots and then enter the autonomic ganglia via the white (medullated) communicating rami. They are the *preganglionic neurons* and, together with the postganglionic (unmyelinated) ones, they comprise the lower motor neurons of the autonomic nervous system (Fig. 26-1).

The cell bodies of the thoracolumbar preganglionic neurons are situated in the lateral horns of the gray

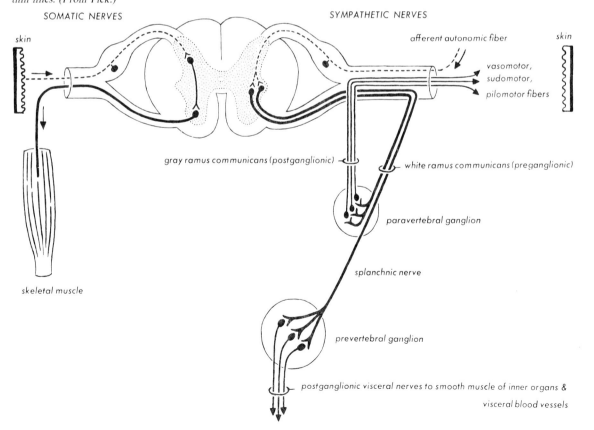

SOMATIC NERVES

SYMPATHETIC NERVES

skin

afferent autonomic fiber

skin

vasomotor,
sudomotor,
pilomotor fibers

gray ramus communicans (postganglionic)

white ramus communicans (preganglionic)

paravertebral ganglion

splanchnic nerve

skeletal muscle

prevertebral ganglion

postganglionic visceral nerves to smooth muscle of inner organs &
visceral blood vessels

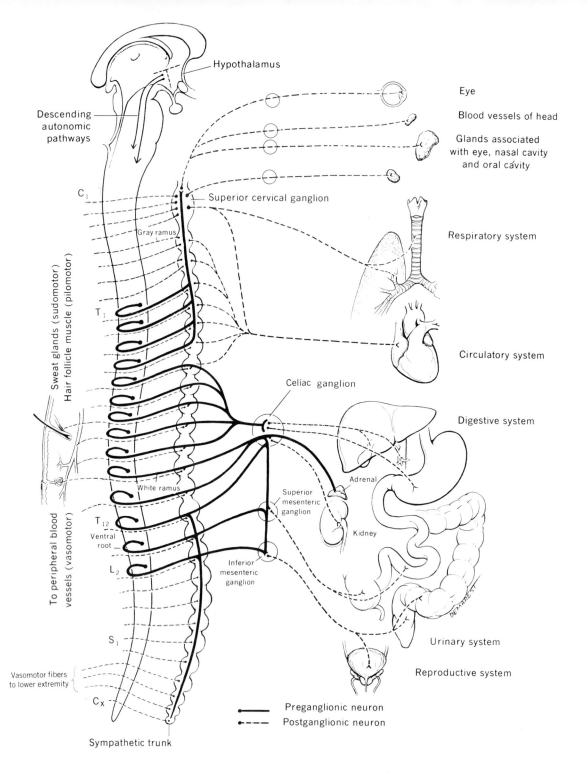

Figure 26-2
The sympathetic (thoracolumbar) division of the autonomic nervous system. Preganglionic fibers extend from the intermediolateral nucleus of the spinal cord to the peripheral auto- *nomic ganglia, and postganglionic fibers extend from the peripheral ganglia to the effector organs, according to the scheme in Fig. 26-1. (From CL Noback, R Demarest, The Human Nervous System, 3d ed, New York, McGraw-Hill, 1981.)*

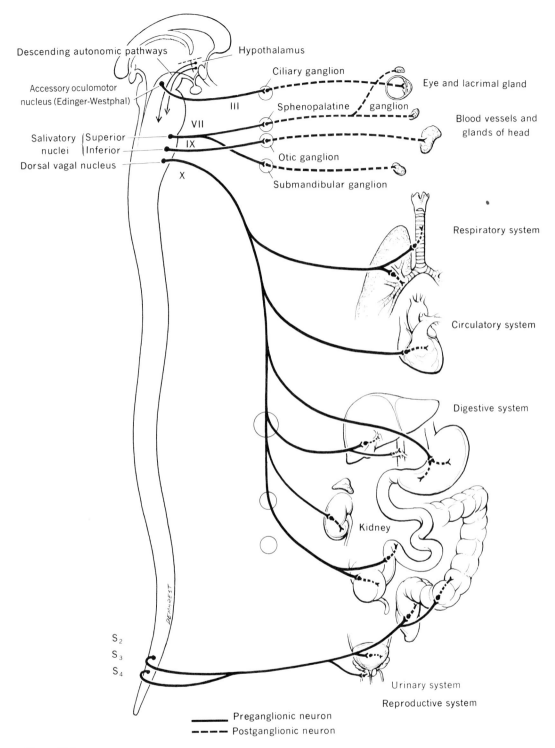

Figure 26-3

The parasympathetic (craniosacral) division of the autonomic nervous system. Preganglionic fibers extend from nuclei of the brainstem and sacral segments of the spinal cord to peripheral ganglia. Short postganglionic fibers extend from the ganglia to the effector organs. The lateral-posterior hypothalamus is part of the supranuclear mechanism for the regulation of parasympathetic activities. The frontal and limbic parts of the supranuclear regulatory apparatus are not indicated in the diagram (see text). (From CL Noback, R Demarest, The Human Nervous System, 3d ed, New York, McGraw-Hill, 1981.)

matter of spinal cord from the first thoracic to the third lumbar segments. Their thinly myelinated axons enter the paravertebral chain of ganglia, which extend from the base of the skull to the coccyx, via the white communicating rami. A preganglionic sympathetic fiber may pass through several ganglia before it finally synapses with a postganglionic neuron (Fig. 26-4), and its terminals make contact with 20 or more postganglionic neurons. In addition, one ganglion cell is supplied by several preganglionic fibers; thus a diffuse discharge of the sympathetic system is possible. Some preganglionic fibers pass through the paravertebral ganglia as splanchnic nerves to synapse in prevertebral ganglia (the celiac, superior, and inferior mesenteric ganglia; see Fig. 26-4); postganglionic fibers form the hypogastric, splanchnic, and mesenteric plexuses, which innervate the glands and smooth muscle of the blood vessels and intestine.

Figure 26-4

The principle of the preganglionic innervation of paravertebral ganglia which are placed beyond the limits of the preganglionic sympathetic outflow from the spinal cord. Preganglionic fibers (heavy lines) emerging from a spinal segment do not synapse exclusively in the corresponding paravertebral ganglion. Some pass as splanchnic nerves to prevertebral ganglia; some fibers enter the sympathetic trunk, in which they pass up or down for a variable number of segments. (From Pick.)

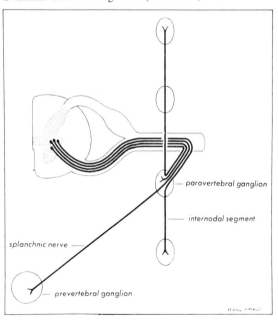

The sympathetic innervation of the adrenal medulla is peculiar in that its secretory cells receive preganglionic fibers directly from the splanchnic nerves. This is an exception to the rule that organs innervated by the autonomic nervous system receive only postganglionic nerves. This unique arrangement can be explained by the fact that the cells of the adrenal medulla are the morphologic homologues of the postganglionic sympathetic nerves, and they secrete epinephrine and norepinephrine, the postganglionic transmitters, directly into the bloodstream.

There are three cervical (superior, middle, and inferior, or stellate), eleven thoracic, and four to six lumbar ganglia. The cranium receives its sympathetic supply from the eighth cervical and first two thoracic cord segments, the fibers of which pass through the inferior and middle cervical ganglia and synapse with the nerve cells of the superior cervical ganglia. Postganglionic fibers from these latter cells follow the internal and external carotid arteries and innervate the blood vessels, smooth muscle, and the sweat, lacrimal, and salivary glands of the cranium. Included are the pupillodilator fibers and those innervating Müller's muscle of the upper eyelid. The arm receives its postganglionic innervation from the upper thoracic segments via the stellate ganglion. The cardiac plexus and other thoracic sympathetic nerves are derived from the upper thoracic segments and the abdominal visceral plexuses, from the fifth to the ninth or tenth thoracic segments. The lower three lumbar and first sacral ganglia, however, have no visceral connections; they supply only the legs.

The nerve terminals, neuromuscular, and neuroglandular junctions of the autonomic nervous system have been more difficult to visualize and to study than the motor end plates of striated muscle. As the postganglionic axons enter an organ, usually via the vasculature, they ramify into many smaller branches. At their ends and in part along their course there are swellings which lie in close proximity to the sarcolemma or gland cell membrane; often the muscle fiber is grooved to accommodate these swellings. At the point of neuroeffector junction the axon is not covered by Schwann cells. The axonal swellings contain vesicles, some of which are clear and others granular. The clear vesicles, on the basis of fluorescence studies, are believed to contain acetylcholine and those with a granular core, catecholamines (Falck, Richardson). For example, the nerves to the dilator of the iris (sympathetic) contain granular vesicles and those to the constrictor (parasympathetic), clear vesicles. A single nerve fiber innervates multiple smooth muscle and gland cells.

Somewhat arbitrarily, anatomists have declared the autonomic nervous system to be purely motor or secretory in function. However, most autonomic nerves are mixed and contain afferent fibers which convey sensory impulses from the viscera and blood vessels. The cell bodies of these sensory neurons lie in the posterior root ganglia; some of their central axons synapse with the lateral horn cells of the spinal cord, subserving visceral reflexes, and others synapse in the dorsal horn; secondary afferents carry sensory impulses to certain brainstem nuclei and the thalamus via the lateral spinothalamic and another polysynaptic tract (see Chap. 7).

PHYSIOLOGIC AND PHARMACOLOGIC CONSIDERATIONS

The function of the autonomic nervous system is to regulate the activities of a group of organs, mainly visceral ones, which possess a high degree of independence. When the autonomic nerves are interrupted, these organs continue to function (the organism survives), but their activities cannot be effectively organized in maintaining homeostasis and adapting to emotional changes and stress.

It was learned long ago that most viscera have a double nerve supply, sympathetic and parasympathetic, and that these two parts of the autonomic nervous system exert opposite effects. For example, the heart is excited by the sympathetic nervous system and inhibited by the parasympathetic. While this statement about double innervation is generally true, it is an oversimplification. Some structures like the sweat glands receive only sympathetic postganglionic fibers, and the adrenal gland, as indicated above, has only a preganglionic sympathetic innervation.

All autonomic functions are mediated through the release of chemical transmitters, the most important of which are acetylcholine (ACh) and norepinephrine (NE). These substances are synthesized at the terminals of axons and stored in presynaptic vesicles until released by the arrival of nerve impulses. ACh is released at the ends of all preganglionic fibers (both in the sympathetic and parasympathetic ganglia) as well as at the ends of all postganglionic parasympathetic and some postganglionic sympathetic fibers. ACh is also the chemical transmitter of nerve impulses to the skeletal muscle fiber. The arrival of nerve impulses releases ACh which traverses the synaptic cleft and attaches to receptor sites on the next neuron, smooth or striated muscle cell, or glandular cell. Removal of ACh is accomplished by its restoration into presynaptic vesicles and destruction locally or in the bloodstream by acetylcholinesterases.

As a general rule, postganglionic sympathetic fibers release NE at their terminals, but here again there

are exceptions. The sweat glands, for example, are innervated by postganglionic sympathetic fibers, but their terminals release ACh. The same is true for the postganglionic sympathetic fibers that innervate the uterus, blood vessels of skeletal muscles, and pilomotor muscles. The NE that is discharged into the synaptic space activates specific receptor sites (*adrenergic receptors*) on the postsynaptic membrane of target cells. The action of this transmitter is terminated by means of an energy-dependent NE pump which restores it to the neurosecretory presynaptic granules. Some NE also diffuses into the bloodstream where it is metabolized to normetanephrine and thence to vanillylmandelic acid (VMA) by means of the action of monoamine oxidase (MAO) and other enzymes such as catechol-O-methyltransferase (COMT). The epinephrine that is released by the adrenal medulla is metabolized to VMA and metanephrine. These catecholamines and their metabolites are excreted in the urine and reflect the functional integrity of the autonomic nervous system. When present in increased amounts, the presence of a pheochromocytoma is suggested.

The adrenal medulla, as has been remarked, represents a special case. Stimulation of the splanchnic nerve (equivalent to a preganglionic sympathetic nerve) releases ACh from its terminals, which in turn depolarizes the chromaffin cells and releases epinephrine and norepinephrine. Thus the sympathetic nervous system and the adrenal medulla act in unison to produce diffuse effects—as one would expect from their role in emergency reactions. The parasympathetic responses (as in the pupil and urinary bladder) tend to be more discrete.

The effects of sympathetic nervous system activation are diverse. The cardiovascular responses consist of arteriolar constriction, tachycardia, enhanced cardiac contractility and renin release, all of which maintain or raise the blood pressure. Other effects are mydriasis, ejaculation, and bronchodilatation. The metabolic effects include lipolysis, glycogenolysis, and release of antidiuretic hormone. The sympathetic nervous system also participates in such functions as regulation of body temperature and salivary secretion. The effects of parasympathetic activation are to slow the sinoatrial rate and atrial-ventricular conduction, stimulate bronchial, salivary, and gastric glands, constrict the pupil, activate smooth muscle cells in the bronchi and intestine, sustain penile erection, and promote sweating.

The particular effect of a catecholamine is determined by the fact that there are two types of receptor with which the agent can react to elicit a response in the effector cell. These receptor sites were classified by Ahlquist as *alpha* and *beta*. In general, the effects of catecholamines on alpha receptors are excitatory, and the effects on beta receptors are inhibitory. This distinction is not absolute, however. The contractility of heart muscle, for example, is increased when its beta receptors are activated; and the inhibitory effects of catecholamines on the gut are mediated by both alpha and beta receptors.

The most important effect of NE is to cause vasoconstriction, by virtue of its action on alpha receptors of vascular smooth muscle. Recently it has been found that NE also acts on receptors that are located on the nerve terminal itself; presumably these presynaptic receptors inhibit the release of neurotransmitter, functioning as a kind of feedback mechanism. It has been suggested that these postsynaptic and presynaptic receptors be designated as $alpha_1$ and $alpha_2$, respectively.

The beta-adrenergic receptor sites can also be subdivided on the basis of the relative selectivity of effects of excitatory drugs and antagonists. $Beta_1$ receptors mediate increased heart rate and contractility and possibly the release of renin; $beta_2$ receptors mediate relaxation of smooth muscle of the bronchi, uterus, and blood vessels. Hyperglycemia and other metabolic responses to catecholamines cannot presently be categorized in this schema.

A remarkable number of new drugs that act on the sympathetic and parasympathetic divisions of the autonomic nervous system have become available in recent years. These agents function in different ways to influence the synthesis and storage and release of the natural neurotransmitters and their activation or blockade at the receptor sites of target tissues. These effects are too numerous to describe in detail, but are summarized in Tables 26-1 and 26-2.

The two divisions of the autonomic nervous system, acting in conjunction with the endocrine glands, with which they are closely related, maintain the homeostasis of the organism. The integration of these two systems is achieved primarily in the hypothalamus. In addition, the endocrine glands are influenced by circulating catecholamines, and some of them are innervated by adrenergic fibers, which terminate not only on blood vessels but in some cases directly on secretory cells. These autonomic-endocrine relations are elaborated in the following pages.

THE CENTRAL NERVOUS SYSTEM REGULATION OF VISCERAL FUNCTION

Among the most important recent advances in neuroanatomy has been the discovery of autonomic regulating mechanisms in the brain. Small, insignificant-appearing nuclei in the walls of the third ventricle beneath the thalami (hypothalamus) and in buried parts of the cerebral cortex, formerly judged to have purely olfactory functions, are now known to control the autonomic nervous system. This is accomplished in two ways—through direct descending nervous pathways in the spinal cord and through the pituitary and thence other endocrine glands.

This supranuclear regulatory apparatus of the autonomic nervous system consists of three main groups of structures: (1) the frontal lobe cortex; (2) the archicortex and medial transitional cortex (the rhinencephalon, or "smell brain," the hippocampal formation, amygdaloid nuclei, olfactory cortex, and cingulate gyrus); and (3) the hypothalamus.

The *frontal lobe cortex*—the least understood and most uniquely human arrangement—appears to be the highest level of integration of autonomic function. Stimulation of one frontal lobe may evoke changes in temperature and sweating in the contralateral arm and leg, and massive lesions here, which usually cause a hemiplegia, may modify these functions in the direction of either inhibition or facilitation. Lesions involving the posterior part of the superior frontal and anterior part of the cingulate gyri (usually bilateral, occasionally unilateral) result in loss of voluntary control of the bladder and bowel (see page 304). The descending spinal pathways subserving bowel and bladder function are believed to lie ventromedial to the corticospinal fibers. Most likely a large contingent of these fibers terminates in the transitional mesocortex (cingulate gyrus) and archicortex (hippocampus) and in the hypothalamus, which in turn send fibers to the brainstem and spinal cord.

The transitional mesocortex and archicortex have now been identified as important parts of the so-called cerebral autonomic centers. Together they have been called the *limbic lobe*, or *visceral brain*. The effects of stimulation and ablation of these structures or parts of them are discussed in Chap. 25. Of central importance in the autonomic regulatory apparatus is the amygdaloid group of nuclei. Electrical stimulation in or near these nuclei in the unanesthetized cat yields a variety of responses in the motor and vegetative spheres. One of these has been referred to as the *fear*, or *flight*, response, in which the animal appears anxious and runs away and hides; another is the *anger*, or *defense*, reaction, characterized by growling, hissing, and piloerection. However,

Table 26-1
Pharmacologic agents which act on the sympathetic nervous system

Agent and site of action	Effects	Clinical usage
Receptor agonists (postsynaptic endings of postganglionic neurons):		
Norepinephrine (alpha effects predominate)	Vasoconstriction (alpha activity) Increases cardiac rate and contractility (beta activity) Stimulates pregnant uterus and sphincters Relaxes bladder and intestine Increases systolic and diastolic blood pressure; if blood pressure rise is excessive, there probably has been denervation	In hypotension due to sympathetic paralysis
Epinephrine (beta effects predominate)	Increases heart rate, cardiac excitability Vasoconstriction of skin and visceral vessels (alpha effect) Vasodilatation in skeletal and heart muscle (total vascular resistance is decreased) Increase in systolic and decrease in diastolic blood pressure	In asthma for bronchodilation In cardiac arrest, to increase excitability With local anesthetic, for vasoconstriction To reverse urticaria and angioneurotic edema Stimulates CNS tremor, anxiety, increased respirations
Dopamine	Both alpha and beta; not established as a peripheral transmitter	In hypotension and congestive failure
Other sympathomimetics:		
Phenylephrine $\rbrace$ Methoxamine	Stimulate alpha receptors	In hypotension during spinal anesthesia
Isoproterenol	Stimulates beta receptors	In cardiac arrhythmias
Metaraminol $\rbrace$ Mephentermine	Indirect action via release of norepinephrine from presynaptic vesicles	For short-term bronchodilation, cardiac stimulation, vasopressor effect, nasal decongestion
Ephedrine	Releases norepinephrine but also has direct action on alpha and beta receptors	In orthostatic hypotension due to postganglionic neuropathy: cardiac and bronchial effects similar to epinephrine, but relaxes uterus; mydriasis
Amphetamine	Direct action	Central analeptic effects predominate
Sympathetic antagonists:		
Alpha adrenoceptor blockers:		
Phentolamine (short-acting)	Inhibit vasoconstrictive effects of norepinephrine	In hypertensive crisis, especially that of pheochromocytoma or that complicating use of MAO drugs
Phenoxybenzamine (long-acting)	Prevent pupillary dilatation	
Prazosin	Mainly postsynaptic alpha$_1$ blocker	
Beta adrenoceptor blockers:		
Propranolol and related drugs	Slows heart rate and reduces force of contraction and excitability	In angina pectoris, arrhythmias, hypertension; decreases sympathetic overactivity in tetanus; suppresses essential tremor

Table 26-1 *(continued)*
Pharmacologic agents which act on the sympathetic nervous system

Agent and site of action	Effects	Clinical usage
Adrenergic drugs acting on CNS:		
Methyldopa (crosses blood-brain barrier and is stored in neurosecretory vesicles of adrenergic neurons)	Stimulates alpha receptors that inhibit sympathetic outflow	Treatment of hypertension
Clonidine	Direct stimulator of CNS alpha receptors	Treatment of hypertension
Ganglion blockers:		
Guanethidine, hexamethonium and related drugs (occupy receptor sites of postsynaptic membranes and stabilize them against ACh)	Selectively block ganglia of sympathetic and parasympathetic nervous system	To reduce blood pressure in hypertensive crises or for hypotensive surgery

Table 26-2
Pharmacologic agents which act on the parasympathetic nervous system

Agent	Site of action and effects	Clinical usage
Acetylcholine	Direct action at receptor site Neurotransmitter to sweat glands (postganglionic sympathetic neurons) Preganglionic transmitter in all ganglia and adrenal medulla Neuromuscular transmitter for skeletal muscle Neurotransmitter at all parasympathetic postganglionic terminals	Percutaneous acetylcholine test of integrity of postganglionic sympathetic fibers
Cholinomimetic drugs:		
Methacholine	Direct action on receptor sites	Test of parasympathetic integrity of pupil
Carbachol ⎫ Bethanecol ⎬	Direct action unaffected by cholinesterases	Stimulation of gastrointestinal tract and detrusor muscle of bladder
Pilocarpine	Direct action on cholinergic effector cells (sweat glands)	In glaucoma as a miotic agent
Cholinergic blocking agents:		
Atropine, scopolamine, and related belladonna alkaloids	Blocks action of ACh at parasympathetic and preganglionic sympathetic synapses; no effect on neuromuscular synapses	To reduce salivary and bronchial secretions; counteract vagal activity on heart and stomach; inhibit overactivity of bladder; dilate pupil
Anticholinesterases:		

Neostigmine (intermediate action)
  Edrophonium (short action)
  Pyridostigmine (long action)
	Inhibits action of cholinesterases on acetylcholine at neuromuscular junctions and at other cholinergic sites	Myasthenia gravis

not only the amygdaloid nuclei are concerned in these reactions. Lesions in the ventromedial nuclei of the hypothalamus (which receives a rich projection of fibers from the amygdaloid nuclei) have also been shown to cause aggressive behavior, and bilateral ablation of neocortical area 24 has produced the opposite state—increased tameness and reduced aggressiveness, at least in some species.

The *hypothalamus* comprises three main groups of nuclei: (1) the *anterior group* includes the supraoptic and paraventricular nuclei; (2) the *middle group* includes the ventromedian, dorsomedian, and tuberal nuclei; and (3) the *posterior group* includes the mammillary bodies and posterior hypothalamic nuclei.

Axons of the supraoptic and paraventricular nuclei pass through the stalk of the pituitary gland (supraopticohypophysial tract) to terminate in its posterior lobe in direct contact with blood vessels. There they release vasopressin (antidiuretic hormone, ADH) and oxytocin, which diffuse rapidly into the blood and are transported to their appropriate target organs (Fig. 26-5).

In the central part of the hypothalamus, crowded around the tuber cinereum, are the many groups of

small cells which are most directly involved in the control of the anterior part of the hypophysis, the portion derived from the epithelial lining of the primitive oral cavity (adenohypophysis). The fine, unmedullated axons of the tuberal nuclei project onto the median eminence of the infundibulum and comprise the tuberoinfundibular system. Cells of this system synthesize, transport, and release small, low-molecular-weight peptides into a specialized portal venous system that connects the mediobasal hypothalamus with the adenohypophysis (Fig. 26-5). These substances, called *hypothalamic releasing factors*, provide for the neural control of the anterior pituitary trophic hormones: growth hormone (GH), ACTH, thyrotropic-stimulating hormone (TSH), luteinizing hormone (LH), follicle-stimulating hormone (FSH), and prolactin.

The hypothalamic releasing factors are probably both stimulating and inhibitory. To date the following have been isolated:

HYPOTHALAMIC-NEUROHYPOPHYSIAL SYSTEM

HYPOTHALAMIC-ADENOHYPOPHYSIAL SYSTEM

Figure 26-5

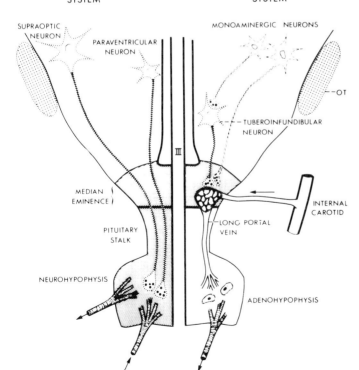

Diagram of the hypothalamic-pituitary axis. Indicated on the left is the hypothalamic-neurohypophysial system consisting of supraoptic and paraventricular neurons, axons of which terminate on blood vessels in the posterior pituitary (neurohypophysis). The hypothalamic-adenohypophysial system is illustrated on the right. Tuberoinfundibular neurons, believed to be the source of the hypothalamic regulatory hormones, terminate on the capillary plexus in the median eminence. (From Martin et al.)

TRH: Thyrotropin-releasing hormone, a tripeptide with a molecular weight of 362.

LHRH: Luteinizing hormone-releasing hormone, consisting of 10 amino acids, stimulates release of the gonadotropic hormones of the hypophysis (FSH and LH).

GHIF: Growth hormone inhibitory factor, also called *somatostatin,* a peptide of 14 amino acids with a disulfide bridge. It inhibits GH secretion but also depresses insulin and glucagon secretion.

These releasing factors are secreted episodically throughout the day and night, some more at night in certain phases of sleep (see page 260). Whether or not hypophysial activity is caused always by an oversecretion of releasing factors or to a decrease in inhibitory factors is unknown.

The neurosecretory neurons of the hypothalamus have been referred to as the "final common pathway" for neuroendocrine communication (Martin and Renaud) or as "neuroendocrine transducers" (Wurtman), possessing, as they do, the capacity to change neuronal (electrical) information into hormone-mediated signals. The feedback mechanism for turning the endocrine system on and off is also effected through these neurons. For example, when we stand up, a baroreceptor mechanism in the lower parts of the body sends a reflex volley of nervous impulses up the spinal cord and brainstem to the supraoptic nerve cells, which are stimulated to increase ADH output and prevent the diuresis that would result from the increased intravascular pressure in the kidneys. The suckling newborn infant on the mother's breast causes prompt release, through the hypothalamus, of prolactin, a hormone that is essential to milk production and secretion. Degeneration of the ovaries with age diminishes the feedback control exerted by estrogens on the tuberoinfundibular system, which then overacts to stimulate the basophil cells of the hypophysis to increase LH and FSH production. Hot flushes and other symptoms of the menopause are associated with overactivity of these pituitary hormones. Current evidence suggests that the release of certain of these hypothalamic hormones may be mediated by catecholamines.

Interaction between the autonomic nervous system and the endocrine glands occurs at a peripheral as well as a central level. The best-known example of this interaction is in the adrenal medulla, as indicated earlier in this chapter. A similar relationship pertains in the pineal gland; release of norepinephrine from postgangli-onic fibers which end on pineal cells has been shown to stimulate several of the enzymes which are involved in the biosynthesis of melatonin. Similarly, the juxtaglomerular apparatus of the kidney and the islets of Langerhans of the pancreas may be considered to function as neuroendocrine transducers, since they convert a neural stimulus (in these cases adrenergic) to an endocrine secretion (renin and insulin, respectively).

Finally, the central role of the hypothalamus in the initiation and regulation of autonomic activity is now generally recognized. Sympathetic responses are most readily obtained by stimulation of the posterior and lateral regions of the hypothalamus. The course taken by the descending sympathetic pathways is not entirely clear. According to Carmel, the fibers from the lateral hypothalamic area at first run in the prerubral field, dorsal and slightly rostral to the red nucleus; they then traverse the lateral tegmentum of the midbrain and pons and descend to the intermediolateral cell column of the spinal cord via the lateral part of the medullary reticular formation. These descending sympathetic fibers are largely or totally uncrossed.

EMERGENCY AND ALARM REACTIONS

Inasmuch as the autonomic nervous system and the endocrine glands, particularly the adrenals, have been accepted for many years as the neural and humoral basis of all instinctive and emotional behavior, it is remarkable how little sound information has been acquired about the role of this apparatus in disease. In chronic anxiety, acute panic reactions, the altered emotionality of depressive psychosis, mania, and schizophrenia, and the many so-called psychosomatic diseases, some of which have an apparent similarity to primitive emotional reactions, no consistent autonomic or endocrine dysfunction has been demonstrated. This has been disappointing, since Cannon, with his emergency theory of sympathoadrenal action, had given us such a promising conception of the neurophysiology of acute emotion and Selye had extended this theory so plausibly to explain all the reactions of human and animal organisms to chronic stressful situations. According to these theories, strong emotion, such as anger or fear, excites the sympathetic nervous system and also the medulla of the adrenal glands, which is under both direct nervous and hormonal control (via the hypothalamohypophysial axis). These sympathoadrenal reactions are brief and capable of sustaining the animal in "flight or fight." Prolonged stressful situations stimulate an excess of ACTH production by the anterior pituitary. This in turn stimulates the adrenal cortex, which elaborates a number of hormones referred to collectively as *steroids.* According to Selye, these more prolonged defensive and adaptive reactions develop in three stages: The first stage is the alarm reaction, i.e., the initial calling forth of the body's defensive forces. The second is the stage of resistance, which develops if the stress is not too strong and if the adaptation is effective. The final stage is exhaustion and death.

Animals deprived of adrenal cortex or human beings with Addison's disease cannot tolerate stress, because they are incapable of mobilizing both the adrenal medulla and adrenal cortex. In animals, exercise, cold, oxygen lack, and surgical injury all are said to evoke the same sympathoadrenal reactions as anger or fear. Some of these reactions are accompanied by adrenal enlargement, thymic and lymphatic hyperplasia, and gastric ulceration and other irreversible tissue changes. Selye's extension of Cannon's theory, although attractive, has received little or no support. Critics have pointed out that the conditions to which the experimental animal has been subjected are so different from human disease that conclusions as to the unity of the two cannot be drawn. More critical studies of the anatomy and physiology of the hypothalamus, hypophysis, adrenal glands and autonomic nervous system are needed before these hypotheses can be fully tested.

An important development in neuroendocrine research has been the demonstration of a multiplicity of hormonal responses to stress, in addition to those involving ACTH and adrenocorticoids. In humans, prolactin or growth hormone, or both, have been found to increase significantly before and during major and minor surgical procedures and a variety of other situations which have in common elements of anxiety and stress. In animals, stress leads to a reduction in TSH levels, a response that does not appear to depend upon ACTH release.

TESTS FOR ABNORMALITIES OF THE AUTONOMIC NERVOUS SYSTEM

With few exceptions, such as testing pupillary reactions and examination of the skin for abnormalities of color and sweating, the neurologist tends not to be precise in evaluating the autonomic nervous system function. Nonetheless, several simple tests can be used to confirm clinical impressions. Some of the more important ones are described below.

TESTS OF VASOMOTOR REACTIONS

Measurement of the skin temperature is a useful index of vasomotor function. Vasomotor paralysis results in vasodilatation of skin vessels and a rise in temperature; vaso-

constriction lowers the temperature. With a skin thermometer one may compare affected and normal areas under standard conditions. The normal skin temperature is usually 31 to 33°C when the room temperature is 26 to 27°C. Vasoconstrictor tone may also be tested by measuring the temperature of the area in question before and after immersing the hands in cold water.

The integrity of the sympathetic reflex arc, which includes baroreceptors in the aorta and carotid sinus and their afferent pathways, vasomotor centers, and the sympathetic and parasympathetic outflow, can be tested in a general way by combining the cold pressor test, Valsalva maneuver, and mental arithmetic test.

Vasoconstriction induces an elevation of the blood pressure and bradycardia. This is the basis of the *cold pressor test.* In normal persons, immersing the hands in ice water for 60 s raises the systolic pressure by 15 to 20 mmHg and the diastolic pressure by 10 to 15 mmHg.

In the *Valsalva maneuver,* the patient exhales into a manometer or against a closed glottis for 10 to 15 s, creating a markedly positive intrathoracic pressure. Normally, this causes a sharp reduction in venous return and cardiac output, so that the blood pressure falls; the effect on the baroreceptors is to cause a reflex tachycardia and peripheral vasoconstriction. With release of intrathoracic pressure, the venous return, stroke volume, and blood pressure return to higher than normal levels; parasympathetic influence then predominates and results in bradycardia.

The stress involved in doing *mental arithmetic* in noisy and distracting surroundings will normally stimulate a mild but measurable increase in pulse rate and blood pressure. This response does not depend upon the afferent limb of the sympathetic reflex arc.

Failure of the heart rate to increase during the positive intrathoracic pressure phase of the Valsalva maneuver points to sympathetic dysfunction, and failure of the rate to slow during the period of blood pressure overshoot points to parasympathetic disturbance. If the response to the Valsalva maneuver is abnormal and the response to the cold pressor test is normal, the lesion is probably in the baroreceptors or their afferent nerves; such a defect has been found in diabetic and tabetic patients. A failure of the pulse rate and blood pressure to rise during mental arithmetic, coupled with an abnormal Valsalva maneuver, suggests a defect in the central or peripheral efferent sympathetic pathways.

The integrity of sympathetic efferent pathways can be assessed further by *tests of sudomotor activity.*

There are several of these. Sweat can be weighed after it is absorbed by small squares of filter paper. Powdered charcoal dusted on the skin will cling to moist areas and not to dry ones. The galvanic skin-resistance test is an easy but not entirely reliable way of measuring sweating. A string galvanometer indicates the resistance offered by the skin to the passage of a weak galvanic current through the skin. Increase in sweating lowers the resistance; anhidrosis raises it. This method can be used to outline the area of a peripheral nerve lesion which reduces sweating. The starch test or a color indicator such as quinizarin (gray when dry, purple when wet) may be used. If the amount of sweating is not sufficient to show by these tests, the patient should be warmed with blankets or a heating cradle and given a diaphoretic such as hot tea or a dose of pilocarpine. Failure to sweat in response to these tests indicates an impairment of the efferent sympathetic pathway, somewhere between the hypothalamus and the skin.

Tearing can be estimated in a rough manner by the Schirmer test, in which one end of a 5-mm-wide and 25-mm-long strip of thin filter paper is inserted into the lower conjunctival sac while the other end hangs over the edge of the lower lid. The moisture of the tears wets the strip of filter paper, producing a moisture front. In normal patients, after 5 min, the moistened area extends over a length of approximately 15 mm. Values below 10 mm are suggestive of hypolacrimia.

Bladder function is best assessed by the cystometrogram, i.e., by measuring intravesicular pressure while sterile saline solution is permitted to flow by gravity into the bladder. Relatively simple apparatus is available for this purpose. The rise of pressure as 500 ml of fluid is allowed to flow gradually into the bladder and the emptying contractions of the detrusor can be recorded by a manometer. The size and motility of the colon can be tested in similar fashion. A quick and simple way of determining bladder atony (prostatic obstruction and overdistention having been excluded) is to measure the residual urine (by catheterization of the bladder) immediately after voluntary voiding or by estimating its volume by intravenous pyelography.

Disorders of gastrointestinal motility are readily demonstrated by radiologic examination. In dysautonomic states a barium swallow may disclose a number of abnormalities, including atonic dilatation of the esophagus, gastric atony and distention, delayed gastric emptying time, and a characteristic small-bowel pattern consisting of an increase in frequency and amplitude of peristaltic waves and rapid intestinal transit. A barium enema may demonstrate colonic distention and a decrease in propulsive activity.

The *topical application of pharmacologic agents* is useful in evaluating pupillary denervation. Part of the rationale behind these special tests is "Cannon's law," or the phenomenon of denervation hypersensitivity, in which an effector organ, 2 to 3 weeks after denervation, becomes hypersensitive to its particular neurotransmitter substance and to related drugs.

The instillation of a 1:1000 solution of epinephrine into the conjunctival sac has no effect on the normal pupil but will cause the sympathetically denervated pupil to dilate. The test is best carried out by the instillation of three drops three times within an interval of 3 min. The pupillary size is checked after 15, 30, and 45 min. As a rule, hypersensitivity to epinephrine is greater with lesions of the postganglionic fibers than of the preganglionic fibers. In lesions which involve central sympathetic pathways, the pupil rarely reacts. If denervation is incomplete, the hypersensitivity phenomenon may not be demonstrable.

The topical application of a 4% cocaine solution as a test for sympathetic denervation may be more reliable. The test should be carried out as described above. Cocaine potentiates the effect of the adrenergic transmitter since it probably prevents the reuptake of epinephrine into nerve endings. A normal response to cocaine consists of pupillary dilatation. In sympathetic denervation caused by lesions of the post- or preganglionic fibers, no change in pupillary size occurs, since no transmitter substance is available. In cases of central sympathetic lesions, slight mydriasis occurs.

A freshly prepared solution of 2.5% methacholine (Mecholyl) can be used in a similar fashion to demonstrate parasympathetic denervation. The normal pupil will not respond to this concentration of methocholine whereas the denervated pupil will constrict.

The intracutaneous injection of 0.05 ml of histamine phosphate in a dilution of 1:1000 normally causes a 1-cm wheal after 5 to 10 min. This is surrounded by a narrow red areola, and this in turn by an erythematous flare which extends 1 to 3 cm from the border of the wheal. A similar triple response follows the release of histamine into the tissue as the result of a scratch. The wheal and the deeply colored red areola are caused by direct action of histamine on blood vessels, while the flare depends upon the integrity of the axon reflex mediated along sensory fibers by antidromic transmission. In familial dysautonomia the flare response is absent. It may also be absent in peripheral neuropathies that involve sympathetic nerves (e.g., diabetes, alcoholic-nutritional disease, Landry-Guillain-Barré syndrome, amyloidosis, porphyria, etc.).

Finally, *the systemic administration of pharmaco-*

logic agents may provide information about the auto-nomic innervation of the heart. These include the infu-sion of methacholine at a steady rate. In dysautonomic states this will produce a drop in blood pressure without an increase in heart rate, at a lower infusion rate than in normal subjects. In cases of familial dysautonomia, methacholine restores temporarily the sense of taste, deep tendon reflexes, and the flare response to hista-mine. The mechanism by which this phenomenon occurs is unknown.

The infusion of norepinephrine causes a rise in blood pressure which is usually more pronounced in dys-autonomic states than with normal subjects for a given infusion rate. In patients with familial dysautonomia, the infusion of norepinephrine also produces erythema-tous blotching of the skin, like that which occurs under emotional stress. Thus, bouts of hypertension and blotching of the skin in dysautonomic children are be-lieved to be due to an exaggerated response to endog-enous norepinephrine.

The infusion of angiotensin II into patients with idiopathic orthostatic hypotension also causes an exag-gerated blood pressure response. The response to metha-choline and norepinephrine has been interpreted as a denervation hypersensitivity to neurotransmitter or re-lated substances. Since angiotensin II is not one of those substances, a different mechanism needs to be invoked, perhaps defective baroreceptor function. Thus, hyper-tension induced by angiotensin II, methacholine, or nor-epinephrine would not lead to compensatory peripheral reflex vasodilatation and bradycardia.

The integrity of autonomic innervation of the heart can be evaluated by the intramuscular injection of atropine, ephedrine, and neostigmine while the heart rate is monitored. Normally, the intramuscular injection of 0.8 mg of atropine causes a parasympathetic block and an increase in heart rate because of unopposed sym-pathetic activity. No such change occurs in cases of sym-pathetic denervation of the heart. Similarly, 25 mg of ephedrine administered intramuscularly results in in-creased heart rate under normal conditions; in cases of sympathetic denervation, this response is absent. Con-versely, 1 mg of neostigmine given intramuscularly re-sults in bradycardia provided the parasympathetic in-nervation of the heart is intact.

CLINICAL DISORDERS OF THE AUTONOMIC NERVOUS SYSTEM

Complete Autonomic Paralysis (*Dysautonomic Poly-neuropathy*)   This relatively rare condition has been ob-served in a few adults and children who over a period of a week or a few weeks developed anhidrosis, orthostatic

hypotension, paralysis of pupillary reflexes, loss of lacri-mation and salivation, impotence, poor bladder and bowel function, reduced gastric acidity (ulcer symptoms may disappear), and loss of certain pilomotor and vaso-motor responses in skin. One of the reported cases had infectious mononucleosis. Although no autopsy studies have been made, it is assumed that both the sympathetic and parasympathetic parts of the autonomic nervous system are affected, mainly at the postganglionic level. Somatic sensory and motor nerve fibers appear to be spared. The CSF protein may be normal or increased. Recovery is complete after a few months. In the few reported cases, corticosteroid therapy, in combination with fluorocortisone acetate (for the hypotension), may have been helpful. It is interesting to compare this dis-ease with botulism where the toxin causes a synaptic block only of the cholinergic systems, both the parasym-pathetic and neuromuscular.

Primary Orthostatic Hypotension   The clinical state known as primary orthostatic hypotension is now known to be caused by at least two diseases. In one, a degener-ative disease of middle and late adult life first described by Bradbury and Eggleston in 1925, the lesions involve mainly the postganglionic sympathetic neurons (Petito and Black). The parasympathetic system is relatively spared. In the other, described by Shy and Drager, the preganglionic lateral horn neurons of the thoracic spinal segments degenerate; extrapyramidal signs are added to the clinical picture later. In both conditions anhidrosis, impotence, and sphincteric disturbances may develop.

The differentiation of these two types of primary orthostatic hypotension, the chronic peripheral postgan-glionic and the central preganglionic, is based on patho-logic and pharmacologic evidence. In the postganglionic type the patients' plasma levels of norepinephrine, while recumbent, are subnormal because of failure of the dam-aged nerve terminals to synthesize or release catechola-mines. In this type there is hypersensitivity to injected norepinephrine, and, on standing, the norepinephrine levels do not rise as they do in normal persons. In the central type, the resting norepinephrine levels in the plasma are normal but on standing, again, there is no rise. However, sensitivity to exogenously administered norepinephrine is normal. In both types the plasma lev-els of dopamine β-hydroxylase, the enzyme that converts dopamine to norepinephrine, are subnormal (Ziegler et al.).

Peripheral Neuropathy with Secondary Orthostatic Hypotension Impairment of autonomic function, of which orthostatic hypotension is the most serious feature, may occur as part of the more common peripheral neuropathies (Landry-Guillain-Barré, infectious mononucleosis, porphyric, diabetic, and alcoholic-nutritional). Disease of the peripheral nervous system may affect the circulation in two ways: baroreceptors may be affected, interrupting normal homeostatic reflexes on the afferent side, or postganglionic sympathetic fibers may be affected in the spinal nerves. The severity of the autonomic failure need not parallel the degree of motor weakness. In some patients with acute polyneuropathy (notably the idiopathic and porphyric types), hypertension may occur, unassociated with underventilation or renal disease. Possibly this is due to overactivity of the sympathetic nervous system.

A particular polyneuropathy with an unusually prominent dysautonomia is that due to amyloidosis (Andrade's disease). Extensive analgesia and thermohypesthesia and to a lesser degree impairment of other forms of sensation may also be present. Motor function is much less affected. Autonomic paralysis affects the sympathetic neurons more than the parasympathetic ones. Iridoplegia (pupillary paralysis) and other glandular and smooth muscle functions are variably disturbed. Some or all of these abnormalities are also observed in Jewish children with the Riley-Day syndrome (familial dysautonomia; see page 914), another form of autonomic and sensory polyneuropathy.

Poisoning with organic phosphate (Parathion), which is an anticholinesterase drug, causes a combination of parasympathetic overactivity and motor paralysis (see page 789). The most severe degree of autonomic disturbance, involving postganglionic sympathetic and parasympathetic function, is produced by ingestion of the rodenticide N-3-pyridylmethyl-N'-p-nitrophenylurea (PNU, Vacor).

Both the primary and secondary types of orthostatic hypotension are discussed more fully in Chap. 17.

SPECIAL RESTRICTED AUTONOMIC SYNDROMES

Bernard-Horner and Stellate Ganglion Syndromes Interruption of the cervical sympathetic fibers in the neck or at any point along the internal carotid arteries (postganglionic fibers), or the removal of the superior cervical ganglion results in miosis, drooping of the eyelid, enophthalmos, and abolition of sweating over one side of the face (see also page 188). The same syndrome may be caused by interruption of the preganglionic fibers from their origin in the intermediolateral cell column of the eighth cervical and first through third thoracic spinal segments, or by interruption of the descending, uncrossed hypothalamospinal pathway in the tegmentum of the brainstem or cervical cord. The common causes of the syndrome are tumorous or inflammatory involvement of cervical lymph nodes, surgical and other types of trauma to cervical structures, neoplastic invasion of the proximal part of the brachial plexus, basal skull fractures, tumor, syringomyelia, or traumatic lesions of the first and second thoracic spinal segments, and infarcts or other lesions of the lateral part of the medulla (Wallenberg's syndrome). There is also an idiopathic variety which may at times be hereditary. If Horner's syndrome develops early in life, the iris on the side of the lesion fails to become pigmented and remains blue or mottled gray-brown and blue. A lesion of the stellate ganglion, e.g., compression by a tumor arising from the superior sulcus of the lung, produces the interesting combination of Horner's syndrome and paralysis of sympathetic reflexes in the arm (hand and arm are dry and warm).

Keane has provided data as to the relative frequency of the lesions causing oculosympathetic paralysis. In 100 successive cases, 67 were of central type due to brainstem strokes, 21 were preganglionic due to trauma or tumors of the neck, and 13 were postganglionic due to miscellaneous causes.

Other Pupillary and Salivary Disturbances A disorder of the oculomotor nerve, in addition to paralyzing four of the extraocular muscles and the levator muscle of the eyelid, causes a dilatation of the pupil, with an abolition of the constriction which normally occurs as a reaction to light; also there may be an associated loss of near vision and accommodation, owing to paralysis of the ciliary muscle. Parasympathetic and sympathetic abnormalities of pupillary function are considered further in Chap. 13.

Diseases which involve the facial, glossopharyngeal, and vagus nerves seldom induce recognizable parasympathetic changes. However, Bell's palsy, or less commonly, head injury, operations on the ear, or surgical resection of the greater superficial petrosal nerve may be followed by imperfect regeneration and misdirection of nerve fibers. For example, fibers which should innervate the salivary glands may reach either the lacrimal or the sweat glands in the preauricular and temporal regions. Eating (or even thinking of good food), with its attendant reflex salivation, then provokes lacrimation (syndrome of crocodile tears) or temporal sweating (auriculotemporal syndrome).

Sympathetic and Parasympathetic Paralysis in Quadriplegia Lesions of the C4 or C5 segments of the spinal cord, if complete, will sever all suprasegmental control of the sympathetic and sacral parasympathetic nervous systems. Thoracic lesions leave much of the descending sympathetic outflow intact, with only sacral parasympathetic control being interrupted. Traumatic necrosis of the spinal cord is the usual cause of these states, but it may happen with infarct necrosis, certain forms of myelopathy, and tumors.

Since all the afferent and efferent autonomic connections with the spinal cord are intact, autonomic reflex discharges may appear as soon as spinal shock wears off. As part of the "mass reflex" of leg flexion and micturition, there may be a rise in blood pressure in association with bradycardia, and sweating and pilomotor reactions in parts below the cervical segments. These reactions may also be evoked by pinprick, passive movement, contact with limbs and abdomen, and pressure on the bladder. An exaggerated vasopressor reaction also occurs when norepinephrine is injected. Tilting the body upright drops the blood pressure, often with some compensatory reaction. Pinching the skin below the lesion causes gooseflesh in adjacent segments. Heating the body results in flushing and sweating over the face and neck, but not the trunk and legs. Bladder and bowel, including their sphincters, are at first flaccid and then become automatic, as spinal reflex control returns. There may be reflex penile erection (priapism) and even ejaculation in the male, and the female may become pregnant even though voluntary control of sexual activity has been abolished.

The Effects of Thoracolumbar Sympathectomy Surgical resection of the thoracolumbar sympathetic trunk, widely used in the 1940s in the treatment of hypertension, has provided the clinician with the only clear-cut example of extensive injury to the peripheral autonomic nervous system, although in primary orthostatic hypotension (see above) a similar defect has long been suspected. In general it may be said that bilateral thoracolumbar sympathectomy results in surprisingly few physiologic changes. Aside from loss of sweating over the denervated areas of the body, the most pronounced abnormality is an impairment of vasomotor reflexes. In the upright posture, syncope is frequent because of the pooling of blood in the splanchnic bed and lower extremities; there is a steady fall in blood pressure to shock levels and little or no pallor, nausea, vomiting, or sweating—the usual accompaniments of syncope. Bladder, bowel, and sexual function are preserved, though in some males the semen is ejaculated into the posterior urethra and bladder. No consistent abnormalities of renal or hepatic function have been found.

Hirschsprung's Disease, or Congenital Megacolon This is a rare disease which affects mainly male infants and children. It is presently ascribed to an absence of ganglion cells in the intramural (Auerbach's) plexus. The parasympathetically denervated segment of the colon is markedly constricted. In the massively dilated portion of the colon, proximal to the constricted portion, the plexus is normal. Some cases of megaloureter are attributed to a similar defect.

Excessive Sweating This sympathetically mediated disorder may be a troublesome complaint in some patients. Its cause is not known. One variety, presumably of congenital origin, affects the palms. In some cases, the hyperhidrosis affects mainly the feet and lower extremities. The social embarrassment of a "succulent hand" or a "dripping paw" is often intolerable. It is taken to be a sign of nervousness, though many persons with this condition disclaim all other neurotic symptoms. Cold, clammy hands are common in individuals with anxiety neurosis, and indeed this has been a useful sign in distinguishing an anxiety state from hyperthyroidism, in which the hands are also moist, but warm. Cervical sympathectomy will relieve the more severe cases of palmar sweating. Shih and Wang relieved the palmar sweating in all except 2 of 457 cases by extirpation of T2 and T3 sympathetic ganglia. As long as the T1 ganglion was left intact there was no Bernard-Horner syndrome. Excessive perspiration is also observed in some cases of peripheral neuropathy, e.g., causalgia and the "burning foot syndrome," in which burning and painful paresthesias and hyperhidrosis are combined. A special type of nonthermoregulatory hyperhidrosis may occur in spinal paraplegics (see page 620).

Anhidrosis in restricted skin areas is a frequent and useful finding in peripheral nerve disease. It is due to the interruption of the postganglionic sympathetic fibers. The loss of sweating corresponds to the area of sensory loss. In contrast, sweating is not affected in spinal root disease for the reason that there is much intersegmental mixing of the preganglionic axons, once they enter the sympathetic chain.

Raynaud's Phenomenon This disorder, characterized by a painful blanching of the fingers on exposure to the cold, is a frequent finding in connective tissue disease,

378

cervical rib, and overuse of the hands in cold weather (rowing, use of a pneumatic drill). It indicates an overactivity of the normal sympathetic vasoconstrictor response, possibly from a partial postganglionic denervation. *Causalgia*, the painful syndrome that follows partial interruption of a peripheral nerve, has been ascribed to the cross stimulation of sensory fibers by efferent sympathetic impulses at the point of artificial synapse where the nerve trunk is injured. Raynaud's phenomenon is described on page 152 and causalgia on page 922.

DISTURBANCES OF BLADDER AND BOWEL FUNCTION

The urinary bladder receives a dual nerve supply, parasympathetic via sacral nerves (mainly the third sacral segment, with lesser contributions from the second and fourth sacral segments) and sympathetic via the hypogastric plexus (lower thoracic and upper lumbar segments). The sympathetic nervous system has relatively little control of bladder function. It supplies mainly the blood vessels in the bladder wall. Afferent fibers for pain and feelings of distension traverse the pelvic nerves (nervi erigentes) and hypogastric nerves, respectively; afferent impulses from the urethra and external sphincter are conducted via the pudendal nerves to the third and fourth sacral spinal segments. Thus, efferent and afferent fibers are conducted through the same nerves. In addition, the external sphincter receives somatic efferent fibers via the third and fourth ventral roots and pudendal nerve (Fig. 26-6).

Emptying of the bladder is effected by the detrusor muscle, which has a reciprocal relationship with the internal sphincter, so that contraction of the detrusor is associated with relaxation of the sphincter and vice versa. The internal sphincter is not a sphincter in the literal sense, since its fibers have no annular organization but arise from the inner longitudinally arranged detrusor muscle fascicles. The internal sphincter probably opens

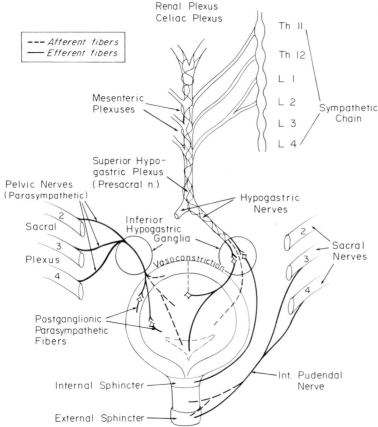

Figure 26-6
Innervation of the urinary bladder and its sphincters.

mechanically, as a result of contractions of the detrusor muscle. The act of micturition is both reflex and voluntary. When the normal person is asked to void, there is first a voluntary relaxation of the perineum, then an increased tension of the abdominal wall, a slow contraction of the vesical muscle itself (the detrusor) with an associated opening of the internal sphincter, and finally a relaxation of the external sphincter (Denny-Brown and Robertson, 1933a). The detrusor contraction is a spinal stretch reflex subject to facilitation and inhibition from higher centers. Voluntary closure of the external sphincter and contraction of the perineal muscles causes the vesical contraction to subside. The abdominal muscles have no power to initiate micturition except when the detrusor muscle is not functioning normally. The voluntary restraint of micturition is a cerebral affair and is mediated by fibers which arise in the frontal lobes (paracentral motor region), descend in the spinal cord just anterior to the corticospinal tracts, and terminate on the efferent vesical neurons in the sacral segments. The action of the upper motor neurons is inhibitory, and in normal circumstances micturition is initiated by variations of this inhibitory effect, which release the segmental mechanisms for control of the bladder (consisting essentially of contraction of the detrusor in response to distention, acting in concert with voluntary facilitation of the abdominal and other muscles). There are said to be other suprasegmental mechanisms in the brainstem, but their exact location and action are not known.

Cerebral lesions which lead to mental confusion are often accompanied by urinary and fecal incontinence (so-called *frontal lobe incontinence*). The patient does not appear to be fully aware of the immediate circumstances and voids in inappropriate places. Usually such a patient is unaware of having voided, and when attention is called to it, he or she may deny responsibility for it or offer an excuse. In addition, discrete lesions of the anteromedial part of the frontal lobes weaken voluntary control of the bladder (see page 304). Unilateral lesions of the paracentral lobule, or of the corticospinal tract at any level from cortex to sacral cord, do not as a rule result in a loss of voluntary control of bladder and bowel.

Transection of the spinal cord, above the level of the sacral segments, at first causes a flaccid paralysis of the bladder and bowel, just as it does of the leg muscles. The bladder rapidly becomes distended, and overflow incontinence follows. Later, as spasticity and heightened spinal reflex activity of the legs develop, the bladder also becomes spastic and contracted because of exaggeration of the stretch reflex. The distension produced by accumulated urine then provokes reflex contraction; this is the *automatic*, or *reflex, bladder*. This state of automa-

ticity may permit relatively complete emptying of the bladder, or emptying may be incomplete as the result of a disturbance in the reciprocal relationship between detrusor contraction and sphincter relaxation ("sphincter-detrusor dyssynergia"). The presence of this latter state can only be established with certainty by simultaneous cystometry and external sphincter electromyography and is of importance in determining rational urologic therapy. If the cord lesion is incomplete and weak voluntary control remains, the patient reports frequency and urgency of urination and difficulty in both initiating and inhibiting bladder action. Sensation of bladder filling and distention may or may not be present, according to whether or not sensory tracts are interrupted.

Posterior root lesions, e.g., tabes dorsalis, impair sensation and also the reflex tone of the detrusor muscle; the bladder is then both insensitive and hypotonic. It overfills without the patient being aware of it, and with a rise in intraabdominal pressure during strain, turning in bed, or stooping, there will be overflowing and dribbling. The urinary stream is feeble. Sacral cord lesions (spina bifida or tumor) or anterior root lesions also leave the bladder partially paralyzed and hypotonic, but in this case (unlike a denervated skeletal muscle), even though completely isolated from spinal control, the bladder does regain tone and becomes capable of some functional activity. However, the isolated bladder does not empty itself completely, and infection from the residual urine always remains a serious hazard.

If the bladder wall is repeatedly overstretched because of the retention of large amounts of urine (as in hysteria or prostatism), the detrusor muscle may be permanently damaged. Thereafter, emptying is incomplete and self-catheterization or urinary diversion becomes necessary.

The colon, rectum, and anal sphincters have an innervation similar to that of the bladder, and their function is disturbed in the same way with central and peripheral lesions. The colon may be hypotonic and distended and the anal sphincters lax. The anal and, in the male, the bulbocavernosus reflex may be abolished. Defecation may be urgent and precipitant in higher spinal lesions. Since the same spinal segments and nearly the same spinal tracts subserve bladder and bowel function, so-called double incontinence is often manifest. However, since the bowel is less often filled and its content is solid, fecal incontinence is usually less troublesome than urinary incontinence.

DISTURBANCES OF SEXUAL FUNCTION

Sexual function in the male, which is not infrequently affected in neurologic disease, is conveniently divided into several parts: (1) sexual impulse, drive, or desire, often referred to as *libido;* (2) penile erection, whereby the act of sexual intercourse can be effected (potency); and (3) ejaculation of semen by the prostate through the urethra, whereby impregnation of the female may be accomplished.

The arousal of libido in man and woman may result from a variety of stimuli, some purely imaginary. Such neocortical influences are transmitted to the limbic system and thence to the hypothalamus and spinal centers. The suprasegmental pathways traverse the lateral funiculi of the spinal cord near the corticospinal tracts to reach sympathetic and parasympathetic segmental centers. Penile erection is effected through sacral parasympathetic motor neurons (S3 and S4) and the nervi erigentes and pudendal nerves. There is evidence also that an outflow from thoracolumbar segments (originating in T12-L1) can mediate psychogenic erections in patients with complete sacral cord destruction. Activation from these segmental centers opens vascular channels between arteriolar branches of the pudendal arteries and the vascular spaces of the corpora cavernosa and corpus spongiosum (erectile tissues) resulting in tumescence. Deturgescence occurs when venous channels open widely. Copulation consists of a complex series of rhythmic thrusting movements of pelvic musculature, and ejaculation involves rhythmic contractions of the prostate, the compressor (sphincter) urethrae, and bulbocavernosus and ischiocavernosus muscles, which are partly under the control of both the sympathetic and parasympathetic centers. Afferent segmental influences arise in the glans penis and reach parasympathetic centers at S3 and S4 (reflexogenic erections). The organization of this neural system and the locations of lesions that can abolish normal potency are shown in Fig. 26-7. Similar neural arrangements exist in females.

The different parts of the sexual act may be affected separately. Loss of libido may depend upon both psychic and somatic factors. It may be complete, as in old age or in medical and endocrine diseases, or it may occur only in certain circumstances or in relation to a certain person. In the latter case, which is usually due to psychological factors, reflexogenic penile erection and even emission of semen may occur nocturnally, and effective sexual intercourse with another person is possible. Sexual desire can on occasion be altered in the opposite direction, i.e., it may be excessive as a sign of neurologic disease. This has been observed in encephalitis and tumors affecting the diencephalon and temporal lobes. Sexual desire on the other hand may be present but penile erection impossible to attain or sustain, a condition called *impotence.* The commonest cause of impotence is a depressive state. It occurs also in patients who suffer disease of the sacral cord segments and their afferent and efferent connections (e.g., cord tumor, tabes, diabetic polyneuropathy). The parasympathetic nerves cannot then be activated to cause tumescence of the corpora cavernosa and corpus spongiosum. Diseases of the spinal cord may abolish psychogenic erections, leaving reflexogenic ones intact. The latter may become overactive, in fact giving rise to sustained erections for long periods of time. This is called *priapism;* it is a reminder that all the neural apparatus for the control of sexual function is organized through the lower spinal segments (sacral 3 and 4 and the nervi erigentes and pudendal nerves) and that the mechanism of erection may function effectively even when completely removed from voluntary control, as in high spinal lesions. Sympathectomy leaves this mechanism for penile erection relatively intact.

Another sexual difficulty may be the premature ejaculation of semen, a common complaint in neurotic individuals, though by no means peculiar to them. After lumbar sympathectomy the semen may be ejected back into the bladder because of paralysis of the periurethral muscle (prostate) at the verumontanum (colliculus seminalis).

Finally, diseases of the testes accompanied by insufficient spermatogenesis or diseases of the seminal vesicles which prevent emission of sperm result in *sterility;* in these cases libido and potency may or may not be normal.

Aberrations of sexual function also occur in the female but are more difficult to analyze. Lack of sexual desire or failure to attain orgasm (frigidity) is much more frequent in the female than in the male, occurring in a significant percentage of neurotic women and in others who exhibit no signs of psychic disorder. States of excessive sexual excitability are known in psychopathic individuals and, rarely, in those who suffer disease of the brain. Fecundity and sterility are often unrelated to the other aspects of sexuality, being the result of diseases of the ovaries, fallopian tubes, and uterus, as well as of other less clearly defined factors.

The genesis of sexual perversions remains obscure. Endocrine, biochemical, and psychological studies have failed to clarify the cause and mechanism. Homosexuality appears to be stamped into the limbic-hypothalamic parts of the nervous system in early life; the brain becomes either male or female. Cerebral disorders of sexual function are discussed further in Chap. 27 and the section on psychiatry.

AUTONOMIC DISTURBANCES WITH LESIONS OF THE BRAINSTEM

With lesions of any type in the lateral tegmentum of the pons and medulla there may be an ipsilateral paralysis of autonomic function in the arm, trunk, and leg. These parts are warm and dry. In addition there may be Horner's syndrome. Rarely, discrete lesions in higher parts of the brainstem, presumably interrupting the hypothalamotegmental sympathetic pathway, may produce the same effects (Carmel).

HYPOTHALAMIC SYNDROMES

Within comparatively recent times the following syndromes consequent to disease of the hypothalamus have been delineated.

Diabetes Insipidus This condition is due to involvement of the supraoptic and paraventricular nuclei, or the supraopticohypophysial tract, interfering with the production of vasopressin or antidiuretic hormone (ADH), and giving rise to the passage of large quantities of dilute urine and secondary polydipsia. Tumors in the diencephalohypophyseal region, basilar meningitis, sarcoidosis, histiocytic disorders, and cerebral (including surgical) trauma are the usual causes.

Inappropriate ADH Secretion In this syndrome there is an increased release of ADH, resulting in excessive retention of water, despite a continued renal excretion of sodium and hypoosmolality of the serum. Reduction of the serum sodium concentration to less than 110 meq/

Figure 26-7
The pathways involved in human penile erection. (From Weiss.)

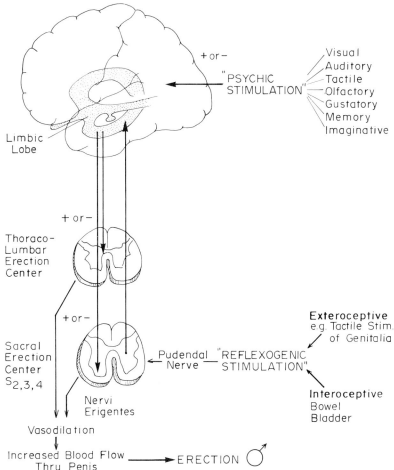

liter is usually accompanied by neurologic signs, consisting of irritability, confusion, muscular weakness, loss of tendon reflexes, and Babinski signs, and in advanced cases, of seizures and stupor. This syndrome was originally described in association with carcinoma of the lung, particularly of the oat-cell type, but it occurs with other forms of carcinoma and lung disease as well as with a variety of disorders that involve the nervous system: idiopathic polyneuritis (Landry-Guillain-Barré), subarachnoid hemorrhage, cerebral infarction, tumor and abscess, meningitis, head trauma, and acute intermittent porphyria. Usually, inappropriate ADH secretion diminishes or disappears once the acute phase of the neurologic disorder subsides. In the case of bronchogenic carcinoma, there is evidence that the tumor tissue itself secretes ADH, but in the neurologic disorders it appears that the ADH is released inappropriately from the supraopticohypophysial system.

Disturbances of Temperature Regulation Lesions in the more anterior parts of the hypothalamus may result in hyperthermia. The heat-dissipating mechanisms of the body are impaired. This often follows operations in the region of the floor of the third ventricle. The temperature rises to 41°C (106°F) or higher and remains elevated until death some hours or days later. Icy coldness of the extremities, dry skin, tachycardia, and tachypnea are also present. Acetylsalicylic acid has little effect on central hyperthermia; the temperature may, however, be reduced by phenobarbital in conjunction with cooling of the body. Lesions in the more posterior parts of the hypothalamus are sometimes attended by hypothermia or poikilothermia. The latter may pass unnoticed unless the patient's temperature is taken after lowering and raising the room temperature. Somnolence and hypotension are often associated.

Adiposogenital Dystrophy (Froehlich's Syndrome) Destruction of the tuberal nuclei and the tuberoinfundibular tracts results in a delay or an arrest of sexual development. This is often combined with obesity. Many cases are idiopathic; craniopharyngioma is the most frequently demonstrated cause. In the *Laurence-Moon-Biedl* syndrome, obesity and hypogenitalism are combined with mental retardation, polydactyly, and retinal pigmentation. In several instances this syndrome has been familial. *Sexual precocity* as a clinical phenomenon is rare and has in several autopsied cases been traced to

an anomalous overdevelopment of tuberal nuclei (hamartoma). The authors have observed this in cases with von Recklinghausen's disease and tuberous sclerosis. Both sexes may be affected; this type of precocious puberty (pubertas precox) evidently has a basis different from that of the sexual precocity in pinealoma, which usually occurs in males.

Disturbances of Appetite In the medial part of the hypothalamus, near the third ventricle, there is a *satiety center* and in the more lateral part, an *appetite, or feeding, center*. Both are important in controlling food intake and body weight. In several mammalian species, including humans, acute bilateral lesions in the lateral hypothalamus render the animal temporarily aphagic. Free feeding ceases for some weeks; then eating begins again, but weight remains subnormal, as though appetite were now at a lower "set point." Abnormal meal patterns, increased motor activity, loss of hydrational control of thirst, and deficits in sodium appetite are also present. Medial lesions have the opposite effects, causing hyperphagia and obesity.

Gastric Hemorrhage and Other Disorders Lesions in or near the tuberal nuclei are sometimes accompanied by superficial erosions, ulcerations, and hemorrhages from the gastric mucosa (Cushing's ulcer). Massive gastrointestinal hemorrhage may occur with any type of acute brain disease. In experimental animals this has been produced most consistently by lesions in or near the tuberal nuclei. However, in human cases coming to autopsy, lesions are usually not found in the hypothalamus; presumably, in these cases, hypothalamic function is impaired, as from a massive brain hemorrhage or epidural hematoma.

Disturbances in sugar metabolism have been produced by experimental lesions in the hypothalamus but are of infrequent occurrence in humans. The transitory hyperglycemia and glycosuria observed in some cases of subarachnoid hemorrhage and stroke can rarely be traced to a lesion in the hypothalamus. The authors have not encountered hypoglycemia with brain disease; if it occurs, it must be extremely rare. Hypothalamic disease may be associated with a variety of cardiac arrhythmias and pulmonary edema.

Emotional and Personality Disorders The role of the hypothalamus and other parts of the limbic system in emotional and behavioral disturbances has been fully discussed in the preceding chapter.

REFERENCES

APPENZELLER O: *The Autonomic Nervous System*, 2d ed. Amsterdam, North-Holland, 1976.

BARTTER FC, SCHWARTZ WB: The syndrome of inappropriate secretion of antidiuretic hormone. *Am J Med* 42:790, 1967.

BROWN GM, MARTIN JB: Neuroendocrine relationships, in Spiegel EA (ed): *Progress in Neurology and Psychiatry*. New York, Grune & Stratton, 1973, pp 193–240.

CANNON WB: *Bodily Changes in Pain, Hunger, Fear and Rage*, 2d ed. New York, Appleton, 1920.

CARMEL PW: Sympathetic deficits following thalamotomy. *Arch Neurol* 18:378, 1968.

DENNY-BROWN D, ROBERTSON EG: On the physiology of micturition. *Brain* 56:149, 1933*a*.

——, ——: The state of the bladder and its sphincters in complete transverse lesions of the spinal cord and cauda equina. *Brain* 56:397, 1933*b*.

FALCK B: Observations on the possibilities of the cellular localization of monoamines by a fluorescence method. *Acta Physiol Scand*, vol 56, suppl 197, 1962.

JOHNSON RH, SPALDING JMK: *Disorders of the Autonomic Nervous System*. Philadelphia, Davis, 1974.

KAADA B: Brain mechanisms related to aggressive behavior, in Clemente CD, Lindsley DB (eds): *Proceedings of the 5th Conference on Brain Function, November 1965, Aggression and Defense: Neural Mechanisms and Social Patterns*. Berkeley, University of California Press, 1967, pp 95–133.

KEANE JR: Oculosympathetic paresis: Analysis of 100 hospitalized patients. *Arch Neurol* 36:13, 1979.

LEWITT PA: The neurotoxicity of the rat poison Vacor. *N Engl J Med* 302:73, 1980.

MARTIN JB, REICHLIN S, BROWN GM: *Clinical Neuroendocrinology*. Philadelphia, Davis, 1977.

——, RENAUD LP: Hypothalamic and extrahypothalamic regulatory mechanisms for hypothalamic hormone secretion, in *Neuroendocrine Relationships*. New York, Raven, 1977.

PETITO CK, BLACK IB: Ultrastructure and biochemistry of sympathetic ganglia in idiopathic orthostatic hypotension. *Ann Neurol* 4:6, 1978.

PICK J: *The Autonomic Nervous System*. Philadelphia, Lippincott, 1970.

RICHARDSON KC: The fine structure of the albino rabbit iris with special reference to the identification of adrenergic and cholinergic nerves and nerve endings in its intrinsic muscles. *Am J Anat* 114:173, 1964.

SELYE H: The general adaptation syndrome and the diseases of adaptation. *J Clin Endocrinol Metab* 6:117, 1946.

SHAND DG, OATES JA: Clinical pharmacology of the autonomic nervous system, in Isselbacher KJ et al (eds): *Harrison's Principles of Internal Medicine*, 9th ed. New York, McGraw-Hill, 1980, chap 72, pp 389–396.

SHIH CJ, WANG YC: Thoracic sympathectomy for palmar hyperhidrosis. *Surg Neurol* 10:291, 1978.

SHY GM, DRAGER GA: A neurological syndrome associated with orthostatic hypotension. A clinical-pathologic study. *Arch Neurol* 2:511, 1960.

THOMPSON PD, MELMON KL: Clinical assessment of autonomic function. *Anesthesiology* 29:724, 1968.

WEISS HD: The physiology of human penile erection. *Ann Int Med* 76:792, 1972.

WICHSER J, VIJAYAN N, DREYFUS PM: Dysautonomia—its significance in neurologic disease. *Calif Med* 117:28, 1972.

WURTMAN RJ: Brain monoamines and endocrine function. *Neurosc Res Program Bull* 9(2):172, 1971.

YOUNG RR, ASBURY AK, CORBETT JL, ADAMS RD: Pure pandysautonomia with recovery. Description and discussion of diagnostic criteria. *Brain* 98:613, 1975.

ZIEGLER MG, LAKE R, KOPIN IJ: The sympathetic nervous system defect in primary orthostatic hypotension. *N Engl J Med* 296:293, 1977.

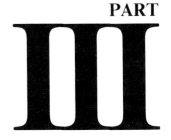

GROWTH AND DEVELOPMENT OF THE NERVOUS SYSTEM AND THE NEUROLOGY OF AGING

The human organism is characterized as much by individual differences as by species similarity. No two persons in the world are identical. Each has unique physical and mental peculiarities, and even in such fundamental matters as the biochemical reactions involved in nutrition, metabolism, and response to drugs there are wide individual variations. The experienced physician accepts these facts, and also certain biologic principles that apply to the majority of the population. Nevertheless, the medical world is constantly confronted with patients who appear to fall at or beyond the limits of normality. Then it must be ascertained whether any given departure is due to disease or represents an exceptional individual variation.

"Normality" in a sense is always a statistical matter a theoretical average with the largest proportion of a population of individuals grouping themselves within a defined distance from a mean. As a general working rule, deviation of a particular biologic trait should compel medical attention only when it falls beyond 2 SD (standard deviations) of the mean. Clinical experience, however, teaches that a deviation beyond this point may still represent no more than an extreme natural variation, although the likelihood of a pathologic process increases.

The extraordinary individuality of human beings appears to be a product of the complexity of their genetic makeup. Residing in the 46 chromosomes are more than 50,000 genes, which subserve not merely such traits as color of the eyes and hair but more complex physical and mental attributes, most of which are polygenic, i.e., the result of multiple gene interactions.

The program of embryologic development and maturation of the nervous system is one of the most complex in the whole realm of biology, and it is not surprising that here we should encounter the highest order of variation. Even a relatively simple function such as learning to walk independently ranges normally from 9 to 20 months of age, and the acquisition of communicative speech and ability

to read vary even more widely. Delays in these and many other functions are potent sources of anxiety to parents which in turn may cause psychic distress and aberrations in behavior in the affected child. They frequently occasion consultation with the pediatrician and pediatric neurologist, who must determine whether a specific developmental delay represents brain disease or an extreme variation of the normal developmental trajectory. Mistakes are often made in attributing slow development purely to environmental influences, since these factors do play a part in modifying genetic traits. Analyzing cases such as these makes up a considerable part of the practice of pediatric neurology.

At the opposite end of the natural life cycle, another set of individual variations become manifest. Some aging people remain hale, hearty, and bright, and others become deaf, tremulous, forgetful, or infirm. The age at which these disabilities set in seems also to be genetically determined. Since the cellular elements of the nervous system are postmitotic, meaning that each individual starts at birth with all the neurons he or she is destined to have and each neuron must last an entire lifetime, one conceives of these special late-life disabilities as neuronal losses through the inexorable effects of aging alone.

Thus, an understanding of pediatric and geriatric neurologic problems involves an intimate knowledge of normal early development, maturation, and aging. One must know in detail the milestones of normal growth and development and the changes that can be attributed to the effects of age, since they provide the background against which all diseases need to be evaluated.

Chapter 27 will deal first with the natural developmental changes in the nervous system and then with the common childhood disorders of nervous functioning which represent failures or deviations of normal development. In Chap. 28 the effects of aging on the nervous system will be considered, followed by a description of the variations in the aging process.

CHAPTER 27

NORMAL DEVELOPMENT AND DEVIATIONS IN DEVELOPMENT OF THE NERVOUS SYSTEM

TIME-LINKED SEQUENCES OF NORMAL DEVELOPMENT

The establishment of a biologic time scale of human development requires observation under standardized conditions of a large number of normal individuals of known ages and testing them for measurable items of behavior. Because of individual variations in the tempo of development, it is equally important to study the growth and development of any *one* individual for a prolonged period. If these observations are to be correlated with stages of neuroanatomic development, the clinical and morphologic data must be expressed in units that are comparable. Early in life, age periods are difficult to ascertain because of the special difficulty in fixing the time of conception. The average human gestational period is 40 weeks (280 days), but to take birth as zero is obviously fallacious, since it may occur with survival as early as 28 or as late as 49 weeks, a time span of 5 months. Conception is the only time when chronological and developmental age correspond, but in practice this can rarely be determined.

After birth, any given item of behavior or structural differentiation must always have two reference points: one to some item of behavior already achieved, the other to units of chronological time or duration of the life of the organism. The former, or biologic scale, assumes special significance in early prenatal life when development is proceeding at such a rapid pace that small units of time weigh heavily, the organism appearing to change literally day by day; in infancy the tempo of development is somewhat slower, but still very rapid in comparison with later childhood.

The neurologist finds it advantageous to organize all knowledge of normal development and disease around each of the time periods given in Tables 27-1 and 27-2.

NEUROANATOMIC BASES OF NORMAL DEVELOPMENT

A large body of knowledge has accumulated concerning the functional and structural status of the nervous system during each of the epochs of life (listed below), and the reader will find it recorded in the references at the end of this chapter. A summary of this information is given in Table 27-2.

EMBRYONAL AND FETAL PERIOD

Knowledge of the nervous system in the germinal and embryonal periods has been derived from the study of a relatively small number of abortuses that have fallen into the hands of anatomists. Neuronal multiplication, neuroblastic differentiation, and migration are already well under way in the first 3 weeks of embryonic life. The germinal cells proliferate rapidly in the matrix layer, next to the surface of the primordial hollow of the neuraxis. They become transformed into bipolar neuroblasts, which migrate, in a series of waves, toward the marginal layer of what is to become the cortex of the cerebral hemispheres. Each step in the differentiation and migration of the neuroblasts proceeds in an orderly fashion, and one stage progresses to the next with remarkable precision. This process of migration is completed by the end of the fifth fetal month; by the end of the sixth fetal month, mitotic figures are no longer observed in the cerebral cortex, which by this time has presumably acquired its full complement of nerve cells.

By the twentieth to twenty-fourth weeks of fetal

life the main cell masses of the brain have acquired their full quota of neurons, estimated variously at 16 to 22 billion. Actually we have little idea of how many nerve cells are to be found in any given nucleus or in the cerebral or cerebellar cortices at different ages. To obtain quantitative data of this type is one of the most pressing needs in neuroanatomy.

Within a few months of midfetal life, the cerebrum, which begins as a small bihemisphered organ with hardly a trace of surface indentation, evolves into a deeply sulcated structure. Every step in the folding of the surface to form fissures and sulci is obedient to order, following a temporal pattern of such precision as to permit a reasonably accurate estimation of age by this criterion alone. The major sylvian, rolandic, and calcarine fissures, for example, take on the adult configuration during the thirtieth to thirty-eighth weeks, and tertiary sulci develop in the last 2 weeks of fetal life.

Concomitantly, subtle changes in neuronal organization are occurring in the cerebral cortex and central ganglionic masses. Neurons become more widely separated as differentiation proceeds, owing to increase in size and complexity of dendrites and axons and enlargement of synaptic surfaces (Figs. 27-1 and 27-2). The familiar cytoarchitectural patterns which demarcate one part of the cerebral cortex from another are already in evidence by the thirtieth week of fetal life, and become definitive at birth and in succeeding months.

Myelination provides another index of the development and maturation of the nervous system and is believed to be related to the functional activity of the fiber systems. The acquisition of myelin sheaths by the spinal nerves and roots by the tenth week of fetal life is associated with the beginning of reflex motor activities. Segmental and intersegmental fiber systems in the spinal cord myelinate soon afterward, followed by ascending and descending fibers to and from the brainstem (reticulospinal, vestibulospinal). The acoustic and labyrinthine systems stand out with singular clarity in myelin-stained preparations by the twenty-eighth to thirtieth weeks, and the spinocerebellar and dentatorubral systems by the thirty-seventh week (Fig. 27-3).

NEONATAL PERIOD AND INFANCY

After birth, the brain continues to grow dramatically. From an average weight of 375 to 400 g at birth it reaches about 1000 g by the end of the first postnatal year. Glial cells derived from the matrix zones continue to divide and multiply during the first 6 months of postnatal life. The visual system begins to myelinate about

Table 27-1
Time scale of stages in human growth and development

Growth period	Approximate age
Prenatal	From 0 to 280 days
Ovum	From 0 to 14 days
Embryo	From 14 days to 9 weeks
Fetus	From 9 weeks to birth
Premature infant	From 27 to 37 weeks
Birth	Average 280 days
Neonate	First 4 weeks after birth
Infancy	First year
Early childhood (preschool)	From 1 to 6 years
Later childhood (prepubertal)	From 6 to 10 years
Adolescence	Girls, 8 or 10 to 18 years
	Boys, 10 or 12 to 20 years
Puberty (average)	Girls, 13 years
	Boys, 15 years

Source: GH Lowrey, *Growth and Development of Children,* 7th ed. Chicago, Year Book, 1978.

Table 27-2
Timetable of growth and nervous system development in the normal embryo and fetus

Age, days	Size (crown-rump length), mm	Nervous system development
18	1.5	Neural groove and tube
21	3.0	Optic vesicles
26	3.0	Closure of anterior neuropore
27	3.3	Closure of postneuropore; ventral horn cells appear
31	4.3	Anterior and posterior roots
35	5.0	Five cerebral vesicles
42	13.0	Primordium of cerebellum
56	25.0	Differentiation of cerebral cortex and meninges
150	225.0	Primary cerebral fissures appear
180	230.0	Secondary cerebral sulci and first myelination appear in brain
180		Further myelination and growth of brain (see text)

the fortieth week, and its myelination cycle proceeds rapidly, being nearly complete a few months after birth. The corticospinal tracts are not myelinated completely until halfway through the second postnatal year. Most of the principal tracts are myelinated by the end of this period. In the cerebrum the first myelin is seen in the posterior frontal and parietal lobes at birth, and the occipital lobes (geniculocalcarine system) myelinate soon thereafter. The myelination of the frontal and temporal lobes proceeds during the first year of postnatal life. Most of the myelination of the cerebrum is completed by the end of the second year (Fig. 27-3).

CHILDHOOD, PUBERTY, AND ADOLESCENCE

Growth of the brain continues, at a much slower rate than before, until 12 to 15 years, when the average adult weight of 1230 to 1275 g in females and 1350 to 1410 g in males is attained. Myelination also continues during this period, but much more slowly. Yakovlev and Lecours, who have checked Flechsig's observations on

Figure 27-1

Cox-Golgi preparations of the leg area of the motor cortex (area 4). Upper row, left to right: 8 months premature; newborn at term; 1 month; 3 months; and 6 months. Lower row, left to right: 15 months; 2 years; 4 years; 6 years. Magnification, 100×; apical dendrites of Betz cells have been shortened, all to the same degree. (Courtesy of Th Rabinowicz, University of Lausanne.)

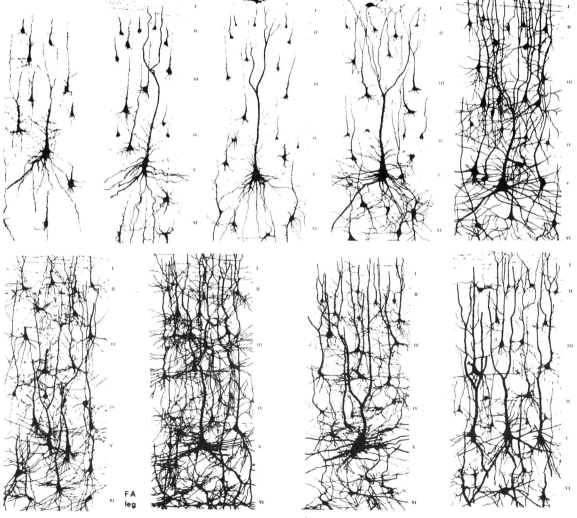

the ontogeny of myelination, have traced the progressive myelination of the middle cerebellar peduncle, acoustic radiation, and bundle of Vicq d'Azyr (mammillothalamic tract) beyond the third postnatal year; the nonspecific thalamic radiations beyond the seventh year; and the reticular formation, great cerebral commissures, and intracortical association areas to the tenth year and beyond (Fig. 27-3). They note, in a study of the fine anatomy, that there is an increasing complexity of fiber systems through late childhood and adolescence and perhaps even into middle adult life. Similarly, in the classic studies of Conel, depicting the cortical architecture at each year from birth to the tenth year of life, the dendritic arborizations and cortical intercellular connections are observed to increase progressively in complexity, thus reducing the "packing density" of neurons (number in any given area).

Interesting questions are (1) whether neurons begin to function only when their axons have acquired a myelin sheath, (2) whether myelination is under the control of the cell body or the axon or of both, and (3) whether a myelin stain yields sufficient information as to the time of onset and degree of the myelination process. At best the correlation can be only approximate. It seems likely that systems of neurons begin to function

before the first appearance of myelin as shown in conventional myelin stains. The whole problem needs to be restudied, using more delicate measures of function and finer staining techniques, as well as the techniques of phase and electron microscopy.

PSYCHOPHYSIOLOGIC DEVELOPMENT

The physiologic and psychological sequences of normal development are as important as the anatomic ones, and there are several outstanding works on these subjects to which reference is made at the end of this chapter (see Peiper, particularly). The main physiologic concepts to emerge are that the human fetus is capable of an amazingly complex series of reflex activities, which appear as early as 5 weeks of postconceptional age. Early there are slow, generalized, patterned movements of the head, trunk, and extremities, evoked by cutaneous and proprioceptive stimuli. Individual movements appear to differentiate from these generalized activities. Reflexes subserving blinking, sucking, grasping, and visceral functions, as well as tendon and plantar reflexes, are all elicitable in late fetal life. They seem to develop *pari passu* with the myelination of peripheral nerves, spinal roots, spinal cord, and brainstem. By the twenty-fourth week of gestation, the neural apparatus is functioning sufficiently to give the fetus some chance of survival if birth occurs at this time. Failure of most infants to sur-

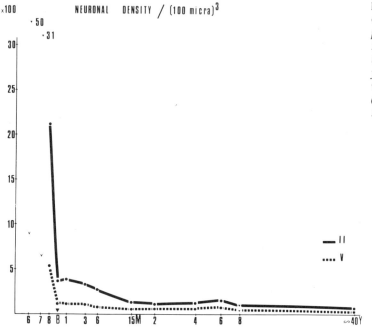

Figure 27-2
Graph of neuronal density in leg area of the precentral convolution (area 4), in cortical layer II (solid line) *and layer V* (broken line), *from the eighth month of fetal life to the fortieth year. Lessening neuronal population coincides with enlargement of cells and dendritic growth. (Courtesy of Th Rabinowicz, University of Lausanne.)*

vive birth at this age is due usually to an inadequacy of pulmonary function. Thereafter, the basic neural equipment matures so rapidly that by the thirtieth week postnatal viability is relatively frequent. It is as though nature were preparing the fetus for the contingency of premature birth by hastening to establish the vital functions necessary for extrauterine existence.

It is in the last trimester of pregnancy that a complete timetable of fetal movements, posture, and reflexes would be of the greatest clinical utility, for only then does the occasion demand that an infant be fully evaluated. Attempts have been made, from an analysis of behavior, reflexes, and tone, to determine whether development has been normal. That there are recognizable differences between newborn infants of sixth, seventh, eighth, and ninth fetal months is stated by Saint-Anne

Dargassies, who has applied the neurologic tests earlier devised by André-Thomas and herself. Her observations are in reference to prevailing postures; control and attitude of head, neck, and limbs; muscular tonus; and grasp and sucking reflexes. These findings are of interest and may well prove to be a means of determining exact age, but many more observations are needed with follow-up data on later development before they can be fully accepted as having predictive value. Part of the difficulty here is the extreme variability of the neurologic functions of the recently born premature infant which literally change from hour to hour.

Even at term, however, there is variability in neurologic functions from one day to the next. These reveal more the traumatic effects of parturition and the effects

Figure 27-3
The myelogenetic cycles. (From Yakovlev and Lecours.)

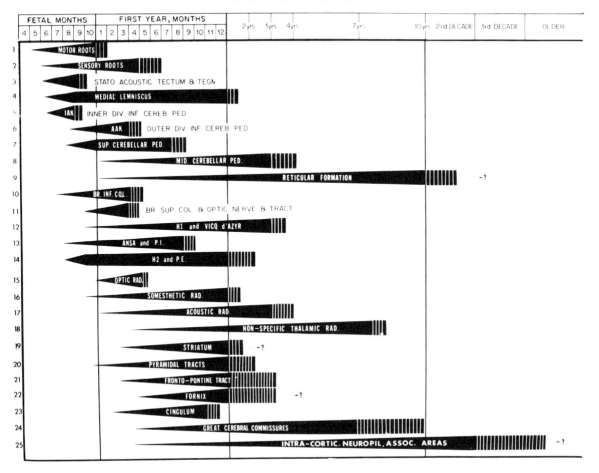

MYELOGENETIC CYCLES

of drugs and anesthesia given the mother than the developmental status of the brain.

At term, vital functions are quickly stabilized, and effective sucking, rooting, and grasping reactions are present. The infant is able to swallow, and the startle reaction (Moro reflex) can be evoked by sound and by extending the neck suddenly. Support and steppage movements can be demonstrated, and incurvation of the trunk on stroking the back. The placing reaction, whereby the dorsal surface of the foot or hand, brought passively into contact with the edge of a table, is lifted automatically and placed on the flat surface, is also present at birth.

That the neonatal automatisms described above depend essentially on the functioning of the spinal cord, brainstem, and possibly diencephalon and pallidum has long been known. In regard to these functions, virtually no difference can be demonstrated in the first weeks of life between a normal infant and one born without cerebral hemispheres. Serious maldevelopment or disease of the cerebrum may be clinically silent at this age. The recognition of injury to the nervous system at this time depends on the demonstration of changes in responsiveness, instability of vital signs, abnormalities of posture and tone, and impairment of the aforementioned reflex movements and automatisms—all of which are under the control of brainstem and spinal cord. In effect, the *Apgar score* is really a numerical rating of brainstem-spinal mechanisms (breathing, heart action, color of skin, tone, and responsivity). Prechtl and his associates have documented the importance of neurologic abnormalities in the neonatal period as predictors of retarded development.

Behavior during the neonatal period, infancy, and early childhood is also the subject of a substantial literature, contributed more by psychologists than neurologists. They have explored particularly the sensorimotor performances of the first year and the language and social development in early childhood. In the first 6 years of life the infant and child traverse far more ground developmentally than they ever will again in a similar interval. From the newborn state, when little more than an amorphous mass of protoplasm with a few postural reflexes, the infant acquires, within a few months, head and hand-eye control; by 6 months, the ability to sit; by 10 months, the strength to stand; by 12 months, the coordination to walk; by 2 years, the agility to run; and by 6 years, mastery of the rudiments of a game of baseball or a musical skill. On the perceptual side the neonate

progresses, in less than 3 months, from a state in which ocular control is tentative and tonic deviation of the eyes occurs only in response to labyrinthine stimulation, to one in which he or she is able to fixate and follow an object. (The latter corresponds to the development of the macula). Much later the child is able to make fine discriminations of color, form, and size. As Gesell remarks in his graphic summarization of the variety, range, and developmental sweep of a child's behavior—at birth the child "reflexly grasps the examiner's finger, with eyes crudely wandering or vacantly transfixed" and by the sixth year the child

> adaptively scans the perimeter of a square or triangle, reproducing each form with directed crayon. The birth cry, scant in modulation and social meaning, marks the low level of language, which in two years passes from babbling to word formation that soon is integrated into sentence structure, and in six years to elaborated syntactic speech with questions and even primitive ideas of causality. In personality makeup . . . the school beginner is already so highly organized, both socially and biologically, that he foreshadows the sort of individual he will be in later years.

The studies of Gesell and Amatruda and of others represent attempts to establish age-linked standards of behavioral development, but the difficulties of using such a rating scale are considerable. The components of behavior which have been chosen as a frame of reference are not likely to be of uniform physiologic value or of comparable complexity, and they have seldom been standardized on large populations of different cultures. Also, the examinations at specified ages are cross-sectional assessments which give little idea of the dynamics of behavioral development. As already stated, temporal patterns of behavior reveal an extraordinary degree of change, emergence, increment, and decrement, and marked variation from one individual to another.

The predictive value of developmental assessment has been the subject of a lively dispute. Gesell has taken the position that the careful observation of a large number of infants, with accurate recording of the age at which various skills are acquired, permits the establishment of norms or averages. From such a framework one can determine the level of developmental attainment, expressed as the development quotient (DQ = developmental age/chronological age) and thus ascertain whether any given child is superior, average, or inferior.

After examining 10,000 infants over a period of 40 years, Gesell concluded that "attained growth is an indicator of past growth processes and a foreteller of growth yet to be achieved." In other words the DQ predicts potential attainment. The other position, taken by Anderson, Kirman, and others is that developmental attainments are of no real value in predicting the level of intelligence but are measures of completely different functions. Illingworth and most clinicians, including the authors, have taken an intermediate position, that the developmental scale in early life is a useful source of information, but it needs always to be combined with a full clinical assessment. When this is done, the clinician has a reasonably certain means of detecting mental retardation and other forms of neurologic impairment.

The trajectory of rapid growth and maturation continues in late childhood and adolescence, though at a slower pace than before. Motor skills attain their maximal precision in the performances of athletes, artists, and musicians, whose peak development is at maturity (age 18 to 21). Capacity for reflective thought and the manipulation of mathematical symbols becomes possible only in adolescence and later. Emotional control, precarious in the school age and all through adolescence, stabilizes in adulthood. We tend to think of all these phenomena as being achieved through the stresses of human relations, which are conditioned and habituated by the powerful influences of social approval. In this extensive and pervasive penetration of the individual by the environment, which is the preoccupation of the child psychiatrist, it is well to remember that the processes of extrinsic and intrinsic organization can be separated only for the purpose of analytical discussion. There is always *interdependence* rather than conflict between them.

MOTOR DEVELOPMENT

When motor development is analyzed in greater detail, it is noteworthy that from the time of birth healthy infants display a wide variety of movements and postures. They blink at light, move their face, jaws, and tongue, turn their head, flex and extend their arms and legs, twist the trunk of the body, and arch it toward the side stimulated (incurvation). When they are placed on their feet, they extend their legs to support the body and make stepping movements as the body is tipped forward and rocked from side to side. From birth, and certainly within days, these seemingly random movements are firmly organized into reflexive-instinctual patterns called *automatisms*. The most testable of the automatisms are blinking at light, tonic deviation of the eyes in response to labyrinthine stimulation (turning of the head), sucking and prehensile movements of the lips in response to labial contact, swallowing, avoidance movements of the head and neck, startle reaction (Moro response) in response to loud noise or dropping of the head into an extended position, grasp reflexes, support and stepping movements, and placing movements (lifting and extension of the foot or hand when the dorsal or lateral surface comes in contact with the edge of a table). As has been remarked, this repertoire of movements depends on reflexes organized at the spinal and brainstem levels. Only the placing reactions and ocular fixation and following movements (the latter are established by the third month) are thought to depend on emerging cortical connections, but even this is debatable. As a corollary, impairment of these automatisms and of body temperature, circulation, and respiration must be interpreted to mean that spinal-brainstem functions and structures are seriously compromised.

At this early age, when little of the cerebrum has begun to function, extensive cerebral lesions may cause no derangement of motor function and may pass unnoticed, and many serious cerebral diseases cannot be diagnosed unless special ancillary methods (sensory evoked potentials, EEG, CT scan) are used. Of testable neurologic functions, disturbances of ocular movement, seizures, tremulousness of the arms, impaired arousal reactions and muscular tone—all of which relate to upper brainstem and diencephalic (cerebral?) mechanisms—provide the most reliable clues to neurologic diseases in the neonatal period.

During early infancy the motor system undergoes a variety of differentiations as visual, auditory, and tactile-motor mechanisms develop. Bodily postures are modified to accommodate these elaborate sensorimotor acquisitions. In the normal infant these emerging motor differentiations and elaborations follow a time schedule prescribed by the maturation of neural connections. Normalcy is expressed by the age of the organism when each and every one of these appear, as shown in Table 27-3.

It is evident from this table that reflex and instinctual motor activities are of maximal importance in the evaluation of early development. Further, in the normally developing organism, some of these activities disappear as others appear. For example, extension of the limbs without a flexor phase, Moro response, tonic neck reflexes, and crossed adduction in response to knee jerk all gradually become less prominent and are usually not elicitable by the sixth month. In contrast, neck-righting reflexes, support reactions, Landau reaction (extending neck and legs when held prone), parachute maneuver,

Table 27-3
Neurological functions and disturbances in infancy

Age	Normal functions	Pathologic signs
Newborn period	Blinking, tonic deviation of eyes on turning head, sucking, rooting, swallowing, yawning, grasping, brief extension of neck in prone position, incurvation response, Moro response, flexion postures of limbs Biceps reflexes present and others variable; infantile type of flexor plantar reflex; stable temperature, respirations and blood pressure; periods of sleep and arousal; vigorous cry	Lack of arousal (stupor or coma) High-pitched or weak cry Abnormal (incomplete or absent) Moro response Opisthotonus Flaccidity or hypertonia Convulsions Tremulous limbs Failure of tonic deviation of eyes on passive movement of head or of head and body
2 months	Supports head Smiles Makes vowel sounds Adopts tonic asymmetric neck postures (tonic neck reflexes) Large range of movements of limbs, tendon reflexes usually present Fixates on and follows a dangling toy Suckles vigorously Period of sleep sharply differentiated from awake periods Support and stepping unelicitable Vertical suspension—legs flex Optokinetic nystagmus elicitable Laughs aloud, shows pleasure	Absence of any or all of the normal functions Convulsions Hypotonia or hypertonia of neck and limbs Vertical suspension—legs extend and adduct
4 months	Good head support, minimal head lag Coos and chuckles Inspects hands Tone of limbs moderate or diminished Turns to sounds Rolls over Grasping, sucking and tonic neck reflexes subservient to volition	No head support Motor deficits Hypertonia No social reactions Tonic neck reflexes present Strong Moro response Absence of symmetric attitude
5-6 months	Babbles Reaches and grasps Vocalizes in social play Discriminates between family and strangers Moro and grasp disappear Tries to recover lost object Begins to sit; no head lag on pull to sit Positive support reaction Tonic neck reflexes gone Landau (holds head above horizontal and arches back when held horizontally) Begins to grasp objects with one hand; holds bottle	Altered tone Obligatory postures Cannot sit or roll over Hypo- of hypertonia Persistent Moro and grasp Cannot sit Persistent tonic neck reflexes No Landau response

Age	Normal functions	Pathologic signs
9 months	Creeps and pulls to stand; stands holding on Sits securely Babbles "Mama," "Dada," or equivalent Sociable; plays "pat-a-cake," seeks attention Drinks from cup Landau present Parachute present Grasps with thumb to forefinger	Fails to attain these motor, verbal and social milestones Persistent automatisms and tonic neck reflexes or hypo- or hypertonia
12 months	Stands alone May walk, or walks if led Tries to feed self May say several single words, echoes sounds Plantar reflexes definitely flexor Throws objects	Retardation Functions at earlier level Persistence of automatisms
15 months	Walks independently (9–16 months), falls easily Moves arms steadily Says several words; scribbles with crayon Requests by pointing Interest in sounds, music, pictures, and animal toys	Retardation at earlier age level Persistent abnormalities of tone and posture Sensory discriminations defective
18 months	Says at least 6 words Feeds self; uses spoon well May obey commands Runs stiffly; seats self in chair Hand dominance Throws ball Plays several nursery games Uses simple tools in imitation Removes shoes and stockings Points to two or three parts of body, common objects, and pictures in book	Cannot walk No words
24 months	Says 2- or 3-word sentences Scribbles Runs well; climbs stairs one at a time Bends over and picks up objects Kicks ball; turns knob Organized play Builds tower of 6 or 7 blocks Toilet training sometimes completed	Retarded in all motor, linguistic, and social adaptive skills

Source: Modified from Gesell et al.

and pincer grasp, which are absent in the first 6 months, begin to appear by the seventh to eighth month and are present in all normal infants by the twelfth month.

Since many functions that are classified as mental at a later period of life have a different anatomic basis than motor functions, it is not surprising that early motor achievements do not correlate closely with childhood intelligence. The converse does not apply, however; delay in the acquisition of motor milestones does correlate with mental retardation. Most retarded children sit, stand, walk, and run at a much later age than normal children, and deviations from this rule are exceptional.

In the period of early childhood, reflex activities are no longer of help in neurologic evaluations, and one must turn to language functions and learned sensory and motor skills, most particularly for the appraisal of cerebral development. These are outlined in Tables 27-4 and 27-5.

SENSORY DEVELOPMENT

Under normal circumstances, sensory development keeps pace with motor development, and at every age sensorimotor interactions are apparent. However, under conditions of disease there are many instances where this generalization does not hold, i.e., motor development remains relatively normal in the face of sensory defects, or vice versa.

The sense organs are fully formed at birth, yet the newborn infant is not very reactive to external stimuli. The neonate does not see, hear, feel, smell or taste as do older children. Although crudely aware of stimuli, the newborn cannot comprehend such stimuli. Moreover, any stimulus-related response is only to the immediate situation; there is no evidence that previous experience with the stimulus has influenced a response, i.e., that learning and memory have taken place. The capacity to attend to a stimulus, to fixate upon it for any period of time, also comes later. Indeed, the length of fixation time is a quantifiable index of perceptual development in infancy.

Information is available about the time at which the infant makes the first interpretable responses to each of the different modes of stimulation. The most nearly perfect senses in the newborn are those of touch and pain. A series of pinpricks causes distress, whereas an abrasion of the skin seems not to do so. The sense of touch clearly plays a role in feeding behavior. Newborn

Table 27-4

Developmental achievements of the normal preschool child

Age	Observed items	Useful clinical tests
2 years	Runs well Goes up and down stairs, one step at a time Climbs on furniture Opens doors Helps to undress Feeds well with spoon Puts three words together Listens to stories with pictures	Pencil-paper test: scribbles, imitates horizontal stroke Folds paper once Builds tower of six blocks
$2\frac{1}{2}$ years	Jumps on both feet; walks on tiptoes if asked Knows full name; asks questions Refers to self as "I" Helps put away toys and clothes Names animals in book, knows 1 to 3 colors Can complete three-piece form board	Pencil-paper test: copies horizontal and vertical line Builds tower of eight blocks
3 years	Climbs stairs, alternating feet Talks constantly; recites nursery rhymes Rides tricycle Stands on one foot momentarily Plays simple games Helps in dressing Washes hands Identifies five colors	Builds nine-cube tower Builds bridge with three cubes Imitates circle and cross with pencil
4 years	Climbs well; hops and skips on one foot; throws ball overhand; kicks ball Cuts out pictures with scissors Counts four pennies Tells a story; plays with other children Goes to toilet alone	Copies cross and circle Builds gate with five cubes Builds a bridge from model Draws a human figure with two to four parts other than head Distinguishes short and long line
5 years	Skips Names four colors; counts ten pennies Dresses and undresses Asks questions about meaning of words	Copies square and triangle Distinguishes heavier of two weights More detailed drawing of a human figure

infants react vigorously to irritating odors such as ammonia and acetic acid, but discrimination between olfactory stimuli is not evident until much later. Sugar solutions initiate and maintain sucking from birth on, whereas quinine solutions seldom do, and later the latter stimulus elicits avoidance behavior. Hearing in the newborn is manifest within the first few postnatal days. Sharp, quick sounds elicit responsive blinking and sometimes startle. In some infants, the human voice appears to cause similar reactions by the second week. Strong light and objects held before the face evoke reactions in the neonate, and later visual searching is an integrating factor in most projected motor activities.

Although sensation in the newborn infant must be judged largely by motor reactions, so that sensory and motor developments seem to run in parallel, there are discernible maturational stages that constitute sensory milestones, so to speak. This is most apparent in the visual system, which is more easily studied than some of the other senses. Sustained ocular fixation on an object is observable a few hours after birth; at this time, however, it is essentially a reflexive phototropic reaction. This

primitive type of fixation is found in 75 percent of infants at 5 to 10 days of age. So-called voluntary fixation is a later development. Following a moving object horizontally occurs at 50 days, and vertically at 55 days. Following an object moved in a circle is observable at 2.5 months. Preference for a colored stimulus over a gray one was recorded by Staples by the end of the third month. By 6 months the infant discriminates between colors, and saturated colors can be matched at 30 months. Naming of colors comes later. Perception of form, judged by the length of time spent in looking at different visual presentations, is evident at 2 or 3 months of age (Fantz). At this time infants are attracted more to certain patterns than to colors. At 3 months, most infants have discovered their hands and spend considerable time watching their movements. Details concerning the ages at which infants observe color, size, shape, and number are available in the Terman-Merrill and the Stutzman Intelligence Tests (see Gibson and Olum). Perception of size becomes increasingly accurate in the preschool years. An 18-month old child discriminates between pictures of familiar animals and recognizes them equally well if they are upside down.

Visual discriminations are clearly reflected in manual reactions just as auditory discriminations are reflected in vocal responses. Much of early development (first year) involves peering at objects, judging their position, reaching for them, and seizing and manipulating them. The inseparability of sensory and motor functions is never more obvious. Sensory deprivation impedes not only the natural sequences of perceptual awareness of the world about but of all motor activities.

Table 27-5
Useful tests for evaluating learning disabilities in children

Developmental diagnosis (birth to 5 years)	Denver Developmental Test Vineland Social Maturity Test
Developmental diagnosis (school-age children)	Raven's Colored Progressive Matrices Test Wide Range Achievement Test
IQ and mental age (2 years to adult)	Stanford-Binet Wechsler Preschool and Primary Scale Wechsler Intelligence Test for Children
Language	Peabody Picture Vocabulary Tokens Test
Developmental Gerstmann's syndrome (finger agnosia, right-left disorientation, dysgraphia, dyscalculia)	Finger-Recognition Test Benton right-left discrimination test
Visuomotor integration	Figure-copying test
Visual memory	Benton Visual Retention Test Bender Gestalt Test
Intersensory integration	Birth auditory-visual integration test

Source: Kinsbourne, 1980.

THE DEVELOPMENT OF INTELLIGENCE

The subject of intellectual endowment and development has already been touched upon in Chap. 20. There it was pointed out that intelligence is modifiable by training, practice, and schooling but that it is much more a matter of native endowment. Intelligent parents tend to beget intelligent children, and stupid ones, stupid children, and this seems to be not simply a question of environment and stimulus to learn. It is evident early in life that some individuals have a superior intelligence and maintain this superiority all through life.

Much of the uncertainty about the relative influence of heredity and environment in determining intelligence relates to our imprecise definitions of this state.

Authoritative writers have defined intelligence variously as the capacity to acquire new knowledge, to solve problems, and to perfect through experience new and more efficient modes of adaptation, and as the totality of capacities of observing, understanding, thinking, and remembering as means of learning and of acting purposefully and rationally.

Even a superficial analysis of these definitions discloses that they include a multiplicity of functions, which probably accounts for a lack of unanimity about the mechanism(s) of intelligence. Kurt Goldstein argued that intelligence is a unitary mental capacity, impairment of which gives rise to a fundamental disorder (*Grundstörung*)—a loss of "abstract attitude." By this he meant an incapacity to deal with objects at a conceptual level and an undue dependence on their immediate, concrete attributes. Everyday experience, however, teaches us that people regarded as intelligent are not all alike. As a corollary, it is not always abstract tasks that suffer most when intelligence is impaired. Indeed, as Zangwill has pointed out, even abstraction may not be a unitary function. Other theoreticians, like Karl Spearman, believed that intelligence is comprised of a general (*g*), or core, factor and a series of special (*s*) factors, such as verbal and arithmetic ability, memory, capacity for abstract thinking, practical skills in manipulating objects, geographic or spatial sense, and certain social adaptations (see Chap. 20). Still others think of intelligence as a mosaic of specific abilities. Not only do individuals appear to vary in these native abilities, but the superior ones are found to use them with greater speed and efficiency. According to this view, individuals gifted in only one ability would not be considered intelligent, only talented in the particular field. Physicians in their daily experience tend to accept this latter view of intelligence as consisting of a series of special abilities, and to recognize among their patients wide individual differences, manifest in their daily activities, their capacity to give a history, and to follow instructions.

If one accepts the view that intelligence consists of a mosaic of many specific abilities (this idea is suggested also by its seemingly polygenic inheritance), then how do these abilities develop in infancy and childhood? Admittedly, their origins are difficult to detect. Measurements of the individual abilities of infants and young children are so heavily weighted toward sensory and motor functions, which have only an uncertain relation to intelligence, that they give untrustworthy predictions of the latter. Even up to the sixth year results of so-called intelligence tests are relatively unreliable and have only a modest correlation with later school performance. Nonetheless, the first hints of something beyond simple sensorimotor reactions and reflex patterns do begin to emerge at 8 to 9 months of life when infants begin to crawl and explore. Now for the first time they separate themselves from the mother. As soon as they stand and walk, this fascinating world begins to open before them. Now for the first time, learning proceeds rapidly, as the mother attaches names to objects and helps the baby manipulate them. At about 14 to 15 months the child begins to declare its independence as a social organism by saying "no" to every request. Gradually the child acquires verbal facility (learning what words mean), memory, color and spatial perception, concept of number, and the practical use of tools, each at a particular time according to a schedule set largely by the maturational state of the brain. In these early achievements individuals differ greatly, and they are much influenced by their parents and other individuals in their environment. The rate of learning, adaptability, understanding, and tolerance of restrictions, and, later, the acquisition of knowledge, capacity to work, and personality structure vary enormously, as will be pointed out below. Neurologists who need a quick and practical method of ascertaining whether an infant or preschool child is measuring up to normal standards for a particular age will find Tables 27-4 and 27-5 useful. The main items are drawn from Gesell and Amatruda and from the Denver Developmental Test.

A variety of intelligence tests, designed to measure special abilities (see Table 27-5), demonstrate the child's increasing success in learning with age. Starting at 6 to 7 years there is a steady improvement in scores that parallels chronological age up to about 13 years, and thereafter the rate of advance diminishes. By 16 to 17 years performance reaches a plateau and remains more or less constant through early adult life. From about the thirtieth year, test scores diminish slowly throughout the remainder of life. Individuals with high or low IQs at 6 years tend to maintain their rank at 10, 15 and 20 years, unless the early scores were impaired by anxiety, poor motivation, or gross lack of opportunity to acquire the necessary tools to take such tests (language skill in particular). Even then, reliance upon performance tasks, which largely eliminate verbal or mathematical skill, will display similar individual differences. Effective performance on tests of whatever type obviously requires interest and motivation on the part of the subject.

The reliability of intelligence tests and their validity as measures of an aggregate of abilities that predict scholastic success, quality of work performance, etc., have been heatedly debated in recent years. Some critics claim these tests to be only measures of achievement which in themselves are dependent on motivation and opportunity. While no one would disagree that a factor of achievement enters into intelligence tests, the most persuasive argument for them as tests of native abilities is that individuals drawn from a fairly homogeneous environment tend to maintain the same position on the intelligence scale throughout their lifetime.

THE DEVELOPMENT OF LANGUAGE

Closely tied to the development of intelligence is the acquisition of language. Indeed, facility with language is one of the best indices of intelligence (Lenneberg). The acquisition of speech and language by the infant and child has been observed methodically by a number of eminent scientists, and their findings provide a background for the understanding of a number of derangements in the development of these functions.

First, there is the *babbling* and *lalling stage*, during which the infant a few weeks old emits a variety of cooing and then babbling sounds in the form of vowel-consonant (labial and nasogutteral) combinations. At first this appears to be a purely self-initiated activity, being the same in normal and deaf infants. However, a study of the latter shows that auditory modifications begin within a period of 2 to 3 months; without auditory sense the babblers do not produce the variety of random sounds of the normal infant, nor do they begin to imitate the sounds in their environment. Thus motor speech activity is stimulated and reinforced predominantly by auditory sensations, which become linked to the kinesthetic ones arising from the speech musculature. It is not clear whether the capacity to hear and understand the spoken word precedes or follows the first motor speech. Possibly it varies from one infant to another, but the dependence of motor-speech development on hearing is undeniable. Comprehension seems to postdate the first verbal utterance in most infants.

Soon babbling merges with *echo speech*, in which short sounds are repeated parrotlike; then gradually longer syllable groups are repeated correctly as the praxic function of the speech apparatus develops. By the end of 12 months the first recognizable words appear. Initially these are attached directly to persons and objects and are used increasingly to designate the object. The word then becomes the symbol, and this substitution greatly facilitates speaking and later thinking about people and objects. To learn to say a spoken name, it is necessary to form a link between the auditory association (Wernicke's) area in the superior temporal gyrus of the dominant hemisphere and the center for motor patterns of speech (Broca's area). Similarly, to learn the name of a seen object requires the formation of a link between the visual association region of the occipital lobe and Wernicke's area. It is known that nouns are learned first, then verbs and other parts of speech. Through experience and correction from parents and siblings vocal behavior is gradually shaped to conform to that of the social group in which the child is raised.

During the second year of life, word combinations are learned. They form the propositions which, according to Hughlings Jackson, are the very essence of language. The average child of 18 months can form a phrase of $1\frac{1}{2}$ words and at 2 years of 2 words, at $2\frac{1}{2}$ years of 3 words, and at 3 years of 4 words. Pronunciation of words undergoes a similar progression; 90 percent of children can articulate all vowel sounds by the age of 3 years. At a slightly later age the consonants *p, b, m, h, w, d, n, t,* and *k* are enunciated; *ng* by the age of 4 years; *y, j, zh,* and *wh* by 5 to 6 years; and *f, l, v, sh, ch, s, v,* and *th* by 7 years. Girls acquire articulatory facility somewhat earlier than boys. The vocabulary increases each year. At 18 months the young child knows 6 to 20 words; by 24 months, 50 to 200 words; by 3 years, 200 to 400 words; and by 4 years, the child is normally capable of telling stories with little distinction between fact and fancy. By 6 years, the average child knows several thousand words. Also by that age the child can indicate spatial and temporal relationships and starts to inquire about causality. The understanding of spoken language always exceeds the child's speaking vocabulary; that is to say, the child understands more than he or she says.

The next stage of language development is reading. Here there must be an association of graphic symbols with the auditory, visual, and kinesthetic images of words already acquired. Usually the written word is learned by associating it with the spoken word rather than with the seen object. The superior gyrus of the temporal lobe (Wernicke's area) and contiguous parietooccipital areas of the dominant hemisphere are essential to the establishment of these cross-modal associations. Writing is learned soon after reading, the auditory-visual symbols of words being linked to cursive movements of the hand. The traditional beginning of public school instruction at 6 years is based not on arbitrary decision but on the empirically determined age at which the nervous system of the average child is ready to execute the tasks of reading, writing, and soon thereafter of calculating.

Once language is fully acquired it is integrated into all aspects of complex action and behavior. Every movement of volitional type is activated by a spoken command or the individual's own phrasing of an intended action. Every plan for the solution of a problem must be cast into language, and the final result is analyzed in verbal terms. Thinking and language are inseparable.

Anthropologists see in all this a grander scheme wherein the individual recapitulates the language development of the human race. They point out that in primitive peoples, language consisted of gestures and the utterance of simple sounds expressing emotion, and that over periods of time, movements and sounds became the conventional signs and verbal symbols of concrete objects and then of the abstract qualities of objects. Historically, signs and spoken language were the first means of human communication; graphic records appeared much later. The American Indian, for instance, never reached the level of syllabic written language. Writing commenced as pictorial representation, and only much later were alphabets devised. The reading and writing of words are comparatively late achievements.

For further details concerning communicative and cognitive abilities and methods of assessment, the reader should consult the monograph by Minifie and Lloyd.

THE DEVELOPMENT OF PERSONALITY

The term *personality* encompasses all the physical and psychological traits that distinguish one individual from every other one.

The notion that one's physical characteristics are determined by inheritance is a fundamental tenet of neurobiology. One has but to observe the resemblances between parent and child to confirm this view. Only the extent of human variation occasions surprise. Just as no two persons are physically identical, not even monozygotic twins, so too do they differ in body chemistry or any other quality one chooses to measure. These qualities, together with certain predilections to disease, explain why any one person may have an unpredictable reaction to a pathogenic agent. Strictly speaking, the normal person is an abstraction, just as is a typical example of any disease.

However, it is in other, seemingly nonphysical attributes that individuals display the greatest differences. Here reference is made to their variable place on a scale of energy, capacity for effective work, intellectual power (which also makes them susceptible to different degrees

of training and education), sensitivity, temperament and emotional responsivity, agressivity or passivity, character, and tolerance to stress. The composite of these qualities constitutes the human personality.

THE ROOTS OF SOCIAL BEHAVIOR

Perhaps it is not obvious to the student and young physician that social behavior, like neurologic and psychological functions in general, depends to a great extent on the development and maturation of the brain. Involved also are genetic factors. Obviously, environment plays a role, for one cannot adapt to society except in the presence of other people; i.e., social interaction is necessary for the emergence of many basic biologic traits. One must think of personality as a series of intrinsic forces continuously emerging and being altered by the forces of the social environment.

The roots of social behavior are traceable to certain instinctive patterns, and the progressive elaboration of one's social attributes is induced by conditioned emotional reactions. Pleasure accompanies behavior demanded by evolution (e.g., the sexual act, necessary for reproduction, and eating, for health and nutrition), and anxiety and fear protect the organism against conditions that lead to maladaptation.

At a higher level of social interaction between an individual and the family unit and community, we see more clearly the workings of another principle—that biologic evolution merges with, and is finally superseded by, cultural evolution. The latter is uniquely human. Only human beings are able to alter their environment in a systematic fashion. The future can be anticipated and planned. Of the primate family only human beings are able to think and communicate by symbols. Language enables us to think through the consequences of an action before attempting it, to abstract from the concrete to the general situation, and to analyze the relationships between the elements of a problem without the necessity of actually manipulating the elements. Language is also the agency whereby the experiences of the past are made available for understanding current problems. Thus we build continuously on our cultural heritage.

THE DEVELOPMENT OF THE COMPONENTS OF PERSONALITY

As William James once remarked, "The baby upon entering this world, assailed by sensations from the eyes, ears, nose, skin and entrails, all at once must feel it as one blooming, buzzing confusion," and the ways in which our nervous system brings these sensations to order during development are nothing short of miraculous.

With respect to patterns of behavior, the neonate is virtually a pulp with no sense of identity, and seemingly unconscious of self. By the second year the child begins to announce his or her independence by refusing to comply with the wishes of others, and the words *I, me,* and *you* are added to the vocabulary. Continued stresses in human relations condition and habituate the child. Individual differences in energy, curiosity, aggressivity, tolerance of change, warmth of emotional response, already apparent, will persist throughout life, but, as was said, it is the interpenetration of environmental forces which complete social development.

Freudian formulations present emotional development as a series of predictable modifications of the sexual instinct. The energy of the sexual impulse, called libido, is traced back to the earliest sensory pleasures that attend the activities of the oral and genital parts of the body. Successively the sexuality of the child expands to include many of the relationships to the mother, to other members of the same sex, and finally to the opposite sex. Powerful forces repress the sexual impulse, such as social custom, but always with the risk, so it is argued, that the energy of the sexual drive may be displaced into other channels of thought and action, with unwholesome alterations of behavior. Personality development is thus regarded as a process of sexual maturation, the final purpose of which is to ensure procreation and the installment of the individual as an integral part of a new family unit.

There are many who believe that the Freudian emphasis on sexuality provides far too restricted a theory of human personality. While the tie to the mother can be conceived of as derived from the nursing act, it is likely that body contact with the mother soon becomes less important than touch, smell, sight, and sound as determinative factors in the infant's behavior. Further, many others in the infant's environment, e.g., siblings, father, teacher, begin to figure in special nonsexual ways in the child's development.

In the formation of personality, especially the part concerned with feeling and emotional sensitivity, basic temperament surely plays a part. By nature, some children, from the beginning, seem to be happy, cheerful, and unconcerned about immediate frustrations, and others are the opposite. By the third month of life, Birch and his associates recognize individual differences in activity-passivity, regularity-irregularity, intensity of action, approach-withdrawal, adaptivity-unadaptivity, high-low threshold of response to stimulation, positive-negative mood, high-low selectivity, and high-low distractibility. Ratings on these qualities at this early age were found by these authors to correlate with the results of examinations made at 5 years. Not all psychologists agree with these observations; some insist that the mother's behavior is of crucial importance in teaching such patterns. The problem is made even more complicated by the possibility that the character of the infant may influence the mother's reactions. One may presume that the more common aspects of personality, i.e., worry about one's health and other matters, anxiety or serenity, timidity or boldness, the power of instinctual drives and need of satisfaction, sympathy for others, sensitivity to criticism, and degree of disorganization resulting from adverse circumstances, are genetically determined. Identical twins raised apart are remarkably alike in many personality traits and have the same IQs, within one or two points.

SOCIAL ADAPTATION

In the long series of human interactions, first with parents, then siblings, other children, and finally a widening circle of individuals in the classroom and community at large, the capacity to cooperate, to subjugate one's own egocentric needs to those of the group, to lead or be led appear as other secondary modes of response, i.e., secondary to some of the basic impulses of anger, fear, self-protection, love, and pleasure already described.

The sources of these social reactions are more obscure than those of temperament and intelligence. The ubiquity of aggressive behavior in children, for example, is often cited as an argument for an innate aggressive instinct. But to a large extent this is a derived mode of behavior. The ascription of aggressive behavior to instinct alone is an example of a common tendency to explain infantile behavior by a prior assignment of adult motives. To elaborate the point, in a normal child aggression usually originates in innate curiosity or takes the form of a defense reaction to frustration and failure. In both instances, aggression is an appropriate reaction. Its frequency in an abnormal child may be related to defects in the germ plasm, as in the case of brain malformations, and also to environmental factors which expose the infant and child to faulty identification models. Moreover, the frequency of display of aggressive behavior is a function of the culture in which the child is reared. While aggression is encouraged in some cultures as a desirable manifestation of energetic and vigorous action, becoming unacceptable only if assaultive and violent, it may not be condoned at all in other cultures. The capacity for aggression is indeed inherent in human impulse, as it is in all animals, but its frequency of evocation and display are determined by other factors.

The greatest demands and frustrations in social development are likely to occur in late childhood and adolescence. The difficulties of children tend first to be exposed by an inability to take their places in a classroom. Adolescents, half emancipated from family ties, have trouble as they seek recognition and respect of their peers. For the first time they think seriously of what they are and what they will be. In search of personal identity they become more critical of their parents and turn increasingly to interaction with larger social groups for a sense of belonging. If their relationship with their parents is firmly established and if the parents meet their doubts and criticisms with sympathetic understanding, this temporary unsettling of their primary family position leads later to a resynthesis of their relations with the family on a firm and lasting basis. The development of adult gonadal function and the further evolution of psychosexual impulses cause the adolescent to experience a bewildering array of new sensations. These latter lead to a surge of interest in physical sex and psychological sensitization to new aspects of interpersonal relations. An increasing capacity for abstract thought paves the way for advanced education and creativity and for increasing concern about the meaning and value of human existence.

These types of social adjustment continue as long as life continues. As social roles change, as intellectual and physical capacities first advance and later recede, new challenges demand new adaptations. The success of these adaptations is enhanced if started from a solid base of accomplishment in a secure work role, from a position as a member of a stable family unit, with a religion or a philosophy of life. Conditions that thwart the development of proper attitudes toward family, work, and health often become major causes of maladjustment in later life.

FAILURES AND DISHARMONIES OF NORMAL NEUROLOGIC DEVELOPMENT

DELAY IN MOTOR DEVELOPMENT AND CEREBRAL PALSY

Delay in motor development often accompanies mental retardation, in which case it is part of the syndrome of delayed maturation, but the most severe forms of delayed motor development, associated with spasticity and athetosis, are invariably manifestations of particular prenatal and paranatal diseases of the brain.

Assessment of developmental abnormalities of the motor system is assisted by several maneuvers which elicit postures and certain combinations of reflexes. Some of the most useful are the following:

1. The *Moro response* is the infant's response to startle and can be evoked by suddenly withdrawing support of the head and letting the neck extend. A loud noise, slapping the bed, or jerking one leg will have the same effect, causing first an elevation and abduction of the arms followed by a clasping movement to the midline. Present in all newborns and infants up to 4 or 5 months of age, its absence designates a profound disorder of the motor system. An absence or inadequate Moro response on one side is found in hemiplegia, brachial plexus palsy and fractured clavicle. Persistence of the Moro response beyond 4 or 5 months of age is noted only in infants with severe neurologic defects.

2. The asymmetric *tonic neck reflex* (extension of arm and leg on the side to which the head is passively turned and flexion of the opposite limbs), if it is obligatory and sustained, is a sign of pyramidal or extrapyramidal motor abnormality at any age. Fragments of the reflex such as brief extension of one arm may be elicited in 60 percent of normal infants at 1 to 2 months of age, and the infant may spontaneously adopt these postures up to 6 months. Barlow reports having obtained this reflex in 25 percent of mentally retarded infants at 9 to 10 months of age.

3. The *placing reaction* (described above, under Psychophysiologic Development) is present in all normal newborns. Its absence or asymmetry under 6 months of age indicates a motor abnormality.

4. The *"parachute response"*—dropping the infant held prone in the horizontal position toward the bed to evoke extension of the arms as if to break the fall—is elicitable in most 9-month-old infants. If asymmetrical, it means a unilateral motor abnormality.

5. In the *Landau maneuver* the infant, if suspended horizontally in the prone position, will extend the neck and trunk and will break the trunk extension when the neck is passively flexed. This reaction is present by 6 months. Delay in a hypotonic child is indicative of a fault in the motor apparatus.

The detection of gross delays or abnormalities of motor development in the neonatal or early infantile period of life is little aided by tests of tendon and plantar reflexes. Arm reflexes are always rather difficult to obtain in infants, and a normal neonate may have a few beats of ankle clonus. The plantar response is always wavering and uncertain in pattern. A consistent extension of the great toe and fanning of the toes on stroking the side of the foot is abnormal at any age.

The early discovery of cerebral palsy is hampered by the fact that the corticospinal tract is not myelinated until 18 months of age, allowing at best only quasivoluntary movements. A congenital hemiparesis, for example, may not be evident until many months have passed. It then becomes manifest by subtle signs such as the holding of the hand in a fisted posture or inefficiency in reaching for objects and in transferring them from one hand to the other. Later the leg is seen to be less active as the infant crawls, steps, and places the foot. Early hand dominance should always raise the suspicion of a motor defect. Spasticity is most evident in attempts to passively abduct the arm, extend the elbow, and dorsiflex and supinate the wrist. In the leg, passive flexion of the knee is the best maneuver to elicit the characteristic catch and yielding resistance, but the time of appearance and degree of spasticity are always variable from patient to patient. The stretch reflexes are hyperactive, and the plantar reflex may be extensor on the affected side. With bilateral hemiplegia the same abnormalities are detectable, but there is greater likelihood of pseudobulbar involvement with delayed, poorly enunciated speech. Also, intelligence is more likely to be impaired (in 40 percent of hemiplegias and 70 percent of quadriplegias). In diparesis or diplegia, hypotonia gives way to spasticity with the same delayed motor development except that it is confined to the legs.

Hypotonia presages developmental motor delay and other abnormalities in a rather large group of infants. Lifting the infant and passive manipulation of the limbs encounter little muscle reactivity. In the legs the laxity results in a frog-leg posture along with unusual mobility of ankles and hips. Hypotonia, if generalized and accompanied by a complete absence of tendon reflexes will usually be due to Werdnig-Hoffmann disease (see Chap. 50). Those infants who will later manifest a central motor defect can sometimes be recognized by the postures assumed by the limbs when the infant is lifted. In the normal infant the legs are flexed, slightly rotated externally, and there are vigorous kicking movements; the hypotonic infant with pyramidal or extrapyramidal disease may extend the legs or rotate them internally with dorsiflexion of the feet and toes. Often the extended legs are raised anteriorly 30 to 45° and exceptionally they are firmly flexed, but in either instance relatively few movements are made.

When hypotonia is a forerunner of an extrapyramidal motor disorder, as may happen, the first hint of abnormality may be an opisthotonic posturing of the head and neck. However, the irregular involuntary movements of chorea do not appear in the upper extremities before 5 to 6 months, and often they are so slight as to be overlooked. They increase as the months pass and by 12 months assume a more athetotic character, often combined with tremor. Tone in the affected limbs is by then increased but may be interrupted by passive manipulation.

When hypotonia is a prelude to a cerebellar motor defect, the ataxia becomes apparent only in the first reaching movements. Tremulous irregular movements of the trunk and head are seen with attempts to sit without support. Still later, in attempting to stand, there is unsteadiness of the entire body.

The other common causes of hypotonia (muscular dystrophies and congenital myopathies, polyneuropathies, Down's syndrome, Praeder-Willi syndrome, and spinal cord injuries) are described in other chapters.

Systemic diseases in infancy pose special problems in the evaluation of the motor system. The achievement of motor milestones is delayed by illnesses such as congenital heart disease (especially cyanotic forms), cystic fibrosis, renal and hepatic diseases, infections, and surgical procedures. Under such conditions one does well to deal with the immediate illnesses and defer pronouncements about the status of cerebral function. The brain proves to be simultaneously affected in 25 percent of patients with congenital heart disease and an even higher proportion of patients with rubella and Coxsackie B infections. In a disease such as cystic fibrosis, where the brain is not affected, it is advisable to depend more on the analysis of language development than of locomotion, for the muscular activity may be enfeebled.

DELAYS IN SENSORY DEVELOPMENT

Failure to see and to hear are the most important sensory inadequacies of the infant and child. When both senses are affected, the usual cause is a severe cerebral defect. Only at a later age, when the infant becomes more testable, will it be apparent that the trouble is not with the sensory apparatus per se but with the central integrating mechanisms of the brain.

Failure of development of visual function is usually revealed in a disorder of ocular movements. Any defects in the refractive apparatus or visual acuity result in wandering, jerky movements of the eyes. The retinae may be abnormal in such cases, as in congenital hypoplasia of the optic nerves (optic disks are extremely small). The optic disks may be atrophic, but it should be pointed out that the infantile optic disks tend naturally to be more pale than those of an older child. Faulty vision becomes increasingly apparent in older infants when the normal sequences of hand inspection and visuomanual coordinations fail to emerge. Retention of pupillary light reflexes in a sightless child signifies a defect in the geniculocalcarine tracts and/or occipital lobes.

With respect to retardation of auditory function, again there is the difficulty in evaluating hearing in an infant. Usually, after a few weeks have passed, alert parents have noticed a brisk startle to loud noises, and a harkening to other sounds. During examination a tinkling bell brought from behind the infant usually results in head turning and visual searching, but a lack of these responses warns only of the most severe hearing defects. Slight degrees of deafness, enough to interfere with auditory learning, require special testing for their elicitation. To make the problem more difficult, in some conditions such as kernicterus, a peripheral as well as a central disorder may be present. Computerized auditory-evoked responses should be particularly helpful in confirming such abnormalities, but as yet we have not had wide experience with the test. After the first months impaired hearing becomes more obvious and interferes with language development, as will be described further on.

MENTAL RETARDATION WITHOUT EVIDENT CEREBRAL DISEASE

The symptom complex of failure of intellectual development and associated behavioral abnormalities (variously referred to as mental retardation, subnormality or deficiency; amentia; or oligophrenia) stands as the single largest neurologic disorder in every civilized society, estimated to affect 2.5 to 3 percent of the total population. Using any one of a number of indices of social and psychological failure, two somewhat overlapping groups are recognized: (1) The severely impaired, corresponding to the categories of idiot (IQ < 20) and low-grade imbecile (IQ = 20 to 45) in older classifications, also called the *pathological mentally retarded*, make up only 10 percent of the subnormal population. (2) The less severely impaired (IQ = 45 to 70), corresponding to high-grade imbecile or "feeble-minded" and far more numerous than the first, are also referred to as the *subcultural mental retardates*. In addition there are the simpletons (morons or "debiles") and "borderline" defectives, who are not generally classified as mentally retarded. The American Association on Mental Deficiency has suggested yet another grouping of mental retardation: *profound* (IQ < 25), *severe* (IQ = 25 to 39), *moderate* (IQ = 40 to 54), and *mild* (IQ = 55 to 69). The group of pathologically retarded overlaps the group of subculturally retarded as shown in Fig. 27-4.

There has been much criticism of the use of the IQ and similar tests in defining such groups, for admittedly they are essentially measures of scholastic and social efficiency. Certainly such scores are meaningless for the idiots who have no language and lack altogether the capacity to reason, but their status is so obvious that there

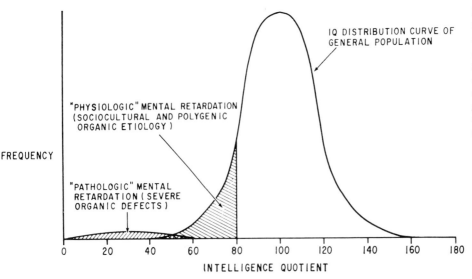

IQ DISTRIBUTION CURVE OF GENERAL POPULATION

"PHYSIOLOGIC" MENTAL RETARDATION (SOCIOCULTURAL AND POLYGENIC ORGANIC ETIOLOGY)

FREQUENCY

"PATHOLOGIC" MENTAL RETARDATION (SEVERE ORGANIC DEFECTS)

0   20   40   60   80   100   120   140   160   180

INTELLIGENCE QUOTIENT

Figure 27-4
Gaussian curve of intelligence and its skewing by the group of mental retardates with diseases of the brain. The shaded areas indicate the two groups of mentally retarded. (See text for discussion.)

is no problem in diagnosis. Nonetheless, for the others, if drawn from a fairly homogeneous population, the scores have a 0.8 correlation with other indices of subnormality.

Each of these two groups exhibits several distinctive features. Members of the pathologic group (approximately 600,000 in the United States) require constant care, and the majority are found in special institutions, whereas only about 3 percent (180,000) of the mildly retarded are institutionalized. Males predominate in the pathologic group; females, in the subcultural group. The former often show other neurologic signs, while the latter do not. The former differ also in being physically subnormal and infertile. The parents of members of the pathologic group are usually normal, but siblings may be defective, whereas in the subcultural group parents and siblings are often subnormal to varying degrees.

The pathologic type of subnormality, often consequent to major developmental derailment, chromosomal abnormality, or an exogenous factor, will be discussed more fully in Chap. 43. The remainder of this discussion will be confined to the larger subcultural form of mental retardation.

Clinical Features   Two clinical types can be recognized. In one, the essential characteristic is that almost from birth the infant is backward in all aspects of development. There is a tendency to sleep more, to be less demanding of nourishment, to suck poorly and regurgitate, and to move less. Parents often comment on how good the baby is, how little he or she troubles them by crying. As the months pass every achievement is late. The baby is more hypotonic and turns over, sits unsupported, and walks later than the normal infant. Yet despite these obvious motor delays, there is later no sign of paralysis, ataxia, chorea, or athetosis. These babies do not smile at the usual time, and take little notice of the mother or other persons or objects in their environment. They are inattentive to visual and often to auditory stimuli, to the point where questions are raised about blindness or deafness. Certain phases of normal development such as hand-regard may persist beyond the sixth month, when it normally is replaced by other activities. Mouthing (putting everything in mouth) and slobbering, which should end by 1 year of age, persist. There are only fleeting signs of interest in toys, and the impersistence of attention becomes increasingly prominent. Vocalizations are scant, often guttural, piercing, or high-pitched and feeble.

In the second type, early motor milestones (supporting head, rolling over, sitting, standing, and walking) may be attained at their normal times, yet the infant is later inattentive and slow in learning. It seems as

though motor development had somehow escaped the disordered developmental process. Aimless overactivity may also occur and, like the persistence of rhythmic movements, grinding of the teeth (bruxism), hypotonia, and microcephaly, should raise suspicion of mental backwardness.

Because the developmental sequence of motor function may be normal, even to the point where the baby acquires a few words by the end of the first year, the examiner may be misled into thinking that the mentally retarded infant was first normal and then deteriorated. Indeed it can even be shown that various test procedures yield lower scores with progressing age (from 3 years onward), but the reason for this is not a decline in ability but the fact that the tests are not comparable. In the first three years the tests are weighted toward sensorimotor functions and after that toward perception, memory, and concept formation. Interestingly, language reflects both groups of functions, needing a certain maturation of the auditory and motor apparatus at the start and highly specialized cognitive skills for continued development.

When studied more carefully in this regard, the mentally retarded infant produces a normal or increased amount of sound, and the early vocalizations do not differ from those of the normal infant. At this point, however, the difference becomes obvious. Whereas the healthy infant has done with babbling by 24 months, the retardate does not replace babbling by formed words, phrases, or sentences and does not chant or imitate the noises of vehicles or animals. If these latter vocalizations do occur in sequence, they come at a much later time than normal. In the subnormal, as in the normal child, the understanding of spoken words is superior to the ability to speak them. If the backward child does form words and sentences, their semantic content remains simple, and as Lenneberg points out, "the sophistication of wit, drama or propaganda are beyond his comprehension." A total absence of speech is observed only in severe mental retardation. If the mental age is 5 years or beyond, language production and comprehension are essentially normal.

Members of both groups of subcultural retardates exhibit a number of noteworthy features that have medical and social implications (Reissman). They tend to be sickly, and the more severely retarded among them have poor physique and are often undersized. Deviant behavior is frequent (6.6 percent incidence in normal children, 28.6 percent in the retarded, and 58.3 percent in the epileptic retarded, according to Rutter et al.). Most often deviant behavior takes the form of aggressivity, especially in the temporal lobe epileptics; other aspects that prove to be sources of medical complaint are restlessness, repetitive activity, explosive rage reactions and tantrums, obsessive behavior, stereotyped play, and the seeking of sensory experiences in unusual ways (Chess and Hassibi). The parents of a large proportion of children with deviant behavior fall in the lowest segment of the population socially and economically; in other words, the parents may be incompetent to maintain stable homes and to find work. Abandonment, neglect, and child abuse (battered-child syndrome) are frequent in this group. The majority of afflicted children must be put in special classes or schools, and special measures must be taken to reduce the tendency to truancy, pauperism, sociopathy, and criminality.

An endless debate is centered on matters of causation—whether the marginally subnormal are products of societal discrimination and lack of training and education or of faulty germ plasm which prevents successful competition, or of malnutrition, infections, or other exogenous factors. Surely both environmental factors and genetic causes are at work (Penrose).

Pathologic Features The cerebra of the subcultural group of mental retardates have defied interpretation. No visible lesions have been described, unlike the pathologic group, in which malformations and a variety of destructive lesions are fairly obvious (see Chap. 43). Even in the severely retarded there are cerebra (5 to 10 percent) which do not differ from normal for age by gross and microscopic criteria. Admittedly, a few such specimens are underweight by approximately 10 percent, but one cannot presently interpret what this means.

It is certain that a new methodology will be needed if the cerebra of the subcultural retardates and the subnormal extreme of the general population (the part that falls more than 2 SD below the mean) are to be differentiated from the highly superior and genius segment (more than 2 SD above the mean). Differences might be expected in terms of number of neurons in thalamic nuclei and cortex, in dendritic-axonal connectivity, in synaptic surfaces, elements which are not being assayed by the conventional techniques of tissue neuropathology. The observations of Huttenlocher, who finds a marked sparsity of dendritic arborization in Golgi-Cox preparations, and of Purpura, who finds an absence of short, thick spines on dendrites of cortical neurons and

other abnormalities of dendritic spines, are the first steps in this new direction.

Diagnosis Infants should be considered at risk for mental subnormality when there is a family history of mental deficiency, low birth weight in proportion to length of gestation (small-for-date babies), marked prematurity, maternal infections early in pregnancy (especially rubella), and toxemia of pregnancy.

In early life, certain behavioral characteristics are of greater predictive value than psychological tests. Prechtl and his associates have found that a low Apgar score, flaccidity, underactivity, and asymmetrical neurologic signs are the earliest indices of subnormality in the infant. Slow habituation of orienting reactions to novel auditory and visual stimuli is an early warning of mental retardation.

In the first year or two of life, suspicion of mental retardation is based largely on clinical impression, but it should always be validated by psychometric procedures. Most pediatric neurologists utilize some of the tests described by Gesell and Amatruda or the Denver Developmental Screening Scale from which a developmental quotient (DQ) is calculated. Unfortunately significant lowering of the DQ occurs only in the most flagrant cases of mental retardation, for the reason that early sensorimotor delays are more heavily weighted than are impairments of cognitive skills. Mental testing becomes increasingly effective if done later in childhood, at a time when some language has been attained.

For testing of preschool children, the Wechsler Preschool and Primary Scale of Intelligence are used, and for school-age children, the Wechsler Intelligence Scale for Children. Normal scores for age eliminate mental retardation as a cause of poor achievement, and special cognitive defects may be revealed by poor results on a particular subtest. Retarded children not only have low scores but exhibit more scatter of subtest scores. They also achieve greater success with performance than with verbal items. The physician must know the conditions of testing, for poor scores may be due to fright, inadequate motivation, lapses in attention, or a subtle sensory defect (auditory or visual) rather than a developmental lag of the cerebrum.

The EEG, in addition to exposing subclinical seizures, shows a high incidence of other abnormalities in the mentally retarded. Presumably this is due to a greater degree of immaturity of the cerebrum at any given age. However, a normal EEG is of relatively little help.

Differential diagnosis involves severe malnutrition, neglect and deprivation, chronic systemic disease, deafness, blindness, and possibly childhood psychosis. Of particular importance is the differentiation of a group of patients who are normal for a variable period after birth and then manifest a progressive disease of the nervous system. This type of disorder is representative of a group of hereditary metabolic diseases which will be discussed in Chap. 37. Of importance also is a seizure disorder which can impair cerebral function (see Chap. 15).

Management Since there is little or no possibility of treating the condition(s) underlying the mental retardation and since there is no way of restoring function to a nervous system that is developmentally subnormal or diseased, the medical objective is to assist in planning for the patient's training, education, and social and occupational adjustments. The parents must be guided in forming realistic attitudes and expectations. Psychiatric counseling may help the family to maintain a gentle but firm support of the patient so that he or she learns all the self-help skills, acquires self-control, good work habits, and a congenial personality.

Most individuals with an IQ over 60 and no other handicaps can be trained to live an independent life. Special schooling may enable such patients to realize their full potential. Social factors that cause underachievement must be sought and eliminated, if possible. Later there is need of advice about possible occupational attainments.

If the IQ is below 20, institutionalization is almost inevitable, for few families can provide long-term custodial care. Well-run institutions are usually better than community homes because they offer many more facilities (medical, educational, recreational). Often institutionalization is necessary even when the IQ is between 20 and 50. Patients in the latter group, if stable in character and relatively well adjusted socially, may work under supervision, but rarely do they become vocationally independent. For the more severely retarded, special training in the basics of hygiene and self-care are the most that can be expected.

When a decision concerning institutionalization needs to be made, great care must be exercised. While the severe degrees of retardation are all too apparent by the first or second year, the less severely affected are difficult to recognize early. As was said above, psychological tests alone are not trustworthy. The method of assessment suggested many years ago by Fernald still has a ring of soundness: (1) physical examination, (2) family background, (3) developmental history, (4) school progress, (5) examination in schoolwork, (6) practical knowledge, (7) social behavior, (8) industrial efficiency, (9) moral reactions, and (10) intelligence as measured by psychological tests. All these data except (5) and (10)

can be obtained by a skillful physician during the initial medical and neurologic examination.

RESTRICTED DEVELOPMENTAL ABNORMALITIES

DISORDERS IN THE DEVELOPMENT OF SPEECH AND LANGUAGE

In the pediatric age period and extending into adult life an interesting assortment of developmental language disorders has been uncovered. A high percentage of such patients come from families in which similar speech disorders and ambidexterity and left-handedness are frequent. Males predominate; in some series, male-to-female ratios as high as 10:1 have been reported.

Developmental disorders of language are actually far more frequent than acquired disorders, i.e., aphasia. The former include developmental speech delay, congenital deafness with speech delay, cleft-palate speech, developmental word deafness, dyslexia (special reading disability), and stuttering. Here the various stages of language development, described in an earlier section of this chapter, often are not attained at the usual age and may not even be achieved by adult life. Disorders of this type are probably due to slowness in the normal processes of maturation rather than to an acquired disease. Visible lesions are probably not to be expected in most cases, though it must be admitted that the brains of such individuals have rarely been studied by proper methods. Of particular interest in this regard is the case of developmental dyslexia described by Galaburda and Kemper, in which whole-brain serial sections showed a wider left cerebral hemisphere, an area of polymicrogyria in the left temporal language zones, and a mild cortical dysplasia in the limbic, primary, and association cortex of the left hemispheres. The same uncertainty surrounds the anatomic bases of stammering, stuttering, and other articulatory disorders. These conditions are often misunderstood by parents, teachers, and physicians. The unfortunate child or adult is judged to be feebleminded or lazy. Another frequent error is to assume that the condition is due to psychological factors, since nervousness, depression, poor sleep, and headaches frequently appear in such persons. Many of these emotional disturbances are probably secondary.

Developmental Speech Delay More than 95 percent of infants say their first words at 10 to 12 months and their first phrases before their second birthday, and when this does not happen, it becomes a cause of parental concern. In clinics where speech delay or retarded speech development (no words by 18 months, no phrases by 30 months) is studied systematically, 35 to 50 percent of such children have been found to have mental retardation or "cerebral palsy." Hearing deficit explains many of the other cases, and the remainder represent what appears to be a slowness in the maturation of the motor speech areas or, rarely, an acquired lesion in these parts. Only in this small latter group is it appropriate to speak of the language disorder as aphasia, a term that refers to a derangement or loss of language due to cerebral disease.

In the majority of cases of delayed speech there is no clear evidence of an acquired lesion in the motor speech areas. It is this group of cases, which includes otherwise normal children who talk late (they deviate from their age norm well beyond 2 SD), that proves the most puzzling. Here it is virtually impossible to draw the line between normal and abnormal. Prelanguage speech continues into the period when words and phrases should normally be used in propositional speech. The combinations of sounds are close to the standard of normal vowel-consonant combinations of the 1- to 2-year-old, and they may even be strung together as in a sentence. Yet as time passes, only a few understandable words may be uttered, even by the third or fourth years. Often one discovers a family history of delayed speech, and three out of four such patients will be boys. When speech does begin, as always happens, it may overlap the early stages of spoken language, and the child progresses rapidly to speaking in full sentences. Not infrequently, however, articulation is infantile and the content of speech impoverished semantically and syntactically. During all this period of speech delay, the understanding of words and intelligence progress normally. Sometimes, however, the child distinguishes speech sounds poorly. Motor speech delay does not presage mental backwardness. (It is said that Albert Einstein did not speak until the age of 4 and lacked fluency at 9.) Later the patient with delayed speech may be found to have dyslexia and dysgraphia, a combination that is inherited as an autosomal dominant trait, more frequently in boys than girls.

Aphasia, when it develops as the result of an acquired lesion (vascular, traumatic) is essentially motor and lasts but a few months. It may be accompanied by a right-sided hemiplegia. An interesting acquired example, possibly encephalitic, has been described by Landau and Kleffner in association with seizures and bitemporal fo-

cal discharges in the EEG. There may later be full recovery when the seizures are controlled.

Congenital Deafness Motor speech delay due to congenital deafness, whether peripheral (loss of pure-tone acuity) or central (pure-tone threshold normal by audiogram) may at first be difficult to discern. One suspects faulty hearing when there are in the background the well-known antecedents of deafness—congenital rubella, erythroblastosis fetalis, meningitis, and bilateral ear infections—which account for 75 percent of cases. (It is estimated that 3 million American children have hearing defects; 0.1 percent of the school population is deaf and 1.5 percent hard of hearing.) The parents' attention may be drawn to a defect in hearing when the infant does not heed loud noises, does not turn the eyes to sound sources outside the immediate visual fields, and fails to react to music, but in other instances it is the delay in speech that calls attention to it.

The deaf child makes the transition from crying to cooing and babbling at the usual age of 3 to 5 months. After the sixth month, however, the child becomes much quieter, and the usual repertoire of babbling sounds becomes stereotyped and unchanging though still uttered with pleasant voice. A more conspicuous failure comes somewhat later, when babbling fails to give way to word formation. Should deafness develop within the first few years of life, after speech has been acquired, the child gradually loses speech but can be retaught by the lip-reading method. The speech, however, is harsh, poorly modulated, and unpleasant and accompanied by many peculiar throat noises of a snorting or grunting kind. Unlike the mentally retarded child, social and other acquisitions appear at the expected times in the congenitally deaf child, who seems eager to communicate and makes known all needs by gesture or pantomime—often very cleverly. In fact, the deaf child may attract attention by vivid facial expression, motions of lips, nodding, or head shaking. The Leiter performance scale, which makes no use of sounds, will show that intelligence is normal. The deafness can be demonstrated at an early age by careful observation of the child's responses to sounds and by free-field audiometry, but the full range of hearing cannot be accurately tested before the age of 3 or 4 years. The recording of auditory-evoked brainstem potentials, the testing of reaction to sounds by the psychogalvanic reflex technique, and testing of the labyrinths, which are frequently unresponsive in deaf-mutes, may be helpful. Early diagnosis is important in order to obtain possible hearing aids and appropriate language training.

In contrast to children in whom deafness is the only abnormality, the imbecile or moron is defective in all actions and talks little because he or she has nothing to say. Autistic children may also be mute, and if they speak, echolalia is prominent and the personal *I* is avoided. Blind children of normal intelligence tend to speak slowly and fail to acquire imitative gestures.

Congenital Word Deafness This disorder, also called *developmental receptive dysphasia, auditory imperception,* or *central deafness* may be difficult to distinguish from peripheral deafness. Usually the parents have noted that the word-deaf child responds to loud noises and music, though obviously this does not assure perfect hearing, particularly for high tones. The word-deaf child does not understand what is said, and delay and distortion of speech are evident.

It is supposed that the auditory apparatus of the dominant temporal lobe fails to discriminate between the complex acoustic patterns of words and to associate them with visual images of people and objects—a theory that cannot be either affirmed or refuted at this time. One observation stands out, that the child, despite intact pure-tone hearing, does not seem to hear word patterns properly and fails to reproduce them in natural speech. In other ways the child may be bright, but more often than not this auditory imperception of words is associated with hyperactivity, inattentiveness, bizarre behavior, or perceptual defects incident to focal brain damage, particularly in the temporal lobes. Deaf children may chatter incessantly. Often they adopt a language of their own design which the parents come to understand. This peculiar type of speech is known as *idioglossia*. It is also observed in children with marked articulatory defects.

Little is known about congenital word deafness, perhaps because of its rarity. Speech habilitation of the bright word-deaf child should follow along the same lines as that of the congenitally deaf. Such a child learns to lip-read quickly and is clever at acting out his or her own ideas.

Congenital Inarticulation This condition represents a slightly different developmental defect, in which the child seems unable to coordinate the vocal, articulatory, and respiratory apparatus for the purpose of speaking. It too occurs more often in boys than girls, and again there is often a family history of the disorder, although the data are not quite sufficient to establish the pattern of inheritance. The incidence is 1 in every 200 children. The motor, sensory, emotional, and social attainments correspond to the norms for age, although in a few of the cases, a minority in the authors' opinion, there has been some indication of cranial nerve abnormality in the first months of life (ptosis, facial asymmetry, strange neonatal cry, and altered phonation).

In children with congenital inarticulation, the "prelanguage" sounds are probably abnormal, but this aspect of the speech disorder has not been well studied. Babbling tends to be deficient, and in the second year the vocalizations do not show vowel-consonant combinations that resemble the spoken words of the parents. In attempting to say something, the child makes noises that do not sound at all like language, and in this way the child is unlike the late talker already described. Again the understanding of language is entirely normal; the comprehension vocabulary is average for age, and the child can appreciate syntax as indicated by correct responses to questions by nodding or head shaking and by the execution of complex spoken commands. Usually such patients are shy but otherwise quick in response, cheerful, and without behavior disorder. While some of these children are bright, a combination of congenital inarticulation disorder and mild mental dullness is not uncommon. Speech correction should be attempted (by a trained therapist) if many of the spontaneous utterances are intelligible. However, if the child makes no sounds that resemble words, the therapeutic effort should be directed toward a modified school program and mental hygiene, and speech habilitation should wait until some words are acquired.

Studies of the cerebra of such patients are not available, and it is doubtful if they would show any abnormality by the usual techniques of neuropathologic examination. Occasionally, suspicion of a lesion is raised by focal changes in the EEG or a slight widening of the temporal horn of the left ventricle. Delayed speech is often attributed to "tongue-tie," i.e., a short lingual frenulum, but we have never been convinced of this. Also psychologists have attributed speech retardation to overprotectiveness or excessive pressure by the parents. We are inclined to believe that these are the results rather than the cause of the delay.

The whole subject is well reviewed in the monograph *The Child with Delayed Speech,* edited by Rutter and Martin.

Other Articulatory Defects These are most common in preschool children, having an incidence of 15 percent. There are a number of varieties of deficient articulation. One is *lisping,* in which the *s* sound is replaced by *th,* e.g., *thimple* for *simple.* Another common condition in early childhood, *lallation,* or *dyslalia,* is characterized by multiple substitutions or omissions of consonants. Milder degrees consist of a difficulty in pronouncing only one or two consonants. For example, the letter *r* may be incorrectly pronounced, so that it sounds like *w* or *y*; *running a race* becomes *wunning a wace* or *yunning a yace*. In severe forms speech may be almost unintelligible. The child seems to be unaware that his or her speech differs from that of others and is distressed at not being understood. These and similar abnormalities of speech are often present in normal children and are referred to as "infantilisms," but why do they persist in some individuals? It has been suggested that the development of language is so rapid that there is sometimes a partial failure of the corrective mechanism of both hearing and imitation.

Of importance is the fact that in more than 90 percent of children these abnormalities disappear by the age of 8 years, either spontaneously or in response to speech therapy. The latter is best started if these conditions persist to the fifth year. Presumably the natural cycle of motor speech acquisition has been only delayed developmentally, not arrested. Such abnormalities are more frequent among the feebleminded than in normal children; with mental defect many consonants are persistently mispronounced. Worster-Drought has described a congenital form of spastic bulbar speech in which words are spoken slowly, with stiff labial and lingual movements, hyperactive jaw and facial reflexes, and sometimes mild dysphagia and dysphonia. The limbs may be unaffected, in contrast to most children with "cerebral palsy."

The speech disorder resulting from *cleft palate* is easily recognized. Many of these patients also have a harelip; the two abnormalities together interfere with sucking and later in life with the enunciation of labial and guttural consonants. The voice has an unpleasant nasality, and often, if the defect is severe, there is an audible escape of air through the nose.

Aside from these special types of developmental language disorder, there are many other common defects in speech that handicap individuals throughout their lives. Word blocking, multiple substitution of words, inability to complete spoken sentences, and word cluttering are observed in many adults and make their speech inefficient and unpleasant to hear. These abnormalities are often associated with specific language defects.

Congenital Word Blindness (Developmental Dyslexia)

This is a condition that becomes manifest in an older child who fails in the first grade to master the written or printed word. Several excellent books have been written on the subject, to which the interested reader is referred for a detailed account (see References).

The main problem is an inability to read words, and also to spell and to write them despite the ability to see and recognize letters. There is no loss of the ability to recognize the meaning of objects, pictures, and diagrams. Often the ingredients of reading failure are present before the child enters school and can be anticipated by difficulty in copying, color naming, and formation of number concepts, and by the persistent reversal of letters. The writing appears to be defective because of faulty perception of form and a kind of constructional and directional apraxia. Not infrequently there is an associated vagueness about the serial order of letters in the alphabet and months in the year, as well as difficulty with numbers (acalculia) and an inability to spell and to read music. Some dyslexic children have already had trouble in learning to speak and in acquiring clear articulation. For this reason Ingram sees all these motor and perceptual speech difficulties as parts of a complex of congenital language defect.

Lesser degrees of dyslexia are more common than the severe ones and are found in a large segment of the school population. Some 10 percent of school children have some degree of this disability, but the problem is complex, because the condition is unquestionably influenced by the way reading is taught. However, only a small number are unable to read at all after many years in school.

This form of language disorder, unattended by other neurologic signs, is strongly familial, being almost in conformity with an autosomal dominant pattern and again more frequent in the male. There is a statistically higher incidence of left-handedness among these persons.

The steady drill of a cooperative child by a skillful teacher over an extended period (many hours per week) slowly overcomes the handicap and enables an otherwise intelligent child to follow successfully a regular program of education.

In the study of the dyslexic and dysgraphic child as well as in some whose speech is essentially normal, a number of other apparently congenital developmental abnormalities have been documented, such as (1) inadequate perception of space and form (poor performance on form boards) and in tasks requiring construction, etc., (2) inadequate perception of size, of distance, and also of temporal sequences and rhythms, and (3) inability to imitate sequences of movements gracefully, and extreme degrees of clumsiness in all motor tasks and games (the clumsy-child syndrome described by Gubbay et al.). Less fully studied than other developmental disorders, they represent, nonetheless, when present in pure form with normal intelligence, an inordinate delay in one phase of neurologic development. These disorders may also occur in brain-injured children; hence there may be considerable difficulty in separating simple delay or arrest in development from a pathologic process in the brain. Probably all that is said about dyslexia applies to the kindred state of *acalculia*, where no amount of classroom work helps the child learn arithmetic. Often this is associated with dyslexia.

Precocious Reading and Calculating In contrast, unusually precocious reading and calculation abilities have also been identified. A child 2 or 3 years old may read with the skill of an average adult. Extraordinary facility with numbers (mathematical prodigies) and vivid memory capacity (eidetic imagery) are similar traits. Here one observes presumably an extraordinary overdevelopment of these single faculties. Occasionally one of these special abilities will be observed in a child with a mild form of autism. He may exhibit a prodigious skill in a mathematical trick but have no capacity to solve mathematical problems or to understand the meaning of numbers (a mild degree of "idiot savant").

Stuttering and Stammering These difficulties occur in an estimated 1 to 2 percent of the school population. Often such conditions disappear in late childhood and adolescence, and only about 1 in every 300 individuals suffers from a persistent stammer or stutter.

Stammering and stuttering are difficult to classify. In some respects they belong to the developmental disorders, but they differ from them in being largely centered in articulation. Essentially both take the form of a spasm of the articulatory muscles upon attempting to speak. The spasm may be tonic and result in a complete blocking of speech (sometimes referred to as stammering) or clonic, i.e., a series of spasms interrupting the emission of consonants, usually the first syllables of a word (stuttering). There is no valid reason to distinguish between these two forms of the disorder, since they are intermingled, and the terms *stammer* and *stutter* are now used synonymously. Certain sounds, particularly *p* and *b*, offer greater difficulty than others; *paper boy* comes out *p-p-paper b-b-boy*. The severity of the stutter is increased by excitement and stress, as when speaking before others, and is reduced when the stutterer is relaxed and alone or when singing. When severe, the spasms may overflow into other groups of muscles such as those of the face, neck, arms. The stuttering muscles show no fault in performing nonlinguistic actions.

Males are affected four times as often as females. The time of onset of stuttering is mainly at two periods in life—between 2 and 4 years, when speech is beginning, and between 6 and 8 years, when the evolution of language extends to reciting, reading aloud, and writing in the classroom. However, there may be a later onset. Many afflicted children have an associated difficulty in reading and writing. If stuttering is mild, it tends to develop or to be present only during periods of emotional stress, and it usually disappears spontaneously during adolescent or early adult years. If severe, it persists all through life, regardless of treatment, but tends to improve as the patient grows older.

Theories of causation are legion. Slowness in developing hand and eye preference, or an enforced change from left- to right-hand use has been a popular explanatory principle of which Orton was a leading advocate. However, these associations seem to apply to only a minority of stutterers (Hécaen and de Ajuriaguerra). The disappearance of mild stuttering with advancing age has been attributed incorrectly to all manner of treatment (hypnosis, progressive relaxation, speaking in rhythms, temporarily changing the speech activity in different ways) and used to bolster particular theories of causation. Since stuttering may reappear at times of emotional strain, a psychogenesis has been proposed, but, as Orton points out, if there are any neurotic tendencies in the stutterer, they are secondary rather than primary. We have observed that many stutterers, probably as a result of this impediment to free social intercourse, do become increasingly fearful of talking and develop feelings of inferiority. By the time adolescence and adulthood are reached, emotional factors are so prominent that many physicians have mistaken stuttering for neurosis. Usually there is little or no evidence of any personality deviation before the onset of stuttering, and psychotherapy, though helpful in relieving emotional tension and assisting the patient's adjustment to the condition, has not in our experience had a consistent effect on the underlying defect. A strong family history in many cases and male dominance lend support to a genetic origin of the disorder, but the inheritance does not follow a readily discernible pattern.

The essential character of stuttering has been difficult to define in physiologic terms. There is no detectable weakness or ataxia of the speech musculature, which functions normally in all other commonplace acts. Stuttering differs from an apraxia in that the muscles of speech, when called upon to perform the specific act of speaking, go into spasm. The spasms are not invoked by other actions (possibly the others are not as complex or voluntary), and only in this way does stuttering differ from the intention spasm of athetosis. In fact, stuttering appears to represent a special category of movement disorder, much like writer's cramp, another nonpsychogenic motor disorder of unknown cause which is induced by writing and a few other specialized learned actions.

Careful observation of the speech of small children and of adults as well discloses that stuttering may rarely appear as the result of a lesion in motor speech areas.

Because of its course the therapy of stuttering is difficult to evaluate. Many methods have been tried but have had no lasting value. As remarked above, all speech-fluency disturbances are modifiable by various environmental circumstances. Thus a certain proportion of stutterers will become more fluent under certain therapeutic conditions, such as reading aloud. Yet a smaller proportion will stutter more severely at this time. Again, a majority of stutterers will be adversely affected by talking on the telephone; a small minority are helped by this device. Some stutterers are more fluent under conditions of mild alcohol intoxication. Nearly every stutterer is fluent while singing.

On the whole, the therapy of speech-fluency disorders has been a frustrating effort. Nearly any environmental stimulus whose occurrence is strictly contingent upon dysfluencies will modify their frequency in the experimental situation. This fact has led to the adoption of a number of such stimuli, most notably contingent white noise and delayed auditory feedback, as therapeutic measures. Schemes such as the encouragement of associated muscular movements ("penciling," etc.) and the adoption of a "theatrical" approach to speaking have been advocated. Common to all such efforts has been a difficulty in achieving carry-over into the natural speaking environment. Progressive relaxation, hypnosis, and tranquilization help temporarily. A few controlled studies with antidopaminergic drugs, particularly haloperidol, have shown promising results in a minority of severe stutterers.

Another special developmental disorder, *cluttering, or cluttered, speech,* is characterized by uncontrollable speed of speech, which results in truncated, dysrhythmic, and often incoherent utterances. It is as though the child is too hurried to take the trouble to pronounce each word carefully and to compose sentences. Omissions of consonants, elisions, improper phrasing, and inadequate intonation occur. It is closely related to other motor speech impediments.

AUTISM AND CHILDHOOD PSYCHOSIS

The term *autism,* introduced by Kanner in 1943, refers to another remarkable disharmony of development wherein children, despite excellent motor skill (normal motor milestones and facile use of hands), are unable to mature socially, i.e., to form any emotional bonds with parents and other individuals, and often to learn to speak. It is the discrepancy between their excellent motor skill on the one hand and the global asociality, lack of or restricted communicative speech, and certain other eccentricities of behavior on the other that sets them apart from the more common mental retardates. Severely autistic children cannot be disciplined. They do not heed words or react to other human beings; hence they are essentially uneducable. A minority acquire some language but use it little in communication. The mildest degree of the disease allows an uneven development of cognitive and social abilities.

When the biographies of a group of autistic children are examined, two courses of development are perceived. One group appears to have been entirely normal until 18 to 24 months of age, at which time an alarming regression begins, sometimes in temporal relation to an injury or an upsetting experience. The other group appears to have been abnormal from the first months of life. Their level of activity is reduced, they cry little, and are indifferent to their surroundings. Toys are ignored or are held tenaciously. In contrast motor development proceeds normally or even precociously. Later an unusual sensitivity to all modes of sensory stimulation may be displayed.

Regardless of the mode of onset, older autistic children exhibit a striking disregard for other persons; they make no eye contact and are no more interested in another person than in an article of furniture. Preferred toys are either manipulated cleverly or are ignored. Insistence on constancy of environment may reach the point where such patients become distraught if even a single object in their room has been moved in their absence. If speech does develop, it is highly automatic and words are spoken without feeling. Reading capacity and calculation may greatly exceed expressive speech. Elaborate stereotypes of movement, such as whirling of the body, spinning of objects, and toe walking are frequent. Certain objects such as spinning toys or running water have a strange fascination.

The outcome of childhood autism is discouraging, according to Eisenberg, who has followed a large number through adolescence into adulthood. One-third of the patients never speak, another third acquire a rudimentary language devoid of communicative value, and only in the remainder does an affected, stilted, colorless speech develop. As many as a third of all such patients, as they grow older, begin to manifest other visuoperceptive and auditory defects, indicative of a variety of cerebral diseases. This is not surprising, since autism is a rather imprecise syndrome. Hence any group of such patients is often contaminated with a variety of other encephalopathic states. Yet in purest form it probably represents a unique metabolic (or other) disease. Moreover, we have the impression that many patients show milder degrees of this disorder, evolving as eccentric, mirthless, flat personalities unable to adapt socially but possessing certain unusual aptitudes (arithmetic ability, factual knowledge of history or science well beyond age norms).

The basis of pure childhood autism is as much a mystery today as it was when Kanner described it. Most of these children are physically normal, have a head of average size, and have no somatic defects or other neurologic abnormalities. The EEG may be normal or show slight immaturity. The pneumoencephalogram and CT scan reveal ventricles of average size and no atrophy of the brain. In a few the temporal horn of the left lateral ventricle is enlarged. There is usually no familial tendency, though we have seen the disease in identical twins and in brothers and a familial subgroup is known to exist. Only two or three rather inadequate postmortem examinations have been recorded and have shown no lesions.

The implication that these children or adults are truly autistic, i.e., have a rich inner psychic life or dream world that is out of relation to reality, is an assumption totally without foundation. Despite many claims to the contrary, there is no evidence of psychogenesis. Although this disorder has been referred to as "childhood schizophrenia," the afflicted individuals do not resemble schizophrenics when they reach adolescent and adult years.

Whether there is, quite apart from autism, a form of schizophrenia that affects infants and young children has been difficult to decide. Schizophrenic parents have been known to beget children who from the beginning are aloof, impersonal, withdrawn, and asocial in their daily contact. They may be rigid, resistive, and show abnormal reactions to stimuli (overreaction, avoidance, unnatural fear), inexplicable anxiety, hallucinations, mutism and bizarre postures, hyperactivity, rocking, and spinning. Such states, called *childhood psychosis* or childhood schizophrenia, have been well described by Lauretta Bender.

Psychotherapy is of no proven value. Currently there is interest in determining whether behavior-modification methods have anything to offer. Lithium carbonate, phenytoin, dextroamphetamine and other of the antipsychotic drugs sometimes result in improvement in behavior.

"MINIMAL BRAIN DYSFUNCTION" SYNDROMES

A large portion of ambulatory pediatric neurology consists of children referred because of failure in school. The question asked is whether they have a brain disease or the sequelae of brain injury that alters behavior, interferes with learning, or causes clumsiness.

When a large number of such cases is analyzed, fully 80 to 85 percent prove to have no major signs of neurologic disease (Barlow). Perhaps 5 percent are mentally retarded, and another 5 percent show some evidence of cerebral palsy. In the group without neurologic signs, the IQ is normal though there are a larger number of borderline cases than in the general population. More of the boys are found to be hyperactive and inattentive and to have trouble in learning to read and write. Many are clumsy. More of the girls have trouble with numbers and arithmetic. Dyslexia has already been discussed. The other causes of school failure are grouped under the hyperactivity and the learning disability syndromes, which are discussed below.

HYPERACTIVITY SYNDROME

Human infants exhibit astonishing differences in amount of activity almost from the first days of life. Some babies are constantly on the move, wiry, and hard to hold, and others are placid and as slack as a sack of meal. Irwin, who studied motility in the neonate, found a difference of 290 times between the most and least active in terms of amount of movement per 24 h.

Once walking and running begin, children normally enter a period when they are extremely active, more so than at any other period of life. The degree of activity, which again varies widely from one child to another, seems not to be correlated with the age of achieving motor milestones or with great motor skill at a later time. The male is more active than the female, and the black child tends to be more precocious in motor development and more active than the white. Children with cerebral defects tend to exhibit hyperactivity more often than normal children.

Again, two groups can be discerned: In one the infants are overactive from birth, sleeping less and feeding poorly, and by the age of 2 years the syndrome is obvious. In the other, at the preschool age (4 to 6 years), it becomes apparent that these children are unable to sit quietly. Seldom do they remain in one position for more than a few seconds, even when watching television. They cannot attend to any task no matter how interesting. As a rule there is also an abnormal impulsivity and often intolerance of all measures to control the activity.

Once in school, such children are disruptive. They cannot sit at their desks, take turns in reciting, be quiet, or control their own impulses. The teacher finds it impossible to discipline them and often insists that the parents seek medical consultation. Sometimes it is discovered that one or more males in a previous generation had the same problem. Some children are so hyperactive that they cannot attend regular school. Their behavior verges on the "organic driveness" that has been known to occur in children whose brains have been injured by encephalitis. Most are less active and can be managed in special ways.

In the majority of cases, the natural course of this disorder is for the hyperactivity to subside gradually by puberty or soon thereafter. Mild degrees of mental retardation and epilepsy and other special disabilities are conjoined in many patients. Dislocation in educational and social adjustment may render the child prone to truancy and a variety of sociopathic trends in late childhood and adolescence.

There has been a tendency in recent years to consider children with the hyperkinetic syndrome as having minimal brain disease. "Soft neurologic signs" such as right-left confusion, mirror movements, minimal choreic instability, awkwardness, finger agnosia, tremor, and borderline hyperreflexia are said to be more frequent. These signs, however, are seen so often in normal children that their attribution to disease is invalid. Schain and others have therefore substituted the term *minimal brain dysfunction*, which in essence does no more than restate the problem. Lacking altogether are accurate clinicoanatomic and clinicopathologic correlative data.

The treatment of the hyperactive child can proceed intelligently only after medical and psychological explorations have elucidated the context in which the hyperactivity occurs. If the child is principally hyperactive and inattentive in school and less so in an unstructured environment, it may be that mental retardation or dyslexia, which prevents scholastic success, is a source of frustration and anger. The child then turns to other activities and becomes occupied in ways that disturb the classroom. Another possibility is that the hyperactive child may have failed to acquire self-control because of a disorganized home life, and the overactivity is but one manifestation of anxiety or intolerance of constraint. Clearly problems such as these require a modification of the educational program.

For intelligent overactive children who have failed to control their impulses even with parental assistance and who at all times have boundless energy, require little sleep, exhibit a wriggling restlessness (the choreiform syndrome of Prechtl and Stemmer) and incessant exploratory activity that repeatedly gets them into mischief, even to their own dismay, medical therapy is in order—dextroamphetamine in doses of 2.5 to 5 mg tid or methylphenidate, 5 to 10 mg tid. Strangely, these two drugs, which are stimulants, have a quieting effect on these children. In contrast, phenobarbital has the opposite effect on them. If these pharmacologic agents control the activity and improve school performance (they can be continued for a number of years), then there is no need to alter the child's school program. If the child is not helped, lithium, chlorpromazine or phenytoin should be tried. Psychotherapy may be needed over brief periods for the child and the child's family. Remedial education should be reserved for recalcitrant cases.

LEARNING DISABILITY

School is obviously the most challenging event in the child's life and, since it is compulsory, serves to evince in many children dramatic behavioral disorders.

Timid and easily frightened children, despite attempts at kindergarten attendance, may not tolerate separation from their mothers and may refuse to go to school. In others this first step may be achieved, but from the beginning there is failure in all scholastic tasks, even when the child has an apparently normal intelligence. Neuropsychiatric opinion is then sought to ascertain whether the child cannot or will not learn. If the former is evidenced, it must be decided whether the disability is due to a limitation of cognitive functions, a specific reading or calculating disability, or an inattentiveness and overactivity syndrome. Seizures and anticonvulsive medications often are an additional source of trouble. In other words, the role of the child neurologist is to help decide whether the difficulty reflects a general or a restricted cerebral impairment. Reading and writing failure are singled out most often because they are among the first scholastic tasks which the child must master and are of fundamental importance in all later school-work.

Often, upon clinical analysis, it is discovered for the first time that mental retardation has been present since birth or early life but ignored by unobservant parents. In others intelligence is normal, and a specific dyslexia or other language problem becomes unmasked when the child is confronted for the first time by demanding tasks. The language problems need to be corrected by special educational methods.

The study of such children should be supplemented by a number of tests of intelligence, language, memory, perception, attention, visual memory, and auditory-visual integration. Kinsbourne (1980) has listed those which are most useful (Table 27-3).

ENURESIS

Voluntary sphincteric control develops according to a predetermined time scale. Usually normal children stop soiling themselves before they can remain dry, and day control precedes night control. Some children are toilet-trained by their second birthday, but there are wide variations. Many children have not acquired full sphincteric control until the fourth year. Constant dribbling usually indicates spina bifida, but in the boy one must look also for obstruction of the bladder neck and in the girl for an ectopic ureter entering the vagina.

When a child of 5 years or older wets the bed nearly every night and is dry by day, the child is said to have *nocturnal enuresis.* This condition afflicts approximately 10 percent of children between 4 and 14 years of age, boys more than girls, and continues in many cases to be a problem even into adolescence and adulthood. Although mentally retarded children are notably late in acquiring sphincter control (some never do), the majority of enuretic individuals are normal in other respects.

The cause of this condition is disputed. Often there is a family history of the same complaint. Some psychiatrists have insisted that overzealous parents "pressure" the child until he develops a complex about his bedwetting. Punishment, shaming, rewards, etc., doubtless have this effect, but the underlying condition is believed by most neurologists to be a delay in the maturation of higher control of spinal reflex centers during sleep. As indicated on page 271, Gastaut and Broughton have uncovered a number of abnormalities of bladder function in the enuretic child. These and other aspects of this disorder are discussed in Chap. 18.

SOCIOPATHY AND NEUROSIS

During the formative years, when children or adolescents seek tribe approval, every blemish, every physical abnormality becomes a cross to bear. On the neurologic side, a stammer or stutter, dyslexia, hyperactivity, etc., not only place them apart but also interfere with the training and education to which their intelligence enti-

tles them. When forced in their schoolwork beyond their capacities in language and speech, they may become rebellious and aggressive or give up completely and divert themselves in other ways. Not infrequently, social development, which may revolve more around classmates than family, is thwarted or misguided.

Extremes of egocentricity, lack of understanding of the feelings, needs, and actions of other members of one's social group, and an inability to judge one's own strengths and weaknesses stand as the central issues in the development of psychoneurosis. Such difficulties usually become manifest by adolescence. Indeed *neurosis* may be defined in such terms; *psychosis* refers only to a more global disorganization of thinking and behavior, but again revealed to a maximal degree in social relationships. In later life neurotic persons habitually attempt to preserve their egocentric ways in each newly formed social circle. If socially rejected for this or other reasons, anxiety and unhappiness often result. The complete detachment of the child with psychosis, the amorality of the constitutional sociopath, the major disturbances in thinking of the schizophrenic, and the mood swings of the manic-depressive have also expressed themselves in many instances by adolescence. Here one confronts one of the key problems in psychiatry—the extent to which neurosis, sociopathy, and psychosis have their roots in derangements in the affective and social life of the individual during the processes of personality development. In other words, in what measure are they determined by early life experiences, and to what extent are they genetically determined?

The answers to these questions cannot be given with finality. Experienced clinicians tend to believe that genetic factors are actually more important than environmental ones. The discovery that unusually tall males with severe acne vulgaris and aggressive psychopathic behavior may have a karyotype of XYY chromosomes in an example of a possible genetic relationship. Further, there is no critical evidence to show that deliberate alteration of the familial and social environment or mental hygiene measures now so popular have ever prevented a neurosis, psychosis, or sociopathy. Admittedly, counseling of parents is helpful in managing behavior and adjustment problems of adolescents, but children identified as high-risk individuals because of early truancy, conflict with the law, and general maladjustment, if transferred to a more stable and supportive environment, have as a group not turned out much better than others left alone. Here data are meager, however, and a completely con-

trolled study has probably never been attempted. For
this reason the mental hygiene movement continues to
be supported in the United States.

Many patients concern the physician, other than
those who develop frank neurosis or psychosis, for civilized society is filled with countless unhappy, maladjusted individuals who cannot be called either neurotic
or psychotic. It is with reference to these persons that
one seeks explanations in terms of psychogenesis and
looks for early signs of psychopathic trends. Adolescent
turmoil often seems to stem from parental neglect, poor
child-parent relations, or unstable home environment
that has engendered either defiance or excessive dependency. The result may be either a failure of emancipation or an early rupture of family ties, both with a lasting
effect on social maturation. Similarly, sexual deviations
of the adolescent and young adult are often ascribed to
lack of early guidance and instruction. Certainly, the
adolescent is not helped by the ambivalence of Western
society, which evinces interest in sex but then imposes
sanctions on its expression. Actually, little is known
about the early conditioning that inculcates traits of
masculinity and femininity (see page 1045). Hormonal
factors play but a minor part. Whether or not sexual
perversions are due to early patterning of the brain is
unsettled. Ignorance of sex and impoverishment of human relations also seem to account for many sexual misadventures.

The sensitivity of adolescents to the good opinion
of their peers obviously renders them psychologically
vulnerable. If in addition they happen to be endowed
with limited intelligence and a physical defect, the
ground for persistent and indomitable feelings of inferiority are laid, especially if there is repeated failure in
competition. The individualization of education and vocational training for such adolescents is essential, to permit the talented to exploit their abilities and those with
handicaps to be directed into activities that constructively develop personality.

It is during the period of late childhood and adolescence, when personality is least stable, that transient
symptoms, many resembling the psychopathologic states
of adult life, are most frequent and difficult to interpret.
Some of these behavioral disorders represent the early
signs of schizophrenia or manic-depressive disease, but
many have a way of disappearing as adult years are
reached, so that one can only surmise that they were but
expressions of adolescent turmoil (see Chap. 55).

REFERENCES

ANDERSON LD: The predictive value of infancy tests in relation to intelligence at five years. *Child Dev* 10:203, 1939.

ANDRÉ-THOMAS, CHESNI Y, SAINT-ANNE DARGASSIES S: *The Neurological Examination of the Infant.* London, Medical Advisory Committee, National Spastics Society, 1960.

ANDREWS G, HARRIS M: *Clinics in Developmental Medicine, no 17: The Syndrome of Stuttering.* London, Heinemann, 1964.

BARLOW C: *Mental Retardation and Related Disorders.* Philadelphia, Davis, 1977.

BAYLEY H: Comparisons of mental and motor test scores for age 1-15 months by sex, birth order, race, geographic location and education of parents. *Child Dev* 36:379, 1965.

BENDER L: *A Visual-Motor Gestalt Test and Its Use.* New York, American Orthopsychiatric Association, 1938.

———: The life course of schizophrenic children. *Biol Psychiatry* 2:165, 1970.

BENTON AL: *Revised Visual Retention Test.* New York, Psychological Corporation, 1974.

———: Right-left discrimination. *Pediatr Clin North Am* 15:747, 1968.

BIRCH HG, BELMONT L: Auditory-visual integration in normal and retarded readers. *Am J Orthopsychiatry* 34:852, 1964.

BRECKENRIDGE ME, MURPHY MN: *Growth and Development of the Young Child.* New York, Saunders, 1963.

CHESS S: Diagnosis and treatment of the hyperactive child. *NY State J Med* 60:2379, 1960.

———, HASSIBI M: Behavioral deviations in mentally retarded children. *J Am Acad Child Psychiatry* 9:282, 1970.

CONEL J: *The Postnatal Development of the Human Cerebral Cortex,* vols 1-8. Cambridge, Mass, Harvard, 1939-1967.

CRITCHLEY M, CRITCHLEY EA: *Dyslexia Defined.* Springfield, Ill, Charles C Thomas, 1978.

EISENBERG L: The autistic child in adolescence. *Am J Psychiatry* 112:607, 1965.

ELLINGSON RG: The incidence of EEG abnormality among children with mental disorder of apparently nonorganic origin. *Am J Psychiatry* 111:263, 1954.

FANTZ RL: The origin of form perception. *Sci Am* 204:66, 1961.

FERNALD WE: Standardized fields of inquiry for clinical studies of borderline defectives. *Ment Hyg* 1:211, 1917.

FRANKENBERG WK, DODDS JB, FANDAL AW: *Denver Developmental Screening Test,* rev ed. Denver, University of Colorado Medical Center, 1970.

GALABURDA AM, KEMPER TL: Cytoarchitectonic abnormalities in developmental dyslexia. *Ann Neurol* 6:94, 1979.

GESELL A, AMATRUDA CS: *Developmental Diagnosis: Normal and Abnormal Child Development,* 2d ed. New York, Hoeber-Harper, 1954.

——— et al: *The First Five Years of Life: The Preschool Years.* New York, Harper & Row, 1940.

GIBSON EJ, OLUM J: Experimental methods of studying perception in children, in Mussen P (ed): *Handbook of Research Methods in Child Development.* New York, Wiley, 1960, chap 8.

GOLDSTEIN K: *Language and Language Disturbances: Aphasic Symptom Complexes and Their Significance for Medicine and Theory of Language.* New York, Grune & Stratton, 1948.

GUBBAY SS et al: Clumsy children: a study of apraxic and agnosic defects in 21 children. *Brain* 88:295, 1965.

HÉCAEN N, DE AJURIAGUERRA J: *Left-handedness.* New York, Grune & Stratton, 1964.

HUTTENLOCHER PR: Dendritic development in neocortex of children with mental defect and infantile spasms. *Neurology* 24:203, 1974.

ILLINGWORTH RS: *The Development of the Infant and Young Child, Normal and Abnormal,* 3d ed. Edinburgh, Livingstone, 1966.

INGRAM TTS: Developmental disorders of speech, in Vinken PJ, Bruyn W (eds): *Handbook of Clinical Neurology,* vol 4. Amsterdam, North-Holland, 1969, chap 22, pp 407–442.

IRWIN OC: Can infants have IQ's? *Psychol Rev* 49:69, 1942.

KAGAN J, MOSS HA: *Birth to Maturity: A Study of Psychological Development.* New York, Wiley, 1962.

KANNER I: Early infantile autism. *J Pediatr* 25:211, 1944.

KINSBOURNE M: Developmental Gerstmann's syndrome: A disorder of sequencing. *Pediatr Clin North Am* 15:771, 1968.

————: Disorders of mental development, in Menkes JH (ed): *Textbook of Child Neurology,* 2d ed. Philadelphia, Lea & Febiger, 1980, chap 13, pp 636–666.

KIRMAN BH: Early disturbances of behavior in relation to mental defection. *Br Med J* 2:1215, 1958.

LANDAU WM, KLEFFNER FR: Syndrome of acquired aphasia with convulsive disorder in children. *Neurology* 7:523, 1957.

LENNEBERG EH: *Biological Foundations of Language.* New York, Wiley, 1967.

LOWREY GH: *Growth and Development of Children,* 7th ed. Chicago, Year Book, 1978.

MINIFIE FD, LLOYD LL: *Communicative and Cognitive Abilities—Early Behavioral Assessment.* Baltimore, University Park Press, 1978.

ORTON ST: *Reading, Writing and Speech Problems in Children.* New York, Norton, 1937.

PEIPER A: *Cerebral Function in Infancy and Childhood.* New York, Consultants Bureau, 1963.

PENROSE LS: *The Biology of Mental Defect.* London, Sidgwick & Jackson, 1954.

PIAGET J: *The Origins of Intelligence in Children.* New York, International Universities Press, 1952.

PRECHTL HFR: Prognostic value of neurological signs in the newborn. *Proc R Soc Med* 58:3, 1965.

————, BEINTEMA D: *Little Club Clinics in Developmental Medicine,* no 12: *The Neurological Examination of the Full Term Newborn Infant.* London, Heinemann, 1964.

————, STEMMER CJ: The choreiform syndrome in children. *Dev Med Child Neurol* 4:119, 1962.

PURPURA DP: Dendritic spine "dysgenesis" and mental retardation. *Science* 186:1126, 1974.

Raven's Colored Progressive Matrices. New York, Psychological Corporation, 1947–1963.

RENZI E, VIGNOLA LA: Token test: A sensitive test to detect receptive disturbances in aphasics. *Brain* 85:665, 1962.

RIESSMAN F: *The Culturally Deprived Child.* New York, Harper & Row, 1962.

RIMLAND B: *Infantile Autism.* New York, Appleton-Century-Crofts, 1964.

RUTTER M, MARTIN JAM (eds): *Clinics in Developmental Medicine,* no 43: *The Child with Delayed Speech.* London, Heinemann, 1972.

————, GRAHAM P, YULE W: *Clinics in Developmental Medicine,* nos 35, 36: *A Neuropsychiatric Study in Childhood.* London, Heinemann, 1970.

SCHAIN RJ: *Neurology of Childhood Learning Disorders,* 2d ed. Baltimore, Williams & Wilkins, 1977.

SPEARMAN C: *Psychology Down the Ages.* London, Macmillan, 1937.

STAPLES R: Responses of infants to color. *J Exp Psychol* 15:119, 1932.

TIZARD J, O'CONNOR N: The employability of high-grade mentally defectives. *Am J Ment Defic* 54:563, 1950.

WORSTER-DROUGHT C: Congenital suprabulbar paresis. *J Laryngol Otol* 70:453, 1956.

YAKOVLEV PI, LECOURS AR: The myelogenetic cycles of regional maturation of the brain, in Minkowski A (ed): *Regional Development of the Brain in Early Life.* Oxford, Blackwell, 1967, pp 3–70.

ZANGWILL OL: Psychopathology of dementia. *Proc R Soc Med* 57:914, 1964.

CHAPTER 28
THE NEUROLOGY OF AGING

As was remarked in the preceding chapter, standards of growth, development, and maturation are recognized as providing a frame of reference against which every pathologic process in early life must be viewed. However, it has been less appreciated that at the other end of the life cycle neurologic deficits must be judged in a similar way, against a background of normal aging changes. The earliest of these changes begins long before the acknowledged period of senescence and continues throughout the remainder of life. For some reason, perhaps because of man's irrepressible egotism or wish for immortality, there has been an unwillingness to accept aging and involution as normal and inevitable phases of life. Not a few medical scientists and physicians believe that all changes in senescence are but the cumulative effect of injury and disease.

As a first generalization, it may be said that the length of life itself, the span of the natural life cycle, is one of the organism's most integral characteristics, genetically programmed in some mysterious way by some kind of biological death clock. The rat survives for 2 years; the rhesus monkey, for 20 to 25 years; the African elephant, for 70 to 75 years; and the Galapagos tortoise, for 100 years. Many years ago the German physiologist Max Rubner pointed out that the total number of calories burned per gram of body weight and the total number of heartbeats in the lifetime of each of these mammals and of humans are about the same, despite the great differences in their size and life span. Further, the span of animal and human life correlates roughly with the size of the brain. These observations are intriguing, but their relevance to the aging process is not clear.

Despite all the publicity about medical science having lengthened life, this has been mainly a statistical feat, a reflection of the reduction of fatal infectious diseases and infant mortality; these accomplishments in medicine and public health have merely enabled more people to reach an apparently immutable upper age limit. In fact, since biblical times, when human beings were allotted three score years and ten, human life has not lengthened greatly. For most persons the clock inevitably runs down by the seventy-fifth year, and it seems to make little difference whether one inhabits a luxurious urban apartment or a primitive hut. Only a relatively small proportion of individuals survives much beyond this. There is little firm evidence to support the popular belief that tucked away in the remote mountain regions of the Caucasus, Peru, or Kashmir are small groups of people who live active lives for as long as 120 years or more.

This issue of life expectancy is obscured by the fact that with advancing age there is a steady, inexorable susceptibility to fatal disease. The probability of death doubles about every 8 years, as we grow older. It has been estimated that if the major causes of death in late adult life and the senium—cancer, coronary occlusion, stroke—were eliminated, life expectancy would be extended by about 20 years. Interestingly, delay in growth by undernutrition in early life has been shown to delay aging in animals, and also the vulnerability to disease in their senescence. Whether overnutrition has the opposite effect is not known. It has also been observed that whole-body irradiation hastens aging and increases susceptibility to disease and death.

For a long time the general process of aging has been measured by calculation of the mortality rate, which correlates more or less with age. This fact, derived by the English actuary Gompertz in 1825 from crude biologic data, states that the probability of death increases in logarithmic ratio to age, a formulation which is found to apply to many species. Expressed graphically, the correlation of mortality rate and age assumes the configuration shown in Fig. 28-1.

To the biologist and physician, death is not the main consideration. What is more meaningful are indexes of vitality, of resistance to disease, and of organ efficiency. In fact, *senescence* is defined in just such terms, i.e., the progressive lowering of biologic efficiency and capacity of the organism to maintain itself as an efficient machine. A semantic distinction is drawn between the process of aging, or senescence, and the state of being aged, or *senility*. The process of decline or decay that occurs in all organ systems of the body after middle life is called *involution;* unexpected, premature decay of any given tissue or cell population has been termed *abiotrophy.*

The composite of bodily changes due to senescence, such as the cessation of bodily growth, wrinkling of the skin, graying of hair, loss of teeth, atrophy of gonads, blunting of sensory acuity, stooped posture, loss of muscular strength and endurance, rigidity of mind, and forgetfulness are known to every observant person. Biologists have measured many of these changes. Estimates of structural and functional decline that accompany aging, from 30 to 75 years, are given in Table 28-1. It appears that all structures and functions share in the aging process. It is equally evident, however, that senescence and waning vitality have different times of manifestation and rates of progress in different organs, and that there are wide individual variations as well.

AGING IN THE NERVOUS SYSTEM

Of all the age-related changes, those in the nervous system are of paramount importance. Actors portray old people as feeble, idle, obstinate, given to reminiscing,

and walking slowly with a stoop and shuffling steps, with the hands tremulous and the voice soft and quavering. In doing so they have selected some of the principal effects of age on the nervous system. The lay as well as the medical observer is inclined to interpret the changes of advanced age as a kind of second childhood. "Old men are boys again," said Aristophanes. While roughly correct, this view of old age comes largely from certain resemblances, superficial at best, of the senile dement and the helpless young child.

The most consistent neurologic changes in octogenarians, according to Critchley and others, are presbyopia, presbycusis (especially for high tones), diminution in the sense of smell, reduced rate and amount of motor activity, slowed reaction time, slowness and narrowed compass of perception (inapperception of the aged), small pupils with restricted pupillary reflexes, limited range of upward gaze, tendency to flexed posture of trunk and limbs, diminution of vibratory sense in toes and feet, impairment of fine coordination and agility,

Figure 28-1
Correlation of mortality rate and age. (After Medawar.)

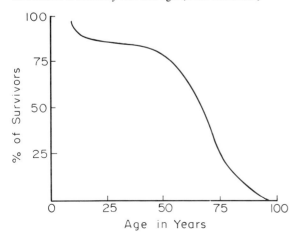

Table 28-1
Physiologic and anatomic deterioration with age

	Percent decrease
Brain weight	10
Blood flow to brain	20
Speed of return of blood acidity to equilibrium after exercise	83
Cardiac output at rest	30
Number of glomeruli in kidney	44
Glomerular filtration rate	31
Number of fibers in nerves	37
Nerve-conduction velocity	10
Number of taste buds	64
Maximum O_2 utilization wth exercise	60
Maximum ventilation volume	47
Vital capacity	44
Power of hand grip	45
Maximum work rate	30
Basal metabolic rate	16
Body water content	18
Body weight (males)	12

Source: Shock.

reduced muscular power, thinness of leg muscles, and reduced or absent Achilles reflexes.

Probably the most detailed information as to the effects of age on the nervous system comes from the measurement of cognitive functions. Perception, memory, and general intelligence all decline, starting from early adult life and progressing into the senium. On a large sample of the population, regression is linear, but the losses are not uniform and predictable. Performance on certain subtests of the Wechsler Adult Intelligence Scale—vocabulary, fund of information, comprehension, object assembly, and picture completion—holds up better than on digit symbol, block design, similarities, reversal of digits, picture arrangement, and arithmetic.

The effects of age on mental abilities are extremely variable. A few individuals may retain exceptional mental power and perform creative work until late life. Verdi, for example, composed *Otello* at the age of 73 years and *Falstaff* at 79. Humboldt wrote the five volumes of his *Kosmos* between the ages of 76 and 89 years; Goethe produced the second part of *Faust* when he was more than 70 years old; and Galileo and Laplace continued to make scientific contributions in their eighth decades. It must be pointed out, however, that most of these accomplishments were continuations of lines of endeavor that were begun in early adult life. Indeed, little that is new and original is started after the fortieth year. High intelligence, well-organized work habits, and sound judgment compensate for the progressive deficiencies of this period.

Personality Changes in the Aged   These are less easily measured, but nevertheless certain trends are observable and may seriously disturb the life of an aged person and those around him or her. Many old people become opinionated, self-centered, rigid, and conservative; the opposite qualities—undue pliancy, vacillation, and the uncritical acceptance of ideas—are observed in a few. Many elderly persons seem to lack self-confidence and require a strong probability of success before undertaking certain tasks. Whereas environment plays a part in molding these traits, Kallman's studies of senescent monozygotic twins suggest that genetic factors are more important. Aggressive individuals with much energy and a diversity of interests, leading to a wide range of social interactions, appear to resist better the ravages of age than those with the opposite tendencies. But this may be effect rather than cause. Those with depressive tendencies are more easily overwhelmed by the prospects of the

senium and adopt an attitude of hopelessness, fear, suspicion, and worry. This may explain the threefold increase in suicides in late middle life and old age. Certainly the agitated depression is the most frequent psychiatric disease of these periods of life.

One of the weaknesses of all studies of the aged has been the bias of population selection. Many of the reported observations have been restricted to decrepit individuals in homes for the aged. Examination of functionally intact old people of comparable age, such as that of Kokmen and his colleagues, reveals fewer deficits, limited mainly to forgetfulness of names, diminished vibratory sense in the feet, diminished ankle jerks, and slight loss of agility.

Morphologic Basis of Involutional Changes in the Nervous System   This has never been fully established. From early adult life to the senium, the weight of the average male brain declines from 1375 to 1232 g, a loss of nearly 150 g. This is based presumably on a degeneration of neurons and replacement gliosis. The loss amounts to 30 to 35 percent for lumbosacral anterior horn cells, sensory ganglion cells, and Purkinje cells. Not all neuronal groups behave equally in this regard. The locus ceruleus loses about 35 percent of its neurons between youth and old age, whereas the vestibular nuclei and inferior olives maintain a constant number of cells throughout life. A progressive loss, decade by decade, of the cells and myelinated fibers of the spinal cord has been convincingly demonstrated by Morrison.

The neuronal population in the neocortex is progressively depleted in the seventh, eighth, and ninth decades. The greatest loss appears to be among the small neurons of the second and fourth layers (external and internal granular laminae) in the frontal and superior temporal regions. Concomitantly, as Scheibel et al. have shown, there occurs a progressive loss of neuronal dendrites as well as a decline in the number of spines on the dendrites that remain. Particularly affected in this way are the horizontal dendrites of the third and fifth layers.

With advancing age, there is an increasing tendency for "senile plaques" to appear in the cerebral cortex and basal ganglia. These are loose aggregates of amorphous argentophilic material containing amyloid. They occur in increasing numbers in the senile, and by the ninth decade of life few cerebra are without them. However, as shown by Tomlinson and his colleagues, relatively few plaques are present in the cerebra of mentally intact old people, in contrast to the large numbers in the Alzheimer disease-senile dementia group. Similarly, neurons showing Alzheimer's neurofibrillary change are rare in the neocortex of the mentally sound individuals.

Several investigators cite the Alzheimer type of fibrillary change, senile plaques, and amyloid deposits as the principal alterations of the aging process in the human nervous system. Roth et al. determined a correlation of 0.8 between the incidence of these changes and the degree of dementia. These authors and others have used this finding to support the argument that the Alzheimer disease-senile dementia complex simply represents an acceleration of the natural aging process in the brain. We take an opposite position—that these changes represent an *acquired age-linked disease,* analogous to certain cerebrovascular diseases. In support of this latter view are the observations that (1) *Homo sapiens* is the only animal species in which Alzheimer fibrillary changes and senile plaques are found in the aging brain (a few plaquelike structures, but no neurofibrillary changes, have been seen in an old dog or monkey); it seems to us unbiologic that human aging should differ from that of all other animal species. (2) Some of the most severe forms of Alzheimer's disease occur in middle adult life, long before the senium. (3) These histopathologic changes in variable form occur in a number of human diseases (dementia pugilistica or the punch-drunk state, Down's syndrome, postencephalitic Parkinson's disease, progressive supranuclear palsy) and can be reproduced in the experimental animal by such toxins as aluminum, vincristine, vinblastine, and colchicine. We decided, therefore, to present Alzheimer disease under degenerative diseases (see Chap. 42), where the entire subject will be discussed further.

Increasing accumulation of lipofuscin granules (see below) sometimes extreme in degree, accompanies advancing age, being especially prominent in thalamic and certain other neurons. Amyloid bodies, formed by astrocytes, increase in number. Granulovacuolar changes are a regular finding in the aging hippocampi regardless of the mental state of the individual. Clearly these are aging effects. In addition, slight thickening and hyalinization of the walls of small blood vessels and pericapillary fibrosis also become more evident in the aging brain, and there is a natural inclination to assume this to be the basis of the reduced blood flow that several workers have reported. Such changes are probably not primary but secondary to reduced circulatory need (the so-called vascular atrophy of involuting organs). There is no evidence that the aforementioned aging changes, which are often referred to as arteriosclerotic, depend on any recognized form of vascular disease.

Many biochemical studies have been made of the effects of aging on cerebral tissues. As would be expected, the substances found in neurons and their med-

ullated fibers diminish in proportion to the loss of these cellular components. DNA, RNA, cerebrosides, and other components of myelin diminish in the brains of aged, mentally intact humans and old animals; intracellular enzymes also diminish. In the intact organism the cerebral uptake of oxygen and glucose are reduced in advanced age. The problems raised by all these studies is whether the changes reflect a primary effect of aging or merely the loss of neurons and gliosis. (See Samorajski and Ordy for critical review of the biochemistry of aging.) More recently, Bowen and his colleagues assayed choline acetyltransferase in the temporal lobes of the brains of patients with Alzheimer's disease, vascular disease, and normal controls of the same age. They found a significant reduction in all except the control patients, but it corresponded more or less to neuronal loss. It was not decided whether the enzyme changes were merely a reflection of cell depletion or represented a change of significance.

AGING CHANGES IN THE MUSCULATURE

With advancing age, skeletal muscles lose cells (fibers), and a gradual reduction in their weight more or less parallels that of the brain. Atrophy of muscle and diminution in peak power and endurance are the clinical expressions of these changes. Our own studies indicate that the wasting involves several processes, some principally myopathic, others denervative from loss of motor neurons. The muscle fibers that are lost are gradually replaced by endomysial connective tissue and fat cells. The surviving fibers are generally thinner than normal (disuse atrophy?), but groups of fibers all at the same stage of atrophy undoubtedly relate to loss of motor innervation. Reduced conduction velocities of nerves may be taken as another index of loss of motor and sensory axons. All these changes are more marked in the legs than elsewhere.

CHANGES IN LUNGS, HEART, KIDNEYS, SKIN AND SUPPORTING TISSUES, AND ENDOCRINE GLANDS

A textbook of neurology is not the place to itemize these age-linked alterations. It need only be pointed out that each system undergoes a significant regression that seems to be due to age alone and not to any known disease. In many instances the effects of aging in these organs have not been as well studied as those in the nervous system; apparently the diseases in these other organs are so much more dramatic and interesting than the biologic changes due to aging that the latter have been ignored to a large extent. Moreover, little is known of the extent to which these extracerebral changes are determinative of those in the nervous system, either the neuronal aging or the age-linked degenerative diseases.

THE CELLULAR BASIS OF AGING

Many mechanisms are presumed to be involved in the aging process of the cellular constituents of the various bodily organs. Recent investigative efforts have been directed along these lines: (1) the decline in functional efficiency and finally the deterioration and death of highly specialized nondividing cells such as the neuron and to some extent the muscle fiber; (2) the failure of cell multiplication and of mitosis in tissues composed of dividing cells; and (3) the progressive alteration of the structural protein collagen which constitutes about 40 percent of the body protein and serves as the binding substance of the skin, muscle, bones, and blood vessels.

LIFE SPAN AND AGING OF SPECIALIZED CELLS

As was said, nerve and muscle cells, which cease early to divide and are in near-maximum number at birth, must last the lifetime of the individual. Once destroyed, whether by aging or disease, they are never replaced. Obviously the life span is not the same for every cell; some survive longer than others. If a significant number die early, functional deficits result. It seems that the outfall of neurons begins at the end of the period of growth and maturation, and it accelerates in the last decades of life. The point at which functional deficits appear varies for each system, depending upon its "safety factor," i.e., a protective excess of cells that must be lost before symptoms appear. Whether cells falter functionally before their final disintegration is unknown. It seems likely that they do.

The cytologic events that lead to the death of nondividing cells are little understood. In humans as well as in animals, accumulation of lipofuscin in the cytoplasm is a phenomenon of such constancy that it can be used as a reliable cytologic index of age. Called "wear and tear" or "age" pigment, these yellow granules of lipochrome, or lipofuscin, form in the cytoplasm of both nerve and muscle cells, in close relation to lysosomes. Simultaneously with their formation the cell diminishes in volume, due presumably to the loss of other cytoplasmic components such as Nissl bodies (the main cytoplasm RNA of neurons) and mitochondria. The nucleus becomes smaller with infolding of the nuclear membrane and alteration of the nucleolus. Histochemical stains reveal a depletion of oxidative as well as phosphorylative and presumably other enzymes. Neurons lose dendrites and thereby reduce their synaptic surface (Scheibel et al.). All these changes have been observed in cultured cells.

Considering the ubiquitous nature of these morphologic changes, it is remarkable that we know so little of their pathogenesis. They have been attributed to progressive exhaustion of cell catalysts (enzymes and coenzymes), but this explanation only restates the problem in rather speculative biochemical terms. It is generally believed that the accumulation of lipofuscin is the result of oxidation of lipids, polymerized with protein and unsaturated peptides, which are released when a cell ages or undergoes necrosis for any reason. According to this view, any factor (e.g., hemorrhage into fatty tissue) which increases the ratio of tissue oxidant to antioxidant favors the accumulation of lipofuscin. Biologic antioxidants such as vitamins C and E, glutathione, cysteine, and sulfhydryl proteins are said to counteract the process.

The concept of lipoidal degeneration of neurons, long a favorite topic of neuropathologists, has its advocates and opponents. The older idea was that the accumulation of lipofuscin was a stage in a degenerative process. An equally tenable view, now more favored, is that the sequestration of lysosomes and lipofuscin is a protective mechanism against neuronal degeneration.

LOSS OF CAPACITY FOR CELL GROWTH AND MULTIPLICATION

The studies of Hayflick and his colleagues on the innate capacity of cells to divide in tissue culture may shed light on this problem. They found that fibroblasts can divide only a finite number of times (contrary to Alexis Carrel's original claim that chicken heart cells, nourished in tissue culture, could continue to live and divide forever). Fibroblasts of a human infant divide about 50 times, those of a 20-year-old about 30 times, and those of an 80-year-old about 20 times. Probably glial cells, leukocytes, and liver cells also possess a limited, genetically determined capacity for mitosis. Toward the end of the life cycle of cultured cells, chromosomal aberrations and peculiarities of cell division appear in some cells. Whether or not these types of cell abnormalities are a characteristic feature of human aging has not been settled. Only if neoplastic transformation takes place (the normal 46-chromosome diploid cell becomes "mixoploid," with 50 to 350 abnormal chromosomes) do cells attain the immortality postulated by Carrel.

Hayflick sees in this aging process and finite lifetime of normal cells a deterioration of the genetic program that "orchestrates" the development of cells. He has postulated that with age the DNA protein-synthesizing apparatus of the dividing cells fall prey to an ever-increasing number of copying errors (as might occur with radiation). The faulty templates serve as faulty models for the production of more faulty enzymes, leading eventually to death of the cell.

AGING OF COLLAGEN

Only brief reference need be made to the lack of turnover of deposited collagen and to the stiffening of collagen with age. By simple mechanical and chemical tests Verzar has shown that aging collagen contracts more slowly when heated and shows a decrease in solubility of amino acids and extractable elastins, an increase in content of aspartic and glutamic acid and amide nitrogen, and a decrease in glycine, proline, and valine. Thus collagen, like nondividing cells, undergoes aging changes in its molecular structure that progressively diminish its integrity and function.

AGE-RELATED DISEASES

The fundamental processes of aging, outlined above, operate during all of adult life, and if the person survives long enough, he or she will succumb to the ultimate failure of normal cells to divide or function. However, few people die of old age alone. Most of them die of diseases, to which they are rendered increasingly susceptible by the aging processes. The most common of these are tumor, vascular diseases of the heart and brain, fractures of the hip, infections (chiefly pulmonary), and in our opinion, Alzheimer's disease. While these diseases increase in frequency with advancing age, the relationship is anything but specific.

Cerebral atherosclerosis is, of course, a frequent finding in the elderly. It does not parallel age with any degree of precision, being severe in some 30- to 40-year-old individuals and absent altogether in some octogenarians. In the normotensive it tends to occur in scattered, discrete plaques mostly in the cervical arteries and basal parts of the cerebral arterial system. In the hypertensive it is more diffuse and extends into finer branches of the cerebral and cerebellar arteries. Superficial cerebral softenings (thrombotic and embolic, old and recent) have been found in about half of all individuals over 70 years

who have been examined postmortem. Even without atherosclerosis, which is obviously a disease, the basal arteries undergo other changes in the aged, being rather large and tortuous and much more opaque than the arteries of a younger person.

While the skull thickens with age, the condition known as hyperostosis frontalis interna (Stewart-Morel Morgagni syndrome) is exclusively a disease of older women. It is said to be joined frequently with obesity and hirsutism. Its neurologic implications are vague, and there has always been a temptation to ascribe more to it than it deserved. At autopsy, aside from close attachment of the dura and opacity of the underlying pia-arachnoid (milk spots), we have observed no consistent neuropathologic lesion.

Likewise, most tumors occur with increasing frequency in early and middle adult life. Only in the most advanced age period does the incidence tend to fall. The cytoplasmic events leading to neoplasia must relate to the process of cell division. Postmitotic cells rarely give rise to tumors. One evidence of this neoplastic tendency is that in experimental animals exposed to gamma radiation increasing numbers of tumors develop in many organs, and there is a linear relation between intensity of exposure and frequency of tumor. One class of endocrine tumors appears to form during periods of intensified functional demands, e.g., hypophyseal adenomas with atrophy of gonads and adrenals during late adult life. Reference has already been made to the chromosomal aberrations that appear in older dividing cells. An example is the trisomy of Down's syndrome, which occurs with increasing frequency from the gametes of the aging mother.

As to the older person's intolerance of infection, it may well relate to the failure of the aging organism to adapt to change, rather than to any failure of the inflammatory process. Older people are slower in adjusting to high and low atmospheric temperatures, but their levels of antibodies, production of leukocytes, and vigor of cellular immune response are all suprisingly well maintained.

In every major illness in the elderly, the exigencies of disease cannot be met efficiently because of a combination of organ inadequacies, no single one of which is of sufficient severity to be manifest clinically. The sum total of these organ deficits constitutes a kind of Gestalt of senility. The long list of diseases found in the elderly at autopsy reflects the increasing susceptibility to disease with age. However, the contributing effects of the aging processes are relatively inapparent, which is the reason the student so often asks, during the autopsy of the elderly person, "But what was the cause of death?"

DEGENERATIVE DISEASES OF THE NERVOUS SYSTEM IN THE AGED

GENERALIZED DEGENERATIVE DISEASE— ALZHEIMER-SENILE DEMENTIA COMPLEX (ASDC)

To be distinguished from the slight shrinkage and loss of weight of the brain that occurs in the majority of older people are the severe degrees of diffuse cerebral atrophy that evolve relatively rapidly in the senile or presenile periods. The latter states are invariably associated with dementia and the underlying pathologic changes prove most frequently to be *Alzheimer's disease.* For reasons that have been given (see above, under "Aging in the Nervous System"), this disease and other age-linked degenerative diseases will be described in Chap. 42.

RESTRICTED DEGENERATIVE DISORDERS

Abnormalities of Gait Human motor agility actually begins to fail in early adult life, even by the thirtieth year, and it seems to be related to a gradual failure of neuromuscular control as well as to changes in joints and other structures. The reality of this motor decrement is best appreciated by professional baseball or tennis players who retire at 35 or soon thereafter because their legs give out and cannot be kept in condition by training. They cannot run as well as younger colleagues even though the coordination of their arms in hitting a ball may still be preserved. The older person becomes less confident in walking; touching the handrail in descending stairs is now needed to prevent a misstep. Standing on one leg while putting on pants becomes difficult. Handwriting tends to worsen, and choking on food is more frequent. Doubtless this complex of motor failures is based on the aforementioned neuronal losses in the spinal cord, cerebellum, and cerebrum.

A small proportion of the aging population suffers an inordinate deterioration of gait while remaining relatively competent in other ways. In all likelihood, this is an age-linked degenerative disorder of the brain, since most instances of it are sooner or later accompanied by mental changes. As indicated in Chap. 6, the gait in the older person is shorter of step, slower, and more

guarded. All the movements are less graceful, more inelastic. The patient looks to the ground and finds it difficult to walk and converse at the same time. The posture of the body is more flexed. The old soldier must now remind himself repeatedly to maintain his bearing. Gradually as the steps shorten, the feet barely clear the ground and finally are merely shuffled forward, a state referred to as *marche à petit pas* (the short-stepped gait). In some instances the patient upon arising from a chair finds it difficult to initiate the first step even though while lying in bed there is no difficulty in moving the legs. After a tremulous pause the first step is finally taken, and the next ones proceed in the customary shuffle. Taking a patient's arm and walking alongside with reminders to keep step with a military cadence may improve the gait disorder at this stage. Other patients may ascribe the trouble to a loss of confidence or a fright from a bad fall and may ask for gait training, which will not help them, and the inexperienced physician may suspect a functional disorder.

In the clinical analysis of such patients one should search for evidence of posterior column or cerebellar ataxia and the spastic ataxia of cervical spondylosis, all of which may unbalance the patient. One recognizes, in several features of the gait disorder, elements of Parkinson's syndrome. Obesity and hypertrophic arthritis of hips and knees or an old hip fracture add to any gait difficulty. In its most advanced form the capacity for upright stance and walking is completely lost, and the patient eventually lies curled up in bed in a state of *cerebral paraplegia in flexion* (Fig. 6-1).

The basis of this peculiar gait is probably a combined frontal lobe–basal ganglionic degeneration, the anatomy of which has never been fully clarified. No treatment or physiotherapeutic measures have proved effective in our hands. L-Dopa has been useful only in Parkinson's syndrome.

Other Restricted Motor Abnormalities in the Aged These are too numerous to be more than cataloged. They inform us of the many ways in which the motor system can deteriorate. Compulsive, repetitive movements are the most frequent: mouthing movements, stereotyped grimacing, protrusion of the tongue, side-to-side or to-and-fro tremor of the head, odd vocalizations such as sniffing, snorting, and bleating. In some respects these disorders resemble tics (voluntary movements to relieve tension), but careful observation shows that they are not really voluntary. Haloperidol and other drugs of this class have an unpredictable therapeutic effect, seeming at times to benefit the patient only by the superimposition of a drug-induced rigidity. The differential diagnosis must raise for consideration one of the phenothiazine faciocervical dyskinesias.

Old age is thought always to carry a liability to tremulousness, and, indeed, one sees such patients from time to time in the clinic. The head, the chin, or the hands tremble and the voice quavers, yet there is not the usual slowness of movement, immobility, facial impassivity, or flexed posture which would give the condition a parkinsonian stamp. Some instances are clearly familial, having appeared or worsened only late in life. Cessation of fast-frequency action tremors in response to alcohol and beta-adrenergic blocking agents also support the idea that certain cases are familial in nature (see page 71). The relation to senility is always open to doubt. Charcot, in a review of over 2000 elderly inhabitants at the Salpetrière, could find only about 30 with tremor.

Spastic dysphonia, a disorder of middle and late life characterized by a spasm of all throat muscles on attempted speech, has been discussed on page 336. *Blepharoclonus* or *blepharospasm,* a somewhat similar involuntary movement of the eyelids, is described on page 76.

GERONTOLOGIC NEUROLOGY

This special branch of medicine embraces the scientific study of all the changes in the nervous system that are attributable to the aging process and all the neurologic diseases in the aging organism. Unlike pediatric neurology, these disciplines have not aroused much interest. The young physician is more excited by disease than by the seemingly immutable changes due to aging and questions whether medicine has a significant role to play in the care of the neurologic disorders of the elderly.

The authors would answer this question affirmatively and would point out that the majority of all neurologic patients seen in practice are elderly, especially if one includes vascular diseases of the brain. Furthermore many of their diseases are preventable or therapeutically controllable. Since aging does not occur simultaneously in all organs and tissues, patients need help and advice about certain of these effects at a time when most of their organs are functionally intact. Some of the chemical involutions (vitamin B_{12} deficiency; diabetes mellitus) and many of the common restricted involutional changes (presbyopia, etc.) may be corrected—and others can be turned to assets. The forgetfulness of the aged and their deafness serve to excuse many of their shortcomings and to spare them effort and annoyance.

Some physicians hesitate to interpret any change as due to involution until the patient is past the biblical three score years and ten or may avoid the diagnosis altogether because it implies an incurable condition. Their reasoning is faulty in both instances. Many involutions like presbyopia can be demonstrated in their larval stages in the twenties, and by the mid-forties failing visual accommodation is almost universal. The disorder of uric acid metabolism causing gout is manifested before the age of 40 years in an appreciable percentage of all those afflicted. Many restricted involutions or abiotrophies, after rapid progress for a few years, become arrested and compensated for in many ways.

In a more general way gerontology should present the medical view of what is needed for ideal care of the elderly. There has been too little planning for them. One of the tragedies of urban civilization is the insufficiency of suitable homes and medical institutions. Many old people, as they become decrepit, are treated as though insane and incarcerated in ways not conducive to happiness or long survival. In rural and primitive cultures such individuals were cared for by their relatives in their own homes, but this has become impossible in small city apartments. Conventional psychotherapy helps little, and moving them into a strange environment and giving sedative medication only increases their confusion.

The high incidence of arterial disease, neoplasia, and infectious diseases in the elderly have traditionally spared the younger generation the responsibility for the care of their parents. In the nineteenth century, when pneumonia was more frequently lethal than now, Osler referred to it as the "old man's friend," for, as in Ecclesiastes, he considered death as a kindness to the old and feeble. As medical science brings these and other diseases under control, more and more elderly persons will burden our society and the need for their care will increase.

REFERENCES

BEHNKE JA, FINCH CE, MOMENT BG (eds): *The Biology of Aging.* New York, Plenum, 1978.
BLESSED G, TOMLINSON BE, ROTH M: The association between quantitative measures of dementia and of senile change in the cerebral grey matter of elderly subjects. *Br J Psychiatry* 114:797, 1968.
BOWEN DM et al: Accelerated aging or selective neuronal loss as an important cause of dementia. *Lancet* 1:11, 1979.
CARREL A: On the permanent life of tissues outside of the organism. *J Exp Med* 15:516, 1912.
CORSELLIS JAN: Aging and the dementias, in Blackwood W, Corsellis JAN (eds): *Greenfield's Neuropathology,* 3d ed. London, Arnold, 1976, chap 18, pp 796-848.

CRITCHLEY M: Neurologic changes in the aged. *J Chron Dis* 3:459, 1956.

HARTROFT WS, PORTA EA: Ceroid. *Am J Med Sci* 250:324, 1965.

HAYFLICK L: The cell biology of human aging. *N Engl J Med* 295:1302, 1976.

KALLMANN FJ: Genetic factors in aging: Comparative and longitudinal observations on a senescent twin population, in Hoch PH, Zubin J (eds): *Psychopathology of Aging.* New York, Grune & Stratton, 1961.

KAY DWK, BEAMISH P, ROTH M: Old age mental disorder in Newcastle-upon-Tyne: I. A study of prevalence. *Br J Psychiatry* 110:146, 1964.

KOKMEN E et al: Neurologic manifestations of aging. *J Geront* 32:411, 1977.

MEDAWAR PB: The definition and measurement of senescence, in Wolstenholme GEW, Cameron MP (eds): *Ciba Foundation Colloquia on Aging,* vol 1. Boston, Little, Brown, 1955, pp 4–15.

MORRISON LR: *The Effect of Advancing Age upon the Human Spinal Cord.* Cambridge, Mass, Harvard, 1959.

OBRIST WD: The EEG of normal aged adults. *Electroenceph Clin Neurophysiol* 6:235, 1954.

ROTH M, TOMLINSON BE, BLESSED G: Correlation between scores for dementia and counts of senile plaques in cerebral grey matter of elderly subjects. *Nature* 209:109, 1966.

SAMORAJSKI T, ORDY JM: The neurochemistry of aging, in Gaitz CM (ed): *Aging and the Brain.* New York, Plenum, 1976, pp 41–63.

SCHEIBEL M, LINDSAY RD, TOMIYASU U, SCHEIBEL AB: Progressive dendritic changes in aging human cortex. *Exp Neurol* 47:392, 1975.

SHOCK NW: The physiology of aging. *Sci Am* 206:100, 1962.

TOMLINSON BE, BLESSED G, ROTH M: Observations on the brains of nondemented old people. *J Neurol Sci* 7:331, 1968.

VERZAR F: The aging of collagen. *Sci Am* 208:104, 1963.

WELLS CE: *Dementia,* 2d ed, *Contemporary Neurology Series.* Philadelphia, Davis, 1977.

PART

IV

THE MAJOR CATEGORIES OF NEUROLOGIC DISEASE

CHAPTER 29

DISEASES OF THE MENINGES AND DISTURBANCES OF CEREBROSPINAL FLUID CIRCULATION, INCLUDING HYDROCEPHALUS

Lumbar puncture and examination of the cerebrospinal fluid (CSF) as a diagnostic aid in neurology was discussed in Chap. 2, and the primary inflammatory diseases of the pia-arachnoid (leptomeninges) and ependyma of the ventricles will be considered in Chap. 31. Further, in many chapters to follow, the ways in which the CSF reflects the basic pathologic processes in a wide variety of metabolic and degenerative diseases will be remarked upon. The latter raise so many interesting and important problems that we considered it advantageous to discuss in one place the mechanisms involved in the chemical and cytological changes that occur in the CSF as a result of disease. Also, it is appropriate to discuss in this chapter some of the basic facts about the formation, circulation and absorption of the CSF, as well as the disturbances of CSF circulation, particularly hydrocephalus and meningeal hydrops.

A few historical points will call to mind how recent is our knowledge of the physiology, chemistry, and cytology of the CSF. Although the lumbar puncture was introduced by Quincke in 1891, it was not until 1912 that Mestrazat made the first correlations between various diseases and the cellular and chemical changes in the CSF, and only in 1937 did Merritt and Fremont-Smith publish their classic monograph on the CSF changes in all types of disease. Most of our detailed knowledge of CSF cytology has accumulated in the last 15 years, since the introduction of the millipore filter. The studies of Dandy in 1919 and of Weed in 1935 provide the basis of our knowledge of CSF formation, circulation, and absorption; and the studies of Pappenheimer and of Ames and their colleagues and the monographs of Davson and of Fishman are the outstanding recent contributions.

PHYSIOLOGY OF THE CSF

FORMATION

The introduction of the ventriculocisternal perfusion technique by Pappenheimer and his colleagues made possible the accurate measurement of the rate of formation and absorption of the CSF. It is now well established that the mean rate of CSF formation is 0.35 ml/min, or 500 ml/day. Since the total volume of CSF ranges from 90 to 150 ml, the CSF as a whole is renewed four or five times daily.

The choroid plexuses are the source of most of the CSF. The thin-walled vessels of the plexuses allow passive diffusion of substances from the blood plasma; in addition, the choroidal epithelial cells contain organelles, indicating their capacity for secretory function, i.e., "active transport." The blood vessels in the subependymal regions and the pia also contribute to the CSF, and some substances enter the CSF as readily from the meninges as from the choroid plexuses. Thus, electrolytes equilibrate with the CSF at all points in the ventricular and subarachnoid spaces, and the same is true of glucose. The transport of sodium, the main cation of the CSF, is under the influence of sodium-potassium-activated adenosine triphosphate and carbonic anhydrase. Electrolytes enter the ventricles more readily than the subarachnoid space (water does the opposite). The penetration of certain other drugs and metabolites is in direct relation to their lipid solubility. Ionized compounds, such as the amino acids, being relatively insoluble in lipids, enter the CSF slowly, unless facilitated by a membrane transport system. The latter is influenced by the small difference in pH between blood and CSF. Certain hydrophilic molecules, such as sugars, are able to enter the CSF and the intercellular fluid only if they have a molecular configuration that conforms to that of a stereospecific carrier transport system.

Diffusion gradients appear to determine the entry of serum proteins into the CSF and also the exchanges of CO_2. Water diffuses as readily from blood to CSF and the intercellular spaces as in the reverse direction. This explains the rapid effects of intravenously injected hypotonic and hypertonic fluids.

Studies using radioisotopic tracer techniques have shown that the various constituents of the CSF (see Table 2-1) are in dynamic equilibrium with the blood. Similarly, the CSF in the ventricles and subarachnoid spaces is in equilibrium with the intercellular fluid of the brain, spinal cord, and olfactory and optic nerves. The terms *blood-CSF barrier* and *blood-brain barrier* are used to indicate the relative or absolute exclusion of many substances in the blood from the CSF and from the intercellular fluid of the brain and spinal cord. The site of the barrier varies for the different plasma constituents. One is the endothelium of the choroidal and brain capillaries; another is the plasma membrane and the adventitia (Rouget cells) of the vessels; a third is pericapillary, the foot processes of astrocytes. Large molecules such as albumin (molecular weight of 69,000) are prevented from entry by the capillary endothelium, and this is the barrier also for such molecules as are bound to albumin, e.g., aniline dyes (trypan blue) and bilirubin. Thus it is that aniline dyes injected into the blood will not penetrate nervous tissues but will do so if injected into the subarachnoid space (the barriers are thus circumvented). Metallic ions attached to serum proteins tend to deposit on the plasma membrane and in the perithelium. The various substances formed in the nervous system during its metabolic activity diffuse rapidly into the CSF. Thus the CSF has a kind of "sink action," to use Davson's term, by which the products of brain metabolism are removed to the bloodstream as CSF is absorbed.

ABSORPTION

The absorption of CSF is through the arachnoid villi. These structures are most numerous over the superior surfaces of the cerebral hemispheres (the large ones in the adult are called Pacchionian granulations) but are also present at the base of the brain and around the spinal nerve roots. These arachnoid villi penetrate meningeal veins and dural sinus walls, and have been thought to act as functional valves which permit "bulk flow" of CSF into the vascular lumen unidirectionally. However, the most recent electron microscopic studies show the arachnoid villi to have a continuous membranous covering. The latter is extremely thin, and CSF flows through the villi at a linearly increasing rate with CSF pressures above 68 mmH₂O. Certain substances such as penicillin and organic acids and bases are also absorbed by the choroid plexus; the bidirectional action of these cells is rather like that of the tubule cells of the kidneys. Some substances have been shown in pathological specimens to pass between the ependymal cells of the ventricles and to enter subependymal capillaries and venules.

CIRCULATION

Harvey Cushing aptly termed the CSF the "third circulation," comparable to that of the blood and lymph. The pathways it traverses are well known. From the principal site of CSF formation in the ventricles it flows downward under a decreasing gradient of pressure, through the basal foramens of Magendie and Luschka, to the perimedullary and perispinal subarachnoid spaces, and thence up over the brainstem to the basal and ambiens cisterns, and finally to the superior and lateral surfaces of the cerebral hemispheres, where most of it is absorbed. The gradient of pressure is highest in the ventricles and diminishes successively along the subarachnoid pathways. Arterial pulsations of the choroid plexuses help drive the fluid from the ventricular system. Strain-gauge manometer recordings have shown the arterial pulse pressure to be 60 mmH₂O in the lateral ventricle, 50 mmH₂O in the cisterna magna, and 30 mmH₂O in the lumbar subarachnoid space.

VOLUME AND PRESSURE

Systemic circulatory factors maintain the volume and pressure of the CSF. When the heart stops, the CSF pressure falls to zero. Normally the CSF pressure is in equilibrium with the capillary pressure which is influenced only by circulatory changes that alter arteriolar tone. Rises in arterial pressure cause little or no increase of pressure at the capillary level and hence no increase in CSF pressure. The inhalation of CO_2, which decreases blood pH and arteriolar resistance, increases the CSF pressure by increasing cerebral blood flow and capillary pressure; and hyperventilation, which reduces P_{CO_2}, has the opposite effect of increasing the pH and vascular resistance, thereby decreasing CSF pressure. Here CSF pressures clearly relate to blood flow and blood volume.

In contrast to arterial blood pressure, venous pressure exerts an immediate effect on CSF pressure by increasing the volume of blood in the veins, venules, and dural sinuses. Jugular compression, as indicated in Chap. 2, causes an immediate rise of intracranial CSF pressure, and this is rapidly transmitted to the lumbar subarachnoid space (Queckenstedt test), unless there is a spinal subarachnoid block. The Valsalva maneuver, which partially blocks cerebral and spinal venous return, has the same effect as jugular compression. Abdominal compression distends the lower spinal veins and will increase the lumbar CSF pressure below the point of subarachnoid block. The intracranial pressure rises in heart failure, when venous pressure becomes elevated, and with obstructing mediastinal tumors. Removal of CSF causes a temporary lowering of intracranial pressure, and this may persist for days after a lumbar puncture that has resulted in a CSF leak.

FUNCTION

The primary function of the CSF appears to be a mechanical one; it serves as a kind of water jacket for the spinal cord and brain, protecting them from potentially injurious blows against the spinal column and skull. As pointed out by Fishman, the 1400-g brain only weighs 50 g when weighed in water, and so the brain virtually floats in its CSF jacket. It is to maintain the relatively constant volume-pressure relationships of the CSF that many of the physiologic and chemical mechanisms described above are committed. Since the brain and spinal cord have no lymphatic channels, the CSF through its "sink action" (see above) serves to remove the waste products of cerebral metabolism. The composition of the CSF is maintained within narrow limits, despite major alterations in the blood; thus the CSF, along with the intercellular fluid of the brain helps to maintain a stable chemical environment for neurons and their medullated fibers. There is no reason to believe that the CSF is actively involved in the metabolism of the cells of the brain and spinal cord.

PATHOLOGIC CHANGES IN CSF VOLUME, PRESSURE, AND CIRCULATION

The intact cranium and vertebral canal together with the relatively inelastic dura form a rigid container, and an increase in any of the intracranial contents, viz., brain, blood, or CSF, will elevate the intracranial pressure. Further, if one of these three elements increases in volume, it must be at the expense of the other two. This is known as the Monro-Kellie hypothesis (Fig. 29-1). Some increase in brain volume does not immediately raise the intracranial pressure because it can be accommodated for a time by diminution in the volume of intracranial blood (particularly that in veins and dural sinuses), reduction in the volume of CSF, stretching of the dura, and plasticity of the brain. Only when the capacity of these compensatory mechanisms is surpassed does the intracranial pressure rise.

Blockage of venous outflow, hydrocephalus, brain swelling, tumor masses, clots of blood, and increased volume of CSF are the recognized causes of elevated intracranial pressure. Each of these types of increased intracranial pressure has its special mechanisms and clinical and pathologic features.

TENSION HYDROCEPHALUS

Essentially this is a condition in which there is an obstruction to the flow of CSF at some point between its principal site of origin, in the lateral ventricles, and the cerebral subarachnoid space, where most of it is absorbed. Because of the obstruction, CSF accumulates within the ventricles under increasing pressure, enlarging the ventricles and expanding the hemispheres. In the infant the head increases in size because of separation of the sutures of the cranial bones. This is called *manifest* or *overt hydrocephalus.*

Unfortunately, the term hydrocephalus (literally, "water head") is frequently applied to the passive enlargement of the ventricles consequent to cerebral atrophy, i.e., *hydrocephalus ex vacuo*, and to the ventricular enlargement in undeveloped brains, a state known as *colpencephaly*. Reference to these conditions as hydrocephalic is such common practice that it is unlikely to change; hence the authors believe it preferable to use the term *tension hydrocephalus* for the obstructive types in which the CSF is or has been under increased pressure.

The site of the obstruction in tension hydrocephalus varies. One foramen of Monro may be blocked by a tumor with expansion of one lateral ventricle. If the obstruction is in the aqueduct of Sylvius, the third and both lateral ventricles dilate, and if it is in the fourth ventricle, the dilatation includes the aqueduct of Sylvius. Occlusion of the basal foramens of Magendie and Luschka or of the subarachnoid space around the medulla, pons, and midbrain results in enlargement of the entire ventricular system, including the fourth ventricle. However, if the obstruction is at the mesencephalic level, the accumulation of CSF around the brainstem may prevent the fourth ventricle from enlarging as much as the other ventricles.

Dandy introduced the unfortunate terminology of *communicating* and *noncommunicating* (*obstructive*) *hydrocephalus.* By communicating, he referred to the fact that a dye injected into the lateral ventricle would diffuse readily into the lumbar subarachnoid space and that air injected into the lumbar subarachnoid space would pass into the ventricular system; in other words, the ventricles are in communication with the spinal subarachnoid space. In obstructive hydrocephalus, it was

assumed, they are not. The distinction between these two types is not fundamental. All forms of tension hydrocephalus are obstructive, and the obstruction is never complete. Even with an intraventricular obstruction such as aqueductal stenosis, air and radionuclide injected into the lumbar subarachnoid state will reflux into the third and lateral ventricles. Complete aqueductal occlusion is incompatible with survival for more than 1 to 2 days. The authors suggest that a more appropriate terminology is one in which a prefix indicates the site of the presumed obstruction, i.e., *meningeal-obstructive, aqueductal-obstructive,* or *third ventricular-obstructive tension hydrocephalus.*

A matter of considerable practical as well as theoretical interest is whether a meningeal obstruction over the cerebral hemispheres, at the site of the arachnoidal villi, or a blockage of the dural sinuses into which the CSF is absorbed can result in tension hydrocephalus.

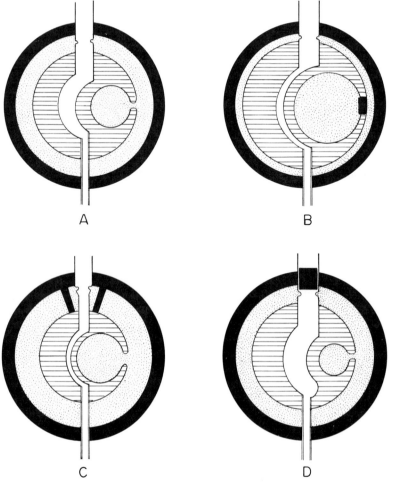

Figure 29-1
A. *Schematic representation of the three components of the intracranial contents: the incompressible brain tissue* (shaded); *the vascular system, open to the atmosphere; and the CSF* (dotted). B. *With ventricular obstruction.* C. *With obstruction at or near the points of outlet of the CSF.* D. *With obstruction of the venous outflow. (Redrawn from Foley.)*

Russell in her own large neuropathological material and in her review of the world's literature could not find a single well-documented example, and one of the authors (R.D.A.) has had a similar experience. Moreover, experiments in animals in which all draining veins had been occluded resulted in a tension hydrocephalus with enlarging lateral ventricles in only a few cases, and in these the investigator could not be sure that a basal meningeal obstruction or brain atrophy from ischemic necrosis had not been produced inadvertently. Yet Gilles and Davidson believe that tension hydrocephalus in children may be due to congenital absence or deficient number of arachnoidal villi, and Rosman and Shands have reported an instance which they attributed to increased intracranial venous pressure. Our hesitancy in accepting such examples stems from the difficulty that the pathologist has in judging the patency of the basal subarachnoid space. The latter is much more reliably visualized by radiologic than neuropathologic means. Theoretically, if the obstruction is high, near the superior sagittal sinus, the CSF should accumulate under pressure outside as well as inside the brain, and the ventricles should not enlarge at all or only very late. The authors remain skeptical of any exceptions to this concept. One could designate this type of increased intracranial pressure as an external hydrocephalus, but most of the reported cases that have been so designated have proved to be cases of subdural hygroma or abscess.

An increase in the rate of formation or decrease in the rate of absorption would be expected to cause an accumulation of CSF and increased intracranial pressure. An overproduction of CSF is the presumed cause of tension hydrocephalus in cases of papilloma of the choroid plexus, but usually with tumors of this type there is an associated ventricular obstruction, either of the third or fourth ventricle or of one lateral ventricle. Air studies in the latter cases have been characteristic, showing both a generalized dilatation of the ventricular system and basal cisterns (due to increased CSF volume?) and an asymmetrical enlargement of the lateral ventricles, due to obstruction of one foramen of Monro.

An increased resistance to CSF outflow has been demonstrated by infusion manometrics in patients with pseudotumor cerebri (Mann et al.). Reabsorption of CSF is also decreased in the Landry-Guillain-Barré syndrome (with CSF protein levels in the range of 750 to 1500 mg per 100 ml) and in patients with thrombosis of dural sinuses (one form of which was inappropriately called "otitic hydrocephalus" by Symonds).

As indicated above, venous congestion that complicates heart failure and superior mediastinal obstruction also raises the CSF pressure, again without enlargement of the ventricles. Spinal cord tumors are occasionally accompanied by increased intracranial pressure, probably because of high CSF protein levels which by colloid-osmotic pressure increase the volume of CSF. Also, certain hormones and drugs may result in intracranial hypertension; these include estrogens, adrenocortical steroids, parathormone, vitamin A, tetracycline, and, rarely, phenothiazines. The mechanisms by which these latter substances increase CSF pressure are poorly understood. In most of the benign forms of intracranial hypertension the ventricles remain normal in size or are small.

Clinical Picture of Hydrocephalus This varies with the age of onset. As remarked above, two major syndromes are recognized, one in which the head enlarges (*overt* hydrocephalus), the other in which the head remains of normal size (*occult* hydrocephalus).

The cranial bones fuse by the end of the second year, and for the head to enlarge, the tension hydrocephalus must develop before this time, usually in the first few months of life. Up to 5 years of age (and very rarely beyond this time) increased intracranial pressure will separate the sutures (diastasis) without significant macrocephaly. Tension hydrocephalus of mild degree also molds the shape of the skull in early life, and in radiographs the inner table is unevenly thinned, an appearance referred to as "beaten silver" or as convolutional or digital markings. The frontal regions are unusually prominent (bossed) and the skull tends to be brachicephalic, except in the Dandy-Walker syndrome, where, because of bossing of the occiput from enlargement of the posterior fossa, the head is dolichocephalic. With marked enlargement of the skull the face looks relatively small and pinched and the skin over the cranial bones is tight and thin, revealing prominent distended veins.

Congenital, or Infantile, Hydrocephalus of Overt Type The usual causes of this disorder are (1) matrix hemorrhages in premature infants, (2) fetal and neonatal infections, (3) Arnold-Chiari malformation, (4) aqueductal stenosis and atresia, and (5) the Dandy-Walker syndrome.

Usually, in this type of hydrocephalus, the head enlarges rapidly and soon surpasses the 97th percentile. The anterior and posterior fontanels are tense when the patient is in the upright position. The infant is fretful, feeds poorly, and may vomit. With continued enlargement of the brain, a torpor sets in and the infant appears languid, uninterested in the immediate surroundings, and unable to sustain activity. Later it is noticed that the upper lids are retracted and the eyes tend to turn down; upward gaze is paralyzed and the scleras above the irises are visible. This is the so-called setting-sun sign and has been incorrectly attributed to downward pressure of the frontal lobes on the roofs of the orbits. The fact that it disappears on shunting the lateral and third ventricles indicates that it is due to hydrocephalic pressure on the mesencephalic tegmentum. Gradually the infant adopts a posture of flexed arms and flexed or extended legs. Signs of corticospinal tract affection are usually elicitable. Movements are feeble and sometimes the arms are tremulous. There is no papilledema, but later the optic disks become pale and vision is reduced. If the hydrocephalus becomes arrested, the infant or child is retarded but often surprisingly verbal. Because the head is so large, the child cannot hold it up and must remain in bed. If the head is only moderately enlarged, the child may be able to sit but not stand, or can stand but not walk. If ambulatory, the child is clumsy. Acute exacerbations of hydrocephalus, or an intercurrent febrile illness, may cause stupor or coma.

The special features of congenital hydrocephalus with Arnold-Chiari malformation, aqueductal stenosis and atresia, and the Dandy-Walker syndrome will be discussed in Chap. 43.

Occult Tension Hydrocephalus In this form of hydrocephalus the increased intracranial pressure is evenly transmitted throughout the subarachnoid spaces and causes papilledema. Bifrontal and biooccipital headaches are prominent, but not invariable. Mental and physical activity are gradually reduced. The clinical picture is predominantly one of bilateral frontal lobe disorder. Inattentiveness, distractibility, inability to plan activity or to sustain any type of complex mental function are characteristic. The immediate responses to verbal and other stimuli are normal, though memory may be slightly impaired. Conspicuous by their absence are apraxia, agnosia, or aphasia. The gait gradually deteriorates. At first the gait is only slightly uncertain; later there is a shortening of step and a mild clumsiness that sometimes looks suspiciously parkinsonian or, if more incoordinate, like cerebellar ataxia. Later still, the patient cannot walk at all without assistance and may even need help in standing. Lastly there is sphincteric incontinence of the "frontal lobe" type (see page 304). Grasping and sucking are variable; plantar reflexes are sometimes extensor.

Occult hydrocephalus due to tumor growth will be discussed further in Chap. 30.

Normal Pressure Hydrocephalus In nonprogressive meningeal and ependymal diseases the hydrocephalus may stabilize or "compensate," meaning that the formation of CSF equilibrates with absorption. Formation diminishes, perhaps because of compression of choroid plexus, and the absorption increases in proportion to the CSF pressure. Once equilibrium is attained, the intracranial pressure gradually falls, though it maintains the same diminishing gradient from ventricle to basal cistern to cerebral subarachnoid space. A stage is reached where the pressure reaches a normal level of 150 to 180 mmH$_2$O while the patient still manifests the cerebral effects of the hydrocephalic state. The name that has been given to this condition by Adams et al. is *normal pressure hydrocephalus* (NPH). With the large ventricles the lower pressure continues to exert a force against the tracts in the cerebral white matter that exceeds the effects of a higher pressure with small ventricles.

A triad of clinical findings is characteristic of NPH—a slowly progressive gait disorder, impairment of mental function, and sphincteric incontinence (a frontal lobe dementia). Grasp reflexes in the feet and falling attacks may occur. Headaches are no longer a complaint and may never have been present, and there is no papilledema. The measurement of CSF pressure over a prolonged period may show intermittent rises of pressure, possibly corresponding to the A waves of Lundberg.[1] According to Katzman and Hussey the infusion of normal saline into the lumbar subarachnoid space at a rate of 0.76 ml/min for 30 to 60 min provokes a rise in pressure (300 to 600 mmH$_2$O) that is not observed in normal individuals. Drainage of large amounts of CSF may result in clinical improvement for a few days.

This syndrome of NPH may follow subarachnoid hemorrhage from ruptured aneurysm or head trauma, meningitis (tubercular, syphilitic, or other), Paget's disease of the base of the skull, and mucopolysaccharidosis of the meninges and achondroplasia, but in at least a third of our cases it is presumably due to an asymptomatic fibrosing meningitis of unknown etiology.

---

[1] Lundberg (1960) recorded intraventricular pressures over long periods of time in patients with brain tumors. He described three types of pressure waves which he designated as A, B, and C, all separable from arterial and respiratory pulsations. Only the A waves were considered to be clinically significant; they consisted of rhythmic rises of pressure occurring every 15 to 30 min, or more protracted fluctuations in pressure. Their physiologic basis is obscure.

The verification of the diagnosis of NPH and the selection of patients for ventriculoatrial or ventriculoperitoneal shunt has presented difficulties. The CT scan (enlarged ventricles without convolutional atrophy) and radionuclide cisternography (reflux into ventricles and delayed pericerebral diffusion) have been the most helpful ancillary examinations. The saline infusion ("flush") test discloses the manometric response during a 1-h infusion of normal saline (at a rate of 0.76 ml/min) into the spinal subarachnoid space; theoretically, this test should quantitate the adequacy of CSF absorption, but it has yielded unpredictable results. Pneumocencephalography, with air entering the ventricles but not the cerebral subarachnoid space, is helpful but may worsen the clinical state.

The authors have obtained gratifying success, often a complete restoration of mental function and gait, in more than a hundred patients, by effecting a ventriculoatrial shunt. As a group, these patients all had the clinical triad described above, and their lateral ventricular span at the level of the anterior horns was in excess of 50 mm. Deviations from this syndrome—such as the occurrence of dementia without gait disorder, or gait disorder with a clear mind, or the presence of apraxias, aphasias, and other focal cerebral signs—all exclude NPH. Uncertainties of diagnosis increase with advancing age owing to the frequent association of senile dementia and the complications of vascular disease.

The neuropathologic effects of tension hydrocephalus have been described by Adams and Sidman and by Penfield and Elvidge. Ventricular expansion is maximal in the frontal horns, explaining the hydrocephalic impairment of frontal lobe functions. The central white matter yields to pressure while the cortical gray matter, thalami, basal ganglia and brainstem structures remain normal. There is an increase in the content of tissue fluid adjacent to the lateral ventricles. Medullated fibers and axons are injured, but not to the extent that one might expect from the degree of compression; minor degrees of astrocytic gliosis and loss of oligodendrocytes in the affected tissue are present in decreasing degree away from the ventricles, and represent a hydrocephalic atrophy of the brain which is permanent. The ependyma is denuded, and the choroid plexuses are flattened and fibrotic.

Treatment The development of sterilizable one-way valves has opened the way to successful treatment of tension hydrocephalus. The valve can be set at a desired pressure so the CSF will escape directly into the bloodstream whenever the pressure level is exceeded. Although relatively simple as a surgical procedure, there are complications, the main ones being postoperative subdural hygromas or hematomas (if the ventricular pressure is reduced too rapidly, allowing the bridging dural veins to stretch and rupture); infection of the valve and catheter, sometimes with septicemia; and occlusion of the tip of the catheter in the ventricle. The authors have found that the complication rate can be considerably reduced by placing the catheter in the anterior horn of the right ventricle, where there is no choroid plexus, and by the use of the sterilizable Hakim valve. Once the ventricles are shunted they diminish in size within 3 or 4 days, even when the hydrocephalus has been present for a year or more. This indicates that the so-called hydrocephalic compression of the cerebrum is largely reversible. Clinical improvement occurs within a few weeks, the gait disturbance being slower to reverse than the mental disorder. Cerebral atrophy from Alzheimer's disease and related conditions is not altered by ventriculoatrial shunting. Of course, if the hydrocephalus is caused by an operable tumor, surgical removal is the procedure of choice.

The treatment of infantile and childhood hydrocephalus utilizes the same shunting procedures. Whether or not to shunt all hydrocephalic infants soon after birth has not been settled. In several large series of cases that have been treated in this way, the number surviving with normal mental function has been small. The use of diamox to inhibit CSF formation by suppressing the enzyme carbonic anhydrase has not been successful in our hands.

BENIGN INTRACRANIAL HYPERTENSION (MENINGEAL HYDROPS, PSEUDOTUMOR CEREBRI)

This is a disease of obscure origin, particularly frequent in fat adolescent girls and young women, in whom increased intracranial pressure develops over a period of weeks or months. Headache is the usual symptom; others complain of blurred vision, a vague dizziness, diplopia, or a trifling numbness of the face on one side. It is then discovered that they have flagrant papilledema, which immediately raises the specter of a brain tumor. The CSF pressure is elevated, usually in the range of 250 to 450 mmH$_2$O. Aside from the papilledema, there is remarkably little to be found on neurological examination—perhaps a unilateral or bilateral abducens palsy, nystagmus on lateral gaze, or a minor sensory change. Exceptionally, in children, an otherwise typical Bell's palsy may be associated (Chutorian et al.). Visual field testing usually shows slight peripheral constriction with enlargement of the blind spots. Mentation and alertness are preserved, and the patient seems surprisingly well.

As has been remarked, most of the patients are young women, practically all of them obese, but the condition may occur in children and in adult males. The cause is not known. Recent studies of the CSF in this disorder have revealed an increase in outflow resistance and slight decrease in formation. CT scans and pneumoencephalograms have shown the ventricles to be normal in size or small. If the intracranial hypertension is left untreated or fails to respond to the measures outlined below, the real danger is loss of vision. Fortunately this complication occurs in only a small proportion of patients. Vision needs to be checked frequently, so as not to overlook the earliest signs of impaired acuity. Sometimes vision is lost abruptly, either without warning or following one or more episodes of visual obscuration.

Treatment   The first step is to make sure that there is no underlying tumor or other space-occupying lesion. Formerly, when reliance was placed on pneumoencephalography and arteriography, the authors observed an occasional patient whose illness had been diagnosed as benign intracranial hypertension because of negative radiologic findings only to find, after some months or a year had passed, that the ventricles were enlarging and there was an aqueductal stenosis, an astrocytoma, a ventricular cysticercosis, or metastatic tumor. These errors in diagnosis are less frequent since the advent of CT scanning.

At least a third of our patients with pseudotumor cerebri have recovered after repeated lumbar punctures and drainage of sufficient CSF to maintain the pressure at normal levels. The lumbar punctures were repeated daily at first and then at increasing intervals according to the level of pressure. Evidently this was sufficient to restore the balance between CSF formation and absorption. In another group of patients, the CSF pressure remains elevated month after month, and the papilledema becomes chronic. It is the management of this group of patients that is most controversial. Prednisone (40 to 60 mg/day) or oral hyperosmotic agents such as glycerol (15 to 60 mg four to six times daily) or acetazolamide (250 mg tid) to reduce CSF formation all have their advocates. We have observed a gradual recession of papilledema and a lowering of CSF pressure with administration of glycerol and/or prednisone, but it was always

difficult to decide whether this represented the effects of treatment or the natural course of the disease. Greer, who has reported on 110 patients, 11 of which were treated with these agents, decided that they were of no value. In his series, 12 percent continued to have raised intracranial pressure 5 months after the diagnosis was made.

In patients with protracted high intracranial pressure and papilledema, especially in those with a measurable impairment of vision that does not respond to the usual therapeutic measures, a lumbar thecoperitoneal shunt should be performed. Not more than 10 percent of our patients have needed this surgical procedure. It is quite safe and effective, although in very obese patients there is a tendency for the shunt to close. In the past 25 years, we have not had the need to perform a single subtemporal decompression, the procedure that was formerly used when vision was threatened.

INTRACRANIAL HYPOTENSION

"Lumbar Puncture Headache" (see also page 120)   This is a well-known phenomenon, attributable to lowering of the intracranial pressure by leakage of CSF through the needle tract into the paravertebral muscles and other tissues. Actually the syndrome includes more than headache. There may be pain at the base of the skull posteriorly and in the neck and upper thoracic spine, stiffness of the neck, and nausea and vomiting. At times the signs of meningeal irritation are so prominent as to raise the question of postlumbar puncture meningitis, although lack of fever usually excludes this possibility. In the infant or child, stiffness of the neck may be accompanied by irritability, unwillingness to move, and refusal of food. Most characteristic is the relation of the headache to upright posture and its relief within a few minutes after assuming the recumbent position. The use of a 22-bore needle, the performance of a single clean tap, and keeping the patient prone in bed for 6 to 12 h after the puncture, reduce the likelihood of the headache. Once started, the headache may last for days or even a week or more. The CSF pressure is in the range of 0 to 50 mmH$_2$O. Forcing fluids, intravenous infusion of hypotonic fluids (1000 to 2000 ml of 5% glucose) are helpful. Analgesic medication is required only if the patient must get up to care for him- or herself or to travel.

Aside from this condition there are few adverse effects of lumbar puncture and these are relatively rare: transient cranial nerve palsy (usually the sixth), bacterial meningitis, spinal subdural or epidural abscess, injury of a lumbar root and sciatic pain, damage to an intervertebral disk, and inadvertent injection of air with aseptic pleocytosis.

Less well known is a syndrome of *spontaneous intracranial hypotension.* The authors have observed several patients in whom the same syndrome as that which follows lumbar puncture occurred after straining, a nonhurtful fall, or for no known reason. The CSF pressure is low or not measurable, and the fluid may contain 20 to 50 mononuclear cells per milliliter. Presumably there has been a tear in the delicate arachnoid surrounding a nerve root, with continuous leakage of CSF. The site of the leak usually cannot be ascertained, except for the one into the paranasal sinuses (CSF rhinorrhea). Recumbency for a few days permits the pressure to build up, and there has been no recurrence in the cases the authors have encountered.

The use of a one-way valve and a ventriculoatrial or ventriculoperitoneal shunt may also result in a low-pressure syndrome. Usually the valve setting is too low, and readjustment to maintain a higher pressure corrects this.

MENINGEAL AND EPENDYMAL REACTIONS

Tha anatomy of the pia-arachnoid (which forms the double membrane surrounding the brain, optic nerves, and spinal cord), the ependyma of the ventricles, and their connection via the foramens of Luschka and Magendie, account for the fact that whatever foreign agent enters the subarachnoid space (SAS) or the ventricles has free access to the other spaces containing CSF. The pia provides a relative barrier, at least to bacteria, between the SAS and the brain and spinal cord. The arachnoidal membrane is a bacterial barrier between the SAS and the subdural space. The dura is tightly adherent to the inner periosteum of the cranial bones, so that there is no cranial epidural space, and the inner side of the dura has no true endothelial lining. There is, however, a wide space between the dura that surrounds the spinal cord and the vertebral bodies. Because of these barriers, the subarachnoid, subdural, and epidural spaces can be affected separately by diseases. The subarachnoid-ventricular spaces are the ones most frequently involved.

PIA-ARACHNOID-EPENDYMAL-CHOROIDAL REACTIONS TO INFECTION

Various bacteria and other infectious agents may gain entrance to the ventricles and SAS, and having done so,

they diffuse readily throughout all of the compartments containing CSF. They excite a chemical and cellular reaction that is mediated mainly through the capillaries and venules of the vascular pia and choroid plexuses. The blood-CSF barrier becomes more permeable, and neutrophilic leukocytes, lymphocytes, plasma cells, and monocytes enter the subarachnoid space. Foreign substances are phagocytized by histiocytes (macrophages) and may be isolated in granulomas by foreign-body giant cells. The more chronic of these reactions lead to fibroblastic proliferation, often with obliteration of the subarachnoid spaces and the development of hydrocephalus. The delicate lining of the ventricles and the fronds of the choroid plexuses, composed of a single layer of cuboidal cells, are regularly damaged. Bacteria or chemical agents may penetrate the tissue beneath the ependyma and excite a focal histiocytic-microglial reaction that erupts into the ventricle. The ependymal cells are shed or are overgrown by subependymal microgliacytes and astrocytes, and the end stage of the process is a granular ependymitis. The aqueduct may become stenotic as part of this subependymal gliosis, and the choroid plexuses may become fibrotic. Some foreign materials drain from the ventricles into subependymal veins.

Structures lying within and next to the cerebrospinal SAS are vulnerable to these reactions. The roots of cranial and spinal nerves, which have no true perineurium, may be injured. The subpial cerebral and cerebellar cortices, the subpial tracts of the spinal cord, and the subpial fibers of the optic nerves, although protected against ingress of bacteria, are nevertheless susceptible to their toxins. The histologic changes in these structures are more subtle, but no less real, than those in the SAS, and are reflected in the encephalopathy and myelopathy that may accompany chronic meningitis. Pial veins may become thrombosed, and cerebral and spinal cord infarction may result. Later, the walls of meningeal arteries become thickened and their lumens narrowed. The thin arachnoidal membrane may be transgressed, particularly in children, and the subdural space is invaded; subdural exudates and vascular and fibroblastic reactions result.

The clinical correlates of these reactions, exemplified best by bacterial meningitis, are shown in Table 29-1.

Table 29-1

Pathologic-clinical correlations in acute, subacute, and chronic meningitis

I. In acute meningitis:

A. *Pure pia-arachnoiditis*: headache, stiff neck, Kernig and Brudzinski signs. These signs depend on the activation of protective reflexes which shorten the spine and immobilize it (extension of the neck and flexion of the hips and knees reduce stretch on inflamed spinal structures; resistance to forward flexion of the neck and extension of the legs involves maneuvers which oppose these postural reflexes).

B. *Subpial encephalopathy*: confusion, stupor, coma, and convulsions are related to this lesion. The tissue beneath the pia is not penetrated by bacteria; hence the change is probably toxic. Cerebral infarction due to cortical vein thrombosis may underlie these symptoms in some cases.

C. *Inflammatory or vascular involvement of cranial nerve roots*: ocular palsies, facial weakness, and deafness are the main clinical signs. *Note*: Deafness may also be due to middle ear infection, to extension of meningeal infection to the inner ear, or to toxic effects of antimicrobial agents.

D. *Thrombosis of meningeal veins*: focal convulsions, focal cerebral defects such as hemiparesis, aphasia (rarely prominent), etc., may appear during the first three or four days, but more often after the first week or two of meningeal infection.

E. *Ependymitis, choroidal plexitis*: it is doubtful if there are any recognizable clinical effects aside from those of the associated hydrocephalus.

II. In more subacute and chronic forms of meningitis:

A. *Tension hydrocephalus*, due at first to purulent exudate around the base of the brain, later to meningeal fibrosis, and rarely to aqueductal stenosis. *In adults*, there are variable degrees of impairment of consciousness, decorticate postures (arms flexed, legs extended), grasp and sucking reflexes, and sphincteric incontinence. CSF pressure may at first be elevated; as the ventricles enlarge and the choroid plexuses are compressed, it may fall to within limits of normal (low-pressure hydrocephalus). *In infants and young children*, main signs are enlarging head, inability to look upward (eyes turn down and lids retract on effort to look up—"sunset" sign); in mildest form, only psychomotor retardation, unsteadiness of gait, and incontinence.

B. *Subdural effusion*: impaired alertness, refusal to eat, vomiting, immobility, bulging fontanels, and persistence of fever despite clearing of CSF. In infants, the effusion causes an exaggerated transillumination. If fever is present but CSF pressure is normal, and if one-sided cerebral signs are clearly in evidence, thrombophlebitis is the leading possibility.

C. *Extensive venous or arterial infarction*: unilateral or bilateral hemiplegia, decorticate or decerebrate rigidity, cortical blindness, stupor or coma with or without seizures.

III. Late effects or sequelae:

A. *Meningeal fibrosis around optic nerves or around spinal cord and roots*: blindness and optic atrophy, and spastic paraparesis with sensory loss in the lower segments of the body (opticochiasmatic arachnoiditis and meningomyelitis, respectively).

B. *Chronic meningoencephalitis with hydrocephalus*: dementia, stupor or coma, and paralysis (general paralysis of the insane). If lumbosacral posterior roots are chronically damaged, tabes dorsalis results.

C. *Persistent hydrocephalus in the child*: blindness, arrest of all mental activity, bilateral spastic hemiplegia.

CHEMICAL REACTIONS OF THE MENINGES

The installation of chemical agents into the CSF always carries the risk of inducing some of the reactions described above. If the substance diffuses rapidly into the blood, as occurs with spinal anesthetic, no harm is done. Agents such as *Pantopaque*, which are used to visualize the subarachnoid space, may cause meningeal reactions and even granuloma formation, and should always be removed after the test. We have observed rare cases of arachnoiditis with spinal cord compression and fatal hydrocephalus as a reaction to Pantopaque that had not been removed.

Chemical contaminants of spinal anesthetics have had deleterious effects on spinal roots and meninges, optic nerves, and basal meninges of the brain. The authors have seen more than 40 cases of serious *neurologic damage from spinal anesthesia* when the latter was dispensed from vials that were kept in sterilizing detergent solutions. Usually, in these cases, the anesthetic effect was inadequate, and immediately following the instillation of the anesthetic agent there was back pain and rapidly progressive lumbosacral root syndrome (areflexic paralysis and anesthesia of legs and paralysis of sphincters). The CSF protein rose rapidly with slight pleocytosis.

Another delayed, chronic effect—a postspinal anesthesia myeloencephalopathy—may occur. Months or even years after spinal anesthesia there is a gradual onset of spastic-ataxic paraparesis and sensory disturbance, hydrocephalus, and blindness. When care is taken to avoid contamination of the spinal anesthetic, these complications can be prevented.

Recurrent hemorrhage into the ventricles or subarachnoid space gives rise to two other interesting clinical-pathologic syndromes: *postmeningeal hemorrhage hydrocephalus* and *meningeal hemosiderosis*. The former has been described in the preceding section, in relation to normal pressure hydrocephalus. With reference to the latter, as blood hemolyzes, iron-containing compounds are liberated into the subarachnoid and intraventricular spaces. The iron, possibly in the form of ferritin, diffuses into the brain and spinal cord for a distance of several millimeters. It is highly toxic and causes neuronal death and a reactive gliosis. The astrocytes are seen to be encrusted with iron particles. The cerebellar cortex, especially the Purkinje cells, are depleted, and the patient becomes *ataxic*. *Mental dullness* and *corticospinal signs* are also a part of the clinical picture. Ferritin injected into the subarachnoid space of experimental animals has a similar pathologic effect. However, the syndrome is difficult to analyze because the repeated subarachnoid hemorrhages that induce the hemosiderotic syndrome may also cause a communicating hydrocephalus. Also, the original hemorrhagic lesion contributes to the symptomatology.

REFERENCES

ADAMS RD, et al: Symptomatic occult hydrocephalus with "normal" cerebrospinal fluid pressure: A treatable syndrome. *N Engl J Med* 273:117, 1965.

———, SIDMAN R: *Introduction to Neuropathology*. New York, McGraw-Hill, 1968, pp 85-86.

AMES A, SAKANOUE M, ENDO S: Na, K, Ca, Mg and Cl concentrations in choroid plexus fluid and cisternal fluid compared with plasma ultrafiltrate. *J Neurophysiol* 27:672, 1964.

BARROWS LJ, HUNTER FT, BANKER BQ: The nature and clinical significance of pigments in the cerebrospinal fluid. *Brain* 78:59, 1955.

CHUTORIAN AM, GOLD AP, BRAUN CW: Benign intracranial hypertension and Bell's palsy. *N Engl J Med* 296:1214, 1977.

DANDY WE: Experimental hydrocephalus. *Ann Surg* 70:129, 1919.

DAVSON H: *Physiology of the Cerebrospinal Fluid*. Boston, Little, Brown, 1967.

FISHMAN RA: *Cerebrospinal Fluid in Diseases of the Nervous System*. Philadelphia, Saunders, 1980.

FOLEY J: Benign forms of intracranial hypertension—"toxic" and "otitic" hydrocephalus. *Brain* 78:1, 1955.

GILLES FH, DAVIDSON RI: Communicating hydrocephalus associated with deficient dysplastic parasagittal arachnoid granulations. *J Neurosurg* 35:421, 1971.

GREER M: Benign intracranial hypertension, in Vinken PJ, Bruyn GW (eds): *Handbook of Clinical Neurology*, vol 16. Amsterdam, North-Holland, 1974, chap. 4, pp 150-166.

HAKIM S, ADAMS RD: The special clinical problem of symptomatic hydrocephalus with normal cerebrospinal fluid pressure. *J Neurol Sci* 2:307, 1965.

HUSSEY F, SCHANZER B, KATZMAN R: A simple constant-infusion manometric test for measurement of CSF absorption: II. Clinical studies. *Neurology* 20:665, 1970.

KATZMAN R, HUSSEY F: A simple constant-infusion manometric test for measurement of CSF absorption: I. Rationale and method. *Neurology* 20:534, 1970.

LUNDBERG N: Continuous recording and control of ventricular fluid pressure in neurosurgical practice. *Acta Psychiatr Scand*, 36(suppl 149):1960.

MANN JD, JOHNSON RN, BUTLER AB, BASS NH: Impairment of cerebrospinal fluid circulatory dynamics in pseudotumor cerebri and response to steroid treatment. *Neurology* 29:550, 1979.

MERRITT HH, FREMONT-SMITH F: *The Cerebrospinal Fluid*. Philadelphia, Saunders, 1937.

MESTREZAT W: *Le Liquide céphalorachidien normal et pathologique: Valeur clinique de l' examen chimique; Syndromes humoraux dans les diverses affections*. Paris, Maloine, 1912.

PAPPENHEIMER JR, HEISEY SR, JORDON EF, DOWNER J: Perfusion of the cerebral ventricular system in unanesthetized goats. *Am J Physiol* 203:763, 1962.

PENFIELD W, ELVIDGE AR: Hydrocephalus and the atrophy of cerebral compression, in Penfield W (ed): *Cytology and Cellular Pathology of the Nervous System*. New York, Hoeber, 1932, pp 1203-1217.

QUINCKE H: Die Lumbarpunktion des Hydrocephalus, *Klin Wochenschr* 28:929, 965, 1891.

ROSMAN NP, SHANDS KN: Hydrocephalus caused by increased intracranial venous pressure: A clinicopathological study. *Ann Neurology* 3:445, 1978.

RUSSELL DS: *Observations on the Pathology of Hydrocephalus*. London, HM Stationery Office, 1949.

SYMONDS CP: Otitic hydrocephalus. *Brain* 54:55, 1931.

WEED LH: Certain anatomical and physiological aspects of the meninges and cerebrospinal fluid. *Brain* 58:383, 1935.

WILFERT CM: Mumps meningoencephalitis with low cerebrospinal fluid glucose, prolonged pleocytosis and elevation of protein. *N Engl J Med* 280:855, 1969.

CHAPTER 30

INTRACRANIAL NEOPLASMS

Speaking generally, tumors of the central nervous system constitute a bleak but vitally important chapter of neurologic medicine. Also, in general, it may be said of them that they occur in great variety; produce neurologic symptoms because of size, location, and invasive qualities; usually destroy the tissues in which they are situated and displace those around them; are a frequent cause of increased intracranial pressure; and are often lethal. This dismal state of affairs is beginning to change, however, thanks to advances in anesthesiology, microneurosurgical techniques, and the use of pharmacologic agents.

For the student of medicine the most important facts to assimilate are that (1) many types of tumor occur in the cranial cavity and spinal canal, and that certain ones are much more frequent than others (see Table 30-1); (2) some of these tumors, such as the craniopharyngioma, meningioma, and schwannoma, have a disposition to grow in particular parts of the cranial cavity, thereby evincing certain syndromes; (3) their growth rates and invasiveness vary, some like the glioblastoma being highly malignant, invasive, and rapidly progressive and others like the meningioma being benign, slowly progressive, and compressive. These pathologic peculiarities are important, for they have valuable clinical implications—frequently providing the explanation of slowly or rapidly evolving clinical states, and good or poor prognosis after surgical excision.

INCIDENCE OF CNS TUMORS AND THEIR TYPES

In 1977 there were an estimated 385,000 deaths from cancer in the United States. Of these the number of patients dying of primary tumors of the brain seems comparatively small (ca. 8800) but another 85,000 patients (22 percent) who die of cancer have intracranial metastases at the time of autopsy. Thus, in somewhat more than 20 percent of all patients with cancer, the brain and its coverings will be involved by neoplasm at some time in the course of the illness. Among causes of death from intracranial disease, tumor is exceeded in frequency only by stroke.

It is difficult to obtain accurate statistics of the types of intracranial tumors, for most of them have been obtained from university hospitals and specialized neurosurgical centers, which attract the more easily diagnosed and treatable forms. From the figures quoted above (collected by Posner and Chernick) secondary tumors of the brain should greatly outnumber primary ones, yet in the large reported series (those of Zülch, Cushing, Olivecrona, and Zimmerman) only 3 to 6 percent are of this type. Even in the autopsy statistics of municipal hospitals, where one would expect a more natural selection of cases, the figures for metastatic growths tend to err on the low side since the brain is frequently not examined in cancer patients, and many of the patients with more benign tumors may have found their way to specialized neurosurgical services.

With these reservations concerning natural incidence the figures in Table 30-1 might be taken as representative.

CAUSATION

The many thoughtful studies of brain tumors have shed little light on their origin. Certainly an analysis of case records has yielded no clue as to why a tumor should begin to grow in the brain during adult life. Antecedent head injury, infection, metabolic and other systemic dis-

440

ease, and exposure to toxins and radiation have all been invoked as causative factors, but there is no conclusive evidence that any of them play a part.

Johannes Müller (1838), in his atlas *Structure and Function of Neoplasms*, first enunciated the appealing idea that tumors might originate in embryonic cells left in the brain during development. This idea was elaborated by Cohnheim (1878), who postulated that the cause of tumors was an anomaly of the embryonic anlage. Tumors would be expected to form, he stated, at sites where there are rapid differentiations of germ layers and complex migrations of cells. How easy it would be for a defective or incomplete migration to leave embryonic cells in the wrong place; and their unnatural environment might encourage neoplasia. Ribbert, in 1918, extended this hypothesis by postulating that the multipotentiality of some of these embryonic cells would favor blastomatous growth. Also implicit in this histogenetic theory is the idea that the degree of anaplasia, or its opposite, differentiation, depends on the status of the cell rests.

This Cohnheim-Ribbert theory seems most applicable to tumors originating in the hypophysial region, such as craniopharyngiomas, teratomas, lipomas, and chordomas. Ostertag (1936) suggested that gliomas might have a similar dysontogenetic origin (i.e., from

Table 30-1

Types of intracranial tumor in the combined series of Zülch, Cushing, and Olivecrona expressed in percentage of total (approximately 15,000 cases)

Tumor	Percent of total
Gliomas:	
Glioblastoma multiforme	20
Astrocytoma	10
Ependymoma	6
Medulloblastoma	4
Oligodendrocytoma	5
Meningioma	15
Pituitary adenoma	7
Neurinoma	7
Metastatic carcinoma	6
Craniopharyngioma, dermoid, epidermoid, teratoma	4
Angiomas	4
Sarcomas	4
Unclassified (mostly gliomas)	5
Miscellaneous (pinealoma, chordoma, granuloma)	3
Total	100

rests of glioblasts), but such rests have never been identified in the normal brain, and no proof of this concept has been forthcoming. Possibly this embryonic rest theory might account for tumors that sometimes arise in the brain of a patient with von Recklinghausen's neurofibromatosis, with Bourneville's tuberous sclerosis, or with Hippel-Lindau hemangioblastomatosis; or it might account for certain midline tumors at sites of closure of the neural tube (polar spongioblastoma; retinoblastoma; gliomas of optic nerve, hypothalamus, periaqueductal region, cerebellum, and spinal cord). However, even in the case of the medulloblastoma, where this embryonic rest theory is invoked most often, one cannot be sure that the neoplasm arises from primitive neuroblasts of the posterior medullary velum. A histogenic theory of brain tumors is implicit in the classification of Bailey and Cushing (1926), which is based on the known or assumed embryology of nerve and glial cells; this has remained the basis of most modern classifications of tumors of central neurogenic origin.

The factor of age is important in the biology of brain tumors. Medulloblastomas, polar spongioblastomas (piloid astrocytomas), and pinealomas occur mainly before the age of 20 years, and meningiomas and glioblastomas are most frequent around the age of 50 years. Heredity figures importantly in retinoblastomas, neurofibromas, and hemangioblastomas. Gliomas have also been reported occasionally in more than one member of a family, but most authorities discount the operation of a genetic factor. Only in the gliomas associated with neurofibromatosis and tuberous sclerosis is there significant evidence of an hereditary determinant.

The discovery that carcinogens, notably hydrocarbons and nitrosamines, could cause a variety of gliomas has cast serious doubt on the validity of the dysontogenetic theory. Examining the origins of these experimental tumors, Zimmerman and others found that the cells which were proliferating to form the tumor were well-differentiated adult elements, not embryonic remnants. A normal astrocyte, oligodendrocyte, microgliocyte, or ependymocyte is transformed into a neoplastic cell, and as it multiplies, the daughter cells become variably dedifferentiated, the more so as the degree of malignancy increases. Certain animal viruses have similar effects. While these experimental studies provide interesting animal examples that bear on the pathogenesis of tumors in general, there is no evidence that human gliomas necessarily develop in this manner. However, one cannot altogether dismiss these possibilities, because curious inclusion bodies have been observed in human tumors (proven not to be viral by electron microscopy), and because collections of lymphocytes and mononuclear cells (conceivably resulting from infection or autoimmune reactions) have been noted—findings which suggest an infective origin.

PATHOPHYSIOLOGY

Certain principles of physics and physiology govern the production of symptoms by tumor growth. The cranial cavity has a restricted volume, and the three elements contained therein—the brain (about 1400 g), CSF (75 ml), and blood (75 ml)—are relatively incompressible. According to the Monro-Kellie hypothesis, the total bulk of the three elements is at all times constant, and any increase in the volume of one of them must be at the expense of one or both of the others; a diminished volume of one is met with a compensatory increase in the others (see Fig. 29-1). A tumor growing in one part of the brain must displace blood or CSF or both, and atrophy of the brain is attended by an increase in CSF.

The pressure of the CSF in the lumbar subarachnoid space serves as a gauge of the intracranial pressure because this space is continuous with the intracranial one. An increased volume of cerebral mass will result in an elevated CSF pressure. However, it must be remembered that the latter is largely maintained by the pressure under which the blood is delivered to the brain. In circulatory collapse in patients with tumors, the elevated CSF pressure falls, and at death it is zero.

When considered in more detail, an intracranial growth first decreases the amount of CSF in both the ventricles and subarachnoid space. Some of this fluid is displaced through the foramen magnum to the spinal subarachnoid space, and some through the optic foramens to the perioptic subarachnoid space. Soon, however, the limits of this adjustment are surpassed, and the pressure throughout the ventriculosubarachnoid spaces begins to rise. The elevation in pressure can be measured through a needle in the lumbar subarachnoid space, the cisterna magna, or lateral ventricle. The elevation of perioptic pressure impairs the venous drainage from the optic nerve head and retina, which manifests itself by papilledema ("choked disk").

Presumably the venules in the cerebral tissue adjacent to the tumor are compressed, with resulting elevation of capillary pressure, particularly in the cerebral white matter. Microvascular transudative factors, that cause a weakening of the blood-brain barrier may also contribute to the vasogenic type of edema. The latter is the postulated basis of the regional swelling, also called *localized cerebral edema*, that surrounds the tumor (see further on).

Any general increase in venous pressure retards the absorption of CSF and results in an increase in the volume of the latter. The pressure in the subarachnoid space must always be maintained at a level above that in the venous sinuses in order for CSF absorption to occur. If the increase in venous and CSF pressure occurs slowly, it is compensated at least partially by dilatation of arteries and arterioles; if the increase is rapid, the arterial blood pressure must rise also—usually the systolic more than the diastolic. As a rule this is accompanied by bradycardia (carotid sinus reflex). These circulatory adjustments are initiated by venous stasis and the accumulation of CO_2 in the vasomotor centers of the medulla and carotid bodies. The respiratory centers also become affected, for increases in intracranial pressure usually cause an irregularity and, finally, an arrest of respiration.

BRAIN EDEMA

This is a most important aspect of tumor growth, but it also assumes importance in cerebral trauma, infarction, abscess, and hypoxia—as well as in certain toxic and metabolic states. Brain edema is such a prominent feature of cerebral neoplasm that this is a suitable place to summarize what is known about it.

For a long time it has been recognized that conditions which lead to peripheral edema, such as hypoalbuminemia (nephrosis) and increased venous pressure (cardiac failure), do not have a similar effect on the brain. In contrast, lesions which alter the blood-brain barrier cause rapid swelling of brain tissue. But the latter is usually part of some other pathologic process such as tumor, trauma, infarction, hypoxia, or hypoosmolality, and to refer to the brain swelling in all these circumstances as brain edema misdirects thinking from the primary pathologic process. Klatzo's classification has one advantage in that it is based at least partly on pathogenesis. He specifies two categories, *vasogenic* edema and *cytotoxic* edema; Fishman accepts these two categories but adds a third which he calls *interstitial*. An example of the latter is said to be obstructive hydrocephalus, in which CSF seeps into the periventricular tissues and occupies the space between cells. Most neuropathologists use the term *interstitial* to refer to any increase in the extravascular intercellular compartment of the brain. This would include vasogenic edema.

Vasogenic edema is the type seen in the vicinity of tumor growths and other localized processes as well as in toxic injuries of blood vessels (e.g., lead encephalopathy). It is confined to the cerebral white matter. Presumably there is increased permeability of the capillary endothelial cells so that plasma enters the extracellular spaces (Fig. 30-1A). The heightened permeability has been attributed to a defect in the tight endothelial cell junctions, but current evidence indicates that increased vesicular transport across the endothelial cells is a more important factor (Fig. 30-1A). Experimentally, the increase in permeability has been shown to vary inversely with the molecular weight of various markers; inulin (molecular weight 5000) enters the intercellular space more readily than albumin (molecular weight 70,000). The particular vulnerability of white matter to vasogenic edema is not understood; probably it is related to some peculiarity of the vessel walls. The accumulation of plasma filtrate, with its high protein content, in the extracellular spaces and between layers of the myelin sheaths would be expected to alter the ionic balance of nerve fibers, impairing their function.

Cytotoxic edema is exemplified by hypoxic injury, in which all the cellular elements (neurons, glia, and endothelial cells) imbibe fluid and swell, with a corre-

Figure 30-1

A. *Schematic representation of the astrocytes and endothelial cells of the capillary wall in the normal state (above) and in vasogenic edema (below). Heightened permeability in vasogenic edema is due partly to a defect in tight endothelial junctions but mainly to active vesicular transport across endothelial cells. B. Cytotoxic edema, showing swelling of the endothelial, glial, and neuronal cells, at the expense of the extracellular fluid space of the brain. (From Fishman.)*

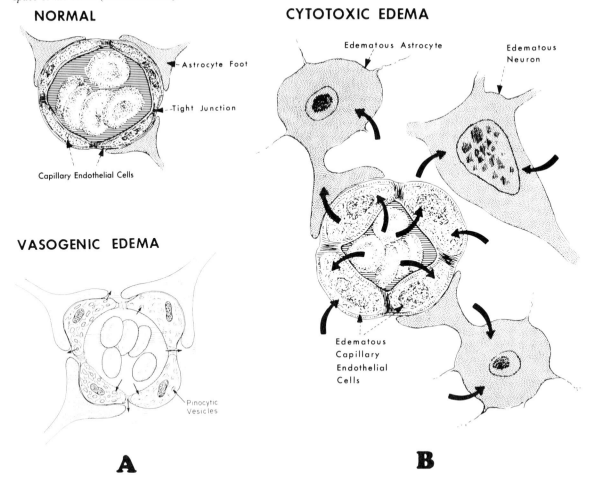

sponding reduction in the extracellular-fluid space. The effect of oxygen deprivation is to cause a failure of the ATP-dependent sodium pump within cells; sodium accumulates within cells, and water follows (Fig. 30-2*B*). Interesting, however, is the fact that several of the most frequent metabolic and nutritional encephalopathies such as normotensive uremia, hepatic coma, and vitamin B_1 and B_{12} deficiencies, are not attended by either vasogenic or cytotoxic edema.

Our view of *interstitial edema*, wherein the extracellular fluid space is enlarged without demonstrable vascular or cell injury, is rather different from that of Fishman. We would place acute hyponatremia and water intoxication in this category and not in the cytotoxic one, as Fishman does. The hypoosmolality of the blood alters the ionic concentration in the extracellular spaces (interstitial fluid), and this in turn causes the brain cells to lose intracellular osmoles, particularly potassium. If this latter compensation is adequate, brain volume is preserved and intracellular osmolality comes to reach equilibrium with the plasma; if not, there is brain swelling.

Most patients with brain tumors have regional swelling of tissue of the vasogenic type, apparently secondary to the elaboration of a transudative factor and to the compressive effects of the mass on surrounding veins. Once pressure is raised in a particular region of the brain, it begins to cause displacement and herniation which allow other vascular and pressure factors to come into play; if respiratory difficulty and secondary hypotension occur, there is an added cytotoxic edema.

BRAIN HERNIATIONS

The problem of brain herniations is of great importance in all mass lesions, and the underlying principles must be understood. Such phenomena become possible because the cranial cavity is subdivided into several compartments by sheets of relatively rigid dura (the falx cerebri which divides the supratentorial space into right and left halves, and the tentorium which separates the cerebellum from the occipital lobes). The pressure from a mass within any one compartment, therefore, is not evenly distributed. This causes shifts or herniations of brain tissue from one compartment where the pressure is high to another where it is lower. There are three well-known herniations, the *subfalcial, temporal lobe-tentorial, and cerebellar-foramen magnum* (Fig. 30-2), and several less familiar ones (cerebellar-tentorial, diencephalic-sella

turcica and orbital frontal-middle cranial fossa). Herniation of swollen brain through an opening in the calvarium, in relation to craniocerebral injury or operation, is yet another (transcalvarial) type.

The *subfalcial herniation*, in which the medial part of one frontal or parietal lobe is pushed under the falx, is frequent, but little is known of its clinical manifestations. The most important herniation is the *temporal lobe-tentorial* one, which was described originally by Adolf Meyer, and whose clinical significance was first appreciated by Vincent et al. and by Jefferson. Here the medial part of one temporal lobe (usually the uncus) is forced into the oval-shaped tentorial opening through which the midbrain passes. The uncal hernia pushes the midbrain and subthalamus to the opposite side and against the opposite free edge of the tentorial opening, exerting great pressure on the midbrain and subthalamic structures and on the vessels which encircle and enter them. The hemiparesis that results from compression of the cerebral peduncle by the tentorium is ipsilateral to

Figure 30-2

Mass shifts associated with a parietal lobe tumor. Top. The cingulate gyrus is displaced under the falx, toward the opposite side. Middle. The inferomedial parts of the temporal lobe are forced into the posterior fossa through the tentorial hiatus, alongside the brainstem (temporal lobe-tentorial herniation or pressure cone). Bottom. The cerebellar tonsils are pressed into the foramen magnum, displacing the medulla caudally. The gyri overlying the tumor are flattened. (From Kautzky and Zülch.)

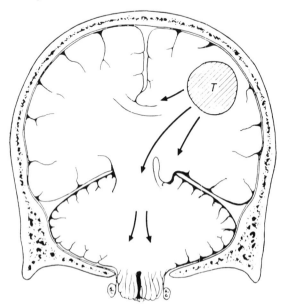

the cerebral lesion and thus constitutes a false localizing sign (crus phenomenon, or syndrome; see Table 30-2).

Plum and Posner subdivide the effects of supratentorial mass lesions on the upper brainstem into two types—a "central or transtentorial" and an "uncal." In the former a rostral-caudal displacement is believed to occur with visible depression of the anterior choroidal artery in the arteriogram; in the latter the displacement is mainly lateral, away from the expanding lesion. Clinically the central syndrome is said to be characterized by the early occurrence of stupor, followed by irregular and then Cheyne-Stokes respiration; by small pupils with full eye movements and later by paralysis of vertical and contralateral gaze; by contralateral hemiplegia and homolateral paratonic rigidity (gegenhalten), giving way to stiffness of the muscles of the neck and decerebrate and decorticate postures as coma deepens. In the uncal syndrome, third nerve palsy on the side of the lesion (ptosis, dilatation of pupil, then ophthalmoplegia) is said to precede disturbances of consciousness, but the latter develop rapidly, and the sequence of respiratory changes (Cheyne-Stokes breathing, central hyperpnea, quiet irregular breathing and finally arrest) is accompanied by bilateral corticospinal tract signs (ipsilateral or contralateral hemiplegia with bilateral Babinski signs) and decerebrate rigidity. In both syndromes the functional deterioration is believed to proceed from diencephalon to midbrain, pons, and finally medulla.

As stated in Chap. 16, the authors find it difficult to distinguish the central from the lateral syndrome and are more impressed with the functional importance of lateral than downward displacement. Early changes in consciousness in the so-called central syndrome are difficult to differentiate from the direct effects of the primary lesion, admitting only that third nerve or nuclear signs do not always precede disturbances of consciousness. We are inclined therefore to subsume all these neurologic changes under a single lateral or uncal syndrome and to emphasize the following clinicopathologic correlations and mechanisms (Table 30-2).

The *cerebellar-foramen magnum herniation* or *pressure cone*, first described by Cushing in 1917, con-

Table 30-2
Temporal lobe–tentorial (uncal) herniation

Pathologic change	Mechanism	Clinical disorders
Injury to outer fibers of ipsilateral oculomotor nerve	Strangulation of nerve between herniating tissue and medial petroclinoid ligament; less often, downward pressure and entrapment of nerve between posterior cerebral and superior cerebellar arteries	Ptosis and pupillary dilatation (Hutchinson's pupil), ophthalmoplegia later
Creasing of contralateral cerebral peduncle (Kernohan's notch)	Pressure of laterally displaced midbrain against sharp edge of tentorium	Hemiplegia ipsilateral to herniation (*false localizing sign*) and bilateral corticospinal tract signs
Lateral flattening of midbrain and zones of necrosis and secondary hemorrhages in tegmentum and base of subthalamus, midbrain, and upper pons (Duret hemorrhages)	Crushing of midbrain between herniating temporal lobe and opposite leaf of tentorium and vascular occlusion (hemorrhages around arterioles and veins)	Cheyne-Stokes respirations; stupor-coma; bipyramidal signs; decerebration; dilated, fixed pupils and alterations of gaze (facilitated oculocephalic reflex movement giving way to loss of all response to head movement and labyrinthine stimulation)
Unilateral or bilateral infarction (hemorrhagic) of occipital lobes	Compression of posterior cerebral artery against the tentorium by herniating temporal lobe	Usually none detectable during coma; homonymous hemianopia (unilateral or bilateral) with recovery
Rising intracranial pressure and hydrocephalus	Lateral flattening of aqueduct and blockage of perimesencephalic subarachnoid space	Increasing coma, rising blood pressure, bradycardia

sists of downward displacement of the inferior mesial parts of the cerebellar hemispheres (mainly the ventral paraflocculi or tonsillae) through the foramen magnum, behind the cervical cord. The displacement may be bilateral or unilateral, in the case of one-sided cerebellar lesions. It may be caused by centrally placed frontal tumors or by general swelling of the brain. Sometimes it is associated with temporal lobe-tentorial herniation which is usually caused by laterally placed cerebral hemispheric or surface lesions (particularly in the temporal region). The herniating cerebellar tissue may swell and become infarcted; but whether it does or not, the lethal effects of this herniation are the result of medullary compression.

The clinical manifestations are less well delineated than those of the temporal lobe-tentorial herniation. Cushing considered the typical signs of cerebellar herniation to be episodes of tonic extension and arching of the neck and back and extension and internal rotation of the limbs, with respiratory disturbances, cardiac irregularity (bradycardia or tachycardia), and loss of consciousness. Later other signs were added—pain in the neck, stiff neck, head tilt, paresthesias in shoulders, dysphagia, loss of tendon reflexes, autonomic effects, cardiac dysrhythmia, and respiratory arrest. It is important to determine which of these signs are due to the cerebellar herniation per se and which to the attendant intracranial pressure effects and hydrocephalus. We would suggest that head tilt, stiff neck, arching of neck, and paresthesias over the shoulders are attributable to the herniation, and that tonic extensor spasms of the limbs and body (so-called cerebellar fits) and coma are due to the compressive effects of the cerebellar lesion or hydrocephalus on upper brainstem structures. Respiratory arrest is the most feared and often a fatal effect of medullary compression.

Elevation of intracranial pressure from a mass lesion or hydrocephalus, if severe, causes a depression of cerebral function. This is manifested clinically by reduced speed of psychocerebral activities, apathy, drowsiness, inattentiveness, and impaired registration of presented material and events—and electrically by a diffuse decrease in the frequency of brain waves. The rate of cerebral blood flow also is slowed.

A knowledge of the effects of elevated intracranial pressure, localized vasogenic edema, and of herniations and displacements of tissue are absolutely essential to an understanding of the clinical behavior of intracranial growths. The symptoms of intracranial tumors are more often related to these effects than to direct invasion of neurologic structures, and many false localizing signs (unilateral or bilateral abducens palsy, ipsilateral or bilateral corticospinal tract signs, etc.) are due to these mechanical changes as well.

CLINICAL AND PATHOLOGIC CHARACTERISTICS OF BRAIN TUMORS

It should be stated at the outset that tumors of the brain may exist with hardly any symptoms. Often a slight bewilderment, slowness in comprehension, or loss of capacity to sustain continuous mental activity is the only deviation from normal function, and specific signs of cerebral disease are wholly lacking. In some patients, on the other hand, there is some early indication of cerebral disease in the form of a seizure or other dramatic symptom, but the evidence for a time may not be clear enough to warrant the diagnosis of a cerebral tumor. In a third group, the existence of a brain tumor can be assumed because of the presence of increased intracranial pressure, with or without localizing signs of the tumor. In a fourth group, the symptoms are so definite as to make it probable not only that there is intracranial neoplasm, but also that it is located in a particular region. In fact, these localized growths may create certain unique syndromes seldom evinced by any other disease.

In the further exposition of this subject, intracranial tumors are considered in relation to the common clinical circumstances in which they are likely to be found, as follows:

1. Patients who present with general impairment of cerebral function or a seizure.

2. Patients who present with unmistakable evidence of increased intracranial pressure.

3. Patients who present with specific intracranial tumor syndromes.

PATIENTS WHO PRESENT WITH GENERAL IMPAIRMENT OF CEREBRAL FUNCTION, HEADACHES, OR SEIZURES

These are the patients who give the most trouble in diagnosis and about whom decisions are often made with a great degree of uncertainty. Their initial symptoms are vague, and not until some time has elapsed will signs of focal brain disease appear; when they do, they are not always of accurate localizing value. Altered mental function, headache, dizziness, and seizures are the usual manifestations in this group of patients.

Changes in Mental Function Practically every patient in this group will show some alteration of mental function, but in order to learn of it one must often obtain the observations of a person who knows the patient intimately. A lack of persistent application to the tasks of the day, an undue irritability, emotional lability, a peculiar inertia, faulty insight, forgetfulness, reduced range of mental activity, indifference to common social practices, lack of initiative and spontaneity—all of which may be falsely attributed to worry, anxiety, or depression—are the usual abnormalities. We have sought a convenient term for this complex of symptoms, which is the most common type of mental disturbance encountered with neurologic disease, but none seems appropriate. There is both a reduction in the amount of thought and action, and a slowing of reaction time. MacCabe refers to this condition as "mental asthenia," which has the merit of distinguishing it from depression. We prefer to call it *psychomotor asthenia.* Much of this change in behavior is accepted by the patient with forebearance; if any complaint is made, it is of being weak, tired, or dizzy (nonrotational). Inordinate drowsiness, apathy, equanimity, or stoicism may be prominent features of this state. Within a few weeks or months these symptoms become more prominent. When questioned, a long pause precedes each reply, and at times the patient may not bother to respond at all. Or at the moment the examiner decides that the patient has not heard the question and prepares to repeat it, an appropriate answer is given, usually in few words. Moreover, the responses are often more intelligent than one would expect, considering the torpid mental state. There are, in addition, patients who are confused or demented (see Chaps. 19 and 20). The dullness and somnolence increase gradually and finally, as increased intracranial pressure supervenes, they progress to stupor or coma.

Mental symptoms of this type cannot be ascribed to disease in any particular part of the brain, but the tumors most likely to cause them are the ones that interfere with long association fiber systems of the cerebral white matter (frontal, temporal, and corpus callosum gliomas); growths which are limited to the cortex and subcortical white matter are less likely to affect the mind. Much of the drowsiness, torpor, inertia, lack of spontaneity, and general restriction of mental horizon is related to increased intracranial pressure and is unrelated to the site and nature of the lesion.

Headaches These are an early symptom in about one-third of "tumor patients," and are variable in nature. In some the pain is slight, dull in character, and episodic; in others it is severe and either dull or sharp, but also transitory or intermittent. If there are any characteristics of the headache, they would be its nocturnal occurrence, its presence on first awakening, and perhaps its deep nonpulsatile quality. However, these are not specific attributes, since migraine, hypertensive vascular headaches, etc., may also begin in the early morning hours or on awakening. Tumor patients do not always complain of the pain even when it is present but may betray its existence by placing their hands on their forehead and looking distressed. When headache appears later in the course of the psychomotor asthenia syndrome, it serves to clarify the diagnosis, but not nearly as much as does the occurrence of a seizure.

The mechanism of the headache is not known. In the majority of instances, the CSF pressure is normal during the first weeks when the headache is present, and one can attribute it only to local swelling of tissues and to distortion of blood vessels in or around the tumor. Later the headache appears to be related to generalized rises in intracranial pressure. Tumors above the tentorium cause headache on the side and in the vicinity of the tumor, in the orbital frontal, temporal, or parietal region; those in the posterior fossa usually cause ipsilateral retroauricular or occipital headache. With elevated intracranial pressure, bifrontal and bioccipital headache is the rule, regardless of the location of the tumor.

Vomiting This symptom appears in about one-third of the patients with a tumor syndrome of this type and usually accompanies the headache. It is more frequent with tumors of the posterior fossa. The most persistent vomiting that we have observed was in a patient with a low brainstem glioma and in another with a subtentorial meningioma. Some patients may vomit unexpectedly and forcibly, without preceding nausea (projectile vomiting), but others suffer both nausea and great pain. Usually the vomiting is not related to the ingestion of food; often it occurs before breakfast.

No less frequent is the complaint of *giddiness* or *dizziness.* As a rule it is not described with accuracy and consists of an unnatural sensation in the head, coupled with feelings of strangeness and insecurity when the position of the head is altered. Frank positional vertigo may be a symptom of a tumor in the posterior fossa (see Chap. 14).

Seizures The occurrence of focal or generalized seizures is the other major manifestation of cerebral tumor. They have been observed, in various series, in 20 to 50 percent of all patients with cerebral tumors. The occurrence of a seizure for the first time during adult years and the existence of a localizing aura are always suggestive of tumor. The localizing significance of seizure patterns has already been discussed (see page 214). There may be one seizure or many, and they may follow the other symptoms or precede them by weeks or months or, exceptionally, by several years in cases of astrocytoma, oligodendrocytoma, or meningioma.

Management The management of patients who present any of the aforementioned symptoms requires brief discussion. Any impairment of intellectual function—especially if accompanied by recurrent headache that is different from the patient's customary headaches or by a seizure, appearing for the first time—justifies a careful review of the patient's general medical status. In obtaining further data, one must rely heavily on the observations of other members of the family. A thorough neurologic examination must follow, with careful inspection of optic fundi, and with testing of visual fields, motor, reflex, and sensory functions in the limbs, alertness, memory, visuospatial orientation, facility in language (speaking, reading, writing, and understanding the spoken word), and calculation. Sooner or later, regional or localizing symptoms and signs will be discovered, but nearly always they are slight and subtle; it is only by repeated examinations that one will note the earliest stages of a hemiparesis, aphasia, visual field defect, hemianesthesia, etc. Signs of increased intracranial pressure may become manifest and establish the diagnosis of tumor with reasonable certainty even before focal or lateralizing signs are detectable.

Choosing the appropriate time for performing diagnostic tests requires balanced clinical judgment. Since many of the symptoms described above could be due to any number of diseases, it is wise to observe the patient for a time with repeated examinations and not to proceed precipitously with a series of expensive and difficult procedures. As the clinical picture begins to unfold, a CT scan and plain films of skull and chest should always be obtained (to help exclude metastatic carcinoma), and lumbar puncture, EEG, and radionuclide scans should be performed, preferably after admitting the patient to a hospital. Perimetry, audiograms, and vestibular and psychometric tests are also helpful in the study of many of these patients. Pneumoencephalography and arteriography should be reserved for those in whom the clinical syndrome is already strongly suggestive of tumor and then only if the CT scan has not clarified the problem

sufficiently. These procedures are too costly and hazardous to be used routinely in every "tumor suspect."

The cerebral tumors which are most likely to produce the syndrome described above are the following: glioblastoma multiforme, astrocytoma, oligodendroglioma, ependymoma, metastatic carcinoma, meningioma, and primary reticulum cell sarcoma.

Glioblastoma multiforme The glioblastoma multiforme accounts for 15 to 20 percent of all intracranial tumors, for about 55 percent of all tumors of the glioma group, and for more than 90 percent of gliomas of the cerebral hemispheres in adults. Although predominantly cerebral in location, similar tumors may be observed in the brainstem, cerebellum, or spinal cord. The peak incidence is in middle adult life, but no age group is exempt. According to Zülch, the incidence in men is twice that in women.

The glioblastoma has been known since the time of Virchow and was definitively recognized as a glioma by Bailey and Cushing in their histogenetic classification. It is highly malignant, infiltrates the brain extensively, and may attain enormous size before attracting medical attention. It may extend to the meningeal surface or the ventricular wall, which probably accounts for the increase in CSF protein (more than 100 mg per 100 ml in many cases), as well as for an occasional pleocytosis of 10 to 100 cells or more, mostly lymphocytes. At autopsy about 50 percent of glioblastomas are bilateral or occupy more than one lobe of a hemisphere; between 3 and 6 percent show multicentric foci of growth. The tumor has a variegated appearance, being a mottled gray, red, orange, or brown, depending on the degree of necrosis and presence of hemorrhage, recent or old. It is highly vascular, and in an arteriogram one can often see a network of abnormal vessels, mistaken at times for a hemangioma, and displacement of normal vessels as an effect of the tumor mass (*mass lesion*). Some part of one lateral ventricle is often distorted, and both lateral and third ventricles are displaced contralaterally, which may be demonstrated by CT scan (Fig. 30-3). The vessels in the tumor are excessively permeable to radioactive phosphorus, arsenic, mercury, and technetium, which explains the diagnostic usefulness of radioactive scanning techniques.

The characteristic histologic findings are great cellularity with pleomorphism of cells and hyperchromatism of nuclei; identifiable astrocytes with fibrils in combination with astroblasts in many cases; tumor giant cells and cells in mitosis; a hyperplasia of endothelial cells of small vessels; and necrosis, hemorrhage, and thrombosis of vessels. Originally regarded as derived from and composed of primitive embryonal cells, this tumor is now generally thought to arise from mature astrocytes. For this reason, Kernohan and Sayre have suggested that the term *glioblastoma* be replaced by *malignant astrocytoma, grade 3 or 4*. Russell and Rubinstein agree, and we have found this way of classifying gliomas clinically useful. However, there is little to be gained by changing the name of the tumor, particularly since there are instances in which the cells are so undifferentiated that a derivation from astrocytes is not demonstrable.

Clinically, the diffuse cerebral symptoms and seizures (present in 30 to 40 percent of cases) usually give way in a few weeks or months to a more definite frontal, temporal, parieto-occipital, or callosal syndrome. Seldom, however, do the symptoms and signs point to one lobe, and often one is satisfied to be able to specify the general region of the hemisphere which is involved. MacCabe's observation that 10 percent of glioblastomas begin with mental symptoms matches our own experience.

In a minority of patients (4 percent, according to Frankel and German) the onset of symptoms may be sudden. The usual explanation is hemorrhage or the rapid expansion of a cyst within the tumor. The CSF is

occasionally bloody under these circumstances. We have also observed patients in whom the clinical picture evolved within 2 to 3 weeks and, with unsuccessful surgery, ended fatally soon afterward. However, in most cases, symptoms have been present for 3 to 6 months before the diagnosis is established. The rapid development of focal cerebral symptoms is usually related to cerebral edema, hemorrhages, and necrosis rather than tumor infiltration. Indeed, it is remarkable how large and extensive the tumor may become before it deranges cerebral function.

The natural history of glioblastoma is well known. Less than a fifth of all patients survive for 1 year after the onset of symptoms, and only about 10 percent beyond 2 years. Cerebral edema, temporal lobe–tentorial herniation, midbrain compression, midbrain and pontine hemorrhages, and increased intracranial pressure are usually the immediate causes of death.

An unusual variant of this tumor is *gliomatosis cerebri*, in which an entire hemisphere, or the entire brain is diffusely infiltrated, without a discrete tumor mass being seen. Many small series of such cases have been reported since Nevin introduced this term in 1938, but no clear-cut clinical picture has emerged. Impair-

Figure 30-3

Glioblastoma multiforme. A. Unenhanced CT scan showing a large lesion of the hemisphere encroaching on the lateral ventricle. B. Enhanced view.

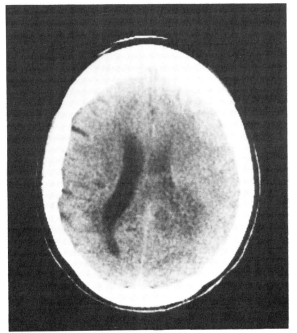

A

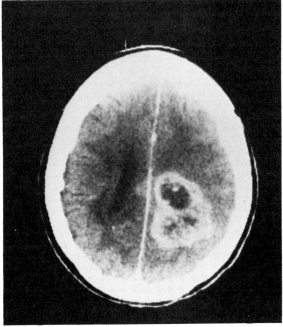

B

ment of intellect, headache, and seizures are the major manifestations and do not set these cases apart from the usual forms of glioblastoma where the tumor may also be more widespread than the macroscopic picture suggests. Also, we find it difficult if not impossible to differentiate, on clinical grounds alone, gliomatosis cerebri from degenerative and slow virus diseases of the cerebrum (see Chap. 42).

The treatment of glioblastomas is rather unsatisfactory. At operation only part of the tumor can be removed, but such a procedure may prevent rapid demise. The multicentricity of these tumors defies the scalpel. In patients whose condition is relatively good, stereotaxic needle biopsy is a relatively safe way of establishing diagnosis. Radiation therapy in daily doses up to 5000 rads in 3 to 4 weeks increases natural survival by 2 to 3 months. Dexamethasone improves neurologic functioning. Several series of reported cases comparing (1) surgical excision, (2) surgical excision and radiation, (3) surgical excision, radiation, and antitumor drugs, and (4) radiation or (5) drug treatment alone show the combination of excision-radiation-drugs to be slightly advantageous. Survival beyond 2 years occurs but is exceptional; most of the patients die in approximately 12 months. The trend of therapy is away from craniotomy, but the antineoplastic drugs procarbazine, bleomycin, BCNU (carmustine) and CCNU (lomustine), vincristine, and methotrexate have been disappointing.

Astrocytoma This tumor may occur anywhere in the brain or spinal cord. Favored sites are the cerebrum, cerebellum, hypothalamus, optic nerve and chiasm, and pons. It is a slowly growing tumor of infiltrative character with a tendency to form large cavities or pseudocysts. Other tumors of this category are noncavitating, grayish white, firm, and relatively avascular, almost indistinguishable from normal white matter, with which they merge imperceptibly. Calcium deposits may occur in parts of the tumor and may be seen in plain films of the skull. The CSF is acellular, and the only abnormality is the increased pressure and protein content in some cases. The tumor may distort the lateral and third ventricles and displace the anterior and middle cerebral arteries (seen in CT scans and arteriograms; see Fig. 30-4). Microscopically the tumor tissue is composed of well-differentiated astrocytes of fibrillary, protoplasmic, or transitional type. Many cerebral astrocytomas eventually undergo malignant degeneration and present as mixed astrocytomas and glioblastomas.

In about half the patients with astrocytoma, the opening symptom is a focal or generalized seizure, and between 60 and 75 percent of patients have recurrent seizures in the course of their illness. The onset of focal seizures in individuals 20 to 60 years of age should always arouse suspicion of a cerebral astrocytoma. Other subtle cerebral symptoms follow after months, sometimes after years. Headaches and signs of increased intracranial pressure are relatively late occurrences.

The temporal lobe gliomas have given particular difficulty in diagnosis when mental symptoms precede seizures. Slight character and personality changes, moodiness, pseudoneurotic symptoms, and episodes suggestive of schizophrenia may precede or follow the onset of temporal lobe seizures. Hemiparesis, in frontal gliomas, may present only as a slight drift of the outstretched arm, a mild limp, and enhanced tendon reflexes, and may remain slight in degree for a long time. Language difficulties and sensory changes are also frequently slight and subtle.

Seizures, headaches, and the mental symptoms described above may be present for several years, in some instances for 10 years or even longer, before the diagno-

Figure 30-4
Enhanced CT scan showing a large astrocytoma of the left cerebral hemisphere, distorting the lateral and third ventricles. Mental symptoms and recurrent generalized seizures had been present for many years before the diagnosis was made.

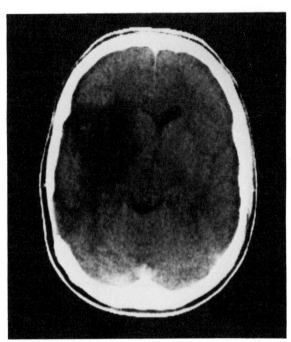

sis is made. In contrast to glioblastoma, the average survival period after the first symptom is 67 months in cases of cerebral astrocytoma, and 89 months in cerebellar ones. The cystic astrocytoma of the cerebellum is particularly benign. It declares itself in children by some combination of gait unsteadiness, unilateral cerebellar signs, and increased intracranial pressure (headaches, vomiting), and some patients are alive and well as long as 30 years after excision of the cyst. In such cases, of course, accuracy of the original diagnosis of neoplasm is always open to question. The astrocytomas of the pons, hypothalamus, optic nerves, and chiasm are discussed in more detail later on in this chapter.

Excision of a part of the cerebral astrocytoma and particularly removing the cystic part may allow survival in a functional state for many years.

Oligodendroglioma This tumor was first identified by Bailey and Cushing in 1926, and described more fully by Bailey and Bucy in 1929. They considered it to be benign. It is relatively infrequent, constituting about 5 to 7 percent of all intracranial gliomas. In some cases the tumor may be recognized macroscopically because of its pinkish gray multilobular form, its relative avascularity and firmness (slightly tougher than surrounding brain), and its tendency to encapsulate and to form calcium and small cysts. Most oligodendrogliomas, however, are indistinguishable grossly from other gliomas. The type cell has a small, round nucleus and halo of unstained cytoplasm. The cell processes are few and stubby, and are visualized only with silver carbonate stains. Microscopic calcifications are observed frequently mainly in relation to zones of necrosis. Probably half the tumors generally classified as oligodendrogliomas are in fact mixed types (oligodendroglioma-astrocytoma).

The most common sites are the frontal lobes (40 to 70 percent), often deep in the white matter with little or no surrounding edema; other parts of the cerebrum, third ventricle, brainstem, cerebellum, and spinal cord are less frequent sites. By extending to the pial surface or ependymal wall, the tumor may metastasize distantly in ventriculosubarachnoid spaces, accounting for 11 percent of Palmeter and Kernohan's series of gliomas with meningeal dissemination (less frequent than medulloblastoma and glioblastoma). Malignant degeneration (evidenced by greater cellularity and by numerous and abnormal mitoses) occurs in about a third of cases; this more malignant form is called oligodendroblastoma. Rarely the tumor converts to a glioblastoma.

The typical oligodendroglioma grows slowly, and the interval between the first symptom and surgical intervention varies from 28 to 70 months. As with astrocytomas, the first symptom in more than half the patients is a focal or generalized seizure; eventually 70 percent of patients develop seizures. In patients whose illness began with seizures, Weir and Elvidge found that an average of 7.3 years had elapsed before the patient came to surgery. Approximately 15 percent of patients enter the hospital with early symptoms and signs of increased intracranial pressure; but even by the time surgery is performed, only about half of all cases have increased intracranial pressure, and only about one-third have focal cerebral signs (hemiparesis). Much less frequent syndromes are unilateral extrapyramidal rigidity, cerebellar ataxia, Parinaud's syndrome, and meningeal oligodendrogliosis (cranial-spinal nerve palsies, hydrocephalus, lymphocytes in CSF). Calcium is seen in plain films of the skull in approximately half the cases.

Surgical excision is the treatment of choice. The mean postoperative survival time in the large series of Weir and Elvidge was 5 years, comparable to that of supratentorial astrocytomas. A number of operated patients have had malignant recurrences within a few months of operation.

Ependymoma and ependymoblastoma This tumor proves to be more complex and variable than other gliomas. Correctly diagnosed by Virchow as early as 1863, its origin from ependymal cells was suggested by Mallory, who found the typical blepharoplasts (small, darkly staining dots, related to ciliation of these cells) in a sacral tumor. Two types were recognized by Bailey and Cushing: one type was the ependymoma, and the other, with more malignant and invasive properties, was the ependymoblastoma. More recently a myxopapillomatous type, localized exclusively in the filum terminale of the spinal cord, has been identified (see Chap. 35). Kernohan and Sayre include choroid plexus papillomas with the ependymomas, because of their common origin in the anlage of the lining cells of the ventricular cavities.

Ependymomas are of glioepithelial origin, arising from ependymal cells (also called neuroectodermal cells) with their characteristic cilia and blepharoplasten, and subependymal astroctyes. As one might expect, the tumors arise from the walls of the ventricles and either grow into the ventricle or adjacent brain tissue. Favorite sites are the fourth, third, and lateral ventricles, and caudal part of the spinal cord. Grossly, those in the fourth ventricle are grayish pink, firm, cauliflower-like growths; those in the cerebrum, arising from the wall of the lateral ventricle, may be large (several centimeters in diameter), reddish gray, softer, and more clearly demarcated from adjacent tissue than astrocytomas, but they are not encapsulated. The tumor cells tend to form canals and rosettes, the presence of which are useful in histologic diagnosis.

Approximately 5 percent of all intracranial gliomas are of this type; the percentage is higher in children (10 to 12 percent). About 40 percent of the infratentorial ependymomas occur in the first decade of life, a few as early as the first year. The supratentorial ones are more evenly scattered through all age groups. In Zülch's series, 120 were supratentorial and 64 infratentorial.

The *symptomatology* depends on the location of the growth. The fourth ventricle is the commonest intracranial site and the clinical manifestations of a tumor in this location will be described later in this chapter. Cerebral ependymomas resemble the other gliomas in their clinical expression. Seizures occur in approximately one-third of the cases. Other localizing cerebral symptoms and signs are not in any way peculiar to this type of tumor. The duration of symptoms from first symptom to operation ranges from 4 weeks, in the most malignant types, to 7 to 8 years. Unlike the medulloblastoma, which almost always runs a rapid course, the ependymoma may have either a short or long course, but it is the latter that serves as a useful clue to diagnosis. In the follow-up study of 101 cases in Norway, where ependymomas comprised 1.2 percent of all primary intracranial tumors (and 32 percent of intraspinal tumors), the postoperative survival was poor. Within 1 year 47 percent died, but 13 percent were alive after 10 years. Postoperative irradiation extended the survival period (Mørk and Løken).

Meningioma   This is a benign tumor, first illustrated by Matthew Bailie, in his *Morbid Anatomy* (1787), and first recognized by Bright, in 1831, to originate from the dura mater or arachnoid. It was analyzed from every point of view by Harvey Cushing and was the subject of one of his most important monographs. Meningiomas comprise about 15 percent of all intracranial tumors and have their highest incidence in the seventh decade.

The precise origin of meningiomas is still moot. According to Rubinstein, they may arise from dural fibroblasts, but most of them come from arachnoidal cells, in particular from those packing the arachnoid villi. Since these clusters of arachnoidal cells penetrate the dura in largest number in the vicinity of venous sinuses,

these are the sites of predilection. Grossly the tumor is firm, gray, and sharply circumscribed, and it takes the shape of the space in which it grows; i.e., some tumors are flat and plaquelike, others are round and lobulated. They may indent the brain and acquire the pia-arachnoid as part of their capsule, but always they are sharply demarcated from the brain tissue. Rarely, they arise from arachnoidal cells within the choroid plexus, forming intraventricular meningiomas. Microscopically the cells are relatively uniform with round or elongated nuclei, visible cytoplasmic membrane, and a characteristic tendency to encircle one another, forming whorls and *psammoma bodies*. Cushing and Eisenhardt subdivided meningiomas into many subtypes depending on the character of the stroma and their relative vascularity, but the validity of such a classification is debatable.

The most common sites are the sylvian region, superior parasagittal surface of frontal and parietal lobes, olfactory grooves, lesser wings of the sphenoid bones, tuberculum sellae, superior surface of cerebellum, cerebellopontine angles, and spinal canal. Inasmuch as they extend to the dural surface, they often invade and erode the cranial bones or excite an osteoblastic reaction. Sometimes they give rise to an exostosis on the external surface of the skull. Some meningiomas, such as those of the olfactory groove, sphenoid wing, and tuberculum sellae, may express themselves by highly distinctive syndromes that are diagnostic in themselves; these will be described further on in this chapter. The following remarks apply only to meningiomas of the parasagittal, sylvian, and other surface areas.

Small meningiomas, less than 2.0 cm in diameter, are often found at autopsy in middle-aged and elderly persons, without having caused symptoms. Only when they exceed a certain size and indent the brain do they alter function. The size that must be reached before symptoms appear varies with the size of the space in which they grow and the surrounding anatomic arrangements. Small tumors in the floor of the third ventricle are more likely to be symptomatic than small ones that lie over the cerebrum. Focal seizures are often an early sign. The parasagittal frontal-parietal meningioma may cause a slowly progressive spastic weakness and/or numbness of the opposite leg, and later of both legs. The sylvian tumors are manifested by a variety of signs in accord with their topography.

Meningiomas may evince neurologic signs for 10 to 15 years before diagnosis is established, attesting to their slow rate of growth. Some tumors reach enormous size before coming to medical attention. A few may be detected in plain films or in CT scans in individuals with unrelated neurologic diseases. Increased intracranial pressure eventually occurs, but it is less frequent in the overall group of meningiomas than in gliomas.

Diagnosis is greatly facilitated by the ready visualization of meningiomas with isotopic and contrast-enhanced CT scanning (Fig. 30-5) and by arteriography, which reveals the prominent vascularity as a "blush." The EEG is less altered than in gliomas. The CSF protein is usually elevated.

Surgical excision should afford permanent cure in all accessible surface tumors. A few show malignant, invasive qualities. There may be recurrence if removal is incomplete. The most dangerous ones lie beneath the hypothalamus, along the medial part of the sphenoid bone and parasellar region, or anterior to the brainstem. By invading adjacent bone they become inoperable. Carefully planned radiation therapy is beneficial both in cases where the tumor is inoperable and in those in which the tumor is incompletely removed (Leibel et al.).

Reticulum cell sarcoma (microglioblastoma) Essentially this is a histiocytic sarcoma, and it may originate in any part of the reticuloendothelial system. The meningeal and perivascular histiocytes and the microgliocytes, the representatives of this system in the brain, are its natural sources. This class of tumors was systematically delineated by Ewing and later by Parker and

Jackson. The earliest primary intracranial examples were reported by Yuile (1938) and by Kinney and Adams (1943). The article by Schaumburg, Plank, and Adams summarizes the literature up to 1973.

The tumor may arise in any part of the cerebrum or cerebellum and may be either monofocal or multifocal. It forms a pinkish gray, soft, ill-defined, infiltrative mass, difficult at times to distinguish from a malignant glioma. Perivascular and meningeal spread results in shedding of cells into the CSF. The tumor is highly cellular, with little tendency to necrosis. The nuclei are oval or bean-shaped with scant cytoplasm. Mitotic figures are numerous. The stainability of reticulum and microglial cells, the latter by silver carbonate, serves to distinguish this tumor microscopically.

The reticulum cell sarcoma grows as rapidly as the glioblastoma, and the interval between the first symptom and operation has been approximately 3 months. Focal cerebral signs predominate over headache and other signs of increased intracranial pressure. In children the tumor may simulate the cerebellar symptomatology of medulloblastoma. Lymphocytic and mononuclear pleocytosis in the CSF is more frequent than with gliomas, and tumor cells may be seen.

Figure 30-5

Contrast-enhanced CT scans. A. Falx meningioma. B. Sphenoid wing meningioma.

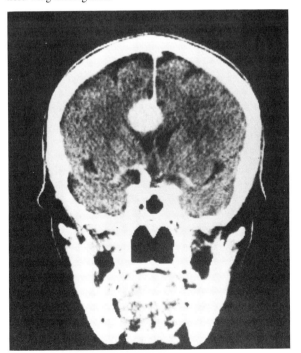

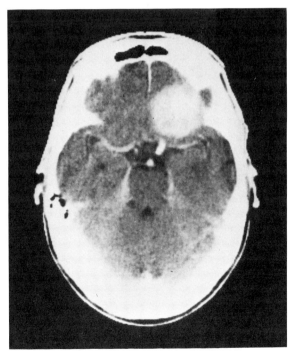

A

B

This tumor should be suspected in individuals who have been given immunosuppressant drugs for long periods of time, a circumstance which appears to favor its development. It is sometimes a complication of obscure medical conditions such as iridocyclitis and idiopathic parotitis (Mikulicz syndrome). Its frequency is increasing in our clinics.

Craniotomy and biopsy are necessary for diagnosis. Radiation therapy is highly effective. One of our patients had only a small recurrence after 5 years, and others have survived several years.

Metastatic carcinoma Of the secondary intracranial tumors only metastatic carcinoma occurs with high frequency. Occasionally one encounters a rhabdomyosarcoma, Ewing's tumor, chorioepithelioma, lymphoma, carcinoid, etc., but these tumors occur so infrequently that their cerebral metastases seldom become a matter of diagnostic concern. Intracranial metastases are of three main patterns—those to the skull and dura, those to the brain itself, and those of the craniospinal meninges (*carcinomatous meningitis*).

Metastases to the skull and dura can occur with any tumor that metastasizes to bone, but are particularly common with carcinoma of the breast and prostate. These secondary deposits often occur without metastases to the brain itself and are believed to reach the skull via Batson's vertebral venous plexus—a valveless system of veins that runs the length of the vertebral column from the pelvic veins to the large venous sinuses of the skull, bypassing the systemic circulation. Metastatic tumors of the convexity of the skull are usually asymptomatic (only rarely do they extend to the brain), but those of the base may involve the cranial nerve roots or the pituitary body. Bony metastases are readily recognized on bone scans and plain skull films, which should always include Towne views. Occasionally, a carcinoma metastasizes to the subdural surface and compresses the brain, like a subdural hematoma.

Carcinomas reach the brain by hematogenous spread. About a third of them come from the lung, and half this number from the breast; melanoma is the third most frequent metastasizing tumor (brain metastases at autopsy in 75 percent of all cutaneous melanomas, according to Amer et al.); the gastrointestinal tract (stomach, colon, or rectum) and kidney are the next most common sources. Carcinoma of the gallbladder, liver, thyroid, testicle, uterus, ovary, pancreas, etc., account for the remainder. Carcinoma of the prostate, esophagus, oropharynx, or skin (except for melanocarcinoma)

rarely metastasize to the brain. In more than 70 percent of cases, the metastases are multiple and are scattered through both the cerebrum and cerebellum; often they lie near the surface in the gray and subcortical white matter and meninges. Hypernephroma and thyroid carcinoma have a slightly greater tendency to form solitary metastases than other tumors, and as with chorioepithelioma and some lung, renal, and melanotic tumors, the metastases are likely to be hemorrhagic. The tumor tissue generally has all the gross and microscopic features of any carcinomatous implant; it forms a circumscribed mass, usually solid but sometimes cystic, and excites rather little glial reaction but much regional vasogenic edema (Fig. 30-6).

The usual clinical picture in metastatic carcinoma of the brain does not differ from that of glioblastoma multiforme. Headache, focal weakness, mental and behavioral abnormalities, seizures, ataxia, aphasia, and signs of increased intracranial pressure—all inexorably progressive—are the common clinical manifestations. However, a number of unusual syndromes also occur. One that presents particular difficulty in diagnosis is a widespread *carcinomatous encephalopathy* with headache, nervousness, depressed mood, trembling, mental confusion, and forgetfulness, a picture very much like that of general paresis. *Carcinomatosis of the cerebellum*

Figure 30-6

Contrast-enhanced CT scan showing a large solitary metastasis (choriocarcinoma) with surrounding edema.

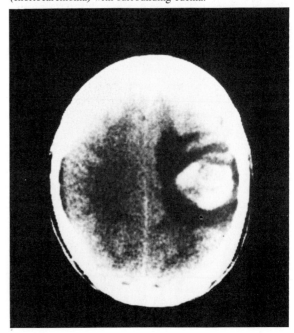

with headache, dizziness, and ataxia (the latter being brought out only by having the patient walk) is another condition that is difficult to diagnose during life. Sometimes the onset of neurologic symptoms is abrupt rather than insidious. Some cases of sudden onset can be explained by bleeding into the tumor, but others cannot be explained in this way. There is also no ready explanation for the spontaneous improvement that sometimes occurs in cases of abrupt onset.

Widespread dissemination of tumor cells throughout the meninges and ventricles (carcinomatous meningitis) has been the pattern in about 4 percent of neurologic metastases in our cases of adenocarcinoma of breast, lung, and gastrointestinal tract, melanoma, and childhood leukemia. Headache, backache, radicular pain, cranial nerve palsies, and dementia have been the principal manifestations. Half the patients develop hydrocephalus. Tumor cells have been identified by cytocentrifugation and millipore filtering in about one-half of our last 100 patients at the Massachusetts General Hospital (Hochberg). Elevation of protein and low glucose levels are other common CSF findings. In 40 percent of cases there was evidence of one or more parenchymal lesions by CT scan, and in some cases CT scan showed enhancement of the cerebral cortex in addition. Treatment consists of radiation therapy to the symptomatic areas, followed by the intrathecal administration of methotrexate or cytarabine, but these measures rarely alter the progressive deterioration. Survival after diagnosis is rarely longer than several weeks or months.

When these several syndromes due to metastatic tumor are fully developed, diagnosis is relatively easy. If only headache and vomiting are present, a common error is to explain these symptoms on a psychological basis. One should make such a diagnosis only if the patient has the standard symptoms of some psychiatric illness. A CT scan, before and after the injection of a contrast agent, is the single most sensitive test for the presence of intracerebral metastases (Fig 30-6). Lumbar puncture, chest films, sedimentation rate (increased in 70 percent of cases of metastatic carcinoma but not in glioblastoma), and other radiologic examinations (gastrointestinal series, barium enema, and pyelograms if symptoms point to visceral involvement) are advisable. Metastatic disease must be distinguished from a primary tumor of the brain and from the neurologic syndromes which sometimes accompany carcinoma but which are not due to the invasion or compression of the nervous system by tumor, i.e., polyneuropathy (especially with carcinoma of the lung), polymyositis, spinocerebellar degeneration (ovarian and other carcinomas), and certain cerebral disorders (multifocal leukoencephalopathy, "limbic encephalitis"). These latter syndromes are discussed fur-

ther on, under "Remote Effects of Neoplasia on the Nervous System."

The treatment of secondary tumor of the nervous system is undergoing change. The CT scan is revealing an increasing number of solitary parenchymatous metastases. If there is no evidence of tumor metastases in other organs and the patient is in good condition, surgical excision followed by radiation is now being undertaken frequently. For multiple metastases radiation therapy and steroids nearly always result in some improvement. Certain drugs—more effective in some tumors than others—are showing promising results:

Testicular carcinoma	*cis*-Platinum
Nasopharyngeal carcinoma	*cis*-Platinum
	Methotrexate
	Bleomycin
Non-Hodgkin's lymphoma	High-dose methotrexate
Chorioepithelioma and Wilms's tumor	High-dose methotrexate
Estrogen-receptive breast carcinoma	Tamoxiphen

Some of these drugs, such as methotrexate, can be injected intrathecally or into the ventricle via a subcutaneous reservoir in meningeal carcinomatosis.

Despite all these therapeutic measures, survival is only slightly prolonged. The average period of survival with therapy is about 6 months. Between 15 and 30 percent live for a year and 5 to 10 percent for 2 years. The patients with bone metastases live longer than those with parenchymatous and meningeal metastases.

Lymphomas of the nervous system Included under this heading are all tumors composed of cells that reside in lymph nodes, i.e., lymphocytes, lymphoblasts, histiocytes and reticulum cells, plasma cells, and the progenitors of these cells (stem cells). Since the brain and spinal cord have no lymphatic system and none of the cellular elements listed above, one would not expect tumors originating from such cells to form in the CNS. There is one exception, however, and that is the histiocytic sarcoma or reticulum cell sarcoma which derives from histiocytes or mononuclear leucocytes and microgliactyes, as pointed out above. Any one of the lymphomas may invade the epidural space from bone, especially in the spinal canal (see Chap. 35).

As a rule, lymphomas of other organs (Hodgkin's

disease, lymphocytic and lymphoblastic lymphomas, plasmacytomas and reticulum cell sarcomas) do not metastasize to the brain. In our large series of cases and in a review of over 10,000 autopsies we observed only a half dozen instances where patients with Hodgkin's disease also had deposits of tumor cells in the brain, and there were no intracerebral metastases of multiple myeloma or plasmacytoma. However, we have observed a fair number of cases of lymphoblastoma of the meninges (with cranial and spinal nerve involvement or one or more cerebral foci). Some had or soon developed lymphatic leukemia and lymphadenopathy. Of course in childhood leukemias the craniospinal leptomeninges are often involved and require intrathecal drugs and radiation. Sometimes lymphoblastic infiltrates appear in the brain quite rapidly during a "blast crisis" and produce a variety of perplexing neurologic pictures. Response to radiotherapy may be quite dramatic. When methotrexate is administered intraventricularly to patients with posterior fossa tumors and evidence of ventricular obstruction, it may cause a necrotizing encephalopathy that may be difficult to distinguish from leukemic infiltrates or hemorrhage (Shapiro et al.).

Sarcomas of the brain These are malignant tumors composed of cells derived from mesenchymal tissues (fibroblasts, rhabdomyocytes, lipocytes, osteoblasts, smooth muscle cells). They take their names from their histogenetic derivation, viz., fibrosarcoma, rhabdomyosarcoma, osteogenic sarcoma, and sometimes from the tissue of which the cells are a part, viz., adventitial sarcomas, hemangiopericytoma. A special group, the histiocytic sarcomas, have been described above under reticulum cell sarcoma, and another is associated with glioblastoma, i.e., gliosarcoma. A new entity called neoplastic angioendotheliosis probably should be included in this group (see further on).

All these tumors are relatively rare. Occasionally one or more deposits of these types of tumors will occur as a metastasis from a sarcoma in another organ. Others are primary in the cranial cavity and exhibit as one of their unique properties a tendency to metastasize to nonneural tissues, which happens infrequently in primary glial tumors. In the gliosarcoma group it would seem that a meningeal fibrosarcoma has been induced by an oncogenic agent in a glioma, or vice versa. The peak incidence is at about the same age as in gliomas (fifth and sixth decades). Temporofrontal-basal location is noted in 40 percent.

The so-called *monstrocellular sarcomas*, so named for the giant cell of spindle form, are highly malignant, rapidly growing, necrotizing masses which compress the brain but are encapsulated. Survival after extirpation and radiation seldom exceeds 12 months according to Distelmaier who reviewed 27 German cases. The hemangiopericytomas and adventitial sarcomas originate in adventitial perithelia of the meningeal vessels and are more variable in their course.

Distressing is the fact that a few sarcomas have developed 5 to 10 years after gamma irradiation, or in one instance after proton beam irradiation, of the brain.

Neoplastic angioendotheliosis or *angioendotheliomatosis* is a condition in which anaplastic malignant cells are found in capillaries and larger vessels in one or several regions of the brain and other organs. The neoplastic cells are thought to be endothelial cells. A confusing clinical picture with apathy, language difficulties, gait disorder, weight loss evolving over several weeks or months has been noted in several of our cases. When examined there may be slight focal or lateralizing signs and papilledema. Operation and biopsy confirm the diagnosis. Peripheral nerves may be involved; the CSF is under increased pressure, and the protein is raised. The condition ends fatally in a few months. The first case was reported by Strouth et al. in 1965, and Dolman et al. have reviewed the literature. We have observed several cases and have the impression that the condition represents hematogenous spread of tumor cells from another organ rather than endotheliosis.

Tumors of infective origin (granulomas and parasitic cysts) *Tuberculoma* is much less frequent in the United States than it was 30 to 40 years ago, and *gumma* has become almost nonexistent. In fact, a patient with syphilis and a positive serologic reaction of the CSF has a greater chance of having two diseases—a cerebral neoplasm and asymptomatic neurosyphilis—than of having a gumma. Tuberculomas may occur in any part of the brain, but in children they are more likely to develop in the posterior fossa, i.e., in the cerebellum or brainstem, than in the cerebrum. Often there are a small number of cells and an increase of protein in the CSF because the lesion usually lies contiguous to the meninges; it may at any time give rise to a tuberculous meningitis with its typical CSF formula (50 to 300 cells, mostly lymphocytes; elevated protein; decreased glucose and chloride). With the CT scan a presumed tuberculoma in a tuberculous patient may be treated with antituberculous drugs and observed to disappear.

In parts of South America and in certain other underdeveloped parts of the world, tuberculoma and gumma are more frequent, and one can usually obtain clues as to their nature from the presence of similar disease in other parts of the body, especially the lungs, and characteristic changes in the CSF. In addition, *Cysticercus cellulosae* and *hydatid cysts* are common lesions and should always be suspected when seizures, increased intracranial pressure, or diffuse cerebral symptoms develop in the adult. Radiographs of the skull and skeletal muscles (e.g., thigh) may reveal characteristic calcific deposits in cysticercosis. *Cryptococcus* and other fungal granulomas and *Schistosoma japonicum* infection may also present as space-occupying cerebral lesions. All these disorders are discussed further in Chap. 31.

PATIENTS WHO PRESENT WITH SIGNS OF INCREASED INTRACRANIAL PRESSURE

A certain number of patients when first seen show the characteristic symptoms and signs of increased intracranial pressure [periodic bifrontal and bioccipital headaches which awaken the patient during the night or are present upon awakening, vomiting that may or may not be expected (projectile), mental torpor, unsteady gait, sphincteric incontinence, and papilledema]. The physician confronted with this clinical problem is forced to take immediate action because a critical rise in intracranial hypertension may occur at any time and result in coma, respiratory arrest, and death. Admission to a hospital with a neurosurgical service is mandatory; nevertheless all the medical aspects of the patient's problem should be explored first.

   Three questions demand immediate answers: (1) Does the patient have a space-occupying intracranial lesion? (2) Where in the cranial cavity is it situated? (3) What is its nature? With respect to the first question, it is well to keep in mind that a number of medical conditions, which are discussed in other parts of this text, may simulate an intracranial growth that causes only the general symptoms of increased intracranial pressure. These are (1) benign intracranial hypertension or pseudotumor cerebri (page 435), (2) hypertensive encephalopathy (page 582), (3) chronic pulmonary disease with hypercapnia and hypoxia (page 731), (4) chronic meningitis or adhesive arachnoiditis and/or aqueductal stenosis (page 477), (5) thrombosis of cerebral veins and dural sinuses (page 486), (6) some endocrinopathies (adrenal tumor, Addison's disease, or hypoparathyroidism; page 741), (7) excessive vitamin A and tetracycline therapy in children, (8) withdrawal from corticosteroid therapy in children, (9) toxic pseudotumor from chlordecone or Kepone therapy (Sanborn et al.), and sometimes (10) corticosteroid therapy.

   Another condition that can simulate intracranial neoplasm is a *supratentorial* or *infratentorial arachnoid cyst* (localized pseudotumor). This lesion, which is probably congenital, presents clinically at all ages but may only become evident in adult life, when it gives rise to symptoms of increased intracranial pressure and sometimes to focal cerebral signs as well. In infants and young children, macrocrania and extensive unilateral transillumination are characteristic features. Usually these cysts overlie the sylvian fissure, less often other parts of the cerebral convexity; occasionally they are interhemispheric or lie under the cerebellum. They may attain a large size, to the point of enlarging the middle fossa and elevating the lesser wing of the sphenoid, but they do not communicate with the ventricle. The cysts are readily recognized on the nonenhanced CT scan, which shows a well-circumscribed deficiency with the density of CSF. Such cases should also be studied by angiography, so as not to overlook a chronic subdural hematoma, which is often associated and which may not be visualized on the CT scan.

True and False Localizing Signs   If the clinical findings permit the exclusion of the aforementioned causes of increased intracranial pressure, there is reasonable certainty that the patient has an intracranial growth. The problem then is to search for signs that will localize the lesion. In doing this, several pitfalls must be avoided. One common source of error is to place undue reliance on a sign which proves to have no localizing value whatsoever. One should distrust any symptom or sign which develops late, after headache and increased intracranial pressure have been established, for it often turns out to be a *false localizing sign*. Under these circumstances drowsiness, slowness in response, inattentiveness, and emotional blunting can be found as often with cerebellar as with cerebral growths. Unsteadiness of gait, urinary incontinence, and psychomotor asthenia may occur as part of a communicating hydrocephalus from any cause. Unilateral or bilateral abducens palsy [due to stretching of the sixth nerve(s)] is another common false localizing sign, and reference has already been made to the ptosis, dilated pupil, ipsilateral hemiparesis, and bilateral Babinski signs that result from temporal lobe herniation. Jacksonian and generalized seizures and ipsilateral or bilateral corticospinal signs may be observed in the advanced stages of a cerebellar tumor.

   Early and sometimes relatively slight focal signs that may be easily overlooked are sometimes the most reliable guides to the localization of the tumor. Examples of useful early signs are a mild weakness or stiffness and hyperreflexia of an arm and leg in a frontal tumor; ataxia of gait (but not of limbs) and head tilt in cerebellar tumors; paralysis of upward gaze and Argyll-Robertson pupillary phenomenon in pinealomas; pale optic disks and chiasmal field defects in craniopharyngiomas; and homonymous visual inattention and sensory extinction in posterior cerebral tumors (see page 310).

The tumors most likely to cause increased intracranial pressure without conspicuous focal or lateralizing signs are medulloblastoma, ependymoma of the fourth ventricle, hemangioblastoma of the cerebellum, pinealoma, colloid cysts of the third ventricle, and craniopharyngioma. In addition, in some of the cerebral gliomas discussed in the preceding section, particularly those of the corpus callosum and frontal lobes, increased intracranial pressure may occasionally precede focal cerebral signs.

Medulloblastoma This is a rapidly growing embryonic tumor which arises in the posterior part of the cerebellar vermis and neuroepithelial roof of the fourth ventricle of children, and rarely in the cerebellum or cerebrum of adults. The tumor frequently fills the fourth ventricle and infiltrates its floor. Seedings of the tumor may be seen on the walls of the third and lateral ventricles, on the meningeal surfaces of the cisterna magna, and around the spinal cord. The tumor is solid, grayish pink in color, and fairly well demarcated from the adjacent brain tissue. It is very cellular, and the cells are small and closely packed with hyperchromatic nuclei, little cytoplasm, many mitoses, and a tendency to form clusters or pseudorosettes.

The origin of this tumor has never been settled. One theory is that it is derived from the fetal remnants of the external granular layer of the cerebellum; another is that it arises from cell rests in the posterior medullary velum. Bailey and Cushing introduced the name *medulloblastoma* in 1926. Medulloblasts as such have never been identified in the fetal or adult human brain, but the term is retained for no other reason than its familiarity.

The majority of the patients are children 4 to 8 years of age and males outnumber females 3:2 or 3:1 in the many reported series. As a rule, symptoms have been present for 1 to 5 months before the diagnosis is made. The clinical picture is distinctive. Typically, the child becomes listless, vomits repeatedly, and has a morning headache. The first diagnosis which suggests itself may be gastrointestinal disease or abdominal migraine. Soon, however, a stumbling gait, frequent falls, and a squint

lead to a neurologic examination and the discovery of papilledema. The latter is present in all except a small number of patients by the time they come to the attention of a neurologist, except when the tumor is located laterally in the cerebellum, as it usually is in adults. Dizziness (positional) and nystagmus are frequent. A small proportion of patients have a slight sensory loss on one side of the face, and a mild facial weakness; bilateral abducens palsies are frequent. Head tilt, the occiput being tilted back and away from the side of the tumor, indicates the presence of cerebellar herniation. Rarely, signs of spinal root and subarachnoid metastases precede cerebellar signs. Extraneural metastases (cervical lymph nodes, lung, liver, bone) may occur, usually after craniotomy which allows tumor cells to reach scalp lymphatics. Decerebrate attacks ("cerebellar fits") may appear in the late stages of the disease.

The tumor is highly radiosensitive. Also, the results of systemic or intrathecal administration of methotrexate and vincristine have been encouraging in some cases. With surgery, radiation of the entire neuraxis, and chemotherapy, there is a 5-year survival in more than two-thirds of cases.

The *neuroblastoma* of childhood is a tumor of nearly identical histologic type arising in the adrenals and metastasizing widely. Usually it remains extradural if it invades the cranial and spinal cavities. A peculiar polymyoclonia with opsoclonus may complicate the disease. Its neuropathologic basis is unsettled (viral cerebellitis?).

Ependymoma and papilloma of the fourth ventricle *Ependymomas,* as pointed out earlier in this chapter, arise from the walls of the ventricles. About 70 percent of them originate in the fourth ventricle, according to Fokes and Earle (Fig. 30-7). The clinical syndrome produced by these latter tumors is much like that of the medulloblastoma except for the longer course and the lack of early cerebellar signs. Fourth ventricular ependymomas occur mostly in childhood, less often in adult life. In Henschen's series of 68 cases, 28 occurred in the first decade, 10 in the second, and 30 after the age of 20 years. Males have been affected almost twice as often as females. The tumor usually arises from the floor of the fourth ventricle, extends through the foramina of Luschka or Magendie and may invade the medulla. Symptoms may be present for 1 or 2 years before diagnosis and operation. About two-thirds of the patients come to notice because of increased intracranial pressure; in the rest, vomiting, difficulty in swallowing, paresthesias of extremities, abdominal pain, vertigo, and head tilt are prominent manifestations. The tumor is not very sensitive to x-ray, and surgical removal offers the only hope of survival. Prolongation of life is sometimes attained through ventriculoatrial shunting of CSF.

Papillomas of the choroid plexus are about one-fifth as frequent as ependymomas. They arise mainly in the lateral and fourth ventricles, occasionally in the third. The two most authoritative articles (by Laurence et al. and by Matson and Crofton) give the ratios of lateral/third/fourth ventricular locations as 50:10:40. The tumor, which takes the form of a giant choroid plexus, has as its cellular element the plexus epithelium, which is closely related embryologically to the ependyma.

Essentially these are tumors of childhood. Fully 50 percent cause symptoms in the first year of life and 75 percent in the first decade. In the younger patients hydrocephalus proves to be the presenting syndrome, often aggravated acutely by hemorrhage; there may be papilledema, an unusual finding in a hydrocephalic child. Headaches, lethargy, stupor, spastic weakness of legs, unsteadiness of gait, and diplopia are more frequent in the older child. Sometimes patients present with a syndrome of the cerebellopontine angle (see further on),

where the tumor presumably arises from choroid plexus that projects into the lateral recess. One consequence of the tumor is said to be increased CSF formation, which contributes to the hydrocephalus (see page 433). Treatment is by surgical excision, but palliative shunting may be needed first if the patient's condition does not permit surgery.

Hemangioblastoma of the cerebellum This tumor is also referred to on page 850. Dizziness, ataxia of gait or of the limbs on one side, symptoms and signs of increased intracranial pressure, and in some instances an associated retinal angioma and polycythemia and spinal cord involvement constitute the neurologic syndrome. Dominant inheritance is well known. The angiographic picture is characteristic: a tightly packed cluster of small vessels forming a mass 1.0 to 2.0 cm in diameter. Craniotomy with opening of the cerebellar cyst and excision of the mural hemangioblastomatous nodule may be curative. Those in the spinal cord are frequently associated with a syringomyelic lesion (greater than 70 percent of cases), may be multiple, and are located mainly in the posterior columns. A retinal hemangioblastoma may be

Figure 30-7
Ependymoma of the fourth ventricle. A. Contrast-enhanced CT scan in a 4-year-old girl who presented with signs of increased intracranial pressure. Note hydrocephalus and end of shunt tube in left lateral ventricle. B. An ependymoma growing out of the fourth ventricle.

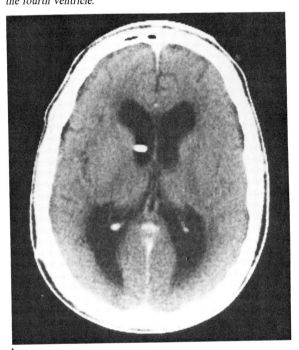

A

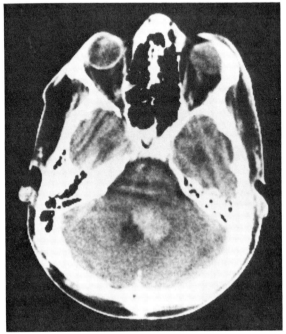

B

the initial finding and may lead to blindness if not treated by laser beam. The children of a parent with a hemangioblastoma of the cerebellum should be examined regularly for an ocular lesion or a renal cell carcinoma (another complication).

Pinealoma There has been much uncertainty as to the proper classification of pineal tumors. Originally they were all thought to be composed of pineal cells, hence true pinealomas, a term suggested by Krabbe. Globus and Silbert believed that the tumors originated from embryonic pineal cells. But later Russell repudiated these ideas of histogenesis and declared the majority to be atypical teratomas, resembling seminoma of the testicle. Today several types are recognized—the germinoma (atypical teratoma), the pinealoma (pineocytoma and pineoblastoma), the true teratoma with cellular derivatives of all three germ layers, and the glioma.

The *germinoma*, which makes up more than half of all pineal tumors, is a firm, discrete, mass that usually reaches 3 to 4 cm in greatest diameter. It compresses the superior colliculi and sometimes the superior surface of the cerebellum, and narrows the aqueduct of Sylvius. Often it extends anteriorly into the third ventricle and may then compress the hypothalamus. A separate atypical teratoma or germinoma, unrelated to the pineal gland, may also arise in the floor of the third ventricle; this has been referred to as an ectopic pinealoma or *suprasellar germinoma*. Microscopically, these tumors are composed of large, spherical epithelial cells separated by a network of reticular connective tissue which contains many lymphocytes. The gliomas have the usual morphologic characteristics of an astrocytoma of varying degrees of malignancy. Children, adolescents, and young adults—males more than females—are affected. Rarely does one see a patient with a pineal tumor which has developed after the thirtieth year of life.

In some cases the clinical syndrome consists solely of symptoms and signs of increased intracranial pressure. Beyond this, the most characteristic localizing signs—an inability to look upward (Parinaud's syndrome) and slightly dilated pupils which react on accommodation but not to light—are related to hydrocephalus (dilatation of the posterior part of the third ventricle compressing the tegmentum of the upper midbrain) and not to the local pressure effects of the tumor. Sometimes an ataxia of the limbs, choreic movements, or spastic weakness appears in the later stages of the

illness, but it is uncertain whether such symptoms are due to compression of the superior cerebellar peduncles and other midbrain structures, or to hydrocephalus. Precocious puberty occurs in males. Diagnosis is made by CT scan which reveal anterior displacement of the aqueduct of Sylvius and posterior part of the third ventricle (Fig. 30-8). The CSF may contain tumor cells and lymphocytes.

Formerly judged to be inoperable, the use of the operating microscope now makes excision by a supracerebellar or transtentorial approach feasible. Operation for purposes of excision and histologic diagnosis is advised because each type of pineal tumor needs to be managed differently. Moreover one may occasionally find an arachnoidal cyst that needs only excision. The atypical teratomas should be removed insofar as possible, and whole neuraxis radiation should be given for cerebrospinal metastases. In our practice several patients who had gliomas removed survived more than 5 years. A combination of atrioventricular shunt and radiation of the tumor is favored in some clinics. If the tumor rapidly decreases in size, one can assume that it is a dysgerminoma. Stereotaxic biopsy is being used to an increasing degree and may obviate surgical exploration which carries a small but significant mortality (Pecker et al.). Ventriculoatrial or ventriculoperitoneal shunt is required in the majority of cases.

Figure 30-8
Contrast-enhanced CT scan showing a pineal dysgerminoma.

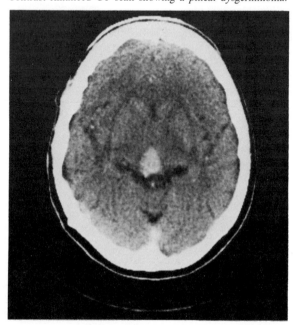

Colloid (paraphysial) cyst and other tumors of the third ventricle The most important of these is the colloid tumor, which is derived, it is generally believed, from ependymal cells of a vestigial structure of the third ventricle known as the paraphysis. The cysts that form in this structure are always situated in the anterior portion of the third ventricle between the interventricular foramens and are attached to the roof of the ventricle. The cysts vary in size from 1 cm to 3 to 4 cm in diameter, are oval or round with a smooth external surface, and are filled with a glary, gelatinous material containing a variety of mucopolysaccharides. The wall is composed of a layer of epithelial cells, some ciliated, and surrounded by a capsule of fibrous connective tissue. Although congenital, these cysts practically never declare themselves clinically until adult life, when they block the third ventricle and produce an obstructive hydrocephalus.

This tumor should be suspected in patients who present with intermittent severe bifrontal-biooccipital headaches, sometimes modified by posture ("ball valve" obstruction of the third ventricle), or with crises of headache and obtundation, "frontal lobe" incontinence, unsteadiness of gait, bilateral paresthesias, dim vision, and weakness of the legs with sudden falls ("drop attacks"). Some of the patients have no headache and present with the symptoms of low-pressure hydrocephalus. The treatment for many years has been surgical excision, but recently satisfactory results have been obtained by ventriculoatrial shunt of the CSF, leaving the benign growth untouched. Decompression of the cyst by aspiration under stereotaxic control has also been used.

Other tumors found in the third ventricle and giving rise mainly to obstructive symptoms are craniopharyngiomas, papillomas of the choroid plexus, and ependymomas.

Craniopharyngioma (suprasellar epidermoid cyst, Rathke pouch or hypophysial duct tumor, adamantinoma, ameloblastoma) This is a congenital tumor, generally believed to originate from *cell rests* (remnants of Rathke's pouch) at the junction of the infundibular stem and pituitary. By the time the tumor has attained a diameter of 3 to 4 cm, it is almost always cystic. Usually it lies above the sella turcica, depressing the optic chiasm and extending up into the third ventricle. Less often it is subdiaphragmatic, i.e., within the sella, where it compresses the pituitary body and erodes one part of the wall of the sella or a clinoid process; but seldom does it balloon the sella like a pituitary adenoma. Large tumors may obstruct the flow of CSF. The tumor is oval, round, or lobulated and has a smooth surface. The wall of the

cyst and the solid parts of the tumor consist of cords and whorls of epithelial cells (often with intercellular bridges and keratohyalin) separated by a loose network of stellate cells. The cyst contains dark albuminous fluid, cholesterol crystals, and calcium deposits; the calcium can be seen in plain films of the suprasellar region in 70 to 80 percent of cases. The sella beneath the tumor tends to be flattened and enlarged. The majority of the subjects are children, but the tumor is not infrequent in adults, and some of our own patients have been up to 60 years of age.

The presenting syndrome may be one of increased intracranial pressure, but more often it takes the form of a combined hypopituitary-hypothalamic-chiasmal derangement in which case it would be more appropriately placed in the next section of this chapter. The symptoms are often subtle and longstanding. In children, adiposity, delayed physical and psychical development (Froehlich or Lorain syndrome—see page 382), headaches, vomiting, dim vision with chiasmal field defects, optic atrophy, and papilledema comprise the clinical picture. In adults, waning libido, amenorrhea, slight spastic weakness of one or both legs, headache without papilledema, and mental dullness and confusion are the usual manifestations. Later drowsiness, ocular palsies, diabetes insipidus, and disturbance of temperature regulation—indicating hypothalamic involvement—may occur.

In the *differential diagnosis* of the several tumor syndromes described in this section, a careful clinical analysis is often more important than laboratory procedures. Arteriography and electroencephalography are not as helpful as in cerebral tumors. The procedures which are likely to give the most useful information are the CT scan (Fig. 30-9), the air encephalogram or ventriculogram, and the Pantopaque or metrizamide ventriculogram (injection of radiopaque fluid into a lateral ventricle). Modern neurosurgical techniques reinforced by corticosteroid therapy before and after surgery, and careful control of temperature and water balance postoperatively permit excision of the tumor in the majority of cases. The mortality rate in the best neurosurgical clinics ranges from 5 to 8 percent. Stereotaxic aspiration is sometimes a useful palliative procedure. Radiotherapy is a useful adjunct in solid, nonresectable tumors.

In certain marginal states of hydrocephalus the administration of acetazolamide (Diamox) in doses of 250 mg three or four times a day may be beneficial, but only surgical shunting of CSF has given lasting results.

PATIENTS WHO PRESENT WITH SPECIFIC INTRACRANIAL TUMOR SYNDROMES

In this group of tumors general cerebral symptoms and the signs of increased intracranial pressure occur late or not at all. The physician arrives at the correct diagnosis by localizing the lesion accurately from a set of neurologic findings and by reasoning that the etiology must be neoplastic because of the afebrile, steadily progressive nature of the illness. Special radiographic studies of the skull, CSF examination, and, depending on the location of the disease, either CT scanning or arteriography will usually confirm the clinical impression.

Tumors which produce these unique intracranial syndromes are craniopharyngioma (described above), acoustic neuroma and other tumors of the cerebellopontine angle, pituitary adenomas and nonneoplastic enlargements of the sella, meningiomas of the sphenoid ridge and olfactory groove, glioma of the optic nerve

Figure 30-9
Contrast-enhanced mass, which proved to be a craniopharyngioma, filling the entire suprasellar cistern. The patient was a 50-year-old man with a 10-month history of headaches and a chiasmal-optic nerve defect.

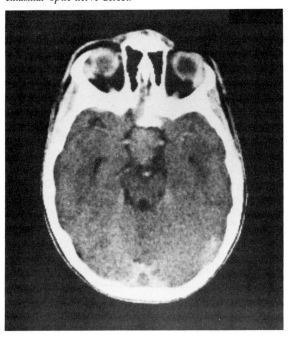

and chiasm, pontine glioma, chordoma, and other erosive tumors at the base of the skull.

Acoustic Neuroma (Schwannoma, Neurofibroma) This tumor was first described as a pathologic entity by Sandifort in 1777, first diagnosed clinically by Oppenheim in 1890, and first recognized as a surgically treatable disease around the turn of the century. Cushing's monograph (1917) was a milestone, and the papers of House and Hitselberger and of Ojemann et al. provide excellent descriptions of the modern diagnostic tests and surgical treatment, as well as a comprehensive bibliography.

Acoustic neuroma occurs occasionally as part of von Recklinghausen's neurofibromatosis, and then it is more likely to occur at an earlier age, to be bilateral, and sometimes to be combined with multiple meningiomas. The usual acoustic neuroma in adults, unassociated with von Recklinghausen's disease, presents as a solitary tumor. Being essentially a schwannoma, it must originate in nerve, usually just distal to the junction between the nerve root and the medulla, i.e., at the point where the axons of the nerve become enveloped in Schwann cells. The point at which this occurs is actually in the internal auditory foramen, several millimeters outside the brainstem. The examination of small tumors reveals that they practically always originate on the vestibular division of the eighth nerve just within the internal auditory canal; as they grow, they extend into the posterior fossa to occupy the angle between the cerebellum and pons (cerebellopontine angle). In their lateral position they are so situated as to compress the seventh, fifth, and less often the ninth and tenth cranial nerves which they implicate in various combinations. Later they displace and compress the pons and lateral medulla and obstruct the CSF circulation.

Certain biologic data assume clinical importance. The highest incidence is in the fifth decade, and the sexes are equally affected. Familial occurrence marks only the tumors which are a part of von Recklinghausen's disease.

The earliest symptoms reported by the patients in the series of Ojemann et al. were loss of hearing (33 of 46 patients), headache (4 of 46), disturbed sense of balance (3 of 46), unsteadiness of gait (3 of 46), and facial pain, tinnitus, and facial weakness—each in a single case. Some patients sought medical advice soon after the appearance of the initial symptom, some late, after other symptoms had occurred. Usually, by the time of the first neurologic examination, the clinical picture was quite complex. One-third of the patients were troubled by vertigo associated with nausea, vomiting, and pressure in the ear. The vertiginous symptoms resembled those of

Ménière's disease, but differed in that discrete attacks separated by normalcy were rare. Usually the vertigo coincided more or less with hearing loss and tinnitus (hissing sound like a kettle, bells, high-pitched ringing, or machinery-like roaring). By then, many of the patients were also complaining of unsteadiness, especially on rapid changes of position (e.g., in turning), and this may have interfered with work and other activities. A few of our patients ignored their deafness for many months or years, or attributed it to some other disease, and in them the presenting syndrome consisted of impaired mentation (psychomotor asthenia), imbalance, and sphincteric incontinence. Hearing loss, slight facial weakness, and numbness of a cheek were then the only clinical findings that permitted an acoustic neuroma to be distinguished from some other cause of low-pressure hydrocephalus.

To summarize, the neurologic findings at the time of examination in the above-mentioned series of 46 patients were as follows: eighth nerve involvement (auditory and vestibular) in 45 of 46, facial weakness including disturbance of taste (26 of 46), sensory loss over face (26 of 46), gait abnormality (19 of 46), and unilateral ataxia of limbs (9 of 46). Inequality of reflexes and eleventh and twelfth nerve palsies were present in only a few patients. Signs of increased intracranial pressure appeared late, and were present in not more than 25 percent of our patients. These findings are comparable to those reported by House and Hitselberger.

Audiologic evaluation includes the tuning fork test, pure tone audiogram, speech audiometry, auditory fatigue and recruitment tests, and vestibular tests, all of which have been described in Chap. 14. In combination they permit localization of the deafness and vestibular disturbance to the cochlear and vestibular nerves rather than their end organs in 80 to 90 percent of cases. Radiographs of the internal auditory meatus show enlargement on the affected side in most of the patients. The CSF protein is raised in two-thirds of the patients (over 100 mg per 100 ml in one-third). In patients with loss of hearing, stapedial foot plate puncture can be done and a perilymph protein in excess of 1200 mg per 100 ml has been found in all cases (one cannot use this procedure if there is retained hearing, for it may cause deafness). The contrast-enhanced CT scan (Fig. 30-10) will detect practically all acoustic neuromas that are larger than 2.0 cm in diameter and that project further than 1.5 cm into the cerebellopontine angle (Davis et al.). Smaller intracanalicular tumors are more reliably detected by tomography of the internal auditory canal and by Pantopaque or metrizamide cisternography.

The tumor is usually 2 to 3.5 cm in greatest diam-

eter and oval in shape, conforming to the shape of the space in which it grows; and its surface is smooth, firm, and whitish in color. It is always encapsulated. The spindle-shaped cells of which it is composed, arranged in bundles and palisades, allow ready identification. Mononuclear giant cells and hyperchromatism may suggest malignant change, but mitoses are not present. Hemorrhage and necrosis occur frequently.

The treatment is surgical excision. Neurosurgeons who have had the largest experience with these tumors favor the microsurgical suboccipital transmeatal operation (Ojemann). In most instances the facial nerve can be preserved, and in some, the cochlear nerve as well. In the hands of a skillful otologic surgeon, small tumors can be removed safely by the translabyrinthine approach, if no attempt is to be made to save hearing.

Neurinoma or schwannoma of the trigeminal or gasserian ganglion, and meningioma of the cerebellopontine angle may in some instances be indistinguishable from an acoustic neuroma. They should always be considered if early tinnitus, deafness, and lack of re-

Figure 30-10
Contrast-enhanced CT scan showing a large acoustic neuroma that had produced an obstructive hydrocephalus.

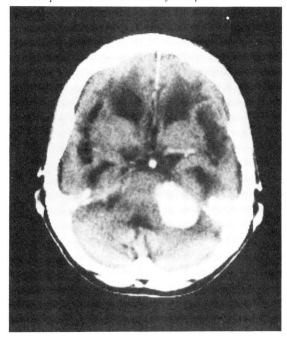

sponse to caloric stimulation ("dead labyrinth") are not the initial symptoms of the cerebellopontine angle syndrome. A true *cholesteatoma (epidermoid) of the temporal bone* may simulate this syndrome, but usually the facial weakness is early and severe, facial twitching is prominent, and deafness is of conductive type and associated with complete loss of labyrinthine function. Other cranial nerve signs, cerebellar ataxia, and increased intracranial pressure are absent. Other disorders that enter into the differential diagnosis are glomus jugulare tumor (see below), basal meningioma, metastatic cancer, syphilitic meningitis, arachnoid cyst, schwannomas of other cranial nerves, vascular malformations, and plasmacytoma of the petrous bone. All these disorders may produce a cerebellopontine angle syndrome, but are more likely to cause only unilateral lower cranial nerve palsies and their temporal course differs (page 474). Occasionally, a tumor that originates in the pons or in the fourth ventricle (ependymoma, astrocytoma, papilloma, medulloblastoma) but grows eccentrically may present as a cerebellopontine angle syndrome.

The *glomus jugulare tumor* is of particular interest. It is a purplish red, highly vascular tumor composed of large epithelioid cells in an alveolar pattern and an abundant capillary network. The tumor is believed to be derived from minute clusters of nonchromaffin paraganglioma cells (glomus bodies) found mainly in the adventitia of the dome of the jugular bulb (*glomus jugulare*) immediately below the floor of the middle ear, but also in multiple other sites in and around the temporal bone. These clusters of cells are part of the chemoreceptor system that includes also the carotid, vagal, ciliary, and aortic bodies. The typical syndrome consists of partial deafness, facial palsy, dysphagia, and unilateral atrophy of the tongue, combined with a vascular polyp in the external auditory meatus and a palpable mass below and anterior to the mastoid eminence, often with a bruit. Other neurologic manifestations are phrenic nerve palsy, numbness of the face, Horner's syndrome, cerebellar ataxia, and temporal lobe epilepsy. The jugular foramen is eroded (visible by x-ray), and the CSF protein may be elevated. Women are affected more than men, and the peak incidence is during middle adult life. The tumor grows slowly over a period of many years, sometimes 10 to 20 or more. Treatment consists of radical mastoidectomy and removal of as much tumor as possible, followed by radiation. The combined intracranial and extracranial two-stage operation has resulted in cure of

many cases (Gardner et al.). A detailed account of this tumor will be found in the article by Kramer.

Pituitary Adenomas   Tumors arising in cells of the anterior pituitary are of considerable interest to neurologists because they often cause visual and other symptoms related to involvement of structures bordering upon the sella turcica. Pituitary tumors are age-linked; they become increasingly numerous with each decade and by the eightieth year, small adenomas are found in more than 20 percent of pituitary glands. Only a small proportion of these enlarge the sella and account for the 6 to 8 percent of pituitary tumors listed in all series of intracranial neoplasms.

On the basis of conventional staining methods, cells of the normal pituitary gland have for many years been classified as chromophobe, acidophil, and basophil, these types being present in a ratio of 5:4:1. Adenomas of the pituitary are most often composed of chromophobe cells (4 to 20 times as common as acidophil cell adenomas); the incidence of basophil cell adenomas is uncertain. Recent histologic studies, utilizing immunofluorescent and immunoperoxidase staining techniques, have been concerned with defining the nature of the cytoplasmic granules of pituitary cells—both of the normal gland and of pituitary adenomas. These methods have shown that either a chromophobe or an acidophil cell may produce prolactin, growth hormone (GH), or thyroid-stimulating hormone (TSH), whereas the basophil cells produce ACTH, β-lipotropin, luteinizing hormone (LH), and follicle-stimulating hormone (FSH).

Pituitary tumors usually arise as discrete nodules in the anterior part of the gland (adenohypophysis). The tumors are reddish gray, soft (almost gelatinous) and often partly cystic. Most often the adenomatous cells are arranged diffusely, with little stroma and few blood vessels; less frequently the architecture is sinusoidal or papillary in type. Variability of nuclear structure, hyperchromatism, cellular pleomorphism and mitotic figures are interpreted as signs of malignancy. Tumors of less than 1 cm in diameter are referred to as "microadenomas," and originally they are confined to the sella. As the tumor grows, it first compresses the pituitary gland; then, as it extends upward and out of the sella, it compresses the optic chiasm; and later, with continued growth, it may extend into the cavernous sinus, third ventricle, temporal lobes, or posterior fossa. Recognition of an adenoma when it is still confined to the sella is of considerable practical importance, since total surgical removal of the tumor or proton-beam therapy are possible at this stage, with prevention of further damage to normal glandular structure and the chiasm. Penetration of the diaphragma sellae by the tumor and invasion of

the surrounding structures makes treatment more difficult.

Pituitary adenomas come to medical attention because of endocrine abnormalities or visual disorder. The
latter usually proves to be a complete or partial bitemporal hemianopia which has developed gradually. Early,
the upper parts of the visual fields may be affected predominantly. A small number of patients will be almost
blind in one eye and have a temporal hemianopia in the
other. Bitemporal central hemianopic scotomata are a
less frequent finding. If the visual disorder is of long
standing, the optic nerve heads are visibly atrophic. In 5
to 10 percent of cases, compression of the cavernous sinus causes some combination of ocular palsies. Other
neurologic abnormalities, rare to be sure, are seizures
from indentation of the temporal lobe, CSF rhinorrhea,
and diabetes insipidus, hypothermia, and somnolence
from hypothalamic compression.

The development of sensitive (radioimmunoassay)
methods for the measurement of pituitary hormones has
made possible the detection of adenomas at an early
stage of their development and the delineation of several
endocrine syndromes.

Amenorrhea-galactorrhea syndrome As a rule,
this syndrome becomes manifest during the child-bearing years. Usually menarche had occurred at the appropriate age; primary amenorrhea is rare. A common history is that the patient took birth control pills, only to
find, when she stopped, that the menstrual cycle did not
reestablish itself. On examination, there may be no abnormalities other than galactorrhea. Serum prolactin
levels are increased (usually in excess of 100 ng/ml). In
general, the longer the duration of amenorrhea and the
higher the serum prolactin level, the larger will be the
tumor. The elevated prolactin levels distinguish this disorder from idiopathic galactorrhea, in which serum prolactin levels are normal.

Males with prolactin-secreting tumors rarely have
galactorrhea and usually present with a larger tumor
and complaints such as headache, impotence, and visual
abnormalities. In normal persons, the serum prolactin
level rises markedly in response to the administration of
chlorpromazine or thyrotropin-releasing hormone
(TRH); patients with a prolactin-secreting tumor fail to
show such a response. With large tumors that compress
normal pituitary tissue, thyroid and adrenal function
will also be impaired.

Acromegaly This disorder is due to an overproduction of growth hormone (GH) occurring after puberty; prior to puberty, an oversecretion of GH produces gigantism. The diagnosis of this disorder, which is
often long delayed, is made on the basis of the characteristic clinical changes, the finding of elevated serum GH
values (> 10 ng/ml), and the failure of the GH level to
rise in response to the administration of glucose or TRH.

Cushing's disease Described in 1932 by Harvey
Cushing, this condition is only about one-fourth as frequent as acromegaly. The cause is in the pituitary gland
in 70 to 80 percent of cases and in the adrenal gland in
the remainder. The syndrome is the result of elevated
blood levels of adrenal corticosteroids which have profound effects on the body, including truncal obesity, hypertension, weakness, amenorrhea, hirsutism, abdominal
striae, glycosuria, osteoporosis, and in some cases a
characteristic psychosis (page 1061). In most cases, the
syndrome is due to an increased secretion of ACTH by
the pituitary, in which instance it is referred to as Cushing's disease. Although Cushing originally attributed the
disease to basophil adenomata, the pathologic change
may consist only of hyperplasia of basophilic cells or a
nonbasophilic adenoma. Seldom is the sella turcica enlarged, and visual symptoms are therefore rare. When
the sella is enlarged, there may be pressure laterally on
structures in the cavernous sinus. A venous sinogram
(injecting contrast medium in a frontal vein to fill the
cavernous sinuses) and the CT scan are of value in the
diagnosis of the pituitary tumors, and the body scan, of
adrenal tumors. The diagnosis of Cushing's disease is
made by demonstrating an increased level of plasma and
urinary cortisol, and the suppression of ACTH and
cortisol levels after high doses of dexamethasone (2 mg
orally every 6 h). A low level of ACTH in the blood,
increased cortisol in the blood and increased free cortisol
in the urine, and nonsuppression of adrenal function after administration of dexamethasone are evidence of an
adrenal source of the Cushing syndrome—usually an adrenal tumor, less often a micronodular hyperplasia.

Diagnosis of pituitary adenoma This is likely
when a chiasmal syndrome is combined with an endocrine syndrome of either hypopituitary or hyperpituitary
type. Laboratory data confirmatory of endocrine disor-
der(s), as described above, and a ballooned sella turcica
in plain films of the skull make diagnosis virtually certain. Patients who are suspected of harboring a pituitary
adenoma, but in whom the plain films are normal,
should have thin-section polytomography in both coronal and lateral planes. Local bulging, asymmetry, or ero-

sion of the sella may betray the presence of a tumor. CT scans, using thin-slice techniques, will demonstrate most pituitary tumors, even some microadenomas.

Conditions other than pituitary adenomas may sometimes expand the sella. Enlargement may be due to intrasellar craniopharyngioma, carotid aneurysm, or cysts of the pituitary gland. Intrasellar, epithelial-lined cysts are rare lesions. They originate from the apical extremity of Rathke's pouch, which may persist as a cleft between the anterior and posterior lobes of the hypophysis. Rarer still are intrasellar cysts that have no epithelial lining and contain thick, dark brown fluid, the product of intermittent hemorrhages. Both of these types of intrasellar cyst may compress the pituitary gland and mimic the effects of pituitary adenomas. Most often the enlargement is of nontumorous type (so-called empty sella). In connection with the latter it is to be noted that there are wide variations in the size of the sella which dictate caution in the interpretation of a slight enlargement.

Nontumorous enlargement of the sella ("empty" sella) results from a defect in the dural diaphragm, which may occur without obvious cause or may follow surgical excision of a pituitary adenoma or a pituitary apoplexy (hemorrhage and/or necrosis in a rapidly growing pituitary adenoma). The arachnoid over the defective diaphragma sellae will bulge through the hole, and the sella then enlarges gradually, apparently as a result of the pressure and pulsations of the CSF acting on the walls of the sella turcica. In the process, the pituitary gland becomes flattened, sometimes to an extreme degree, but the functions of the gland are usually unimpaired. Downward herniation of the optic chiasm occurs occasionally, and may cause visual disturbances simulating those of a pituitary adenoma. *Bitemporal hemianopia with a normal sella* usually means that the causative lesion is a saccular aneurysm of the circle of Willis or a meningioma of the tuberculum sellae.

All radiographic changes associated with nontumorous enlargement of the sella occur below the plane of the diaphragma sellae. CT scans and plain films (using thin-slice techniques) are good screening procedures. However, in all cases of suspected pituitary adenoma, the most definitive diagnostic study is pneumoencephalography with thin section laminography. This procedure will demonstrate intrasellar air, in cases of nontumorous enlargement, as well as the air-soft tissue interface with the flattened pituitary gland or with the pituitary tumor.

The *treatment* of choice of the intrasellar pituitary adenoma or one that has only a small suprasellar protrusion is proton beam radiation. This form of radiation can be focused precisely on the tumor and will destroy it. At the time of writing, Kjellberg had treated over 900 patients at the Massachusetts General Hospital without a single fatality, and in recent years virtually no complications. A single brief transcranial exposure is all that is necessary. The endocrine abnormalities must be corrected by hormone replacement therapy. Unfortunately, proton beam therapy is available in only two centers in the United States. Elsewhere, the major form of treatment is surgical, using a transsphenoidal microsurgical approach, with an attempt at total removal of the tumor and preservation of normal pituitary function. Surgical removal of tumor tissue is followed by radiation therapy. The administration of the dopamine agonist, bromocriptine, which acts as a prolactin inhibitor, may be the only therapy needed or is a useful adjunct in the treatment of the amenorrhea-galactorrhea syndrome and acromegaly. The serotonin antagonist, cyproheptadine, is effective in some cases of Cushing's disease. For microadenomas without enlargement of the sella one may temporize and follow the patient.

Large extrasellar extensions of a pituitary growth must be removed by craniotomy, followed by radiation therapy.

The *pituitary apoplexy syndrome*, described by one of the authors (R.D.A.) with Brougham and Heusner, is characterized by the acute onset of ophthalmoplegia, bilateral amaurosis, drowsiness or coma, with either subarachnoid hemorrhage or pleocytosis and elevated protein in the CSF. It may threaten life, and needs to be treated by dexamethasone (6 to 12 mg every 6 h) and (if there is no improvement after 24 to 48 h) by transnasal decompression of the sella. Some pituitary adenomas are cured by this accident.

Meningioma of the Sphenoid Ridge This tumor is situated over the lesser wing of the sphenoid bone (Fig. 30-5). As it grows, it may expand medially to involve structures in the wall of the cavernous sinus, anteriorly into the orbit, or laterally into the temporal bone. Fully 75 percent are in women and the average age at the time of onset is 50 years. Most prominent among the symptoms are a slowly developing unilateral exophthalmos, slight bulging of the bone in the temporal region, and radiologic evidence of thickening or erosion of the lesser wing of the sphenoid bone. Variants of the clinical syndrome include hyposmia, oculomotor palsy, the syndrome of Tolosa-Hunt (see Table 46-2), blindness and optic atrophy in one eye, sometimes with anosmia and papilledema of the other eye (Foster Kennedy syndrome), mental changes, uncinate fits, and increased intracranial pressure. Sarcomas arising from the skull bones, metastatic carcinoma, orbitoethmoidal osteoma, benign giant cell bone cyst, tumors of the optic nerve, and angiomas of the orbit must be considered in the differential diagnosis. Auscultation of the skull, plain skull films with laminography, bone scans, and carotid arteriography are helpful in differentiating these lesions. The tumor is resectable without further injury to the optic nerve, if the tumor has not invaded the bone and the operating microscope is used during the dissection.

Meningioma of the Olfactory Groove This tumor originates in arachnoidal cells along the cribriform plate. The diagnosis depends on the finding of ipsilateral or bilateral anosmia, ipsilateral or bilateral blindness, often with optic atrophy on one side and papilledema on the other (Kennedy syndrome), and mental changes. The tumors may reach enormous size before coming to the attention of the physician. The anosmia, if unilateral, is rarely if ever reported by the patient. The unilateral visual disturbance may consist of a slowly developing central scotoma. Abulia, confusion, forgetfulness, and inappropriate jocularity (witzelsucht) are the usual psychic disturbances (see page 302). The patient may be indifferent to or joke about his or her blindness. Usually there are radiographic changes along the cribriform plate, and often an extremely high CSF protein level (200 to 400 mg per 100 ml). Except for the largest tumors, extirpation is possible.

Glioma of the Brainstem Astrocytomas of the brainstem (formerly called *bipolar spongioblastomas*) are relatively slow-growing, firm, infiltrating growths which insinuate themselves between tracts and nuclei. They produce a variable clinical picture, depending on their exact location in the medulla, pons, and midbrain. As a rule this tumor begins in childhood (peak age of onset is 7 years, 80 percent appearing before the twenty-first year), and symptoms have usually been present for 3 to 5 months before coming to medical notice. In 90 percent of cases the initial manifestation is a palsy of one or more cranial nerves, most often the sixth and seventh on one side. Long tract signs follow—hemiparesis, unilateral ataxia, ataxia of gait, paraparesis, hemisensory syndromes, gaze disorders, hiccoughs. In the other cases the symptoms occur in the reverse order, i.e., long tract signs precede the cranial nerve abnormalities. The combination of cranial nerve palsy and crossed motor and/or sensory tract signs always indicates brainstem disease. Headache, vomiting, and papilledema usually occur late in the course of the illness. The course is slowly progressive over several years unless some part of the tumor

becomes more malignant (glioblastoma multiforme) in which instance the illness may terminate fatally within months. In some 50 or more fatal cases at the Massachusetts General Hospital, more than half were glioblastomas and had resulted in death within a few months. Patients with pontine astrocytoma may survive for 5 or more years. The main clinical problem is to differentiate this disease from a pontine form of multiple sclerosis, a vascular malformation of the pons, and a brainstem encephalitis. Vertebral angiography and CT scanning to visualize the fourth ventricle, aqueduct, and the prepontine subarachnoid space are helpful in diagnosis. In a few instances surgical exploration is necessary to establish the diagnosis (inspection and possibly biopsy). The treatment is radiation, and if intracranial pressure is increased, a ventriculoatrial (rarely ventriculocisternal) shunt.

Glioma of the Optic Nerves and Chiasm This tumor, like the brainstem glioma, occurs most frequently during childhood and adolescence. In 85 percent of cases the tumor appears before the age of 15 years (average 3.5) and is twice as frequent in girls as in boys (see Cogan). The initial symptoms are dimness of vision with constricted fields, followed by bilateral field defects of homonymous, heteronymous, and sometimes bitemporal type; blindness; and optic atrophy with or without papilledema. Ocular proptosis is the other main symptom. Hypothalamic signs (infantilism, adiposity, polyuria, somnolence, and genital atrophy) occur occasionally. CT scans (Fig. 30-11) and ultrasound examination will usually reveal the tumor, and radiographs will show an enlargement of the optic foramen (greater than 7.0 mm). With this finding and the lack of ballooning of the sella or suprasellar calcification, one can exclude pituitary adenoma, Hand-Schüller-Christian disease, and craniopharyngioma. In adolescents and young adults, the medial sphenoid, olfactory groove, and intraorbital meningiomas are other tumors that cause blindness and proptosis. The treatment is surgical excision or radiation, depending on the exact location. Both gliomas and nontumorous gliotic (hamartomatous) lesions of the optic nerves may occur in von Recklinghausen's disease, and the latter are sometimes impossible to distinguish from tumors.

Chordoma This is a soft, jellylike, grayish pink growth which arises from remnants of the primitive notochord, most often along the clivus (from dorsum sellae to foramen magnum) and in the sacrococcygeal region. It is a rare tumor that affects males more than females, usually in early or middle adult years, and should always be suspected in syndromes involving multiple cranial nerves or the cauda equina. About 40 percent of chordomas occur in each of these two extremities of the neuraxis, and the rest are found at any point in between. The tumor is made up of cords or masses of large cells with granules of glycogen in their cytoplasm, and often with multiple nuclei and intracellular mucoid material. They are locally invasive, but do not metastasize. The neurologic syndrome is remarkable in that all or any combination of cranial nerves from the second to twelfth on one or both sides may be involved. Associated signs in the series of Kendell and Lee were facial pain, conductive deafness, and cerebellar ataxia, the result of pontomedullary and cerebellar compression. The tumors at the base of the skull may destroy the clivus and bulge into the nasopharynx, causing nasal obstruction, discharge, and sometimes dysphagia. Thus, chordoma is one of the

Figure 30-11
Glioma of the optic chiasm. The contrast-enhanced CT scan shows the tumor directly above the dorsum sellae. The patient was a 7-year-old girl with neurofibromatosis who presented with severe visual loss and bilateral optic atrophy.

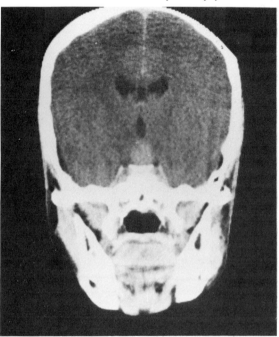

lesions that may present both as an intracranial and extracranial mass, the others being meningioma, neurofibroma, glomus jugulare tumor, and carcinoma of sinuses or pharynx. Midline (Wegener's) granulomas must be differentiated. The treatment of the chordoma is surgical excision and radiation.

Nasopharyngeal Growths Which Erode the Base of the Skull These are rather common in a general hospital, and they arise from the mucous membrane of the paranasal sinuses or the nasopharynx near the eustachian tube, i.e., the fossa of Rosenmueller (*transitional cell carcinoma, Schmincke tumor*). In addition to symptoms of nasopharyngeal or sinus disease, which may not be prominent, facial pain and numbness (trigeminal), abducens palsy, and other cranial nerve palsies may occur. Diagnosis depends on inspection and biopsy of a nasopharyngeal mass, biopsy of an involved cervical lymph node, and radiologic evidence of erosion of the base of the skull. Bone scan, CT scan, and pneumoencephalography are helpful in diagnosis. Biopsy is confirmatory. The treatment is radiation. Carcinoma of the ethmoid or sphenoid sinuses and postradiation neuropathy, coming on years after the treatment of a nasopharyngeal tumor, may produce a similar clinical picture.

Other Tumors of the Base of the Skull There exist a large number and variety of tumors, rather rare to be sure, that derive from cellular elements of tissues at the base of the skull, paranasal sinuses, ears, etc., and which give rise to certain distinctive syndromes. Included in this category are osteomas, chondromas, chordomas, ossifying fibromas, giant cell tumors of bone, lipomas, epidermoids, teratomas, glomus tumors, mixed tumors of the parotid gland, and hemangiomas and cylindromas of the sinuses and orbit. Most of these tumors are benign, but some have a potential for malignant change, becoming sarcomatous and carcinomatous. To the group must be added well-known malignant tumors which metastasize to basal skull bones or involve them as part of a multicentric neoplasia, e.g., reticulum cell sarcoma, Ewing's sarcoma, plasmacytoma, and leukemic deposits.

Details of pathology, embryogenesis, and symptomatology of these various tumors are far too numerous to include in a textbook devoted to principles of neurology. Table 30-3, taken from Bingas' large neurosurgical service in Berlin, summarizes the known facts about each of these tumors, and his authoritative article in the *Handbook of Clinical Neurology* is recommended as a reference and bibliographic source.

Modern radiologic technology serves now to clarify many of the diagnostic problems posed by these tumors. Since many of them arise in, erode, or invade

Table 30-3
The most important clinical syndromes caused by tumors of the base of the skull

Site of lesion	Eponym	Clinical symptoms	Etiology
Anterior part of the base of the skull		Olfactory disturbances (uni- or bilateral anosmia), possibly psychiatric disturbances, seizures.	Tumors which have invaded the anterior part of the base of the skull from the frontal sinus or the ethmoid bone, osteomas. Meningiomas of the olfactory groove.
Superior orbital fissure	Rochon-Duvigneau; syndrome of the pterygopalatine fossa (Behr) and the base of the orbit (DeJean) commencing with a lesion of the maxillary and pterygoid rami and evolving into the superior orbital fissure syndrome.	Lesions of the third, fourth, sixth, and first division of the fifth nerve with ophthalmoplegia, pain and sensory disturbances in the area of V_1; often exophthalmos, some vegetative disturbances.	Tumors: meningiomas, osteomas, dermoid cysts, giant cell tumors, tumors of the orbit, nasopharyngeal tumors, more rarely optic nerve gliomas, eosinophilic granulomas, angiomas, local or neighboring infections, trauma.
Apex of the orbit	Jacod-Rollet (often combined with the syndrome of the superior orbital fissure); infraclinoid syndrome of Dandy.	Visual disturbances, central scotoma, papilledema, optic nerve atrophy; occasional exophthalmos, chemosis.	Optic nerve glioma, infraclinoid aneurysm of the internal carotid artery, trauma, orbital tumors, Paget's disease.
Cavernous sinus	Foix-Jefferson; syndrome of the sphenopetrosal fissure (Bonnet and Bonnet) corresponding in part to the cavernous sinus syndrome of Raeder.	Ophthalmoplegia due to lesions of the third, fourth, sixth, and often fifth nerves, exophthalmos, vegetative disturbances. Jefferson distinguished three syndromes: (1) the anterior-superior, corresponding to the superior orbital fissure syndrome; (2) the middle, causing ophthalmoplegia and lesions of V_1 and V_2; (3) the caudal, in addition affecting the whole trigeminal nerve.	Tumors of the sellar and parasellar area, infraclinoid aneurysms of the internal carotid artery, nasopharyngeal tumors, fistulae of the sinus cavernosus and the carotid artery (traumatic), tumors of the middle cranial fossa, e.g. chondromas, meningiomas, and neurinomas.
Apex of the petrous temporal bone	Gradenigo-Lannois	Lesions of the fifth and sixth nerves with neuralgia, sensory and motor disturbances, diplopia.	Inflammatory processes (otitis), tumors such as cholesteatomas, chondromas, meningiomas, neurinomas of the gasserian ganglion and trigeminal root, primary and secondary sarcomas of the base of the skull.
Sphenoid and petrosal bones, (petrosphenoidal syndrome)	Jacod	Ophthalmoplegia due to loss of function of the third, fourth, and sixth nerves, amaurosis, trigeminal neuralgia possibly with sensory signs.	Tumors of the sphenoid and petrosal bones and middle cranial fossa, nasopharyngeal tumors, metastases.

Table 30-3 (*continued*)
The most important clinical syndromes caused by tumors of the base of the skull

Site of lesion	Eponym	Clinical symptoms	Etiology
Jugular foramen	Vernet	Lesions of ninth, tenth, and eleventh nerves with disturbance of deglutition, curtain phenomenon, sensory disturbances of the tongue, soft palate, pharynx and larynx, hoarseness, weakness of the sternocleidomastoid and trapezius.	Tumors of the glomus jugulare; neurinomas of eighth, ninth, tenth, and eleventh nerves; chondromas, cholesteatomas, meningiomas, nasopharyngeal and ear tumors; infections, angiomas, rarely trauma.
Anterior occipital condyles	Sicard-Collet (Vernet-Sargnon)	Loss of twelfth nerve function (loss of normal tongue mobility) in addition to the symptoms of the jugular foramen.	Tumors of the base of the skull, ear, parotid; leukemic infiltrates; aneurysms, angiomas, and inflammations.
Retroparotid space (retropharyngeal syndrome)	Villaret	Lesions of the lower group of nerves (Sicard-Collet) and Bernard-Horner syndrome with ptosis, miosis, and enophthalmos.	Tumors of the retroparotid space (carcinomas, sarcomas), trauma, inflammations.
Half of the base of the skull	Garcin (Guillain-Alajouanine-Garcin); also described by Hartmann in 1904.	Loss of function of all twelve cranial nerves of one side; in many cases, isolated cranial nerves spared; rarely signs of raised intracranial pressure or pyramidal tract symptoms.	Nasopharyngeal tumors, primary tumors of the base of the skull, leukemic infiltrates of basal meninges, trauma, metastases.
Cerebellopontine angle		Loss of function of eighth nerve (hearing loss, vertigo, nystagmus), cerebellar disturbances, lesions of the fifth, seventh, and possibly ninth, twelfth, cranial nerves. Signs of raised intracranial pressure, brainstem symptoms.	Acoustic neuromas (raised protein in CSF), meningiomas, cholesteatomas, metastases, cerebellar tumors, neurinomas of the caudal group of nerves and the trigeminal nerve, vascular processes such as angiomas, basilar aneurysms.

Source: Adapted from Bingas.

bone, polytomography may reveal an osseous lesion that corresponds to the implicated nervous structures. CT scan is capable also of determining the absorptive values of the tumor itself, and when the lesion is analyzed in this way, an etiologic diagnosis sometimes becomes possible. For example, the absorptive value of lipomatous tissue is different from that of brain tissue, glioma, blood, and calcium. Finally, bone scans (technetium and gallium) display active destructive lesions with remarkable fidelity.

Tumors of the Foramen Magnum Tumors in the region of the foramen magnum are of particular importance because of the difficulties in differentiation from diseases such as multiple sclerosis, Arnold-Chiari malformation, syringomyelia, and bony abnormalities of the craniocervical junction. Erroneous diagnosis is a serious matter since the majority of such tumors are benign and extramedullary, i.e., potentially resectable and curable. If unrecognized, they terminate fatally by causing medullary-spinal compression.

Although not numerous (about 1 percent of all intracranial and intraspinal tumors), sizable series have been collected by several investigators (see Cohen for complete bibliography). In each series neurofibromas (schwannomas or neurilemmomas) and meningiomas are the most common types; others (rare) are teratomas, dermoids, granulomas, cavernous hemangiomas, hemangioblastomas, lipomas, and epidural carcinomas.

Pain in the suboccipital or posterior cervical region, mostly on the side of the tumor, is usually the first and by far the most prominent complaint. It may in some instances extend into the shoulder and even the arm. The latter distribution of pain is more frequent with tumors arising in the spinal canal and extending intracranially than the reverse. For uncertain reasons the pain may radiate down the back, even to the lower spine. Both spine and root pain can be distinguished, the latter due to involvement of either the C_2 or C_3 root or of both. Weakness of one shoulder and arm progressing to the ipsilateral leg and then to the opposite leg and arm is a relatively early and consistent occurrence caused by tumor encroaching upon corticospinal tracts. Occasionally both upper limbs are involved alone; surprisingly, there may be atrophic weakness of hand or forearm or even intercostal muscles with diminished tendon reflexes well below the level of the tumor, an observation made originally by Oppenheim. Whether these latter findings are due to compromise of circulation (descending spinal artery or venous obstruction) or hydromyelia is unsettled. Involvement of sensory tracts to the limbs also occurs; more often it is posterior column sensibility that is impaired on one or both sides with patterns of progression similar to the motor paralysis. Sensation of intense cold in the neck and shoulders has been another unexpected complaint and also "bands" of hyperesthesia round the neck and back of head. Segmental bibrachial sensory loss has been demonstrated in a few of the cases and Lhermitte's sign (electric-like sensations down the spine and limbs on neck flexion) has been reported frequently. Cranial nerve signs most frequently seen, and indicative of cranial extensions, are: dysphagia, dysphonia, and drooping shoulder (due to vagal, hypoglossal, and spinal accessory involvement); nystagmus, episodic diplopia, sensory loss over face, unilateral or bilateral facial weakness, and a Horner syndrome.

The clinical course of such lesions often extends for 2 years or longer, with deceptive and unexplained fluctuations. With dermoid cysts of the upper cervical region, as in the case reported by Adams and Wegner, complete and prolonged remissions from quadriparesis may occur. Of diagnostic value are the finding of an elevated CSF protein and arrest or deformity of the Pantopaque or air column in myelography.

Tumors of the foramen magnum should be suspected in patients with persistent occipital neuralgia, or those who carry a diagnosis of spinal multiple sclerosis, Arnold-Chiari malformation, and chronic adhesive arachnoiditis. Treatment is surgical excision (see Hakuba et al.).

REMOTE EFFECTS OF NEOPLASIA ON THE NERVOUS SYSTEM

In recent years there has been delineated an unusual group of neurologic disorders which occur in patients with carcinoma or some other type of neoplasia, even though the nervous system has not been directly invaded or compressed by the tumor. Some of these disorders, namely polyneuropathy, polymyositis, and the myasthenic-myopathic syndrome of Eaton-Lambert are described on pages 905, 953, and 902, respectively. Here a few remarks will be made about several other degenerative and inflammatory lesions that involve the spinal cord, cerebellum, brainstem, and cerebral hemispheres.

CARCINOMATOUS CEREBELLAR DEGENERATION

This nonmetastatic effect of carcinoma is quite uncommon. In reviewing this subject in 1970, we were able to find only 41 pathologically verified cases. The actual incidence is obviously higher than this reported figure indicates. At the Cleveland Metropolitan General Hospital, in a series of 1700 consecutive autopsies in adults, there were 5 instances of cerebellar degeneration associated with neoplasm.

In most of the reported cases, the underlying carcinoma has been in the lung (44 percent), a figure which reflects the high incidence of this tumor. However, the conjunction of ovarian carcinoma and lymphoma (17 and 14 percent respectively) is higher than would be expected on the basis of the frequency of these malignancies. Carcinomas of the breast, uterus, bowel, and other viscera have accounted for the remaining cases.

Characteristically, the cerebellar symptoms have an insidious onset and steady progression over a period of weeks to months; in about half the cases, the cerebellar signs are recognized before those of the associated neoplasm. Ataxia of gait and of the limbs, affecting arms and legs more or less equally, dysarthria, and nystagmus are the usual manifestations. In addition, there are certain symptoms and signs not ordinarily considered to be cerebellar in nature, notably diplopia, vertigo, and disorders of ocular motility—findings which serve to distinguish carcinomatous from alcoholic and other varieties of cerebellar degeneration. Occasionally myoclonus and opsoclonus may be associated. The CSF may show a mild pleocytosis and increase of protein, or it may be entirely normal. Pathologically, there are diffuse and approximately equally severe degenerative changes in all portions of the cerebellar cortex and deep cerebellar nuclei, associated with perivascular and meningeal clusters of inflammatory cells. In some cases there are associated degenerative changes in the spinal cord, involving the posterior columns and corticospinal tracts. The pathogenesis of this disorder is quite obscure.

PROGRESSIVE MULTIFOCAL LEUKOENCEPHALOPATHY

This is a rare, subacutely evolving, fatal disease of the brain, occurring mainly in adults with chronic lymphoproliferative or myeloproliferative disease, less frequently with tuberculosis, sarcoid, and other nonneoplastic granulomatous disorders. Since it now seems reasonably certain that this neurologic complication of neoplasm has a viral etiology, it is considered with other viral infections, on page 524.

"ENCEPHALITIS" AND "CHRONIC POLIOMYELITIS" IN ASSOCIATION WITH CARCINOMA

The occurrence of encephalomyelitic changes in association with carcinoma, usually of a bronchus, has been described by several authors (Henson et al.; Corsellis et al.). Clinically, the illness has been characterized initially by a disturbance of affect, usually severe anxiety or depression, visual and auditory hallucinations, and convulsive seizures—and later, in a few weeks, by the fairly abrupt impairment of recent memory, and, to a lesser degree, of other intellectual functions. The CSF is usually abnormal, as it is in the cases of carcinomatous cerebellar degeneration. The EEG may show paroxysmal activity and slow waves or both, particularly over one or both temporal lobes ("limbic encephalitis").

The pathologic changes in these cases have been most prominent in the thalami or in the inferomedial portions of the temporal lobes (uncus, amygdaloid nuclei, hippocampus, parahippocampal gyrus), localizations that would explain the defect in retentive memory.

Microscopically, the changes have consisted of an extensive loss of nerve cells, accompanied by an astrocytic proliferation, small patches of necrosis, and a marked perivascular inflammatory reaction. Foci of lymphocytic infiltration have been observed in the leptomeninges as well. A similarity between these changes and those produced by the herpes simplex virus at once suggests itself, and in all probability some of the reported cases are examples of the latter disease.

In other cases, the aforementioned pathologic changes involve the cerebral hemispheres more diffusely. Rarely, the encephalitic changes are confined to the brainstem. In yet others, no pathologic changes are demonstrable in the brain, even though there had been a prominent dementia during life.

A slowly progressive inflammatory anterior horn cell degeneration has been observed very rarely in patients with systemic tumor. One of our patients had Hodgkin's disease, and the other a squamous cell carcinoma of the bronchus.

CARCINOMATOUS MYELOPATHY

In addition to the subacute degeneration of spinal cord tracts that may occur with cerebellar degeneration (see above) there has been described, in association with neoplasm elsewhere in the body, a rapidly progressive form of degeneration that affects the spinal cord primarily (Mancall and Rosales). The latter disorder has been characterized by a rapidly ascending sensorimotor deficit that terminates fatally in a matter of days or weeks and by a roughly symmetrical necrosis of both the grey and white matter of most of the cord. This form of necrotizing myelopathy is distinctly rare, and its status as a remote effect of carcinoma is uncertain.

CONCLUDING REMARKS

The physician's responsibilities in this field of intracranial tumors are (1) to provide a diagnosis (tumor cases must be distinguished from all others); (2) to exclude the possibility that the intracranial mass is part of a general disease which would contraindicate surgery, i.e., metastatic carcinoma, syphilis, tuberculosis, etc.; (3) to exclude the several pseudotumor syndromes; (4) to maintain the patient in the best possible condition, until surgery can be undertaken (fluids, electrolytes, corticosteroid therapy, etc.); and (5) to assist the surgeon in the postoperative medical management.

Tumors of the spinal cord and peripheral nerves are discussed in Chaps. 35 and 45, respectively.

REFERENCES

ADAMS RD, WEGNER W: Congenital cyst of the spinal meninges as cause of intermittent compression of the spinal cord. *Arch Neurol Psychiatry* 58:57, 1947.

ALLEN JC, ROSEN G: Transient cerebral dysfunction following chemotherapy for osteogenic sarcoma. *Ann Neurol* 3:441, 1978.

AMER MH et al: Malignant melanoma and central nervous system metastases. *Cancer* 42:660, 1978.

ANTUNES JL et al: Prolactin-secreting pituitary tumors. *Ann Neurol* 2:148, 1977.

BAILEY P: *Intracranial Tumors*. Springfield, Ill, Charles C Thomas, 1933.

———, BUCY PC: Oligodendrogliomas of the brain. *J Path Bacteriol* 32:735, 1929.

———, CUSHING H: *A Classification of Tumors of the Glioma Group on a Histogenetic Basis with a Correlated Study of Prognosis*. Philadelphia, Lippincott, 1926.

BELLUR SN, CHANDRA V, McDONALD LW: Association of meningiomas with extraneural primary malignancy. *Neurology* 29:1165, 1979.

BINGAS B: Tumors of the base of the skull, in Vinken PJ, Bruyn GW (eds): *Handbook of Clinical Neurology*, vol 17. Amsterdam, North-Holland, 1974, chap 4, pp 136–233.

BRODKEY JS: Hypersecreting pituitary tumors, in *Contemporary Neurosurgery*. Baltimore, Williams & Wilkins, 1979, lessons 18 and 19.

BROUGHAM M, HEUSNER AP, ADAMS RD: Acute degenerative changes in adenomas of the pituitary body—with special reference to pituitary apoplexy. *J Neurosurg* 7:421, 1950.

COGAN DG: Tumors of the optic nerve, in Vinken PJ, Bruyn GW (eds): *Handbook of Clinical Neurology*, vol 17. Amsterdam, North-Holland, 1974, chap 9, pp 350–374.

COHEN L: Tumors in the region of the foramen magnum, in Vinken PJ, Bruyn GW (eds): *Handbook of Clinical Neurology*, vol 17. Amsterdam, North-Holland, 1974, chap 21, pp 719–730.

COPPETO JR, ROBERTS M: Fibrosarcoma after proton-beam pituitary ablation. *Arch Neurol* 36:380, 1979.

CORSELLIS JAN, GOLDBERG GJ, NORTON AR: Limbic encephalitis and its association with carcinoma. *Brain* 91:481, 1968.

CUSHING H: Some experimental and clinical observations concerning states of increased intracranial tension. *Am J Med Sci* 124:375, 1902.

———: *The Pituitary Body and Its Diseases*. Philadelphia, Lippincott, 1912.

———: *Tumors of the Nervus Acusticus and Syndrome of the Cerebellopontine Angle*. Philadelphia, Saunders, 1917.

———: *Intracranial Tumors: Notes Upon a Series of 2000 Verified Cases with Surgical-Mortality Percentages Pertaining Thereto*. Springfield, Ill, Charles C Thomas, 1932.

———, EISENHARDT L: *Meningiomas*. New York, Hafner, 1962.

DAVIS KR, PARKER SW, NEW PFJ: Computed tomography of acoustic neuroma. *Radiology* 124:81, 1977.

DISTELMAIER P: Clinical differential and radiologic pictures of primary sarcomas of the brain. *Nervenarzt* 48:405, 1977.

DOLMAN C, SWEENEY VP, MAGIL A: Neoplastic angioendotheliosis. The case of the missed primary. *Arch Neurol* 36:5, 1979.

DRAYER B et al: Diagnostic approaches to pituitary adenomas. *Neurology* 29:161, 1979.

FISHMAN RA: *Cerebrospinal Fluid in Diseases of the Nervous System*. Philadelphia, Saunders, 1980.

FOKES EC JR, EARLE KM: Ependymomas: Clinical and pathological aspects. *J Neurosurg* 30:585, 1969.

FRANKEL SA, GERMAN WJ: Glioblastoma multiforme. A review of 219 cases with regard to natural history, pathology; diagnostic methods and history. *J Neurosurg* 15:489, 1958.

GARDNER G et al: Combined approach surgery for removal of glomus jugulare tumors. *Laryngoscope* 87:665, 1977.

GLOBUS JH, SILBERT S: Pinealomas. *Arch Neurol Psychiatry* 25:937, 1931.

HAKUBA A et al: Jugular foramen neurinomas. *Surg Neurol* 11:83, 1979.

HARPER CG, STEWART-WYNNE EG: Malignant gliomas in adults. *Arch Neurol* 35:731, 1978.

HASEGALOA H et al: Enhancement of CNS penetration of methotrexate by hyperosmolar intracarotid mannitol or carcinomatous meningitis. *Neurology* 29:1280, 1979.

HENSCHEN T: Tumoren des Zentralnervensystems und seiner Hüllen, in Lubarsch O, Henke F, Rössle R (eds): *Handbuch der speziellen pathologischen Anatomie und Histologie*, vol 13. Berlin, Springer, 1955, part 3, pp 413-1040.

HENSON RA, HOFFMAN HL, URICH H: Encephalomyelitis with carcinoma. *Brain* 88:449, 1965.

HOCHBERG FH: Neurological aspects of systemic tumors, in Isselbacher KJ et al (eds): *Update I: Harrison's Principles of Internal Medicine*, 9th ed. New York, McGraw-Hill, 1981.

——— et al: Quality and duration of survival in glioblastoma multiforme. *J Am Med Assoc* 241:1016, 1979.

HOUSE WF, HITSELBERGER WE: Acoustic tumors, in Vinken PJ Bruyn GW (eds): *Handbook of Clinical Neurology*, vol 17. Amsterdam, North-Holland, 1974, chap 18, pp 666-692.

JEFFERSON G: The tentorial pressure cone. *Arch Neurol Psychiatry* 40:837, 1938.

KAUFMAN B, PEARSON OH, CHAMBERLIN WB: Radiographic features of intrasellar masses and progressive, asymmetrical non-tumorous enlargement of the sella turcica, the "empty" sella, in *Diagnosis and Treatment of Pituitary Tumors*, International Congress Series no. 303. Amsterdam, Excerpta Medica, 1973, pp 100-129.

KAUTZKY R, ZÜLCH KJ: *Neurologisch-neurochirurgische Röntgendiagnostik und andere Methoden zur Erkennung intrakranieller Erkrankungen*. Berlin, Springer Verlag, 1955.

KENDELL BE, LEE BCP: Cranial chordomas. *Br J Radiol* 50:687, 1977.

KERNOHAN JW, SAYRE GP: *Atlas of Tumor Pathology,* fasc. 35: *Tumors of the Central Nervous System.* Washington, Armed Forces Institute of Pathology, 1952.

KINNEY TD, ADAMS RD: Reticulum cell sarcoma of the brain. *Arch Neurol Psychiatry* 50:552, 1943.

KJELLBERG RN: A system of therapy of pituitary tumors: Bragg peak proton hypophysectomy, in Seydel HG (ed): *Tumors of the Nervous System.* New York, Wiley, 1975, pp 145–174.

KLATZO I: Neuropathological aspects of brain edema. *J Neuropathol Exp Neurol* 26:1, 1967.

KRAMER W: Glomus jugulare tumors, in Vinken PJ, Bruyn GW (eds): *Handbook of Clinical Neurology,* vol. 18. Amsterdam, North-Holland, 1975, chap 19, pp 435–455.

LACOUR F, TREVOR R, CAREY M: Arachnoid cyst and associated subdural hematoma. *Arch Neurol* 35:84, 1978.

LASSMAN LP: Tumors of the pons and medulla, in Vinken PJ, Bruyn GW (eds): *Handbook of Clinical Neurology,* vol 17. Amsterdam, North-Holland, 1974, chap 19, pp 693–706.

LAURENCE KM, HOARE RD, TILL K: The diagnosis of choroid plexus papilloma of the lateral ventricle. *Brain* 84:628, 1961.

LEIBEL SA et al: The treatment of meningiomas in childhood. *Cancer* 37:2709, 1976.

MacCABE JJ: Glioblastoma, in Vinken PJ, Bruyn GW (eds): *Handbook of Clinical Neurology,* vol 18. Amsterdam, North-Holland, 1975, chap 2, pp 49–71.

MANCALL EL, ROSALES RK: Necrotizing melopathy associated with visceral carcinoma. *Brain* 87:639, 1964.

MATSON DD, CROFTON FDL: Papilloma of choroid plexus in childhood. *J Neurosurg* 17:1002, 1960.

MEYER A: Herniation of the brain. *Arch Neurol Psychiatry* 4:387, 1920.

MØRK SJ, LØKEN AC: Ependymoma—a followup study of 101 cases. *Cancer* 40:907, 1977.

NEVIN S: Gliomatosis cerebri. *Brain* 61:170, 1938.

OJEMANN RG: Acoustic neuroma, in *Contemporary Neurosurgery.* Baltimore, Williams & Wilkins, 1979, lesson 20.

———, MONTGOMERY W, WEISS L: Evaluation and surgical treatment of acoustic neuroma. *N Engl J Med* 287:895, 1972.

OLIVECRONA H: The surgical treatment of intracranial tumors, in *Handbuch der Neurochirurgie,* vol IV. Berlin, Springer-Verlag, 1967, pt 4, pp 1–301.

OSTERTAG B: *Einteilung und Charakteristik der Hirngewächse; ihre natürliche Klassifizierung Zum Veerständniss von Sitz, Ausbreitung und Gewebsaufbau.* Jena, Fischer, 1936.

PALMETER FE, KERNOHAN JW: Meningeal gliomatosis. *Arch Neurol Psychiatry* 57:593, 1947.

PECKER J et al: Contribution of stereotaxic techniques in the diagnosis and treatment of tumors in the pineal region. *Rev Neurol* 134:287, 1978.

POSNER J, CHERNICK NL: Intracranial metastases from systemic cancer. *Adv Neurol* 19:575, 1978.

PLUM F, POSNER JB: *Diagnosis of Stupor and Coma,* 3d ed. Philadelphia, Davis, 1980.

RIBBERT H: *Geschwulstlehre.* Bonn, Verlag Cohen, 1904.

RIO HORTEGA P DEL: Pineal gland, in Penfield W (ed): *Cytology and Cellular Pathology of the Nervous System,* vol 2. New York, Hoeber-Harper, 1932, chap 14, pp 635–704.

RUBINSTEIN LJ: *Tumors of the Central Nervous System,* fasc. 6, 2d series, Atlas of Tumor Pathology. Washington, Armed Forces Institute of Pathology, 1972.

RUSSELL DS: The pinealoma: Its relationship to teratoma. *J Pathol Bacteriol* 56:145, 1944.

———, RUBINSTEIN LJ: *Pathology of Tumours of the Nervous System,* 4th ed. London, E Arnold, 1977.

SANBORN GE, SELHORST JB et al: Pseudotumor cerebri and insecticide intoxication. *Neurology* 29:1222, 1979.

SCHAUMBURG HH, PLANK CR, ADAMS RD: The reticulum cell sarcoma: Microglioma group of brain tumors. *Brain* 95:199, 1972.

SHAPIRO WR, CHERNIK NL, POSNER JB: Necrotizing encephalopathy following intraventricular instillation of methotrexate. *Arch Neurol* 28:96, 1973.

STROUTH JC et al: Neoplastic angioendotheliosis. *Neurology* 15:644, 1965.

TOMLINSON BE, PERRY RH, STEWART-WYNNE EG: Influence of site of origin of lung carcinomas on clinical presentation and central nervous system metastases. *J Neurol Neurosurg Psychiatry* 42:82, 1979.

VICTOR M, FERRENDELLI JA: The nutritional and metabolic diseases of the cerebellum: Clinical and pathological aspects, in Fields WS, Willis WD Jr (eds): *The Cerebellum in Health and Disease.* St. Louis, Warren H Green, 1970, chap 16, pp 412–449.

VINCENT C, DAVID M, THIEBAUT, F: Cône de pression temporal. *Rev Neurol* 2:116, 1930.

WAGA S, MORIKAWA A, SAKAKURA M: Craniopharyngioma with midbrain involvement. *Arch Neurol* 36:319, 1979.

WEIR B, ELVIDGE AR: Oligodendrogliomas: An analysis of 63 cases. *J Neurosurg* 29:500, 1968.

YUILE CL: A case of primary reticulum cell sarcoma of the brain. *Arch Pathol* 26:1036, 1938.

ZIMMERMAN HM: Brain tumors: Their incidence and classification in man and their experimental production. *Ann NY Acad Sci* 159:337, 1969.

ZÜLCH KJ: *Brain Tumors, Their Biology and Pathology,* 2d ed. New York, Springer, 1965.

CHAPTER 31

NONVIRAL INFECTIONS OF THE NERVOUS SYSTEM

This chapter is concerned mainly with the pyogenic or bacterial infections of the central nervous system (CNS), i.e., bacterial meningitis, intracranial thrombophlebitis, brain abscess, epidural abscess, and subdural empyema. The granulomatous infections of the CNS, notably tuberculosis, syphilis, and certain fungus infections, will also be discussed in some detail. In addition, brief consideration will be given to the CNS effects of certain rickettsias, protozoa, and worms; and to sarcoid, a granulomatous disease of uncertain etiology.

A number of other infectious diseases of the nervous system are more appropriately discussed elsewhere in this book. Diseases due to bacterial exotoxins—diphtheria, tetanus, botulism—are considered with other toxins of the nervous system (Chap. 41). Leprosy, which is essentially a disease of the peripheral nerves, is considered in Chap. 45, which deals with that category of disease. Viral infections of the nervous system, because of their frequency and importance, have been allotted a chapter of their own (Chap. 32).

PYOGENIC INFECTIONS OF THE CENTRAL NERVOUS SYSTEM

All pyogenic infections of the cranial contents originate in one of two ways, by hematogenous spread (emboli of bacteria or infected thrombi) or by extension from cranial structures (ears, paranasal sinuses, osteomyelitic foci in the skull, penetrating cranial injuries, or congenital sinus tracts). In a small number of cases, infection is iatrogenic, being introduced by a lumbar puncture needle. In animals, a needle placed in the subarachnoid space during an experimental bacteremia may cause localization of bacteria at the site of injury. Whether or not this occurs in bacterial infections of humans is not known.

Concerning the hematogenous pathway surprisingly little is known, for human autopsy material seldom divulges information on this point, and animal experiments involving the injection of virulent bacteria into the bloodstream have yielded somewhat contradictory results. In most instances of bacteremia or septicemia, the nervous system seems not to be infected; yet in certain cases, a bacteremia due to pneumonia is the only apparent forerunner of meningitis. In chronic pulmonary diseases, septic emboli have been seen in the pulmonary veins, from which they may reach the cerebral arteries; and in acute and subacute bacterial endocarditis, bacterial emboli are found in cerebral and meningeal arteries. The ideal site of lodgment of these emboli for the production of meningitis—whether in choroid plexuses, or in meningeal or superficial cerebral vessels—has not been ascertained.

With respect to the formation of brain abscess, the notable feature about the cerebral tissues is their resistance to infection. Direct injection of virulent bacteria into the brain of an animal seldom results in abscess formation. In fact, this condition has been successfully produced only by injecting the culture medium along with the bacteria or by causing necrosis of the tissue at the time it is inoculated with bacteria. In humans, infarction of brain tissue by arterial occlusion (embolism) or venous occlusion (thrombophlebitis) appears to be the common and perhaps necessary antecedent.

The cranial epidural and subdural spaces are noticeably invulnerable to blood-borne infective agents, in contrast to the spinal epidural space, which is a considerably more frequent site of suppuration. Furthermore, the cranial bones and the dura mater (which serves essentially as the inner periosteum of the skull) protect the cranial cavity against the ingress of bacteria. This protective mechanism may fail if suppuration occurs in the middle ear, mastoid cells, or frontal, ethmoid, and sphenoid sinuses. Two pathways from these sources have been demonstrated: (1) infected thrombi may form in diploic veins and spread along these vessels into the dural sinuses (into which they flow) and from there in retrograde fashion along the meningeal veins into the brain; and (2) an osteomyelitic focus may form, with erosion of the inner table of bone and invasion of the dura, subdural space, pia-arachnoid, and even the brain substance. Each of these pathways has been visualized in some fatal cases of epidural abscess, subdural empyema, leptomeningitis, cranial venous sinusitis and meningeal thrombophlebitis, and brain abscess. However, in many cases coming to autopsy, the pathway of infection cannot be determined.

A hematogenous infection in the course of a bacteremia usually permits a single type of virulent organism to gain entry to the cranial cavity (in the adult the most common organisms are pneumococcus, meningococcus, *Haemophilus influenzae*, *Listeria monocytogenes*, staphylococcus, and streptococcus; in the neonate, *Escherichia coli* and group B streptococcus); in the infant and child, *H. influenzae* is the most frequent meningeal pathogen. In contrast, when septic material embolizes from infected lungs or congenital heart lesions, or extends directly from ears or sinuses, more than one type of bacterial flora common to these organs may be transmitted. Such "mixed infections" pose difficult problems in therapy. Occasionally, however, in these latter conditions, when active suppuration has occurred, the demonstration of the causative organisms may be unsuccessful, even from the pus of an abscess.

BACTERIAL MENINGITIS (LEPTOMENINGITIS)

This condition consists essentially of an infection of the pia and arachnoid and the fluid in the space which they enclose. Since the subarachnoid space is continuous around the brain, spinal cord, and the optic nerves, an infective agent (or tumor cells or blood) gaining entry to any one part of the space may extend rapidly to all of it, even its most remote recesses; in other words, meningitis is always *cerebrospinal*. Infection also reaches the ventricles of the brain, either directly or by reflux through the foramens of Magendie and Luschka.

Bacterial Meningitis as a Biological Phenomenon The effect of bacteria or other microorganisms in the subarachnoid space is to cause an inflammatory reaction in the pia and arachnoid, in the cerebrospinal fluid

(CSF), and in the ventricles, involving structures that lie within or adjacent to these spaces.

The first effect is hyperemia of the meningeal vessels; very shortly thereafter there occurs a migration of neutrophils into the subarachnoid space. The subarachnoid exudate rapidly increases, particularly over the base of the brain, and extends into the sheaths of cranial and spinal nerves and, for a very short distance, into the perivascular spaces of the cortex. During the first few days, polymorphonuclear leukocytes, many of them containing phagocytized bacteria, are the predominant cells. Within a few days lymphocytes and histiocytes gradually increase in relative and absolute number. During this time there is exudation of fibrinogen and other blood proteins. In the latter part of the second week plasma cells appear and subsequently increase in number. At about the same time the cellular exudate is disposed in two layers—an outer one, just beneath the arachnoid membrane, made up of polymorphonuclear leukocytes and fibrin, and an inner one, next to the pia, composed largely of lymphocytes, plasma cells, and macrophages. Although fibroblasts begin to proliferate very early, they are not conspicuous until later when they take part in the organization of the exudate, resulting in fibrosis of the arachnoid and walling off of pockets of exudate.

During the process of resolution the inflammatory cells disappear in almost the same order as they appear. Neutrophils begin to disintegrate by the fourth to fifth day, and after a few weeks they vanish. Lymphocytes, plasma cells, and macrophages disappear more slowly and may remain in small numbers for several months. The completeness of resolution depends to a large extent on the stage at which the infection is arrested. If it is controlled in the very early stages, there may not be any residual change in the arachnoid, but following an infection of several weeks' duration there is a permanent fibrous overgrowth of the meninges resulting in thickened, cloudy, or opaque arachnoid membrane and often in adhesions between the pia and arachnoid and even the arachnoid and dura.

The pathogenesis of the exudative reaction in the subarachnoid space does not differ from that caused by pyogenic organisms in other tissues. Bacteria or their toxins act as an irritant and induce vascular congestion and increased permeability of venules and capillaries (the first visible cellular exudate is around small veins). Leukocytosis and the migration of neutrophils probably are related to the formation in the meninges of chemical substances which attract these cells in order to destroy the bacteria and toxic substances. Fibrinogen appears very early and is converted to fibrin after a few days, when neutrophils or other cells degenerate and liberate thrombin. Lymphocytes migrate from the blood vessels and are probably the source of the plasma cells which appear later; these cells produce antibodies. The conversion of meningeal histiocytes to macrophages is evidently a response to degeneration of other cellular elements, such as neutrophils and lymphocytes. Productive fibrosis, at first cellular and later fibrous, is the result of subacute and chronic inflammation.

From the earliest stages of the meningitis, changes are found in the small- and medium-sized subarachnoid arteries. The endothelial cells swell, multiply, and crowd into the lumen. This reaction appears within 48 to 72 h and increases in the following days. The adventitial connective tissue sheath becomes infiltrated by neutrophils. Foci of necrosis of the arterial wall sometimes occur. Neutrophils and lymphocytes migrate to beneath the intima, often forming a conspicuous layer. Later there is subintimal fibrosis. This is a striking feature of nearly all types of subacute and chronic infections of the meninges, and notably of tuberculous meningitis.

In the veins, swelling of the endothelial cells and infiltration of the adventitia also occur. The subintimal infiltration is not observed, but there may be a diffuse infiltration of the entire wall. It is in veins so affected that focal necrosis of the vessel wall and mural thrombi are most often found. Thrombophlebitis does not usually develop before the end of the second week of the infection. The unusual prominence of these vascular changes is possibly related to their anatomic peculiarities. The adventitia of the subarachnoid vessels is actually formed by an investment of the arachnoid membrane which is invariably involved by the infectious process. Thus in a sense the vessel wall is affected from the beginning by an inflammatory process arising within itself. The much more frequent occurrence of thrombosis in veins than in arteries is probably accounted for by the thinner walls and the slower current (possibly stagnation) of blood in the former.

Although the spinal and cranial nerves are surrounded by purulent exudate from the beginning of the infection, the perineurial sheaths become infiltrated by inflammatory cells only after several days. Exceptionally in some nerves there is infiltration of the endoneurium, and degenerating myelinated fibers with fatty macrophages and proliferating Schwann cells and fibroblasts may be demonstrated. More often there is little or no damage to nerve fibers. Occasionally cellular infiltrations may be found in the optic nerves or olfactory bulbs, but the more common finding is a proliferation of glial cells beneath the pia, similar to that in the brain tissue.

The outer arachnoid membrane tends to serve as an effective barrier to the spread of infection, but some reaction in the subdural space may occur, nevertheless. This happens more often in infants (subdural effusions) than in adults. Although as a rule there are no large quantities of subdural pus, small amounts of fibrinous exudate are frequently found in microscopic sections which include the cranial and more particularly the spinal dura.

When fibrinopurulent exudate accumulates in large quantities around the spinal cord, it blocks off the spinal subarachnoid space. Hydrocephalus is produced by exudate in the foramens of Magendie and Luschka or in the subarachnoid space around the pons and midbrain, interfering with the flow of CSF from the cisterna magna and lateral recesses to the basal cisterns and convexities (noncommunicating hydrocephalus). In the latter stages fibrous subarachnoid adhesions are an additional and sometimes the most important factor interfering with the circulation of CSF. An infrequent late sequela of bacterial meningitis is *chronic adhesive arachnoiditis* or *chronic meningomyelitis.*

In the early stages of meningitis very little change in the substance of the brain can be detected. After several days microglia and astrocytes increase in number, at first in the outer zone and later in all layers of the cortex. The associated nerve cell changes may be very slight. Obviously some disorder of the cortical neurons must be present from the beginning of the infection to account for the stupor or coma and convulsions so often observed, but several days must elapse before any change can be demonstrated microscopically. It is impossible to say whether or not these cortical changes are due to the diffusion of toxins from the meninges, to a circulatory disturbance, or to some other factor. The changes are not due to the presence of bacteria in the substance of the brain, and should therefore be regarded as a noninfectious encephalopathy. Ischemic necrosis of the cerebral cortex is in some cases the result of cerebral thrombophlebitis, but in others, with quite extensive cortical necrosis, no thrombosed veins are found.

In the early stages of meningitis there may be relatively little change in the ependyma and the subependymal tissues, but in the later stages conspicuous changes are invariably found. The most prominent finding is infiltration of the subependymal perivascular spaces and often of the tissues with neutrophilic leukocytes, and later by lymphocytes and plasma cells. There may be desquamation of ependymal cells. Microglia and astrocytes proliferate, the latter sometimes overgrowing and burying remnants of the ependymal lining. We believe that the bacteria pass through the ependymal lining and set up this inflammatory reaction. It is favored by a developing hydrocephalus which stretches and breaks the ependymal lining. The glial changes are secondary to damage of subependymal tissues.

The choroid plexus is at first congested, but within a few days becomes infiltrated with neutrophils and lymphocytes, and eventually may be covered with exudate. As in the case of the meningeal exudate, lymphocytes, plasma cells, and macrophages later predominate. Eventually there is organization of the exudate covering the plexus.

The reader may wonder at this long digression into matters that are more pathologic than clinical, but only by consideration of the morphologic features of meningitis can one come to understand the basis of the clinical state. The meningeal and ependymal reactions to bacterial infection and the clinical correlates of these reactions are summarized in Table 29-1.

Types of Bacterial Meningitis Almost any bacterium gaining entrance to the body may produce meningitis, but by far the most common are *Haemophilus influenzae*, *Neisseria meningitidis*, and *Diplococcus pneumoniae*, which account for 80 to 90 percent of cases. Less frequent causes are *Staphylococcus aureus* and group A streptococci, usually in association with brain abscess, epidural abscess, head trauma, neurosurgical procedures, or cranial thrombophlebitis; *Escherichia coli;* group B streptococci (in newborns); and the other Enterobacteriaceae such as *Klebsiella, Proteus,* and *Pseudomonas*, which are usually a consequence of lumbar puncture, spinal anesthesia, or shunting procedures to relieve hydrocephalus. Rare meningeal pathogens include *Salmonella, Shigella, Clostridium,* and *Neisseria gonorrhoeae*. Two unusual ones are *Listeria monocytogenes*, which is easily confused with diphtheroids, and *Mima polymorpha*, which may be difficult to distinguish from *Haemophilus* and *Neisseria*.

Epidemiology Pneumococcal, *H. influenzae,* and meningococcal meningitis have a worldwide distribution, occurring mainly during the fall, winter, and spring, and predominating in males. Each has a relatively constant seasonal incidence, although epidemics of meningococcal meningitis seem to occur roughly in 10-year cycles. *H. influenzae* meningitis is encountered almost exclusively in children between 2 months and 7 years of age. There are between 12,000 and 15,000 cases each year in the United States. Meningococcal meningitis occurs most often in children and adolescents, but is also encountered throughout much of adult life, with a sharp decline in incidence after the age of 50. Pneumococcal meningitis predominates in the very young and in adults over 40 years of age.

Pathogenesis All three of the common meningeal pathogens are inhabitants of the nasopharynx in a significant part of the population and depend upon antiphagocytic capsular or surface antigens for survival in the tissues of the infected host; all express their pathogenicity largely in the form of extracellular proliferation. It is evident from the frequency with which the carrier state is detected that nasal colonization is not a sufficient explanation of infection of the meninges. The factors which predispose the colonized patient to bloodstream invasion, which is the usual route by which bacteria reach the meninges, are obscure but include antecedent viral infections of the upper respiratory passages or, in the case of the pneumococcus, infections in the lung. Once blood-borne, the factors which lead to meningeal localization of bacteria are unknown, but it is evident that pneumococci, *H. influenzae*, and meningococci possess a unique predilection for the meninges. It has been postulated that the entry of bacteria into the subarachnoid space is facilitated by disruption of the blood-CSF barrier by trauma, circulating endotoxin, or an initial viral infection of the meninges.

Avenues other than the bloodstream by which bacteria can gain access to the meninges include congenital neuroectodermal defects, craniotomy sites, diseases of the middle ear and paranasal sinuses, and severe cranial trauma, notably skull fractures, and, in cases of recurrent infection, dural tears from remote minor or major trauma. Occasionally a brain abscess may rupture into the subarachnoid space or ventricles, thus infecting the meninges. The isolation of anaerobic streptococci, *Bacteroides*, or *Actinomyces*, or a mixture of microorganisms from the CSF, should suggest the possibility of a brain abscess with an associated meningitis.

In most patients the precise route by which bacteria infect the meninges cannot be determined.

Clinical Features *Adults and older children* The early clinical effects of acute pyogenic meningitis are fever, severe headache, generalized convulsions, a disorder of consciousness (i.e., drowsiness, confusion, stupor, and coma), and stiffness of the neck (resistance to passive movement) on forward bending. Flexion at the hip and knee in response to forward flexion of the neck (Brudzinski sign) and inability to completely extend the legs (Kernig sign) are of the same nature as stiff neck, but less reliable. Diagnosis may offer difficulty only when the initial manifestations are pain in the neck or abdomen, or a confusional state or delirium.

Any circumstance which prolongs the meningitis increases the risk of injury to all the structures enumerated above; this fact accounts for many of the clinical features in the subacute and chronic varieties of meningeal infection. The potential pathologic-clinical relations of acute, subacute, and chronic meningitis are summarized in Table 29-1.

The symptoms which compose the meningitic syndrome are common to the three main types of bacterial meningitis, but certain clinical features correlate with particular types of meningitis. *Meningococcus meningitis* should always be suspected during epidemics of meningitis under the following circumstances: when the evolution is extremely rapid, when the onset is attended by a petechial or purpuric rash or by large ecchymoses and lividity of the skin of lower parts of the body, and when circulatory collapse has occurred. Since a petechial rash accompanies approximately 50 percent of meningococcus infections, its presence dictates immediate institution of therapy for a neisserian infection, even though similar rashes may be observed with certain viral and occasionally with other bacterial meningitides. *Pneumococcus meningitis* is usually preceded by an infection in the lungs, ears, or sinuses, and the heart valves may be affected. In addition, a pneumococcus etiology should be suspected in patients suffering from alcoholism, sickle-cell disease, and basal skull fracture and also following splenectomy. *H. influenzae* meningitis usually follows upper respiratory and ear infections in the child.

Other specific bacterial etiologies are suggested by certain unusual clinical settings. Meningitis in the presence of furunculosis or following a neurosurgical procedure should raise the possibility of coagulase-positive staphylococcal infection. Ventriculovenous shunts, inserted for control of hydrocephalus, are particularly prone to infection with coagulase-negative staphylococci. Brain abscess, myeloproliferative or lymphoproliferative disorders, defects in cranial bones (tumor, osteomyelitis), collagen diseases, metastatic cancer, and therapy with immunosuppressive agents are clinical conditions which favor the invasion of the craniospinal cavities by such pathogens as Enterobacteriaceae, *Listeria*, *Herellea*, and *Pseudomonas*.

The signs of meningeal irritation—stiff neck, Kernig's sign, and Brudzinski's sign—may be absent in the very young or the deeply stuporous or comatose patient. Signs of focal cerebral disease, although seldom prominent, are most frequent in pneumococcal and influenzal meningitis. Seizures are encountered most often with *H. influenzae* meningitis, but it is difficult to ascertain their significance since young children may convulse with fevers of any cause. Some of the more transitory focal cerebral signs may represent postictal phenomena (Todd's paralysis); others may be related to an unusually intense focal meningitis. Stable, focal cerebral lesions developing most often in the second week of the meningeal infection, are consequent to vasculitis—usually occlusion of cerebral veins—and infarction of cerebral tissue. Cranial nerve abnormalities are particularly frequent with pneumococcal meningitis, the result of invasion of the nerve by the infective agent as it traverses the subarachnoid space.

Infants and newborns Acute bacterial meningitis in this age group poses a number of special problems. Infants, of course, cannot complain of headache, and stiff neck may be absent. Fever, irritability, drowsiness, vomiting, convulsions, and a bulging fontanel are the usual manifestations. A high index of suspicion and liberal use of the lumbar puncture needle are the keys to early diagnosis.

The problems in the neonate are even more formidable. More often than not, the signs of meningeal irritation are absent, and one has only the nonspecific signs of a systemic illness—hyperirritability, lethargy, feeding difficulty, respiratory distress, and fever (or hypothermia)—to suggest the presence of meningeal infection. Signs of meningeal irritation do occur, but only late in the course of the illness. Again, lumbar puncture is crucial, and it must be performed before any antibiotics are administered for other neonatal infections. An antibiotic regimen sufficient to control a septicemia may allow a meningeal infection to smolder and to flare up after antibiotic therapy has been discontinued.

A number of other facts about the natural history of neonatal meningitis are noteworthy. It is more common in males than in females, in a ratio of about 3:1. Obstetrical abnormalities in the third trimester (premature birth, prolonged labor, premature rupture of fetal membranes) occur frequently in mothers of infants who develop meningitis in the first weeks of life. The most significant factor in the pathogenesis of the meningitis is maternal infection (usually a urinary tract infection or perinatal fever of unknown cause). The infection in both mother and infant is most often due to gram-negative enterobacteria, particularly *E. coli*, and group B streptococci, and less often to *Pseudomonas*, *Listeria*, *Staphylococcus aureus* or *albus*, and group A streptococci. Analysis of postmortem material indicates that in most cases infection occurs at or near the time of birth, although clinical signs of infection may not become evident until several days or a week later.

Spinal Fluid Examination As has already been indicated, the lumbar puncture is an indispensable part of the examination of patients with the symptoms and signs of meningitis, or of any patient in whom this diagnosis is suspected.

Pleocytosis of the spinal fluid is diagnostic. The number of leukocytes in the CSF ranges from 1000 to 100,000 per cubic millimeter, but the usual number is from 1000 to 10,000. Occasionally, in pneumococcal and influenzal meningitis, the CSF may contain a large number of bacteria but few if any neutrophils for the first few hours. Cell counts above 50,000 per cubic millimeter raise the possibility of a brain abscess having ruptured into the ventricles. Neutrophilic leukocytes predominate (85 to 95 percent of the total), but an increasing proportion of mononuclear cells is found as the infection continues, especially in partially treated meningitis. In the early stages, careful cytologic examination may disclose that some of the mononuclear cells are myelocytes or young neutrophils. Later, as treatment takes effect, the proportions of lymphocytes, plasma cells, and histiocytes steadily increase.

The spinal fluid *pressure* is so consistently elevated (above 180 mmH$_2$O) that a normal or low pressure on the initial lumbar puncture in a case of suspected bacterial meningitis should raise the suspicion that the needle is partially occluded or the spinal subarachnoid space is blocked. Pressures over 400 mmH$_2$O always suggest brain swelling and potential cerebellar herniation.

The *protein* levels are higher than 45 mg per 100 ml in 90 percent of the cases, and most fall in the range of 100 to 500 mg per 100 ml. The *glucose* content is depressed, usually to a level lower than 40 mg per 100 ml, or less than 40 percent of the blood glucose concentration (measured concomitantly), provided the latter is less than 250 mg per 100 ml. However, in atypical or *culture-negative cases,* other conditions associated with a depressed CSF glucose should be considered. These include hypoglycemia from any cause; sarcoidosis of the central nervous system; fungal or tuberculous meningitis; and some cases of subarachnoid hemorrhage, meningeal carcinomatosis, or gliomatosis. Chloride levels in the CSF are usually low (less than 700 mg per 100 ml), reflecting dehydration and low serum chloride levels.

Gram stain of the spinal fluid sediment permits identification of the causative agent in most cases of bacterial meningitis; pneumococci and *H. influenzae* are identified more readily than meningococci. Small numbers of gram-negative diplococci in leukocytes may be indistinguishable from fragmented nuclear material which may also be gram-negative and of the same shape. In such cases, a thin film of uncentrifuged CSF may lend itself more readily to morphologic interpretation than a smear of sedimented CSF. The commonest error in reading Gram-stained smears of CSF is misinterpretation of precipitated dye or debris as gram-positive cocci, or a confusion of pneumococci with *H. influenzae.* The latter organisms may stain heavily at the poles so that they resemble gram-positive diplococci, and older pneumococci often lose their capacity to take a gram-positive stain.

Cultures of the spinal fluid are best obtained by collecting the fluid in a sterile tube, and immediately inoculating plates of blood, chocolate, and MacConkey agar, and tubes of thioglycolate (for anaerobes) and at least one other broth; the advantage of using broth media is that large amounts of CSF can be cultured. Cultures are positive in 70 to 90 percent of cases of bacterial meningitis.

During the past decade counterimmunoelectrophoresis (CIE) has proved to be a valuable adjunct in the diagnosis of bacterial meningitis. This is a sensitive technique that permits the detection of bacterial antigens in the CSF in a matter of 30 to 60 min. It is particularly useful in patients with partially treated meningitis, in whom the CSF still contains bacterial antigens but in whom no organisms can be detected on a smear or grown in culture. Two recently developed serological methods, radioimmunoassay (RIA) and latex particle agglutination (LPA), and an enzyme-linked immunosorbent assay (ELISA) may be even more sensitive than CIE.

Measurements of CSF lactic dehydrogenase (LDH) appear to be of prognostic and diagnostic value in bacterial meningitis. A rise in total LDH activity is consistently observed in patients with bacterial meningitis; most of this is due to fractions 4 and 5, which are derived from granulocytes. LDH fractions 1 and 2, which are presumably derived from brain tissue, are only slightly elevated in bacterial meningitis, but rise sharply in patients who die or who develop neurologic sequelae. Thus the test may be helpful in singling out the patient who is most at risk. CSF lysozymal enzymes, derived from leukocytes, meningeal cells, or plasma, may also be increased in meningitis, but the clinical significance of this observation is unknown. CSF levels of lactic acid (determined by either gas chromatography or enzymatic analysis) are also consistently elevated in bacterial and fungal meningitides (above 35 mg per 100 ml) and may be helpful in distinguishing these disorders from viral meningitides, in which lactic acid levels remain normal.

Other Laboratory Findings In addition to CSF cultures, blood cultures should always be obtained because they are positive in 40 to 60 percent of patients with *H. influenzae* and meningococcal and pneumococcal meningitis, and they may provide the only definite clue as to the causative agent (if CSF cultures are negative). Routine cultures of the pharynx are as often misleading as helpful because pneumococci, *H. influenzae*, and meningococci are such common inhabitants of healthy persons. In contrast, *cultures of the nasopharynx* may be helpful in diagnosis; the finding of typable, encapsulated *H. influenzae* or groupable meningococci may provide the clue to the etiology of the meningeal infection. Contrariwise, the absence of such findings makes an *H. influenzae* and meningococcus etiology unlikely. The *leukocyte count* in the blood is generally elevated, and usually there is a shift to the left. Most meningitic patients are sufficiently ill to require determination of blood urea nitrogen and serum electrolytes. These may be abnormal because of severe dehydration. In addition, inappropriate secretion of antidiuretic hormone (ADH) with resultant severe hyponatremia may occur.

Radiologic Studies Patients with bacterial meningitis should have radiographs of the chest, skull, and sinuses as soon as possible after admission to the hospital. Chest films are particularly important because they may disclose a silent area of pneumonitis or abscess. Sinus and skull films may provide clues to the presence of cranial osteomyelitis, paranasal sinusitis, and mastoiditis. If there is a suspicion of a brain abscess or subdural empyema (or hygroma), a CT scan will settle the matter.

Recurrent Bacterial Meningitis This is probably observed most frequently in patients who have had some type of ventriculovenous shunting procedure for the treatment of hydrocephalus. The patient with recurrent bacterial meningitis of inapparent origin should always be suspected of having a congenital neuroectodermal sinus or a fistulous connection between the nasal sinuses and the subarachnoid space. The fistula in these latter cases is more often traumatic than congenital in origin (a previous basal skull fracture), although the interval between injury and the initial bout of meningitis may be several years. The site of trauma is in the frontal or ethmoid sinuses or the cribriform plate, and *Diplococcus pneumoniae* is the usual pathogen. Often it proves to be

one of the higher serologic types, reflecting the predominance of such strains in nasal carriers. These cases have a good prognosis; mortality is much lower than in ordinary cases of pneumococcal meningitis.

Cerebrospinal fluid rhinorrhea is present in most of the cases of posttraumatic type, but it may be transient and difficult to demonstrate except by injecting a dye such as carmine red or radioactive albumin into the spinal subarachnoid space and watching for its appearance in nasal secretions. Another method of detecting CSF rhinorrhea is by measuring the glucose concentration of nasal secretions. The usual mucous secretions contain little glucose, but in CSF rhinorrhea the amount of glucose approximates that in CSF. Attempts to demonstrate CSF rhinorrhea should be made only after the acute infection has subsided; if evidence of a fistula is found, surgical repair should be considered.

Prognosis The overall mortality rate of *H. influenzae* and meningococcal meningitis has remained fixed at 5 to 15 percent for many years. In pneumococcal meningitis the rate is considerably higher (15 to 30 percent). Fulminating meningococcemia, with or without meningitis, also has a high mortality rate because of the associated vasomotor collapse and infective shock, associated with adrenocortical necrosis (Waterhouse-Friderichsen syndrome). A disproportionate number of deaths occur in infants and in the aged. Mortality rate is highest in neonates, from 40 to 75 percent in the reported series; at least half of those who recover show serious neurologic sequelae. The presence of bacteremia, coma, seizures, and a variety of concomitant diseases, including alcoholism, diabetes mellitus, multiple myeloma, and head trauma, all worsen the prognosis. The triad of pneumococcal meningitis, pneumonia, and endocarditis has a particularly high fatality rate.

It is often impossible to explain the death of the patient, or at least to trace it to a single specific mechanism. The effects of overwhelming infection, with bacteremia and hypotension or brain swelling and cerebellar herniation, are clearly implicated in the deaths of some patients during the initial 48 h. These events may occur in bacterial meningitis of any etiology; however, they are more frequent in meningococcal infection (Waterhouse-Friderichsen syndrome). Some of the deaths occurring later in the course of the illness are attributable to respiratory failure, often consequent to aspiration pneumonia.

Relatively few patients who recover from meningococcal meningitis show residual neurologic defects, whereas such defects are encountered in at least 10 percent of children with *H. influenzae* meningitis and up to 30 percent of patients with pneumococcal meningitis. The acute complications of bacterial meningitis, the intermediate and late neurologic sequelae, and the pathologic basis of these effects, are summarized in Table 29-1.

Differential Diagnosis The diagnosis of bacterial meningitis is not difficult, providing a high index of suspicion is maintained. All febrile patients with lethargy, headache, or confusion of sudden onset, even if only low-grade fever is present, should be subjected to lumbar puncture. It is particularly important to think of meningitis in febrile, confused alcoholic patients. Too often one incorrectly ascribes the symptoms to intoxication, delirium tremens, or hepatic encephalopathy until examination of the CSF reveals a meningitis.

It needs to be reemphasized that bacterial meningitis can be diagnosed definitively only by examination of the CSF. Spontaneous subarachnoid hemorrhage, chemical meningitis (following lumbar puncture, spinal anesthesia, or myelography), and viral, tuberculous, leptospiral, and fungal meningoencephalitis often enter into the differential diagnosis. Also to be considered are Behçet's disease, which is characterized by recurrent oral-pharyngeal mucosal ulceration, uveitis, orchitis, and meningitis; and Mollaret's meningitis, which consists of recurrent episodes of fever and headache, in addition to signs of meningeal irritation. The CSF in both of these recurrent types of meningitis may contain large numbers of polymorphonuclear leukocytes, but no bacteria, and the glucose content is not reduced.

The other intracranial suppurative diseases and their differentiation from bacterial meningitis are considered later in this chapter.

Treatment Bacterial meningitis is a medical emergency. The following therapeutic regimens are recommended:

1. For adults with pneumococcal or meningococcal meningitis, penicillin G, at least 12 to 15 million units intravenously each day in four to six divided doses; for children the daily dose of penicillin G should be 200,000 to 300,000 units per kilogram of body weight. For children over 2 months of age with *H. influenzae* or uncomplicated meningitis of unknown etiology, chloramphenicol is now the drug of choice, because of the emergence of ampicillin-resistant strains, worldwide. Chloramphenicol should be given in doses of 100 mg/kg per day intravenously in a continuous infusion or in divided doses for 2 or 3 days, then 50 mg/kg by the same route. Alternatively, ampicillin may be used (400 mg/kg intravenously in divided doses; adults should receive 12 g/day), but only when the organisms have been shown to be susceptible to this drug.

In adult patients with any of these types of bacterial meningitis who are allergic to the penicillins, chloramphenicol in a dosage of 6 g/day intravenously may be used. Cephalosporins are not recommended for the treatment of meningitis.

2. For meningitis due to Enterobacteriaceae, the drug of choice is gentamicin in dosage of 5 mg/kg per day administered intravenously in divided dosages at 6-h intervals. However, except in infants, therapeutic success with this drug may depend upon intrathecal administration, since adequate CSF concentrations are obtained only by this route. For this reason, ampicillin is preferred, if the offending organism proves to be sensitive to this drug. *Pseudomonas* meningitis should also be treated with gentamicin, as outlined above, with the addition of carbenicillin in large doses intravenously.

3. Meningitis due to *Staph. aureus* should be treated with a penicillinase-resistant penicillin (oxacillin or nafcillin, in a dosage of 10 to 12 g/day), or methicillin, in a dosage of 18 to 20 g/day, intravenously.

Foci of infection in the paranasal sinuses or mastoids, an infected ventriculovenous shunt, or a cranial osteomyelitis should be identified, so that appropriate surgical treatment may be carried out when the acute episode of meningitis has subsided.

Duration of therapy Most cases of bacterial meningitis should be treated for a period of 10 to 14 days except when there is a persistent parameningeal focus of infection. Antibiotics should be administered in full doses parenterally (preferably intravenously) throughout the period of treatment. Treatment failures with several drugs, notably ampicillin, may be attributable to oral or intramuscular administration, resulting in inadequate concentration in the CSF. Repeated lumbar punctures are not necessary to assess the effects of therapy as long as there is progressive clinical improvement. The CSF glucose may remain low for many days after other signs of infection have subsided, and should occasion concern only if bacteria are present and the patient remains febrile and ill.

Prolongation of fever is due usually to subdural effusion(s), sinus thrombosis, mastoiditis, intercurrent infection, phlebitis, or rarely to abscess of the brain; and it requires continuation of therapy for a longer period. Bacteriologic relapse after treatment is discontinued requires immediate reinstitution of therapy.

Adrenocortical steroids The few controlled studies available have demonstrated that steroids exert no beneficial effects in pyogenic meningitis. These drugs should not be used except possibly in overwhelming meningococcal sepsis.

Other forms of therapy Intrathecal administration of enzymes, to lyse excessive subarachnoid cellular exudate which may be responsible for spinal block or hydrocephalus in the subacute stages of bacterial meningitis, is not of proven value. There is also no evidence to support the idea that repeated drainage of CSF is therapeutically effective. In fact, increased CSF pressure in the acute phases of bacterial meningitis is largely a consequence of cerebral edema, and the lumbar puncture may predispose to cerebellar herniation and death. Mannitol and urea have been employed with apparent success in some cases of severe brain swelling with unusually high initial CSF pressures (over 400 mmH$_2$0). Acting as osmotic diuretics, these agents enter cerebral tissue slowly, and their net effect is to decrease brain water and sodium. The administration of these agents may be associated to some extent with the occurrence of a late rebound phenomenon. Neither agent has been studied in controlled fashion. An adequate but not excessive amount of parenteral fluids should be given, and anticonvulsants should be prescribed when seizures are present. In children, care should be taken to avoid hyponatremia and water intoxication—a cause of brain swelling.

Complications vary with the type of organism and the duration of the meningeal infection before therapy is begun. Meningococcal meningitis tends to subside rapidly. Regression tends to be slower with pneumococcal meningitis. The patient may remain stuporous for days, even after fever subsides and CSF is clearing. There is also a higher incidence of mild aphasia, hemiparesis, unilateral seizures, and other focal cerebral signs, which eventually disappear. The child with a severe influenzal meningitis is at high risk of developing lasting complications (hydrocephalus, hemiplegia, blindness, deafness), especially if there has been a delay in instituting therapy. Subdural effusions should be drained repeatedly by subdural taps; if persistent after infection has subsided, surgical removal may be necessary.

SUBDURAL EMPYEMA

Subdural empyema is an intracranial suppurative process, usually on one side, between the inner surface of the dura and the outer surface of the arachnoid. The term subdural abscess, among others, has been applied to this condition, but the proper name is *empyema,* indicating suppuration in a preformed space. Contrary to prevailing opinion, subdural empyema is not a rarity (about one-fifth as frequent as cerebral abscess). It is distinctly more common in males, a feature for which there is no plausible explanation.

Source of Infection The infection usually gains entry to the subdural space from the frontal or ethmoid sinuses, or, less often, from the middle ear and mastoid cells. Infection takes place by direct extension through bone and dura, or as a result of thrombophlebitis involving the venous sinuses, particularly the superior longitudinal sinus. Rarely the subdural infection is metastatic, from infected lungs, and it is hardly ever secondary to bacteremia or septicemia. Occasionally it extends from a brain abscess.

In cases of sinus origin, streptococci (nonhemolytic and viridans) are the most common organisms, followed by anaerobic streptococci or *Bacteroides.* Less often *Staph. aureus, E. coli, Proteus,* and *Pseudomonas* are causative. In about half the cases, no organisms can be cultured or seen on Gram stain. The factors that lead to a subdural empyema rather than to a cerebral abscess are not understood.

Pathology A collection of subdural pus, in quantities of a few milliliters to 100 to 200 ml, lies over the cerebral hemisphere. In advanced cases, pus spreads into the interhemispheric fissure, and occasionally it is found in the posterior fossa, covering the cerebellum. It is often mistaken for meningitis. The arachnoid, when cleared of exudate, is cloudy, and thrombosis of meningeal veins may be seen. The underlying cerebral hemisphere is depressed, as in subdural hematoma, and in fatal cases there is often an ipsilateral temporal lobe pressure cone. Microscopic examination discloses various degrees of organization of the exudate on the inner surface of the dura, and infiltration of the underlying arachnoid with small numbers of neutrophilic leukocytes, lymphocytes, and mononuclear cells. The thrombi in cerebral veins seem to begin on the sides of the veins nearest the subdural exudate. The superficial layers of the cerebral cortex undergo ischemic necrosis, which probably accounts for the unilateral seizures and other signs of disordered cerebral function.

Symptomatology and Laboratory Findings Usually the history includes reference to chronic sinusitis or mastoiditis with a recent flare-up and evidence of local pain and increase in purulent nasal or aural discharge. In sinus cases, the pain is usually over the brow or between the eyes, and it is associated with tenderness on pressure over these parts, and sometimes orbital swelling. General malaise, fever, and headache—at first localized, then severe and generalized and associated with vomiting—are the first indications of intracranial spread. They are followed in a few days by drowsiness and increasing stupor, rapidly progressing to coma. At about the same time, focal neurologic signs appear, the most important of which are unilateral motor seizures, hemiplegia, hemianesthesia, aphasia, and paralysis of lateral conjugate gaze. Fever and leukocytosis are always present and the neck is stiff.

The usual CSF findings are an increased pressure, pleocytosis in the range of 50 to 1000 per cubic millimeter, polymorphonuclear cells predominating, elevated protein concentration (75 to 300 mg per 100 ml) and normal glucose values. If the patient is stuporous or comatose, there is risk in performing a lumbar puncture because it may aggravate a threatening pressure cone of the temporal lobe. Instead, one should proceed with other diagnostic procedures (see below).

Diagnosis Skull films usually demonstrate a sinus infection or mastoiditis, and in addition may reveal an osteomyelitis of the frontal bone. The single most useful procedure is the CT scan. If this is not available, carotid arteriography, which discloses inward displacement of meningeal vessels and contralateral shift of the anterior cerebral arteries, is useful. A lateral frontal burr hole with exposure of the dura reveals pus under increased pressure.

Several conditions need to be distinguished clinically from subdural empyema, particularly cerebral thrombophlebitis and brain abscess (see below), acute herpes simplex encephalitis (page 519), acute necrotizing hemorrhagic leukoencephalopathy (page 661), and focal embolic encephalomalacia due to bacterial endocarditis (see further on in this chapter).

Treatment This consists of immediate drainage through enlarged multiple frontal burr holes, or through an osteoplastic flap in cases of interhemispheric or posterior fossa empyema. The surgical procedure should be coupled with appropriate antibiotic therapy, which consists of the intravenous administration of 20 million units of penicillin per day plus chloramphenicol, 2 to 4 g/day. Bacteriologic findings may dictate a change to more appropriate drugs. Without such massive antimicrobial therapy and surgery, most patients will die, usually within 7 to 14 days, often while the unsuspecting physician and surgeon are waiting for better localization of an assumed cerebral abscess, the most common mistaken diagnosis. On the other hand, patients who are treated promptly may make a surprisingly good recovery, including full or partial resolution of their focal neurologic deficits within a few months.

EXTRADURAL ABSCESS

This condition is almost invariably associated with osteomyelitis in a cranial bone and originates from an infection in the ear or paranasal sinuses, or from a surgical procedure, particularly if the frontal sinus or mastoid had been opened or a foreign body had been used (e.g., dural graft, tantalum button over a burr hole, or Crutchfield tongs). Rarely, the infection is metastatic or spreads outward from a dural sinus thrombophlebitis. Pus and granulation tissue accumulate on the outer surface of the dura, separating it from the cranial bone. The symptoms are those of a local inflammatory process: frontal or auricular pain, purulent discharge from sinuses or ear, and fever and local tenderness. Sometimes the neck is slightly stiff. Localizing neurologic signs are usually absent. Rarely, the fifth and sixth cranial nerves are involved with infections of the petrous part of the temporal bone, producing an abducens palsy, pain in the eye and temple, and impaired sensation in the face (Gradenigo's syndrome), or a focal seizure may occur. The CSF is usually clear and under normal pressure but may contain a few lymphocytes and neutrophils (20 to 100 per milliliter) and slightly raised protein concentration. Treatment consists of antibiotics aimed at the appropriate pathogen(s)—often *Staph. aureus*. Later, the diseased bone in the frontal sinus or the mastoid, from which the extradural infection had arisen, may have to be removed and the wound packed to ensure adequate drainage. Results of treatment are usually good.

Spinal Epidural Abscess This type of abscess possesses unique clinical features and constitutes an important neurologic and neurosurgical emergency. It is discussed in Chap. 35.

The dural sinuses drain blood from all of the brain into the jugular veins. The largest and most important of these channels, and the ones usually involved by infection, are the transverse, cavernous, and longitudinal sinuses. A complex system of lesser sinuses and cerebral veins connects these large sinuses to one another as well as to the paranasal sinuses, diploic and meningeal veins, and veins of the face and scalp.

Usually there is evidence that thrombophlebitis of the large dural sinuses has extended from a manifest infection of the middle ear and mastoid cells, the paranasal sinuses, or skin around the upper lip, nose, and eyes. These cases are frequently complicated by other forms of intracranial suppuration, including meningitis, extradural and subdural empyema, and brain abscess. Occasionally infection may be introduced by direct trauma to large veins or dural sinuses. A variety of organisms, including all the ones that ordinarily inhabit the paranasal sinuses and skin of the nose and face, may give rise to intracranial thrombophlebitis. Streptococci and staphylococci are most often incriminated.

Lateral Sinus Thrombophlebitis   In lateral sinus thrombophlebitis, which usually follows chronic infection of the middle ear, mastoid, or petrous bone, the earache and mastoid tenderness are succeeded, after a period of a few days to weeks, by generalized headache and papilledema. If the thrombophlebitis remains confined to the transverse sinus, there are no other neurologic signs. Spread to the jugular bulb may give rise to the syndrome of the jugular foramen (see Table 46-1), and involvement of the superior sagittal sinus, to seizures and focal cerebral signs. Fever, as in all forms of intracranial thrombophlebitis, tends to be high and intermittent, and other signs of toxemia may be prominent. Infected emboli may be released into the bloodstream, causing petechiae in the skin and mucous membranes, and pulmonary sepsis. The CSF is usually normal, but may show a small number of cells and elevation of protein content.

As a diagnostic aid, compression of the jugular veins separately during the Queckenstedt maneuver will demonstrate failure of the CSF pressure to rise when the vein ipsilateral to the involved lateral sinus is compressed (Tobey-Ayer test). If compression of the jugular vein causes swelling of the veins of the face and retina, it indicates obstruction of the opposite jugular vein or its transverse sinus (Crowe test). Neither of these tests is entirely reliable because anatomic anomalies of the large veins are frequent. Also, some danger attaches to compression of the jugular vein in the face of increased intracranial pressure. For these reasons, one usually resorts to jugular venography as the definitive diagnostic procedure. When the intracranial pressure is greatly elevated, the suspicion of cerebellar abscess is raised, but this process is usually characterized by other neurologic signs—especially nystagmus to the side of the lesion, and ipsilateral ataxia of the arm and leg.

Cavernous Sinus Thrombophlebitis   This condition is usually secondary to infections of the ethmoid, sphenoid, or maxillary sinuses or of the skin around the eyes and nose. In addition to headache, high fluctuating fever, and signs of toxemia, there are characteristic local effects. Obstruction of ophthalmic veins leads to chemosis, proptosis, and edema of the ipsilateral eyelids, the forehead, and the nose. The retinal veins become engorged and may be followed by retinal hemorrhages and papilledema. Involvement of the third, fourth, sixth and ophthalmic division of the fifth cranial nerves, which lie in the lateral wall of the cavernous sinus, leads to ptosis, ocular palsies, and pain and sensory loss around the eye and in the forehead. If the sympathetic plexus around the carotid artery which lies in the sinus is involved, a complete internal and external ophthalmoplegia results. Within a few days, spread through the circular sinus to the opposite cavernous sinus results in bilateral symptoms. The posterior part of the cavernous sinus may be infected via the superior and inferior petrosal veins without the occurrence of orbital edema or ophthalmoplegia. The CSF is usually normal unless there is an associated meningitis or subdural empyema. The only effective therapy in the fulminant variety, associated with thrombosis of the anterior portion of the sinus, has been antimicrobial therapy aimed at coagulase-positive staphylococci, and occasionally gram-negative pathogens as well. Anticoagulants have been used occasionally, but their value has not been proved. Cavernous sinus thrombosis must be differentiated from mucormycosis, which may cause a similar clinical picture in uncontrolled diabetics (described later in this chapter), other fungus infections (aspergillus), carcinomatous invasion of the sphenoid bone, and sphenoid wing meningioma.

Thrombophlebitis of the Superior Longitudinal Sinus   Although occasionally this may be asymptomatic, the typical clinical syndrome is one of unilateral convulsions and hemiplegia, first on one side of the body, then on the other, due to extension of the thrombophlebitis into the superior cerebral veins. Because of the localization of function in the cortex that is drained by the sinus, the paralysis takes the form of a crural monoplegia, or, less often, of a paraplegia. A cortical sensory loss may occur in the same distribution. Homonymous hemianopia or quadrantanopia, aphasia, paralysis of conjugate gaze, and urinary incontinence (in bilateral cases) have also been observed. Headache, papilledema, and increased intracranial pressure may accompany these signs. The diagnosis can be corroborated by direct jugular venography or by demonstrating a failure of the superior sagittal sinus to fill during the late venous phase of the carotid arteriogram. Treatment consists of large doses of antibiotics and temporization until the thrombus recanalizes. Recovery from paralysis may be complete, or the patient may be left with seizures and varying degrees of spasticity in the legs.

It should be reiterated that all types of thrombophlebitis, especially those related to ear and paranasal sinus infection, may be associated with other forms of intracranial suppuration, namely bacterial meningitis, subdural empyema, or brain abscess. Therapy in these complicated forms of infection must be individualized. As a rule, the best plan is to institute antibiotic treatment of the intracranial disease and to decide, after it has been brought under control, whether surgery on the offending ear or sinus is necessary. To operate on the primary focus before medical treatment has taken hold is to court disaster. In cases complicated by bacterial meningitis, the treatment of the latter usually has to take precedence over the surgically treatable diseases, like brain abscess and subdural empyema.

Aseptic Thrombosis of Intracranial Venous Sinuses
This may develop after sinus and ear infections, and may lead to an obscure increase in intracranial pressure because of the occlusion of the superior sagittal or a lateral sinus. The most common type occurs in children and adolescents with otitis media. The symptoms include headache, vomiting, papilledema, and bilateral sixth nerve palsies. There is no fever; there are no signs of toxemia; CSF is normal except for raised pressure. Symonds referred to this condition as "otitic hydrocephalus," but pointed out later that hydrocephalus is a misnomer, as there is no dilatation of the ventricles. Conditions which predispose to aseptic thrombosis are postpartum and postoperative states, which are often characterized by thrombocytosis and hyperfibrinogenemia; congenital heart disease and marasmus in infants; sickle cell disease; and primary or secondary polycythemia. The diagnosis of aseptic venous or sinus thrombosis

in the absence of one of these conditions usually proves to be incorrect.

BRAIN ABSCESS

Pathogenesis   With the exception of a small proportion of cases (about 10 percent) in which infection may be introduced from the outside (compound fractures of the skull, intracranial operations), brain abscess is always secondary to a focus of suppuration elsewhere in the body. Approximately 40 percent of all brain abscesses are secondary to disease of the paranasal sinuses, middle ear, and mastoid cells. Of those originating in the ear, about one-third lie in the anterolateral part of the cerebellar hemisphere, and the remainder lie in the middle and inferior parts of the temporal lobe, above the tegmen tympani. Infections of the nasal cavity and its accessory sinuses account for a small number of brain abscesses. The sinuses most frequently implicated are the frontal and sphenoidal, and the abscesses derived from them are in the frontal and temporal lobes, respectively.

Otogenic and rhinogenic abscesses reach the nervous system in one of two ways. One is by direct extension, in which the bone of the middle ear or nasal sinuses becomes the seat of an osteomyelitis, with subsequent inflammation and penetration by infected material of the dura and leptomeninges, and the creation of a suppurative tract into the brain. Alternately (or concomitantly), infection may spread along the walls of veins. Also, thrombophlebitis of the pial veins and dural sinuses, by infarcting brain tissue, renders the latter more vulnerable to invasion by infectious material. The close anatomic relationship of the lateral (transverse) sinus to the cerebellum explains the frequency with which this portion of the brain is infected via the venous route. The spread along venous channels also explains how an abscess may sometimes form at a considerable distance from the primary focus in the middle ear or paranasal sinuses.

About one-third of all brain abscesses are metastatic, i.e., hematogenous. The majority of these are traceable to a primary septic focus in the lungs or pleura (bronchiectasis, empyema, lung abscess, or bronchopleural fistula). Other metastatic abscesses are traceable to a cardiac abnormality—either infected valves or a congenital defect which permits infected emboli to short-circuit the pulmonary circulation and reach the brain. Occasional cases are associated with infected pelvic organs, skin, tonsils, abscessed teeth, and osteomyelitis of noncranial bones.

In about 20 percent of all cases of brain abscess, the source cannot be ascertained (Murphy et al.). Brain abscess is almost never a consequence of bacterial meningitis. Metastatic abscesses are most likely to occur in the distal territory of the middle cerebral arteries, and they are frequently multiple, in contrast to otogenic and rhinogenic abscesses (Fig. 31-1).

A careful distinction should be made between the neuropathologic effects of subacute and acute bacterial endocarditis. *Subacute bacterial endocarditis* (SBE), i.e., the type caused by the implantation of streptococci of low virulence (alpha and gamma streptococci) on valves previously damaged by rheumatic fever, or on a patent ductus arteriosus or ventricular septal defect, seldom if ever gives rise to brain abscess. The cerebral lesions of SBE, which may be the initial clinical manifestations, are due to the embolic occlusion of vessels by fragments of vegetations and bacteria, which cause infarction of brain tissue and a restricted inflammatory response around the involved blood vessels and in the overlying meninges. The CSF contains a moderate number of polymorphonuclear leukocytes and frequently red cells as well, but the glucose content is never lowered and suppuration in the brain or in the subarachnoid space does not occur. It is theorized that the chronicity of the streptococcal infection allows the body to develop an immunity to the organisms. The meningeal pleocytosis is associated with headache, stiff neck, and alterations of consciousness.

In contrast to SBE, the more fulminant, *acute bacterial (ulcerative) endocarditis*—i.e., the type which is caused by *Staph. aureus*, hemolytic streptococcus, or the pneumococcus, and which may involve previously normal valves—frequently gives rise to multiple small abscesses in the brain (and in other organs of the body). Purulent meningitis may also develop, or there may be infarcts or meningocerebral hemorrhages, secondary to ruptured mycotic aneurysms. Rarely do the miliary abscesses progress to large ones, however. Rapidly evolving cerebral signs in patients with acute endocarditis (delirium, confusional state, mild focal cerebral signs) are nearly always caused by embolic infarction or hemorrhage.

It is estimated that about 5 percent of cases of congenital heart disease are complicated by brain abscess (Cohen, Newton). In children, more than 60 percent of cerebral abscesses are associated with congenital heart disease (Matson). The abscess is usually solitary; this fact, coupled with the potential correctability of the underlying cardiac abnormality, makes the recognition of brain abscess in congenital heart disease a matter of considerable practical importance. For some unknown reason, brain abscess associated with congenital heart disease is rarely seen before the third year of life; infarction of the brain due to thrombosis of arteries or veins is

the usual neurologic complication in the first 2 years of life. The tetralogy of Fallot is by far the most common anomaly associated with brain abscess, but the latter may occur with any type of right-to-left shunt which allows venous blood returning to the heart to enter the systemic circulation, without first passing through the lungs. The filtrating effect of the lungs is thus prevented, and pyogenic bacteria or infected emboli from a variety of sources may gain access to the brain, where, aided by the effects of venous stasis and perhaps of infarction, an abscess is established. At least this is the current theory of its mechanism.

Etiology The most common organisms causing brain abscess are streptococci, many of which are anaerobic or microaerophilic. These organisms are often found in combination with other anaerobes, notably *Bacteroides* and diphtheroids, and may be combined with Enterobacteriaceae, such as *E. coli* and *Proteus*. Staphylococci are also a common cause of brain abscess, but pneumococci, meningococci, and *H. influenzae* are rarely so. In addition to *Bacteroides* and anaerobic streptococci, *Actinomyces, Nocardia, Veillonella, Candida*, and other fungi have been isolated. The bacterial species varies with the site of the abscess; staphylococcal abscesses are usually a consequence of penetrating head trauma or of bacteremia; enteric organisms are almost always associated with otitic infections; while anaerobic streptococci are commonly metastatic from the lung.

Pathology Localized inflammatory exudate, septic thrombosis of vessels, and aggregates of degenerating leukocytes represent the early reaction to bacterial invasion of the brain. Surrounding the necrotic tissue is edematous tissue with macrophages, astroglia, microglia, and many small veins—some of which show endothelial hyperplasia, and are filled with fibrin and cuffed with polymorphonuclear leukocytes. At this stage, which is rarely observed postmortem, the necrotic tissue is poorly circumscribed and tends to spread by a coalescence of inflammatory foci. The loose term *cerebritis* is frequently applied to this local suppurative encephalitis or immature abscess.

Within several days, the intensity of the reaction begins to subside, and the infection tends to become delimited. The center of the abscess takes on the character of pus; at the periphery, fibroblasts proliferate from the adventitia of newly formed blood vessels to form a wall of granulation tissue which is readily identified within 2 weeks of the onset of the infection. As the abscess becomes more chronic, the granulation tissue is replaced by collagenous connective tissue. The inner layer of this wall is made up of degenerating neutrophils and fibrin, and the outer layer merges with a zone of altered tissue in which there are lymphocytes and plasma cells, some lying free and others cuffing the vessels, small foci of necrosis, thrombosed small vessels, and edema of the white matter. Thus, the abscess appears to be delimited and in a reparative phase, but there is still evidence of infection remote to it. Occlusion of the more peripheral vessels could conceivably result in extension of the abscess toward the satellite necrotic zones. It has also been noted, in both experimental animals and humans, that the capsule of the abscess is not of uniform thickness, frequently being thinner in its deeper portions. All these factors account for the propensity of cerebral abscesses to spread deeply into the white matter, to produce daughter abscesses or a chain of abscesses, and in some instances to culminate in a catastrophic rupture into the ventricles.

Clinical Manifestations   Headache is the most frequent initial symptom of intracranial abscess. Other presenting symptoms, roughly in order of their frequency, are drowsiness and confusion; focal or generalized seizures; and focal motor, sensory, or speech disorders. In patients who harbor chronic ear, sinus, or pulmonary infections, a recent reactivation of the infection frequently precedes the onset of cerebral symptoms. In patients without an obvious focus of infection, headache or other cerebral symptoms may appear abruptly on a background of mild, general ill health or congenital heart disease. In some patients, bacterial invasion of the brain substance may be asymptomatic or may be attended only by a transitory focal neurologic disorder, as may happen when a septic embolus lodges in a brain artery. Sometimes stiff neck accompanies generalized headache, suggesting the diagnosis of meningitis (especially a partially treated one).

These early symptoms may improve in response to antimicrobial agents, but within a few days or weeks, recurrent headache, slowness in mentation, focal or generalized convulsions, and obvious signs of increased intracranial pressure provide evidence of an inflammatory mass in the brain. Localizing neurologic signs become evident sooner or later, but like papilledema, they occur relatively late in the course of the illness.

The nature of the focal neurologic signs will, of course, depend on the location of the abscess. In *temporal lobe abscess*, headache in the early stages is usually on the same side as the abscess and is localized to the frontotemporal region. If the abscess lies in the dominant hemisphere, there is characteristically an anomic aphasia (inability to name objects—see page 332). An upper homonymous quadrantanopia may be demonstrable, due to interruption of the inferior portion of the optic radiation; this may be the only sign in abscess of the right temporal lobe. Contralateral motor or sensory defects in the limbs tend to be minimal, though weakness of the lower face is often observed.

In *cerebellar abscess*, headache in the postauricular or suboccipital region is usually the first symptom and may at first be ascribed to the infection in the mastoid cells. Coarse nystagmus, weakness of conjugate gaze to the side of the lesion, and a cerebellar ataxia of the ipsilateral arm and leg are present. The ataxia may be difficult to demonstrate if the patient is very ill. As a general rule, the signs of increased intracranial pressure are more prominent with cerebellar abscesses than with cerebral ones. Mild contralateral or bilateral corticospinal tract signs are evidence of brainstem compression; in the late stages, consciousness becomes impaired and is an ominous sign.

In *frontal lobe abscess*, headache, drowsiness, inattention, and general impairment of mental function are prominent. Hemiparesis with unilateral motor seizures and motor disorder of speech are the most frequent neurologic signs. An abscess of the *parietal lobe* will give a series of characteristic focal disturbances (see page 312). The main manifestation of an *occipital lobe lesion* is a homonymous hemianopia. All of the aforementioned focal signs may be obscured by drowsiness, stupor, and inattentiveness, and one must be persistent in searching for them.

While *fever* is characteristic of the invasive phase of cerebral abscess (suppurative encephalitis), the temperature may return to normal as the abscess becomes encapsulated. The same is true of leukocytosis. In the early stages of abscess formation, the CSF pressure is moderately increased, the cell count ranges from 20 to 300 per cubic millimeter, occasionally higher or lower, with 10 to 80 percent neutrophils, and the protein content is only modestly elevated, rarely more than 100 mg per 100 ml. Glucose values are not lowered and the fluid is sterile, unless there is a concomitant suppurative meningitis. Later, the CSF pressure rises markedly. In a small number of cases there are no spinal fluid abnormalities.

It is apparent from this review of the clinical features that the picture of brain abscess is far from stereo-typed. Whereas headache may be the most prominent feature in most patients, seizures or certain focal signs may predominate in others, and a considerable number of patients will present with the signs of increased intra-cranial pressure. Attempts have made by some authors to divide the clinical course of brain abscess into three or four distinct stages, with the implication that these fol-low one another in a predictable sequence. Such a con-cept does not coincide with our experience. In many in-stances the symptoms evolve swiftly, new ones being added day by day. In patients with metastatic brain ab-scesses, the duration of the illness, from the first symp-tom to the time of death, is 5 to 14 days in half the cases (Gates et al.). In others, the invasive stage of cerebral infection is inconspicuous, and the course is so indolent that the entire clinical picture does not differ from that of brain tumor. Another impressive feature of cerebral abscess is the unpredictability with which the symptoms may evolve, particularly in children. Thus, a patient whose clinical condition seems to have stabilized, may be found in a matter of hours or a day or two, to be in an advanced or irreversible state of coma.

Diagnosis The diagnosis of brain abscess depends on (1) a demonstrated source of infection in the middle ear, mastoid, sinuses, lungs or heart, or the presence of a right-to-left cardiac shunt; (2) evidence of increased in-tracranial pressure; (3) focal cerebral or cerebellar signs; and (4) a characteristic CSF reaction in most cases (see above). Lumbar puncture may be dangerous when intra-cranial pressure is obviously elevated, in which case one depends on the information provided by a series of other diagnostic maneuvers:

1. Plain films of the chest and skull are the most important procedures in disclosing a possible pulmonary or paracranial source of infection. In the adult, a shift in the pineal gland, and in infants, separation of the cranial sutures indicate increased intracranial pressure.

2. Radioactive technetium scanning is an ex-tremely sensitive means of detecting intracranial suppu-ration. Practically all abscesses larger than 1 cm produce positive scans. This method is particularly helpful in de-tecting multiple abscesses, which are often not shown by arteriography. The CT scan has become increasingly im-portant in the diagnosis of intracranial abscess (Fig. 31-1). Suppurative encephalitis appears as an area of decreased density, and fully formed abscesses show a central low-density core and a contrast-enhanced regu-lar or irregular capsule. There is little likelihood of cere-bral abscess if the CT and radionuclide scans are nega-

Figure 31-1
A. *Multiple brain abscesses associated with bacterial endocar-ditis (Staphylococcus aureus) in a 55-year-old man. The large* *abscess in the left hemisphere shows a characteristic ring en-hancement. B. Contrast-enhanced CT scan 4 months after insti-tution of antibiotic treatment. The abscesses have resolved.*

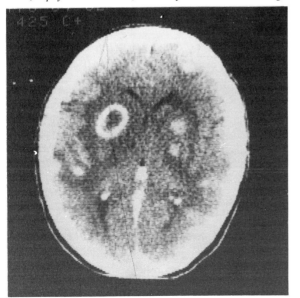

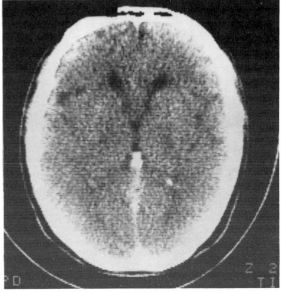

A

B

3. The EEG usually demonstrates a focus of high-voltage slow (delta) activity over the cerebral abscess, and may be used to follow its development or regression after therapy.

4. Arteriography may provide evidence of a cerebral mass by showing displacement of the anterior, middle, or posterior cerebral arteries. This technique is accurate in localizing only about 60 percent of abscesses, and may be unreliable early in the course of disease before liquefaction and encapsulation have occurred. Also, in cyanotic congenital heart disease, arteriography increases the risk of vascular occlusion. For these reasons, arteriography has been largely supplanted by scanning procedures.

5. Ventriculography may disclose deformities of the ventricles. Not infrequently the placement of the ventricular needle has resulted in penetration of a parietooccipital metastatic abscess.

When the classic clinical picture is present and the scanning procedures, radiographs, and EEG corroborate the presence of a mass lesion, the diagnosis is easy. If there is no apparent source of infection and there are only signs and symptoms of a mass lesion, the diagnosis includes glioma, metastatic carcinoma, subdural hematoma, and cerebral hemorrhage. Sometimes only surgical exploration will settle the issue. Once the inflammatory nature of the intracranial mass has been established, brain abscess must be distinguished from subdural empyema and intracranial thrombophlebitis with hemorrhage and infarction of brain (see earlier section in this chapter), herpes simplex encephalitis (page 519), and acute hemorrhagic leukoencephalitis (page 661).

Treatment During the stage of acute suppurative encephalitis, intracranial operation accomplishes little, and probably causes only additional traumatization and swelling of brain tissue and dissemination of the infection. Some cases of acute intracranial suppuration can be cured at this stage by the adequate administration of antibiotics. Even without bacteriologic examination of the intracerebral mass, certain antibiotics can be used. The best regimen consists of 20 million units of penicillin G and 4 to 6 g chloramphenicol, each drug being given intravenously in divided daily doses. This choice of antimicrobial agents is based on the fact that anaerobic streptococci and *Bacteroides* are the preponderant causative organisms. If there is evidence of staphylococcal infection, adequate amounts of penicillinase-resistant penicillin should be added. The initial elevation of intracranial pressure and threatening temporal lobe or cerebellar herniation should be managed by intravenous injection of urea or mannitol followed by dexamethasone, 6 to 12 mg every 6 h. If improvement does not begin promptly and progress steadily, it becomes necessary to needle the abscess for precise etiologic diagnosis (by Gram stain and culture).

Persistence or progression of high intracranial pressure manifested by deepening stupor and threat of herniation indicates the need for surgical intervention, regardless of the stage of the abscess. Likewise, clear-cut evidence of a mass lesion which is not improving with antimicrobial therapy is an indication for surgery. The usual methods of treatment are aspiration of the abscess or unroofing of the abscess and drainage. If superficial and well capsulated, total excision should be attempted; if deep, aspiration and the injection of antimicrobial agents into the abscess are the only treatment, which may have to be repeated. The combination of antimicrobial therapy and surgery has greatly reduced the mortality from brain abscess. The least satisfactory results are obtained in multiple metastatic abscesses. Neurologic residua occur in about 30 percent of surviving patients. Of these, focal epilepsy is one of the most troublesome. Following successful treatment of a cerebral abscess in a patient with congenital heart disease, correction of the cardiac anomaly is indicated to prevent recurrence.

TUBERCULOUS MENINGITIS

In the United States the incidence of tuberculous meningitis, which reflects the incidence of tuberculosis in general, has decreased sharply in recent decades. At the Cleveland Metropolitan General Hospital, for example, the incidence of tuberculous meningitis during the years 1959-1963 was between 4.4 and 8.4 per 10,000 admissions (a decade earlier it was 5.8 to 12.9 per 10,000 admissions). By contrast, at the K. E. M. Hospital in Bombay, during the period 1961 to 1964, the incidence of this disease (in children) was 400 per 10,000 admissions, and similar figures have been reported from other parts of India. In the past decade, there has been a further reduction in the incidence of tuberculosis and tuberculous meningitis. We only see about one or two new cases of tuberculous meningitis each year, and lately, practically all of them have been in adults. Nevertheless, in the economically depressed countries, tuberculosis remains a health problem of very serious proportions.

PATHOGENESIS

Tuberculous meningitis is caused by the acid-fast organism *Mycobacterium tuberculosis*. Rich described two stages in the pathogenesis of the meningitis—first a bacterial seeding of the meninges and underlying brain with the formation of minute tubercles, followed by the rupture of one or more of the foci and the discharge of bacteria into the subarachnoid space.

PATHOLOGIC FINDINGS

Small discrete white tubercles are scattered over the convexities and base of the cerebral hemispheres. The brunt of the pathologic process falls on the basal meninges, where a thick, gelatinous exudate accumulates, obliterating the pontine and interpeduncular cisterns and extending to the meninges around the medulla, the floor of the third ventricle and subthalamic region, the optic chiasm, and the under surfaces of the temporal lobes. By comparison, the convexities are little involved. Microscopically, the meningeal tubercles are like those in other parts of the body, consisting of a central zone of caseation, surrounded by epithelioid and some giant cells, lymphocytes, plasma cells, and connective tissue. The exudate is composed of fibrin, lymphocytes, plasma cells, and other mononuclear cells, some polymorphonuclear leukocytes, and areas of caseation necrosis. The ependyma and choroid plexus are studded with minute glistening tubercles. The exudate surrounds the spinal cord. Unlike the pyogenic meningitides, the inflammatory exudate is not confined to the subarachnoid space but frequently spreads along the pial vessels and invades the underlying brain, so that the process is truly a meningoencephalitis.

Other pathologic changes depend upon the chronicity of the pathologic process and recapitulate the changes that occur in the subacute and chronic forms of the pyogenic meningitides (Table 29-1). Cranial nerves are involved by the inflammatory exudate as they traverse the subarachnoid space. Arteries become inflamed and occluded, with infarction of brain. Blockage of the basal cisterns frequently results in a meningeal obstructive type of hydrocephalus. Noncommunicating hydrocephalus, due to marked ependymitis with blocking of the CSF in the aqueduct or fourth ventricle, is a less common occurrence.

CLINICAL FEATURES

Tuberculous meningitis occurs in persons of all ages. Formerly it was more frequent in young children than in other age groups but now it is more frequent in the adult, at least in the United States. The early manifestations are usually headache, lethargy, confusion, and fever associated with stiff neck and Kernig and Brudzinski signs. In young children and in infants, apathy, hyperirritability, vomiting, and seizures are the usual symptoms, and stiff neck may not be prominent or may be absent altogether.

Characteristically, these symptoms evolve less abruptly in tuberculous than in pyogenic meningitis, usually over a period of a week or two, sometimes longer. Because of the inherent chronicity of the disease, signs of cranial nerve involvement (usually ocular palsies, less often facial palsies or deafness) may be present at the time of admission to the hospital. Occasionally the disease may present with a focal neurologic deficit, such as hemiparesis, or with signs of raised intracranial pressure, and rarely with symptoms referable to the spinal cord and nerve roots.

In most patients with tuberculous meningitis there is evidence of active tuberculosis elsewhere, usually in the lungs, occasionally in bone or kidney. In some patients only inactive pulmonary lesions are found, and in others there is no evidence of tuberculosis outside of the nervous system. In the previously mentioned Cleveland series, which comprised 35 patients, active pulmonary tuberculosis was found in 19, inactive in 6, and involvement of the nervous system alone in 9; only 2 of the 35 patients had nonreactive tuberculin tests (Hinman).

The course of the illness, if untreated, is characterized by confusion and progressively deepening stupor and coma, coupled with cranial nerve palsies, pupillary abnormalities, focal neurologic deficits, raised intracranial pressure and decerebrate postures, and an invariably fatal outcome within 4 to 8 weeks of the onset.

LABORATORY STUDIES

Again, the most important is the lumbar puncture, which should be performed before the administration of antibiotics. The CSF is usually under increased pressure and contains between 50 and 500 white cells per cubic millimeter, rarely more. Early in the disease there may be a more or less equal number of polymorphonuclear leukocytes and lymphocytes, but after several days, lymphocytes predominate. Protein content of the CSF is always elevated, between 100 to 200 mg per 100 ml in most cases, but much higher if CSF blockage occurs around the spinal cord. Glucose is reduced to levels below 40 mg per 100 ml, but rarely to the very low values observed in pyogenic meningitis; the glucose falls slowly and a reduction may only become manifest several days after the patient has been admitted to the hospital.

The demonstration of tubercle bacilli in smears of CSF sediment, stained by the Ziehl-Neelsen method, is a function not only of their number but also of the persistence with which they are sought. There are effective means of culturing the tubercle bacilli; but since their quantity is usually small, attention needs to be paid to proper technique. The amount of CSF submitted to the laboratory is critical; the more that is cultured, the greater the chances of recovery of the organism. Usually growth in culture is not recognized for 3 to 4 weeks. For this reason, if a presumptive diagnosis of tuberculous meningitis has been made, treatment should be instituted immediately without waiting for the results of bacteriologic study.

Other diagnostic procedures (CT scan, ventriculography, arteriography) may be necessary in patients who present with or develop raised intracranial pressure, hydrocephalus, or focal neurologic deficits. The CT scan will demonstrate hydrocephalus. As mentioned earlier this is usually of the meningeal obstructive variety in which cases infusion of contrast material may show an enhancement pattern in the basal cisterns, a finding which suggests a CSF block at or below the tentorium. Angiography may demonstrate major vascular occlusive disease and hydrocephalus.

OTHER FORMS OF CNS TUBERCULOSIS

Tuberculomas are tumorlike masses of tuberculous granulation tissue which form in the parenchyma of the brain. The larger ones may produce symptoms of a space-occupying lesion. In the United States and other affluent countries, tuberculomas are rarities; but in underdeveloped countries they constitute from 5 to 30 percent of all intracranial mass lesions. Because of their proximity to the meninges, the CSF often contains a small number of lymphocytes and increased protein. Tuberculomas may be multiple.

The spinal cord may be affected in a number of ways in the course of tuberculous infection. The inflammatory meningeal exudate may invade the underlying parenchyma, producing the signs of posterior and lateral column disease, in addition to spinal block. Spinal cord symptoms that accompany vertebral caries (Pott's paraplegia) are usually due to compression by an epidural mass of granulation tissue, and, less frequently, to the mechanical effects of angulation of the vertebral column.

TREATMENT

The treatment of tuberculous meningitis consists of the administration of a combination of drugs—isoniazid (INH), rifampin (RMP), and ethambutol (EMB)—given for a prolonged period, 18 to 24 months as a general rule (although it may not be necessary to give all three drugs for the entire period). INH is the single most effective drug. It acts by interfering with DNA synthesis and with the intermediary metabolism of the tubercle bacillus. It can be given in a single daily dose of 5 mg/kg in adults and 10 mg/kg in children. Its most important adverse effects are neuropathy (see page 900) and hepatitis. The former can be prevented by the administration of 50 mg pyridoxine daily. In patients who develop hepatitis, INH should be discontinued.

Rifampin and ethambutol act by interfering with RNA synthesis. The usual dose of RMP is 600 mg daily for adults, 15 mg/kg for children. Ethambutol is given in a single daily dose of 15 mg/kg. These drugs have replaced para-aminosalicylic acid (PAS) and streptomycin in the treatment of tuberculous meningitis. RMP and EMB can only be given orally or by stomach tube. INH may be given parenterally, in the same dosage as with oral use. *Corticosteroids* should be used only in patients whose lives are threatened by the effects of subarachnoid block, and only in conjunction with other antituberculous drugs. Intracranial tuberculoma calls for a course of chemotherapy, as outlined above. Under the influence of these drugs, the tuberculoma(s) may decrease in size and ultimately disappear, as judged by the CT scan; if they do not, excision may be necessary. Patients with Pott's paraplegia should also be explored surgically after an initial course of chemotherapy, and an attempt should be made to excise the tuberculous focus.

The overall mortality of patients with CNS tuberculosis is still significant (about 10 percent), infants and the elderly being at greatest risk. Early diagnosis, as one might expect, enhances the chances of survival. Between 20 and 30 percent of survivors manifest a variety of neurologic sequelae, the most important of which are retarded intellectual development, psychiatric disturbances, recurrent seizures, visual and oculomotor disorders, deafness, and hemiparesis. A detailed account of these has been given by Wasz-Höckert and Donner.

SARCOIDOSIS
(Besnier-Boeck-Schaumann Disease)

The infectious etiology of sarcoidosis has never been established, but the disease may suitably be considered at this point because of its close resemblance pathologically and clinically to tuberculosis and other granulomatous infections. The essential lesion in sarcoidosis consists of focal collections of epithelioid cells surrounded by a rim of lymphocytes; frequently there are giant cells, but caseation is lacking. The sarcoid tubercles may be found in all organs and tissues including the nervous system, but the most frequently involved are the mediastinal and peripheral lymph nodes, lungs, liver, skin, phalangeal bones, eyes, and parotid glands.

Sarcoidosis may affect the nervous system in several ways. As indicated on page 904, isolated sarcoid granulomas may involve peripheral or cranial nerves, giving rise to a subacute or chronic neuropathy of asymmetric type (see Jefferson). Of the cranial nerves, the facial is the most frequently involved, usually as part of the uveoparotid syndrome. Involvement of the meninges, brain, and spinal cord may also occur, but is equally infrequent. In Scadding's series of 275 patients, for example, only 3 developed central nervous system (CNS) lesions; in other large series the incidence of CNS involvement was greater [10 of 145 patients studied by Mayock et al. (see below)].

In the CNS, sarcoidosis takes the form of a granulomatous infiltration of the meninges and underlying parenchyma, most prominent at the base of the brain. The disease process is subacute or chronic in nature, mimicking other granulomatous lesions and neoplasm. Visual disturbances, due to lesions in and around the optic nerves and chiasm, and polydipsia, polyuria, somnolence, or obesity, due to involvement of the pituitary and hypothalamus, are the usual features. Hydrocephalus, seizures, cranial nerve palsies, and corticospinal and cerebellar signs are other common manifestations. In rare cases, the spinal meninges and cord are infiltrated, imparting a picture of adhesive arachnoiditis; in others, focal cerebral signs, due presumably to large focal deposits of sarcoid in the brain, are observed. The spinal fluid in cases of CNS sarcoid shows a slight lymphocytic pleocytosis (10 to 200 cells per cubic millimeter, mostly lymphocytes) and moderate increase in protein content and gamma globulin. The spinal form may be associated with CSF block.

As to the relative frequency of affection of different parts of the nervous system, Mayock and his associates, in a personal series of 145 cases of sarcoidosis, observed neurologic signs in 23 cases (16 percent); as indicated above, the CNS was involved in 10 cases; in the remainder the signs were indicative of cranial or peripheral nerve involvement. In a combined series of 625 patients with sarcoidosis, peripheral and/or central nervous system involvement was found in 32 (5.1 percent).

The diagnosis of CNS sarcoidosis is made on the basis of the clinical features together with clinical and biopsy evidence of sarcoid granulomas in other tissues (uveal tract, skin, lungs, bones). Test material for the Kveim reaction is not generally available, although this diagnostic test is still under investigation in several centers. Delayed hypersensitivity skin reactions are frequently depressed. Mild anemia and elevated sedimentation rate are common in active disease. Differential diagnosis includes epidemic parotitis, leprosy, cryptococcosis, syphilis, and tuberculosis.

Administration of corticosteroids is the only known effective therapy. Prednisone, in divided daily doses of 40 mg, is given for 2 weeks, followed by 2-week periods in which the dose is reduced by 5 mg until a maintenance dose of 20 to 10 mg is reached. Therapy should be continued for at least 6 months, and in many cases for several years.

NEUROSYPHILIS

The incidence of neurosyphilis, like that of CNS tuberculosis, has declined dramatically in the past three decades. In the United States, for instance, the rate of first admissions to mental hospitals because of neurosyphilis fell from 4.3 per 100,000 population (in 1946) to 0.4 per 100,000 (in 1960). Nevertheless, new cases of neurosyphilis and incompletely treated old ones are still being seen from time to time. Furthermore, the number of reported cases of early syphilis has actually increased in the last decade, so that one may logically anticipate an increase in late syphilis, including neurosyphilis.

ETIOLOGY AND PATHOGENESIS

Syphilis is caused by a slender, spiral, motile organism, the *Treponema pallidum*. The biologic characteristics of this organism and the natural history of the disease which it produces are described in *Harrison's Principles of Internal Medicine*, which should be read as an introduction to the following discussion. In this chapter, only some basic facts regarding the neurosyphilitic infection will be considered. These facts have been reasonably well established by clinical and postmortem observation, and without knowledge of them it is not possible to treat patients with syphilis intelligently.

1. *The treponeme usually invades the CNS within 3 to 18 months of inoculation with the organism.* If the nervous system is not involved by the end of the second year, as shown by completely negative CSF, there is only 1 chance in 20 that the patient will develop neurosyphilis as a result of the original infection; and if the CSF is negative at the end of 5 years, the likelihood of developing neurosyphilis falls to 1.0 percent.

2. *The initial event in the neurosyphilitic infection is a meningitis which occurs in about 25 percent of all cases of syphilis.* Usually this meningitis is asymptomatic and can only be discovered by lumbar puncture.

Exceptionally, it is more intense and causes cranial nerve palsies, convulsions, apoplectic phenomena (due to associated vascular lesions), and symptoms of increased intracranial pressure. As a corollary, the occurrence of these symptoms in a young adult should always suggest the possibility of neurosyphilis and requires examination of the CSF.

3. *This meningitis may persist in an asymptomatic state and ultimately, after a period of years, cause parenchymal damage.* In some cases, however, there may be a natural subsidence of the meningitis—a spontaneous cure.

4. *All forms of neurosyphilis begin as a meningitis, and a more or less active meningeal inflammation is the invariable accompaniment of all forms of neurosyphilis.* The early clinical syndromes are meningitis and meningovascular syphilis; the late ones are vascular syphilis (1 to 12 years) followed by general paresis, tabes dorsalis, optic atrophy, and meningomyelitis. *These latter are pathologic sequences which result from chronic syphilitic meningitis.* These sequences and their interrelationships are illustrated in Fig. 31-2.

The intermediate pathologic stages in the trans-

Figure 31-2
Diagram of the evolution of neurosyphilis.

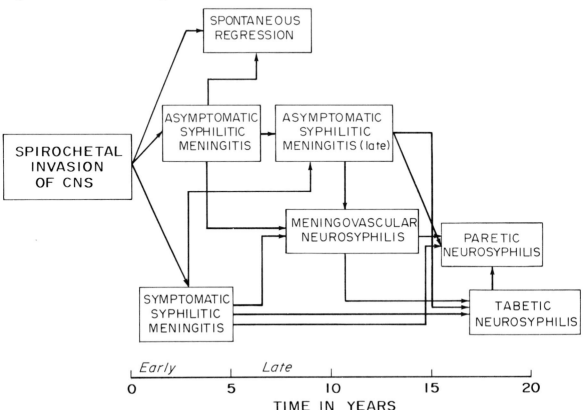

formation of asymptomatic syphilitic meningitis to the late forms of parenchymal neurosyphilis are unknown. Syphilis is by far the most chronic form of meningitis affecting human beings, and many of the pathologic changes thought to be peculiar to syphilis of the nervous system are simply due to the chronicity of the meningeal reaction. Confirmation of this view comes from the study of the brain and spinal cord in the more chronic cases of tuberculous and cryptococcus meningitis. Inflammation and thrombosis of subarachnoid arteries, meningoencephalitis, ependymitis, and meningomyelitis, resembling closely the lesions of neurosyphilis, can be found in these chronic forms of meningitis.

5. From a clinical point of view, *asymptomatic neurosyphilis is the most important form of neurosyphilis.* If all cases of asymptomatic neurosyphilis were discovered and adequately treated, the symptomatic varieties of neurosyphilis could be prevented. Conversely, if not treated or inadequately treated a certain proportion of patients with asymptomatic neurosyphilis will develop meningovascular syphilis, general paresis, tabes, etc. Since asymptomatic neurosyphilis can be recognized only by the changes in the CSF, it is axiomatic that all patients with late syphilis must have a lumbar puncture and spinal fluid examination.

6. *So-called vascular syphilis is usually, if not always, meningovascular syphilis.* In all types of meningitis—that is, bacterial, fungal, treponemal—it is common to find an inflammatory reaction in the walls of subarachnoid arteries. In the more chronic stages of meningitis, fibrous thickening of the vessel wall occurs with narrowing of the lumen and thrombotic occlusion.

7. Clinical syndromes such as syphilitic meningitis, meningovascular syphilis, general paresis, tabes dorsalis, optic atrophy, and meningomyelitis are abstractions which at autopsy seldom exist in pure form. Since all of them have a common origin in a meningitis there is usually a combination of two or more syndromes, e.g., meningitis and vascular syphilis, taboparesis, etc. Just why the most intense meningeal reaction and consequent parenchymal damage is in the cerebral hemispheres in one case, and around the optic nerves or spinal cord in another, is not known. Even though the patient's symptoms may have been referable to only one part of the nervous system, postmortem examination usually discloses diffuse changes in both brain and spinal cord, which were of insufficient severity to be detected clinically.

8. *The CSF is a sensitive indicator of the presence of active neurosyphilitic infection.* It reflects the presence of meningeal inflammation. The finding of pleocytosis and an increased total protein in the CSF

corresponds to the infiltration of the pia-arachnoid with lymphocytes and plasma cells at autopsy. Occasionally postmortem examination shows a slight to moderate cellular infiltration of the meninges in patients whose CSF during life contained no cells; in such cases the total protein is usually elevated.

The *abnormalities of the CSF which are commonly found in neurosyphilis are* (a) 200 to 300 cells per cubic millimeter, mostly lymphocytes and a few plasma cells and other mononuclear cells, (b) elevation of protein, particularly the globulin fraction, from 40 to 200 mg per 100 ml, (c) an increase in gamma globulin, and (d) positive serologic tests. The glucose content is usually normal.

The serologic diagnosis of syphilis depends on the demonstration of one of two types of antibodies—nonspecific (reagin) antibodies and specific treponemal antibodies. The common tests for reagin are the Kolmer, which uses a complement fixation technique, and the Venereal Disease Research Laboratory (VDRL) slide test, which uses a flocculation technique. These reagin tests in the CSF, if positive, are diagnostic of neurosyphilis. However, these tests are negative in a significant proportion of patients with late syphilis and in those with neurosyphilis in particular (*seronegative syphilis*). In such patients it is essential to employ tests for specific treponemal antibodies, such as the fluorescent treponemal antibody absorption (FTA-ABS) test and the treponema immobilization test (TPI), which are positive in practically every instance of neurosyphilis.

The earliest changes in the CSF consist of pleocytosis and an elevation of protein. These may occur in the first few weeks of the infection before the serologic tests become positive. Later, the CSF changes may vary. With either spontaneous or therapeutic remission of the disease, the cells disappear first; next the total protein returns to normal; and then the gamma globulin levels are reduced. The positive serologic tests are the last to revert to normal. Frequently the CSF serology remains positive, despite repeated courses of therapy and the subsidence of all signs of inflammatory activity (see below). The *blood serology* is positive if there is an abnormal CSF, but rare exceptions to this rule have been recorded.

9. *The CSF is an almost infallible guide, probably even more than the clinical symptomatology, in the diagnosis, treatment and prognosis* of the disease. If the CSF is negative in a patient with manifestations of neu-

rosyphilis, it may be safely concluded that the syphilitic inflammation in the nervous system is burned out and that further progression of the disease probably will not occur. In cases with progressive neurologic symptoms and a completely negative CSF, postmortem examination usually discloses a nonsyphilitic neurologic disease. If treatment restores the CSF to normal, particularly the cell count and protein, arrest of the clinical symptoms almost always occurs. A return of cells and elevation of protein precedes or accompanies the clinical relapse.

10. *The clinical syndromes and pathologic reactions of congenital syphilis are similar to those of the acquired forms.* All the aforementioned biologic events are equally applicable to congenital and acquired neurosyphilis (see page 858).

PRINCIPAL TYPES OF NEUROSYPHILIS

Asymptomatic Neurosyphilis In this condition, there are no symptoms or physical signs except, in some cases, abnormal pupils (see page 188). The diagnosis is based entirely on the CSF findings without which the case would be regarded as latent syphilis, or if other viscera are affected, as cardiovascular syphilis, gumma, etc. The abnormality in the CSF varies, as mentioned in paragraph 8 above. Cases coming accidentally to autopsy have shown only lymphocytic, plasma cell, and mononuclear infiltrates of the pia, a sparse granular ependymitis, and slight infiltrations of meningeal vessels.

Meningeal Syphilis Symptoms of meningeal involvement may occur at any time after inoculation, but most often within the first 2 years. The commonest symptoms are headache, stiff neck, cranial nerve palsies, convulsions, and mental confusion. Occasionally the symptoms consist of headache, papilledema, nausea, and vomiting, due to the presence of increased intracranial pressure. The patient is afebrile, unlike the one with tuberculous meningitis. The CSF is always abnormal, often more so than in asymptomatic neurosyphilis. Obviously the meningitis is more intense in this type and may be associated with hydrocephalus. The prognosis, with adequate treatment, is good. The symptoms usually disappear within days to weeks, but if the CSF remains abnormal, it is likely that some other form of neurosyphilis will subsequently develop.

Meningovascular Syphilis This form of neurosyphilis should always be considered when a young person has one or several cerebrovascular accidents, i.e., a sudden development of hemiplegia, aphasia, sensory loss, visual disturbance or mental confusion. The commonest time of occurrence of meningovascular syphilis is 6 to 7 years after the original infection, but it may be as early as 6 months or as late as 10 to 12 years. The CSF almost always shows some abnormality, usually an increase in cells, protein content, and gamma globulin, as well as a positive serologic test. Patients in middle or late life with stroke and a positive serologic test in the CSF will usually be found at autopsy to have atherothrombotic or embolic infarction, rather than meningovascular syphilis. The changes in the latter disorder consist not only of meningeal infiltrates but also inflammation of arteries as well as productive fibrosis that leads to narrowing and finally occlusion. The vascular lesion was first described by Heubner, hence *Heubner's arteritis.* In some cases of vascular syphilis there is a meningoencephalitis as well.

The neurologic signs which remain after 6 months will usually be permanent, but adequate treatment will prevent further apoplectic episodes. If repeated cerebrovascular accidents occur despite adequate therapy, one must always consider the possibility of nonsyphilitic vascular diseases of the brain.

Paretic Neurosyphilis (General Paresis, General Paralysis of the Insane, Dementia Paralytica, Syphilitic Meningoencephalitis) The general setting of this form of cerebral syphilis is a long-standing meningitis; as was remarked above, some 15 to 20 years usually separate the first symptoms from the original infection.

The history of the disease is entwined with some of the major developments of neuropsychiatry. Haslam in 1798 and Esquirol at about the same time first delineated the clinical state. Bayle in 1822 commented on the arachnitis and meningitis, and Calmeil, on the encephalitic lesion. Nissl and Alzheimer added details to the pathologic descriptions. The syphilitic nature of the disease was suspected by Lasègue and others long before Schaudinn's discovery of the spirochete and was finally affirmed by Noguchi in 1913. Kraepelin's monograph, *General Paresis* (1913), is one of the classic reviews (see Merritt et al. for these and other historical references).

Once a major cause of insanity, accounting for some 4 to 10 percent of admissions to asylums, general paresis is now a rarity. The discovery of penicillin has provided the means of eradicating the disease. The famous dictum of Krafft-Ebing that general paresis is a product of syphilization and civilization is no longer applicable. Blacks are as susceptible as whites except for the West Indian natives, who are notoriously resistant. Pregnancy appears to protect the female but the incidence in women who have never been pregnant is nearly the same as in males. Since syphilis is aquired mainly in late adolescence and early adult life, the middle years (30 to 50) are the usual time of onset of the paretic symptoms. Congenital paresis blights early mental development in half the cases, and results in late childhood and adolescent regression in both normal and mentally retarded children.

Symptomatology The clinical picture, in its fully developed form, is one of progressive mental and physical dissolution, and includes dementia, dysarthria, myoclonic jerks, action tremor, seizures, hyperreflexia, Babinski signs, and Argyll-Robertson pupils. However, more importance attaches to diagnosis at an earlier stage when few of these manifestations are conspicuous. The insidious onset of memory defect, impairment of reasoning, and reduction in critical faculties, along with minor oddities of deportment and conduct, irritability, and lack of interest in personal appearance are not too different from the syndrome of dementia already outlined in Chap. 20. One can appreciate how elusive the disease may be, at any one point in its early evolution. Indeed, with the currently low index of suspicion of the disease, diagnosis at this *preparalytic stage* is more often accidental than deliberate.

Classical writings have stressed the development of delusional systems, most dramatically in the direction of megalomania, which are evident to family and friends and not at all to the individual involved. Typically, the patient conceives ambitious schemes to aggrandize a fortune or to enhance social prestige. The delusions are viewed by the patient in an uncritical fashion that obscures their extravagance and worthlessness. When thwarted, the patient may become quarrelsome and obstinate. Another warning of imminent dissolution is an obvious disregard for social conventions and moral standards.

Flagrant and elaborate delusional systems are altogether exceptional in the early or preparalytic phase, in the authors' experience. More usual has been a simple dementia with weakening of intellectual capacities, forgetfulness, disorders of speaking and writing, and vague concerns about health. The first hint of a syphilitic encephalitis may be facial quivering, tremulousness of the hands, indistinct hurried speech, myoclonus, and seizures, reminiscent of delirium or acute viral encephalitis. As the deterioration continues into the *paralytic stage*, intellectual function decays completely, and aphasias, agnosias, and apraxias intrude themselves. Wilson

(quoting Kraepelin) estimated that two-thirds of the patients at this stage become psychotic, either with expansive-grandiose or depressive-hypochondriacal delusions, and one-third continue with a simple dementia. Even in the past, however, the much-discussed megalomania with its release of boundless energies, extreme boastfulness, ridiculous claims of supernatural power, of being King, Emperor, or God never appeared in more than 30 percent of the cases.

Physical dissolution progresses concomitantly—poor carriage, debility, muscular hypotonia, unsteadiness, dysarthria, and tremor of the tongue and hands. All these disabilities lead eventually to a bedridden state; hence, the term *paretic* is quite applicable. Other symptoms are hemiplegia, hemianopia, aphasia, cranial nerve palsies, seizures with prominent focal signs of unilateral frontal or temporal lobe disease also known as Lissauer's cerebral sclerosis. Agitated, delirious, depressive, and schizoid psychoses were special psychiatric syndromes that could be differentiated from the so-called functional psychoses by the mental decline, the neurologic signs, and the CSF findings.

We have elaborated the neuropsychiatric features of this disease, even though rare nowadays, because it manifests so uniquely a chronic frontotemporoparietal encephalitis and creates a picture unlike that of most of the degenerative diseases discussed in Chap. 42. Also it is well to remember that many of our ideas about the brain and the mind were shaped historically by this disease.

The blood serology is positive in nearly all cases. The CSF is invariably abnormal, usually with 10 to 200 lymphocytes, plasma cells, and mononuclear cells per cubic millimeter, a total protein of 40 to 200 mg per 100 ml, an elevated gamma globulin, and strongly positive serologic tests.

The pathologic changes consist of meningeal thickening, brain atrophy, ventricular enlargement, and granular ependymitis. Microscopically, the perivascular spaces are filled with lymphocytes, plasma cells, and mononuclears; nerve cells have disappeared; there are numerous rod-shaped microgliacytes and plump astrocytes; iron is deposited in mononuclear cells; and with special stains spirochetes are visible in the cortex. The changes are most pronounced in the frontal and temporal lobes. Meningeal fibrosis with obstructive hydrocephalus is probably present in many cases.

The prognosis in early cases is fairly good; 35 to

40 percent will make some occupational readjustment, and the disease will be arrested but leave the patient economically dependent in another 40 to 50 percent. Without treatment there is progressive mental enfeeblement, and death occurs within 3 to 4 years.

Tabetic Neurosyphilis (Tabes Dorsalis) This type of neurosyphilis, classically described by Duchenne in his monograph *L'Ataxie locomotrice progressive* (1858), usually develops 15 to 20 years after the onset of the infection. The major symptoms are lightning pains, ataxia, and urinary incontinence; the chief signs are absent knee and ankle reflexes, impaired vibratory and position sense in feet and legs, and a Romberg sign. The ataxia is due purely to the sensory defect. Muscular power, by contrast, is fully retained in most cases. The pupils are abnormal in over 90 percent of cases, usually Argyll-Robertson type, and the majority of patients exhibit ptosis or some degree of ophthalmoplegia. Optic atrophy is frequent. The lancinating or lightning pains (present in over 90 percent of cases) are, as their name implies, sharp, stabbing, and brief, like a flash. They are more frequent in the legs than elsewhere, but roam over the body from face to feet, sometimes playing persistently on one spot "like the repeated twanging of a fiddle string," as Wilson remarked. They may come in bouts lasting several hours or days. "Pins and needles" feelings, coldness, numbness, tingling, and other paresthesias are also present and are associated with variable impairment of tactile, pain, and thermal sensation. The bladder is insensitive and hypotonic, resulting in unpredictable overflow incontinence. Constipation and megacolon as well as impotence are other expressions of dysfunction of the sacral roots and cord.

In the established phase of the disease, now seldom seen, ataxia is the most prominent feature. The patient totters and staggers while standing and walking. In mild form it is best seen as the patient tries to walk between obstacles, attempts to walk a straight line, turns suddenly, or halts. To correct the instability the patient places the feet wide apart, flexes the body slightly and contracts the extensor muscles repeatedly as he or she sways (*la danse des tendons*). In moving forward, the patient flings the leg abruptly in a piece, and the foot strikes the floor with a resounding thump. The patient clatters along in this way with eyes glued to the floor. If vision is blocked, the patient is rendered helpless. When the ataxia is severe, walking becomes impossible despite relatively normal strength of the leg muscles. Trophic

lesions, perforating ulcers of feet, and Charcot joints are characteristic complications of the tabetic state.

With regard to Charcot joints, they occur in 1 to 10 percent of tabetics. Most often they affect the hips, knees, and ankles but sometimes they are seen in the lumbar spine or upper limbs. The process generally begins as an osteoarthritis which, with repeated injury to the insensitive joint, progresses to destruction of the articular surfaces. Osseous architecture disintegrates, with fractures, dislocations, and subluxations, some of which occasion discomfort. We have observed the arthropathy to occur as frequently in the burned-out as in the active phase of tabes; hence it is only indirectly related to the syphilitic process. Although the basic abnormality appears to be repeated injury to an anesthetic joint, the process need not be painless. Presumably an incomplete hypalgesia is enough to interfere with protective mechanisms.

Visceral crises represent another interesting manifestation of this disease. The gastric ones are the best known. The tabetic is seized abruptly with epigastric pain that spreads around the body or up over the chest. There may be a sense of thoracic constriction, and nausea and vomiting—the latter repeated until nothing but blood-tinged mucus and bile are raised. The symptoms may last for several days; a barium swallow sometimes demonstrates pylorospasm. The attack subsides as quickly as it came, leaving the patient exhausted, with a soreness of the epigastric skin. Intestinal crises with colic and diarrhea, pharyngeal and laryngeal crises with gulping movements and dyspneic attacks, rectal crises with painful tenesmus, and genitourinary crises with strangury and dysuria are all less frequent but well-documented types.

In 5 to 10 percent of cases the CSF is normal when the patient is first examined (so-called burned-out tabes). In the others it is abnormal, but often less so than in general paresis.

Pathologic study reveals a striking thinning and grayness of the posterior roots, principally lumbosacral, and a thinness of the spinal cord due mainly to the degeneration of the posterior columns. Only a slight outfall of neurons is observed in the dorsal root ganglia, and the peripheral nerves are essentially normal. For many years there was an argument as to whether the spirochete first attacked the posterior columns of the spinal cord (Spielmeyer), or the posterior root as it pierced the pia (Obersteiner and Redlich), or the more distal part of the radicular nerve where it acquires its arachnoid and dural sheaths (Nageotte), or the dorsal root ganglion cell. Our observations of rare "active cases" have shown the inflammation to be all along the root, and the dorsal ganglion cell loss and posterior column degeneration are secondary.

The hypotonia, areflexia, and ataxia relate to destruction of proprioceptive fibers in the sensory roots, and the ataxia is also purely sensory. The hypotonia and insensitivity of the bladder are due to deafferentation at S2 and S3 levels, and the same is true of the impotence and obstipation. Lightning pains and visceral crises cannot be fully explained but are probably attributable to incomplete posterior root lesions at different levels. Analgesia and joint insensitivity relate to the partial loss of A-δ and C fibers in the roots.

If the CSF is negative and there is no evidence of cardiovascular or other types of syphilis, no further antisyphilitic treatment is necessary. If positive, the patient should be treated with penicillin as described below. Residual symptoms in the form of lightning pains, gastric crises, Charcot joints, or urinary incontinence frequently continue long after all signs of active neurosyphilitic infection have disappeared. These should be treated symptomatically rather than by antisyphilitic drugs (see below under "Treatment").

Syphilitic Optic Atrophy This takes the form of progressive blindness beginning in one eye and then involving the other. The usual finding is a constriction of the visual fields but scotomata may occur in rare cases. The optic disks are grayish white. Other forms of neurosyphilis, particularly tabes dorsalis, not infrequently coexist. The CSF is almost invariably positive though the degree of abnormality may be slight in some cases. The prognosis is poor if vision in both eyes is greatly reduced. If only one eye is badly affected, sight in the other eye can usually be saved. In exceptional cases visual impairment may progress, even after the CSF becomes negative. The pathologic changes consist of a perioptic meningitis with subpial gliosis and fibrosis replacing degenerated optic nerve fibers. Exceptionally there are vascular lesions with infarction of central parts of the nerve.

Spinal Syphilis There are several types of spinal syphilis other than tabes. Two of them, syphilitic meningomyelitis (sometimes called Erb's spastic paraplegia, because of the predominance of bilateral corticospinal tract signs) and spinal meningovascular syphilis, are observed from time to time, though less often than tabes. Spinal meningovascular syphilis may occasionally take the form of an anterior spinal artery syndrome. In meningomyelitis there occurs a subpial loss of myelinated fibers and gliosis, as a direct result of the chronic fibrosing meningitis. Gumma of the spinal meninges and cord also occurs, but is rare. Progressive muscular atrophy (syphilitic amyotrophy) is a very rare disease of

questionable syphilitic etiology. The same is true of syphilitic hypertrophic pachymeningitis or arachnoiditis, which allegedly gives rise to radicular pain and amyotrophy of the hands, and signs of long tract involvement in the legs (syphilitic amyotrophy with spastic-ataxic paraparesis). In all these syndromes there is an abnormal CSF, unless of course the neurosyphilitic infection is burned out.

The prognosis in spinal neurosyphilis is uncertain. There is improvement or at least an arrest of the disease process in most instances, though a few may progress slightly after the treatment is begun. A steady advance of the disease in the face of a negative CSF usually means that the original diagnosis was incorrect and that the patient suffers from some other disease, e.g., a spinal form of multiple sclerosis.

Syphilitic Nerve Deafness This may occur in either early or late syphilitic meningitis and may be combined with other syphilitic syndromes. We have had little experience with this disorder.

TREATMENT

Penicillin is the treatment of choice for all varieties of neurosyphilis, both asymptomatic and symptomatic. The dosage recommended by the United States Public Health Service is 6.0 to 9.0 million units, either as benzathine penicillin G (3.0 million units at intervals of 7 days) or aqueous procaine penicillin G (600,000 units daily for 10 to 15 days). The authors favor the use of the procaine penicillin G in much larger dosage, 12 to 18 million units over a period of 21 to 24 days. Erythromycin and tetracycline, in doses of 0.5 g every 6 h for 20 to 30 days, are suitable substitutes in patients who are sensitive to penicillin. The so-called Jarisch-Herxheimer reaction, which occurs after the first dose of penicillin and is a matter of concern in the treatment of primary syphilis, is usually of little consequence in neurosyphilis; it consists usually of no more than a mild temperature elevation and leukocytosis.

Certain symptoms of neurosyphilis, especially tabetic neurosyphilis, are unpredictably and often little influenced by treatment with penicillin and require other measures. Lightning pains may respond to phenytoin, or to carbamazepine. Analgesics may be helpful, but opiates must be avoided. Neuropathic (Charcot) joints require bracing or fusion. Atropine and phenothiazine derivatives are said to be useful in the treatment of visceral crises.

In all forms of neurosyphilis, the patient should be reexamined every 3 months and the CSF should be retested after a 6-month interval. If after 6 months the patient is free of symptoms and the CSF abnormalities have been reversed (disappearance of cells, reduction in protein, gamma globulin, and serology titers), no further treatment is indicated. Further follow-up should include another clinical examination at 9 and 12 months and another lumbar puncture at the end of a year. Satisfactory progress is judged by absence of symptoms and further improvement in the CSF. These procedures should be repeated every 6 months until the CSF becomes completely negative. In the opinion of most syphilologists, a persistent weakly positive serologic (VDRL) test after the cells and protein levels have returned to normal does not constitute an indication for further treatment. According to the Dattner-Thomas concept of neurosyphilitic activity, such a CSF assures that the disease is quiescent or arrested. Others are not convinced of the reliability of this concept and prefer to give more penicillin. If at the end of 6 months there are still an increased number of cells and an elevated protein in the fluid, another full course of penicillin should be given. Clinical relapse is almost invariably attended by recurrence of cells and increase in protein levels. Rapid clinical progression in the face of a negative CSF suggests the presence of a nonsyphilitic disease of the brain or cord.

Finally it may be said that the neurologist finds the various forms of neurosyphilis of more theoretical than practical importance. No other disease portrays more vividly the effects of a chronic, continuously active cerebrospinal meningitis on the entire neuraxis.

FUNGAL INFECTIONS OF THE NERVOUS SYSTEM

Fungal infections of the CNS are much less common than bacterial ones, although their pathologic and clinical effects are not unlike. Fungi may give rise to meningitis and meningoencephalitis, intracranial thrombophlebitis and brain abscess. A large number of fungal diseases may involve the nervous system, but only a few do so with any regularity—cryptococcosis, coccidioidomycosis, mucormycosis, nocardiosis (brain abscess), and, to a lesser extent, candidiasis and aspergillosis.

GENERAL FEATURES

Fungal infections of the CNS may arise without obvious predisposing cause, but frequently they complicate some other disease process (organ transplantation, leukemia, lymphoma or other malignancy, diabetes, collagen vascular disease). The mechanisms that are operative in the latter situation are not fully understood, but the most obvious factors are interference with the body's normal flora and immunologic responses. Thus fungal infections tend to occur in patients with leukopenia or insufficient antibodies, particularly in those being treated for prolonged periods with antibiotics, corticosteroids, and other immunosuppressant drugs, cytotoxic agents, and antimetabolites. Infections that are related to impairment of the body's protective mechanisms are referred to as *opportunistic,* and include not only fungal infections, but those due to certain bacteria (*Pseudomonas* and other gram-negative organisms), viruses (cytomegalovirus, *H. simplex,* varicella-zoster), and protozoa (*Toxoplasma*). It follows that these types of infection should always be considered and sought in the aforementioned clinical situations.

Fungal meningitis develops insidiously as a rule, over a period of several days or weeks, like tuberculous meningitis, and the symptoms and signs are also much the same. Involvement of cranial nerves, arteritis with thrombosis and infarction of brain, and communicating or obstructive hydrocephalus frequently complicate the course of fungal meningitis, as they do all chronic meningitides. Often the patient is afebrile.

The spinal fluid changes in fungal meningitis are also like those of tuberculous meningitis. Pressure is elevated to a varying extent, pleocytosis is moderate, usually less than 1000 cells per cubic millimeter, and lymphocytes predominate. Exceptionally, in acute cases, more than 1000 cells per cubic millimeter and a predominant polymorphonuclear response are observed. Glucose is subnormal, and protein is elevated—sometimes to very high levels.

Specific diagnosis can only be made from smears of the CSF sediment and from cultures. The CSF examination should also include a search for tubercle bacilli and abnormal white cells, because of the frequent concurrence of fungal infection and tuberculosis, leukemia, or lymphoma.

Some of the special features of the more common fungal infections are indicated below.

CRYPTOCOCCOSIS (TORULOSIS, EUROPEAN BLASTOMYCOSIS)

Cryptococcosis (formerly called *torulosis*) is the most frequent fungal infection of the CNS. The cryptococcus is a common soil fungus, found in the roosting sites of birds, especially pigeons. Usually the respiratory tract is the portal of entry, less often skin and mucous membranes. The pathologic changes are those of a granulomatous meningitis; but, in addition, small granulomas and cysts form within the cerebral cortex, and sometimes large granulomas and cystic nodules form deep in the brain. The cortical cysts contain a gelatinous material and large numbers of organisms; the solid granulomatous nodules are composed of fibroblasts, giant cells, aggregates of organisms, and areas of necrosis.

Cryptococcus meningitis has a number of distinctive clinical features as well. Most cases evolve subacutely, like other fungal infections or tuberculosis. The disease may be fatal within a few weeks if untreated. In other cases, however, headaches, fever and stiff neck are lacking altogether and the patient presents with symptoms of gradually increasing intracranial pressure due to hydrocephalus, or with dementia, cerebellar ataxia, spastic paraparesis, or other focal neurologic deficit. Rarely, a granulomatous lesion forms in one part of the brain, and the only clue to the etiology of the cerebral tumor is a lung lesion and CSF abnormality. Meningovascular lesions, presenting as strokes, may be superimposed on the clinical picture. As a rule, the course is steadily progressive over a period of several weeks or months, but in a few patients it may be remarkably indolent, lasting for years, during which there may be periods of clinical improvement and normalization of the CSF. Lymphoma, Hodgkin's disease, leukemia, carcinoma, and other debilitating diseases which alter the immune responses are predisposing factors in as many as half the cases in general hospitals.

The principal diseases that must be considered in differential diagnosis are tuberculous meningitis (distinguished by fever and organisms in CSF); granulomatous cerebral vasculitis (distinguished by normal glucose values in CSF); multifocal leukoencephalopathy (distinguished by negative CSF); unidentifiable forms of viral meningoencephalitis (normal CSF glucose values); and lymphomatosis or carcinomatosis of meninges (neoplastic cells in CSF).

Specific diagnosis depends upon finding *Cryptococcus neoformans* in the CSF. These are spherical cells, 5 to 15 μm in diameter, which retain the Gram stain and are surrounded by a thick refractile capsule. Large volumes of CSF (20 to 40 ml) may be needed to find the organism. India-ink preparations are distinctive and diagnostic in experienced hands. The carbon particles fail to penetrate the capsule, producing a wide halo around the doubly refractile wall of the yeast. In most cases the organisms grow readily in Sabouraud's glucose agar at room temperature and at 37°C, but in some cases they

cannot be identified by smear or culture, and the only evidence for infection is a positive latex agglutination test for the cryptococcal antigen in the CSF (Snow and Dismukes). The latter test, if negative, excludes cryptococcus meningitis with a 95 percent reliability.

Treatment This consists of the intravenous administration of amphotericin B, beginning with 5 mg daily, and increasing this dose by small increments to 1.0 mg/kg, at which point the drug may be given every second day, to a total of 2.0 to 3.0 g. If this regimen fails to control the meningeal infection, then 0.5 mg of the drug should be injected intrathecally on alternate days, in conjunction with intravenous therapy. Renal tubular acidosis frequently complicates amphotericin B therapy. Administration of the drug should be discontinued if the blood urea nitrogen reaches 40 mg per 100 ml, and resumed when it approaches normal levels. Mortality rate, even in the absence of other disease, is about 40 percent. A recent prospective collaborative study has shown that the addition of flucytosine (150 mg/kg daily) to amphotericin B results in fewer failures or relapses, more rapid sterilization of the CSF, and less nephrotoxicity than the use of amphotericin B alone (Bennett et al.).

MUCORMYCOSIS

This is a malignant infection of cerebral vessels with one of the *Mucorales*. It occurs as a rare complication of diabetic acidosis, and even less frequently in patients with leukemia and lymphoma, particularly those treated with corticosteroids and cytotoxic agents.

The cerebral infection begins in the nasal turbinates and paranasal sinuses, spreads from there along invaded vessels to the retroorbital tissues (where it results in proptosis, ophthalmoplegia, and edema of the lids and retina), and proceeds to the brain, causing hemorrhagic infarction at various sites. Numerous hyphae are present within the thrombi and vessel wall, often extending into the surrounding parenchyma. Usually the cerebral form of mucormycosis is rapidly fatal. Rapid correction of hyperglycemia and acidosis and treatment with amphotericin B have resulted in recovery in some patients.

Candidiasis (moniliasis), aspergillosis, and *nocardiosis* are other fungal infections that occur in patients debilitated by alcoholism and drug addiction; leukemia and renal transplantation, and the treatment associated with these disorders, are other common antecedents. An important condition predisposing to nocardial brain abscess is pulmonary nocardial infection associated with alveolar proteinosis. Other common antecedents of candida sepsis are severe burns and total parenteral nutrition. This organism may occasionally cause a meningoencephalitis of subacute evolution with multiple small granulomas in the cerebral tissues. No special features distinguish these fungal infections from others; meningitis, meningoencephalitis and cerebral abscess, usually multiple, are the modes of clinical presentation. Diagnosis in each case depends on identification of the specific organism in the CSF. Aspergillosis has presented as a chronic sinusitis with osteomyelitis at the base of the skull and cranial nerve palsies in several of our cases, and as brain abscess(es) and spinal epidural granuloma in others.

COCCIDIOIDOMYCOSIS

This is a common infection in southwestern United States. Usually it causes only a benign, influenza-like illness with pulmonary infiltrates that mimic those of nonbacterial pneumonia, but in a few individuals (0.05 to 0.2 percent) it progresses to the disseminated form of the disease, of which meningitis may be a part. The pathologic reactions in the meninges and CSF and the clinical features are very much like those of tuberculous meningitis. *Coccidioides immitis* is recovered with difficulty from the CSF, but readily from the lungs, lymph nodes, and ulcerating skin lesions.

Treatment consists of the intravenous administration of amphotericin B, coupled with a device implanted into the lateral ventricle which permits injection of the drug for a period of years (Ommaya reservoir). Even with the most diligent treatment, only about half the patients with meningeal infections survive.

A similar type of meningitis may occasionally complicate *histoplasmosis*, *blastomycosis*, and *actinomycosis*. None of these meningitides possesses any specific features. Penicillin is the drug of choice in actinomycosis and amphotericin B in the others.

INFECTIONS CAUSED BY RICKETTSIAS, PROTOZOA, AND WORMS

RICKETTSIAL DISEASES

Rickettsias are obligate intracellular parasites which appear microscopically as pleomorphic coccobacilli. They are maintained in nature by a cycle which involves an animal reservoir, an insect vector (lice, fleas, mites, and ticks), and humans. Epidemic typhus is an exception, involving only lice and human beings. At the time of the First World War, and before, the rickettsial diseases, typhus in particular, were remarkably prevalent and of the utmost gravity. In Eastern Europe, between 1915 and 1922, there were an estimated 30 million cases of typhus, with 3 million deaths. Now the rickettsial diseases are of minor importance, the result of insect control by DDT and other chemicals and the therapeutic effectiveness of broad-spectrum antibiotics. In the United States these diseases are quite rare. About 200 cases of spotted fever (the most common rickettsial disease) occur each year, with a mortality of 5 percent or less. Neurologic manifestations occur in only a small portion of these cases, and neurologists may not encounter a single instance in a lifetime of practice. For this reason, the rickettsial diseases are discussed here only briefly. (A comprehensive account will be found in *Harrison's Principles of Internal Medicine*).

The following are the major rickettsial diseases:

1. Small pockets of *epidemic typhus* are present in many underdeveloped parts of the world. It is transmitted from lice to humans and from person to person.

2. *Murine* (*endemic*) *typhus* is present in the same areas as Rocky Mountain spotted fever (see below). It is transmitted from rats to humans by rat fleas.

3. *Scrub typhus* or *tsutsugamushi fever* is confined to eastern and southeastern Asia. It is transmitted by mites from infected rodents or humans.

4. *Rocky Mountain spotted fever* was first described in Montana but is most common in Long Island, Tennessee, Virginia, North Carolina, and Maryland. It is transmitted by special varieties of ticks.

5. *Q fever* has a worldwide distribution (except for the Scandinavian countries and the tropics). It is transmitted in nature by ticks but also by inhalation of dust and handling of materials infected by the causative organism, *Coxiella burnetii*.

With the exception of Q fever, the clinical manifestations and pathologic effects of the rickettsial diseases are much the same, varying only in severity. Typhus may be taken as the prototype. The incubation period varies from 3 to 18 days. The onset is usually abrupt with fever that rises to extreme levels over several days, and with headache and prostration. A macular rash, which resembles that of measles and involves the trunk and extremities, appears on the fourth or fifth febrile day. An important diagnostic sign in scrub typhus is the necrotic ulcer and eschar at the site of attachment of the infected mite. Delirium, followed by progressive stupor and coma, sustained fever, and occasionally focal neurologic signs and optic neuritis, characterize the untreated cases. Stiffness of the neck is noted only rarely, and the CSF may be entirely normal or show only a modest lymphocytic pleocytosis. Q fever, unlike the other rickettsioses, is not associated with an exanthem or agglutinins for the *Proteus* bacteria (Felix-Weil reaction), and the main symptoms are those of a low-grade meningitis. Patients who survive the illness usually recover completely; a few are left with residual neurologic signs.

The rickettsial lesions are scattered diffusely throughout the brain, affecting gray and white matter alike. The changes consist of swelling and proliferation of endothelial cells of small vessels and a microglial reaction, with the formation of so-called microglial or typhus nodules.

Treatment This consists of the administration of chloramphenicol or tetracycline, which are highly effective in all rickettsial diseases. If these drugs are given early, coincident with the appearance of the rash, symptoms abate dramatically and little further therapy is required. Cases which are recognized late in the course of the disease require considerable supportive care, including the administration of corticosteroids, whole-blood transfusions and intravenous albumin, to overcome the effects of toxemia, anemia, and hypoproteinemia.

AMEBIC MENINGOENCEPHALITIS

This disease is caused by free-living flagellate amebas, usually of the genus *Naegleria*. It is acquired by swimming in ponds or lakes, although a large outbreak in Czechoslovakia followed swimming in a chlorinated indoor swimming pool. Most of the cases in this country have occurred in the southeastern states. In 1978, the Federal Center for Disease Control recorded 123 cases worldwide with only three survivors.

The onset of the illness is abrupt, with severe headache, fever, nausea and vomiting, and stiff neck. The course of the illness is inexorably progressive—with seizures, increasing stupor and coma and focal neurologic signs—and the outcome is practically always fatal, usually within a week of onset. The reaction in the CSF is like that of acute bacterial meningitis—increased pressure, a large number of polymorphonuclear leukocytes, and an increased protein and decreased glucose content. The diagnosis depends on eliciting a history of swimming in fresh warm water, particularly extended underwater swimming, and on finding viable trophozoites in a

wet preparation of unspun spinal fluid. Gram stains and ordinary cultures do not reveal the organism.

Autopsy discloses a purulent meningitis and numerous microabscesses in the underlying cortex.

Treatment with the usual antiprotozoal agents is ineffective. Because of the in vitro sensitivity of *Naegleria* to amphotericin B, this drug should be used, as outlined for the treatment of cryptococcal meningitis.

TOXOPLASMOSIS

This disease is caused by *Toxoplasma gondii*, a tiny (2 to 5 μm) obligate intracellular parasite that is readily recognized in Wright- or Giemsa-stained preparations. Infection in humans is either congenital or acquired. Congenital infection is the result of parasitemia in the mother, who happens to be pregnant at the time of her initial (asymptomatic) toxoplasma infection. (Mothers can be assured, therefore, that there is no risk in producing a second infected infant.) Several modes of transmission of the acquired form have been described—the eating of raw beef, contact with cat feces, and the handling of uncooked mutton (in Western Europe).

The congenital infection has attracted more attention, because of the severe destructive effects upon the neonatal brain. Signs of active infection—fever, rash, seizures, hepatosplenomegaly—may be present at birth. More often, chorioretinitis, hydrocephalus or microcephaly, cerebral calcification and psychomotor retardation are the major manifestations. These may become evident soon after birth, or only several weeks or months later. Most infants succumb, others survive with varying degrees of the aforementioned abnormalities.

Although serologic surveys indicate that toxoplasma infection is widespread and frequent (about one-third of American city dwellers have specific antibodies), cases of clinically evident active infection are rare.

The medical literature contains about 45 well-documented cases of acquired toxoplasmosis (Townsend et al.), and it is noteworthy that in half of them there was an underlying systemic disease (malignant neoplasms, renal transplants, collagen vascular disease) that had been treated intensively with immunosuppressive agents. Frequently the neurologic manifestations of toxoplasma were misinterpreted as being related to the disease with which toxoplasmosis was associated and an opportunity for effective therapy was missed. The clinical picture varies. There may be a fulminating, widely disseminated infection with a rickettsia-like rash, encephalitis, myocarditis, and polymyositis. The neurologic signs may consist only of myoclonus and asterixis, suggesting a metabolic encephalopathy; more often, there are the signs of a meningoencephalitis, i.e., seizures, mental confusion, signs of meningeal irritation, coma, and a lymphocytic pleocytosis and increased protein in the CSF. The brain in such cases shows necrotic lesions with free and encysted *T. gondii*, scattered throughout the white and gray matter. Rarely, large areas of necrosis manifest themselves as one or more mass lesions.

Specific diagnosis depends of the finding of organisms in CSF sediment and occasionally in biopsy specimens of muscle or lymph node. A presumptive diagnosis can be made on the basis of a Sabin-Feldman dye test titer of 1:512 or more, a rise in titer, or a positive IgM indirect fluorescent antibody test. Patients with a presumptive diagnosis should be treated with sulfadiazine (4 g initially, then 2 to 6 g daily) and pyrimethamine (100 to 200 mg initially, then 25 mg daily). Leucovorin, 2 to 10 mg daily should be given to counteract the antifolate action of pyrimethamine. Treatment should be continued for at least 4 weeks.

OTHER DISEASES DUE TO PROTOZOA

A number of these are of importance in tropical countries. One is *cerebral malaria*, which complicates about 2 percent of cases of *falciparum malaria;* this is a rapidly fatal disease, characterized by headache, seizures, hemiplegia, aphasia, hemianopia, cerebellar ataxia, and other focal neurologic signs, delirium, and coma. Capillaries are filled with malarial parasites, and the brain is dotted with small foci of necrosis surrounded by glia (Durck's nodes). Usually the neurologic symptoms occur in the second or third week of the infection, but they may occur as the initial manifestation. Useful laboratory findings are anemia and parasitized RBCs. The CSF may be under increased pressure and contain a few white blood cells. The glucose content is normal. These data confirm the diagnosis. With *Plasmodium vivax* infections there may be drowsiness, confusion, and seizures, without invasion of brain by the parasite. Quinine and related drugs are curative if the cerebral symptoms are not pronounced, but once coma and convulsions supervene, there is a strong probability of fatality. CSF pressure should be relieved by appropriate measures.

Trypanosomiasis is a common disease in equatorial Africa and in Central and South America. The African type ("sleeping sickness") is caused by *Trypanosoma brucei* and is transmitted by several species of the tsetse fly. The infection begins with a chancre at the site of inoculation and localized lymphadenopathy. Later, episodes of parasitemia occur, and at some time during this stage of dissemination, usually in the second year of the infection, the trypanosomes give rise to a diffuse meningoencephalitis, which expresses itself clinically as a chronic progressive neurologic syndrome, consisting of a vacant facial expression, ptosis and ophthalmoplegia, dysarthria and then muteness, seizures, progressive apathy, stupor, and coma.

The South American variety of trypanosomiasis (Chagas' disease) is caused by *Trypanosoma cruzi*, and is transmitted from infected animals to humans by the bite of reduviid bugs. The sequence of local lymphadenopathy, hematogenous dissemination, and chronic meningoencephalitis is like that of African trypanosomiasis.

Treatment is pentavalent arsenicals, which have proven most effective in the African form of the disease.

TRICHINOSIS

This disease is caused by the intestinal nematode *Trichinella spiralis*. Infection in humans results from the ingestion of uncooked or undercooked pork (occasionally bearmeat) containing the encysted larvae of *T. spiralis*. The larvae are liberated from their cysts by the gastric juices and develop into adult male and female worms in the duodenum and jejunum. After fertilization, the female burrows into the intestinal mucosa, where she deposits several successive batches of larvae. These make their way via the lymphatics, regional lymph nodes, thoracic duct, and bloodstream into all parts of the body. The new larvae penetrate all tissues, but survive only in muscle, where they become encysted and eventually calcify. Animals are infected in the same way as humans, and the cycle can be repeated only if a new host ingests the encysted larvae. The most authoritative review of this subject is that of Gould (1970).

The early symptoms of the disease, beginning a day or two after the ingestion of pork, are those of a mild gastroenteritis. These are followed by symptoms attributable to invasion of muscle by larvae. The latter symptoms begin about the end of the first week and may last for 4 to 6 weeks. Low-grade fever, pain and tenderness of muscles, edema of the conjunctivae and eyelids, and fatigue are the usual manifestations. Muscle weakness may be present, and if severe, tendon reflexes may be lost. The weakness may be generalized or limited to certain groups of muscles, e.g., ocular muscles with diplopia and strabismus, tongue muscles with dysarthria. The muscles most susceptible to invasion are the diaphragm, extraocular, tongue, laryngeal, jaw, intercostal, neck, back, abdominal, and limb muscles, in that order.

Heavy infestation may be associated with central nervous system disorder. Headache, stiff neck, and a mild confusional state are the usual symptoms. Delirium, coma, hemiplegia, and aphasia occur occasionally. The spinal fluid is usually normal, but may contain a moderate number of lymphocytes and rarely, parasites.

An eosinophilic leukocytosis usually appears when the muscles are invaded. Serologic (precipitin) test and skin test become positive early in the third week. The heart is often involved, manifested by tachycardia and electrocardiographic changes. These findings may aid in the diagnosis, which can be confirmed by finding the larvae in muscle biopsy, using the technique of low-power scan of the wet tissue pressed between two glass slides.

Trichinosis is seldom fatal. Most cases recover completely, although myalgia may persist for several months. Recurrent seizures and focal neurologic deficits may persist indefinitely. The latter are based on a trichina encephalitis (the filiform larvae may be seen in cerebral capillaries and in cerebral parenchyma) and emboli from mural thrombi arising in infected heart muscle.

In the treatment of trichinosis, thiabendazole, an antihelminthic agent, and corticosteroids are of particular value. Thiabendazole, 25 mg/kg twice daily for 5 to 7 days, is effective in both the enteral and parenteral phases of the disease, preventing larvae reproduction (therefore useful in patients known to have ingested trichinous meat) and interfering with the metabolism of muscle-dwelling larvae. Fever, myalgia, and eosinophilia respond well to the antiinflammatory and immunosuppressant effects of prednisone (40 to 60 mg daily), and a salutary effect has been noted on the cardiac and neurologic complications as well.

OTHER HELMINTHIC INFECTIONS

Cysticercosis, the larval or intermediate stage of infection with the pork tapeworm, *Taenia solium,* may involve the nervous system. The symptoms are related to encystment of the larvae. When the cysticerci are widely distributed, the symptoms may be those of a meningoencephalitis. Cystic nodules of varying size may be scattered throughout the brain and mimic the symptoms of brain tumor or other cerebral disorders. A racemose formation of organisms may block the ventricular system. In South American countries this is one of the commonest causes of epilepsy. It should also be suspected in patients presenting with headache and other signs of increased intracranial pressure. Usually multiple calcified

lesions are seen in the cerebrum and thigh and leg muscles. There is no medical therapy. Surgical removal of ventricular cysticerci may relieve hydrocephalus.

Infection with *Echinococcus* may occasionally affect the brain. The usual sources of infection are water and vegetables contaminated by canine feces. After ingestion, the ova hatch and the freed embryos migrate, primarily to lung and liver, but sometimes to brain (approximately 2 percent of cases), where a large solitary (hydatid) cyst may be formed.

Cerebral coenuriasis is an uncommon infestation by larvae (*Coenurus cerebralis*) of the tapeworm *Multiceps multiceps.* It occurs mainly in sheep-raising areas where there are many dogs, the latter being the definitive hosts. The larvae form grapelike cysts, most often in the posterior fossa, which obstruct the spinal fluid pathways and cause signs of increased intracranial pressure.

The nervous system may also be invaded directly by certain worms (ascaris, filaria) and flukes (schistosoma, paragonimus). These diseases are virtually nonexistent in the United States.

SCHISTOSOMIASIS

The ova of trematodes seldom involve the nervous system, but when it is involved, the infecting organism is usually *Schistosoma japonicum* or, less often, *S. haematobium* or *S. mansoni. S. japonicum* has a tendency to localize in the cerebral hemispheres and *S. mansoni* in the spinal cord. The cerebral lesion centers on invaded blood vessels and takes the form of a necrotizing parenchymal focus infiltrated by eosinophils and giant cells with deposits of calcium.

Schistosomiasis is widespread in tropical regions, especially in Egypt, and North American neurologists have little contact with it. An estimated 3 to 5 percent of patients develop neurologic symptoms several months after exposure and early gastrointestinal symptoms. Headaches, convulsions (either focal or generalized), and other cerebral signs appear. With numerous lesions of larger size, headache and papilledema may appear. Also, granulomatous lesions may implicate the spinal cord, causing a transverse myelitis. There is a pleocytosis of CSF often with an increase in eosinophils, increased protein content, and sometimes increased pressure. Biopsy of liver, rectal mucosa, skin tests, and complement fixation tests confirm the diagnosis. Treatment consists of antimony preparations (Fuadin) in doses of 2.2 g given intravenously every 2 to 3 days for 15 doses. Surgi-

cal excision of granulomatous tumors is sometimes indicated.

REFERENCES

ADAMS RD, KUBIK CS, BONNER FJ: The clinical and pathological aspects of influenzal meningitis. *Arch Pediatr* 65:354,
1948.

BENNETT JE et al: A comparison of amphotericin B alone and
combined with flucytosine in the treatment of cryptococcal
meningitis. *N Engl J Med* 301:126, 1979.

BERMAN PH, BANKER BQ: Neonatal meningitis: A clinical and
pathological study of 29 cases. *Pediatrics* 38:6, 1966.

BHANDARI YS, SARKARI NBS: Subdural empyema: A review of
37 cases. *J Neurosurg* 32:35, 1970.

BREWER NS et al: Brain abscess: A review of recent experience.
Ann Intern Med 82:571, 1975.

CARPENTER RR, PETERSDORF RG: The clinical spectrum of
bacterial meningitis. *Am J Med* 33:262, 1962.

COHEN MM: The central nervous system in congenital heart
disease. *Neurology* 10:452, 1960.

COONROD JD, DANS PE: Subdural empyema. *Am J Med* 53:85,
1972.

GALBRAITH JG, BARR VW: Epidural abscess and subdural empyema, in Thompson RA, Green JR (eds): *Advances in Neurology*, vol 6. New York, Raven Books, 1974, pp 257-267.

GARFIELD J: Management of supratentorial intracranial abscess: A review of 200 cases. *Br Med J* 2:7, 1968.

GATES EM et al: Metastatic brain abscess. *Medicine* 29:71,
1950.

GOULD SE: *Trichinosis in Man and Animals*. Springfield, Ill,
Charles C Thomas, 1970.

HAND LW, SANFORD JP: Posttraumatic bacterial meningitis.
Ann Intern Med 72:869, 1970.

HEINEMAN HS et al: Intracranial suppurative disease. *J Am
Med Assoc* 218:1542, 1971.

HINMAN AR: Tuberculous meningitis at Cleveland Metropolitan General Hospital. *Am Rev Respir Dis* 94:465, 1966.

JEFFERSON M: Sarcoidosis of the nervous system. *Brain* 80:540,
1957.

KANE CH, MOST H: Schistosomiasis of the central nervous system. *Arch Neurol Psychiatry* 59:141, 1948.

KUBIK CS, ADAMS RD: Subdural empyema. *Brain* 66:18, 1943.

LEWIS JL, RABINOVICH S: The wide spectrum of cryptococcal
infection. *Am J Med* 53:315, 1972.

MATHIES AW: Penicillins in the treatment of bacterial meningitis. *J R Coll Physicians* 6:139, 1972.

MATSON DD: *Neurosurgery of Infancy and Childhood*. Springfield, Ill, Charles C Thomas, 1969, p 716.

MAYOCK RL et al: Manifestations of sarcoidosis. *Am J Med*
35:67, 1963.

MERRITT HH, ADAMS RD, SOLOMON H: *Neurosyphilis*. New
York, Oxford, 1946.

MURPHY FK, MACKOWIAK P, LUBY J: Management of infections affecting the nervous system, in Rosenberg RN (ed):
The Treatment of Neurological Diseases. New York, Spectrum, 1979, pp 249-376.

NAGEOTTE J: Pathogénie du tabes dorsale. *Presse Med* 2:1179,
1902.

NEWTON EM: Hematogenous brain abscess in cyanotic congenital heart disease. *Q J Med* 25:201, 1956.

OBERSTEINER H, REDLICH E: Über das Wesen und Pathogenese
der tabischen Knitenstrangs Degeneration. *Arb Hirnanato-
mischen Institut* 2:158, 1894; 3:192, 1895.

O'LAUGHLIN JM: Infections in the immunosuppressed patient.
Med Clin North Am 59:495, 1975.

SCADDING JG: *Sarcoidosis*. London, Eyre and Spottiswoode,
1967.

SCHMIDT RP, GONYEA EF: Neurosyphilis, in Baker AB, Baker
LH (eds): *Clinical Neurology*. New York, Harper & Row,
1980, chap 19.

SMITH BH: Infections of the dura and its venous sinuses, in
Baker AB, Baker LH (eds): *Clinical Neurology*. New York,
Harper & Row, 1971, chap 14.

SNOW RM, DISMUKES WE: Cryptococcal meningitis. *Arch Intern Med* 135:1155, 1975.

SPIELMEYER W: Zur Pathogenese der Tabes. *Z Ges Neurol Psychiatr* 84:257, 1923; 91:672, 1924; 97:287, 1925.

SWARTZ MN: Anaerobic bacteria in central nervous system infections. *J Fl Med Assoc* 57:19, 1970.

————, DODGE PR: Bacterial meningitis: A review of selected
aspects. *N Engl J Med* 272: 725, 779, 842, 898, 1965.

TANDON PN, PATHAK SN: Tuberculosis of the central nervous
system, in Spillane JD (ed): *Tropical Neurology*. London,
Oxford, 1973, pp 37-62.

THOMPSON RA: Clinical features of central nervous system fungus infection, in Thompson RA, Green JR (eds): *Advances
in Neurology*, vol 6. New York, Raven Books, 1974, pp
93-100.

TOWNSEND JJ et al: Acquired toxoplasmosis. *Arch Neurol*
32:335, 1975.

WASZ-HÖCKERT O, DONNER M: Results of the treatment of 191
children with tuberculous meningitis. *Acta Paediatr* 51(suppl
141):7, 1962.

WEISS W et al: Prognostic factors in pneumococcal meningitis.
Arch Intern Med 120:517, 1967.

WILSON SAK: *Neurology*. London, William Woods, 1940.

YOSHIKAWA TT et al: Role of anaerobic bacteria in subdural
hematoma. *Am J Med* 58:99, 1975.

CHAPTER 32

VIRAL INFECTIONS OF THE NERVOUS SYSTEM

The notion that certain viruses are neurotropic, i.e., have a selective affinity for the nervous system, is no longer tenable. With the possible exception of rabies, viral infections of the nervous system are invariably complications of generalized viral infections. Considering the frequency of the latter, invasion of the nervous system is a relatively uncommon occurrence; nevertheless, it may be of overriding clinical importance. Many of the common viruses (herpes simplex, measles, varicella, for example), which cause only insignificant systemic illnesses, can have a devastating effect upon the nervous system. In other words, the neural aspects of viral infection may assume a clinical importance that is quite disproportionate to the systemic illnesses of which they are a part, and the term *neurotropic* should be used only in this qualified sense.

The characteristics of viruses and of immune reactions are not appropriate topics of discussion in a textbook of neurology. The reader is referred to Chap. 176 in the ninth edition of *Harrison's Principles of Internal Medicine*.

PATHWAYS OF INFECTION

Viruses gain entrance to the body by one of several pathways. The most common viruses—mumps, measles, varicella—enter via the respiratory passages. Polioviruses and other enteroviruses enter by the oral route; herpes simplex enters mainly via the oral or genital mucosal route. Other viruses are acquired by inoculation, as a result of the bites of animals (e.g., rabies) or mosquitoes (*arthropod-borne* or arbovirus infections). The fetus may be infected transplacentally by the rubella virus and cytomegalovirus.

Following entry into the body, the virus multiplies locally and in secondary sites, and usually gives rise to a viremia. Most viral particles are cleared from the blood by monocytes and other elements of the reticuloendothelial system, but if the viremia is massive or other factors are favorable, they will invade the CNS via the cerebral capillaries and the choroid plexus. Clearance of virus from CNS tissues is accomplished by humoral immune globulins and secretory IgA antibodies produced by thymus-derived lymphocytes.

Another pathway of infection is along peripheral nerves; centripetal movement of virus is accomplished by retrograde axoplasmic flow. Herpes simplex and rabies viruses and possibly herpes zoster virus utilize this peripheral nerve pathway, which explains why the initial symptoms of rabies and the rare B virus infection of monkeys (*herpes simiae*) occur locally, at a segmental level that corresponds to the animal bite. Experimentally it has been shown that viruses may spread to the CNS by penetrating the olfactory mucosa, but the role of this pathway in human infection is not certain. Of these different routes of infection, the hematogenous one is by far the most important. The steps in the hematogenous spread of infection are illustrated diagramatically in Fig. 32-1.

MECHANISMS OF VIRAL INFECTIONS

Viruses, once they invade the nervous system, have diverse clinical and pathologic effects. One reason for this diversity is that different cell populations within the CNS vary in their susceptibility to infection with different viruses. Thus, some infections are confined to meningeal cells, in which case the clinical manifestations will be those of a benign aseptic meningitis (see below). Other viruses will involve parenchymal cells of the brain or spinal cord, giving rise to the more serious disorders of encephalitis and poliomyelitis, respectively. In some

ENTRY INTO HOST
  Inoculation
  Respiratory
  Enteric

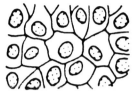

GROWTH IN EXTRANEURAL TISSUES
  Primary sites
    subcutaneous tissue and muscle, lymph
    nodes, respiratory or gastrointestinal
    tracts
  Secondary sites
    muscle, vascular endothelium, bone
    marrow, liver, spleen, etc.

MAINTENANCE OF VIREMIA
  Sufficient input
  Adsorption to red cells
  Growth in white cells
  Decreased clearance by RES

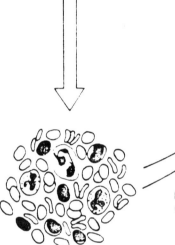

Normally phagocytozed by
reticuloendothelial system

CROSSING FROM BLOOD TO BRAIN

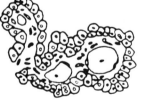

CHOROID PLEXUS TO CSF
  Growth in choroid plexus
  Passage through choroid plexus

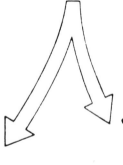

SMALL VESSELS TO BRAIN
  Transport by infected leukocytes
  Infection of vascular endothelium
  Diffusion across normal cells and
    membranes
  Passage through areas of permeability

Figure 32-1
*Steps in the hematogenous spread of virus to
the central nervous system. (Courtesy of RT
Johnson.)*

viral infections the susceptibility of particular cell groups is even more specific. In poliomyelitis, for example, there is a particular vulnerability of motor neurons of cranial and spinal nerves; and in rabies, of neurons of the trigeminal ganglia, cerebellum, and limbic lobes. Furthermore, the pathologic effects of viruses upon susceptible cells vary greatly. In acute encephalitis, susceptible neurons are invaded directly by virus, and the cells undergo lysis, with an appropriate glial and inflammatory reaction. In the disease known as progressive multifocal leukoencephalopathy (PML), there appears to be a selective lysis of oligodendrocytes, resulting in foci of demyelination. In acute disseminated (postexanthem) encephalomyelitis, the destruction of myelin has a different mechanism, possibly an immune response focused on viral antigens on the surfaces of oligodendrocytes. In herpes zoster and in certain instances of herpes simplex, the virus remains latent in cells for long periods until immunity falls, particularly in old age, or some other factor triggers an outbreak of acute infection. In certain congenital infections, e.g., rubella and cytomegalovirus, the virus persists in nervous tissue for months or years. In still other circumstances, a protracted viral infection simulating degenerative disease occurs only after a long incubation period (*slow virus* infections) and excites no inflammatory reaction.

CLINICAL SYNDROMES

The number of viruses that affect the nervous system is legion. Among the enteroviruses alone, more than 40 distinct serologic types have been associated with CNS disease, and additional types from this family of viruses and others are still being discovered. There is no need to consider these viruses individually, since there are only a limited number of ways in which they express themselves clinically. Five syndromes recur with regularity and should be familiar to all neurologists: (1) acute anterior poliomyelitis; (2) herpes zoster ganglionitis; (3) acute aseptic (nonsuppurative or "lymphocytic") meningitis; (4) acute encephalitis or meningoencephalitis; and (5) chronic infections due to "slow viruses" and unconventional agents, simulating degenerative disease.

SYNDROME OF ACUTE ANTERIOR POLIOMYELITIS

This syndrome is almost invariably the result of infection by one of the three types of poliovirus. Illnesses that are clinically indistinguishable from poliovirus infections can be caused by other enteroviruses, such as Coxsackie viruses and echoviruses, but the latter are less common

and the associated paralysis is rarely significant. The important (paralytic) disease in this category is poliomyelitis, and the remainder of the discussion will be concerned with it alone.

Poliomyelitis has ceased to be a scourge in areas where vaccination is common, but its lethal and crippling effects are still fresh in memory. As recently as the summer of 1955, when New England experienced its last epidemic, 3950 cases of acute poliomyelitis were reported in Massachusetts alone, and 2771 of these were paralytic. Now paralytic poliomyelitis is a rarity in the United States; the authors have not seen a bona fide instance for many years. Nevertheless, isolated cases are still being reported among unvaccinated persons, particularly in parts of the world where a vaccination program has not been started or sustained, and of course the paralytic residua of previous epidemics are everywhere around us. It is necessary, therefore, to review the main features of the disease.

ETIOLOGY AND EPIDEMIOLOGY

The disease is caused by a small RNA virus of the picornavirus group. Three antigenically distinct types have been defined, and infection with one does not protect against the others. The disease has a worldwide distribution, but epidemics, when they occurred, were more frequent in the north temperate zone, in regions of excellent sanitation, than elsewhere. The peak incidence of infection was in the months of July through September.

Poliomyelitis is a highly communicable disease. The main reservoir of infection is the human intestinal tract, and the main route of infection is fecal-oral, as with other enteric pathogens. The virus multiplies in the pharynx and intestinal tract, and during the incubation period, which is from 1 to 3 weeks, virus can be recovered from both of these sites. The virus penetrates the intestinal wall and is borne in the blood to all parts of the body. In only a small fraction of infected patients is the nervous system invaded. It is estimated that between 95 to 99 percent of infected patients are asymptomatic or experience a nonspecific illness. It is the latter type of patient—the carrier with inapparent infection—that is most important in the spread of the virus from one person to another.

CLINICAL MANIFESTATIONS

As indicated above, the large majority of infections are unaccompanied by any symptoms (*inapparent infec-*

tion), or there may be only mild systemic symptoms with pharyngitis or gastroenteritis or flulike symptoms (so-called *minor illness* or *abortive poliomyelitis*). These mild forms of poliomyelitis correspond to the period of viremia and dissemination of the virus, and in most cases they give rise to an effective immune response, which accounts for their failure to cause meningitis or poliomyelitis. In the relatively small proportion of patients in whom the nervous system is invaded, the illness still has a wide range of severity, from a mild attack of aseptic meningitis (*nonparalytic* or *preparalytic poliomyelitis*) to the most severe forms of paralytic disease (*paralytic poliomyelitis*). These latter forms are described below.

Nonparalytic or Preparalytic Poliomyelitis The prodromal symptoms in this form of the illness are those of the minor illness, mentioned above. Listlessness, generalized, nonthrobbing headache, fever of 38 to 40°C, stiffness and aching in the muscles, sore throat in the absence of upper respiratory infection, anorexia, nausea, and vomiting are the usual manifestations. These symptoms may subside to a varying extent, to be followed after 3 to 4 days by recrudescence of headache and fever and by symptoms of nervous system involvement (so-called dromedary or biphasic form). More often the second phase of the illness blends with the first. Tenderness and pain in the muscles, tightness of the hamstrings (*spasm*), and pain in the neck and back become increasingly prominent. Other manifestations of nervous system involvement include irritability, restlessness, and emotional instability. The occurrence of the latter symptoms is frequently a prelude to paralysis. Added to these symptoms are stiffness of the neck on forward flexion, Kernig and Brudzinski signs, and the characteristic CSF findings of *aseptic meningitis*. The cell count is between 25 and 500 per cubic millimeter, occasionally higher; neutrophils predominate in the first few days of the illness, then lymphocytes; protein is elevated, rarely to more than 150 mg per 100 ml; and the glucose content is normal.

The symptoms described above may constitute the entire illness. In such instances, fever and other systemic manifestations subside in a matter of days, although the signs of meningeal irritation may persist for a week or two and the CSF protein may not return to normal for 4 to 5 weeks. Alternately, the preparalytic symptoms may be followed by paralytic ones. The weakness becomes manifest while the fever is at its height, or, just as fre-

quently, weakness occurs as the temperature is falling and the general clinical picture seems to be improving.

The clinical patterns of preparalytic and paralytic poliomyelitis vary to some extent, depending upon the age of the patient. The diphasic or dromedary course is common in children, but unusual in patients over 15 years of age. Symptoms tend to develop more rapidly in younger patients, and the interval between onset of symptoms and paralysis tends also to be shorter in this group. On the other hand, pain in the muscles is a more prominent feature in adolescents and adults than in young children.

Paralytic Poliomyelitis The conventional division of paralytic poliomyelitis into spinal, bulbar, and encephalitic types is a convenient descriptive device, but it has no valid pathologic basis, as will be indicated further on. Clinically, one or other of these forms may predominate, but more often they occur in combination.

Muscle weakness may develop rapidly, attaining its maximum severity in 48 h or even less, or it may advance more slowly, or in stuttering fashion, for a week or longer. As a general rule, there is no progression of weakness after the temperature has been normal for 48 h. The distribution of spinal paralysis is quite variable. In children under 5 years of age, the most common but by no means the only form is a weakness of one leg; in older children, weakness of an arm or both legs is usual, and in the 16 to 65-year-old group, an asymmetric weakness of all four limbs. The most widespread weakness occurs in infants. Rarely there may be an acute symmetrical paralysis of the muscles of the trunk and limbs, like that of the Landry-Guillain-Barré syndrome.

Coarse fasciculations are frequently seen as the muscles weaken; they are transient as a rule, but occasionally they persist. Abdominal, cremasteric, and tendon reflexes are diminished and lost as the weakness of abdominal and limb muscles evolves. Patients frequently complain of paresthesias in the affected limbs, but objective sensory loss is not demonstrable. Retention of urine is a common occurrence in adult patients, but does not persist. Atrophy of muscle can be detected within 3 weeks of onset of paralysis, and is permanent.

More or less pure bulbar affection may be seen in children, particularly in those in whom tonsils and adenoids had been removed. Adults with bulbar symptoms almost always have spinal involvement as well. Any of the cranial muscles may be weakened, but the most frequently involved are the muscles of deglutition, because of affection of the nucleus ambiguus. The other great hazards of bulbar disease are the disturbances of respiration and vasomotor control—hiccough, shallowness and progressive slowing of respiration, cyanosis, hypertension, and ultimately hypotension and circulatory collapse. When these symptoms are added to paralysis of phrenic and intercostal musculature, the fatality rate is between 25 and 75 percent.

Restlessness and agitation, anxiety and fear of death, somnolence, confusion, stupor, and coma are the symptoms usually referred to as encephalitic. They are probably related to pathologic changes in the high brainstem and hypothalamus, as indicated in the following section.

PATHOLOGIC CHANGES AND CLINICOPATHOLOGIC CORRELATIONS

In fatal infections, nonparalytic as well as paralytic, lesions are found in the cerebral cortex, brainstem, and spinal cord. As far as the pathologist is concerned, therefore, all cases of poliomyelitis are also encephalitic. The cerebral lesions, however, are confined to the precentral gyrus and are usually of insufficient severity to cause symptoms. The brunt of the disease is borne by the hypothalamus, thalamus, motor nuclei of the brainstem and surrounding reticular formation, vestibular nuclei and roof nuclei of the cerebellum, and the gray matter of the spinal cord, particularly the neurons of the anterior and intermediate columns. In these areas, nerve cells are destroyed; a leukocytic reaction is present for only a few days but mononuclear cells and microglia persist as perivascular accumulations for many months. The initial inflammatory response may at times be so severe as to cause small foci of tissue necrosis and petechial hemorrhages.

The nature of the histopathologic changes and their relationship to the clinical findings have been studied most carefully by Bodian, both in experimental animals and in humans, and the following account is based largely on his observations.

The earliest visible alterations, in response to invasion of the CNS by virus, is central chromatolysis of the cytoplasmic Nissl substance of the nerve cells, along with an inflammatory reaction. These changes are accompanied by a multiplication of virus in the CNS, and both precede the onset of paralysis by a day or by several days. Changes in the nerve cells proceed rapidly; progressive dissolution of cytoplasmic Nissl substance is followed by disintegration of the nucleus and then by complete lysis or necrosis of the cell.

It is of interest that while poliovirus has been readily isolated from CNS tissue of fatal cases, it can rarely be recovered from the CSF during clinical disease. This is in contrast to the closely related Coxsackie and echo picornaviruses which have been isolated frequently from the CSF during neurologic illnesses.

Bodian's observations in experimental animals indicate that the infected motor neurons continue to function until the stage of severe chromatolysis is reached. Furthermore, if damage to the cell has attained only the stage of central chromatolysis, complete morphologic recovery can be expected. Cells are either destroyed quickly in the first few days of the disease, or are restored to morphologic normality—a process that takes a month or longer. After this time it can be shown that the degree of paralysis and atrophy is closely correlated with the number of motor nerve cells that have been destroyed; where limbs remain atrophic and paralyzed, less than 10 percent of neurons survive in corresponding cord segments.

The variability of the clinical signs and symptoms depends mainly on the variation in severity of the nerve cell injury and inflammatory response in different regions. Only when the pathologic changes reach a certain threshold of severity, exceeding the margin of safety of the particular cell population involved, is a clinical effect observed.

As mentioned previously, the nerve cell changes and inflammatory reaction in the cerebral cortex are of insufficient severity to cause the so-called encephalitic changes (restlessness, anxiety, confusion, stupor, etc.). The latter seem to be related to the presence of severe brainstem lesions, including those in the hypothalamus. Also, hypotension and hypoxia may be responsible for these symptoms.

Lesions in the motor nuclei of the brainstem may be associated with paralysis in corresponding muscles, but only if the lesions are severe in degree. In fatal cases it is usual to find lesions in all brainstem nuclei (except those of the basis pontis and inferior olives); yet paralytic symptoms in corresponding muscles are rarely recorded, except in those of the face, larynx, and pharynx. This testifies to the wide margin of safety in the oculomotor, motor trigeminal, and hypoglossal nuclei.

The three regions of the brainstem most severely affected are the reticular formation, vestibular nuclei, and roof nuclei of the cerebellum. Vertigo, nystagmus, ataxia, and tremor are probably related to the latter lesions, but these clinical manifestations are distinctly uncommon. Symptoms of nausea and vomiting may also be due to lesions in these nuclei. The disturbances of swallowing, respiration, and vasomotor control are related to lesions in the medullary reticular formation, including the region of the nucleus ambiguus.

Atrophic, areflexic paralysis of muscles of the

trunk and limbs relates, of course, to destruction of neurons in the corresponding segments of the spinal cord gray matter, more specifically of cells in the anterior and intermediate horns. Impairment of sensation practically never occurs in poliomyelitis, although mild, spotty lesions are observed frequently in the dorsal horns. The common symptoms of stiffness and pain in the neck and back are usually attributed to "meningeal irritation"; probably they are related to the mild inflammatory exudate in the meninges and to lesions of varying severity in the dorsal root ganglia and dorsal horns. Also it is likely that these lesions account for the muscle pain and paresthesias in parts that later become paralyzed. Abnormalities of autonomic function are probably attributable to lesions of autonomic pathways in the reticular substance of the brainstem and in the lateral horn cells in the spinal cord.

TREATMENT

Patients with suspected acute poliomyelitis should be kept in bed and hospitalized if signs of nervous system involvement are detected. Careful observation of swallowing function, vital capacity, pulse, and blood pressure is necessary in anticipation of respiratory and circulatory complications.

If the neurologic signs are limited to those of meningeal irritation and muscle pain, the administration of aspirin or other mild analgesics and the application of hot packs provide relief. If paralysis of limb muscles develops, foot boards, hand and arm splints, and knee and trochanter rolls should be used to prevent foot drop and other deformities.

Respiratory failure may be caused by paralysis of the intercostal and diaphragmatic muscles or by depression of the respiratory centers in the brainstem. Either type calls for the use of a mechanical respirator, preferably a positive-pressure respirator, and this also requires a tracheotomy. The management of the respirator patient and of the pulmonary and circulatory complications does not differ from that of patients with other neurologic diseases, such as myasthenia gravis or acute ascending polyneuropathy, and it is best carried out in special respiratory care units.

PROGNOSIS

The overall mortality rate of acute paralytic poliomyelitis is between 5 and 10 percent, higher in adults and with increasing age, and higher in very young children and infants. If the patient survives the acute stage, paralysis of respiration and deglutition usually recover completely; in only a small fraction of such patients is chronic respirator care necessary. Many patients also recover completely from muscular weakness, and most of them improve to some extent. The return of muscle strength occurs mainly in the first 3 to 4 months and is the result of enlargement of motor units by reinnervation and by morphologic restitution of partially damaged nerve cells. Slow recovery of slight degree may then continue for a year or more, the result of hypertrophy of undamaged muscle. Branching of axons of intact motor cells with reinnervation of muscle fibers of denervated motor units may also play a part.

PREVENTION

This, of course, has proved to be the most significant aspect of treatment, and one of the outstanding accomplishments of modern medicine. The cultivation of poliovirus in cultures of human embryonic tissues, the achievement of Enders and his associates, made possible the development of vaccines which offer effective and long-lasting immunity. The first of these was the injectable Salk vaccine, containing formalin-inactivated virulent strains of the three viral serotypes. Since 1960, this vaccine has been almost completely replaced by the Sabin type, which consists of attenuated live virus, administered orally in two doses 8 weeks apart; boosters are required at 1 year of age and before starting school. Since 1965, the reported annual incidence of poliomyelitis has been less than 0.01 per 100,000 (compared to an annual incidence of 24 cases per 100,000 during the years 1951 to 1955). Very rarely, poliomyelitis may follow vaccination (0.02 to 0.04 cases per million doses). Equally rare are instances of postvaccinial encephalomyelitis. The only obstacle to complete prevention of the disease is inadequate utilization of the vaccine. Significant segments of the population in areas with low public-health standards are not being immunized. Conceivably, if there is an increasing lack of immunity, outbreaks of poliomyelitis could occur once again.

SYNDROME OF HERPES ZOSTER

Herpes zoster (zona, "shingles") is a common viral infection of the nervous system, occuring at an overall rate of 3 to 5 cases per 1000 persons per year, and at a much higher rate with advancing age. It is characterized clinically by radicular pain, a vesicular cutaneous eruption, and, less often, by segmental sensory loss and motor palsies. The pathologic changes consist of an acute inflammatory reaction in isolated spinal or cranial sensory ganglia, the posterior gray matter of the spinal cord, and the adjacent leptomeninges. The neurologic implications of the segmental distribution of the rash were recognized by Richard Bright, as long ago as 1831. The inflammatory changes in the corresponding ganglia and related portions of the spinal nerves were first described by von Barensprung in 1862 and were later studied extensively by Head and Campbell. The concept that varicella and zoster are caused by the same agent was introduced by von Bokay, in 1909, and was established more recently by Weller and his associates (1954, 1958). The common agent, referred to as varicella or varicella-zoster (VZ) virus, is a DNA virus that is similar in structure to the virus of herpes simplex. These and other historical features of herpes zoster are reviewed by Denny-Brown et al. and by Weller et al.

PATHOLOGY AND PATHOGENESIS

The pathologic changes in herpes zoster are unique and consist of (1) an inflammatory reaction in several unilateral adjacent sensory ganglia of the spinal or cranial nerves, frequently of such intensity as to cause necrosis of all or part of the ganglion, with or without hemorrhage; (2) an inflammatory reaction in the spinal roots and peripheral nerve contiguous to the involved ganglion; (3) a poliomyelitis which closely resembles acute anterior poliomyelitis, but is readily distinguished by its unilaterality, segmental localization, and greater involvement of the posterior horn, posterior root, and dorsal root ganglion; and (4) a relatively mild leptomeningitis, largely limited to the involved spinal or cranial segments and nerve roots. These pathologic changes are the substratum of the neuralgic pains, the pleocytosis in the CSF, and the local palsies that may attend and follow the zoster infection.

The pathogenesis of herpes zoster is not fully understood, but the most widely accepted hypothesis is that it represents a spontaneous reactivation of varicella virus infection, which becomes latent in the sensory ganglia following the primary infection with chickenpox (Hope-Simpson). This hypothesis is consistent with the differences in the clinical manifestations of chickenpox and herpes zoster, even though both are caused by the same virus. Chickenpox is highly contagious, has a well-marked seasonal incidence (winter and spring) and a tendency to occur in epidemics. Zoster, on the other hand, is not communicable (except to a person who has not had chickenpox), occurs sporadically throughout the year, and shows no increase in incidence during epidemics of chickenpox. In patients with zoster, there is practically always a past history of chickenpox. In rare instances of herpes zoster in infants such a history may be lacking, but in these latter cases there usually has been prenatal maternal contact with the VZ virus.

Although the VZ virus has not been recovered from sensory ganglia of asymptomatic individuals, it has been recovered from the segmental sensory ganglia of patients who have died during the course of an active zoster infection. Also the closely related viruses of herpes simplex have been obtained from human trigeminal and sacral ganglia (Baringer). The supposition is that in both varicella and zoster infections the virus makes its way from the cutaneous vesicles, along the sensory nerves to the ganglion, where it remains latent until activated, at which time it progresses down the axon to the skin. Multiplication of the virus in epidermal cells causes swelling, vacuolization and lysis of cell boundaries, leading to the formation of vesicles and Lipschutz inclusion bodies. Alternately, the ganglia could be infected during the viremia of chickenpox, but then one would have to explain why only one or a few sensory ganglia become infected. Reactivation of virus is attributed to waning immunity, which would explain the increasing incidence of zoster with aging (increasing lack of exposure to children with chickenpox) and with lymphomas, administration of immunosuppressive drugs and radiation therapy.

CLINICAL FEATURES

As has been indicated, the incidence of herpes zoster rises with age. Hope-Simpson has estimated that if a cohort of 1000 people lived to 85 years of age, half would have had on attack of zoster and 10 would have had two attacks. The notion that one attack of zoster provides lifelong immunity is only relatively correct (recurrent herpes, however, is usually due to the simplex virus). The sexes are equally affected as are both sides of the body. Zoster occurs in about 10 percent of patients with lymphoma and 25 percent of patients with Hodgkin's disease—particularly in those who have undergone splenectomy and received radiotherapy. Conversely, about 5 percent of patients who present with herpes zoster are found to have a concurrent malignancy (about twice the number that would be expected).

The vesicular eruption is usually preceded for several days by itching, tingling, or burning sensations in the involved dermatome(s), and sometimes by malaise and fever as well. Or there is severe localized pain which may be mistaken for pleurisy, appendicitis, or cholecystitis until the diagnosis is clarified by the appearance of vesicles (nearly always within 72 to 96 h). The rash consists of tense clear vesicles on an erythematous base, the contents of which becomes cloudy after a few days (due to accumulation of inflammatory cells) and dry, crusted, and scaly after 5 to 10 days. In a small number of patients the vesicles are confluent and hemorrhagic, and healing is delayed for several weeks. In most cases, pain and dysesthesia last for 1 to 4 weeks; but in the others (7 to 33 percent of cases, in different series) the pain persists for months or in different forms even for years, and presents a difficult problem in management. Impairment of superficial sensation in the affected dermatome(s) is common and, in about 5 percent of patients, segmental weakness and atrophy are added. In the majority of patients the rash and sensorimotor signs are limited to the territory of a single dermatome, but in some, particularly those with cranial or limb involvement, two or more contiguous nerves are involved. Rarely (and usually in association with malignancy) the rash is generalized, like that of chickenpox. The CSF frequently shows a mild pleocytosis, mainly lymphocytic, and an elevated protein content. The diagnosis can be confirmed by direct immunofluorescence of a biopsied skin lesion, using antibody to VZ virus.

Virtually any dermatome may be involved in herpes zoster, but some regions are far more frequently involved than others. The thoracic dermatomes, particularly T5 to T10, are the most common sites, accounting for more than two-thirds of all cases, followed by the craniocervical regions. In the latter cases the disease tends to be more severe, with greater pain, more frequent meningeal signs, and involvement of the mucous membranes.

There are two rather characteristic cranial herpetic syndromes—so-called ophthalmic herpes and geniculate herpes. In *ophthalmic herpes,* which accounts for 10 to 15 percent of all cases of herpes zoster, the rash and pain are in the distribution of the first division of the trigeminal nerve, and the pathologic changes are centered in the gasserian ganglion. The main hazard in this form of the disease is herpetic involvement of the cornea and conjunctiva, with corneal anesthesia and residual scarring. Palsies of extraocular muscles, ptosis, and mydriasis are frequently associated, indicating that the third, fourth, and sixth cranial nerves are affected in addition to the gasserian ganglion.

A less common cranial nerve syndrome consists of a facial palsy in combination with a herpetic eruption of the external auditory meatus, with or without tinnitus, vertigo, and deafness. Ramsay Hunt attributed this syndrome to herpes of the geniculate ganglion, despite the fact that pathologic confirmation of such a lesion has not been forthcoming, either in Hunt's time or since then. One of the authors (R.D.A.) found the geniculate ganglion only slightly affected in a man who died 64 days after the onset of a so-called Ramsay Hunt syndrome (during which time he had recovered from the facial palsy); there was, however, a neuritis of the facial nerve, a finding that provided an explanation for the facial palsy.

Herpes zoster of the palate, pharynx, neck, and retroauricular region (herpes occipitocollaris) depends upon herpetic infection of the ganglia of the vagus and glossopharyngeal nerves and of the upper cervical roots. Herpes zoster in this distribution may be associated with the Ramsay Hunt syndrome. Encephalitis and myelitis are rare but well-described complications of herpes zoster in this location. Granulomatous angiitis is another rare complication of herpes zoster infection; it is due apparently to the direct invasion of vessels by virus from neighboring nerves (Linnemann and Alvira).

The notion that a Bell's palsy or pain in the distribution of a trigeminal or intercostal nerve, without subsequent rash, is due to herpetic ganglionitis without spread to the skin (zoster sine herpete) is purely speculative. In practically none of such cases can an antibody response to VZ virus be demonstrated.

TREATMENT

There is no specific treatment for herpes zoster; about all that can be done during the acute stage is to blunt the pain with analgesics and with lotions or powders applied to the skin lesions. The administration of corticosteroids has been shown to shorten the duration of pain, and probably carries no hazard in patients with uncomplicated zoster. Corticosteroids are contraindicated in patients with neoplasms or other immunodeficient states because of the increased danger of dissemination of the lesions. In these latter patients a course of adenine arabinoside may be worthwhile; it has been shown that immunosuppressed patients who receive this drug in the first 6 days of the disease have a more rapid clearance of virus from vesicles and less pain than nontreated controls (Whitley et al.). On the other hand, cytosine arabinoside is ineffective in these circumstances. The effect of adenine arabinoside upon the incidence and severity of postherpetic neuralgia remains to be determined. In cases of ophthalmic zoster, the application of idoxuridine (IDU) to the eye, either in a 0.1% solution every hour or a 0.5% ointment four or five times a day, is recommended by some ophthalmologists.

The management of postherpetic pain and dysesthesia can be a trying matter for both the patient and the physician. It would appear that incomplete interruption of nerves results in a hyperpathic state where every stimulus excites pain. Sometimes, a course of phenytoin or carbamazepine ablates the pain, particularly if it is of lancinating type. It should be emphasized that postherpetic neuralgia eventually subsides even in the most severe and persistent cases. Until this happens, the physician must exercise skill and patience in the medical management of chronic pain (see page 100), and avoid the temptation of subjecting the patient to one of the many surgical measures that have been advocated for this disorder. Excision or undercutting the involved region of skin, section of the spinal nerves or roots, and cordotomy have generally proved to be ineffective, or at best given only temporary relief. Many of the patients with the most persistent complaints will have all the symptoms of a depressive state and will be helped by appropriate antidepressive medications.

THE SYNDROME OF ASEPTIC MENINGITIS

The term *aseptic meningitis* was first introduced to designate what was thought to be a specific disease, but it is now applied to a symptom complex that can be produced by any one of numerous infective agents, the majority of which are viral. Since aseptic meningitis is rarely fatal, the precise CNS changes are uncertain, but are presumably limited to the meninges. Conceivably, there may be some minor changes in the brain itself (as in experimental poliomyelitis in primates) but these are of insufficient severity to cause neurologic symptoms and signs.

In outline, *the clinical syndrome of aseptic meningitis consists of fever, headache, and other signs of meningeal irritation, and a lymphocytic and mononuclear pleocytosis of the cerebrospinal fluid (CSF)*. Usually the temperature is elevated, from 38 to 40°C. Headache, perhaps more severe than that associated with other febrile states, is the most frequent symptom. A variable degree of drowsiness, confusion, or even stupor and coma may occur, but as a rule the derangement of consciousness is mild in degree. Photophobia and pain on movement of the eyes are common complaints. Stiffness of the neck and spine on forward bending attest to the presence of meningeal irritation, but at first it may be so

slight as to pass unnoticed. Here the Kernig and Brudzinski signs help very little, for they are often absent in the presence of a manifest viral meningitis. Other symptoms and signs are infrequent; these include sore throat, nausea and vomiting, vague weakness, pain in the back and neck, paresthesias in an extremity, isolated strabismus and diplopia, a slight inequality of reflexes, or a wavering Babinski sign. In general, then, the symptoms are mild, and at times the meningitis is entirely asymptomatic. An erythematous papulomacular, nonpruritic rash, confined to the head and neck or generalized, may be a prominent feature (particularly in children) of aseptic meningitis that is caused by certain echoviruses and Coxsackie viruses. An enanthem, taking the form of grayish white spots on the buccal mucosa, may occur with echovirus infections.

The CSF findings consist of pleocytosis (mainly mononuclear, except in the first day of the illness, when more than half the cells may be neutrophils), small and variable increase in protein, and no demonstrable microorganisms by smear and bacterial culture. The concentration of glucose in the CSF is normal; this is important because a low glucose value in conjunction with a lymphocytic or mononuclear pleocytosis usually signifies tuberculous or fungal meningitis, or certain noninfectious disorders such as metastatic carcinoma, lymphoma, or sarcoid of the meninges; rarely, the CSF glucose is low in mumps meningitis or that caused by one or two other viruses. Since the CSF glucose level may be normal in the early stages of tuberculous or cryptococcal meningitis, this determination should be repeated at intervals until the diagnosis is established or the patient is definitely convalescent.

CAUSES OF ASEPTIC MENINGITIS

The majority of cases of aseptic meningitis are due to viral infections. Of these the most common are the enteroviral infections—echovirus, Coxsackie, and nonparalytic poliomyelitis, which make up 75 percent of cases in which a specific viral cause can be established. Mumps is the next most common, followed by herpes simplex (type 2), lymphocytic choriomeningitis (LCM), and adenovirus infections. The California virus, which is an arthropod-borne (arbo) virus, is responsible for a small number of cases (the arboviruses cause frank encephalitis or meningoencephalitis, as a rule). All these viral infections, together with leptospirosis, comprise about 95 percent of cases of aseptic meningitis of established etiology.

Among the less common diseases of viral origin, the icteric stage of infectious hepatitis is rarely preceded by mild meningitis, the nature of which becomes evident when the jaundice appears. Infectious mononucleosis (Epstein-Barr virus) and rarely a nonbacterial pneumonia (caused by *Mycoplasma pneumoniae)* may produce what appears to be a primary meningitis.

It should be noted that in every published series of cases from virus isolation centers, a specific cause cannot be established in a third or more of cases of presumed viral origin.

DIFFERENTIAL DIAGNOSIS OF VIRAL MENINGITIS

Clinical distinctions between the many viral forms of aseptic meningitis cannot be made with a high degree of reliability, but useful leads can be obtained by attention to certain details of the clinical history and physical examination. It is important to inquire about immunizations, past history of infectious disease, family outbreaks, insect bites, contact with animals, and areas of recent travel. The presence or absence of an epidemic, the season during which the illness occurs, and the geographic location are other helpful data.

The picorna viruses (polioviruses, echoviruses, and Coxsackie viruses) are by far the commonest causes of viral meningitis. Because they grow in the intestinal tract and are spread mainly by the fecal-oral route, family outbreaks are usual and the infections are most common among children. A number of echovirus and Coxsackie virus infections are associated with exanthemata, and group A Coxsackie viruses may in addition be associated with the grayish vesicular lesions of herpangina of the pharyngeal mucosa. Pleurodynia, a brachial neuritis, pericarditis, and orchitis are characteristic of group B Coxsackie virus infections. Pain in the back and neck and in the muscles should always suggest poliomyelitis. As has been stated, lower motor neuron weakness may occur with echovirus and Coxsackie virus infections, but it is mild and transient in nature. The peak incidence of enteroviral infections is in August and September. This is true also of infections due to arboviruses, but as a general rule the latter cause encephalitis rather than meningitis.

Mumps meningitis occurs sporadically throughout the year, but the highest incidence is in late winter and spring. Males are affected three times more frequently than females. Other manifestations of mumps infection—parotitis, orchitis, oophoritis, and pancreatitis—may or may not be present. It should be noted that orchitis is not specific for mumps but occurs occasionally with group B Coxsackie virus infections, infectious mononucleosis, and lymphocytic choriomeningitis. A definite past history of mumps aids in excluding the disease, since an attack confers lifelong immunity.

The natural host of the LCM virus is the common house mouse, *Mus musculus.* Humans acquire the infection by contact with food or dust that is contaminated by mouse excreta. The meningitis may be preceded by respiratory symptoms (sometimes with pulmonary infiltrates) of a week's duration. The infection is particularly common in late fall and winter, presumably because mice enter dwellings at that time.

The infectious agent in leptospirosis is a spirochete, but the clinical syndrome which it produces is indistinguishable from viral meningitis. Infection is acquired by contact with soil or water contaminated by the urine of rats, and also of dogs, swine, and cattle. Although leptospirosis may appear in any season, its incidence in the United States shows a striking peak in August. The presence of conjunctival suffusion, a transient blotchy erythema, severe leg and back pain, and pulmonary infiltrates should suggest leptospiral infection.

Wild rodents may also be the source of encephalomyocarditis virus infection, and cats, of course, of catscratch disease. The latter has recently been found to induce a localized cranial arteritis (Selby and Walker).

The presence of sore throat, generalized lymphadenopathy, transient rash, and mild icterus are suggestive of infectious mononucleosis. Icterus is a prominent manifestation of viral hepatitis.

Aside from viral isolation and serologic tests, few laboratory examinations are helpful. The peripheral white cell count is often normal, but leukopenia may be present. However, it accompanies so many of the diseases responsible for aseptic meningitis that rarely is it a useful finding. Eosinophilia should suggest a parasitic infection, and in most cases infectious mononucleosis can be identified by the blood smear and specific serologic tests. LCM produces an intense pleocytosis in the CSF. Counts above 1000 mononuclear cells per cubic millimeter are most often due to LCM, but may also occur with mumps and with echovirus 9; in the latter, neutrophils may predominate in the CSF for a week or longer. Serologic reactions of CSF should be interpreted with caution because inflammation of many types can produce a false positive reaction; infectious mononucleosis and lupus erythematosus often evoke false positive serum reactions for syphilis. Liver function tests are abnormal in many patients with infectious mononucleosis, leptospiral infections, and anicteric hepatitis; hepatic abnormalities are not regularly present in the other entities under consideration. In a majority of patients with *Mycoplasma pneumoniae* infections, cold agglutinins appear in the serum toward the end of the first week of the illness.

NONVIRAL FORMS OF ASEPTIC MENINGITIS

Three other categories of disease may cause an apparently sterile, predominantly lymphocytic or mononuclear reaction in the leptomeninges: (1) bacterial infections lying adjacent to the meninges, (2) specific meningeal infections or parainfectious diseases in which the organism is difficult or impossible to isolate, and (3) neoplastic invasion (usually lymphoma or carcinoma). The recognition of these is of great importance, since they require vigorous antibiotic therapy or some other form of treatment.

In respect to the first category, a smoldering paranasal sinusitis or mastoiditis may produce a CSF picture of aseptic meningitis because of intracranial extension (epidural or subdural infection), or a brain abscess, the localizing signs of which are minimal or absent, may deceive the clinician into making a diagnosis of aseptic meningitis (see Chap. 31). Also it must be remembered that antibiotic therapy given for a systemic or pulmonary infection may suppress a coexistent meningitis to the point where mononuclear cells predominate, glucose is near normal, and organisms are not detected in the CSF. A mistaken diagnosis of aseptic meningitis may then be made on the basis of the CSF examination. The true state of affairs becomes evident only when the patient worsens and bacteria again appear in the CSF. Careful attention to the history of recent antimicrobial therapy sometimes permits recognition of these cases before symptoms recur.

Syphilis, cryptococcosis, and tuberculosis are the important members of the second group. Acute syphilitic meningitis may be asymptomatic or symptomatic; in the latter case there will be both the clinical and CSF picture of aseptic meningitis except that the condition is usually afebrile. In former times acute syphilitic meningitis was likely to develop as a neurorecurrence after inadequate arsenic therapy, but now it may be the first manifestation of a florid syphilitic infection (see page 496). Tuberculous meningitis, in its initial stages, may occasionally masquerade as an innocent aseptic meningitis; the diagnosis may be difficult because the tubercle bacillus is frequently not seen in stained smears, and cultures require several weeks. Similarly, the diagnosis of cryptococcus is missed occasionally because the organisms may be present in such low numbers as to be overlooked in smears. Lymphocytic meningitis may occur as a complication of Q fever, a rickettsial disease.

Children with scarlet fever or streptococcus pharyngitis rarely have been noted to develop meningeal signs and pleocytosis, the result of a sterile serous inflammation that does not involve invasion of the meninges by organisms. The same may occur in subacute bacterial endocarditis.

In the third (neoplastic) group, leukemias and lymphomas are the most common sources of meningeal reactions. In children, a leukemic meningitis with cells (lymphoblasts or myeloblasts) in the CSF numbering in the thousands occurs frequently in the late stages of the illness. In adults, a pleocytosis with lymphocyte or lymphoblast counts reaching as high as 4000 per cubic millimeter may complicate lymphomas with or without leukemia. In these disorders and in carcinomatous "meningitis" (from lung, breast, stomach, melanoma, or other source) great numbers of neoplastic cells may extend through the leptomeninges, involving cranial and spinal nerve roots, and produce a picture of meningoradiculitis with normal or low CSF glucose values. Gliomatous infiltration of the ependyma and meninges may have the same effect. Millipore filter preparations usually permit identification of the tumor cells.

Finally, in a number of other chronic or acutely recurring diseases of obscure origin, the CSF formula corresponds to that of aseptic meningitis: (1) Behçet's disease (see below); (2) Vogt-Koyanagi disease and Harada's disease with various combinations of uveitis, depigmentation of hair and skin around the eyes, loss of eyelashes, dysacousis, and deafness; (3) Mollaret's recurrent meningitis with recurrent bouts of fever, accompanied by the signs of aseptic meningitis, from which the patient recovers rapidly and spontaneously and for which no cause is ever determined; and (4) allergic or hypersensitivity meningitis, occurring in the course of serum sickness and diseases of connective tissue such as lupus erythematosus.

Behçet's disease, distinguished originally by the clinical triad of relapsing iridocyclitis, meningitis, and recurrent ulcers of the mouth and genitalia, is now known to be a systemic disease with a much wider range of symptons, including erythema nodosum, thrombophlebitis, polyarthritis, ulcerative colitis and a number of neurologic manifestations. The latter occur in about 30 percent of patients (Chajek and Fainaru) and include meningoencephalitis, cranial nerve (particularly abducens) palsies, cerebellar ataxia, and corticospinal tract signs. There may be episodes of brainstem dysfunction, resembling minor strokes. The neurologic symptoms usually have an abrupt onset and are accompanied by as many as 3000 polymorphonuclear cells per cubic millimeter in the CSF, along with elevated protein but normal glucose values. The neurologic symptoms usually clear completely in several weeks but have a tendency to recur. Rarely the clinical picture is that of a progressive confusional state and dementia (see the recent review of Lehner and Barnes for a detailed account of clinical and immunological features).

In summary, the history of the illness, the associated clinical findings, and the laboratory tests usually provide the clues to the diagnosis of nonviral forms of aseptic meningitis. Most important is to keep in mind the possibility of tuberculosis, cryptococcosis, syphilis, inadequately treated pyogenic meningitis, and brain abscess—all of which may simulate aseptic meningitis. These diseases present pressing diagnostic problems, for they may take the life of the patient if they are not recognized and treated. In contrast, the various viral forms of aseptic meningitis are usually self-limiting and benign.

THE SYNDROME OF ACUTE ENCEPHALITIS

From the foregoing discussion it is evident that the separation of the clinical syndrome of aseptic meningitis and encephalitis is not always easy. In some patients with aseptic meningitis, drowsiness or confusion may be present. Conversely, in some patients with encephalitis the cerebral symptoms may be mild or inapparent, and only the meningeal symptoms and CSF abnormalities may be manifest. These facts make it difficult to place complete reliance on statistical data from various virus laboratories about the relative incidence of meningitis and encephalitis. Although the same spectrum of viruses causes both meningitis and encephalitis, some cause only benign disease. It is our impression that many cases of enteroviral infection and practically all cases of mumps and LCM are little more than examples of intense meningitis. Rarely have they caused death with postmortem demonstration of cerebral lesions, and surviving patients seldom have residual neurologic signs.

*The core of the encephalitis syndrome is an acute febrile illness with evidence of meningeal involvement, added to which are various combinations of the follow-*ing symptoms and signs: *convulsions, delirium, confusion, stupor, or coma; aphasia or mutism; hemiparesis with asymmetry of tendon reflexes and Babinski signs; involuntary movements, ataxia, and myoclonic jerks; nystagmus, ocular palsies, and facial weakness.* Some one or other of these groups of findings predominate in certain types of encephalitis, as will be pointed out below, but always the clinical diagnosis, in the setting of a febrile aseptic meningitis, rests on the demonstration of derangement of the function of the cerebrum, brainstem, or cerebellum. Death occurs in 5 to 20 percent of patients with acute viral encephalitis. Residual signs such as mental deterioration, amnesic defect, personality change, and hemiparesis are seen in about 20 percent of patients. These overall figures fail to reflect, however, the wide variation in mortality and the incidence of residual neurologic abnormalities that follow infection by different viruses. In herpes simplex encephalitis, for example, the mortality is about 50 percent; neurologic sequelae have been observed in 80 to 90 percent of patients with eastern equine encephalitis and in only 5 to 10 percent of those with western equine infections.

ETIOLOGY

Whereas numerous viral, bacterial, fungal, and parasitic agents are listed as causes of the encephalitis syndrome, only the viral ones are considered here, for it is to these that one usually refers when the term *encephalitis* is used. The nonviral forms of encephalitis are considered in Chap. 31.

As with aseptic meningitis, the number of viruses that can cause an encephalitis or a postinfectious allergic reaction is large, and one might suppose that the clinical problems would be infinitely complex. However, the types of viral encephalitis that occur with sufficient frequency to be of diagnostic importance are relatively few, and many of them have a characteristic geographic and seasonal incidence. In the United States, *eastern equine encephalitis,* as the name implies, has been observed mainly in the Eastern states; there have been only two recognized outbreaks of this disease in New England, each in the early autumn. *Western equine encephalitis* is fairly uniformly distributed throughout the country. *St. Louis encephalitis,* another arthropod-borne, late-summer encephalitis, also has a widespread distribution; in the Far West it occurs mainly in rural areas, whereas elsewhere it has been observed in urban epidemics; curiously it is rarely encountered along the West Coast. *Venezuelan equine encephalitis,* which is common in South and Central America, is practically confined to the southwestern part of the United States. *California virus encephalitis* predominates in the Midwestern states. *Rabies* infections occur nationwide, but mostly in the Middle West and along the West Coast. Japanese B encephalitis, Russian spring-summer encephalitis, Murray Valley encephalitis (Australian X disease), and many other viral encephalitides are unknown in the United States.

Infectious mononucleosis, which is a frequent cause of meningoencephalitis in adolescents and young adults, has no particular seasonal incidence or geographic distribution. The same is true of *herpes simplex encephalitis.* Definite cases of epidemic (lethargic) encephalitis have not been observed in the acute form since 1930, though patients with residual symptoms (Parkinson's syndrome) are still to be seen in neurology clinics.

Encephalitis or encephalomyelitis that follows measles, rubella, chickenpox, or rabies vaccination by a few days to a week represents a disordered immune reaction of nervous tissue to a preceding viral infection, and is considered with the demyelinative diseases, in Chap. 36.

ARTHROPOD-BORNE (ARBO)VIRUS ENCEPHALITIS

The arbovirus infections that occur in the United States and their geographic range have been listed above. There are alternating cycles of viral infection in mosquitoes and vertebrate hosts; the uninfected mosquito may become infected by taking a blood meal from a viremic host (horse or bird) or, if infected, will inject virus into the host, including humans. The seasonal incidence of these infections is limited to the summer and early fall, when mosquitoes are biting. In the equine encephalitides, regional deaths in horses usually precede human epidemics. In St. Louis encephalitis, the urban bird or animal or possibly the human becomes the intermediate host. These encephalitides occur in epidemics that appear to be related to the migration of infected birds. California virus infections are endemic because of the cycle of infection in small rodents.

The clinical manifestations of the various arbovirus infections are indistinguishable one from the other, although they do vary with age. In infants, there may be only an abrupt onset of fever and convulsions. In older children the onset is usually less abrupt, with complaints of headache, listlessness, nausea or vomiting, drowsiness, and fever for several days before medical attention is sought. Convulsions, confusion and stupor, and stiff neck then become prominent. Photophobia, diffuse myalgia, and tremor (sometimes of the intention type) may be observed in this age group and in adults. Reflex asymmetry, hemiparesis, extensor plantar signs, and sucking and grasping reflexes may also occur.

The CSF findings are much the same as in aseptic meningitis. The fever and neurologic signs subside after 4 to 14 days, unless death supervenes or destructive CNS changes have occurred.

The pathologic changes consist of widespread degeneration of single nerve cells with neuronophagia as well as scattered foci of inflammatory necrosis involving both the gray and white matter. The brainstem is relatively spared. In eastern equine encephalitis the destructive lesions may be massive, involving the major part of a lobe or hemisphere, but in the other arbovirus infections the foci are microscopic in size. Perivascular cuffing by lymphocytes, mononuclear leukocytes, and plasma cells and a patchy infiltration of the meninges with similar cells are the other histopathologic hallmarks of viral encephalitis.

Of the arbovirus infections in the United States, eastern equine encephalitis is the most serious since a large proportion of those infected develop encephalitis, and of the latter, about two-thirds die or are left with severe disabling abnormalities—mental retardation, emotional disorders, recurrent seizures, blindness, deafness, hemiplegia, and speech disorders. Fortunately, eastern equine encephalitis is also the least frequent of the arbovirus infections. The mortality rate in other arbovirus infections varies from 2 to 12 percent in different outbreaks, and the incidence of serious sequelae is about the same.

HERPES SIMPLEX ENCEPHALITIS (ACUTE INCLUSION BODY ENCEPHALITIS)

This rather remarkable form of acute encephalitis is the only one which occurs sporadically throughout the year and in patients of all ages and in all parts of the world. It is due almost always to the type 1 herpes simplex virus. The type 1 virus is also the cause of the common herpetic lesions of the oral mucosa, but rarely have these lesions been associated with acute herpes simplex encephalitis. The type 2 virus may also cause acute encephalitis, but only in the neonate, and is related to genital herpetic infection in the mother. Type 2 infection in the adult may cause an aseptic meningitis, and sometimes a polyradiculitis or myelitis, again in association with a recent genital herpes infection.

The initial symptoms, which evolve over several days, are in most cases like those of any other acute encephalitis, viz., fever, headache, seizures, confusion, stupor, and coma. In some patients there are additional symptoms that betray the propensity of this disease to involve the inferomedial portions of the frontal and temporal lobes. These latter manifestations include olfactory or gustatory hallucinations, anosmia, temporal lobe seizures, a brief period of bizarre or psychotic behavior, aphasia, and hemiparesis. Very rarely a disproportionate affection of memory can be recognized, but usually this only becomes evident later, in the convalescent stage of the illness. Swelling and herniation of one or both temporal lobes through the tentorium may occur, leading to deep coma and respiratory arrest during the first 24 to 72 h.

The CSF shows a pleocytosis, usually less than 200 cells per cubic millimeter, mainly lymphocytes and mononuclear cells. The protein content is increased in most cases. Red cells, sometimes numbering in the thousands, and xanthochromia are found in some cases, reflecting the hemorrhagic nature of the lesions. Rarely, the CSF glucose levels may be reduced to slightly less than 40 mg per 100 ml, creating confusion with tuberculous and fungal meningitides. The herpes simplex virus has been isolated from the CSF in only a few patients. A rising titer of neutralizing antibodies can be demonstrated from the acute to the convalescent stage, but this is not of diagnostic help in the acutely ill patient, and may not be etiologically significant in patients with recurrent herpes infections of the oral mucosa.

The exact incidence of mortality from this disease is unknown, because of the limitations of presently available diagnostic methods, but is estimated to be from 30 to 70 percent. Many of the survivors are left with severe mental sequelae, in the form of a Korsakoff's psychosis or global dementia, as well as with seizures and dysphasia. The prognosis is not hopeless, however; some patients recover to the point where they can resume an independent or even a normal life.

The lesions take the form of an intense hemorrhagic necrosis of the inferior and medial parts of the temporal lobes and the orbital parts of the frontal lobes. This distribution of lesions is so characteristic that the diagnosis can be made by simple inspection. Cases described in past years as *acute necrotizing encephalitis* were probably instances of herpes simplex encephalitis. In the acute stages of the disease, intranuclear eosinophilic inclusions are found in neurons and glial cells, in addition to the usual microscopic abnormalities of acute encephalitis.

The *diagnosis* may be difficult. Acute herpes sim-

plex encephalitis must be distinguished from acute hemorrhagic leukoencephalitis (page 661) and from subdural empyema, cerebral abscess, thrombophlebitis, and septic embolism (Chap. 31). The EEG changes, consisting of high-voltage sharp waves in the temporal regions, are hardly specific but may be helpful when they are periodic and change pattern frequently. The CT scan is helpful in some cases (Fig. 32-2); low-density, nonenhancing areas with surrounding edema and sometimes with scattered areas of hemorrhage occupy the inferior parts of the frontal and temporal lobes. At present, the only certain way to establish the diagnosis of acute herpes simplex encephalitis is by fluorescent antibody study and by viral culture of cerebral tissue obtained by brain biopsy.

Until recently there has been no specific *treatment* for herpes simplex encephalitis. Antiviral agents such as idoxuridine and cytosine arabinoside (cytarabine) have proved to be ineffective in controlled studies and both may seriously suppress bone marrow function. A collaborative study, sponsored by the National Institutes of Health, has indicated that the antiviral agent, adenine arabinoside, significantly reduces both the mortality and morbidity from herpes simplex encephalitis (Whitley et al.). Recent clinical experience also seems to indicate

Figure 32-2

Herpes simplex encephalitis. Contrast-enhanced scan showing asymmetrical areas of hemorrhage and necrosis involving inferior portions of the frontal and temporal lobes.

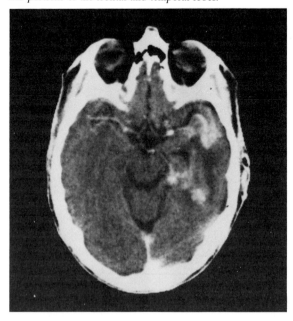

that early treatment with adenine arabinoside increases the chances of survival. The use of this latter agent, as well as corticosteroids for brief periods, in order to control brain swelling and prevent herniation, thus appears to be justified. In some instances it is desirable to do a brain biopsy in order to confirm the diagnosis, but the authors do not consider this procedure to be necessary in every suspected case. If the diagnosis is reasonably certain, there is no harm in proceeding at once with treatment.

ENCEPHALITIS LETHARGICA (VON ECONOMO'S DISEASE, SLEEPING SICKNESS)

This disease first occurred in the wake of the pandemic of influenza that began during World War I, and continued for about 10 years. No disease just like it had occurred before 1914. Although the viral agent was never identified, the clinical and pathologic features were typical of viral infection. The unique symptoms were pronounced somnolence, from which the disease takes its name, and ophthalmoplegia. A small proportion of the patients were overly active rather than somnolent, and manifested a disorder of movement in the form either of chorea or myoclonus. Headache, dizziness, fatigability, or frank confusional psychosis were common features. In contrast, paralysis (hemiplegia), cortical sensory loss, aphasia, disorders of hearing and vision, and convulsions were virtually unknown. The onset was acute or subacute, and the symptoms persisted for several weeks. Lymphocytic pleocytosis in the CSF was found in half the patients, together with variable elevation of the protein level. More than 20 percent of the victims died within a few weeks, and many survivors were left with varying degrees of impairment of mental function. Also, after an interval of months or years (sometimes as long as 25 years) a high proportion of survivors developed the syndrome of parkinsonism, as described on page 807. In fact, this is the only form of encephalitis known to cause an immediate or delayed extrapyramidal syndrome of this type (a similar though not identical syndrome may follow Japanese B encephalitis). Myoclonus, dystonia, oculogyric crises (page 179) and other muscle spasms, bulimia, obesity, reversal of sleep pattern, and, in children, a psychopathic personality with compulsive behavior, were other distressing sequelae.

The pathology was typical of a viral infection (nerve cell destruction and neuronophagia, perivascular cuffing with lymphocytes and mononuclear cells, and meningeal infiltrations of similar cells), localized principally to regions of the midbrain, subthalamus, and hypothalamus. In the patients who died years later of Parkinson's syndrome, depigmentation of the substantia nigra and locus ceruleus, fibrillary changes in the nerve cells of substantia nigra, oculomotor and adjacent nuclei, and nerve cell destruction and gliosis were the only findings.

Few if any new cases have been seen in the United States and western Europe since 1930. The only treatment available for the survivors consists of administration of L-dopa and other antiparkinsonian drugs, as outlined on page 810.

The importance of encephalitis lethargica relates to (1) the unique clinical syndromes and sequelae (Parkinson's syndrome, tics, sleep disorder, oculogyric crises, psychopathic behavioral states) and (2) its place as the first slow virus infection of the nervous system in human beings.

RABIES

This disease stands apart from other acute viral infections by virtue of the long latent period following introduction of the virus and its distinctive clinical and pathologic features. Human cases of this disease are rare: only five cases were reported in 1979 in the United States, and in some countries (Australia, Hawaii, Great Britain) no cases have ever been reported. Its importance derives from the fact that in the past almost every case of rabies was fatal, and the survival of the inoculated individual depended upon the institution of specific therapeutic measures before the infection became established. Furthermore, each year 20,000 to 30,000 individuals are treated with rabies vaccine because of contacts with animals that might have been rabid, and although the incidence of complications of rabies vaccination is much lower than before (see below), serious reactions continue to be encountered.

Etiology Practically all cases of rabies follow inoculation of the virus through the skin by an animal bite. The most commonly rabid species are skunks, foxes, bats, and racoons, among wild animals, and dogs and cats among domestic ones. Because rabid animals commonly bite without provocation, the nature of the attack should be determined. Also, the prevalence of animal rabies virus varies widely in the United States, and local presence of the disease should be assessed. As indicated earlier, the virus spreads along peripheral nerves to reach the nervous system.

Clinical Features The incubation period is usually several months, but may be as short as 14 to 21 days, especially in cases with multiple deep bites around the face and neck. The initial neurologic symptoms (following a 2- to 4-day prodromal period of fever, headache, and malaise) consist of severe anxiety and speech and psychomotor overactivity, followed by dysphagia (hence salivation and "frothing at the mouth"), spasms of throat muscles induced by attempts to swallow water (hence hydrophobia), dysarthria, numbness of the face, and spasms of facial muscles—to which are added generalized seizures and a confusional psychosis. This localization indicates the intensive involvement of the tegmental medullary nuclei in the *rabid* form of the disease. A less common *paralytic form*, due to spinal cord affection, may accompany or replace the state of excitement. Once these neurologic symptoms become established, death ensues within 2 to 7 days.

Pathologic Features The disease is distinguished by the presence of cytoplasmic eosinophilic inclusions, the Negri bodies. They are most prominent in the pyramidal cells of the hippocampus and the Purkinje cells, but have been seen in nerve cells throughout the CNS. In addition there may be widespread perivascular cuffing and meningeal infiltration with lymphocytes and mononuclear cells and small foci of inflammatory necrosis, as one sees in other viral infections. The focal collections of microglia in this disease are referred to as *Babes' nodules*.

Treatment Bites and scratches should be thoroughly washed with soap and water and, after all soap has been removed, cleansed with benzyl ammonium chloride (Zephiran), which has been shown to inactivate virus. Wounds that have broken the skin require tetanus prophylaxis, as described on page 783.

After a bite by a seemingly healthy animal, surveillance of the animal for a 10-day period is necessary. Should signs of illness appear in the animal, it should be killed and the brain sent, under refrigeration, to a government-designated laboratory for appropriate diagnostic tests. Wild animals, if captured, should be killed and the brain examined in the same way.

If the animal is found by fluorescent-antibody or other tests to be rabid or if the patient was bitten by a wild animal that escaped, the patient should receive *postexposure prophylaxis*. Human rabies immune globulin (HRIG), which avoids the complications of equine antirabies serum, should be given in a dose of 20 units per kilogram of body weight (one-half infiltrated around the wound and one-half intramuscularly). This provides passive immunization for 10 to 20 days, allowing time for active immunization. For the past decade duck embryo vaccine (DEV) has been used for the latter purpose and has greatly reduced the danger of serious allergic reactions in the CNS (encephalomyelitis). DEV is given subcutaneously in doses of 1.0 ml according to the following schedule: two doses per day for 7 days, then one dose per day for 7 days, followed by a single dose 10 and 20 days later, for a total of 23 doses over a 34-day period. Then, 10 days after the last dose, serum antibodies should be determined at a governmental laboratory.

Recently a rabies vaccine, grown on a human cell line, has been licensed by the Food and Drug Administration. The new vaccine reduces the doses needed to just 6 (from the 23 needed with DEV) and promises to increase the rate of antibody response and to reduce even further the allergic reactions by eliminating foreign protein. Recent improvements in intensive care of respiratory paralysis and failure of other vital functions have resulted in survival of proven cases of rabies encephalitis.

CHRONIC VIRAL INFECTIONS SIMULATING DEGENERATIVE DISEASE

The idea that viral infections may lead to chronic disease, especially of the nervous system, has been entertained for half a century, but only recently has it been firmly established. The following indirect and direct evidence support this view: (1) the demonstration of a slowly progressive noninflammatory degeneration of nigral neurons long after an attack of encephalitis lethargica; (2) the finding of inclusion bodies in cases of subacute and chronic sclerosing encephalitis; (3) the discovery of chronic degenerative diseases in sheep caused by a viruslike transmissible agent (scrapie) and by a conventional RNA virus (visna) (it was in relation to these that Sigurdsson first used the term *slow infection*, to indicate long incubation periods, during which the animals appeared well); (4) the demonstration by electron microscopy of viral particles in the lesions of multifocal leukoencephalopathy and, later, isolation of the virus from the lesions; and (5) the transmission of kuru and subacute spongiform encephalopathy (*Creutzfeldt-Jakob* disease) to chimpanzees. The late onset of motor system disease after poliomyelitis may also represent a slow infection, but this remains to be proved. Claims have also been made by several Soviet scientists for a viral causation of multiple sclerosis, amyotrophic lateral sclerosis, epilepsia partialis continua, and other degenerative diseases, but the evidence is questionable.

The slow infections of the nervous system are of two general types: (1) those due to conventional viruses, viz., subacute sclerosing panencephalitis, progressive rubella panencephalitis, and progressive multifocal leukoencephalopathy, and (2) those due to unconventional agents, viz., kuru and subacute spongiform encephalopathy (and mink encephalopathy and scrapie in sheep). Although the agents producing these latter disorders are transmissable and capable of replication, they are insensitive to the various forms of physicochemical treatment that inactivate conventional viruses, they do not cause an immune response, and viral particles have not been seen in infected tissue. These unconventional agents have been referred to as *subacute spongiform encephalopathy agents* and as *slow viruses*, but they probably represent a new type of transmissible agent.

The aforementioned slow infections so perfectly simulate degenerative disease that notions about many other diseases of white and gray matter of the brain, presently classified as degenerative, are being altered. One of the most exciting prospects in medical neurology is thus unfolding before us.

SUBACUTE SCLEROSING PANENCEPHALITIS (SSPE)

This disease was first described by Dawson in 1934, under the title "inclusion body encephalitis," and extensively studied by Van Bogaert, who named it *subacute sclerosing leukoencephalitis*. The condition affects children and adolescents for the most part, rarely appearing beyond the age of 18 years. The illness evolves in several stages. Initially there is a decline in proficiency at school, temper outbursts and other changes in personality, difficulty with language, and loss of interest in usual activities. These soon give way to the second stage, in which there occurs a severe and progressive intellectual deterioration, in association with focal or generalized seizures, widespread myoclonus, and visual disturbances (in some patients), due to progressive chorioretinitis. As the disease advances, rigidity, hyperactive reflexes, Babinski signs, progressive unresponsiveness, and signs of autonomic dysfunction appear. In the final stage the child lies insensate, virtually "decorticated." The course is usually steadily progressive, death occurring within a few months or years. In some cases the course is more prolonged, with one or more remissions.

The EEG shows a characteristic abnormality consisting of periodic (every 3 to 4 s) bursts of high-voltage slow and sharp waves. The CSF contains few or no cells, but the protein is increased, particularly the gamma globulin. High levels of neutralizing antibody to measles

(rubeola) virus have been found in serum and CSF, but the virus has been isolated from the brain tissue in only a few instances. Recently, Hall et al. found that SSPE patients lack antibody to one viral protein (M protein), despite high antibody titers to the other viral proteins—the result, probably, of a failure of the host's brain cells to synthesize M protein.

The lesions involve the cerebral cortex and white matter of both hemispheres and the brainstem. The cerebellum is usually spared. Destruction of nerve cells, neuronophagia, and perivenous cuffing by lymphocytes and mononuclear cells indicate the viral nature of the infection. In the white matter there is degeneration of medullated fibers (myelin and axis cylinders), accompanied by perivascular cuffing with mononuclear cells and fibrous gliosis (sclerosing encephalitis). Eosinophilic inclusions, the histopathologic hallmark of the disease, are found in the cytoplasm and nuclei of neurons and glial cells. Virions, thought to be measles nucleocapsids, have been observed in inclusion-bearing cells examined with the electron microscope.

The differential diagnosis includes the childhood and adolescent dementing diseases such as lipid storage diseases (Chap. 37) and Schilder's disease (page 660). In presumptive cases of SSPE, the findings of periodic complexes in the EEG, elevated gamma globulin in the CSF, and elevated measles-antibody titers in the serum and CSF are sufficient to make the diagnosis. To date, no effective treatment has been available, although recently it has been reported that the long-term administration of amantadine may bring about sustained remissions and prolong survival (Robertson et al.).

Lyon and his associates have described a condition closely related to SSPE, which they call *acute measles encephalitis of delayed type*. Three months after a measles infection their patient, a 6-year-old boy, developed epilepsia partialis continua of the right arm, progressing to a state of continuous clonic seizures of the right arm and leg and both sides of the face. High levels of measles antibodies appeared in the serum and CSF. The patient died after remaining in coma for nearly a year and an autopsy revealed a severe polioencephalitis with widespread pannecrosis of the cerebral cortex and a communicating hydrocephalus. Tubular inclusions of the type seen in SSPE were found in nerve cell nuclei. A similar clinical picture has been described in children contracting measles when under treatment with immunosuppressive drugs.

PROGRESSIVE RUBELLA PANENCEPHALITIS

Generally the deficits associated with congenital rubella infection are nonprogressive at least after the second or third year of life (page 857). Recently, however, there have been descriptions of children with the congenital rubella syndrome in whom a progressive neurologic deterioration occurred after a stable period of 8 to 19 years (Townsend et al.; Weil et al.). At the time of writing, 10 cases of this late-appearing, progressive syndrome have been described—one of them apparently related to acquired rather than congenital rubella (see review by Wolinsky).

The clinical syndrome in these cases has been quite uniform. On a backgound of the fixed stigmata of congenital rubella, there occurs initially a deterioration in behavior and school performance, often associated with seizures, and soon thereafter, a progressive impairment of mental function (dementia). Clumsiness of gait is an early symptom, followed by a frank ataxia of gait and then of the limbs. Spasticity and other corticospinal tract signs, dysarthria, and dysphagia ensue. Pallor of the optic disks, ophthalmoplegia, spastic quadriplegia, and mutism mark the final phase of the illness.

The CSF shows a mild lymphocytic pleocytosis, a modest elevation of protein, and a marked increase in the proportion of gamma globulin (35 to 52 percent of the total protein), which assumes an oligoclonal pattern when analyzed by agarose gel electrophoresis. The CSF and serum rubella-antibody titers are elevated.

Pathologic examination of the brain of two patients showed a widespread, progressive subacute panencephalitis mainly affecting the white matter. No inclusion-bearing cells were seen. Thus it appears that rubella virus infection, acquired in utero, persists in the nervous system for years, before rekindling a chronic active infection.

Analogies have been drawn between this disorder and the chronic encephalitis associated with the rubeola virus (SSPE). The latter disorder has not been associated with maternal infection, however; furthermore, myoclonus and EEG abnormalities are not as prominent as in SSPE, and inclusion bodies that characterize SSPE have not been observed in the patients with progressive rubella panencephalitis.

PROGRESSIVE MULTIFOCAL LEUKOENCEPHALOPATHY (PML)

This disorder, observed originally by the authors in 1952, has been fully described morphologically by As-

trom, Mancall, and Richardson (Astrom et al.; Richardson). It is characterized by the occurrence of widespread demyelinative lesions, mainly of the cerebral hemispheres, but also of the brainstem and cerebellum, and rarely of the spinal cord. The lesions vary greatly in size and severity—from microscopic foci of demyelination to massive foci of destruction of both myelin and axis cylinders involving the major part of a cerebral hemisphere. There are distinctive abnormalities of the glial cells. Many of the reactive astrocytes in the lesions are gigantic and contain deformed and bizarre-shaped nuclei and mitotic figures, changes that are seen otherwise only in malignant glial tumors. Also, at the periphery of the lesions, the nuclei of oligodendrocytes are greatly enlarged and contain abnormal inclusions. Vascular changes are lacking, and inflammatory changes are usually insignificant.

Clinical Features An uncommon disease of late adult life, PML rarely occurs independently but usually in a setting of chronic neoplastic disease (mainly chronic lymphocytic leukemia, Hodgkin's disease, lymphosarcoma, myeloproliferative disease) or, less often, of nonneoplastic granulomatosis, such as tuberculosis or sarcoid. A number of cases have occurred in patients receiving immunosuppressive drugs for renal transplantation and for other reasons. The neurologic disorder evolves over a period of several days to weeks. Hemiparesis progressing to quadriparesis, visual field defects, cortical blindness, aphasia, ataxia, dysarthria, dementia, confusional states, and coma are the typical manifestations. Seizures and cerebellar ataxia are rare. In most cases death occurs in 3 to 6 months from the onset of neurologic symptoms. The CSF is usually normal. Angiography and pneumoencephalography have been uninformative, but the CT scan in several personally observed cases has localized the lesions (which appear as low-density, nonenhancing areas) with striking accuracy.

Pathogenesis Waksman's original suggestion (quoted by Richardson), that PML could be due to viral infection of the CNS in patients with diseases producing impaired immunologic responses, has proved to be correct. ZuRhein and Chou, in 1965, demonstrated by electron microscopy the presence of particles resembling papovaviruses in the inclusion-bearing oligodendrocytes in a lesion of a case of PML. Since then, two serologic types of papovaviruses have been isolated from the brains of patients with PML (Padgett et al.; Weiner et al.)—a virus antigenically similar to simian virus 40 (SV 40) and a new papovavirus, the JC virus, the latter being much more frequent. This aspect of the subject has been reviewed by Walker.

Treatment The disease is generally believed to be untreatable and to end fatally in 3 to 20 months. One spontaneous remission has been reported, and five cases have reportedly responded to cytoarabine therapy or to carmustine. The most impressive report is that of Peters et al., in which the clinical picture was typical and the virus was demonstrated in brain biopsy by a fluorescent antibody technique and electron microscopy. After intravenous and intrathecal administration of cytoarabine, the lesions regressed (on CT scan), as did many of the symptoms of cerebral deficit.

DISEASES DUE TO SUBACUTE SPONGIFORM
ENCEPHALOPATHY AGENTS

This category of diseases, as indicated earlier, includes scrapie in sheep, and kuru and so-called Creutzfeldt-Jakob disease in humans.

Kuru, first described in the Fore natives of New Guinea, was the first slow infection documented in human beings. Clinically the disease takes the form of an afebrile, progressive cerebellar ataxia, with abnormalities of extraocular movements, weakness progressing to immobility, incontinence in the late stages, and death within 3 to 6 months of onset. The remarkable epidemiologic and pathologic similarities between kuru and scrapie were pointed out by Hadlow (1959), who suggested that kuru might be transmitted to subhuman primates. This was accomplished in 1966 by Gajdusek, Gibbs, and Alpers; a kurulike syndrome was transmitted to chimpanzees after a latency of 18 to 36 months. Since then the disease has been transmitted from one chimpanzee to another, and to other primates, by both neural and nonneural tissues. The transmissible agent has not been visualized, however.

Naturally occurring kuru has become extinct because of the cessation of ritual cannibalism, by which the disease had been transmitted. In this ritual, infected tissue was ingested and rubbed over the body of the victim's kin (women and young children of either sex) permitting absorption of the infective agent through conjunctivae, mucous membranes, and abrasions in the skin.

Subacute Spongiform Encephalopathy (Heidenhain's Disease, Creutzfeldt-Jackob Disease) These terms refer to a distinctive cerebral disease, in which a rapidly progressive and profound dementia is associated with cerebellar ataxia and diffuse myoclonic jerks. The major neuropathologic changes are in the cerebral and cerebellar cortex; the outstanding features of the lesions are widespread neuronal loss and gliosis accompanied by a striking vacuolation or spongy state of the affected regions—hence the designation *subacute spongiform encephalopathy* (SSE). Less severe changes in a patchy distribution are found in cases of short duration.

These changes, both clinical and pathologic, occur so regularly and with such remarkable uniformity from case to case that they doubtless form a nosologic entity. It is frequently referred to as Creutzfeldt-Jakob disease, an inappropriate term in the authors' opinion, since it seems to us unlikely that SSE and the somewhat ill-defined syndrome(s) described by Creutzfeldt and Jakob can truly be the same disease. Pending further knowledge, at any rate, we believe that they should be kept distinct from one another, or at least, whenever one speaks of Creutzfeldt-Jakob disease, it should be specified whether subacute spongiform encephalopathy is meant or the slower progressive dementia with signs of pyramidal and extrapyramidal affection originally described by Creutzfeldt and Jakob (the latter condition is discussed fully on page 805). Preciseness in definition of these states is of greater importance now than before, since it was shown by Gibbs et al. that brain tissue from patients with SSE, injected into chimpanzees, can transmit the disease after an incubation period of a year or longer.

Pathology As already indicated, the disease affects principally the cerebral and cerebellar cortex, generally in a diffuse fashion, although in some cases the occipitoparietal regions are almost exclusively involved, as in those described by Heidenhain. The degeneration and disappearance of nerve cells is associated with extensive astroglial proliferation; ultrastructural studies have shown that the microscopic vacuoles which give the tissue its typically spongy appearance are located within the cytoplasmic processes of glial cells and dendrites of nerve cells. Despite the fact that the disease is due to a transmissible agent, possibly a virus, the lesions show no evidence of an inflammatory reaction.

Epidemiology and pathogenesis The disease appears in all parts of the world and in all seasons, with an annual incidence approaching one case per million of population. Although the reported incidence of SSE is somewhat higher in urban than in rural areas, temporospatial clustering of cases has not been observed, at least in the United States. A small proportion of all series of cases is familial—6 to 9 percent of 170 cases reported by Brown et al., and 15 percent of 1435 cases analyzed by Masters et al. The mode of transmission of the disease remains unclear. The occurrence of familial cases suggests a genetic susceptibility to infection, although the possibility of common exposure to the transmissible agent cannot be dismissed. The only clearly demonstrated mechanism of spread of SSE is iatrogenic, having occurred after corneal transplantation in one case and after implantation of infected depth electrodes in several others. Individuals exposed to scrapie-infected sheep and to patients with SSE are not disproportionately affected by the disease.

Clinical features Transmissible SSE is in most cases a disease of late middle age, although it can occur in young adults. The sexes are affected equally. In the large series reported by Brown et al. and by Bernoulli et al., prodromal symptoms, consisting of fatigue, depression, weight loss, and disorders of sleep and appetite and lasting for several weeks, were observed in about one-third of the patients.

The early stages of the disease are characterized by a great variety of clinical manifestations, but the most frequent are changes in behavior, in emotional response, and in memory and reasoning, together with abnormalities of cerebellar function and of vision such as distortions of the shape and alignment of objects or actual impairment of visual acuity. In some instances cerebellar ataxia precedes mental changes. Hallucinations, delusions, confusion, and other evidence of delirium are frequently seen in the early phases of the disease. Characteristically, the disease progresses rapidly, so that obvious deterioration may be seen from week to week and even day to day. Sooner or later, in almost all cases, myoclonic contractions of various muscle groups appear, perhaps unilaterally at first, but later becoming generalized. These are associated with a striking startle response, mainly to a loud noise. In general, the myoclonic jerks are sensitive to sensory stimuli of all sorts, but they occur spontaneously as well. Twitches of individual fingers are typical. Ataxia and dysarthria are likewise prominent. These changes gradually give way to stupor and coma, but the myoclonic contractions may continue to the end. The EEG pattern is distinctive, changing over the course of the disease from one of diffuse and nonspecific slowing to one of high voltage synchronous sharp waves followed by "burst suppression" on an increasingly flat background. Blood and CSF are normal.

The disease is invariably fatal, usually in less than a year from the onset. In about 10 percent of patients, the illness begins with almost strokelike suddenness and

runs its course rapidly, in a matter of a few weeks or months. A small number of patients have been reported to survive for 2 to 10 years, but these cases should be accepted with caution; in many of them, SSE appears to have been superimposed on Alzheimer's or Parkinson's or other chronic disease.

Differential diagnosis The diagnosis of most cases of subacute spongiform encephalopathy presents no difficulty. Not infrequently, however, we have been surprised by a "typical" case that proves to be some other disease. The early stages of a toxic or metabolic-nutritional encephalopathy, or a carcinomatous meningitis, or even Schilder's disease may mimick subacute spongiform encephalopathy. Contrariwise, the early mental changes of SSE may be misinterpreted as an atypical or unusually intense emotional reaction to environmental factors or as one of the major psychoses. Patients who present in the later stages of SSE may for a time be mistaken for Alzheimer's or Pick's disease, or the Parkinson-amyotrophic lateral sclerosis-dementia syndrome, until the rapidly evolving clinical picture clarifies the issue. SSPE (see above) in its fully developed form resembles SSE, but the former is chiefly a disease of children or young adults, and the CSF shows elevation of gamma globulin (IgG), whereas the latter is essentially a disease of middle age and the presenile period, and the CSF is normal. Cerebral lipidosis in children or young adults can result in a similar combination of myoclonus and dementia, but the clinical course in such cases is extremely indolent, and there are retinal changes that do not occur in SSE.

Management No specific treatment is known. Antiviral agents have been ineffective. In view of the transmissibility of the disease from humans to primates and iatrogenically from patient to patient, certain precautions should be taken in the medical care of and handling of materials from patients with SSE (Gajdusek et al., 1977). The transmissible agent is resistant to boiling, formalin, alcohol, and ultraviolet radiation, but can be inactivated by autoclaving and by certain disinfectants (phenolics, permanganate, iodine, hypochlorite). Workers exposed to infected materials should wash thoroughly with ordinary soap. Needles, glassware, needle electrodes, and other instruments should be immersed in appropriate disinfectants or incinerated and discarded. The isolation of affected patients is not necessary.

All aspects of the slow transmissible diseases of the nervous system have recently been reviewed in a two-volume publication, edited by Prusiner and Hadlow.

VIRAL INFECTIONS OF THE DEVELOPING NERVOUS SYSTEM

Viral infections of the fetus, notably rubella and cytomegalovirus, and herpes simplex infection of the newborn are important causes of CNS abnormalities. They are considered in Chap. 43, under "Developmental Diseases of Infancy and Childhood."

REFERENCES

ASTROM KE, MANCALL EL, RICHARDSON EP: Progressive multifocal leukoencephalopathy. *Brain* 81:93, 1958.

BARINGER JR: Human herpes simplex virus infections, in Thompson RA, Green JR (eds): *Advances in Neurology*, vol 6. New York, Raven, 1974, pp 41-51.

BERNOULLI CC et al: Early clinical features of Creutzfeldt-Jakob disease (subacute spongiform encephalopathy), in Prusiner SB, Hadlow WS (eds): *Slow Transmissible Diseases of the Nervous System*. New York, Academic, 1979, vol 1, pp 229-251.

BODIAN D: Histopathologic basis of clinical findings in poliomyelitis. *Am J Med* 6:563, 1949.

BROWN P et al: Creutzfeldt-Jakob disease in France. *Ann Neurol* 6:430, 438, 1979.

CHAJEK T, FAINARU M: Behçet's disease: Report of 41 cases and a review of the literature. *Medicine* 54:179, 1975.

DAWSON J: Cellular inclusions in cerebral lesions of epidemic encephalitis. *Arch Neurol Psychiatry* 31:685, 1934.

DENNY-BROWN D, ADAMS RD, FITZGERALD PJ: Pathologic features of herpes zoster: A note on "geniculate herpes." *Arch Neurol Psychiatry* 51:216, 1944.

DRACHMAN DA, ADAMS RD: Herpes simplex and acute inclusion-body encephalitis. *Arch Neurol* 7:45, 1962.

ENDERS JF, WELLER TH, ROBBINS FC: Cultivation of Lansing strain of poliomyelitis virus in cultures of various human embryonic tissues. *Science* 109:85, 1949.

GAJDUSEK DC et al: Precautions in medical care of, and in handling of materials from, patients with transmissible virus dementia (Creutzfeldt-Jakob disease). *N Engl J Med* 297:1253, 1977.

———, GIBBS CJ JR, ALPERS M: Experimental transmission of a Kuru-like syndrome to chimpanzees. *Nature:* 209:794, 1966.

GIBBS CJ JR et al: Creutzfeldt-Jakob disease (spongiform encephalopathy): Transmission to the chimpanzee. *Science* 161:388, 1968.

HADLOW WJ: Scrapie and kuru. *Lancet* 2:289, 1959.

HALL WW, LAMB RA, CHOPPIN PW: Measles and SSPE virus proteins: Lack of antibodies to the M protein in patients with subacute sclerosing panencephalitis. *Proc Natl Acad Sci USA* 76:2047, 1979.

HEIDENHAIN A: Klinische und anatomische Untersuchungen über eine eigenartige organische Erkrankung des Zentralnervensystems im Praesenium. *Z Gesamte Neurol Psychiatr* 118:49, 1929.

HOPE-SIMPSON RE: The nature of herpes zoster: A long-term study and a new hypothesis. *Proc R Soc Med* 58:9, 1965.

HORSTMANN DM: Clinical aspects of acute poliomyelitis. *Am J Med* 6:592, 1949.

JOHNSON KP, BYINGTON DP, GADDIS L: Subacute sclerosing panenccphalitis, in Thompson RA, Green JR (eds): *Advances in Neurology*, vol 6. New York, Raven, 1974, pp 77-86.

———, ROSENTHAL MS, LERNER PI: Herpes simplex encephalitis: The course in five virologically proven cases. *Arch Neurol* 27:103, 1972.

JOHNSON RT: Pathophysiology and epidemiology of acute viral infections of the nervous system, in Thompson RA, Green JR (eds): *Advances in Neurology*, vol 6. New York, Raven, 1974, pp 27-40.

———, GIBBS CS JR: Koch's postulates and slow infections of the nervous system. *Arch Neurol* 30:36, 1974.

———, NARAYAN O, WEINER LP: The relationship of SV 40-related viruses to progressive multifocal leukoencephalopathy, in Robinson WS, Fox CF (eds): *Mechanisms of Virus Disease*. Menlo Park, Calif, WA Benjamin, 1974, pp 187-197.

LEHNER T, BARNES CG (eds): *Behçet's Syndrome: Clinical and Immunological Features*. New York, Academic, 1980.

LEPOW ML et al: A clinical, epidemiologic, and laboratory investigation of aseptic meningitis during the four-year period 1955-1958. *N Engl J Med* 266:1181, 1188, 1962.

LINNEMANN CC JR, ALVIRA MM: Pathogenesis of varicella-zoster angiitis in the CNS. *Arch Neurol* 37:239, 1980.

LYON G, PONSOY G, LEBON P: Acute measles encephalitis of the delayed type. *Ann Neurol* 2:322, 1977.

MASTERS CL et al: Creutzfeldt-Jakob disease: Patterns of worldwide occurrence and the significance of familial and sporadic clustering. *Ann Neurol* 5:177, 1979.

MOLLARET P: La méningite endothélial-leucocytaire multi-récurrente bénigne. *Rev Neurol* 133:225, 1977.

PADGETT BL et al: Cultivation of papova-like virus from human brain with progressive multifocal leukoencephalopathy. *Lancet* 1:1257, 1971.

PETERS ACB et al: Progressive multifocal leukoencephalopathy. *Arch Neurol* 37:497, 1980.

PRUSINER SB, HADLOW WJ (eds): *Slow Transmissible Diseases of the Nervous System*. New York, Academic, 1979.

RICHARDSON EP JR: Progressive multifocal leukoencephalopathy. *N Engl J Med* 265:815, 1961.

ROBERTSON WC JR, CLARK DB, MARKESBERY WR: Review of 38 cases of subacute sclerosing panencephalitis: Effect of amantadine on the natural course of the disease. *Ann Neurol* 8:422, 1980.

SELBY G, WALKER GL: Cerebral arteritis in cat-scratch fever. *Neurology* 29:1413, 1979.

TOWSEND JJ et al: Progressive rubella panencephalitis: Late onset after congenital rubella. *N Engl J Med* 292:990, 1975.

VON ECONOMO C: *Encephalitis Lethargica.* New York, Oxford, 1931.

WALKER DL: Progressive multifocal leukoencephalopathy: An opportunistic viral infection of the central nervous system, in Vinken PJ, Bruyn GW (eds): *Handbook of Clinical Neurology,* vol 34. Amsterdam, North-Holland, 1978, pp 307-329.

WEIL ML et al: Chronic progressive panencephalitis due to rubella virus simulating subacute sclerosing panencephalitis. *N Engl J Med* 292:994, 1975.

WEINER LP et al: Isolation of virus related SV 40 from patients with progressive multifocal leukoencephalopathy. *N Engl J Med* 286:385, 1972.

WELLER TH, COONS AH: Fluorescent antibody studies with agents of varicella and herpes zoster propagated in vitro. *Proc Soc Exp Biol Med* 86:789, 1954.

——, WITTON HM, BELL EJ: Etiologic agents of varicella and herpes zoster. *J Exp Med* 108:843, 1958.

WHITLEY RJ et al: Adenine arabinoside therapy of herpes zoster in the immunosuppressed (NIAID collaborative antiviral study). *N Engl J Med* 294:1193, 1976.

WOLINSKY JS: Progressive rubella panencephalitis, in Vinken PJ, Bruyn GW (eds): *Handbook of Clinical Neurology,* vol 34. Amsterdam, North-Holland, 1978, chap 17.

VAN BOGAERT, L: Une leuco-encéphalite sclérosante subaigue. *J Neurol Neurosurg Psychiatry* 8:101, 1945.

ZURHEIN GM, CHOU SM: Particles resembling papova-viruses in human cerebral demyelinative disease. *Science* 148:1477, 1965.

CHAPTER 33
CEREBROVASCULAR DISEASES

Among all the neurologic disorders of adult life, the cerebrovascular diseases clearly rank first in frequency and urgency. At least 50 percent of the neurologic problems in a general hospital are of this type. At some time or other every physician will be required to examine patients with cerebrovascular disease and should at least know something of the common types—particularly those in which there is reasonable prospect of successful medical or surgical intervention. There is also another advantage to be gained from the study of this group of diseases, for they have traditionally provided one of the most instructive approaches to neurology. As our colleague C. M. Fisher has remarked, house officers and students literally learn neurology "stroke by stroke." The focal ischemic lesion has divulged some of the most important ideas about the function of the human brain.

INCIDENCE OF CEREBROVASCULAR DISEASES

Stroke is the third commonest cause of death in the United States. In 1977 there were 83,000 deaths from this cause; in addition about 1 million persons survived strokes, but were left disabled. Interestingly the incidence has been falling for the past 20 years. In Rochester, Minnesota, Garraway et al. found a reduction of 45 percent in cerebral infarction and hemorrhage when the period 1970-1974 was compared with 1945-1949. Both sexes shared in the reduced incidence. The incidence of coronary heart disease and malignant hypertension had also fallen. There had been no change in the frequency of aneurysmal rupture, however. Probably this diminution in the incidence of stroke is related to a reduced incidence of cerebral embolism from heart disease and improved control of hypertension.

DEFINITION OF TERMS

The term *cerebrovascular disease* designates any abnormality of the brain resulting from a pathologic process implicating blood vessels. *Pathologic process* is given an inclusive meaning, viz., any lesion of the vessel wall, occlusion of the lumen by thrombus or embolus, rupture of a vessel, altered permeability of the vascular wall, and increased viscosity or other change in the quality of the blood. The pathologic change may be considered not only in terms of its grosser aspects—thrombosis, embolism, rupture of a vessel—but also in terms of the more basic or primary disorder, i.e., the formation of atherosclerosis, hypertensive arteriosclerotic change, arteritis, aneurysmal dilation, and developmental malformation. Equal importance attaches to the parenchymal changes in the brain. These are of two types—ischemia, with or without infarction, and hemorrhage—and unless they occur, the vascular lesion usually remains silent. The only exceptions to this statement are the local pressure effects of an aneurysm, vascular headache (migraine, hypertension, temporal arteritis), multiple small vessel disease with progressive ischemic deficits (as in cerebral giant cell arteritis), and increased intracranial pressure (as occurs occasionally in hypertensive encephalopathy, giant cell arteritis, and venous sinus thrombosis). The many types of cerebrovascular diseases are listed in Table 33-1.

More than any other organ, the brain depends from minute to minute on an adequate supply of oxygenated blood. In Stokes-Adams attacks, for example, unconsciousness occurs within 10 s of the beginning of asystole, and in animal experiments the complete stoppage of blood flow for longer than 3 min produces irreversible damage. Brain tissue deprived of blood undergoes *ischemic necrosis or infarction* (also referred to as a zone of *softening* or *encephalomalacia*). Obstruction of an artery by thrombus or embolus is the usual cause, but failure of the circulation and hypotension from cardiac decompensation or shock, if severe and sufficiently prolonged, can also produce ischemic damage.

Table 33-1
Causes of cerebral abnormalities from disease of cerebral arteries and veins

1. Atherosclerotic thrombosis
2. Transient ischemic attacks
3. Embolism
4. Ruptured saccular aneurysm or AV malformation
5. Arteritis
    a. Meningovascular syphilis, arteritis secondary to pyogenic and tuberculous meningitis, rare infective types (typhus, schistosomiasis, malaria, trichinosis, mucormycosis, etc.)
    b. Connective tissue diseases (polyarteritis nodosa, lupus erythematosus), necrotizing arteritis, Wegener's arteritis, temporal arteritis, Takayasu's disease, granulomatous or giant cell arteritis of the aorta, and giant cell granulomatous angiitis of cerebral arteries
6. Cerebral thrombophlebitis: secondary to infection of ear, paranasal sinus, face, etc.; with meningitis and subdural empyema; debilitating states, postpartum, postoperative, cardiac failure, hematologic disease (polycythemia, sickle-cell disease), and of undetermined cause
7. Hematologic disorders: polycythemia, sickle-cell disease, thrombotic thrombocytopenic purpura, thrombocytosis, etc.
8. Trauma to carotid artery
9. Dissecting aortic aneurysm
10. Systemic hypotension with arterial stenoses: "simple faint," acute blood loss, myocardial infarction, Stokes-Adams syndrome, traumatic and surgical shock, sensitive carotid sinus, severe postural hypotension
11. Complications of arteriography
12. Neurologic migraine with persistent deficit
13. With tentorial, foramen magnum, and subfalcial herniations
14. Miscellaneous types: fibromuscular dysplasia, radioactive or x-ray irradiation, lateral pressure of intracerebral hematoma, unexplained middle cerebral infarction in closed head injury, pressure of unruptured saccular aneurysm, local dissection of carotid or middle cerebral artery, complication of oral contraceptives
15. Undetermined cause as in children and young adults: moyamoya; multiple, progressive intracranial arterial occlusions (Taveras).

Cerebral infarcts vary greatly in the amount of congestion and hemorrhage that are found within the softened tissue. Some infarcts are devoid of blood and therefore pallid (*pale infarction*); others show mild congestion (dilatation of blood vessels and escape of red blood cells), especially in their margins; still others show an extensive extravasation of blood from all the small vessels in the infarcted gray matter (red or *hemorrhagic infarction*). Some infarcts are all of one type, either pale or hemorrhagic; others are mixed. The reason for the simultaneous occurrence of pale and red infarctions, always, it seems, in cases of cerebral embolism, is not known. The hypothesis which we favor attributes red infarction to the fragmentation and distal migration of embolic material from its original site of arrest, allowing blood to seep through the damaged blood vessels into parts of the infarct originally deprived of blood.

In hemorrhage, blood leaks from the vessel (usually a small artery) directly into the brain, one of the ventricles, or the subarachnoid space. Once the leakage is arrested, the blood slowly disintegrates and is absorbed over a period of weeks and months. The mass of clotted blood causes physical disruption of the tissue and pressure on the surrounding brain.

THE STROKE SYNDROME

So distinctive is the mode of presentation of cerebrovascular disease that the diagnosis is seldom in doubt. The common mode of expression is the *stroke*, defined as a sudden, nonconvulsive, focal neurologic deficit. In its more severe form the patient becomes hemiplegic and even comatose, an event so dramatic that it has been given its own designation, namely *apoplexy, stroke, shock,* or *cerebrovascular accident (CVA)*. In its mildest form it may consist of only a trivial neurologic disorder insufficient even to arouse concern or demand medical attention. There are all gradations of severity between these two extremes, but in all forms the denominative feature of the stroke is the *temporal profile* of neurologic events. It is the abruptness with which the neurologic deficit develops—literally a matter of seconds, minutes, hours, or at most a few days—that stamps the disorder as vascular. Embolic strokes characteristically begin suddenly and the deficit reaches its peak almost at once. Thrombotic strokes may have the same abrupt onset, but many are comparatively slower and evolve over a period of several minutes, hours, or days, usually in saltatory fashion, i.e., in a series of steps, rather than smoothly. In cerebral hemorrhage related to hypertension, the deficit is from its moment of onset steadily progressive over a period of minutes or hours. The other important aspect of the temporal profile is the arrest and then regression of the neurologic deficit in all except the fatal strokes. Not infrequently an extensive deficit from embolism reverses itself dramatically within a few hours or a day or two. More often, and this is the case in most thrombotic strokes, improvement takes place gradually over weeks and months, and the residual disability is considerable. A gradual downhill course over a period of several days or weeks will usually be traced to a nonvascular disease. The only exceptions are multiple arteriolar and venular occlusions (platelet thrombosis, arteritis, lupus erythematosus, and hypertensive arteriolar sclerosis).

The neurologic deficit reflects both the location and size of the infarct or hemorrhage. Hemiplegia stands as the classic sign of all cerebrovascular diseases, whether in the cerebral hemisphere or brainstem, but there are many other manifestations as well, occurring in an almost infinite number of combinations. These include mental confusion, numbness and sensory deficits of many types, aphasia, visual field defects, diplopia, dizziness, dysarthria, and so forth. The neurovascular syndromes which they form enable the physician to locate the lesion—sometimes so precisely that the arterial branch that has been affected may be specified—and to indicate whether the lesion is an infarct or hemorrhage. These many neurovascular syndromes will be described in the section that follows.

It would be incorrect to assume that every cerebrovascular illness expresses itself in a clearly delineated stroke. Sometimes neither the patient nor the family can date the onset of the illness. Certain vascular symptoms may be so mild as to pass unnoticed, and are presented as complaints only when their cumulative effects become manifest. Furthermore, dominant hemispheric lesions may cause aphasic disturbances which hamper history taking, and nondominant ones may induce an anosognosia, which leaves the patient unaware of any deficits.

New laboratory methods for the demonstration of both the cerebral lesion and the offending vessel(s) have virtually revolutionized clinical study of the stroke patient. Computerized tomography (CT scan) demonstrates and accurately localizes small hemorrhages, hemorrhagic infarcts, subarachnoid clots around aneurysms, regions of infarct necrosis, and ventricular deformities. Radionuclide scanning successfully visualizes many hematomas and some infarcts in their subacute stage (days to weeks), although not in their late ones. Atheromatous plaques and stenoses of large vessels, particularly the carotid arteries, can frequently be detected by the use of ultrasound and Doppler flow studies. Arteriography demonstrates stenoses and occlusions of the larger vessels (both thrombotic and in some instances embolic) as well as aneurysms and vascular malformations. This

technique may also demonstrate hematomas, but only the larger ones, and then by displacement of vessels (mass effect). Lumbar puncture indicates whether or not blood has entered the subarachnoid space (aneurysm, vascular malformation, hypertensive hemorrhage, and some instances of hemorrhagic infarction), but the CSF is clear in pale infarction from thrombosis and embolism. In many stroke cases the CT scan, which entails no risk to the patient, has supplanted arteriography and lumbar puncture, both of which are sometimes hazardous.

RISK FACTORS

Several factors are known to increase the patient's liability to stroke. The most important of these are diabetes and hypertension. Diabetes hastens the atherosclerotic process in both large and small arteries; hypertension does the same, in addition to being the most readily recognized factor in the genesis of primary intracerebral hemorrhage. Furthermore, it now appears that systolic blood pressure is as important as diastolic pressure in producing these adverse effects (Rabkin et al.). The cooperative study of the Veterans Administration has convincingly demonstrated that the long-term control of hypertension decreases the incidence of both atherothrombotic infarction and intracerebral hemorrhage. It is also possible that smoking, obesity, and hyperlipidemia constitute risk factors. As for embolic strokes, the most important risk factors are structural cardiac disease and arrhythmias, particularly auricular fibrillation. The interactions between diabetes and hypertension on the one hand and intracerebral hemorrhage and atherothrombotic infarction on the other, and the association of cardiac disease and cerebral embolism are considered further on in this chapter, in relation to each of these categories of cerebrovascular disease.

Public health measures designed to detect and eliminate these risk factors provide the most intelligent, long-range approach to the treatment of cerebral vascular disease.

THE ISCHEMIC STROKE

The effects on brain tissue of arterial occlusion by thrombus or embolus vary, depending upon the location of the occlusion with relation to available collateral and anastomotic channels. If the obstruction lies proximal to the circle of Willis, the anterior and posterior communi-

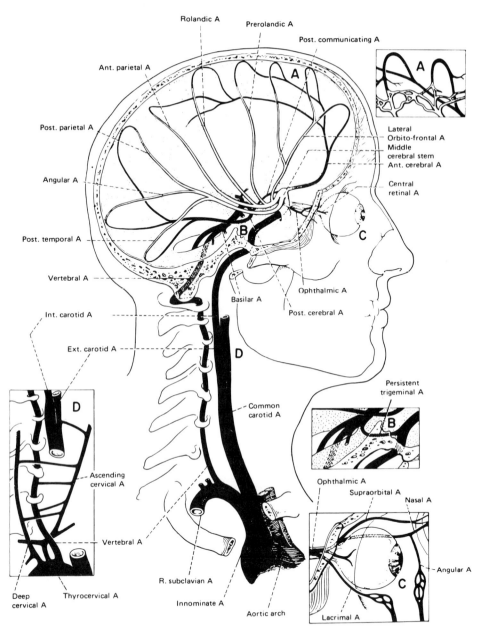

Figure 33-1

Arrangement of the major arteries on the right side carrying blood from the heart to the brain. Also shown are collateral vessels that may modify the effects of cerebral ischemia. For example, the posterior communicating artery connects the internal carotid and the posterior cerebral arteries, and may provide anastomosis between the carotid and basilar systems. Over the convexity, the subarachnoid interarterial anastomoses linking the middle, anterior, and posterior cerebral arteries are shown, with insert A illustrating that these anastomoses are a continuous network of tiny arteries forming a border zone between the major cerebral arterial territories. Occasionally a persistent trigeminal artery connects the internal carotid and basilar arteries proximal to the circle of Willis, as shown in insert B. Anastomoses between the internal and external carotid arteries via the orbit are illustrated in insert C. Wholly extracranial anastomoses from muscular branches of the cervical arteries to vertebral and external carotid arteries are indicated by insert D.

532

cating arteries of the circle may be and often are adequate to prevent infarction. In occlusion of the internal carotid artery in the neck, there may be retrograde anastomotic flow from the external carotid artery through the ophthalmic artery or via smaller external-internal connections (Figs. 33-1 and 33-2). With blockage of the vertebral artery the anastomotic flow may be via the deep cervical, thyrocervical, or occipital artery, or retrograde from the other vertebral artery. If the occlusion is in the stem portion of one of the cerebellar arteries (Fig. 33-3) or one of the cerebral arteries, i.e., distal to the circle of Willis (Fig. 33-1), then a series of meningeal interarterial anastomoses that connect many branches of these arteries may carry sufficient blood into the compromised territory to lessen (rarely prevent) ischemic damage. A capillary anastomotic system also exists between adjacent arterial branches, and although it may reduce the size of the ischemic field, particularly of the penetrating arteries, it is probably inconsequential in preventing infarction. Thus in the event of occlusion of a major arterial trunk, the extent of infarction ranges from none at all to the entire vascular territory of that vessel. Between these two extremes are countless variations in the extent of infarction, and its degree of completeness.

Additional *ischemia-modifying factors* are operative in determining the extent of necrosis. The speed of occlusion assumes importance; gradual narrowing of a vessel allows time for collateral channels to open. The level of blood pressure may influence the result; hypotension at a critical moment may render anastomotic channels ineffective. Hypoxia and hypocapnia would obviously have a deleterious effect. Altered viscosity and osmolality of the blood and hypoglycemia are potentially important factors, but difficult to evaluate. Finally, anomalies of vascular arrangement (of neck vessels, circle of Willis, and surface arteries) and the existence of previous vascular occlusions must influence the final outcome.

The specific neurologic deficit obviously relates to the location and size of the infarct or focus of ischemia. The territory of any artery, large or small, deep or superficial, may be involved. When an infarction lies in the territory of a carotid artery, unilateral signs predominate, as would be expected: hemiplegia, hemianesthesia, hemianopia, aphasia, and agnosias of certain types are the usual consequences. In the territory of the basilar artery the signs of infarction are bilateral; quadriparesis, hemiparesis, or hemisensory or bilateral sensory impairment occur in conjunction with cranial nerve palsies and other abnormalities of segmental functions subserved by the brainstem and cerebellum. The importance, therefore, of whether the symptoms and signs indicate a unilateral or bilateral lesion is obvious.

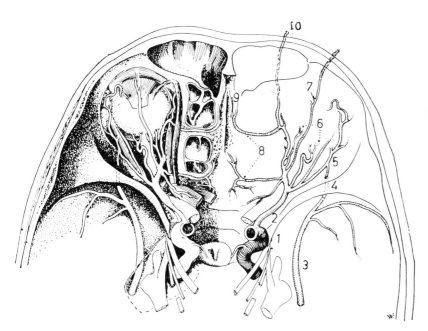

Figure 33-2
Diagram of orbital arteries: (1) internal carotid; (2) ophthalmic; (3) middle meningeal; (4) anastomosis; (5) lacrimal; (6) ocular (including central retinal); (7) supraorbital; (8) anterior and posterior ethmoidal; (9) anterior meningeal; (10) supratrochlear. (From Krayenbühl and Yasargil.)

NEUROVASCULAR SYNDROMES

For reasons already given, the clinical picture that results from an occlusion of any one artery differs in minor
ways from one patient to another. There is sufficient uniformity, however, to justify a study of the typical syndrome of each major artery. The following descriptions
apply particularly to infarction and ischemia due to embolism and thrombosis. Although hemorrhage within a
specific vascular territory may give rise to many of the
same effects, the total clinical picture is apt to differ because in its deep extension the hemorrhage involves the
territory of more than one artery and by its mass effect
may cause an increase in intracranial pressure.

INTERNAL CAROTID ARTERY

The territory supplied by this vessel and its main
branches is shown in Fig. 33-4. The clinical manifestations of atherosclerotic thrombotic disease of this artery
are the most variable of any cerebrovascular syndrome,
as one might infer from what was said above. Occlusion
is not infrequently silent, owing to the efficacy of the
willisian collaterals; but in other instances it may cause
a massive infarction involving the anterior two-thirds or
all of the cerebral hemisphere, including the basal ganglia, and lead to death in a few days. Most often the
infarct involves all or some part of the middle cerebral
territory; but when the anterior communicating artery is
very small, the ipsilateral anterior cerebral territory is
affected as well. If the two anterior cerebral arteries arise
from a common stem on one side, infarction may involve the territories of both. When the posterior cerebral

Figure 33-3
*Diagram of the brainstem showing the principal vessels of the
vertebral-basilar system. The letters and arrows on the right
indicate the levels of the four cross sections which follow: A =
Fig. 33-16; B = Fig. 33-15; C = Fig 33-14; D = Fig. 33-13.*
Although vascular syndromes of the pons and medulla

*have been designated by sharply outlined shaded areas, one
must appreciate that since satisfactory clinicopathologic studies
are scarce, the diagrams do not always represent established
fact. The frequency with which infarcts fail to produce a well-
recognized syndrome and the special tendency for syndromes to
merge with one another must be emphasized.*

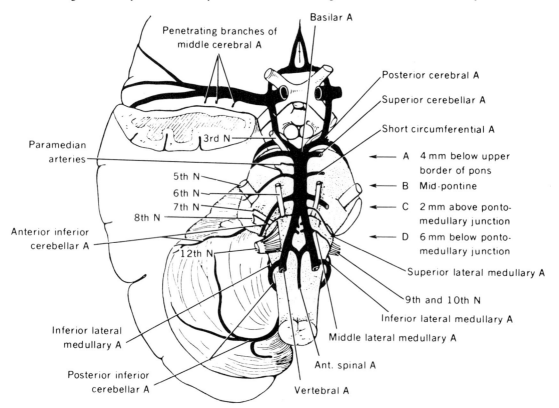

artery receives its main supply from the internal carotid rather than the basilar artery, its territory is included in the infarction. Not infrequently the territory of the anterior choroidal artery is also affected. If one internal carotid artery had been occluded at an earlier time, occlusion of the other one may cause bilateral cerebral infarction. The clinical effects in such cases may include coma with quadriplegia and continuous horizontal "metronomic" conjugate eye movements.

Symptomatic occlusion of the internal carotid artery usually produces a picture resembling that of middle cerebral artery occlusion—contralateral hemiplegia, hemihypesthesia, and aphasia (with involvement of the dominant hemisphere). When the anterior cerebral territory is included, there will be added some or all of the clinical features of the latter (see further on). Such patients are usually stuporous or semicomatose, because of the sheer mass of swollen, necrotic brain. Headache, usually located above the eyebrow, may also occur with either thrombosis or embolism of the carotid artery. The headache associated with occlusion of the middle cerebral artery is usually more lateral, at the temple, and that of posterior cerebral occlusion is in or behind the eye.

When the circulation of one carotid artery has been compromised, the most distal parts of the middle and anterior cerebral territories come to lie in the zone of maximal ischemia. This region is situated between the two vascular territories rather than in the center of each one; but the heavier involvement tends to fall in the distal territory of the middle cerebral artery. The zone of damage forms an elongated sickle-shaped strip of variable width from the frontal to the occipital poles. This tendency for a certain number of carotid infarcts to occupy the distal rather than central part of the sylvian region is a product of vascular arrangements that alter the pattern of ischemia. The distal zone also proves to be the most vulnerable in transient ischemic attacks with stenosis of the carotid artery. These attacks usually take the form of weakness or paresthesias of the arm, and only when the ischemia is more extensive do they include the face and tongue. Frequent sparing of the posterior part of the hemisphere is reflected in a low incidence of posterior types of aphasia and persistent homonymous hemianopia.

The internal carotid artery nourishes the optic nerve and retina as well as the brain (Figs. 33-1 and 2). Transient monocular blindness occurs as an intermittent symptom prior to the onset of stroke in approximately 25 percent of cases of symptomatic carotid occlusion. Yet central retinal artery occlusion is relatively rare, presumably because of efficient collateral supply.

Whereas most cerebral arteries can be evaluated only indirectly, by analysis of the clinical effects of occlusion, more direct means are available for the evaluation of the common and internal carotid arteries in the neck. With severe atherosclerotic stenosis at the level of the carotid sinus, with or without a superimposed thrombus, stethoscopy frequently discloses a bruit. Occasionally the bruit is due to stenosis at the origin of the external carotid artery and can then be misleading. If the bruit is heard at the angle of the jaw, the stenosis usually lies in the carotid sinus; if heard lower in the neck, it is in the common carotid or subclavian artery. The duration of the bruit is important—bruits which extend into diastole are almost invariably associated with a tight stenosis. One must be careful to distinguish bruits in the neck from transmitted aortic valve murmurs. An additional sign of carotid occlusion is the presence of a bruit on the opposite side, heard best by placing the bell of the stethoscope over the eyeball; presumably the murmur is accounted for by augmented circulation through the patent but irregularly narrowed vessel. Pulsation may be palpably reduced or absent in the common carotid artery in the neck, in the external carotid artery in front of the ear, and in the internal carotid artery in the lateral wall of the pharynx. In the presence of a unilateral internal carotid occlusion, compression of the normal common carotid should be avoided because it may precipitate unconsciousness, seizures, or an EEG change. Central retinal artery pressure is reduced on the side of a carotid occlusion or severe stenosis. A diastolic retinal pressure (determined by ophthalmic dynamometry) of less than 20 mmHg usually means that the common or internal carotid artery is occluded. The state of the arterial channels over the face may also suggest carotid occlusion. The supraorbital and supratrochlear pulses (on the upper orbital rim) become prominent as these vessels dilate to carry blood through the orbit via the ophthalmic artery into the upper carotid. The occurrence of retinal emboli, either shining or plain reddish in appearance, is another sign of carotid disease (crystalline cholesterol may be sloughed from an atherosclerotic ulcer).

Other neurologic and nonneurologic signs of carotid occlusion include pulseless arms (as in pulseless disease, see below); faintness in arising from the horizontal position or recurrent loss of consciousness when walking; headache and neck pain; transient blindness, either unilateral or bilateral; dimness of vision with exercise; premature cataracts; retinal atrophy and pigmentation; atrophy of the iris; leukomas; peripapillary arterio-

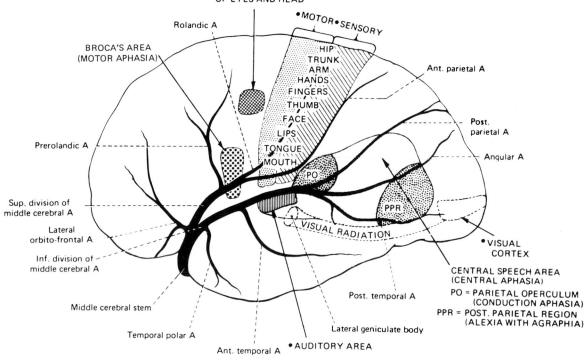

Figure 33-4

Diagram of a cerebral hemisphere, lateral aspect, showing the branches and distribution of the middle cerebral artery and the principal regions of cerebral localization. Below is a list of the clinical manifestations of infarction in the territory of this artery and the corresponding regions of cerebral damage.

Signs and symptoms	Structures involved
Paralysis of the contralateral face, arm, and leg	Somatic motor area for face and arm and the fibers descending from the leg area to enter the corona radiata
Sensory impairment over the contralateral face, arm, and leg (pinprick, cotton touch, vibration, position, two-point discrimination, stereognosis, tactile localization, barognosis, cutaneographia)	
Motor speech disorder	Broca's area of the dominant hemisphere
"Central" aphasia, word deafness, anomia, jargon speech, agraphia, acalculia, alexia, finger agnosia, right-left confusion (the last four comprise the Gerstmann syndrome)	Central language area and parietooccipital cortex of the dominant hemisphere
Apractagnosia (amorphosynthesis), anosognosia, hemiasomatognosia, unilateral neglect, agnosia for the left half of external space, "dressing apraxia," "constructional apraxia," distortion of visual coordinates, inaccurate localization in the half field, impaired ability to judge distance, upside-down reading, visual illusions	Usually nondominant parietal lobe. Loss of topographic memory is usually due to a nondominant lesion, occasionally to a dominant one.
Homonymous hemianopia (often superior homonymous quadrantanopia)	Optic radiation deep to second temporal convolution
Paralysis of conjugate gaze to the opposite side	Frontal contraversive field or fibers projecting therefrom
Avoidance reaction of opposite limbs	Parietal lobe

Figure 33-4 (*continued*)

Signs and symptoms	Structures involved
Miscellaneous: frontal ataxia	Frontopontine tract (?)
Loss or impairment of optokinetic nystagmus	Supramarginal or angular gyrus
Limb-kinetic apraxia	Premotor or parietal cortical damage
Mirror movements	Precise location of responsible lesions not known
Cheyne-Stokes respiration, contralateral hyperhidrosis, mydriasis (occasionally)	
Capsular (pure motor) hemiplegia	Upper portion of the posterior limb of the internal capsule and the adjacent corona radiata.

venous anastomoses in the retinae; optic atrophy; claudication of jaw muscles; perforation of the nasal septum; saddle nose deformity; facial atrophy (unilateral or bilateral); indolent infections of the face; abnormal facial pigmentation; and loss of hair.

Pulseless disease, which is expressed by various combinations of the above abnormalities, was originally reported from Japan by Takayasu, who observed it mainly in young women. They were found to be suffering from granulomatous arteritis of unknown cause which tended to involve all branches of the arch of the aorta to cranium and arms. Earlier examples had been recognized for several decades in Western Europe. In the Occident, by far the most frequent cause of pulseless disease, both partial and complete, is atherosclerotic thrombosis. Some of these have been incorrectly called Buerger's disease of the brain.

MIDDLE CEREBRAL ARTERY

This artery through its *cortical branches* supplies the lateral part of the cerebral hemisphere (Fig. 33-4). Its territory encompasses (1) the cortex and white matter of the lateral and inferior aspects of the frontal lobe including the motor areas 4 and 6, contraversive centers for lateral gaze, motor speech area of Broca (dominant hemisphere); (2) cortex and white matter of the parietal lobe including the sensory cortex and the angular and supramarginal convolutions; and (3) superior parts of the temporal lobe and insula. The *penetrating branches* of the middle cerebral artery supply the putamen, part of the head and body of the caudate nucleus, the outer globus pallidus, the posterior limb of the internal capsule, and the corona radiata (Fig. 33-5).

The middle cerebral artery may be occluded in its stem, blocking the flow in deep penetrating as well as the superficial cortical branches, or its major branches may be occluded individually. The classic picture of total occlusion is contralateral hemiplegia, hemianesthesia, and homonymous hemianopia; in addition there is aphasia

with left hemispheric lesions (Fig. 33-4) and amorphosynthesis with right-sided ones (see page 310). In the beginning the patient is dull or stuporous. Once established, the motor, sensory, and language deficits remain static or improve very little as months and years pass. If globally aphasic, seldom does the patient ever again communicate effectively. Occlusion of branches of the middle cerebral artery give rise to only parts of the symptom complex.

Occlusion of the stem of the middle cerebral artery by a thrombus, contrary to former teaching, is relatively infrequent. Pathologic studies have shown that most carotid occlusions are thrombotic, whereas most middle cerebral occlusions, particularly of the cortical branches, are embolic (Fisher, 1975). Most emboli tend to drift into superficial cortical branches; not more than 1 in 20 will enter penetrating basal branches. The distal territory of the middle cerebral artery may also be rendered ischemic by failure of the systemic circulation, especially if the carotid artery is stenotic; this may simulate embolic branch occlusions.

An embolus entering the middle cerebral artery often lodges in one of its two main divisions, the superior (supplying the rolandic and prerolandic areas) or inferior (temporoparietal areas). Major infarction in the territory of the superior division causes a dense sensorimotor deficit in the contralateral face, arm, and leg and mimics the syndrome of stem occlusion, except that there is less impairment of alertness. If the occlusion is lasting (not merely transient ischemia with fragmentation of the embolus), there will be slow improvement, and after a few months the patient will be able to walk with a spastic leg, while the motor deficits of the arm and face remain severe. With left-sided lesions there is initially a global aphasia which changes to a predominantly motor aphasia, with improvement in comprehension of spoken and written words and the emergence of a hesitant, grammatically simplified, dysmelodic speech. Embolic occlusion, limited to one of the branches of the superior division, produces a highly circumscribed in-

537

farct that further fractionates the syndrome. With occlusion of the ascending frontal branch the motor deficit is limited to the face and arm with little affection of the leg, and the latter, if weakened at all, soon improves; and with left-sided lesions an initial mutism and mild comprehension defect give way, within days to weeks, to grammatically appropriate speech, slightly dysmelodic, with normal comprehension (see Chap. 22). Embolic occlusion of the rolandic branches results in sensorimotor paresis with severe dysarthria but little evidence of aphasia. It resembles a pure motor stroke from lacunar infarction (see further on). Embolic occlusion of ascending parietal and other posterior branches of the superior division may cause no sensorimotor deficit, but only a con-

duction aphasia (page 330) and bilateral ideomotor apraxia. Improvement can be expected within a few weeks to months.

The inferior division of the middle cerebral artery is occluded less often than the superior one, but again nearly always by embolism. The usual result in left-sided lesions is a Wernicke's aphasia (see page 329). After remaining static for weeks to months, improvement can be expected. In less extensive infarcts from branch occlusions (superior parietal, angular, or posterior temporal), the deficit in comprehension of spoken and written language may be especially severe. Again, after a few months the deficits usually improve, often to the point where they are evident only in self-generated efforts to read and copy visually presented material. With either right or left hemisphere lesions there is usually a homonymous hemianopia and with right-sided ones an amorphosynthesis.

ANTERIOR CEREBRAL ARTERY

This artery through its cortical branches supplies the anterior three-quarters of the medial surface of the cerebral

Figure 33-5
Diagram of a cerebral hemisphere, coronal section, showing the territories of the major cerebral vessels.

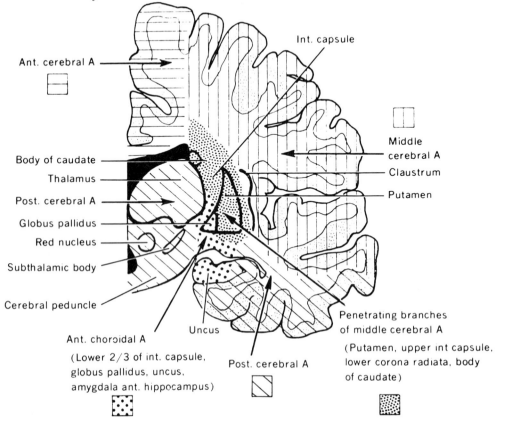

Int. capsule

Ant. cerebral A

Middle
cerebral A

Body of caudate

Claustrum

Thalamus

Putamen

Post. cerebral A

Globus pallidus

Red nucleus

Subthalamic body

Cerebral peduncle

Penetrating branches
of middle cerebral A

Uncus

Ant. choroidal A

(Lower 2/3 of int. capsule,
globus pallidus, uncus,
amygdala ant. hippocampus)

Post. cerebral A

(Putamen, upper int capsule,
lower corona radiata, body
of caudate)

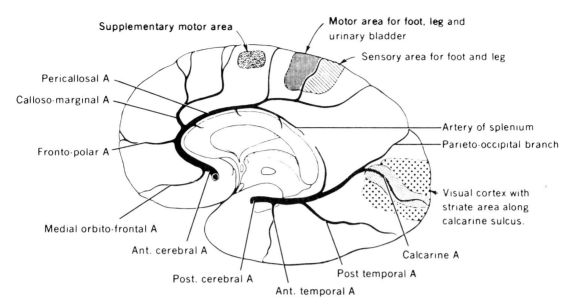

Figure 33-6

Diagram of a cerebral hemisphere, medial aspect, showing the branches and distribution of the anterior cerebral artery and the principal regions of cerebral localization. Below is a list of the clinical manifestations of infarction in the territory of this artery and the corresponding regions of cerebral damage.

Signs and symptoms	Structures involved
Paralysis of opposite foot and leg	Motor leg area
A lesser degree of paresis of opposite arm	Involvement of arm area of cortex or fibers descending therefrom to corona radiata
Cortical sensory loss over toes, foot, and leg	Sensory area for foot and leg
Urinary incontinence	Posteromedial part of superior frontal gyrus
Contralateral grasp reflex, sucking reflex, gegenhalten (paratonic rigidity), "frontal tremor"	Medial surface of the posterior frontal lobe (?)
Abulia (akinetic mutism), slowness, delay, lack of spontaneity, whispering, motor inaction, reflex distraction to sights and sounds	Uncertain localization—probably inferomedial lesion near subcallosum
Impairment of gait and stance (gait "apraxia")	Inferomedial frontal-pallidal (?)
Mental impairment (perseveration and amnesia)	Localization unknown
Miscellaneous: dyspraxia of left limbs	Corpus callosum
Tactile aphasia in left limbs	Corpus callosum
Cerebral paraplegia	Motor leg area bilaterally (due to bilateral occlusion of anterior cerebral arteries)

Note: Aphasia and hemianopia do not occur, although the occasionally observed abulia and echolalia may at first appear to be aphasia.

hemisphere, including the medial-orbital surface of the frontal lobe, the frontal pole, a strip of the lateral surface of the cerebral hemisphere along the superior border, and the anterior four-fifths of the corpus callosum. The deep branches which arise near the circle of Willis run chiefly to the anterior limb of the internal capsule and to the inferior part of the head of the caudate nucleus (Figs. 33-5, 33-6, and 33-7).

Again the clinical picture will depend on the location and size of the infarct which in turn relates to the site of the occlusion, the pattern of the circle of Willis, and the other ischemia-modifying factors mentioned above. Well-studied cases of infarction in the territory of this artery are not numerous; hence the syndromes are imperfectly known.

Occlusion of the stem of the artery proximal to its connection with the anterior communicating artery is usually well tolerated since adequate collateral flow will come from the anterior cerebral artery of the opposite side. Maximal disturbance occurs when both arteries arise from one anterior cerebral stem, in which case there will be infarction of the medial parts of both cerebral hemispheres. This results in paraplegia, incontinence, and abulic and aphasic symptoms.

Figure 33-7

Corrosion preparations with plastics demonstrating penetrating branches of the anterior and middle cerebral arteries. (1) Lateral lenticulostriate arteries. (2) Heubner artery and medial lenticulostriate arteries. (3) Anterior cerebral artery. (4) Internal carotid artery. (5) Middle cerebral artery. (From Krayenbühl and Yasargil.)

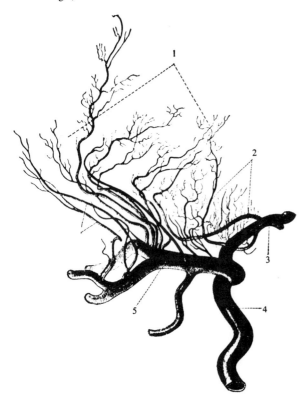

Complete infarction due to occlusion of one anterior cerebral artery distal to the anterior communicating artery results in a sensorimotor deficit of the opposite foot and leg and a lesser degree of paresis of the arm with sparing of the face. Urinary incontinence, contralateral grasp and sucking reflexes, and paratonic rigidity (gegenhalten) may be evident. With a left-sided occlusion there may be a sympathetic apraxia of the left arm and leg. Also, transcortical motor aphasia may occur with occlusions of Heubner's branch of the left anterior cerebral artery. Alexander and Schmitt cite cases in which a right hemiplegia (predominant in leg) with grasping and groping responses of the right hand and buccofacial apraxia are accompanied by a diminution or absence of spontaneous speech, agraphia, labored telegraphic speech, and a limited ability to name objects and to compose word lists, but striking preservation of repetition of spoken and written sentences (transcortical motor aphasia). Disorders of behavior that may be overlooked in routine clinical examination are abulia, presenting as a slowness and lack of spontaneity in all reactions; a tendency to speak in whispers; and distractibility. As would be expected, branch occlusions of the anterior cerebral artery produce only fragments of the total syndrome, usually a spastic weakness or cortical sensory loss in the opposite foot and leg.

ANTERIOR CHOROIDAL ARTERY

A few incomplete clinicopathologic studies are the basis of our present knowledge of the syndrome caused by occlusion of this artery. It is said to consist of contralateral hemiplegia, hemihypesthesia, and homonymous hemianopia due to involvement of the posterior limb of the internal capsule and white matter posterolateral to it, through which the geniculocalcarine tract passes. In the reported cases, however, the clinical syndrome has usually fallen short of what is expected on anatomic grounds. Indeed, the proof that such a syndrome exists has yet to be obtained since for a time the anterior choroidal artery was being surgically ligated, for the purpose of abolishing the tremor and rigidity of unilateral Parkinson's disease, without these ischemic effects having occurred.

VERTEBRAL-BASILAR AND POSTERIOR CEREBRAL ARTERIES

Posterior Cerebral Artery In about 70 percent of cases both posterior cerebral arteries arise from the basilar, and only thin posterior communicating arteries join this system to the internal carotids. In 20 to 25 percent, one posterior cerebral artery comes from the basilar and the other from the internal carotid; in the remainder both come from the carotids.

The configuration and branches of the *circular or proximal segment of the posterior cerebral* artery are illustrated in Figs. 33-8 and 33-9. The interpeduncular branches arising just above the basilar bifurcation supply the red nuclei, subthalamic nuclei (of Luys), substantiae nigrae, medial parts of the cerebral peduncles, oculomotor nuclei, reticular substance of the upper brainstem, decussation of the brachia conjunctiva (superior cerebellar peduncles), medial longitudinal fasciculi, and medial lemnisci. The thalamoperforate branches arise more distally, near the junction of the posterior cerebral and posterior communicating arteries, and supply the inferior, medial, and anterior parts of the thalamus; the thalamogeniculate branches arise still more distally, opposite the lateral geniculate body, and supply the geniculate body and the central and posterior parts of the thalamus. Medial branches from the posterior cerebral, as it encircles the midbrain, supply the lateral part of the cerebral peduncle, lateral tegmentum and corpora quadrigemina, and pineal gland. Posterior choroidal branches run to the posterosuperior thalamus, choroid plexus, hippocampus, and psalterium (decussation of fornices).

The terminal or *cortical branches of the posterior cerebral artery* supply the inferomedial part of the temporal lobe and the medial occipital lobe, including visual areas 17, 18, and 19 (see Figs. 33-6, 33-8, and 33-9).

Potentially, occlusion of the posterior cerebral artery can produce a greater variety of clinical effects than occlusion of any other artery, because both the upper brainstem, which is crowded with important structures, and the temporal and occipital lobes lie within its domain. Obviously the site of the occlusion and arrangement of the circle of Willis will in large measure determine the location and extent of the resulting infarct. For example, occlusion proximal to the posterior communicating artery may be asymptomatic if the collateral flow is adequate (A, Fig. 33-8; see also Fig. 33-9). Even distal to the posterior communicating artery, an occlusion may cause relatively little damage providing that the collateral flow through border zone collaterals from anterior and middle cerebral arteries is sufficient.

For convenience of exposition it is helpful to divide the various posterior cerebral artery syndromes into three groups: (1) anterior and proximal (involving interpeduncular and perforating thalamic branches), (2) cortical (inferior temporal and medial occipital), and (3) bilateral.

Anterior and proximal syndromes (Figs. 33-9 and 33-10) Thalamic syndrome of Déjerine and Roussy (see also page 100) follows infarction of the sensory relay nuclei in the thalamus, the result of occlusion of thalamogeniculate branches. There is a severe sensory loss, both deep and cutaneous, of the opposite side of the body, accompanied by a transitory hemiparesis. A homonymous hemianopia may be conjoined. In some instances there is a dissociation of sensory loss, with pain and thermal sensation being more affected than touch, vibration, and position, or only one part of the body is rendered anesthetic. After an interval, sensation begins to return and the patient may then be afflicted with pain and hyperpathia in the affected parts. There may also be distortion of taste, athetotic posturing of the hand, and depression of mood. Such conditions may persist for years.

Central midbrain syndromes are due to occlusion of paramedian branches on one or both sides. The clinical changes include Weber's syndrome (oculomotor palsy with contralateral hemiplegia), paralysis of vertical gaze, stupor or coma, and movement disorders, most often ataxic tremor which may be contralateral, i.e., on the side of hemiparesis (see below). Hemiplegia from infarction of the cerebral peduncle is relatively rare.

Anteromedial-inferior thalamic syndrome follows occlusion of the thalamoperforate branches. Here the main effect is an extrapyramidal movement disorder (hemiballismus or hemichoreoathetosis). Deep sensory loss, hemiataxia, or tremor may be added in various combinations. Hemiballismus is due usually to occlusion of a small branch to the corpus Luysii or its connections with the pallidum.

Cortical syndromes Classically, occlusion of branches to the temporal and occipital lobes gives rise to a homonymous hemianopia because of involvement of the primary visual receptive area (calcarine or striate cortex), or of the converging geniculocalcarine fibers. It may be incomplete and then involves the upper quadrants of the visual fields more than the lower ones (see Chap. 12). Macular or central vision may be spared because of collateralization of the occipital pole from distal branches of the middle (or anterior) cerebral arteries. Posterior cortical infarcts of the dominant hemisphere cause alexia (with or without agraphia), anomia (amnesic aphasia), and rarely an impairment of memory (see pages 292 and 308). The anomias (dysnomias) are most severe for colors, but the naming of other visually pre-

sented material such as pictures, musical notes, mathematical symbols, and manipulable objects may also be
impaired. The patient may treat objects as familiar, that
is, describe their functions and use them correctly, while
having forgotten their names. Color dysnomia and amnesic aphasia are more often present in this syndrome
than is alexia. The defect in retentive memory is of varying severity and may or may not improve with the passage of time. Nondominant hemisphere lesions may be
accompanied by topographic disorientation and dysnomia for faces (so-called prosopagnosia).

A complete proximal arterial occlusion leads to a
syndrome that combines anterior and proximal syndromes and cortical syndromes in part or totally. The
vascular lesion may be either an embolus or an atherosclerotic thrombus.

Bilateral cortical syndrome This may occur as a
result of successive infarctions or from a single embolic
or thrombotic occlusion of the upper basilar artery,
especially if the posterior communicating arteries are
unusually small.

Bilateral lesions of the occipital lobes, if extensive,
cause total blindness of the *cortical* type, i.e., a bilateral
homonymous hemianopia, sometimes accompanied by
unformed visual hallucinations. The pupillary reflexes
are preserved, and funduscopically the optic disks are
normal. Often the patient is unaware of being blind and

may in fact deny it, even when it is pointed out. More
frequently the lesions are incomplete, and a sector or
sectors of the visual fields remain intact. When the rem-
nant is small, vision appears to fluctuate from moment
to moment, as the patient attempts to capture the image
in the island of intact vision. Hysteria may be suspected
because of such inconsistencies. In bilateral lesions that
are confined to the occipital poles, there may be a loss of
only central vision (homonymous central scotomas).
With other lesions of the occipital pole there may be
homonymous paracentral scotomas, or the occipital
poles may be spared, leaving the patient with only central ("gun barrel") vision.

With bilateral lesions that involve the inferomedial portions of the temporal lobes, the impairment of
memory may be severe (Korsakoff's amnesic state). This
syndrome and its accompaniments are fully described in
Chaps. 20 and 21.

Vertebral Artery The vertebral arteries are the chief
arteries of the medulla; each supplies the lower three-
fourths of the pyramid, the medial lemniscus, all or
nearly all the retroolivary region (the lateral medullary
region), the restiform body, and the posterior inferior
part of the cerebellar hemisphere (Figs. 33-11 and 33-
12). The relative sizes of the vertebral arteries vary a
good deal, and in approximately 10 percent of cases, one
vessel is so small that the other is essentially the only
artery of supply to the brainstem. In these latter cases, if
collateral flow from the carotid system via the circle of
Willis is unavailable, occlusion would be equivalent to
occlusion of the basilar artery or both vertebral arteries.

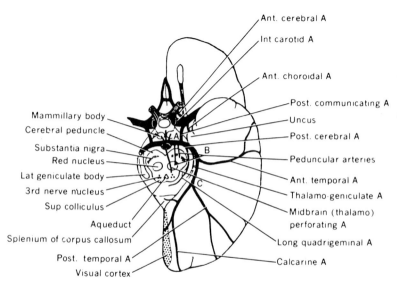

Figure 33-8
*Inferior aspect of the brain with the
branches and distribution of the posterior
cerebral artery and the principal anatomic
structures shown. On page 543 are listed the
clinical manifestations produced by infarction in its territory and the corresponding
regions of damage.*

Labels on figure:
Ant. cerebral A
Int carotid A
Ant. choroidal A
Post. communicating A
Uncus
Post. cerebral A
Peduncular arteries
Ant. temporal A
Thalamo-geniculate A
Midbrain (thalamo) perforating A
Long quadrigeminal A
Calcarine A

Mammillary body
Cerebral peduncle
Substantia nigra
Red nucleus
Lat geniculate body
3rd nerve nucleus
Sup colliculus
Aqueduct
Splenium of corpus callosum
Post. temporal A
Visual cortex

Figure 33-8 (*continued*)

Signs and symptoms	Structures involved
Peripheral territory	
Homonymous hemianopia	Calcarine cortex or optic radiation; hemiachromatopsia may be present. Macular or central vision tends to be preserved because occipital striate area is usually spared.
Bilateral homonymous hemianopia, cortical blindness, unawareness or denial of blindness; achromatopsia, failure to see to-and-fro movements, inability to perceive objects not centrally located, apraxia of ocular movements, inability to count or enumerate objects	Bilateral occipital lobe possibly with involvement of parietooccipital region
Dyslexia without agraphia, color anomia	Dominant calcarine lesion and posterior part of corpus callosum
Memory defect	Lesion of inferomedial portions of temporal lobe bilaterally or on the dominant side only
Topographic disorientation and prosopagnosia	Usually nondominant calcarine and lingual gyri
Simultagnosia	Dominant visual cortex
Unformed visual hallucinations, metamorphopsia, teleopsia, illusory visual spread, paliopsia, distortion of outlines, photophobia	Calcarine cortex
Central territory	
Thalamic syndrome: sensory loss (all modalities), spontaneous pain and dysesthesias, choreoathetosis, intention tremor, spasms of hand, mild hemiparesis	Posteroventral nucleus of thalamus in territory of thalamogeniculate artery. Involvement of the adjacent subthalamic body or its pallidal connections results in hemiballismus and choreoathetosis.
Thalamoperforate syndrome: (1) superior, crossed cerebellar ataxia; (2) inferior, crossed cerebellar ataxia with ipsilateral third nerve palsy (Claude's syndrome)	Dentatothalamic tract and issuing third nerve
Weber's syndrome—third nerve palsy and contralateral hemiplegia	Third nerve and cerebral peduncle
Contralateral hemiplegia	Cerebral peduncle
Paralysis or paresis of vertical eye movement, skew deviation, sluggish pupillary responses to light, slight miosis and ptosis (retraction nystagmus and "tucking" of the eyelids may be associated)	Supranuclear fibers to third nerve, high midbrain tegmentum ventral to superior colliculus (interstitial nucleus of Cajal, nucleus of Darkschewitsch, and posterior commissure)
Contralateral, ataxic or postural tremor	Dentatothalamic tract (?) after decussation. Precise site of lesion unknown
Decerebrate attacks	Damage to motor tracts between red and vestibular nuclei

Note: Tremor in repose has been omitted because of the uncertainty of its occurrence in the posterior cerebral artery syndrome. Peduncular hallucinosis may occur in thalamic-subthalamic ischemic lesions, but the exact location of the lesion is unknown.

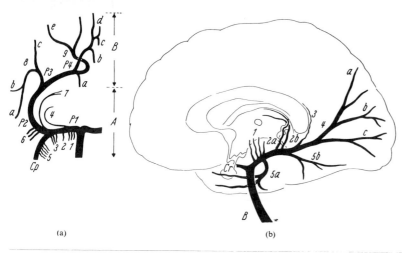

Figure 33-9
The posterior cerebral and basilar arteries.
(From Krayenbühl and Yasargil.)

Posterior cerebral artery	Regions of vascular supply

Figure 33-9A

(A) Circular or proximal segment
    (1) Paramedian arteries (interpeduncular, intercrural, perforating) — Substantia nigra, red nucleus, mammillary body, oculomotor nerve, trochlear nerve
    (2) Quadrigeminal arteries — Quadrigeminal bodies
    (3) Thalamic arteries (medial and lateral) — Central nucleus, medial nucleus, ventrolateral nucleus of the thalamus, pulvinar, lateral geniculate body, internal capsule (posterior portion)
    (4) Medial posterior choroidal arteries
    (5) Premammillary arteries (of the posterior communicating artery) — Epithalamus, pineal gland, tela choroidea of the prosencephalon
    (6) Peduncular artery — Tuber cinereum, cerebral peduncle, ventral nuclei of the thalamus, nuclei of the hypothalamus, chiasm
    (7) Lateral posterior choroidal arteries (anterior and posterior) — Hippocampal gyrus, lateral geniculate body, pulvinar, dentate fascia, hippocampus, anterior basal cortex of the temporal lobe, choroid plexus of the temporal horn, trigone, dorsolateral nuclei of the thalamus

(B) Cortical or distal segment
    (8) Lateral occipital artery
        (a) Anterior temporal arteries — Laterobasal aspects of the temporal and occipital lobe
        (b) Middle temporal arteries
        (c) Posterior temporal arteries
    (9) Medial occipital artery
        (a) Dorsal callosal artery — Splenium
        (b) Posterior parietal artery — Cuneus, precuneus
        (c) Occipitoparietal artery
        (d) Calcarine arteries — Calcarine gyrus, occipital pole
        (e) Occipitotemporal artery — Laterobasal occipital lobe

Figure 33-9B

(B) Basilar artery
Cr Posterior communicating artery
(1) Thalamic arteries
(2a) Medial posterior choroidal artery
(2b) Lateral posterior choroidal artery
(3) Dorsal callosal artery
(4) Medial occipital artery
    (a) Posterior parietal arteries
    (b) Occipitoparietal arteries
    (c) Calcarine arteries
(5a) Anterior and middle temporal arteries
(5b) Posterior temporal artery

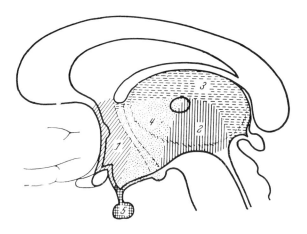

Figure 33-10

Diagram of the vascularization of the diencephalon. Distribution of (1) the anterior cerebral artery, (2) the posterior cerebral artery, (3) the anterior and posterior choroidal arteries, (4) the posterior communicating artery, and (5) the internal carotid artery. (From Krayenbühl and Yasargil.)

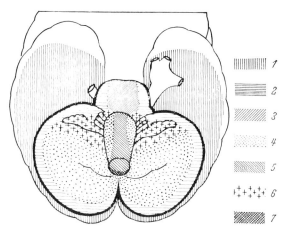

Figure 33-12

Regions supplied by the posterior segment of the circle of Willis, basal view: (1) posterior cerebral artery; (2) superior cerebellar artery; (3) paramedian arteries of the basilar artery and spinal artery; (4) posterior inferior cerebellar artery; (5) vertebral artery; (6) posterior inferior cerebellar artery; (7) dorsal spinal artery. (From Krayenbühl and Yasargil.)

Figure 33-11

Regions of supply by the posterior segment of the circle of Willis, lateral view: (1) posterior cerebral artery; (2) superior cerebellar artery; (3) basilar artery and superior cerebellar artery; (4) posterior inferior cerebellar artery; (5) vertebral artery (posterior inferior cerebellar artery, anterior spinal artery, posterior spinal artery).

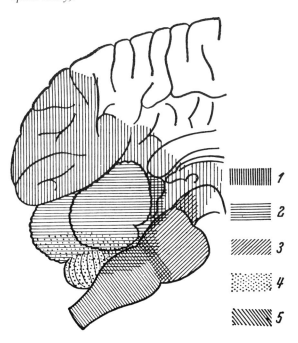

The posterior inferior cerebellar artery is usually a branch of the vertebral artery, but can have a common origin with the anterior inferior cerebellar artery from the basilar artery. It is necessary to keep these anatomic variations in mind when considering the effects of vertebral artery occlusion.

The results of vertebral occlusion are quite variable. When there are two good-sized arteries, occlusion on one side may occur without any recognizable symptoms and signs or pathologic changes. If the subclavian artery is blocked proximal to the origin of the vertebral artery, exercise of the arm on that side may draw blood from the vertebral-basilar system into the arm, sometimes resulting in the symptoms of basilar insufficiency. Fisher originally referred to this as the *subclavian steal* syndrome. If the occlusion of the vertebral artery is so situated as to block the arteries supplying the *lateral medulla*, a characteristic syndrome may result; this is probably the most frequent consequence of occlusion of one vertebral artery (see below). When the branch to the anterior spinal artery is blocked, collateral influx from the corresponding branch to the anterior spinal artery is usually sufficient to prevent infarction of the cervical cord. If the branch to the pyramid is occluded, that part of the pyramidal tract may be infarcted unless collateral flow is adequate. Any of these branches may become occluded in its course as well as at its origin from the vertebral artery and have similar effects. Rarely, occlusion of the vertebral artery or one of its medial branches produces an infarct which involves the medullary pyramid, the medial lemniscus, and the emergent hypoglossal fibers [causing contralateral paralysis of arm and leg (face spared), contralateral loss of position and vibration sense, and ipsilateral paralysis and atrophy of the tongue]. This is the *medial medullary syndrome* (Fig. 33-13). Occlusion of a vertebral artery low in the neck is usually compensated by anastomotic flow to the upper part of the artery via the thyrocervical, deep cervical, and occipital arteries, or influx from the anterior part of the circle of Willis.

The *lateral medullary syndrome* (Fig. 33-13) is produced by infarction of a wedge of lateral medulla lying posterior to the inferior olivary nucleus. The classic syndrome, as outlined by Fisher, Karnes, and Kubik, reflects the involvement of the spinothalamic tract (*contralateral* impairment of pain and thermal sense over half the body, sometimes the face); descending sympathetic tract (*ipsilateral* Horner's syndrome of miosis, ptosis, decreased sweating); issuing fibers of the ninth and tenth nerves (hoarseness, dysphagia, ipsilateral paralysis

of the palate and vocal cord, diminished gag reflex); vestibular nuclei (nystagmus, oscillopsia, vertigo, nausea, vomiting); olivocerebellar and/or spinocerebellar fibers and, sometimes, restiform body (*ipsilateral* ataxia of limbs, falling to the ipsilateral side); descending tract and nucleus of the fifth nerve (pain, numbness, impaired sensation over ipsilateral half of the face); nucleus and tractus solitarius (loss of taste); cuneate and gracile nuclei (numbness of *ipsilateral* arm and hiccup). This syndrome, one of the most striking in neurology, is almost always due to ischemic necrosis. Although occlusion of the posterior inferior cerebellar artery is usually stated to be the cause of the lateral medullary syndrome, careful studies have shown that in 8 out of 10 cases it is the vertebral artery that is occluded; in the remainder, either the posterior inferior cerebellar artery or rarely one of the lateral medullary arteries is occluded. Infarction in the *posterior medullary region* causes ipsilateral cerebellar ataxia and, rarely, hiccup. The symptoms associated with isolated infarction of the inferior part of the cerebellum include sudden severe dizziness, nausea, vomiting, ataxia, and nystagmus—a picture that mimics acute labyrinthine disorder.

Basilar Artery The branches of the basilar artery may be conveniently grouped as follows: (1) paramedian, 7 to 10 in number, supplying a wedge of pons on either side

Figure 33-13

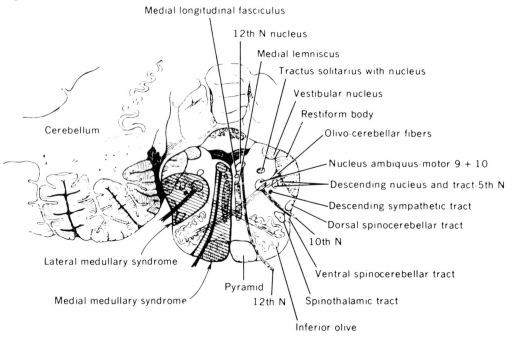

Medial longitudinal fasciculus
12th N nucleus
Medial lemniscus
Tractus solitarius with nucleus
Vestibular nucleus
Restiform body
Olivo-cerebellar fibers
Nucleus ambiguus-motor 9 + 10
Descending nucleus and tract-5th N
Descending sympathetic tract
Dorsal spinocerebellar tract
10th N
Ventral spinocerebellar tract
Spinothalamic tract
12th N
Pyramid
Medial medullary syndrome
Lateral medullary syndrome
Cerebellum
Inferior olive

Figure 33-13 (*continued*)

Signs and symptoms	*Structures involved*
1. Medial medullary syndrome (occlusion of vertebral artery or branch of vertebral or lower basilar artery)	
a. On side of lesion	
(1) Paralysis with atrophy of half the tongue	Issuing twelfth nerve
b. On side opposite lesion	
(1) Paralysis of arm and leg sparing face	Pyramidal tract
(2) Impaired tactile and proprioceptive sense over half the body	Medial lemniscus
2. Lateral medullary syndrome (occlusion of any of five vessels may be responsible—vertebral, posterior inferior cerebellar, or superior, middle, or inferior lateral medullary arteries)	
a. On side of lesion	
(1) Pain, numbness, impaired sensation over half the face	Descending tract and nucleus of fifth nerve
(2) Ataxia of limbs, falling to side of lesion	Uncertain—restiform body, cerebellar hemisphere, olivocerebellar fibers, spinocerebellar tract (?)
(3) Vertigo, nausea, vomiting	Vestibular nuclei and connections
(4) Nystagmus, diplopia, oscillopsia	Vestibular nuclei and connections
(5) Horner's syndrome (miosis, ptosis, decreased sweating)	Descending sympathetic tract
(6) Dysphagia, hoarseness, paralysis of vocal cord, diminished gag reflex	Issuing fibers ninth and tenth nerves
(7) Loss of taste (rare)	Nucleus and tractus solitarius
(8) Numbness of ipsilateral arm, trunk, or leg	Cuneate and gracile nuclei
(9) Hiccup	Uncertain
b. On side opposite lesion	
(1) Impaired pain and thermal sense over half the body, sometimes face	Spinothalamic tract
3. Total unilateral medullary syndrome (occlusion of vertebral artery); combination of medial and lateral syndromes	
4. Lateral pontomedullary syndrome (occlusion of vertebral artery); combination of medial and lateral syndromes	
5. Basilar artery syndrome (the syndrome of the lone vertebral artery is equivalent); a combination of the various brainstem syndromes plus those arising in the posterior cerebral artery distribution. The clinical picture comprises bilateral long-tract signs (sensory and motor) with cerebellar and cranial nerve abnormalities.	
a. Paralysis or weakness of all extremities, plus all bulbar musculature	Corticobulbar and corticospinal tracts bilaterally
b. Diplopia, paralysis of conjugate lateral and/or vertical gaze, internuclear ophthalmoplegia, horizontal and/or vertical nystagmus	Ocular motor nerves, apparatus for conjugate gaze, medial longitudinal fasciculus, vestibular apparatus
c. Blindness, impaired vision, various visual field defects	Visual cortex
d. Bilateral cerebellar ataxia	Cerebellar peduncles and the cerebellar hemispheres
e. Coma	Tegmentum of midbrain, thalami
f. Sensation may be strikingly intact in the presence of almost total paralysis. Sensory loss may be syringomyelic or the reverse or involve all modalities	Medial lemniscus, spinothalamic tracts or thalamic nuclei

of the midline; (2) short circumferential, 5 to 7 in number, supplying the lateral two-thirds of the pons and the middle and superior cerebellar peduncles; (3) the long circumferential, 2 on each side (the superior and anterior inferior cerebellar arteries), which run laterally around the pons to reach the cerebellar hemispheres (Figs. 33-11 and 33-12); and (4) several paramedian branches at the bifurcation of the basilar artery into the posterior cerebral arteries supplying the medial subthalamic zone; here a branch on one side distributes branches that cross the midline so that the occlusion of such a stem vessel may cause bilateral infarction. The other branches of the posterior cerebral artery have been described above.

The picture of basilar occlusion due to thrombosis may arise in several ways: (1) occlusion in the basilar artery itself, usually in the lower third at the site of an atherosclerotic plaque; (2) occlusion of both vertebral arteries; and (3) occlusion of a single vertebral artery, when there is only one of adequate size. It must be emphasized that thrombosis frequently involves only a branch of the basilar artery rather than the trunk (*basilar branch occlusion*). When the obstruction is embolic, the embolus usually lodges at the upper bifurcation of the basilar or in one of the posterior cerebral arteries, since if it is small enough to pass through the vertebral artery, it easily traverses the length of the basilar artery, which is of greater diameter than either vertebral artery.

The syndrome of *basilar artery occlusion* as outlined by Kubik and Adams, reflects the involvement of a large number of structures: corticospinal and corticobulbar tracts, cerebellum, middle and superior cerebellar peduncles, medial and lateral lemnisci, spinothalamic tracts, medial longitudinal fasciculi, pontine nuclei, vestibular and cochlear nuclei, descending hypothalamospinal sympathetic fibers, and the third through eighth cranial nerves (the nuclei and their segments within the brainstem).

The *complete basilar syndrome* comprises bilateral long tract signs (sensory and motor) with variable cerebellar and cranial nerve abnormalities and other segmental disorders of the brainstem. Often the patient is comatose because of ischemia of the reticular activating system. In the presence of the full syndrome, it is usually not difficult to make the correct diagnosis. The aim should be, however, to recognize basilar insufficiency long before the stage of total deficit has been reached. The early manifestations occur in many combinations.

Occlusion of branches at the bifurcation of the basilar results in a remarkable number of complex syndromes that include, in various combinations, somnolence, visual hallucinations, disorders of ocular movement (convergence spasm, paralysis of vertical gaze, retraction nystagmus, pseudoabducens palsy, retraction of upper eyelids), skew deviation of the eyes, an agitated delirious state, Korsakoff's amnesic defects and visual defects. These have been reviewed by Caplan as "top of the basilar" syndromes.

The main signs of thrombosis of the *superior cerebellar artery* are severe ipsilateral cerebellar ataxia (middle and/or superior cerebellar peduncles); nausea and vomiting; slurred speech (pseudobulbar); and loss of pain and thermal sensation over the extremities, body, and face of the opposite side (spinothalamic tract). Partial deafness, static tremor of the ipsilateral upper extremity, ipsilateral Horner's syndrome, and bulbar myoclonus have also been reported.

With occlusion of the *anterior inferior cerebellar artery* the extent of the infarct is extremely variable. The size of this artery and the territory it supplies vary inversely with the size and territory of supply of the posterior inferior cerebellar artery. The principal findings are vertigo, nausea, vomiting, nystagmus, tinnitus; ipsilateral cerebellar ataxia (inferior cerebellar peduncle, or restiform body), ipsilateral Horner's syndrome, and paresis of conjugate lateral gaze; and contralateral loss of pain and temperature sense of the arm, trunk, and leg (lateral spinothalamic tract). If the occlusion is close to the origin of the artery, the corticospinal fibers may also be involved, producing a hemiplegia. Occlusion of the *artery to the retroolivary space* will result in infarction of the spinothalamic fibers, the adjacent pontine nuclei, and the pontocerebellar fibers on one side of the pons. If the infarct extends deeper, to reach the tegmentum, as it occasionally does, paralysis of conjugate lateral gaze and a contralateral sensory deficit will result.

Another cardinal manifestation of brainstem involvement is a "crossed" or "alternate" cranial nerve and long tract sensory or motor deficit. These "crossed" syndromes, which may involve cranial nerves III through XII, are listed in Table 46-2. Although the finding of bilateral neurologic signs strongly suggests brainstem involvement, it must be emphasized that in many instances of infarction within the basilar territory the signs are limited to one side of the body, without cranial nerve involvement, indicating occlusion of a branch of the basilar artery, not of the main trunk.

It is impossible from motor signs alone to distinguish a hemiplegia of pontine origin from one of cerebral origin. With brainstem lesions, as with cerebral lesions, a flaccid paralysis gives way to spasticity after a few days or weeks, and there is no satisfactory explana-

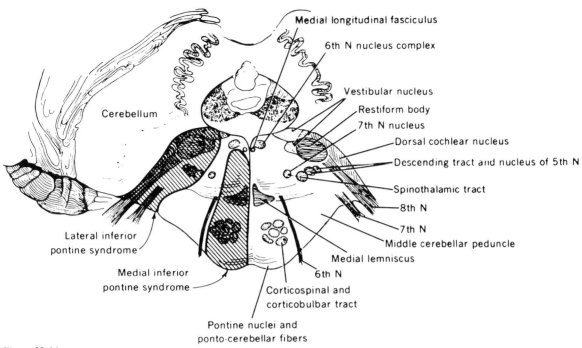

Labels in figure:
Medial longitudinal fasciculus
6th N nucleus complex
Vestibular nucleus
Restiform body
7th N nucleus
Dorsal cochlear nucleus
Descending tract and nucleus of 5th N
Spinothalamic tract
8th N
7th N
Middle cerebellar peduncle
Medial lemniscus
6th N
Corticospinal and corticobulbar tract
Pontine nuclei and ponto-cerebellar fibers
Medial inferior pontine syndrome
Lateral inferior pontine syndrome
Cerebellum

Figure 33-14

Signs and symptoms	*Structures involved*
1. Medial inferior pontine syndrome (occlusion of paramedian branch of basilar artery)	
a. On side of lesion	
(1) Paralysis of conjugate gaze to side of lesion (preservation of convergence)	Paraabducens "center" for lateral gaze
(2) Nystagmus	Vestibular nuclei and connections
(3) Ataxia of limbs and gait	Middle cerebellar peduncle (?)
(4) Diplopia on lateral gaze	Abducens nerve
b. On side opposite lesion	
(1) Paralysis of face, arm, and leg	Corticobulbar and corticospinal tract in lower pons
(2) Impaired tactile and proprioceptive sense over half of the body	Medial lemniscus
2. Lateral inferior pontine syndrome (occlusion of anterior inferior cerebellar artery)	
a. On side of lesion	
(1) Horizontal and vertical nystagmus, vertigo, nausea, vomiting, oscillopsia	Vestibular nerve or nucleus
(2) Facial paralysis	Seventh nerve
(3) Paralysis of conjugate gaze to side of lesion	Paraabducens "center" for lateral gaze
(4) Deafness, tinnitus	Auditory nerve or cochlear nucleus
(5) Ataxia	Middle cerebellar peduncle and cerebellar hemisphere
(6) Impaired sensation over face	Descending tract and nucleus fifth nerve
b. On side opposite lesion	
(1) Impaired pain and thermal sense over half the body (may include face)	Spinothalamic tract
3. Total unilateral inferior pontine syndrome (occlusion of anterior inferior cerebellar artery); lateral and medial syndromes combined	

tion for the variability in this period of delay or for the occurrence in some cases of spasticity from the onset of the stroke. Localization depends upon coexisting neurologic phenomena. With a lower brainstem hemiplegia the eyes may deviate to the side of the paralysis, just the opposite of supratentorial lesions. The pattern of sensory disturbance may be helpful. A dissociated sensory deficit over the face or half the body usually indicates a lesion within the brainstem, while a sensory loss over one side of the body involving all modalities indicates a lesion in the thalamus or deep in the white matter of the parietal lobe. When position sense, two-point discrimination, and tactile localization are affected relatively more than pain, temperature, and tactile sense, a cortical lesion is suggested; the converse suggests a brainstem localization. Bilaterality of both motor and sensory manifestations is almost certain evidence that the lesion lies infratentorially. When hemiplegia or hemiparesis and sensory loss are coextensive, the lesion lies supratentorially. Additional manifestations which point unequivocally to a brainstem site are whirling dizziness, diplopia, cerebellar ataxia, Horner's syndrome, and deafness. The several

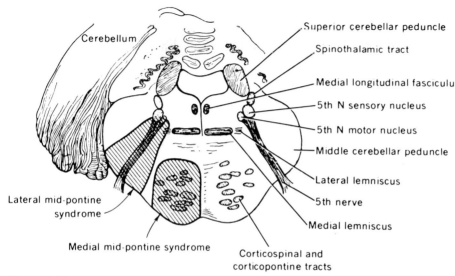

Figure 33-15

Signs and symptoms	Structures involved
1. Medial midpontine syndrome (paramedian branch of midbasilar artery	
a. On side of lesion	
(1) Ataxia of limbs and gait (more prominent in bilateral involvement)	Middle cerebellar peduncle
b. On side opposite lesion	
(1) Paralysis of face, arm, and leg	Corticobulbar and corticospinal tract
(2) Deviation of eyes	
(3) Variably impaired touch and proprioception when lesion extends posteriorly. Usually the syndrome is purely motor.	Medial lemniscus
2. Lateral midpontine syndrome (short circumferential artery)	
a. On side of lesion	
(1) Ataxia of limbs	Middle cerebellar peduncle
(2) Paralysis of muscles of mastication	Motor fibers or nucleus of fifth nerve
(3) Impaired sensation over side of face	Sensory fibers or nucleus of fifth nerve

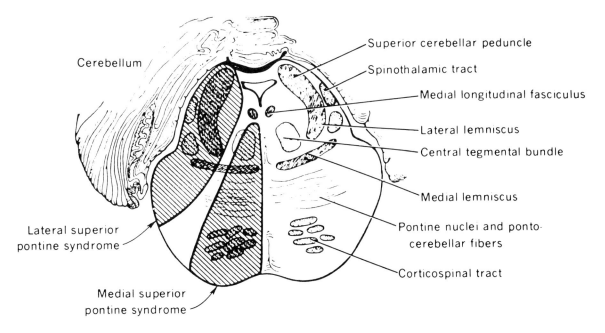

Labels on figure:
Cerebellum

Superior cerebellar peduncle
Spinothalamic tract
Medial longitudinal fasciculus
Lateral lemniscus
Central tegmental bundle
Medial lemniscus
Pontine nuclei and ponto-cerebellar fibers
Corticospinal tract

Lateral superior pontine syndrome

Medial superior pontine syndrome

Figure 33-16

Signs and symptoms	Structures involved
1. Medial superior pontine syndrome (paramedian branches of upper basilar artery	
a. On side of lesion	
(1) Cerebellar ataxia	Superior and/or middle cerebellar peduncle
(2) Internuclear ophthalmoplegia	Medial longitudinal fasciculus
(3) Rhythmic myoclonus of palate, pharynx, vocal cords, respiratory apparatus, face, oculomotor apparatus, etc.	Central tegmental bundle
b. On side opposite lesion	
(1) Paralysis of face, arm, and leg	Corticobulbar and corticospinal tract
(2) Rarely touch, vibration, and position senses are affected	Medial lemniscus
2. Lateral superior pontine syndrome (syndrome of superior cerebellar artery)	
a. On side of lesion	
(1) Ataxia of limbs and gait, falling to side of lesion	Middle and superior cerebellar peduncles, superior surface of cerebellum, dentate nucleus
(2) Dizziness, nausea, vomiting	Vestibular nucleus ⎫
(3) Horizontal nystagmus	Vestibular nucleus ⎬ Territory of descending branch to middle cerebellar peduncle from superior cerebellar artery
(4) Paresis of conjugate gaze (ipsilateral)	Uncertain
(5) Loss of optokinetic nystagmus	Uncertain
(6) Skew deviation	Uncertain ⎭
(7) Miosis, ptosis, decreased sweating over face (Horner's syndrome)	Descending sympathetic fibers
b. On side opposite lesion	
(1) Impaired pain and thermal sense on face, limbs, and trunk	Spinothalamic tract
(2) Impaired touch, vibration, and position sense, more in leg than arm (there is a tendency to incongruity of pain and touch deficits)	Medial lemniscus (lateral portion)

brainstem syndromes illustrate the important point that the cerebellar system, spinothalamic tract, trigeminal nucleus, and sympathetic fibers can be involved at different levels, and neighborhood phenomena must be used to identify the exact site.

A myriad of proper names have been applied to the brainstem syndromes (see Table 46-2). Most of these syndromes were originally described in relation to tumors and other nonvascular diseases. The diagnosis of vascular disorders in this region of the brain is not greatly facilitated by a knowledge of these eponymic syndromes, and it is much more profitable to memorize the anatomy of the brainstem. The principal syndromes to be recognized are the full basilar, vertebral, anterior inferior cerebellar, superior cerebellar, pontomedullary, and those of the medial medullary branches. Other syndromes can usually be identified as fragments of the major ones.

LACUNAR STATE

As one might surmise, small penetrating branches of the cerebral arteries may become occluded, and the resulting infarct may be so small or so situated as to cause no symptoms whatsoever. As the softened tissue is removed it leaves a small cavity or lacune. Early in the twentieth century, Pierre Marie described the occurrence of multiple small cavities of this type and referred to the state as *état lacunaire*. He distinguished them from a fine loosening of tissue around thickened vessels that enter the anterior and posterior perforated spaces, an appearance to which he referred as *état criblé*. Pathologists have not always agreed on these distinctions, but Fisher and Adams have taken the position that the lacunar state is due always to occlusion of small arteries, 50 to 150 μm in diameter, and the cribriform state to mere thickening of vessels.

Interestingly, in our pathologic material, there has always been a strong correlation of the lacunar state with a combination of hypertension and atherosclerosis, and to a lesser degree with diabetes. One may hypothesize that the basis of the lacunar state is unusually severe atherosclerosis that has involved not just the large arteries, as it usually does, but has extended into their finest branches.

When Fisher examined a series of such lesions in serial section, from a basal parent artery up to and through the lacune, he found atheroma and thrombosis to be the basic abnormality in some and a lipohyalin

degeneration and occlusion of small vessels in others. In some instances the latter changes had resulted in false aneurysm formation, resembling the Charcot-Bouchard aneurysms of brain hemorrhage (see further on). Usually 4 to 6, sometimes up to 10 to 15 lacunes are found in any given specimen. They tend to be situated in the caudate and lenticular nuclei, the thalami, basis pontis, and cerebral and cerebellar white matter. The cavities range from 2 to 15 mm in diameter, and whether or not they cause symptoms depends entirely on their location.

Fisher has delineated some of the more frequent symptomatic forms. If the lacune lies in the territory of a lenticulostriate artery, i.e., in the internal capsule or corona radiata, it may cause a *pure motor hemiplegia* or a *pure hemisensory syndrome*. Such deficits tend to evolve in a relatively leisurely fashion over as long a period as 2 to 3 days, raising the possibility of a small hemorrhage. The CT scan and arteriogram usually show nothing. The weakness in pure motor hemiplegia involves the face, arm, and leg. Recovery, which may begin within hours, days, or weeks, is often nearly complete. Similarly, with a lacune of the thalamus or parietal white matter, presenting as a pure *hemisensory* defect, no other neurologic abnormalities coexist. The course and outcome are much the same as in a pure hemiplegia. In the midbrain the most frequent lacunar syndrome is a hemiparesis with cerebellar ataxia on the same side as the weakness. In the basis pontis the syndrome may be one of pure motor hemiplegia, mimicking that of internal capsular infarction; or a combination of dysarthria and clumsiness of one hand may occur. Surely other syndromes are occurring but have yet to be defined. Some of the brainstem syndromes may blend with basilar branch syndromes, and these, too, are in need of precise definition. Multiple lacunar infarcts, involving the corticospinal and corticobulbar tracts, are of course the usual cause of pseudobulbar palsy.

CLASSIFICATION OF CEREBROVASCULAR DISEASES

In classifying the cerebrovascular diseases it is most practical, from the clinical viewpoint, to preserve the classic division into thrombosis, embolism and hemorrhage; our descriptions will follow this scheme. The causes of each of the "big three," as well as the criteria for diagnosis and the confirmatory laboratory tests, will be considered in the corresponding section. This plan has the disadvantage of not providing a niche for disorders such as reversible ischemia, hypertensive encephalopathy, and venous thrombosis; but these will be taken up in separate sections.

The frequency of the different types of cerebrovascular disease has been difficult to ascertain. Obviously clinical diagnosis is not always correct, and clinical services are heavily weighted with acute strokes and nonfatal cases. An autopsy series inevitably includes many old vascular lesions, particularly infarcts, whose exact nature cannot always be determined, and there is a bias also toward large fatal lesions (usually hemorrhages).

Table 33-2 summarizes the findings of the Harvard Cooperative Stroke Registry which now includes 756 successive patients, each of whom was examined by a physician knowledgeable about strokes and subjected when necessary to all appropriate laboratory aids (four-vessel arteriography, CT scan, CSF examination). For comparison, we have included an autopsy series of 179 successive cases of cerebral vascular disease, examined during the year 1949 by Fisher and Adams.

Interestingly, in both series the ratio of infarcts to hemorrhages was 4:1 and embolism accounted for approximately one-third of all strokes. The incidence of aneurysms and vascular malformations was higher at the Massachusetts General Hospital because such cases had been referred there. The initial diagnosis by the Stroke Registry group corresponded to the final diagnosis (resulting from further clinical study, neuroradiologic tests, surgery, and autopsy) in 85 percent of cases. Hypertensive hemorrhages, aneurysms, and vascular malformations were correctly diagnosed in nearly every case. The most frequent sources of error were (1) mistaking a small embolic occlusion for a lacune or vice versa, (2) confusing a thrombotic infarct for an embolic infarct or vice versa, and (3) misdiagnosing a recurrent ischemic attack as a transient embolic occlusion. An earlier problem of mistaking a small hypertensive hemorrhage for an infarct has been virtually eliminated by the CT scan.

ATHEROTHROMBOTIC INFARCTION

Most cerebrovascular disease can be attributed to atherosclerosis and hypertension; until ways are found to prevent or control them, the problems related to vascular disease of the brain will not cease to be major causes of morbidity.

Hypertension and atherosclerosis interact in a variety of ways. Atherosclerosis, by reducing the resilience of large arteries, induces systolic hypertension. Atherosclerotic stenosis of the renal arteries, by causing ischemia of the kidneys, raises the blood pressure. Hypertension in turn worsens atherosclerosis, seemingly "driving" it into the walls of small arteries. Also, it leads to a disorganization of the walls of small branch arteries (0.5 mm or less) in which all the coats of the vessel become impregnated with a kind of hyaline-lipid material, a process that Fisher has called *lipohyalinosis*. The segment so affected may weaken and allow the formation of a small dissecting aneurysm (Charcot-Bouchard aneurysm) which some neuropathologists hold responsible for the hypertensive brain hemorrhage. Lipohyalinosis also results in thrombosis of small penetrating arteries, leading to the aforementioned lacunar state.

The identity of the atheromatous process in brain arteries and that in the aorta, coronary, and other arteries cannot be questioned. In general the process in the cerebral arteries runs parallel to but is somewhat less severe than that in the aorta, heart, and lower limbs. There are many exceptions to this rule, however, and not infrequently a brain artery becomes occluded when there is not the slightest clinical evidence of coronary disease or ischemia of the legs. Although atheromatosis is known to have its onset in childhood and adolescence, only in the middle and late years of life is it likely to have clinical effects. Hypertension, hyperlipemia, and diabetes aggravate the process.

There is a tendency for atheromatous plaques to form at branchings and curves of the cerebral arteries.

Table 33-2
Major types of cerebrovascular diseases and their frequency

	Harvard stroke series* (756 successive cases)	BCH autopsy series† (179 cases)
Atherosclerotic thrombosis	244 (32%)	21 (12%)
Lacunes	129 (18%)	34 (18.5%)
Embolism	244 (32%)	57 (32%)
Hypertensive hemorrhage	84 (11%)	28 (15.5%)
Ruptured aneurysms and vascular malformations	55 (7%)	8 (4.5%)
Indeterminate		17 (9.5%)
Other‡		14 (8%)

* Compiled by J. Mohr, L. Caplan, D. Pessin, P. Kistler, and G. Duncan at Massachusetts General Hospital and Beth Israel Hospital, Boston.

† Compiled by C. M. Fisher and R. D. Adams in an examination of 780 brains during the year 1949 at Mallory Institute of Pathology, Boston City Hospital.

‡ Hypertensive encephalopathy, cerebral vein thrombosis, meningovascular syphilis, and polyarteritis nodosa.

The most frequent sites are in the internal carotid artery at the carotid sinus, in the cervical part of the vertebral arteries and at their junction to form the basilar, at the main bifurcation of the middle cerebral arteries, in the posterior cerebral arteries as they wind around the midbrain, and in the anterior cerebral arteries as they curve over the corpus callosum. It is rare for the cerebral arteries to develop plaques beyond their first major branching. Also it is rare for the cerebellar and ophthalmic arteries to show atheromatous involvement, except in conjunction with hypertension. The common carotid and vertebral arteries, at their origins from the aorta, are frequent sites of atheromatous deposits. However, because of abundant collateral arterial pathways, occlusions of brachiocephalic, common carotid, and vertebral arteries are not commonly associated with cerebral ischemia.

The atheromatous lesions develop and grow silently for 20 or 30 or more years, and only in the event of a secondary and seemingly accidental thrombotic complication do they become symptomatic. Although atheromatous plaques may narrow the lumen of an artery, causing stenosis, complete occlusion is always the consequence of thrombosis. In general, the more severe the atheromatosis the more likely the thrombotic complication, but the two phenomena do not always run in parallel. A patient with only scattered atheromatous plaques may have many thrombosed vessels, and another with marked atherosclerosis may have few or none.

Degeneration or hemorrhage into the wall of the sclerotic vessel (from rupture of vasovasorum) may damage the endothelium. Platelets and fibrin then adhere to the damaged part of the wall and form delicate, friable clots, or a subintimal atheromatous deposit may slough, spewing crystalline cholesterol emboli into the lumen and occluding small distal vessels. Presumably a thrombus does not occlude the lumen completely from the first moment; total blockage may happen only after several hours. In some instances thrombotic particles may form and break off repeatedly, thus becoming an important source of cerebral embolism. Once the lumen of the artery is completely occluded, the thrombus may propagate distally and proximally to the next branching points and block an anastomotic channel.

These several events in the atherosclerotic-thrombotic process probably account for the prodromal ischemic attacks—intermittent blockage of the circulation and variable impairment of function in the vascular territory often proceeding to permanent ischemic effects.

Not infrequently several arteries are affected by stenosis and thrombosis; then it becomes difficult to decipher the interplay of hemodynamic factors that lead to symptoms both transitory or persistent. Some of the possibilities have been outlined by one of the authors (R.D.A.) in a study of hemodynamic mechanisms in stroke. The evolution of the thrombotic process is sufficiently prolonged to explain the clinical state known as *stroke in evolution;* and when the hemodynamic disturbance stabilizes, the stage of *completed stroke* is reached. These different stages, so denominated by Fisher, acquire significance in relation to therapy and prognosis.

CLINICAL PICTURE

In general, the evolution of the clinical phenomena incident to thrombosis is more variable than that of embolism and hemorrhage. We have observed that in approximately 75 percent of cases the main part of the stroke (paralysis or other deficit) is preceded by minor signs or one or more transient attacks of focal neurologic dysfunction (Table 33-3). In a sense, these herald the oncoming vascular catastrophe. *A history of such prodromal episodes is of paramount importance in establishing the diagnosis of cerebral thrombosis.* (Only rarely and for unclear reasons are embolism and cerebral hemorrhage preceded by a transient neurologic disorder). In carotid and middle cerebral artery disease the transient warning attacks consist of monocular blindness, hemiplegia, hemianesthesia, speech disturbance, confusion, etc. In the vertebral-basilar system, the prodromata take

Table 33-3

Development of the clinical picture in 125 cases of cerebral thrombosis

Clinical development	No. of cases	Percent
Transient ischemic attacks progressing to a major or minor persistent neurologic deficit	53	42
Stepwise development of a stroke, with or without transient ischemic attacks	23	18
Stroke developing as a single event: Abrupt (hours), with or without fluctuations	14	11
Slow, gradual (a few days), with or without minor fluctuations	7	6
Transient ischemic attacks only	17	14
Development of a limited stroke followed by transient ischemic attacks	11	9

the form of episodes of dizziness, diplopia, numbness, impaired vision in one or both visual fields, and dysarthria. These will be described more fully under "transient ischemic attacks" (TIAs). Such attacks last from a few minutes to several hours; usually the duration is less than 10 min. Those of several hours' duration are usually due to embolism. The final stroke may be preceded by one or two attacks or a hundred or more, and it may follow the onset of the attacks by hours, weeks, or months. When there are no prodromal ischemic attacks, one must use other criteria in diagnosing the cerebrovascular process as one of thrombosis.

The main part of the thrombotic stroke, whether or not preceded by warning attacks, develops in one of several ways. Most often there is a single attack, and the whole illness evolves within a few hours. More telling diagnostically is a "stuttering," intermittent progression of neurologic deficits extending over several hours or days. Again, a partial stroke may occur, even with temporary improvement for several hours, after which there is rapid progression to the completed stroke. Several fleeting episodes may be followed by a longer one and a day or two later by a major stroke. Several parts of the body may be involved at once, or only one part, such as a limb or one side of the face, the other parts becoming involved serially in steplike fashion until the stroke is fully developed. All these various modes of development indicate cerebral thrombosis, and their temporal dispersion reflects *thrombosis in evolution*. It might be commented that each of the transient attacks and the abrupt episodes of progression reproduce the temporal profile of the stroke in miniature. The principle of intermittency seems to characterize the thrombotic process from beginning to end.

Even more frequent than the modes of onset outlined above is the occurrence of the thrombotic stroke during sleep; the patient awakens paralyzed during the night or in the morning. Unaware of any difficulty, he or she may arise and fall helplessly to the floor with the first step. This is the story in fully 60 percent of our patients with thrombotic strokes and in a certain number with embolic ones as well. Most deceptive of all are the cases in which the neurologic disorder has evolved over 1 to 2 weeks in a slow, gradual fashion. One's first impulse is to make a diagnosis of brain tumor, abscess, or subdural hematoma. Some cases of this type have even come to surgery only to disclose infarct necrosis of the brain. This error can usually be avoided by analyzing minutely the course of the illness, which will disclose an uneven, saltatory progression; and if the clinical data are incomplete, observation for a few days or weeks will reveal the stroke profile more clearly. Actually there are very

few cases—and these are usually instances of pure motor hemiplegia—in which the evolution of a thrombotic stroke was truly gradual over a period of days or weeks.

Arterial thrombosis is not usually accompanied by headache, but the latter does occur in some cases. Usually the pain is located on one side of the head in carotid occlusion, at the back of the head or simultaneously in forehead and occiput in basilar occlusion, and behind the ipsilateral ear in vertebral occlusion. The headache is not as violent as in intracerebral or subarachnoid hemorrhage, and there is no stiffness of the neck. The mechanism is unclear. Presumably it is related to the disease process within the vessel since it may antedate the other manifestations of the stroke.

Hypertension is more often present than not in patients with atherothrombotic infarction. Diabetes mellitus is common also. Often there is evidence of vascular disease in other parts of the body: a history of coronary occlusion or angina pectoris, an ECG abnormality, intermittent claudication, or an absence of one or several pulses in the lower limbs. The retinal arteries may show uniform or focal narrowing, increase and irregularity of the light reflex, and arteriovenous "nicking," but these findings are to be correlated with hypertension rather than atherosclerosis. The same is true of hemorrhages and exudates. The patient is more often elderly, but may be in the fourth decade or younger when stricken.

LABORATORY FINDINGS

The CSF pressure is normal in patients with atherothrombotic infarction unless the infarct is massive and the damaged tissue swells. Then it may, exceptionally, lead to high pressure and fatal temporal lobe–tentorial or cerebellar–foramen magnum herniation. Cerebral thrombosis never causes blood to enter the CSF. Frequently the CSF protein is elevated (usually 50 to 100 mg per 100 ml). Rarely is the total protein in excess of 100 mg per 100 ml; when it is, a faint xanthochromia (1 to 2 on a scale of 10) may be perceived and some other diagnosis must be considered. A small number of polymorphonuclear leukocytes (3 to 8 per cubic millimeter) is common in the first few days. Rarely, and for unexplained reasons, a brisk, transient pleocytosis (400 to 2000 polymorphonuclear leukocytes per cubic millimeter) occurs on about the third day. A persistent pleocytosis, however, suggests a chronic meningitis (syphilis, tuberculosis, cryptococcosis), granulomatous arteritis, septic embolism, thrombophlebitis, or a nonvascular process. Occasionally, the serological test for syphilis may be helpful. Meningovascular syphilis occurring during the first few years of a syphilitic infection is an uncommon but well-recognized entity. Always there are increased protein, pleocytosis, and a positive VDLR or other serologic test in both blood and CSF (see page 496). If the CSF is bloody, a positive test for neurosyphilis is not valid since the syphilitic reagin may have been carried into the spinal fluid by the contaminated blood. Skull films are not informative, as a rule, and the calcified pineal gland will not be shifted unless severe cerebral swelling has occurred. Then the patient is usually stuporous or comatose.

Serum cholesterol or triglycerides, or both, are elevated in some cases, but normal values are not helpful. The EEG is only of limited value in indicating infarction or distinguishing it from hemorrhage. In extensive cerebral infarction the brain waves in overlying leads may be of slightly lower frequency and lower voltage than normal. High-voltage slow waves (3 to 5 per second) favor hemorrhage. Arteriography is the definitive diagnostic procedure for the demonstration of arterial thrombosis or stenosis and also provides information about collateral flow. Injection of radiopaque fluid into the major cervicocerebral arteries via a catheter introduced into the femoral artery is preferred to direct puncture of the common carotid artery. Arteriography carries a slight risk, and in patients with vessels narrowed by atherosclerosis the infarction may be extended. It should be used, therefore, when the diagnosis of vascular disease is uncertain, when surgery is possible, or when anticoagulant therapy is being contemplated in an indefinite case. Radionuclide scans and positron emission techniques often show the infarct before it becomes visible in CT scans. Scintillation counting over the two sides of the skull after the intravenous injection of radioactive material may provide a comparative index of circulation in the two carotid systems. CT scanning usually shows the necrotic tissue within a few days and later demonstrates cavitation (Figs. 33-17 and 33-18). Lacunar infarcts are usually too small to be seen.

COURSE AND PROGNOSIS

When the patient is seen early in the course of cerebral thrombosis, it is difficult to give an accurate prognosis. One must ask where the patient stands in the stroke pro-

Figure 33-17
Ischemic infarction of the midbrain due to basilar artery occlusion. Unenhanced CT scan, 72 h after onset, shows a large area of decreased attenuation (necrotic tissue) sparing only the colliculi.

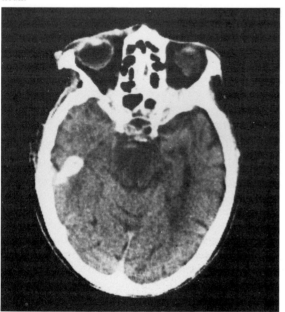

Figure 33-18
Large hemispheric ischemic infarct with prominent gyral enhancement ("luxury perfusion") 2 weeks after stroke.

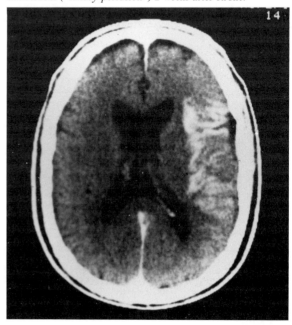

cess at the time of the examination. Is worsening to be anticipated or not? No rules have yet been formulated which allow one to predict the course with confidence. A mild paralysis today may become a disastrous hemiplegia tomorrow, or the patient's condition may only worsen temporarily for a day or two. In basilar artery occlusion, dizziness and dysphagia may progress in a few days to total paralysis and deep coma. The course of cerebral thrombosis is so often progressive that a cautious attitude on the part of the physician is justified in what appears to be a mild case.

As indicated above, progression of the stroke is most often due to increasing stenosis of the involved artery by mural thrombus. In some instances, extension of the thrombus along the vessel may block side branches and hinder anastomotic flow. In the basilar artery, thrombus may gradually build up along its entire length. In the carotid system, thrombus at times propagates distally from the site of origin in the neck to the supraclinoid portion, and possibly into the anterior cerebral artery, preventing collateral flow from the opposite side. In middle cerebral occlusion, retrograde thrombosis may extend back to the mouth of the anterior cerebral, perhaps secondarily infarcting the territory of that vessel. Embolic particles from the site of an incompletely thrombosed artery may precipitate an abrupt change.

Several other circumstances influence the *immediate prognosis* in cerebral thrombosis. In the case of large infarcts, swelling of the infarcted tissue may occur, followed by tentorial herniation and death of the patient in 2 to 4 days. Even smaller infarcts of the inferior surface of the cerebellum may cause fatal herniation into the foramen magnum. Milder degrees of swelling and increased intracranial pressure, though causing an apparent progression for 2 to 3 days, do not prove fatal. In extensive basilar infarction associated with deep coma, the patient seldom lives for more than a few days. If coma or stupor is present from the beginning, survival is largely determined by the success in keeping the airway clear, preventing aspiration pneumonia, and in maintaining fluid and electrolyte balance. Respiratory and urinary infections are constant dangers, and once they begin, there is usually a rapid decline in the patient's condition as body temperature rises.

As for the *eventual or long-term prognosis* of the neurologic deficit, there are many possibilities. Improvement is the rule if the patient survives. The patient with a lacunar infarct and pure motor hemiparesis fares well. Recovery from small infarcts may start within hours or a day or two, and restoration may be complete within a week. In cases of severe deficit there may be no significant recovery whatsoever, and after months of assiduous effort at rehabilitation, the patient may remain bereft of speech and understanding, with the upper extremity still useless and the lower extremity serving only as an uncertain prop in attempting to walk. Between these two extremes there is every gradation of recovery. The longer the delay before recovery begins, the poorer the prognosis becomes. If recovery does not begin in 1 or 2 weeks, the outlook is gloomy both for motor activity and speech. Constructional apraxia, uninhibited anger (with left temporal lesions), nonsensical logorrhea and placidity, unawareness of the paralysis and neglect (with nondominant lesions), all tend to diminish and may disappear within a few weeks. A hemianopia which has not cleared in a few weeks will usually be permanent, although reading and color discrimination may continue to improve. In lateral medullary infarction, difficulty in swallowing may be protracted, lasting 4 to 8 weeks or longer; yet relatively normal function is nearly always restored finally. Aphasia, dysarthria, cerebellar ataxia, and walking may improve for a year or longer, but for all practical purposes it may be said that whatever motor paralysis remains after 5 to 6 months will probably be permanent.

Characteristically, the paralyzed muscles are flaccid in the first days or weeks following a stroke, and the tendon reflexes may be unchanged, slightly increased, or decreased. Gradually spasticity develops, and the tendon reflexes become brisker. The arm tends to assume a flexed adducted posture, whereas the leg is usually extended. Function is rarely if ever restored after the slow evolution of spasticity. Conversely, the early development of spasticity in the arm, or the appearance of a grasp reflex may presage a favorable outcome. In some patients with extensive temporoparietal lesions the hemiplegia remains flaccid; the arm dangles and the slack leg must be braced to stand. If the internal capsule is not interrupted completely in a stroke that involves the lenticular nucleus or thalamus, the paralysis may give way to hemichoreoathetosis, hemitremor, or hemiataxia, depending upon the particular anatomy of the lesion. Bowel and bladder control usually returns, and sphincteric disorders persist only in a few cases. Often the hemiplegic limbs are at first tender and ache on manipulation. Nevertheless, physiotherapy should be initiated early in order to prevent pseudocontracture of muscles and periarthritis at shoulder, elbow, wrist, knuckles, knee, and ankle—frequent complications and often the source of pain and added disability, particularly in relation to the shoulder. A characteristic atrophy of bone and pain in the hand may accompany the shoulder pain (shoulder-hand syndrome). An annoying feeling of dizziness and unsteadiness often persists after damage to the vestibular system in brainstem infarcts.

Recurrent convulsive (epileptic) seizures are an uncommon sequela of thrombotic strokes. This is in contrast to embolic cortical infarcts, which are followed by recurrent focal or generalized seizures in more than 20 percent of patients.

Many patients complain of fatigability and are depressed. The explanation of these symptoms is uncertain; some are expressions of a reactive depression. Only a few patients become serious *behavior problems* or are psychotic after a stroke, but paranoid trends, ill temper, stubbornness, and peevishness are common.

Finally, in regard to prognosis, it must be mentioned that having had one thrombotic stroke, the patient is at risk in the ensuing months and years of having a stroke at the same or another site, especially if there is hypertension or diabetes mellitus. Myocardial infarction is also frequent; it is more often the cause of death than is another stroke.

TRANSIENT ISCHEMIC ATTACKS OF CEREBRAL ORIGIN

It has already been pointed out that when transient ischemic attacks (TIAs) precede a stroke, they almost always stamp the process as thrombotic. Furthermore, neuropathologic studies inform us that these attacks are linked almost exclusively to atherosclerotic thrombosis. There would seem to be little doubt that these attacks are due to transient focal ischemia, and they might be referred to as temporary strokes which fortunately reverse themselves. They belong, therefore, under the heading of atherosclerotic thrombotic disease, but are discussed separately here because of their clinical importance. Corresponding to the higher incidence of atherosclerosis in persons with hypertension and in the entire male population, about two-thirds of all patients with TIAs are men or hypertensive, or both.

CLINICAL PICTURE

TIAs can reflect the involvement of virtually any cerebral or cerebellar artery, deep or superficial: a common carotid, internal carotid, middle cerebral, anterior cerebral, ophthalmic, vertebral, basilar, posterior cerebral, the cerebellar arteries, and the penetrating branches to the basal ganglia and brainstem. If the posterior cerebral arteries are included in the vertebral-basilar system, ischemic episodes are slightly more common in that system than in the carotid. TIAs may precede, accompany, or follow the development of a stroke, or they can occur by themselves without leading to a stroke, a fact which makes any form of therapy difficult to evaluate.

TIAs may last a few seconds up to 12 to 24 h; most of them last 2 to 15 min, and an attack of more than 30 min is uncommon. There may be only a few attacks or several hundred. Between attacks, the neurologic examination may disclose no abnormalities. A stroke may occur after the first or second episode or only after hundreds of attacks have occurred over a period of weeks or months. Not infrequently the attacks gradually cease and no important paralysis occurs. So far it has not been possible to distinguish the cases in which a stroke will not develop from those in which it will, except in a general way. About 20 percent of infarcts that follow TIAs occur within a month after the first attack, and about 50 percent within a year (Whisnant et al., 1973).

The neurologic features of the transient episode indicate the territory or artery involved and are fragments borrowed from the stroke which may be approaching. In the *carotid system*, attacks reflect involvment of cerebral hemisphere and eye. The visual disturbance is ipsilateral; the sensorimotor disturbance is contralateral. Individual attacks tend to involve either the eye or the brain. Usually the initial attacks are ocular and the later ones are hemispheric. It is almost unknown for the eye and the brain to be involved simultaneously. In the hemispheric attacks, ischemia occurs foremost in the distal territory of the middle cerebral artery and adjacent border zone, producing weakness or numbness of the opposite hand and arm. However, many different combinations may be seen: face and lips, or lips and fingers, fingers alone, hand and foot, etc. Less common manifestations include headache, confusion, aphasia and difficulty in calculation (when the dominant hemisphere is involved), and other temporoparietal disturbances. In ocular attacks, transient monocular blindness is the usual symptom. Many of the latter episodes evolve swiftly and are described as a shade falling smoothly over the visual field until the eye is completely but painlessly blind. The attack clears slowly and uniformly. Uncommonly, it may take the form of a wedge of visual loss; sudden generalized blurring; or rarely, a bright light. Transient attacks of monocular blindness are usually more stereotyped than hemispheric attacks.

The clinical picture of transient attacks in the vertebral-basilar system is diverse, since such varied motor-sensory traffic in the brainstem and thalamus is sustained by the blood carried in these vessels. Dizziness, diplopia (vertical or horizontal), dysarthria, bifacial numbness, and weakness or numbness of part or all of one or both sides of the body (i.e., a disturbance of the long motor or sensory tracts bilaterally) are the hallmarks of vertebral-basilar involvement. Transient vertigo or diplopia (or headache) as solitary symptoms should not be interpreted as a TIA. Also, some patients with dizziness will prove to have carotid TIAs; hence this symptom is not a reliable indicator of the vascular circuit which is involved, according to Ueda et al. Other manifestations, in their approximate order of frequency, include headache, staggering, veering to one side, a feeling of cross-eyedness, dark vision, blurred vision, tunnel vision, partial or complete blindness, pupillary change, ptosis, paralysis of gaze, speechlessness, and dysphagia. Less common symptoms include noise or pounding in the ear or in the head, pain in the head or face, peculiar head sensations, vomiting, hiccups, memory lapse, confused behavior, drowsiness, transient unconsciousness (rare), impaired hearing, deafness, a feeling of movement of a part, hemiballismus, peduncular hallucinosis, and forced deviation of the eyes.

The attacks may be identical or they may vary in detail, although maintaining the same basic pattern. For example, weakness or numbness may involve fingers and face in some episodes, and fingers only in others; or dizziness alone may occur in some attacks, while in others diplopia is added to the picture. In basilar artery disease each side of the body may be affected alternately. All the involved parts may be affected simultaneously, or a march or spread from one region to another can occur in a period of 10 to 60 s, but more often in a few minutes, much slower than in a seizure. The individual attack may cease abruptly or fade gradually.

MECHANISM

Ophthalmoscopic observations of the retinal vessels made during episodes of transient monocular blindness show either arrest of the blood flow in the retinal arteries and breaking up of the venous columns to form a "box-car" pattern, or white material temporarily blocking the retinal arteries. This indicates that in ischemic attacks a temporary, complete or relatively complete cessation of blood flow occurs locally, possibly associated with microembolism. TIAs have been attributed to cerebral vasospasm or to transient episodes of systemic arterial hypotension with resulting compromise of the intracranial circulation, but neither of these mechanisms has been established. Although dropping the blood pressure to 80 mmHg or less by tilting the patient upright may cause EEG changes, it has not in the authors' experience

reproduced the attacks. Vasodilator drugs have been without effect. There is good evidence that the attacks can be abolished by anticoagulant drugs, but the mechanism of this effect is not known. Whatever the exact cause of TIAs, they are intimately related to vascular stenosis due to atherosclerosis and thrombosis in the majority of cases.

The onset of attacks in a small proportion of patients has been clearly related to standing up after lying or sitting. In the majority of cases, attacks bear no relation to position or activity, although in general they are likely to occur when the patient is up and around rather than lying down. They have been encountered in relation to exercise, outbursts of anger or joy, and during bouts of coughing. Transient symptoms present on awakening from sleep usually indicate that a stroke is in the offing.

Platelet emboli to the brain from sites of atherosclerosis is frequently suggested as an explanation of TIAs. This may indeed be the cause of attacks in many cases but it is difficult to understand, in attacks of identical pattern, how successive emboli from a distance would enter the same arterial branch each time. Moreover, one would expect the involved cerebral tissue to be at least partially damaged, leaving some residual signs. When only a single transient episode has occurred, the factor of recurrence does not assist in the diagnosis, and cerebral embolism must then be strongly considered. In some cases of documented embolism, the deficit fluctuates from normal to abnormal repeatedly for as long as 36 h, giving the appearance of TIAs; in others, a deficit of several hours' duration occurs, fulfilling the traditional criterion of TIAs. These cases should be considered as symptomatically short-lived strokes when the ipsilateral carotid artery territory is found normal arteriographically. A single transitory episode, especially if it lasts longer than 1 h, and *multiple episodes of different pattern* suggest embolism and must be clearly distinguished from brief (2 to 15 min) *recurrent attacks of the same pattern*, which suggest atherosclerosis and thrombosis. Recurrent seizures and attacks of syncope and vertigo must also be clearly distinguished from TIAs, using the criteria outlined in Chaps. 15, 17, and 14, respectively.

The routine of four-vessel arteriography has shed some light on the problem. Almost a fifth of the 95 patients with "carotid TIAs" in the Massachusetts General Hospital series (Pessin et al.), and a somewhat larger proportion of the Winston-Salem series (Ueda et al.) had open carotid arteries with neither stenosis nor ulceration. In most of the cases with arteriographically normal carotids the ischemic attacks exceeded 1 h in duration, suggesting embolism from the heart or great vessels; but there was also a small number of brief ischemic attacks that were unexplained by arteriography. Of course a small atheromatous ulceration may not be seen in the arteriogram. The majority of those with bruits had stenoses with more than 50 percent reduction in the lumen.

TREATMENT OF ATHEROTHROMBOTIC INFARCTION AND TRANSIENT ISCHEMIC ATTACKS

The treatment of atherothrombotic disease may be divided into four parts: (1) management in the acute phase, (2) measures to restore the circulation and arrest the pathologic process, (3) physical therapy and rehabilitation, and (4) measures to prevent further strokes and progression of vascular disease.

MANAGEMENT IN THE ACUTE PHASE

Rarely is the patient who has had a stroke seen within a few minutes of onset. This may happen when a patient is in the hospital for another reason. If the common or internal carotid artery is thrombosed, immediate surgical removal of the clot or the performance of a bypass procedure may restore function. We have had a small number of such cases who have recovered completely within hours. Usually several hours have elapsed before the diagnosis is established. If the interval is longer than 12 h, opening the occluded vessel is of little value.

If the patient is stuporous or comatose, care follows along the lines indicated in Chap. 16.

MEASURES TO RESTORE THE CIRCULATION AND ARREST THE PATHOLOGIC PROCESS

Once a thrombotic stroke has developed fully, no therapy so far devised is of any value in restoring the damaged cerebral tissue or its function. *To be effective, therapy must be preventive.* The diagnosis of thrombosis must be made at the earliest possible stage, and the full catastrophe circumvented by all means presently available. These measures will be instituted at various stages of the process, when only transient ischemic attacks are occurring, or at any point in the progression of a throm-

bosis-in-evolution, or when almost the full neurologic deficit has appeared. Even when persistent signs and symptoms have appeared, it is conceivable that some of the tissue affected, particularly at the edges of the infarct, has not been irreversibly damaged and will survive if blood flow can be increased.

The following therapeutic methods are being used at present or have been tried in the recent past.

Medical Therapy On the assumption that decrease in the cerebral circulation resulting from the upright position can aggravate cerebral ischemia, patients with a major stroke as the result of ischemic infarction should remain horizontal in bed for the first few days. When walking begins, special attention should be given to maintenance of the systemic circulation (avoid standing quietly for prolonged periods, sit with the feet up, etc.). The treatment of previously unappreciated hypertension is preferably deferred until later, when the neurologic deficit has stabilized. Elevating the foot of the bed in the acute stage may be beneficial. It is of great importance that the blood pressure be maintained [correction of blood loss, use of metaraminol bitartrate (Aramine) or levarterenol bitartrate (Levophed) in myocardial infarction with vascular collapse, avoidance of autonomic blocking agents, etc.]. Injections of epinephrine have been recommended as a means of raising the systemic blood pressure above the usual levels. Although this enhances cerebral blood flow and might be beneficial, a systematic trial in thrombotic cases has not been undertaken. One would fear that it might cause hemorrhage into the infarcted tissue. Anemia must be corrected. Polycythemia, if severe, may slow the circulation locally and must be treated.

Anticoagulant Drugs These may prevent transient ischemic attacks and an impending stroke. Anticoagulants also may halt the advance of a progressive thrombotic stroke, but not in all cases. In deciding whether or not to use anticoagulants, one faces the question of where in the course of the stroke the patient stands when first examined. Will the course be benign or disastrous? As was stated above, there are no reliable rules for predicting this at the present time. Anticoagulants are not of value in the fully developed stroke, whether this be in the patient with a lacunar infarct or in the patient with a devastating hemiplegia, aphasia, etc. Whether anticoagulants prevent the recurrence of a thrombotic stroke when given for a prolonged period is a question that has never been answered satisfactorily, and the incidence of complicating hemorrhage limits the value of anticoagulants in these cases.

The use of anticoagulant drugs makes an accurate clinical diagnosis imperative. Intracranial hemorrhage must be ruled out by CT scan, or if this technique is not available, by examination of the CSF; it must be remembered, however, that a clear fluid does not necessarily exclude hemorrhage (see "Laboratory Findings," above). Estimation of prothrombin activity and coagulation time are desirable before therapy is started, but if this is not feasible, the initial doses of anticoagulant drugs can usually be given safely if there is no evidence of active bleeding anywhere in the body. Severe hypertension is not necessarily a contraindication to anticoagulant therapy. There is no reliable evidence that complications are more frequent in the presence of hypertension if the prothrombin activity is maintained at 25 percent of normal or higher, and therefore the authors have not withheld anticoagulant therapy in these patients; however, when the blood pressure is greater than 220/120 mmHg, an attempt is made at the same time to lower the pressure gradually with hypotensive agents, exercising care not to prejudice further the circulation in the region of the infarct by too great a reduction in the systemic pressure. As has been stated, it is preferable to avoid reduction of the blood pressure in the 2-week period immediately following a thrombotic stroke. Other contraindications to anticoagulant therapy are bleeding peptic ulcer, uremia, hepatic failure, and the prospect of poor compliance by the patient.

When anticoagulant therapy is instituted in the prodromal or early phase of a stroke, heparin is administered intravenously in a dose of approximately 50 mg every 4 h, or by continuous drip in patients with a progressing stroke or with transient ischemic attacks occurring more than once in 2 days. Heparin therapy is maintained for one to 2 weeks while warfarin (Coumadin) therapy is being instituted, and the latter may be continued for many months (see below). Coumadin can be used alone from the beginning when transient ischemic attacks occur less than once every few days.

Coumadin therapy is relatively safe provided the prothrombin activity is maintained at 15 to 17 s (normal 12 s), and the level is determined regularly (once a day, for the first 10 days, then three times a week, and finally once every 1 or 2 weeks). Therapy can be prolonged for months and years, but the tendency now is not to give Coumadin for indefinite lengths of time. There are data to suggest that the greatest usefulness of Coumadin is in the first 2 to 4 months following the onset of the ischemic attack(s); after that the risk of intracranial hemorrhage increases greatly and the benefits of anticoagulant therapy are less clear (Sandok et al.). Coumadin overdosage may cause hemorrhage into the brain or subdural space or into the kidney, nose, bowel, skin, or mus-

cle; fresh plasma and vitamin K_1 should be administered immediately.

Antiplatelet Drugs Several other drugs which prevent clotting by reducing platelet adhesiveness are under study and show promise of preventing thrombotic and embolic strokes. Aspirin (600 mg twice daily) can be substituted for Coumadin. Dipyridamole (Persantine) in doses of 50 mg every 8 h and sulfinpyrazone (Anturane), in doses of 200 mg every 8 h, may also prove to be useful. Aspirin inhibits platelet aggregation and reduces thromboxane (A_2), a vasoconstricting prostaglandin, and also prostacyclin, a vasodilating prostaglandin. Dipyridamole acts by inhibiting platelet phosphodiesterase so that cyclic AMP is not catabolized, and sulfinpyrazole is believed to inhibit the "platelet release reaction," interfering with platelet adherence to endothelial cells.

Aspirin and sulfinpyrazone have been evaluated by the Canadian Cooperative Study Group in 585 patients with threatened stroke, followed for an average period of 26 months. All the patients had had at least one cerebral or retinal ischemic attack in the previous 3 months. The cases were randomized and the trials were double-blind. Aspirin reduced the risk of recurrent ischemic attacks, stroke or death by 19 percent and the risk of stroke or death by 31 percent, but this latter effect was sex-dependent: in men the risk of stroke or death was reduced 48 percent, whereas no significant trend was observed among women. Sulfinpyrazone did not reduce ischemic attacks and diminished the risk of strokes or death by only 10 percent. Because of the small sample size of this trial and other considerations, several epidemiologists (Lilienfeld, Kurtzke) have not accepted the major conclusions of the Canadian study and believe that the therapeutic efficacy of aspirin remains to be proved.

Surgery Arterial stenosis or an ulcerating plaque in the neck and thorax in patients with recurrent ischemic attacks is frequently amenable to surgical management, employing thromboendarterectomy or bypass grafts. Most often it is the carotid sinus region that lends itself to such therapy. Other sites suitable for surgical management include the common carotid, innominate, and subclavian arteries. Operation on the vertebral artery at its origin has not proved beneficial.

Before operation the existence of the lesion and its extent must be determined by arteriography, a procedure that carries a risk of worsening the stroke or producing focal signs (see below). If the patient is in good medical condition, has normal vessels on the contralateral side, and normal cardiac function, these lesions can usually be dealt with safely by endarterectomy. The overall morbidity and mortality should not exceed 3 percent. When a thrombus in the internal carotid artery extends to the siphon, the surgical approach depends on some form of bypass grafting (transcranially—external carotid to middle cerebral). The latter procedure as well as temporal-middle cerebral and other extracranial-intracranial arterial anastomoses are technically feasible and currently under active study. Surgery may also be done early in the course of thrombosis-in-evolution, as remarked above. When total infarction has occurred, surgery will be ineffective even though patency of the vessel is restored.

Concerning the relative value of anticoagulants and surgery in the treatment of patients with TIAs, there is still a wide divergence of opinion. In fact, currently available data have not completely settled the question as to whether any specific treatment is worthwhile. Toole and his colleagues have reported on 225 patients observed for periods of 3 to 14 years (average 5.5 years). Of those patients, 82 had died, 21 of cerebral infarction, 52 of heart disease, and 9 of other causes. Of 56 untreated patients, 11 (19 percent) had had cerebral infarctions of which 4 were fatal; of the 45 patients treated medically, 10 (24 percent) had had cerebral infarctions of which 3 were fatal; of 124 patients treated surgically, 27 (21 percent) had postoperative cerebral infarctions of which 7 were fatal. About the same number of patients in the medical and surgical groups continued to have TIAs.

Whisnant and his colleagues followed 199 patients with TIAs, some of whom were untreated and the rest treated with anticoagulants. The survival rate in the two groups was approximately the same, which is not surprising, since the primary cause of death in all patients with TIAs is myocardial infarction. The group receiving anticoagulants had fewer strokes than the untreated group but the difference was small and not significant statistically. Among patients with vertebral-basilar TIAs, those treated with anticoagulants had definitely fewer strokes, starting at 3 months after the onset of attacks. However, the risk of intracranial hemorrhage was at least four times greater in the anticoagulant-treated group.

Surgical therapy, as has been indicated, is applicable only to the group of carotid artery cases with ex-

tracranial stenosis and ulcerated plaques. This group constitutes less than 20 percent of all patients with TIAs (Marshall). Despite the data quoted above, the authors have the distinct impression that well-executed surgery in appropriately chosen cases stops the TIAs, and that the prognosis is better than if no treatment is given. We continue to use anticoagulants in nonsurgical carotid and all vertebrobasilar cases.

Some of the problems in the management of patients with TIAs are discussed further in the final section of this chapter (page 590).

Therapy for Cerebral Edema   In the first few days following major cerebral infarction, cerebral edema may threaten life. In such instances, dexamethasone in intramuscular doses of 4 to 6 mg every 4 to 6 h may be useful. Mannitol, 50 g intravenously in acute situations, and glycerol in oral doses of 30 ml every 4 to 6 h or daily intravenous doses of 50 g dissolved in 500 ml 2.5 saline solution are other available forms of therapy. Apart from their effects on edema, the value of these agents in improving the neurologic deficit remains questionable.

Cerebral Vasodilators and Thrombolytic Agents   Despite experimental evidence that some of these vasodilators increase cerebral blood flow, as measured by the nitrous oxide method, none of them has proved beneficial in carefully studied human stroke cases at the stage of transient ischemic attacks or thrombosis-in-evolution, or in the established stroke. Vasodilators may be harmful rather than beneficial, at least on theoretical grounds, since by lowering the systemic blood pressure or by dilating vessels to normal brain tissue they reduce the intracranial anastomotic flow. The thrombolytic agents, fibrinolysin and profibrinolysin activator, have also not proved helpful in cases of transient ischemia, thrombosis-in-evolution, and established stroke.

PHYSICAL THERAPY AND REHABILITATION

Beginning within a few days, the paralyzed limbs should at intervals be carried through a full range of passive movement, to a total of 50 times a day. The purpose is to avoid contracture (and periarthritis), especially at the shoulder, elbow, and ankle. Soreness and aching in the paralyzed limbs should not be allowed to interfere with exercises. Most patients can be moved from bed to chair after a week or so, depending on the severity of the illness. Nearly all hemiplegics regain the ability to walk to some extent, usually within a 3- to 6-month period, and this should be a primary aim in rehabilitation. The presence of deep sensory loss, in addition to hemiplegia, is the main limiting factor. A short or long leg brace is often required. Speech therapy is not of proven value but should be tried; at least it improves the morale of the patient. Physical therapy seems not to benefit patients with cerebellar ataxia. As motor function improves, and if mentality is preserved, instruction in the activities of daily living, using various special devices, can assist the patient in becoming at least partly independent in the home.

PREVENTIVE MEASURES

As has already been indicated, the primary objective in the treatment of atherothrombotic disease is prevention. Efforts to find patients at risk depend on clinical and laboratory methods, the latter to screen large populations for hypertension, diabetes, hyperlipidemia, and coronary artery disease in the period of life when strokes are frequent. The carotid vessels, being readily accessible, need always to be studied for the presence of a bruit; the latter quite reliably indicates a stenosis though not all stenoses cause a bruit. However, there is still uncertainty as to how to proceed in patients with asymptomatic bruits. In several current publications it is recommended that such patients be subjected to ocular plethysmography, Doppler analysis and ultrasound study of the carotid artery, and carotid angiography, and that endarterectomy be performed if stenosis is found (see Thompson et al. for review). Our practice has been different; we follow such patients closely and await the first symptom or sign of neurologic disorder before proceeding to invasive studies or surgery. The recent population study by Heyman et al. has shed some light on this problem. These authors found that cervical bruits in men were a risk for death from ischemic heart disease. They also found that the presence of asymptomatic bruits in men (but not in women) does indeed carry an increased risk of stroke but, more importantly, that the subsequent stroke often fails to correlate in its angioanatomic locus and laterality with the cervical bruit. They concluded that asymptomatic cervical bruits do not in themselves justify invasive diagnostic procedures or surgical correction of underlying extracranial arterial lesions.

For patients who have had a stroke and are functional, preventive measures consist of avoiding situations in which strokes are likely to occur: (1) particular care should be taken to maintain the systemic blood pressure, oxygenation, and intracranial blood flow during surgical procedures, especially in elderly patients; (2) hypotensive agents, whether given therapeutically or for diagnostic procedures, should be administered with caution; (3) in the elderly patient, in whom deep sleep might contribute to a state of cerebral ischemia, oversedation should be avoided; (4) systemic hypotension, severe ane-

mia, and polycythemia should be treated promptly; and (5) rapid diuresis may be contraindicated.

The ultimate solution of the problem of cerebrovascular disease lies in more fundamental fields, namely the prevention or alleviation of hypertension and atherosclerosis.

EMBOLIC INFARCTION

In most cases of cerebral embolism, the embolic material consists of a fragment which has broken away from a thrombus within the heart. Less frequently the source is intraarterial, from an atheromatous plaque that has damaged the endothelium or ulcerated into the lumen of the carotid sinus, or from the distal (intracranial) end of a thrombus in the internal carotid artery. Embolism due to fat, tumor cells, or air is a rare occurrence and seldom enters into the differential diagnosis of stroke. The embolus usually becomes arrested at a bifurcation or other site of narrowing of the lumen, and ischemic infarction follows. The infarction is pale, hemorrhagic, or mixed; hemorrhagic infarction, as pointed out earlier, nearly always indicates embolism. Any region of the brain may be affected, but the territory of the middle cerebral artery is most frequently involved, especially the upper division. The two hemispheres are approximately equally affected. Large embolic masses will block large vessels (sometimes the carotids in the neck), while tiny fragments may reach vessels as small as 0.2 mm in diameter, in which case the stroke may clear in a few days and the infarct be so small as to almost escape detection at autopsy. Often, embolic material remains arrested and plugs the lumen solidly, but in many cases it breaks up into fragments which enter smaller vessels and disappear completely, so that careful pathologic examination fails to reveal their final location. The anatomic diagnosis must then be made by inference, e.g., absence of a vascular occlusion at the proper site to explain the infarct, absence of atherosclerosis or other cause of occlusion in the cerebral vessel, presence of a source of emboli and infarcts in other organs such as kidneys and spleen, the occurrence of hemorrhagic infarction, and finally, the clinical history.

Because of the rapidity with which occlusion develops in embolism, there is not much time for collateral influx to become established. Thus, sparing of territory distal to the site of occlusion is not as evident as in thrombosis. However, the *ischemia-modifying factors* mentioned under "The Ischemic Stroke" (see above) are still operative and will influence the size and severity of the infarct.

Brain embolism is essentially a manifestation of heart disease. The commonest cause is *chronic atrial fibrillation* due to atherosclerotic or rheumatic heart disease, the source of the embolus being a mural thrombus within the atrial appendage. Atrial fibrillation due to other types of heart disease (e.g., hypertensive or syphilitic) can, of course, act in the same way. Embolism occurs also during paroxysmal atrial fibrillation or flutter. Patients with atrial fibrillation are five times more liable to stroke than an age-matched population with normal cardiac rhythm. *Mural thrombus* deposited on the damaged endocardium overlying a myocardial infarct is an important source of cerebral emboli, as is a thrombus associated with severe mitral stenosis without atrial fibrillation. *Cardiac catheterization or surgery*, especially valvuloplasty, may disseminate fragments of thrombus or a calcified valve. *Mitral and aortic valve prostheses* are presently associated with embolism in 70 percent of cases. *Paradoxic embolism* can occur when an abnormal communication exists between the right and left sides of the heart, or when both ventricles communicate with the aorta; thus embolic material arising in the veins of the lower extremity or anywhere in the systemic venous tree can bypass the pulmonary circulation and reach the cerebral vessels. Pulmonary hypertension (often from previous pulmonary embolism) favors the occurrence of paradoxic embolism. Subendocardial fibroelastosis, idiopathic myocardial hypertrophy, cardiac myxomas, and cardiac lesions in trichinosis are rare causes of embolism.

The *vegetations of acute and subacute bacterial endocarditis* give rise to several different pathologic pictures in the brain (see page 487). Mycotic aneurysm is a rare complication of septic embolism and may be a source of intracerebral or subarachnoid hemorrhage. *Marantic* or *nonbacterial endocarditis* occasionally causes cerebral embolism and at times produces a baffling clinical picture, especially when associated, as it often is, with carcinomatosis.

The following sources of embolic material are more difficult to prove or are less frequent: (1) Mural thrombus, deposited upon ulcerated atheroma in the arch of the aorta or in the carotid arteries, may break loose and find its way into brain arteries. Massage of the carotid sinus, a favorite site for atherosclerosis, may dislodge mural thrombus, with the production of a hemi-

plegia. This is why carotid massage should not be done in the elderly and only with caution in others. (2) Atheromatous material may be washed out of a large plaque in the aorta or carotid arteries (possibly during arteriography) and carried distally into the branches of the cerebral tree. (3) A prolapsed mitral valve may be a source of emboli, especially in young patients. In a group of 60 patients who had transient ischemic attacks or partial stroke and were under 45 years of age, a prolapsed mitral valve was detected (by echocardiography and a characteristic midsystolic click) in 24 patients, but in only 5 of 60 age-matched controls (Barnett et al.). Recently Rice and his colleagues have described a familial syndrome of premature stroke in association with mitral valve prolapse. (4) The pulmonary veins are a source of cerebral emboli, as indicated by the occurrence of cerebral abscesses in association with pulmonary suppurative disease and by the high incidence of cerebral deposits secondary to pulmonary carcinoma. (5) Surgery of the neck and thorax can be complicated by cerebral embolism. A rare type is that which follows thyroidectomy, in which thrombosis in the stump of the superior thyroid artery extends proximally until a section of it, protruding into the lumen of the carotid, is carried into the cerebral arteries. (6) During arteriography emboli may form on the tip of the indwelling catheter and account for some of the arteriographic accidents.

Cerebral embolism must always have occurred when secondary tumor is deposited in the brain, and cerebral embolism regularly accompanies septicemia. However, a mass of tumor cells or bacteria seldom is large enough to occlude a cerebral artery and produce the picture of stroke. Nevertheless, tumor embolism has been reported secondary to cardiac myxomas and occasionally with other tumors. It must be distinguished from the marantic endocarditis and embolism which occasionally complicate carcinomatosis and other neoplasms. Embolism in the course of septicemia usually indicates the presence of a vegetative endocarditis with thrombus formation. Cerebral fat embolism is related to trauma. As a rule, the emboli are minute and widely dispersed, giving rise first to pulmonary symptoms and then to multiple cerebral petechial hemorrhages; accordingly the clinical picture is not strictly focal, as it is in a stroke. Cerebral air embolism is a rare complication of criminal abortion or of cervical and thoracic operations, and was formerly encountered as a complication of pneumothorax therapy. This condition is usually difficult to separate on clinical grounds from the deficits following hypotension or hypoxia, which frequently coexist.

Not infrequently the diagnosis of cerebral embolism is made at autopsy without finding a source. Possibly the routine search for a thrombotic nidus is not sufficiently thorough, and small thrombi in the atrial appendage, endocardium between the papillary muscles of the heart, aorta and its branches, or pulmonary veins may be overlooked. Nevertheless, in some cases studied most carefully no source of embolic material has been discovered.

CLINICAL PICTURE

Of all strokes, those due to cerebral embolism develop most rapidly, "like a bolt out of the blue." The full-blown picture evolves within several seconds or a minute, exemplifying most strikingly the temporal profile of a stroke. With rare exceptions, there are no warning episodes whatsoever. The embolus strikes at any time of the day or night. Getting up to go to the bathroom is a time of danger.

The neurologic picture will depend on the artery involved and where the obstruction lies. The syndromes related to each angioanatomic territory are the same as those outlined above, under "Neurovascular Syndromes." A large embolus may plug the internal carotid artery or the stem of the middle cerebral artery, producing the full-blown syndromes referable to occlusion of

Table 33-4
Causes of cerebral embolism

1. Cardiac origin
   a. Atrial fibrillation and other arrhythmias (with rheumatic, atherosclerotic, hypertensive, congenital or syphilitic heart disease)
   b. Myocardial infarction with mural thrombus
   c. Acute and subacute bacterial endocarditis
   d. Heart disease without arrhythmia or mural thrombus (mitral stenosis, myocarditis, etc.)
   e. Complications of cardiac surgery
   f. Valve prostheses
   g. Nonbacterial thrombotic (marantic) endocardial vegetations
   h. Prolapsed mitral valve
   i. Paradoxical embolism with congenital heart disease
   j. Trichinosis
2. Noncardiac origin
   a. Atherosclerosis of aorta and carotid arteries (mural thrombus, atheromatous material)
   b. From sites of cerebral artery thrombosis (basilar, vertebral, middle cerebral)
   c. Thrombus in pulmonary veins
   d. Fat, tumor, or air
   e. Complications of neck and thoracic surgery
3. Undetermined origin

these arteries. More often the embolus is smaller and passes into one of the branches of the middle cerebral artery, producing a strikingly focal disorder, such as a motor aphasia, a monoplegia, or a receptive type of aphasia with little or no motor paralysis. In fact, most patients diagnosed as having middle cerebral artery thrombosis prove to have emboli in the middle cerebral artery (or an atherosclerotic thrombosis of the internal carotid artery).

Embolic material entering the vertebral-basilar system occasionally is arrested in the vertebral artery just below its union with the basilar; but, as indicated above, it more often traverses the vertebral and also the basilar artery which is larger, and is not held up until it reaches the upper bifurcation. If arrested here, it abruptly produces deep coma and total paralysis. More often the embolus enters one or both of the posterior cerebral arteries and, by infarcting the visual cortex, causes a unilateral or bilateral homonymous hemianopia. Occasionally it will enter one of the small branches to the subthalamus; one of the "top of the basilar" syndromes results (see above). Embolic infarction of the undersurface of the cerebellum is common, and the resulting swelling of necrotic brain may cause acute, fatal brainstem compression. Embolic material rarely enters the penetrating branches of the pons.

It is important to emphasize that an embolus in its passage along an artery may produce a severe neurologic deficit which is only temporary; symptoms disappear as the embolus fragments and finally passes into a small branch supplying a small or relatively silent part of the hemisphere. In other words, embolism is a common cause of a single evanescent stroke. Also, as has already been pointed out, it can give rise to multiple transient attacks of almost identical or differing pattern.

Although the abruptness with which the stroke develops and the lack of prodromal symptoms point strongly to embolism, it is the total clinical picture upon which the diagnosis is based. If hemorrhage is ruled out, particularly by the use of the CT scan, there remains only thrombosis to be excluded. The presence of atrial fibrillation, a history of myocardial infarction (recent or in the preceding months), or the occurrence of embolism to other regions of the body all support the diagnosis of embolism. This diagnosis merits careful consideration in young persons in whom atherosclerosis is unlikely. Not infrequently the first sign of myocardial infarction is the occurrence of embolism; therefore, it is advisable that an *electrocardiogram be made in all patients with stroke of uncertain origin,* particularly since about 20 percent of myocardial infarctions are of the "silent" variety; and if the ECG does not yield relevant information, Holter monitoring for 24 to 48 h or echocardiographic study of heart valves should be undertaken.

LABORATORY FINDINGS

The findings described above, under "Atherothrombotic Infarction," apply also to embolism, except for hemorrhagic infarction and septic embolism (focal embolic encephalitis). In some 30 percent of cases, or less in some series, cerebral embolism produces a hemorrhagic infarct, but only in a minority of these do red cells enter the CSF (as high as 10,000 red cells per cubic millimeter). In the milder cases of hemorrhagic infarction, a slight xanthochromia (grade 1 to 3 on a scale of 1 to 10) may appear after a few days. CT scan is helpful in showing hemorrhagic infarction, which has been observed within hours of stroke onset (Fig. 33-19). The possibility that an embolic infarct is bloody underlines the danger of administering anticoagulants routinely, without a

Figure 33-19
Contrast-enhanced CT scan showing a large occipital and several small embolic (hemorrhagic) infarcts, 36 h after the onset of cerebral symptoms.

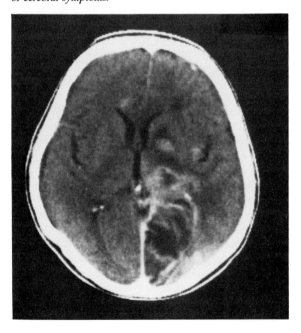

careful examination of the CSF. Also, it is the single exception to the rule that the presence of blood in the CSF of the patient with a stroke is due to an intracerebral hemorrhage, aneurysm, or vascular malformation.

In septic embolism resulting from subacute bacterial endocarditis the white blood cells in the CSF may be increased, usually up to 200 per cubic millimeter, but occasionally much higher; the proportion of lymphocytes and polymorphonuclears varies with the acuteness of the septic process. There may also be an equal number of red blood cells and a faint xanthochromia. The protein values are elevated, but the glucose content is within normal limits. No bacteria are seen or obtained by culture. The CSF formula in acute bacterial endocarditis may be that of subacute endocarditis or of a purulent meningitis.

COURSE AND PROGNOSIS

The remarks made concerning the *immediate prognosis* in cerebral thrombosis apply here as well. Most patients survive the initial insult. Massive brainstem infarction as a result of basilar embolism is almost always fatal. The *eventual prognosis* is determined by the occurrence of further emboli and the gravity of the underlying illness—cardiac failure, myocardial infarction, bacterial endocarditis, malignant growth, etc. In about 80 percent of cases, the first episode of cerebral embolism will be followed by another, frequently with severe damage. Furthermore, there is no certain way of predicting when the second embolus will strike; it may do so within a few days or weeks of the first. The urgency of instituting anticoagulant therapy is thereby emphasized. The *eventual prognosis* regarding the neurologic deficit is also similar to that of "Cerebral Thrombosis" (see above).

TREATMENT

The first three phases of therapy—(1) general medical management in the acute phase, (2) measures directed to restoring the circulation, and (3) physical therapy and rehabilitation—are much the same as described above under "Atherothrombotic Infarction." Attempted embolectomy at the bifurcation of the common carotid artery has usually failed, but should be considered. If pulsation in the temporal artery in front of the ear is present, the embolus has passed beyond that bifurcation, into the internal carotid system, and embolectomy will probably be unsuccessful. The same is true of embolectomy of the middle cerebral artery, a procedure made possible by the development of microvascular surgical techniques. Fibrinolysin therapy has not been effective.

Of prime importance is the *prevention of cerebral*

embolism, and this applies both to patients who have had an episode of embolism and to those who have not but are at risk to do so. There is good evidence that the long-term use of anticoagulants is effective in the prevention of embolism in cases of atrial fibrillation, myocardial infarction, and valve prosthesis. In patients with atrial fibrillation of recent onset, an attempt should be made to restore normal sinus rhythm by the use of electrical cardioversion, but failing in this attempt, prophylactic anticoagulant therapy is recommended.

After cerebral embolism has occurred, the question arises as to the advisability of delaying anticoagulant therapy for several days to avoid further bleeding into a hemorrhagic infarct. It is the authors' practice to first perform a CT scan, or if this is not available, to do a lumbar puncture, in order to rule out gross hemorrhage from the infarct. If the CT scan is normal and the CSF is clear, we proceed with intravenous heparin, followed by Coumadin, since there is always the danger of another embolic episode. Indications are that such therapy is safe, but exceptions to this statement may be expected. Also, in our opinion, the use of anticoagulant therapy in patients with acute myocardial infarction, including those judged to be in the "good risk" category, is advisable. In cerebral embolism associated with subacute bacterial endocarditis, anticoagulant therapy is contraindicated because of the danger of intracranial bleeding, and it is preferable to rely on rapid sterilization of the bloodstream.

Valvuloplasty and amputation of the atrial appendage have substantially reduced the incidence of embolism in rheumatic heart disease. The need for special care in preventing emboli from entering the carotid arteries during the performance of valvuloplasty is appreciated by all cardiac surgeons.

OTHER OCCLUSIVE CEREBROVASCULAR DISEASES

FIBROMUSCULAR DYSPLASIA

This is a segmental, nonatheromatous arterial disease of unknown etiology. The disease is uncommon, but judging from the review of the literature by Houser et al., it is being reported with increasing frequency because of improved diagnostic arteriography.

First described in the renal artery by Leadbetter and Burkland (1938), it is now known to affect other vessels including cervicocerebral ones. Of the latter, the internal carotid artery is involved most frequently followed by the vertebral artery. The radiologic alteration consists of a series of transverse constrictions, giving the

appearance of an irregular string of beads or a tubular narrowing and is observed bilaterally in 75 percent of cases. Usually only the extracranial part of the artery is involved. In the personal series of Houser et al., 42 of 44 patients were women, and 75 percent were over 50 years of age. Cerebral ischemia is the regular consequence of the lesion.

The pathology of this disease is poorly defined. In the narrowed arterial segments there are degeneration of elastic tissue, disruption and loss of the muscular coat, and increase in fibrous tissue. The dilatations are due to atrophy of the vessel wall. Some patients have had atherosclerosis in addition. Usually vascular occlusion is not present, though there may be marked stenosis; hence the cause of the ischemic lesion in the brain is unsettled. The clinical and pathologic separation of this disease from atherosclerosis is incomplete.

SPONTANEOUS DISSECTING ANEURYSMS OF THE INTERNAL CAROTID ARTERY

It is well known that Erdheim's medionecrosis aortica cystica may extend into the common carotid arteries, occluding them and causing massive infarction of the cerebral hemispheres. Weisman and Adams cited examples of this in their study of the neurology of dissecting aneurysms of the aorta in 1944. But in the last 20 years there have been a series of cases in which false aneurysms with dissection of blood between intima and media have been responsible for hemiplegias in children, adolescents, and young adults. Ojemann et al. described such a case and reviewed the literature on this subject; since then Ojemann and Fisher have collected more than 25 such cases at the Massachusetts General Hospital.

Clinically it is of interest that several of the patients have had warning ischemic attacks in the carotid territory for a day or two before the final episode. Headache was a frequent symptom on the homolateral side. The neurologic syndrome sometimes evolved smoothly over a period of minutes to hours or in stepwise fashion. A unilateral Horner syndrome or a new cervical bruit may be important diagnostic clues. Arteriography reveals a long narrow column of dye, beginning 1.5 to 3 cm above the carotid bifurcation and extending to the base of the skull, a picture which Fisher has called the *string sign*. There may be an outpouching at the end of the string. Ojemann has succeeded in opening the vessel and removing the clot from the vessel wall by inserting a catheter with a balloon tip to beyond the dissection and then retracting it. Several of Ojemann's cases have regained normal neurologic status after the dissecting clot was removed, but whether the operation was responsible for the recovery is unclear.

The pathogenesis of the dissection is undetermined. Although the lesion may develop spontaneously, it has been found in relation to external trauma to the head and neck, and to carotid puncture for angiography. In most of the reported cases, cystic medial necrosis was not found on microscopic examination of the involved artery. In some there was a disorganization of the media and internal elastic lamina, but its specificity is in doubt, since Ojemann and his colleagues noted similar changes in some of their control cases. A more thorough study of these vessels in routine autopsy material is needed.

MOYAMOYA DISEASE AND MULTIPLE PROGRESSIVE INTRACRANIAL ARTERIAL OCCLUSIONS

The term *moyamoya* is a Japanese word for a *cloud of smoke* or *haze*, and it has been used in recent years to refer to an *extensive basal cerebral rete mirabile*—a network of small anastomotic vessels at the base of the brain around and distal to the circle of Willis, seen in carotid arteriograms, along with segmental stenosis or occlusion of the terminal parts of both internal carotid arteries.

Nishimoto and Takeuchi collected 111 cases, selected on the basis of these two radiologic criteria. The condition has been observed mainly in infants, children, and adolescents (more than half the cases were less than 10 years of age, and only 4 of 111 cases were more than 40 years). All their patients were Japanese; both males and females were affected, and eight were siblings. The symptom that had led to medical examination was weakness of a limb or arm and leg on one side. The weakness tended to clear rapidly but recurred in some instances. Headache, convulsions, impaired mental development, visual disturbance and nystagmus were less frequent. In older patients, subarachnoid hemorrhage was the most common initial manifestation. Other symptoms and signs were speech disturbance, sensory impairment, involuntary movements, and unsteady gait. Only six of the entire series became worse after the initial illness, and four died. Postmortem examinations have failed to delineate the carotid lesion precisely. The adventitia, media, and internal elastic lamina of the ste-

nosed or occluded arteries were normal in these cases, and only the intima was thickened by fibrous tissue. No inflammatory cells or atheromata were seen. In a few cases, hypoplasia of the vessel with absent muscularis was reported. The rete mirabile consists of a fine network of vessels over the basal surface (in the pia-arachnoid). These latter may be the source of subarachnoid hemorrhage.

This form of cerebrovascular disease is not limited to the Japanese. The authors have observed several such patients, and there are observations of similar cases from other parts of the United States, Western Europe, and Australia.

Opinion is divided as to whether the basal rete mirabile represents a congenital vascular malformation (i.e., a persistence of the embryonal network) or a rich collateral vascularization, secondary to a congenital hypoplasia or acquired stenosis or occlusion of the internal carotid arteries early in life. One part of the symptomatology is traced to the carotid stenosis and another to the rupture of the vascular network.

In the authors' view, the pathologic process is not sufficiently clear to permit separation of moyamoya from the occlusive vascular diseases of children and young adults or from vascular malformations.

The condition described in non-Orientals by Taveras as *multiple progressive intracranial arterial occlusion* occurs in the same age period as moyamoya and has many of the clinical characteristics of the latter. It lacks only the cloud of fine anastomotic channels. Since the vascular pathology of both diseases is incompletely studied, their exact relationship cannot be stated at this time.

STROKES IN CHILDREN AND YOUNG ADULTS

The occurrence of hemiplegia in infants and children is a well-recognized phenomenon. In a series of 555 consecutive postmortem examinations at the Children's Medical Center in Boston, there were 48 cases (8.7 percent) of occlusive vascular disease of the brain (Banker). The occlusions were both embolic (mainly associated with *congenital heart disease*) and thrombotic, and the latter were actually more common in veins than in arteries.

Persistent cerebral ischemia and infarction may occasionally complicate *migraine* (page 122), not only in elderly persons but in young ones as well. In young women the combination of migraine and "the pill" has been particularly hazardous (see below).

In young adults with strokes, one must also consider cerebral embolism from *rheumatic endocarditis,* *bacterial endocarditis,* and the *verrucous endocarditis* that complicates lupus erythematosus (Libman-Sacks syndrome). Stroke in young persons due to either arterial or venous occlusion occurs occasionally in association with *ulcerative colitis* and *regional enteritis*. Evidence points to a hypercoagulable state during exacerbations of the inflammatory bowel disease, but a precise defect in coagulation has not been defined. *Sickle-cell anemia* is an important cause of stroke in black children; acute hemiplegia is the most common manifestation, but all types of focal cerebral disorder have been observed. The pathological findings are those of infarction, large and small, and their basis is assumed to be vascular obstruction associated with the sickling process. Intracranial bleeding (subdural, subarachnoid, and intracerebral) may also complicate sickle-cell anemia, and for some reason there is an increased incidence of pneumococcal meningitis in this disease. *Homocystinuria* and *Fabry's angiokeratosis*, two of the hereditary metabolic diseases described in Chap. 37, may give rise to strokes in children or young adults.

ORAL CONTRACEPTIVES AND CEREBRAL INFARCTION

Transient or prolonged cerebral ischemia has been particularly striking in females during pregnancy and the puerperium, and while taking the contraceptive pill or during estrogen therapy. Fisher has reviewed the literature and has himself analyzed 12 postpartum cases, 9 puerperal cases, 14 contraceptive cases, and 9 cases in which estrogen therapy was being given; arterial thrombosis of obscure type was demonstrated in half of the group.

It now seems clear, particularly from the findings of the Collaborative Group for the Study of Stroke in Young Women, that women who take oral contraceptives in the child-bearing years are at increased risk of developing cerebral infarction. The mechanism is not completely understood. The infarction in these cases is due to arterial occlusion, occurring in both the carotid-middle cerebral and vertebral-basilar territories. In most of the reported fatal cases, the thrombosed artery has been free of atheroma or other disease. This has been taken to indicate that embolism is responsible for the strokes; no source of embolism has been demonstrated, however. Noncerebral venous thrombosis is another, relatively rare complication of "the pill." These observations, coupled with evidence that estrogen alters the coagulability of the blood, suggest that a state of hypercoagulability is the important factor in the genesis of contraceptive-associated infarction.

The vascular lesion underlying cerebral thrombosis in women taking oral contraceptives has been studied by Irey and his colleagues. It consists of intimal hyperplasia of nodular eccentric topography with increased acid mucopolysaccharides and replication of the internal elastic lamina. Similar changes have been found in pregnancy and in humans and animals receiving exogenous steroids including estrogens.

INTRACRANIAL HEMORRHAGE

This is the third most frequent cause of stroke. Although more than a dozen causes of intracranial hemorrhage have been listed (Table 33-5), primary or hypertensive ("spontaneous") intracerebral hemorrhage, ruptured saccular aneurysm and vascular malformation, and hemorrhage associated with bleeding disorders account for most of the hemorrhages which present as strokes. Duret hemorrhages, hypertensive encephalopathy, and brain purpura will not simulate a stroke and are included only for the sake of completeness.

Table 33-5
Causes of intracranial hemorrhage (including intracerebral, subarachnoid, ventricular, and subdural)

1. Primary (hypertensive) intracerebral hemorrhage
2. Ruptured saccular aneurysm
3. Ruptured AV malformation
4. Undetermined cause (normal blood pressure, no aneurysm or AV malformation)
5. Trauma including posttraumatic delayed apoplexy
6. Hemorrhagic disorders: leukemia, aplastic anemia, thrombocytopenic purpura, liver disease, complication of anticoagulant therapy, hyperfibrinolysis, hypofibrinogenemia, hemophilia, Christmas disease, etc.
7. Hemorrhage into primary and secondary brain tumors
8. Septic embolism, mycotic aneurysm
9. With hemorrhagic infarction, arterial or venous
10. With inflammatory disease of the arteries and veins
11. Miscellaneous rare types: after vasopressor drugs, upon exertion, during arteriography, during painful urologic examination, as a late complication of early-life carotid occlusion, complication of carotid-cavernous AV fistula, with anoxemia, migraine, teratomatous malformations. Herpes simplex encephalitis and acute necrotizing hemorrhagic encephalopathy may be associated with up to 2000 red blood cells or more per cubic millimeter in the CSF; tularemia, anthrax, and pseudomonas meningitis and snake venom poisoning may cause bloody CSF.

PRIMARY (HYPERTENSIVE) INTRACEREBRAL HEMORRHAGE

This is the common, well-known brain hemorrhage. Although it occurs sometimes with levels of blood pressure in the normal range (rare) or in the range of only 150/90 to 170/90, in most cases they are much higher. Hypertensive hemorrhage occurs within brain tissue, and rupture of the arteries lying in the subarachnoid space is practically unknown, apart from aneurysm. The extravasation forms a roughly circular or oval mass which disrupts the tissue as the bleeding continues and grows in volume. Adjacent brain tissue is displaced and compressed. If the hemorrhage is large, midline structures are displaced to the opposite side and vital centers are compromised, leading to coma and death. Rupture or seepage into the ventricular system usually occurs, and the CSF becomes bloody in more than 90 percent of cases. A hemorrhage of this type almost never ruptures through the cerebral cortex, and the blood reaches the subarachnoid space via the ventricular system. When the hemorrhage is small and located at a distance from the ventricles, the CSF may remain clear even on repeated examination.

Extravasated blood undergoes a series of changes beginning with the collection of phagocytes at the outer rim and followed by the formation of a brown-orange peripheral zone of hemosiderin-filled macrophages. The mass gradually decreases in size, and after a period of some 2 to 6 months, only an orange-stained cleft (color due to hemosiderin and iron in macrophages) is left at the site of the hemorrhage.

Hemorrhages may be described as massive, small, slit, and petechial. *Massive* refers to hemorrhages several centimeters in diameter; *small* applies to those 1 to 2 cm in diameter; and *slit* refers to a special type of small hypertensive hemorrhage which lies subcortically at the junction of white and gray matter and which in the healing stage becomes narrowed to an elongated, thin, orange cavity.

In order of frequency, the most common sites of hypertensive hemorrhage are (1) the putamen and adjacent internal capsule (50 percent of cases), (2) various parts of the central white matter (frontal lobe, corona radiata, etc., often extensions from the putamen), (3) thalamus, (4) cerebellar hemisphere, and (5) pons. The vessel involved is usually a penetrating artery. The nature of the vascular lesion which leads to arterial rupture is not fully known, but in the few cases studied by serial sections, the hemorrhage appeared to arise from an arterial wall altered by the effects of hypertension, the change referred to in a preceding section as segmental lipohyalinosis.

Clinical Picture This conforms closely to the temporal profile of a stroke, i.e., there is an abrupt onset and rather rapid evolution of symptoms. The stroke usually evolves gradually and steadily over an appreciable length of time, taking minutes, hours, or occasionally days (usually 1 to 24 h) to reach its fully developed form, depending on the speed of bleeding. Hemorrhages that complicate the administration of anticoagulants may evolve at a leisurely pace. Usually there are no warnings or prodromal symptoms. Often headache, dizziness, and epistaxis have not occurred with any consistency, and many patients have felt entirely well. There is no sex or age predilection except that the average age of occurrence is lower than in thrombotic infarction. The incidence of hypertensive cerebral hemorrhage is higher in Negroes than in Caucasians. In the great majority of cases, the hemorrhage has its onset while the patient is up and active; onset during sleep is a rarity. The level of blood pressure is maintained early in the course of the stroke or may even rise higher, so that the existence of hypertension is readily established when the patient is first examined. Hypertension is usually of the "essential" type, but other causes must always be considered—renal disease, renal artery occlusion, toxemia of pregnancy, pheochromocytoma, aldosteronism, ACTH or corticosteroid overdosage, and, rarely, violent exertion or intense excitement. Cardiomegaly is present.

There is ordinarily only one episode of hemorrhage, and recurrence of bleeding from the same site, as occurs in cases of saccular aneurysm, is not encountered. Once bleeding has become arrested, rebleeding in the next few days is not to be anticipated. Blood that has extravasated into cerebral tissue is removed slowly, over a period of weeks and months, during which time symptoms and signs persist. Hence the neurologic deficit is never transitory in intracerebral hemorrhage, as it so often is in thrombosis and embolism; for the same reason, one should not expect rapid improvement in the neurologic deficit from one examination to another.

The neurologic symptoms and signs vary with the site and size of the extravasation. The most common syndrome is the one due to *putaminal hemorrhage*, with implication of the adjacent internal capsule (Fig. 33-20). With large hemorrhages patients lapse almost immediately into stupor and coma with hemiplegia, and their condition visibly deteriorates as the hours pass. More often, however, patients complain of headache or of some other abnormal sensation within the head. In a few minutes the face sags on one side, speech becomes slurred or aphasic, the arm and leg gradually weaken and the eyes tend to deviate away from the side of the paretic limbs. These events occur gradually over a period of 5 to 30 min; this type of evolution is strongly suggestive of intracerebral bleeding. Gradually the paralysis worsens, a Babinski sign appears, the affected limbs become flaccid, painful stimuli are not appreciated, speaking becomes impossible, and confusion gives way to stupor. In the most advanced cases, signs of upper brainstem compression appear—coma, bilateral Babinski signs, deep, irregular, or intermittent respiration, dilated fixed pupils, and, occasionally, decerebrate rigidity.

Thalamic hemorrhage of moderate size also produces a hemiplegia or hemiparesis by compression of the adjacent internal capsule. The sensory deficit equals or outstrips the motor weakness. Aphasia may be present with lesions of the dominant side, and amorphosynthesis with nondominant lesions. A homonymous field defect, if present, usually clears in a few days. Thalamic hemorrhage, by virtue of its extension medially and into the subthalamus, causes a series of ocular disturbances— palsies of vertical and lateral gaze, forced deviation of the eyes downward, inequality of pupils with absence of light reaction, skew deviation with the eye opposite the hemorrhage being displaced downward and medially,

Figure 33-20
An unenhanced CT scan showing the typical picture of a massive primary (hypertensive) hemorrhage in the basal ganglia. The third ventricle and opposite lateral ventricle are compressed by the expanding mass (12 h after onset of stroke).

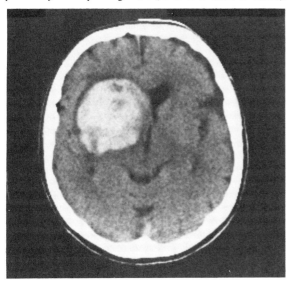

ipsilateral ptosis and miosis, absence of convergence, retraction nystagmus, and tucking in of the eyelids. Retraction of the neck may be prominent.

In *pontine hemorrhage*, deep coma usually ensues in a few minutes, and the clinical picture includes total paralysis, prominent decerebrate rigidity, and small (1 mm) pupils that react to light. Lateral eye movements, evoked by head turning or caloric testing are impaired or absent. Death usually occurs within a few hours, but there are rare exceptions where consciousness is retained and the clinical manifestations indicate a lesion in the tegmentum of the pons, e.g., disturbances of lateral ocular movements, crossed sensory or motor disturbances, small pupils, and cranial nerve palsies, in addition to signs of bilateral corticospinal tract involvement.

Cerebellar hemorrhage usually develops over a period of several hours, and loss of consciousness at the onset is unusual. Repeated vomiting is a prominent feature, along with occipital headache, vertigo, and inability to stand or walk. There is a paresis of conjugate lateral gaze to the side of the hemorrhage, forced deviation of the eyes to the opposite side, or an ipsilateral sixth nerve weakness. Vertical eye movements are retained. Other ocular signs include blepharospasm, involuntary closure of one eye, skew deviation, "ocular bobbing," and small, often unequal pupils which continue to react until very late in the illness. In the early phase of the illness there may be little or no evidence of cerebellar disease; only a minority of cases show nystagmus or cerebellar ataxia of the limbs, although these signs must always be sought. A mild ipsilateral facial weakness and a diminished corneal reflex are common. Dysarthria and dysphagia may be prominent. Contralateral hemiplegia and facial weakness do not occur. Occasionally at the onset there is a spastic paraparesis or a quadriplegia with preservation of consciousness. The plantar reflexes are flexor in the early stages, but extensor later. As the hours pass, and occasionally with unanticipated suddenness, the patient becomes stuporous and then comatose as a result of brainstem compression, at which point reversal of the syndrome, even by surgical therapy, is seldom successful.

It will be noted that in the localization of intracerebral hemorrhages, ocular signs are important. In putaminal hemorrhage the eyes are deviated to the side opposite the paralysis; in thalamic hemorrhage the commonest ocular abnormality is downward deviation of the eyes, and the pupils may be unreactive; in pontine hemorrhage the eyeballs are fixed and the pupils tiny but reactive; and in cerebellar hemorrhage the eyes are deviated laterally to the side opposite the lesion.

Hemorrhage at each of the sites described above is usually massive, and patients survive only a few hours or a few days, succumbing as a result of secondary brainstem disturbance. Once a deep stupor has supervened, patients rarely survive, although some linger in an unresponsive state for a week or two. In some 30 percent of cases, however, the hemorrhage is less extensive, and survival is possible; hemorrhage into the thalamus tends to be somewhat smaller than putaminal or cerebellar hemorrhage.

A *severe headache* is generally considered to be a constant accompaniment of intracerebral hemorrhage, and in many cases it is a prominent and helpful diagnostic point. Nevertheless, in almost 50 percent of our cases headache has been absent or insignificant. *Nuchal rigidity* is frequently found, but again, it is so often absent that failure to find it should by no means detract from the diagnosis. Stiffness of the neck characteristically disappears as coma deepens. *Vomiting* at the onset of intracerebral hemorrhage occurs much more frequently than with infarction. It is important to note that often the patient is alert and responding accurately when first seen. This is true even when the CSF is grossly bloody; thus the adage that hemorrhage into the ventricular system always precipitates coma is quite incorrect. Only if bleeding into the ventricles is massive will coma result. *Cerebral seizures*, usually focal, occur in some 10 percent of cases of supratentorial hemorrhage in the first few days, especially in association with subcortical *slit* hemorrhages. The fundi often show hypertensive changes in the arteries. Rarely, white-centered retinal hemorrhages (Roth spots) or fresh preretinal (subhyaloid) hemorrhages occur, but the latter are much more common with ruptured aneurysm or arteriovenous malformation.

Many of the less precisely localized neurologic manifestations described under cerebral thrombosis are also encountered in intracerebral hemorrhage, including coma, stupor, drowsiness, confusion, Cheyne-Stokes respiration, bilateral or contralateral grasping and sucking reflexes, incontinence of bowel and bladder, and unilateral and bilateral extensor rigidity.

Although the proper interpretation of this array of clinical data allows the correct diagnosis to be established in most cases, the laboratory examinations described below are helpful, especially in the diagnosis of small hemorrhages.

Laboratory Findings Among laboratory methods for the diagnosis of intracerebral hemorrhage, the CT scan occupies the foremost position. This procedure has proved totally reliable in the detection of hemorrhages 1.5 cm or more in diameter situated in the cerebral or cerebellar hemispheres. However, small pontine hemorrhages are visualized less certainly. Hemorrhages are localized with remarkable accuracy, far surpassing that achieved with arteriography. At the same time coexisting hydrocephalus, tumor, cerebral swelling, and displacement of intracranial contents are readily appreciated. The CT scan is particularly useful in the diagnosis of small brain hemorrhages that do not spill blood into the CSF and were heretofore clinically unrecognizable.

Before the introduction of CT scanning the examination of the CSF was the most dependable method for the diagnosis of hemorrhage. In cases of massive hemorrhage, the CSF is often under increased pressure; but in almost half our cases, readings under 200 mmH$_2$O have been obtained. The fluid is usually grossly bloody, although the count may vary from a few thousand cells up to 1 million per cubic millimeter. In smaller hemorrhages into central structures, the CSF contains a lesser amount of blood; in some cases of intracerebral hemorrhage, particularly in those of the *slit* type, it may be entirely clear. In these latter cases, slight xanthochromia may appear after a few days. At times the CSF may be clear grossly, but contains some 200 to 400 red cells per cubic millimeter; it is then difficult to decide if this represents intracranial bleeding or a traumatic tap. These details are mentioned because if a CT scan is unavailable they are critical in making an accurate diagnosis of the type of stroke, prior to the use of therapeutic measures such as anticoagulant drugs or surgical exploration. A traumatic tap, which may greatly complicate the diagnostic problem, can be distinguished from preexisting bleeding by the criteria outlined in Chap. 2.

Lumbar puncture is not completely innocuous, since temporal lobe herniation may be aggravated in cases of massive supratentorial hemorrhage or softening. Despite this danger, the procedure is necessary when CT scanning is not available, if specific therapeutic measures are contemplated, or if any suspicion exists about the presence of meningitis. Skull films early in the course of cerebral hemorrhage may show a shift of the calcified pineal gland, a change rarely seen in infarction. The EEG does not show a typical or diagnostic pattern, but high-voltage, slow waves are the most common finding with hemorrhage into the cerebral hemisphere. Films of the chest will often show cardiomegaly. Urinary abnormalities usually reflect coexisting renal disease, although transient glucosuria has been reported to result specifically from intracranial hemorrhage. The white cell count in the peripheral blood often rises to 15,000 to 20,000 per cubic millimeter, a higher figure than in thrombosis. The sedimentation rate is elevated.

Course and Prognosis The immediate prognosis is grave; some 70 to 75 percent of patients die in 1 to 30 days. Either the hemorrhage extends into the ventricular system, or temporal lobe herniation and midbrain compression occur. Sometimes the hemorrhage itself seeps into vital centers. Gastric erosion and gastrointestinal hemorrhage of neurogenic origin may occur at any time within the first week or so. In patients who survive, i.e., in those with smaller hemorrhages, there can be a surprisingly adequate restitution of function, since, in contrast to infarction, the hemorrhage has to some extent pushed brain tissue aside instead of destroying it. Function may be slow to return, however, because extravasated blood is slow to be resorbed or removed from the tissues. Since rebleeding from the same site is unlikely, the patient may live for many years. In some instances of medium-sized cerebral and cerebellar hemorrhages, the patient survives and his or her condition gradually stabilizes, but papilledema appears after several days of increased intracranial pressure. This does not mean that the hemorrhage is increasing in size or swelling—only that papilledema is slow to develop. Healed scars impinging on the cortex are liable to be epileptogenic.

Treatment *The general medical management of the comatose patient with intracerebral hemorrhage* is the same as for the patients with cerebral thrombosis and embolism and has been outlined on page 246. The management of patients with large intracerebral hemorrhages includes maintaining adequate ventilation, controlled hyperventilation to a Pco_2 of 25 to 30 mmHg, tissue dehydration by the use of mannitol or furosemide (osmolality kept at 305 to 315 mosmol/liter and Na at 150 meq), limited fluid intake to 1200 ml/day given as intravenous infusions of normal saline, and Decadron 4 mg every 6 h.

Surgical removal of the clot in the acute stage, either by evacuation or aspiration, seldom proves beneficial. Possible exceptions are patients who are not comatose and whose hemorrhage lies near the cortical surface, and patients with acute cerebellar hemorrhage, providing that removal of the hematoma is accomplished within the first few days of onset and before coma has supervened. The appearance of papilledema in association with smaller hemorrhages that have stabilized has in many instances dictated unnecessary surgical attempts to evacuate the clot.

Attempts to halt the hemorrhage by lowering the systemic blood pressure through the use of autonomic blocking agents have not been effective, and in many instances the inadvertent occurrence of hypotension has seriously complicated the illness. Artifical hypothermia has been used sporadically, but there are insufficient data to permit appraisal of this procedure.

The *most important measure* is the use of antihypertensive drugs in cases of essential hypertension. When hypotension threatens during surgical procedures, injections of excessive amounts of epinephrine or ephedrine are to be avoided. Toxemia of pregnancy must be detected early.

RUPTURED SACCULAR ANEURYSM

This is the fourth most frequent cerebrovascular disorder—following atherosclerosis, embolism, and hypertensive intracerebral hemorrhage. Saccular aneurysms, or berry aneurysms, as they are called, take the form of small, thin-walled blisters protruding from the arteries of the circle of Willis or its major branches. The aneurysms are located for the most part at bifurcations and branchings (Fig. 33-17) and are generally presumed to be the result of developmental defects in the media and elastica. An alternate theory holds that the aneurysmal process is initiated by focal destruction of the internal elastic membrane, which is produced by hemodynamic forces at the apices of bifurcations (Ferguson). Owing to the local weakness, the intima bulges outward, covered only by adventitia; the sac gradually enlarges until finally rupture occurs. Saccular aneurysms vary in size from 2 mm up to 2 or 3 cm in diameter, averaging 8 to 10 mm. They vary greatly in form. Some are round and connected to the parent artery by a narrow stalk; others are broadbased without a stalk; still others are narrow cylinders. The site of rupture is usually the dome of the aneurysm, which may present one or more secondary sacculations. Enlargement is the result of dilatation of the lumen, but after bleeding, organization of surrounding clot may be an added factor.

In routine autopsies the incidence of ruptured aneurysms is 1.8 percent; of unruptured ones, 2.0 percent, excluding minor outpouchings of 3 mm or less. Saccular aneurysms are rare in childhood, even at routine postmortem examination, and increase in frequency to reach their highest plateau of incidence in persons between 35 and 65 years of age. Therefore, they are not congenitally formed anomalies but develop over the years on the basis of the developmental or acquired arterial defect. There is an increased incidence of congenital polycystic kidney and coarctation of the aorta in association with saccular aneurysm. Hypertension is more frequently present than in the average population, but aneurysms occur in persons with normal blood pressure. Aneurysmal rupture may complicate pregnancy, but pregnancy is not associated with an increased incidence of aneurysmal rupture. Atherosclerosis, although present in the walls of some saccular aneurysms, probably plays no part in their formation or enlargement.

Approximately 90 to 95 percent of saccular aneurysms lie on the anterior part of the circle of Willis (Fig. 33-21). The four most common sites are (1) in relation to the anterior communicating artery, (2) at the origin of the posterior communicating artery from the stem of the internal carotid, (3) at the first major bifurcation of the middle cerebral artery, and (4) at the bifurcation of the internal carotid into middle and anterior cerebral arteries. Other sites include the internal carotid artery in the cavernous sinus, the origin of the ophthalmic artery, the junction of the posterior communicating and posterior cerebral arteries, the bifurcation of the basilar artery,

and the origins of the three cerebellar arteries. In 20 percent of cases there is more than one aneurysm, and they may be situated unilaterally or bilaterally.

There are several types of aneurysm other than saccular, e.g., mycotic, fusiform, diffuse, and globular. The last three are named for their predominant morphologic characteristics and consist of enlargement or dilatation of the entire circumference of the involved vessels, usually the internal carotid, vertebral, or basilar arteries. They are often referred to as arteriosclerotic aneurysms, since they frequently show atheromatous deposition in their walls, but it is likely that they are at least partly developmental in nature. They press on neighboring structures or become occluded by thrombus and rupture only infrequently.

Clinical Picture Prior to rupture, saccular aneurysms are usually asymptomatic. Occasionally, large aneurysms immediately distal to the cavernous sinus may compress the optic nerves or chiasm, third nerve, hypothalamus, or pituitary gland. In the cavernous sinus they may press on the third, fourth, sixth, or ophthalmic division of the fifth cranial nerve (see page 183; see also Fig. 33-22). In the posterior fossa, one or more of the cranial nerves may be compressed adjacent to the brainstem. Rarely they cause headache, but by then other signs will usually have appeared.

When rupture occurs, blood under high pressure is forced into the subarachnoid space (the circle of Willis

Figure 33-21
Diagram of the circle of Willis to show the principal sites of saccular aneurysms. Approximately 90 percent of aneurysms are on the anterior half of the circle.

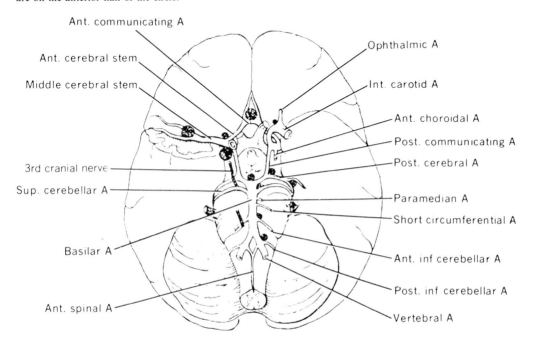

lies in the subarachnoid space), and the resulting clinical events fall into one of three patterns: (1) the patient may be stricken with an excruciating generalized headache and fall unconscious almost immediately; (2) headache may develop as in (1), but the patient remains relatively lucid; (3) rarely, consciousness may be lost quickly without any preceding complaint. Decerebrate rigidity may occur at the onset of hemorrhage in association with unconsciousness. If the hemorrhage is massive, death may ensue in a matter of minutes, hours, or a day or two, so that ruptured aneurysm must be considered in the differential diagnosis of sudden death. Persistent deep coma is accompanied by irregular respirations, attacks of extensor rigidity, and finally respiratory arrest and circulatory collapse. In these rapidly fatal cases, the blood has usually dissected intracerebrally and entered the ventricular system (meningocerebral-ventricular hemorrhage).

In milder cases, consciousness, if lost, may be regained within a few minutes or hours but a residuum of drowsiness, confusion, and amnesia accompanied by severe headache and stiff neck persists for several days. It is not uncommon for the drowsiness and confusion to last 10 days or longer. If the hemorrhage is confined to the subarachnoid space, there are few or no lateralizing neurologic signs.

In most patients there are no warning symptoms; some, however, will have had an episode of headache, or perhaps a transitory unilateral weakness, numbness and tingling, or speech disturbance in the days or weeks preceding the major event. These prodromal symptoms are generally attributed to minor leakage from the aneurysm. Rupture of the aneurysm usually occurs while the patient is active rather than during sleep, and in many instances sexual intercourse or other exertion precipitates the ictus.

Gross lateralizing signs in the form of hemiplegia, hemiparesis, homonymous hemianopia, or aphasia are absent in the majority of cases, but can occur; in the acute stages these disturbances are due to an intracerebral clot or ischemia in the territory of the aneurysm-bearing artery. The initial neurologic deficits may clear in a matter of days, indicating that hemorrhage into brain tissue was not responsible for them. The pathogenesis of such manifestations is not fully understood, but a transitory fall in pressure in the circulation distal to the aneurysm is postulated. Transient deficits, still more evanescent, are not uncommon and constitute reliable telltales of the site of the ruptured aneurysm (see below). A delayed hemiplegia or other deficit may occur 4 to 10 days after rupture. This has been loosely attributed to focal narrowing (*spasm*) of a large artery due to the presence of extravasated blood. Areas of ischemic necrosis of tissue in the territory of the vessel bearing the aneurysm, usually without thrombosis of the vessel, is the usual finding in such cases at autopsy. A subacute hydrocephalus due to blockage of the CSF pathways by blood may appear after 2 to 4 weeks.

Although in most patients the neurologic manifestations do not point to the exact site of the aneurysm, in many instances they provide clues to the localization. Examples follow: (1) Third nerve palsy (ptosis, diplopia, dilatation of pupil, and divergent strabismus) usually indicates an aneurysm at the junction of the posterior

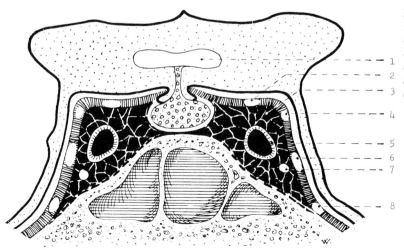

Figure 33-22
Diagram of the cavernous sinus: (1) optic chiasm; (2) oculomotor nerve; (3) cavernous sinus; (4) trochlear nerve; (5) internal carotid artery; (6) ophthalmic nerve; (7) abducent nerve; (8) maxillary nerve. (From Krayenbühl and Yasargil.)

communicating artery and the internal carotid stem; the third nerve passes immediately lateral to this point. (2) Transient paresis of one or both of the lower limbs at the onset of the hemorrhage is suggestive of an anterior communicating aneurysm which has interfered with the circulation in the anterior cerebral arteries. (3) Hemiparesis or aphasia points to an aneurysm at the first major bifurcation of the middle cerebral artery. (4) Unilateral blindness indicates an aneurysm which lies anteromedially in the circle of Willis (at the origin of the ophthalmic artery, at the bifurcation of the internal carotid artery, or in the anterior communicating region). (5) A stage of retained consciousness with akinetic mutism or abulia (sometimes associated with paraplegia) favors an aneurysm of the anterior communicating artery which has caused ischemia of or hemorrhage into one or both of the frontal lobes, hypothalamus, or corpus callosum. (6) The side on which the aneurysm lies may be indicated by a unilateral preponderance of headache or preretinal hemorrhages, occurrence of monocular pain, or lateralization of an intracranial sound heard at the time of rupture of the aneurysm. Sixth nerve palsy, unilateral or bilateral, results from the presence of subarachnoid blood and raised intracranial pressure and is seldom of localizing value. Other neurologic signs which have relatively little localizing value include sucking and grasping reflexes, a Korsakoff type of amnesia which usually clears in 4 to 6 weeks, choreoathetosis, and extensor rigidity.

In summary, the clinical sequence of sudden violent headache, collapse, relative preservation of consciousness, and a paucity of lateralizing signs in the face of massive subarachnoid hemorrhage is diagnostic of a ruptured saccular aneurysm.

Other clinical data may be of assistance in reaching a correct diagnosis. Nuchal rigidity is usually present, but occasionally it is absent, and the main complaint of pain may be referable to the interscapular region or the low back rather than to the head. Examination of the fundi frequently reveals smooth-surfaced, sharply outlined collections of blood which cover the retinal vessels—the so-called preretinal or subhyaloid hemorrhages; Roth spots are seen occasionally. Bilateral Babinski signs are found in the early days following rupture. Fever with the temperature rising to 39°C is common in the first week. The escaping blood occasionally enters the subdural space and produces a hematoma, evacuation of which may be life-saving. Spontaneous intracranial bleeding with normal blood pressure should

always suggest ruptured aneurysm or arteriovenous malformation, a bleeding diathesis, and rarely hemorrhage into a cerebral tumor.

Laboratory Findings Carotid and vertebral angiography is the only certain means of demonstrating an aneurysm and does so in some 85 percent of patients in whom aneurysm appears to be the correct diagnosis on clinical grounds, i.e., in cases of so-called spontaneous subarachnoid hemorrhage.

A CT scan will detect blood within the brain or ventricular system or locally or diffusely in the subarachnoid spaces (Fig. 33-23). When two or more aneurysms are visualized by arteriography, the CT scan may indicate the one which has ruptured by the surrounding clot. Also a coexistent hydrocephalus will be demonstrable.

Usually the CSF is grossly bloody, with red cell counts reaching 1 million per cubic millimeter or even higher. With slight degrees of hemorrhage, there may be only a few thousand cells. It is unlikely that an aneurysm can rupture entirely into brain tissue without some leakage of blood into the subarachnoid fluid, and therefore the diagnosis of ruptured saccular aneurysm should never be made unless blood is present in the CSF. Usually deep xanthochromia is found after centrifugation. The CSF is under greatly increased pressure, as high as 1000 mmH$_2$O, an important finding in differentiating sponta-

Figure 33-23
Unenhanced CT scan from patient with ruptured saccular aneurysm. Blood fills the subarachnoid space over the cerebral hemispheres as well as entering the sulci and interhemispheric fissure.

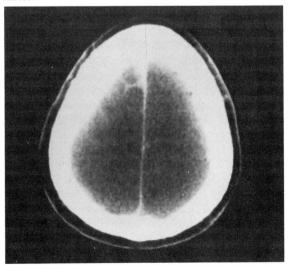

neous subarachnoid hemorrhage from a traumatic tap. The proportion of white to red blood cells in the CSF is usually the same as in the circulating blood, but in some patients a brisk leukocytosis appears within 48 h, reaching 2000 to 3000 cells per cubic millimeter. The protein is elevated, and in some instances glucose is abnormally low.

Skull films are usually negative, though in a few patients they may show erosion of one or both of the anterior clinoid processes from the pressure of an adjacent aneurysm, or calcification in the region of a previous hemorrhage. A calcified pineal gland may be displaced by an intracerebral or subdural clot. In general the skull films yield so little information that they are hardly worthwhile, unless a head injury and skull fracture cannot be excluded.

A transient albuminuria and glycosuria may be present for a few days. Rarely diabetes insipidus occurs. A leukocytosis of 15,000 to 18,000 cells per cubic millimeter is common.

Acute subarachnoid hemorrhage may be associated with ECG abnormalities suggestive of myocardial ischemia. The EEG is of little help in localizing the lesion unless a gross neurologic deficit is present, in which case the localization is probably evident clinically.

Course and Prognosis The outstanding characteristic of this condition is the tendency for the hemorrhage to recur. This threat colors all prognostications, and unfortunately there appears to be no way of determining reliably which cases will bleed again. The cause of recurrent bleeding is not understood, but may be related to naturally occurring mechanisms of clot formation and lysis.

Patients with the typical clinical picture of spontaneous subarachnoid hemorrhage, but in whom the angiogram shows no aneurysm or arteriovenous malformation, have a slightly better prognosis than those in whom the lesion is demonstrated. If negative, it is usually advisable to repeat the arteriogram in 2 weeks, because vascular spasm may have obscured the aneurysm in the first one.

McKissock, Paine, and Walsh found that the patient's state of consciousness at the time of arteriography was the single best criterion of prognosis. Their data, representative of most large series, indicate that of every 100 patients reaching a hospital and coming to arteriography, 17 will be stuporous or comatose, and 83 will appear to be recovering from the ictus. At the end of the next 6 months, 7 of the first 17 patients will have died from the original hemorrhage, and 7 more will have had a fatal recurrence. Of the other 83, 1 will have died of the original hemorrhage and 52 will have had a recurrence, of which 33 will have died. Thus, of the entire 100

patients, at the end of 6 months, 8 will have died of the original hemorrhage, 59 will have had a recurrence, with 40 deaths, making a total of 48 deaths and 52 survivors. Of the survivors in the series of McKissock et al., 36 went back to full work, 12 were partly disabled, and 4 were totally disabled. The disability was due to paralysis, mental deterioration, or epilepsy.

In regard to the recurrence of bleeding, it was found that of every 50 patients seen on the first day of the illness, 5 rebled in the first week (all fatal), 8 in the second week (5 fatal), 6 in the third and fourth weeks (4 fatal), and 2 in the next 4 weeks (2 fatal), making a total of 21 recurrences in 8 weeks (16 fatal). Rerupture did not occur in the first 2 days; thereafter, it occurred at a steady rate for the next 19 days and tapered off abruptly. However, in the case of patients at the Massachusetts General Hospital and the Cleveland Metropolitan Hospital, rerupture in the first 2 days certainly occurs.

Treatment General medical management in the acute stage is similar to that described under "Atherothrombotic Infarction," above. The earlier the case comes under medical purview and the more severe the impairment of consciousness, the less certain are therapeutic measures to be beneficial. Operations on patients who are stuporous or comatose carry an unacceptable risk; the mortality rate approaches 50 percent. The medical program outlined below must be instituted at once in these patients as well as in those whose condition warrants a direct surgical approach. With the advances in neurosurgery (microsurgery and efficient hemostasis) operation is the recommended definitive treatment, once a patient's condition improves. Patients who survive in good condition for several days have the best outlook, and with the passage of time the risk of recurrent bleeding diminishes.

Rational medical measures are based on the assumption that decreasing the arterial blood pressure is the most reasonable way of arresting the hemorrhage and preventing recurrence. Absolute bed rest for 4 to 6 weeks is prescribed, with the head of the bed raised some 15 to 20°. Straining during bowel movement is forbidden, and laxatives or gentle enemas are administered. Coughing and all forms of exertion are avoided. The patient is fed. The duration of the period of bed rest is empiric and not founded on any reliable clinical observations or information about the formation of scar tissue around aneurysms. Sedatives and analgesics are important in aiding relaxation. Hypotensive agents are used to bring high blood pressures to normal. In the presence of severe hypertension, ganglionic blocking agents may be cautiously used to lower the blood pressure to 160/100, great care being exercised not to precipitate excessive hypotension and cerebral infarction. Restlessness should be treated with barbiturates, which also help to lower blood pressure, and pain is controlled by salicylates, codeine, or meperidine. Promazine intramuscularly is used to control nausea and vomiting. Phenytoin or phenobarbital may be prescribed to prevent seizures.

At present, the systemic antifibrinolysin aminocaproic acid (Amicar) is being administered, with the idea of impeding lysis of the clot at the site of aneurysmal rupture. An initial dose of 5 g is given intravenously or orally followed by 1- to 1.25-g doses at hourly intervals, not to exceed 30 g in any 24-h period. The drug is given from the onset of bleeding to the time of operation, but not longer than 3 weeks. This drug, although not yet approved by the FDA for this purpose, seems to have been effective in reducing the incidence of rebleeding. Tranexamic acid, another fibrinolytic agent given intravenously is said to reduce the incidence of rebleeding (Fodstad et al.), but some dispute these findings. With both antifibrinolytic agents there is some risk of venous thrombosis. The patient fares better if antihypertensive medicines are not given concomitantly. To prevent vascular spasm, which may result in a disastrous hemiplegia, reserpine (Serpasil) in a dose of 0.2 mg intramuscularly tid and kanamycin (Kantrex) 1.0 g orally qid are being tried and have given promising results. Nitroprusside and trimethaphan camsylate and blood volume expanders have been given to prevent vascular spasm, but the efficacy of these measures is still under study.

Repeated drainage of the CSF by lumbar puncture is no longer practiced. One lumbar puncture is usually carried out for diagnostic purposes, and thereafter it is performed only for the relief of intractable headache, to detect recurrence of bleeding, or to measure the intracranial pressure prior to surgery.

In maintaining fluid balance, intravenous fluid should be used sparingly and in the proper electrolyte combination (a mixture of equal parts of 5% glucose in water and normal saline solution or balanced electrolytes) in order to minimize the danger of brain swelling. If diabetes insipidus has occurred, it should be treated with vasopressin. Body hypothermia for 2 to 5 days in the stage of acute hemorrhage has been used with uncertain efficacy. Intravenous mannitol may be effective in temporarily reducing the intracranial pressure, but has

been suspected of precipitating or aggravating rebleeding.

After a period of 4 to 6 weeks in bed, the patient is gradually allowed to resume activity and may return to work in 4 months. It seems logical to advise that strenuous physical activity not be resumed.

Surgical Therapy   Apart from occasionally evacuating an associated intracerebral clot or placing a ventriculo-atrial shunt to relieve the stupor and tension hydrocephalus that sometimes develop after aneurysmal rupture (see above), surgical treatment is directed to the prevention of recurrence of hemorrhage. The procedures are either *extracranial* (ligation of the common carotid in the neck) or *intracranial* (clipping or ligating the neck of the aneurysm; wrapping or tamponade of the aneurysmal sac by muscle, fascia, plastic coating, or arterial graft; trapping the aneurysm; ligation of the main feeding vessel proximal to the aneurysm). Occasionally extracranial and intracranial procedures are combined. Because of the aforementioned high mortality if surgery is undertaken early, operation is usually delayed for 1 to 2 weeks after rupture, allowing the patient's condition to stabilize. Before treatment is undertaken, the site, size, and form of the aneurysm must be determined by angiography. At the same time the pattern of the anterior half of the circle of Willis is noted, as it may influence the choice of operative procedure. It has been demonstrated that in patients with middle cerebral and internal carotid-posterior communicating aneurysms surgical treatment is superior to conservative treatment; with anterior communicating aneurysms, the mortality is about the same (McKissock, Richardson, and Walsh, 1962, 1965).

The most informative study of the long-term prognosis in patients who were treated only by a conservative medical program is that of Richardson and Jane. They followed 364 patients for a period of up to 21 years after subarachnoid hemorrhage from an aneurysm of the posterior communicating (29 percent) or anterior cerebral artery (71 percent). Since these patients had a single aneurysm, they would have been candidates for surgery. Of 213 who survived 6 months or more, 61 had another hemorrhage within 10 years. Death occurred in 27 of 41 anterior cerebral aneurysm cases that rebled and in 10 of the 20 posterior communicating cases. Repeat angiograms showed enlargement of the aneurysms. The rebleeding rate is estimated to be 3 percent per year. The authors are convinced that a similar study of surviving surgically treated patients, even with an estimated operative mortality of 5 percent, would fare better. Presently it is our practice to refer all patients whose condition has stabilized to our neurosurgical colleagues for direct ligation.

ARTERIOVENOUS MALFORMATIONS OF THE BRAIN

An arteriovenous (AV) malformation consists of a tangle of dilated vessels which form an abnormal communication between the arterial and venous systems, really an arteriovenous fistula. It is a developmental abnormality, representing persistence of an embryonic pattern of blood vessels, and not a neoplasm, but the constituent vessels enlarge with growth and the passage of time. AV malformations have been designated by a number of other terms, such as angioma and arteriovenous aneurysm, but these are less appropriate; *angioma* suggests a tumor and *aneurysm* is generally reserved for the saccular lesion described above.

Vascular malformations vary in size from a small blemish, a few millimeters in diameter, lying in the cortex or white matter, to a huge mass of tortuous channels comprising an AV shunt of enough magnitude, in rare instances, to raise cardiac output. Hypertrophic dilated *arterial feeders* approach the main lesion, disappear below the cortex, and break up into a network of thin-walled blood vessels which connect directly with draining veins. The latter often form huge, dilated, pulsating channels, carrying away arterial blood. The tangled blood vessels interposed between arteries and veins are abnormally thin and do not have the normal structure of arteries or viens. AV malformations occur in all parts of the brain, brainstem, and spinal cord, but the larger ones are more frequently found in the posterior half of the cerebral hemispheres, commonly forming a wedge-shaped lesion extending from the cortex to the ventricular lining.

AV malformations are more common in males than females. They may occur in more than one member of a family in the same or successive generations. Although the lesion is present from birth, onset of symptoms is most common between 10 and 30 years of age, but occasionally is delayed to as late as age 50 or beyond. In about half the patients, the first clinical manifestation is a cerebral or cerebral-subarachnoid hemorrhage; in 30 percent, a seizure is the first manifestation; and in 20 percent, headache, hemiparesis or other focal neurologic sign. The seizure pattern depends on the site of the lesion; when focal motor in type, the seizure may be followed by a temporary postictal paralysis. When hemorrhage occurs, blood may enter the subarachnoid space almost exclusively, producing a picture identical with that of ruptured saccular aneurysm, but since the AV malformation lies within the cerebral tissue, bleed-

ing is more likely to be partly intracerebral, causing a hemiparesis, hemiplegia, etc., or even death.

Before rupture, chronic nondescript headache is a frequent complaint. Occasionally typical migraine is associated, but this is probably a coincidence. Huge AV malformations may produce a slowly progressive neurologic deficit because of diversion of blood from adjacent brain or compression of neighboring structures by the enlarging mass of vessels. When the vein of Galen is involved, hydrocephalus may result. Not infrequently one or both carotid arteries pulsate unusually forcefully in the neck. A systolic bruit heard over the carotid in the neck, or the mastoid process, or the eyeballs in young adults is almost pathognomonic of angioma. The patient should be exercised in order to bring out a bruit if none is present at rest. A bruit may be heard over a spinal angioma of large size. The blood pressure may be raised or normal, and it is axiomatic that the occurrence of intracranial bleeding with normal blood pressure should lead to the suspicion of an AV malformation, ruptured saccular aneurysm, a bleeding diathesis, or hemorrhage into a tumor. Inspection of the eye grounds may disclose a vascular malformation of the retina, which is coextensive with a malformation of the optic nerve and basal portions of the brain. Skull films occasionally show crescentic linear calcifications in the territory of larger malformations. Most AV malformations are revealed by CT scan if iodine enhancement is used (Fig. 33-24). Arteriography establishes the diagnosis with certainty, and will demonstrate AV malformations larger than 5 mm in diameter. Small ones may be obscured by hemorrhage, and even at autopsy a careful search under the dissecting microscope may be necessary to find them.

Most AV malformations are clinically silent for a long time, but will bleed sooner or later. The first hemorrhage may be fatal, but in more than 90 percent of cases bleeding stops and the patient survives. Recurrence of hemorrhage with a fatal outcome is a constant danger. Once bleeding has occurred the risk of recurrence is approximately 4 percent per year, if no treatment is given; if there has been no previous hemorrhage, the risk is less, perhaps 1 to 2 percent per year. About 50 percent of AV malformations are amenable to block dissection, with an operative mortality rate of approximately 5 percent. For the others a variety of treatment methods have been tried such as obliteration by means of artificial embolization, ligation of feeding arteries, and intravascular resins. One of the authors (R.D.A.) and R. N. Kjellberg have treated more than 200 AV malformations with low-dose focused proton beam. A single treatment is given, and the patient is sent home the following day. Recurrence of hemorrhage appears to be reduced, and in 2 years some of the AV malformations have virtually disappeared (Fig. 33-25). We must follow the cases for several more years to completely evaluate this method of therapy.

OTHER CAUSES OF INTRACRANIAL BLEEDING

Although *intracranial bleeding due to head trauma* does not rightfully fall within the scope of cerebrovascular disease, it must be mentioned here because of the great frequency with which it enters into the differential diagnosis, especially when the history is inadequate or the patient falls and is injured at the onset of the stroke. *Acute extradural* and *acute subdural hemorrhage* must always be considered in the patient who, under unknown circumstances, has rather abruptly developed a neurologic deficit such as hemiparesis or confusion, with or without bloody CSF. In *chronic subdural hemorrhage,* which can occur without known trauma, the in-

Figure 33-24
Contrast-enhanced CT scan showing an AV malformation of the temporal lobe.

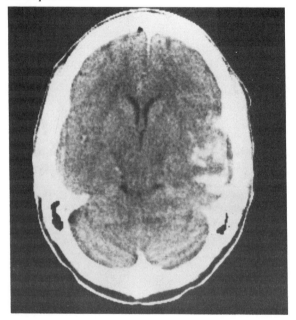

definite picture of drowsiness, confusion, and mild hemiparesis may erroneously be attributed to a stroke, especially in elderly persons. Failure to make the correct diagnosis deprives the patient of lifesaving surgical intervention. There should be no hesitation in subjecting those patients to CT scanning or arteriography, in whom subdural hemorrhage cannot be excluded on clinical grounds. If the patient falls, striking the head at the onset of a stroke, it may be difficult or impossible to decide if the blood in the CSF is due to the stroke or to *cerebral contusion.* Trauma may also cause *acute or delayed intracerebral hemorrhage, acute intracerebellar or infratentorial subdural hemorrhage, acute brain swelling,* and on rare occasions, extensive *focal infarction* of undetermined pathogenesis (see Chap. 34).

Several *hematologic disorders* are commonly complicated by hemorrhage into the brain. The most frequent of these are leukemia, aplastic anemia, and thrombocytopenic purpura. As a rule this complication signals a fatal issue. Other less common causes of intracerebral bleeding are advanced *liver disease* and *lymphoma.* Usually several factors are operative in these cases: reduction in prothrombin or other clotting elements (fibrinogen, factor V), bone marrow suppression by antineoplastic drugs, and disseminated intravascular coagulation. Any part of the brain may be involved, and often the hemorrhagic lesions are multiple. Often there is evidence of abnormal bleeding elsewhere (skin, mucous membranes, kidney) by the time cerebral hemorrhage occurs. Intracranial bleeding is also an important complication of *anticoagulant therapy;* the hemorrhages that develop may occur in the sites of predilection of hypertensive hemorrhage, or elsewhere. They tend to have a leisurely but steady evolution, and at times attempts to control them by reversal of the anticoagulant effects have failed. When precipitated by warfarin therapy, treatment by fresh-frozen plasma and vitamin K is recommended; when associated with aspirin therapy or other agents that affect platelet function, fresh platelet infusions, often in massive amounts, are required to control the hemorrhage.

Occasionally the origin of intracranial hemorrhage cannot be determined clinically and pathologically. In some postmortem cases a careful microscopic search discloses a small AV malformation in the cerebral tissue at one side of the hemorrhage, and on this basis it is suspected that an overlooked vascular malformation may have been the cause of the cerebral hemorrhage in other cases. *Primary* intraventricular hemorrhage, a rare event, is at times due to a vascular malformation or neoplasm of the choroid plexus; more often, such a hemorrhage is the result of paraventricular bleeding, in which blood enters the ventricle immediately, without producing a large parenchymal clot.

Hemorrhage into primary and secondary brain tumors is not rare, and when it is the first manifestation of the neoplasm, diagnosis may be extremely difficult. Choriocarcinoma, melanotic, renal cell, and bronchogenic carcinoma, pituitary adenoma, glioblastoma multiforme, and medulloblastoma may present in this way. Careful inquiry will usually disclose that neurologic symptoms, compatible with intracranial tumor growth, had preceded the onset of hemorrhage. Needless to say, a thorough search should be made in these circumstances for evidence of intracranial tumor or of secondary tumor deposits in other organs. A chest film will show metastatic or primary neoplasm in 75 percent of cases and should be performed in all cases of obscure intracerebral hemorrhage.

Mycotic aneurysm, the result of *septic embolism,* is a rare cause of massive intracranial bleeding. Any part of the circulatory tree may be involved, but usually the aneurysm lies at a forking of a small meningeal branch (about 0.5 mm in diameter) of the middle cerebral artery.

Brain purpura, incorrectly referred to as hemorrhagic encephalitis, consists of multiple petechial hemorrhages scattered throughout the white matter of the brain. This disorder is described on pages 662 and 787. The clinical picture is that of a diffuse cerebral disease. There is never blood in the CSF and the condition should not be confused with a stroke.

Brainstem hemorrhages secondary to temporal lobe herniation are extremely common but never present as a cerebrovascular accident.

Inflammatory diseases of arteries and veins, especially polyarteritis nodosa and lupus erythematosus, are sometimes associated with hemorrhage into the nervous system. In polyarteritis, rupture of a vessel may occur on the basis of hypertension or local vascular disease. Also in lupus erythematosus, hemorrhage may be attributable to hypertension or to disease of the vascular wall of undetermined nature. Bleeding nearly always occurs into the brain tissue rather than the subarachnoid space.

The other rare types of hemorrhage, listed in Table 33-5, are self-explanatory.

Hemorrhages of *intraspinal* origin may be the result of trauma, AV malformations (the usual cause of

PRE

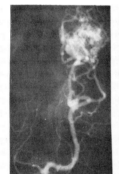
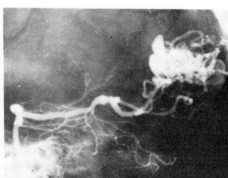

PROTON RX   10/14/77

2.0 YRS POST

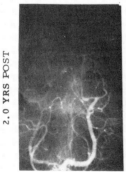
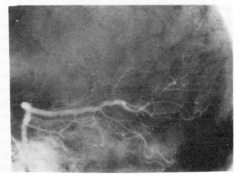

Figure 33-25

Top. *Parietooccipital AV malformation, fed by the posterior cerebral artery, in a 50-year-old woman. The AV malformation had bled and caused small intracerebral and subdural hematomas, with a visual field defect. Bottom. Arteriograms taken 2 years after proton beam treatment. The patient was asymptomatic.*

nontraumatic hematomyelia), or bleeding into tumors. Spinal subarachnoid hemorrhage from an AV malformation may simulate an intracranial subarachnoid hemorrhage, causing headache, stiff neck, and even subhyaloid hemorrhages. Extradural and subdural extravasations may be *spontaneous* (often in relation to rheumatoid arthritis), but much more often are due to trauma or anticoagulants, or both. Extradural spinal hemorrhage causes the rapid evolution of paraplegia, and diagnosis must be prompt if function is to be salvaged by surgical drainage.

HYPERTENSIVE ENCEPHALOPATHY

This term refers to a relatively acute syndrome in which severe hypertension is associated with headache, nausea and vomiting, visual disturbances, convulsions, confusion, stupor, and coma. These symptoms of diffuse cerebral disturbance may be accompanied by focal or lateralizing neurologic signs, either transitory or lasting, which should always suggest cerebral hemorrhage or infarction, i.e., the more common cerebrovascular complications of severe chronic hypertension. Multiple microinfarcts and petechial hemorrhages in one region may result in a mild hemiparesis, aphasic disorder, or rapid failure of vision (retinal lesions). By the time the neurologic manifestations appear, the hypertension has usually reached the malignant stage, with retinal hemorrhages, exudates, and papilledema (*hypertensive retinopathy* grade IV), and evidence of renal and cardiac disease. In many but not all the cases, the CSF pressure and protein values are elevated, the latter to more than 100 mg per 100 ml in some cases. The hypertension may be "essential" or due to chronic renal disease, acute glomerulonephritis, acute toxemia of pregnancy, pheochromocytoma, Cushing's syndrome, or ACTH toxicity. Lowering of the blood pressure with hypotensive drugs may reverse the picture in a day or two. If the hypertension cannot be controlled, the outcome is usually fatal.

Neuropathologic examination may reveal a rather normal-looking brain, but occasionally cerebral swelling or hemorrhages of various sizes, or both, will be found. A cerebellar pressure cone reflects increased volume of tissue and increased pressure in the posterior fossa, and in some instances lumbar puncture may have precipitated a fatality. Microscopically there are widespread minute infarcts in the brain (with a predilection for the basis pontis), the result of fibrinoid necrosis of the walls of arterioles and capillaries, and occlusion of their lumens by fibrin thrombi. Similar vascular changes are found in other organs, particularly the retinae and the kidneys.

Volhard originally attributed the symptoms of hypertensive encephalopathy to vasospasm. This notion was reinforced by Byrom, who demonstrated, in rats, a segmental constriction and dilatation of cerebral and retinal arterioles in response to severe hypertension. However, the observations of Byrom, and of others, indicate that the overdistension of the arterioles, rather than the excessive constriction, may be responsible for the necrosis of the vessel wall (see recent reviews of Auer and of Chester et al.).

The term *hypertensive encephalopathy* should be reserved for the above syndrome and should not be used to refer to chronic recurrent headaches, dizziness, epileptic seizures, transient ischemic attacks, or strokes which often occur in association with high blood pressure.

INFLAMMATORY DISEASES OF BRAIN ARTERIES

Inflammatory diseases of the blood vessels of infectious origin, and their effects upon the nervous system, are considered in detail in Chap. 31. *Meningovascular syphilis, tuberculous meningitis, fungal meningitis*, and the *subacute forms of bacterial meningitis* (*H. influenzae*, staphylococcal, pneumococcal) may be accompanied by inflammatory changes and vascular occlusion of either the cerebral arteries or veins. Occasionally in syphilitic and tuberculous meningitis a stroke may be the first clinical sign of meningitis; more often it develops after the meningeal symptoms are established.

Typhus, schistosomiasis, mucormycosis, malaria, and trichinosis are rare types of infective diseases of the arteries which, unlike the above, are not secondary to meningeal inflammation. In *typhus and other rickettsial diseases*, capillary and arteriolar changes and perivascular inflammatory cells are found in the brain, and presumably they underlie the convulsions, acute psychoses, and coma which characterize the neurologic disorder in these diseases. The internal carotid artery may be occluded in diabetic patients as part of the orbital and cavernous sinus infections with *mucormycosis*. In *trichinosis*, the cause of the cerebral symptoms has not been established. Parasites have been found in the brain; in one of our cases the cerebral lesions were produced by bland emboli arising in the heart and related to a severe myocarditis. In *cerebral malaria* convulsions, coma and sometimes focal symptoms appear to be due to blockage of capillaries and precapillaries by masses of parasitized red blood corpuscles. The neurologic effects of all these diseases are discussed further in Chap. 31.

OTHER INFLAMMATORY AND NONINFLAMMATORY DISEASES OF CRANIAL ARTERIES

Included under this heading is a diverse group of arteritides that have little in common with one another, except their tendency to involve the cerebral vasculature: temporal (giant cell or cranial) arteritis, granulomatous arteritis, polyarteritis nodosa, systemic lupus erythematosus, marantic endocarditis with cerebral embolism, rheumatic arteritis, thrombotic thrombocytopenic purpura, and the cerebrovascular lesions associated with oral contraceptives.

Temporal Arteritis (Giant Cell or Cranial Arteritis) This is an uncommon affliction of elderly persons in which arteries of the external carotid system, particularly the temporal branches, are the seat of a subacute granulomatous inflammation with an exudate of lymphocytes and other mononuclear cells, neutrophilic leucocytes, and giant cells. Usually the most severely affected parts of the artery become thrombosed.

Headache or head pain is the chief complaint, and there may be severe pain, aching, and stiffness in the proximal muscles of the limbs, associated with a markedly elevated sedimentation rate. Thus the clinical picture overlaps that of *polymyalgia rheumatica*. Other less frequent systemic manifestations include fever, anorexia and loss of weight, malaise, anemia, and slight leucocytosis.

Occlusion of branches of the ophthalmic artery results in blindness in one or both eyes in over 25 percent of patients, and occasionally an ophthalmoplegia due to involvement of ocular nerves occurs. An arteritis of the aorta and its major branches, including carotid, subclavian, coronary, and femoral, is found at postmortem examination. Significant inflammatory involvement of intracranial arteries is rare but strokes occur occasionally on the basis of occlusion of the internal carotid and vertebral arteries. The diagnosis should be suspected in elderly patients who develop severe, persistent headache, and depends on finding a tender thrombosed or thickened cranial artery and demonstration of the lesion in a biopsy. The administration of adrenal corticosteroids provides striking relief of the headache and polymyalgic symptoms and also prevents blindness.

Granulomatous Arteritis of the Brain Scattered examples of a small vessel, giant cell arteritis of undetermined etiology, in which only brain vessels are affected, have come to our notice over the years. The clinical state has taken diverse forms, sometimes presenting as a low-grade, nonfebrile meningitis with sterile CSF, followed by one or several infarcts in parts of the cerebrum or cerebellum. In other cases it has masqueraded as a cerebral tumor evolving over a period of weeks, or as a viral encephalitis. Severe headaches, focal cerebral or cerebellar signs of gradual onset (seldom strokelike), CSF pleocytosis and elevated protein, and papilledema (in about half the cases) as a result of increased intracranial pressure has been the most frequently encountered syndrome. In some instances the diagnosis was made after tissue was excised during an operation for a suspected brain tumor, and in others the findings at autopsy came as a distinct surprise.

The affected vessels are in the 100- to 500-μm range and are surrounded and infiltrated by lymphocytes, plasma cells, and other mononuclear cells; giant cells are distributed in small numbers in the media, adventitia, or perivascular connective tissue. Infarction of tissue relates to thrombosis. The meninges are variably infiltrated with inflammatory cells. Usually only a part of the brain has been affected—in one instance the cerebellum, in another one frontal lobe and the opposite parietal lobe. The disease raises questions of sarcoidosis, which is believed at times to be limited to the nervous system, or to the special type of polyarteritis (allergic granulomatous angiitis) described by Churg and Strauss. Unlike the latter disease, however, the lungs and other organs are spared; there is no eosinophilia, increase in sedimentation rate, or anemia. We have the impression that some patients suspected of this disease (those presenting as an aseptic meningitis with multiple infarcts) have responded dramatically to corticosteroid therapy.

In *polyarteritis (periarteritis) nodosa*, there is an inflammatory necrosis of arteries and arterioles throughout the body. The lungs are usually spared, which is the basis of distinguishing this form of vasculitis from allergic granulomatous angiitis, mentioned above. The vasa nervorum are involved frequently by the lesions of polyarteritis, giving rise to a *mononeuropathy multiplex* or to a symmetrical polyneuropathy (see page 903). Involvement of the central nervous system is unusual and takes the form of widespread microinfarcts; macroscopic infarction is a rarity.

There is also another type of small vessel arteritis occurring as a hypersensitivity phenomenon. Often it is associated with an allergic skin lesion. The clinical picture does not resemble that of polyarteritis nodosa; the response to corticosteroids is excellent.

Systemic Lupus Erythematosus The involvement of the nervous system is an important aspect of this disease. In the series reported by Johnson and Richardson, the central nervous system was involved in 75 percent of cases. Cerebral seizures, disturbances of mental function and of consciousness, and signs referable to cranial nerves are the usual neurologic manifestations; most often they develop in the late stages of the disease, but they may occur early and may be mild and transient. Hemiparesis, paraparesis, aphasia, homonymous hemianopia, movement disorders, and derangements of hypothalamic function are less common. The CSF is entirely normal or shows only a mild lymphocytic pleocytosis and increase in protein content—although in some patients, primarily those with myelopathy and peripheral neuropathy, which are rare complications of systemic lupus erythematosus, the protein content may be greatly increased.

Most of the neurologic manifestations can be accounted for by widespread microinfarcts in the cerebral cortex and brainstem, and these in turn are related to destructive and proliferative changes in arterioles and capillaries. The acute lesion is subtle and elusive; it is not a typical fibrinoid necrosis of the vessel wall, like that in hypertensive encephalopathy. There is no cellular infiltration. Thus, the changes do not represent a vasculitis in the strict sense of the word. Other neurologic manifestations are related to hypertension, which frequently accompanies systemic lupus erythematosus and may precipitate cerebral hemorrhage; to endocarditis which may give rise to cerebral embolism; and to treatment with corticosteroids which may precipitate or accentuate seizures and psychosis. In other cases, steroids appear to improve these latter neurologic manifestations.

Marantic Endocarditis and Cerebral Embolism Sterile vegetations, referred to also as *terminal or nonbacterial thrombotic endocarditis*, consist of fibrin and platelets and are loosely attached to the mitral and aortic valves and contiguous endocardium. They are a common source of cerebral embolism (almost 10 percent of all instances of cerebral embolism, according to Barron et al.). The vegetations are usually associated with a malignant neoplasm, but may occur in patients debilitated by other diseases. Except for the setting in which it occurs, marantic embolism has no distinctive clinical features

that permit differentiation from cerebral embolism of other types. The apoplectic nature of marantic embolism distinguishes it from tumor metastases. The hazards of anticoagulants in gravely ill patients with widespread malignant disease probably outweigh the benefits to be derived from this form of treatment.

The lesions of small cerebral arteries observed in patients with rheumatic heart disease and referred to as *rheumatic arteritis* have not been well characterized, clinically or pathologically. The vascular lesions and the microinfarcts that accompany them probably represent cerebral emboli.

Venous Thrombosis Thrombophlebitis of bacterial origin and its main clinical features are described in Chap. 31. There occurs, in addition, bland occlusion of cerebral veins (phlebothrombosis), taking the form of either a brain hemorrhage or infarctive stroke. Diagnosis is difficult except in certain clinical settings known to favor the occurrence of venous thrombosis, such as cyanotic congenital heart disease, the puerperium and possibly the postoperative period, sickle-cell anemia, and polycythemia. A stroke in patients suffering from any one of these conditions is suggestive of venous thrombosis though in some instances—e.g., postpartum strokes—arteries are occluded as often as veins. The slower evolution of the clinical syndrome and its greater epileptogenic potential and hemorrhagic tendency favor venous over arterial thrombosis.

Averback has reported seven cases of venous thrombosis in young adults and emphasizes the diversity of the clinical state. Two of his patients had carcinoma of the breast, and one, ulcerative colitis; both of these conditions are known to be associated with hypercoagulability of blood, stickiness of platelets, and thrombocytosis. In the other four patients, the underlying cause could not be established. Headache, drowsiness, aphasia, and hemiplegia progressed to coma within hours to days. CT scan should be helpful in the diagnosis of the hemorrhagic variety of the disease and the venous phase of the carotid arteriogram should show the occlusion. The CSF pressure is usually increased and may be clear or sanguinous.

Thrombotic Thrombocytopenic Purpura (TTP, Thrombotic Microangiopathy, Moschkowitz's Syndrome) This is yet another uncommon but serious disease of the small blood vessels, observed mainly in young adults. It is characterized pathologically by widespread occlusions of arterioles and capillaries involving practically all organs of the body, including the brain. The nature of the occluding material has not been completely defined. Fibrin components have been identified by immunofluorescent techniques; some investigators have demonstrated disseminated intravascular platelet aggregation, rather than fibrin thrombi.

Clinically, virtually all patients have fever, anemia, symptoms of renal and hepatic disease, and thrombocytopenia—the latter giving rise to the common hemorrhagic manifestations (petechiae and ecchymoses of the skin, retinal hemorrhages, hematuria, gastrointestinal bleeding, etc.). Neurologic symptoms are practically always present, and are the initial manifestation of the disease in about half the cases. Confusion, delirium, seizures, and altered states of consciousness which are sometimes remittent or fluctuating in nature are the usual signs of nervous system disorder and are readily explained by the widespread microscopic ischemic damage in the brain. Gross infarction is rarely observed.

Thrombocytosis and Thrombocythemia   These terms refer to an elevation of platelets above 800,000 per cubic millimeter. The condition is generally considered to be a form of myeloproliferative disorder. Some of the patients have an enlarged spleen, polycythemia, chronic myelogenous leukemia or myelosclerosis. Several patients have been observed on our wards in whom no explanation of the thrombocytosis was found. They presented with recurrent thrombotic episodes, often of minor degree and transient. Plasmapheresis to reduce the platelets and antimitotic drugs to suppress megakaryocytes relieved the neurologic symptoms.

Thromboangiitis Obliterans of Cerebral Vessels (Winiwarter-Buerger Disease)   Despite the large volume of literature on the subject, there is little evidence that this is a recognizable entity. Thin, threadlike, white leptomeningeal arteries and border-zone infarction of the brain have been considered characteristic, but as C. M. Fisher has convincingly demonstrated, these lesions are simply the result of atherosclerosis or embolic occlusion of the carotid or cerebral arteries with *stasis thrombosis* and organization of the more distant cerebral branches. Buerger's disease of the legs has an equally dubious status.

THE DIAGNOSIS OF CEREBROVASCULAR DISEASE

There are two separate aspects of the problem of differential diagnosis: (1) vascular disease must be distinguished from other neurologic illnesses, and (2) the different kinds of vascular disease must be separated from one another. In the following paragraphs many of the important points discussed in the body of the chapter will be summarized.

DIFFERENTIATION OF VASCULAR DISEASE FROM OTHER NEUROLOGIC ILLNESSES

The diagnosis of a vascular lesion rests essentially on recognition of the stroke syndrome, and without evidence of this the diagnosis must always be in doubt. The three criteria by which the stroke is identified should be reemphasized: (1) the temporal profile of the clinical syndrome, (2) evidence of focal brain disease, and (3) the clinical setting. The temporal profile can usually be defined by a clear history of premonitory phenomena, the mode of onset, and the evolution of the neurologic disturbance in relationship to the patient's medical status. If these data are lacking, the course may still be determined by extending the period of observation for a few days or weeks, thus resorting to the clinical rule that the physician's best diagnostic tool is the second and third examination. An inadequate history is the most frequent cause of diagnostic errors.

As has already been stated, the neurologic deficit in a stroke develops suddenly, and later in the illness, if death does not occur, stabilization and some degree of recovery take place. There are few categories of neurologic disease whose temporal profile mimics that of the cerebrovascular disorders. The neurologic deficit of migraine may do so, but the history usually provides the diagnosis. Tumor, infection, inflammation, degeneration, and nutritional disease are not likely to manifest themselves precipitously. In trauma, of course, a sudden insult occurs, but usually the cause is readily discerned. In multiple sclerosis and other demyelinative diseases, there may be a relatively abrupt onset or exacerbation of symptoms, but for the most part they occur in a different age group and clinical setting.

Many thrombotic strokes are preceded by transient ischemic attacks (TIAs) which, if recognized, are diagnostic of vascular disease. It is essential that TIAs be differentiated from cerebral seizures, syncopal attacks, neurologic migraine, and attacks of labyrinthine vertigo, since a failure to do so may result in a series of unnecessary arteriographic studies and even a surgical operation. A stroke developing over a period of several days usually progresses in a stepwise fashion, increments of deficit being added from time to time. A slow, gradual downhill course over a period of 2 weeks or more indicates that the lesion is probably not vascular, but rather a tumor, abscess, granuloma, or subdural hematoma.

In regard to the focal neurologic deficit of cerebrovascular diseases, many nonvascular diseases (tumor, abscess, multiple sclerosis, multifocal leukoencephalitis, etc.) may produce symptoms which are not strikingly different, and the diagnosis usually cannot rest solely on this aspect of the clinical picture. Nonetheless, certain combinations of neurologic signs which comform to a neurovascular pattern, e.g., the lateral medullary syndrome, are seen almost exclusively in occlusive vascular disease.

The presence of *blood in the CSF* always points to a cerebrovascular lesion, provided that trauma and a *traumatic tap* can be excluded. *Headache* is common in cerebrovascular disease; it occurs not only in hemorrhage but also in thrombosis and embolism. *Cerebral seizures* are almost never the premonitory, first, or only manifestation of a stroke but can occur in the first few hours after infarction or intracranial bleeding. *Brief unconsciousness* (5 to 10 min) is rare in stroke cases, being seen only in ruptured aneurysm and basilar artery insufficiency. Certain neurologic disturbances are hardly ever attributable to stroke, e.g., diabetes insipidus, bitemporal hemianopia, parkinsonism, generalized myoclonus, and isolated cranial nerve palsies, and their presence may be of help in ruling out vascular disease.

Finally, the diagnosis of cerebrovascular disease should always be made on positive data, and diagnosis by exclusion is to be deprecated.

A *few conditions are so often confused with cerebrovascular diseases that they merit further consideration.* When a history of trauma is absent, the headache, drowsiness, mild confusion, and hemiparesis of *subdural hematoma* may all too easily be ascribed to a "small stroke," and the patient may fail to receive immediate surgical therapy. In subdural hematoma the symptoms and signs usually develop gradually over a period of days or weeks. The degree of headache, obtundation, and confusion will be disproportionately great in comparison with the focal neurologic deficit, which tends to be indefinite and variable. In addition to the findings on CT scan and arteriography, a fracture line or shift of the pineal in the skull films may point to a subdural hematoma. The CSF may be blood-tinged or xanthochromic when the type of stroke under suspicion would not be expected to show this. Occasionally the EEG is strikingly silent over a subdural hematoma. If the patient has fallen and injured his or her head at the onset of the stroke, it may be impossible to rule out a complicating subdural hematoma on clinical grounds alone.

The reverse diagnostic error will not be made if one remembers that patients with subdural hematoma rarely exhibit a complete hemiplegia, monoplegia, hemianesthesia, homonymous hemianopia, or well-developed aphasia. If these focal signs are present and particularly if they developed suddenly, subdural hematoma is not likely to be the explanation.

A *brain tumor*—especially a rapidly growing glioblastoma multiforme, which may produce a severe hemiplegia within a week or two—can be mistaken for a stroke. Also, the neurologic deficit due to secondary carcinoma may evolve rapidly. However, in both conditions, a detailed history will show that the evolution of symptoms was gradual; and if they progressed in saltatory fashion, seizures will usually have occurred. The standard laboratory procedures should never be omitted in these circumstances. A chest film frequently discloses a primary or secondary tumor, and an increased blood sedimentation rate suggests that a concealed systemic disease process is at work. A lack of detailed history may also be responsible for the opposite diagnostic error, i.e., mistaking a relatively slowly evolving stroke (usually due to internal carotid artery occlusion) for a tumor. Arteriography and CT scanning will usually settle the problem. Rarely a *brain abscess* occurs without an evident antecedent focus of infection and may escape consideration in the differential diagnosis, especially if the patient is elderly.

Senile dementia is often ascribed, on insufficient grounds, to the occurrence of multiple small strokes. If vascular lesions are responsible, evidence of an apoplectic episode, to account for at least part of the syndrome, and of focal neurologic deficit will be disclosed by history and examination. The commonest cause of intellectual deterioration in the elderly patient is Alzheimer's disease or a related degenerative process, and in the absence of a history of episodic development or of focal neurologic signs, it is unwarranted to attribute this syndrome to cerebral vascular disease—in particular, to small strokes in silent areas. *Cerebral arteriosclerosis* is another term that is used carelessly as an explanation for such mental changes, the implication being that ischemia, focal or generalized, irreparably damages the nervous system, producing loss of intellectual function but no other focal neurologic signs. If cerebral arteriosclerosis (atherosclerosis) is actually responsible, there should be evidence of it in the brain (strokes) at some time in the course of the illness, and also in the heart (myocardial infarction, angina pectoris) or legs (intermittent claudication, loss of pulses). Frequently both ischemic infarction and Alzheimer's disease are present, and there may be difficulty in determining to what extent each of them is responsible for the neurologic deficit.

Chronic cerebral seizures occur as the result of stroke in some 20 percent of cases (*postinfarction epi-*

lepsy). When a history of the original stroke is lacking, or if the seizures are not properly observed or leave behind a temporary increase in the neurologic deficit (Todd's paralysis), the diagnosis of another stroke or of a tumor may be made in error.

Fear, anxiety, and depression in patients who have had one small stroke may lead to additional symptoms, such as generalized weakness, paresthesias, headache, or disequilibrium, which suggest to the patient and physician that further vascular lesions have occurred or threaten.

Miscellaneous conditions which occasionally lead to the suspicion of a stroke are Bell's palsy, Stokes-Adams attacks, a severe attack of labyrinthine vertigo, diabetic ophthalmoplegia, acute ulnar, radial, or peroneal palsy, embolism to a limb, and temporal arteritis associated with blindness.

Contrariwise, certain manifestations of stroke may be incorrectly interpreted as indicating other neurologic disorders. In the lateral medullary syndrome, *dysphagia* may be the outstanding feature, and if the syndrome is not kept in mind, a fruitless surgical investigation may be undertaken, looking for an esophageal neoplasm. *Headache* at times occurs as a prodrome of a thrombotic stroke or as an early manifestation of a cerebral or subarachnoid hemorrhage; unless this is appreciated a diagnosis of migraine may be made. *Dizzy spells or brief lapses or intermittent loss of equilibrium* due to vascular disease of the brainstem may be ascribed to Ménière's disease, Stokes-Adams syncope, or paroxysmal tachycardia. A detailed account of the attack will usually avert this error. A strikingly *focal monoplegia of cerebral origin* causing only weakness of the hand or causing only foot drop is not infrequently misdiagnosed as a peripheral lesion.

The differentiation of vascular from other neurologic diseases in the presence of coma offers special problems. If the patient is comatose when first seen and an adequate history is not available, cerebrovascular lesions have to be differentiated from all the other causes of coma described in Chap. 16. In most cases there will be some history to assist in the series of necessary diagnostic deductions.

Differentiation of Thrombosis, Embolism, Hypertensive Hemorrhage, and Ruptured Saccular Aneurysm Although it is difficult to lay down simple, hard-and-fast rules, it is usually possible to distinguish these four conditions at the bedside.

The most important diagnostic criteria of *atherosclerotic thrombosis* are (1) a history of prodromal TIAs, (2) an intermittent or stepwise evolution of the neurologic deficit, with recovery or improvement between worsenings, rather than a steady progression, (3) relative preservation of consciousness unless the upper part of the basilar territory is infarcted, (4) normal CSF, except for modest elevation of protein and occasional pleocytosis with massive infarction, (5) onset during sleep or shortly after arising or during a period of hypotension, (6) evidence of atherosclerosis elsewhere, especially in the coronary and peripheral vessels and the aorta, (7) the advanced age of the patient and the presence of disorders usually associated with atherosclerosis (hypertension, diabetes mellitus, and xanthomatosis), (8) headache of moderate severity (either as a prodromal warning or accompanying the stroke), (9) carotid bruit in the neck, indicating carotid stenosis, and (10) occlusion of the internal carotid artery in the neck as determined by palpation, auscultation, and ophthalmodynamometry.

Cerebral embolism is characterized by (1) abrupt development of the completed stroke—within a few seconds or minutes; (2) absence of prodromal TIAs (*rarely*, one or two transitory episodes occur in the hours before the stroke, especially if the embolus lodges in the carotid artery); (3) a source of emboli, usually in the heart, i.e., atrial fibrillation or other arrhythmia, myocardial infarction, subacute bacterial endocarditis, mitral stenosis, prolapsed mitral valve, valvulotomy or prosthetic valve, marantic endocarditis associated with carcinoma; (4) evidence of recent embolism in other organs, i.e., spleen, kidney, extremities, gastrointestinal tract, or lungs; (5) evidence of recent involvement of several regions of the brain in different cerebrovascular territories; (6) clear CSF except in a small proportion of cases with extensive hemorrhagic infarction; (7) rapid improvement (many embolic strokes produce persistent deficits, but it is not uncommon for an extensive focal deficit to reverse itself in minutes, hours, or days); (8) relative preservation of consciousness in the presence of extensive neurologic deficit, unless the upper part of the basilar territory is involved or massive brain swelling has occurred with temporal lobe–tentorial herniation; (9) occurrence at an age when atherosclerosis is usually not a factor and in the absence of hypertension, diabetes, arteritis, or infection; and (10) localized headache of moderate severity.

The diagnosis of arteritis as a cause of infarction is justifiable only in the following circumstances: (1) evidence of arteritis elsewhere; (2) in young individuals who manifest neither hypertension nor signs of cardiovascular disease; and (3) in individuals with an infection which could affect the meningeal vessels (syphilis, tuberculosis, etc.). *Venous thrombosis with infarction* should be considered when focal neurologic signs develop in the period following parturition or an operation, in the course of meningeal infection, ear or sinus suppuration, and in patients with cachexia, congenital heart disease, polycythemia, or sickle-cell disease.

In *hypertensive cerebral hemorrhage* the diagnosis rests on (1) presence of hypertension; (2) absence of prodromal phenomena; (3) frequent but not invariable occurrence of headache; (4) gradual development of a neurologic deficit over a period of 10 min up to several hours (sometimes the onset is more abrupt); (5) grossly bloody CSF (this also is not invariable for rarely the hemorrhage does not extend to the ventricular system and thus does not reach the CSF); (6) deepening stupor or coma (generally speaking, a patient with an extensive paralysis due to hemorrhage will be stuporous, whereas a hemiplegic stroke which leaves the patient alert and the mind relatively clear proves in nearly all instances to be due to an infarct); (7) onset during waking hours rather than in sleep; and (8) nuchal rigidity, except when deep coma supervenes.

The chief clinical features of *ruptured saccular aneurysms* are (1) sudden onset of severe headache; (2) brief or prolonged loss of consciousness at onset (in the most severe cases coma persists, and the patient dies within a few hours); (3) grossly bloody CSF under increased pressure; (4) relative alertness (after initial episode) and absence of focal neurologic signs (except for third or sixth nerve palsies); (5) preretinal (subhyaloid) hemorrhages (these suggest ruptured aneurysm or AV malformation, although they can occur in massive intracerebral hemorrhage and after trauma); (6) stiff neck on forward flexion, Kernig and Brudzinski signs; (7) transient weakness, numbness, aphasia, or seizure at onset; (8) usually an absence of warning attacks, although there may be a history of one or more transient episodes of headache ("leaks"?); (9) onset during exertion, sexual intercourse, etc.; (10) absence of hypertension in many cases; and (11) presence of coarctation of the aorta and polycystic disease of the kidneys in some cases.

Saccular aneurysm is likely to produce a diffuse subarachnoid hemorrhage without causing significant damage to the cerebral hemispheres. If the CSF is bloody and the patient retains mental clarity or is only mildly confused, aneurysm or cerebellar hemorrhage is the likely diagnosis. If the aneurysm also bleeds into the brain tissue or into the ventricular system, focal neurologic signs and coma ensue, as in intracerebral hemorrhage. Cerebral infarction in the 4- to 10-day period fol-

lowing aneurysmal rupture, is another cause of focal neurologic deficit.

Intracranial hemorrhage from a vascular malformation is a tenable diagnosis under the following circumstances: (1) stroke in a young patient with bloody CSF in the absence of hypertension; (2) antecedent epilepsy, often with transient postictal paralysis; (3) presence of a cervical or cranial bruit sometimes heard by the patient; (4) repeated subarachnoid hemorrhages (sometimes more than five); (5) calcification in the lesion in the skull films; and (6) lateralizing neurologic signs which are more frequent than with aneurysm.

THE COMMON CLINICAL PROBLEMS CREATED BY CEREBROVASCULAR DISEASES

The perceptive physician realizes at once that the diagnosis of cerebrovascular diseases may be ridiculously simple or incredibly difficult. The welter of details that have accumulated about cerebrovascular diseases is hardly reassuring to one who seeks a confident clinical approach to this category of disease. Yet experience teaches that certain diagnostic problems recur with impressive consistency and a planned approach to each of them enables the physician to make a correct diagnosis in 80 to 90 percent of cases, and to take proper action.

THE PATIENT ARRIVING COMATOSE

The most common vascular cause of coma is intracranial hemorrhage, usually one deep in the substance of the brain in a setting of hypertension. Less often it results from the meningocerebral or subarachnoid hemorrhage of a ruptured aneurysm or AV malformation or from occlusion of the basilar artery or both carotid arteries.

The comatose state from hypertensive hemorrhage or from aneurysmal meningocerebral hemorrhage probably reflects disordered function of the upper brainstem. This may be because of transtentorial-temporal herniation from the accumulating mass of blood in one cerebral hemisphere, disruption from pontine hemorrhage, or compression from upward cerebellar herniation in the case of a cerebellar hemorrhage. When temporal lobe–transtentorial herniation has occurred, the brainstem dysfunction may be so complete as to mask the unilateral signs of the basal ganglionic-capsular hemorrhage. The coma is then accompanied by decerebration and bilateral signs. Then the larger pupil, which is usually ipsilateral to the involved hemisphere, may provide the only clue. In these circumstances the CSF will be bloody virtually without exception, but to do a lumbar puncture may worsen the patient's condition. When it is available, CT scanning is the preferred diagnostic step and lumbar puncture should be deferred. Arteriography with corroborative lumbar puncture is a second choice. Urgency of action is no longer of importance, for in coma from all the foregoing causes, the outlook is rather hopeless. Surgical intervention in such cases is occasionally undertaken to relieve intracranial pressure on the chance that some of the functionally inactivated tissue is compressed but not yet destroyed. If such an attempt is decided upon, diagnostic procedures should be prompt and followed by surgical evacuation of the hematoma. Even with early craniotomy, however, the chances of survival and functional restoration are increased very little.

Coma due to ruptured aneurysm may occur without direct bleeding into the brain. The meningeal bleeding (pressure effect?) in the initial moments following rupture may abolish all cerebral and upper brainstem function and cause even a cessation of respiration and fall in heart rate and blood pressure. Death may occur in minutes. In some instances the patient is thought to be dead or dying and may be given artificial resuscitation. This state of deep coma, flaccid limbs, immobile eyes, and fixed pupils may persist for only a few moments, following which more vigorous heart action, rising blood pressure, and spontaneous respirations emerge, along with restoration of tone, reflexes, and eye movements; the coma gradually diminishes and is replaced by stupor and an improving state of consciousness over several hours. This continuously improving state is highly characteristic of ruptured aneurysm and is usually well under way by the time such patients reach a hospital. On examination, subhyaloid hemorrhages are occasionally seen and are diagnostic of ruptured aneurysm. Stiff neck can usually be elicited as the patient begins to awaken, but not when he or she is comatose or stuporous. Unless hemiplegia or other focal signs are present, the lumbar puncture should suffice as an initial diagnostic step. If the patient regains full alertness and has only headache and stiff neck, four-vessel arteriography is undertaken. If stuporous or semicomatose or severely hypertensive, arteriography should be deferred for a few days so that hypertension can be reduced and other later complications of ruptured aneurysm, such as spasm and hydrocephalus, can be sought at the same time as one attempts to visualize the aneurysm.

Infarction due to occlusion of a major cerebral artery may stupefy the patient but rarely causes deep coma unless the infarcted hemisphere herniates transtentorially. Coma from ischemic disease alone occurs in two circumstances, each highly lethal: basilar artery occlusion and bilateral carotid occlusion. In the latter circumstance, a unilateral carotid occlusion occurs on a background of a previous (sometimes asymptomatic) carotid artery occlusion on the other side. The result is bihemispheral cerebral infarction, which leaves the patient deeply comatose, bilaterally paralyzed, with almost unique, continuous, side-to-side ("metronomic") conjugate horizontal eye movements, only transiently interrupted by caloric stimulation or doll's-head maneuver. The diagnosis of basilar artery occlusion poses little problem when the brainstem is severely but incompletely damaged, as evidenced by ocular and other segmental brainstem abnormalities in combination with long tract signs. When there is nearly complete destruction of the brainstem, coma is accompanied by motor signs so symmetric and ocular motility so impaired that the state may be difficult to differentiate from severe drug intoxication on clinical grounds alone. In the latter state, ice-water caloric stimulation and brisk rotation of the head from side to side usually evoke ocular motility. In basilar and carotid artery occulsion the CSF is clear, and arteriography is currently the most direct corroborative diagnostic step. If lumbar puncture is delayed for many hours or days after the onset of a large embolic or thrombotic infarction, a brisk leukocytosis is occasionally found, reflecting the cellular response to the massive necrosis. CT scanning in this setting should suffice to settle any worries of occult abscess in a patient whose ictus had not been witnessed. If a decision is made to treat these cases, carotid endarterectomy is the only choice for carotid cases, while heparinization can be tried for either carotid or basilar cases, but in either event the results are disappointing.

In brief, there is usually little that can be done for the comatose stroke patient, other than to provide general supportive measures.

THE PATIENT WHO PRESENTS WITH A NONCOMATOSE NEUROLOGIC DISORDER OF RECENT ONSET

While the development of a stroke is so dramatically rapid that most other etiologies are readily excluded, there are several characteristic patterns of evolution within the group of stroke illnesses that help the physician to decide whether embolus, thrombosis, parenchymal hemorrhage, or ruptured aneurysm is responsible. A clear history is absolutely essential in differentiating these types of stroke. Their differentiating characteristics and the methods of investigation and management have already been outlined.

THE PATIENT WHO PRESENTS WITH A TRANSIENT ISCHEMIC ATTACK

As has been remarked, no reliable means have yet been developed to predict the outcome at any stage of the stroke process, and a significant percentage of patients develops massive infarction following what seemed initially to be a trivial transient attack. Once it has been determined that the focal neurologic disorder represents a transient ischemic attack, the patient should be subjected to an arteriogram, and *the timing of the arteriogram should reflect the proximity to the most recent TIA:* the more recent the attack, the more urgent the need for the arteriogram; an attack the day of admission warrants an arteriogram that day. In carotid artery disease, endarterectomy appears to halt the symptomatic progress and is warranted at the stage of TIAs or a minor persisting deficit, if it can be determined that the disease is principally located in the carotid sinus in the neck. Cases in which the disease falls heaviest on the intracranial portion of the artery, e.g., at the carotid siphon, and all cases of basilar disease, can only be treated with anticoagulants. It might be argued that arteriography be deferred in patients whose TIAs suggest disease of the basilar territory, since the arteriographic findings presumably would not modify the treatment plan. However, TIAs attributed on clinical grounds to basilar ischemia sometimes prove to be associated with carotid disease. Also, decisions regarding the vigor with which to pursue anticoagulant treatment and the expected outcome are made more easily with arteriographic information, but this is a matter of clinical judgment.

The routine investigation of TIAs by arteriography raises a number of problems. Symptomatic atherothrombosis involving the carotid or basilar artery is sometimes worsened drastically by this procedure. Our experience is similar to that of Faught and his colleagues, that cerebral complications occur in 5 to 10 percent of patients. Fortunately, most are reversible but, even in the best of hands, some 2 to 3 percent will have permanent deficits related to the arteriographic procedure. Increasing use is being made of noninvasive methods, such as ocular plethysmography, Doppler flow studies, and ultrasound imaging of the carotid arteries. These methods yield data that have a high correlation with atherothrombotic carotid disease and are proving useful in the investigation of asymptomatic bruits and other forms of cerebrovascular disease. However, when accurate information is needed urgently for possible carotid surgery, it is our practice to proceed directly to angiography, despite the slight risk involved.

Ischemic disease of the *lacunar type* warrants anticoagulation only in the stage when it simulates TIAs and is better withheld once the stroke is under way or completed, lest the damaged arterial wall that set the stage for the lacunar stroke yields and gives rise to hemorrhage. Many such cases continue to progress over a 2- to 3-day period, often to a total deficit in the affected modality, sensory or motor. This progress is usually smooth, raising fears of a deep hemorrhage, yet the expected coinvolvement of the other modality (sensory with motor or vice versa) does not develop; the issue is easily settled by a normal CT scan, since even small hematomas are easily detected by this method.

THE PATIENT WITH THE INOBVIOUS STROKE

Although hemiplegia is the classic sign of stroke, cerebrovascular disease may present with signs that spare the motor pathways, yet carry the same prognostic and therapeutic implications. Fortunately, only four such inobvious stroke syndromes occur regularly. The first is a leaking aneurysm presenting as a sudden, generalized headache (unlike any experienced in the past), often having developed during exertion, persisting for hours or days. Examination may disclose no abnormalities, except for a slightly stiff neck. Casual urinary and less often fecal incontinence, vague recollection for recent events, and unaccountable delays in answering simple questions may also be present and reflect emerging hydrocephalus in the days after the headache had its onset. Subdural hematoma, anticoagulant-induced frontal pole hemorrhage, brain tumor, and other entities must be included in the differential diagnosis.

A second type of inobvious stroke is cerebellar hemorrhage. Sudden onset of dizziness, repeated uncontrollable vomiting, inability to stand and walk, ipsilateral gaze palsy, ipsilateral facial paresis, and, less often, ipsilateral cerebellar ataxia are often incompletely detected and fail to be assembled into the diagnostic syndrome by the examining physician. Considerate of the patient's misery, the physician often defers testing the patient's ability to stand and walk, and, finding no obvious hemiparesis, he or she may also defer testing ocular movements fully; the mild facial asymmetry easily escapes notice in the setting of vomiting and dizziness. Labyrinthitis, Ménière's disease, alcoholic or drug intoxication, even viral gastroenteritis are some of the labels that have been applied to this syndrome, and little thought is given to impending disaster because the patient seems so alert—until brainstem compression suddenly intervenes, with fatal results. CT scan or lumbar puncture is an essential diagnostic step in the evaluation of all such cases. Evacuation of the hematoma in the acute phase has proved to be the only reliable therapeutic step.

A third inobvious stroke involves the posterior cerebral artery territory. Homonymous hemianopia is often not implicitly appreciated by the patient, whose complaints, if any, center on the need for new eyeglasses, or vague descriptions of blurring of vision. Accompanying deficits in higher cerebral function, including reading, naming of colors or manipulable objects, faces, description of routes on maps, require testing despite the patient's seeming normalcy during conversation. Headache that may accompany embolism in the posterior cerebral artery is often referred to the outer edge of the ipsilateral eyebrow.

The fourth common inobvious stroke is an episode of mild paraphasic speech and slightly impaired auditory comprehension that characterizes certain instances of Wernicke's aphasia due to embolism. The patient is often thought to be confused. Most of them perform satisfactorily at a superficial level in making socially appropriate greetings and gestures, and they may approve readily of the examiner's efforts to shorten the interview by posing questions to be answered yes or no. Scrutiny of their remarks and behavior during history-taking will elicit the deficit.

THE PATIENT WITH A HISTORY OF A RECENT NEUROLOGIC DEFICIT OF VASCULAR TYPE

This is the time when the identification of the patient at risk becomes an important matter, for it offers the best opportunity for medical intercession. Excluding a postconvulsive state, any deficit in neurologic function involving a cerebral or brainstem location that has persisted over a few hours should be taken as evidence of a destructive vascular lesion in the brain even though the deficit appears to have disappeared. Electrolyte disturbance, fever, intoxication with drugs, etc., may often cause a transient relapse, and knowledge of such a prior lesion is of immeasurable value in assessing the significance of any focal cerebral disorder that emerges during a general metabolic derangement. A history of the brief episodic focal deficit compels consideration of TIAs. In such a setting, migraine, seizure, depression, peripheral neuropathies, and other entities arise in the differential diagnosis. Search for extracranial vascular abnormalities including a carotid bruit is useful. If the episodes are recurrent, the similarities between episodes, the arterial

territory implicated by the symptoms, and their duration are all important features to be studied. TIAs that warn of disaster frequently last only seconds to a few minutes, and are often shrugged off by the patient as insignificant. Although some patients experience hundreds of attacks over months before a stroke, most experience few, often only one; and the last and sometimes the only such attack tends to occur within the day(s) before the stroke. The more recent the last attack, the more expeditious should be the attempt to find the source of the prior deficit.

REFERENCES

ADAMS RD: Vascular disease of the brain. *Annu Rev Med* 4:213, 1953.

———, TORVIK A, FISHER CM: Progressing stroke: Pathogenesis, in Siekert RG, Whisnant JP (eds): *Cerebral Vascular Diseases, Third Conference*. New York, Grune & Stratton, 1961, pp 133–150.

ALEXANDER MP, SCHMITT MA: The aphasia syndrome of stroke in the left anterior cerebral artery territory. *Arch Neurol* 37:97, 1980.

AUER LM: The pathogenesis of hypertensive encephalopathy. *Acta Neurochir*, suppl 27, 1978.

AVERBACK P: Primary cerebral venous thrombosis in young adults: the diverse manifestations of an unrecognized disease. *Ann Neurol* 3:81, 1978.

BANKER BQ: Cerebral vascular disease in infancy and childhood: I. Occlusive vascular disease. *J Neuropathol Exp Neurol* 20:127, 1961.

BARNETT HJM et al: Further evidence relating mitral-valve prolapse to cerebral ischemic events. *N Engl J Med* 302:139, 1980.

BARRON KD, SIQUEIRA E, HIRANO A: Cerebral embolism caused by nonbacterial thrombotic endocarditis. *Neurology* 10:391, 1960.

BYROM FB: The pathogenesis of hypertensive encephalopathy. *Lancet* 2:201, 1954.

CANADIAN COOPERATIVE STUDY GROUP: Randomized trial of aspirin and sulfinpyrazone in threatened stroke. *N Engl J Med* 299:53, 1978.

CAPLAN LR: "Top of the basilar" syndrome. *Neurology* 30:72, 1980.

CHESTER EM et al: Hypertensive encephalopathy: A clinicopathologic study of 20 cases. *Neurology* 28:928, 1978.

CHURG J, STRAUSS L: Allergic granulomatosis, allergic angiitis and periarteritis nodosa. *Am J Pathol* 27:277, 1951.

COLLABORATIVE GROUP FOR THE STUDY OF STROKE IN YOUNG WOMEN: Oral contraception and increased risk of cerebral ischemia or thrombosis. *N Engl J Med* 288:871, 1973.

FAUGHT E, TRADER SD, HANNA GR: Cerebral complications of arteriography for transient ischemia and stroke. *Neurology* 29:4, 1979.

FERGUSON GG: Physical factors in the initiation, growth, and rupture of human intracranial saccular aneurysms. *J Neurosurg* 37:666, 1972.

FIELDS WS: *Pathogenesis and Treatment of Cerebrovascular Disease.* Springfield, Ill, Charles C Thomas, 1961.

FISHER CM: Cerebral thromboangiitis obliterans. *Medicine* 36:169, 1957.

———: Lacunes: Small, deep cerebral infarcts. *Neurology* 15:774, 1965.

———: A lacunar stroke: The dysarthria-clumsy hand syndrome. *Neurology* 17:614, 1967.

———: The arterial lesions underlying lacunes. *Acta Neuropathol* 12:1, 1969.

———: Cerebral ischemia—less familiar types. *Clin Neurosurg* 18:267, 1971.

———: The anatomy and pathology of the cerebral vasculature, in Meyer JS (ed): *Modern Concepts of Cerebrovascular Disease.* New York, Spectrum, 1975, pp 1-41.

———: Late-life migraine accompaniments as a cause of unexplained transient ischemic attacks. Can J Neurol Sci 7:9, 1980.

———, KARNES WE, KUBIK CS: Lateral medullary infarction—the pattern of vascular occlusion. *J Neuropathol Exp Neurol* 20:323, 1961.

FODSTAD H et al: Tranexamic acid in the preoperative management of ruptured intracranial aneurysms. *Surg Neurol* 10:9, 1978.

GARRAWAY WM et al: Declining incidence of stroke. *N Engl J Med* 300:449, 1979.

HEYMAN A et al: Risk of stroke in asymptomatic persons with cervical arterial bruits. *N Engl J Med* 302:838, 1980.

HOUSER OW et al: Fibromuscular dysplasia of the cephalic arterial system, in Vinken PJ, Bruyn GW (eds): *Handbook of Clinical Neurology,* vol 11: *Vascular Disease of the Nervous System,* pt 1. Amsterdam, North-Holland, 1972, chap 14, pp 366-385.

HUTCHINSON EC, ACHESON EJ: *Strokes.* Philadelphia, Saunders, 1975.

IREY NS, McALLISTER HA, HENRY JM: Oral contraceptives and stroke in young women: A clinicopathologic correlation. *Neurology* 28:1216, 1978.

JOHNSON RT, RICHARDSON EP: The neurological manifestations of systemic lupus erythematosus. *Medicine* 47:337, 1968.

KRAYENBÜHL H, YASARGIL MG: Radiological anatomy and topography of the cerebral arteries, in Vinken PJ, Bruyn GW (eds): *Handbook of Clinical Neurology,* vol 11: *Vascular Diseases of the Nervous System,* pt 1. Amsterdam, North-Holland, 1972, chap 4, pp 65-101.

KUBIK CS, ADAMS RD: Occlusion of the basilar artery—a clinical and pathological study. *Brain* 69:73, 1946.

KURTZKE JF: Critique of the Canadian "TIA" study, in Price TR, Nelson E (eds): *Cerebrovascular Diseases.* New York, Raven, 1979, pp 243-250.

LEADBETTER WF, BURKLAND CE: Hypertension in unilateral renal disease. *J Urol* 39:611, 1938.

LILIENFELD AM: Critique of "A randomized trial of aspirin and sulfinpyrazone in threatened stroke," in Price TR, Nelson E (eds): *Cerebrovascular Diseases.* New York, Raven, 1979, pp 239-241.

MARSHALL J: Angiography in the investigation of ischemic episodes in the territory of the internal carotid artery. *Lancet* 1:719, 1971.

McKISSOCK W, PAINE KW, WALSH LS: An analysis of the results of treatment of ruptured intracranial aneurysms: A report of 722 consecutive cases. *J Neurosurg* 17:762, 1960.

———, RICHARDSON A, WALSH L: Middle cerebral aneurysms: Further results in the controlled trial of conservative and surgical treatment of ruptured intracranial aneurysms. *Lancet* 2:417, 1962.

———, ———, ———: Anterior communicating aneurysms: A trial of conservative and surgical treatment. *Lancet* 1:873, 1965.

MOHR JP et al: The Harvard Cooperative Stroke Registry: A prospective registry of patients hospitalized with stroke. *Neurology* 28:754, 1978.

NISHIMOTO A, TAKEUCHI S: Moyamoya disease, in Vinken PJ, Bruyn GW (eds): *Handbook of Clinical Neurology,* vol 12: *Vascular Diseases of the Nervous System,* pt 2. Amsterdam, North-Holland, 1972, chap 11, pp 352-383.

OJEMANN RG, FISHER CM, RICH JC: Spontaneous dissecting aneurysms of the internal carotid artery. *Stroke* 3:434, 1972.

PESSIN MS et al: Clinical and angiographic features of carotid transient ischemic attacks. *N Engl J Med* 296:358, 1977.

RABKIN SW, MATHEWSON FAL, TATE RB: Long-term changes in blood pressure and risk of cerebrovascular disease. *Stroke* 9:319, 1978.

RICE GPA et al: Familial stroke syndrome associated with mitral valve prolapse. *Ann Neurol* 7:130, 1980.

RICHARDSON AE, JANE JA: Long-term prognosis in untreated cerebral aneurysms: I. Incidence of late hemorrhage in cerebral aneurysm: Ten year evaluation of 364 patients. *Ann Neurol* 1:358, 1977.

SAHS AD et al: *Intracranial Aneurysms and Subarachnoid Hemorrhage: A Cooperative Study.* Philadelphia, Lippincott, 1969.

SANDOK BA et al: Guidelines for the management of transient ischemic attacks. Mayo Clin Proc 53:665, 1978.

TAKAYASU M: A case with peculiar changes of the central retinal vessels. *Acta Soc Ophthalmol Jpn* 12:554, 1908.

TAVERAS JM: Multiple progressive intracranial arterial occlusions: A syndrome of children and young adults. *Am J Roentgenol* 106:235, 1969.

THOMPSON JE, PALMAN D, TALKINGTON CM: Asymptomatic carotid bruit. *Ann Surg* 188:308, 1978.

TOOLE JF, YUSON CP, JANEWAY R: Transient ischemic attacks: A study of 225 patients. *Neurology* 28:746, 1978.

UEDA K, TOOLE JF, MCHENRY LC: Carotid and vertebral transient ischemic attacks: Clinical and angiographic correlation. *Neurology* 29:1094, 1978.

VETERANS ADMINISTRATION COOPERATIVE STUDY IN ANTIHYPERTENSIVE AGENTS: *J Am Med Assoc* 202:1028, 1967; 213:1143, 1970.

VOLHARD F: Clinical aspects of Bright's disease, in Berglund H et al (eds): *The Kidney in Health and Disease.* Philadelphia, Lea & Febiger, 1935, pp 665-688.

WEISMAN AD, ADAMS RD: The neurological complications of dissecting aortic aneurysm. *Brain* 67:69, 1944.

WHISNANT JP, MATSUMOTO N, ELVEBACK LR: Transient cerebral ischemic attacks in a community: Rochester, Minnesota, 1955 through 1969. *Mayo Clin Proc* 48:194, 1973.

—— et al: Carotid and vertebral-basilar transient ischemic attacks: Effect of anticoagulants, hypertension, and cardiac disorders on survival and stroke occurrence—a population study. *Ann Neurol* 3:107, 1978.

CHAPTER 34

CRANIOCEREBRAL TRAUMA

Among the vast array of neurologic diseases, cerebral trauma ranks high in order of frequency and gravity. The basic process is at once both simple and complex— simple because there is usually no problem about etiologic diagnosis, viz., a blow to the head—and complex because of uncertainty about the pathogenesis of the immediate cerebral disorder and a number of delayed effects that may complicate the injury. About the trauma nothing medical can be done, for it is finished before the physician arrives on the scene. At most there can be an assessment of the factors conducive to further injury and the institution of measures for their avoidance. But of the disastrous intracranial phenomena which are initiated by head injury, several fall within the purview of the physician, for they evolve during the period of medical observation, offering possibilities of both prevention and treatment.

It is a common misconception that craniocerebral injuries are matters of only neurosurgical import and rarely concern the general or specialized neurologic physician. Actually, some 80 percent of head injuries are first seen by a general physician, and probably fewer than 20 percent ever require neurosurgical intervention of any kind—and even this number is decreasing. Often neurologists must take charge of the head-injured patient, or their opinion is sought in consultation. To enact their role effectively they must be familiar with the clinical manifestations and the natural course of the primary brain injury and its complications, and have a sound grasp of the underlying physiologic mechanisms. Such knowledge must be up-to-date and immediately applicable. Matters pertaining to spinal injury are considered in Chap. 35. The present chapter undertakes to review the salient facts concerning injuries to the brain and to outline a clinical approach that the authors have found useful over the years.

DEFINITIONS AND MECHANISMS

The very language which one uses to discuss certain types of head injury divulges a number of misconceptions which have been inherited from previous generations of physicians. Words have crept into the medical vocabulary and have often been retained long after the ideas for which they stood have been refuted—evidence of the disadvantage of the premature adoption of explanatory rather than descriptive terms. The word *concussion*, for example, implies violent shaking and agitation of the brain or the transient functional impairment which results therefrom. Yet despite numerous experiments to demonstrate the physical changes within the nerve cells, axons, or myelin sheaths (vibration effects, formation of intracellular vacuoles, etc.), no convincing confirmation of their existence has been possible. Similarly the word *contusion* meaning a bruising or crushing without interruption of physical continuity, is applied rather indiscriminately to a variety of clinical states, some of which could not depend on a pathologic change of this type, e.g., "minor contusion state or syndrome"— an expression introduced by Wilfred Trotter, who was himself most critical of words that "embalm a fallacious theory."

In all attempts to analyze the mechanism(s) of cerebral trauma one fact stands preeminent—that there must be the sudden application of a physical force of considerable magnitude to the head. Unless the head is struck, the brain suffers no injury—except in the rare and somewhat controversial cases of crush injury to the chest or explosive injury with raised intrapulmonary pressure. A second fact, also readily verified, is that the area of the skull over which the force is exerted is of importance. High-velocity missiles may destroy a small part of the skull and penetrate the cranial cavity without causing significant displacement of the head or brain; injuries in which the skull is compressed between two converging forces may crush the brain. In these two circumstances it is interesting to note that the patient may suffer severe and often fatal injury without immediate loss of consciousness. Hemorrhage, destruction of brain tissue, and, if the patient survives for a time, meningitis or abscess, are the principal pathologic changes created by injuries of these types. They offer little difficulty in understanding. The various types of head injuries are illustrated in Fig. 34-1.

A factor of particular importance in brain injury is the mobility of the head. As will be pointed out below, all concussive injuries relate to a physical force (large blunt object) that imparts motion to the stationary head or a hard surface that arrests the motion of the moving head. These constitute the common civilian head injuries. Termed *blunt head injuries*, they are remarkable in two respects: (1) they frequently induce at least a temporary loss of consciousness; (2) even though the skull is not penetrated and fragments of bone are not driven into its cavity, the brain may suffer gross damage, i.e.,

contusion, laceration, hemorrhage, swelling, herniation, etc. Clinicians as well as experimental physiologists have sought a theory which would bring into plausible form all gross neuropathologic changes (including skull fracture) and the transient paralysis of nervous function (concussion) or the prolonged coma so often observed in fatal cases. It may be said that a comprehensive theory, acceptable to all workers in this field, has yet to be formulated.

The relation of skull fracture to brain injury has been viewed in changing perspective throughout the history of this subject. In early times, fractures dominated the thinking of the medical profession, and cerebral lesions were regarded as secondary. Later it became known that the skull, although rigid, is still flexible enough to yield to a blow that could injure the brain without causing fracture. Therefore, the presence of a fracture, although a rough measure of the violence to

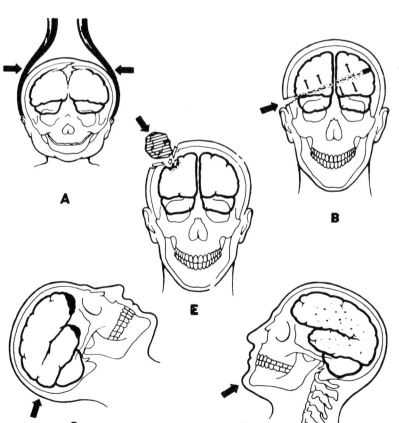

Figure 34-1

Mechanisms of craniocerebral injury. A. Cranium distorted by forceps (birth injury). B. Gunshot wound of the brain. C. Falls (also traffic accidents). D. Blows on the chin ("punch drunk"). E. Injury to skull and brain by falling objects. [From Courville (a study based upon a survey of lesions found in a series of 15,000 autopsies).]

which the brain has been exposed, is no longer considered an infallible index. Even in fatal head injury, autopsy reveals an intact skull in some 20 to 30 percent of cases. Contrariwise many patients suffer skull fractures without serious or prolonged disorder of cerebral function.

The modern trend is to be concerned primarily with the presence or absence of brain injury rather than with the fracture of the skull itself. Nevertheless, fractures cannot be dismissed without a few comments, for they assume importance in indicating the site and possible severity of brain damage, in providing an explanation for cranial nerve palsies, and in creating potential pathways for the ingress of bacteria and air or the egress of cerebrospinal fluid (CSF). Some of the major sites and directions of basal skull fractures are indicated in Fig. 34-2. One can readily perceive the possibilities of injury to cranial nerves in relation to such fractures.

INJURY OF CRANIAL NERVES AND BASAL STRUCTURES BY FRACTURES

The existence of a basal skull fracture may be indicated by signs of cranial nerve damage. Cranial nerves which are particularly liable to trauma are the olfactory, optic, oculomotor, trochlear, first and second branches of the trigeminal, the facial, and the auditory. Anosmia and an apparent loss of taste (actually a loss of perception of aromatic flavors, since elementary modalities of taste—salt, sweet, bitter, sour—remain) are frequent sequelae of head injury, especially of falls on the back of the head. In the majority of cases the anosmia is permanent. If unilateral, it will not be noticed by the patient. The mechanism of these disturbances is believed to be displacement of the brain and tearing of the olfactory nerve filaments in or near the cribriform plate, through which they course.

A fracture in or near the sella may tear the stalk of the pituitary gland, with resulting diabetes insipidus, impotence and reduced libido, and amenorrhea. A fracture of the sphenoid bone may lacerate the optic nerve, with blindness from the beginning. The pupil is dilated and unreactive to a direct light stimulus but still reacts to a light stimulus to the opposite eye (consensual reflex). The optic disk becomes pale, i.e., atrophic, after an interval of several weeks. Partial injuries may result in a troublesome blurring of vision. Injury to the eighth cranial nerve with petrosal fractures causes loss of hearing

and/or postural vertigo and nystagmus immediately after the cranial trauma. The deafness due to nerve injury must be distinguished from deafness caused by rupture of the eardrum or the presence of blood in the middle ear; and the vertigo must be distinguished from post-traumatic nervous giddiness.

In oculomotor nerve injury there is a divergent squint, with loss of internal and vertical movement of the eye and a fixed, dilated pupil. Diplopia—worse on looking down—and compensatory tilting of the head suggest trochlear nerve injury. These ocular nerve disor-

Figure 34-2
The course of fracture lines through the base of the skull. Arrows indicate point of application and direction of force. (From Courville.)

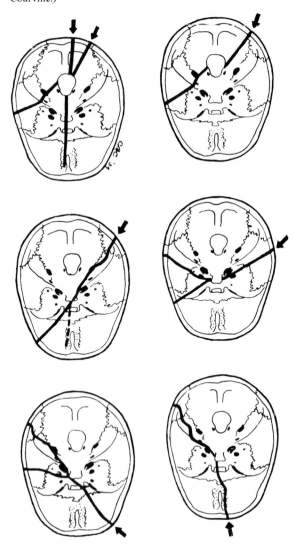

ders must be distinguished from ocular deviations due to direct orbital injuries with displacement of muscle attachments. Direct injury of the facial nerve by a basal fracture may be present immediately after the injury or delayed for several days. This delayed form is usually transitory, and its mechanism is not known. It may be misinterpreted as an important progression of the intracranial traumatic lesion. Injury to the ophthalmic or maxillary divisions of the trigeminal nerve may be the result either of a basal fracture across the middle cranial fossa or of a direct extracranial injury to the branches of the nerves. Numbness and paresthesias over the area of skin supplied by the nerve or a troublesome neuralgia are the sequelae of these injuries.

CAROTID-CAVERNOUS FISTULAE

A basal fracture through the sphenoid and petrous bone may lacerate the internal carotid artery where it lies in the cavernous sinus. Within hours or a few days a severe and disfiguring pulsating exophthalmos develops as arterial blood enters and distends the orbital veins which empty into the sinus. Usually the orbit feels tight and is painful. The eye may become partially or completely immobile because of pressure on the ocular nerves. The sixth nerve is affected most often and the third and fourth less frequently. Also, there may be a loss of vision, due to involvement of the optic nerve; congestion of the retinal veins and glaucoma are additional factors in the visual failure. Surgical therapy is indicated; the several techniques include trapping the torn carotid segment or ligating the carotid artery in the neck (see review by Stern).

Not all carotid-cavernous fistulae are traumatic. They may occur in a number of medical conditions, such as intracavernous saccular aneurysm or in Danlos-Ehlers disease, where the connective tissue is defective; or the cause may be unexplained.

If the skin over the skull fracture is lacerated and the underlying meninges are torn, or if the fracture passes through the posterior wall of a nasal sinus, bacteria or air may enter the cranial cavity with resulting meningitis, abscess, and aerocele (air in the ventricles). Also, CSF may leak into the sinus and present as a watery discharge from the nose (CSF rhinorrhea). Identification of CSF is assisted by testing the nasal discharge for glucose with diabetic test tape (mucus has no glucose) or for the presence of fluorescein or dye injected into the lumbar subarachnoid space. Persistence of the rhinorrhea or the occurrence of repeated episodes of meningitis is often an indication for repair of the torn dura mater over the fissure. Depressed fractures are of

significance only if the underlying dura is lacerated or if the brain is depressed by indentation of bone.

CEREBRAL CONCUSSION

Much has been written about the mechanism of coma in closed or blunt head injury. Certain facts concerning the condition stand out. (1) Concussion, defined as a *usually reversible traumatic paralysis of nervous function*, is always immediate (not delayed even by seconds). (2) Concussive effects on brain function may last for a variable time (seconds, minutes, hours, or longer). To set arbitrary limits on the duration of loss of consciousness, i.e., to consider a brief loss as indicative of concussion and a prolonged loss as indicative of contusion or other traumatic cerebral lesion—as is proposed in some medical circles—is illogical and unsound physiologically, as pointed out by Symonds. Any such difference is quantitative, not qualitative. Admittedly, in the more prolonged states of coma there is a greater chance of finding hemorrhage and contusion, which undoubtedly contribute to the persistence of coma and the likelihood of irreversible change. (3) The optimal conditions for the production of concussive paralysis of brain function, demonstrated originally by Denny-Brown and Russell, is a blunt nonpenetrating injury which causes a change in the momentum of the head; i.e., either movement is imparted to the head by a blow, or movement of the head is arrested by a hard, unyielding surface. These two types of injury are called accelerative and decelerative, respectively.

The mechanism of concussive cerebral paralysis has been interpreted variously throughout medical history, in the light of the scientific knowledge available at a particular time. The favored hypothesis for the better part of a century was vasoparalysis (suggested by Fischer in 1870) or an arrest of circulation by an instantaneous rise in intracranial pressure (proposed by Strohmeyer in 1864 and popularized by Trotter in 1932). Trotter asserted that the brief cerebral anemia induced an immediate paralysis of cerebral function with a tendency to rapid and spontaneous recovery, usually leaving no visible sign of damage to the brain. More prolonged periods of concussive coma were attributed by Trotter to contusion, a proposition for which he adduced no pathologic evidence. Jefferson in his essay on the nature of concussion convincingly refuted these vascular hypotheses; more recently, Shatsky et al., by high-speed cineangiography (1000 frames per second), showed displacement of vessels but no arrest of circulation immediately after impact.

Beginning with the work of Denny-Brown and Russell, the physical factors involved in head and brain injury have been subjected to careful analysis. As indicated above, these investigators determined that the change in momentum of the head is critical in the genesis of concussion. In their experiments, in the monkey and cat, concussion resulted when the head was struck by a heavy mass, as large as or larger than the head, with a velocity greater than 28 ft/s (energy of 17.83 ft·lb). If the head was prevented from moving at the moment of injury, this degree of force invariably failed to produce concussion. Holbourn, in 1943, attempted to solve the paradox of why coma occurs when a freely moving head is struck but does not occur when the head is stationary. From the study of gelatin models under conditions simulating head trauma he deduced that when the head is struck, movement of the round, partly tethered but suspended brain always lags (inertia); but inevitably the brain must rotate, for it occupies a round skull whose motions (because of attachment to the neck) usually describe an arc. Pudenz and Sheldon and later Ommaya et al. (1964) proved the correctness of this assumption by photographing the brain through a lucite calvarium at the moment of the trauma. The cerebral tissue is thus subjected to shearing stresses set up by rotational forces. This provides a reasonable explanation of surface injuries in certain places, i.e., where the swirling brain comes into contact with bony prominences on the inner surface of the skull (petrous ridges, sphenoid wings, orbital ridges). Also such motions of the brain could conceivably explain the immediate loss of consciousness. However, the precise mechanism(s) involved in the genesis of concussion are still not fully explained; explanations in terms of "molecular commotion," direct injury of neurons (Denny-Brown and Russell), neuronal chromatolysis (Groat et al.), and "synaptic breaks" in the gray matter, remain speculative.

Strich, in 1956, studied the brains of five patients who died between 5 and 15 months after severe closed head injuries which had caused protracted coma. Using the Marchi method, she observed a diffuse, uneven degeneration of the cerebral white matter. In these cases, where there had been "no skull fracture, raised intracranial pressure or gross subarachnoid hemorrhage," the clinical state had been attributed to midbrain and subthalamic hemorrhages or softenings, but these latter changes were not found at autopsy. A direct shearing of myelin or axons was postulated. Strich later extended her observations to 20 cases. In cases with more recent lesions she observed ballooning of axis cylinders (end bulbs), a finding which Nevin has confirmed. Symonds saw in these pathologic changes a possible explanation of concussion, i.e., an effect of Holbourn's shearing stresses, which distort and stretch axis cylinders.

While the authors acknowledge the importance of white matter lesions, they do not agree with these interpretations. In our opinion, the Marchi type of degeneration in tracts of cerebrum and brainstem, attributed by Strich to direct shattering of white matter, is probably secondary to focal necroses of cerebral cortex and of tracts in subcortical white matter, corpus callosum, and brainstem. Strich's failure to trace such changes to focal necroses is due, we believe, to the inadequacy of her method of examination. In all such theorizing, one again is faced with the problem of extrapolating from the visible degenerative changes of chronic traumatic encephalopathy to those of acute concussive paralytic injury. These matters cannot presently be resolved.

Much interest in recent years has centered on the *anatomic site of the concussive injury*. Once it became known that the reticular formation of the upper brainstem served as a nonspecific activating system for the cerebral cortex, the possibility suggested itself that it was the site of concussive injury. Foltz and Schmidt showed that in the concussed monkey lemniscal sensory transmission through the brainstem was unaltered, but its effect in activating the upper reticular formation was blocked. They also demonstrated that the electrical activity of the medial reticular formation was depressed for a longer time and more severely than that of the cerebral cortex. These effects on the reticular formation were thought to be analogous to the ones produced by ether and barbiturate anesthesia. It has been suggested that maximal shearing stress occurs at the point where the cerebral hemispheres could most easily rotate on the brainstem, i.e., at the midbrain-subthalamic level. Using the fluorescein technique, Ommaya et al. (1964) found selective changes of the blood-brain barrier in the lower brainstem and spinal cord of concussed animals, i.e., lower than the level of injury postulated by Foltz and Schmidt. Meyer and Denny-Brown believe the cerebral cortex to be directly involved because of the finding in monkeys of a change in the cortical dc potentials immediately after concussive injury.

Formerly it was thought that the initial action of a blunt concussive injury was to excite the nervous system, with evocation of a massive discharge. The "stars" that one sees with a minor head injury and the gasp of the injured animal were cited as expressions of this effect, but continuous electrical monitoring through implanted cortical electrodes at the time of impact and for 10 s afterwards has offered no support for this suggestion. There was no increase in electrical activity and nothing resembling a seizure discharge; instead, cortical activity was briefly suppressed and relatively little altered thereafter.

The *clinical effects of concussion* are invariable: immediate abolition of consciousness, suppression of reflexes (falling to the ground if standing), transient arrest of respiration, a brief period of bradycardia and fall in blood pressure following a momentary rise at the time of impact. If sufficiently intense, death may occur at this moment, presumably from respiratory arrest. Usually the vital signs return to normal and stabilize within a few seconds while the patient remains unconscious. The plantar reflexes are extensor. Then, after a variable period of time, the patient begins to stir, opens the eyes, but is unseeing. Corneal, pharyngeal, and cutaneous reflexes, originally depressed, begin to return; and the limbs are withdrawn from painful stimuli. Gradually contact is made with the environment, and the patient passes successively through stages of obeying only simple commands, of responding to simple questions, and then of amnesia, in which a conversation can be carried on, but recall later is poor. Finally there is full recovery corresponding to the time when the patient can form consecutive memories of current experiences. The time required for the patient to pass through these stages of recovery may be a few minutes or several hours or days, but again, between these extremes Symonds sees only quantitative differences, varying with the intensity of the process. The sequences which he believes to represent lower levels of brain function return first and higher levels, later. To the observer such patients are comatose only from the moment of injury until they open their eyes and begin to speak; for the patients, unconsciousness extends from a time before the injury occurred (*retrograde amnesia*) until they are able to form consecutive memories, viz., at the end of the period of *anterograde amnesia*. The duration of the amnesic period is the best index of the severity of the concussive injury.

Certain interesting biochemical changes attend craniocerebral injury, whether of the purely concussive type or that with gross cerebral lesions, but their significance is uncertain. Acetylcholine and lactate are elevated in the CSF during the first 3 to 4 days after the injury (leakage from damaged brain) and then gradually return to normal. Serum lactate is also raised, presumably because of the ready diffusibility of lactic acid from brain and CSF to blood. Also during the first few days there is sodium retention followed, after this time, by sodium diuresis. However, at the time of sodium reten-

tion there is actually a mild hyponatremia due to simultaneous water retention. Potassium, in contrast, remains in balance throughout this period. Nitrogen loss—amounting to about 10 g/day—is a consistent finding in all types of serious head injury during the first days following trauma.

In fatal cases of head injury, where these concussive effects must have existed, the brain is almost invariably bruised, swollen, and lacerated, and often there is hemorrhage, either meningeal or intracerebral. The prominence of these gross pathologic findings has led to the widely prevalent view that cerebral injuries are largely matters of bruises and hemorrhages and urgent operations. That this can hardly be the case is suggested by the fact that some patients survive head injuries almost as severe as the fatal ones and make an excellent recovery. Years later, postmortem examination discloses old contusions (plaques jaunes) and hemorrhages of approximately the same distribution and extent as those observed in some of the immediately fatal cases. One can only conclude, therefore, that most of the immediate symptoms of severe head injury, both general and localized, depend on invisible and highly reversible changes in the brain, probably of the same nature as those which underlie concussion.

Nevertheless, bruises, lacerations, hemorrhages, and localized swellings of tissues cannot be disregarded, because they are probably responsible for many of the fatalities that occur 12 to 72 h or more after the injury. Of these lesions the most important are the bruising of the surface of the brain beneath the point of impact (*coup lesion*) and the more extensive lacerations and contusions on the side of the brain opposite to the site of the impact (*contrecoup lesion*). The usual sites are shown in Fig. 34-3. Blows to the front of the head usually produce only coup lesions, whereas blows to the back of the head usually cause only contrecoup lesions (sometimes coup lesions as well). Blows to the side of the head produce coup or contrecoup lesions, or both. Irrespective of the site of the impact, the common sites of cerebral contusions are in the frontal and temporal lobes, as illustrated in Fig. 34-4. The inertia of the malleable brain, which causes it to be flung against the side of the skull that was struck, to be pulled away from the contralateral side, and to rotate against bony promontories within the cranial cavity explain these coup-contrecoup contusions. The experimental studies of Ommaya and his colleagues indicate that the effects of linear acceleration of the head are of much less significance than distortions due to rotation. Sparing of the occipital lobes in coup-contrecoup injury is explained by the smooth inner surface of the occipital bones and tentorium.

CLINICAL MANIFESTATIONS OF HEAD INJURY

The physician being called to see a patient who has had a closed (blunt) head injury will generally find the patient in one of three clinical conditions. Each must be dealt with differently. It is usually possible to place such patients in one of these three categories by assessing their mental and general neurologic status when they are first seen and at intervals of time after the accident.

PATIENTS WHO ARE CONSCIOUS OR ARE RAPIDLY REGAINING CONSCIOUSNESS WHEN FIRST SEEN (MINOR HEAD INJURY)

This is the most frequently encountered form of head injury. Roughly two degrees of disturbance of function may have occurred. In one, the patient may not have been unconscious at all, but was only stunned or "saw stars." This injury is insignificant when judged in terms of life and death and brain damage—though as we shall point out below, there is always the possibility of skull fracture or the later development of an epidural or subdural hematoma. Moreover, the patient is still liable to several troublesome posttraumatic symptoms including posttraumatic nervous instability (headache, giddiness, fatigability, insomnia, and nervousness) which may appear at once or within a few days. In the second instance, consciousness may have been temporarily abolished for a few seconds or minutes, viz., concussion. When such patients are first seen, recovery may already be complete, or they may be in one of the stages of recovery described above. Even though mentally clear

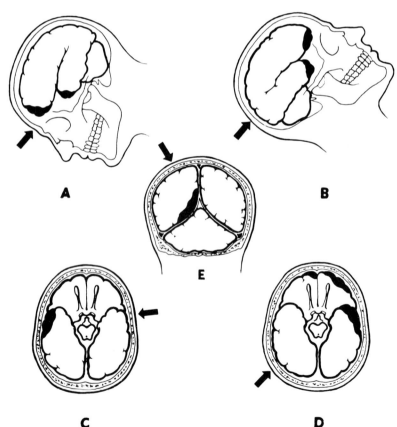

Figure 34-3

Mechanisms of cerebral contusion. Arrows indicate point of application and direction of force; black areas indicate location of contusion. A. Frontotemporal contusion consequent to frontal injury. B. Frontotemporal contusion following occipital injury. C. Contusion of temporal lobe due to contralateral injury. D. Frontotemporal contusion due to injury to opposite temporooccipital region. E. Diffuse mesial temporooccipital contusion due to blow on vertex. (From Courville.)

these patients have amnesia for events immediately preceding and following the injury. Thereafter, headache and other symptoms of posttraumatic nervous instability may be present.

These minor and seemingly trivial head injuries may rarely be followed by a number of puzzling clinical phenomena, some insignificant, others of grave import, which indicate the presence of a pathologic process other than concussion.

Delayed Collapse after Head Injury   Following an accident the injured person, after walking about and seeming to be normal, may turn pale and fall unconscious to the ground. Recovery occurs within a few seconds or minutes. This is a vasopressor syncopal attack, related to pain and emotional upset, and differs in no way from syncope that follows pain and fright without injury. It also happens with injuries that have spared the head, but with head injury it becomes more difficult to interpret.

Denny-Brown has described a more severe type of delayed posttraumatic collapse. In this type, patients appear to be recovering from a blow to the head, which may simply have dazed them or caused a brief period of unconsciousness, when suddenly, after a period of several minutes to hours, they collapse and become unresponsive. The most disquieting feature of this clinical state is a marked bradycardia, which coupled with the lucid interval, raises the specter of an evolving epidural hemorrhage (actually, bradycardia is a late and inconstant sign of epidural bleeding). However, intracranial pressure is not raised, the disorder fails to develop further, and following a brief period of restlessness, vomiting and headache, the patient recovers completely over a period of several days to weeks. Denny-Brown has suggested that this form of delayed posttraumatic collapse is due to a contusion of the medulla, but how this explains the sequence of clinical events is not clear. The authors believe it to be a form of vagal syncope.

Immediate Drowsiness, Headache, and Confusion   This occurs most often in children who after a concussive or nonconcussive head injury seem not to be themselves. They lie down, are drowsy, complain of headache, and may vomit—symptoms that raise the suspicion of an epidural hemorrhage. These symptoms subside after a few hours. There may be minor alterations in the EEG. The intravenous administration of 5% glucose and water is particularly dangerous in this type of cerebral injury and in more serious ones, because it may induce a state of water intoxication. Apparently, under these circumstances, there is an excessive excretion of antidiuretic hormone which causes retention of water.

Occasionally a migraine attack may be induced by a blow to the head, and this can be perplexing for a few

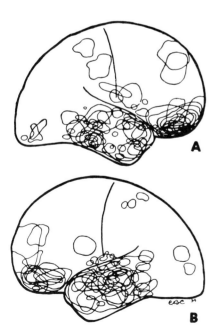
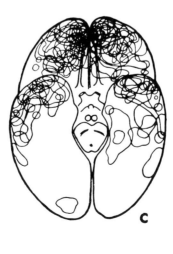

Figure 34-4
Composite drawing showing size and location of contusions found in a series of 40 consecutive cases. The tendency to localize in the subfrontal and temporal regions is clearly indicated. (From Courville.)

hours, especially if it is the first attack of migraine in a child.

Transient Traumatic Paraplegia or Blindness   With falls or blows on top of the head, both legs may become temporarily weak and numb with bilateral Babinski signs and possibly sphincteric incontinence. Blows to the occiput may cause temporary blindness. The symptoms disappear after a few hours. It seems unlikely that these transient symptoms represent a direct localized concussive effect, caused either by indentation of skull against the brain or movement of these parts of the brain against the inner table of the skull. A concussion of the cervical portion of the spinal cord is another suggested but improbable mechanism of transient paraplegia. Possibly the blindness and the paraplegia, which are usually followed by a throbbing vascular type of headache, are examples of migraine provoked by the traumatic event.

Delayed Hemiplegia or Coma   Most of the examples we have seen were male adolescents or young adults who some hours after a relatively minor athletic or road injury developed a massive hemiplegia, hemianesthesia, homonymous hemianopia, and aphasia (with left-sided lesions). Arteriography may reveal a dissecting aneurysm of the common or internal carotid artery. In other instances a mural thrombus in the carotid has shed an embolus to the anterior or middle cerebral artery. The other causes of delayed hemiplegia and coma are an acute epidural and subdural hematoma, and in more severe injuries, an intracerebral hemorrhage or cerebral venous thrombosis. With fractures of large bones there may be, after 24 to 72 h, an acute onset of pulmonary symptoms (dyspnea and hyperpnea) followed by coma with or without focal signs; this sequence is due to cerebral fat embolism, first of the lungs and then of the brain.

Posttraumatic Nervous Instability   See further on, under "Sequelae of Severe Head Injury."

Concussion Complicated by Serious Cerebral Damage In the purely concussive syndrome one is justified in assuming that the cerebrum suffered no serious contusion and no subarachnoid or intracerebral hemorrhage or swelling. The EEG, if taken when the patient is first seen, is normal as is also the CSF. The skull is fractured in only a small proportion of such cases. If the fracture is in the calvarium it is of little or no significance. Frac-

tures at the base, if in the petrous bone, may damage the labyrinth and cochlea, and cause impaired hearing and/or vertigo and nystagmus; other cranial nerves are also commonly damaged as a result of basilar fractures, as described earlier in this chapter.

On rare occasions, a patient who is regaining consciousness when first seen, and who seems at first to belong in the category of minor head injury, will prove to have more serious cerebral damage. While under observation such patients may speak or respond to commands, but later they slip back into coma. Here the resemblance to a pure concussive state ends, for the period of initial coma in such cases is usually prolonged (more than 5 min), and mental clarity is never fully regained. Moreover, the CSF may be bloody and under increased pressure. Contusions and swelling of brain tissue may be demonstrated. In actuality, this type of case falls in the category of head injury described below.

PATIENTS WHO ARE AND HAVE BEEN COMATOSE FROM THE TIME OF HEAD INJURY

Here the central problem, so ably set forth by Symonds, is the relationship between concussion and contusion. In such cases, since consciousness is immediately abolished upon receipt of head injury, one could hardly doubt the existence of concussion, but when hours and days pass without consciousness being fully regained, the other half of the definition of concussion, viz., that the cerebral paralysis be transitory, is not satisfied. Moreover, when the pathologic data in such cases are carefully examined, there are almost invariably cerebral bruises, lacerations, subarachnoid hemorrhage, and scattered intracerebral hemorrhages at the point of injury (coup), on the opposite side (contrecoup), and between them, along the *line of force* of the injury. The tissue around the contusions is swollen, and later the white matter in these regions will appear *demyelinated*. Some blood in the subdural space is not unusual. A temporal lobe–tentorial pressure cone (see page 445) is frequently present with creasing of the opposite cerebral peduncle by the free margin of the tentorium and numerous midbrain hemorrhages and zones of necrosis. The conclusion that prolongation of coma and death are due to the contusive complications seems quite logical. Surely they are not part of pure concussion in which obvious and irreversible lesions do not occur.

The difficulty in separating the effects of concussion and contusion is even greater on the basis of the clinical facts. We have already pointed out that patients with craniocerebral injuries that have caused prolonged coma, bloody CSF, unilateral or focal cerebral signs, and EEG abnormalities may hover on the brink of death for a time and then slowly recover. Moreover, such patients may be restored to a level of virtually normal neurologic function. The question then is how the patient could have recovered from seemingly irreversible cerebral contusions. Symonds interprets the prolonged coma as being a manifestation of a particularly severe concussion and questions whether rapid reversibility is a valid criterion of the concussive state. While agreeing that there are different degrees of concussive paralysis of cerebral functions and that there is no way of deciding at what point concussive coma ceases and gives way to contusive coma, the authors would point out that the pathologic processes of contusion and bleeding also have a certain reversibility. If not too extensive, if there are no hypoxic-hypotensive effects, and if the upper brainstem is not damaged from a temporal lobe pressure cone, a few surface lesions would not be expected to cause severe and lasting cerebral defects. We prefer to believe that in states of protracted cerebral disorder the intensity of the injuring force has produced not only a prolonged concussive effect, but also contusion(s) of the brain. In our opinion it is the latter, with subsequent swelling of tissue, bleeding, herniation and displacement of brainstem, and respiratory disturbances leading to hypoxia and hypotension, that usually account for the fatal effects of head injury and, with survival, account for the persistent neurologic deficits.

In this category of serious head injury, where the patient is in coma when first seen by the physician and has been so from the onset, one must always assume that gross pathologic changes in a state of evolution have been superimposed on concussion. Further, the very acuteness of both processes (concussion and contusion) offers promise of reversibility if life-threatening complications can be averted.

Three clinical subgroups can be recognized: one in which cerebral damage and other bodily injuries are incompatible with survival; a second in which improvement sets in within a few days, followed by recovery with certain residual signs; and a third and relatively small group in which the patients remain permanently comatose, stuporous, or profoundly reduced in their cerebral capacities. Of course there are many degrees of injury that fall between these three arbitrary subgroups.

The first subgroup comprises patients who from the onset are so severely injured that life is obviously endangered. When first seen, such a patient may be in a state of shock with subnormal blood pressure, hypothermia, fast, thready pulse, and pale, moist skin. If this state persists along with deep coma, widely dilated fixed pupils, absent eye movements, corneal and pharyngeal reflexes, flaccid limbs, stertorous and irregular respirations or respiratory failure, death usually follows shortly. Once respiration ceases and the EEG becomes isoelec-

tric, the clinical state corresponds to *brain death* as described on page 234. In those comatose patients in whom the blood pressure and respirations regularize, the degree of cerebral injury can best be evaluated over a period of hours and days by observing the depth of coma, and the temperature, pulse, and blood pressure. Deep coma with subnormal temperature and rising pulse rate are grave prognostic signs. This is true also of a rapidly rising temperature and pulse rate with rapid and irregular respirations. In some fatal cases the fever continues to mount until the end when there is circulatory collapse.

In this category of cerebral injury, where the patients die after surviving for only a few hours or days, postmortem examination almost invariably discloses cerebral contusion, focal brain swelling, hemorrhage, and necrosis of tissue. In 50 consecutive autopsies of such cases summarized in Rowbotham's excellent monograph, all but two showed macroscopic changes. The lesions in these cases consisted of surface contusions (48 percent), lacerations of the cerebral cortex (28 percent), subarachnoid hemorrhage (72 percent), subdural hematoma (15 percent), extradural hemorrhage (20 percent), and skull fractures (72 percent). As a rule, several of these pathologic changes are found in the same case. Moreover, traumatism of extracranial organs and tissues is frequent. In one series of 50 fatal head injuries, there were associated fractures of the limbs in 21 percent, chest injuries in 19 percent, abdominal injuries in 13 percent, and ruptured visceral organs in a few patients. These extracerebral injuries obviously contribute to the fatal outcome.

In respect to the second subgroup, i.e., the relatively less severe and seldom fatal head injuries, all gradations in tempo and degree of completeness of recovery may be observed. In the least severely injured of this group, recovery of consciousness begins in a few hours, but there may be a relapse within the first day or two as the contused brain tissue swells. The CSF is usually bloody, as described further on. Eventually recovery may be complete, but the period of traumatic amnesia covers a span of several days or weeks. Regarding the duration of the concussive effects, it should be repeated that penetrating types of injuries and depressed fractures may occasionally injure the brain without causing concussion at all, but here we are considering only the blunt, closed contusive head injuries.

In the more severely injured of this group, the temperature, pulse, and respirations, although slightly elevated, tend to become stable within a few days, and not long thereafter the level of awareness and responsiveness improves slightly. Still there is danger of a rapid and fatal rise in temperature even after the second and third day. Once the patient begins to speak, there is reasonable certainty of progressive improvement. However, improvement may be distressingly slow, and the patient may remain stuporous or barely arousable for days on end or even several weeks. A substantial risk of developing aspiration pneumonia, meningitis, gastric hemorrhage, and epidural and subdural hemorrhage continues for 2 to 3 weeks.

In this foregoing group, the sequence of clinical events is the same as that described under concussion, except that the time sequence is more protracted. Stupor gives way to a confusional state that may last for weeks, and it may for a short time be associated with aggressive behavior and uncooperativeness (traumatic delirium). The period of traumatic amnesia is proportionately longer than in the less severely injured. It is during the period of recovering consciousness that focal neurologic signs (hemiparesis, aphasia, abulia, etc.) become most obvious, though some may have been discerned even in the comatose state. Once the patient improves to the point of being able to converse, he or she is slow in thinking, unstable in emotional reactions, and faulty in judgment—a state sometimes called "traumatic psychosis" or "traumatic dementia."

Finally there is that small, distressing group of severely brain-injured patients in whom the vital signs become normal, but in whom consciousness never returns. As the weeks pass, the prospects become more bleak. Such patients may still emerge from coma after 6 to 8 weeks and make a surprisingly good recovery, but most of them remain in their traumatic coma for months to years, depending on the adequacy of medical support. Some of those who survive for long periods may open their eyes, but they do not see or recognize even the closest members of their family. They do not speak, or they say only a few words; emotional reactions are inappropriate; food placed in the mouth may be chewed and swallowed ("persistent vegetative state," see page 233). Hemiplegia or quadriplegia are usually demonstrable. Finally, life is mercifully terminated by some medical complication. In some 10 or more such cases that have come to autopsy, the authors have found old contusions and hemorrhages and a few scattered focal cerebral lesions with wallerian degeneration in appropriate regions of the brain; but most importantly, there has been damage to one or other cerebral peduncle and old hemorrhages and zones of necrosis in the thalamus and reticular formation of the upper brainstem. The latter changes may be primary or are secondary to temporal lobe–tentorial herniation. We are surprised that they were not reported in the pathologic material of Strich (see above) and wonder whether the mesencephalon and thalamus were examined with a sufficient number of transverse microscopic sections.

In generalizing about this category of head injury, i.e., patients who are and have been comatose from the time of injury, one has the impression that the effects of contusion, hemorrhage, and brain swelling are most severe about 18 to 36 h after the injury; and, if the patients survive this period, the chances of dying from the complications of craniocerebral trauma (contusions, intracerebral hemorrhage, localized cerebral edema, herniations of the temporal lobe, subdural hemorrhage, hypoxia, and pneumonia) are greatly reduced. The mortality rate of those who reach the hospital in coma is about 20 percent, and most of the deaths occur in the first 12 to 24 h as a result of direct injury to the brain in combination with other nonneurologic injuries. Of those alive at 24 h, the overall mortality falls to 7 to 8 percent; after 48 h, only 1 to 2 percent succumb.

PATIENTS WHO ARE UNCONSCIOUS WHEN FIRST SEEN BUT ARE SAID TO HAVE REGAINED CONSCIOUSNESS AFTER THE ACCIDENT (PRESENCE OF LUCID INTERVAL)

The number of patients in this group is smaller than in the other two, but the category is of great importance because it includes many who are in urgent need of surgical treatment. The initial coma may have lasted only a few minutes, and exceptionally there may have been none at all—in which instance one might wrongly conclude that since there was no concussion there is no possibility of traumatic hemorrhage or other type of brain injury. The following conditions must be considered in every case of this type.

Acute Epidural Hemorrhage   This condition is due as a rule to a temporal or parietal fracture with laceration of the middle meningeal artery and vein. Less often there is a tear in a dural venous sinus. The injury, even when it fractures the skull, may not have produced coma. A typical example is that of a child who has fallen from a bicycle or swing or has suffered some other hard blow to the head and was only momentarily unconscious. A few hours or a day or two later (exceptionally the interval may be several days or a week, especially with venous bleeding), headache of increasing severity develops, along with vomiting, drowsiness, confusion, seizures (which may be one-sided), and hemiparesis with slightly increased tendon reflexes and a Babinski sign. As coma develops, the hemiparesis may give way to bilateral spasticity of the limbs and Babinski signs. There may be aphasia. Respirations become deeper and stertorous, then shallow and irregular, and finally stop. The pulse is often slow (below 60 beats per minute) and bounding, with a concomitant rise in systolic blood pressure. The pupil may dilate on the side of the hematoma. The CSF is usually under increased pressure, though normal and subnormal pressures do not exclude the possibility of an epidural hematoma. The fluid may be clear or bloody, depending on whether or not there is an associated contusion, laceration, or subarachnoid hemorrhage. Death, which is almost invariable if the clot is not removed surgically, comes at the end of a comatose period, rarely if ever in a conscious patient, and is due to respiratory arrest. The visualization of a fracture line across the groove of the middle meningeal artery and knowledge of which side of the head was struck (the clot is usually on that side) are of aid in diagnosis and of lateralization of the lesion. CT scan or carotid arteriography are confirmatory. The surgical procedure consists of placement of several burr holes (a single one may miss the clot), drainage, identification of the bleeding vessel, and ligation. The operative results are excellent, except in the cases with extended fractures and laceration of the dural venous sinuses, in which the epidural hematoma may be bilateral rather than unilateral, as it ordinarily is. If coma, bilateral Babinski signs, spasticity, or decerebrate rigidity supervene before operation, the prognosis for life becomes poor. This usually means that temporal lobe herniation and crushing of the midbrain have already occurred.

Acute and Chronic Subdural Hematoma The problems created by acute and chronic subdural hematomas are so different that they need to be discussed separately. In *acute subdural hematoma*, which may be unilateral or bilateral, the latent interval is usually longer than in epidural hemorrhage—several days or one to two weeks. Headache, drowsiness, sometimes agitation, slowness in thinking, and confusion, all of which progressively worsen, are the most frequent symptoms. Focal or lateralizing signs (mainly hemiparesis) are late and tend to be less prominent than the disturbances of consciousness and mentation. Frequently the acute subdural hematoma is combined with cerebral contusion and laceration, and the clinical effects of these several lesions are difficult to distinguish; there are some patients in whom it is impossible to state before operation whether the clot is epidural or subdural in location. The CT scan visual-

izes the clot accurately in about 90 percent of cases. In less acute hematomas the fluid is isodense with the cortex, and its presence is betrayed by ventricular shift. If bilateral, there is no shift (see Figs. 34-5 to 34-7). Arteriography shows displacement of cerebral arteries inward from the skull. Treatment consists of placing bilateral temporal burr holes and evacuating the clot. The surgical results are less certain than in chronic subdural hematoma. If the clot that is found is too small to explain the coma or other symptoms, there is probably extensive contusion and laceration of the cerebrum. Exceptionally the subdural hematoma forms in the posterior fossa and gives rise to headache, vomiting, pupillary inequality, dysphagia, cranial nerve palsies, and, rarely, stiff neck and ataxia of the trunk and gait, in some combination.

In *chronic subdural hematoma*, the traumatic etiology is less clear. The head injury, especially in elderly persons and in those taking anticoagulant drugs, may be trivial (striking the head against the branch of a tree, or on the mantel of a fireplace during a faint, etc.), and it may have been forgotten completely. A period of weeks

Figure 34-5
Unenhanced CT scan showing acute subdural hematoma with shift of lateral ventricles to opposite side.

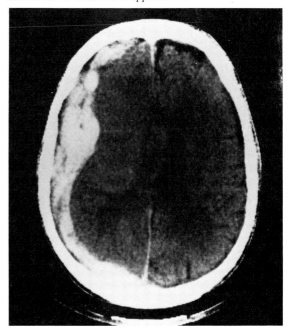

then follows when headaches (not invariable), giddiness, slowness in thinking, confusion, apathy and drowsiness, and rarely a seizure or two are the main symptoms. The initial impression may be that the patient has a vascular lesion or brain tumor or suffers from drug intoxication or a depressive, senile, or other type of psychosis. As with acute subdural hematoma, the disturbance of consciousness (drowsiness, inattentiveness, incoherence of thought and stupor) is more prominent than focal or lateralizing signs. The latter usually consist of hemiparesis and rarely of an aphasic disturbance. Hemianesthesia and homonymous hemianopia are seldom observed, probably because the anatomic structures subserving these functions are deep and not easily compressed (in the case of the geniculocalcarine pathway), and sensory changes are likely to be overlooked in a stuporous, confused patient. Hemiplegia, i.e., complete paralysis of one arm and leg, is usually indicative of a lesion within the cerebral hemisphere, rather than a compressive lesion on its surface. Another important feature of the hemiparesis

is that it may be contralateral or ipsilateral, depending on whether the temporal lobe has herniated through the notch of the tentorium and compressed the contralateral cerebral peduncle against the free edge of the tentorium. As the condition progresses, the patient becomes comatose but often with striking fluctuations of awareness. The ipsilateral pupil dilates (Hutchinson's pupillary sign), owing, it is believed, to direct pressure of the herniating temporal lobe upon the oculomotor nerve. The dilated pupil and ptotic eyelid are more reliable indicators of the side of the hematoma than the hemiparesis, though they too may be misleading in certain cases. Convulsions are seen occasionally, most often in alcoholics or in patients with contusions, but cannot be regarded as a cardinal sign of subdural hematoma. Infants and children may suffer a subdural hematoma and in them enlargement of the head, vomiting, and convulsions are prominent.

Skull films are usually negative except for a shift of a calcified pineal to one side or an occasional unexpected fracture line. The EEG is usually abnormal bilaterally, sometimes with reduced voltage or electrical silence over the subdural hematoma and high-voltage slow waves over the opposite side because of the damping effects of the clot and displacement of the brain, respectively. The cortical branches of the middle cerebral artery are separated from the inner surface of skull,

Figure 34-6

Contrast-enhanced CT scan showing a large right frontal subdural hematoma of 10 days duration. Presence of the clot, which is isodense with the cerebral cortex, is betrayed by the marked ventricular shift.

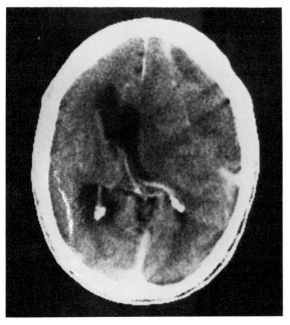

Figure 34-7

Chronic subdural hematomas over both frontal lobes, without shift of the ventricular system. Chronicity results in hypodense appearance.

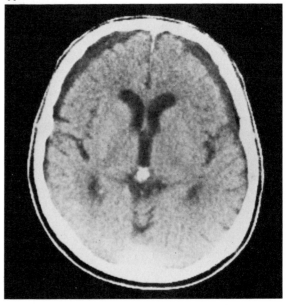

and the anterior cerebral artery may be displaced contralaterally in an arteriogram. The CSF may be clear, bloody, or xanthochromic, depending on the presence or absence of recent or old contusion and subarachnoid hemorrhage; the pressure may be elevated, normal, or subnormal. Of all these diagnostic procedures, the CT scan and arteriography are the most reliable.

The acute, rapidly evolving subdural hematomas are due to tearing of bridging veins, and symptoms are caused by direct compression of the brain by an expanding clot of fresh blood. Unlike the epidural arterial hemorrhage, which is progressive, the bleeding is usually arrested by the rising intracranial pressure.

The chronic subdural hematoma becomes encysted by fibrous membranes (pseudomembranes) which grow from the dura. Some hematomas—probably the ones in which the initial bleeding was slight (see below)—resorb spontaneously. Others expand slowly and act as space-occupying masses. In 1932 Gardner proposed a hypothesis to explain the latter phenomenon, and since then it has been widely accepted that the gradual enlargement of the hematoma is due to the accession of fluid, particularly CSF, which is drawn into the hemorrhagic cyst by its increasing osmotic tension, as red blood cells hemolyse and protein is liberated. The available data do not support this concept. Rabe and his colleagues have demonstrated convincingly that red cell breakdown contributes little, if at all, to the accumulation of fluid in the subdural space. More recently, Weir has shown that there is no significant difference in the osmolalities of fluid samples taken simultaneously from the subdural hematoma, venous blood, and CSF. Why somewhat less than one-half of all subdural hematomas remain solid and nonenlarging and the remainder liquefy and then enlarge, is not known. The experimental observations of Labadie and Glover suggest that the volume of the original clot is a critical factor: the larger its initial size, the more likely that subsequent enlargement will occur. An inflammatory reaction, triggered by the breakdown products of blood elements in the clot, appears to be an additional stimulus for growth as well as for neomembrane formation. According to Rabe et al., the most important factor in the accumulation of subdural fluid is a pathologic permeability of the capillaries in the outer subdural membrane. The CSF plays no discernible role in this process, contrary to the original view of Munro and Merritt. In any event, as the hematoma enlarges, the compressive effects increase. Severe cerebral compression and displacement with temporal lobe-tentorial herniation are the usual causes of death. Treatment consists of placing burr holes and evacuating the clot before deep coma has developed.

Subdural hygromas (collections of blood and CSF in the subdural space) may also form after an injury, as well as after meningitis (in an infant or young child) and pneumoencephalography. It is said that a tear of the arachnoid permits bacteria to enter and excite a serous reaction in the subdural space. Drowsiness, confusion, irritability, and fever are relieved when the subdural fluid is aspirated or drained. Shrinkage of the hydrocephalic brain after ventriculoatrial or ventriculoperitoneal shunting is also conducive to the formation of a subdural hematoma.

Acute Contusional Swelling   Here patients with moderately severe injury, invariably unconscious for more than 5 min at the onset, improve to the point where they are capable of purposive movements of a protective kind but are still confused, mute, and often unresponsive to command, or they may even have begun to respond to forceful commands or to answer a few simple questions when they suddenly relapse into stupor or light coma, raising the suspicion of brain compression from an epidural hemorrhage. Actually, a true lucid interval of normal consciousness has not occurred. However, in the uncomplicated contusion, relapse is seldom profound, and the stupor or light coma can be reversed by the use of dehydrating measures, suggesting that brain swelling is an important factor. The plantar reflex may be extensor on one or both sides and, if unilateral, is always on the side of a hemiparesis. When the abnormal plantar reflexes are not part of a unilateral or bilateral hemiparesis, they usually become flexor by the time the traumatic confusion clears. Pulse and temperature may be slightly elevated for several days. The CSF is often bloody and under increased pressure. [In a series of 200 head injuries, half of which were of a mild type, Russell found 32 with more than 1000 red cells per cubic millimeter. All of the latter had some stiffness of the neck on forward flexion. If there was much blood (more than 100,000 red cells per cubic millimeter), the patient was either comatose or stuporous.]

If improvement resumes after hours or a day or two, one can be assured that serious cerebral compression from dural clots or a delayed cerebral hemorrhage (see below) has not occurred. The threat of temporal lobe-tentorial herniation continues for some days and once this happens the outlook is bleak.

Traumatic Cerebral Hemorrhage   Acute, massive brain hemorrhage may develop as late as a week after a moderate to severe head injury (spätapoplexie), but seldom is there a true lucid interval. This condition, the pathogenesis of which is not well understood, occurs in the elderly patient more than the young. The clinical picture is similar to that of hypertensive brain hemorrhage (deepening coma with hemiplegia, a dilating pupil, bilateral Babinski signs, stertorous and irregular respirations). The problem that cannot be solved, even at postmortem examination, is whether the patient had a fall followed after an interval by the common variety of primary intracerebral hemorrhage or whether a delayed hemorrhage into traumatized brain tissue occurred. Of course, slow venous bleeding might permit a relatively lucid interval of 2 to 3 days between injury and the symptoms of the cerebral hemorrhage, but this is not the explanation of all cases. Coma or confusion, if present from the time of the injury, may obscure the signs of the intracerebral hemorrhage. Craniotomy with evacuation of the clot has given a successful result in a few cases. The wider application of CT scans should help elucidate the pathogenesis and, of course, facilitate diagnosis.

"PUNCH-DRUNK ENCEPHALOPATHY" (DEMENTIA PUGILISTICA)

The cumulative effects of repeated cerebral injuries, observed in boxers who had engaged in many contests over a long period of time, constitute a type of head injury that is difficult to classify. What is referred to is the development, after many years in the ring (sometimes toward the end of the boxer's career, more often a number of years after retirement), of a state of forgetfulness, slowness in thinking and other signs of dementia, and dysarthric speech. Movements are slow, stiff and uncertain, especially those involving the legs, and there is a shuffling, wide-based, unsteady gait. Often there is a parkinsonian syndrome (found in 20 of the 52 case reports of boxers that Roberts abstracted from the literature up to 1969), and sometimes a moderately disabling ataxia. The plantar reflexes may be extensor on one or both sides. The EEG shows slow waves of theta and sometimes of delta type. The pneumoencephalogram in these patients has revealed dilated lateral ventricles and also, according to Spillane, a cavum septi pellucidi, a finding which distinguishes the punch-drunk state from other forms of cerebral atrophy. The clinical syndrome has been analyzed by Roberts, who found it present to some degree in 37 of 224 professional boxers whom he had examined.

A thorough pathologic study of this disorder has been made by Corsellis and his associates. They examined the brains of 15 retired boxers who had shown the punch-drunk syndrome and identified a group of cerebral changes that appear to explain the clinical findings. Mild to moderate enlargement of the lateral ventricles and thinning of the corpus callosum were found in all cases. Also, practically all of them showed a greatly widened cavum septi pellucidi and the septal leaves were grossly fenestrated. Readily identified areas of glial scarring were situated on the inferior surface of the cerebellar cortex, most marked in the folia around the groove formed by the sloping edge of the foramen magnum. In these areas, and well beyond them, Purkinje cells were lost and the granule cell layer was somewhat thinned. Surprisingly, cerebral cortical contusions were found in only a few cases. Notably absent, also, was evidence of previous hemorrhage. Eleven of the fifteen cases showed a varying degree of loss of pigmented cells of the substantia nigra and locus ceruleus, while many of the cells that remained showed Alzheimer's neurofibrillary change; Lewy bodies were not observed, however. The neurofibrillary changes were scattered diffusely through the cerebral cortex and brainstem, but were most prominent in the medial temporal gray matter. Noteworthy was the absence or almost complete absence of senile plaques.

The pathogenesis of the punch-drunk state remains unclear. Meningeal fibrosis and hydrocephalus from repeated small subarachnoid hemorrhages cannot be excluded.

PENETRATING WOUNDS OF THE HEAD (Missiles and Fragments)

All the descriptions in the preceding pages apply to blunt, nonpenetrating injuries of the skull and their effects on the brain. The disorders included in this section are more the concern of the neurosurgeon than the neurologist. In the past, most injuries of this type were a major preoccupation of the military surgeon, but with the increasing amount of violent crime in Western society they have become commonplace on the emergency wards of general hospitals.

Missile injuries, in civilian life, refer essentially to injuries caused by bullets fired from rifles or handguns at high velocities. Air is compressed in front of the bullet so that it has an explosive effect upon entering tissue and causes damage for a considerable distance around the missile tract. *Fragments* or *shrapnel* are pieces of exploding shells, grenades, or bombs, and are the usual causes of penetrating cranial injuries in wartime. The cranial wounds that result from missiles and shrapnel have been classified by Purvis as (1) tangential injuries, with scalp lacerations, depressed skull fractures, and meningeal and cerebral lacerations, (2) penetrating injuries with indriven metal particles and hair, skin, and bone fragments, and (3) through-and-through wounds.

If the brain is penetrated at the lower levels of the brainstem, death is instantaneous from respiratory and cardiac arrest. Fully 80 percent of patients with through-and-through injuries die at once or within a few minutes. If vital centers are untouched, the immediate problem is the continuation of intracranial bleeding and rising intracranial pressure from swelling of the traumatized brain tissue. There is also bleeding from the scalp wound, but this can be staunched without difficulty, and circulatory collapse can be counteracted if the patient reaches the emergency ward alive.

Once the initial complications are dealt with, the surgical problems as outlined by Meirowsky are reduced to three: (1) prevention of infection by rapid and radical (definitive) debridement, followed by the administration of broad spectrum antibiotics, (2) control of increased intracranial pressure and shift of midline structures by removal of clots of blood and the vigorous administration of mannitol or other dehydrating agents and dexamethasone, and (3) the prevention of life-threatening systemic complications.

When first seen, the majority of the patients with penetrating cerebral lesions are comatose. Despite the fact that a small metal fragment may penetrate the skull without causing concussion, this is not true of high-velocity missiles. In a series of 132 cases of the latter type, analyzed by Frazier and Ingham, consciousness was retained at the time of injury in only 22. Of those patients who were unconscious, the depth and duration of coma seemed to depend upon the degree of cerebral necrosis, edema, and hemorrhage. Upon emerging from coma the patient passes through states of stupor, confusion, and amnesia like those which follow severe closed head injuries. Headache, vomiting, vertigo, pallor, sweating, slowness of pulse, and elevation of blood pressure are other common findings. Focal or focal and generalized seizures occur in the early phase of the injury in some 15 to 20 percent of cases.

Recovery may take many months. Frazier and Ingham comment on the "loss of memory, slow cerebration, indifference, mild depression, inability to concentrate, fatigability, nervous irritability, vasomotor and cardiac instability, frequent seizures, headaches and giddiness," all reminiscent of the contusion syndrome of blunt head injury. Every possible combination of focal cerebral symptoms may be caused by such lesions, and there is no point in detailing them further. Useful references are the articles by Feiring and Davidoff, and also those of Russell, and of Teuber, listed at the end of this chapter.

Epilepsy, i.e., recurrent seizures of more or less identical pattern, is the most troublesome sequela. Ascroft and Caviness, in reviewing World War II cases, found that approximately half of all patients with wounds that had penetrated the dura eventually developed epilepsy, most often focal in nature; the figures of Caveness, for the Korean War veterans, are about the same.

CSF rhinorrhea may also occur as an acute manifestation of any penetrating injury that produces a fracture through the frontal, ethmoid, or sphenoid bones. In fact, Cairns has listed these acute cases as a separate group in his classification of CSF rhinorrheas, the other types being (1) a delayed form after craniocerebral injury, (2) a form that follows sinus and cranial surgery, and (3) a spontaneous variety.

Pneumoencephalocele (aerocele) i.e., air entering the cerebral subarachnoid space or ventricles spontaneously or while sneezing or blowing the nose, also indicates an opening from the paranasal sinus through the dura. Feiring and Davidoff cite cases where the air actually entered the cerebral tissue and produced focal signs. This the authors have never seen.

CRUSHING INJURIES OF THE SKULL

Aside from the absence of concussion, these relatively rare cerebral lesions present no special clinical features or neurologic problems not already discussed.

BIRTH INJURIES

These involve a unique combination of physical forces and circulatory-oxygenation factors and are discussed separately in Chap. 43.

SEQUELAE OF SEVERE HEAD INJURY

The signs of focal brain disease, whether due to closed head injuries or to open and penetrating ones, tend always to ameliorate as the months pass. A hemiplegia is often reduced to a minimal hemiparesis or to an ineptitude of voluntary motor function with exaggerated reflexes and an equivocal Babinski sign on that side, and an aphasia to a stuttering or hesitant paraphasia which is not disabling except in a professional person, speaker, or writer. Many of the signs of brainstem disease improve also, often to a surprising extent.

POSTTRAUMATIC EPILEPSY

Epilepsy is the most common sequela of craniocerebral trauma, occurring in about 5 percent of patients with closed head injuries and in as many as 50 percent of patients who had sustained a compound wound of the brain. The basis is nearly always a contusion or laceration of the cortex. Indeed, in cases of pure concussion without contusion or laceration, seizures are not much more frequent than in the general population. The likelihood of epilepsy is said to be greater in parietal and posterior frontal lesions, but it may arise from lesions in any area of the cerebral cortex.

The interval between the head injury and the first seizure varies greatly. About 1 percent of head-injured individuals have one or more seizures (usually generalized) within moments of their injury, and a somewhat larger number within 24 to 48 h (Jennett). These episodes have a good prognosis as far as recurrence of seizures is concerned, and are not ordinarily referred to as posttraumatic epilepsy. The latter term is reserved for the seizures that develop several months after the head injury (1 to 3 months in most cases). Approximately 6 months after injury, half the patients who will develop epilepsy have had their first attack, and by the end of two years the figure rises to 80 percent (Walker). The interval between head injury and development of seizures is said to be longer in children. The longer the interval, the less certain one is of its relationship to the traumatic incident.

The seizures are either of focal character, or generalized with loss of consciousness (grand mal); petit mal is rarely if ever due to trauma. The significance of the different patterns of focal seizures, which vary according to the location of the lesion, has been worked out in detail by Penfield and his associates (see page 214). The frequency of seizures in any given patient varies widely; some patients have only a few, others many, with occasional flurries of status epilepticus. The EEG is of value in diagnosis; a focus of spike or sharp waves is the characteristic finding.

Posttraumatic seizures tend to decrease in frequency as the years pass, and some patients (10 to 30 percent, according to Caveness) eventually stop having them. Individuals who have early attacks (within a week

of injury) are more likely to have a complete remission of their seizures than those whose attacks began a year or so after injury. A low frequency of attacks is another favorable prognostic sign. Alcoholism has an adverse effect on this seizure state. We have observed some 25 patients with posttraumatic epilepsy, in whom seizures had ceased altogether for several years, but then recurred, only in relation to drinking. In these patients the seizures were precipitated by a weekend or only one evening of heavy drinking, and occurred usually in the 12 to 30 h period after the last drink.

Usually the seizures can be controlled by anticonvulsant medications, and relatively few are recalcitrant to the point of requiring excision of the epileptic focus. The surgical results vary according to the methods of selection and techniques of operation. Under the best of neurosurgical conditions, with careful selection of cases, Rasmussen (and Penfield) have been able to eradicate seizures in approximately 50 percent of cases by excision of the focus.

POSTTRAUMATIC NERVOUS INSTABILITY

This troublesome and frequent sequela of head injury has been alluded to above as well as in Chap. 9, on headache. This disorder has also been called the *postconcussional syndrome, posttraumatic headache, traumatic neurasthenia* (Symonds) and *traumatic psychasthenia* (Mapother). Headache is the central symptom, either generalized or localized to the part that had been struck. It is variously described as an aching, throbbing, pounding, stabbing, pressing or bandlike pain and is remarkable for its variability. The intensification of symptoms by mental and physical effort, straining, stooping, and emotional excitement has already been mentioned. Rest and quiet tend to relieve them. Such headaches may present a major obstacle to convalescence. Dizziness, another prominent symptom, is usually not a true vertigo but a giddiness or light-headedness. The patient may feel unsteady, dazed, weak, or faint. However, a certain number of patients describe symptoms which are consonant with labyrinthine disorder. They report that objects in the environment move momentarily, and that looking upward or to the side may cause a sense of unbalance; labyrinthine tests may show either hyperactivity, or the results may be normal. McHugh finds a high incidence of minor abnormalities by electronystagmography both in the concussed patients and in those suffering from whiplash injuries of the neck, but some of the data we find difficult to interpret. Exceptionally, vertigo is accompanied by diminished excitability of both the labyrinth and the cochlea (deafness), and one may assume the existence of direct injury to the nerve or end organ.

The patient with posttraumatic nervous instability is intolerant of noise, emotional excitement, and crowds. Tenseness, restlessness, inability to concentrate, a feeling of nervousness, fatigue, worry, apprehension, and an inability to tolerate the usual amount of alcohol complete the clinical picture. In contrast to this multiplicity of subjective symptoms, intellectual functions and memory show little or no impairment on detailed testing. The resemblance of these symptoms to those of depression is at once apparent. The syndrome, once established, may persist for months or even years, but usually the symptoms lessen as time passes. Strangely, it is almost unknown in children. Its intensity and duration are augmented by compensation problems and litigation, suggesting a psychopathologic process.

EXTRAPYRAMIDAL AND CEREBELLAR DISORDERS

The question of *posttraumatic Parkinson's syndrome* has been discussed many times, usually with the conclusion that it does not exist. Most patients have merely had paralysis agitans or postencephalitic parkinsonism that was brought to light by the head injury. Cerebellar ataxia is a rare consequence of cranial trauma. When present, it is frequently unilateral and is due to injury of the superior cerebellar peduncle. An ataxia of gait may reflect the presence of a communicating hydrocephalus. The one exception to these statements is the punch-drunk syndrome.

POSTTRAUMATIC HYDROCEPHALUS

This is a not uncommon complication of severe head injury. Intermittent headaches, vomiting, confusion, and drowsiness are the initial manifestations, and later there are mental dullness, apathy, and psychomotor retardation. The CSF pressure may by then have fallen to a normal level (low-pressure hydrocephalus). Postmortem examinations have demonstrated an adhesive basilar arachnoiditis, attributed to subarachnoid or ventricular hemorrhage. Since a similar syndrome has been observed occasionally after the rupture of a saccular aneurysm with massive subarachnoid hemorrhage, due presumably to blocking of the aqueduct and fourth ventricle by blood clot or basilar meningeal obstruction, these mechanisms have also been suggested as possible explanations of traumatic hydrocephalus. Response to ventriculoatrial shunt may be dramatic. Zander and Foroglou have had a large experience with this condition and have written informatively about it.

POSTTRAUMATIC PSYCHIATRIC DISORDERS

In all patients with cerebral concussive injury there will be a gap in memory (traumatic amnesia) spanning a variable period from just before the accident to some point following it. This gap is permanent and is filled in only by what the patient is told. In addition, as has already been stated, some degree of impairment of higher cortical function may persist for weeks after moderate to severe head injuries, even after the patient has reached the stage of forming continuous memories. During this period of deranged mentation, the memory disorder is the most prominent feature so that the state resembles alcoholic Korsakoff's psychosis. Pfeifer-Nietleben asserts that this amnesic state is a constant feature of one phase of every prolonged traumatic mental disorder, but to the authors it merely emphasizes the ease with which memory can be tested. Such patients rarely confabulate and usually show abnormalities of registration of events and presented information not seen in the pure amnesic-confabulatory syndrome. Apart from disorientation in place and time there is also a defect in perception and in the ability to synthesize perceptual data. Judgment is grossly impaired. A strong perseverative tendency interferes with action and thought.

These difficulties of obvious organic type were described in detail by Schilder and by Goldstein. The latter author, in his search for underlying psychological mechanisms, settled upon the following factors: (1) a raised threshold of sensory excitation (defective perception), (2) a persistence of or perseveration of response to any stimulus that surpasses the threshold and causes excitation, (3) undue influence on the organism by all external factors, i.e., distractibility, and (4) difficulty in separating figure from background. The latter failure, according to Goldstein, is the most important, for in every perception and every thought process, there must be the selection of a "figure" and the exclusion of all other elements. The authors find this formulation to be an interesting way of phrasing the distractibility, perseveration, and defects in perception, but fail to see the reason for reducing all mental activity to disturbance in figure-background relationships or (in another favorite Goldstein idiom) for reversion from an abstract (higher level) mode of thinking to a lower and more concrete level.

There are other mental and behavioral abnormalities of a more subtle type that remain as sequelae to cerebral injury. As the stage of posttraumatic dementia recedes, the patient may find it impossible to work or to readjust to the family situation. Such patients continue to be abnormally abrupt, argumentative, stubborn, opinionated, and suspicious. These traits, unlike the traumatic mental disorder described above in which there is a certain uniformity, vary with the patient's age, constitution, past experience, and environmental stress. Extremes of age are important. The most prominent behavioral abnormality in children, described by Bowman et al. and by Black et al., is a change in character. They become impulsive, heedless of the consequences of their actions, and lacking in moral sense—much like those who have recovered from encephalitis lethargica. In the older person it is the impairment of intellectual functions that assumes prominence. Even more important is the constitution of the patient. Stable, athletic, tough-fibered individuals take a concussive injury in stride while the sensitive, nervous, complaining types may be so overwhelmed by such an accident that they are unable to expel the incident from their minds. Environmental stress assumes importance as well, for if too much is demanded of the patient soon after injury, irritability, insomnia, and anxiety are enhanced. A calm, supportive environment that does not tax mental energies is conducive to a smooth convalescence.

The tendency is for all such symptoms to subside slowly, even in those in whom an accident has provoked a frank outburst of psychosis, as may happen to a manic-depressive, a paranoid schizophrenic, or a neurotic. These latter were carefully analyzed for the first time by Adolf Meyer.

TREATMENT

PATIENTS WHO WERE ONLY CONCUSSED

Patients with an uncomplicated concussive injury, who have already regained consciousness by the time they are seen in hospital, pose few difficulties in management. They should be detained in hospital until appropriate examinations (radiographs of skull, lumbar puncture, etc.) have been made and proved to be negative, and until the capacity to make consecutive memories has been regained and arrangements have been made for the possible occurrence of delayed complications (subdural and epidural hemorrhage, intracerebral bleeding, and edema).

The group of patients with chronic complaints of

headache, dizziness, and nervousness, the syndrome which we have designated as *posttraumatic nervous instability* is most difficult to manage. Three subgroups can be discerned.

1. A group in which the accident has provoked anxiety or anxious-depressive reactions. Compensation factors loom large in this group especially for the man or woman whose circumstances are marginal, who is uncertain of a job, and who must care for dependents. Such a person is often willing to persist in illness even if compensated at a level considerably below his or her earning capacity, if it provides a modicum of security. Obviously, we are dealing here with matters that have little relation to the physical factors involved in cerebral trauma.

2. A group of patients in whom the *premorbid personality* was of a neurotic or depressive type. The injury to the brain is but one more factor in decompensating a tenuous social and occupational adjustment.

3. A small number of patients, obviously the more severely injured, who upon close examination are found to be *still suffering from a personality change* and *subtle impairments of cognitive function,* i.e., traumatic psychosis or dementia. The anxiety and depression reflect an awareness of their inability to cope with environmental stress.

A rational therapeutic program must be planned in accordance with the basic problem. If there is mainly an anxiety state or anxious depression, the use of drugs, such as meprobamate, chlordiazepoxide or diazepam are useful for the former, and amitriptyline or imipramine for the latter. Simple analgesics, such as aspirin or aspirin-codeine compounds, should be prescribed for the headache and flurazepam or chloral hydrate for insomnia. Any litigation should be ended as soon as possible. To delay settlement usually works to the disadvantage of the patient. Ordinarily the degree of permanent injury can be ascertained within 6 to 9 months, except in a few patients with a prolonged traumatic dementia. Long periods of observation and waiting only reinforce the patient's worries and fears and reduce the motivation to return to work.

THE CONCUSSIVE-CONTUSIONAL INJURY

If the physician arrives on the scene of the accident, a quick examination should be made before the patient is moved in order to determine whether there is dangerous hemorrhage from a scalp laceration or other parts of the body and whether there is a likelihood of a fracture dislocation of the cervical spine, which is occasionally associated with head injury. If the patient is in shock, with cold, clammy skin and feeble pulse, he or she should be covered with warm blankets. In moving an individual with a potential cervical spine injury, the precautions outlined on page 622 should be observed. Bleeding from the scalp can usually be controlled with a pressure bandage, unless an artery is divided, and then a suture becomes necessary.

All such patients should be taken to the hospital, and specifically to an intensive care unit that is fully prepared to deal with them. The first step is to clear the airway and ensure adequate ventilation, by intubation if necessary. To avoid aspiration, the patient should be placed semisupine, with the head on a pillow and turned to one side. If shock is present, it should be controlled by the application of warmth, keeping the head low, and leaving the patient undisturbed for a few minutes. The shock usually comes under control in a few minutes with or without vasopressor drugs or transfusions. Persistent shock is rare in head injury and always raises the suspicion of a ruptured viscera with internal bleeding, extensive fractures, or trauma to the cervical spinal cord.

A quick survey will enable one to estimate the depth of coma, size of pupils, and presence of obvious fractures; if shock is not present, or after the blood pressure has stabilized, a more detailed examination can be performed. The skull should be carefully inspected and palpated. The hair should be cut away from any scalp wounds. Bogginess of the temporal or postauricular region (Battle's sign), bleeding from the nose or ear, and extensive conjunctival edema and hemorrhage are useful signs of underlying skull fracture. However, it should be remembered that rupture of the eardrum or a blow on the nose may also cause bleeding from the ear and nose, respectively. Fracture of the orbital bones may cause displacement of the eye with resulting diplopia; fracture of the jaw causes malocclusion of the teeth, and great discomfort on attempting to open the mouth. Temperature, pulse and blood pressure should be checked and charted hourly and careful notes made of the state of consciousness, pupil size, ocular movements, corneal reflexes, facial movements during grimace, swallowing, tone of limb muscles, movements of limbs, predominant postures, and reflexes. If urine is retained and the bladder is distended, a catheter should be inserted and kept there. If coma persists for more than 48 to 72 h, a nasal tube should be passed and fluids and nourishment given by that route. Intravenous fluids should be administered slowly and not in excessive amounts; the object here is to prevent the development of pulmonary and cerebral edema, the danger of the latter being especially great in children. Lumbar puncture should be done as soon as practicable for diagnostic purposes (immediately if bac-

terial meningitis is suspected), and if the pressure is elevated, it should be lowered to 100 to 150 mmH$_2$O. The practice of daily lumbar punctures has its advocates and its opponents. The authors have tended to use them only if the pressure is elevated and the patient's condition is not improving.

Intravenous hypertonic solutions are of therapeutic value. Urea, 100 ml, or 50 to 100 ml of 25% mannitol may be injected intravenously in an attempt to lower CSF pressure. Ideally the osmolality of the blood should be maintained at 310 to 320 mosmol. Corticosteroids, e.g., dexamethasone (16 to 48 mg/day), have been strikingly effective in reducing brain swelling and permitting vital signs to stabilize. Radiographs of skull and other parts should be obtained after the first day or two, unless there is a suspicion of an epidural hemorrhage, in which case they should be done at once, to visualize a crack across the course of the middle meningeal artery. Restlessness is controlled by sodium phenobarbital or paraldehyde, but only if careful nursing fails to quiet the patient and provide sleep for a few hours at a time.

A practical rating scale by which the state of impaired consciousness can be evaluated hour by hour has been suggested by Teasdale and Jennett (Glasgow scale). It registers three aspects of neurologic function: (1) eye opening (spontaneously, in response to command and to pain), (2) verbal responsiveness (in terms of orientation, confusion, inappropriateness, and incomprehensibility), and (3) motor responsiveness (to command, to localized stimulus, flexion or extension). We find it useful, for it requires little training. A deteriorating scale dictates a change in management. It is useful also in defining the duration of prolonged coma and stupor, and hence, in prognosis.

Once the patient has regained consciousness, the danger of suffocation, aspiration pneumonia, thrombophlebitis, and pulmonary embolism has usually passed. There follows a period of close medical observation, the various proximate and chronic complications being managed if and when they arise, along the lines described earlier in this chapter.

Death from head injury in the first few hours probably cannot be prevented. The advisability of any surgical procedure during this period is much debated. If the patient survives for 1 or 2 or more days but remains in coma, the control of brain swelling and hemorrhage by surgical means must be considered. Should the condition of the patient then begin to deteriorate (pulse rising, temperature rising or falling below normal, state of consciousness worsening, hemiplegia more obvious, plantar reflexes more clearly extensor), a decision must be made concerning an epidural or subdural hemorrhage and increasing brain edema with temporal lobe herniation. Rowbotham, who has had a large experience with cases of this type, recommends a right-sided temporal decompression and two inspection burr holes in the left, one at the sylvian point and one at the parietal eminence, for some of these patients. In his opinion the indications for surgery are (1) retrogression following a period of improvement, which cannot be controlled by lumbar puncture, by oral and rectal hypertonic solutions, or by intravenous dehydration measures; (2) decerebrate rigidity which has its onset after an interval of 24 h (early decerebrate rigidity implies primary brainstem injury), if meningitis is ruled out; (3) persistent coma with a dilated fixed pupil on one side, with no improvement after 12 h; and (4) prolonged unconsciousness associated with persistently high CSF pressure. Not all neurologists and neurosurgeons agree on the value of this plan and would insist on diagnostic CT scans and arteriography as guides. Certainly the removal of a large epidural or subdural hemorrhage, which cannot be diagnosed easily in the comatose patient, may be a lifesaving procedure.

In recent years a striking reduction in the mortality from acute head injuries has been achieved by the application of intensive care together with the free use of tracheostomy. Brain swelling may respond to controlled ventilation, and many of the comatose patients who would otherwise have succumbed to respiratory obstruction, pulmonary infections, or dehydration are thereby saved. Also, greater efforts to evacuate intracranial hematomas as soon as possible seem to have helped. The mortality rate of a group of patients in a state of decerebrate rigidity has been reduced by 50 percent, and the total mortality rate of all hospitalized patients has fallen from about 10 to 3.5 percent. Survivors may be left permanently disabled, but a surprising number return to productive work.

The treatment of the patient with protracted coma has been outlined on page 246. Every patient presents special problems which must be dealt with individually.

SUBDURAL AND EPIDURAL HEMORRHAGES

Treatment of these disorders has been discussed in an earlier part of this chapter.

GENERAL PRINCIPLES OF MANAGEMENT

A head injury has special significance to most persons. Often victims of head injury fear for their sanity and are concerned about their capacity to resume their place in society. In former times, therapeutic measures often involved long discussions of the seriousness of the injury, protracted bed rest, and inactivity, all of which served only to engender greater anxiety. Even worse, these measures were not of proved value. It is now widely acknowledged that the patient does better if the physician minimizes the seriousness of the head injury and reassures the patient about the prognosis of the injury. Early rehabilitation should be encouraged. It may safely begin as soon as the CSF becomes clear, usually within a few weeks except, of course, in the rare cases of protracted coma.

Rehabilitation centers are of great help in restoring morale and reeducating the patient. Rusk and his associates in the New York Rehabilitation Institute were able to return about half of a group of severely head-injured to an independent existence within a year and most of these maintained their improved status after 5 years.

PROGNOSIS

The prognosis of head injury is influenced by several factors. The *age of the patient* is one. Increasing age reduces the chances of survival and of good recovery. Such patients often remain disabled, especially when compensation is involved. Young and middle-aged adults do better, particularly if they are not entitled to compensation. Russell has pointed out that the severity of the injury as measured by the duration of *traumatic amnesia* is a useful prognostic index. If the period of amnesia was less than 1 h, 95 percent of patients were back at work within 2 months; if longer than 24 h, only 80 percent had returned to work within 6 months. About 60 percent of the patients in his series, however, still had symptoms at the end of 2 months, and 40 percent at the end of 18 months. Of the most severely injured (those comatose for several days), many will remain permanently disabled. However, the degree of recovery is often better than one expects; the motor impairment, aphasia, and dementia tend to lessen and may clear. Improvement can continue over a period of 5 or more years. Children seem to recover more completely than adults.

For discussion of trauma of spinal cord, nerve roots, and peripheral nerves, see Chaps. 35 and 45.

REFERENCES

ASCROFT PB: Traumatic epilepsy after gunshot wounds of the head. *Br Med J* 1:739, 1941.

BAKAY L, GLASAUER FE: *Head Injury.* Boston, Little, Brown, 1980.

BLACK P et al: The post-traumatic syndrome in children, in Walker AE, Caveness WF, Critchley M (eds): *The Late Effects of Head Injury.* Springfield, Ill, Charles C Thomas, 1969, chap 14, pp 142-194.

BOWMAN KM, BLAU A, REICH R: Psychiatric states following head injury in adults and children, in Feiring EH (ed): *Brock's Injuries of the Brain and Spinal Cord and Their Coverings,* 5th ed. New York, Springer, 1974, chap 18, pp 570-613.

CAIRNS H: Injuries of frontal and ethmoid sinuses with special reference to CSF rhinorrhea and aerocele. *J Laryngol Otol* 52:289, 1937.

CAVENESS WF: Onset and cessation of fits following craniocerebral trauma. *J Neurosurg* 20:570, 1963.

———: Post traumatic sequelae, in Caveness WF, Walker AE (eds): *Head Injury.* Philadelphia, Lippincott, 1966, chap 17, pp 209-219.

CAVINESS VS JR: Epilepsy and craniocerebral injury of warfare, in Caveness WF, Walker AE (eds): *Head Injury.* Philadelphia, Lippincott, 1966, chap 18, pp 220-234.

CORSELLIS JAN, BRUTON CJ, FREEMAN-BROWNE D: The aftermath of boxing. *Psychol Med* 3:270, 1973.

COURVILLE CB: *Pathology of the Central Nervous System,* pt 4. Mountain View, Calif, Pacific, 1937.

CRITCHLEY M: Medical aspects of boxing. *Br Med J* 1:357, 1957.

DENNY-BROWN D: Delayed collapse after head injury. *Lancet* 1:371, 1941.

———: Disability arising from closed head injury. *J Am Med Assoc* 127:429, 1945.

———, RUSSELL WR: Experimental cerebral concussion. *Brain* 64:93, 1941.

FEIRING EH, DAVIDOFF LM: Gunshot wounds of the brain and their complications, in Feiring EH (ed): *Brock's Injuries of the Brain and Spinal Cord and Their Coverings,* 5th ed. New York, Springer, 1974, chap 9, pp 283-335.

FOLTZ EL, SCHMIDT RP: The role of reticular formation in the coma of head injury. *J Neurosurg* 13:145, 1956.

FRAZIER CH, INGHAM SD: A review of the effects of gunshot wounds of the head based on the observation of 200 cases at U.S. Army General Hospital, No. 11, Cape May, N.J. *Trans Am Neurol Assoc* 45:59, 1919.

GARDNER WJ: Traumatic subdural hematoma with particular reference to the latent interval. *Arch Neurol Psychiatry* 27:847, 1932.

GOLDSTEIN K: *After-Effects of Brain Injuries in War.* New York, Grune & Stratton, 1942.

GROAT RA, WINDLE WF, MAGOUN HW: Functional and structural changes in the monkey's brain during and after concussion. *J Neurosurg* 2:26, 1945.

HOLBOURN AHS: Mechanics of head injury. *Lancet* 2:438, 1943.

JEFFERSON G: The nature of concussion. *Br Med J* 1:1, 1944.

JELLINGER K, SEITELBERGER F: Protracted posttraumatic encephalopathy: Pathology and clinical implications, in Walker AE, Caveness WF, Critchley M (eds): *Late Effects of Head Injury.* Springfield, Ill, Charles C Thomas, 1969, chap 18, pp 168-181.

JENNETT B: *Epilepsy after Blunt Head Injuries.* London, Heinemann, 1962.

———, TEASDALE G: *Management of Head Injuries: Contemporary Neurology,* no 20. Philadelphia, Davis, 1981.

LABADIE EL, GLOVER D: Physiopathogenesis of subdural hematomas. *J Neurosurg* 45:382, 393, 1976.

LEWIN W: Clinical laboratory investigation of head injuries, in Caveness WF, Walker AE (eds): *Head Injury.* Philadelphia, Lippincott, 1966, chap 20, pp 242-259.

MAPOTHER E: Mental symptoms associated with head injury: The psychiatric aspect. *Br Med J* 2:1055, 1937.

MCHUGH HE: Auditory and vestibular disorders in head injury, in Caveness WF, Walker AE (eds): *Head Injury.* Philadelphia, Lippincott, 1966, chap 8, pp 97-105.

MEIROWSKY AM: Penetrating craniocerebral trauma, in Caveness WF, Walker AE (eds): *Head Injury.* Philadelphia, Lippincott, 1966, chap 15, pp 195-202.

MEYER A: The anatomical facts and clinical varieties of traumatic insanity. *Am J Insanity* 60:373, 1904.

MEYER JS, DENNY-BROWN D: Studies of cerebral circulation in brain injury: II. Cerebral concussion. *Electroencephalogr Clin Neurophysiol* 7:529, 1955.

MUNRO D: The diagnosis, treatment and immediate prognosis of cerebral trauma. *N Engl J Med* 210:287, 1934.

———, MERRITT HH: Surgical pathology of subdural hematoma based on a study of 105 cases. *Arch Neurol Psychiatry* 35:64, 1936.

NEVIN NC: Neuropathological changes in the white matter following head injury. *J Neuropathol Exp Neurol* 26:77, 1967.

OMMAYA AK, GRUBB RL, NAUMANN RA: Coup and contrecoup injury: Observations on the mechanics of visible brain injuries in the rhesus monkey. *J Neurosurg* 35:503, 1971.

———, ROCKOFF LD, BALDWIN M: Experimental concussion. *J Neurosurg* 21:249, 1964.

PFEIFER-NIETLEBEN B: Die psychischen Störungen nach Hirnverletzungen, in Bumke O (ed): *Handbuch der Geisteskrankheiten.* 1928, band 7, teil 3, p 415.

PUDENZ RH, SHELDON CH: The lucite calvarium—method for direct observation of the brain. *J Neurosurg* 3:487, 1946.

PURVIS JT: Craniocerebral injuries due to missiles and fragments, in Caveness WF, Walker AE (eds): *Head Injury.* Philadelphia, Lippincott, 1966, chap 10, pp 133-141.

RABE EF, FLYNN RE, DODGE PR: A study of subdural effusions in an infant. *Neurology* 12:79, 1962.

————, YOUNG GF, DODGE PR: The distribution and fate of subdurally instilled human serum albumin in infants with subdural collections of fluid. *Neurology* 14:1020, 1964.

RASMUSSEN T: Surgical therapy of post-traumatic epilepsy, in Walker AE, Caveness WF, Critchley, M (eds): *Late Effects of Head Injury.* Springfield, Ill, Charles C Thomas, 1969, chap 26, pp 277-305.

ROBERTS AH: *Brain Damage in Boxers: A Study of Prevalence of Traumatic Encephalopathy among Ex-professional Boxers.* London, Pitman, 1969.

ROWBOTHAM GF: *Acute Injuries of the Head,* 4th ed. Baltimore, Williams & Wilkins, 1964.

RUSK HA, BLOCK JM, LOWMAN EW: Rehabilitation of the brain-injured patient. A report of 157 cases with long-term follow-up of 118, in Walker AE, Caveness WF, Critchley M (eds): *Late Effects of Head Injury.* Springfield, Ill, Charles C Thomas, 1969, chap 29, pp 327-329.

RUSSELL WR: Cerebral involvement in head injury: A study based on the examination of 200 cases. *Brain* 55:549, 1932.

————: *The Traumatic Amnesias.* London, Oxford, 1971.

SCHILDER P: Psychic disturbances after head injuries. *Am J Psychiatry* 9:155, 1934.

SHATSKY SA et al: High speed angiography of experimental head injury. *J Neurosurg* 41:523, 1974.

SPILLANE JD: Brain injuries in boxers, in Feiring EH (ed): *Brock's Injuries of the Brain and Spinal Cord and Their Coverings,* 5th ed. New York, Springer, 1974, chap 16, pp 529-543.

STERN WE: Carotid-cavernous fistula, in Vinken PJ, Bruyn GW (eds): *Handbook of Clinical Neurology,* vol 24. Amsterdam, North-Holland, 1975, chap 22.

STRICH SJ: The pathology of severe head injury. *J Neurol Neurosurg Psychiatry* 19:163, 1956.

————: The pathology of severe head injury. *Lancet* 2:443, 1961.

SYMONDS CP: Concussion and its sequelae. *Lancet* 1:1, 1962.

————: Concussion and contusion of the brain and their sequelae, in Feiring EH (ed): *Brock's Injuries of the Brain and Spinal Cord and Their Coverings,* 5th ed. New York, Springer, 1974, chap 4, pp 100-161.

TEASDALE G, JENNETT B: Assessment of coma and impaired consciousness. A practical scale. *Lancet* 2:81, 1974.

TEUBER H-L: Effects of brain wounds implicating right or left hemisphere in man, in Mountcastle VB (ed): *Interhemispheric Relations and Cerebral Dominance.* Baltimore, Johns Hopkins, 1962, pp 131-157.

TOGLIA JU: Dizziness after whiplash injury of the neck and closed head injury: Electronystagmographic correlations, in Walker AE, Caveness WF, Critchley M (eds): *Late Effects of Head Injury.* Springfield, Ill, Charles C Thomas, 1969, chap 6, pp 72-83.

TROTTER W: Certain minor injuries of the brain. *Lancet* 1:935, 1924.

————: Injuries of the skull and brain, in *Choyce's System of Surgery.* London, Cassell, 1932, vol 3, p 358.

VAN DER ZWAN A: Late results from prolonged traumatic unconsciousness, in Walker AE, Caveness WF, Critchley M (eds): *Late Effects of Head Injury.* Springfield, Ill, Charles C Thomas, 1969, chap 13, pp 138-141.

WALKER AE: Post-traumatic epilepsy, in Rowbotham GF (ed): *Acute Injuries of the Head,* 4th ed. Baltimore, Williams & Wilkins, 1964, chap 15, pp 486-509.

WEIR B: The osmolality of subdural hematoma fluid. *J Neurosurg* 34:528, 1971.

ZANDER E, FOROGLOU G: Post-traumatic hydrocephalus, in Vinken PJ, Bruyn GW (eds): *Handbook of Clinical Neurology,* vol 24. Amsterdam, North-Holland, 1976, chap 12, pp 231-253.

CHAPTER 35

DISEASES OF THE SPINAL CORD

Diseases of the nervous system may be confined to the spinal cord, where they produce a number of distinctive syndromes. The latter relate to special physiologic and anatomic features of the cord, such as its prominent function in nervous conduction and in relatively primitive reflex activity; its long cylindrical shape; its tight envelopment by meninges; the peripheral location of medullated fibers, next to the pia; the special arrangement of its blood vessels; and its particular relationships to the vertebral column. Because of the frequency and gravity of spinal cord disorders, and the special problems which they raise in diagnosis, we have allotted a separate chapter to them.

In keeping with the general plan of this book, the disorders of the spinal cord are grouped into relatively common syndromes. Some of the anatomic and physiologic considerations pertinent to an understanding of these disorders will be found in Chaps. 3 and 8; others will be discussed in relation to particular spinal cord syndromes.

PARAPLEGIA OR QUADRIPLEGIA DUE TO COMPLETE TRANSVERSE LESIONS OF THE SPINAL CORD

This syndrome is best considered in relation to trauma, its most frequent cause, but it occurs also as a result of infarction or hemorrhage and with rapidly advancing compressive, necrotizing, demyelinative, or inflammatory lesions.

TRAUMA TO THE SPINE AND SPINAL CORD

Throughout recorded medical history, signal advances in the understanding of the physiology of the spinal cord

have coincided with periods of warfare. The first thoroughly documented study of the effects of sudden total cord transection was that of Theodor Kocher in 1896, based on his observations in 15 cases. During World War I, Riddoch—and later, Head and Riddoch—gave the classic description of spinal transection in humans; in France, Lhermitte and Guillain and Barré made additional observations. World War II marked a turning point in the understanding and management of spinal cord injuries. The advent of antibiotics and of rapid and efficient means of transportation permitted the survival of unprecedented numbers of soldiers with spinal cord lesions, and coincidentally provided the opportunity for the long-term observation of these patients. In special centers, exemplified by the Long Beach, Hines, and West Roxbury Veterans Administration Hospitals in the United States and the Stoke Mandeville National Spinal Injuries Center in England, the care and rehabilitation of the paraplegic has been perfected. Studies conducted in these installations have greatly enhanced our knowledge of the functional capacity of the chronically isolated human spinal cord. The contributions of Kuhn, Munro, Comarr, Davis and Martin, Guttmann, and Pollock, listed in the references, are particularly noteworthy.

MECHANISMS OF INJURY

Although trauma may involve the spinal cord alone, it is seldom that the vertebral column is not injured at the same time. Often there is an associated head injury as well, as pointed out in Chap. 34.

A useful classification of spinal injuries is one which divides them into fracture dislocations, pure fractures, and pure dislocations. The relative frequency of these types is about 3:1:1. Except for bullet, shrapnel, and stab wounds, a direct blow to the spine is a relatively uncommon cause of serious vertebral injury. In civilian life, most spinal injuries are the result of *force applied at a distance*. All three types of injury mentioned above are produced by a similar mechanism, usually a vertical compression of the spinal column to which anteroflexion is almost immediately added (anterohyperflexion injury), or, in the neck, the mechanism may be one of vertical compression and retrohyperflexion (commonly referred to as hyperextension). The most important variables in the mechanics of vertebral injury are *the nature of the bones, and the intensity, direction, and point of impact of the force.*

If the cranium is struck by a hard object at high velocity, a skull fracture occurs, the elastic quality of the skull absorbing the force of the injury. If the traumatizing force is relatively soft yet heavy, the spine, and particularly its most mobile (cervical) portion, will be the part injured. If the neck happens to be rigid and straight and the force is applied quickly to the head, the atlas and the odontoid process of the axis may break. If the force is applied less quickly, an element of flexion is added.

When the cervical spine is sharply retroflexed, the spinous and articular processes of the midcervical vertebrae (C4 to C6) are forced together, and these, now acting as a fulcrum, cause a separation between the vertebral body and the adjacent lower intervertebral disk. This results in dislocation, and the cord is caught between the laminae of the lower vertebra and the body of the higher one. Depending upon the intensity of the driving force, the separation may continue, with rupture of the anterior ligament. The posterior ligament may become dislodged from the vertebra below and may then buckle and squeeze the spinal cord backward against the lower vertebra.

In the case of severe forward flexion of the head and neck, the adjacent vertebrae are forced together at the level of maximum stress. The anterior-inferior edge of the upper vertebral body is driven into the one below, sometimes splitting it in two. The posterior part of the fractured body is displaced backward and compresses the cord. Less severe degrees of anteroflexion injury produce only dislocation. Vulnerability to the effects of anteroflexion and retroflexion injuries is increased by the presence of cervical spondylosis or ankylosing spondylitis or a congenital stenosis of the spinal canal.

The spinal cord may be damaged without radiologic evidence of fracture or dislocation, particularly in children, and sometimes one cannot determine the full extent of spinal injury even at autopsy, because of the difficulty in examining the vertebrae. A lateral radiograph of the spine is by far the most satisfactory means of demonstrating the degree of vertebral injury and the tearing of ligaments with dislocation, but one must be careful to avoid full flexion or extension of the neck in order to prevent further injury to the spinal cord.

Another mechanism of cord and root injury, involving extremes of extension and flexion of the neck, is so-called *whiplash* or *recoil injury*. This type of injury is most often the result of an automobile accident. A vehicle struck sharply from behind causes the passenger's head to be whipped back; or if the vehicle stops abruptly, there is sudden forward flexion of the neck, followed by retroflexion. Occipitonuchal muscles and other supporting structures of the neck and head are affected much more often than spinal cord or roots. The exact mechanism of neural injury in these circumstances is not clear; perhaps there is a transient posterior dislocation, or momentary retropulsion of the intervertebral disk into the spinal canal. Again, the presence of cervical spondylosis adds to the hazard of damage to the cord or roots.

A special type of spinal cord injury, occurring most often in wartime, is that in which high-velocity missiles pass through the vertebral canal and damage the spinal cord directly. In some cases they strike the vertebral column without entering the spinal canal but virtually shatter the contents of the dural tube or produce lesser degrees of impairment of spinal cord function. Rarely, a vertebral injury of this type will cause a paralysis of spinal cord function that is completely reversible in a day or two (*spinal cord concussion*). This condition may also be produced by violent falls flat on the back. Little is known of the underlying pathologic changes. The term *concussion*, as applied to spinal cord injury, has led to much confusion because it has been applied indiscriminately to a variety of minor or partial spinal cord injuries in addition to the completely and rapidly reversible form of spinal cord paralysis.

An analysis of 2000 cases of spinal injury, collected from the medical literature by Jefferson, showed that most vertebral injuries occurred at the first to second cervical, fourth to sixth cervical, and eleventh thoracic to second lumbar vertebrae. Industrial accidents most often involved the dorsolumbar vertebrae; accidents in which the individual fell with head down, as in diving into shallow water, affected the cervical region. These are not only the most mobile portions of the vertebral column, but also the regions in which the cervical and lumbar enlargements of the cord greatly reduce the space between neural and bony structures. The thoracic portion of the cord is relatively small and the canal is roomy, and additional protection is provided by the high articular facets (making dislocation difficult) and limitations in anterior movement imposed by the thoracic cage.

In the authors' neuropathologic material, the usual circumstances of spinal injury have been a state of alcoholic intoxication and a fall down a flight of stairs, diving accidents, automobile accidents, crushing industrial injuries, gunshot or stab wounds, and birth injury, in that order of frequency. The majority of these fatal cases had fracture dislocations or dislocations of the cervical spine. As indicated above, this is the most frequently established mechanism of spinal cord injury in civilian life.

PATHOLOGY OF SPINAL CORD INJURY

As a result of squeezing or shearing of the spinal cord, there is destruction of gray and white matter and a variable amount of hemorrhage, chiefly in the more vascular parts. These changes are maximal at the level of injury and one or two segments above and below it. Rarely is the cord cut in two, and seldom is the pia-arachnoid lacerated. The condition is best designated as *traumatic necrosis of the spinal cord.* Separation of such pathologic entities as hematomyelia, concussion, contusion, and hematorrhachis (bleeding into the vertebral canal) is of little value either clinically or pathologically. As a lesion heals, it results in cavitation or a gliotic focus. Progressive meningeal fibrosis and a tension hydromyelia have in rare instances led to a delayed syndrome of spinal deficit.

As with most lesions, the total clinical effect is compounded of an irreversible structural component and a disorder of function, each of which may vary in degree. The extent and permanence of the clinical manifestations are determined by the relative proportions of these two elements.

CLINICAL EFFECTS OF SPINAL CORD INJURY

When the spinal cord is suddenly and completely severed, three disorders of function are at once evident: (1) all voluntary movement in parts of the body below the lesion is immediately and permanently lost; (2) all sensation from the lower (aboral) parts is abolished; and (3) reflex function in all segments of the isolated spinal cord is completely lost. The last effect, called *spinal shock,* lasts for weeks to months and is so dramatic that Riddoch used it as a basis for dividing the clinical effects into two stages: (1) spinal shock or areflexia and (2) heightened reflex activity. The distinction between these stages is not as sharp as this division might imply, but it is nevertheless fundamental. Less complete lesions of the spinal cord may result in little or no spinal shock, and the same is true of lesions that develop slowly.

Spinal Shock or Areflexia   The loss of motor function at the time of injury—quadriplegia (better termed tetraplegia) with lesions of the fourth to fifth cervical vertebrae, paraplegia with lesions of the thoracic vertebrae—is accompanied by atonic paralysis of bladder and bowel, loss of sensibility below the level corresponding to the spinal cord lesion, a state of muscular flaccidity, and complete or almost complete suppression of reflex activity of all spinal segments below the lesion. This condition, in which the neural elements below the lesion fail to perform their normal function because of their separation from higher levels (see further on), involves all skeletal muscles; bladder, bowel, and sexual function; and autonomic control. Vasomotor tone, sweating, and piloerection in the lower parts of the body is lost. The lower extremities lose heat if left uncovered, and they swell if dependent. The skin is dry and pale, and ulcerations may develop over bony prominences. The sphincters of the bladder and the rectum remain contracted (from loss of inhibitory influence of central origin), but the detrusor and smooth muscles are atonic. Urine accumulates until intravesicular pressure is sufficient to overcome the sphincter; then driblets escape (overflow incontinence). There is also passive distention of the bowel, retention of feces, and absence of peristalsis (paralytic ileus). Genital reflexes (penile erection, bulbocavernosus reflex, contraction of dartos muscle) and contraction of the sphincter ani are abolished or profoundly depressed.

The duration of the state of complete areflexia varies greatly. In a small number (5 of Kuhn's 29 patients, for example) it is permanent, or only fragmentary reflex activity is regained many months or years after the injury. Presumably in such patients the spinal segments below the lesion have themselves been injured (vascular?). In others, minimal genital and flexor reflex activity can be detected within a few days of the injury. In the majority of patients, this *minimal reflex activity* appears within a period of 1 to 6 weeks. Noxious stimulation of the plantar surfaces evokes a tremulous twitching and brief flexion or extension movements of the great toes. Contraction of the sphincter ani is elicited by plantar or perianal stimulation, and the genital reflexes reappear at about the same time.

The explanation of the stage of spinal shock, which is brief in submammalian forms and more lasting in higher mammals and especially primates, is believed to be due to sudden interruption of suprasegmental descending fiber systems that keep the spinal motor neurons in a continuous state of subliminal depolarization (ready to respond). Fulton found that in cat and monkey the facilitatory tracts in question are the reticulospinal and vestibulospinal. More recent studies have shown, however, that these tracts are less important in primates and that spinal shock can result from a limited sectioning of the corticospinal tracts. However, this cannot be the complete explanation, at least in humans, for spinal shock does not occur as a result of cerebral and brainstem lesions which interrupt the corticospinal tracts.

Heightened Reflex Activity After a few more weeks, the reflex responses to stimulation, which are initially minimal and transient, become stronger and more easily elicitable, and gradually include additional and more proximal muscle groups. Gradually a typical Babinski pattern of flexion reflexes emerges: dorsiflexion (i.e., physiologic flexion) of the big toe; fanning of the other toes; and later, flexion or slow withdrawal movements of the foot, leg, and thigh (triple flexion). Tactile stimulation of the foot suffices as a stimulus, but pain is more effective. The ankle jerks and then the knee jerks return. Retention of urine and feces becomes less complete, and at irregular intervals urine is expelled by active contraction of the detrusor muscle. Reflex defecation also begins. After several months the withdrawal reflexes become greatly exaggerated (flexor spasms) and are often accompanied by profuse sweating, piloerection, and automatic emptying of bladder (occasionally of rectum). This is the "mass reflex," which is evoked by stimulation of the skin of the legs or by some interoceptive stimulus, such as a full bladder. Varying degrees of heightened flexor reflex activity may last for years, especially if sepsis of bladder or skin intervenes. Heat-induced sweating is defective, but reflex-evoked ("spinal") sweating may be profuse, as indicated above (see Kneiseley). Presumably, in such cases, the lateral horn cells in much of the thoracic cord are still viable and disinhibited. *Above* the level of the lesion, thermoregulatory sweating may be exaggerated and is accompanied by cutaneous flushing, pounding headache, hypertension, and reflex bradycardia. This latter syndrome ("autonomic dysreflexia") is episodic and occurs in response to a specific stimulus, such as a distended bladder or rectum.

Extensor reflexes eventually develop in many of the cases (18 of 22 of Kuhn's patients who survived more than 2 years), *but do not lead to the abolition of the flexor reflexes.* The overactivity of extensor muscles may appear as early as six months after the injury, but only do so, as a rule, after flexor responses are fully developed. Extensor responses are at first manifest in certain

muscles of the hip and thigh, and later of the leg. In a few patients extensor reflexes are organized into support reactions sufficient to permit *spinal standing.* Kuhn observed that extensor movements were at first provoked most readily by a sudden shift from a sitting to a supine position, and later by proprioceptive stimuli (squeezing thigh muscles) and tactile stimuli from wide areas. Marshall, in a study of 44 patients with chronic spastic paraplegia of spinal origin, found all possible combinations of flexor and extensor reflexes; the kind of reflex obtained was determined by the intensity and duration of the stimulus used to elicit it (a mild prolonged noxious stimulus evoked an ipsilateral extensor reflex; an intense brief stimulus, a flexor response).

From these observations one would suspect that the ultimate posture of the legs—flexion or extension—does not depend solely upon the completeness or incompleteness of the spinal cord lesion, as postulated originally by Riddoch. The development of paraplegia in flexion relates also to the level of the lesion, being seen most often with cervical lesions and progressively less often with more caudal ones. Repeated flexor spasms, which are more frequent with higher lesions, and ensuing contractures ultimately determine a fixed flexor posture. Conversely, reduction of flexor spasms by elimination of nociceptive stimuli (infected bladder, decubiti, etc.) favors an extensor posture of the legs. According to Guttmann, the positioning of the limbs during the early stages of paraplegia greatly influences their ultimate posture. Thus, prolonged fixation of the paralyzed limbs in adduction and semiflexion favors subsequent paraplegia in flexion. Placing the patient prone, or placing the limbs in abduction and extension facilitates the development of predominantly extensor postures. Nevertheless, strong and persistent extensor postures are observed only with partial lesions of the spinal cord.

Of some interest is the fact that many patients report subjective sensation below the level of their transection. A wide variety of paresthesias is described, but the most common is a dull, burning pain in the lower back and abdomen, buttocks, and perineum. The pain may be intense and last for a year or longer, after which it gradually subsides. It may persist after rhizotomy but can be abolished by anesthetizing the distal stump of the proximal segment of the spinal cord, according to Pollock and his collaborators. Transmission of sensation over splanchnic afferents to levels of spinal cord above the lesion (which has been suggested) is therefore not the most plausible explanation.

The overactivity of neurons in the isolated segments of the spinal cord is not fully understood. One assumes that suprasegmental inhibitory influences have been removed by the transection so that afferent sensory impulses evoke exaggerated nocifensive and phasic and tonic myotatic reflexes. But isolated neurons also become hypersensitive to neurotransmitters. Since the early experiments of Cannon and Rosenblueth it has been known that section of sympathetic motor fibers leaves the denervated structures hypersensitive to adrenalin, and Cannon and Haimovici found the motor neurons in the isolated spinal segments to be abnormally sensitive to acetylcholine.

Various combinations of residual deficits (lower and upper motor neuron and sensory) may be expected. Complete or incomplete voluntary motor paralysis, a flaccid atrophic paralysis (if appropriate segments of gray matter are destroyed), a spastic weakness of the legs, paraplegia in flexion or extension, and a partial or complete Brown-Séquard syndrome, all with variable sensory impairment in the legs and arms, are some of the resulting clinical pictures. High cervical lesions may result in extreme and prolonged tonic spasms of the legs due to release of tonic myotatic reflexes. Under these circumstances, attempted voluntary contraction may excite intense contraction of all flexor and extensor muscles lasting for several minutes. Segmental damage in low cervical or lumbar gray matter, destroying inhibitory Renshaw neurons, may release activity of anterior horn cells leading to spinal segmental spasticity. Any residual symptoms persisting after six months are likely to be permanent, although in a small proportion of patients some return of function (particularly sensation) is possible after this time. Loss of motor and sensory function above the lesion, coming on years after the trauma, occurs occasionally and is due to cavitation in the proximal segment of the cord (see further on, under "Syringomyelia").

The level of the spinal cord and vertebral lesions can be determined from the clinical findings. A complete paralysis of the arms and legs usually indicates a fracture or dislocation at the fourth to fifth cervical vertebrae. If the legs are paralyzed and the arms can still be abducted and flexed, the lesion is likely to be at the fifth to sixth cervical vertebrae. Paralysis of the legs and only the hands indicates a lesion at the sixth to seventh cervical level. Below the cervical region, the spinal cord segments and roots are not opposite their similarly numbered vertebrae (Fig. 35-1). The spinal cord ends opposite the first lumbar interspace. Vertebral lesions below this point give rise predominantly to cauda equina

Figure 35-1

The relationship of spinal segments and roots to the vertebral bodies and spinous processes. The cervical roots (except C8) exit through foramina above their respective vertebral bodies, and the other roots issue below these bodies. (From W Haymaker, B Woodhall, Peripheral Nerve Injuries, 2d ed, Philadelphia, Saunders, 1953.)

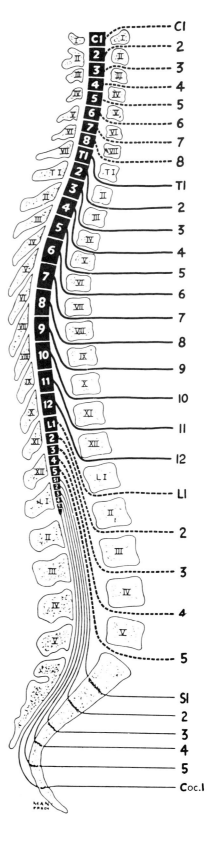

621

syndromes; these carry a better prognosis than injuries to the lower thoracic vertebrae, which involve both cord and multiple roots. In all cases of spinal cord and cauda equina injury the prognosis for recovery is favorable if any movement or sensation is elicitable during the first 48 to 72 h.

Treatment In general, the treatment of spinal injuries is conservative and symptomatic. In all cases of suspected spinal injury, the immediate concern is that there be no movement (especially flexion) of the cervical spine from the moment of the accident. The patient should be placed prone or supine on a firm flat surface (with one person assigned to keeping the head immobile) and should be transported by a vehicle that can accept the litter. Heavy sandbags or similar objects should be placed on each side of the head and neck, and a small hard roll under the nape of the neck.

Once it has been determined that the spinal cord has been injured, corticosteroids may be given, as for brain swelling (page 11), to reduce the swelling of spinal cord tissue. If the spinal cord injury is associated with dislocation of the vertebrae, traction on the neck is necessary to secure proper alignment. This is accomplished by a head halter attached through the head of the bed over a pulley to a weight of 10 to 15 lb, or even better, by the use of Crutchfield tongs which fasten onto the skull. In thoracic crush injuries, hyperextension can be maintained by placing a narrow pillow under the affected area. Traction should be continued for 4 to 6 weeks, and then a brace may be substituted. In practically all centers for the treatment of spinal cord injuries, early fixation and traction of spine have completely replaced decompression by laminectomy. In a few American centers vertebral dislocation and cord compression by bony fragments or disk tissue are still considered to be an indication for decompressive laminectomy and fusion, but there is no compelling evidence that these procedures shorten the rehabilitation of the patient.

The greatest risk to the patient with spinal cord injury is in the first week or 10 days when gastric dilatation, ileus, shock, and infection are the main problems. According to Messard et al., the mortality rate falls rapidly after the first 3 months, and beyond this time 86 percent of paraplegics and 80 percent of quadriplegics are still alive after 10 years.

The aftercare of patients with paraplegia is concerned with management of bladder and bowel disturbances, care of the skin, and maintenance of nutrition.

Decubitus ulcers can be prevented by special skin care. At first continual catheterization is necessary, and then, after several weeks, intermittent catheterization once or twice daily by the "no touch" technique is carried out as a means of encouraging reflex bladder emptying. Close watch is kept for bladder infection, and this is treated promptly should it occur. Morning suppositories and enemas are usually the most effective means of controlling fecal incontinence. Physiotherapy, muscle reeducation, and the proper use of braces are all important in the rehabilitation of the patient. All this is best carried out in special centers for rehabilitation of spinal cord injuries.

The second edition of Guttmann's monograph provides a comprehensive account of the modern management of spinal cord injuries, as well as many other aspects of the subject.

SPINAL CORD INJURY DUE TO ELECTRIC CURRENTS AND LIGHTNING

Among the physical agents that may injure the spinal cord acutely electric currents and lightning should be mentioned. These agents also injure the brain and peripheral nerves, and these effects will be noted briefly. It is the spinal cord, however, that is involved most frequently and severely.

Electrical Injuries In the United States, inadvertent contact with an electric current causes about 1000 deaths annually and many more nonfatal but serious injuries. About one-third of the fatal accidents result from contact with household currents, indicating the vulnerability of most of the population to this type of injury.

The most significant contributing factor to damage of the nervous system is the strength of the current or amperage with which the victim comes in contact, and not the voltage, as is generally believed. The former is derived from the formula:

$$\text{Current strength (amperage)} = \frac{\text{tension (volts)}}{\text{resistance (ohms)}}$$

In any particular case, the duration of contact with the current and the resistance offered by the skin (this is greatly reduced if the skin is moist or immersed in water) may be of critical importance. The physics of electrical injuries is much more complex than these brief remarks indicate (for full discussion see review by Panse).

Any part of the peripheral and central nervous systems may be injured by electric currents and lightning. The effects may be immediate, which is understandable, but of greater interest are the rare instances of neurologic damage which occur many days or months after the accident. The immediate effects are apparently the result of the direct heating of the nervous tissue, but the pathogenesis of the delayed effects is not well understood. Most likely they are secondary to vascular occlusive changes induced by the electric current, a mechanism that also seems to underlie the delayed effects of x-ray irradiation (see below).

Spinal cord sequelae are the most common and occur when the path of the current is from arm to arm or arm to leg. Usually there are pain and paresthesias immediately in the involved limb, but these symptoms are transient. A delayed spinal cord syndrome has been described, most often taking the form of segmental muscular atrophy, occasionally of amyotrophic lateral sclerosis or transverse myelopathy. Unlike the delayed cerebral symptoms, the spinal cord ones may be of gradual onset and slow progression.

When the head is one of the contact points, the patient may become unconscious, or suffer tinnitus, deafness, or headache for a short period following the injury. In a small number of surviving patients, after an asymptomatic interval of varying length, there has been an apoplectic onset of hemiplegia, with or without aphasia, or a striatal or brainstem syndrome, presumably due to thrombotic occlusion of cerebral vessels.

Lightning The factors involved in injuries from lightning are less well defined than those from electric currents, but the effects are much the same. The risk of being struck by lightning is about 30 times greater in rural areas than in cities. Lightning prefers prominences such as trees and hills, so these should be avoided; a person caught in the open should curl up on the ground, lying on one side, with legs close together.

Arborescent red lines or burns on the skin indicate the point of contact of lightning, but the path through the body can be deduced only approximately, from the clinical sequelae. Lightning which strikes the head is particularly dangerous, proving fatal in 30 percent of cases. Death is due to ventricular fibrillation or to the effects of intense desiccating heat on the brain. Persons struck by lightning are initially unconscious, irrespective of where they are struck. In those who survive, consciousness is usually regained rapidly and completely. Rarely, unconsciousness or an agitated-confusional state may persist for a week or two. There is usually a disturbance of motor-sensory function of a limb or all the limbs, which may be pale and cold or cyanotic. These signs also last for only a few minutes to hours, but in some instances the neurologic signs persist, or an atrophic paralysis of a limb or part of a limb makes its appearance after a symptom-free interval. Persistent seizures are surprisingly rare.

MYELITIS

In the nineteenth century, almost every disease of the spinal cord was labeled myelitis. Morton Prince, writing in Dercum's *Textbook of Nervous Diseases* in 1895, referred to traumatic myelitis, compressive myelitis, etc., obviously giving a rather imprecise meaning to the term. Gradually, however, as knowledge of neuropathology accumulated, one disease after another was removed from this category until only the truly inflammatory ones remained.

Today the spinal cord is known to be the locus of a limited number of infective and noninfective inflammatory processes, some causing selective destruction of neurons, others involving the meninges and white matter or leading to a necrosis of both gray and white matter. The currently accepted term for all these diseases is *myelitis*. A distinction is usually drawn between the *acute* variety, in which symptoms develop rapidly and reach their peak of severity within days; the *subacute*, in which the disease evolves over a period of 2 to 6 weeks; and the *chronic*, in which more than 6 weeks elapse between the onset and full development of the clinical picture. Of course there is no sharp distinction between these classes; but in general, the more acute the evolution, the greater the possibility of reversibility, viz., the impermanence of structural change.

Other special terms are used to indicate more precisely the distribution of the inflammatory process: if confined to gray matter, the proper expression is *poliomyelitis*; if to the white matter, *leukomyelitis*. If the whole thickness of the cord is involved, the myelitis is said to be transverse; if the lesions are multiple and widespread over a long vertical extent, the modifying adjectives *diffuse* or *disseminated* are used. The term *meningomyelitis* refers to combined inflammation of meninges and spinal cord, and *meningoradiculitis*, to combined meningeal and root involvement. An inflammatory process limited to the spinal dura is called *pachymeningitis*; and if infected material collects in the epidural space, it is called *epidural abscess* or *granuloma*.

CLASSIFICATION OF INFLAMMATORY DISEASES OF THE SPINAL CORD

  I. Myelitis due to filterable viruses
    A. Poliomyelitis, group B Coxsackie virus, echovirus
    B. Herpes zoster

    C. Rabies
    D. B virus
  II. Myelitis (myelopathy) of unknown etiology
    A. Postinfectious and postvaccinal
    B. Acute and chronic relapsing multiple sclerosis
    C. Necrotic or degenerative
  III. Myelitis secondary to inflammatory diseases of the meninges
    A. Syphilitic myelitis
      1. Chronic meningoradiculitis (tabes dorsalis)
      2. Chronic meningomyelitis
      3. Meningovascular syphilis
      4. Gummatous meningitis including chronic spinal pachymeningitis
    B. Pyogenic or suppurative myelitis
      1. Subacute meningomyelitis
      2. Abscess of spinal cord
      3. Acute epidural abscess and granuloma
    C. Tuberculous myelitis
      1. Pott's disease with spinal cord compression
      2. Tuberculous meningomyelitis
      3. Tuberculoma of spinal cord
    D. Miscellaneous
      1. Parasitic and fungal infections producing epidural granuloma, localized meningitis, or meningomyelitis and abscess
      2. Chronic adhesive arachnoiditis

From this outline it is evident that many different and totally unrelated diseases are under consideration and that a general description cannot possibly encompass such a diversity of pathologic processes. Many of the myelitides are considered elsewhere in this volume in relation to the diseases of which they are a part. Here it is only necessary to comment on the three principal categories and to describe a few of the common subtypes.

MYELITIS DUE TO FILTERABLE VIRUSES

Poliomyelitis and herpes zoster are the important members of this category. The viruses of poliomyelitis have an affinity for neurons of the anterior horn, and those of herpes zoster for the dorsal root ganglia; hence the disturbance of function is in terms of motor and sensory neurons respectively, and not of spinal tracts. There are other forms of poliomyelitic reactions of unknown, presumably viral etiology (see further on, under spinal myoclonus). Affection of the white matter, with sensory and motor paralysis below the level of a lesion, have only been reported in so-called dumb rabies (in contrast to the usual form of "mad" rabies encephalitis), zoster my-

elitis, and an unusual infection transmitted by the bite of a monkey, called the *B virus*, each of which is very rare. As a generalization one may say that any inflammation of the spinal cord that expresses itself by dysfunction of motor and sensory tracts will prove not to be viral in origin, but due rather to one of the disease processes in category II or III. The common types of viral myelitis are described in Chap. 32.

MYELITIS (MYELOPATHY) OF UNDETERMINED ETIOLOGY

These disorders take the form of a leukomyelitis based either on demyelination or necrosis of the tracts in the spinal cord. Varied clinical syndromes are induced, and the basic disease is classified in most textbooks under headings such as postinfectious myelitis, postvaccinal myelitis, acute multiple sclerosis, chronic relapsing multiple sclerosis, necrotizing myelitis, and neuromyelitis optica (Devic's disease). While each of these conditions may affect other parts of the central nervous system as well as the spinal cord, not infrequently the only manifestations are spinal. The distinctions between the aforementioned myelitides are sufficient to justify their separate classification, for in most cases they run true to form; but transitional cases, sharing the attributes of more than one disease, are encountered in any large clinical and pathologic material.

Postinfectious and Postvaccinal Myelitis The characteristic features of these diseases are (1) their temporal relationship to a viral infection (usually one with exanthematous manifestations such as rubeola, varicella, variola, and rarely rubella, influenza, mumps) or a vaccination (antirabies, cowpox); (2) the development of neurologic signs over the period of a few days; and (3) a monophasic temporal course, i.e., a single attack of several weeks' duration with variable degrees of recovery and no recurrence. In most cases these diseases involve the brain as well as the spinal cord (i.e., they are encephalomyelitic); in others the spinal cord is affected predominantly or exclusively.

The usual history in the latter cases is for weakness and numbness of the feet and legs (less often of the hands and arms) and difficulty in voiding to develop over a few days, as the skin rash is fading. Recrudescence of fever may precede or coincide with the onset of neurologic symptoms. Headache and stiff neck may or may not be present. The neurologic symptoms progress for several days after which they remain stationary and then recede slowly. Almost invariably the CSF contains lymphocytes and other mononuclear cells in the range of 20 to 200 (rarely up to 1000) per cubic millimeter with normal or slightly raised protein and normal glucose values. In most cases there are other neurologic signs pointing to lesions in the brainstem, cerebellum, optic nerves, and cerebrum. In some of the cases that followed antirabies inoculation, the peripheral nerves were affected more than the spinal cord; this may happen rarely in the postexanthem cases. Myelitic symptoms that follow antirabies inoculation begin 10 to 20 days after the first treatment and once started, worsen with each subsequent injection. Use of the duck vaccine, which utilizes duck embryo tissues rather than myelinated spinal cord, has almost eliminated this complication.

Most puzzling are autopsy-verified instances of postinfectious myelitis in which the disease developed without an apparent antecedent infection or one which could not be identified (influenza?). Clinical diagnosis in such cases must be based on the time course of the illness and the clinical and CSF findings. There is always uncertainty in such cases as to whether the illness is the opening phase of multiple sclerosis.

The pathologic changes take the form of myriads of subpial and perivenular zones of demyelination, with perivascular and meningeal infiltrations of lymphocytes and other mononuclear cells, and paraadventitial pleomorphic histiocytes and microgliacytes (see page 658).

Once symptoms begin, it is doubtful if any except supportive therapy is of value. One's first impulse, assuming the mechanism to be an autoimmune disorder, is to administer ACTH or prednisone. Probably it is advisable to do so, but there is no evidence that this practice alters the natural course of the illness.

The prognosis must be guarded. Improvement occurs invariably, sometimes to an astonishing degree, but there are examples in which the sequelae have been severe and permanent. The authors have several times given a good prognosis for long-term recovery and assurance of no subsequent relapse only to later witness a recrudescence of symptoms, proving the original illness to have been multiple sclerosis.

Demyelinative Myelitis The lesions of acute multiple sclerosis, presenting as a myelitis, share many of the properties of the postinfectious type, except that the clinical manifestations evolve more slowly, over a period of 1 to 2 weeks or months. Also, their relationship to inoculation or infection is less certain, and in many recorded examples these antecedent events were lacking. Yet as Uchimura and Shiraki have shown in their study of postrabies inoculation in Japan, where myelitis has taken the form of acute multiple sclerosis, the disease does have the monophasic character and some of the pathologic attributes of the postinfectious variety. However, there are other cases which declare by subsequent attacks that the basic illness is one of chronic recurrent demyelination identical to the usual type of multiple sclerosis.

The most typical mode of clinical expression is by a numbness that spreads over one or both sides of the body from the sacral segments to the feet, anterior thighs, and up over the trunk, with coincident weakness and then paralysis of the legs. As the latter becomes complete, the bladder is also paralyzed. The sensorimotor disturbance may extend to involve the arms. Depending on the speed and intensity of the paralysis, elements of spinal shock may supervene. The CSF may be normal or show a pleocytosis, as in the postinfectious variety. Usually the condition is painless and without fever, and the patient recovers with variable residual signs.

There may be difficulty in separating this disease (a severe myelitis of acute multiple sclerosis type with spinal shock) from the ascending Landry-Guillain-Barré polyneuritis and from spinal epidural abscess. With reference to the former, the most helpful finding is a sensory and motor level on the trunk below which all function is abolished; this never really happens in polyneuritis. In the recovery phase of myelitis, the patient enters the stage of minimal reflex activity (see above, under "Trauma to the Spine and Spinal Cord"). Spine ache and tenderness and root pain are features of epidural abscess, along with fever, leukocytosis, increased sedimentation rate, and often a positive bone scan; myelographic block is invariable. Rarely, however, a demyelinative myelitis causes some pain, and the cord may swell sufficiently to interfere with the flow of contrast media. In a few such cases, because of the danger of leaving an epidural abscess undrained, or in the mistaken belief that the swollen cord represented an intramedullary tumor, laminectomy has been performed with negative results.

Treatment with ACTH or corticosteroids, as outlined for multiple sclerosis (page 657), may lead to a regression of symptoms, sometimes with relapse when the injections are discontinued too soon (after 1 to 2 weeks). Other patients, however, show no apparent response, and a few have even continued to worsen while the hormones are being given.

The episode of evolving myelitis in what proves later to be chronic (polyphasic) multiple sclerosis has virtually the same pattern and course as the episode of acute (monophasic) multiple sclerosis. (See Chap. 36 for the description of other clinical variants of acute multiple sclerosis.)

Acute Necrotizing Myelitis In every large medical center, occasional examples of this disorder are to be found among the many patients who present with an acute onset of paraplegia or quadriplegia, sensory loss, and sphincter paralysis. The neurologic signs may erupt in hours, with such precipitancy as to suggest a vascular lesion (myelomalacia from extra- or intravertebral arterial occlusion or hematomyelia from vascular malformation or bleeding diathesis). In other cases the disease evolves at a slower pace, over several days, and some, but not all, are attended by unilateral or bilateral optic neuritis. In the series of cases reported by Bassoe and Hassin, Greenfield and Turner, Kahle and Schaltenbrand, and most recently by Hughes, patients of all ages and both sexes were affected. Sensory disturbance tends to precede motor, and the latter, at first of upper motor neuron type, gives way to a flaccid, areflexic paralysis. A few or several hundred mononuclear cells per cubic millimeter and increased protein may be found in the CSF. The neurologic deficits tend to be lasting. The fatal cases have survived for weeks or months before death from intercurrent infection.

In several cases coming to postmortem examination at variable intervals after the onset, the acute lesion has proved to be a necrotizing hemorrhagic leukomyelitis, not essentially different from the hemorrhagic necrotizing leukoencephalitis described on page 661. For this reason the authors agree with Hughes in classifying it with the demyelinative diseases. Perivenous demyelination and diffuse necrosis of all tissue elements appear related to injury of walls of small vessels and to fibrin thrombi and fibrin exudation. Older lesions leave the spinal cord cavitated or collapsed for a vertical extent of 5 to 20 cm. The optic nerve lesions tend usually to be of demyelinative type, in fact much the same as those of multiple sclerosis. This combination of spinal cord necrosis and optic neuritis appears to correspond to the syndrome described by Devic in 1894 and named neuromyelitis optica. Rarely, postinfectious encephalomyelitis may involve the optic nerves and spinal cord, but most cases, especially where the visual and spinal symptoms are separated by weeks or months, are examples of multiple sclerosis. In one of the authors' cases, in which death occurred many years after the onset of the myelitis, there was an old necrotizing myelitic lesion and many cerebral ones, the latter typical of multiple sclero-

sis. Cases of this type show the overlapping relationship between the necrotic and demyelinative processes.

Under the title of *subacute necrotic myelitis* Foix and Alajouanine and later Greenfield and Turner described a disorder of adult males, characterized by an amyotrophic paraplegia which ran a progressive course over several months. An early spastic state passed into a flaccid, areflexive paralysis. Sensory loss, at first dissociated and then complete, and loss of sphincteric control came on after the paresis. The CSF protein was considerably elevated but there were no cells. Postmortem examinations in their cases and others subsequently reported have shown the lumbosacral segments to be the most severely involved, with progressively less severe affection on passing upward through the thoracic segments. In the affected areas there was severe necrosis of both gray and white matter with appropriate macrophage and astrocytic reactions. The walls of small vessels, which seemed to be relatively increased in number, were thickened, cellular, and fibrotic. Yet their lumens were not occluded. The veins were also thickened and surrounded by lymphocytes, mononuclear cells, and macrophages. These findings have been difficult to interpret. The importance of spinal phlebothrombosis in the pathogenesis has been emphasized, but in the case of Mair and Folkerts only one thrombosed anterior spinal vein was seen; and in the cases of Foix and Alajouanine no thrombosed vessels were found. The authors believe the evidence of venous occlusion to be unconvincing.

MYELITIS SECONDARY TO INFLAMMATORY DISEASES OF THE MENINGES

This class of spinal cord disease is well known and seldom offers any difficulty in diagnosis. The CSF always holds the clue to causation. Often the inflammatory reaction of the spinal meninges is only one manifestation of a generalized disease process. The spinal lesion may involve primarily the pia-arachnoid (leptomeningitis), the dura (pachymeningitis), or the epidural space, e.g., abscess or granuloma; in the latter circumstance, damage to the spinal cord is due to compression and ischemia. Chronic spinal meningitis may involve the pial arteries, and as the inflamed vessels become thrombosed, infarction (myelomalacia) of the spinal cord results. Chronic meningeal inflammation may provoke a progressive constrictive pial fibrosis that virtually strangulates the spinal cord. Spinal roots may in certain instances become progressively damaged, especially the lumbosacral ones that have a long meningeal course. Posterior roots which enter the subarachnoid space near arachnoidal villi (where CSF is resorbed) tend to suffer greater injury than anterior ones (e.g., tabes dorsalis).

Interestingly there are many types of chronic spinal or cerebrospinal meningitis that remain entirely asymptomatic until the spinal cord or roots become involved.

Syphilitic myelitis is discussed on page 499. *Abscess of the spinal cord* (acute bacterial myelitis) is exceedingly rare and probably undiagnosable. It may occur in the course of a staphylococcal septicemia or endocarditis. At times it is a single pyogenic metastasis. *Acute spinal epidural abscess and granuloma* are the most important representatives of this group.

Spinal Epidural Abscess Children or adults may be affected. An injury to the back, often trivial, at the time of a furunculosis or other skin or wound infection or a bacteremia, may permit seeding of the spinal epidural space or of a vertebral body. The latter gives rise to osteomyelitis with extension to the epidural space. *Staphylococcus aureus* is the most frequent etiologic agent, followed by streptococci, gram-negative bacilli, and anaerobic organisms.

The suppurative process is accompanied at first only by fever and pain in the back, followed within a day or several days by radicular pain. Headache and nuchal rigidity are frequently present. After several more days there is the onset of a rapidly progressive paraparesis and paraplegia, associated with sensory loss in the lower parts of the body, sphincteric paralysis, and urinary and fecal retention. Percussion of the spine elicits tenderness over the site of the infection. Examination reveals all the signs of a transverse cord lesion with spinal shock if paralysis is complete. The CSF contains a small number of white cells (usually fewer than 100 per cubic millimeter), both polymorphonuclear leukocytes and lymphocytes—unless the needle penetrates the abscess, when pure pus is obtained. The protein content is relatively high (100 to 400 mg per 100 ml, or more), but the glucose is normal. More importantly, there is a dynamic block (positive Queckenstedt test).

There are other circumstances in which an acute spinal epidural abscess may develop. It may occur in a patient with chronic medical disease(s), in which a septicemia develops. Here the spinal symptoms may be minimal until the onset of the signs of spinal cord compression some weeks later. In other cases organisms may be introduced into the epidural space via a lumbar puncture needle, during epidural or spinal anesthesia, or during a laminectomy for a ruptured lumbar disk. The localization is then over lumbar and sacral roots. In these cases of *cauda equina epidural abscess*, pain may be severe and neurologic symptomatology minimal unless the infection extends upward to the upper lumbar and thoracic segments of the spinal cord.

The foregoing clinical and spinal fluid findings

call for immediate myelography, to determine the level of block and the operative site. If not treated surgically by laminectomy and drainage at the earliest possible moment, the spinal cord lesion, which is due in part to ischemia (compression mainly of veins), becomes more or less irreversible. Antibiotic therapy must also be given. The cauda equina epidural abscess without neurologic signs should be treated with appropriate antibiotics. If osteomyelitis develops, it may require drainage. When osteomyelitis of a vertebral body is the primary abnormality, the epidural extension may implicate only a few spinal sensory and motor roots, leaving long tracts intact. In the cases described by Messer and Litvinoff, stiff neck, fever and deltoid-biceps weakness were the main neurologic abnormalities.

Subacute pyogenic infections and granulomatous infections (tuberculous, fungal) may also arise in the spinal epidural space. The clinical picture is less dramatic, and the diagnosis depends on the demonstration, in a patient with weakness and sensory loss below a certain level on the trunk, of a partial or complete block by contrast myelography. Osteomyelitis may not be seen for a time in plain films, but bone scans are revealing. The treatment depends on the nature of the underlying disease and the general condition of the patient.

Tuberculous Myelitis Solitary tuberculoma of the spinal cord as part of a generalized infection is an extreme rarity. Tuberculous osteitis of the spine with kyphosis (Pott's disease) is more frequent; pus or caseous granulation tissue may be extruded from an infected vertebra and gives rise to an epidural abscess which compresses the cord (Pott's paraplegia). Occasionally a tuberculous meningitis may result in pial arteritis and spinal cord infarction. Paraplegia may appear before the tuberculous meningitis is diagnosed.

All these forms of tuberculosis have become infrequent in the United States and Western Europe. Additional comments will be found on pages 490 to 492.

Meningomyelitis Due to Fungus and Parasitic Diseases A wide variety of fungal and parasitic agents may involve the spinal meninges. They are rare and some do not occur at all in the United States or are limited to certain geographic areas. *Actinomyces, Blastomyces, Coccidioides,* and *Aspergillus* may invade the spinal epidural space via intervertebral foramens or by extension from a vertebral osteomyelitic focus. *Cryptococcus,* which causes meningoencephalitis and rarely a cerebral granuloma, seldom leads to spinal lesions. Hematogenous metastases to the spinal cord or meninges may occur in both blastomycosis and coccidioidomycosis. Occasionally echinococcus infection of the posterior mediastinum may extend to the spinal canal (epidural space) via intervertebral foramens and compress the spinal cord. Schistosomiasis is a recognized cause of myelitis in the Far East and South America; occasionally, it is complicated by compression and necrosis of the spinal cord.

Spinal Arachnoiditis (Chronic Adhesive Arachnoiditis, Meningitis Circumscripta Spinalis) This is a relatively uncommon spinal cord disorder (about one-eighth as frequent as intraspinal tumors, according to Lombardi et al.). It is characterized clinically by a combination of root and spinal cord symptoms which mimic intraspinal tumor. Pathologically there is opacification, thickening, and adhesions of the arachnoidal membranes, the result of proliferation of connective tissue and obliteration of the subarachnoid space. In this sense, the term arachnoiditis is not entirely appropriate, although it seems likely that the connective tissue overgrowth is a reaction to an antecedent arachnoidal inflammation. Some forms of arachnoiditis can be traced to a preceding subarachnoid hemorrhage, and others are known to occur in syphilis or in a subacute therapeutically resistant meningitis. Still others apparently follow the introduction of a variety of substances into the subarachnoid space for diagnostic or therapeutic purposes. These include penicillin and other antibiotics, lipiodol and other contrast media, and (formerly) spinal anesthetics. Repeated corticosteroid injections have also been incriminated. Less convincing are cases attributed to closed spinal injuries. In most cases no antecedent event can be recognized.

Pathologic features Arachnoiditis is usually a diffuse process with a predilection for the thoracic segments. In advanced cases the subarachnoid space is completely obliterated, and the roots and cord are strangulated by the thickened connective tissue. Peripherally placed fibers of the cord are destroyed to a varying extent, and the posterior and lateral columns undergo secondary degeneration. In a few cases the pathologic process is confined to relatively circumscribed portions of the cord, and the subarachnoid space is occupied by loculated collections of fluid that cause a compressive myelopathy, like a meningeal tumor (meningitis serosa circumscripta). The rare association of spinal arachnoiditis and syringomyelic cavitation of the cord will be considered later in this chapter.

Clinical manifestations Spinal arachnoiditis may occur at any age, although the highest incidence of onset of symptoms is between 40 and 60 years; it is rare below the age of 20. Symptoms may occur in close temporal relationship to the acute arachnoidal inflammation or be delayed for weeks, months, or even years. The commonest mode of onset is with pain in the distribution of one or more sensory nerve roots, first on one side, then on both. The pain frequently has a burning or stinging quality, and is persistent. Weakness and atrophy, the results of damage to anterior roots, are less common findings, except in cases involving the cauda equina. Symptoms of root involvement may antedate those of cord compression by months or years. Sooner or later, however, there is involvement of the spinal cord manifested by a slowly progressive spastic ataxia with sphincter disturbances.

Formerly, many examples of adhesive arachnoiditis were observed following spinal anesthesia (immediately or after an interval of weeks or months, or even years). This complication was eventually traced to a detergent which had contaminated vials of procaine. If enough of the contaminant was injected, an areflexic paralysis and sensory loss in the legs and sphincteric paralysis developed within a few days, along with considerable pain. Recovery usually occurred within a year or two. More pernicious, however, was a delayed meningomyelopathy that would develop within a few months up to 5 or more years, causing a spastic paralysis, sensory loss, incontinence of sphincters, and decubiti. Some of the patients died later of blindness and hydrocephalus. There was no effective treatment. This remarkable chemical meningitis has virtually disappeared since anesthetists began to prepare their spinal anesthetic from crystals.

The spinal fluid is abnormal in practically all cases of adhesive arachnoiditis. In some there is a moderate lymphocytic pleocytosis, but the striking findings are those of partial or complete block (positive Queckenstedt test) and elevated protein content, sometimes extreme in degree. The myelographic appearance of arachnoiditis is characteristic (patchy holdup and dispersion of the column of dye and "candle-guttering" appearance) and allows one to make the diagnosis with certainty.

Treatment In the early stages of arachnoiditis, adrenocorticosteroids may be used to control the inflammatory reaction and to prevent progress of the disease, but their value is questionable. Surgery may be effective in cases with localized "cyst" formation and cord compression. Selective posterior rhizotomy may be useful in relieving severe radicular pain. For chronic adhesive arachnoiditis, there is no effective surgical or medical treatment.

OTHER MYELITIDES OF INDETERMINATE CAUSE

The older medical literature contains numerous references to bacterial infections (pneumonia, gonorrhea, and other) that resulted in some type of myelopathy. However, the descriptions are inexact and pathologic verification is lacking so that it is difficult to interpret them. The same is true of myelopathies that follow intravenous injections of contaminated heroin and other drugs. The authors have the impression that some type of angiitis may underlie them. Their rarity does not promise quick solution.

Recently attention has been drawn to a rare but distinctive form of *encephalomyelitis of unknown cause*, characterized clinically by tonic rigidity and intermittent myoclonic jerking of the trunk and limb muscles and by painful spasms evoked by sensory or emotional stimuli (Whitely et al.). Signs of brainstem involvement occur in the late stages of the disease, which is usually progressive over a period of several months or a year or longer; but consciousness is preserved. The CSF may be normal or show a mild lymphocytic pleocytosis and increase in protein content. This is probably the same disorder that has been described by Campbell and Garland under the title of *subacute myoclonic spinal neuronitis*, and more recently by Howell et al.

The brunt of the pathologic process falls on the cervical portion of the spinal cord. Widespread loss mainly of internuncial neurons with relative sparing of the anterior horn cells, neuronophagia of internuncial neurons, reactive gliosis and microglial proliferation, conspicuous lymphocytic cuffing of small blood vessels, and scanty meningeal inflammation are the main findings. Involvement of the white matter is less conspicuous.

The pathophysiology of the rigidity in these cases is not well understood, but may be due to the impaired function (or destruction) of Renshaw cells, with the release of tonic myotatic reflexes. The painful spasms and dysesthesias relate in some way to neuronal lesions in the posterior horns of the spinal cord and dorsal root ganglia. Comparable states of rigidity and spasms of the limbs may be seen with various lesions of the cervical spinal cord, notably trauma (see above) and glioma, due to interruption of descending medullary-spinal inhibitory tracts, and as has been indicated on page 75, myo-

clonic jerking of the trunk and limbs may be due to neuronal damage that is limited to the spinal cord.

The disorder under discussion needs to be differentiated clinically from the syndrome of *continuous muscle fiber activity* of Isaacs and the "*stiff man*" *syndrome* of Moersch and Woltmann (see Chap. 52).

VASCULAR DISEASES OF THE SPINAL CORD

In comparison to the brain, the spinal cord is an uncommon site of vascular disease. The spinal arteries are not susceptible to atherosclerosis, and emboli rarely lodge there. As was stated above, in relation to chronic meningeal infections, an endarteritis involving vessels on the surface of the cord may lead to thrombosis and infarction. Polyarteritis nodosa may have a similar effect, although this disease is more often localized to the peripheral than to the central nervous system. Very rarely the spinal cord is affected in lupus erythematosus, but a vascular basis has not been established. Transient or lasting ischemia of the cervical segments has been observed by the authors as a complication of arteriography. Occlusion of vertebrospinal branches results in lesions in the upper cervical segments, of the thyrocervical branches of the carotid in lesions in the middle cervical segments, and of the costocervical branches of the carotid in lesions of lower cervical segments. Recovery after several days is the rule.

Of all the vascular disorders of the spinal cord, infarction and bleeding are the only ones that occur with any regularity. An understanding of these disorders requires some knowledge of the blood supply of the spinal cord.

VASCULAR ANATOMY OF THE SPINAL CORD

The blood supply of the spinal cord is derived from a paired series of segmental vessels arising from the aorta and from branches of the subclavian and internal iliac arteries (Fig. 35-2). The most important branches of the subclavian are the vertebral arteries, the segmental branches of which form the rostral origins of the anterior median and posterior lateral spinal arteries and constitute the major blood supply to the cervical cord. The thoracic and lumbar cord are nourished by segmental arteries arising from the aorta and internal iliac arteries;

segmental branches of the lateral sacral arteries supply the sacral cord.

A typical segmental artery divides into an anterior and posterior ramus (Fig. 35-3). Each posterior ramus gives rise to a spinal artery which enters the vertebral foramen, pierces the dura, and supplies the spinal ganglion and roots through its anterior and posterior radicular branches. The spinal cord is not supplied by these radicular arteries, but by *anterior and posterior medullary arteries*, which arise separately from the spinal arteries at irregular intervals. There are six to eight important anterior medullary arteries and a somewhat larger number of posterior medullary arteries and, for all practical purposes, these are the only sources of blood to the spinal cord. The most consistent and important of the anterior medullary arteries is the *artery of Adamkiewicz*, which usually approaches the cord on the left side with the anterior roots of a cord segment between T10 and L3. This artery may be occluded at its origin by atherosclerosis or arteritis. In any individual patient, however, one cannot predict the precise area supplied by this or any other anterior medullary artery, or what proportion of cord will be infarcted if one of these vessels is occluded.

The anterior medullary arteries form the single anterior median spinal artery, which runs the full length of the cord in the anterior sulcus and gives off direct penetrating branches via the central (sulcal) arteries. These penetrating branches supply most of the anterior gray columns and the ventral portions of the dorsal gray columns (Fig. 35-3). The peripheral rim of white matter of the anterior two-thirds of the cord is supplied from a pial network which also originates from the anterior median spinal artery. Thus, the branches of the anterior median spinal artery supply roughly the ventral two-thirds of the spinal cord. The posterior medullary arteries form the paired posterior spinal arteries which supply the dorsal third of the cord by means of direct penetrating vessels and a plexus of pial vessels (similar to that of the ventral cord, with which it anastomoses freely). Within the cord substance, then, there is a "watershed" area of capillaries where the penetrating branches of the anterior median spinal artery (via the central sulcal arteries) meet the penetrating branches of the posterior spinal arteries and the branches of the circumferential pial network. All spinal segments, because of the variable size of collateral arteries, do not have the same abundance of circulatory protection. Hence a hypoten-

sive crisis, as in diabetic acidosis, poliomyelitis, anesthesia, etc., may result in ischemic necrosis of certain segments, usually the upper thoracic, leading to interruption of sensorimotor tracts. This may explain the occasional occurrence of sensory symptoms in poliomyelitis.

Figure 35-2

Anterior view of spinal cord with its segmental blood supply from the aorta. See text for details. (From Herrick and Mills.)

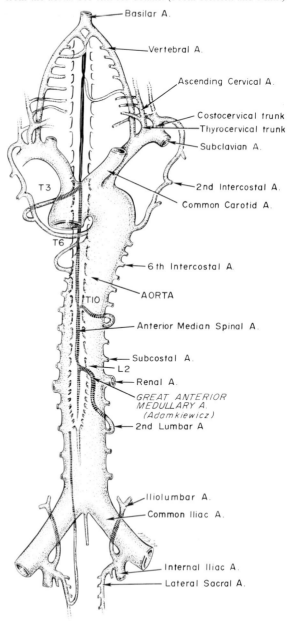

INFARCTION OF SPINAL CORD (MYELOMALACIA)

Ischemic softening of the spinal cord usually involves the territory of the anterior spinal artery, i.e., a variable vertical extent of the ventral parts (anterior two-thirds) of the spinal cord. The resulting clinical abnormalities are generally referred to as the *anterior spinal artery syndrome*, first described by Spiller in 1909. Atherosclerosis and thrombotic occlusion of the anterior spinal artery itself is not common, however, and infarction in the territory of this artery is more often secondary to disease of important medullary arteries (see above) or to disease of the aorta—either advanced atherosclerosis or a dissecting aneurysm, which occludes or shears the impor-

secting aneurysm, which occludes or shears the important segmental spinal arteries at their origins. Nonetheless, we have seen a number of possible instances in adolescents and young adults in whom no aortic or spinal arterial disease could be demonstrated. Cardiac surgery, which requires clamping of the aorta for more than 30 min, and aortic arteriography may occasionally be complicated by infarction in the territory of the anterior spinal artery. Occasionally, polyarteritis nodosa or emboli arising from severely atheromatous aortas may occlude spinal medullary arteries. Infarction may be associated with an arteriovenous (AV) malformation of the spinal cord. According to Antoni, who reported several cases, the blood is shunted away from spinal cord tissue through the AV fistula. Hughes considers this the most common cause of symptoms in AV malformations and points out that many of the cases in Wyburn-Mason's

Figure 35-3

Representative cross section of lumbar vertebra and spinal cord with its blood supply at level of an anterior medullary artery. The shaded zones in the posterior part of the cord, ventral part of the cord, and margins of the ventral cord represent the regions of blood supply of the posterior spinal arteries, central (sulcal) arteries, and pial plexus, respectively. Borders of these three zones, appearing as white in the diagram, represent watershed areas. (From Herrick and Mills.)

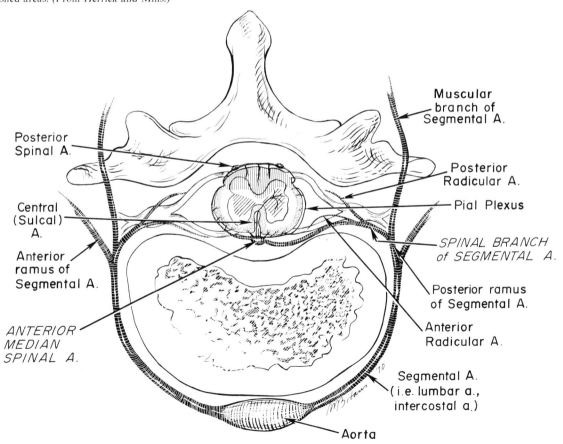

monograph on vascular malformations of the spinal cord were of this type.

The clinical manifestations will of course vary with the level of infarction, but common to all cases is the *development of motor paralysis and dissociated sensory loss* below the level of the lesion, accompanied by paralysis of sphincteric function. The symptoms may develop instantaneously or over an hour or two, surely much more rapidly than in the myelitides. Pain is sometimes a complaint, either diffuse in a segment of the body (e.g., legs) or more often radicular, corresponding to the upper level of the lesion. Paralysis is usually bilateral, occasionally unilateral, and is rarely complete. Except in high cervical lesions, the sensory changes are dissociated; i.e., pain and temperature sensations are lost (due to interruption of the spinothalamic tracts), but vibration and position sense are unimpaired (sparing of posterior columns). Initially the limbs are flaccid and areflexic, as in spinal shock from other abrupt transverse lesions, followed after several weeks by the development of spasticity, hyperactive tendon reflexes, clonus and Babinski signs, and some degree of voluntary bladder control (unless sacral segments have been infarcted). Dissecting aneurysm of the aorta—which announces itself by intense interscapular and/or chest pain (occasionally it is painless), widening of the aorta, and circulatory obstruction to the legs or arms and various organs—gives rise to a number of neurologic syndromes. The most common syndromes are (1) paralysis of both legs and sphincters with sensory loss usually below T6 (Weisman and Adams), (2) obstruction of a brachial artery with sensorimotor neuropathy in the limb, and (3) obstruction of a common carotid artery with hemiplegia.

Rarely, ischemic infarction of the cord is confined to the gray matter. In these cases there is also an abrupt onset of muscle weakness in the legs, but no pain or sensory loss. In a few cases, ischemia of internuncial motor neurons has resulted in intensely painful *segmental spasm and spinal myoclonus.*

Arteriography was formerly an occasional cause of acute myelopathy, and the authors have observed a number of such cases. Killen and Foster reviewed 43 examples of this accident in 1966. The onset of sensorimotor paralysis is immediate, and the effects, often permanent. The syndrome of painful spasms, spinal myoclonus and rigidity has also been observed under these conditions. Vascular spasm and occlusion result in infarct necrosis. The frequency of this complication has

been reduced by the introduction of less toxic contrast media.

Treatment in all forms of spinal cord infarction is symptomatic with attention, in the acute stage, to the care of bladder, bowel, and skin; after 10 to 14 days, more active rehabilitation measures can be started.

HEMORRHAGE INTO THE SPINAL CORD (HEMATOMYELIA) AND SPINAL CANAL (HEMATORRHACHIS)

Hemorrhage into the spinal cord is also rare, compared to the frequency of cerebral hemorrhage. The apoplectic onset of symptoms that involve tracts (motor or sensory or both) in the spinal cord, associated with blood and xanthochromia in the spinal fluid, are the identifying features of hematomyelia. Aside from trauma, hematomyelia is usually traceable to a vascular malformation or bleeding disease, and particularly to the administration of anticoagulants. Bleeding into the epidural or subdural space may have the same causes and give rise to a rapidly evolving compressive myelopathy. Like epidural abscess, this represents a neurologic emergency and calls for immediate myelographic localization and surgical evacuation.

Recent advances in the techniques of selective spinal angiography and microsurgery have permitted the visualization and treatment of vascular lesions with a precision not imaginable a decade or two ago (see Djindjian). These angiographic procedures have made it possible to distinguish between the several types of vascular malformations and hemangioblastomas and to localize them accurately to the spinal cord, epidural or subdural space, or the vertebral bodies.

The clinical picture in many of the vascular malformations is one of intermittent progression over a long period of time (weeks, months, years). Paresis and sensory disturbances appear first in the legs and later in the arms. Acute exacerbations may be accompanied by subarachnoid bleeding. (Such cases tend to progress more slowly than the subacute necrotizing myelitis of Foix and Alajouanine.)

Logue has summarized his experience with a special group of largely venous AV malformations of the thoracolumbosacral cord in elderly men. All had developed a sensorimotor paralysis with sphincteric disturbances which had progressed over months to a year or more to partial or complete paraplegia. Arrest of the disease and often some improvement was achieved by excising the angioma nidus and ligating the "feeder vessels," thereby reducing the venous bed. Ischemia and venous compression of neural elements is believed to be the mechanism of spinal cord damage. Care must be taken to distinguish such malformations from the spinal hemangioblastomas of Lindau's disease, which tend to lie on the posterior surface of the cord and to cause syringomyelic cavitation.

In the Klippel-Trénaunay syndrome, a vascular malformation of the spinal cord is associated with a cutaneous vascular nevus; when the malformation lies in the low cervical region, there may be enlargement of finger, hand, or arm (the hemangiectatic hypertrophy of Parkes Weber). Some of these vascular lesions have been treated by defining and ligating their feeding vessels. In other cases it has been possible to extirpate the entire lesion.

The authors have had under their care several patients with the familial telangiectasia of Osler-Rendu-Weber disease, who developed acute hemorrhagic lesions of the spinal cord. The cord lesions cause partial syndromes and are usually followed by considerable recovery of function. The CSF may or may not be sanguineous. Rarely, this same disease is responsible for a hemorrhagic lesion of the brain.

UNEXPLAINED CASES

The aforementioned diseases do not account for all the cases of acute spinal paraplegia or quadriplegia. The authors have observed a number of children or adolescents who developed such a syndrome within a few hours, from which there was only slight recovery, if any. The CSF and the radiographic pictures obtained during myelography are normal. One cannot determine whether or not these are instances of myelitis or ischemic necrosis.

THE SYNDROME OF SUBACUTE OR CHRONIC SPINAL ATAXIA WITH PARAPARESIS

The gradual development of ataxia and weakness of the legs is the common manifestation of several diseases. A syndrome of this type, which begins insidiously in late childhood or adolescence and progresses steadily over many years, is usually indicative of spinocerebellar degeneration (Friedreich's ataxia) or one of its variants. In early adult life, multiple sclerosis is the most frequent cause; syphilitic meningomyelitis and spinal arachnoiditis are uncommon causes. In middle and late adult life, subacute combined degeneration of the cord (vitamin B_{12} deficiency), combined system disease of the nonpernicious anemia type, a late demyelinative myelopathy,

cervical spondylosis, and tumor are the important diagnostic considerations.

FRIEDREICH'S ATAXIA

See pages 816 to 818.

MULTIPLE SCLEROSIS

Ataxic paraparesis is probably the most common manifestation of multiple sclerosis. Asymmetric affection of the limbs, and signs of cerebral, optic nerve, brainstem, and cerebellar involvement provide the important confirmatory evidence for the diagnosis of this disease. Nevertheless, purely spinal involvement may occur, no lesions being found outside the spinal cord, even at autopsy. A frequent problem in diagnosis is posed by the older adult patient who is not known to have had multiple sclerosis in earlier life (previous episodes having been subclinical or forgotten). Such cases must be differentiated from cervical spondylosis and tumor. Of aid in the diagnosis is the finding of monoclonal bands of IgG in the CSF, and the demonstration by evoked potential studies of lesions in the optic nerves and in the auditory and tactile tracts of the brainstem (see Chap. 36).

SYPHILITIC MENINGOMYELITIS

Here, as in multiple sclerosis, the degree of ataxia and spastic weakness is variable. A few patients have an almost pure state of spastic weakness of the legs, requiring differentiation from motor system disease and familial spastic paraplegia. Such cases, formerly called Erb's spastic paraplegia and attributed to meningovascular syphilis, are now recognized as being nonspecific. In others, sensory ataxia and other posterior column signs predominate, and ventral roots are involved in the chronic meningeal inflammation. There may be signs of segmental amyotrophy, hence the term *syphilitic amyotrophy of the upper extremities with spastic paraplegia*. As indicated earlier, spinal arteries may become thrombosed, converting a chronic spastic paraparesis to a flaccid one, with urinary retention and sensory loss. The confirmation of diagnosis depends on the finding of a lymphocytic pleocytosis, an elevated protein and gamma globulin, and a positive serologic reaction in the CSF. Apparently, in rare instances, a late and advancing form of the disease may appear in a known syphilitic patient after the

CSF has become negative. Treatment and other aspects of this disease are discussed on pages 499 and 500.

SUBACUTE COMBINED DEGENERATION (SCD) OF SPINAL CORD

This form of spinal cord disease, due to vitamin B_{12} deficiency, is fully described in Chap. 38. Almost invariably it begins with symptoms and signs of posterior column involvement, followed within a matter of several weeks or months by affection of the corticospinal tracts. Of particular importance is the fact that SCD is a treatable disease and that the degree of reversibility is dependent upon the duration of symptoms before specific treatment is begun. There is a premium, therefore, on early diagnosis.

COMBINED SYSTEM DISEASE OF NONPERNICIOUS ANEMIA TYPE

A more common intrinsic disease of the spinal cord, affecting the posterior and lateral columns (in this sense, *a combined system disease)*, is not associated with pernicious anemia. In this syndrome, in distinction to SCD, signs of corticospinal tract disease precede those of the posterior columns and are more prominent throughout the illness, which is slowly and chronically progressive. Little is known of its pathologic basis or cause.

Progressive spastic or spastic-ataxic paraparesis of a chronic, irreversible type may also develop *in conjunction with chronic, decompensated liver disease* (see page 735); in certain cases of *adrenoleukodystrophy*, particularly in the symptomatic heterozygote, i.e., the female carrier (page 696); and in *adhesive spinal arachnoiditis*, which has been discussed in the preceding section on myelitis.

CERVICAL SPONDYLOSIS WITH MYELOPATHY

It has been stated, correctly in our opinion, that this is the most frequently observed myelopathy in general hospitals. Basically a degenerative disease of the spine, involving the lower cervical vertebrae, it narrows the spinal canal and intervertebral foramens and causes progressive injury of the spinal cord or roots, or both.

Historical Note   Key, in 1838, probably gave the first description of a spondylotic bar. In two cases of compressive myelopathy with paraplegia, he found "a projection of the intervertebral substance, or rather the pos-

terior ligament of the spine, which was thickened and presented a firm ridge which had lessened the diameter of the canal by nearly a third. The ligament, where it passes over the posterior surface of the intervertebral substance, was found to be ossified." In 1892, Horsley performed a cervical laminectomy in such a patient, in whom a subacutely evolving paraplegia had been precipitated by trauma: a "transverse ridge of bone" was found to be compressing the spinal cord at the level of the sixth cervical vertebra. Thereafter, operations were performed in many cases of this sort, and the tissues removed at operation were repeatedly misidentified as benign cartilaginous tumors or "chondromata." In 1928, Stookey described in detail the pathologic effects upon the spinal cord and roots of these "ventral extradural chondromas."

Also of historical importance is Gowers' original account, in 1892, of *vertebral exostoses,* in which he described osteophytes that protrude from the posterior surface of the vertebral bodies and encroach upon the spinal canal, causing slow compression of the cord, as well as bony overgrowth in the intervertebral foramina, giving rise to radicular pain. Gowers correctly predicted that these lesions would offer a more promising field for the surgeon than other kinds of vertebral tumors.

Schmorl and his associates, beginning in 1929, drew attention to the rupture of the nucleus pulposus into the adjacent vertebral body (Schmorl's nodules) and into the spinal canal, but little clinical significance was attributed to these lesions. Peet and Echols, in 1934, were probably the first to suggest that the so-called chondromata represented protrusions of intervertebral disk material. This idea gained wide credence after the publication, in the same year, of the classic article on ruptured intervertebral disk by Mixter and Barr. Although the latter names are usually associated with the lumbar disk syndrome, 4 of their original 19 cases were instances of cervical disk disease.

Strangely, there was little awareness of the frequency and importance of spondylotic myelopathy for many years after these basic observations were made. All the interest was in the acute ruptured disk. Finally it was Russell Brain, in 1948, who put it on the neurologic map, so to speak. He drew a distinction between acute rupture and protrusion of the cervical disk (often traumatic and more likely to compress the nerve roots than the spinal cord), and chronic spinal cord and root compression, consequent upon disk degeneration and associated osteophytic outgrowths (*hard disk*) and changes in joints, ligaments, and bones. In 1957, Payne and Spillane documented the importance of a smaller-than-normal spinal canal in the genesis of myelopathy in patients with cervical spondylosis. These reports were followed by a flood of writings on the subject (see Wilkinson), yet few of our standard textbooks of neurology contain adequate accounts of it. Nurick's review of the natural history of cervical spondylosis and the results of surgical therapy is a useful modern reference.

Symptomatology In outline, the most characteristic syndrome consists of a triad of (1) painful, stiff neck, (2) brachialgia, and (3) spastic weakness with variable ataxia of the legs. As in other clinical states with multiple components, they may occur separately or in several combinations and sequences. These symptoms and the underlying degenerative changes have proved to be remarkably frequent, as indicated below.

With reference to the first of these symptoms, in any sizable group of patients beyond 50 years of age, some 40 percent will be found to have some kind of an abnormality of the neck, usually crepitus or pain, with restriction of lateral flexion and rotation (less often of extension). Pallis et al. (1954) in a survey of 50 patients, all of them over 50 years and none with neurologic complaints, found that 75 percent showed radiologic evidence of narrowing of the cervical spinal canal due to posterior osteophytosis or narrowing of the intervertebral foramina due to osteoarthritis at the neurocentral and apophyseal joints; about half of the patients with radiologic abnormalities showed physical signs of root or cord involvement (changes in the tendon reflexes in the arms, briskness of reflexes and impairment of vibratory sense in the legs, and occasional Babinski signs). The occasional occurrence of a Babinski sign in older individuals who had never complained of neurologic symptoms may be explained by an otherwise silent osteophyte. Thus, Savitsky and Madonick found a Babinski sign in 4.3 percent of 2500 nonneurologic hospital patients; this sign was four times more frequent in persons over 50 years of age as in those under 50.

In patients with only shoulder and arm symptoms as well as in those in whom these symptoms are combined with a disorder of the legs, pain is the most frequent symptom. It is centered in the back of the neck, often radiating to an area above the scapula. When brachialgia is also present it takes several forms: a stabbing pain in the pre- or postaxial border of the limb, extending to the elbow, wrist, or fingers; or a persistent dull ache in the forearm or wrist, sometimes with burning. In rare instances the pain is referred substernally. Some patients also complain of paresthesias, most often in one or two digits, a part of the palm, or in a longitudinal band along the forearm. Slight clumsiness or weakness of the hand is another complaint. The biceps and supinator reflexes may be depressed, sometimes in association with an increase in the triceps reflex. The hand or

forearm muscles undergo atrophy if chronically weakened. In cases with sensory loss, pain and temperature appear to be affected more than touch.

The third part of the triad, the myelopathy, most often presents as a complaint of weakness of one leg and a slight unsteadiness of gait. The whole leg feels stiff and heavy and gives out quickly after exercise. Mobility of the ankle is often reduced, and the advancing toe and lateral border of the shoe scrape the floor. On examination spasticity is more evident than weakness, and the tendon reflexes are increased (ankle jerks may not share in this change in the elderly). Although the patient may believe only one leg to be affected, it is commonly found that both plantar reflexes are extensor, the one on the side of the stiffest leg being more clearly so. Less often both legs are equally affected. As to the sensory disorders, numbness, tingling, and prickling of the soles of the feet and around the ankles are the most frequent complaints. Impaired vibratory sensation, pattern recognition, touch from the hip down, and postural sense in the toes and feet are the most conspicuous sensory findings (indicating a lesion of the posterior columns). Less often there is loss of pain and temperature. These sensorimotor defects tend also to be asymmetrical. Rarely the pattern is that of a partial Brown-Séquard syndrome (page 114). Neck flexion may induce electrical feelings down the spine (Lhermitte's sign). Paresthesias and dysesthesias in lower extremities and trunk may be the principal complaints.

As the myelopathy progresses both legs weaken further and become more spastic. Sphincteric control may then be altered; slight hesitancy or precipitancy of micturition are the usual complaints, and frank incontinence is infrequent. In its more advanced form walking must be aided by cane(s) or walker, and in rare cases all locomotion ultimately becomes impossible.

Pathogenesis The particular vulnerability of the lower cervical spine to degenerative change has no ready explanation. Perhaps it is related in some way to the high degree of mobility of the lower cervical vertebrae, which is accentuated by their situation next to the relatively immobile thoracic spine.

The obvious mechanism of spinal cord injury would seem to be simple compression. When the spinal canal is diminished in its anterior-posterior dimension at one or several points to less than 9 to 10 mm, the available space for the spinal cord is insufficient. However, the presence and degree of cord injury correlates poorly with the anteroposterior dimensions of the spinal canal. The range of the latter in symptomatic cervical spondylosis is from 8 to 15 mm (normal 17 to 18 mm). One must consider, therefore, the effects of the natural motions of the spinal cord during flexion and extension of the neck. Adams and Logue confirmed the observation of O'Connell that during full flexion and extension of the neck the cervical cord and dura move up and down. The spinal cord is dragged over protruding osteophytes, and conceivably this type of intermittent trauma progressively injures the spinal cord. Also it has been shown that the spinal cord, displaced posteriorly by osteophytes, will be compressed by the infolding ligamentum flavum each time the neck is extended (Stoltmann and Blackwood). Segmental ischemic necrosis resulting from intermittent compression of arteries to the spinal cord or from compression (spasm?) of the anterior spinal artery has also been postulated. Most neuropathologists favor the idea of intermittent cord compression between osteophytes anteriorly and ligamentum flavum posteriorly. Trauma from sudden extreme extension, as in a fall or chiropractic manipulation, or from a lesser degree of retraction of the head during myelography, a tooth extraction, or a tonsillectomy, may be an additional factor— particularly in patients with congenitally narrow canals.

Pathologic Changes The fundamental lesion is a tearing of the annulus fibrosus, with extrusion of disk material into the spinal canal. The disk becomes covered with fibrous tissue, partly calcified or covered with bone. Another common lesion is bulging of the annulus without extrusion of nuclear material. This may also be associated with the formation of osteophytes and transverse bony ridges. The latter, unlike ruptured disks which occur chiefly at the C5-C6 or C6-C7 interspaces, may extend two or three interspaces higher and occur at several levels. The adjacent dura mater may be thickened and adherent to the posterior longitudinal ligament. The underlying pia-arachnoid is also thickened. This series of pathologic changes is frequently ascribed to hypertrophic osteoarthritis. However, in lesser degree, the osteophyte formation and ridging are so frequently observed in patients who have no other signs of arthritic disease that this explanation is surely incorrect. Subclinical trauma is far more likely, in the authors' opinion.

When the root is compressed by osteophytic overgrowth, the dural sleeve is thickened, and the root fibers degenerate. Usually the fifth, sixth, or seventh cervical

roots are affected in this way, both the anterior and posterior, or only the anterior. A small neuroma may appear proximal to the site of anterior root compression.

The spinal cord is flattened and the dura ridged. The root lesions may have led to secondary wedge-shaped areas of degeneration in the lateral parts of the posterior columns at higher levels. The most marked changes in the spinal cord are at the level(s) of compression. There may be zones of demyelination at the points of attachment of the dentate ligaments (which tether the spinal cord to the dura) and zones of necrosis in posterior and lateral columns, as well as loss of nerve cells. The latter lesions, often asymmetrical, are attributed by Hughes to ischemia.

Differential Diagnosis When pain and stiffness in the neck, brachialgia, and sensorimotor reflex changes in the arms are combined with signs of myelopathy, there is little difficulty in diagnosis. When the neck and arm changes are inconspicuous or absent, the diagnosis becomes difficult. The myelopathy must then be distinguished from the late, progressive form of spinal multiple sclerosis (page 653). Since posterior osteophytes and other bony alterations are frequent in the sixth and seventh decades, the question which must be answered is whether the cervical spondylosis bears any relationship to the neurologic abnormality. The problem is resolved by the finding of some degree of sensorimotor or reflex change corresponding to the level of the spinal abnormalities, a point which always favors spondylotic myelopathy. A lack of such corresponding changes, an elevation of CSF gamma globulin, and signs of lesions in the optic nerves and brainstem argue for demyelinative myelopathy. Myelography becomes critical in such cases. An air myelogram with polytomography to show the position of the spinal cord with reference to the spondylotic abnormality during flexion and extension of the neck is the most helpful diagnostic procedure. Contrast myelography with the patient supine and lateral views taken during flexion and extension of neck are also useful in settling the problem.

It is said that spondylotic myelopathy may simulate amyotrophic lateral sclerosis (amyotrophy of arms and spastic weakness of the legs). This has seldom proved to be a problem in our experience. We have observed but few patients with spondylotic myelopathy who exhibited a purely motor syndrome, i.e., one in which there was no cervical or brachial pain and no sensory symptoms in the arms or impairment of vibratory or position sense (posterior column sensation) in the legs. A pure spastic paraparesis without cervicobrachial amyotrophy may also occur in multiple sclerosis, liver failure, hereditary spastic paraplegia with or without de-mentia, and adrenoleukodystrophy (page 696).

Subacute combined degeneration of the spinal cord due to vitamin B$_{12}$ deficiency (page 717), *combined system disease* of nonpernicious anemia type (see above), and spinal cord tumor (discussed later in this chapter) are always listed among the conditions that might be confused with spondylotic myelopathy. Adherence to the diagnostic criteria for each of these disorders should eliminate the possibility of error in most instances.

The special problems attendant upon spondylotic radiculopathy are discussed on pages 148 and 635.

Treatment The slow, intermittently progressive course of cervical myelopathy with long periods of relatively unchanging symptomatology makes it difficult to evaluate therapy. Assuming that the prevailing opinions of the mechanisms of the cord and root injury are correct, then the use of a soft collar to restrict anterior-posterior motions of the neck seems reasonable. This form of treatment alone may be sufficient to control the discomfort in the neck and arms. Rarely in our experience has brachialgia been sufficiently severe and persistent to require radicular decompression.

Many of our patients have been dissatisfied with this passive approach and dislike or refuse to wear a collar continuously. If posterior osteophytes have narrowed the spinal canal at several interspaces, a posterior decompressive laminectomy with severance of the dentate ligaments, to untether the spinal cord, helps to prevent further injury. The results of such a procedure are fairly satisfactory. In fully two-thirds of the patients, improvement in the function of the legs occurs; in most of the others, progression of the myelopathy is halted. The operation carries some risk, and rarely an acute quadriplegia—due, presumably, to manipulation of the spinal cord and damage to nutrient spinal arteries—has followed the surgical procedure. When one or two interspaces are the site of osteophytic overgrowths, their removal by an anterior approach, as devised by Cloward, has given even better results and carries less risk.

OTHER SPINAL ABNORMALITIES WITH MYELOPATHY

The spinal cord is obviously vulnerable to any vertebral maldevelopment or disease that encroaches upon the spinal canal or compresses its nutrient arteries. Some of the common ones are listed below.

Anomalies at the Craniocervical Junction Of these, congenital *fusion of the atlas and foramen magnum* is the most common. McCrae, who reviewed the radiologic findings in over 100 patients with bony abnormalities at the craniocervical junction, found a partial or complete bony union of atlas and foramen magnum in 28 cases. He found also that whenever the anteroposterior diameter of the canal behind the odontoid process was less than 19.0 mm, there were signs of spinal cord compression. Fusion of the second and third cervical vertebras is a common anomaly as well, but does not seem to be of clinical significance.

Platybasia and basilar invagination Platybasia refers to a flattening of the base of the skull (the angle formed by intersection of the plane of the clivus and the plane of the anterior fossa is greater than 135°). Basilar impression or invagination means an upward bulging of the margins of the foramen magnum; if the occipital condyles, which bear the thrust of the spine, are displaced above the plane of the foramen magnum, basilar invagination is present. Each of these abnormalities may be congenital or acquired (as in Paget's disease), and frequently they are conjoined. They give rise to a characteristic shortness of the neck and a combination of cerebellar and spinal signs.

Abnormalities of the odontoid process These were found in 17 of McCrae's series. There may be complete separation of the odontoid from the axis or chronic *atlantoaxial dislocation* (atlas displaced anteriorly with relation to the axis). These abnormalities may be congenital or the result of injury, and are known causes of acute or chronic spinal cord compression.

Rheumatoid arthritis is another cause of atlantoaxial dislocation. The ligaments that attach the odontoid to the atlas and to the skull are weakened by the destructive inflammatory process. The subsequent dislocation of the atlas on the axis may remain mobile or become fixed and give rise to an intermittent or persistent mild to moderate paraparesis or quadriparesis. Similar effects may result from a forward subluxation of C4 on C5 (see Nakano et al.).

In all the congenital anomalies of the foramen magnum and the high cervical spine there is a high incidence of syringomyelia. McCrae found, at the Montreal Neurological Institute, that 38 percent of all patients with syringomyelia and syringobulbia showed such bony anomalies. All patients whose symptoms might be explained by a lesion in the cervicocranial region (particularly where multiple sclerosis and foramen magnum tumor are suspected) should have careful radiologic examination.

In mucopolysaccharidosis IV, or the Morquio syndrome, a nearly invariable feature is absence or severe hypoplasia of the odontoid process. This abnormality, combined with laxity or redundancy of the ligaments, results in atlantoaxial subluxation and compression of the spinal cord. Affected children refuse to walk or develop spastic weakness of the limbs. Early in life they excrete an excess of keratan sulfate (Chap. 37), but this may no longer be detectable in adult life. We have also seen a true pachymeningiopathy with great thickening of the basal cisternal and high cervical dura and spinal cord compression in certain mucopolysaccharidoses. Surgical decompression and spinal immobilization may be curative (McKusick).

Achondroplasia occasionally results in great thickening of the vertebral bodies, neural arches, laminae, and pedicles because of increased periosteal bone formation. The spinal canal is narrowed in the thoracolumbar region, often with kyphosis. It may lead to a progressive spinal cord or cauda equina syndrome. Excessive bone proliferation from *fluorosis* (high fluoride content of drinking water) is reported to have produced a spastic paraparesis with sensory loss below the level of compression and radiculopathy (segmental pain and paresthesias).

Paget's Disease (Osteitis Deformans) Involvement of vertebrae may result in narrowing of the spinal canal and a clinical picture of spinal cord compression. Alkaline phosphatase values are high and the typical bone changes in this disease are seen in radiographs. Usually other parts of the skeleton are also involved, which facilitates diagnosis. The level of the lesion is determined by myelography. Posterior surgical decompression, leaving the pedicles intact, is indicated if there is sufficient stability of the vertebral bodies to prevent collapse. Calcitonin should be administered. Neurologic disturbances in Paget's disease and the results obtained by the use of daily injections of porcine or synthetic salmon calcitonin over a 6- to 12-month period are described by Chen et al.

Paget's disease of the skull may cause neurosensory deafness, occasionally compression of an optic nerve, with loss of sight, and lower cranial neuropathies

(weak, atrophic tongue; dysphagia; dysphonia; pain at base of occiput). The latter effects may be combined with spinal and cerebellar abnormalities, due to basilar invagination.

Spinal cord compression does not occur in ankylosing spondylitis, except as a complication of trauma. Signs of cervical root compression are frequently attributed to ankylosing spondylitis, but in such cases (including the ones originally described by Bechterew, in 1893) the underlying bone disease proves to be osteoarthritis. A cauda equina syndrome is a bona fide but rare complication of ankylosing spondylitis (Mathews).

INTRASPINAL TUMORS

Tumors which involve the spinal cord are considerably less frequent than those which involve the brain; in the Mayo Clinic series of 8784 primary tumors of the central nervous system, only 15 percent were intraspinal (Sloof et al.). In distinction to brain tumors, the majority of intraspinal ones are benign and produce their effects mainly by compression of the spinal cord, rather than by invasion. Thus, a large proportion of intraspinal tumors are amenable to surgical removal, and their early recognition, before irreversible neurologic changes have occurred, becomes a matter of utmost importance.

Anatomic Considerations Neoplasms and other space-occupying lesions within the spinal canal can be conveniently divided into two groups: (1) those which arise within the substance of the spinal cord and invade and destroy tracts and central gray structures (*intramedullary*), and (2) those which arise outside the spinal cord (*extramedullary*), either in the vertebral bodies and epidural tissues (extradural), or in the leptomeninges or roots (intradural). In a general hospital, the relative frequency of spinal tumors in these different locations is about 5 percent intramedullary, 40 percent intradural-extramedullary, and 55 percent extradural. This percentage of extradural lesions is higher than that encountered in more specialized neurosurgical clinics (e.g., Elsberg's figures of 7, 64, and 29 percent respectively), which do not include many of the extradural lymphomas, metastatic carcinomas, etc., seen in general hospitals.

The commonest *extramedullary tumors* are the neurofibromas and meningiomas, which together constitute about 55 percent of all intraspinal neoplasms. They are more often intradural than extradural. Neurofibromas have a predilection for the thoracic region, whereas meningiomas are more evenly distributed over the vertical extent of the cord. The other extramedullary tumors are sarcomas, vascular tumors, chordomas, and epidermoid and similar tumors, in that order of frequency.

Secondary growths (carcinoma, lymphoma, and myeloma) are more often extradural than intradural and arise from hematogenous deposits or extend from tumors of the vertebral bodies or from extraspinal sources, via intervertebral foramina.

Intramedullary tumors of the spinal cord have the same cellular origins as those arising in the brain (Chap. 30), although the proportions of particular cell types differ. Ependymomas (many of which arise from the filum terminale) make up about 60 percent of the spinal cases, and astrocytomas about 25 percent. The latter is the commonest intramedullary tumor, if one excludes the filum terminale. Oligodendrogliomas are much less common. The remainder (about 10 percent) consists of a diverse group of nongliomatous tumors: lipomas, epidermoids, dermoids, teratomas, hemangiomas, and hemangioblastomas. The hemangioma is a common source of spontaneous hematomyelia. As has already been indicated there is a frequent association between intramedullary tumors (both gliomatous and nongliomatous) and syringomyelia. The basis of this relationship remains obscure.

Intramedullary growths both invade as well as compress and distort fasciculi in the adjacent white matter. As the cord enlarges from the tumor growing within it or is compressed by a tumor from without, the free space around the cord is consumed, and the CSF below the lesion becomes isolated or loculated from the remainder of the circulating fluid above the lesion. This is indicated eventually by Froin's syndrome (xanthochromia and clotting of CSF), a positive Queckenstedt test, and interruption of flow of a contrast medium in the subarachnoid space (myelogram).

Symptomatology Patients with spinal cord tumor are likely to manifest one of three clinical pictures, either (1) a purely sensorimotor spinal tract syndrome, or (2) a painful radicular-spinal cord syndrome, or (3) rarely, a syringomyelic syndrome.

Sensorimotor spinal tract syndromes The predominant clinical picture relates to compression and less often to invasion and destruction of spinal cord tracts. The onset of the compressive symptoms is usually gradual and the course progressive over a period of weeks and months. The initial disturbance is likely to be motor, and the distribution asymmetric. With cervical lesions, a common sequence of motor impairment is first an arm, followed by the ipsilateral leg, contralateral leg, and finally the opposite arm. With thoracic lesions, one leg usually becomes weak and stiff before the other one. Subjective sensory symptoms of the dorsal column type (tingling paresthesias) have the same pattern. Pain and

temperature are more likely to be affected than touch, vibration, and position senses, and initially the sensory disturbance is contralateral to the maximum motor weakness (Brown-Séquard syndrome). Nevertheless the posterior columns are also frequently involved. The bladder and bowel usually become paralyzed coincident with motor paralysis of the legs. If the compression is relieved, there is recovery from these sensory and motor symptoms in the reverse order of their affection; the first part affected is the last to recover, and sensory symptoms disappear before motor ones.

Radicular-spinal cord syndrome The syndrome of spinal cord compression is often combined with radicular pain, i.e., pain in the distribution of a sensory nerve root. It is described as knifelike or as a dull ache with superimposed sharp stabs of pain which are intensified by coughing, sneezing, or straining, and which radiate in a distal direction, i.e., away from the spine. Segmental sensory changes (paresthesias, impaired perception of pinprick and touch) or motor disturbances (cramp, atrophy, fascicular twitching, and loss of tendon reflex) and an ache in the spine, in addition to the radicular pain, are the usual manifestations of a cord compression-irritative root lesion. Tenderness of spinous processes over the growth is found in half the patients. These segmental changes, particularly the sensory ones, often precede the signs of spinal cord compression by months or years if the lesion is benign. The latter consist of (1) an asymmetric spastic weakness of the legs with thoracolumbar lesions and of the arms and legs with cervical lesions, (2) a sensory level on the trunk below which perception of pain and temperature is reduced or lost, (3) posterior column signs, and (4) a spastic bladder under weak voluntary control.

No single symptom is unique to intramedullary tumors. Pain is the most common symptom and is almost invariably present with tumors of the filum terminale. Ependymomas and astrocytomas, the two most common intramedullary tumors, usually give rise to a mixed sensorimotor tract syndrome, but if they initially involve the central gray matter, a *syringomyelic syndrome* may result. Rarely, for reasons that are difficult to understand, an extramedullary tumor may give rise to a syringomyelic syndrome as well.

The diagnosis is established by radiographs of the spine (erosion of vertebrae, widened spinal canal), lumbar puncture (elevated CSF protein and signs of block), and electromyography, which demonstrates the fasciculations and denervation resulting from involvement of motor roots. The most important diagnostic procedure is the contrast myelogram which permits precise localization of the lesion. No doubt the CT scan will assume increasing importance as a diagnostic method, as techniques for visualizing the spinal cord improve.

Special spinal syndromes Unusual clinical syndromes may be found in patients with *tumors near the foramen magnum.* They may produce a quadriparesis with pain in the back of the head and stiff neck, weakness and atrophy of the hands and dorsal neck muscles, and variable sensory changes, or, if spread occurs intracranially, there may be signs of cerebellar and lower cranial nerve involvement. These types of tumor are described fully in Chap. 30. Lesions at the level of the lowermost thoracic and the first lumbar vertebrae may result in *mixed cauda equina and spinal cord symptoms.* A Babinski sign means that the spinal cord is involved above the fifth lumbar segment. *Lesions of the cauda equina* alone, always difficult to separate from those of the lumbosacral plexuses and multiple nerves, are usually attended in the early stages by pain which is variously combined with an asymmetric, atrophic, areflexic paralysis, radicular sensory loss, and sphincteric disorder. These must be distinguished from *lesions of the conus medullaris* (lower sacral segments of the spinal cord) in which there are early disturbances of the bladder and bowel (urinary retention and constipation), back pain, hypesthesia or anesthesia over the sacral dermatomes, a lax anal sphincter with loss of anal and bulbocavernosus reflexes, impotence, and sometimes weakness of leg muscles. Sensory abnormalities may precede motor and reflex changes by many months. *Pain and stiffness of the back* may antedate signs of spinal cord disease or dominate the clinical picture in some extramedullary tumors. The back pain is usually worse when the patient lies down, or may become worse after several hours in the recumbent position and be improved by sitting up. *In children,* severe back pain associated with spasm of paravertebral muscles is often prominent initially; scoliosis and spastic weakness of the legs come later. Because of this somewhat unusual clinical presentation and the rarity of intraspinal lesions in childhood, spinal cord tumors in this age group may be overlooked.

Differential Diagnosis Several problems may arise in the diagnosis of spinal cord tumors, in addition to the ones mentioned above. In their early stages they must be distinguished from other diseases which cause pain over certain segments of the body, i.e., those affecting the gallbladder, kidney, stomach and intestinal tract, pleura, etc. The localization of the pain to a dermatome, its intensification by sneezing, coughing, and straining, the finding of segmental sensory changes and minor alterations of motor, reflex, or sensory function in the legs will usually provide the clues to the presence of a spinal cord–radicular lesion. Examination of the CSF, spine films, and myelography will settle the diagnosis in most instances.

If symptoms and signs of disorder of sensorimotor tracts are present, there is still the problem of locating the segmental level of the lesion. At first the sensory and motor deficits may be most pronounced in those parts of the body farthest removed from the lesion, i.e., in feet or lumbosacral segments. Later the levels of the sensory and motor deficits ascend, but they may continue to be below the lesion. In determining the level of the lesion, the location of the root pain and atrophic paralysis is of greater help than the upper level of hypalgesia.

Once vertebral and segmental levels of the lesion are settled, there remains the necessity of determining whether the lesion is extradural, intradural-extramedullary, or intramedullary, and whether the lesion is neoplastic. This is important from the standpoint of etiologic diagnosis. If there is a visible or palpable spinal deformity or radiographic evidence of vertebral destruction, one may confidently assume an extradural localization. Even without these changes one still suspects an extradural lesion if root pain developed early and is bilateral, if pain and aching in the spine are prominent and percussion tenderness is marked, if motor symptoms below the lesion precede sensory ones, and sphincter disturbances are late. However, to distinguish between intradural-extramedullary lesions and intramedullary lesions on clinical grounds alone may be impossible. The presence of radicular pain and early CSF blockage (positive Queckenstedt test and high protein) favor an extramedullary localization. The findings of segmental amyotrophy and sensory loss of dissociated type point to an intramedullary lesion.

Extradural tumors need to be differentiated from cervical spondylosis; from tuberculous granuloma and other chronic pyogenic, fungal, or syphilitic granulomatous lesions; and from secondary carcinoma (most often from breast, lung, prostate and kidney), myeloma, or lymphoma. In the region of the lower back, i.e., over the cauda equina, one must distinguish between tumor and protruded intervertebral disk. In this location, an extradural tumor may produce mainly sciatic and low back pain with little or no motor, sensory, reflex, or sphincteric disturbances. Here, the most important diagnostic measure is myelography. With intradural-extramedullary lesions the important diagnostic considerations are meningioma, neurofibroma, meningeal carcinomatosis, cholesteatoma and teratomatous cyst, a meningomyelitic process or adhesive arachnoiditis. Contrast myelography and the study of cells in the CSF by millipore-filter techniques are the most useful laboratory aids. Intramedullary lesions are usually gliomas or vascular malformations. The definition of the latter lesions by means of selective spinal angiography has been discussed in an earlier section of this chapter. In general, a negative Queckenstedt test, normal or relatively low protein in the CSF, and a negative myelogram will serve to rule out intraspinal tumors or granulomatous lesions.

Treatment   This varies with the nature of the lesion and the clinical condition of the patient. Intradural-extramedullary tumor should be removed as soon as possible after diagnostic myelography. Laminectomy, decompression, excision under the operating microscope, and radiotherapy constitute the treatment of intramedullary gliomas. Such patients may improve and lead useful lives for a decade or longer. Epidural growths of carcinoma and lymphoma are best managed by the use of radiotherapy, endocrine therapy (for carcinoma of breast and prostate), the administration of antineoplastic drugs (for certain lymphomas and myelomas) and the use of analgesics for pain. Sometimes laminectomy and decompression are necessary for diagnosis and prevention of irreversible compressive effects and infarction of the spinal cord. With tuberculous caries, immobilization of the spine in hyperextension and appropriate chemotherapy are indicated, and laminectomy should be reserved for exceptional cases with complete and irreversible spinal block. The management of other forms of spinal cord and cauda equina compression are considered in relation to the specific compressive lesions.

RADIATION INJURY OF THE SPINAL CORD

Delayed necrosis of the spinal cord and brain are well-recognized sequelae of radiotherapy for tumors in these regions. The peripheral nerves are much more resistant to x-ray irradiation although we have observed, as have others, a delayed, progressive, sensorimotor effect many years after radiation, e.g., in the distribution of the brachial plexus after radiation for breast carcinoma. Lower motor neuron lesions may also follow radiation injury to anterior horn cells.

Radiation Myelopathy   This, the most common complication of radiotherapy, is a chronic progressive myelopathy which follows, after a characteristic latent period, the radiation of malignant tissues in the vicinity of the spinal cord. The incidence of this complication is difficult to determine because many patients die of their malignant disease before the cord lesion matures, but is estimated to be between 2 and 3 percent (Palmer).

The neurologic disorder first appears many months after the course of radiation therapy, practically always after 6 months and usually between 12 and 15 months (latent periods as long as 60 months have been reported). The onset is insidious, usually with sensory symptoms—paresthesias and dysesthesias of the feet or a Lhermitte's sign, and similar symptoms in the hands in cases of cervical cord damage. Local pain is notably absent initially, in distinction to spinal tumors. In some cases, the sensory abnormalities are transitory, but more often additional signs make their appearance and progress slowly over a period of several weeks or months, with involvement of the corticospinal and spinothalamic pathways, often taking the form of a Brown-Séquard syndrome, but later of a transverse myelopathy, with a spastic paraplegia, sensory level on the trunk and sphincteric disturbances. Reagan et al. describe yet another myelopathic radiation syndrome, that of a slowly evolving amyotrophy with paresis, atrophy of muscles, and areflexia in parts of the body supplied by anterior horn cells of the irradiated spinal segments. Most patients die within a year of onset of the neurologic disease.

The CSF in radiation myelopathy is normal except for a slight elevation of protein content in some cases. Also, myelography discloses no abnormalities. This is an important point to establish, because a mistaken diagnosis of intraspinal tumor may lead to further irradiation of an already damaged cord.

In the spinal cord, corresponding with the level of the irradiated area, is an irregular zone of coagulation necrosis, involving both white and gray matter, the former to a greater extent than the latter. Varying degrees of secondary degeneration involve the ascending and descending tracts. Vascular changes—necrosis of arterioles or hyaline thickening of their walls, with thrombotic occlusion of their lumens—are prominent in the most severely damaged portions of the cord. Most authors have attributed the parenchymal lesion to the blood vessel changes; others believe that the degree of vascular change is insufficient to explain the parenchymal change (Malamud et al.; Burns et al.). Certainly the parenchymal changes in the cord are not specific for infarction; the insidious onset and slow, steady progression of the clinical disorder is also difficult to explain on a vascular basis.

It needs to be stressed that radiation myelopathy

is an iatrogenic disease and is preventable. The tolerance of the adult human spinal cord to radiation, taking into account the volume of tissue irradiated, the duration of the irradiation, and total dose, has been determined by Boden and by Pallis et al. (1961). The latter authors have recommended that for treatment times of 42 days, no more than 3300 rads be given to fields greater than 10-cm cord length, and no more than 4300 rads to fields less than 10 cm long. The limits proposed by Boden are about 20 percent higher. It is noteworthy that in the cases reported by Sanyal et al. the amount of radiation exceeded these limits.

DYSRAPHIC AND CONGENITAL TUMOR SYNDROMES

See Chap. 43.

SYNDROME OF SEGMENTAL SENSORY DISSOCIATION WITH BRACHIAL AMYOTROPHY (Syringomyelic Syndrome)

This syndrome is most often ascribable to syringomyelia (i.e., a central cavitation of the spinal cord of undetermined cause), but a similar clinical syndrome may sometimes be observed in association with other pathologic states, such as intramedullary cord tumors, traumatic myelopathy, postradiation myelopathy, spinal arachnoiditis, infarction (myelomalacia) and bleeding (hematomyelia), and rarely with extramedullary tumors, cervical spondylosis, and cervical necrotizing myelitis.

SYRINGOMYELIA

Syringomyelia (from the Greek *syrinx*, "pipe" or "tube") may be defined as a chronic progressive degenerative disorder of the spinal cord, characterized clinically by brachial amyotrophy and segmental sensory loss of dissociated type, and pathologically by cavitation of the central parts of the spinal canal, usually involving the cervical region but extending upward in some cases into the medulla oblongata (syringobulbia) or downward into the thoracic or even the lumbar segments. In approximately 15 percent of cases studied post mortem, an intramedullary tumor (astrocytoma, hemangioblastoma, ependymoma) has been found in or near some part of the syrinx.

Historical Note Although pathologic cavitation of the spinal cord was recognized as early as the sixteenth century, the term *syringomyelia* was first used to describe this process in 1827 by Ollivier d'Angers (cited by Ballantine et al.). Later, following the recognition of the central canal as a normal structure, it was assumed by Virchow (1863) and by Leyden (1876) that cavitation of the spinal cord had its origin in an abnormal expansion of the central canal, and they renamed the process *hydromyelia*. Cavities in the central portions of the spinal cord, unconnected with the central canal, were recognized by Hallopeau (1870); Simon suggested in 1875 that the term *syringomyelia* be reserved for such cavities and that the term *hydromyelia* be restricted to dilatation of the central canal itself. Thus a century ago the stage was set for an argument about pathogenesis that has not been settled to the present day.

Pathogenesis One theory of pathogenesis, of which Gardner is the most convincing protagonist, is that normal flow of CSF is prevented by a congenital failure of opening of the outlets of the fourth ventricle. As a result, a pulse wave of CSF pressure, generated by systolic pulsations of the choroid plexus, is transmitted into the cord from the fourth ventricle through the central canal. According to this theory, the syrinx consists essentially of a greatly dilated central canal or a ramifying diverticulum from the central canal, which dissects along gray matter and fiber tracts. The frequency with which syringomyelia is linked to malformations at the craniocervical junction, i.e., to lesions that could interfere with normal flow of CSF, has lent credence to this theory.

There are many instances, however, where Gardner's hydrodynamic theory does not explain the syringomyelia. In some cases the foramens of Luschka and Magendie are found to be patent, and other abnormalities of the posterior fossa or foramen magnum are also not in evidence. Cases have been observed in which two well-developed cavities, one at a cervical and another at a lumbar level, were unconnected by any patent channel. Furthermore, in many cases, histologic sections of the tissue between the fourth ventricle and the syrinx in the spinal cord have failed to demonstrate any connection (Hughes; Feigin et al.).

Gardner's theory has been questioned on other grounds. Ball and Dayan have calculated the pulse-pressure wave transmitted into the cord to be of so low an order as to be most unlikely to produce a syrinx. These authors have suggested a somewhat different mechanism. In their view, the CSF, under increased pressure because of subarachnoid obstruction at the craniocervical junction, tracks into the spinal cord along the Virchow-Robin spaces. Over a prolonged period of time, small pools of fluid coalesce to form a syrinx, which originally forms independently of the central canal but eventually becomes connected with it. A blastomatous formation in the spinal cord, akin to tuberous sclerosis or central von Recklinghausen's disease but with a tendency for the abnormal tissue to cavitate, is another suggested explanation of syrinx formation. Feigin et al. have suggested that edema is a major pathogenetic factor, induced by angiomatous malformations, neoplasms, trauma, arachnoiditis, etc. This hardly exhausts the list of hypotheses, but none of them have been confirmed, and there is no point in enumerating all of them here. Nevertheless, in at least one type of syringomyelia, it appears that there is an important relationship between basal cranial, cervical spine, and cerebellospinal malformations and hydrosyringomyelia, and that disturbed hydrodynamics of CSF is an important factor in the pathogenesis.

Irrespective of its mode of origin, the syrinx first occupies the central gray matter of the *cervical* portion of the spinal cord, where it interrupts the crossing pain and temperature fibers in the anterior commissure at several successive cord segments. As the cavity enlarges it extends symmetrically or asymmetrically into the posterior and anterior horns and eventually into the lateral and posterior funiculi of the cord. It may enlarge the spinal cord and even widen the interpedicular spaces. The cavity is lined with astrocytic glia and a few thick-walled blood vessels, and the fluid in the cavity is clear or xanthochromic and has a relatively low protein content, like CSF.

The cavitation is always to be found in the cervical portion of the cord and the thoracic and lumbar portions are involved less often, usually by extension from the cervical region. Either a cavity or a glial septum may extend asymmetrically into the medulla oblongata, usually in the vicinity of the descending root of the fifth cranial nerve (syringobulbia).

Clinical Features Syringomyelia is a sporadic disease, perhaps more frequent in males than in females. Familial occurrence is very rare. Symptoms may begin in late childhood or adolescence, but more often in early adult life, and progress irregularly, often being arrested for long periods of time. The precise clinical picture depends upon the cross-sectional and vertical extent of cord destruction, but certain features are fundamental and the clinical diagnosis can hardly be made without them. These features are *segmental* weakness and atrophy of the hands and arms with loss of tendon reflexes, and *segmental* anesthesia of dissociated type (loss of pain and temperature sense and preservation of sense of touch) over the neck, shoulders, and arms; and thoracic

kyphoscoliosis is almost invariably added. The dissociated sensory loss is caused by stretching and destruction of the ventral commissural fibers (i.e., decussating nociceptive and thermal fibers) with sparing of the uncrossed fibers for touch and proprioception (see Fig. 7-1A). The restriction of the lesion, early in the disease, to the gray matter of the cervical or cervicothoracic segments accounts for the "cape" or "vest" distribution of sensory loss. With extension of the lesion into the posterior columns, tactile, position, and vibration sense are affected as well; extension into the ventrolateral funiculi, with involvement of the spinothalamic pathways, causes analgesia of the trunk and legs. Corticospinal tract signs in the legs tend to appear relatively late in the course of the disease and are attributable to extension of the syrinx into the lateral columns of the cord or into the decussation of the corticospinal tracts at the first cervical segment, or to compression of these tracts by a distended syrinx. The amyotrophy is due to involvement of the anterior horns. Analgesia and thermoanesthesia account for painless infections, ulcers, injuries and burns; Charcot joints, also common in this disease, result from injury of the denervated joint tissue. Areflexia without atrophy may occur, due to involvement of the afferent limb of the reflex arc; but far more frequently, areflexia and amyotrophy are combined, due to destruction of anterior gray matter. A useful clinical rule is that a neurologic disease which leaves all deep tendon reflexes in the arms intact is probably not syringomyelia.

Pain, often severe, is a frequent symptom in syringomyelia. It usually has a deep aching or boring quality, but may be lancinating in nature. Paradoxically, the pain may be most intense in an analgesic limb, i.e., one in which perception of pinprick is completely lost (anesthesia dolorosa).

Horner's syndrome may result from ipsilateral involvement of cells in the intermediolateral cell column of the eighth cervical to first thoracic segments of the spinal cord. If the syringomyelic cavity enlarges the spinal cord, a spinal subarachnoid block may result, and prolonged pressure by the distended cord may cause widening of the spinal canal and erosion of pedicles. The kyphoscoliosis, which may antedate other evidence of disease by several years, is thought to result from asymmetric weakness of paravertebral muscles. Congenital malformations at the cervicocranial junction, which are frequently conjoined, may result in a short neck, low hairline, and other dysplastic features.

As mentioned above, a syrinx in the brainstem

(*syringobulbia*) usually extends into the lateral tegmentum of the medulla, being so placed as to result in nystagmus and sensory impairment over one or both sides of the face. Unilateral palatal and vocal cord paralysis, as well as weakness and atrophy of one side of the tongue, are other clinical signs which call attention to lesions at this level of the neuraxis. Syringobulbia never occurs without syringomyelia.

Other Forms of Syringomyelia Syringomyelia in relation to ependymoma, astrocytoma, and particularly to hemangioblastoma has already been mentioned. There is in addition a frequent association of cavitation of the spinal cord with myelomeningocele and type I Arnold-Chiari malformation (see Chap. 43), platybasia or basilar impression, and other congenital defects at the cervicocranial junction. It has also been described in association with adhesive arachnoiditis in the posterior fossa, leading to an obstruction to the flow of CSF and to hydrocephalus (*communicating syringomyelia*). Some of these latter cases have been traced to an antecedent meningitis, but in others the cause of the arachnoiditis has not been apparent. In a certain proportion of these cases, an abnormal descent or ectopia of the cerebellar tonsils has been demonstrated by myelography in the supine position, and in this particular group decompression of the posterior fossa at the foramen magnum has improved or arrested the progress of symptoms (Hankinson).

Syringomyelic cavitation may also occur as a rare complication of spinal arachnoiditis. The syrinx in the few reported cases has been in the cervical cord, usually above the upper level of the arachnoiditis, and the cavity has contained clear watery fluid with a low content of protein.

Progressive central cavitation of the spinal cord has also been observed in a small number (1 or 2 percent) of patients who survive traumatic paraplegia (Barnett et al.). The symptoms begin between 1 and 15 years after the original trauma and take the form of an ascending lesion of the central gray matter, involving the portion of the cord above the point of original trauma. Downward cavitation can occur as well, but the latter lesion will of course be clinically silent. At first the symptoms are unilateral, but later bilateral, and eventually the signs indicate involvement of the uppermost level of the cervical cord. Postmortem examinations have shown the lesion to be a syrinx, lined with a glial network and containing CSF. The pathogenesis of this delayed posttraumatic syringomyelia is obscure.

Treatment This is in general not satisfactory. The fact that the disease process may remain stationary for months or years makes evaluation of any mode of therapy difficult. Decompression of a distended syrinx may alleviate the symptoms and signs resulting from local compression of ascending and descending spinal tracts, but relief is seldom lasting. Reducing the pressure within the cavity by occluding the upper end of the central canal (a procedure advocated by Gardner), opening the spinal cord cavity, or placing a ventriculosubarachnoid shunt have given unpredictable results. Unroofing the spinal cord by removing the posterior rim of the foramen magnum and the cerebellar tonsils arrested the neurologic symptoms in 75 percent of Hankinson's cases (see above). Radiotherapy, based on the belief that symptoms result from a gliomatous malformation of the cord which subsequently cavitates, is probably worthless unless there is an underlying tumor.

CONCLUDING REMARKS

In conclusion, it is always well to remind oneself that of the more than 30 diseases of the spinal cord, effective means of treatment are available for only a few—spondylosis, extramedullary spinal cord tumors, syphilis (meningomyelitis and tabes), epidural abscess, hematoma and granuloma (tuberculous, fungal), and subacute combined degeneration and other forms of nutritional myelopathy. The physician's major responsibility is to determine whether the patient has one of the treatable diseases.

REFERENCES

ADAMS CBT, LOGUE V: Studies in cervical spondylotic myelopathy. *Brain* 94:569, 1971.

ANTONI N: Spinal vascular malformations (angiomas) and myelomalacia. *Neurology* 12:795, 1962.

BAKER AS et al: Spinal epidural abscess. *New Engl J Med* 293:463, 1975.

BALL MJ, DAYAN AD: Pathogenesis of syringomyelia. *Lancet* 2:799, 1972.

BALLANTINE HT, OJEMANN RG, DREW JH: Syringohydromyelia, in Krayenbühl H, Maspes PE, Sweet WH (eds): *Progress in Neurological Surgery*, vol 4. New York, S Karger, 1971, pp 227-245.

BARNETT HJM, FOSTER JB, HUDGSON P: *Syringomyelia*. Philadelphia, Saunders, 1973.

BASSOE P, HASSIN GB: Myelitis and myelomalacia. *Arch Neurol Psychiatry* 6:32, 1921.

BODEN G: Radiation myelitis of the cervical spinal cord. *Br J Radiol* 21:464, 1948.

BOSHES B: Trauma to the spinal cord, in Baker AB, Baker LH (eds): *Clinical Neurology.* New York, Harper & Row, 1980, chap 35.

BRADSHAW P: Some aspects of cervical spondylosis. *Q J Med* 26:177, 1957.

BRAIN WR: Discussion on rupture of the intervertebral disc in the cervical region. *Proc R Soc Med* 41:509, 1948.

————, NORTHFIELD D, WILKINSON M: The neurological manifestations of cervical spondylosis. *Brain* 75:187, 1952.

BURNS RJ, JONES AN, ROBERTSON JS: Pathology of radiation myelopathy. *J Neurol Neurosurg Psychiatry* 35:888, 1972.

CAMPBELL AMG, GARLAND H: Subacute myoclonic spinal neuronitis. *J Neurol Neurosurg Psychiatry* 19:268, 1956.

CANNON WB, HAIMOVICI H: The sensitization of motoneurons by partial denervation. *Am J Physiol* 126:731, 1939.

————, ROSENBLUETH A: *The Supersensitivity of Denervated Structures.* New York, Macmillan, 1949.

CHEN JR et al: Neurologic disturbances in Paget disease of bone: Response to calcitonin. *Neurology* 29:448, 1979.

CLOWARD RB: A new method of diagnosis and treatment of cervical disc disease. *Clin Neurosurg* 8:93, 1962.

COMARR AE: The practical urological management of the patient with spinal cord injury. *Br J Urol* 31:1, 1959.

DAVIS L, MARTIN J: Studies upon spinal cord injuries: The nature and treatment of pain. *J Neurosurg* 4:483, 1947.

DJINDJIAN R: Angiomas of the spinal cord, in Vinken PJ, Bruyn GW (eds): *Handbook of Clinical Neurology,* vol 32. Amsterdam, North-Holland, 1978, chap 16.

ELKINGTON J ST C: Arachnoiditis, in Feiling A (ed): *Modern Trends in Neurology.* New York, Hoeber-Harper, 1951, pp 149-161.

ELSBERG CA: *Surgical Diseases of the Spinal Cord, Membranes and Nerve Roots: Symptoms, Diagnosis and Treatment.* New York, Hoeber-Harper, 1941.

FEIGIN I, OGATA J, BUDZILOVICH G: Syringomyelia: The role of edema in its pathogenesis. *J Neuropathol Exp Neurol* 30:216, 1971.

FOIX C, ALAJOUANINE T: La myélite nécrotique subaiguë. *Rev Neurol* 2:1, 1926.

FRYKHOLM R: Cervical nerve root compression resulting from disc degeneration and root sleeve fibrosis. *Acta Chir Scand Suppl,* vol 160, 1951.

GARDNER WJ: Hydrodynamic mechanism of syringomyelia: Its relationship to myelocele. *J Neurol Neurosurg Psychiatry* 28:247, 1965.

GILBERT RW, KIM JH, POSNER JB: Epidural spinal cord compression from metastatic tumor: Diagnosis and treatment. *Ann Neurol* 3:40, 1978.

GREENFIELD JG, TURNER JWA: Acute and subacute necrotic myelitis. *Brain* 62:227, 1939.

GUILLAIN G, BARRÉ JA: Les plaies de la moelle épinière par blessures de guerre. *Presse Med* 24:497, 1916.

GUTTMANN L: Clinical symptomatology of spinal cord lesions, in Vinken PJ, Bruyn GW (eds): *Handbook of Clinical Neurology,* vol 2. Amsterdam, North-Holland, 1969, chap 9, pp 178-216.

————: *Spinal Cord Injuries: Comprehensive Management and Research.* Oxford, Blackwell, 1976.

HANKINSON J: Syringomyelia and the surgeon, in Williams D (ed): *Modern Trends in Neurology,* vol. 5. London, Butterworth, 1970, chap 7, pp 127-148.

HEAD H, RIDDOCH G: The automatic bladder: Excessive sweating and some other reflex conditions in gross injuries of the spinal cord. *Brain* 40:188, 1917.

HERRICK M, MILLS PE JR: Infarction of spinal cord. *Arch Neurol* 24:228, 1971.

HOWELL DA, LEES AJ, TOGHILL PJ: Spinal internuncial neurones in progressive encephalomyelitis with rigidity. *J Neurol Neurosurg Psychiatry* 42:773, 1979.

HUGHES JT: *Pathology of the Spinal Cord,* 2d ed. Philadelphia, Saunders, 1978.

————, BROWNELL B: Cervical spondylosis complicated by anterior spinal artery thrombosis. *Neurology* 14:1073, 1964.

JEFFERSON G: Discussion on spinal injuries. *Proc R Soc Med* 21:625, 1927.

KAHLE W, SCHALTENBRAND G: Zür Klinik und Pathologie der Myelitis necroticans diffusa. *Dtsch Z Nervenheilkd* 173:234, 1955.

KILLEN DA, FOSTER JH: Spinal cord injury as a complication of contrast angiography. *Surgery* 59:962, 1966.

KNEISELY LW: Hyperhydrosis in paraplegia. *Arch Neurol* 34:536, 1977.

KOCHER T: Die Verletzungen der Virbelsäule zugleich als Beitrag zur Physiologie des menschlichen Rückenmarcks. *Mitt Grenzgeb Med Chir* 1:415, 1896.

KUHN RA: Functional capacity of the isolated human spinal cord. *Brain* 73:1, 1950.

LHERMITTE J: *La section totale de la moelle épinière.* Bourges, Imprimerie V Tardy, 1919.

LOGUE V: Angiomas of the spinal cord: Review of the pathogenesis, clinical features, and results of surgery. *J Neurol Neurosurg Psychiatry* 42:1, 1979.

LOMBARDI G, PASSERINI A, MIGLIAVACCA F: Spinal arachnoiditis. *Br J Radiol* 35:314, 1962.

MAIR WGP, FOLKERTS JF: Necrosis of spinal cord due to thrombophlebitis (subacute necrotic myelitis). *Brain* 76:563, 1953.

MALAMUD N, BOLDREY EB, WELCH WK, FADELL EJ: Necrosis of brain and spinal cord following x-ray therapy. *J Neurosurg* 11:353, 1954.

MARSHALL J: Observations on reflex changes in the lower limbs in spastic paraplegia in man. *Brain* 77:290, 1954.

MATHEWS WB: The neurologic complications of ankylosing spondylitis. *J Neurol Sci* 6:561, 1968.

McCRAE DL: Bony abnormalities in the region of the foramen magnum: Correlation of the anatomic and neurologic findings. *Acta Radiol* 40:335, 1953.

McKUSICK VA, NEWFELD EF, KELLY TE: The mucopolysaccharide storage diseases, in Stanbury JB et al (eds): *The Metabolic Basis of Inherited Disease*, 4th ed. New York, McGraw-Hill, 1978, chap 53, pp 1282–1308.

MESSARD L et al: Survival after spinal cord trauma. *Arch Neurol* 35:78, 1978.

MESSER HD, LITVINOFF J: Pyogenic cervical osteomyelitis. *Arch Neurol* 33:571, 1976.

MIXTER WJ, BARR JS: Rupture of the intervertebral disc with involvement of the spinal canal. *N Eng J Med* 211:210, 1934.

MUNRO D: The rehabilitation of patients totally paralyzed below the waist. *N Engl J Med* 234:207, 1946.

NAKANO KK et al: The cervical myelopathy associated with rheumatoid arthritis: Analysis of 32 patients, with 2 postmortem cases. *Ann Neurol* 3:144, 1978.

NURICK S: The cervical spine and paraplegia, in Williams D (ed): *Modern Trends in Neurology*, vol 6. London, Butterworth, 1975, pp 167–182.

O'CONNELL JEA: Cervical spondylosis. *Proc R Soc Med* 49:202, 1956.

PALLIS C, JONES AM, SPILLANE JD: Cervical spondylosis. *Brain* 77:274, 1954.

———, LOUIS S, MORGAN RL: Radiation myelopathy. *Brain* 84:460, 1961.

PALMER JJ: Radiation myelopathy. *Brain* 95:109, 1972.

PANSE F: Electrical lesions of the nervous system, in Vinken PJ, Bruyn GW (eds): Handbook of Clinical Neurology, vol. 7. Amsterdam, North-Holland, 1970, chap 13, pp 344–387.

PANT SS, BHARGAVA AN, SINGH MM, DHANDA PC: Myelopathy in hepatic cirrhosis. *Br Med J* 1:1064, 1963.

PAYNE EE, SPILLANE JD: The cervical spine: An anatomicopathological study of 70 specimens (using a special technique) with particular reference to the problem of cervical spondylosis. *Brain* 80:571, 1957.

PEET MM, ECHOLS DH: Herniation of the nucleus pulposus: A cause of compression of the spinal cord. *Arch Neurol Psychiatry* 32:924, 1934.

POLLOCK LJ et al: Pain below the level of injury of the spinal cord. *Arch Neurol Psychiatry* 65:319, 1951.

———: Spasticity, pseudospontaneous spasm, and other reflex activities late after injury to the spinal cord. *Arch Neurol Psychiatry* 66:537, 1951.

REAGAN TJ, THOMAS JE, COLBY MY: Chronic progressive radiation myelopathy. *J Am Med Assoc* 203:128, 1968.

RIDDOCH G: The reflex functions of the completely divided spinal cord in man, compared with those associated with less severe lesions. *Brain* 40:264, 1917.

SANYAL B et al: Radiation myelopathy. *J Neurol Neurosurg Psychiatry* 42:413, 1979.

SAVITSKY N, MADONICK MJ: Statistical control studies in neurology; Babinski sign. *Arch Neurol Psychiatry* 49:272, 1943.

SCHMORL G: Zur pathologischen Anatomie der Wirbelsaule. *Klin Wochenschr* 8:1243, 1929.

SLOOF JH, KERNOHAN JW, MacCARTY CS: *Primary Intramedullary Tumors of the Spinal Cord and Filum Terminale.* Philadelphia, Saunders, 1964.

SPILLER WG: Thrombosis of the cervical anterior median spinal artery; syphilitic acute anterior poliomyelitis. *J Nerv Ment Dis* 36:601, 1909.

STOLTMANN HF, BLACKWOOD W: The role of the ligamenta flava in the pathogenesis of myelopathy in cervical spondylosis. *Brain* 87:45, 1964.

STOOKEY B: Compression of the spinal cord due to ventral extradural cervical chondromas. *Arch Neurol Psychiatry* 20:275, 1928.

UCHIMURA I, SHIRAKI H: A contribution to the classification and pathogenesis of demyelinating encephalomyelitis. *J Neuropathol Exp Neurol* 16:139, 1957.

WEISMAN AD, ADAMS RD: The neurological complications of dissecting aortic aneurysm. *Brain* 67:69, 1944.

WHITELY AM et al: Progressive encephalomyelitis with rigidity. *Brain* 99:27, 1976.

WILKINSON M: *Cervical Spondylosis*, 2d ed. Philadelphia, Saunders, 1971.

WYBURN-MASON R: *Vascular Abnormalities and Tumors of the Spinal Cord and Its Membranes.* St Louis, Mosby, 1944.

ZIEVE L, MENDELSON DF, GOEPFERT M: Shunt encephalomyelopathy. *Ann Intern Med* 53:53, 1960.

CHAPTER 36

MULTIPLE SCLEROSIS AND ALLIED DEMYELINATIVE DISEASES

It has long been the practice to set apart a group of diseases of the brain and spinal cord in which destruction of myelin (demyelination) is a prominent feature. To define these diseases precisely is difficult if not impossible, for the simple reason that there is probably no disease in which myelin destruction is the primary or exclusive pathologic change. The whole idea of a demyelinative disease is, more or less, an abstraction which serves merely to focus attention on one of the more striking and distinctive features of a pathologic process.

The commonly accepted criteria of a demyelinative disease are ① destruction of the myelin sheaths of the nerve fibers, ② a relative sparing of the other elements of nervous tissue, i.e., of axis cylinders, nerve cells, and supporting structures, ③ an infiltration of inflammatory cells in the adventitial sheaths of blood vessels, ④ a particular distribution of lesions, often perivenous, either in multiple small disseminated foci or in larger foci spreading from one or more centers, and ⑤ a relative lack of wallerian, or secondary, degeneration of fiber tracts (an expression of the relative integrity of the axis cylinders in the lesions).

The diseases included in the following classification conform approximately to the above criteria. Like all classifications that are not based on etiology, this one has its shortcomings, in that it is somewhat arbitrary and inconsistent. In some of the diseases here classified as demyelinative, there is a more or less equal affection of both axis cylinders and myelin. Furthermore, a number of diseases in which demyelination is a prominent feature are not included. In some cases of anoxic encephalopathy, for example, the myelin sheaths of the radiating nerve fibers in the deep layers of the cerebral cortex or in ill-defined patches in the convolutional and central white matter are destroyed, while most of the axis cylinders are spared. A relatively selective degeneration of

myelin may also occur in some small ischemic foci due to vascular occlusion. In subacute combined degeneration of the cord (SCD), associated with pernicious anemia, myelin may be affected earlier and to a greater extent than axis cylinders; and the same is true of progressive multifocal leukoencephalopathy (PML), central pontine myelinolysis, and Marchiafava-Bignami disease. Some of these disorders and several others are no longer classified as demyelinative diseases because their etiology is known. Because PML has proved to be a viral infection of oligodendrocytes in immune-deficient subjects, and because SCD is due to vitamin B_{12} deficiency, these disorders are more appropriately included with the viral and nutritional diseases, respectively. Other diseases are not categorized as demyelinative because they lack the characteristic perivascular inflammatory lesion, and exhibit pathologic features which are judged to be more fundamental than the demyelination.

In the language of neurology, therefore, the term *demyelination* has acquired a special meaning; if it is to retain its value, it should be used in the restricted sense indicated above and not as a synonym for complete degeneration of nerve fibers or necrosis of white matter, even though in a section stained for myelin the lesions may look alike. In this latter, more general sense there are few diseases of the central nervous system to which the term *demyelinating* would not apply.

CLASSIFICATION OF THE DEMYELINATIVE DISEASES

I. Multiple sclerosis (disseminated or insular sclerosis)
   A. Chronic relapsing encephalomyelopathic form
   B. Acute multiple sclerosis
   C. Neuromyelitis optica

II. Acute disseminated encephalomyelitis
  A. Following measles, chickenpox, smallpox, and rarely mumps, rubella, and influenza
  B. Following rabies or smallpox vaccination
III. Schilder's diffuse cerebral sclerosis (encephalitis periaxalis diffusa) and concentric sclerosis of Baló
IV. Acute and subacute necrotizing hemorrhagic encephalopathy
  A. Acute encephalopathic form (hemorrhagic leukoencephalitis of Hurst)
  B. Subacute necrotic myelopathy?
  C. Acute brain purpura (acute pericapillary encephalorrhagia)?

MULTIPLE SCLEROSIS

Multiple sclerosis (MS), referred to by the British as *disseminated sclerosis* and by the French as *sclerose en plaques,* is among the most venerable of neurologic diseases and one of the most important, by virtue of its frequency, chronicity, and tendency to attack young adults. It is characterized clinically by episodes of focal disorder of the optic nerves, spinal cord, and brain, which remit to a varying extent and recur over a period of many years. The clinical manifestations are protean, being determined by the varied location and extent of the foci of demyelination; nevertheless, the lesions tend to have a predilection for certain portions of the nervous system, resulting in characteristic complexes of symptoms and signs which can often be readily recognized.

Classical features include motor weakness, paresthesiae, impaired vision, diplopia, nystagmus, dysarthria, intention tremor, ataxia, impairment of deep sensation, bladder dysfunction, paraparesis, and alteration in emotional responses. Diagnosis may be uncertain at the onset and in the early years of the disease, when symptoms and signs point to a lesion in only one locus of the nervous system. Later, as the disease disseminates through the cerebrospinal axis, diagnostic accuracy approaches 100 percent. A long period of latency (1 to 10 years or longer) between a minor initial symptom, which may not even come to medical attention, and the subsequent development of more characteristic symptoms and signs may delay the diagnosis. In most cases the initial manifestation(s) improve partially or completely, to be followed, after a variable interval, by the recurrence of the same abnormalities or the appearance of new ones referable to other parts of the nervous system. In as many as half the patients, the disease presents as an intermittently progressive illness, and sometimes as a steadily progressive one. As a general clinical rule, the diagnosis of multiple sclerosis is not secure unless there is a history of remission and relapse and evidence on examination of more than one discrete lesion of the CNS.

PATHOLOGIC FINDINGS

Before being sectioned, the brain generally shows no evidence of disease, but the surface of the spinal cord may feel uneven. Sectioning of the brain and cord discloses numerous scattered lesions which are slightly depressed below the cut surface and stand out from the surrounding white matter by virtue of their pinkish gray color (due to loss of myelin). The lesions may vary in diameter from less than 1 mm to several centimeters; they affect principally the white matter of the brain and spinal cord and do not extend beyond the root entry zones of the cranial and spinal nerves. Because of their sharp delineation they are called plaques. Frequently they encroach on the cerebral gray matter, but do not destroy nerve cells, and often they are located in the paraventricular areas of the brain in relation to the veins in the walls of the lateral ventricles. The lesions appear to have a predilection for myelin where it abuts pial veins, hence the frequent involvement of tracts of the spinal cord, brainstem, and optic nerves and chiasm.

The histologic appearance of the lesion depends on its age. Relatively recent lesions show a partial or complete destruction and loss of myelin throughout a zone formed by the confluence of many small predominantly perivenous foci, with sparing of axis cylinders and a degeneration of oligodendroglia, neuroglial reaction, and perivascular and paraadventitial infiltration with mononuclear cells and lymphocytes. Later, large numbers of microglial phagocytes infiltrate the lesions, and astrocytes in and around the lesions increase in number and size. Long-standing lesions, on the other hand, will show thickly matted, relatively acellular fibroglial tissue, with only occasional perivascular lymphocytes and macrophages; in such lesions intact axis cylinders may still be found. Sparing of axis cylinders prevents wallerian degeneration. However, in old lesions with loss of many axis cylinders there may be descending and ascending degeneration of long fiber tracts in the spinal cord. Remyelination is believed to take place on undamaged axons. All gradations of pathologic change between these two extremes may be found in lesions of diverse size, shape, and age, consistent with the extended clinical course.

Cruveilhier (circa 1835), in his classic original description of the disease, attributed it to suppression of sweat and since that time there has been endless speculation about the etiology. Many of the early theories appear ludicrous in the light of present-day concepts, and others are only of historical interest. There is no point in enumerating them here; complete accounts are to be found in the reviews of McAlpine and his associates (1972), DeJong (1970), Prineas (1970), R. T. Johnson (1975, 1978), and Portersfield (1977).

Although the precise cause or causes of multiple sclerosis remain undetermined, a number of epidemiologic facts have been clearly established and will eventually have to be incorporated in any etiologic hypothesis. The disease has a prevalence of less than 1 per 100,000 in equatorial areas; 6 to 14 per 100,000 in southern United States and southern Europe; and 30 to 80 per 100,000 in Canada, northern Europe, and northern United States. A less well-defined gradient exists in the Southern Hemisphere. Kurland's studies indicate that there is a threefold increase in prevalence and a fivefold gradient in mortality rate between New Orleans (30°N latitude) on the one hand, and Boston (42°N) and Winnipeg (50°N) on the other. An exception to these patterns appears to exist in Japan, where the prevalence rates are reportedly very low and uniform from north to south, but case ascertainment in the Japanese surveys was almost certainly less complete than in others. The increasing risk of developing multiple sclerosis with increasing latitude has been confirmed most recently by Kurtzke et al., who have studied a series of unprecedented size (5305 undoubted cases of multiple sclerosis and matched controls). In the United States, blacks are at lower risk than whites at all latitudes, but both races show the same south-to-north gradient in risk, indicating the importance of an environmental factor, regardless of race (Kurtzke et al.).

Several studies indicate that persons who migrate from a high-risk to a low-risk zone carry with them at least part of the risk of their country of origin, even though the disease may not become apparent until 20 years after migration. Such a pattern has been demonstrated both in South Africa and in Israel. Dean determined that the prevalence in native-born white South Africans was 3 to 11 per 100,000, whereas the rate in immigrants from northern Europe was about 50 per 100,000, only slightly less than in the nonimmigrating natives of those countries. The data of Dean and Kurtzke further indicate that in persons who had immigrated before the age of 15 the risk was similar to that of

native-born South Africans, whereas in persons who had immigrated after that age, the risk was similar to that of their birthplace. Alter et al. found that in the descendants of European immigrants born in Israel the risk of multiple sclerosis was low, similar to that of other native-born Israelis, whereas among recent immigrants the incidence in each national group approached the incidence in the land of birth. Again the critical age of immigration appeared to be about 15 years. These epidemiologic studies and others have shown that multiple sclerosis is associated with particular localities rather than with a particular ethnic group in those localities, and emphasize the importance of environmental factors in the genesis of the disease.

A familial tendency toward multiple sclerosis is now recognized. McAlpine and others have calculated that for a first-degree relative of a patient with multiple sclerosis the risk of developing the disease is at least 5 to 15 times greater than for a member of the general population, and the risk is greater for siblings than for parents. Within families with more than one affected member, no consistent genetic pattern has emerged. The concordance rate for twins is higher than for other siblings, but differences between monozygotic and dizygotic pairs of twins have not been statistically significant, a finding that argues against a major genetic factor in the etiology of multiple sclerosis. There is a tendency to consider all diseases with an increased familial incidence as hereditary, but instances of the same condition in several members of a family may simply reflect exposure to a common environmental agent. Paralytic poliomyelitis, for example, is about eight times more common in immediate family members than in the population at large.

The low conjugal incidence of multiple sclerosis supports the view that common exposure to this disease occurs early in life. In order to test this hypothesis, Schapira, et al. determined the periods of common exposure (common habitation periods) among members of families with two or more cases. From this they calculated the mean common exposure to have occurred before 14 years of age, with a latency of about 21 years—figures that are in general agreement with those derived from the migration studies quoted above.

The incidence of multiple sclerosis in children is very low; only 0.3 to 0.4 percent of all cases occur during the first decade. Beyond this time, the risk of first developing symptoms of the disease rises steeply with age, reaching a peak at 30 to 35 years, then falling off sharply and becoming low in the sixth decade. It has been pointed out that multiple sclerosis has a unimodal age-specific onset curve, similar to the age-specific onset curves of many infectious diseases. These epidemiologic data suggest an infectious (presumably viral) etiology of multiple sclerosis (see below).

About two-thirds of cases of multiple sclerosis have their onset between 20 and 40 years of age. In a smaller number the disease appears to develop in late adult life (late fifties and sixties). In these latter patients, early symptoms may have been forgotten or never declared themselves clinically (we have found the typical lesions of multiple sclerosis by chance in autopsied individuals who had no reported neurologic abnormalities). The incidence of multiple sclerosis is higher in women than in men (1.7:1), but the significance of this fact is unclear.

Studies in Norway and Sweden have suggested that the risk of developing multiple sclerosis is somewhat greater in farmers than in urban dwellers; studies of American Army personnel have suggested the opposite (Beebe et al.). Several surveys in Great Britain have intimated that the disease is more frequent in higher than in lower socioeconomic groups. Relationships to numerous other environmental factors (surgical operations, anesthesia, exposure to household pets) have been proposed but are unsupported by firm evidence.

All these epidemiologic data indicate that multiple sclerosis is related to some environmental factor which is encountered in childhood and which, after years of latency, either evokes the disease or contributes to its causation. In the past decade, speculation has grown that this factor is an infection, presumably viral. A large body of indirect evidence has been marshaled in support of this idea, based on the demonstration, in patients with multiple sclerosis, of alterations in humoral and cell-mediated immunity to viral agents [see reviews of R. T. Johnson (1975, 1978), Lampert, and K. P. Johnson et al.]. However, a virus has never been isolated from the tissues of patients with multiple sclerosis, despite innumerable attempts to do so, and no satisfactory viral model of multiple sclerosis has been produced experimentally.

If the initial insult to the nervous system is a viral or viral-like infection, then some secondary factor must be operative in later life to initiate the neurologic disease and to cause exacerbations. The most popular view holds that this secondary mechanism is an autoimmune reaction, attacking myelin, and in its most intense form,

destroying all tissue elements, including axis cylinders. Again, the evidence is largely circumstantial. An analogy has been drawn between the lesions of multiple sclerosis and those of disseminated encephalomyelitis, which is almost certainly an autoimmune disease of delayed hypersensitivity type (see further on). Elevated levels of antibodies to measles and to other viruses (herpes simplex, varicella-zoster, Epstein-Barr, vaccinia, rubella) have been found in the serum and CSF of patients with multiple sclerosis. The significance of these findings is unclear. Certainly multiple sclerosis occurs in patients who have never had an attack of measles and have no antibodies to this disease, and multiple sclerosis patients have no immunity to measles. Contrariwise, elevated levels of antibodies to measles and other viruses are found in a significant proportion of normal control subjects, and in a variety of diseases other than multiple sclerosis (lupus erythematosus, rheumatoid arthritis, chronic liver disease).

Another line of evidence, seemingly established by several investigators, is that the T lymphocytes in the blood disappear during attacks of multiple sclerosis, although they are known to be present in fresh multiple sclerotic plaques. Since these cells are responsible for cell-mediated immune reactions, this finding supports the idea that an autoimmune mechanism is operative.

Recent interest has centered about the finding that certain histocompatibility (HLA) antigens are more frequent in patients with multiple sclerosis than in control subjects, redirecting attention to the importance of genetic factors in this disease. It has been suggested that the HLA antigens which are overrepresented in multiple sclerosis (HLA-A3, -B7, and -Dw2) are markers for a multiple sclerosis "susceptibility gene"—possibly an immune response gene—and that possession of these antigens are related to the severity and tempo of progression of the disease (see review of Jersild). These antigens may prove to be important in determining the frequency and expression of the disease, but at the moment their exact role remains to be established.

PRECIPITATING FACTORS

A variety of events occurring immediately before the initial symptoms or exacerbations of multiple sclerosis have been regarded as precipitating factors. The most commonly invoked are infection, trauma, and pregnancy. The incidence of influenza or other infections preceding the onset or exacerbations of the disease varies in different series from 5 to 50 percent. The possible role of physical injury in precipitating multiple sclerosis is difficult to assess. McAlpine and Compston found that the incidence of trauma within a 3-month period preceding the onset of multiple sclerosis was slightly greater than in a random control group of hospital patients. Furthermore, there appeared to be a relationship between the site of the injury (e.g., the jaw, following dental extraction; or a limb) and the site of initial symptoms, particularly in patients who developed symptoms within a week of injury. Other forms of trauma (including lumbar puncture and surgical procedures) that occur after the onset of the neurologic disorder have not been shown to have an adverse effect on the course of the illness. Although there is a definite increase of exacerbations during the pregnancy year (i.e., in the 9 months of pregnancy and the 3 months that follow), most of these occur in the latter period, suggesting a relationship to the stresses of labor and the increased fatigue during the puerperium, rather than to pregnancy itself.

CLINICAL MANIFESTATIONS

The conventional view of multiple sclerosis as a disease which strikes young people at a time when they are enjoying perfect health is not altogether correct. Often the history discloses that fatigue, lack of energy, weight loss, and vague muscle and joint pains had been present for several weeks or months before the onset of neurologic symptoms. Nor is it generally appreciated that the neurologic disorder frequently has a sudden, even apoplectic, onset. McAlpine et al. (1972), who analyzed the mode of onset in 219 patients, found that in about 20 percent the neurologic symptoms were fully developed in a matter of minutes, and, in a similar number, in a matter of hours. In about 30 percent the symptoms evolved more slowly, over a period of a day or several days, and in another 20 percent more slowly still, over several weeks to months. In the remaining 10 percent the symptoms had an insidious onset and slow, steady progression over months and years.

Early Symptoms and Signs Weakness and/or numbness in one or more limbs are the initial symptoms in about one-half the patients. Symptoms of tingling of the extremities and tight bandlike sensations around the trunk or limbs are commonly associated and are probably the result of involvement of the posterior columns of the spinal cord. The resulting clinical syndromes vary from mere dragging or poor control of one or both legs to a spastic or ataxic paraparesis, or both. The tendon reflexes later become hyperactive with extensor plantar reflexes, the abdominal reflexes disappear, and varying degrees of deep and superficial sensory loss may be associated. It is a useful adage that the patient with multiple sclerosis presents with symptoms in one leg and signs in both. The patient will complain of weakness, incoordi-

nation, or numbness and tingling in one lower extremity and prove to have bilateral Babinski signs and other evidence of bilateral corticospinal and posterior column disease. Passive flexion of the neck may induce a tingling, electriclike feeling down the back and, less commonly, down the anterior thighs. This phenomenon is known as Lhermitte's sign, although it is more a symptom than a sign and was originally described by Babinski in a case of cervical cord trauma. Lhermitte's contribution was to draw attention to this phenomenon as a frequent manifestation of multiple sclerosis.

In about 25 percent of all patients (and in a larger proportion of children) the initial manifestation is an episode of *retrobulbar neuritis.* Characteristically, the syndrome is one of rapid evolution, over a period of several hours to days, of partial or total loss of vision in one eye. Usually a scotoma can be demonstrated involving the macular area, but a wide variety of other field defects may occur, even hemianopic ones, sometimes homonymous (see page 174). In some patients, both optic nerves are involved, either simultaneously or within a few days to weeks of one another. In about half the patients, if serial examinations are made, some evidence of swelling of the optic nerve head (papillitis) will be observed. The occurrence of papillitis depends upon the proximity of the demyelinating lesion to the nerve head. Subtle manifestations of optic nerve affection such as atrophy of retinal nerve fibers (page 170) and abnormalities of the visual evoked response (page 26) should always be sought in patients who have no visual symptoms but are suspected of having multiple sclerosis. It will be recalled that the optic nerve is in fact a tract of the brain, and involvement of the optic nerves is therefore consistent with the rule that lesions of multiple sclerosis occur only in the central nervous system.

About one-third of patients with optic neuritis recover completely, one-third improve to a considerable extent, and one-third show little or no improvement. When improvement occurs, it begins usually within 2 weeks of onset, as is true of most acute manifestations of multiple sclerosis. Once improvement in neurologic function begins, it may continue for several months. It should be noted that about 35 to 40 percent of patients who develop optic neuritis will develop other signs of multiple sclerosis within 15 years. The risk is somewhat lower if the initial attack of optic neuritis occurs in childhood, and somewhat higher if the attack occurs in adult life. The longer the period of observation, the greater will be the proportion of patients who develop other signs of multiple sclerosis.

It is unclear whether optic neuritis that occurs alone and is not followed by other evidence of demyelinating disease is simply a form of multiple sclerosis with only an isolated lesion or a manifestation of some other disease process, such as postinfectious encephalomyelitis. No pathologic basis for optic neuritis other than demyelinative disease has so far been established, though it is known that compression of an optic nerve by a tumor or mucocele will sometimes cause a central scotoma.

Other initial manifestations of multiple sclerosis, in descending order of frequency, are unsteadiness in walking, brainstem symptoms (diplopia, vertigo, vomiting), and disorders of micturition. Onset with discrete manifestations, such as hemiplegia, trigeminal neuralgia or other pain syndromes, facial paralysis, deafness, or seizures occurs in a small proportion of cases. More often than not the disease presents with more than one of the aforementioned symptoms.

Not infrequently the disease begins with nystagmus and ataxia, with or without weakness and spasticity of the limbs, a syndrome that reflects involvement of the cerebellar and corticospinal tracts and their connections. Ataxia of cerebellar type can be recognized by scanning speech, rhythmic instability of the head and trunk, intention tremor of the arms and legs, and incoordination of voluntary movements, as described in Chap. 4. The combination of nystagmus, scanning speech, and intention tremor is known as *Charcot's triad,* but most neurologists agree that, while this group of symptoms is often seen in the advanced stages of the disease, it is a rare mode of presentation. The most severe forms of cerebellar ataxia, in which the slightest attempt at voluntary movement of the trunk or limbs precipitates a violent and uncontrollable ataxic tremor, are observed among patients with multiple sclerosis. The responsible lesion probably lies in the tegmentum of the midbrain and involves the dentatorubrothalamic tracts. Cerebellar ataxia may be mixed with sensory ataxia, due to involvement of the posterior columns of the spinal cord. In many cases of this type the signs of spinal cord involvement ultimately become predominant; in others, the cerebellar signs predominate.

Diplopia is another common presenting complaint. It is due most often to involvement of the medial longitudinal fasciculus, producing an internuclear ophthalmoplegia (see page 177). The latter is characterized by paresis of the medial rectus on attempted lateral gaze, with a coarse nystagmus in the abducting eye; in multiple sclerosis, this abnormality is usually bilateral. As a corollary, the presence of bilateral internuclear ophthalmoplegia in a young adult is virtually diagnostic of multiple sclerosis. Other palsies of gaze, due to interruption of supranuclear connections, or palsies of individual ocular muscles, due to involvement of the third or sixth cranial nerves in their intramedullary course, also occur—but less frequently. Other manifestations of brainstem involvement include myokymia or paralysis of facial muscles, deafness, tinnitus, unformed auditory hallucinations (because of involvement of cochlear connections), and vertigo and vomiting (vestibular connections). The occurrence of transient facial anesthesia or of trigeminal neuralgia in a young person should always suggest the diagnosis of multiple sclerosis, with involvement of the intramedullary fibers of the fifth cranial nerve. In the most severe forms of the disease, all or some of the aforementioned brainstem symptoms may be combined with quadriplegia, pseudobulbar palsy, and cerebellar ataxia.

Symptoms of bladder dysfunction—including hesitancy, urgency, frequency, and incontinence—occur commonly with spinal cord involvement. Urinary retention, due to affection of sacral segments (Fig. 26-6), is less frequent. In males, these symptoms are often associated with impotence, a symptom which the patient may not report unless specifically questioned in this regard. About 5 percent of patients with multiple sclerosis, at some time during the course of their disease, will have a seizure or recurrent seizures, presumably as the result of lesions in the cerebral cortex or subjacent white matter.

Traditional teaching has overemphasized the frequency of euphoria, a pathologic cheerfulness or elation which seems inappropriate in the face of the obvious neurologic deficit. Some patients do show this mental abnormality, the result probably of lesions of the white matter of the frontal lobes, often in association with other signs of cerebral impairment. In some instances it is manifestly a part of the syndrome of pseudobulbar palsy. There are, however, a much larger number of patients who are depressed, irritable, and short-tempered as a reaction to the disabling features of the disease. Other psychological deficits, such as loss of retentive memory or a global dementia, also occur in a relatively small proportion of patients, usually in the late stages of the disease.

Dull, aching pain in the low back is a common complaint, but its relation to the lesions of multiple sclerosis is uncertain. Sharp, burning pains in the legs and girdle pains—presumably caused by demyelinative foci involving the root entry zones—occur infrequently. These symptoms may precede the onset of sensory signs or appear at any time in established cases of the disease.

Abrupt attacks of neurologic deficit, lasting a few seconds or minutes and sometimes recurring many times daily, are an infrequent but well-recognized feature of multiple sclerosis. Usually the attacks occur in the course of the illness, rarely as an initial manifestation. The clinical manifestations are referable to any part of the central nervous system but most often consist of dysarthria and ataxia; paroxysmal pain and dysesthesia in a limb; flashing lights; or tonic flexion of the hand, wrist, and elbow with extension of the lower limb. The cause of these transitory phenomena is uncertain. They are variously attributed to movement, temporary rise in body temperature, and transversely spreading ephaptic activation of axons within a lesion (Halliday and McDonald). Carbamazepine is usually effective in controlling the attacks.

In the established stage of the disease, when diagnosis has become virtually certain, a number of clinical syndromes are observed to occur with regularity. Approximately one-half of the patients will manifest a clinical picture of *mixed* or *generalized type* with signs pointing to involvement of optic nerves, brainstem, cerebellum, and spinal cord. Another 30 to 40 percent will exhibit varying degrees of spastic ataxia and deep sensory changes in the extremities, i.e., essentially a *spinal form of the disease*. A predominantly *cerebellar* or *pontobulbar-cerebellar form* will be noted in only about 5 percent of cases and an *amaurotic form* in a like number. Thus the mixed cerebrospinal and spinal ones together have comprised at least 80 percent of our clinical material.

A number of interesting variants of multiple sclerosis have come to our attention over the years and have given rise to difficulties in diagnosis. Several times we have been consulted by a young woman or man with typical tic douloureux; only their young age, and bilaterality of the pain in some of them, raised the suspicion of multiple sclerosis, confirmed later by sensory loss in the face and other neurologic signs. Severe thoracic or lumbosacral pain consisting mainly of thermal and algesic dysesthesias were sources of puzzlement in two other patients until other lesions developed. In several patients the occurrence of a right hemiplegia and aphasia first raised the probability of a cerebrovascular lesion, only to be followed by spinal cord lesions. In others, a slowly evolving hemiplegia had led to the diagnosis of a cerebral glioma.

Twice we have seen coma during relapse, and in each instance it continued to death. In one case it oc-

curred in a 64-year-old woman who had had two previous episodes of nondisabling spinal multiple sclerosis at 30 and 44 years. A confusional psychosis with drowsiness was the reported initial syndrome in another patient whom we later saw with a relapse involving cerebellum and spinal cord. Another unusual syndrome is one of slow intellectual decline with slight cerebellar ataxia. A 10-year slowly progressive cerebellar ataxia in an adolescent girl who later developed internuclear ophthalmoplegia was another perplexing variant. A rapid onset of ascending paralysis of bladder and bowel, legs, and trunk with severe pain in sacral parts, areflexia, and 1600 mononuclear cells per cubic millimeter of CSF occurred in another of our patients and lasted 2 years before she began to walk; earlier she had had diplopia and retrobulbar neuritis. Repeatedly, seemingly more in recent years, we have observed patients whose illness satisfied all the criteria for the diagnosis of multiple sclerosis, except for the onset of symptoms in the sixth or seventh decade. Presumably we were witnessing the late deteriorative phase of the illness, and the earlier symptoms had been forgotten or were never recognized (see above under "Etiology").

Two other variants of multiple sclerosis merit more extended discussion. They are acute multiple sclerosis and neuromyelitis optica.

Acute Multiple Sclerosis Occasionally multiple sclerosis takes a highly malignant form. A combination of cerebral, brainstem, and spinal manifestations evolve over a few weeks rendering the patient stuporous or comatose, or decerebrate with prominent cranial nerve and corticospinal abnormalities. Death may end the illness within a few weeks to months without any remission having occurred. At autopsy the lesions (unlike those of acute disseminated encephalomyelitis) are of macroscopic dimensions, typical of the acute plaques of multiple sclerosis. The only difference is that many plaques are of the same age and the confluence of many perivenous zones of demyelination is more obvious. Two of our most striking examples of this rapidly fatal form were in a 6-year-old girl and a 16-year-old boy, both of whom died within 5 weeks of the onset of symptoms. Another was a 30-year-old man who lived 2 months. In none of them had there been a preceding exanthem or inoculation.

Nonfatal clinical cases of similar type in children, adolescents, and young adults are admitted to the Massachusetts and Cleveland Metropolitan General Hospitals once or twice a year. Some have responded to ACTH, and others worsened while receiving this medication. Many have made an astonishing recovery after several months, and a few have then remained well for 25 to 30 years. Others have relapsed and the subsequent clinical course was typical of multiple sclerosis.

It seems to the authors that more than one disease is being included in the clinical category of acute multiple sclerosis. One type conforms in its temporal profile to a rather protracted form of acute disseminated encephalomyelitis—an acute monophasic illness extending over 4 to 8 weeks akin to some of the Japanese postrabies-inoculation cases (Shiraki and Otani). Others subsequently prove to be typical polyphasic multiple sclerosis. Only the clinical course presently separates the two types.

Neuromyelitis and Neuromyelitis Optica The conjunction of peripheral nerve and spinal cord affection has been commented upon since the latter part of the last century. A number of morbid states such as porphyria, pellagra, beriberi, syphilis, and intoxication with lead or alcohol were said to have this combined effect. Austregesilo, for example, reported in 1932 on an outbreak of neuromyelitis in Brazil in which a mild peripheral neuritis was followed in 1 to 4 months by an ascending myelitis with bulbar symptoms. The authors, not having seen such cases, have reason to be skeptical of the diagnosis, for it is not always easy to separate neuropathic from myelitic manifestations on clinical grounds alone, and there are but few if any adequate pathologic studies. The one exception has been polyarteritis nodosa, where the common peripheral nerve lesions may be complicated by ischemic damage to the spinal cord. Wilson has reviewed the rather confusing literature on this subject.

Simultaneous or successive involvement of optic nerves and spinal cord has been more convincingly documented. The combination was remarked upon by Clifford Albutt in 1870, and Gault (1894), stimulated by his teacher Devic, devoted his thesis to the subject. Devic endeavored to crystallize medical thought about a condition that has come to be known as *neuromyelitis optica*. Its principal features are acute to subacute onset of blindness of one or both eyes preceded or followed within days or weeks by a transverse or ascending myelitis (Beck). As stated on page 626, the lesions in the spinal cord and sometimes the optic nerves are usually of necrotizing type leading eventually to cavitation; and, as

would be expected, the clinical effects are more likely to be permanent than those of demyelination. Many of the patients have been children, and in a number of instances they suffered only a single episode of neurologic illness.

While it is true that cases corresponding to this prototype are seen on occasion in every large medical center, and at all age periods, the isolation of such an entity on clinical grounds alone has been unsatisfactory. Most of our patients have proven by subsequent clinical developments, and in a few instances by autopsy, to have chronic relapsing multiple sclerosis. In one notable example, where hemiplegia and aphasia were followed within 2 weeks by a necrotizing myelitis from which there was no recovery, the patient then developed typical attacks of multiple sclerosis, including retrobulbar neuritis. At autopsy more than 15.0 cm of the spinal cord had been destroyed, reducing it to collapsed membranes. Elsewhere the lesions were typically demyelinative. Also, acute disseminated encephalomyelitis may occasionally present as a neuromyelitis optica.

One must conclude that *neuromyelitis optica* is usually a form of multiple sclerosis, but other types of demyelinative disease, namely acute disseminated encephalomyelitis, acute multiple sclerosis, and acute necrotizing hemorrhagic leukoencephalitis and leukomyelitis may on occasion present this clinical syndrome.

Cerebrospinal Fluid In about 25 percent of patients, particularly those with an acute onset or exacerbation, there may be a slight mononuclear pleocytosis (usually less than 50 cells per cubic millimeter) in the CSF. In rapidly progressive cases of neuromyelitis optica (see above) and in certain instances of severe demyelinative disease of the brainstem, the total cell count may reach or exceed 100 and rarely 1000 cells per cubic millimeter, and with the high cell counts the greater proportion may be polymorphonuclear leucocytes. This pleocytosis is in fact the only measure of activity of the disease. Other laboratory tests (except for myelin basic protein, see below) do not reflect the activity of the disease.

Also, in about 25 percent of patients, the total protein content of the CSF is increased. The increase is slight, however, and a level of more than 100 mg per 100 ml is so unusual that the possibility of another diagnosis should be entertained. On the other hand, in the more chronic forms of multifocal demyelination the proportion of gamma globulin (essentially IgG) is increased (above 12 to 13 percent of the total protein) in about two-thirds of patients. It has been shown that the gamma globulins in the CSF of patients with multiple sclerosis are synthesized in the CNS (Tourtellotte) and that they migrate in agarose electrophoresis as abnormal discrete populations, so-called oligoclonal bands. A simple method for demonstrating these bands has been described, using readily available commercial reagents and apparatus (Johnson et al., 1977). Such bands also appear in the CSF of patients with syphilis, Guillain-Barré polyneuritis and subacute sclerosing panencephalitis—disorders that should not be difficult to distinguish from multiple sclerosis on clinical grounds. The demonstration of oligoclonal bands in the CSF and not in the blood can be particularly helpful in the diagnosis of early or atypical cases of multiple sclerosis.

It has been shown also, by the use of a sensitive radioimmunoassay, that the CSF contains high levels of myelin basic protein during acute exacerbations of multiple sclerosis, and that these levels are lower in slowly progressive multiple sclerosis and normal during remissions of the disease (Cohen et al.). Thus the assay is a useful measure of activity of multiple sclerosis; unfortunately, the method is not simple and is being carried out in only a few laboratories.

When cells, total protein, gamma globulin, and oligoclonal bands are all taken into account, some abnormality will be found in almost every case of multiple sclerosis. At present the measurement of gamma globulins and oligoclonal bands in the CSF are the only reliable laboratory tests of multiple sclerosis.

Other Laboratory Tests   When the clinical data point to only one lesion in the CNS, as often happens in the early stages of the disease or in the late spinal form, a number of delicate physiologic tests may establish the existence of other asymptomatic lesions. These tests include visual, auditory, and tactile evoked responses, perceptual delay on visual stimulation, electrooculography to show a lag in contraction of an ocular muscle, altered blink reflexes, and a change in flicker fusion of visual images. Halliday and McDonald report abnormalities in one or more of these tests in 50 to 90 percent of a series of multiple sclerosis patients.

PATHOPHYSIOLOGY

The observations of delayed optic nerve conduction of patterned visual stimuli in patients with normal visual acuity and normal fields have reopened the matter of the pathophysiology of demyelination. When the latter process is acute, there is obviously a functional block in nerve fiber conduction, but the remarkable reversibility (recovery) is more difficult to understand. Surely it could not be due to remyelination. More likely, recovery is due to subsidence of the edema in and around the lesion. Remyelination probably does occur, but it is a slower process and its functional effects in the CNS are un-

known. A slowing of optic nerve conduction, if it is present in an eye with normal vision, may account for the reduction in flicker fusion and in perception of multiple visual stimuli (Halliday and McDonald).

CLINICAL COURSE AND PROGNOSIS

The intermittency of the clinical manifestations, the disease advancing in a series of attacks each permitting less and less remission, is one of the most important clinical attributes of the disease. Some patients will have a complete remission after the initial attack, or rarely there may be a series of exacerbations, each with complete remission; such exacerbations may be severe enough to have caused quadriplegia and pseudobulbar palsy. The relapse rate is 0.3 to 0.4 attacks per year according to the calculations of McAlpine and Compston, and the interval between the opening symptom and the first relapse is highly variable. It was within 1 year in 30 percent of McAlpine's cases and within 2 years in another 20 percent. A further 20 percent relapsed in 5 to 9 years and another 10 percent in 10 to 30 years. Not only is the length of this latent interval remarkable, but also the fact that the pathologic process can remain potentially active for such a long time.

After a number of years there is an increasing tendency for the patient to enter a phase of slow, steady, or fluctuating deterioration of neurologic function, attributable to the cumulative effect of increasing numbers of lesions, but in about 10 percent of cases the course of the disease is steadily progressive from the beginning. In these latter cases the disease usually takes the form of a spastic paraparesis and probably represents the most frequent type of obscure myelopathy observed by the authors, as pointed out on page 625.

The duration of the disease is exceedingly variable. A small number of patients die within several months or years of the onset, but the average duration is in excess of 20 years. A 60-year appraisal of the resident population of Rochester, Minnesota, revealed that 74 percent of patients with multiple sclerosis survived 25 years as compared to 86 percent of the general population. At the end of 25 years, one-third of the surviving patients were still working and two-thirds were still ambulatory (Percy et al.). These latter data are not in accord with other statistical analyses that give a worse prognosis. Patients with mild and quiescent forms of the disease are, of course, less likely to come to the attention of physicians working with chronically ill patients.

DIAGNOSIS

In the usual forms of multiple sclerosis, i.e., in those with a relapsing and remitting course and evidence of disseminated lesions in the CNS, the diagnosis of multiple sclerosis is rarely in doubt. Only meningovascular syphilis, certain rare forms of cerebral arteritis, and lupus erythematosus could possibly simulate relapsing multiple sclerosis, and each of these has its own characteristic diagnostic features. Difficulties are most likely to arise when the standard clinical criteria of multiple sclerosis are lacking, as occurs in the acute initial attack of the disease and in cases with an insidious onset and slow, steady progression.

As has been stated, the initial attack of multiple sclerosis may mimic acute labyrinthine vertigo or tic douloureux. Careful neurologic examination of such patients usually discloses the signs of a brainstem lesion; the CSF examination may be particularly helpful in these circumstances. Extensive brainstem demyelination of subacute evolution, involving tracts and cranial nerves sequentially, may be mistaken for a pontine glioma. The course of the illness settles the matter; symptoms of brainstem multiple sclerosis remit as a rule, and to a surprisingly complete degree in many cases. During epidemics of poliomyelitis, the acute onset of multiple sclerosis with limb weakness and CSF pleocytosis was sometimes mistaken for paralytic poliomyelitis, but this is no longer a practical consideration.

Disseminated encephalomyelitis (see further on) is an acute illness with widely scattered lesions, but is self-limited and monophasic; furthermore, fever, stupor, and coma, which are characteristic, rarely occur in multiple sclerosis.

The purely spinal form of multiple sclerosis, presenting as a progressive spastic paraparesis with varying degrees of posterior column involvement, is a special source of diagnostic difficulty. Such patients require careful evaluation for the presence of spinal cord compression due to neoplasm or cervical spondylosis. Radicular pain at some point in the illness is a frequent manifestation of the latter disorders and is rare in multiple sclerosis. Pain in the neck, immobility of the cervical spine, and severe muscle wasting due to spinal root involvement, as is sometimes seen in spondylosis, are almost unknown in multiple sclerosis. As a general rule, loss of abdominal reflexes and disturbances of bladder function occur early in the course of demyelinative myelopathy, but late or not at all in cervical spondylosis.

The CSF protein in the latter condition is apt to be significantly elevated and the proportion of gamma globulin normal, in distinction to multiple sclerosis. Slowed or altered visual, auditory, and somatic sensory evoked potentials may be demonstrated in the majority of patients without deafness, optic atrophy, or a history of optic neuritis, and provide proof of dissemination of lesions. The highest court of appeal is myelography, and every patient with progressive spastic paraparesis in whom the neurologic signs are limited to the spinal cord should be investigated by this method.

Amyotrophic lateral sclerosis (ALS) and subacute combined degeneration (SCD) of the cord should not be confused with multiple sclerosis. ALS can be identified by the presence of muscle wasting, fasciculations, and the total absence of sensory involvement. SCD is characterized by the symmetric involvement of the posterior and lateral columns of the spinal cord, low serum level of vitamin B_{12}, gastric achlorhydria, megaloblastic marrow and macrocytic anemia in many cases, and defective absorption of vitamin B_{12} (Schilling test; see page 719).

The presence of *nystagmus* and disorders of ocular movement should always be sought in patients with progressive spastic paraparesis, since such an association might establish the diagnosis of multiple sclerosis. It is important to remember that ingestion of barbiturates and phenytoin is a common cause of nystagmus. The possibility that an anxious or sleepless patient with a nondemyelinative spinal cord disease has taken a barbiturate should always be borne in mind.

Platybasia and basilar impression of the skull should also be considered in the differential diagnosis, but patients with these conditions have a characteristic shortening of the neck, and careful radiographs of the base of the skull will be diagnostic. Neurologic syndromes resulting from the Arnold-Chiari malformation (without meningomyelocele) and from tumors of the cerebellopontine angle and other parts of the posterior fossa and foramen magnum, have been misdiagnosed as multiple sclerosis. In each of these instances, a solitary, strategically placed lesion may give rise to a variety of neurologic symptoms and signs referable to the brainstem, cerebellum, lower cranial nerves, and upper cervical cord, and may give the impression of dissemination of lesions. It is an excellent clinical rule that a diagnosis of multiple sclerosis should not be made when all the patient's symptoms and signs can be explained by a lesion in one region of the neuraxis.

Confusion may occasionally arise with the hereditary ataxias, which are generally distinguished by their familial incidence and other associated genetic traits; by their insidious onset and slow, steady progression; and by their symmetry and stereotyped clinical pattern. Intactness of abdominal reflexes and sphincteric function, and the presence of pes cavus, kyphoscoliosis, and cardiac disease are other features that favor the diagnosis of a heredodegenerative disorder.

Careful clinical appraisal will usually lead to accurate diagnosis, but the label of "multiple sclerosis" should not be attached to a patient until the evidence is unequivocal. Once such a label is applied, it tends to stick; and since the diagnosis of multiple sclerosis will explain almost any subsequent neurologic event, attention may be directed away from consideration of another, perhaps treatable, disease.

TREATMENT

As one might expect, numerous forms of treatment have been proposed, and many have been thought to be successful because of the remitting nature of the disease. Only ACTH and prednisone have proved to have a beneficial effect on the disease, on the basis of controlled clinical trials. Under the influence of these agents, recovery from acute relapses appears to be hastened, particularly from an attack of optic neuritis. However, a substantial group of patients with acute exacerbations fail to respond to this type of treatment. Also, there is no evidence that ACTH and steroids have a significant effect upon the ultimate degree of improvement, or that they prevent the recurrence of the disease, so there is no justification for treatment over a period of many months or years. The reports concerning the effectiveness of intrathecal prednisolone are conflicting, and it is not to be recommended.

A variety of dosage schedules have been employed. It seems important that a high dose be used initially to be effective. We give ACTH intravenously in a dose of 80 units in 500 ml dextrose and water for 3 days, followed by 40 units of gel intramuscularly every 12 h for 7 days. The dose is then reduced by 10 units every 3 days. Many patients who show improvement on this therapy continue to improve or maintain their previous improvement even though the medication is gradually reduced and discontinued. Other patients have a recurrence of symptoms as the dose is reduced and need to be maintained on small doses of ACTH (20 to 40 units) every other day for a period of several months. Because of the risk of potassium depletion, the patients are given potassium supplements in a daily dose of 60 meq/liter. Euphoria or depression may be severe enough to terminate medication, and a sedative drug may be necessary because of the complaints of nervousness and difficulty in sleeping. The occurrence of peripheral edema due to sodium retention can be treated with mild diuretics and salt restriction. Gastrointestinal bleeding and the activa-

tion of tuberculosis and diabetes should always be considered as possible complications of treatment. Hirsutism and acne cannot be prevented but disappear when the medication is stopped. When it is impractical to administer ACTH, comparable amounts of oral prednisone may be substituted.

A variety of other treatments have been tried without convincing or verifiable results. Immunosuppressive drugs such as azothiaprine, cyclophosphamide, and cytosine arabinoside have been given to small groups of patients, but the results are uninterpretable. Some of these drugs are also antiviral agents. A low-fat diet was recommended on the basis of the low incidence of new cases of multiple sclerosis during famines in wartime. There are no statistically valid control studies. The same may be said of gluten-free diets. Linoleate supplementation of the diet is still under study.

General measures include the provision of an adequate period of bed rest and convalescence to ensure maximum recovery from the initial attack or exacerbation, prevention of excessive fatigue and infection, the use of all possible rehabilitative measures to postpone the bedridden stage of the disease (braces, chairs, ramps, lifts, cars with manual controls, etc.), and meticulous attention to the prevention of bedsores in the bedridden patient by the use of alternating pressure mattresses, silicone gel pads, and other special devices. The use of belladonna alkaloids and bethanechol chloride in the treatment of bladder dysfunction can be helpful. Antibiotics and acidifying drugs to suppress urinary tract infections should also be employed. Severe constipation is best managed with properly spaced enemas. Often a program of bowel training can be successfully undertaken. Injections of dilute solutions of phenol intrathecally and crushing of the obturator nerves are sometimes of value in the management of severe spasticity and flexor spasms. Some patients with lesser degrees of spasticity have benefitted from dantrolene sodium or baclofen (Lioresal).

The importance of an understanding and sympathetic physician in the care of patients with a chronic incapacitating neurologic disease of this kind cannot be overemphasized. From the beginning, when the patients first inquire about the nature of their disease, they require advice about their daily routine, marriage, pregnancy, the use of drugs, inoculations, etc. The term *multiple sclerosis* should not be introduced unless the diagnosis is certain, and then it should be qualified by a balanced explanation of the symptoms, stressing always the optimistic aspects of the disease. Some patients consider the uncertainty of the prognosis worse than the true disability, and need repeated assurance that the disease will not shorten their life or impair their mind.

ACUTE DISSEMINATED ENCEPHALOMYELITIS (Postinfectious, Postexanthem, Postvaccinal Encephalomyelitis; Acute Perivascular Myelinoclasis)

These terms, used to refer to the neurologic sequelae of infectious fevers, were introduced into medicine in the late nineteenth century, but it wasn't until about 50 years ago that Perdrau, Greenfield, and others identified a pathologic reaction type common to a number of exanthems and vaccination. The current view of this entity is that it represents an acute demyelinative disease, distinguished pathologically by numerous foci of demyelination that are scattered throughout the brain and spinal cord; these foci vary from 0.1 to 1 mm in diameter and invariably surround small and medium-sized veins. The axons and nerve cells are more or less intact. Equally distinctive is the inflammatory reaction; the reacting cells consist of pleomorphic microglia, which correspond to the zones of demyelination, and of lymphocytes and mononuclear cells, which cuff the vessels. Multifocal meningeal infiltration is another invariable feature but is rarely severe in degree.

The clinical manifestations reflect the diffuse involvement of the brain and spinal cord and of the meninges. There is an acute onset of confusion, somnolence, and often convulsions, with headache, fever, and stiffness of the neck. Ataxia, myoclonic movements, and choreoathetosis may be observed. In the more severe cases, stupor, coma, and, at times, decerebrate rigidity may occur in rapid succession. With spinal cord involvement there is partial or complete paraplegia or quadriplegia, diminution or loss of tendon reflexes, sensory impairment, and paralysis of bladder and bowel.

An acute encephalitic, myelitic, or encephalomyelitic process of this type may occur concurrently with or, more often, shortly after the onset of the exanthem of measles, smallpox, and chickenpox and very rarely with mumps, influenza, and rubella. A similar illness occurs following vaccination against rabies and smallpox and reportedly after the administration of tetanus antitoxin. Some cases, clinically and pathologically indistinguishable from these two categories of acute disseminated encephalomyelitis, appear to develop without any clearly defined preceding illness, vaccination, or inoculation.

The disease has grave significance because of the substantial death rate (10 to 20 percent) and the approximately equal incidence of persistent neurologic defects in patients who survive. There may be only slight motor disturbances or spastic paraplegia and impairment of sphincter control. In children, recovery from the acute stage is sometimes followed by a permanent disorder of behavior, mental retardation, or epilepsy. As in most acute diseases of the nervous system, the functional derangement during the acute stage is out of all proportion to the permanent structural damage.

The pathogenesis of disseminated encephalomyelitis is still unclear, despite its obvious association with viral infections. Usually a definite interval separates the onset of disseminated encephalomyelitis from the onset of the rash; also, the pathologic changes are quite different from those of viral infections and rarely has virus been recovered from the brains of patients with disseminated encephalomyelitis. For these reasons it is thought that the latter disorder represents an immune-mediated complication of infection, rather than a direct viral infection of the CNS. A laboratory model of the disease, experimental allergic encephalomyelitis (EAE), can be produced by inoculating animals with a combination of sterile brain tissue and adjuvants. The experimental animals show the characteristic perivenular demyelinative and inflammatory lesions of the human disease, presumably the result of a cell-mediated immune reaction to myelin proteins.

POSTVACCINAL ENCEPHALOMYELITIS

Since late in the nineteenth century it has been known that a severe form of encephalomyelitis may complicate the injection of rabies vaccine (neuroparalytic accident). Until quite recently, the vaccine in common use consisted of killed rabies virus produced in rabbit brain tissue; encephalomyelitis occurred in about 1 in 750 patients inoculated with this vaccine, and in 20 percent of cases this complication proved fatal. The alternative duck embryo vaccine, which contains no nerve tissue, causes fewer and less severe side effects, and is now used exclusively except in patients who are allergic to avian tissue.

Encephalomyelitis following vaccination against smallpox has been known since 1860, but only isolated instances were recognized until 1922, when the first major outbreak of postvaccinal encephalomyelitis occurred. The disease may appear at any time between the second and twenty-fifth days after vaccination, but usually between the tenth and thirteenth days (end of pustular stage). The disease occurs about once in 4000 vaccinations and about 20 times more frequently after primary vaccination than after revaccination. Smallpox vaccination is no longer recommended as part of routine pediatric immunization schedules in the United States. The occurrence of the disease, as might be expected, parallels the number of persons vaccinated when smallpox threatens, but there is good evidence that the incidence of postvaccinal encephalomyelitis varies considerably from time to time and from one place to another. The source of material used for the vaccine seems to have no bearing on its occurrence.

The onset of postvaccinal encephalomyelitis is generally abrupt—with headache, drowsiness, fever, vomiting, and sometimes with convulsions. There may be stiffness of the neck and other signs of meningeal irritation. Typically, signs of spinal cord involvement appear soon afterward, with flaccid weakness or paralysis, usually involving all four limbs; occasionally hemiplegia may occur. Tendon reflexes disappear, and the plantar responses become extensor. Sphincter control is often lost, and sensory loss, though variable, may be extensive and severe. Nystagmus, ocular palsies, and pupillary changes indicate brainstem involvement, and stupor and deepening coma point to diencephalic or cerebral lesions; these signs have a serious prognosis. Variations of this clinical picture are common. One patient may suffer a predominantly encephalitic illness with convulsions and coma and little evidence of cord damage; in another, hemiplegia or a pure transverse myelitis may occur, without headache, neck stiffness, or clouding of consciousness. The site of vaccination has no influence on the neurologic syndrome, and the florid skin lesions in the form of a generalized vaccinia or erythematous rash do not increase the likelihood of neuroparalytic accident. The CSF almost invariably shows a moderate increase in protein and cells, predominantly lymphocytes, but in rare cases it has been normal.

The association of the neurologic disorder with vaccination usually leaves the diagnosis in little doubt, and the characteristic combination of encephalitic and myelitic features will help to distinguish the condition from meningitis, viral encephalitis, and poliomyelitis. Rarely, an atypical case may mimic any one of these disorders. On occasion, the disease may suggest involvement of nerve roots and peripheral nerves and resemble acute inflammatory polyneuritis (Landry-Guillain-Barré syndrome).

The mortality rate is high, between 30 and 50 percent, but varies from one outbreak to another. If recovery occurs it may be surprisingly complete. However, a significant proportion of patients show residual neurologic signs, intellectual impairment, and psychoneurotic behavior.

POSTINFECTIOUS ENCEPHALOMYELITIS

This syndrome occurs most often in association with measles. Clinically evident neurologic complications occur in 1 in 800 to 1 in 1000 cases. Prior to widespread immunization against measles, an epidemic in a large city might have included 100,000 cases and resulted in a substantial number of neurologic complications. The mortality among patients with such complications ranges from 10 to 20 percent; about an equal number are left with persistent neurologic damage. Patients without clinically apparent neurologic residua may undergo significant and sometimes permanent changes in behavior. The neurologic complications of measles alone provide sufficient justification for immunization against the disease.

The incidence of encephalomyelitis following smallpox complications is approximately 2.5 cases per 1000, somewhat less following chickenpox, and much less after rubella. An acute encephalomyelitic reaction probably occurs in association with mumps, but the latter disease is often complicated by a true viral meningoencephalitis, which may be difficult to differentiate from a postinfectious process in the living patient.

The encephalomyelitic syndrome generally begins 2 to 4 days after the appearance of the rash. In fact the rash may be fading and other symptoms improving when the patient suddenly develops a recrudescence of fever, convulsions, stupor, and deepening coma. Less commonly, the patient may develop hemiplegia or evidence of cerebellar disease, and occasionally a transverse myelitis, sphincteric disturbances, or other signs of spinal cord involvement. Choreoathetotic movements are seen infrequently. In many cases the disease is much less severe and the patient suffers a transient encephalitic illness with headaches, confusion, and signs of meningeal irritation. The CSF, as in postvaccinal encephalomyelitis, almost invariably shows a lymphocytic pleocytosis and increase in protein content.

Differential Diagnosis It needs to be emphasized that not all the neurologic complications of measles and other exanthems are truly encephalomyelitic; in some cases cerebrovascular disease (particularly thrombophlebitis), acute toxic hepatoencephalopathy (Reye's syndrome), or hypoxic encephalopathy may be responsible.

Infectious mononucleosis, herpes simplex encephalitis and other forms of encephalitis may all mimic postinfectious encephalomyelitis. In a child the first attack of seizures in what will prove to be idiopathic epilepsy may at first raise suspicion of encephalitis or postinfectious encephalomyelitis.

Prevention and Treatment   The incidence of postinfectious and postvaccinal encephalomyelitis has declined significantly in the past decade. Paradoxically, this has resulted from the initiation of widespread immunization against measles and from the discontinuation of immunization against smallpox. The universal use of duck embryo vaccine for rabies prophylaxis may well eliminate the encephalomyelitic complications of rabies vaccination, and the selective use of smallpox vaccination in travelers and high-risk populations should further reduce the risk of encephalomyelitis from this disease.

The use of high-potency steroids appears to be the treatment of choice, although controlled trials of this treatment have not been carried out. Steroids, given soon after the appearance of neurologic signs, modify the severity of experimental allergic encephalomyelitis, and this provides the logic for their use in the human counterpart of this disease.

SCHILDER'S DIFFUSE CEREBRAL SCLEROSIS (Schilder's Disease, Encephalitis Periaxalis Diffusa)

The term *diffuse sclerosis* was probably first used by Strümpell (1879) to describe the hard texture of the freshly removed brain of an alcoholic; later the term was applied to widespread cerebral gliosis of whatever cause. In 1912, Schilder described an instance of what he considered to be "diffuse sclerosis." This was the case of a 14-year-old girl with progressive mental deterioration and signs of increased intracranial pressure, terminating fatally after 19 weeks. Postmortem examination disclosed the presence of large, well-demarcated areas of demyelination in the white matter of both cerebral hemispheres, as well as a number of smaller demyelinative foci, resembling the common lesions of multiple sclerosis. Because of the similarities of the pathologic changes to those of multiple sclerosis (prominence of the inflammatory reaction and relative sparing of axis cylinders) Schilder called this disease *encephalitis periaxalis dif-*

fusa, bringing it in line with *encephalitis periaxalis scleroticans*, a term that Marburg had used to describe a case of acute multiple sclerosis. Unfortunately, Schilder in subsequent publications used the same term for two conditions of different type (one appears to have been a familial leukodystrophy and the other a subacute encephalitis) and seriously confused the subject for many years. In the ensuing years the terms *Schilder's disease* and *diffuse sclerosis* were used to describe many different conditions. Some resembled Schilder's original descriptions; others differed with respect to familial occurrence and widespread symmetric destruction and gliosis of the white matter, often with metachromatic bodies and globoid bodies representing catabolic products of myelin; and still others (e.g., subacute encephalitides, vascular encephalopathies) seemed to have no connection with either of these categories.

One group of entities that can be readily culled from the overall category of diffuse sclerosis are the leukodystrophies, including the adrenoleukodystrophy of boys and young men, the globoid-body leukodystrophy of Krabbe, sudanophilic leukodystrophy, and the metachromatic leukodystrophy of Greenfield, which involves peripheral nerves as well as central nervous system tissue. These are a group of diseases usually of genetic origin but sometimes occurring sporadically, characterized clinically by progressive visual failure, mental deterioration, and spastic paralysis; and pathologically by massive and more or less symmetrical destruction of the white matter of the cerebral hemispheres. In each entity there is unquestionably a specific inherited biochemical defect in the metabolism of myelin proteolipids. These inherited metabolic diseases are discussed further in Chap. 37.

If one sets aside the hereditary forms of metabolic leukodystrophy and the varied childhood disorders of cerebral white matter that have indiscriminately been included under the rubric of "Schilder's disease" or "diffuse sclerosis," there remains a characteristic group of cases that does indeed correspond to Schilder's original description. These latter cases are nonfamilial and are most frequently encountered in children or young adults. Clinically they are characterized by a progressive course which may be steady and unremitting or punctuated by a series of episodes of rapid worsening. In rare instances the disease may become arrested for many years, or the patient may even improve slightly for a time. Dementia, homonymous hemianopia, cortical blindness, cortical deafness, varying degrees of hemiplegia and quadriplegia and pseudobulbar palsy are the usual clinical findings. The CSF may show changes similar to those in chronic relapsing multiple sclerosis. Death occurs in most patients within a few months or years, but some survive for a decade or longer. In the differential diagnosis, cerebral neoplasm is the main consideration.

The characteristic lesion in these cases is a large, sharply outlined, asymmetrical focus of myelin destruction often involving an entire lobe or cerebral hemisphere, typically with extension across the corpus callosum and affection of the opposite hemisphere. In some cases both hemispheres may be symmetrically involved. A careful examination of the optic nerves, brainstem, and spinal cord will often disclose the typical discrete lesions of multiple sclerosis. Histologically, the large single focus as well as the smaller disseminated ones, show the characteristic features of multiple sclerosis.

Poser's review of the literature, in 1957, uncovered 105 cases which could be designated as Schilder's diffuse sclerosis, in the original sense of the term. In 33 of these, the only lesions were the extensive areas of demyelination involving the centrum ovale; most of the patients in this group were children, and the disease had a tendency to take an acute or subacute progressive course. In 72 patients, isolated demyelinative plaques were found in other parts of the CNS, in addition to the large foci in the cerebral white matter; the age of onset in this latter group was similar to that of chronic, relapsing multiple sclerosis, and frequently the illness ran a protracted and remitting course.

It is apparent that diffuse cerebral sclerosis of this type must be closely related to multiple sclerosis, and may indeed be a variant of it, as Schilder originally proposed. The treatment of this form of juvenile cerebral multiple sclerosis is the same as that outlined for multiple sclerosis.

The *concentric sclerosis of Baló* is probably a variety of Schilder's disease, which it resembles in its clinical aspects and in the overall distribution of its lesions. The distinguishing feature is the occurrence of alternating bands of destruction and preservation of myelin in a series of concentric rings. The occurrence of lesions in this pattern suggests the centrifugal diffusion of some factor that is damaging to myelin. A similar pattern of lesions, although far less extensive, is seen in occasional cases of chronic relapsing multiple sclerosis.

Adrenoleukodystrophy, in which there is a combination of adrenal atrophy, bronzing of the skin, and leukodystrophy, is closely related to but nevertheless distinct from Schilder's disease. The neurologic picture and the cerebral lesion are indistinguishable from Schilder's disease, but the sex-linked male inheritance and the adrenal atrophy are unique (see page 696 for further description of this metabolic disorder).

ACUTE NECROTIZING HEMORRHAGIC ENCEPHALOMYELITIS (Acute Hemorrhagic Leukoencephalitis of Weston Hurst)

This, the most fulminant form of demyelinative disease, affects mainly young adults but also children. It is almost invariably preceded by a respiratory infection of indeterminate cause and of variable duration (1 to 14 days). The neurologic symptoms appear abruptly, beginning with headache, fever, stiff neck, and confusion. These are followed in short order by signs of disease of one or both cerebral hemispheres and brainstem—focal seizures, hemiplegia or quadriplegia, pseudobulbar paralysis, and progressively deepening coma. Leukocytosis is usually present, sometimes reaching 30,000 cells per cubic millimeter, and the sedimentation rate is elevated. The CSF is often under increased pressure; cells vary in number from a few lymphocytes to a polymorphonuclear pleocytosis of up to 3000 cells per cubic millimeter; red cells may be present in variable numbers; protein content is increased, but glucose values are normal. Many cases terminate fatally in 2 to 4 days but some survive somewhat longer. Patients with a similar clinical picture and who are thought to have the same disease on the basis of brain biopsy examinations have recovered with almost no residual symptoms.

Acute encephalitis due to herpes simplex or other viruses, brain abscess, subdural empyema, and focal embolic encephalomalacia are the important considerations in the differential diagnosis.

The pathologic findings are distinctive. On sectioning the brain, the white matter of one or both hemispheres is seen to be destroyed almost to the point of liquefaction. The involved tissue is pink or yellowish gray and flecked with multiple small hemorrhages. Similar changes are often found in the brainstem and cerebellar peduncles and rarely in the spinal cord. Such lesions are readily visualized in CT scans, particularly the ones in the cerebral hemispheres (Fig. 36-1). On histologic examination one finds widespread necrosis of small blood vessels, necrosis of brain tissue around the vessels with intense cellular infiltration, multiple small hemorrhages, and a violent inflammatory reaction in the meninges. The pathologic picture resembles that of disseminated encephalomyelitis in its perivascular distribution, with the added feature of more widespread necrosis and a tendency of lesions to form large foci in the cerebral hemispheres. The vascular alterations account for the exudation of fibrin into the vessel wall and surrounding tissue.

It is probable that certain patients showing an explosive myelitic illness are suffering from a necrotizing lesion of similar type, but pathologic evidence in support of this view has been difficult to obtain.

The etiology of this condition remains obscure, but the resemblance to other demyelinating diseases should be emphasized. The similarities of the histologic changes to those of disseminated encephalomyelitis, noted above, suggest that the two diseases are related forms of the same fundamental process. The observations of Behan et al., that the lymphocytes of a patient with postinfectious encephalomyelitis and of another with acute necrotizing hemorrhagic encephalitis underwent transformation to lymphoblasts in response to a pure encephalitogenic myelin basic protein, support the view that delayed hypersensitivity mechanisms are operative in both diseases. Also it is noteworthy that

Figure 36-1
Acute necrotizing hemorrhagic leukoencephalitis, mainly bifrontal.

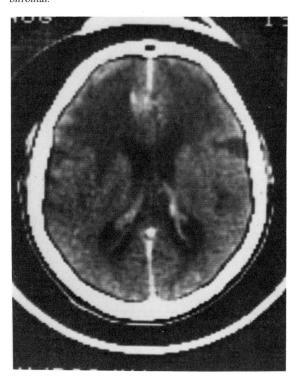

among the small number of patients who have recovered from what appeared to be a typical necrotizing hemorrhagic encephalitis, a few have gone on to develop typical multiple sclerosis. These points of similarity are sufficient to suggest that corticosteroids should be used in the treatment of acute necrotizing hemorrhagic encephalopathy; in several personally observed patients, we have had the impression that they produced a favorable result.

BRAIN PURPURA (PERICAPILLARY ENCEPHALORRHAGIA)

This is another hemorrhagic condition, sometimes confused with acute necrotizing hemorrhagic encephalopathy. The lesions in brain purpura are always small, 0.1 to 2.0 mm in diameter, and are confined to the white matter, particularly the corpus callosum, centrum ovale, and middle cerebellar peduncles. Each lesion is situated around a small blood vessel, usually a capillary. In this paraadventitial area both the myelin and axis cylinders are destroyed, and the lesion is usually though not always hemorrhagic. Fibrin exudation, perivascular and meningeal infiltrates of inflammatory cells, and widespread necrosis of tissue are not observed; in these respects brain purpura differs fundamentally from acute necrotizing hemorrhagic encephalitis. The etiology of brain purpura is quite obscure. It may complicate virus pneumonia and arsenical intoxication, or there may be no associated disease.

REFERENCES

ADAMS RD, KUBIK CS: The morbid anatomy of the demyelinative diseases. *Am J Med* 12:510, 1952.

ADAMS RD, RICHARDSON EP JR: The demyelinative diseases of the human nervous system: A classification; a review of salient neuropathologic findings; comments on recent biochemical studies, in Folch-Pi J (ed): *Chemical Pathology of the Nervous System.* New York, Pergamon, 1961, pp 162–196.

ALTER M et al: The prevalence of multiple sclerosis in Israel among immigrants and native inhabitants. *Arch Neurol* 8:253, 1962.

AUSTREGESILO A: Les neuromyelites aigues et subaigues. *Rev Neurol* 2:543, 1932.

BECK GM: A case of diffuse myelitis associated with optic neuritis. *Brain* 50:687, 1927.

BEEBE GW et al: Studies on the natural history of multiple sclerosis: III. Epidemiologic analyses of the Army experience in World War II. *Neurology* 17:1, 1967.

BEHAN PO et al: Delayed hypersensitivity to encephalitogenic protein in disseminated encephalomyelitis. *Lancet* 2:1009, 1968.

Cohen SR, Herndon RM, McKhann GM: Radioimmuno-assay of myelin basic protein in spinal fluid. *N Engl J Med* 295:1455, 1976.

Coxe WS, Luse SA: Acute hemorrhagic leukoencephalitis. *J Neurosurg* 20:584, 1963.

Dean G: The multiple sclerosis problem. *Sci Am* 233:40, July 1970.

———, Kurtzke JF: On the risk of multiple sclerosis according to age at immigration to South Africa. *Bri Med J* 3:725, 1971.

DeJong RN: Multiple sclerosis: History, definition and general considerations, in Vinken PJ, Bruyn GW (eds): *Handbook of Clinical Neurology*, vol 9. Amsterdam, North-Holland, 1970, chap 3, pp 45-62.

Halliday AM, McDonald WI: Pathophysiology of demyelinating disease. *Br Med Bull* 33:21, 1977.

Jersild C: The HLA system and multiple sclerosis. *Birth Defects* 14:123, 1978.

Johnson KP, Arrigo SC, Nelson BS, Ginsberg A: Agarose electrophoresis of cerebrospinal fluid in multiple sclerosis. *Neurology* 27:273, 1977.

——— et al: Comprehensive viral immunology of multiple sclerosis: Clinical, epidemiological, and CSF studies. *Arch Neurol* 37:537, 610, 616, 1980.

Johnson RT: The possible viral etiology of multiple sclerosis, in Friedlander WJ (ed): *Advances in Neurology*, vol 13. New York, Raven, 1975, pp 1-46.

———: Current knowledge of multiple sclerosis. *South Med J* 71:2, 1978.

Kurland LT: The frequency and geographic distribution of multiple sclerosis as indicated by mortality statistics and morbidity surveys in the United States and Canada. *Am J Hyg* 55:457, 1952.

Kurtzke JF, Beebe GW, Norman JE Jr: Epidemiology of multiple sclerosis in U.S. veterans: I. Race, sex, and geographic distribution. *Neurology* 29:1228, 1979.

Lampert PW: Autoimmune and virus-induced demyelinating diseases. *Am J Pathol* 91:176, 1978.

McAlpine D, Compston MD: Some aspects of the natural history of disseminated sclerosis. *Q J Med* 21:135, 1952.

——— Lumsden CE, Acheson ED: *Multiple Sclerosis: A Reappraisal*. Edinburgh, Churchill-Livingstone, 1972.

McDonald WI, Halliday AM: Diagnosis and classification of multiple sclerosis. *Br Med Bull* 33:4, 1977.

Percy AK et al: Multiple sclerosis in Rochester, Minnesota: A 60-year appraisal. *Arch Neurol* 25:105, 1971.

Portersfield JS (ed): Multiple sclerosis. *Br Med Bull* 33:1977.

Poser CM: Diffuse-disseminated sclerosis in the adult. *J Neuropathol Exp Neurol* 16:61, 1957.

———, van Bogaert L: Natural history and evolution of the concept of Schilder's diffuse sclerosis. *Acta Psychiatr Neurol Scand* 31:285, 1956.

Prineas JW: The etiology and pathogenesis of multiple sclerosis, in Vinken PJ, Bruyn GW (eds): *Handbook of Clinical Neurology*, vol 9. Amsterdam, North-Holland, 1970, chap 6, pp 107-160.

Schapira K, Poskanzer DC, Miller H: Familial and conjugal multiple sclerosis. *Brain* 86:315, 1963.

Schilder P: Zur Kenntniss der sogennanten diffusen Sklerose. *Z Gesamte Neurol Psychiatr* 10:1, 1912.

Shiraki H, Otani S: Clinical and pathological features of rabies postvaccinal encephalomyelitis in man, in Kies MW, Alvord EC Jr (eds): *"Allergic" Encephalomyelitis*. Springfield, Ill, Charles C Thomas, 1959, p 58.

Tourtellotte WW: Cerebrospinal fluid in multiple sclerosis, in Vinken PJ, Bruyn GW (eds): *Handbook of Clinical Neurology*, vol 9. Amsterdam, North-Holland, 1970, chap 11, pp 324-382.

Wilson SAK: Neuromyelitis, in *Neurology*, 2d ed. Baltimore, Williams & Wilkins, 1955, vol 1, pp 233-236.

CHAPTER 37

THE INHERITED METABOLIC DISEASES
OF THE NERVOUS SYSTEM

Advances in biochemistry have led to the discovery of such a large number of metabolic diseases of the nervous system that it taxes the memory even to keep their names in mind. Largely this has resulted from the application by Dent of a paper chromatographic method for the analysis of amino acids in blood and urine. More recently, high-pressure gas-liquid chromatography and mass spectroscopy have continued to reveal previously unknown diseases and the basic biochemistry of old ones.

Through these innovative methodologies, mass screening and prevention are now becoming practicable, and the physician's role is changing as a consequence. No longer must the physician wait until a disease of the nervous system has declared itself by symptoms and signs, by which time the lesion may have become irreversible. Now it is possible to find patients who, though asymptomatic, are at risk, and to introduce dietary and other measures to prevent injury to the nervous system. To assume this responsibility intelligently requires some knowledge of genetics, of biochemical screening methods, and of public health measures.

These metabolic diseases, which numbered more than 100 at the time this chapter was last revised, are heredofamilial, and most of them become manifest in infancy and childhood. Only a few appear as late as adolescence or adult life; many damage the nervous system so severely that survival to adult years is impossible. As a group, these diseases—along with embryologic anomalies (Chap. 43) and birth injuries, epilepsy, disharmonies of development and learning disabilities (Chap. 27)—make up the bulk of the problems with which the pediatric neurologist must contend.

The clinical syndromes by which these metabolic diseases declare themselves vary in accordance with the nature of the biochemical defect and the stage of maturation of the nervous system at which it acts. In phenylketonuria, for example, there is a rather diffuse but specific effect on the cerebral white matter, but only during the period of active myelination. Once the maturational processes are complete, the biochemical abnormality becomes relatively harmless. Even more important is the level of function that has been achieved by the developing nervous system when the disease strikes. A derangement of nervous function in a neonate or infant, when much of the cerebrum is inactive, is much less obvious than one in an older child; and, as the disease evolves, the clinical manifestations are influenced always by the continuing maturation of the untouched elements in the nervous system.

Because of the overriding importance of the age factor and the tendency of certain pathologic processes to appear in particular epochs of life, the authors believe that it is logical to group the inherited metabolic diseases not according to their major syndromes of expression, as we have done in other parts of the book, but in relation to periods of life: the neonatal period; infancy (1 to 12 months); early childhood (1 to 4 years); late childhood, adolescence, and adult life. Only in the latter two age periods will we return to a syndromic ordering of diseases.

THE NEUROLOGY OF NEONATAL METABOLIC DISEASES

A small number of progressive metabolic diseases become manifest in the first few days of life. The importance of these diseases relates not to their frequency (they constitute but a small fraction of diseases that compromise function of the nervous system in the first weeks of life) but to the fact that they must be recognized promptly if the child is to be prevented from dying or from the worse fate of lifelong idiocy. These threats give a new sense of urgency to medical action in pediatric neurology.

The mechanism(s) of the neonatal metabolic diseases, while not fully understood, can be traced in most instances to an inborn enzymatic defect. The cells of all organs are to some extent exposed to the failure of a metabolic pathway, the lack of an essential substrate, or to the accumulation of a harmful metabolite. It is the nervous system, however, that is most consistently affected, perhaps because of its protracted growth and maturation, which extend for years after birth. Although the diseases of this period are genetic, the pattern of heredity is such that neither parent is clinically abnormal, viz., recessive. Often the heterozygous status of the parents cannot be detected. Moreover, the mother's normal metabolism usually protects the fetus in utero; only after birth does the faulty metabolism induced by the abnormal gene begin to exert its deleterious effects on brain function and structure.

Two approaches to the neonatal metabolic disorders are possible—one, to screen every newborn, using a battery of biochemical tests of blood and urine; the other, to undertake in the days following birth a detailed neurologic assessment that will detect the earliest signs of these diseases. Unfortunately the biochemical tests are costly, and not all have been simplified to the point where they can be adapted to a mass screening program; and many of the commonly used clinical tests at this age have yet to be validated as signs of disease.

THE NEUROLOGIC ASSESSMENT OF NEONATAL METABOLIC DISEASE

As was pointed out in Chap. 27, the neonate, in terms of nervous functioning, is essentially a brainstem-spinal preparation. The pallidum and motor and visual cortices are only beginning to be myelinated and their contribution to the totality of neonatal behavior cannot be very great. Neurologic examination, to be informative, must therefore be directed to evaluating diencephalic-midbrain, cerebellar-lower brainstem, and spinal functions. The integrity of these functions in the neonate are most reliably assessed by noting the following:

1. The state of alertness and attention (stimulus responsivity and capacity to make contact), as well as sleep patterns and EEG—diencephalic mechanisms

2. Movements and postures of neck, trunk, and limbs such as reactions of support, extension of neck and trunk, flexion movements and steppage—lower brainstem (reticulospinal), cerebellar, and spinal mechanisms

3. Reflex organization of eye movements—tegmental midbrain and pontine mechanisms

4. Certain reflexive reactions such as startle (evoked by removal of support—Moro reaction), and placing reactions of foot and hand—upper brainstem-spinal mechanisms with cortical facilitation

5. Control of respiration and body temperature; regulation of thirst, fluid balance, and appetite—hypothalamus-brainstem-spinal mechanisms

Derangement of these functions is manifested as an impairment of alertness and arousal, disturbances of ocular movement (oscillations of the eyes, nystagmus, loss of tonic conjugate deviation of the eyes in response to vestibular stimulation, i.e., to rotation of the infant), tremors, clonic jerkings, tonic spasms, opisthotonus, reduced or absent movements of the limbs, irregular or chaotic breathing, hypothermia or poikilothermia, bradycardia, circulatory difficulties, poor color, and seizures.

In most instances of neonatal metabolic disease the pregnancy and delivery have proceeded without mishap. The infant is of a size and weight expected for the duration of pregnancy, and there are no signs of a developmental abnormality. Furthermore, the infant continues to be normal in the first few days of life. The first hint of trouble may be food intolerance, diarrhea, and vomiting. The infant becomes fretful and fails to gain weight and thrive.

The first definite indication of disordered nervous functioning is likely to be the occurrence of seizures. These take the form of unpatterned clonic or tonic contractions of one side of the body, sudden arrest of respiration, turning of the head and eyes to one side, or twitching of the hands and face. They may occur singly or in clusters, and in the latter instance are associated with unresponsiveness, immobility, and arrest of respiration. While seizures are occurring, certain other automatic activities such as sucking, grasping, Moro reaction, and support and steppage are suppressed.

The other clinical manifestations, according to authorities such as Prechtl and Beintema, and Joppich and Schulte, can be subdivided roughly into three groups, each of which constitutes a kind of syndrome: (1) hyperkinetic-hypertonic, (2) apathetic-hypotonic, or (3) hemi- or unilateral syndromes. Prechtl and Beintema, from a study of more than 1500 newborns, found that if any one of the three syndromes is revealed consistently by clinical examination the chances are two out of three that by the seventh year the child will be abnormal neurologically. Other neurologic signs such as facial palsy, grasping, excessive floppiness, and impairment of sucking—while sometimes indicative of serious disease of the nervous system—they find to be less dependable; also, being rare, these signs will identify but few brain-damaged infants. It is not the single neurologic sign but groups of them that are held to be the most reliable indexes of brain abnormality, and the three mentioned above are important even though their anatomic and physiologic bases are little understood.

In our observations of neonatal metabolic disease we have endeavored to determine if particular diseases consistently manifest themselves by one or other of the three syndromes; this we are unable to affirm. In hypocalcemia-hypomagnesemia, the hyperkinetic-hypertonic syndrome prevails, but most of the other diseases tend usually to induce the apathetic-hypotonic state. The hyperactive-hypertonic syndrome, if present at all, represents the initial phase of the illness and carries a less

ominous prognosis. Conversely, the apathetic-hypotonic state represents a more severe and potentially dangerous condition regardless of cause. We have not been confident in the recognition of the hemi- or unilateral syndromes in any of the metabolic diseases. Even more discouraging has been the frequent overlapping of the three syndromes, and seizures may occur in all of them. Clearly what is needed is a new neonatal neurologic semiology utilizing every possible type of stimulus-response test including visual, auditory, and somatosensory evoked potentials; also needed are ways of accurately quantifying more of the natural activities of this age period. Even the *brain death syndrome* in which all brainstem-spinal reflexes are abolished, has not been fully defined in the neonate.

THE NEONATAL METABOLIC DISEASES AND THEIR ESTIMATED FREQUENCY

In Massachusetts a state-sponsored screening program for all newborns has been in operation for more than 15 years. The data on 16 metabolic diseases have been collated by our colleague H. L. Levy and are summarized in Table 37-1. Some of these disorders can be recognized

Table 37-1
Metabolic disorders and their estimated frequency among newborn infants in Massachusetts

Disorders	Total screened	Total detected	Frequency
Phenylketonuria*	981,361	67	1:15,000
Atypical phenylketonuria†	981,361	57	1:17,000
Iminoglycinuria	332,143	34?‡	1:10,000?‡
Cystinuria†	332,143	21	1:16,000
Hartnup disease	332,143	18	1:18,000
Histidinemia	332,143	18	1:18,000
Galactosemia*	550,000	5	1:110,000
Maple syrup urine disease*	842,004	5	1:170,000
Argininosuccinic acidemia*	332,143	5	1:70,000
Cystathioninemia	332,143	3	1:110,000
Homocystinuria*	449,615	3	1:150,000
Hyperglycinemia (nonketotic)*	332,143	2	1:170,000
Propionic acidemia*	332,143	1	1:300,000
Hyperlysinemia†	332,143	1	1:300,000
Hyperornithinemia†	332,143	1	1:300,000
Fanconi syndrome†	332,143	1	1:300,000

*Disorders with definite clinical complications.
†Disorders that may or may not be associated with clinical disease.
‡Number of cases and incidence for iminoglycinuria may be falsely high since carriers for this disorder who have only hyperglycinemia later in life may have iminoglycinuria as young infants.
Source: Levy.

by simple color reactions in the urine; these are listed in Table 37-2.

To this group should be added other inherited hyperammonemic syndromes and pyridoxine dependency, as well as certain nonfamilial metabolic disorders that make their appearance in the neonatal period—hypocalcemia and hypomagnesemia with tetany, hypoglycemia, cretinism, and congenital adrenal hyperplasia.

It is important to note that the three most frequently identified hereditary metabolic diseases—phenylketonuria, hyperphenylalaninemia, and histidinemia—are ones that do not become clinically manifest in the neonatal period. This is fortunate, for it allows time to introduce preventive measures before the first symptoms become manifest. A number of others, which can be recognized either by screening or by early signs, are synopsized below.

Pyridoxine Dependency   This is a rare disease, inherited as an autosomal recessive trait. It is characterized by the early onset of convulsions, sometimes in utero, failure to thrive, hypertonia-hyperkinesia, irritability, tremulous movements ("jittery baby"), exaggerated auditory startle (*hyperacusis*), and later, if untreated, by psychomotor retardation. The specific laboratory abnormality is an increased excretion of xanthurenic acid in response to a tryptophane load. The neuropathology has been studied in only a few cases. In one of our patients, a $13\frac{1}{2}$-year-old boy with mental retardation, pale optic disks, and spastic legs, the brain weight was 350 g below normal. There was a decreased amount of central white matter in the cerebral hemispheres and a depletion of neurons in the thalamic nuclei and cerebellum, with gliosis (Lott et al.). Treatment with 50 to 100 mg vitamin B_6 terminates seizures, and daily doses of 40 mg permit normal development.

Galactosemia   Inheritance of this disorder is autosomal recessive in type. The biochemical abnormality consists of a defect in galactose-1-phosphate uridyl transferase (G-1-PUT), the enzyme that catalyzes the conversion of galatose-1-phosphate into galactose uridine diphosphate. At least seven forms of galactosemia have been described, based on the degree of completeness of the metabolic block. The onset of symptoms is in the first days of life, after ingestion of milk; vomiting and diarrhea are followed by a failure to thrive. Drowsiness, inattention, hypotonia, and diminution in vigor of neonatal automatisms then become evident. The fontanelles may bulge, the liver and spleen become enlarged, the skin yellows in excess of neonatal jaundice, and anemia develops. Cataracts may be present due to galactitol accumulation. Surviving infants show retarded psychomotor development, visual impairment, and residual cirrhosis, sometimes with splenomegaly and ascites. In one such patient, who died at 8 years, the main change in the brain was slight micrencephaly with fibrous gliosis of the white matter and some loss of Purkinje and granule cells in the cerebellum, with gliosis (Crome). The diagnostic laboratory tests are an elevated blood galactose level, low glucose, galactosuria, and deficiency of G-1-PUT in red and white blood cells and in liver cells. The treatment consists essentially of a diet containing milk substitutes.

Table 37-2
Urinary screening tests for metabolic defects

Disease	Ferric chloride	DNPH	Benedict's	Nitroprusside reaction
Phenylketonuria	Green	+	−	−
Maple syrup urine disease	Navy blue	+	−	−
Tyrosinemia	Pale green (transient)	+	±	−
Histidinemia	Green-brown	±	−	−
Propionic acidemia	Purple	+	−	−
Methylmalonic aciduria	Purple	+	−	−
Homocystinuria	−	−	−	+
Cystinuria	−	−	−	+
Galactosemia	−	−	+	−
Fructose intolerance	−	−	+	−

Hyperglycinemia Two forms have been delineated: a ketotic and a nonketotic.

Ketotic hyperglycinemia (propionic acidemia), is an autosomal recessive disease, expressed clinically by episodes of vomiting, lethargy, coma, convulsions, hypertonia, and respiratory difficulty. The onset is in the neonatal or early infantile period and in time psychomotor retardation is evident. Death occurs usually within a few months. Propionic acid, glycine, various forms of fatty acids, and butanone are elevated in the serum. Milk protein and casein hydrolysate induce ketotic attacks.

Ketotic hyperglycinemia can occur with a number of organic acidurias of infancy. The most important of these are methylmalonic acidemia, isovaleric acidemia, and lactic acidemia. Each of these disorders presents in early infancy with profound metabolic acidosis and intermittent lethargy and coma, with early death in about half the patients and developmental retardation in those who survive. Rare subtypes of *methylmalonic acidemia* respond to vitamin B_{12}. In *isovaleric acidemia*, which is characterized by a striking odor of stale perspiration, marked restriction of dietary protein may prevent attacks of ketoacidosis and permit relatively good psychomotor development. Numerous metabolic defects, most commonly of pyruvate decarboxylase and pyruvate dehydrogenase, are responsible for the accumulation of lactic and pyruvic acids. The latter enzymatic defect has also been demonstrated in recurrent cerebellar ataxia and athetosis and in Leigh's disease, which are described further on in this chapter, and in some cases of Friedreich's ataxia (Chap. 42).

In the *nonketotic form* there are high levels of glycine but no acidosis, and the effects on the nervous system are more devastating. In the 30 or more reported cases (the authors have seen several) the neonate is hypotonic and listless and has difficulty breathing, dysconjugate eye movements, and seizures. A few survive to infancy but are extremely retarded and helpless. Spongy degeneration of the brain has been reported, both in this disease and in the ketotic form (Shuman et al.). There is no treatment.

Inherited Hyperammonemic Syndromes These are a series of diseases caused by inborn deficiencies of the enzymes of the Krebs-Henseleit urea cycle and designated as carbamyl phosphate synthetase deficiency (type I hyperammonemia), ornithine carbamyl transferase deficiency (type II hyperammonemia), citrullinemia, argini-

nosuccinic aciduria, and hyperargininemia. Hyperornithemia and hyperlysinemia are closely related disorders. A detailed account of these inherited hyperammonemic syndromes is contained in the reviews by Hsia and by Shih (1978).

The inheritance of each of these disorders is autosomal recessive in type except for type II hyperammonemia, which is an X-linked dominant trait. Their clinical manifestations are a common expression of an accumulation of ammonia or of urea cycle intermediates in the brain, and they differ only in severity, in accordance with the degree of completeness of the enzymatic deficiency and with the age of the affected individual.

In the most severe forms of these disorders, the infants are asymptomatic at birth and for the first few days of life, after which they refuse their feedings, vomit, and rapidly become inactive, lethargic, and lapse into an irreversible coma. Profuse sweating, focal or generalized seizures, rigidity with opisthotonus, and respiratory distress have been observed in the course of the illness.

Hyperammonemia develops after the onset of protein feeding. Diagnosis is established by the finding of hyperammonemia, as high as 1500 μg per 100 ml in types I and II hyperammonemia. The precise biochemical diagnosis requires testing of the blood and urine amino acids or assays for specific enzymes in red cells or liver biopsies. The primary hyperammonemias need to be distinguished from the organic acidurias, including methylmalonic aciduria (see above), in which hyperammonemia can occur as a secondary metabolic abnormality.

In older infants and children, the symptoms are less severe and are compatible with survival. Difficulty with feeding can occur, and attempts to enforce feeding or periods of constipation (which increases ammonia production in the bowel) may be accompanied by bouts of vomiting and screaming. Alternating hypertonia and hypotonia, seizures, and periods of stupor and coma are the other major manifestations. With survival, signs of motor and mental retardation become evident, and the patient is vulnerable to repeated infections. In about half of the patients with argininosuccinic aciduria, there is an excessive dryness and brittleness of the hair (trichorrhexis nodosa).

In all the neonatal hyperammonemic diseases, the liver cell appears inadequate in one or more of its many metabolic functions, but how the enzymatic deficiencies or other disorders of amino acid metabolism affect the brain remains uncertain. It must be assumed that in some of them the saturation of the brain by ammonia impairs the oxidative metabolism of cerebral neurons, and when blood levels increase (from protein ingestion, constipation, etc.), episodic coma or a more chronic impairment of cerebral functions occurs—as it does in cirrhosis of the liver and in portal-systemic encephalopathy. The treatment of acute hyperammonemic syndromes is directed at removal of ammonium (by peritoneal dialysis, exchange transfusions, and administration of amino or keto acids). In more chronic cases treatment is directed at decreasing the ammonium load (by dietary protein restriction, and administration of oral antibiotics, enemas, and lactulose).

Maple Syrup Urine Disease and Variants These conditions are the result of some inborn errors of branched-chain amino acid catabolism. Maple syrup urine disease may be taken as the prototype of the group. The pattern of inheritance is autosomal recessive. Normal at birth, the infant begins to feed poorly toward the end of the first week, followed by the appearance of hypotonicity-apathy, diminished neonatal automatisms, convulsions, severe ketoacidosis, and often coma and death toward the end of the second to the fourth week. Milder forms of the disease present with feeding difficulties that begin somewhat later in the early infantile period, followed by recurrent infections; episodic acidosis and coma; and retarded psychomotor development with clumsiness, ataxia, and Babinski signs. The urine smells like maple syrup and gives a positive 2,4-dinitrophenylhydrazine (DNPH) test.

Other important laboratory findings are elevation of plasma and urine levels of leucine, isoleucine, valine, and keto acids. Secondary accumulation of a derivative of α-hydroxybutyric acid probably accounts for the maple syrup odor. The neuropathologic findings are uncertain; there appears to be a pallor and loss of myelin and gliosis of the cerebral white matter. Treatment by restriction of foods containing branched-chain amino acids (leucine, isoleucine, and valine) allows reasonably normal mental development.

Sulfite Oxidase Deficiency This is an extremely rare disorder of sulfur metabolism, manifested clinically during the neonatal period by seizures, reduced level of responsivity, and spasms with opisthotonus. With survival into infancy episodic confusion and stupor give way to seizures, mental retardation and ataxia. Shih et al. (1977) have identified sulfite, thiosulfite, and S-sulfocysteine in the urine. Cerebral atrophy with loss and destruction of white matter and gray matter (cerebral cortex, basal ganglia, and cerebellar nuclei) have been observed in one postmortem examination. Theoretical therapeutic possibilities, as yet untried, are increasing the intake of molybdenum or lowering dietary intake of sulfur amino acids.

DIAGNOSIS OF NEONATAL METABOLIC DISEASES

An important clue, of course, is provided by a family history of an earlier neonatal disease or of a prior unexplained death in the same sibship or in a male maternal relative.

The history that protein foods are rejected by the infant, or even a history among relatives of dislike of protein or feeding difficulties in infancy, should raise the suspicion of an inherited hyperammonemic disorder. A mass screening program may disclose a biochemical abnormality; this is the optimal state of affairs especially if the information becomes available before symptoms appear.

A number of nonhereditary metabolic diseases must be distinguished from the above. Hypocalcemia is one of the most frequent causes of neonatal seizures; tetany, spasms, and tremulous movements are usually present. This disorder is easily corrected, with excellent prognosis. Symptomatic hypoglycemic reactions are frequent in neonates. Premature and dysmature infants are the most susceptible. With blood sugar levels of less than 30 mg per 100 ml in the mature infant, and less than 20 mg per 100 ml in the premature, there are convulsions, tremulousness, and drowsiness. Maternal toxemia and diabetes mellitus are predisposing factors. Other causes are adrenal insufficiency, galactosemia, and an idiopathic form due to islet cell hyperplasia. The damaging effects of untreated hypoglycemia are well documented in the report of Koivisto and associates. Cretinism and idiopathic hypercalcemia must also be recognized.

The hereditary metabolic diseases must also be distinguished from a number of other catastrophic disorders that occur at or soon after birth, such as asphyxia, perinatal ventricular hemorrhage with the respiratory distress syndrome of hyaline membrane disease, other hypotensive-hypoxic states, erythroblastosis fetalis with kernicterus, neonatal bacterial meningitis, meningoencephalitis (herpes simplex, cytomegalic inclusion disease, listeriosis, rubella, syphilis, and toxoplasmosis), and hemorrhagic disease of the newborn.

THE HEREDITARY METABOLIC DISEASES OF EARLY INFANCY

The hallmark of all the hereditary metabolic diseases is psychosensorimotor regression. However, those that have their onset in the first year of life pose extraordinary problems in neurologic diagnosis. If the onset is in the first postnatal months, before the infant has had time to develop a complex repertoire of behavior, the first signs of disease may take the form of subtle delays in maturation rather than of psychomotor regression. Departures from normalcy include a lack of interest in surroundings, a lack of visual engagement, poor head control, an inability to sit up at the usual time, and poor hand-eye coordination. Of course, embryologic maldevelopment of the brain may have similar effects, and even systemic diseases and other visceral malformations such as cystic fibrosis of the pancreas, renal disease, biliary atresia and congenital heart disease, chronic infection, malnutrition and seizures (with drug therapy) may appear to impede psychomotor development. Diagnosis becomes somewhat easier in the second half of the first year, especially if development in the first half had proceeded normally. Then an observant mother can perceive loss of certain early acquisitions, attesting to the progressive nature of the disease.

The most distinctive members of this category are the so-called lysosomal storage diseases. Here the enzymes necessary for the degradation of specific glycosidic or peptide linkages in the intracytoplasmic lysosomes are genetically deficient, causing the lysosomes to become engorged with material that they would ordinarily degrade, with eventual damage to the cell. The type of enzyme deficiency and accumulated metabolite, as well as the tissue distribution of the undegradable substrate, impart a distinctive biochemical and clinical character to the disease. The concept of lysosomal storage diseases, introduced by Hers in 1965, has excited great interest among neurologists because of the potential for prenatal diagnosis and detection of carriers.

There are now more than 40 "storage" diseases in which the biochemical abnormalities have been determined. They are listed in Table 37-3, which is an updated version of the table which appeared originally in Kolodny's (1976) review. In addition to the sphingolipidoses, which are the lysosomal storage diseases most likely to be encountered in the first year of life, the table includes the storage diseases that are encountered in childhood and adolescence, to be considered later in the chapter.

The inherited metabolic diseases of infancy are listed below, followed by a brief summary of the clinical-pathologic features of each of them:

1. Tay-Sachs disease (G_{M2} gangliosidosis) and variants such as Sandhoff-Jatzkewitz disease

2. Infantile Gaucher's disease

3. Infantile Niemann-Pick disease

4. Infantile G_{M1} generalized gangliosidosis

5. Krabbe's globoid-body leukodystrophy

6. Farber's lipogranulomatosis

7. Pelizaeus-Merzbacher and other sudanophilic leukodystrophies

8. Spongy degeneration (Canavan-Van Bogaert disease)

9. Alexander's disease

10. Alper's disease

11. Leigh's subacute necrotizing encephalomyelopathy

12. Congenital lactic acidosis

13. Zellweger's encephalopathy

14. Lowe's oculorenalcerebral disease

15. Kinky-hair or steely-hair disease

In the following descriptions, which are brief, we have italicized the characteristic clinical signs and the corroborative laboratory tests.

TAY-SACHS DISEASE (G_{M2} GANGLIOSIDOSIS)

This is an autosomal recessive disease, mostly of Jewish children of Eastern European background. Onset is in the first weeks and months of life and almost always by the fourth month. The first manifestations are an abnormal *startle to acoustic stimuli*, listlessness, and irritability, followed by a *delay in psychomotor development* or regression (4 to 6 months), with loss of ability to roll over and sit. At first *axial hypotonia* is prominent, followed by *spasticity* and other corticospinal tract signs, visual failure, and *cherry-red spots* in the retinas in more than 90 percent of patients. In the second year, there are tonic-clonic or minor motor seizures and an increasing size of the head (diastasis of sutures) with relatively normal ventricles; in the third year, dementia, decerebration, blindness, and cachexia; death occurs at 3 to 5 years. The EEG becomes abnormal in the early stages (paroxysmal slow waves with multiple spikes). Occasionally one observes basophilic granules in leukocytes and vacuoles in lymphocytes. The basic enzymatic abnormality, a *deficiency of hexosaminidase A*, can be detected in white blood cells and in cultured fibroblasts (the latter is diagnostic in amniotic fluid and in serum and tears of heterozygotes).

Table 37-3
Lysosomal storage diseases

	Enzyme deficiency	Accumulated metabolite
Sphingolipidoses:		
G_{M1} gangliosidosis	G_{M1} ganglioside β-galactosidase	G_{M1} ganglioside, galactose-containing oligosaccharides
Type 1—infantile, generalized		
Type 2—juvenile		
G_{M2} gangliosidosis:		
Tay-Sachs disease	Hexosaminidase A	G_{M2} ganglioside
Sandhoff-Jatzkewitz disease	Hexosaminidases A and B	G_{M2} ganglioside, globoside
Variant	Activator factor	G_{M2} ganglioside
Sulfatidoses:		
Metachromatic leukodystrophy	Aryl sulfatase A	Sulfatide
Multiple sulfatase deficiency	Aryl sulfatases A, B, C; steroid sulfatase; iduronate sulfatase, heparan N-sulfatase.	Sulfatide, steroid sulfate, heparan sulfate, dermatan sulfate
Krabbe's disease	Galactocerebroside β-galactosidase	Galactocerebroside
Fabry's disease	α-Galactosidase	Ceramide trihexoside
Gaucher's disease:		
Infantile form	Total β-glucosidase	Glucocerebroside
Adult form	Membrane-bound β-glucosidase	Glucocerebroside
Niemann-Pick disease	Sphingomyelinase	Sphingomyelin
Farber's disease	Ceramidase	Ceramide
Mucopolysaccharidoses:		
Hurler-Scheie syndrome	α-Iduronidase	Dermatan sulfate, heparan sulfate
Hunter's syndrome	Iduronate sulfatase	Dermatan sulfate, heparan sulfate
Sanfilippo syndrome:		
Type A	Heparan N-sulfatase	Heparan sulfate
Type B	α-N-Acetylglucosaminidase	Heparan sulfate
Type C	Acetyl CoA: α-glucosaminide N-acetyltransferase	Heparan sulfate
Morquio syndrome	N-Acetylhexosamine-6-sulfate sulfatase	Keratan sulfate, chondroitin-6-sulfate
Maroteaux-Lamy syndrome	Aryl sulfatase B	Dermatan sulfate
β-Glucuronidase deficiency	β-Glucuronidase	Dermatan sulfate, heparan sulfate
Mucolipidoses:		
Type 1	α-N-Acetylneuraminidase	Sialyloligosaccharides
Type 2 (I-cell disease)	Cellular deficiency of many lysosomal enzymes; increased levels of same enzymes extracellularly	Mucopolysaccharide, glycolipid
Type 3 (pseudo-Hurler polydystrophy)		
Type 4	Unknown	Mucopolysaccharide, ganglioside
Other diseases of complex carbohydrates:		
Fucosidosis	α-Fucosidase	Fucose-containing sphingolipids and glycoprotein fragments
Mannosidosis	α-Mannosidase	Mannose-containing oligosaccharides
Aspartylglycosaminuria	Aspartylglycosamine amide hydrolase	Aspartyl-2-deoxy-2-acetamidoglycosylamine
Other lysosomal storage diseases:		
Wolman's disease	Acid lipase	Cholesterol esters, triglycerides
Acid phosphatase deficiency	Lysosomal acid phosphatase	Phosphate esters
Neuronal ceroid lipofuscinosis	Unknown	Ceroid-lipofuscin-like pigments

Source: Modified from Kolodny, 1976.

The brain is large, sometimes twice the normal weight. In addition there is loss of neurons and gliosis, and remaining nerve cells throughout the central nervous system are distended with glycolipid. Under the electron microscope the particles of stored material appear as membranous cytoplasmic bodies. Retinal ganglion cells distended with the same material, together with fat-filled histiocytes, cause the whitish gray rings around the fovea, where there are no nerve cells (allowing the vascular choroid to appear as a red spot).

In Sandhoff's disease, which affects non-Jewish infants, there is a deficiency of both hexosaminidase A and B, moderate hepatosplenomegaly, and coarse granulations in bone marrow histiocytes. The clinical and pathologic picture is the same as in Tay-Sachs disease except for the signs of visceral lipid storage.

INFANTILE GAUCHER'S DISEASE

This is an autosomal recessive disease, without ethnic predominance. The onset is usually before 6 months and frequently before 3 months, with a more rapid course than Tay-Sachs disease (most patients with infantile Gaucher's disease are dead by 1 year and 90 percent by 2 years). There is rapid loss of head control, of ability to roll over and sit, and of purposeful movements—along with apathy, irritability, frequent crying, and difficulty in sucking and swallowing. Progression is slower in some cases with acquisition of single words by the first year, bilateral corticospinal signs (Babinski signs and hyperactive reflexes), persistent *retroflexion of the neck*, and *strabismus*. Laryngeal stridor and trismus, reduction in reaction to stimuli, smallness of the head, rare seizures, normal optic fundi, *enlarged spleen* and slightly enlarged liver, poor nutrition, skin and scleral pigmentation, and sometimes lymphadenopathy complete the clinical picture.

The important laboratory findings are an *increase in serum acid phosphatase and characteristic histiocytes (Gaucher cells) in marrow* smears and liver biopsies. A *deficiency of glucocerebrosidase* in leukocytes and hepatocytes is diagnostic; glucocerebroside accumulates in the involved tissues. The characteristic pathologic features are the Gaucher cells (20 to 60 μm with wrinkled appearance of the cytoplasm and eccentricity of the nucleus) in marrow, lungs, and other viscera; a few of these cells can also be found in the brain, where the main abnormality is a loss of nerve cells, particularly in the bulbar nuclei, and a reactive gliosis.

INFANTILE NIEMANN-PICK DISEASE

This also is an autosomal recessive disease. Two-thirds of the reported cases have been of Ashkenazi Jewish parentage. The onset of symptoms is between 3 and 9 months of age, frequently with marked *enlargement of liver, spleen, and lymph nodes;* rarely there is jaundice and ascites. *Cerebral deterioration* is definite by the end of the first year, often earlier; the usual manifestations are loss of spontaneous movements, disinterest in the environment, axial hypotonia with bilateral corticospinal signs, *blindness* and *amaurotic nystagmus,* and *a macular red spot* (in about one-quarter of the patients). Seizures occur relatively late. There is no acoustic myoclonus, and head size is normal or slightly reduced. Loss of tendon reflexes and slowed nerve conduction have been reported, but are rare. Protuberant eyes, mild hypertelorism, pigmentation of oral mucosa and dysplasia of dental enamel have also been reported in rare instances. Most patients succumb to intercurrent infection by the end of the second year. *Vacuolated histiocytes ("foam cells") in the bone marrow and vacuolated blood lymphocytes* are the important laboratory findings; a *deficiency of sphingomyelinase* in leukocytes, cultured fibroblasts, and hepatocytes is diagnostic. Neurons are decreased in number and many of the remaining ones are pale, ballooned, and granular. The most prominent changes may be seen in the midbrain, spinal cord, and cerebellum. The white matter is little affected. The retinal cell changes are similar to those in the brain. The foamy histiocytes (Niemann-Pick cells) that fill the viscera contain sphingomyelin and cholesterol; the distended nerve cells contain mainly sphingomyelin.

INFANTILE, GENERALIZED (TYPE I) G_{M1} GANGLIOSIDOSIS (FAMILIAL NEUROVISCERAL LIPIDOSIS, PSEUDO-HURLER'S DISEASE)

This is probably an autosomal recessive disease, and is without ethnic predominance. The infants appear abnormal at birth, with *dysmorphic facial features* like those of the mucopolysaccharidoses (depressed and wide nasal bridge, frontal bossing, hypertelorism, epicanthi, puffy eyelids, long upper lip, gingival and alveolar hypertrophy, macroglossia, low-set ears). Other indications of the disease are an early onset of impaired awareness and receptivity; reduced responsivity in the first days or weeks of life; *no psychomotor development* after 3 to 6 months; hypotonia and later hypertonia with lively tendon reflexes and Babinski signs. Seizures are frequent. The head size is variable (microcephaly more than macrocephaly). *Loss of vision, coarse nystagmus and strabismus, macular cherry-red spots* in half the cases, flexion pseudocontractures of elbows and knees, kyphoscoliosis, and *enlarged liver and sometimes spleen* are the other important clinical findings. Radiographic abnormalities include subperiosteal bone formation, midshaft widening, demineralization, and hypoplasia and beaking of the thoracolumbar vertebras. Vacuoles are seen in 10 to 80 percent of blood lymphocytes, and foam cells in the urinary sediment. A *deficiency of* G_{MI} *ganglioside β-galactosidase* and accumulation of G_{MI} ganglioside in the brain and viscera are the specific biochemical abnormalities. Neurons and glial cells throughout the CNS are swollen with G_{MI} ganglioside. In addition, the epithelial cells of the renal glomeruli, the histiocytes of the spleen, and the liver cells contain a modified keratan sulfate and a galactose-containing oligosaccharide. The changes in the bone are like those seen in the Hurler form of mucopolysaccharidosis. The disease should be suspected in a child who has the facial features of mucopolysaccharidosis and severe neurologic abnormalities.

GLOBOID CELL LEUKODYSTROPHY (KRABBE'S DISEASE)

This is an autosomal recessive disease without ethnic predilection. The onset is usually before the sixth month and often before the third month (10 percent after 1 year). *Generalized rigidity*, loss of head control, diminished alertness, frequent vomiting, hyperirritability and bouts of inexplicable crying, and spasms induced by stimulation are early manifestations. With increasing muscular tone *opisthotonic recurvation* of neck and trunk develop. Later signs are adduction of legs, flexion of arms, clenching of fists, Babinski signs, and hyperactive reflexes. In other cases tendon reflexes are depressed or lost. Blindness and optic atrophy supervene. Convulsions occur but are difficult to distinguish from tonic spasms. The head size is normal or rarely slightly increased. In the last stage, which may occur one to several months after the onset, the child is blind and usually deaf, opisthotonic, irritable, and cachectic. Most patients are dead by the end of the first year, and survival beyond two years is unusual.

The EEG shows nonspecific slowing without spikes, and the *CSF protein is usually elevated* (70 to 450 mg per 100 ml).

Clinical signs of neuropathy are difficult to detect, except for decrease or loss of tendon reflexes, but *EMG evidence of denervation and decrease in motor nerve conduction velocity* are frequent findings.

The deficient enzyme in Krabbe's disease is *galactocerebroside β-galactosidase* (cerebrosidase), resulting in the accumulation of galactocerebroside, particularly in the cerebral white matter. Gross examination of the brain discloses a marked reduction in the cerebral white matter, which feels firm and rubbery. Microscopically, there are widespread myelin degeneration and gliosis in the cerebrum, brainstem, spinal cord, and nerves; the characteristic globoid cells (abnormal, large histiocytes containing accumulated metabolite) and Schwann cells with tubular or crystalloid inclusions are present in electron-microscopic preparations.

LIPOGRANULOMATOSIS (FARBER'S DISEASE)

This is a very rare disorder that is probably genetic, affecting both sexes and without any particular racial predilection. The onset is in the first weeks of life, with *hoarse cry* (fixation of laryngeal cartilage), respiratory distress, and sensitivity of the joints—followed by the characteristic *periarticular* and *subcutaneous swellings* and *progressive arthropathy* leading to ankylosis. Usually there is severe psychomotor retardation, but a few patients have appeared neurologically normal. Inanition and recurrent infections lead to death in the first 2 years. The diagnostic abnormality is a *deficiency of ceramidase* leading to accumulation of ceramide. There is widespread lipid storage in neurons and in granulomas in the skin, and accumulation of PAS-positive macrophages in periarticular and visceral tissues.

SUDANOPHILIC LEUKODYSTROPHIES AND PELIZAEUS-MERZBACHER DISEASE

These are a heterogeneous group of disorders, which have in common a defective myelination of the cerebrum, brainstem, cerebellum, spinal cord, and peripheral nerves. Morphologic peculiarities and genetic features separate a certain group called *Pelizaeus-Merzbacher disease*; other types are artificially delineated, and as a result a relatively meaningless terminology has been introduced.

Pelizaeus-Merzbacher Disease This is predominantly an X-linked disease of childhood and adolescence which includes other closely related pathologic entities with different modes of inheritance. Onset may be in the first months of life or later in childhood. The first signs are *abnormal movements of the eyes* (rapid, irregular, often asymmetrical pendular nystagmus) and intermittent shaking movements of the head (like spasmus nutans), followed by *ataxia*; intention tremor; choreiform or athetotic movements of arms; and slow psychomotor development with failure to sit, stand, and walk. Seizures occur occasionally. In cases developing later, pendular nystagmus, choreoathetosis, corticospinal signs, dysarthria, cerebellar ataxia, and mental deterioration are the major manifestations. Patients may survive to the second and third decade. One group of cases resembles Cockayne's syndrome with photosensitivity of skin, dwarfism, cerebellar ataxia, corticospinal signs, cataracts, retinitis pigmentosa, and deafness. Pathologically, islands of preserved myelin give a tigroid pattern of degenerated and intact myelin in the cerebrum.

Unclassified Sporadic and Familial Sudanophilic Leukodystrophies There are two types of disorder, one early and the other of late onset, affecting both sexes. In the former, onset is before 3 months with survival of less than 2 years; in the latter type, onset is from 3 to 7 years, and the course is chronic. *Psychomotor regression; spastic paralysis; incoordination; blindness* and optic atrophy; seizures (rare); *severe microcephaly;* and absence of skeletal, visceral, and hematologic evidence of the metabolic abnormality are the main features. No characteristic laboratory abnormalities are known. Widespread diffuse degeneration of medullated fibers with phagocytosis of sudanophilic-degeneration products of myelin and gliosis are the major pathologic changes.

SPONGY DEGENERATION OF INFANCY (CANAVAN-VAN BOGAERT-BERTRAND DISEASE)

This is an autosomal recessive disease. Of 48 affected families reported to date, 28 were Jewish. Onset is early, often recognizable in the first 3 months of life. There is either a lack of or rapid *regression of psychomotor development, loss of sight and optic atrophy,* lethargy, difficulty in sucking, irritability, reduced motor activity, hypotonia followed by spasticity of limbs with corticospinal signs, and *enlarged head* (due to macrocephaly). There are no visceral or skeletal abnormalities. Seizures occur in some cases. An interesting but unexplored aspect of the disease is the occurrence of blond hair and light complexion in affected members, in contrast to the darker hair and complexion of their normal siblings (Banker and Victor). The CSF is usually normal, but the protein is slightly elevated in some cases; there are no diagnostic biochemical abnormalities. The characteristic pathologic changes are an increase in brain volume (and weight), spongy degeneration in the deep layers of the cerebral cortex and subcortical white mat-

ter, widespread loss of myelin involving the convolutional more than the central white matter, loss of Purkinje cells, and hyperplasia of Alzheimer type II astrocytes throughout the cerebral cortex and basal ganglia. Adachi et al. have demonstrated an abnormal accumulation of fluid in astrocytes and between splitting myelin lamellae, and have suggested that the loss of myelin is secondary to these changes.

The disease has to be distinguished clinically from G_{M2} gangliosidosis, Alexander's disease, Krabbe's disease, and nonprogressive megalencephalopathy, and pathologically from a variety of disorders that are characterized by vacuolation of nervous tissue.

ALEXANDER'S DISEASE

The classification of this rare disease is uncertain. A familial incidence has not been reported, and no metabolic fault has been defined. It shares certain features with the leukodystrophies and gray matter diseases, both clinically and pathologically. The onset is in infancy with *a failure to thrive, psychomotor retardation, and seizures.* An early and progressive *macrocephaly* has been a consistent feature. Pathologically, there are severe destructive changes in the cerebral white matter, most intense in the frontal lobes. Eosinophilic hyaline bodies, most prominent just below the pia and around blood vessels, are seen throughout the cerebral cortex, brainstem, and spinal cord. These have been identified as *Rosenthal fibers* and probably represent glial degradation products.

ALPER'S DISEASE

This disease, known also as progressive infantile poliodystrophy (Christensen), probably has a number of different etiologies, including hypoxia and hypoglycemia. Nevertheless, a familial form (probably autosomal recessive) is known, with a certain uniformity of clinical features—*seizures* and *diffuse myoclonic jerks* from early infancy, followed by incoordination of movements; *progressive spasticity* of limb, trunk, and cranial muscles; blindness and optic atrophy; growth retardation and increasing microcephaly; and finally, virtual decortication. Some instances of terminal jaundice and fatty degeneration or cirrhosis of the liver have been described, but these may have been the effects of anticonvulsant drugs. There are no diagnostic laboratory tests. Pathologic investigations reveal a marked atrophy of the cerebral convolutions and cerebellar cortex with loss of nerve cells and fibrous gliosis. Hypoxic and hypotensive encephalopathies need always to be considered in the differential diagnosis.

SUBACUTE NECROTIZING
ENCEPHALOMYELOPATHY (SNE, LEIGH'S DISEASE)

This is a familial disorder of autosomal recessive type with a wide range of clinical manifestations. The onset, in more than half the cases, is in the first year of life, mostly before the sixth month. Loss of head control and other recent motor acquisitions, hypotonia, poor sucking, anorexia and vomiting, irritability and continuous crying, generalized seizures and myoclonic jerks constitute the usual clinical picture. If the onset is in the second year, there are difficulties in walking, ataxia, dysarthria, intellectual regression, tonic spasms, *characteristic respiratory disorders* (episodic hyperventilation, periods of apnea, gasping, sobbing without cry), *external ophthalmoplegia and abnormal eye movements* (irregular, rolling, pendular nystagmus), *paralysis of deglutition,* and abnormal movements of the limbs (jerky, choreiform, ataxic). Peripheral nerves are involved in some cases (areflexia, weakness, atrophy, and slowed conduction velocity). In some children the course is quite protracted, with exacerbation of neurologic symptoms in association with nonspecific infections. CSF is usually normal, but protein may be elevated.

The pathologic changes take the form of bilaterally symmetric foci of necrosis and spongiform degeneration, vascular proliferation, and gliosis in the thalami, midbrain, pons, medulla, and spinal cord. Demyelinative lesions are present in the peripheral nerves. In their distribution and histologic appearance the CNS lesions of SNE resemble those of Wernicke's disease, except that the former tend to be more extensive—sometimes involving the striatum—and they tend to spare the mammillary bodies.

Leigh's disease is characterized by a number of biochemical abnormalities. Pincus and his colleagues (1972) have described a substance in the patient's urine, blood, and CSF that inhibits thiamine pyrophosphate—*ATP phosphoryl transferase,* an enzyme that catalyzes the formation of thiamine triphosphate (TTP) from thiamine pyrophosphate. However, this abnormality has not been found consistently. The administration of massive doses of thiamine chloride has reportedly caused a dramatic improvement in the neurologic status of some patients, but the effect has not been sustained.

Pyruvate metabolism appears to be altered in this disease, as indicated by the finding of alaninuria, pyruvic acidemia, and lactic acidemia in many cases. The original suggestion by Hommes et al., that the enzymatic deficiency in SNE is one of pyruvate carboxylase, has not been substantiated. From the observations of De-Vivo and his colleagues, it appears that the biochemical abnormality in SNE is a defect in the activation mechanism of the pyruvate dehydrogenase complex of enzymes. Their findings suggest that dichloroacetate may be useful in the treatment of this disease.

CONGENITAL LACTIC ACIDOSIS

This is a very rare disease of the neonatal period or early infancy, of unproven genetic etiology. The symptoms have consisted of *psychomotor regression* and *episodic hyperventilation, hypotonia* and *convulsions,* with intervening periods of normalcy, and of *choreoathetosis* in a few of the reported cases. Death usually occurs before the third year. The important laboratory findings are *acidosis with high lactate levels* and hyperalininemia. The defect is probably in the pyruvate dehydrogenase complex of enzymes, which function in the oxidative decarboxylation of pyruvate to acetyl CoA. The few cases that have been examined postmortem have shown necrosis and cavitation of the globus pallidus and cerebral white matter. Possibly this disorder is a variant of Leigh's disease. It needs to be distinguished from the several diseases of infancy that are complicated by lactic acidosis.

ZELLWEGER'S CEREBROHEPATORENAL DISEASE

This disease, also very rare, is inherited as an autosomal recessive trait. It has its onset in the neonatal period or early infancy, and leads to death usually within a few months. Motor inactivity and hypotonia, *peculiar facies* (high forehead, shallow orbits, hypertelorism, highly arched palate, abnormal helices of ears, retrognathia), poor visual fixation, *multifocal seizures,* swallowing difficulties, flexion fixation of the limbs, *cataracts,* abnormal retinal pigmentation, *hepatomegaly,* and hepatic dysfunction are the usual manifestations. There are no distinctive biochemical abnormalities. Pathologically, there are dysgenesis of the cerebral cortex and degeneration of white matter, as well as a number of visceral abnormalities—cortical renal cysts, hepatic fibrosis, intrahepatic biliary dysgenesis, agenesis of the thymus, and iron storage in the reticuloendothelial system.

LOWE'S OCULOCEREBRORENAL DISEASE

Here the mode of inheritance is X-linked recessive. The clinical abnormalities comprise *bilateral cataracts* and *glaucoma,* large eyes with megalocornea and buphthalmos, corneal opacities and blindness, pendular nystagmus, hypotonia and absent or depressed tendon reflexes, corticospinal signs without paralysis, slow movements of the hands, high-pitched cry, occasional seizures, and *psychomotor regression.* Later the frontal bones become prominent and the eyes sunken. Death is often from *renal failure.* Laboratory findings include demineralization of bones and typical rachitic deformities, anemia, metabolic acidosis, and generalized aminoaciduria. The neuropathologic changes are nonspecific; inconstant atrophy and poor myelination have been described in the brain, and tubular abnormalities in the kidneys. Differential diagnosis is from Zellweger's disease.

KINKY-HAIR OR STEELY-HAIR DISEASE (MENKES' DISEASE)

This is a rare disorder, inherited as a sex-linked recessive trait. Poor feeding and failure to gain weight, instability of temperature (mainly *hypothermia*) and *seizures* become apparent in early infancy. The hair is normal at birth, but the secondary growth is lusterless and depigmented; strands of hair break easily and feel like steel wool, and under the microscope they appear twisted (*pili torti*). Radiologic examination shows *metaphyseal spurring,* mainly of the femora, and subperiosteal calcifications of the shafts. Arteriography discloses *tortuosity and elongation of the cerebral and systemic arteries,* and occlusion of some of them. There is no discernible neurologic development, and rarely does the child survive beyond the second year.

The manifestations of this disease are attributable to a profound deficiency of copper. The *basic defect is in the absorption of copper from the gastrointestinal tract* (Danks et al.). Further, since copper fails to cross the placenta, a severe reduction of serum and hepatic copper is evident from birth. In this sense, the abnormality of copper metabolism is the opposite of that in Wilson's disease. Parenteral administration of cupric salts restores the serum and hepatic copper, but its effect on the clinical symptoms remains to be determined.

DIAGNOSIS OF INHERITED METABOLIC DISEASES OF INFANCY

It will be recognized, from the foregoing synopses, that many of the neurologic manifestations of the inherited metabolic diseases of infancy are nonspecific and are common to most or all of the diseases in this group. In general, in the early stages of all these diseases there is a loss of postural tone and a paucity of movement, without paralysis or loss of reflexes; later there is spasticity with hyperreflexia and Babinski signs. Equally nonspecific are features such as irritability and prolonged crying; poor feeding, difficulty in swallowing, inanition and retarded growth; failure of regarding, fixation of gaze and following (often misinterpreted as blindness); and tonic spasms, clonic jerks, and focal and generalized seizures.

In general terms, the differentiation of the inherited metabolic diseases of infancy rests upon four types of data: (1) a few highly characteristic neurologic and ophthalmic signs; (2) the presence of an enlarged liver and spleen; (3) special dysmorphic features of the face; and (4) the results of certain relatively simple laboratory tests, such as radiographs of the thoracolumbar spine, hips, and long bones, smears of peripheral blood and bone marrow, CSF examination, and certain biochemical estimations. Attention to these particular clinical and laboratory features, tabulated below, permits the correct diagnosis in most cases.

Neurologic signs that are more or less specific to certain metabolic diseases include the following:

1. Acousticomotor obligatory startle: Tay-Sachs disease

2. Abolished tendon reflexes with definite Babinski signs: Krabbe's globoid-body leukodystrophy, occasionally Leigh's disease, and (beyond infancy) metachromatic leukodystrophy

3. Peculiar eye movements, pendular nystagmus, head rolling: Pelizaeus-Merzbacher disease, Leigh's disease; later, hyperbilirubinemia and Lesch-Nyhan's hyperuricemia (see further on)

4. Marked rigidity, opisthotonus, and tonic spasms: Krabbe's, infantile Gaucher's, or Alper's disease

5. Intractable seizures and generalized or multifocal myoclonus: Alper's disease

6. Intermittent hyperventilation: Leigh's disease and congenital lactic acidosis (in nonprogressive familial agenesis of vermis)

Ocular abnormalities of specific diagnostic value include the following:

1. Rapid pendular nystagmus: Pelizaeus-Merzbacher disease, rarely Krabbe's leukodystrophy

2. Macular cherry-red spots: Tay-Sachs disease and Sandhoff variant, some cases of infantile Niemann-Pick disease, and rarely lipofuscinosis

3. Corneal opacification: Lowe's disease, infantile G_{MI} gangliosidosis; later, the mucopolysaccharidoses

4. Cataracts: galactosemia, Lowe's disease, Zellweger's disease (also congenital rubella)

Other medical findings of specific diagnostic value:

1. Dysmorphic facies: generalized G_{MI} gangliosidosis, Lowe's disease, Zellweger's disease, some early cases of mucopolysaccharidosis and mucolipidosis

2. Enlarged liver and spleen: infantile Gaucher's disease and Niemann-Pick disease; one type of hyperammonemia; Sandhoff's disease; later, the mucopolysaccharidoses and mucolipidoses.

3. Enlarging head without hydrocephalus (macrocephaly): spongy degeneration of Canavan-van Bogaert, some cases of Tay-Sachs disease, Alexander's disease

4. Beaking of vertebral bodies in x-rays: G_{MI} gangliosidosis (and mucopolysaccharidoses, fucosidosis, mannosidosis, and the mucolipidoses)

5. Multiple arthropathies and raucous dysphonia: Farber's disease

6. Storage granules and vacuolated lymphocytes: Niemann-Pick disease, generalized G_{MI} gangliosidosis

7. Abnormal histiocytes in marrow smears: Gaucher cells, foamy histiocytes in Niemann-Pick disease, generalized G_{MI} gangliosidosis and closely related diseases, Farber's disease

8. Colorless, friable hair: Menkes' disease

INHERITED METABOLIC DISEASES OF LATE INFANCY AND EARLY CHILDHOOD

Included here are the diseases that become manifest between the ages of 1 and 4 years. Diagnosis is less difficult than in the neonate and young infant. Ascertainment of a morbid process in the nervous system is reliably revealed by a loss of ability to walk and to speak, which usually parallel a regression in other high-level (quasi-intellectual) functions. Embryologic anomalies, prenatal diseases, and birth injuries can be excluded with certainty if psychomotor development was normal in the first year or two. Diseases characterized by seizures and myoclonus may prove more difficult to interpret, for the seizures may occur at any age from a variety of antecedent or immediate neurologic causes, and, if frequent, may cause a significant impairment of psychomotor function. The effects of anticonvulsant medications may add to the impairment of diencephalocortical function.

Unfortunately, most of the slowly advancing metabolic diseases of the second year may be so subtle in their effects that the physician cannot be sure for a time whether a regression of intellectual functions or the first appearance of mental retardation is taking place. To distinguish the two is more difficult if the parents have been unobservant. Repeated examination and testing will usually settle the matter. Suspicion of a progressive encephalopathy is heightened by the presence of certain ocular, visceral, and skeletal abnormalities, as described below.

The following are inherited metabolic diseases which occur most frequently in this age period:

1. Many of the milder disorders of amino acid metabolism

2. Metachromatic leukodystrophy

3. Late infantile G_{MI} gangliosidosis

4. Late infantile Gaucher's disease and Niemann-Pick disease

5. Neuroaxonal dystrophy

6. The mucopolysaccharidoses

7. Mucolipidoses

8. Fucosidosis

9. Mannosidoses

10. Aspartylglycosaminuria

11. Bielschowsky-Jansky "ceroid" lipofuscinosis

12. Cockayne's disease

THE AMINOACIDURIAS

As was pointed out in the first part of this chapter, only a few of the many aminoacidurias declare their existence in the neonatal and early infantile period of life. More often the only clinical manifestation is a simple lag in psychomotor development which, if mild, does not become evident until the second and third years, or later. Like other members of this class of biochemical disorders, the aminoacidurias do not derange growth, development, and maturation in utero or interfere with parturition. No physical sign betrays their presence in early life. The only possibility of detection is by screening all newborns. The relative frequency of these diseases is indicated in Table 37-1, and the practical tests for their identification are summarized in Table 37-2.

The aminoacidurias of the late infantile and early

childhood period—phenylketonuria (PKU) and Hartnup disease—will be described here because of their clinical importance, and because they exemplify different types of biochemical defect. Reference will also be made to other aminoacidurias, described in the first part of this chapter, which, like Hartnup disease, cause intermittent ataxia. Only passing reference will be made to the other aminoacidurias which are exceedingly rare or have only an uncertain effect upon the nervous system. A detailed account of these disorders can be found in the monograph of Stanbury et al. and the review of Swaiman et al. (see references).

The Phenylketonurias   These are the most frequent of all the aminoacidurias, and interestingly were the first to be discovered, by Følling in 1934. One must refer to the phenylketonurias in the plural, for there are (1) the usual type and a mild variant thereof, in which phenylalanine tolerance is reduced and mental retardation invariable if the disease is not treated early in life, and (2) other types, in which there is hyperalininemia without phenylketonuria and without effect on the nervous system. Phenylketonuria is transmitted as an autosomal recessive trait. All infants born of untreated phenylketonuric mothers are mentally retarded from birth because they are exposed to the metabolic abnormality in utero.

In the classic form of PKU, the lag in *psychomotor development* can usually be recognized in the latter part of the first year; by 5 to 6 years, when IQ can be estimated, it is usually under 20, occasionally 20 to 50, and only exceptionally above 50. *Hyperactivity*, aggressivity, clumsy gait, fine tremor of the hands, poor coordination, odd posturings, *repetitious digital mannerisms*, rhythmias, and slight corticospinal tract signs are the usual clinical manifestations. Athetosis, dystonia, and frank cerebellar ataxia occur, but are relatively rare. Seizures are common in the severely retarded. The majority of patients are blue-eyed and fair in color. A musty body odor (due to phenylacetic acid excretion) is commonly noted. Two-thirds are slightly microcephalic. The fundi are normal, and there is no visceral enlargement or skeletal abnormality.

The finding of *high levels of serum phenylalanine* (higher than 20 mg per 100 ml) and of *phenylpyruvic acid in the urine* is diagnostic of PKU. The addition of 3 to 5 drops of 10 percent ferric chloride to 1 ml of urine yields an emerald green color, which reaches a peak intensity in 3 to 4 min and fades in 20 to 40 min. In contrast, the green-brown color in the urine of patients with

histidinemia is permanent. In maple syrup urine disease, addition of ferric chloride gives a navy-blue color; ketones or salicylates in the urine yield a purple color.

The fundamental biochemical abnormality is a deficiency of the hepatic enzyme phenylalanine hydroxylase; the failure of conversion of phenylalanine to tyrosine results in the excretion of phenylpyruvic acid by affected individuals. Pathologic examination shows poor staining of myelin in the cerebral hemispheres; reduction in size and dendritic arborization of cortical neurons is demonstrable in some cases.

Low phenylalanine diets have been used in the treatment of PKU, and may improve intellectual development if instituted in infancy or early childhood. Once the neurologic picture unfolds, diet has no effect on the mental status, but may improve behavior. Prolonged dietary treatment has many untoward effects, and should be supervised by physicians experienced in its use. Dietary treatment is contraindicated in children with the enzyme defect (hyperalininemia), but without phenylketonuria.

The late form of maple syrup urine disease, histidinemia, and hydroxyprolinemia evolve in much the same fashion as PKU, and raise similar problems in diagnosis and therapy.

Hartnup Disease   This disease, named after the family in which it was first observed, is probably transmitted by an autosomal recessive gene. The onset of symptoms is in late infancy or early childhood. The clinical features consist of an *intermittent red, scaly rash over the face, neck, hands, and legs*, resembling that of pellagra; episodic personality disorder in the form of *emotional lability*, uncontrolled temper, and confusional-hallucinatory psychosis; *episodic cerebellar ataxia* (unsteady gait, intention tremor, and dysarthria); and occasionally spasticity, vertigo, nystagmus, ptosis, and diplopia. Episodes of disease are triggered by exposure to sunlight, emotional stress, and sulfonamide drugs. Attacks last for about 2 weeks, followed by variable periods of relative normalcy. The frequency of attacks diminishes with maturation.

The basic metabolic fault is a *transport error of neutral amino acids, with excretion of greatly increased amounts of these amino acids in the urine* and feces; the *excretion of large amounts of indicans,* mainly indoxyl sulfate, particularly after oral L-tryptophan loading; and an abnormally high excretion of nonhydroxylated indole metabolites. The pathologic basis of the disease is undetermined. Differential diagnosis includes a large number of intermittent and progressive cerebellar ataxias of childhood, described below.

Treatment consists of avoidance of sunlight and of

sulfonamide drugs. Because of the similarities between pellagra and Hartnup disease, the usual practice is to give nicotinic acid, 25 mg daily, but the value of this measure has not been established.

Other Intermittent Metabolic Ataxias In addition to Hartnup disease, a number of other metabolic diseases give rise to episodic ataxias *of early childhood.* These are (1) mild forms of maple syrup urine disease and the congenital hyperammonemias (type II hyperammonemia, citrullinemia, argininosuccinic aciduria, hyperornithinemia), which have been described in an earlier part of the chapter; (2) Leigh's necrotizing encephalomyelopathy and hyperalininemia, also described earlier; and (3) hyperalininemia and hyperpyruvic acidemia (Lonsdale et al., Blass et al.).

In all these conditions the ataxia is highly variable from time to time, and it may follow a burst of seizures (as in argininosuccinic aciduria). The seizures are treated always with anticonvulsant drugs, which may at first be held responsible for the ataxia. In time, however, it becomes apparent that the ataxia lasts a week or two, and bears no relationship to the medicine. Indeed, seizures and ataxia are both due to the common biochemical abnormality. Between attacks, in all the intermittent ataxias, the patient's movements are relatively normal, but most of the affected children are slow in learning and remain backward mentally to a varying degree.

PROGRESSIVE CEREBELLAR ATAXIAS OF EARLY CHILDHOOD

The problems in diagnosis of the *persistent early-childhood ataxias* are first, to make certain that ataxia exists; and second, to differentiate cerebellar ataxia from the sensory ataxia of peripheral nerve disease. Since cerebellar ataxia is more a disorder of voluntary than of postural movements, the ataxia is usually not detected until intentional (projected) movements become part of the child's repertoire of motor activity. As indicated in Chap. 27, the earliest signs become manifest in the arms when the infant reaches for an object and brings it to the mouth, or transfers it from hand to hand. A jerky, wavering, tremulous movement then appears; in sitting, a titubation of the head and a tremor of the trunk may be apparent. Once walking begins, apart from the usual clumsiness of the toddler, there is the same incoordination of movement. Sensory ataxia is always difficult to distinguish, but is rare at this age and nearly always accompanied by weakness and absence of tendon reflexes. By the fourth or fifth year, when sensory testing becomes possible, the presence or absence of a proprioceptive disturbance can be demonstrated.

The group of persistent and progressive cerebellar ataxias is heterogeneous and of varied etiology, and some of them merge with Friedreich's ataxia, Lévy-Roussy syndrome, and other adolescent-adult hereditary ataxias. These disorders are discussed in the chapter on degenerative diseases since neither their cause nor pathogenesis is completely known. There are many other childhood ataxias that probably belong in the category of degenerative disease—some in which cerebellar ataxia is the most prominent abnormality, and some in which other neurologic abnormalities are more prominent. To describe each one in detail would be inappropriate in a book on principles of neurology, and they will only be tabulated here. A more complete list of these disorders and appropriate references to each of them will be found in Ford's monograph. The following are noteworthy:

1. A disequilibrium and dyssynergia syndrome of Hagberg and Janner: early-life onset of relatively pure cerebellar ataxia, with psychomotor retardation.

2. Cerebellar ataxia with diplegia, hypotonia, and mental retardation (also called *Foerster's atonic diplegia*): this is either a fetal disease or birth injury, and the neuropathology is uncertain.

3. Agenesis of the cerebellum: early cerebellar ataxia (with or without mental retardation) and episodic hyperventilation (Norman's family with granule-cell degeneration falls in this category).

4. Cerebellar ataxia with cataracts and oligophrenia: onset from childhood to as late as adult years (Marinesco-Sjögren disease).

5. Cerebellar ataxia and retinal degeneration.

6. Cerebellar ataxia with cataracts and ophthalmoplegia, or with cataracts and mental as well as physical retardation.

7. Familial cerebellar ataxia with mydriasis.

8. Familial cerebellar ataxia with deafness and blindness, and a similar combination called retino-cochleodentate degeneration, referring to loss of neurons in these three structures.

9. Familial cerebellar ataxia with choreoathetosis, corticospinal tract signs, and mental and motor retardation (Gökay and Tükel).

In none of the above-mentioned syndromes has a biochemical abnormality been established, so their metabolic nature can only be inferred. The persistent cerebellar ataxias of childhood in which a metabolic fault has been demonstrated are (1) Refsum's disease, (2) abetalipoproteinemia (Bassen-Kornzweig syndrome), (3) ataxia-telangiectasia, and (4) possibly Friedreich's ataxia (Chap. 42). Refsum's disease is discussed fully on page 912. The Bassen-Kornzweig syndrome more often has its onset in late than in early childhood, and is more appropriately described in the following section of this chapter.

Ataxia-Telangiectasia This is a relatively frequent childhood ataxia, inherited as an autosomal recessive trait. The onset of the disease coincides, more or less, with the acquisition of walking, which is awkward and unsteady. Later, by the age of 4 to 5 years, the limbs become ataxic, and choreoathetosis, grimacing, and dysarthric speech are added. The eye movements become jerky, and there is also apraxia for voluntary gaze (patient turns the head and not the eyes). By the age of 9 to 10 years some intellectual decline appears, and signs of mild polyneuropathy are evident. The characteristic telangiectatic lesions appear at 3 to 5 years of age or later, and are most apparent in the outer parts of the bulbar conjunctivae, over the ears, on exposed parts of the neck, on the bridge of the nose and cheeks in a butterfly pattern, and in the flexor creases of the forearms. The disease is progressive, and death occurs usually in the second decade from intercurrent bronchopulmonary infection or neoplasia (usually lymphoma, less often glioma).

The significant abnormalities in the CNS are severe degeneration in the cerebellar cortex; loss of myelinated fibers in the posterior columns, spinocerebellar tracts, and peripheral nerves; degenerative changes in the posterior roots and cells of the sympathetic ganglia; and loss of anterior horn cells at all levels of the spinal cord. In a few cases, vascular abnormalities, like the mucocutaneous ones, have been found scattered diffusely in the white matter of the brain and spinal cord. Also, there may be a loss of pigmented cells in the substantia nigra and locus ceruleus, and cytoplasmic inclusions (Lewy bodies) in remaining cells (Agamanolis and Greenstein).

An absence or decrease in immunoglobulin (IgA) has been found in practically every patient. This deficiency, shown by McFarlin and his associates to be due to decreased synthesis, is associated with hypoplasia of the thymus, failure of delayed hypersensitivity reactions, lymphopenia, and slow response to the formation of circulating antibodies. Probably this immunodeficient state accounts for the striking susceptibility of these patients to recurrent pulmonary infections and bronchiectasis.

METACHROMATIC LEUKODYSTROPHY

This is one of the sphingolipid storage diseases (Table 35-3). The basic abnormality is the absence of the enzyme aryl sulfatase A, a deficiency of which prevents the conversion of sulfatide to the cerebroside and results in an accumulation of the former. The disease is transmitted as an autosomal recessive trait, and usually becomes manifest between the first and fourth years of life (variants have their onset in late childhood and even in adult life). It is characterized clinically by *progressive impairment of motor function* in combination with *mental regression*. Usually the tendon reflexes are at first brisk, but later, as peripheral nerves become involved, the *reflexes are decreased and lost*. Instead, there may be hypotonia and areflexia from the beginning, or spasticity throughout the illness with hyporeflexia and slowed conduction velocities. Signs of mental regression may be apparent from the onset or appear after the motor disorder has become established. Later there is impairment of vision, sometimes with squint and nystagmus; intention tremor in the arms and dysarthria; dysphagia and drooling; and optic atrophy (one-third of patients), sometimes with grayish degeneration around the macula. Seizures are rare. Head size is usually normal, but rarely there is macrocephaly. Progression to a bedridden quadriplegic state without speech or comprehension occurs over a 1- to 3-year period, somewhat more slowly in late-onset types.

There is widespread degeneration of myelinated fibers in the cerebrum, cerebellum, spinal cord, and peripheral nerves. The presence of metachromatic granules in glial cells and engorged macrophages is characteristic, and enables the diagnosis to be made from a biopsy of the peripheral nerves (the stored material, sulfatide, stains brown-orange rather than purple with aniline dyes). Sulfatides are also PAS-positive in frozen sections.

The diagnostic laboratory findings are an elevated CSF protein (75 to 250 mg per 100 ml) and a marked *decrease or absence of aryl sulfatase A* in the urine; methods are available also for detecting this abnormality in white blood cells, in serum, and in cultured fibroblasts. Assaying the aryl sulfatase A activity in cultured fibroblasts and amniotic fluid cells permits the identification of carriers and prenatal diagnosis of the disease.

The differential diagnosis is from neuroaxonal dystrophy (see below), early cases of Déjérine-Sottas polyneuropathy, late-onset Krabbe's disease, and childhood forms of Gaucher's disease and Niemann-Pick disease.

NEUROAXONAL DYSTROPHY (DEGENERATION)

This is a rare disease transmitted as an autosomal recessive trait. The onset is usually in the second year of life (rarely after third or fourth year), with *progressive difficulty in walking*, weakness, and diminished or *absent tendon reflexes*. Later there are corticospinal and pseudobulbar signs, with hyperactive reflexes and Babinski signs; loss of sight with optic atrophy; and *diminished sensitivity to pain* over limbs and trunk. *Mental deterioration* coincides with motor impairment. Effective communicative speech is never achieved; head circumference is normal or slightly reduced; seizures are infrequent. Death occurs in 3 to 8 years, in a decorticate state. CSF is normal; nerve conduction velocities and EMG may betray the presence of anterior horn cell and peripheral nerve disease. There are no biochemical or blood cell abnormalities.

Pathologic examination reveals eosinophilic spheroids of swollen axoplasm in the posterior columns and nuclei of Goll and Burdach and in Clarke's column of cells, substantia nigra, subthalamic nuclei, and central nuclei of brainstem and cerebral cortex, and increased iron-containing pigment in the basal ganglia (like Hallervorden-Spatz disease). The differential diagnosis is mainly from metachromatic leukodystrophy.

LATE INFANTILE AND EARLY CHILDHOOD GAUCHER'S DISEASE AND NIEMANN-PICK DISEASE

Although Gaucher's disease usually develops in early infancy, some cases may begin in childhood. The onset is between 5 and 8 years and the course progressive over 3 to 5 years. The clinical picture is one of *mental deterioration, ataxia,* and *spastic weakness* of the limbs, with normality of vision; another group (northern Sweden) has shown progressive mental deterioration starting at 5 to 6 years, with rigidity of the limbs, grimacing, trismus, poor abduction of the eyes, and jerky eye movements. Diagnosis is established by the finding of *splenomegaly,* Gaucher cells, glucocerebroside storage, and deficient activity of glucocerebrosidase. Adult Gaucher's disease is only rarely accompanied by neurologic abnormalities. (Note: Gaucher cells are not entirely specific; similar cells have been observed in chronic granulocytic leukemia and at least one other ill-defined metabolic storage disease.)

Late infantile or childhood Niemann-Pick disease causes *mental retardation,* seizures, *dysarthria,* and *paralysis of vertical eye movements;* a special syndrome called *juvenile dystonic lipidosis* features extrapyramidal symptoms and paralysis of vertical eye movements. The syndrome of "the sea-blue histiocyte" (liver, spleen, and bone marrow contain histiocytes with sea-blue granules) in which there is retardation in mental and motor development, grayish macular degeneration, and, in one instance, posterior column and pyramidal degeneration, may be another variant. In the latter, several types of glycolipids were found in the liver and spleen, and the urinary level of mucopolysaccharides was increased. Sphingomyelin is increased in the viscera in Niemann-Pick disease.

LATE INFANTILE-CHILDHOOD G_{MI} GANGLIOSIDOSIS

In so-called type 2, or "juvenile," G_{MI} gangliosidosis the onset is between 12 and 24 months, with survival for 3 to 10 years. The first sign is usually *difficulty in walking* (poor gait, frequent falls), followed by awkwardness of arm movements, disappearance of speech, severe *mental regression,* gradual development of *spastic quadriparesis* and pseudobulbar palsy (dysarthria, dysphagia, drooling), and seizures. Retinal changes are variable—usually they are absent, but macular red spots may be seen at the age of 10 to 12 years; vision is usually retained, but squints (comitant) are common. There is a facial dysmorphism which resembles that of Hurler's disease, and the liver and spleen are enlarged. Important laboratory findings are hypoplasia of thoracolumbar vertebral bodies, mild hypoplasia of the acetabula, and the presence in the marrow of histiocytes with clear vacuoles or wrinkled cytoplasm. Leukocytes and cultured skin fibroblasts show a *deficiency* or absence *of β-galactosidase* activity. G_{MI} ganglioside accumulates in the cerebral neurons.

BIELSCHOWSKY-JANSKY DISEASE

Designated by these names is a rare form of lipid storage disease which is inherited as an autosomal recessive trait. The onset of symptoms is between 2 and 4 years, after normal or slightly retarded earlier development, with survival to 4 to 8 years of age. In some cases the onset is even later (see below). The first neurologic manifestations are usually *seizures* (petit mal or grand mal) *and myoclonic jerks* evoked by proprioceptive and other sensory stimuli, including voluntary movement and emotional excitement. *Incoordination,* tremor, ataxia, and spastic weakness with lively tendon reflexes and Babinski signs, *deterioration of mental faculties,* and dysarthria proceed to dementia and eventually to mutism. In patients with relatively late onset, dementia is the cardinal manifestation. Visual failure may occur early in some cases because of *retinal degeneration* and pigmentation (degeneration of rods and cones), but in others vision is normal. The electroretinogram is isoelectric if vision is affected. Abnormal inclusions (translucent vacuoles) are seen in 10 to 30 percent of circulating lymphocytes, and azurophilic granules occur in neutrophils; EEG spikes are induced by photic stimuli. In early-onset cases there may be microcephaly.

Pathologic examination shows neuronal loss in the cerebral and cerebellar cortices (granule and Purkinje cells), and curvilinear storage particles in the neurons, with some properties of lipofuscin. Inclusions are also observed in cutaneous nerve twigs and endothelial cells, which permits diagnosis during life (electron microscopy of skin or conjunctival biopsies). In the differential diagnosis, one needs to consider late infantile G_{M1} gangliosidosis, idiopathic epilepsy, Alper's disease and Batten-Spielmeyer-Vogt disease (see further on).

MUCOPOLYSACCHARIDOSES

This is a group of diseases in which a lipid storage process in neurons and a deposit of polysaccharides in connective tissues are combined. As a consequence there is a conjunction of neurologic and skeletal abnormalities that are virtually unique. The nervous system may also be involved secondarily as a result of skeletal deformities and thickening and hyperplasia of connective tissue at the base of the brain, leading to obliteration of the subarachnoid space and obstructive hydrocephalus. Depending on the degree of visceral-skeletal and neurologic changes, at least seven different subtypes are recognized (see Table 37-3).

Hurler's Disease (MPS I, MPS IH) This, the classic form, is inherited as an autosomal recessive trait. The onset is toward the end of the first year. *Mental retardation* is severe, and *skeletal abnormalities* are prominent (dwarfism; gargoyle facies; large head with synostosis of longitudinal suture; kyphosis; broad hands with short, stubby fingers; flexion contractures at knees and elbows). Conductive deafness and corticospinal signs are

usually present. Protuberent abdomen, hernias, *enlarged liver and spleen,* valvular heart disease, chronic rhinitis, respiratory infections, and *corneal opacities* are the common medical findings. The biochemical abnormalities consist of the accumulation of *dermatan* and *heparan sulfate* in the tissues and their *excretion in the urine,* due probably to *absence of activity* of α-L-*iduronidase.* Also, there is an increase in the ganglioside content in the brains of these patients.

Hunter's Disease (MPS II) Unlike the Hurler and other types, Hunter's disease is transmitted as an X-linked trait. The clinical syndromes are alike, except that Hunter's disease is milder: mental retardation is less severe than in the Hurler type, deafness is less common, and *corneal clouding is usually absent.* Probably there are two forms of the syndrome—a more severe form in which the patients do not survive beyond the midteens, and a less severe form, with survival to middle age and with relatively normal intelligence. Excessive amounts of dermatan and heparan sulfate are excreted in the urine. The basic abnormality is a *deficiency of iduronate sulfatase activity.*

Sanfilippo's Disease (MPS III) This form is inherited as an autosomal recessive trait. The onset is between 2 and 3 years of age, with progressive intellectual deterioration. The patients are of short stature, but in other respects the physical changes are fewer and less severe than in the Hunter and Hurler syndromes. Three types of Sanfilippo's disease, designated A, B, and C, are distinguished on the basis of different enzymatic defects (see Table 37-3); patients of all three types excrete excessive amounts of heparan sulfate in the urine.

Morquio Syndrome (MPS IV) This form of the disease is characterized by marked *dwarfism* and *osteoporosis.* Skeletal deformity may cause compression of the spinal cord and medulla in some cases. Also, because of hypoplasia of the odontoid process, there may be atlantoaxial dislocation. The dura around the cervical cord and inferior surface of the cerebellum may be thickened. Intelligence is affected only slightly or not at all. *Corneal opacities may be present.* The mode of inheritance is autosomal recessive. Patients excrete large amounts of keratan sulfate and chondroitin-6-sulfate in the urine; the *enzymatic deficiency* is one of N-acetylhexosamine-6-sulfate sulfatase.

Scheie's Disease (MPS V, MPS IS) This form of the disease is also inherited as an autosomal recessive trait. It differs from the Hurler type in that the patients are of normal intelligence and height. Some have a carpal tunnel syndrome. *Corneal clouding* is the main abnormality. Other skeletal and visceral abnormalities are the same as in Hurler's disease, as are the pathologic biochemical defects. There is no plausible explanation for the phenotypic differences between the Hurler and Scheie forms.

Maroteaux-Lamy Syndrome (MPS VI) This syndrome also is inherited as an autosomal recessive trait. There are severe skeletal deformities, but intelligence is normal. Hepatosplenomegaly is often present. Large amounts of dermatan sulfate are excreted in the urine, as a result of an aryl sulfatase B deficiency.

β-Glucuronidase Deficiency (MPS VII) This is a rare and more recently described type of mucopolysaccharidosis. The clinical features still have to be sharply delineated. Short stature, progressive thoracolumbar gibbus, hepatosplenomegaly, and the bony changes of dysostosis multiplex (as in the Hurler syndrome) are the main clinical features. There is excessive excretion of dermatan and heparan sulfate, the result of a deficiency of β-glucuronidase.

MUCOLIPIDOSES AND OTHER DISEASES OF COMPLEX CARBOHYDRATES

In recent years several new diseases have been described, in which there is abnormal accumulation of mucopolysaccharides, sphingolipids, and glycolipids in visceral, mesenchymal, and neural tissues. Patients with these diseases manifest many of the clinical features of Hurler's disease, but in contrast to the mucopolysaccharidoses, normal amounts of mucopolysaccharides are excreted in the urine. G_{M1} gangliosidosis, described above, is frequently classified with the mucolipidoses. The other members of this category are briefly described below.

Mucolipidoses At least three and possibly four closely related forms have been described. In *mucolipidosis I (lipomucopolysaccharidosis)* the morphologic features are those of gargoylism, with slowly progressive mental retardation. Cherry-red spots in the maculae, corneal opacities, and ataxia have been noted in some patients. Vacuolation of lymphocytes, marrow cells, hepatocytes and Kupfer cells in the liver, and metachromatic changes in the sural nerve have been described.

In *mucolipidosis II ("I-cell" disease)*, the most common of the four forms, there is an early onset of psychomotor retardation, which is severe by the second year. *Abnormal facies and periosteal thickening* (like that of G_{M1} gangliosidosis and Hurler disease) are evident in the first postnatal months. *Gingival hyperplasia* is prominent, and the *liver* and *spleen are enlarged;* but corneal opacities and deafness are not found. Death occurs by the third to eighth year, of heart failure.

There is vacuolation of lymphocytes, Kupfer cells, and cells of the renal glomeruli. Bone-marrow cells are finely vacuolated and contain refractile cytoplasmic granules (hence the term *inclusion-cell,* or *I-cell, disease*). A deficiency of several lysosomal enzymes required for the catabolism of mucopolysaccharides, glycolipids, and glycoproteins has been described.

In mucolipidosis III (pseudo-Hurler polydystrophy) the biochemical abnormalities are like those of I-cell disease, but there are clinical differences. In the former, symptoms do not begin until after 2 years of age and are relatively mild. Retardation of growth, fine corneal opacities, and valvular heart disease are the major manifestations.

In recent years, yet another variant, so-called mucolipidosis IV, has been described (see Tellez-Nagel et al.). Clouding of the corneas is noticed soon after birth, and profound retardation is evident by the age of 1. Skeletal deformities, enlargement of liver and spleen, seizures or other neurologic abnormalities are notably lacking. Ultrastructural examination of conjunctival and skin fibroblasts has demonstrated lysosomal inclusions of material similar to lipids and mucopolysaccharides, which remain to be characterized.

Mannosidosis This is another rare hereditary disorder with poorly differentiated symptomatology. The onset is in the first 2 years, with *Hurler-like facial* and *skeletal deformities, mental retardation* and slight motor disability. Corticospinal signs, loss of hearing, *gingival hyperplasia,* and spokelike opacities of the lens (but no corneal clouding) may be present. The liver and spleen are enlarged in some cases. Radiographs show beaking of the vertebral bodies and poor trabeculation of long bones. Vacuolated lymphocytes and granulated leukocytes are characteristic. The urinary mucopolysaccharides are normal. *Mannosiduria is diagnostic,* caused by a defect in α-mannosidase. Mannose-containing oligosaccharides accumulate in nerve cells, spleen, liver, and leucocytes (Kistler et al.).

Fucosidosis This also is a rare disorder with neurologic deterioration beginning at 12 to 15 months, progressing to spastic quadriplegia, decerebrate rigidity, absence of mental activity, and death within 4 to 6 years. *Hepato-*

megaly, splenomegaly, enlarged salivary glands, thick skin, excessive sweating, normal or typical gargoyle facies, *beaking of the vertebral bodies,* and vacuolated lymphocytes have been described. A variant of this disease has been described with slower progression and survival into late childhood and adolescence, coarse facial features, skeletal deformities, and the dermatologic changes of Fabry's disease (angiokeratoma corporis diffusum).

Aspartylglycosaminuria   This disease is characterized by the early onset of psychomotor regression; delayed, inadequate speech; severe behavioral abnormalities (*bouts of hyperactivity* mixed with apathy and hypoactivity or psychotic manifestations); *progressive dementia*; clumsy movements; corticospinal signs; rarely corneal clouding; retinal abnormalities and cataracts; coarse facies, low bridge of nose, thick lips, epicanthi, thickening of skin; enlarged liver; and hernias in some. Radiographs show minimal *beaking of the vertebral bodies*, and vacuolated lymphocytes are seen in the blood.

Autosomal recessive inheritance is probably the basis of this entire group of diseases. Diagnostic methods applicable to amniotic fluid and cells are being developed so that prenatal diagnosis will be possible, prompted by the occurrence of the disease in an earlier child. Neurons are vacuolated rather than stuffed with granules, much like the lymphocytes and liver cells. The specific biochemical abnormalities, as far as they are known, are indicated in Table 37-3.

COCKAYNE'S SYNDROME

This disorder is probably inherited as an autosomal recessive trait. The onset is in late infancy after apparently normal early development. The main clinical findings are evident *stunting of growth* by the second and third years; *photosensitivity of the skin*; microcephaly; *retinitis pigmentosa, cataracts,* blindness and pendular nystagmus; nerve deafness; *delayed psychomotor* and speech development; *spastic weakness* and *ataxia of limbs* and gait; occasionally athetosis; amyotrophy with abolished reflexes and slowed nerve conduction velocities; wizened face, sunken eyes, prominent nose, prognathism, anhydrosis, and poor lacrimation (resembling progeria and bird-headed dwarf). Some cases show calcification of the basal ganglia. The CSF is normal, and there are no diagnostic biochemical findings.

Pathologic examination shows a small brain, striatocerebellar calcifications, leukodystrophy like that of Pelizaeus-Merzbacher disease, and a severe cerebellar cortical atrophy. The pathogenesis is unknown. The variability in clinical and pathologic manifestations of reported cases suggests that not all of them are representative of the same disease.

OTHER DISEASES

Krabbe's globoid-body leukodystrophy and *Leigh's* necrotizing encephalomyelopathy may begin in late infancy or early childhood. They have been described in the preceding section of this chapter. Familial striatocerebellar calcification (Fahr's disease) and Lesch-Nyhan disease may also become manifest in this age period, but usually they have a later onset and are therefore described with the diseases of later childhood, in the following section.

DIAGNOSIS

The metabolic disorders of late infancy and early childhood present many of the same diagnostic problems in diagnosis as those in early infancy. Some symptoms—simple psychomotor regression, unsteady gait, seizures, progressive quadriplegia—are common to most of the diseases in this group and are therefore of little specific diagnostic value. On the other hand, certain neurologic, skeletal, dermal, ophthalmic, and laboratory findings, or groups of findings, are highly distinctive and often diagnostic. These signs are listed below:

1. Evidence of involvement of peripheral nerves (weakness, hypotonia, areflexia, sensory loss, slowed conduction velocities) in conjunction with lesions of the central nervous system—metachromatic leukodystrophy, Krabbe's leukodystrophy, neuroaxonal dystrophy, and Leigh's disease (rare)
2. Ophthalmic signs
   a. Corneal clouding—several of the mucopolysaccharidoses (Hurler, Scheie, Morquio, Maroteaux-Lamy), mucolipidoses, aspartylglycosaminuria (rare)
   b. Cherry-red macular spot—G_{M2} gangliosidosis, G_{M1} gangliosidosis (rare), lipomucopolysaccharidosis, occasionally Niemann-Pick disease
   c. Retinal degeneration with pigmentary deposits—Bielschowsky-Jansky lipid storage disease, G_{M2} gangliosidosis, syndrome of sea-blue histiocytes
   d. Optic atrophy and blindness—metachromatic leukodystrophy, neuroaxonal dystrophy, Behr's disease (page 827)
   e. Cataracts—Marinesco-Sjögren syndrome, Fabry's disease, mannosidosis
   f. Telangiectasia and optic apraxia—ataxia telangiectasia
   g. Impairment of vertical eye movements—late infantile

Niemann-Pick disease, juvenile dystonic lipidosis, sea-blue histiocyte syndrome

   h. Jerky eye movements, limited abduction—late infantile Gaucher disease

3. Extrapyramidal signs—late-onset Niemann-Pick disease (rigidity, abnormal postures), juvenile dystonic lipidosis (dystonia, choreoathetosis), ataxia telangiectasia (athetosis), Sanfilippo mucopolysaccharidosis

4. Facial dysmorphism—Hurler, Scheie, Morquio, and Maroteaux-Lamy forms of mucopolysaccharidosis, aspartylglycosaminuria, mucolipidoses, G_{M1} gangliosidosis, mannosidosis, fucosidosis (some cases)

5. Dwarfism and spine deformities, arthropathies—Hurler and Morquio mucopolysaccharidoses, Cockayne's syndrome

6. Enlarged liver and spleen—Niemann-Pick disease, Gaucher disease, all mucopolysaccharidoses, fucosidosis, mucolipidoses, G_{M1} gangliosidosis

7. Alterations of skin—photosensitivity (Cockayne's syndrome and one form of porphyria); papular nevi (Fabry's disease); telangiectasia of ears, conjunctiva, chest (ataxia telangiectasia); ichthyosis (Sjögren-Larsen disease)

8. Beaked thoracolumbar vertebras—all mucopolysaccharidoses, mucolipidoses, mannosidosis, fucosidosis; aspartylglycosaminuria

9. Deafness—mucopolysaccharidoses, Cockayne's syndrome

10. Hypertrophied gums—mucolipidoses, mannosidosis

11. Vacuolated lymphocytes—all mucopolysaccharidoses, mucolipidoses, mannosidosis, fucosidosis

12. Granules in neutrophils—all mucopolysaccharidoses, mucolipidoses, mannosidosis, fucosidosis

INHERITED METABOLIC ENCEPHALOPATHIES OF LATE CHILDHOOD AND ADOLESCENCE

Unavoidably one must refer here to certain inherited metabolic diseases, already described, that permit survival to late childhood and adolescence and even to adult life. But there are others that only become manifest in this age period, after a normal early childhood. There is a tendency for them to be less severe and less rapidly progressive, an attribute shared by many diseases with a dominant mode of inheritance. Nonetheless, there are diseases, such as the Wilson-Westphal-Strümpell hepatocerebral degeneration, in which the onset of neurologic symptoms is always after the tenth year and even after the thirtieth year of life in a rare instance, and the mode of inheritance is recessive in type. However, in the latter instance, manifestations of the disease have existed since early childhood in the form of a ceruloplasmin deficiency with early cirrhosis and splenomegaly; only the neurologic disorder is of late onset. This brings us to another principle—that the pathogenesis of the cerebral lesion may involve a factor(s) once removed from the basic abnormality, here cirrhosis of the liver.

The diseases in this category are of more particular interest to neurologists than the preceding ones, for they evince familiar neurologic abnormalities such as epilepsy, polymyoclonia, dementia, cerebellar ataxia, choreoathetosis, dystonia, tremor, spastic-ataxic paraparesis, blindness, deafness, and stroke. These manifestations appear much the same in late childhood and adolescence as they do in adult life, and the neurologist whose experience has been mainly with adult patients feels quite comfortable with them.

Diseases in this age period have a diversity of manifestations, yet each disease has certain characteristic patterns of neurologic expression, as though the pathogenetic mechanism were acting selectively on particular systems of neurons. Such affinities between the disease process and certain anatomic structures raise questions of *pathoclisis*, i.e., specific vulnerability of certain neuron systems to certain morbid agents. Stated in another way, for each disease there is a common and stereotyped clinical syndrome and a small number of variants; conversely, certain other symptoms and syndromes are rarely observed with a given disease. At the same time, however, it is clear that more than one disease may cause the same syndrome.

In deference to these principles, the diseases in this section are grouped according to their common mode of clinical expression, as follows:

1. The progressive cerebellar ataxias of childhood and adolescence

2. The parkinsonian or extrapyramidal motor syndrome

3. The syndrome of dystonia and generalized athetosis

4. Familial polymyoclonias

5. The syndrome of bilateral hemiplegia, cerebral blindness and deafness, and other manifestations of focal cerebral disorder

6. Strokes in association with inherited metabolic diseases

7. Metabolic polyneuropathies

8. Personality changes and behavioral disturbances as manifestations of inherited metabolic diseases

It is of advantage to memorize these groupings, for knowledge of them facilitates clinical diagnosis.

Variants seen personally by the authors will be mentioned in the descriptions of the diseases themselves. One word of caution—it is a mistake to assume that the diseases in the aforementioned categories affect one and only one particular part of the nervous system, or to assume that they are exclusively neurologic. Once the biochemical abnormality is discovered, it is usually found to implicate cells of certain other organs and tissues; whether or not the effects of such involvement become symptomatic is often a quantitative matter.

THE PROGRESSIVE CEREBELLAR ATAXIAS OF CHILDHOOD AND ADOLESCENCE

It has already been pointed out that there is a large group of diseases, some with (but most without) a known metabolic basis, in which an acute, episodic, or chronic disorder of coordination begins early in life. Apparently the anatomic peculiarities of the cerebellar cortex render it especially susceptible to a number of morbid processes. The acute forms are essentially nonmetabolic and are observed in postinfectious encephalomyelitis, in postconvulsive, postmeningitic and posthyperthermic states, and with drug intoxication. The ataxias of hereditary metabolic disease are episodic (see above) or chronic. Most of these begin in infancy and childhood. In the later age periods the number of ataxias of proven metabolic type diminishes markedly, and those that begin in adult life are rare. Friedreich's ataxia and its variants are the most frequent of these, but although hereditary there is only presumptive evidence of a metabolic defect (Chap. 42). Of the other cerebellar ataxias of late childhood and adolescence only the Bassen-Kornzweig acanthocytosis falls in the category of a truly metabolic disease—and one could perhaps add Refsum's disease and ataxia telangiectasia. Refsum's disease is so clearly a polyneuropathy (cerebellar features only in exceptional cases) that it is presented in Chap. 45. Ataxia telangiectasia is encountered in later childhood, but the ataxia may begin in the second year of life, so that it has been described in the preceding section with the ataxias of early childhood.

Bassen-Kornzweig Acanthocytosis (Abetalipoproteinemia) The delineation of this disease excited great interest, for it promised to be a breakthrough into a hitherto obscure group of "degenerative" disorders. In the authors' experience, however, it is an extremely rare disease. Not more than two dozen cases are on record, and

several reports are based on the study of the same case. Further, the resemblance to Friedreich's ataxia is not so close that an experienced clinician would be likely to confuse the two.

The inheritance of this disease is autosomal recessive in type. At the onset, between 6 and 12 years (range 2 to 17 years) the initial symptoms have been *weakness of the limbs with areflexia* and an *ataxia of sensory (tabetic) type*, to which a cerebellar component is added later. *Steatorrhea* (raising suspicion of celiac disease) often precedes the weak, unsteady gait. Later, vision may fail because of *retinal degeneration* (similar to retinitis pigmentosa), which is present in more than 50 percent of cases. Kyphoscoliosis and pes cavus in association with sensory loss, ataxia, and Babinski signs are other elements in the clinical picture. Cranial muscles may also be weak. The neurologic disorder is relatively slowly progressive—by the second to third decade the patient is usually bedridden.

The diagnostic laboratory findings are spiky or *thorny red blood cells* (*acanthocytes*), low sedimentation rate, and marked *lowering of low-density serum lipoproteins* (cholesterol, phospholipid and β-lipoprotein levels are all subnormal). Pathologic study has revealed an absorptive block in the intestinal mucosa with foamy, vacuolated epithelial cells, diminished numbers of myelinated nerve fibers in sural nerve biopsies, depletion of Purkinje and granule cells in all parts of the cerebellum, loss of fibers in posterior columns and spinocerebellar tracts, loss of anterior horn cells, loss of ganglion cells in the retina, and muscle fiber loss and fibrosis of myocardium. It has been proposed that the basic defect is an inability of the body to synthesize proteins of cell membranes, specifically because of impaired absorption of fat from the small intestine through the mucosa. The administration of a low-fat diet and high doses of vitamin A and E may prevent progression of the neurologic disorder (Illingworth et al.).

There are doubtless many other conditions of metabolic type where cerebellar ataxia figures importantly in the clinical picture. The Cockayne syndrome and Marinesco-Sjögren disease, already described under the metabolic disorders of early childhood, persist into later childhood and adolescence, or may even have their onset in this later period. Some patients with cerebral gigantism are clumsy and awkward. Cerebrotendinous xanthomatosis (see further on) combines spastic weakness and pseudobulbar palsy with cerebellar ataxia. The Prader-Labhart-Willi children have a broad-based gait and are clumsy in addition to being obese, genitally deficient, and diabetic. One family of five males with a syndrome of hyperuricemia, spinocerebellar ataxia, and deafness was reported by Rosenberg et al.; the enzymatic defect of Lesch-Nyhan disease was not present, however.

THE PARKINSONIAN OR EXTRAPYRAMIDAL MOTOR SYNDROME

Reference here is to the relatively pure motor disorder described in Chap. 4, in which strength remains relatively intact and corticospinal signs are absent, but in which effectiveness of movement is nonetheless impaired by the patient's disinclination to use the affected parts (hypokinesia), by slowness, and by rigidity and tremor. Dystonic postures and spasms of gaze may be conjoined.

When these symptoms have their onset in middle or late adult life, they always indicate paralysis agitans (Parkinson's disease). Formerly they occurred in adolescents and young adults as delayed but progressive manifestations of von Economo's encephalitis lethargica, but since this disease became extinct (about 1930), it is no longer encountered in this age group.

The development of an extrapyramidal syndrome in late childhood and adolescence should always suggest (1) Wilson-Westphal-Strümpell hepatocerebral degeneration and (2) Hallervorden-Spatz disease.

Hepatolenticular Degeneration (Wilson's Disease, Westphal-Strümpell Pseudosclerosis) The classic description of "progressive lenticular degeneration: a familial nervous disease associated with cirrhosis of the liver" was given by S. A. K. Wilson in 1912. A similar neurologic disorder had been described previously by Gowers (1906) under the title of "tetanoid chorea" and by Westphal (1883) and Strümpell (1898), as "pseudosclerosis," but the latter authors had not recognized the association with cirrhosis. The clinical studies of Hall (1921) and the histopathologic studies of Spielmeyer (1920), who reexamined the liver and brain tissues of Westphal's and Strümpell's cases, clearly established that the pseudosclerosis described by the latter authors was the same disease as the lenticular degeneration described by Wilson. Interestingly, none of these authors had recognized the golden-brown (Kayser-Fleischer) corneal ring, the one pathognomonic sign of the disease. The corneal abnormality was first recognized by Kayser in 1902, and in the following year Fleischer related it to pseudosclerosis. Haurowitz first demonstrated the greatly increased copper content of the liver and brain in 1930, but this discovery was generally neglected until Mandelbrote (1948) found, quite by chance, that the urinary excretion of copper was elevated in Wilson's disease, and that it was increased further by the injection of the chelating agent BAL (British antilewisite). In 1952, Scheinberg and Gitlin made the important discovery that ceruloplasmin, the serum enzyme that binds copper, is consistently reduced in Wilson's disease. These authors postulated that the inherited defect is an inability to synthesize ceruloplasmin, but how this leads to excessive tissue deposition of copper is not understood. An alternate hypothesis is that the impairment of ceruloplasmin synthesis is secondary to an intrahepatic defect in copper metabolism. (See review by Adams for a full historical account and references.)

Clinical features The disease is transmitted as an autosomal recessive trait, and the incidence is about 1 per 200,000 of the general population. The onset of neurologic symptoms is usually in the second and less often in the third decades, and rarely beyond that time.

In all instances the first expression of the disease (often asymptomatic) is a deposition of copper in the liver and other tissues, leading eventually to multilobular cirrhosis and splenomegaly (Scheinberg and Sternlieb). This may give rise to symptoms in childhood—attacks of jaundice, unexplained hepatosplenomegaly, or hypersplenism with thrombocytopenia and bleeding.

The first neurologic manifestations are *tremor* of a limb or of the head, slowness of movement, *dysarthria*, *dysphagia*, hoarseness, and occasionally choreic movements or dystonic postures of the limbs. Exceptionally an abnormality of behavior (argumentative; excessive emotionality), or a gradual impairment of intellectual faculties precedes other neurologic signs. As the disease progresses, the "classic syndrome" evolves: dysphagia and drooling; *rigidity* and slowness of movements of the limbs; flexed postures; fixity of facial muscles with mouth constantly agape, giving an appearance of grinning or a "vacuous smile"; dysarthria; and a tremor in repose which increases when the limbs are outstretched (coarse, "wing-beating" tremor). Usually an element of cerebellar ataxia and intention tremor of variable degree are added. In this and other ways the syndrome differs from classic parkinsonism.

As the neurologic disease progresses, the *Kayser-Fleischer rings* become more evident. They take the form of a rusty-brown discoloration of the deepest layer of the cornea (Descemet's membrane). They may not be seen in children in the hepatic stage of the disease (25 percent of cases) but are invariably present once neurologic signs are present. A slit-lamp examination may be necessary for their detection, particularly in brown-eyed patients. The disability becomes greater because of increasing rigidity and tremor. The patient becomes mute, immobile, and slowed mentally (late and variable effect).

The diagnosis is virtually certain when there is a similar syndrome in a sibling, or when an extrapyramidal syndrome of this type is conjoined with liver disease and the corneal rings. Variants of the above syndrome that the authors have seen are an early choreoathetosis (like Sydenham's chorea); prominent dystonic postures; a cerebellar ataxia with minimal rigidity; a syndrome of coarse action or action and intention tremor, resembling a cerebellar degeneration; an akinetic mute state with profound rigidity; and, as was remarked, a dementia, character change, or psychosis with relatively few extrapyramidal signs. Action myoclonus has been described.

In these variants the finding of a *low serum ceruloplasmin* level (less than 20 mg per 100 ml), low serum copper (less than 80 μg per 100 ml), and *increased urinary copper excretion* (more than 100 μg Cu in 24 h) corroborate the diagnosis in most cases. Early in the course of the illness the most reliable diagnostic finding is *high copper content in a biopsy of liver tissue* (more than 250 μg Cu per gram dried weight). Persistent aminoaciduria is present in most but not all patients. Liver function tests are only minimally altered until late in the illness, and the cirrhosis may not always be evident in a liver biopsy (some regenerative nodules are large, and the biopsy may be taken from one of them).

Neuropathologic changes These vary with the rate of progress of the disease. Exceptionally, in the rapidly advancing and fatal form, there is frank cavitation in the lenticular nuclei, as was observed in Wilson's original cases. In the more chronic form there is only shrinkage and a light-brown discoloration of the lenticular nuclei. Nerve cell loss and some degree of degeneration of myelinated fibers in lenticular (putaminal and pallidal) nuclei, substantia nigra, and dentate nuclei are usually apparent. More striking, however, is a marked hyperplasia of protoplasmic astrocytes (Alzheimer type II cells) in the cerebral cortex, basal ganglia, brainstem nuclei, and cerebellum.

Treatment This consists of (1) administration of sulfurated potash, 20 mg tid with meals to prevent absorption of copper; (2) reduction of dietary copper to less than 1 mg/day, which can usually be accomplished by avoidance of copper-rich foods (liver, mushrooms, cocoa, chocolate, nuts, and shellfish); and (3) administration of the copper chelating agent D-penicillamine (1 to 2 g/day) by mouth. If sensitivity to the latter develops (rash, arthralgia, fever, leukopenia), temporary reduc-

tion of dosage or a course of cortisone may bring the reaction under control. Severe reactions (lupus-like syndrome; nephrotic syndrome) occur occasionally and require discontinuation of the drug. Reinstitution of drug therapy should be undertaken, using low dosages and small, widely spaced increases. The D-penicillamine needs to be continued for the patient's lifetime.

Under the influence of treatment, neurologic signs almost always improve, Kayser-Fleischer rings disappear, and liver function tests may return to normal, although the abnormalities of copper metabolism remain unchanged. In moderately severe and advanced cases, clinical improvement may not begin for several weeks or months despite full doses of D-penicillamine, and it is important not to discontinue the drug during this period.

Hallervorden-Spatz Disease This disease is also known as *pigmentary degeneration of the globus pallidus, substantia nigra, and red nucleus.* It is inherited as an autosomal recessive trait and begins in late childhood or early adolescence, and progresses slowly over a period of 10 to 20 years. The early signs are motor, both *corticospinal* (spasticity, hyperreflexia, Babinski signs) and *extrapyramidal* (rigidity, dystonia, and choreoathetosis). General deterioration of intellect is conjoined. In individual cases, ataxia and myoclonus have been described at some phase of the illness. The spasticity and rigidity are predominantly paraplegic in distribution, but in some instances they begin in the bulbar muscles, interfering with speech and swallowing, as happens in Wilson's disease. Eventually the patient becomes almost completely inarticulate and unable to walk. Optic atrophy has been mentioned in a few reports, but we have not observed it.

There is no known biochemical test by which the diagnosis can be corroborated. The deposits of iron in basal ganglia have not been associated with demonstrable abnormality of serum iron or of iron metabolism. It has, however, been reported that there is a high uptake of radioactive iron in the region of the basal ganglia following intravenous injection of labeled ferrous citrate (Vakili et al.; Szanto and Gallyas). This technique may prove to be useful in diagnosis.

The neuropathology proves to be the most distinctive attribute of the disease. There is an intense brown pigmentation of the globus pallidus, substantia nigra, especially the anteromedial parts, and red nucleus. Granules and larger amorphous deposits of iron mixed with calcium stud the walls of small blood vessels; others lie free in the tissue. A loss of neurons and medullated fibers occurs in the most affected regions. Another unique feature is the presence of swollen axon fragments, which resemble those of neuroaxonal dystrophy; for this reason some authors regard Hallervorden-Spatz disease as a juvenile form of neuroaxonal dystrophy. However, iron deposits are not a conspicuous finding in the latter disease, which leaves this interpretation in doubt.

No treatment is known to be effective. One of our patients was temporarily improved on L-dopa, but the effect was slight. The use of chelating agents to reduce iron storage has not helped.

Differential Diagnosis Disorders which need to be differentiated from Wilson's and Hallervorden-Spatz disease are Chédiak-Higashi disease, juvenile paralysis agitans, Huntington's chorea, status dysmyelinatus, and Lafora-body disease, Leigh's disease and other rare, presumably biochemical, disorders of unknown type. Several of the latter have come to our attention, simulating the neurological picture of Wilson's disease but without evidence of liver involvement or copper abnormality.

In Chédiak-Higashi disease (which is characterized by massive granulation of leukocytes in blood and marrow, and by partial albinism) there is a variety of neurologic symptoms in approximately half the reported cases. Mental retardation, seizures, chronic polyneuropathy, cerebellar ataxia, and Parkinson's syndrome have been mentioned. The polyneuropathy, however, is the main clinical problem.

In families known to have *Huntington's chorea*, children may be afflicted. The age of onset may be as early as 1 to 4 years, but more often it is between 5 and 14 years. About 5 percent of all cases of Huntington's chorea are of this juvenile type. Surprisingly, slow decay in intellect is attended by rigidity of the limbs, short-stepped gait, and flexion hypertonia of the trunk, rather than a movement disorder. Nevertheless, choreoathetosis does occur in some cases, and not all juvenile cases are rigid. Speech may be slurred. Ocular movements are full except for upward gaze. A less frequent abnormality is a decreased velocity of conjugate ocular movements, so that the eyes move as though floating in an oil bath. The tendon reflexes are not exaggerated, but there are occasional reports of Babinski signs. Generalized seizures have occurred in some cases. Other neurologic abnormalities in the childhood syndrome are abnormal behavior, withdrawal and negativism, and catatonic posturing. Irritability and emotionality may raise the question of Sydenham's chorea. Myoclonic jerks have also been reported, and cerebellar ataxia occurs in some families. See Chap. 42 for a discussion of the neuropathology and treatment.

Juvenile paralysis agitans was described by Ramsay Hunt in 1917. From the descriptions the resemblance to Parkinson's syndrome is close. The course was slowly progressive. Familial incidence (two brothers aged 10 and 19) was reported by van Bogaert, but most cases have been sporadic. Postmortem examination has shown shrinkage of the lenticular nuclei and loss of large cells in the pallidum. In an anatomic specimen from van Bogaert's laboratory (1930) (age of onset was 7 years), cell loss was noted in both the substantia nigra and pallidum. There was no evidence of encephalitis lethargica and the pathologic findings differed from those of paralysis agitans, Wilson's disease, Hallervorden-Spatz disease, and Huntington's chorea. The authors are puzzled about this entity and have had no personal experience with it upon which to rely.

The *status dysmyelinatus* of Vogt and Vogt represents another obscure disease in which all myelinated fibers and nerve cells in the lenticular nuclei (both striatofugal and pallidofugal) disappear. The principal clinical features are extrapyramidal rigidity and, later, athetosis. Eventually the child becomes helpless, with limbs contorted in weird postures and deformed by spasms. At one phase it is said to resemble Parkinson's disease.

In isolated late-life cases of *Lafora-body disease* (see further on in this chapter), there may be rigidity, akinesia, and tremor; but usually myoclonus, seizures, and dementia dominate the picture. Rarely *Leigh's disease* gives rise to a slowly evolving extrapyramidal rigidity in late childhood or adolescence. Cavitation of putamens may be seen in the lenticular nuclei in CT scans.

The differential diagnosis of the above diseases presents certain difficulties. Hallervorden-Spatz disease and its variants cannot always be recognized for want of a satisfactory laboratory test; some cases presently included in this category may have some other disease. The similarities between the diseases included under the rubric of Parkinson's syndrome are in general smaller than the differences. Wilson's disease, for example, shares certain signs with Parkinson's disease, yet the appearance of each is quite distinctive. The special qualities of the facial expression in Wilson's disease—as well as the dysarthria, severe ataxic tremor, and some degree of cerebellar ataxia —are not readily confused with Parkinson's disease. Furthermore, in several of the diseases in this category there may be myoclonus and extrapyramidal signs such as choreoathetosis, dystonia, etc., which are essential parts of the syndromes described below. Hence one must not insist that each disease conform strictly to a unique clinical syndrome.

THE SYNDROME OF DYSTONIA AND GENERALIZED ATHETOSIS

As indicated in Chap. 4, the authors find the differences between dystonia and athetosis recondite. If one examines many patients with involuntary movements of these types, every gradation between the two is seen, and not infrequently the quicker, unpatterned involuntary movements of chorea and ballismus as well. Even tremor and myoclonus may complicate the composite movement disorder. With reference to muscular tone in patients with athetosis and dystonia, there are unpredictable accessions of hypertonia and hypotonia.

A number of rare inherited metabolic diseases are characterized by the syndrome of athetosis and dystonia.

The Lesch-Nyhan Syndrome and Hyperuricemia This rare form of metabolic disease is inherited as an X-linked recessive trait. Although it carries the name of Lesch and Nyhan (1964), the occurrence of uricemia in association with spasticity and choreoathetosis in early childhood had been described in 1959 by Catel and Schmidt. Essentially it is an *hereditary choreoathetosis with self-mutilation* and *hyperuricemia*. The compulsive self-mutilation, mainly of the lips, occurs early (during the second and third year), and spasticity, choreoathetosis, and tremor come later. Speech is delayed; once attained, it is dysarthric through life. Mental retardation is moderately severe. In patients over 10 years of age, gouty tophi appear on the ears, and there is increasing risk from gouty nephropathy. The serum levels of uric acid are in the range of 7 to 10 mg per 100 ml. Deficient activity of the enzyme hypoxanthine-guanine-phosphoribosyl transferase (HGPRT) has been found in all definite cases of this disease. As a result of this deficiency, hypoxanthine is either excreted or catabolized to xanthine and uric acid.

In the differential diagnosis, one must consider mental retardation with nonspecific hand biting and mutilation, athetosis from *birth trauma*, and encephalopathies with chronic renal disease. *Hyperuricemia* has also been reported in one family with spinocerebellar ataxia and deafness, and in another with autism and mental retardation, both without the enzymatic defect of Lesch-Nyhan disease.

Treatment with allopurinol, a xanthine oxidase inhibitor which blocks the last steps of uric acid synthesis, reduces the uric acid in the Lesch-Nyhan disease and prevents the uricosuric nephropathy, but has no effect on CNS symptoms.

Familial Calcification of Vessels in Basal Ganglia and Cerebellum (Hypoparathyroidism and Fahr's Syndrome)

Ferruginization and calcification of vessels in the basal ganglia occur to a slight degree in many otherwise normal persons (and in other mammals). When it occurs early in life and is of such degree as to be visible in plain films of the skull, it must always be regarded as abnormal. An adult case of this type was described by Fahr, so that his name is sometimes attached to this disorder, but it was known long before his publication appeared, and his account added little to our knowledge of the condition.

Many authors have called attention to familial forms of calcification of the basal ganglia and cerebellum, in which choreoathetosis and rigidity are prominent. In some of our patients there was a unilateral athetosis (arm and leg) which gradually was replaced by a parkinsonian syndrome, or there was a double athetosis which persisted. Other of our patients have been either mentally retarded, or intellectually intact. The familial form of calcification, inherited as an autosomal recessive trait, usually has its onset in adolescence and early adult life. The serum calcium levels are usually normal, and there is no explanation of the calcification.

In hypoparathyroidism (idiopathic or acquired) and pseudohypoparathyroidism (a rare familial disease characterized by the symptoms and signs of hypoparathyroidism in association with distinctive skeletal and developmental abnormalities) not only does diminution in ionized serum calcium induce tetany and seizures, but choreoathetosis may be added. The latter symptom is presumably due to calcification of the basal ganglia, which occurs in about one-half of the patients. Also, in some instances there are signs of a cerebellar lesion.

Finally, it should be pointed out that in the middle-aged and elderly, small calcifications of the basal ganglia are only rarely associated with clinical signs of basal ganglia disease or with abnormalities of calcium or phosphorus. Such calcifications are being detected with increasing frequency by CT scanning, which is far more sensitive for this purpose than plain roentgenograms of the skull (Fig. 37-1).

Other Metabolic Disorders Associated with Choreoathetosis and Dystonia Exceptionally, lipofuscinosis, metachromatic leukodystrophy of tardive type, Niemann-Pick disease, Hallervorden-Spatz disease, and Wilson's disease may present with a syndrome of which dystonia or athetosis is an important component. Usually the other elements in the clinical picture are detectable, so that the correct diagnosis is seldom in doubt for long. Dal Canto et al. have described a *variant of neuronal lipofuscinosis* in which a boy and girl of unrelated non-

Jewish parents developed severe choreoathetosis and dystonia at 6 to 7 years of age. Intellectual deterioration, gait abnormality, and seizures were the other clinical features. Cerebral biopsy showed intraneuronal inclusions consisting of *curvilinear bodies*. These observations support the notion of nosologic heterogeneity among the nonglycolipid neuronal storage disorders.

A form of *familial paroxysmal choreoathetosis* was recognized by Mount and Reback in 1940, and the subject has more recently been reviewed by Lance (see Chap. 4). Its metabolic basis has not been established. The authors have observed attacks of this kind also in children with "cerebral palsy" who became intoxicated with phenytoin; lowering the dose terminated the attacks. Clearly the metabolic effect of phenytoin on a damaged nervous system was capable of evoking this syndrome. Perhaps some unknown metabolite has a similar effect in other cases.

A *nonprogressive familial choreoathetosis* with onset in early childhood has been described by Pincus and Chutorian. Cerebellar signs are usually conjoined, but the intellect is spared. This syndrome is thought to be inherited as an autosomal recessive trait, but the metabolic fault, if one is present, is unknown.

Figure 37-1
Idiopathic basal ganglionic calcification in a 25-year-old woman who had no symptoms or signs of cerebral disease.

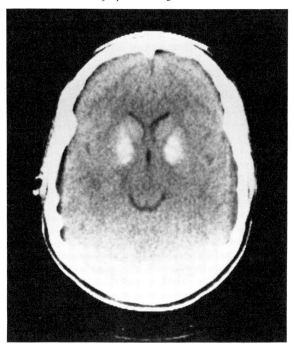

In terms of metabolic pathologies, those of acquired type are much more common than inherited ones. A prototype of athetosis is known to follow hypoxic encephalopathy of birth, leading to *état marbré* of the basal ganglia. This is the double athetosis syndrome that usually does not become manifest until after the first year of life and persists thereafter (page 854). The Rh and ABO blood incompatibilities which induce erythroblastosis fetalis and kernicterus may occasion a bilateral athetosis at about the same period of life, but are distinguished by deafness and paralysis of upward gaze (see page 855). The same is true of the Crigler-Najjar form of hereditary hyperbilirubinemia, wherein kernicterus (with ataxia or athetosis) may rarely appear as late as childhood or adolescence. The defect is one of glucuronide-bilirubin conjugation (Schmid and McDonagh).

FAMILIAL POLYMYOCLONIAS

As was stated in Chap. 5, the term *myoclonus* is applied to many conditions not at all alike, but here we refer to exceedingly brief, random, arrhythmic twitches of parts of muscles, muscles, and groups of muscles, differing from choreoathetosis by virtue of their brevity.

A movement disorder of this type may be mixed with any of the aforementioned syndromes of athetosis and dystonia, but may, in certain conditions, stand as a relatively pure syndrome. The many acquired forms of polymyoclonia, such as subacute sclerosing panencephalitis, have been mentioned in Chap. 5. Here we are concerned with those of known or presumed metabolic origin.

Myoclonic Encephalopathy of Infants   Under this title Kinsbourne originally described a form of widespread, continuous myoclonus (except during deep sleep) affecting male and female infants, whose development had been normal until the onset of the disease (9 to 20 months). The myoclonus evolves over a week or less, affects all the muscles of the body, and interferes seriously with all the natural muscular activities of the child. The eyes are notably affected by rapid (up to 8 per second) irregular conjugate movement ("dancing eyes"). The child is irritable and speech may cease. All laboratory tests are normal.

ACTH and dexamethasone, the latter in doses of 1.5 to 4.0 mg/day, suppress the myoclonus and permit developmental progress. Some patients have recovered, and have been mentally slow and mildly ataxic afterward. Others have required corticosteroid therapy for 5 to 10 years, with relapse whenever it is discontinued. Ordinary anticonvulsants have no effect.

A similar syndrome has been observed in conjunction with neuroblastoma.

Familial Progressive Myoclonus Three major categories of familial polymyoclonus of late childhood and adolescence have been delineated: (1) Lafora- or amyloid-body type, (2) juvenile cerebroretinal degeneration, and (3) a more benign degenerative disease (dyssynergia cerebellaris myoclonica of Hunt and paramyoclonus of Friedreich).

Lafora-body polymyoclonus The identification of this disease, which is inherited as an autosomal dominant trait, is based on the postmortem finding of large basophilic cytoplasmic bodies in the dentate, brainstem, and thalamic neurons. They have been shown by Yokoi et al. to be composed of a glucose polymer, chemically but not structurally related to glycogen. Possibly some of the cases of familial myoclonus epilepsy reported by Unverricht and Lundborg (see page 74) were of this type, but since they had no pathologic data, one cannot be sure.

Beginning in late childhood and adolescence, in a previously normal individual, the disease announces itself by a seizure (petit mal or grand mal) or by many myoclonic jerks, or both. The illness may at first be mistaken for ordinary epilepsy, but within a few months it becomes evident that it is far more serious. The myoclonus becomes widespread and can be initiated by noise, startle, excitement, or the persistence of certain motor activities. An evoked train of myoclonic jerks may progress to a generalized seizure with loss of consciousness. As the disease advances, the myoclonus interferes increasingly with the patient's activities until function is seriously impaired. Close examination may also reveal an alteration in muscle tone and a slight degree of cerebellar ataxia. At this time, or even before the onset of myoclonus and seizures, the patient may exhibit irritability, odd traits of character, uninhibited or impulsive actions, or experience visual hallucinations. Later there is progressive failure in all cognitive functions. Deafness has been an early sign in a few cases. Rigidity, hypotonia, impaired tendon reflexes, acrocyanosis, and rarely corticospinal tract signs are late findings. Finally the patient becomes cachectic and bedfast, and succumbs to intercurrent infection. Most cases do not survive beyond their twenty-fifth birthday. Nonetheless there are isolated reports of Lafora-body disease in which symptoms began as late as 40 years, with death at 50 years.

No abnormalities of blood, urine, or CSF have been detected. Inclusion bodies have been seen in liver biopsies even though liver function was normal. The EEG shows diffuse slow waves and spikes. Pathological examinations have shown a slight loss of granule and Purkinje cells, and loss of neurons in the dentate nuclei, inner segment of globus pallidus, and cerebral cortex— in addition to the Lafora bodies. The latter may also be seen in the retina, myocardium, and striated muscles.

Anticonvulsant drugs help in the control of the seizures, but have no effect on the basic process.

Juvenile cerebroretinal degeneration (lipofuscinosis) This is one of the most slowly advancing forms of the lipidoses. Earlier it was thought to be similar to Tay-Sachs disease, except for the retinal lesion, which in the juvenile form involves not only the retinal ganglion cells but the rods and cones as well.

In a review of more than 200 reported cases of lipid storage disease, Kolodny (1972) has divided them into three subtypes; (1) Jansky-Bielschowsky form, which begins with seizures at the age of 2 to 4 years, (2) Spielmeyer-Sjögren type, which begins with visual symptoms at 4 to 10 years, and (3) the Kufs type which begins in late childhood, adolescence, or adult years with alterations of personality and progresses to dementia.

The salient clinical features of (1) and (2) are myoclonus, seizures, and visual loss. The maculae are the site of the first lesions; they appear as yellowish gray areas of degeneration, in contrast to the cherry-red spot and the encircling gray ring of Tay-Sachs disease. At first the pigment is fine, like dust; later it agglomerates to resemble more the bone-corpuscular shapes in retinitis pigmentosa. The liver and spleen are not enlarged, and there are no osseous changes. The usual development of these and other manifestations of the disease has been outlined by Sjögren, who has had experience with a large number of cases in Sweden. He divides the illness into five stages:

1. Visual impairment, sometimes preceding retinal changes by months.

2. After approximately 2 years, the onset of generalized seizures and myoclonus, often with irritability, poor control of emotions, and stuttering, jerky speech.

3. Gradual intellectual deterioration (poor memory, reduced mental activity, inattentiveness). By this stage the movements have usually become slow, stiff, and tremulous, resembling somewhat those of Parkin-

son's disease—to which are added elements of cerebellar ataxia and intention tremor, coming in this way to resemble Wilson's disease.

4. Stage of severe dementia in which the patient needs assistance to get about, no longer speaks, and may scream when disturbed or forced to move. The muscles are wasted, though the tendon reflexes are lively and the plantar reflexes are extensor.

5. Finally the patient lies curled up in bed, blind and speechless, with strong extensor plantar reflexes, occasionally adopting dystonic postures. Mercifully the illness ends in 10 to 15 years.

In the early stages the EEG picture of random, high-voltage, triphasic waves is diagnostic; later, as the seizures and myoclonic jerks become less frequent and finally cease, only delta waves are seen. The electroretinographic waveforms are lost if the retina is affected. The lateral ventricles are slightly dilated. The CSF is normal. No enzymatic defect has been demonstrated.

The Kufs type, which develops later (15 to 25 years), is often unattended by visual or retinal changes, and is even slower in its evolution. Personality change and seizures, usually with some degree of myoclonus, are the principal abnormalities. As the disease progresses, cerebellar ataxia, spasticity and rigidity, or athetosis, or mixtures thereof, are combined with dementia. Van Bogaert (personal communication) has noted that relatives of these patients may have retinal changes without neurologic accompaniments.

Of all the lipidoses, the juvenile cerebroretinal type has defied biochemical definition. There is no deficiency in hexosaminidase activity in the serum nor increase in gangliosides in the brain. Zeman et al. have shown that the cytoplasmic inclusions are autofluorescent and give a positive histochemical reaction for ceroid or lipofuscin, but accumulation of this latter substance is a nonspecific aging phenomenon. Under the electron microscope the stored particles are curvilinear, and give a fingerprint pattern quite unlike that of lipofuscin.

Late form of G_{M2} gangliosidosis In recent years there have been a number of reports of children or adolescents who developed a dementia and polymyoclonus with variable cerebellar ataxia and cherry-red macular spots. The biochemical abnormality is similar to that of Tay-Sachs disease. The progression of the disease is slow, over a period of many years.

Late Gaucher's disease with polymyoclonia A type of Gaucher's disease is occasionally encountered in which seizures, severe diffuse myoclonus and gradual impairment of intellectual function begins at 10 to 15

years or later. The spleen is enlarged. The biochemical abnormality is the same as that described in Gaucher's disease of early onset.

Benign familial polymyoclonia This, the third major polymyoclonus syndrome of childhood, adolescence, and early adult life, should be listed as a degenerative disease, for it has not been associated with any biochemical abnormalities. The inheritance is autosomal dominant in type, and in some families the disease has been traced through several generations.

The onset of the illness is with shocklike myoclonic contractions in the muscles of the shoulders and upper arms. As the years pass, all truncal and appendicular muscles are implicated, and finally the face, eyes, tongue, and palate are affected. Parts of a muscle may be involved (fasciculations), or whole muscles and groups of muscles. The frequency of the myoclonic jerks is highly variable. Some are rhythmic, but extreme variability is the rule; there are times when they are barely detectable, and others when they are so strong as to seriously interfere with all activities and even throw the patient out of a chair or bed. The myoclonus may begin at any age from infancy to adult life. Some of the most benign forms may virtually subside for a few years only to reappear later.

Mentation is usually preserved until late, when it may become impaired. In a few patients, dementia has been a prominent feature. If any other neurologic abnormality develops, it is likely to be a cerebellar ataxia, which was the combination described by Hunt as *dyssynergia cerebellaris myoclonica* (page 820). A few have had choreoathetosis. Some patients have seizures, but many do not. A form of polymyoclonia associated with nerve deafness has also been reported. The neuropathologic basis of this illness is unsettled.

BILATERAL HEMIPLEGIA, CEREBRAL BLINDNESS AND DEAFNESS, AND OTHER MANIFESTATIONS OF DECEREBRATION

This is the syndrome by which most of the chronic familial leukodystrophies are expressed. There are several varieties, some of unquestionable metabolic origin and others of uncertain status. Cerebral gray matter diseases (poliodystrophies) have a slightly different mode of presentation than the leukodystrophies—seizures, myoclonus, chorea, choreoathetosis, and tremor being prominent in the former. Clinically, the diagnosis of the

Table 37-4
Differential diagnosis of poliodystrophies of infancy

	Tay-Sachs	Niemann-Pick	Gaucher's	Alper's	Subacute necrotizing encephalopathy
Age of onset	4–6 months	Under 6 months	Under 6 months	Under 1 year	Under 1 year, rarely late childhood
Rate of progression	Rapid Death 2–3 years	Rapid Death before 3 years	Very rapid Death before 2 years	Rapid Death before 3 years	Usually rapid Death before 3 years
Ethnic group	Almost all Jewish	50% Jewish	65% Jewish		
Genetic	Recessive	Recessive	Recessive Rarely, dominant		Recessive
Head size	Enlarges late	Normal	Normal	Reduces late	Normal
Skin and/or systemic	Normal	Hepato-splenomegaly Xanthoma of skin, rare	Hepato-splenomegaly	Normal	Normal
Eye	Cherry-red macula Optic atrophy	Cherry-red macula Optic atrophy	Normal	Normal	Optic atrophy
Seizures	Frequent, but late	Rare	Rare	Onset with seizures Myoclonus and other types	Seizures late and rare
Neurologic signs	Early: flaccid paresis Late: spastic paresis Dementia: early Hyperacusis	Spastic paresis Early: dementia	Early: retroflexion of head Strabismus Bulbar palsy Spastic paralysis Early: dementia	Spastic paresis Dementia Cortical blindness and deafness	Bulbar palsy Weak, infrequent cry Flaccid paresis with immobility
Blood	Absent fructose-1-phosphate-aldolase ↑ SGOT ↑ Vacuolated lymphocytes	↑ Vacuolated lymphocytes ↑ Serum lipids ↑ SGOT	↑ Acid phosphatase	Normal	Normal
Urine	Normal	Normal	Normal	Normal	Normal
CSF	Normal	Normal		Normal	Normal
Biopsy	+ Rectal	"Foam cells"—bone marrow	Gaucher cells—bone marrow		
X-ray		Diffuse pulmonary infiltrates Demineralization of bone			
Electroretinogram	Normal				

Source: Modified from AL Drew, Jr, in S Carter, AP Gold (eds), *Neurology of Infancy and Childhood*, New York, Appleton-Century-Crofts, 1974.

Table 37-5
Differential diagnosis of leukodystrophies of infancy

	Krabbe's	Metachromatic leukodystrophy	Spongy degeneration	Palizaeus-Merzbacher	Schilder's
Age of onset	3–6 months	1–2 years, rarely late childhood	0–4 months	6–24 months	5–10 years
Rate of progression	Rapid Death by 2 years	Slow Death by 3–5 years	Rapid Death by 3 years	Slow May survive to adult life	Abrupt onset Death in months to years
Sex or ethnic group			Most Jewish	Predominantly males	
Genetic	Recessive	Recessive	Recessive	Sex-linked recessive	Adrenoleuko-dystrophy form—X-linked recessive
Head size	Normal	Enlarges late	Enlarges early	Normal	Normal
Skin or systemic	Normal	Normal	Normal	Normal	Bronzing with adrenal atrophy
Eye	Late: optic atrophy	Late: optic atrophy	Optic atrophy blindness	Slow optic atrophy	Optic neuritis or optic atrophy
Seizures	Tonic spasms	Rare	Uncommon	Late	Rare, late
Neurologic signs	Spastic paresis Nystagmus Head retraction Bulbar palsy Dementia	Changes in gait Ataxia Combined upper and lower motor neuron signs Bulbar palsy Blindness } late Deafness Dementia	Hypotonia→spastic diplegia→decerebrate rigidity	Pendular nystagmus Titubation of head and other cerebellar signs in early childhood Spastic diplegia, late childhood Slow dementia	Early spastic paralysis Dementia Late: cortical blindness, deafness, aphasia, pseudobulbar palsy
Miscellaneous		Reduced nerve conduction			EEG diffuse delta waves
Blood	Normal	Normal	Normal	Normal	Normal or ↓ cortisol
Urine	Normal	Metachromatic bodies	Normal	Normal	Normal
CSF	↑ Protein (150–300 mg/100 ml)	Normal or ↑ protein up to 200 mg/100 ml	↑ Pressure Normal or ↑ protein up to 200 mg/100 ml	Normal	Normal or ↑ gamma globulin
Biopsy	Brain	Sural nerve	Brain		
X-ray		Nonfilling of gallbladder	Suture separation		

Source: Modified from AL Drew, Jr, in S Carter, AP Gold (eds), *Neurology of Infancy and Childhood,* New York, Appleton-Century-Crofts, 1974.

leukodystrophies is based on identification of symptoms and signs which are attributable to the interruption of tracts (corticospinal, corticobulbar, cerebellar peduncular, sensory, medial longitudinal fasciculi), and visual pathways (optic nerve, optic tract, geniculocalcarine), with infrequency or absence of seizures, myoclonus, and spike and wave abnormalities in the EEG.

The syndrome of progressive spasticity and rigidity with spastic dysarthria and pseudobulbar palsy poses a difficult problem. One's first impulse is to assume a corticospinal disorder, especially if tendon reflexes are brisk, but frequently the plantar reflexes are flexor and the facial reflexes not excessively brisk. Unsteadiness of gait and sudden breaks or interruptions of speech suggest a cerebellar defect; unusual postures and a more plastic type of rigidity, an extrapyramidal disorder. Such combinations, with mental backwardness and dementia, characterize the mild and late forms of metachromatic leukodystrophy—which may be taken as an example of a leukoencephalopathy with only a slight degree of neuronal storage. However, these may be observed in other less-well-characterized degenerative diseases, such as the one reported by Willvonseder et al., in which a mild dementia, spastic dysarthria, paresis of vertical eye movements, gait disturbance, and splenomegaly came on during early adult life. Here abnormalities of copper metabolism were found (slightly decreased serum ceruloplasmin, copper turnover values in the range of those of heterozygous carriers of Wilson's disease, but no increase in urinary copper excretion). The authors have seen several such patients.

Sudanophilic Leukodystrophy with Bronzing of Skin and Adrenal Atrophy (Adrenoleukodystrophy) This combination of leukodystrophy and Addison's disease, originally included under the rubric of Schilder's disease, is now set apart as an independent metabolic encephalopathy.

The onset varies from 4 to 16 years and only males are affected (probably sex-linked recessive). The signs of either the adrenal insufficiency or the cerebral lesion may be the first to appear. In the case of Siemerling and Creutzfeldt, the first recorded example of this disorder, *bronzing of the skin* of the hands appeared at 4 years of age; *quadriparesis, with dysarthria and dysphagia* (pseudobulbar palsy) became evident at 7 years; a single seizure occurred at 8 years; and by 9 years, shortly before death, the patient was *decerebrate* and unrespon-

sive. In personally observed cases, the first abnormalities appeared at 9 to 10 years and took the form of episodic vomiting, a change in personality, and decline in scholastic performance, with silly, inappropriate giggling and crying. After a time, severe vomiting and even an episode of circulatory collapse occurred, following which the gait became unsteady and arms ataxic, with an action or intention tremor. Only then may increasing pigmentation of the oral mucosa and the skin around nipples and over elbows, knees, and scrotum become evident. *Cortical blindness* follows in some instances. In the late stages, bilateral hemiplegia (at first asymmetrical), pseudobulbar paralysis, blindness, deafness, and impairment of all higher cerebral functions occur.

Griffin et al. have described a spinal-neuropathic form of the disease (*adrenomyeloneuropathy*). In their patients evidence of adrenal insufficiency was present since early childhood, but only in the third decade did a progressive spastic paraparesis and a relatively mild polyneuropathy develop. Recently, Moser et al. have drawn attention to a neonatal form and to a purely spinal form (*progressive spastic paraparesis*) in the heterozygote (female carrier).

The important laboratory findings are low sodium and chloride and elevated potassium levels—reflecting the atrophy of the adrenal glands. The latter results in reduced excretion of corticosteroids, low serum cortisol levels, and lack of rise in 17-hydroxyketosteroids after ACTH stimulation. The CSF protein may be elevated.

Massive degeneration of the myelin occurs, often asymmetrically in various parts of the cerebrum, brainstem, optic nerves, and sometimes spinal cord. Degradation products of myelin are visible in macrophages in recent lesions, viz., sudanophilic demyelination. Axis cylinders are damaged, but to a lesser degree. The cortex of the adrenal glands is atrophic, and the cells and invading histiocytes contain an abnormal lipid material. The testes show marked interstitial fibrosis and atrophy of the seminiferous tubules. Electron microscopically, the macrophages of the brain and adrenals and the Leydig cells of the testes show characteristic lamellar cytoplasmic inclusions. Igarashi and his associates have isolated an abnormal *long-chain fatty acid in cholesterol esters* from both the *brain* and *adrenals*. This type of fatty acid abnormality has not been described in other pathologic conditions, and may represent the unique biochemical abnormality in this disease.

Adrenal replacement therapy may prolong life, and occasionally effects a partial neurologic remission. Trials of dietary control with avoidance of long-chain fatty acids are underway.

Familial Orthochromic Leukodystrophy This is a diffuse, symmetrical cerebral, cerebellar, and spinal degeneration of white matter without visceral lesions. It is believed to be inherited as an autosomal recessive trait but the data are meager.

The age of onset has varied from 1 to 15 years. Some of the sporadic cases reported in the adult were probably examples of cerebral multiple sclerosis, but we have seen orthochromic or metachromatic leukodystrophy begin as late as middle adult life. In all cases, the clinical picture is one of intellectual decline with spastic weakness; hyperreflexia; Babinski signs; and stiff, short-stepped gait. As the disease progresses over 3 to 5 years, there is a loss of vision and speech, then hearing, and finally a state of virtual decerebration. Variants not seen by us include cases wth sudanophilic dystrophy and striatocerebellar calcification and those with microcephaly, large ears, hypertelorism, and epicanthal folds, who later developed quadriparesis, optic atrophy, and mild choreoathetosis.

In some of these cases it is impossible to distinguish this demyelinative disease from that of Pelizaeus-Merzbacher and of Cockayne, described in the preceding section.

Cerebral Sclerosis of Scholz This is a closely related white-matter disease which begins in childhood and is characterized by cerebral blindness, deafness, aphasia, and spastic quadriparesis. Choreoathetosis has been described in a few cases.

Polycystic White Matter Degeneration This disease of early or late childhood is probably transmitted as an autosomal recessive trait, and causes quadriparesis, blindness, deafness, and loss of speech and other higher cerebral functions. Seizures may be present but are infrequent.

Cerebrotendinous Xanthomatosis This rare disease is probably transmitted by an autosomal recessive gene. It usually begins in late childhood, with *cataracts* and *xanthomata of tendon sheaths and lungs*. As it progresses, mild mental retardation (the earliest neurologic manifestation) gives way to dementia, unsteady ataxic or *ataxic-spastic gait, dysarthria*, and *dysphagia*. In the late stages (after 5 to 15 years) the patient becomes bedfast and helpless; death occurs at 20 to 30 years of age. In other cases the clinical course is much more benign. Neuropathologic examination shows masses of crystalline cholesterol deposits in the brainstem and cerebellum and sometimes in the spinal cord, with symmetrical destruction of myelin in the same areas.

The serum cholesterol levels have been normal in five of seven cases and in the others was as high as 450 mg per 100 ml. The tendon xanthomas contain cholesterol of which 4 to 9 percent is cholestanol (dihydrocholesterol). Cholestanol levels in the serum and red cells are increased. The CT scan visualizes the cerebellar and brainstem deposits of cholesterol.

This disease should not be confused with that described by *Wolman*, in which there is an hereditary malabsorption syndrome with hepatosplenomegaly, calcification of the adrenal glands, lymph node enlargement, and storage of cholesterol esters and triglycerides in the tissues (Crocker et al.). Neurologic symptoms are usually limited to impaired intellectual development.

STROKES IN ASSOCIATION WITH INHERITED METABOLIC DISEASES

On page 568 it was remarked that strokes occur from time to time in infants and children (childhood hemiplegias) with a number of poorly understood vascular pathologies. Two metabolic diseases must always be considered in the differential diagnosis of such cases: homocystinuria and Fabry's disease.

Homocystinuria This aminoaciduria is inherited as an autosomal recessive trait and simulates Marfan's disease. Tall, slender habitus, great length of limbs, sometimes scoliosis and arachnodactyly (long, spidery fingers and toes), thin and rather weak muscles, knock-knees, highly arched feet, and kyphosis are the main skeletal features. Sparse, blond, brittle hair and malar flush are often noted, and there may occur a *dislocation of one or both lenses* (usually downward), giving the iris a tremulous appearance. The only neurologic abnormality is *mental retardation*, which sets this syndrome apart from Marfan's disease, in which intellect is unimpaired.

The basis of the vascular lesions is uncertain. An abnormality of platelets, favoring clot formation and thromboses of cerebral arteries has been suggested. A number of reported cases have died of coronary occlusions during adolescence, and a myocardial lesion may also occur and be the source of emboli to cerebral arteries.

Homocystine is elevated in the blood, CSF, and urine. There is an inherited cystathionine synthase deficiency that results in an inadequacy of cystathionine formation, a substance essential to many tissues, including the brain. This may be the explanation of the mental retardation. The infarcts in the brain are clearly related to thrombotic and embolic arterial occlusions. The administration of a low-methionine diet and large doses of pyridoxine (a cystathionine synthase coenzyme) reduces the excretion of homocystine, but is of uncertain clinical benefit.

Fabry's Disease (Anderson-Fabry Disease, Hereditary Dystopic Lipidosis)   This disease, also known as *angiokeratoma corporis diffusum*, is inherited as an X-linked recessive trait. It occurs in its complete form in men and in incomplete form in female carriers. The primary deficit is in the enzyme α-galactosidase, which results in an accumulation of ceramide trihexoside in endothelial, perithelial, and smooth muscle cells of the blood vessels, as well as in renal tubular and glomerular cells and other viscera and in nerve cells in many parts of the nervous system (hypothalamic and amygdaloid nuclei, substantia nigra, reticular and other nuclei of the brainstem, anterior and intermediolateral horns of the spinal cord, sympathetic and dorsal root ganglia). The disease becomes manifest clinically in childhood or adolescence, with intermittent lancinating pains and dysesthesias of the extremities. Later, the diffuse vascular involvement leads to hypertension, renal damage, cardiomegaly, and myocardial ischemia. Thrombotic infarctions occur in the brain during early adult years. Garcin et al. have reviewed the neurologic and neuropathologic findings in this disease. Its painful neuropathic character is discussed on page 913.

PERSONALITY CHANGES AND BEHAVIORAL DISTURBANCES AS MANIFESTATIONS OF INHERITED METABOLIC DISEASES

Although rare among the large numbers of maladjusted, neurotic, psychopathic, and psychotic adolescents, certain metabolic diseases may derange mind and behavior, and the management of the metabolic diseases is so different that one must take pains to identify them.

All the metabolic diseases of late childhood and adolescence share the property of deranging behavior, thinking, feelings, and emotional reactions. The most obvious and easily detectable of these derangements are in the cognitive sphere, i.e., reduction in the capacity to retain experiences and assimilate new information, to solve problems, and to make progress in scholastic pursuits and in verbal and arithmetic skills. More pro-

nounced forms of these impairments are recognized as neurologic deficits such as "the amnesic state," aphasia, dyscalculia, and visual-perceptual disorientation. Each of these phenomena has its own anatomy in the cerebrum, as was pointed out in Chap. 21, and the state known as dementia comprises various degrees and combinations of them.

In early childhood, when the composite of intellectual functions is but little developed, it is difficult to decide upon qualities of mind. Slowness in learning, in acquiring language functions, etc., may be interpreted loosely as mental retardation. At this age these abilities have not developed sufficiently to permit recognition of a regression in intellectual functions. Only in late childhood do mental retardation and dementia become clearly distinguishable.

Far less tangible are subtle changes in personality and behavior, which must always be judged against the standards of the cultural group of which the patient is a member. The occurrence in adolescence of scholastic failure, withdrawal from the parental circle, unwillingness to accept parental and societal standards, abuse of drugs, bizarre thinking, somatic delusions, hallucinations, and depressed mood, all raise difficult questions about adolescent maladjustment, sociopathy, schizophrenia, or manic-depressive disease.

The principle that most neuropsychiatrists follow in selecting from the large mass of maladjusted adolescents those with a metabolic brain disease, is that the latter will sooner or later cause a regression in cognitive or intellectual functions. Schizophrenia and manic-depressive psychoses and the sociopathies and character disorders do so little or not at all. This is not to say that personality changes and emotional disturbances do not occur in the metabolic encephalopathies; of course they do. However, their recognition depends on the demonstration of failing memory, impaired thinking, inability to learn, and loss of verbal and arithmetic capacities, many of which are measured quantitatively in intelligence tests.

If one reviews all the diseases described in this chapter which demonstrate early regression of cognitive function associated with personality change and alteration of behavior, and which are for a time unaccompanied by other neurologic abnormalities, the following merit special consideration:

1. Wilson's disease

2. Hallervorden-Spatz pigmentary degeneration

3. Lafora-body myoclonic epilepsy

4. Late-onset cerebroretinal lipofuscinosis (Kufs' form)

5. Some of the mucopolysaccharidoses

6. Adolescent Schilder's disease (sudanophilic leukodystrophy), with or without adrenal atrophy

7. Metachromatic leukodystrophy

8. Cerebrotendinous xanthomatosis

9. Non-wilsonian copper disorder with dementia, spasticity, and paralysis of vertical eye movements

10. Childhood Huntington's chorea

In each of the above diseases, dementia and personality disorder may gradually develop and persist for many months, even a year or two, before other neurologic signs appear. Special problems in diagnosis are raised by each. Personality and behavioral change may so predominate that cognitive losses seem subordinate. The latter need to be sought in a carefully elicited history and review of mental status. One must look also for the earliest signs of movement disorders and other neurologic abnormalities which greatly clarify the diagnostic problem. Often a psychogenesis is incorrectly assumed and prolonged psychoanalytic study, completely fruitless, has been undertaken.

ADULT FORMS OF INHERITED METABOLIC DISEASES

The increasing range and precision of biochemical and cytologic tests have brought to light a number of inherited metabolic diseases which sometimes have their onset in adult life. Such disorders are uncommon but nevertheless important because they must be considered in the differential diagnosis of degenerative diseases and atrophies, for which explanations are beginning to be found.

In the last few years the authors have personally observed or otherwise come to know of examples of the following diseases, the onset of which was in late adolescence or adult life.

1. Metachromatic leukoencephalopathy
2. Adrenoleukodystrophy
3. Kuf's form of lipofuscinosis
4. G_{M2} gangliosidosis
5. Wilson's disease
6. Leigh's disease
7. Gaucher's disease
8. Niemann-Pick disease
9. Polysaccharide encephalopathy
10. Polyneuropathies (Andrade's disease, porphyria, Refsum's disease)

In the encephalopathic forms of these diseases the diagnosis was usually made only after symptoms had been present for months or years and the disease was in most instances mistaken for some other condition. One of our patients with metachromatic leukodystrophy, a 30-year-old man, began failing in college and was later unsuccessful in holding a job because of carelessness and mistakes in his work and indifference (clearly traceable to a mild dementia), irritability, and stubbornness. Only when Babinski signs and loss of tendon reflexes in the legs were detected was the diagnosis entertained for the first time. By then he had been ill for nearly 10 years. One of our patients with Wilson's disease had twice been committed to a psychiatric hospital for paranoid tendencies and fighting with his family; the presence of a tremor and mild rigidity of the limbs had been attributed at first to phenothiazine drugs. In some of Griffin's cases of adrenomyeloneuropathy a spastic weakness of the legs and sensory ataxia progressing over several years were the main clinical manifestations; a spinocerebellar degeneration was suspected. One of our patients with Kufs' lipofuscinosis began to deteriorate mentally in early adult life and later showed an increasing rigidity with athetotic posturing of limbs and difficulty in walking; he succumbed to his disease after more than 10 years. Cerebellar ataxia, polymyoclonus, and progressive blindness have been observed in several adolescents and adults with a variant of G_2 gangliosidosis; cherry-red macular spots provided the clue to diagnosis. Several such cases have been reported recently, particularly among the Japanese (Miyatake). Dementia, optic atrophy, mild cerebellar ataxia and corticospinal signs have been features of several personally observed patients with Leigh's disease who survived in a relatively helpless state for nearly 20 years. One of our patients, an adolescent with severe diffuse myoclonus and seizures and slight intellectual deterioration, was found after several years to have one of the rare variants of Gaucher's disease; he is still alive. Another with dementia, rigidity, choreoathetosis, slight cerebellar ataxia and Babinski signs had a variant of Niemann-Pick disease. We also have under observation a family with Gaucher's disease, several members of which developed seizures, cerebellar ataxia, and mild blunting of the intellect in early adult life. We have had the experience of finding laboratory evidence of adrenal insufficiency in several young men with white matter lesions of the frontal lobes and other parts of the cerebrum; there was no bronzing of the skin, and earlier a diagnosis of multiple sclerosis or Schilder's disease had been made.

These rare forms of inherited metabolic disease are notable for their chronicity and for the early prominence of a particular neurologic symptom or syndrome. Once the disease is established, however, there is nearly always evidence of involvement of multiple neuronal systems, reflected in a subtle or overt dementia, character disorder, or signs referable to cerebellar, pyramidal, extrapyramidal, visual, and peripheral nerve structures. This multiplicity of neuronal system involvement is much more a feature of hereditary metabolic disease than of degenerative disease, and the finding of such involvement should always stimulate a search for an inherited metabolic disorder. The dictum that tract involvement (corticospinal, cerebellar, peduncular, sensory, optic nerve) indicates a leukodystrophy and that "gray matter" signs (seizures, myoclonus, dementia, retinal lesions) indicate a poliodystrophy is useful but not absolute. Some of the lysosomal storage diseases affect both galactolipids (galactocerebrosides and sulfatides) as well as gangliosides; hence both white and gray matter are involved.

In concluding this last section, which classifies the inherited metabolic diseases in accordance with their salient clinical characteristics, the careful reader will appreciate its artificiality. Nearly every one of the diseases of each category may present some neurologic abnormality other than the ones we have emphasized, so that the potential number of variations is almost limitless. However, it is hoped that the plan adopted here—of thinking of these diseases in reference to age periods and syndromic relationships—will facilitate the development of a clinical approach to this new and extremely difficult part of neurologic medicine.

REFERENCES

ADACHI M, et al: Electron microscopic and enzyme histochemical studies of the cerebellum in spongy degeneration. *Acta Neuropathol* 20:22, 1972.

ADAMS RD: Hereditary hepatocerebral degeneration of Wilson-Westphal-Strümpell with reference to acquired hepatocerebral degeneration, in Bammer HG (ed): *Future of Neurology.* Stuttgart, Georg Thieme Verlag, 1967, pp 45-69.

AGAMANOLIS DP, GREENSTEIN JI: Ataxia-telangiectasia. *J Neuropathol Exp Neurol* 38:475, 1979.

ALPERS BJ: Diffuse progressive degeneration of cerebral gray matter. *Arch Neurol Psychiatry* 25:469, 1931.

BANKER BQ, VICTOR M: Spongy degeneration of infancy, in Goodman RM, Motulsky AG (eds): *Genetic Diseases among Ashkenazi Jews.* New York, Raven, 1979, pp 210-216.

BLASS JP, AVIGAN J, UHLENDORF BW: A defect in pyruvate decarboxylase in a child with intermittent movement disorder. *J Clin Invest* 49:423, 1970.

CARTER S, GOLD AP (eds): *Neurology of Infancy and Childhood.* New York, Appleton-Century-Crofts, 1974.

CATEL W, SCHMIDT J: Uber familiare gichtische Diathese in Verbindung mit zerebalen und renalen Symptomen bei einen Kleinkind. *Dtsch Med Wochenschr* 84:2145, 1959.

CHRISTENSEN E, KRABBE KH: Poliodystrophia cerebri progressiva. *Arch Neurol Psychiatry* 61:28, 1949.

COWEN D, OLMSTEAD EV: Infantile neuroaxonal dystrophy. *J Neuropathol Exp Neurol* 22:175, 1963.

CROCKER AE et al: Wolman's disease: Three new patients with a recently described lipidosis. *Pediatrics* 35:627, 1965.

CROME L: A case of galactosaemia with the pathological and neuropathological findings. *Arch Dis Child* 37:415, 1962.

DAL CANTO MC, RAPIN I, SUZUKI K: Neuronal storage disorder with chorea and curvilinear bodies. *Neurology* 24:1026, 1974.

DANKS DM et al: Menkes kinky-hair syndrome. An inherited defect in the intestinal absorption of copper with widespread effects. *Birth Defects Orig Artic Series* 10(10):132, 1974.

DAWSON JR: Cellular inclusions in cerebral lesions of epidemic encephalitis. *Arch Neurol Psychiatry* 31:685, 1934.

DEVIVO DC et al: Defective activation of the pyruvate dehydrogenase complex in subacute necrotizing encephalomyelopathy (Leigh disease). *Ann Neurol* 6:483, 1979.

DREW AL JR: The degenerative and demyelinating diseases of the nervous system, in Carter S, Gold AP (eds): *Neurology of Infancy and Childhood.* New York, Appleton-Century-Crofts, 1974, chap 4, pp 57-89.

FAHR T: Idiopathische Verkalkung der Hirngefässe. *Zentralbl Allg Pathol* 50:129, 1930-1931.

FOLEY J: Calcification of the corpus striatum and dentate nuclei occurring in a family. *J Neurol Neurosurg Psychiatry* 14:253, 1951.

FØLLING A: Uber Ausscheidung von Phenylbrenztraubensaure in den Harn als Stoffwechselanomalie in Verbindung mit Imbezillität. *Hoppe-Seyler's Z Physiol Chem* 227:169, 1934.

FORD FR: *Diseases of the Nervous System in Infancy Childhood and Adolescence,* 6th ed. Springfield, Ill, Charles C Thomas, 1973.

GARCIN R et al: Les aspects neurologiques de l'angiokeratose de Fabry: A propos de deux cas. *Presse Med* 75:435, 1967.

GOKAY, FK, TUKEL K: Uber Fälle von familiaren cortico-striato-cerebellaren Syndrome. *Schweiz Med Wochenschr* 78:1043, 1948.

GRIFFIN JW et al: Adrenomyeloneuropathy: A probable variant of adrenoleukodystrophy. *Neurology* 27:1107, 1977.

HERS HG: Inborn lysosomal diseases. *Gastroenterology* 48:625, 1965.

HOLMES LB et al: *Mental Retardation: An Atlas of Diseases with Associated Physical Abnormalities.* New York, Macmillan, 1972.

HOMMES FA, POLMAN HA, REERINK JD: Leigh's encephalo-myelopathy: An inborn error of gluconeogenesis. *Arch Dis Child* 43:423, 1968.

HSIA YE: Inherited hyperammonemic syndromes. *Gastroenterology* 67:347, 1974.

HUNT JR: Dyssynergia cerebellaris myoclonica. *Brain* 44:490, 1921.

IGARASHI M et al: Fatty acid abnormality in adrenoleukodystrophy. *J Neurochem* 26:851, 1976.

ILLINGWORTH DR, CONNOR WE, MILLER RG: Abetalipoproteinemia. Report of two cases and review of therapy. *Arch Neurol* 37:659, 1980.

JOPPICH G, SCHULTE FJ: *Neurologie des Neugeborenen.* Berlin, Springer-Verlag, 1968.

KINSBOURNE M: Myoclonic encephalopathy in infants. *J Neurol Neurosurg Psychiatry* 25:271, 1962.

KISTLER JP et al: Mannosidosis. *Arch Neurol* 34:45, 1977.

KOIVISTO M, BLENCO-SEQUIROS M, KRAUSE U: Neonatal symptomatic hypoglycemia. A follow up of 151 children. *Dev Med Child Neurol* 14:603, 1972.

KOLODNY EH: Clinical and biochemical genetics of the lipidoses. *Semin Hematol* 9:251, 1972.

————: Current concepts in genetics. Lysosmal storage diseases. *N Engl J Med* 294:1217, 1976.

LANCE JW: Familial paroxysmal dystonic choreoathetosis and its differentiation from related syndromes. *Ann Neurol* 2:285, 1977.

LESCH M, NYHAN WL: A familial disorder of uric acid metabolism and central nervous system function. *Am J Med* 36:561, 1964.

LEVY HL: Newborn screening for metabolic disorders. *N Engl J Med* 288:1299, 1973.

————, MADIGAN PM, SHIH V: Mass metabolic disorder screening program. *Pediatrics*, 49:825, 1972.

LONSDALE D et al: Intermittent cerebellar ataxia associated with hyperpyruvic acidemia, hyperalininemia and hyperalininuria. *Pediatrics* 43:1025, 1969.

LOTT IT et al: Vitamin B$_6$-dependent seizures: Pathology and chemical findings in brain. *Neurology* 28:47, 1978.

MCFARLIN DE et al: The immunological deficiency state in ataxia-telangiectasia. *Res Publ Assoc Res Nerv Ment Dis* 49:275, 1971.

MELCHIOR JC et al: Familial idiopathic cerebral calcifications in childhood. *Am J Dis Child* 99:787, 1960.

MIYATAKE T et al: Adult type neuronal storage disease with neuraminidase deficiency. *Ann Neurol* 6:232, 1979.

MOSER HW et al: Adrenoleukodystrophy: Studies of the phenotype, genetics and biochemistry. *Johns Hopkins Med J* 147:217, 1980.

MOUNT LA, REBACK S: Familial paroxysmal choreoathetosis: Preliminary report on a hitherto undescribed clinical syndrome. *Arch Neurol Psychiatry* 44:841, 1940.

PINCUS JH: Subacute necrotizing encephalomyelopathy (Leigh's disease): A consideration of clinical features and etiology. *Dev Med Child Neurol* 14:87, 1972.

————, CHUTORIAN A: Familial benign chorea with intention tremor: A clinical entity. *J Pediatr* 70:724, 1967.

PRADER A, LABHART A, WILLI H: Ein syndrom von Adipositas, Kleinwuchs, Kryptochismus und Oligophrenie nach Myatonieartigem Zustand in Neugeborenenalter. *Schweiz Med Wochenschr* 86:1260, 1956.

PRECHTL H, BEINTEMA D: *The Neurological Examination of the Full-Term Newborn Infant.* London, Spastics Society, 1964.

ROSENBERG AL et al: Hyperuricemia and neurologic deficits: A family study. *N Engl J Med* 282:992, 1970.

SALAM M: Metabolic ataxias, in Vinken PJ, Bruyn GW (eds): *Handbook of Clinical Neurology,* vol 21. Amsterdam, North-Holland, 1975, chap 32, pp 573-585.

SASS-KORTSAK A, BEARN AG: Wilson's disease (hepatolenticular degeneration), in Stanbury JB et al (eds): *The Metabolic Basis of Inherited Disease,* 4th ed. New York, McGraw-Hill, 1978, pp 1103-1116.

SCHAUMBURG HH et al: Adrenomyeloneuropathy: A probable variant of adrenoleukodystrophy. *Neurology* 27:1114, 1977.

SCHEINBERG IH, GITLIN D: Deficiency of ceruloplasmin in patients with hepatolenticular degeneration (Wilson's disease). *Science* 116:484, 1952.

————, STERNLIEB I: Wilson's disease. *Ann Rev Med* 16:119, 1965.

SCHMID R, MCDONAGH AF: Hyperbilirubinemia, in Stanbury JB, Wyngaarden JB, Fredrickson DS (eds): *The Metabolic Basis of Inherited Diseases,* 4th ed. New York, McGraw-Hill, 1978, chap 51, pp 1238-1243.

SHIH VE: *Laboratory Techniques for the Detection of Hereditary Metabolic Disorders,* Long JW (ed). Cleveland, Ohio, CRC Press, 1973.

————: Urea cycle disorders and other congenital hyperammonemic syndromes, in Stanbury JB, Wyngaarden JB, Fredrickson DS (eds): *The Metabolic Basis of Inherited Disease,* 4th ed. New York, McGraw-Hill, 1978, pp 362-386.

———— et al: Sulfite oxidase deficiency. *N Engl J Med* 297:1022, 1977.

SHUMAN RM, LEECH RW, SCOTT CR: The neuropathology of the nonketotic and ketotic hyperglycinemias: Three cases. *Neurology* 28:139, 1978.

SIEMERLING E, CREUTZFELDT HG: Bronzkrankheit und sklerosierende Encephalomyelitis (Diffuse Sklerose). *Arch Psychiatr Nervenkr* 68:217, 1923.

SJÖGREN T: Die juvenile amaurotische Idiotie: Klinische und erblichkeitsmedizinische Untersuchungen. *Hereditas* 14:197, 1931.

STANBURY JB, WYNGAARDEN JB, FREDERICKSON DS (eds): *The Metabolic Basis of Inherited Disease,* 4th ed. New York, McGraw-Hill, 1978.

SWAIMAN KF, MENKES JH, PRENSKY AL: Metabolic disorders of the central nervous system, in Swaiman KF, Wright FS (eds): *The Practice of Pediatric Neurology.* St Louis, Mosby, 1975, chap 27, pp 359-479.

SZANTO J, GALLYAS F: A study of iron metabolism in neuropsychiatric patients: Hallervorden-Spatz disease. *Arch Neurol* 14:438, 1966.

TELLEZ-NAGEL I et al: Mucolipidosis IV. *Arch Neurol* 33:828, 1976.

VAKILI S et al: Hallervorden-Spatz syndrome. *Arch Neurol* 34:729, 1977.

VAN BOGAERT L: Contribution clinique et anatomique a l'étude de la paralysie agitante juvenile primitive. *Rev Neurol* 2:315, 1930.

————: Le cadre des xanthomatoses et leurs differents types: Xanthomatoses secondaires. *Rev Med* 17:433, 1962.

VOGT C, VOGT O: Zur Lehre der Erkrankungen des striaren Systems. *J Psychol Neurol* 25:627, 1920.

WILLVONSEDER R et al: A hereditary disorder with dementia, spastic dysarthria, vertical eye movement paresis, gait disturbance, splenomegaly, and abnormal copper metabolism. *Neurology* 23:1039, 1973.

WILSON SAK: Progressive lenticular degeneration: A familial nervous disease associated with cirrhosis of the liver. *Brain* 34:295, 1912.

YOKOI S, NAKAYAMA H, NEGESHI T: Biochemical studies on tissues from a patient with Lafora disease. *Clin Chim Acta* 62:415, 1975.

ZEMAN W et al: The neuronal ceroid-lipofuscinoses (Batten-Vogt syndrome), in Vinken PJ, Bruyn GW (eds): *Handbook of Clinical Neurology*, vol 10. Amsterdam, North-Holland, 1970, chap 25, pp 588-679.

CHAPTER 38

DISEASES OF THE NERVOUS SYSTEM
DUE TO NUTRITIONAL DEFICIENCY

Among nutritional disorders, those of the nervous system occupy a position of special interest and importance. The early studies of beriberi, at the turn of the century, were largely responsible for the discovery of thiamine, and, consequently, for the modern concept of deficiency disease. Despite the notable achievements in the science of nutrition which followed the discovery of vitamins, diseases due to nutritional deficiency—and particularly those of the nervous system—still represent a worldwide health problem of serious proportions. In Far Eastern communities, where the diet consists mainly of raw (as opposed to parboiled), highly milled rice, there is still a significant incidence of beriberi. In other underdeveloped countries, deficiency diseases are endemic, the result of chronic dietary deprivation. It comes as a surprise to many physicians to learn that deficiency diseases are also common in the United States and other parts of the Western world. Mainly this is due to the prevalence of alcoholism. Dietary faddism and impaired absorption of dietary nutrients (which occurs in patients with sprue, pernicious anemia, or surgical exclusion of portions of the gastrointestinal tract) account for a relatively small number of cases. Occasionally, manifestations of nutritional deficiency may be induced by the use of vitamin antagonists or certain drugs, such as isonicotinic acid hydrazide, which is used in the treatment of tuberculosis and which interferes with the enzymatic function of pyridoxine.

GENERAL CONSIDERATIONS

The term *deficiency* will be used throughout this chapter in its strictest sense, to designate disorders that result from *the lack of an essential nutrient or nutrients in the diet, or from a conditioning factor which increases the need for these nutrients.*

The most important of these nutrients are the vitamins, and more specifically, certain members of the B group—thiamine, nicotinic acid, pyridoxine, pantothenic acid, and cyanocobalamin (vitamin B_{12}). Most deficiency diseases cannot be related to the lack of a single vitamin (pernicious anemia or vitamin B_{12} deficiency being a notable exception); usually the effects of deficiency of several vitamins can be recognized. This truism should neither obscure the fact that certain manifestations of deficiency disease (e.g., the ocular palsies of Wernicke's disease) are indeed related to a deficiency of a specific nutrient, nor diminish the need to identify such relationships.

Nutritional diseases of the nervous system are however, not simply a matter of vitamin deprivation. Practically always, these diseases are associated with the general signs of undernutrition, such as circulatory abnormalities, and loss of subcutaneous fat and muscle bulk. Furthermore, a total lack of vitamins, which occurs in starvation, is not associated with beriberi or pellagra; a certain amount of food is necessary for the production of these syndromes. An excessive intake of carbohydrate relative to the supply of thiamine favors the development of a thiamine deficiency state. Deficiency diseases in general, including those of the nervous system, are influenced by factors such as exercise, growth, pregnancy, and infection, and by disorders of the liver and the gastrointestinal tract which might interfere with the synthesis and the absorption of essential nutrients.

As has been mentioned, alcoholism is an important factor in the causation of nutritional diseases of the nervous system, at least in the United States. Alcohol acts mainly by displacing food in the diet, but also by adding carbohydrate calories (alcohol is burned almost entirely as carbohydrate), thus increasing the need for thiamine. There is also evidence that alcohol impairs the absorption of thiamine and other vitamins from the gastrointestinal tract.

In infants and young children, a reduction of protein and caloric intake (so-called protein-calorie malnutrition or PCM) has a devastating effect upon body growth; even those with milder degrees of PCM may be permanently stunted. Whether or not PCM also hinders the growth of the brain, with consequent effects upon intellectual and behavioral development, cannot be answered as readily. The data bearing on this subject are discussed in the last part of this chapter.

Deficiency diseases of the nervous system may occur in pure form and will be so described, but usually they occur in various combinations. Stated another way, the nutritional disorders are characterized by involvement of both the central and peripheral nervous systems, an attribute which this category of disease shares with the hereditary metabolic disorders.

The following are the deficiency diseases to be discussed in this chapter:

1. Wernicke's disease and Korsakoff's psychosis

2. Nutritional polyneuropathy (neuritic beriberi)

3. Deficiency amblyopia (nutritional optic neuropathy; "tobacco-alcohol" amblyopia)

4. The neurologic aspects of pellagra (with some remarks on spinal spastic ataxia and nicotinic acid deficiency encephalopathy)

5. The syndrome of amblyopia, painful neuropathy and orogenital dermatitis (Strachan's syndrome)

6. Subacute combined degeneration of the spinal cord (vitamin B_{12} deficiency)

In addition, attention will be drawn to several distinctive neurologic disorders which are probably nutritional in origin, but in which the etiology is not proved. These are (1) "alcoholic" cerebellar degeneration, (2) central pontine myelinolysis, and (3) primary degeneration of the corpus callosum (Marchiafava-Bignami disease).

Finally, some comments will be made about the relationship of protein-calorie malnutrition to mental retardation, the neurologic disorders associated with gastrointestinal defects, and the vitamin-responsive hereditary diseases.

THE WERNICKE-KORSAKOFF SYNDROME

DEFINITION OF TERMS

Wernicke's disease and Korsakoff's psychosis are common nuerologic disorders which have been recognized since the 1880s. *Wernicke's disease* (polioencephalitis hemorrhagica superioris) is characterized by nystagmus, abducens and conjugate gaze palsies, ataxia of gait, and mental confusion. These symptoms usually have an abrupt onset and may occur singly or, more often, in various combinations. Wernicke's disease is due to nutritional deficiency, more specifically to a deficiency of thiamine and is observed mainly though not exclusively in alcoholics.

Korsakoff's psychosis (amnesic or amnestic-confabulatory psychosis; psychosis polyneuritica) refers to a unique mental disorder in which retentive memory is impaired out of all proportion to other cognitive functions, in an otherwise alert and responsive patient. This disorder, like Wernicke's disease, is usually associated with alcoholism and malnutrition, but it may be a symptom of various other disorders that have their basis in lesions of the diencephalon or the temporal lobes. Thus, classical instances of Korsakoff's psychosis may be observed in patients with third ventricular tumors, infarction (or surgical resection) of the inferomedial portions of the temporal lobes, or as a sequela of herpes simplex encephalitis. A transient impairment of retentive memory of the Korsakoff type may be the salient manifestation of temporal lobe epilepsy, concussive head injury, and so-called transient global amnesia; a permanent abnormality of this sort characterizes certain instances of anoxic encephalopathy and Alzheimer's disease.

In the alcoholic, nutritionally deficient patient, Korsakoff's psychosis is usually associated with Wernicke's disease. Stated in another way, Korsakoff's psychosis is the psychic manifestation of Wernicke's disease. For this reason, and others to be elaborated later, this symptom complex should be called *Wernicke's disease* with or without Korsakoff's psychosis, or the *Wernicke-Korsakoff syndrome*, if both components are present.

HISTORICAL NOTE

In 1881, Carl Wernicke first described an illness of sudden onset, characterized by paralysis of eye movements, ataxia of gait, and mental confusion. Swelling of the optic disks and retinal hemorrhages were also said to be present. His observations were made in three patients, of whom two were alcoholics and one was a young woman with persistent vomiting following the ingestion of sulfuric acid. In each of these patients there was progressive stupor and coma, culminating in death. The pathologic changes described by Wernicke consisted of punctate hemorrhages, primarily affecting the gray matter around the third and fourth ventricles and aqueduct of Sylvius; he considered these changes to be inflammatory in nature and confined to the gray matter, hence his designation "polioencephalitis hemorrhagica superioris."

In the belief that Gâyet had described an identical disorder in 1875, the term *Gâyet-Wernicke* is used frequently by French authors. Such a designation is hardly justified insofar as the lesion in Gâyet's patient consisted of a single hemorrhagic focus that occupied practically all of the pons (it was probably an instance of hemorrhagic leukoencephalitis); also the clinical features differed from those of Wernicke's patients in all essential details.

In a similar vein, a number of early writers, beginning with Magnus Huss in 1852, made casual reference to a disturbance of memory in the course of chronic alcoholism. However, the first comprehensive account of this disorder was given by the Russian psychiatrist S. S. Korsakoff, in a series of articles published between 1887 and 1891 (for English translation and commentary, see references). Korsakoff stressed the relationship between polyneuropathy and the disorder of memory (psychosis polyneuritica), which, he proposed, represented "two facets of the same disease." But he also made the point, generally disregarded by subsequent authors, that neuritis need not accompany the characteristic amnesic syndrome. Korsakoff's observations of the neuritic and mental aspects of the syndrome were made in both alcoholic and nonalcoholic patients. His clinical descriptions are remarkably complete and have hardly been excelled to the present day.

It is of interest that the relationship between Wernicke's disease and Korsakoff's polyneuritic psychosis was appreciated neither by Wernicke nor by Korsakoff. Murawieff, in 1897, first postulated that a single cause was responsible for both. The intimate clinical relationship was established by Bonhoeffer in 1904, who stated that in all cases of Wernicke's disease he found neuritis and an amnesic psychosis. Confirmation of this relationship on pathologic grounds came much later.

CLINICAL FEATURES

The incidence of Wernicke's disease and Korsakoff's psychosis cannot be stated with precision, but they are common disorders, judging from our experience. At the Cleveland Metropolitan General Hospital, for example, in a consecutive series of 3548 autopsies in adults, lesions of the Wernicke-Korsakoff syndrome were found in 77 cases (2.2 percent). The disease affects males and

females about equally and the age of onset is fairly evenly distributed, between 30 and 70 years.

The triad of clinical features described by Wernicke—ophthalmoplegia, ataxia, and mental confusion—is still diagnostically useful. Any one of them may be the initial manifestation. Often the disease begins with ataxia, followed in a few days or weeks by mental confusion; or there may be the simultaneous onset of ataxia and ocular symptoms with or without confusion. A description of each of the major manifestations follows.

Ocular Abnormalities The diagnosis of Wernicke's disease is made most readily on the basis of the ocular signs. These consist of (1) nystagmus that is both horizontal and vertical, (2) weakness or paralysis of the external rectus muscles, and (3) weakness or paralysis of conjugate gaze. Usually these abnormalities are combined.

The palsy of conjugate gaze varies from merely a nystagmus on extreme gaze to a complete loss of ocular movement in that direction. This applies to both horizontal and vertical movements, abnormalities of the former being somewhat more frequent. Paralysis of downward gaze is an unusual manifestation, but internuclear ophthalmoplegia is common. Next to nystagmus, the most frequent ocular abnormality is a lateral rectus weakness, which is always bilateral but not necessarily symmetrical, and which is accompanied by diplopia and internal strabismus. With complete paralysis of the lateral rectus muscles, nystagmus is initially absent in the abducting eyes, but it becomes evident as the weakness improves. In advanced stages of the disease there may be a complete loss of ocular movements, and the pupils, which are usually spared, may become miotic and nonreacting. Ptosis, small retinal hemorrhages, involvement of the near-far focusing mechanism, and evidence of optic neuropathy occur occasionally, but we have never observed papilledema in this disease.

Ataxia Essentially the ataxia is one of stance and gait, and in the acute stage of the disease it may be so severe that the patient cannot stand or walk without support. Lesser degrees of this disorder are characterized by a wide-based stance and by a slow, uncertain, short-stepped gait; in its mildest form the ataxia can be brought out only by tandem walking. In contrast to the gross disorder of locomotion is the relative infrequency of a clear-cut intention tremor. When present, it is more likely to be brought out by heel-to-knee than by finger-to-nose testing. Scanning speech is present only rarely.

Disturbances of Consciousness and Mentation These are present in all but 10 percent of patients. At least three types of deranged mental function can be recognized:

1. About 15 percent of patients show the signs of alcohol withdrawal, i.e., hallucinations and other disorders of perception, confusion, agitation, tremor, and overactivity of autonomic nervous system function. These symptoms are evanescent in nature and usually mild in degree.

2. By far the commonest derangement of mental function is a *global confusional state.* Typically, the patient is apathetic, inattentive, and indifferent to the surroundings. Spontaneous speech is minimal and many questions are unanswered, or the patient may suspend the conversation in the middle of a sentence and drift off to sleep—although he or she can be aroused from this state without difficulty. In spite of the fact that drowsiness is common, stupor or coma are distinctly rare as initial events in the illness. The questions that are answered by the patient betray disorientation in time and place, misidentification of those around, and an inability to grasp the meaning of the illness or immediate situation. Many of the patient's remarks are irrational and lack consistency from one moment to another. If the patient's interest and attention can be maintained long enough to ensure adequate testing, one finds that memory and learning ability are also impaired. Under the influence of thiamine or of an adequate diet, the patient rapidly becomes more alert and attentive and more capable of taking part in mental testing. Then the most prominent abnormality is one of retentive memory (Korsakoff's psychosis).

3. Some patients are alert and responsive from the time they are first seen, and already show the characteristic features of Korsakoff's amnesic psychosis. In yet others Korsakoff's psychosis is the only manifestation of the syndrome, and no ocular or ataxic signs can be discerned. The memory disorder, which constitutes the chronic and truly crippling aspect of the Wernicke-Korsakoff syndrome, is described below.

The Amnesic State The general features of the amnesic, or Korsakoff's, syndrome have been discussed in Chap. 20. In the alcoholic, nutritionally depleted patient the syndrome is highly stereotyped. Invariably there is a

permanent gap in the patient's memory of the acute phase of the illness, attributable no doubt to the impairment of registration and general confusion which are so prominent during that period.

As indicated in Chap. 20, the core of amnesic disorder is an impairment of learning (anterograde amnesia) and of past memories (retrograde amnesia). The defect in learning is never complete but may be very severe in degree. The patient may be incapable, for example, of committing to memory three simple facts (such as the examiner's name, the date, and the time of day) despite countless attempts; they can repeat each fact as it is presented, indicating that they understand what is wanted of them and that "registration" is intact, but by the time the third fact is repeated, the first may have been forgotten. Since the adaptation to new situations requires the formation of new memories and their integration with past experience, it is this learning defect that renders patients helpless in society and capable of performing only the most habitual tasks.

The anterograde amnesia is always coupled with a *disturbance of past memory.* As a rule, the latter disorder is also severe in degree, though rarely complete, and covers a period that antedates the onset of the illness by several years. Characteristically, isolated events and information from the past are retained, but these are related without regard for the intervals which separated them or for their proper temporal sequence. Usually the patient "telescopes" events, sometimes the opposite. This aspect of the memory disorder becomes prominent after the acute stage of the illness has passed and some improvement in memory function has occurred, and may account for certain instances of confabulation (see below).

It is probably true that memories of the recent past are more severely impaired than those of the remote past, but this is not to say that remote memories are intact. Memories of the distant past are not as readily tested as more recent ones and are therefore difficult to compare. It is our impression, based on observations of patients whose past history could be obtained in detail, that memories of the distant past are impaired in practically all cases of Korsakoff's psychosis and seriously impaired in some of them.

It should be emphasized that all the manifestations of Korsakoff's psychosis cannot be explained in terms of memory loss alone. Formal psychological testing, using Wechsler's Adult Intelligence Scale, discloses a characteristic though nonspecific pattern of impairment of cognitive functions. The most consistent failure is with the digit symbol task, and to a lesser degree, with arithmetic and block design. Applying the customary interpretations to these tests, the defects are in learning ability in a new situation, spatial organization, and visual and verbal abstraction. However, patients have a relatively normal capacity to reason with data immediately before them—i.e., in circumstances where memory function is not the major factor.

Using a battery of tests of perceptual functions, Talland has demonstrated a number of defects in Korsakoff patients which could not be attributed to a primary abnormality in learning or memorizing. Whereas patients showed no deficit in immediate apprehension, they were greatly handicapped if the task was changed and a new "mental set" required, especially if the first task was continued. It seemed that patients were excessively dependent upon the immediate sensory input; their inability to detach themselves from it by imagery or to change their orientation toward it prevented them from assimilating a diversity of newly presented material. In addition, Korsakoff patients showed serious defects in the formation of concepts. Talland proposed that the inability to adopt new attitudes of orientation to a situation is the basic abnormality in both the perceptual and conceptual deficits.

Confabulation is generally considered to be an indispensable attribute of Korsakoff's psychosis. The validity of this view depends largely on how one defines confabulation, but there is no uniformity of opinion on this point. Some patients simply do not confabulate, no matter how broadly one interprets this term. In our experience, confabulation is associated with two phases of Korsakoff's psychosis: the initial phase, in which profound general confusion dominates the disease; and the convalescent phase in which the patient recalls fragments of past experience in a distorted fashion. Events that were separated by long intervals are juxtaposed or related out of sequence, so that the narrative has an implausible or fictional aspect. Whether this disorder is regarded as confabulation or as a particular defect of retentive memory is academic. In the chronic, stable state of the disease, confabulation is usually absent.

The statement is often made that the Korsakoff patient fills gaps in memory with confabulation. In the sense that gaps in memory exist and that whatever the patient supplies in place of the correct answers fills these gaps, the statement is incontrovertible. It is hardly explanatory, however. The implication that confabulation is a deliberate attempt to hide the memory defect, out of embarrassment or for other reasons, is probably not correct. In fact, the opposite seems to pertain: as the patient improves and becomes more aware of a defect in memory, the tendency to confabulate becomes less.

Prognosis Once the symptoms of Korsakoff's psychosis are established, complete or almost complete recovery occurs in only about 20 percent of patients. Of the remainder, some improve slightly, to the point where they can find their way to their room or dining hall; others improve somewhat more, so they are eventually able to carry out routine household or institutional tasks under supervision. Improvement may begin within a few weeks after the amnesic syndrome is recognized and treated, but in the majority of cases the onset of improvement is delayed for 1 to 3 months, and the maximum degree of recovery may not be attained for a year, or longer.

Other Clinical Abnormalities Signs of *peripheral nerve disease* are found in more than 80 percent of patients with Wernicke's disease. In the majority of cases the neuropathic affection is mild in degree and does not account for the disorder of gait, but it may be so severe that stance and gait cannot be tested. In a small number of cases, retrobulbar neuropathy is added. Although peripheral neuropathy is a common finding in Wernicke's disease, overt signs of beriberi heart disease are rare. However, indications of *disordered cardiovascular function* such as tachycardia, exertional dyspnea, postural hypotension, and minor electrocardiographic abnormalities are frequent; an occasional patient may die suddenly, following slight exertion. These patients may show an elevation of cardiac output out of proportion to oxygen consumption, associated with low peripheral vascular resistance—abnormalities that revert to normal after the administration of thiamine. *Postural hypotension* and syncope are common findings in Wernicke's disease and are probably due to impaired function of the autonomic nervous system, more specifically to a defect in the sympathetic outflow (Birchfield). In the chronic stage of the disease, many patients demonstrate an *impaired capacity to discriminate between odors.* The studies of Mair et al. suggest that this deficit is attributable, not to a lesion of the peripheral olfactory system or to the rapid decay of memory stores, but to a lesion of the medial dorsal nucleus and its neocortical connections.

Ancillary Findings Vestibular function, as measured by the response to standard ice-water caloric tests, is universally impaired in the acute stage of Wernicke's disease (Ghez). To this abnormality of function, which is bilateral and more or less symmetrical, the term *vestibular paresis* may be applied. It probably accounts for the severe disequilibrium in the initial stage of the illness. The *CSF* in uncomplicated cases of the Wernicke-Korsakoff syndrome is normal or shows only a modest elevation of the protein content. Protein values above 100 mg per 100 ml or a CSF pleocytosis should suggest the presence of a complicating illness—subdural hematoma and meningeal infection being the most common.

Blood pyruvate is consistently elevated in untreated cases of Wernicke's disease. The usefulness of this estimation as an index of thiamine deficiency is limited, however, mainly because of its lack of specificity. This shortcoming has been overcome to a large extent by the introduction of the *blood transketolase assay* as an index of thiamine deficiency. Transketolase, one of the enzymes of the hexose monophosphate shunt, requires thiamine pyrophosphate as a cofactor. The estimation of transketolase activity in red cell hemolysates (Dreyfus and Moniz) requires the incubation of samples of hemolyzed whole blood with an excess of ribose-5-phosphate substrate, both in a plain buffered medium and in a medium containing an excess of thiamine pyrophosphate (TPP). The sedoheptulose-7-phosphate (S7P) elaborated after an incubation period of 30 min at 38°C is then measured spectrophotometrically, and the results are expressed as micrograms of S7P produced per milliliter of hemolysate per hour. The difference in enzymatic activity between the tube containing plain medium and the tube containing excess thiamine pyrophosphate, expressed in percent, is designated as the *TPP effect*.

In normal adult human control subjects, transketolase values range from 90 to 140 μg S7P per milliliter per hour and the TPP effect from 0 to 10 percent, depending upon the degree of vitamin supplementation. Before specific treatment with thiamine, patients with Wernicke's disease show a marked reduction in their transketolase activity (as low as one-third of normal values) and a striking TPP effect (up to 50 percent). Restoration of these values toward normal occurs within a few hours of the administration of thiamine, and completely normal values are usually attained within 24 h.

An interesting abnormality of transketolase has recently been described by Blass and Gibson. They found that transketolase in fibroblasts from four alcoholics with Wernicke-Korsakoff disease bound TPP less avidly than did the transketolase from control lines. Presumably this defect in transketolase would be insignificant if the diet were adequate, but would be deleterious if the diet were low in thiamine. These findings, if corroborated, would implicate an hereditary factor in the genesis of Wernicke-Korsakoff disease, and would explain why only a small proportion of nutritionally deficient alcoholics develop this disease.

Only about half the patients with Wernicke-Kor-

sakoff disease show EEG abnormalities, consisting of diffuse slow activity, mild to moderate in degree. Total cerebral blood flow and cerebral oxygen and glucose consumption may be greatly reduced in the acute stages of the disease, and these defects may still be present after several weeks of treatment (Shimojyo et al.). These observations indicate that profound reductions in brain metabolism need not be reflected in EEG abnormalities or in depression of the state of consciousness, and that the latter is a function of the location of the lesion, not the overall degree of metabolic defect.

COURSE OF THE ILLNESS

The mortality rate in the acute phase of Wernicke's disease was 17 percent in our series of patients. Most of the fatalities were attributable to infection (pneumonia, pulmonary tuberculosis, and septicemia being the most common) and decompensated liver disease due to cirrhosis. Some deaths undoubtedly were due to thiamine deficiency that had reached an irreversible stage.

Patients who recover respond to specific treatment (administration of thiamine) in a fairly predictable manner. The most dramatic improvement is in the *ocular manifestations*. Recovery often *begins* within hours after the administration of thiamine, and practically always within several days. This effect is so constant that a failure of the ocular palsies to respond to thiamine should raise doubts about the diagnosis of Wernicke's disease. Sixth nerve palsies, ptosis, and vertical gaze palsies recover completely, within a week or two in most cases, but vertical nystagmus may occasionally persist for several months. Horizontal gaze palsies recover completely as a rule, but in 60 percent of cases a fine horizontal nystagmus remains as a permanent sequela of the disease. In this respect, horizontal nystagmus is unique among the ocular signs.

In comparison to the ocular signs, improvement of *ataxia* is somewhat delayed. In most patients improvement is noted within a week, and in most of the remainder, within 1 to 3 weeks after treatment is begun. About 40 percent of patients recover completely from ataxia. The remainder recover incompletely or not at all, and are left with a slow, shuffling, wide-based gait and inability to walk tandem. The residual gait disturbances and horizontal nystagmus provide a means of identifying obscure and chronic cases of dementia as alcoholic-nutritional in origin.

Vestibular function, as disclosed by caloric testing, improves at about the same rate as the ataxia of stance and gait, i.e., over a period of weeks or months, and recovery is usually but not always complete.

The symptoms that constitute the *global confusional state* are always reversible. In about 15 percent of patients these symptoms improve rapidly and completely, in a matter of a week or two. In the remainder, the symptoms of apathy, drowsiness, and global confusion improve more slowly, and as they recede, the defect in memory and learning (Korsakoff's psychosis) stands out more clearly. The memory disorder, once it becomes established, recovers in only a small proportion of patients, as has been indicated above, in the discussion of the amnesic state.

It is apparent, from the foregoing account, that the symptoms of Wernicke's disease and Korsakoff's psychosis do not comprise separate diseases; rather, the changing ocular and ataxic signs and the transformation of the global confusional state into an amnesic syndrome are successive stages in the recovery of a single disease process. Of 186 patients in our series who presented with Wernicke's disease and survived the acute illness, 157 (84 percent) showed this sequence of clinical events. As a corollary, a survey of alcoholic patients with Korsakoff's psychosis in a state mental hospital disclosed that in most of them the illness had begun with the symptoms of Wernicke's disease, and that most of them still showed the ocular or cerebellar stigmata, or both, of Wernicke's disease many years after the onset.

NEUROPATHOLOGIC FINDINGS AND CLINICAL-PATHOLOGIC CORRELATION

Patients who die in the acute stages of Wernicke's disease show symmetrical lesions in the paraventricular regions of the thalamus and hypothalamus, the mammillary bodies, the periaqueductal region of the midbrain, and floor of the fourth ventricle, particularly in the regions of the dorsal motor nuclei of the vagus and vestibular nuclei, and the superior vermis. Lesions are consistently found in the mammillary bodies, less consistently in other areas. The microscopic changes are characterized by varying degrees of necrosis of parenchymal structures, though it is seldom complete. The tissue appears loose and vacuolated. Within the area of necrosis, nerve cells are lost, but usually some remain; some of these are damaged, but others are intact. These changes result in a prominence of the blood vessels, although in some cases there is a true endothelial proliferation. In the areas of parenchymal damage there is a density of cells, representing astrocytic and microglial proliferation. These alterations are most intense in the center of the lesion, shading off toward the periphery. Discrete hemorrhages were found in only 20 percent of our cases, and many of them appeared to be agonal in nature. The cerebellar changes consist of a degeneration

of all layers of the cortex, particularly of the Purkinje cells; usually this lesion is confined to the superior parts of the vermis, but in advanced cases the cortex of the most anterior parts of the anterior lobes is involved as well.

Correlation of the clinical manifestations with the anatomic localization of lesions indicates that the ocular muscle and gaze palsies are attributable to lesions of the sixth and third nerve nuclei and adjacent tegmentum, and the nystagmus to lesions in the regions of the vestibular nuclei. The latter lesions are also responsible for the loss of caloric responses and probably for the gross disturbance of equilibrium that characterizes the initial stages of the disease. The lack of significant destruction of nerve cells in these lesions accounts for the rapid improvement and the high degree of recovery of oculomotor and vestibular function. The persistent ataxia of stance and gait is due to the lesion of the superior vermis of the cerebellum; ataxia of individual movements of the legs is attributable to an extension of the lesion into the anterior parts of the anterior lobes. Hypothermia, an occasional occurrence in Wernicke's disease, is probably attributable to lesions in the posterior and posterolateral nuclei of the hypothalamus, since these nuclei are commonly affected in Wernicke's disease and experimentally placed lesions in these parts have been shown to cause hypothermia in monkeys.

The neuropathologic changes in patients who die in the chronic stages of the disease, when the amnesic symptoms predominate, are very much the same as the changes in patients who die in the acute stages of Wernicke's disease. Apart from the expected differences with respect to the age of the glial and vascular reactions, the only important difference has to do with the involvement or lack of involvement of the medial dorsal nucleus of the thalamus and perhaps of the posterior nucleus as well. These structures were consistently involved in patients who had shown Korsakoff's psychosis during life; they were not involved in patients who had had no symptoms of Korsakoff's psychosis, although the mammillary bodies were involved in all of them. These observations suggest that the lesions responsible for the memory disorder are those of the medial thalami, rather than of the mammillary bodies, as is frequently stated.

The lesion responsible for the olfactory deficit is uncertain. It may be in the mammillary nuclei, ventromedial nucleus of the hypothalamus, or dorsomedial nucleus of the thalamus, all of which are thought to function as relay nuclei in the central connections that mediate olfactory sensation (Mair et al.).

McEntee and Mair have pointed out that the paraventricular lesions of the Wernicke-Korsakoff syndrome lie in the monoamine-containing pathways, and have presented evidence that levels of 3-methoxy-4-hydroxyphenylglycol, the primary brain metabolite of norepinephrine, are decreased in the CNS of patients with Korsakoff's psychosis. They found further that the administration of clonidine, a putative alpha-noradrenergic agonist, seemed to improve the disorder of memory in these patients. On the basis of these observations, McEntee and Mair have theorized that damage to ascending norepinephrine-containing neurons in the brainstem and diencephalon may be the basis for the amnesia in Korsakoff's psychosis.

THE NUTRITIONAL DEFECT IN WERNICKE'S DISEASE AND KORSAKOFF'S PSYCHOSIS

For many years it was believed that Wernicke's disease was due to the toxic effects of alcohol. The first steps in the identification of Wernicke's disease as a nutritional disorder were taken when it was recognized to be a complication of gastric carcinoma and other disturbances of the alimentary tract, and of hyperemesis gravidarum. Shortly after the appearance of these reports, Alexander and his colleagues drew attention to the similarity of the pathologic changes in pigeons deprived of B vitamins and the changes observed in Wernicke's disease; it then became evident that the lesions in many thiamine-deficient mammalian species also bore such a resemblance.

Thiamine is the specific nutritional factor responsible for most if not all the symptomatology of Wernicke's disease. Ophthalmoplegia, nystagmus, and ataxia can be reversed by the administration of thiamine alone, although horizontal nystagmus and ataxia may persist in mild form for months or years after their onset. The marked sensitivity of the ophthalmoplegia to the administration of thiamine accounts for the rapid disappearance of this sign after a meal or two, and the quality of prompt reversibility suggests that the symptoms are due more to a biochemical abnormality than to structural change.

Many of the initial mental symptoms—apathy, drowsiness, listlessness, inattentiveness, and inability to concentrate and to sustain a conversation—clear rapidly under the influence of thiamine alone. With respect to memory defect and confabulation, the specific role of thiamine is less certain. The amnesic symptoms recover slowly and incompletely, and at much the same rate both in patients who are given a full diet and all vitamins from the outset, and in those who receive a deficient diet, supplemented only with thiamine. These observations suggest that the memory loss is due to a structural lesion rather than to a reversible biochemical process.

INFANTILE BERIBERI

This term designates an acute and frequently fatal disease of infants, which until recently was very common in rice-eating communities of the Far East. It affects only breast-fed infants, usually in the second to the fifth months of life. Acute cardiac symptoms dominate the clinical picture, but neurologic symptoms (aphonia, strabismus, nystagmus, spasmodic contraction of facial muscles, and convulsions) have been described in many cases. This syndrome can be reversed dramatically by the administration of thiamine, so that some authors prefer to call it *acute thiamine deficiency in infants.*

Infantile beriberi bears no consistent relationship to beriberi in the mother. Infants of mothers with overt signs of beriberi may be quite normal. Conversely, mothers of infants with beriberi are themselves frequently free of the disease. The levels of thiamine in the breast milk of such mothers has not been determined, however. The absence of beriberi in the mothers of affected infants suggested that infantile beriberi might be due to a toxic factor in breast milk, but such a factor, if it exists, has never been isolated.

In the few neuropathologic studies that have been made of this disorder, changes like those of Wernicke's disease in the adult have been described.

TREATMENT OF THE WERNICKE-KORSAKOFF SYNDROME

Wernicke's disease constitutes a medical emergency, and its recognition demands the immediate administration of thiamine. The prompt use of thiamine prevents the progression of the disease and reverses those lesions that have not yet progressed to the point of fixed structural change. In patients who show only ocular signs and ataxia, the administration of thiamine is crucial in preventing the development of an amnesic psychosis.

Although 2 to 3 mg of thiamine may be sufficient to modify the ocular signs, much larger doses are usually employed—50 mg intravenously and 50 mg intramuscularly, the latter dose being repeated each day until the patient resumes a normal diet. The administration of thiamine frequently has diagnostic as well as therapeutic value, as indicated above.

The further management of Wernicke's disease involves the use of a balanced diet and all the B vitamins, since the patient is usually deficient in more than thiamine alone. It is also good practice to give B vitamins to all alcoholic patients, particularly those being treated with parenteral glucose. Characteristically, such patients have subsisted on a diet low in thiamine and disproportionately high in carbohydrate, and often gastroenteritis and diarrhea are associated. In these circumstances the patient's reserve of thiamine may be exhausted after 7 or 8 weeks; the administration of glucose at this time may precipitate Wernicke's disease or cause an early form of the disease to progress rapidly.

A problem in management may arise once the patient has recovered from Wernicke's disease and the amnesic psychosis becomes prominent. The onset of recovery of mental function may be delayed for several weeks or even months, and then it proceeds very slowly over a period of many months. The extent to which the amnesic symptoms will recover cannot be predicted accurately during the acute stages of the illness; one must guard against the premature commitment of the patient to a mental hospital.

NUTRITIONAL POLYNEUROPATHY
(Neuropathic Beriberi)

Most physicians have a somewhat bemused notion about beriberi, which they recall as an ill-defined, predominantly cardiac disorder occurring among the rice-eating people of the Orient. In fact, beriberi is a rather distinct clinical entity which is not restricted to any particular part of the world. Essentially it is a disease of the heart and of the peripheral nerves (which may be affected separately), with or without edema, the latter feature providing the basis for the classical division into wet and dry forms. The cardiac manifestations range from tachycardia and exertional dyspnea to acute and rapidly fatal heart failure. The latter is the most dramatic manifestation of beriberi, but is uncommon. Here we will be concerned with the affection of the peripheral nerves, or *neuropathic beriberi*, as it will be designated.

That beriberi is essentially a degenerative disorder of the peripheral nerves was established in the latter part of the nineteenth century by the classical studies of Eijkman and of Pekelharing and Winkler. Only after beriberi gained acceptance as a nutritional disease (this followed Funk's discovery of vitamins in 1911) was it

suspected that the neuropathy of alcoholics was also nutritional in origin. The similarity between beriberi and alcoholic neuropathy was commented upon by several authors, but it was Shattuck, in 1928, who first seriously discussed the relationship of the two disorders. He suggested that "polyneuritis of chronic alcoholism was caused chiefly by failure to take or assimilate food containing a sufficient quantity of vitamin B . . . and might properly be regarded as true beriberi." Convincing evidence that "alcoholic neuritis" is not due to the neurotoxic effect of alcohol was supplied by Strauss. He allowed 10 patients to continue their daily consumption of whiskey while they were given a well-balanced diet supplemented with yeast and vitamin B concentrates; improvement occurred in all the patients. Our own observations are supportive of Strauss' contention that all alcoholic polyneuropathy is nutritional.

The nutritional factor(s) responsible for the neuropathy of alcoholism and beriberi have not been precisely defined. Because of the difficulties in producing peripheral neuropathy in Mammalia by means of a thiamine-deficient diet, several authors have questioned whether thiamine is the antineuritic vitamin. Very few of the animal experiments undertaken to settle this point are satisfactory from a nutritional and pathologic point of view. Nevertheless, several studies in birds and in humans do indeed indicate that uncomplicated thiamine deficiency may result in peripheral nerve disease. The necessity of either accepting or rejecting the specific role of thiamine became less urgent when it was demonstrated, both in animals and in humans, that a deficiency of pyridoxine or of pantothenic acid could result in degeneration of the peripheral nerves.

PATHOLOGIC FEATURES

The essential pathologic change is axonal degeneration with destruction of both axon and myelin sheath, but variable amounts of segmental demyelination may also occur. The latter change may be difficult to discern in myelin-stained sections of whole nerve trunks, but can be observed in teased nerve fibers stained with osmium. The most pronounced changes are observed in the distal parts of the longest and largest myelinated fibers in the crural and, to a lesser extent, in the brachial nerves. In advanced cases the degenerative changes involve the anterior and posterior nerve roots. The vagus and phrenic nerves and paravertebral sympathetic trunks may be implicated in advanced cases.

Anterior horn and dorsal root ganglion cells undergo chromatolysis, indicating axonal damage. Degenerative changes in the posterior columns are seen in some cases, and are probably secondary to the changes in the posterior roots.

CLINICAL FEATURES

The symptomatology of nutritional polyneuropathy is diverse. In fact, many patients are asymptomatic, and evidence of peripheral nerve affection is found only on examination. In the latter circumstance the neuropathic signs are mild in degree, consisting only of thinness and tenderness of the leg muscles, loss or depression of the Achilles reflexes and perhaps of the patellar reflexes as well, and at times a patchy blunting of pain and touch sensation over the feet and shins.

The majority of patients, however, are symptomatic—weakness, paresthesias, and pain being the usual complaints. The symptoms are insidious in onset and slowly progressive, although occasionally they seem to evolve or to worsen rapidly over a matter of days. The initial symptoms are often referred to the distal portion of the limbs and progress proximally if the illness remains untreated. The legs may be affected exclusively; they are always affected earlier and more severely than the arms. Usually some aspect of motor disability constitutes the chief complaint, but in about one-quarter of the patients the main complaints are pain and paresthesias. The discomfort takes many forms: a dull constant ache in the feet or legs; sharp and lancinating pains, momentary in duration, like those of tabes dorsalis; cramping sensations in the muscles of the feet and calves; "tightness" of the calves; or bandlike feelings around the legs. Coldness of the feet is a common complaint, but it is purely subjective. Far more distressing are feelings of heat or "burning"; these affect the soles mainly, less frequently the dorsal aspects of the feet. They fluctuate in severity or they may be intermittent in nature; characteristically, they are worsened by contactual stimuli. In severe cases patients cannot bear to have the bedclothes touch their feet, nor can they bear to walk, despite the relative preservation of motor power. The term *burning feet* has been applied to this syndrome, but is not particularly apt, since the patient complains not only of "burning" but of other types of paresthesia and pain, and these symptoms may involve the hands as well as the feet.

Examination discloses varying degrees of motor, sensory, and reflex loss. As the symptoms suggest, the signs are symmetrical, usually more severe in distal than in proximal portions of the limbs, and often confined to the legs. The disproportionate affection of motor power may be striking, taking the form of a foot and wrist drop, but even in these patients the proximal muscles are usually affected. Involvement of thigh muscles is indicated by difficulty in arising from a squatting position. In other patients, all the leg muscles are affected more or less equally, and in still others the proximal muscles are disproportionately weakened. Absolute paralysis of the legs is observed only rarely; immobility due to contractures at the knees and ankles is a more common occurrence. Tenderness of muscles on pressure is a highly characteristic finding. This is elicited most readily in the muscles of the feet and calves, but all muscles of the limbs may be painful on pressure—even if they show only minimal weakness. Deep tendon reflexes in the legs are almost always lost, even when weakness is slight in degree. In the arms, tendon reflexes are sometimes retained, despite a loss of strength in the hands. In a small number of patients, particularly those in whom pain and paresthesias are prominent, the reflexes may be of greater than average briskness.

Excessive sweating of the soles and dorsal aspects of the feet, and of the volar surfaces of the hands and fingers, is a common manifestation and hypotension a rare manifestation of alcoholic neuropathy. These symptoms are indicative of involvement of the peripheral sympathetic nerve fibers.

Sensory loss or impairment usually involves all the modalities, although one may be affected out of proportion to the others. One cannot predict from the patient's symptoms which mode of sensation might be affected disproportionately. In cases with impairment of superficial sensation (i.e., of touch, pain, and temperature), the border between normal and impaired sensation is not sharp but shades off gradually over a considerable vertical extent of the limbs.

Patients in whom pain is the outstanding symptom do not constitute a distinct group in terms of their neurologic signs. Pain and dysesthesias may be prominent symptoms in cases with severe or very slight degrees of motor, reflex, and sensory loss. The term *hyperesthetic* is used commonly to designate the exquisitely painful form of neuropathy but is not well chosen, as pointed out on page 97; the term implies a heightened receptiveness of the nervous system or an increased response of the receptors to tactile and painful stimuli.

Actually, in patients with severe "hyperesthesia" one is usually able, by using finely graded stimuli, to demonstrate an elevated threshold to painful, thermal, and tactile stimuli in the "hyperesthetic" zone. Once the stimulus is perceived, however, it has a severely painful, diffuse, or unpleasant quality (hyperpathia).

In most cases, nutritional polyneuropathy involves only the limbs; the abdominal, thoracic, and bulbar musculature is spared. In patients with severe neuropathy, hoarseness and weakness of the voice and dysphagia due to affection of the vagus nerves may be added to the clinical picture.

An idea of the incidence of the motor, reflex, and sensory abnormalities and the combinations in which they occur can be obtained from Table 38-1, derived from the study of 189 nutritionally depleted alcoholic patients. The legs were affected in all cases and exclusively in 132 (70 percent) of the 189 cases. In the remaining 57 cases, both the arms and legs were involved; in these cases the neuropathic signs were severe in degree and almost always more severe in the legs than in the arms. In no case were the arms alone affected. Only 66 (35 percent) of the 189 patients showed the clinical picture of polyneuropathy in its entirety—i.e., a symmetrical impairment or loss of tendon reflexes, sensation, and motor power affecting legs more than the arms, and the distal more than the proximal segments of the limbs. In the remaining patients the motor-reflex-sensory signs occurred in various combinations, as indicated in Table 38-1. In about two-thirds of the patients with sensory abnormalities, both superficial and deep sensation were impaired more or less equally; 25 percent showed a predominant affection of superficial sensation (touch, pain, and temperature); and in the remaining 10 percent, deep sensation (deep pressure, vibratory and position sense)

Table 38-1

Neuropathic abnormality	Legs (189 cases)	Arms (57 cases)
Loss of reflexes alone	45 (24)*	6 (10)†
Loss of sensation alone	10 (5)	10 (18)
Weakness alone	—	5 (9)
Weakness and sensory loss	2 (1)	10 (18)
Reflex and sensory loss	40 (21)	2 (3)
Sensory, motor, and reflex loss	66 (35)	17 (30)
Data incomplete	26 (14)	7 (12)

*Figures in parentheses indicate percent of 189 cases.
†Figures in parentheses indicate percent of 57 cases.

was seemingly impaired to a greater extent. Usually vibratory and position sense were involved together, but in some cases one or the other was selectively affected.

The CSF is usually normal, although a modest elevation of protein content is found in a small number of cases. Sensory and motor nerve conduction velocities are reduced to a varying degree and the electromyogram of paralyzed muscles reveals denervation (see Chap. 44). In the alcoholic patient, skin changes (dryness and scaliness, pigmentation over the forehead and malar eminences, acne vulgaris, rhinophyma, or frank lesions of pellagra), folic acid–deficiency anemia, and liver disease frequently coexist.

TREATMENT AND PROGNOSIS

The first consideration in treatment is to supply adequate nutrition in the form of a balanced diet supplemented with B vitamins. It is equally important to make certain that the patient eats the prescribed diet. If persistent vomiting or other gastrointestinal complications prevent the patient from eating, then parenteral feeding becomes necessary; the vitamins may be given intramuscularly or added to intravenous fluids. A suitable parenteral preparation is Berroca-C, one ampul daily.

Where pain and sensitivity of the feet are the major complaints, the pressure of bedclothes may be avoided by placing a cradle support over the legs. Aching of the limbs may be related to their immobility, in which case they should be moved passively on frequent occasions. Acetylsalicylic acid, in a dosage of 0.3 to 1.0 g (5 to 15 grains) every 4 h, usually is sufficient to control hyperpathia; occasionally codeine in doses of 15 to 30 mg has to be added. Opiates and the addicting synthetic analgesics should be avoided, particularly if the pain is chronic in nature. Some of our patients with severe burning pain (similar to causalgia) in the feet have been helped by blocking the lumbar sympathetic ganglia.

The regeneration of peripheral nerves, which may take many months, will be of no avail if the muscles which they innervate have been allowed to undergo contracture and the joints to become fixed. During the day, the patient's legs should be positioned so that the soles rest firmly against a footboard, in order to prevent shortening of the heel cords. In cases of severe paralysis, molded splints should be applied to the arms, hands, legs, and feet during periods of rest. Pressure on the heels and elbows can be avoided by padding the splints and by turning the patient frequently or by asking the patient to turn. As soon as the patient's general condition permits, the limbs must be passively moved through a full range of movement several times daily. Gentle massage is also useful. As function returns, more vigorous physiotherapeutic measures can be undertaken.

Recovery from nutritional polyneuropathy is a slow process. In the mildest cases there may be a considerable restoration of motor function in a few weeks. In severe forms of the disease, several months may pass before the patient is able to walk unaided. The slowness of recovery creates a special problem for the alcoholic patient. In the alcoholic, the great danger to continued recovery is the resumption of drinking. Suitable arrangements must therefore be made for close supervision during the long and tedious convalescence.

DEFICIENCY AMBLYOPIA (Nutritional Optic Neuropathy, "Tobacco-Alcohol Amblyopia")

These terms refer to a characteristic form of visual impairment that results from nutritional deficiency. The defect in vision is due not to an abnormality of the cornea or other parts of the refractive mechanism (hence the term *amblyopia*), but to a lesion of the optic nerve, more or less confined to the region of the papillomacular bundle.

Typically, the patient complains of dimness or blurring of vision for near and distant objects, evolving gradually over a period of several days or weeks. Examination discloses a reduction in visual acuity due to the presence of central or centrocecal scotomata, which are larger for colored than for white test objects. Pallor of the temporal portion of the optic disk is observed in some cases. These abnormalities are practically always bilateral and roughly symmetrical. Untreated, they may progress to irreversible optic atrophy. With nutritious diet and vitamin supplements, improvement occurs in all but the most chronic cases, the degree of recovery depending upon the severity of the amblyopia and particularly upon its duration before therapy is instituted.

The nutritional basis of this form of amblyopia was established beyond doubt during World War II and the Korean War, when innumerable instances were observed in prisoners-of-war who had been confined for prolonged periods under conditions of severe dietary deprivation. Fisher has described the optic nerve lesions in four such patients who died of unrelated causes be-

tween 8 and 10 years after the onset of amblyopia. The optic nerves in each of these cases showed distinct loss of myelin and axis cylinders, restricted to the region of the papillomacular fibers. Three of the four cases also showed demyelination of the posterior columns of the spinal cord, no doubt an expression of the associated sensory polyneuropathy.

In the Western world, an amblyopia indistinguishable clinically and pathologically from that observed in prisoners of war is observed sporadically, mainly among undernourished alcoholics. This is generally referred to as *tobacco-alcohol amblyopia*—with the implication that the amblyopia is due to the toxic effects of alcohol or tobacco, or both. Actually, the evidence is overwhelming that so-called tobacco-alcohol amblyopia is nutritional in origin. The specific nutrient responsible for deficiency amblyopia has not been established, however. There is evidence in humans and in animals that under certain conditions a deficiency of any one of several B vitamins—thiamine, vitamin B_{12}, and perhaps riboflavin—may cause degenerative changes in the optic nerves—a situation that pertains in the peripheral nerves as well.

In the 1960s, a popular theory held that the combined effects of vitamin B_{12} deficiency and chronic poisoning by cyanide (generated in tobacco smoke) were responsible for "tobacco amblyopia." Vitamin B_{12} deficiency is a rare but undoubted cause of optic neuropathy, but the notion that cyanide or other substances in tobacco smoke have a damaging effect upon the optic nerves is supported neither by logic nor by experimental data. The arguments leading to this conclusion have been fully marshaled in two reviews (Potts; Victor, 1970) to which the reader is referred for a more detailed account than can be presented here.

PELLAGRA

In the early 1900s, pellagra attained epidemic proportions in the southern part of the United States and in the alcoholic population of large urban centers. Since 1940, the prevalence of pellagra has diminished greatly, both in alcoholics and nonalcoholics, probably because of the general practice of enriching bread with niacin. In its fully developed form, pellagra affects the skin, alimentary tract, and hematopoietic and nervous systems. Only the effects upon the nervous system will concern us here.

The most clearly defined neurologic manifestations are the *cerebral* ones. In the early stages the symptoms may be mistaken for those of psychoneurosis. Insomnia, fatigue, nervousness, irritability, and feelings of depression are common complaints; examination may disclose mental dullness, apathy, and an impairment of memory. Sometimes an acute confusional psychosis dominates the clinical picture. Pellagra may not only produce insanity but occasionally may result from it, by virtue of anorexia and the refusal of food that accompanies certain mental illnesses. The manifestations of *spinal cord involvement* have not been clearly delineated, perhaps because the patient's mental state often precludes accurate testing; in general, the signs are referable to both the posterior and lateral columns, predominantly the former. Signs of *peripheral nerve affection* are relatively less common and are indistinguishable from those of neuropathic beriberi.

A *spinal spastic syndrome* occurs occasionally in nutritionally depleted patients. The main clinical signs are spastic weakness of the legs, with absent abdominal and increased tendon reflexes, clonus, extensor plantar responses, and a loss of position and vibratory senses. This syndrome is said to occur by itself, but in our experience it has been associated with other nutritional disorders, such as Wernicke's disease, deficiency amblyopia, and peripheral neuropathy. In prisoner-of-war camps, the "spastic syndrome" was observed in association with mental and emotional changes, dimness of vision, and at times with widespread muscular rigidity, delirium, coma, and death. Unfortunately, this syndrome has never been studied pathologically so that it is impossible to state whether the lesions are the same as or different from those of pellagra.

NICOTINIC ACID DEFICIENCY ENCEPHALOPATHY

Under this title Jolliffe et al. in 1940 described an acute cerebral syndrome in alcoholic patients, consisting of clouding of consciousness progressing to coma, extrapyramidal rigidity and tremors ("cogwheel" rigidity) of the extremities, and uncontrollable grasping and sucking reflexes. Most of their patients showed overt manifestations of nutritional deficiency, such as Wernicke's disease, pellagra, scurvy, and polyneuropathy. These authors concluded that the encephalopathy represented an acute form of nicotinic acid deficiency, since most of their patients recovered when treated with a diet of low vitamin B content supplemented by intravenous glucose and saline and large doses of nicotinic acid. Sydenstricker and his colleagues (1938) had previously reported the salutary effects of nicotinic acid on the unresponsive state of elderly undernourished patients, and Spillane (1947) described a similar syndrome and response to nicotinic acid in the indigent Arab population of the Middle East.

The status of this syndrome and its relation to pellagra are uncertain. The clinical and nutritional features were never delineated precisely and the pathologic basis never determined. It is unlikely that new information will be forthcoming, for the syndrome seems to have disappeared. Virtually nothing has been written about it in the past 30 years, and during this time we have been unable to find any convincing examples—despite the systematic examination of large numbers of undernourished patients in the alcoholic populations of Boston and Cleveland.

PATHOLOGIC CHANGES AND PATHOGENESIS

These are most readily discerned in the large cells of the motor cortex, the cells of Betz—although the same changes are seen to a lesser extent in the smaller pyramidal cells of the cortex, the large cells of the basal ganglia, the cells of the cranial motor and dentate nuclei, and the anterior horn cells of the spinal cord. The affected cells appear swollen and rounded, with eccentric nuclei and loss of the Nissl particles. These changes were originally designated by Adolf Meyer as "central neuritis" and are frequently referred to as "axonal reaction" because of their similarity to the changes which occur in anterior horn cells whose axons are severed. It has never been decided whether or not the central neuritis of pellagra is the same as the axonal reaction and whether it is, in fact, dependent on injury to the axons of the Betz cells. One argument against this possibility is the frequency with which the motor tracts are interrupted in the brain and spinal cord without an axonal reaction appearing in their cells of origin. Furthermore, in pellagra the cortical nerve cell changes are not always associated with corticospinal tract lesions; this may mean that the cytoplasmic alterations reflect a purely biochemical abnormality in the axon which only reaches the stage of visible myelin degeneration in certain of the more acute or severe cases. On the other hand, the changes described as central neuritis may represent a primary cytolytic degeneration of the motor cell.

The spinal cord lesions in pellagra take the form of a symmetrical degeneration of the dorsal columns, especially of Goll, and to a lesser extent of the corticospinal tracts. Such a posterior column degeneration, affecting a specific system of fibers, is likely to be secondary to degeneration of the posterior roots or ganglion cells, rather than a primary degeneration. The reason for the corticospinal tract degeneration is not clear; it has been speculated that this change is secondary to the pyramidal cell degeneration, but there are serious objections to this idea, as has already been indicated.

The few studies that have been made of the peripheral nerves in pellagra have disclosed changes like those in alcoholics and other patients with nutritional deficiency.

It has been known since 1937, when Elvehjem and his coworkers showed that nicotinic acid cured black tongue, a pellagralike disease in dogs, that this vitamin is effective in the treatment of pellagra. Many years before, Goldberger had demonstrated the curative effects of dietary protein and proposed that pellagra was caused by a lack of specific amino acids. Now it is known that pellagra may result from a deficiency of either nicotinic acid or of tryptophan, the amino acid precursor of nicotinic acid. This explains the frequent occurrence of pellagra in persons who subsist mainly on corn, which contains only small amounts of tryptophan and of niacin—some of the niacin being in bound form and unavailable to the organism.

It should be pointed out that in experimental subjects only the cutaneous-gastrointestinal-neurasthenic manifestations of pellagra have been produced by the feeding of tryptophan- or niacin-deficient diets; neurologic symptoms were not produced by these diets (Goldsmith). As a corollary, only the dermal, gastrointestinal, and neurasthenic manifestations respond to treatment with niacin and tryptophan; neurologic disturbances in pellagrins have proved to be recalcitrant to prolonged treatment with nicotinic acid, although the peripheral nerve disorder may subsequently respond to treatment with thiamine. In monkeys, degeneration of peripheral nerves as well as the unique cerebral cortical changes of pellagra were induced by a deficiency of pyridoxine (Victor and Adams, 1956), and Vilter and his colleagues have produced polyneuropathy in human subjects rendered pyridoxine-deficient; these subjects also showed seborrheic dermatitis, glossitis (indistinguishable from that of niacin deficiency), cheilosis, angular stomatitis, and conjunctivitis. The foregoing observations indicate that certain lingual and cutaneous manifestations that are characteristic of pellagra may be produced by a deficiency of pyridoxine, and that the neurologic manifestations of pellagra are most likely due not to niacin but to pyridoxine deficiency and perhaps to a deficiency of other B vitamins.

THE SYNDROME OF AMBLYOPIA, PAINFUL NEUROPATHY, AND OROGENITAL DERMATITIS
(Strachan's Syndrome)

There remains to be considered a neurologic syndrome which is almost certainly nutritional in origin but which does not conform clinically to the classical deficiency diseases, beriberi and pellagra. This syndrome was originally described by Strachan (1897), a medical officer in Jamaica. The main symptoms in his patients were pain, numbness, and paresthesias of the extremities; objectively there was ataxia of gait, weakness, wasting, and loss of deep tendon reflexes and sensation in the limbs. Dimness of vision and impairment of hearing were common findings as were soreness and excoriation of the mucocutaneous junctions of the mouth. This disorder, originally known as "Jamaican neuritis," was quickly recognized in other parts of the world, particularly in the undernourished populations of tropical countries. Subsequently, many cases of this syndrome were observed in the besieged population of Madrid during the Spanish Civil War, and later among prisoners of war in the Middle and Far East.

The clinical descriptions from these varied sources are not entirely uniform, but certain features are common to all of them, and others occur with sufficient frequency to allow the delineation of a neurologic syndrome and its identification with the one described by Strachan. Essentially, the disorder is one of the peripheral and optic nerves. The former is characterized mainly by sensory symptoms and signs and the latter by failing vision which may go on to complete blindness and pallor of the optic disks. Deafness and vertigo are in general rare complications, but in some outbreaks among prisoners of war these symptoms were common enough to earn the epithet "camp dizziness." In all these respects the syndrome differs from beriberi. Along with the neurologic signs there may be varying degrees of stomatoglossitis, corneal degeneration, and genital dermatitis (the orogenital syndrome). These mucocutaneous lesions are distinct from those of pellagra—at least from the classic form of the disease.

There have been only a few neuropathologic studies of *Strachan's syndrome*. Aside from the changes in the papillomacular bundle of the optic nerve, the most consistent abnormality has been a loss of medullated fibers in each column of Goll adjacent to the midline. Fisher has interpreted this change to indicate a systemized degeneration of the central processes of the bipolar sensory neurons of the dorsal root ganglions. The fact that the primary sensory neuron is the chief site of this disease is consistent with the predominantly sensory symptomatology. The authors find it difficult to see the line which separates nutritional amblyopia and polyneuropathy from Strachan's syndrome.

Cruickshank has described still another neurologic disorder in Jamaican natives, characterized by the gradual onset of spastic paraplegia, frequently with loss of vibration and position sense, and sometimes with deafness and optic and peripheral neuropathy. The spinal cord of these cases has shown patchy widespread demyelination of the posterior and lateral columns as well as anterior horn cell changes, secondary to the degeneration of the peripheral nerves. Also, there were prominent inflammatory changes around the vessels and in the arachnoid of the spinal cord. Although a substantial proportion of Cruickshank's patients subsisted on a poor diet, the nutritional etiology of this disorder is still unproven, and the causal significance of treponemal infection and of toxins has not been fully assessed.

THE NEUROLOGIC MANIFESTATIONS OF VITAMIN B₁₂ DEFICIENCY

The spinal cord, brain, optic nerves, and peripheral nerves may all be involved in pernicious anemia. The part that is usually affected first and often exclusively is the spinal cord. The term *subacute combined degeneration* (SCD) is generally used to designate the spinal cord lesion in pernicious anemia, to distinguish it from other forms of so-called combined system disease, in which the posterior and lateral columns are affected. Pernicious anemia and its neurologic manifestations are distinctive insofar as they result not from a dietary lack of vitamin B_{12}, but from the inability to transfer minute amounts of this nutrient across the intestinal mucosa— "starvation in the midst of plenty," as Castle has aptly put it. This is referred to as a *conditioned deficiency*, insofar as it is conditional upon a lack of intrinsic factor in the gastric secretion.

CLINICAL MANIFESTATIONS

Symptoms of nervous system disease occur in the majority of patients with pernicious anemia. The patient first notices general weakness and paresthesias, consisting of tingling, "pins and needles" feelings, or other vaguely described sensations. The paresthesias tend to be constant, to progress steadily, and to be the source of much distress. They are localized to the distal parts of all four limbs in a symmetric distribution; occasionally the lower

extremities are involved before the upper ones. As the illness progresses, stiffness and weakness of the limbs, especially of the legs, develop, which combined with a defect in postural sensation, produce a weak, unsteady gait and awkwardness of the limbs. If the disease remains untreated, an ataxic paraplegia with variable degrees of spasticity and contracture may develop.

Early in the course of the illness, when only paresthesias are present, there may be no objective signs. Later, examination discloses a disorder of the posterior and lateral columns of the spinal cord, predominantly of the former. Loss of vibration sense is by far the most consistent sign; it is more pronounced in the legs than in the arms, and frequently it extends over the trunk. Position sense is usually impaired as well. The motor signs include loss of strength, spasticity, changes in tendon reflexes, clonus, and extensor plantar responses. These signs are usually limited to the legs. At first the patellar and Achilles reflexes are found to be diminished as frequently as they are increased, and they may even be absent. With treatment the reflexes may return to normal or become hyperactive. The gait at first is predominantly ataxic, later ataxic and spastic.

Loss of superficial sensation below a segmental level on the trunk may occur in isolated instances, implicating the spinothalamic tracts, but such a finding should always suggest the possibility of some other disease of the spinal cord. The defect of cutaneous sensation may take the form of a blunting of touch, pain, and temperature sensation over the limbs in a distal distribution, implicating the *peripheral nerves*, but such findings are also uncommon.

The nervous system involvement in subacute combined degeneration is roughly symmetrical and a definite asymmetry of motor or sensory findings maintained over a period of weeks or months should always cast doubt on the diagnosis.

Mental signs are frequent, ranging from irritability, apathy, somnolence, suspiciousness, and emotional instability to a marked confusional or depressive psychosis, or intellectual deterioration. *Visual impairment* may occasionally be the earliest or sole manifestation of pernicious anemia; examination discloses roughly symmetrical centrocecal scotomata and optic atrophy in the most advanced cases.

The CSF is usually normal; in some cases there is a moderate increase of the protein.

NEUROPATHOLOGIC CHANGES AND PATHOGENESIS

The pathologic process takes the form of a diffuse though uneven degeneration of white matter of the spinal cord and occasionally the brain. The earliest histologic event is a swelling of myelin sheaths, characterized by separation of myelin lamellae and formation of intramyelinic vacuoles. This is followed by a coalescence of small foci of tissue destruction into larger ones, imparting a vacuolated, sievelike appearance to the tissue. The myelin sheaths and axis cylinders are both involved in the degenerative process, the former more obviously and perhaps earlier than the latter. There is relatively little fibrous gliosis in the early lesions, but in more chronic ones, particularly those in which considerable tissue is destroyed, the gliosis is pronounced. The changes begin in the posterior columns of the lower cervical and upper thoracic segments of the cord and spread from this region up and down the cord, as well as forward into the lateral and anterior columns. The lesions are not limited to specific systems of fibers within the posterior and lateral funiculi but are scattered irregularly through the white matter. For this reason, the term *combined system disease*, which is used frequently to designate the myelopathy of pernicious anemia, is not entirely appropriate.

In rare instances, foci of spongy degeneration are found in the optic nerves and chiasm and in the central white matter of the brain. It has been shown that there is a loss of myelin in peripheral nerves, but there is no unequivocal evidence that axis cylinders are significantly affected.

Recently it has been shown that monkeys who were sustained on a vitamin B_{12}-deficient diet for a prolonged period developed neuropathologic changes indistinguishable from those of SCD in humans (Agamanolis et al., 1976). The time required for the production of CNS changes in monkeys—33 to 45 months—is comparable to the time required to deprive humans of their stores of vitamin B_{12}. It is noteworthy that the monkeys did not become anemic, despite the prolonged period of vitamin B_{12} deficiency. Also, in distinction to the human condition, involvement of the optic nerves was particularly severe in the monkeys and probably preceded the degeneration of the spinal cord. The optic nerve lesion appeared first in the papillomacular bundles, in the retrobulbar portions of the nerves, and subsequently spread caudally and beyond the confines of this bundle. These changes are much the same as those of "tobacco-alcohol amblyopia" (see above). The peripheral nerves were not affected in experimental vitamin B_{12} deficiency.

Pathogenesis   This is not well understood. It has been proposed that impairment of DNA synthesis in vitamin B_{12} deficiency accounts for the hematologic abnormalities and particularly for the production of megaloblasts; however, since neurons do not divide, this factor does not appear to be operative in regard to the CNS. One of the better-understood functions of vitamin B_{12} is its role as a coenzyme in the methylmalonyl CoA–mutase reaction. In this reaction, which is a key step in propionate metabolism, methylmalonyl CoA is transformed to succinyl CoA, which subsequently enters the Krebs cycle. It has been shown that impairment of this metabolic step may lead to production of abnormal fatty acids (Cardinale et al.). Since fatty acids are important building blocks of cell membranes and of myelin, it is conceivable that this biochemical abnormality may in some way be responsible for the nervous system lesions.

Clinical-Pathologic Correlation   The paresthesias, impairment of deep sensation, and ataxia are due to lesions in the posterior columns, and these may also account for the loss of tendon reflexes. Weakness, spasticity, increased tendon reflexes, and Babinski signs depend on involvement of the corticospinal tracts. The spinothalamic tract may be involved in the pathologic process, which explains the occasional finding of a sensory level on the trunk. The distal and symmetrical impairment of superficial sensation that occurs in some cases is best explained by involvement of peripheral nerves.

TREATMENT

This consists of the administration of vitamin B_{12}, as soon as the diagnosis has been established.

Theoretically, a few micrograms of parenteral vitamin B_{12} are adequate, but in practice much larger doses are used. The most important factor influencing the response to treatment is the duration of symptoms before treatment is begun; other factors such as age, sex, presence of arteriosclerosis and hypertension, and the degree of anemia are relatively unimportant. The greatest improvement occurs in those patients whose disturbance of gait has been less than 3 months in duration, and recovery may be complete if therapy is instituted within a few weeks after the onset of symptoms. In practically all instances at least partial improvement is effected, although in the long-standing cases often the best that can be accomplished is arrest of progression. All neurologic symptoms and signs may improve, mostly during the first 3 to 6 months of therapy, and then, at a slower tempo, during the ensuing year or even longer.

The chief obstacle to *early diagnosis* is the lack of parallelism which may exist between the hematologic and neurologic signs. This occurs particularly in patients who have received folic acid, which serves to maintain a hematologic remission for an indefinite period while the neurologic signs worsen, often to an irreversible stage. Under these circumstances the most reliable diagnostic procedure is the Schilling test.

DISEASES OF THE NERVOUS SYSTEM OF PROBABLE NUTRITIONAL ORIGIN

The disorders comprising this category will be discussed only briefly because their nutritional etiology has not yet been proved. They are found mainly in alcoholics, but their relationship to alcohol is probably not fundamental, since each of them has been observed in nonalcoholic patients as well. The belief that these disorders are nutritional in origin is based on the following indirect evidence: (1) Usually a prolonged period of undernutrition, associated with a significant loss of weight, precedes the neurologic illness. In some of these cases the amount of alcohol consumed need not be large, but the dietary deprivation is always severe. (2) Examination, at the onset of the illness, discloses physical evidence of undernutrition as well as the presence of neurologic disorders of known nutritional etiology. (3) Certain attributes of the neuropathologic changes, namely their symmetry and constancy of localization, are precisely the features that characterize neurologic disorders of known nutritional etiology.

"ALCOHOLIC" CEREBELLAR DEGENERATION

This term refers to a common and uniform type of cerebellar degeneration in alcoholics. This disorder is about twice as frequent as Wernicke's disease and far more frequent in men than in women (ratio of 11:1). It is characterized clinically by a wide-based stance and gait, varying degrees of instability of the trunk, and ataxia of the legs, the arms being affected to a lesser extent and often not at all. Infrequent signs are nystagmus, dysarthria, and a tremor of the fingers or hands which resembles a parkinsonian tremor but appears only when the limbs are placed in certain sustained postures. Recently it has been demonstrated that the instability of the trunk in these cases consists of a specific 3-Hz rhythmic swaying in the anteroposterior direction. In contrast, patients with lesions of the cerebellar hemispheres show only

slight postural instability without directional preponderance (Mauritz et al.).

In most cases, the cerebellar syndrome evolves subacutely, over a period of several weeks or months, after which it remains unchanged for many years. In some instances, it evolves more rapidly and in still others more slowly, but in these cases also the disease stabilizes eventually. Occasionally, the cerebellar disorder progresses in a saltatory manner, the symptoms worsening in relation to a severe infectious illness or an attack of delirium tremens.

The *pathologic changes* consist of a degeneration of all the neurocellular elements of the cerebellar cortex, but particularly of the Purkinje cells, and are restricted to the anterior and superior aspects of the vermis and, in advanced cases, to the anterior parts of the anterior lobes. The cerebellar atrophy is readily visualized by CT scan (Fig. 38-1).

Two particular forms of this syndrome have not been emphasized sufficiently. In one, an instability of

Figure 38-1

CT scan from a patient with alcoholic cerebellar degeneration, showing enlargement of the ambiens and quadrigeminal cisterns and atrophy of the folia of the anterior lobe.

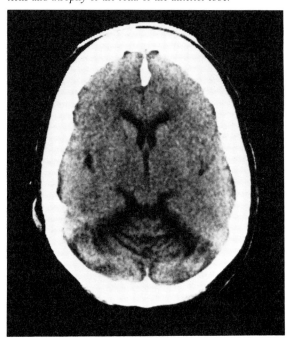

station and gait are the main symptoms, individual movements of the limbs being unaffected; the pathologic changes in such cases are restricted to the anterior-superior portions of the vermis. A second type is acute and transient in nature; the cerebellar symptoms, except for their reversibility, are identical to those which characterize the chronic, fixed form of the disease. In this transient type, the derangement is only one of function ("biochemical lesion") and has probably not progressed to the point of fixed structural changes.

These forms of cerebellar disease, and particularly the restricted and reversible varieties, cannot be distinguished from the cerebellar manifestations of Wernicke's disease either on pathologic or on clinical grounds. As a general rule, the cerebellar manifestations of Wernicke's disease tend to be more abrupt in onset, less severe, and more likely to improve than those which occur apart from Wernicke's disease—but these distinctions are hardly fundamental. The cerebellar manifestations of Wernicke's disease may be very severe, comparable to the most advanced instances of so-called alcoholic cerebellar degeneration.

It is our opinion that the cerebellar ataxia of Wernicke's disease and that which is referred to as alcoholic cerebellar degeneration represent the same disease process, the former term being used when the cerebellar abnormalities are associated with ocular and mental signs, and the latter when the cerebellar syndrome occurs alone. Alcoholic cerebellar degeneration is in all likelihood due to nutritional deficiency and not to the toxic effects of alcohol or other causes, for reasons that have already been indicated. Insofar as the ataxia may resolve under the influence of thiamine alone (see above, under Wernicke's disease) it is likely that a deficiency of this vitamin is responsible for the cerebellar lesion.

CENTRAL PONTINE MYELINOLYSIS

In 1950, the authors observed a rapidly evolving quadriplegia and pseudobulbar palsy in a young alcoholic man who entered the hospital 10 days earlier with symptoms of alcohol withdrawal. Postmortem examination several days later disclosed a large, essentially demyelinative lesion occupying the central part of the basis pontis. Over the next 5 years, one of us (R.D.A.) had the opportunity to study three other cases pathologically, and in 1959 these four cases became the subject of a communication by Adams, Victor, and Mancall, titled *Central Pontine Myelinolysis*. This term was chosen because it denotes both the specific anatomic localization of the disease and its essential pathologic attribute: the remarkable unsystematic dissolution of the sheaths of medullated fibers. Once attention was focused on this distinctive lesion, many other reports appeared. The exact incidence of this disease is not known, but in a series of 3548 consecutive autopsies in adults, the typical lesion was found in 9 cases or 0.25 percent (see recent review of Wright et al.).

The Lesion of Central Pontine Myelinolysis (CPM) One is compelled to define this disease in terms of its pathologic anatomy because the latter stands as its most certain feature. Transverse sectioning of the fixed brainstem discloses a grayish discoloration and fine granularity in the center of the basis pontis. The lesion may be only a few millimeters in diameter, or it may occupy almost the entire basis pontis. There is always a rim of intact myelin between the lesion and the surface of the pons. Posteriorly it may reach and involve the medial lemnisci and, in the most advanced cases, other tegmental structures as well. Very rarely the lesion encroaches on the midbrain, but inferiorly it has never been seen to extend as far as the medulla. Particularly large pontine lesions may be associated with identical myelinolytic foci symmetrically distributed in the thalamus, striatum, internal capsule, lateral geniculate body and cerebral cortex. We have studied one such case (Wright et al.), and at the time of writing are aware of 11 similar cases in the medical literature.

Microscopic examination discloses the fundamental abnormality—destruction of the medullated sheaths throughout the lesion with relative sparing of the axis cylinders and intactness of the nerve cells of the pontine nuclei. These changes always begin and are most severe in the geometric center of the lesion, where they may proceed to frank necrosis of tissue. Reactive phagocytes and glial cells are in evidence throughout the demyelinative focus, but no oligodendrocytes are seen. Signs of inflammation are conspicuously absent.

This constellation of pathologic findings provides easy differentiation of the lesion from infarction and the inflammatory demyelinations of multiple sclerosis and postinfectious encephalomyelitis. The lesion vaguely resembles that of Marchiafava-Bignami disease (see below), with which it is rarely associated. Wernicke's disease is not infrequently associated with CPM, but the topography and character of the lesions bear no resemblance to the latter condition.

Clinical Features Central pontine myelinolysis occurs only sporadically, with no hint of a genetic factor. The two sexes are affected equally. The cases do not fall into any one age period. Whereas the cases first reported were in adults, there are now reports of the disease in more than 20 children.

The outstanding clinical characteristic of CPM is its invariable association with some other serious, often life-threatening disease. In more than half the cases it has appeared in the late stages of chronic alcoholism, often in association with Wernicke's disease and polyneuropathy. The other medical conditions and diseases with which CPM has been conjoined are chronic renal disease in which there was a severe degree of weight loss or prolonged periods of nausea and vomiting; hepatic failure; advanced lymphoma, carcinoma, and cachexia from a variety of other causes; severe bacterial infections, dehydration, and electrolyte disturbances; acute hemorrhagic pancreatitis; and pellagra.

In the majority of cases of CPM there are no symptoms or signs that betray the pontine lesion, presumably because it is so small, extending only 2 to 3 mm on either side of the median raphe and involving only a few corticopontine or pontocerebellar fibers. In others, the presence of CPM is obscured by coma from a metabolic or other associated disease. In only a small proportion of cases, exemplified by the first patient whom we observed, can CPM be recognized during life. In this patient, a serious alcoholic with delirium tremens and pneumonia, there evolved, over a period of several days, a flaccid paralysis of all four limbs and an inability to chew, talk, or swallow. Pupillary reflexes, movements of the eyes and lids, corneal reflexes, and facial sensation were spared. In some instances, however, conjugate eye movements have been limited, and there may be nystagmus. With survival for several days reflexes may return; in several patients, spasticity and extensor posturing of the limbs on painful stimulation have been reported. Mutism with paralysis, i.e., one form of the "locked-in syndrome," has been described, but this is only another interpretation of the paralytic state of pseudocoma. To summarize, whenever a patient gravely ill with a general medical disease develops a quadriplegia, pseudobulbar palsy, and pseudocoma over a period of several days, one is justified in making a clinical diagnosis of CPM. However, from the available data this will be possible in less than a third of the cases in which the disease is demonstrated in postmortem material. The demonstrated capacity of the CT scan to visualize the pontine lesion (Anderson et al.) should increase the possibility of making a premortem diagnosis.

Brainstem infarction due to basilar artery embolism or thrombosis may be a source of confusion to the clinician. Sudden onset or steplike progression of the clinical state, more extensive involvement of tegmental structures of the pons as well as midbrain and thalamus are the distinguishing characteristics of vertebral-basilar disease.

Massive pontine demyelination in acute or chronic relapsing multiple sclerosis rarely produces a pure basis pontis syndrome. Other features of this disease provide the clues to correct diagnosis.

Etiology and Pathogenesis Nutritional deficiency is the most commonly invoked cause of CPM, because it is observed so frequently in chronic wasting diseases and particularly in malnourished alcoholics, often with Wernicke's disease. Nevertheless there are cases in which it is difficult to incriminate a nutritional factor. In recent years, attention has been drawn to the possible role of hyponatremia in the genesis of CPM. Severe hyponatremia (< 130 meq/liter) was present in all our patients and in all 15 patients in the series of Burcar et al. That a derangement of serum sodium is important in the pathogenesis of this disease has been demonstrated recently by Laureno. Dogs were made severely hyponatremic (100 to 115 meq/liter) by repeated injections of vasopressin and intraperitoneal infusions of water. The hyponatremia and profound weakness were corrected by infusion of hypertonic (3%) saline, following which the dogs developed a rigid quadriparesis and showed, at autopsy, pontine and extrapontine lesions that were indistinguishable in their distribution and histologic features from those of the human disease.

Extant data provide no support for theories that attribute the disease to other electrolyte disorders, or to toxic factors. The pontine lesion does not correspond to any known effect of ischemia, hypoxia, or compressive effect of temporal lobe herniation, each of which has been proposed as the cause of CPM.

Nor has a coherent theory been advanced to explain the unique localization of the lesion. The pathoclisis hypothesis of Vogt, proposed by Berry and Olszewski, hardly seems credible, since fibers of all sizes and of different functional systems are indiscriminately affected. The notion that the center of the basis pontis is a zone where the circulation is marginal is not acceptable, because the tissue around the median raphi lies between two paramedian arteries, and in unilateral vascular lesions is usually spared. The suggestion of Landers et al. that this region might be affected by stasis in the pontine veins, the result of obstruction in the galenic venous system superiorly, is negated by the lack of hemorrhages, the sparing of the more vascular tegmentum of the pons, and the integrity of nerve cells within the lesion. All one can say at the present time is that a specific region or zone of the brain, the center of the basis pontis, has a special susceptibility to some acute metabolic fault, analogous to the selective vulnerability of the corpus callosum and anterior commissure in Marchiafava-Bignami disease.

MARCHIAFAVA-BIGNAMI DISEASE (PRIMARY DEGENERATION OF THE CORPUS CALLOSUM)

In 1903, the Italian pathologists Marchiafava and Bignami described a unique alteration of the corpus callosum, based on their autopsy findings in three alcoholic patients. In each case, coronal sectioning of the fixed brain disclosed a pink-gray discoloration of the central portion of the corpus callosum, throughout the longitudinal extent of this structure. Microscopically, the lesion proved to be confined to the middle lamina (which makes up about two-thirds of the thickness of the corpus callosum), in which there was a loss of myelin with relative preservation of the axis cylinders; macrophages were abundant in the altered zone. The clinical observations in these patients were few and incomplete; in two of them, a chronic, ill-defined psychosis had been present and in all three, seizures and coma had occurred terminally.

Bignami, in 1907, described another case in which the lesion in the corpus callosum was accompanied by a similar lesion in the central portion of the anterior commissure. These early reports were followed by a spate of articles which confirmed and amplified the original clinical and pathologic findings. By 1931 about 40 cases of this disorder had been described in the Italian literature (Mingazzini). With one exception, all the reported cases were in males and all of them were insatiable drinkers. They drank red wine for the most part, but other forms of liquor also.

The first report of this disease outside of Italy was by King and Meehan, in 1936. Remarkably, their patient had been born in Italy. Since then, however, the disease has been described in patients native to France, Germany, Switzerland, England, and North and South America, and the notion that it has a special racial predisposition or geographic restriction has had to be abandoned.

Pathologic Features Marchiafava-Bignami disease, like central pontine myelinolysis, is more readily defined by its pathologic than its clinical features. The principal alteration, as has repeatedly been emphasized, is in the middle portion of the corpus callosum, which on gross examination appears somewhat rarefied and sunken and reddish or gray-yellow in color, depending on its age. In the anterior portion of the corpus callosum, the lesion tends to be most severe in the midline, but in the splenium, the opposite may pertain. The most chronic lesion takes the form of a centrally placed yellow cleft or cavity, with collapse of the surrounding tissue and reduction in thickness of the corpus callosum. Microscopically, corresponding to the gross lesions, one observes clearly demarcated zones of demyelination, with relative sparing of the axis cylinders and an abundance of fatty macrophages. Inflammatory changes are absent.

Less consistently, lesions of a similar nature are found in the central portions of the anterior and posterior commissures, and the brachia pontis. These zones of myelin destruction are always surrounded by a rim of intact white matter. The predilection of this disease process for commissural fiber systems has been stressed, but it certainly is not confined to these fibers. Symmetrically placed lesions have been observed in the columns of Goll, superior cerebellar peduncles, and cerebral hemispheres, involving the centrum semiovale and extending, in some cases, into the convolutional white matter. As a rule, the internal capsule and corona radiata, subcortical arcuate fibers, and cerebellum are spared. In several cases, the lesions of deficiency amblyopia (see above) have been observed and in others, the lesions of Wernicke's disease.

Clinical Features The disease affects persons in middle and late adult life. With few exceptions, all the patients have been males and severe chronic alcoholics. The clinical features of the illness are otherwise quite variable, and a clear-cut syndrome of uniform type has not emerged. Many patients have presented in a state of terminal stupor or coma, which has precluded a detailed neurologic assessment. In others, the clinical picture was dominated by the manifestations of chronic inebriation and alcohol withdrawal—tremor, seizures, hallucinosis, and delirium tremens. In some patients, following the subsidence of these symptoms, no signs of neurologic disease could be elicited, even in the end stage of the disease which lasted for several days to weeks. In yet another group, a progressive dementia has been described, evolving slowly over a 3- to 6-year period before death. Emotional disorders leading to acts of violence, marked apathy, moral perversions, and sexual misdemeanors have been noted frequently in these patients. Dysarthria, slowing and unsteadiness of movement, transient sphincteric incontinence, hemiparesis, and apractic or aphasic disorders were superimposed. An impressive feature of these varied neurologic deficits has been their tendency toward remission. The last stage of the disease is characterized by physical decline, seizures, stupor, and coma.

In two cases that have come to our attention, the clinical manifestations were essentially those of bilateral frontal lobe disease: motor and mental slowness; apathy; prominent grasping and sucking reflexes; gegenhalten; incontinence; and a slow, hesitant, wide-based gait. In both of these cases, the neurologic abnormalities evolved over a period of about 2 months, and both patients recovered from these symptoms within a few weeks of hospitalization. Death occurred several years later, as a result of liver disease and subdural hematoma, respectively. In each case, autopsy disclosed an old lesion typical of Marchiafava-Bignami disease, confined to the central portion of the corpus callosum.

In view of the great variability of the clinical picture, and the obscuration in many patients of subtle mental and neurologic abnormalities by the effects of chronic inebriation, the *diagnosis* of Marchiafava-Bignami disease is understandably difficult. In fact, the diagnosis is rarely made during life. The occurrence, in a chronic alcoholic, of a frontal lobe syndrome or a symptom complex that points to a diagnosis of Alzheimer's disease or frontal or corpus callosum tumor, but in whom the symptoms remit, should suggest the diagnosis of Marchiafava-Bignami disease. Possibly the CT scan will disclose some unsuspected instances of this disease (Fig. 38-2).

Pathogenesis and Etiology Originally, Marchiafava-Bignami disease was attributed to the toxic effects of alcohol, but this is an unlikely explanation, in view of the prevalence of alcoholism and the rarity of corpus callosum degeneration. Further, the distinctive callosal lesions have not been observed with other neurotoxins. More importantly, undoubted examples of Marchiafava-Bignami disease have occurred in abstainers, so that alcohol cannot be an indispensable factor. A nutritional etiology has been invoked, for reasons given in the introduction to this section (see page 719), but a precise nutritional factor has not been defined. The mechanisms involved in the selective necrosis of particular areas of white matter remain to be elucidated. Enzymatic failure by virtue of vitamin deficiency, "edema damage," and a "vasocirculatory" defect have all been suggested, but these notions are purely speculative.

PROTEIN-CALORIE MALNUTRITION (PCM) AND MENTAL RETARDATION

The reader might gather from the foregoing descriptions that the nervous system is rarely affected by deranged nutrition except when subjected to the influence of chronic alcoholism, and then the essential problem is an unbalanced diet with an inadequacy of B vitamins in the face of an adequate or near-adequate caloric intake. It is true that the CNS resists the effects of starvation better than other organs. Nonetheless there is increasing evidence that severe dietary deprivation during critical phases of brain development may result in permanent impairment of cerebral function and mental retardation. Inasmuch as there are an estimated 100 million children in the world who are undernourished and suffer from varying degrees of protein, calorie, and other dietary inadequacies this is potentially one of the most pressing problems in medicine and society.

Two overlapping syndromes have been defined in

Figure 38-2
CT scan from a 43-year-old man with Wernicke's disease. Although the ophthalmoparesis and disequilibrium improved rapidly under the influence of thiamine, he remained very apathetic, with prominent grasping and sucking reflexes, apraxias, and palilalia. The scan showed an area of decreased attenuation between the anterior horns of the lateral ventricles, in the genu of the corpus callosum, suggesting a diagnosis of Marchiafava-Bignami disease. Also, the quadrigeminal cistern is enlarged, suggesting atrophy of the superior vermis.

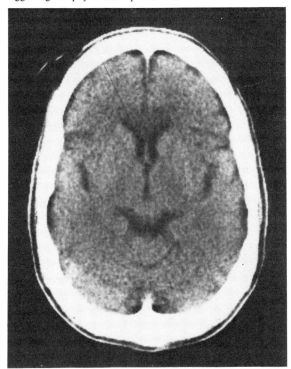

malnourished infants and children: kwashiorkor and marasmus. *Kwashiorkor* is a syndrome of weanling children consisting of edema (and sometimes ascites), hair changes (sparsity and depigmentation), and stunting of growth due to protein deficiency. The edema is due to hypoalbuminemia, and there is in addition an abnormal pattern of blood amino acids as well as a fatty liver. Sometimes there are skin changes suggestive of pellagra or riboflavin deficiency, but no signs of polyneuropathy or subacute combined degeneration of the cord are pre-sent. *Marasmus* consists of an extreme degree of cachexia and growth failure in early infancy. Infants with marasmus usually have been weaned early or were never breast-fed. Common to both groups of children is an apathy and indifference to the environment, combined with irritability when handled or moved. The children are underactive, and even after being started on an adequate diet their tendency is to follow with the eyes rather than to move. At one stage of early convalescence a small number of the kwashiorkor children passes through a phase of rigidity and tremor which has not been explained.

Of great interest is whether the children who are rescued from these states of undernutrition by proper

Table 38-2
Mechanisms whereby malabsorption may be related to neurological disease

Gastrointestinal defect	Substance malabsorbed	Associated neurological disorder
Localized gastric lesions:		
Pernicious anemia	Vitamin B_{12}	Neuropathy, myelopathy, etc.
Congenital IF deficiency	Vitamin B_{12}	Neuropathy, myelopathy, etc.
Partial gastrectomy	Vitamin B_{12}	Neuropathy, myelopathy, etc.
	Vitamin D	Osteomalacic myopathy
Localized lesions of small intestine:		
Predominantly proximal	? Water-soluble vitamins	? Hypovitaminosis B
	Vitamin D	? Osteomalacic myopathy
	Folic acid	Probably none
Predominantly distal	Vitamin B_{12}	Neuropathy, myelopathy, etc.
Bacterial contamination of small bowel (jejunal diverticulosis, blind-loop syndrome, strictures)	Vitamin B_{12}	Neuropathy, myelopathy, etc.
Congenital absorptive defect	"Neutral" amino acids	Hartnup disease
	Tryptophan	"Blue diaper" syndrome
	Methionine	"Oast-house" urine disease
	Folic acid	Mental retardation, seizures, ataxia, choreoathetosis
	Vitamin B_{12}	Neuropathy, myelopathy
Transmucosal transport disorders associated with steatorrhoea:	Fat-soluble vitamins	Xerophthalmia
Endocrine causes		Keratomalacia
Postirradiation		? Osteomalacic myopathy
Drug-induced		
Defective synthesis of chylomicrons	? Vitamin E (carrier lipoprotein not synthesized in liver)	Bassen-Kornzweig disease
Infiltration of villous cores	Fats (defective chylomicron release)	Encephalopathy of Whipple's disease
Competition for essential nutrients (e.g. fish tapeworm)	Vitamin B_{12}	Neuropathy, myelopathy, etc.

Source: Pallis and Lewis.

feeding are left with an underdeveloped or damaged brain. This subject has been studied extensively in many species of animals, as well as in humans, by clinical, biochemical, and neuropathologic methods. The literature is too large to review here, but excellent critiques have been provided by Winick, Birch et al., Latham, and Dodge et al.

In contrast to the devastating effect of PCM upon body growth, the brain weight is only slightly reduced. Nevertheless, on the basis of experiments in dogs, pigs, and rats, it is evident that early (prenatal and early postnatal) malnutrition retards cellular proliferation in the brain. All cells are affected, including oligodendroglia, with a proportional reduction in myelin. Also, the process of dendritic branching may be retarded by early malnutrition. A limited number of studies in humans suggest that PCM has a similar effect upon the brain during the first 8 months of life. In animals, varying

degrees of recovery from the effects of early malnutrition are possible if normal nutrition is reestablished during the vulnerable periods. Presumably this is true for humans as well, although it remains to be proved. In every series of severely undernourished infants and young children who have been followed for many years, a variable percentage have been left mentally backward to a modest degree; the majority recover, however. Unfortunately, the neurologic and intellectual consequences of PCM have defied accurate assessment because of the difficulty of isolating the effects of malnutrition from those of infection, social deprivation, and other factors. The relative importance of these various factors is still under study.

Table 38-3
Vitamin-responsive inherited disorders affecting the nervous system

Vitamin	Disorder	Therapeutic dose	Enzymatic defect	Neurologic manifestations
Thiamine (B$_1$)	Branched-chain ketoaciduria	5–20 mg	Branched-chain keto acid decarboxylase	Lethargy, coma
	Lactic acidosis	5–20 mg	Pyruvate carboxylase	Mental retardation
	Pyruvic acidemia	5–20 mg	Pyruvate dehydrogenase	Cerebellar ataxia
Pyridoxine (B$_6$)	Homocystinuria	>25 mg	Cystathionine synthase	Mental retardation, cerebrovascular accidents, psychoses
	Infantile convulsions	10–50 mg	Glutamic acid decarboxylase	Seizures
	Xanthurenic aciduria	5–10 mg	Kynureninase	Mental retardation
Cobalamin (B$_{12}$)	Methylmalonic aciduria	1000 μg	5′-Deoxyadenosylvitamin B$_{12}$ synthesis	Lethargy, coma
	Methylmalonic aciduria, homocystinuria, and hypomethioninemia	>500 μg	5′-Deoxyadenosylvitamin B$_{12}$ and methylvitamin B$_{12}$ synthesis	Developmental arrest, cerebellar ataxia
Folic acid	Megaloblastic anemia	<0.05 mg	Intestinal malabsorption	Mental retardation
	Formiminotransferase deficiency	>5 mg	Formiminotransferase	Mental retardation
	Homocystinuria and hypomethioninemia	>10 mg	N^5,N^{10}-Methylenetetrahydrofolate reductase	Schizophrenic syndrome
Biotin	β-Methylcrotonyl-glycinuria	↑ 5–10 mg	β-Methylcrotonyl CoA carboxylase	Mental retardation
	Propionic acidemia	↑ 5–10 mg	Propionyl CoA carboxylase	Lethargy, coma
Nicotinamide	Hartnup disease	>400 mg	Intestinal malabsorption of tryptophan	Cerebellar ataxia

Source: Rosenberg.

NUTRITIONAL DEFICIENCIES SECONDARY TO DISEASES OF THE GASTROINTESTINAL TRACT

The vitamins that are known to be essential to the normal functioning of the central and peripheral nervous systems cannot be synthesized by the human organism. Each is ingested as an essential part of the normal diet and absorbed at certain points in the gastrointestinal tract. Impairment or failure of absorption due to diseases of the gastrointestinal tract gives rise to several malabsorption syndromes. In these diseases, the site of the block in transport from the intestinal lumen varies; it may be at the surface of the enterocytes or at their interface with the lymphatic channels and portal capillaries.

Table 38-2, which is modified from Pallis and Lewis, lists the malabsorptive diseases and their relationships to the intestinal abnormalities. From personal experience we have found the most frequent neurological complication of intestinal malabsorption, e.g., sprue (idiopathic steatorrhea), to be a symmetrical sensorimotor polyneuropathy, similar to that of beriberi. Polyneuropathy and subacute combined degeneration of the cord, manifesting themselves many years after gastrectomy, are encountered only rarely.

VITAMIN-RESPONSIVE NEUROLOGIC DISEASES

While humans lack the capacity to synthesize essential vitamin molecules, they are able nonetheless to use them in a series of complex chemical reactions involved in intestinal absorption, transport in the plasma, entry into the organelles of many organs, activation of the vitamin into coenzyme, and finally in their interaction with certain specific apoenzyme proteins. This compels consideration of another aspect of nutrition wherein one or more of these steps in vitamin utilization may be defective as a result of a genetic abnormality. The signs of vitamin deficiency result, under these circumstances, not from vitamin deficiency in the diet but from a genetically deranged control mechanism. In some instances the defect is only quantitative, and by loading the organism with a great excess of the vitamin in question, the biochemical abnormality can be overcome. Rosenberg has listed these hereditary vitamin-responsive diseases, which we have simplified for the reader who is interested in this subject. The diseases of this category, being of hereditary type, have already been described in the previous chapter.

REFERENCES

ADAMS RD, VICTOR M, MANCALL EL: Central pontine myelinolysis. *Arch Neurol Psychiatry* 81:154, 1959.

AGAMANOLIS DP et al: Neuropathology of experimental vitamin B_{12} deficiency in monkeys. *Neurology* 26:905, 1976.

———— et al: An ultrastructural study of subacute combined degeneration of the spinal cord in vitamin B_{12} deficient rhesus monkeys. *J Neuropathol Exp Neurol* 37:273, 1978.

ANDERSON TL et al: Computerized tomography in central pontine myelinolysis. *Neurology* 29:1527, 1979.

BIGNAMI A: Sulle alterazione del corpo calloso e della commissura anteriore ritrovate in un alcoolista. *Policlinico* (sez prat) 14:460, 1907.

BIRCH HG et al: Relation of kwashiorkor in early childhood and intelligence at school age. *Pediatr Res* 5:579, 1971.

BIRCHFIELD RE: Postural hypotension in Wernicke's disease: A manifestation of autonomic nervous system involvement. *Am J Med* 36:404, 1964.

BLASS JP, GIBSON GE: Abnormality of a thiamine-requiring enzyme in patients with Wernicke-Korsakoff syndrome. *N Engl J Med* 297:1367, 1977.

BURCAR PJ, NORENBERG MD, YARNELL PR: Hyponatremia and central pontine myelinolysis. *Neurology* 27:223, 1977.

CARDINALE GJ, CARTY TJ, ABELES RH: Effect of methylmalonyl coenzyme A, a metabolite which accumulates in B_{12} deficiency, on fatty acid synthesis. *J Biol Chem* 245:3771, 1970.

CRUICKSHANK EK: Neuromuscular disease in relation to nutrition. *Fed Proc*, vol 20, pt 3, suppl 7, March 1961, p 345.

DODGE PR, PRENSKY AL, FEIGIN R: *Nutrition and the Developing Nervous System*. St Louis, Mosby, 1975.

DREYFUS PM, MONIZ R: The quantitative histochemical estimation of transketolase in the nervous system of the rat. *Biochim Biophys Acta* 65:181, 1962.

FISHER CM: Residual neuropathological changes in Canadians held prisoners of war by the Japanese. *Can Serv Med J* 11:157, 1955.

GHEZ C: Vestibular paresis: A clinical feature of Wernicke's disease. *J Neurol Neurosurg Psychiatry* 32:134, 1969.

GOLDSMITH GA: Niacin-tryptophan relationships in man and niacin requirement. *Am J Clin Nutr* 6:479, 1958.

JOLLIFFE N et al: Nicotinic acid deficiency encephalopathy. *J Am Med Assoc* 114:307, 1940.

KING LS, MEEHAN MC: Primary degeneration of the corpus callosum (Marchiafava's disease). *Arch Neurol Psychiatry* 36:547, 1936.

LANDERS JW, CHASON JL, SAMUEL VN: Central pontine myelinolysis. A pathogenetic hypothesis. *Neurology* 15:969, 1965.

LATHAM MC: Protein-calorie malnutrition in children and its relation to psychological development and behavior. *Physiol Rev* 54:541, 1974.

LAURENO R: Experimental pontine and extrapontine myelinolysis. *Ann Neurol* 7:117, 1980.

LEVENTHAL CM et al: A case of Marchiafava-Bignami disease with clinical recovery. *Trans Am Neurol Assoc* 90:87, 1965.

MAIR RG et al: Odor discrimination and memory in Korsakoff's psychosis. *J Exp Psychology* 6:445, 1980.

MARCHIAFAVA E, BIGNAMI A: Sopra un alterazione del corpo calloso osservata in soggetti alcoolisti. *Riv Patol Nerv* 8:544, 1903.

MAURITZ KH, DICHGANS J, HUSCHMIDTA A: Quantitative analysis of stance in late cortical cerebellar atrophy of the anterior lobe and other forms of cerbellar ataxia. *Brain* 102:461, 1979.

McENTEE WJ, MAIR RG: Memory enhancement in Korsakoff's psychosis by clonidine: Further evidence for a noradrenergic deficit. *Ann Neurol* 7:466, 1980.

MINGAZZINI G: *Der Balken*. Berlin, Springer, 1922.

PALLIS CA, LEWIS PD: *The Neurology of Gastrointestinal Disease*. London, Saunders, 1974.

POTTS AM: Tobacco amblyopia. *Surv Ophthalmol* 17:313, 1973.

ROSENBERG LE: Vitamin-responsive inherited diseases affecting the nervous system, in Plum F (ed): *Brain Dysfunction in Metabolic Disorders*, vol 53. New York, Raven, 1974, pp 263–270.

SHATTUCK GC: Relation of beriberi to polyneuritis from other causes. *Am J Trop Med Hyg* 8:539, 1928.

SHIMOJYO S, SCHEINBERG P, REINMUTH OM: Cerebral blood flow and metabolism in the Wernicke-Korsakoff syndrome. *J Clin Invest* 46:849, 1967.

SPILLANE JD: *Nutritional Disorders of the Nervous System*. Baltimore, Williams & Wilkins, 1947.

STRACHAN H: On a form of multiple neuritis prevalent in the West Indies. *Practitioner* 59:477, 1897.

STRAUSS MB: Etiology of "alcoholic" polyneuritis. *Am J Med Sci* 189:378, 1935.

SYDENSTRICKER VP et al: Treatment of pellagra with nicotinic acid: Observations in 45 cases. *South Med J* 31:1155, 1938.

TALLAND GA: *Deranged Memory*. New York, Academic, 1965.

VICTOR M: Tobacco amblyopia, cyanide poisoning and vitamin B_{12} deficiency: A critique of current concepts, in Smith SL (ed): *Miami Neuroophthalmology Symposium*. Hallandale, Fla, Huffman, 1970, vol 5, chap 3, pp 33–48.

—— : Polyneuropathy due to nutritional deficiency and alcoholism, in Dyck PJ, Thomas PK, Lambert EH (eds): *Peripheral Neuropathy*. Philadelphia, Saunders, 1975, pp 1030–1066.

——, ADAMS RD: Neuropathology of experimental vitamin B_6 deficiency in monkeys. *Am J Clin Nutr* 4:346, 1956.

——, ——: On the etiology of the alcoholic neurologic diseases: With special reference to the role of nutrition. *Am J Clin Nutr* 9:3/9, 1961.

——, ——, COLLINS GH: *The Wernicke-Korsakoff Syndrome: A Clinical and Pathological Study of 245 Patients, 82 with Post-Mortem Examinations*. Philadelphia, Davis, 1971.

——, ——, MANCALL EL: A restricted form of cerebellar degeneration occurring in alcoholic patients. *Arch Neurol* 1:577, 1959.

——, LAURENO R: Neurologic complications of alcohol abuse: Epidemiologic aspects, in Schoenberg BS (ed): *Advances in Neurology*, vol 19. New York, Raven, 1978, pp 603–617.

——, MANCALL EL, DREYFUS PM: Deficiency amblyopia in the alcoholic patient: A clinicopathologic study. *Arch Ophthalmol* 64:1, 1960.

——, YAKOVLEV PI: SS Korsakoff's psychic disorder in conjunction with peripheral neuritis: A translation of Korsakoff's original article with brief comments on the author and his contribution to clinical medicine. *Neurology* 5:394, 1955.

VILTER RW et al: The effect of vitamin B_6 deficiency induced by desoxypyridoxine in human beings. *J Lab Clin Med* 42:335, 1953.

WINICK M: *Malnutrition and Brain Development*. New York, Oxford, 1976.

WRIGHT DG, LAURENO R, VICTOR M: Pontine and extrapontine myelinolysis. *Brain* 102:361, 1979.

CHAPTER 39

THE ACQUIRED METABOLIC DISORDERS
OF THE NERVOUS SYSTEM

An important segment of neurologic medicine, and one seen with great frequency in general hospitals, consists of a number of diverse disorders, in which the disturbance of cerebral function is consequent upon a failure in some other organ system—heart (and circulation), lungs (and respiration), kidneys, liver, pancreas, and the endocrine glands. Unlike the diseases presented in Chap. 37, wherein a genetic abnormality affects many organs and tissues, including the brain, here the cerebral disorders are strictly secondary to derangements of the visceral organs themselves.

Relationships of this type, between a primary acquired disease of some thoracic or abdominal organ and the brain, have rather interesting implications. In the first place, recognition of the neurologic syndrome may guide one to the diagnosis of the visceral disease; indeed, the neurologic symptoms may be more informative and significant than the symptoms referable to the organ primarily involved. Then too, neurologists must have an understanding of the underlying medical disorder, for this may provide the means of controlling the neurologic part of the disease. In other words, the therapy for what appears to be a neurologic disease lies squarely in the field of internal medicine—a clear reason why every neurologist should be well trained in internal medicine. Lastly, and of more theoretical importance, the investigation of the acquired metabolic diseases promises new insights into the chemistry and pathology of the brain. To select a single example, the discovery of the episodic encephalopathy that is associated with portacaval shunt (Eck fistula) has opened a new and still unclear area in brain chemistry, pertaining to the effect of ammonium ions on glutamic acid and glutamine metabolism; and it has brought to light a curious histopathologic change—a relatively pure hyperplasia of protoplasmic astrocytes. Each visceral disease affects the brain in a somewhat different way, and since the pathogenic mechanism is

not completely understood in any one of them, the study of these metabolic diseases promises rich rewards to the neurological scientist.

Table 39-1 outlines those syndromes which represent the most common clinical expressions of the acquired metabolic diseases.

Table 39-1
Classification of the acquired metabolic disorders of the nervous system

I. Metabolic diseases presenting as a syndrome of episodic confusion, stupor, or coma
   A. Hypoxic-hypotensive encephalopathy
   B. Hypercapnia
   C. Hypoglycemia
   D. Hyperglycemia
   E. Hepatic failure and Eck fistula
   F. Uremia
   G. Other metabolic encephalopathies: acidosis due to diabetes mellitus and renal failure (see also inherited forms of acidosis in Chap. 37); hyponatremia and hypernatremia; hypokalemia and hyperkalemia; Addison's disease; myxedema; hypercalcemia
II. Metabolic diseases presenting as a progressive extrapyramidal syndrome
   A. Acquired hepatocerebral degeneration
   B. Kernicterus
   C. Hypoparathyroidism
III. Metabolic diseases presenting as cerebellar ataxia
   A. Hyperthermia
   B. Hypothyroidism
IV. Metabolic diseases causing psychosis or dementia
   A. Cushing's disease and steroid encephalopathy
   B. Thyroid psychoses
   C. Hyperparathyroidism
   D. Pancreatic encephalopathy (?)
   E. Whipple's disease

METABOLIC DISEASES PRESENTING AS A SYNDROME OF EPISODIC CONFUSION, STUPOR, OR COMA

The *syndrome of impaired consciousness*, its general features, the terms used in describing it, and the mechanisms involved in its genesis have been discussed in Chap. 16, which should be reread as an introduction to this section.There it was pointed out that metabolic disturbances are frequent causes of impaired consciousness, and that their presence has always to be considered when there are no focal or lateralizing signs of cerebral disease and the CSF is clear. Intoxication with alcohol and other drugs figures prominently in the differential diagnosis.

HYPOXIC-HYPOTENSIVE ENCEPHALOPATHY

Here the basic disorder is a lack of oxygen to the brain, the result of failure of the heart and circulation or of the lungs and respiration. Often both are responsible and one cannot say which predominates, hence the ambiguous allusion in clinical records to "cardiorespiratory failure."

Hypoxic encephalopathy in various forms and degrees of severity is one of the most frequent and disastrous cerebral accidents encountered in the emergency and recovery rooms of every general hospital. The medical conditions which most often lead to it are (1) suffocation (from drowning, strangulation, aspiration of vomitus or blood, compression of trachea by a surgical pack or hemorrhage or foreign body in the trachea); (2) carbon monoxide (CO) poisoning, in which respiration fails first and then the cardiovascular system; (3) diseases which paralyze the respiratory apparatus (Landry-Guillain-Barré syndrome and poliomyelitis) or damage the CNS diffusely (trauma and vascular disease of the brain, encephalopathies of children, and epilepsy), again with respiratory failure being the initial factor, preceding cardiac failure; and (4) myocardial infarction, hemorrhage, shock and circulatory collapse, cardiac arrest during inhalation or spinal anesthesia, infective and traumatic shock, in all of which cardiac action is paralyzed before respiration.

The terms *anoxic, anemic,* and *stagnant,* introduced by Barcroft to designate the various forms of anoxia, still appear in medical writings but have limited clinical value, since the ultimate effect of all three is the same, namely to deprive the brain tissue of its critical oxygen supply. *Anoxic anoxia* implies a reduced arterial pressure of oxygen, as might occur at high altitudes or with pulmonary disease, in which oxygen cannot cross the alveolar capillary membrane. In *anemic anoxia* there is insufficient hemoglobin to bind and transport the oxygen (CO poisoning, profound anemia). *Stagnant anoxia* is more appropriately designated *ischemic anoxia*, since circulatory failure, the underlying cause, never results in hypoxia alone; here the blood may contain sufficient oxygen, but cerebral blood flow (CBF) is insufficient to supply the cerebral tissues. Seldom is there a need to use the term *histotoxic anoxia*, which refers to chemical interference with the cellular utilization of oxygen, as occurs when cyanide blocks the cytochrome system.

Clinical Features Mild degrees of hypoxia induce only inattentiveness, poor judgment, and motor incoordination; there are no lasting effects. With severe hypoxia or anoxia, as occurs with cardiac arrest, consciousness is lost within seconds, but recovery will be complete if breathing, oxygenation of blood, and cardiac action are restored within 3 to 5 min. If the state of complete ischemic anoxia persists beyond this time, serious and permanent injury to the brain results, particularly to those parts which are most susceptible because of the marginal efficiency of their circulation (globus pallidus, cerebellum and parts of the cerebral cortex, especially the hippocampus and parietooccipital lobes in "border-zone regions"). As shown by Ames and his colleagues, one of the reasons for the irreversibility of the lesion is swelling of the endothelium and blockage of circulation into the ischemic cerebral tissues (no reflow phenomenon). Clinically, however, it is difficult to judge the precise degree of hypoxia since slight heart action or an imperceptible blood pressure may serve to maintain the circulation to some extent. Hence some individuals have made an excellent recovery after cerebral hypoxia that allegedly lasted 8 to 10 min or longer. Subnormal body temperatures, as might occur when the body is immersed in ice water, greatly prolong the tolerated period of hypoxia. *An important clinical rule is that degrees of hypoxia which at no time abolish consciousness rarely if ever cause permanent damage to the nervous system.* Also, generally speaking, anoxic patients who demonstrate intact brainstem function (as indicated by normal pupillary light and ciliospinal responses, intact doll's-head eye movements and oculovestibular reflexes) have a good outlook for recovery of consciousness and perhaps all of their faculties. Conversely, absence of these reflex activities, particularly a fixity of the pupils to light, implies a hopeless outlook.

The most severe degrees of oxygen lack, most often caused by circulatory collapse (ischemic anoxia), are manifested by a state of complete unawareness and unresponsiveness with abolition of all brainstem reflexes.

Natural respiration cannot be sustained; only the *cardiac action and blood pressure are maintained.* No electrical activity is seen in the EEG (it is isoelectric). This is the *brain death syndrome* (Chap. 16). When caused by hypoxia-hypotension it is always irreversible. At autopsy one finds that most if not all the cerebral, cerebellar, and brainstem tissues, and in some instances even the spinal cord, have been destroyed.

When this syndrome of brain death occurs, one must consider the advisability of discontinuing all supportive measures (respiratory aid, vasopressor agents, etc.). Such victims often become donors of vital organs. One must exercise extreme caution in concluding that the patient has irreversible brain damage, because anesthesia, drug intoxication, and hypothermia may also cause deep coma and an isoelectric EEG, but permit recovery. Such cases have been brought increasingly to public attention because of ethical and moral issues that surround the question of discontinuing medical therapy. In the authors' experience, the vital functions of patients with brain death syndrome usually cannot be sustained for more than several days; in other words, the problem settles itself and is not nearly so difficult as the one in which the patient has suffered severe but somewhat lesser degrees of cerebral damage, as described below.

Patients who have suffered severe but lesser degrees of hypoxia will have stabilized breathing and heart action when first seen; yet they may be profoundly comatose, with eyes slightly divergent and motionless but with reactive pupils, the limbs inert and flaccid or intensely rigid, and tendon reflexes diminished. Within a few minutes after cardiac action and breathing have been restored, generalized convulsions and also isolated or grouped twitches of muscles (myoclonus) may supervene. The seizures, if severe and recurrent, double or treble the oxygen need of the cerebral tissues, a deficiency that can only be corrected by neurogenic hypertension and metabolic cerebral vasodilatation (Plum and Posner). If the damage is severe, coma persists and decerebrate postures may be present or occur upon pinching the limbs, and bilateral Babinski signs can be evoked. In the first 24 to 48 h death may terminate this state in a setting of rising temperature, deepening coma, and circulatory collapse. Tragically, however, the individual may survive for an indefinite period in a state which is variously referred to as *cortical death, irreversible coma,* or *persistent vegetative state* (see Chap. 16).

In this lesser degree of injury, the cerebral and cerebellar cortices are partly or completely destroyed, but brainstem-spinal structures survive. Some patients remain mute, unresponsive, and unaware of their environment for weeks, months, or years. Long survival is usually attended by some degree of improvement, but the patient appears to have lost all knowledge of the present situation, past memories, power of reasoning, capacity for meaningful social interaction and independent existence. One has only to observe such patients and their families to appreciate the gravity of the problem, the heartache, the waste of hospital facilities, and the tremendous expense of medical care. The only person who does not suffer is the patient. The medical profession is searching for criteria that will accurately predict this hopeless state early in the comatose period, but the data are as yet insecure. If intoxication can be excluded, the presence of fixed dilated pupils and paralysis of eye movement for 24 to 48 h, along with marked slowing of the EEG, usually signifies irreversible cerebral damage. We have not observed deep coma of this type, lasting 5 days or more, to be attended by full recovery. The question of what to do with such cases of protracted coma is a societal and not a medical problem. The most that can be expected of the neurologist is to state the level and degree of brain damage, its cause, and the prognosis. Of course one prudently avoids heroic, lifesaving therapeutic measures once the state is established.

With still lesser degrees of injury the patients improve after a period of coma. Consciousness is regained and then various degrees of confusion, visual agnosia, or any one of several types of abnormal movement (action or intention myoclonus, extrapyramidal rigidity, choreoathetosis) becomes manifest. Some of these patients quickly pass through this acute hypoxic phase and proceed to make a full recovery; others are left with a permanent degree of disability. The permanent neurologic sequelae or *posthypoxic syndromes* that we have observed most frequently are (1) *persistent coma or stupor* and, with lesser degrees of cerebral injury, (2) dementia with or without extrapyramidal signs, (3) *visual agnosia,* (4) *extrapyramidal (parkinsonian) syndrome with mental enfeeblement,* (5) *choreoathetosis,* (6) *cerebellar ataxia,* (7) *intention or action myoclonus,* and (8) *Korsakoff's amnesic state. Seizures* may or may not continue to be a problem. These several sequelae do not occur in pure form; they overlap in various combinations.

A relatively uncommon and unexplained phenomenon is *delayed postanoxic encephalopathy.* Initial improvement, which appears to be complete, is followed after a variable period of time (2 to 10 days, sometimes longer) by a relapse, characterized by apathy, confusion, irritability, and occasionally agitation or mania. A few patients have recovered from this second episode, but in most of the reported cases there has been further progression of the neurologic syndrome, with weakness, shuffling gait, diffuse rigidity and spasticity, coma, and death after 1 to 2 weeks. Postmortem examination of these cases has shown the major abnormality to be a widespread cerebral demyelination. Exceptionally, there is yet another delayed syndrome in which an episode of hypoxia is followed by a slow, deteriorative state, that progresses for weeks to months until the patient is mute, rigid, and helpless. In such cases the basal ganglia are affected more than the cerebral cortex and white matter (Dooling and Richardson).

The essential *mechanism* in hypoxic encephalopathy is a lack of oxygen and an arrest of all aerobic metabolic processes necessary to sustain the Krebs (tricarboxylic acid) cycle and the electron-transport system. Deprived of their intrinsic source of energy, neurons proceed to catabolize themselves in an attempt to maintain their activity, and in so doing are damaged to such a degree that they cannot survive. The accumulation of catabolic products in the interstitial tissue contributes to the parenchymal damage. The phenomenon of delayed neurologic deterioration after anoxia is not understood but may be due to the blockage or exhaustion of some enzymatic process during the period when brain metabolism is restored or even increased (as in hyperthermia or possibly with seizures or increased motor activity).

Diagnosis depends on (1) the history of the hypoxic event and evidence of reduced oxygenation of arterial blood (in general, a Po_2 of less than 50 mmHg causes confusion and less than 25 mmHg, coma) or CO intoxication (the latter is indicated by a cherry-red color of the skin or a characteristic spectroscopic band for only a few minutes to hours after the episode), blood pressures below 70 systolic, or cardiac arrest; (2) the typical clinical sequence of events outlined above after a possible hypoxic episode has terminated. Renal damage (anuria) and myocardial infarction may also have occurred, and provide corroborative evidence of hypoxia.

Treatment is directed mainly to the prevention of a critical degree of hypoxic injury. After a clear airway is secured, cardiopulmonary resuscitation, open-chest surgery, and the use of a cardiac defibrillator or pacemaker all have their place, and every second counts in their prompt utilization. Once cardiac and pulmonary function are restored, there is some evidence that reducing cerebral metabolic requirements by continuous hypothermia for 48 to 72 h and by barbiturate medication may prevent the delayed worsening referred to above. Oxygen may be of value during the first hours, but it is probably of little use after the blood becomes well-oxygenated. Dexamethasone intravenously in doses of 6 to 12 mg every 6 h helps combat brain (cellular?) swelling. Seizures should be controlled by the methods indicated on page 229. If the seizures are severe, continuous, and unresponsive to drugs, controlled respiration and curare may need to be used. Often the seizures cease after a few days. If they persist, they are often myoclonic, in which case mephobarbital (Mebaral), in divided doses up to 500 mg/day, phenobarbital, 300 mg/day, or clonazepam, 8 to 12 mg daily in divided doses, may be useful in their control. Keeping the patient at bed rest for 10 days, even if consciousness has been regained in 24 to 48 h, may help to prevent the delayed form of postanoxic encephalopathy.

HYPERCAPNIA (AND HYPOXIA) IN PULMONARY DISEASE

Chronic emphysema, chronic fibrosing lung disease, and in some instances a seeming inadequacy of the respiratory center lead to chronic respiratory acidosis, with an elevation of Pco_2 and a reduction in arterial Po_2. Secondary polycythemia, cor pulmonale, and heart failure often accompany these diseases of the lungs, and pulmonary infection may be superimposed.

The clinical syndrome comprises *headache, papilledema, mental dullness, drowsiness, confusion, and coma, asterixis* and a kind of *action tremor and coarse twitching* of all muscles that are in a state of sustained contraction. The headache tends to be generalized or frontal or occipital in location, intense, persistent for hours, and of a steady, aching type; nocturnal occurrence is a feature in some cases. The papilledema is bilateral, but may be slightly more in one eye than the other, and hemorrhages may encircle the choked disk. The visual acuity is undiminished and the visual fields are full. The tremor is best seen in the outstretched fingers and has all the characteristics of a fast-frequency, slightly arrhythmic action tremor. It continues all through voluntary movement and increases slightly with effort, sometimes being misinterpreted as an intention tremor. In addition there is inability to maintain a fixed posture or a voluntary movement because of brief interruptions of muscle-action potentials (asterixis).

Intermittent drowsiness, indifference and inattention to the environment, reduction of psychomotor activity, imperception of sequences of events, and forgetfulness constitute the more subtle manifestations of this syndrome and may prompt the family to seek medical help. Such symptoms may last only a few minutes or hours and one cannot count on their presence at the time of a particular examination.

In fully developed cases, the CSF is under increased pressure. PCO_2 may exceed 75 mmHg, and the O_2 saturation of arterial blood ranges from 85 percent to as low as 40 percent. The EEG reveals slow activity, in the delta or theta range, sometimes bilaterally synchronous. The mechanism of the cerebral disorder is said to be CO_2 narcosis, but the biochemical details are not known. The danger of administering morphine, which depresses the respiratory center (now insensitive to CO_2), and the danger of oxygen inhalation, which removes the sole stimulus to the respiratory center, are now widely recognized; patients treated in this way have lapsed into coma and some have died.

Forced ventilation with an intermittent positive-pressure device, using room air or oxygen if hypoxia is severe, the treatment of heart failure with digitalis and diuretics, venesection to reduce the viscosity of the blood, and antibiotics to combat pulmonary infection have been the most effective therapeutic measures; often they result in a surprising degree of improvement that may be maintained for months or years. If stupor or coma persist, the arterial O_2 level should be checked; it may be critically reduced. On the other hand, the pH of the CSF may be very low, in the range of 7.15 to 7.25. In CO_2 narcosis it is easier to correct the acidosis of the blood than of the CSF, which tends to lag.

Unlike pure hypoxic encephalopathy, prolonged coma due to hypercapnia is exceptional, and in our experience has not led to irreversible brain damage. Papilledema and jerky, intermittent lapses of posture (asterixis) are features of diagnostic import. The syndrome is apt to be mistaken for brain tumor, a confusional psychosis of other type, or a disease causing chorea or myoclonus. The latter must be distinguished from other metabolic diseases presenting as chronic extrapyramidal syndromes, as described later in this chapter.

HYPOGLYCEMIC ENCEPHALOPATHY

This condition is a rather infrequent but important cause of confusion, convulsions, stupor, and coma; and it merits separate consideration as a metabolic disorder of the brain. The essential biochemical abnormality is a critical lowering of blood glucose. At a level of 30 mg per 100 ml the cerebral disorder takes the form of a confusional state, and one or more seizures may occur; at a level of 10 mg per 100 ml there is profound coma

which may result in irreparable injury to the brain if not corrected by the administration of glucose.

The normal brain has a glucose reserve of 1 to 2 g (30 μmol per 100 g of tissue), mostly in the form of glycogen. Since glucose is utilized by the brain at a rate of 60 to 80 mg/min, the glucose reserve will sustain cerebral activity for only about 90 min, once blood glucose is no longer supplied. Glucose is transported from the blood to the brain by a carrier system. Once glucose enters the brain, it either undergoes glycolysis or is stored as glycogen. Of the glucose taken up by the brain, 85 to 90 percent is oxidized; the remainder goes into amino acid pools and is utilized in the formation of proteins and other substances (notably neurotransmitters, particularly GABA).

The brain is the only organ, besides the heart, that suffers severe functional and structural disorder under conditions of hypoglycemia. The pathophysiology of the cerebral disorder has not been fully elucidated (see Ferrendelli; also, Wilkinson and Prockop). The suggestion that it results in a rapid depletion and inadequate production of high-energy phosphate compounds has not been corroborated; some other glucose-dependent biochemical process must be involved. When blood glucose falls, the central nervous system may utilize nonglucose substrates to a variable extent for its metabolic needs, especially keto acids and intermediates of glucose metabolism, such as lactate, pyruvate, fructose, and other hexoses. In the neonatal brain, which has a higher glycogen reserve, keto acids account for a considerable proportion of cerebral energy requirements, and this also happens after prolonged starvation. Hypoglycemia also activates the adrenal glands and the autonomic nervous system to induce a corrective gluconeogenesis. If convulsions occur, they do so during a period of confusion; the convulsions have been attributed to an altered integrity of neuronal membranes and depressed GABA levels.

Etiology The most common causes of hypoglycemic encephalopathy are (1) accidental or deliberate overdose of insulin or an oral diabetic agent, (2) an islet cell, insulin-secreting tumor of the pancreas, (3) depletion of liver glycogen that occasionally follows a prolonged alcoholic debauch or some form of acute liver disease such as acute nonicteric hepatoencephalopathy of childhood (Reye's syndrome), (4) glycogen storage disease of infancy, and (5) an idiopathic state in the neonatal period. In the past, hypoglycemic encephalopathy was a rather frequent complication of "insulin shock" therapy of schizophrenia. In functional hyperinsulinism the hypoglycemia is rarely of sufficient severity or duration to damage the central nervous system.

Clinical Features As the level of blood glucose descends, to about 30 mg per 100 ml, the initial symptoms appear—nervousness, hunger, flushed facies, sweating and trembling, headache, palpitation, anxiety and these gradually give way to confusion, drowsiness, and occasionally excitement or overactivity. In the next stage, forced sucking, grasping, motor restlessness, muscular spasms, and finally decerebrate rigidity occur, in that sequence. Myoclonic twitching and convulsions may develop in some patients, but are by no means the rule. Blood levels of approximately 10 mg per 100 ml are associated with deep coma, dilation of pupils, pale skin, shallow respiration, slow pulse, and hypotonicity of limb musculature—the so-called medullary phase of hypoglycemia. If glucose is administered before this medullary phase appears, the patient is restored to normalcy, retracing the aforementioned steps in reverse order. However, once the medullary phase is reached, and particularly if it persists for a time before the hypoglycemia is corrected by intravenous glucose or spontaneously by the so-called gluconeogenic activities of the adrenal glands and liver, recovery is delayed for a period of days or weeks and may be incomplete.

The EEG is altered as the blood glucose falls, but the correlations are inexact. There is a decrease in the frequency of brain waves diffusely, in the theta or delta range. During recovery sharp waves may appear and coincide in some cases with seizures.

A huge dose of insulin that produces intense hypoglycemia, even of relatively brief duration (30 to 60 min), is more dangerous than a series of less severe hypoglycemic episodes from smaller doses of insulin, possibly because the former impairs or exhausts essential enzymes. This condition cannot then be overcome by large quantities of glucose intravenously.

The major clinical differences between hypoglycemic and hypoxic encephalopathy lie in the setting and the mode of evolution of the neurologic disorder. The effects of hypoglycemia usually unfold more slowly, over a period of 30 to 60 min, rather than in seconds or a few minutes. The recovery phase and sequelae of the two conditions bear close resemblance. A severe and prolonged episode of hypoglycemia may result in permanent impairment of intellectual function as well as other neurologic residua, like those which follow severe anoxia. We have also observed protracted coma and a relatively pure Korsakoff's amnesic state. However, one should not be hasty in *prognosis*, for slow improvement may continue for 1 to 2 years. *Recurrent hypoglycemia*, as with an islet cell tumor, may masquerade for some time as an episodic confusional psychosis or convulsive illness, and diagnosis awaits a period of demonstrably low blood glucose or hyperinsulinism.

In addition to hypoglycemic stupor and coma, lesser degrees and more chronic forms of low blood glucose may produce two other distinct but not mutually exclusive syndromes, according to Marks and Rose, who have written an authoritative monograph on the subject. One of these syndromes, termed *subacute hypoglycemia*, is characterized by drowsiness and lethargy, diminution in psychomotor activity, deterioration of social behavior, and confusion. Oral or intravenous glucose will immediately alleviate the symptoms. In the other syndrome, termed *chronic hypoglycemia*, there is a gradual deterioration of intellectual functions, raising the question of dementia; and in some reported instances tremor, chorea, rigidity, cerebellar ataxia, and rarely signs of lower motor neuron involvement (*hypoglycemic amyotrophy*) are added. The latter feature has not been seen by the authors, who can only refer the reader to the report by Tom and Richardson.

These subacute and chronic forms of hypoglycemia have been observed in conjunction with islet cell hypertrophy and islet cell tumors of the pancreas, carcinoma of the stomach, fibrous mesothelioma, carcinoma of the cecum and hepatoma. Supposedly an insulin-like substance is elaborated by these nonpancreatic tumors.

Functional or reactive hypoglycemia is the most ambiguous of all syndromes related to low blood glucose. This condition may precede diabetes mellitus or accompany peptic ulcer. The rise of insulin in response to a carbohydrate meal is delayed, but then causes an excessive fall in blood glucose, to 30 to 40 mg per 100 ml. The symptoms are malaise, fatigue, nervousness, headache, tremor, etc., which may be difficult to distinguish from anxious depression. This syndrome is proved by excessive reaction to insulin, low blood glucose during symptomatology, and response to oral glucose. Treatment, which consists of a high protein-low carbohydrate diet, should be reserved for those patients whose symptom complex correlates with hypoglycemia as documented by a 5-h glucose tolerance test.

Pathologically, in all forms of hypoglycemic encephalopathy, the major damage is to the cerebral cortex. Cortical nerve cells degenerate and are replaced by microgliacytes and astrocytes. The distribution of lesions is similar though not identical to that in hypoxic encephalopathy. (It appears that the cerebellar cortex is less vulnerable to hypoglycemia than to hypoxia.)

Treatment of all forms of hypoglycemia obviously consists of correction of the hypoglycemia at the earliest possible moment. It is not known whether hypothermia or other measures will increase the safety period in hypoglycemia or alter the outcome.

HYPERGLYCEMIA

Two syndromes have been defined, mainly in diabetics: (1) hyperglycemia with ketoacidosis and (2) hyperosmolar nonketotic hyperglycemia.

In diabetic acidosis the familiar picture is one of dehydration, fatigue, weakness, headache, abdominal pain, stupor or coma, and Kussmaul type of breathing. Usually the condition has developed over a period of days in a known diabetic. Insulin has often been omitted. Usually the blood glucose level is found to be more than 400 mg per 100 ml, the pH of the blood is less than 7.20, the Pco_2 is 10 meq/liter or less, and the bicarbonate is less than 10 meq/liter. Ketone bodies and β-hydroxybutyric acid are elevated in blood and urine, and there is a marked glycosuria. The prompt administration of insulin, correction of the acidosis by molar lactate, and repletion of body fluids restore cerebral function over a period of hours.

Of considerable interest is a small proportion of patients, such as those reported by Young and Bradley, in whom deepening coma and cerebral edema develops as the blood level of glucose falls. The basis of this condition, which is indicated by rising CSF pressure, is ascribed by Prockop to an accumulation of fructose and sorbitol in the brain. The latter substance is a polyol formed during hyperglycemia, which crosses membranes slowly and causes a shift of water into the brain and an intracellular edema. According to Fishman, the increased polyols in the brain in hyperglycemia are not present in sufficient concentration to be important osmotically; they may have other metabolic effects related to the encephalopathy. Attempts at therapy by the administration of urea, mannitol, salt-poor albumin and dexamethasone have been unsuccessful though recoveries are reported.

In hyperosmolar nonketotic hyperglycemia the blood glucose is extremely high, over 1000 mg per 100 ml, but ketoacidosis does not develop. The effects on the brain are rather like those of hypernatremia. Modern appreciation of the neurological syndrome is generally credited to Wegierko who published descriptions of it in 1956 and 1957. Most of the patients are elderly diabetics, but some were not previously known to have been diabetic. An infection, enteritis, pancreatitis or drugs known to upset diabetic control (thiazides, prednisone, phenytoin) lead to severe polyuria, fatigue, confusion,

stupor and coma. If testable when first seen, focal signs such as seizures, weakness of one side, a homonymous visual field defect, or a hemisensory defect suggest the possibility of a stroke. Plasma osmolality usually is around 350 mosmol per kilogram of water. There is also hemoconcentration of blood cells and prerenal azotemia. Many of the patients are in shock when first seen, and the mortality rate has been as high as 40 percent. Fluids should be replaced cautiously, using isotonic saline and probably parenteral potassium. Correction of the markedly elevated blood glucose requires only small amounts of insulin (10 units regular insulin intravenously), since these patients often do not have insulin resistance.

HEPATIC STUPOR AND COMA (HEPATIC OR PORTAL-SYSTEMIC ENCEPHALOPATHY)

Chronic hepatic insufficiency with portacaval shunting of blood is often punctuated by episodes of stupor, coma, and other neurologic symptoms—a state that may be referred to as hepatic encephalopathy. This state complicates all varieties of liver disease. Less widely known is the fact that a portal-systemic shunt (Eck fistula) may be attended by the same clinical picture, in which case the liver may be entirely normal. Also, there are a number of hereditary hyperammonemic syndromes of childhood, outlined in Chap. 37, which may lead to episodic coma with or without seizures. Reye's syndrome, a special type of acute nonicteric hepatic encephalopathy of children, is also associated with very high levels of ammonium in the blood (see further on in this chapter).

Clinical Features The clinical picture of hepatic encephalopathy consists essentially of a derangement of consciousness, presenting first as mental confusion with increased or decreased psychomotor activity, followed by progressive drowsiness, stupor, and coma. The confusional state, before coma intervenes, is frequently combined with a characteristic intermittency of sustained muscle contraction, imparting an irregular "flapping" movement to the outstretched hands. The latter phenomenon, which was originally described in patients with hepatic stupor by Adams and Foley, and called asterixis (from the Greek sterein, "to fasten" or "to support"), is now recognized as a sign of various metabolic encephalopathies. The EEG is a sensitive and reliable indicator of impending hepatic coma, becoming abnormal during the earliest phases of the disordered mental state. The usual EEG abnormality consists of paroxysms of bilaterally synchronous slow waves, in the delta range, which at first are interspersed with alpha activity and which later, as the coma deepens, displace all normal activity. A small number of patients show only random high-voltage asynchronous slow waves. A variable, fluctuating rigidity of the trunk and limbs, grimacing, suck and grasp reflexes, exaggeration or asymmetry of tendon reflexes, Babinski signs, and focal or generalized seizures round out the clinical picture.

The syndrome of hepatic or portal-systemic encephalopathy evolves over a period of days to weeks and often terminates fatally. In other patients, the syndrome does not advance beyond the stage of mild mental dullness and confusion, with asterixis and EEG changes. In this relatively mild form it must be differentiated from other acute confusional psychoses and deliria. If the metabolic disorder persists for months and years, a mild dementia and a disorder of posture and movement may gradually appear (grimacing, tremor, dysarthria, ataxia of gait, choreoathetosis), and the condition must then be distinguished from other dementing and extrapyramidal syndromes (see below).

The blood ammonium levels, if measured repeatedly, usually exceed 200 μg per 100 ml, and the severity of the neurologic and EEG disorders parallels the ammonium levels. With treatment the fall in the level of ammonium precedes clinical improvement. Once recovery occurs, an intolerance to ammonium can be demonstrated by an oral dose of 6.0 g NH_3Cl, which raises the blood ammonium and sometimes produces mild symptoms.

Neuropathologic Changes The striking finding in patients who die in a state of hepatic coma is a diffuse increase in the number and size of the protoplasmic astrocytes in the deep layers of the cerebral cortex, lenticular nuclei, thalamus, substantia nigra, cerebellar cortex, and red, dentate, and pontine nuclei, with little or no visible alteration in the nerve cells or other parenchymal elements. These abnormal glial cells are generally referred to as Alzheimer type II astrocytes having been described originally by von Hösslin and Alzheimer in 1912, in a case of Westphal-Strümpell pseudosclerosis (familial hepatolenticular degeneration). These astrocytic alterations occur to some degree in all patients who die of progressive liver failure, and the degree of this glial abnormality is roughly parallel to the intensity and duration of the neurologic disorder. The clinical and EEG features, as well as the astrocytic hyperplasia, though highly characteristic of hepatic coma, are not specific features of this metabolic disorder. Nevertheless, taken together in a setting of liver failure, these manifestations constitute a distinctive clinicopathologic entity.

Pathogenesis of Hepatic Encephalopathy This is not fully understood, but the most plausible hypothesis relates it to an abnormality of nitrogen metabolism, wherein ammonium (NH_4), or perhaps some other amine(s), which are formed in the bowel by the action of urease-containing organisms on dietary protein and are carried to the liver in the portal circulation, fail to be converted into urea, either because of hepatocellular disease or portal-systemic shunting of blood, or both. As a result, these substances reach the systemic circulation, where they interfere with cerebral metabolism in some obscure way. One theory is that the effect of hyperammonemia is to deplete the brain of α-ketoglutarate (by reductive amination of α-ketoglutarate to glutamate, and amidation of the latter to glutamine), leading eventually to a depletion of high-energy phosphate compounds and to a decrease in cerebral metabolism and oxygen utilization. An alternate theory is that CNS function in cirrhotic patients is impaired by short-chain fatty acids (from the diet or from bacterial metabolism of carbohydrate). Still another suggestion (Fischer and Baldessarini) is that biogenic amines (octopamine) which arise in the gut and bypass the liver act as false neurotransmitters, displacing the putative transmitters norepinephrine and dopamine. However, it has been shown in rats that the intraventricular infusion of large amounts of octopamine, causing up to 90 percent reduction of brain dopamine and norepinephrine concentrations, fails to alter the animals' alertness and activity (Zieve and Olsen). Hypoxia, hypokalemia and metabolic alkalosis, and the use of sedative-hypnotic drugs predispose the cirrhotic patient to hepatic encephalopathy. Excessive dietary intake of protein, gastrointestinal hemorrhage, and constipation are the most important precipitating events.

Despite the incompleteness of our understanding of the role of disordered ammonium metabolism in the genesis of hepatic coma, an awareness of this relationship has provided the few effective means of treating this disorder: restriction of dietary protein; mechanical cleansing of the colon; oral administration of neomycin or kanamycin, which suppresses the urease-producing organisms in the bowel; and the use of lactulose, an inert sugar that acidifies the colonic contents. Should these measures not control the protein intolerance, surgical exclusion of the bowel may be undertaken, but this operation carries a prohibitively high risk of mortality. The salutary effects of these therapeutic measures, the common attribute of which is the lowering of blood ammonium, lend strong support to the theory of *ammonium intoxication*.

More recent methods of treatment, the practicality of which remains to be established, include the use of keto analogues of essential amino acids and of bromocriptine. Theoretically, the keto analogues should provide a nitrogen-free source of essential amino acids (Maddrey et al.), and bromocriptine, a dopamine agonist, should enhance dopaminergic transmission. Morgan and her associates have recently described clinical improvement as well as an increase in cerebral blood flow and oxygen consumption in patients with chronic hepatic encephalopathy who were treated with bromocriptine.

In *acute hepatitis*, delirious, confusional, and comatose states also occur, but their mechanisms are still unknown. Ammonium may be elevated, but usually not to a degree that would be expected to affect central nervous system function.

Reye's Syndrome (Reye-Johnson Syndrome) As indicated above, this is a special type of nonicteric hepatic encephalopathy, occurring in children and adolescents, and characterized by acute brain swelling in association with fatty infiltration of the viscera, particularly of the liver. Although individual cases of this disorder had been described for many years, its recognition as a clinical-pathologic entity dates from 1963, when a large series was reported from Australia by Reye and his colleagues and from the United States by Johnson et al. The disorder is not uncommon and tends to occur in outbreaks (286 cases were reported to the Center for Disease Control during a 4-month period in 1974).

Most cases occur in childhood, boys and girls being equally affected, but rare instances have been observed in the third decade. In most cases the encephalopathy is preceded for several days to a week by fever, symptoms of upper respiratory infection, and protracted vomiting. These are followed by the rapid evolution of stupor and coma, associated in many cases with focal and generalized seizures, signs of sympathetic overactivity (tachypnea, tachycardia, mydriasis), decorticate and decerebrate rigidity, and loss of pupillary, corneal, and vestibuloocular reflexes. Initially there is a metabolic acidosis, followed by a respiratory alkalosis (rising arterial pH and falling P_{CO_2}). The CSF is usually under increased pressure and is acellular; glucose values may be low, reflecting the hypoglycemia. SGOT and blood ammonia levels are increased, sometimes to an extreme degree. The EEG is characterized by diffuse arrhythmic delta activity, progressing to electrocerebral silence in patients who fail to survive (about 35 percent).

Lesser degrees of cerebral involvement are also observed from time to time. The authors have seen children who became acutely confused, frightened, or mute; the liver was not enlarged and only the high levels of SGOT and modest elevation of serum ammonium provided clues to the nature of the illness. Recovery was complete within a few days. Such cases usually are found among more severe cases during epidemics of influenza.

The major *pathological findings* are cerebral edema, often with cerebellar herniation, and infiltration of hepatocytes with fine droplets of fat (mainly triglycerides); the renal tubules, myocardium, skeletal muscle, pancreas, and spleen are infiltrated to a lesser extent. There are no inflammatory lesions in the brain, liver, or other organs. The pathogenesis of this disorder remains obscure. The antecedent infections so far identified have been influenza and varicella.

Treatment is purely supportive (mechanically assisted ventilation, administration of hypertonic glucose and corticosteroids, and measures to lower the serum ammonium).

UREMIC ENCEPHALOPATHY

Episodic confusion and stupor and other neurologic symptoms may accompany any form of severe renal disease—acute or chronic. In addition, a number of neurologic syndromes complicate chronic hemodialysis and kidney transplantation. Chronic polyneuropathy is the most common neurologic complication of renal failure and is discussed on page 906.

The cerebral symptoms attributable to the uremic state are best discerned in normotensive individuals in whom renal failure develops rapidly. Toxic nitrogenous and other products accumulate in the blood, rising day by day to high levels. Apathy, fatigue, inattentiveness, and irritability are usually the initial symptoms; later, confusion, disturbances of sensory perception, hallucinations, and stupor supervene. Characteristically these symptoms fluctuate from day to day, or even from hour to hour. In some patients these symptoms may come on rather abruptly and progress rapidly to a state of coma. In others, mild visual hallucinations and a disorder of attention may persist for several weeks in relatively pure form.

Clouding of the sensorium is practically always associated with a variety of motor phenomena, which usually occur early in the course of the encephalopathy, sometimes when the patient is still mentally clear. The patient begins to twitch and jerk, and may convulse. The twitches involve parts of muscles, whole muscles, or limbs, are lightning quick, arrhythmic, asynchronous on the two sides of the body, and incessant during wakefulness and sleep. At various times the term fasciculation, arrhythmic tremor, myoclonus, chorea, asterixis, or convulsion is applicable to a particular abnormality of movement. At other times they are difficult to classify. The authors prefer to speak of the condition as the *uremic twitch-convulsive syndrome*.

Because of the similarity of this syndrome to tetany, one is prompted to measure serum calcium and magnesium, and of course hypocalcemia and hypomagnesemia do occur in uremia. But often the values for these ions are normal, and the administration of calcium and magnesium salts has little effect. The resemblance of uremic encephalopathy to hepatic and other metabolic encephalopathies has been stressed by Raskin and Fishman, yet the authors are more impressed with differences than similarities. We have observed the twitch-convulsive syndrome in association with a variety of diseases such as widespread neoplasia, delirium tremens, diabetes with necrotizing pyelonephritis, and lupus erythematosus, where the blood urea nitrogen was only modestly elevated, but always the factor of renal failure was ultimately discovered. Glaser and his colleagues produced a state of twitching and convulsions in rats by the injection of urea alone.

As the uremia worsens, the patient lapses into a quiet coma. Unless the accompanying metabolic acidosis is corrected, Kussmaul breathing appears and gives way, before death, to Cheyne-Stokes breathing.

Since uremia is so frequently associated with hypertension, a major problem arises in distinguishing the cerebral effects of uremia per se from those of severe hypertension. Volhard was the first to make this distinction; he introduced the term *pseudouremia* to designate the cerebral effects of malignant hypertension and to separate them from *true uremia*. The name *hypertensive encephalopathy*, by which pseudouremia is now generally known, was first used by Oppenheimer and Fishberg. The clinical picture of the latter disorder and its pathophysiology are fully discussed on page 582.

Opinions vary as to the cause of uremic encephalopathy and the twitch-convulsive syndrome. It would appear that every level of the central nervous system is affected from spinal cord to cerebrum. The authors have been unable to detect a lesion in the brain or spinal cord other than a mild hyperplasia of protoplasmic astrocytes in some cases, but never of the degree observed in hepatic encephalopathy. Cerebral edema is notably absent. Restoration of renal function completely corrects the neurologic syndrome, attesting to an abnormality at a subcellular level. Whether caused by the retention of organic acids, elevation of phosphate in CSF (claimed by Harrison et al.), or by the action of other toxins has never been settled.

In the *treatment* of uremic encephalopathy the

nature of the renal disease assumes paramount importance, for if it is irreversible and progressive the prognosis is poor without dialysis or renal transplantation. Convulsions, which occur in about 35 percent of cases, often preterminally, respond to relatively low plasma concentrations of anticonvulsants, the reason being that serum albumin is depressed in uremia, reducing the amount of phenytoin that is bound to albumin and increasing the unbound, therapeutically active portion. Phenobarbital is also useful in the treatment of uremic convulsions, but care must be taken to avoid sedation. One must be cautious in prescribing drugs in the face of renal failure, for inordinately high, toxic blood levels may result. Examples are gentamicin (vestibular damage), kanamycin (cochlear damage) nitrofurantoin, isoniazid, and hydralazine (peripheral nerve damage).

The "Dysequilibrium Syndrome" This term refers to a group of symptoms that may occur during and following hemodialysis or peritoneal dialysis. The symptoms include headaches, nausea, muscular cramps, nervous irritability, agitation, drowsiness, and convulsions. The headache, which may be bilateral and throbbing, or resemble common migraine, develops in approximately 70 percent of patients, while all the other symptoms are observed in 5 to 10 percent, usually in those undergoing rapid dialysis or in the early stages of a dialysis program. The symptoms tend to occur in the third or fourth hour of dialysis and last for several hours. Sometimes the symptoms appear 8 to 48 h after completing dialysis. Originally these symptoms were attributed to the rapid lowering of serum urea, leaving the brain with a higher concentration of urea than the serum, and resulting in a shift of water into the brain to equalize the osmotic gradient (*reverse urea syndrome*). Now the condition is attributed to a shift of water into the brain which is akin to water intoxication, and to inappropriate secretion of antidiuretic hormone.

The symptoms of subdural hematoma, which occurs in 3.3 percent of patients undergoing dialysis, may be mistakenly attributed to the dysequilibrium syndrome.

Dialysis Encephalopathy (Dialysis Dementia) This is another subacutely progressive syndrome that complicates chronic hemodialysis. Characteristically the condition begins with a hesitant, stuttering dysarthria, dysphasia and sometimes apraxia of speech, to which are added facial and then generalized myoclonus, focal and generalized seizures, personality and behavioral changes, and intellectual decline. The EEG is invariably abnormal, taking the form of paroxysmal and sometimes periodic sharp wave or polyspike and wave activity (up to 500 μV and lasting 1 to 20 s) intermixed with abundant theta and delta activity. The CSF is normal, except for increased protein in a few cases.

At first the myoclonus and speech disorders are intermittent, occurring during or immediately after dialysis and lasting for only a few hours, but gradually they become more persistent and eventually permanent. Once established, the syndrome usually is steadily progressive over a 1- to 15-month period (average survival of 6 months in the 42 cases analyzed by Lederman and Henry). However, there is some variability in the clinical picture. Some patients have a waxing and waning course and survive for several years; in others the symptoms are transient. We have observed two patients in whom a syndrome, indistinguishable from the one described above, occurred between 1 and 2 weeks after successful renal transplantation, at a time when they were not being dialyzed and were receiving only small doses of immunosuppressant drugs. Both these patients recovered spontaneously. Nadel and Wilson, and others, have observed a dramatic reversal of the clinical symptoms and EEG abnormalities in patients with dialysis encephalopathy who were given diazepam, suggesting that some of the symptoms and EEG changes in dialysis dementia represent a form of seizure disorder.

No consistent neuropathologic changes have been found in the fatal cases, and the pathogenesis of this syndrome is still obscure. Current speculation centers on the role of aluminum. Alfrey and his associates found that the cerebral gray matter of patients who died from dialysis encephalopathy contained a much greater amount of aluminum than tissue from dialysis patients without encephalopathy. The aluminum may be derived from the dialysate or orally administered aluminum gels, or both. These authors suggested that dialysis encephalopathy represents a form of aluminum intoxication, a view that has received support from recent observations that interruption of aluminum intake may reverse the symptoms of encephalopathy (Poisson et al., Rozas and Port).

Other Complications of Kidney Transplantation The greatly increased risk of developing reticulum cell sarcoma has already been mentioned (page 453). Wernicke's encephalopathy and central pontine myelinolysis

have also been observed. Systemic fungal infections are found at autopsy in about 45 percent of patients who have had renal transplants and long periods of immunosuppressive treatment, and in about one-third of these patients the CNS is involved. *Aspergillus, Candida, Nocardia,* and *Histoplasma* are the usual organisms, in that order of frequency (page 500). Other CNS infections that have complicated transplantation are toxoplasmosis and cytomegalic inclusion disease.

Other Metabolic Encephalopathies Limitations of space permit only brief reference to other important metabolic disturbances that present as episodic confusion, stupor, or coma. *Metabolic acidosis* due to diabetes mellitus or renal failure produces a syndrome typified by drowsiness, stupor, and coma with dry skin and Kussmaul breathing (page 238). Acidosis in infancy and childhood may occur in the course of hyperammonemia, isovaleric acidemia, maple syrup urine disease, hyperglycinemia, etc. (Chap. 37). High-voltage, slow activity predominates in the EEG, and correction of the acidosis restores nervous function to normal, provided that coma has not persisted for too long a time and has not become complicated by hypoxia or hypotension. There is no recognizable neuropathologic change in uncomplicated acidotic coma.

Extreme degrees of *hyperosmolality* of the blood may develop in the course of diabetes mellitus (blood glucose greater than 400 mg) and in *hypernatremic dehydration,* resulting in both instances in alterations of the state of consciousness, ranging from lethargy and stupor to deep coma. Delirium, muscle twitches or jerks, and seizures may occur. In some cases the movement disorder resembles chorea and myoclonic twitching, like that of uremia. Frequently the seizures occur during the period of rehydration, which needs to be accomplished cautiously, using polyionic solutions. *Hyponatremia,* usually with water intoxication, is another cause of episodic lethargy, confusion, delirium, stupor, and coma, especially in infants. Muscle weakness and cramps, myoclonus and asterixis are other manifestations. Encephalopathy due to *Addison's disease* (adrenal insufficiency) may be attended by episodic confusion, stupor, or coma without special identifying features; its basis remains unclear. Hypotension and diminished cerebral circulation and hypoglycemia are the most readily recognized metabolic abnormalities, and measures which correct these conditions appear to have been beneficial in some instances.

In children more than adults, cholera being an exception, extremely *severe diarrhea* may be attended by an encephalopathy. Irritability, weakness, headache, seizures, stupor, and coma may develop over a period of 2 to 3 days and carry a grave prognosis unless promptly relieved. Presumably this is a metabolic encephalopathy due to loss of fluids and electrolytes and can be corrected by their replacement. In the more protracted illness of *typhoid fever*, approximately half the patients are delirious and a small number will exhibit meningism and become comatose with twitching and seizures, or spasticity and hyperactive reflexes in the legs—all transitory symptoms. In none of the infective diarrheas have there been definite lesions in the brain at autopsy, and the nature of such encephalopathic disorders is poorly understood.

METABOLIC DISEASES PRESENTING AS PROGRESSIVE EXTRAPYRAMIDAL SYNDROMES

These syndromes are usually of mixed type, i.e., they include a number of extrapyramidal symptoms in various combinations, and may emerge as part of an acquired chronic hepatocerebral degeneration or chronic hypoparathyroidism, or as a sequela of kernicterus, or of hypoxic or hypoglycemic encephalopathy. The basal ganglionic-cerebellar symptoms that result from severe *anoxia* and *hypoglycemia* have been described in the preceding section and in Chap. 4. *Kernicterus* is considered on page 855, with the special neurologic diseases of infancy and childhood, and calcification of the basal ganglia and cerebellum (chronic parathyroid deficiency) on page 690, with the inherited metabolic disorders. It must be realized, however, that acquired hypoparathyroidism may lead to calcification of the basal ganglia (see below under diseases presenting as cerebellar ataxia). Hyperthyroidism is accompanied by chorea in 2 percent of patients, according to Weiner and Klawans. They ascribe the chorea to a disturbance of dopamine metabolism. The acquired form of hepatocerebral degeneration remains to be discussed here.

ACQUIRED (NON-WILSONIAN) HEPATOCEREBRAL DEGENERATION

Patients who survive an episode or several episodes of hepatic coma are occasionally left with residual neurologic abnormalities, such as tremor of the head or arms, asterixis, grimacing, choreic movements and twitching of the limbs, dysarthria, ataxia of gait, or impairment of intellectual function; and these symptoms may worsen with repeated attacks of stupor and coma. In other patients with chronic liver disease, permanent neurologic abnormalities become manifest in the absence of discrete episodes of hepatic coma. In either event, patients thus

afflicted deteriorate neurologically over a period of years. Examination of the brain of such patients discloses foci of destruction of nerve cells and other parenchymal elements in addition to a widespread transformation of astrocytes, changes that are very much the same as those of Wilson's disease.

Probably the first to describe this acquired type of hepatocerebral degeneration was van Woerkom (1914), whose report appeared only two years after Wilson's classic description of the familial form. Since then, there have been sporadic reports of the acquired disease. A full account of these as well as of our own extensive experience with this disorder is contained in the article by Victor, Adams and Cole, listed in the references.

Clinical Features The first symptom may be a tremor of the outstretched limbs, fleeting arrhythmic twitches of the face and limbs (resembling either myoclonus or chorea) or a mild unsteadiness of gait with action tremor. As the condition evolves over months or years a rather characteristic dysarthria, mild ataxia, wide-based, unsteady gait, and choreoathetosis, mainly of the face, neck, and shoulders, are joined in a common syndrome. Mental function is slowly altered, taking the form of a simple dementia with lack of concern and indifference to the illness. A coarse rhythmic tremor of the arms, appearing with certain sustained postures, mild corticospinal tract signs, and diffuse EEG abnormalities complete the clinical picture. Other less-frequent signs are muscular rigidity, grasp reflexes, tremor in repose, nystagmus, asterixis, and action or intention myoclonus. In essence, each of the neurologic abnormalities that characterizes chronic hepatocerebral degeneration may also be observed in patients with hepatic coma, the only difference being that the abnormalities are evanescent in the latter and irreversible in the former.

As a rule, all measurable hepatic functions are altered, but the neurologic disorder correlates best with an elevation of serum ammonium (usually greater than 200 μg per 100 ml). Unlike Wilson's disease, where the cirrhosis usually remains occult for a long time, there is no question about its presence in the acquired syndrome; jaundice, ascites, and esophageal varices are manifest in most of the acquired cases. Wilson's disease, which enters into the differential diagnosis, is usually not difficult to differentiate on clinical grounds, although the distinction in some cases requires the critical evidence of familial occurrence, Kayser-Fleischer rings (never found in the acquired type), and certain biochemical determinations (serum ceruloplasmin and copper levels, urinary copper excretion—see page 688).

Pathologic Findings The chronic cerebral symptoms, like the transient ones, may occur with all varieties of chronic liver disease. Portal-systemic shunts are always sent. Occasionally the liver is normal and an Eck fistula has formed as a result of a thrombosis or surgical ligation of the portal vein.

The cerebral lesion is localized more regularly in the cortex than is the case in Wilson's disease. In some specimens an irregular gray line of necrosis or gliosis can be observed throughout both hemispheres, with a predilection for the parietal and occipital regions, and the lenticular nuclei may appear shrunken and discolored. These lesions resemble hypoxic ones, but tend to spare the hippocampus, globus pallidus, and deep folia of the cerebellar cortex—the sites of predilection in anoxic encephalopathy. Microscopically, a widespread hyperplasia of protoplasmic astrocytes is visible in the deep layers of the cerebral cortex, in the cerebellar cortex, as well as in thalamic and lenticular nuclei and many other nuclear structures of the brainstem. In the necrotic lesions the medullated fibers and nerve cells are destroyed, with marginal fibrous gliosis; at the corticomedullary junction, in the striatum (particularly in the superior pole of the putamen) and in the cerebellar white matter, polymicrocavitation may be prominent. Protoplasmic astrocytic nuclei contain periodic acid–Schiff (PAS) positive glycogen granules. Nerve cells may appear swollen and chromatolyzed, taking the form, we believe, of the so-called Opalski cells. The similarity of the neuropathologic lesion in the familial (Wilson's) and acquired forms of the liver disease suggests a common hepatogenesis.

Pathogenesis It is evident that a close relationship exists between the acute transient form of hepatic encephalopathy (hepatic coma) and the chronic, largely irreversible hepatocerebral syndrome. As stated above, the latter syndrome frequently develops on a background of repeated episodes of hepatic coma; in these patients it is often impossible to identify the point at which the reversible illness ends and the permanent one begins, so imperceptibly does one blend into the other. This intimate relationship is reflected in the pathologic findings as well; the astrocytic hyperplasia and PAS-positive inclusions are identical in both forms of the disease, and the distribution of the destructive lesions follows closely the distribution of the astrocytic change. Also, both dis-

orders are characterized by hyperammonemia, episodic in one and persistent in the other. Reducing the serum ammonium by the measures that are effective in acute hepatic encephalopathy will cause a recession of many of the chronic neurologic abnormalities, not completely but to an extent that the patient is able to function better.

All these considerations allow one to theorize about the genesis of the acquired form of hepatocerebral degeneration and its relation to hepatic coma. As has been postulated above, episodic stupor or coma, reflected pathologically by a diffuse astrocytic hyperplasia, is a metabolic disorder secondary to the rapid accumulation of ammonium in the blood. A prolongation of this effect would lead to a chronic and largely irreversible neurologic syndrome based on parenchymal lesions. One may theorize further that the symptoms in both forms of the disease have their basis in a parenchymal lesion of similar mechanism, being transitory and invisible (at least by light microscopy) in one and permanent and microscopically evident in the other. Stated in another way, the damage to parenchymal elements might simply represent the most severe degree of a pathologic process which in its mildest form is reflected in an astrocytic hyperplasia alone.

METABOLIC DISEASES PRESENTING AS CEREBELLAR ATAXIA

CEREBELLAR ATAXIA ASSOCIATED WITH MYXEDEMA

The association of myxedema and cerebellar ataxia has been mentioned sporadically in medical writings since the latter part of the nineteenth century. Interest in this problem was revived in recent years by Jellinek and Kelly, who described six such cases. All of them showed an ataxia of gait; in addition, ataxia of the arms and dysarthria were present in four instances, and nystagmus in two. Cremer et al. have reported a similar clinical experience, based on a study of 24 patients with either primary or secondary hypothyroidism.

There have been only a few reports of the pathologic changes, and these are far from satisfactory. The myxedematous patient described by Price and Netsky had also been a serious alcoholic, and the clinical signs (ataxia of gait and of the legs) and pathologic changes (loss of Purkinje cells and gliosis of the molecular layer, most pronounced in the vermis) cannot be distinguished from those due to alcoholism and malnutrition. Scattered throughout the nervous system of their case were unusual glycogen-containing bodies, similar but not identical to corpora amylacea. These structures, designated *myxedema bodies* by Price and Netsky were also observed in the cerebellar white matter of a second case of myxedema; there were no other neuropathologic changes, however, and this patient had shown no ataxia during life.

It is difficult to know whether these peculiar bodies have anything to do with myxedema. If they do, it should be possible to demonstrate them in more than two cases. We have not seen them in one carefully studied case of myxedema, nor have they been described by others. Thyroid medication corrects the defect in motor coordination, raising doubt as to whether there could be a visible structural lesion underlying it.

The authors have had no experience with this condition, but wonder whether the attribution of the faulty gait and ataxia of movement to a cerebellar change might not be in error. Theoretically, the slowness of muscle relaxation (a characteristic of hypothyroidism) might interfere with the timing of muscle actions during a coordinated movement, thus simulating ataxia.

THE EFFECTS OF HYPERTHERMIA ON THE CEREBELLUM

The damaging effects of hyperthermia, like those of anoxia, involve the brain diffusely. In the case of hyperthermia, however, the changes are disproportionately severe in the cerebellum. The acute manifestations of profound hyperthermia are coma and convulsions, frequently complicated by shock and renal failure. Patients who survive the initial stage of the illness frequently show signs of widespread cerebral affection, such as confusion, dementia, and pseudobulbar and spastic paralysis. These abnormalities tend to resolve gradually, leaving the patient with a more or less pure disorder of cerebellar function.

The most extensive account of the pathologic effects of hyperthermia is that of Malamud et al. These authors studied 125 fatal cases of heat stroke, but their observations are equally applicable to hyperthermia of other types. They found that the alterations in the cerebellum were more striking, more consistent, and more rapid in development than in any other part of the brain. In patients who survived less than 24 h, the changes consisted mainly of a loss of some of the Purkinje cells and swelling, pyknosis, and disintegration of those which remained. In cases surviving longer, there was almost complete degeneration of the Purkinje cells, with gliosis throughout the cerebellar cortex, as well as degeneration of the dentate nuclei. The changes in the cerebellar cortex were equally pronounced in the hemispheres and vermis.

HYPOPARATHYROIDISM

This condition and pseudohypoparathyroidism (page 690) were mentioned in relation to the hereditary metabolic disorders. Formerly, the usual cause of hypoparathyroidism was surgical removal of the parathyroid glands during subtotal thyroidectomy, but there were always idiopathic cases as well. With the more widespread use of radiation and drug therapy for thyroid disease, the surgical group has become small in proportion to the idiopathic one. The latter occurs in pure form—presumably an agenesis of parathyroid glands with unmeasurable levels of parathormone in the blood, or as part of the DiGeorge syndrome of agenesis of thymus and parathyroids, organs embryologically derived from the third and fourth branchial clefts. Hypoparathyroidism is also part of a familial disorder in which there is a deficiency of thyroid, ovarian, and adrenal function, pernicious anemia, and other defects based presumably on a derangement of autoimmune mechanisms. In all instances the low levels of parathormone and normal responses to injected hormone permit recognition of a primary defect in parathyroid glands and distinguish it from all other conditions in which there is hypocalcemia and hyperphosphatemia.

The clinical manifestations, mainly attributable to the effects of hypocalcemia, are tetany, muscle cramps, convulsions, laryngeal spasm, and paresthesias. Children with this disease state may be irritable and show personality changes. In the adult patients, calcium deposits occur in the basal ganglia, dentate nuclei, and cerebellar cortex. We have observed in such patients unilateral tremor, a restless choreoathetotic hand, bilateral rigidity, slowness of movement and flexed posture resembling Parkinson's syndrome, and ataxia of limbs and of gait—all in various combinations. Interestingly, the multiple skeletal and developmental abnormalities that characterize both pseudo- and pseudo-pseudohypoparathyroidism (short stature, round face, short neck, stocky body build, shortening of metacarpal and metatarsal bones and phalanges from premature epiphyseal closure) are rarely seen in pure hypoparathyroidism.

METABOLIC DISEASE PRESENTING AS PSYCHOSIS AND DEMENTIA

The point has already been made that milder degrees of episodic stupor and coma, if persistent, may present as a state of protracted confusion that is impossible to distinguish from dementia. Chronic portal-systemic encephalopathy, the syndromes of chronic hypoglycemia, chronic hypercalcemia, and dialysis encephalopathy all fall within this category. Clouding of the sensorium, inattentiveness, inaccurate perceptions and interpretations, the attributes that usually allow a confusional state to be distinguished from a dementia, are no longer dependable. If the onset is rapid rather than gradual (over weeks and months) and if any therapeutic maneuver reverses the condition, restoring full mental clarity, the conclusion is justified that one is dealing with a confusional state; but on strict clinical analysis at any one time in the active phase of the disease the distinction may be impossible.

In general hospitals, an episodic confusional state lasting days and weeks in the course of a medical illness or following an operation should always raise the suspicion of one of the aforementioned metabolic states. Usually, however, all of them can be excluded, and one falls back on a rather unsatisfactory interpretation—that a combination of drugs, fever, toxemia, and unspecifiable metabolic disorders is responsible.

In the *endocrine encephalopathies,* which are described below, the clinical phenomena are even more abstruse. Confusional states may be combined with agitation, hallucinations, delusions, anxiety, and depression, and the time span of the illness may be in terms of weeks and months, rather than days. Certain aspects of the endocrine psychoses are discussed further on pages 1059 to 1061.

CUSHING'S DISEASE AND CORTICOSTEROID PSYCHOSES

Derangement of higher nervous function by the administration of ACTH or corticosteroid agents has become the prototype of all iatrogenic psychoses. The same symptoms have been reported in Cushing's disease.

Our experience with this neurologic condition comes mainly from observations of patients receiving ACTH or prednisone for a variety of neurologic and medical diseases. At low dose levels there is usually no psychic effect other than a sense of well being and decreased fatigability. At higher dose levels (80 units per day for ACTH and 60 to 100 mg/day for prednisone) approximately 10 to 15 percent of patients become overly active, emotionally labile, and unable to sleep. Unless the dose is promptly reduced, there follows a progressive shift in mood, usually toward euphoria and hypomania—but sometimes toward depression, and then inattentiveness, distractibility, and mild confusion. The EEG becomes less well-modulated and slower frequencies begin to appear. Frank hallucinations and delusions are expressed by a minority of patients, giving the illness a truly psychotic stamp, and raising suspicions of schizophrenia or manic-depressive disease. In nearly all instances, however, this mixture of confusion and mood change in association with disordered cognitive function distinguishes the iatrogenic corticosteroid psychosis. Withdrawal of medication relieves the symptoms, but full recovery may take several days to a few weeks. Later, as with all confusional states and deliria, the patient's recollection of events during the illness is fragmentary.

The neurologic basis of this condition is poorly understood. The ascription of it to premorbid personality traits or a disposition to psychiatric illness is plausible, but lacks convincing documentation. Part of the difficulty is the lack of knowledge of the role of these endocrine agents in normal cerebral metabolism. We have no information as to how they act to reduce the volume of the edematous cerebral tissue around a tumor or the volume or the tumor growth itself. Critical studies of cellular or subcellular metabolism and morphologic changes are lacking. Cerebral "atrophy" (ventricular enlargement) has been shown radiologically in patients with Cushing's disease and after a prolonged period (years) of corticosteroid therapy, but its basis also is unexplained. In some cases treatment has led to reversal of symptoms and reduction in ventricular size, documented by repeated CT scans.

THYROID ENCEPHALOPATHIES: THYROTOXIC AND MYXEDEMATOUS PSYCHOSES AND CRETINISM

Hyperthyroidism The neurology of thyrotoxicosis has proved to be peculiarly elusive. Allusions to psychosis are widely recorded in the medical literature and some thyrotoxic patients have been observed with mental confusion, seizures, manic or depressive attacks, delusions, and chorea in various combinations with muscular weakness and atrophy, periodic paralysis, and myasthenia. We have some ideas about the ocular and neuromuscular disorders, but few or none about these cerebral conditions. Treatment of the hyperthyroidism gradually restores the mental state to normal, leaving one with no explanation of what had happened to the CNS.

Hypothyroidism The myxedematous patient as a rule is slow to react, and psychomotor activity is reduced; but only in exceptional cases have we observed a major change in cerebral function. When we have observed such a change, drowsiness, inattentiveness, and apathy have predominated. In two personally observed cases the somnolence was so extreme that the patients could not stay awake long enough to be fed or examined. They were in a state of hypothermic stupor, but exhibited no other neurologic abnormality. The extreme somnolence can be reversed within a few weeks by thyroid medication.

Cretinism This form of severe hypothyroidism, occurring during intrauterine life (hypothyroidism in mother and fetus) or postnatally as an hereditary or acquired thyroid disease, is one of the correctable forms of metabolic cerebral disease. Although frequent in goitrous regions in which there is a lack of iodine, there are also a number of genetically determined defects in thyroxin synthesis that have come to light in recent years (Stanbury et al.). The thyroid gland in sporadic cretinism is either absent or represented by cysts, indicating a failure of development or a destructive lesion.

As a rule, the symptoms and signs of congenital thyroid deficiency are not recognizable at birth, but become apparent only after a few weeks; and more often the condition is first diagnosed between the sixth and twelfth months of life. Physiologic jaundice tends to be severe and prolonged (up to 3 months), and this, along with widening of the posterior fontanelle and mottling of the skin, should raise suspicion of the disease. In typical cases the face is pale and puffy; the skin dry; the hair coarse, scanty, and dry; the eyelids thickened; the heavy lips parted by the enlarged tongue; the forehead low; and the base of the nose broad. There are fat pads above the clavicles and in the axillae. The abdomen is protuberant, often with an umbilical hernia, and the head is small—a physical appearance that prompted William Boyd to remark: "What was intended to be created in the image of God has turned out to be the pariah of nature, all for the want of a little thyroid."

In the latter part of the first year, *stunting of growth and delay in psychomotor development* become evident. Untreated, the child is severely retarded but placid and good natured; such children sleep contentedly for longer periods than normal children. Sitting, standing, and walking are delayed. Movements are slow, and if reflexes can be obtained, their relaxation time is clearly delayed. The body temperature is low, and the extremities are cold and cyanotic. Although the head is small, the fontanelles may not close until the sixth or seventh year, and there is delayed ossification. If the hypothyroidism in the mother was present in the first trimester of pregnancy, cochlear development is imperfect, and there is *congenital deafness.* The gait is slow and the

movements are stiff and awkward, manifestations of a *spastic paraparesis.*

The electrocardiogram is of low voltage; the EEG is slower than normal with less alpha activity; the CSF contains an excess of protein (50 to 150 mg per 100 ml) and the serum T_3 and T_4, protein-bound iodine, and radioactive iodine uptake are all subnormal. Serum cholesterol is increased (300 to 600 mg per 100 ml).

At autopsy the brain, though small, is normally formed. A reduction in number of nerve cells was described by Marinesco, especially in the fifth cortical layer, but others have not confirmed this finding. The use of Golgi techniques has shown less than the usual interneuronal distances (packing density increased as in the immature cortex) and a deficiency of neuropil. The latter change is due to a poverty of dendritic branchings and crossings, and presumably there is a decrease of the synaptic surfaces of cells (Eayrs). Thyroid hormone appears to be essential, not for neuronal formation and migration, but for dendritic-axonic development and organization.

If the condition is recognized early and treated consistently with potent thyroid hormones, statural and mental development can be stimulated to normal or near-normal levels. Extent of recovery depends on the severity of the hypothyroidism and its duration before treatment was begun, and adequacy of therapy. In most patients, some degree of mental backwardness persists throughout life.

Hyperparathyroidism We have not been much impressed with the effects of this endocrine disorder upon the nervous system. The neuromuscular effects are the most definite, and consist of weakness and reversible electrophysiologic disturbances of nerve and muscle (see page 975). When serum calcium levels reach 15 mg per 100 ml or higher, the patient sinks into a quiet state of inattentiveness, drowsiness, lethargy, and confusion. Stupor, coma, and death may be caused by extreme degrees of hypercalcemia such as occur occasionally in cases of excessive vitamin D administration and metastatic carcinoma of bones.

PANCREATIC ENCEPHALOPATHY

This term was introduced by Rothermich and Von Haam in 1941 to describe a relatively uniform clinical state observed in patients with acute abdominal symptoms referable to pancreatic disease. As to the latter, there is usually a sudden development of midabdominal pain (on a background of biliary tract disease or alcoholism), associated with vomiting, upper abdominal tenderness, and rigidity. An elevation of serum amylase occurs later and may last for a few days. The encephalopathy consists of an agitated, confused state, sometimes with hallucinations and clouding of consciousness, dysarthria, and changing rigidity of the limbs—all of which fluctuate over a period of hours or days. Coma and quadriplegia have been reported. At autopsy there are a variety of lesions; two cases have had central pontine myelinolysis, and others have had small foci of necrosis and edema, petechial hemorrhages, and "demyelination" scattered through the cerebrum, brainstem, and cerebellum. These have been uncritically attributed to the action of released lipases and proteolases from the action of pancreatic enzymes. Rothermich and Von Haam were struck with the resemblance of the syndrome to what was described at that time as acute nicotinic acid deficiency (page 715).

The status of this entity, in the authors' opinion, is uncertain. Pallis and Lewis express reservations and suggest that before such a diagnosis can be seriously entertained in a patient with acute pancreatitis, one should exclude delirium tremens, cerebral circulatory insufficiency from shock, renal failure, hypoglycemia, diabetic acidosis, hyperosmolality syndrome, hypokalemia, and hypocalcemia or hypercalcemia—any one of which may complicate the underlying disease(s).

WHIPPLE'S DISEASE

This is a rare disorder, predominantly of middle-aged men, which may give rise to a number of neurologic syndromes. Weight loss, fever, anemia, steatorrhea, abdominal pain and distension, arthralgia, lymphadenopathy and hyperpigmentation are the usual systemic manifestations. Bacterial infection has been postulated repeatedly as the cause of the disease, but this has never been proved. Biopsy of the jejunal mucosa, which discloses macrophages filled with PAS-positive material, is diagnostic. PAS-positive histiocytes have also been identified in the CNS, either in periventricular, hypothalamic and tuberal foci, or diffusely scattered in the brain, and are apparently responsible for the neurologic manifestations. The latter most often take the form of a slowly progressive dementia, like that of Alzheimer's disease; visual impairment, ophthalmoplegia and myoclonus have been noted less often (Schochet and Lampert).

REFERENCES

ADAMS RD, FOLEY JM: The neurological disorder associated with liver disease. *Res Publ Assoc Res Nerv Ment Dis* 32:198, 1953.

ALFREY AC, LEGENDRE GR, KAEHNY WD: The dialysis encephalopathy syndrome: Possible aluminum intoxication. *N Engl J Med* 294:184, 1976.

AMES A et al: Cerebral ischemia: II. The no-reflow phenomenon. *Am J Pathol* 52:437, 1968.

BARCROFT R: *The Respiratory Function of the Blood.* London, Cambridge, 1925.

CREMER GM, GOLDSTINE NP, PARIS J: Myxedema and ataxia. *Neurology* 19:37, 1969.

DEVIVO DC, KEATING JP: Reye's syndrome. *Adv Pediatr* 22:175, 1976.

DOOLING EC, RICHARDSON EP JR: Delayed encephalopathy after strangling. *Arch Neurol* 33:196, 1976.

EAYRS JT: Influence of the thyroid on the central nervous system. *Br Med Bull* 16:122, 1960.

FERRENDELLI JA: Cerebral utilization of nonglucose substrates and their effect on hypoglycemia, in Plum F (ed): *Brain Dysfunction in Metabolic Disorders,* vol 53. New York, Raven Press, 1974, pp 113-120.

FISCHER JE, BALDESSARINI RJ: Pathogenesis and therapy of hepatic coma, in Popper H, Schaffner F (eds): *Progress in Liver Disease.* New York, Grune & Stratton, 1976, chap 23, pp 363-397.

FISHMAN RA: *Cerebrospinal Fluid in Diseases of the Nervous System.* Philadelphia, Saunders, 1980, p 95.

GLASER GH: Brain dysfunction in uremia, in Plum F (ed): *Brain Dysfunction in Metabolic Disorders,* vol 53. New York, Raven Press, 1974, pp 173-201.

HARRISON TR, MASON MF, RESNIK H: Observations on the mechanism of muscular twitchings in uremia. *J Clin Invest* 15:463, 1936.

HAYMOND MW et al: Metabolic response to hypertonic glucose administration in Reye syndrome. *Ann Neurol* 3:207, 1978.

HOYUMPA AM JR et al: Hepatic encephalopathy. *Gastroenterology* 76:184, 1979.

JELLINEK EH, KELLY RE: Cerebellar syndrome in myxedema. *Lancet* 2:225, 1960.

JOHNSON GM, SCURLETIS TD, CARROLL NB: A study of sixteen fatal cases of encephalitis-like disease in North Carolina children. *NC Med J* 24:464, 1963.

LEDERMAN RS, HENRY CE: Progressive dialysis encephalopathy. *Ann Neurol* 4:199, 1978.

MADDREY WC et al: Effects of keto analogues of essential amino acids in portal-systemic encephalopathy. *Gastroenterology* 71:190, 1976.

MALAMUD N, HAYMAKER W, CUSTER RP: Heat stroke: A clinicopathologic study of 125 fatal cases. *Mil Surg* 99:397, 1946.

MARINESCO G: Lesions en myxedème congénitale avec idiotie. *L'Encéphale* 19:265, 1924.

MARKS R, ROSE FC: *Hypoglycemia.* Oxford, Blackwell, 1965.

MORGAN MY et al: Successful use of bromocriptine in the treatment of chronic hepatic encephalopathy. *Gastroenterology* 78:663, 1980.

Nadel AM, Wilson WP: Dialysis encephalopathy: A possible seizure disorder. *Neurology* 26:1130, 1976.

Naville F: Diplegia and thyroid disturbance in defective children. *Schweiz Arch Neurol Psychiatr* 13:559, 1923.

Oppenheimer BS, Fishberg AM: Hypertensive encephalopathy. *Arch Intern Med* 41:264, 1928.

Pallis CA, Lewis PD: *The Neurology of Gastrointestinal Disease*. London, Saunders, 1974.

Plum F, Posner JB: *Diagnosis of Stupor and Coma*, 3d ed. Philadelphia, Davis, 1980.

———, ———, Hain RF: Delayed neurological deterioration after anoxia. *Arch Int Med* 110:18, 1962.

Poisson M, Mashaly R, Lafforgue B: Progressive dialysis encephalopathy. *Ann Neurol* 6:88, 1979.

Price TR, Netsky MG: Myxedema and ataxia: Cerebellar alterations and "neural myxedema bodies." *Neurology* 16:957, 1966.

Prockop LD: Hyperglycemia: Effects on the nervous system, in Vinken PJ, Bruyn BW (eds): *Handbook of Clinical Neurology*, vol 27: *Metabolic and Deficiency Diseases of the Nervous System*, pt I. Amsterdam, North-Holland, 1976, pp 79-99.

Raskin NH, Fishman RA: Neurologic disorders in renal failure. *N Engl J Med* 294:143, 204, 1976.

Reye RDK, Morgan G, Baral J: Encephalopathy and fatty degeneration of the viscera: A disease entity in childhood. *Lancet* 2:749, 1963.

Rothermich NO, Von Haam E: Pancreatic encephalopathy. *J Clin Endocrinol* 1:872, 1941.

Rozas VV, Port FK: Progressive dialysis encephalopathy: Prevention through control of aluminum levels in water. *Ann Neurol* 6:88, 1979.

Schochet SS Jr, Lampert PW: Granulomatous encephalitis in Whipple's disease. Electron microscopic observations. *Acta Neuropathologica* 13:1, 1969.

Stanbury JB, Wyngaarden JB, Fredrickson DS (eds): *The Metabolic Basis of Inherited Disease*, 4th ed. New York, McGraw-Hill, 1978.

Tom MI, Richardson JC: Hypoglycaemia from islet cell tumor of pancreas with amyotrophy and cerebrospinal nerve cell changes. *J Neuropathol Exp Neurol* 10:57, 1951.

Tyler HR: Neurological disorders seen in renal failure, in Vinken PJ, Bruyn BW (eds): *Handbook of Clinical Neurology*, vol 27: *Metabolic and Deficiency Diseases of the Nervous System*, pt I. Amsterdam, North-Holland, 1976, pp 321-348.

van Woerkom W: La cirrhose hepatique avec alterations dans les centres nerveux evoluant chez des sujets d'age moyen. *Nouvelle Iconographie de la Salpêtrière* 7:41, 1914.

Victor M, Adams RD, Cole M: The acquired (non-Wilsonian) type of chronic hepatocerebral degeneration. *Medicine* 44:345, 1965.

Volhard F: Clinical aspects of Bright's disease, in Berglund H et al (eds): *The Kidney in Health and Disease*. Philadelphia, Lea & Febiger, 1935, chap 29, pp 665-673.

von Hösslin C, Alzheimer A: Ein Beitrag zur Klinik und pathologischen Anatomie der Westphal-Strümpellschen Pseudosklerose. *Z Gesamte Neurol Psychiatr* 8:183, 1912.

Wegierko J: Typical syndrome of clinical manifestations in diabetes mellitus with fatal termination in coma without ketotic acidemia: So-called third coma. *Pol Tyg Lek* 11:2020, 1956.

Weiner WJ, Klawans HL: Hyperthyroid chorea, in Vinken PJ, Bruyn BW (eds): *Handbook of Clinical Neurology*, vol 27: *Metabolic and Deficiency Diseases of the Nervous System*, pt I. Amsterdam, North-Holland, 1976, pp 279-281.

Wilkinson DS, Prockop LD: Hypoglycemia: Effects on the nervous system, in Vinken PJ, Bruyn BW (eds): *Handbook of Clinical Neurology*, vol 27: *Metabolic and Deficiency Diseases of the Nervous System*, pt I. Amsterdam, North Holland, 1976, chap 4, pp 53-78.

Wilson SAK: Progressive lenticular degeneration: A familial nervous disease associated with cirrhosis of the liver. *Brain* 34:295, 1912.

Young E, Bradley RF: Cerebral edema with irreversible coma in severe diabetic ketoacidosis. *N Engl J Med* 276:665, 1967.

Zieve L, Olsen RL: Can hepatic coma be caused by a reduction of brain noradrenaline or dopamine? *Gut* 18:688, 1977.

CHAPTER 40

ALCOHOL AND ALCOHOLISM

Intemperance in the use of alcohol creates many problems in modern society, the importance of which can be judged by the repeated emphasis they receive in contemporary writings, both literary and scientific. These problems may be divided into three categories: psychological, medical, and sociological. The main psychological problem is why a person drinks excessively, often with full knowledge that such action will result in personal physical injury and irreparable harm to the family. The medical problem embraces all aspects of alcoholic habituation as well as the diseases which result from the abuse of alcohol. The sociological problem consists of the effects of sustained drinking on the patient's work, family, and community.

These several problems engendered by excessive drinking cannot be separated from one another, and the physician must therefore be conversant with all aspects of the subject. He or she may be asked to help the patient conquer the tendency to alcoholism or to diagnose and to treat the numerous diseases to which the patient is subject; often the physician must admit or commit the patient to a general or mental hospital, according to the nature of the presenting clinical disorder; and lastly, the physician may be required to enlist the aid of available social agencies when their services are needed by either the patient or the patient's family.

Alcoholism has been defined as both a chronic disease and a disorder of behavior, characterized in either context by drinking of alcohol to an extent that interferes with the drinker's health, interpersonal relations, or means of livelihood. Reduced to pharmacologic terms, it is addiction to alcohol.

The causation of alcoholism remains obscure, despite a great deal of theorizing on the subject. The writings of Roebuck and Kessler and of Schuckit and Haglund, listed in the references, provide a critical overview of the many etiologic theories. An important recent contribution to this subject is that of Goodwin et al. They studied 55 men with alcoholic biologic parents and 55 controls whose biologic parents were not alcoholics. All of the subjects had been adopted before the age of 6 weeks and had no knowledge of their biologic parentage. Twenty percent of the offspring of biologic alcoholic parents had become alcoholics by the age of 25 to 29 years, versus 5 percent of the controls. Thus there appears to be a genetic factor in the development of alcoholism, in addition to sociocultural and psychological factors.

The incidence of alcoholism in the United States cannot be stated precisely. In 1971 the Department of Health, Education and Welfare estimated that about 9 million men and women (7 percent of the adult population) "manifested the behavior of alcohol abuse and alcoholism." It requires little projection of the imagination to conceive the havoc wrought by alcohol in terms of decreased productivity, increased incidence of suicide, accidents, crime, mental and physical disease, and disruption of family life.

PHARMACOLOGY AND METABOLISM OF ALCOHOL

Ethyl alcohol, or ethanol, is the active ingredient in beer, wine, whiskey, gin, brandy, and other less common alcoholic beverages. In addition, the stronger spirits contain enanthic ethers, which give the flavor but have no important pharmacologic properties, and impurities such as amyl alcohol (fusel oil) and acetaldehyde, which act like alcohol but are more toxic. Contrary to popular opinion, the content of B vitamins in American beer and other liquors is so low as to have little nutritional value.

Alcohol is absorbed unaltered from the gastrointestinal tract, about 25 percent from the stomach and the rest from the upper small intestine. Its presence may be detected in the blood within 5 min after ingestion, and the maximum concentration is reached in 30 to 90 min. The ingestion of milk and fatty foods impedes and water facilitates its absorption. The rate of absorption increases after Billroth I and II gastrectomies; in these cases maximum blood alcohol concentrations are higher and are attained faster than in subjects with intact stomachs. In habituated persons the blood alcohol concentration rises somewhat faster and reaches a higher maximum than in abstainers.

Alcohol is carried chiefly in the plasma and enters the various organs of the body—as well as the CSF, urine, and pulmonary alveolar air—in concentrations which bear a constant relationship to the concentration in the blood. It is eliminated chiefly by oxidation, less than 10 percent being excreted chemically unchanged in the urine, perspiration, and breath. The energy liberated by the oxidation of alcohol (7 kcal/g) can be utilized as completely as that of fats, sugars, and proteins, which it replaces isodynamically. It should be emphasized that alcohol cannot be stored in the body or used in the replacement of destroyed tissue. Therefore, unless the chronic drinker takes an adequate amount of protein (which he or she frequently fails to do), muscle bulk is lost and other tissues are damaged.

The metabolism of alcohol is accomplished mainly in the liver, where several enzyme systems (located in different subcellular compartments of the hepatocyte) can independently oxidize alcohol to acetaldehyde. In the most important of these systems alcohol dehydrogenase (ADH) plays a key role; it is an enzyme which is found in the cell sap or soluble fraction of the hepatocyte and which utilizes nicotinamide adenine dinucleotide (NAD) as the cofactor. This reaction leads to the formation of acetaldehyde and the reduction of NAD to NADH. A second pathway for oxidation of alcohol involves catalase, which is located in the peroxisomes and mitochondria; a third utilizes the "microsomal ethanol oxidizing system" (MEOS), located mainly in the microsomes of the endoplasmic reticulum. The MEOS, which is dependent upon reduced nicotinamide adenine dinucleotide phosphate (NADPH), does not account for much of the alcohol metabolized in normal circumstances, but it may be responsible for the increased rate of alcohol metabolism observed in chronic alcoholics.

The exact steps in the metabolism of acetaldehyde are still the subject of debate. Most likely it is converted by acetaldehyde dehydrogenase to acetylcoenzyme A (acetyl CoA), via acetate. This reaction, which is accomplished mainly in the mitochondria, also requires NAD

as a cofactor. Alternatively, it is possible that alcohol is converted directly to acetyl CoA, which in turn could yield acetate. In either event, acetyl CoA and acetate (the end products of alcohol metabolism in the liver) are metabolized further through well-established normal pathways, with eventual release of carbon dioxide and water.

Acetaldehyde has a number of unique biochemical effects which are not produced by alcohol alone, and this has led to speculation that acetaldehyde might be responsible for the manifestations of alcoholic intoxication and addiction. This idea has its basis in the observation that aldehydes condense with certain amines (norepinephrine, epinephrine, and serotonin) to form alkaloids, the molecular structure of which is similar to a number of highly addictive plant alkaloids, such as morphine. Because of this similarity, it has been suggested that the addictive properties of ethanol are related to the formation of alkaloids from acetaldehyde, generated during the metabolism of ethanol. Although the notion that addiction to alcohol and to opiates depends upon a common biochemical pathway is an attractive one, it is not consistent with either clinical observations or pharmacologic data (Seevers).

There are important reasons for believing that acetaldehyde does not play a significant role in alcoholic intoxication and that ethanol itself, rather than its initial metabolite, is the major addicting agent in alcoholism. The rate of acetaldehyde metabolism is very rapid and greatly exceeds the rate of oxidation of ethanol to acetaldehyde, and for this reason, acetaldehyde levels in the blood remain low even in the face of high blood alcohol levels. It is unlikely that these low blood acetaldehyde concentrations have serious toxic effects, considering the high doses of acetaldehyde required to produce such effects in animals.

For all practical purposes it may be accepted that once absorption is ended and an equilibrium established with the tissues, ethyl alcohol is oxidized at a constant rate, independent of its concentration in the blood (about 150 mg alcohol per kilogram of body weight per hour, or about 1 oz 90-proof whiskey per hour). Actually, slightly more alcohol is burned per hour when the initial concentrations are very high, but this increment is of little clinical significance. On the other hand, the rate of oxidation of acetaldehyde does depend on its concentration in the tissues. This fact is of importance in connection with the drug disulfiram (Antabuse), which raises the tissue concentration necessary for the metabolism of a certain amount of acetaldehyde per unit of time. The patient taking both Antabuse and alcohol will accumulate an inordinate amount of acetaldehyde, resulting in nausea, vomiting, and hypotension, sometimes pronounced in degree and even fatal. This pharmacologic principle underlies the treatment of alcoholism with Antabuse. Certain other drugs, notably the sulfonylureas, metronidazole, and furazolidone, have effects like those of disulfiram, but of lesser degree.

Very few factors are capable of increasing the rate of alcohol metabolism. There is some evidence that repeated ingestion of alcohol facilitates its metabolism in both normal and alcoholic subjects. Insulin, amino acids, and fructose enhance ethanol metabolism, but none of these has proved to be important in the treatment of alcohol intoxication. Starvation slows the rate of alcohol metabolism in the liver, although this varies greatly in degree from one person to another.

PHYSIOLOGIC EFFECTS OF ALCOHOL

HEART AND CIRCULATION

There appears to be a direct action on the excitability and contractility of heart muscle. With intoxicating doses there is a rise in cardiac rate and output, a rise in systolic and pulse pressures, and a cutaneous vasodilatation at the expense of splanchnic constriction. Curiously, peripheral vasodilatation, increased heart rate, and decreased blood pressure in response to alcohol are much more prominent in Orientals than whites (Ewing et al.), perhaps providing a physiologic explanation for the purportedly low rate of alcoholism among the former. Some investigators have suggested that prolonged intoxication may have a damaging effect on cardiac and skeletal muscle, a degeneration of fibers supposedly due to suppression of myophosphorylase activity. Increased sweating and vasodilatation cause a loss of body heat and a fall in temperature.

GASTROINTESTINAL SYSTEM

In low concentrations, by whatever route it is administered, alcohol stimulates the gastric glands to produce acid, apparently by releasing gastrin from the antral region and possibly by causing the mucosa to form or release histamine. With the ingestion of alcohol in concentrations of more than 10 to 15 percent the secretion of mucus is increased, the stomach mucosa becomes congested and hyperemic, and the secretion of acid then becomes depressed. Clinically these changes account for the state known as acute gastritis. The increase in appetite following ingestion of alcohol is due to the stimulation of the end organs of taste and to a general sense of well-being. Similarly, the reviving effect of alcohol in fatigue states is a cerebral one and is not the result of a direct stimulating effect on muscle or other organs.

LIVER

Alcohol has a number of important effects on liver function. With respect to lipid metabolism it can cause hypertriglyceridemia and lead also to a fatty liver. It interferes with carbohydrate metabolism and can produce hypoglycemia by impairing gluconeogenesis. However, a significant lowering of blood glucose will occur only if the hepatic store of glycogen has been depleted. In certain circumstances alcohol can also interfere with the peripheral utilization of glucose, resulting in hyperglycemia. When alcohol is oxidized, there is a simultaneous generation of reduced nicotinamide adenine dinucleotide (NADH); as a consequence, pyruvate is converted to lactate. Thus, prolonged alcohol ingestion may result in increased levels of serum lactate and occasionally in lactic acidosis.

RENAL AND ENDOCRINE EFFECTS

The inhibitory action of lactic acid on the renal excretion of uric acid may result in a secondary hyperuricemia. Other renal effects are low serum levels of phosphate and magnesium, presumably because of the increased tubular excretion of these ions. There are also an increased urinary excretion of ammonium and a titratable acidity following alcohol ingestion owing to a mild degree of both metabolic and respiratory acidosis. The former is presumably the result of an accumulation of acid metabolites and the latter the effect of the direct action of alcohol on the respiratory center.

Alcohol has a well-known effect on the renal excretion of water. The ingestion of 4 oz of 100-proof bourbon whiskey results in a diuresis qualitatively indistinguishable from that which follows the drinking of large amounts of water. This diuresis is most likely a result of the transient suppression of the release of antidiuretic hormone (ADH) from the supraopticohypophysial system, since a relatively small amount of alcohol injected directly into a carotid artery evokes a prompt diuresis without a detectable rise in the concentration of alcohol in the systemic blood. Alcohol does not alter the sensitivity of the kidney tubules to endogenous or exogenous ADH (Pitressin) and has no discernible effect on renal hemodynamic function in normal persons. The degree of diuresis seems to be more closely related to the duration of the rising blood alcohol level than to the rate of increase or the absolute level attained if the period of alcohol intoxication is sustained. Diuresis occurs only during the initial phase of alcohol administration and does not persist during prolonged drinking.

It has been demonstrated that the administration of alcohol to normal young men for periods up to 4 weeks decreases the rate of production and the plasma concentration of testosterone (Gordon et al.). These abnormalities of testosterone metabolism have been traced to both a central (hypothalamus-pituitary) and gonadal effect of alcohol and are independent of nutritional deficiency and liver disease.

HEMATOPOIETIC EFFECTS

Alcohol has a direct effect upon cells of the bone marrow. Human volunteers who were given alcohol in doses equaling half their caloric intake for several weeks manifested an increase in vacuolation of red and white cell precursors, particularly of the former. In addition, there was a depression of the platelet count. Serum iron fell, but only during the withdrawal period. All these hematologic defects occurred despite excellent nutrition and concomitant administration of folic acid (Lindenbaum and Lieber).

BEHAVIORAL EFFECTS AND THE PHENOMENON OF TOLERANCE

Apart from the derangements noted above, the obvious effects of acute, nonlethal doses of alcohol are those exerted on the nervous system, constituting the characteristic symptoms and signs of *alcohol intoxication*. It is now generally accepted that alcohol is not a stimulant of the central nervous system, but a depressant. Some of the early effects of alcohol, manifested by garrulousness, aggressiveness, and excessive activity and increased electrical excitability of the cerebral cortex—all of which suggest stimulation—are due to the inhibition of certain subcortical structures (high brainstem reticular formation?) which ordinarily modulate cerebral cortical activity. Similarly, the initial hyperactivity of tendon reflexes may represent a transitory escape of spinal motor neurons from higher inhibitory centers. With increasing amounts of alcohol, however, the depressant action spreads to involve the cerebral and cortical neurons, as well as other brainstem and spinal neurons.

All manner of motor performance—whether the simple maintenance of a standing posture, the control of speech and eye movements, or highly organized and complex motor skills—is adversely affected by alcohol. The movements involved in these acts are not only slower than normal but also more inaccurate and random in character and therefore less adapted to the accomplishment of specific ends.

Alcohol also impairs the efficiency of mental function by interfering with the learning process, which is slowed and rendered less effective. The facility of forming associations, whether of words or of figures, tends to be hampered and the power of attention and concentration is reduced. The person is not as versatile as usual in directing thought along new lines appropriate to the problems at hand. Finally, alcohol impairs the faculties of judgment and discrimination and, all in all, the ability to think and reason clearly.

A scale relating various degrees of clinical intoxication to blood alcohol levels in *nonhabituated* persons has been constructed by Miles. At a blood alcohol level of 30 mg per 100 ml, a mild euphoria was detectable, and at 50 mg per 100 ml, a mild incoordination. At 100 mg per 100 ml, ataxia was obvious; at 200 mg per 100 ml there was confusion and a reduced level of mental activity; at 300 mg per 100 ml, the subjects were stuporous; and a level of 400 mg per 100 ml was accompanied by deep anesthesia and could prove fatal. These figures are valid, provided the alcohol content in the blood rises steadily over a 2-h period.

It should be emphasized that such a scale has virtually no value in the chronic alcoholic patient, for it does not take into account the adjustment which the organism makes to alcohol, i.e., the phenomenon of tolerance. It is common knowledge that a habituated person can drink more and show fewer effects than the moderate drinker or abstainer. This phenomenon accounts for the surprisingly large amounts of alcohol that can be consumed by the chronic drinker without significant signs of drunkenness. In such individuals, there is a very narrow margin between the doses associated with low blood alcohol levels and sobriety and the doses associated with high blood levels and drunkenness. One must question the validity, therefore, of a single estimation of alcohol concentration as a reliable index of drunkenness.

The organism is capable of adapting to alcohol after a very short exposure. If the alcohol concentration in the blood is raised very slowly, few symptoms appear, even at quite high levels. Contrariwise, the degree of intoxication is more severe when there is a rapid peak in blood alcohol levels. It would appear that the important factor in this rapid adaptability is not so much the height of the blood alcohol level, but the length of time the alcohol has been present in the body. It has also been shown that if the dosage of alcohol which just causes blood levels to be high is held constant, the blood alcohol concentration falls and clinical evidence of intoxication disappears. The cause of this fall in alcohol concentration is not clear.

The biochemical mechanisms that underlie tolerance are not known. There is little evidence that an enhanced rate of alcohol metabolism can adequately account for the degree of tolerance observed in alcoholics. An increased degree of neuronal adaptation to alcohol is a more likely explanation. It would appear that alcohol has an important physicochemical effect on the cell membrane, inhibiting the active transport of sodium and potassium ions. A satisfactory biochemical theory remains to be formulated, however. Removal of alcohol from the habituated nervous system results in another disturbance in neuronal function, presumably an overactivity (see further on).

CLINICAL EFFECTS OF ALCOHOL ON THE NERVOUS SYSTEM

Although alcohol may alter the function of practically every organ system, the important clinical effects are on the digestive organs and the nervous system. The former—gastritis, cirrhosis, pancreatitis—are considered in *Harrison's Principles of Internal Medicine.* Only the effects on the nervous system will be considered here.

A large number of neurologic disorders are associated with alcoholism. The factor common to all of them, of course, is the abuse of alcohol, but the mechanism by which alcohol produces its effects varies widely from one group of disorders to another. The classification which follows is based for the most part on known mechanisms.

 I. Alcohol intoxication—drunkenness, coma, excitement ("pathological intoxication"), "blackouts"
 II. The abstinence or withdrawal syndrome—tremulousness, hallucinosis, "rum fits," delirium tremens
 III. Nutritional diseases of the nervous system secondary to alcoholism
  A. Wernicke-Korsakoff syndrome

  B. Polyneuropathy
  C. Optic neuropathy ("tobacco-alcohol amblyopia")
  D. Pellagra
 IV. Diseases of uncertain pathogenesis, associated with alcoholism
  A. Cerebellar degeneration
  B. Marchiafava-Bignami disease
  C. Central pontine myelinolysis
  D. "Alcoholic" cardiomyopathy and myopathy
  E. Alcoholic deteriorated state (alcoholic dementia)
  F. Cerebral atrophy
  G. Fetal alcohol syndrome
 V. Neurologic disorders consequent upon Laennec's cirrhosis and portal-systemic shunts
  A. Hepatic stupor and coma
  B. Chronic hepatocerebral degeneration

ALCOHOL INTOXICATION

The manifestations of alcohol intoxication are so commonplace that they require no elaboration. They consist of varying degrees of exhilaration and excitement, loss of restraint, irregularity of behavior, loquacity and slurred speech, incoordination of movement and gait, irritability, drowsiness, and, in advanced cases, stupor and coma.

Pathological Intoxication On rare occasions alcohol has an excitatory rather than a sedative effect. This reaction has been referred to as *pathological,* or *complicated, intoxication* and as *acute alcoholic paranoid state.* Since all forms of intoxication are pathologic "atypical intoxication" would be a more appropriate designation. Nevertheless, pathological intoxication is the term that has survived. The boundaries of this syndrome have never been clearly drawn. In the past, variant forms of delirium tremens and epileptic phenomena as well as psychopathic and criminal behavior were indiscriminately included. Now the term is generally used to designate an outburst of blind fury with assaultive and destructive behavior. Often the patient is subdued only with difficulty. The attack terminates with deep sleep, which occurs spontaneously or in response to sedation, and on awakening the patient has no memory of the episode. Allegedly this reaction may follow the ingestion of a small amount of alcohol, but in our experience the amount has always been substantial. Unlike the usual forms of alcohol intoxication and withdrawal, pathological intoxication has not been produced in experimental subjects, and the diagnosis depends upon these rather arbitrary anecdotal criteria.

Pathological intoxication has been ascribed to many factors, the common ones being constitutional differences in the susceptibility to alcohol, preexistent craniocerebral trauma or other brain disease and an underlying "hysterical or epileptoid temperament." There are no meaningful data to support any of these beliefs. An analogy may be drawn between pathological intoxication and the paradoxic reaction that occasionally follows the administration of barbiturates.

The diagnosis of pathological intoxication may have important legal implications. A person suffering from alcoholism or the usual forms of drunkenness is considered responsible for any harmful actions, whereas a person with pathological intoxication is considered insane at the time and therefore not responsible. The main disorders that need to be distinguished from pathological intoxication are temporal lobe seizures that occasionally take the form of an outburst of rage and violence, and the explosive episodes of violence that characterize the behavior of certain sociopaths. The diagnosis in these cases may be difficult and depends on eliciting the other manifestations of temporal lobe epilepsy or sociopathy.

"Blackouts" In the language of alcoholics, this term refers to transient episodes of amnesia which accompany severe degrees of intoxication. When sober again, the patient cannot recall events that had occurred during the drinking episode, even though the state of consciousness, as observed by others, was not grossly altered during that time. The nature and significance of such episodes are unclear. Some psychiatrists deny that a loss of memory has occurred and view the blackout as a form of malingering; others speak of "repression," which prevents conscious awareness of painful memories. These views are purely speculative. It is widely held that the occurrence of blackouts is an early and serious prognostic sign of alcoholism. In our experience, blackouts may occur at any time in the course of alcoholism, and they may occur also in relation to isolated episodes of drinking in persons who never become alcoholics. The salient fact is that a degree of intoxication has occurred that prevented the formation of memories for the period of intoxication, and rarely will the amount of alcohol consumed in moderate social drinking produce this effect.

Alcoholic Stupor and Coma As has already been indicated, the symptoms of alcoholic intoxication are the result of the depressant action of alcohol on cerebral and spinal neurons. In this respect alcohol acts on nerve cells in a manner akin to the general anesthetics. Unlike the latter, however, the margin between the dose of alcohol that produces surgical anesthesia and that which dangerously depresses respiration is a very narrow one, a fact which adds an element of urgency to the diagnosis and treatment of alcoholic narcosis. One must also be alert to the possibility that barbiturates or other sedative-hypnotic drugs have potentiated the depressant effects of alcohol.

The signs of alcohol intoxication are distinctive and most forms present no problem in diagnosis or management. On the other hand, coma due to alcohol may present difficulties in differential diagnosis. It should be stressed that the diagnosis of alcoholic coma is made not merely on the basis of a flushed face, stupor, and the odor of alcohol, but only after the careful exclusion of all other causes of coma (see Table 16-3).

Treatment of Alcohol Intoxication Mild to moderate degrees of intoxication require no special treatment. Certain time-honored remedies such as a cold shower, strong coffee, forced activity, or induction of vomiting may be helpful, but there is no evidence that any of them influences the rate of disappearance of alcohol from the blood. Alcoholic stupor is also a relatively brief, self-limited state, and if the vital signs are normal no special therapeutic measures are necessary. *Pathological intoxication* may require the use of restraints and the parenteral administration of phenobarbital sodium (200 mg subcutaneously) or amobarbital sodium (500 mg intramuscularly), repeated once in 30 to 40 min if necessary.

Coma due to alcohol intoxication represents a medical emergency. The main object of treatment is to prevent respiratory depression and the complications it engenders. The management of the comatose patient is described on page 246. One would like to lower the blood alcohol level as rapidly as possible, but the administration of fructose or of insulin and glucose for this purpose is of little practical value. Analeptic drugs such as amphetamine, pentylenetetrazol (Metrazol), and various mixtures of caffeine and picrotoxin are antagonistic to alcohol only insofar as they are powerful cerebral cortical stimulants and overall nervous system excitants; they do not hasten the combustion of alcohol. The use of hemodialysis should be considered in patients with extremely high blood alcohol concentrations ($>$ 500 mg per 100 ml), particularly if accompanied by acidosis, and in those who have concurrently ingested methanol or ethylene glycol or some other dialyzable drug.

Methyl, Amyl, and Isopropyl Alcohols and Ethylene Glycol Poisoning with alcohols other than ethyl alcohol is a relatively rare occurrence. *Amyl alcohol* (fusel oil) and *isopropyl alcohol* are used as industrial solvents and in the manufacture of varnishes, lacquers, and pharmaceuticals, in addition to the use of isopropyl alcohol as a rubbing alcohol. Intoxication may follow the oral ingestion of these alcohols or inhalation of their vapors. The effects of both these alcohols are much like those of ethyl alcohol, but much more toxic.

Methyl alcohol (methanol, wood alcohol), the major ingredient of antifreeze and many combustibles, is used in the manufacture of formaldehyde; as an industrial solvent; and as an adulterant of alcoholic beverages, a practice that provides the most common source of methyl alcohol intoxication. The oxidation of methyl alcohol to formaldehyde and formic acid proceeds relatively slowly; thus, signs of intoxication do not appear for several hours or may be delayed for a day or longer. Many of the toxic effects are like those of ethyl alcohol, but in addition methyl alcohol poisoning may produce serious degrees of acidosis and damage to the retinal ganglion cells, giving rise to scotomata and varying degrees of blindness, dilated unreactive pupils, and retinal edema. The most important aspect of treatment is the intravenous administration of large amounts of sodium bicarbonate. Hemodialysis may be a useful adjunct because of the slow rate of oxidation of methanol.

Ethylene glycol, an aliphatic alcohol, is a commonly used industrial solvent and the major constituent of antifreeze. In the latter form it is sometimes consumed by alcoholics, with disastrous results. At first the patient merely appears drunk, but severe confusion, convulsions, and coma follow in rapid succession. Acidosis and CSF pleocytosis are other characteristic features. Death from cardiopulmonary failure is the usual outcome. The acidosis of salicylism and methanol intoxication need to be distinguished.

THE ABSTINENCE OR WITHDRAWAL SYNDROME

Included under this title is the symptom complex of tremulousness, hallucinations, seizures, and confusion, i.e., delirium. Although a sustained period of chronic inebriation is the most obvious factor in the causation of these symptoms, they become manifest only *after a period of relative or absolute abstinence* from alcohol—hence the designation *abstinence,* or *withdrawal,* syndrome. Each of the major manifestations of the withdrawal syndrome may occur in more or less pure form and will be so described, but usually they occur in various combinations. The prototype of the patients afflicted with these symptoms is the spree, or periodic, drinker, although the steady drinker is not immune if, for some reason, he or she stops drinking.

Tremulousness   By far the most common manifestation of the abstinence syndrome is tremulousness, commonly referred to as "the shakes" or "the jitters," combined with general irritability and gastrointestinal symptoms, particularly nausea and vomiting. These symptoms first appear after several days of drinking, in the morning, after a night's abstinence. The patient "quiets the nerves" with a few drinks and then is able to drink for the rest of the day without distress. The symptoms return on successive mornings with increasing severity. The usual spree lasts about 2 weeks, but the duration varies greatly. It is terminated usually because of increasing severity of recurrent tremor and vomiting, but for other reasons as well, such as lack of funds, weakness, self-disgust, injury, illness, or collapse. The symptoms then become greatly augmented, reaching their peak intensity 24 to 36 h after the complete cessation of drinking.

At this stage, the patient presents a distinctive clinical picture. The face is deeply flushed, the conjunctivas are injected, and there is usually tachycardia, anorexia, nausea, and retching. The patient is fully awake, startles easily, and complains of insomnia. He or she is inattentive and disinclined to answer questions, and may respond in a rude or perfunctory manner. The patient may be mildly disoriented in time and have a poor memory for events of the last few days of the drinking spree, but shows no serious confusion, being generally aware of immediate surroundings and the nature of his or her illness.

Generalized tremor is the most obvious feature of this illness. It is of fast frequency (six to eight oscillations per second), slightly irregular, and variable in its severity, tending to diminish when the patient is in quiet surroundings and to increase with motor activity or emotional stress. The tremor may be so violent that the patient cannot stand without help, speak clearly, or eat without assistance. Sometimes there is little objective evidence of tremor, and the patient complains only of being "shaky inside."

The flushed facies, anorexia, tachycardia, and tremor subside to a large extent within a few days, but the overalertness, tendency to startle easily, and jerkiness of movement may persist for a week or longer and the feeling of uneasiness may not leave the patient completely for 10 to 14 days. An attempt should be made to keep the patient in the hospital for this length of time. To discharge the patient after a few days increases the likelihood that he or she will turn to alcohol to suppress the still-present tenseness and sleeplessness.

Hallucinosis Symptoms of disordered perception occur in about one-quarter of the tremulous patients. The patient may complain of "bad dreams"—nightmarish episodes associated with disturbed sleep, which are difficult to separate from real experience. Sounds and shadows may be misinterpreted, or familiar objects may be distorted and assume unreal forms. Although these are not hallucinations in the strict sense of the term, they represent the most common forms of disordered sense perception in the alcoholic.

True hallucinations may be purely visual in type, mixed visual and auditory, tactile, or olfactory, in that order of frequency. There is little evidence to support the popular belief that certain visual hallucinations (bugs, pink elephants) are specific to alcoholism. Actually, the hallucinations comprise the totality of visual experience. They are more often animate than inanimate; persons or animals may appear singly or in panoramas, shrunken or enlarged, natural and pleasant, or distorted, hideous, and frightening.

Acute and Chronic Auditory Hallucinosis A special type of alcoholic psychosis, consisting essentially of an auditory hallucinosis, has been recognized for many years. Kraepelin referred to this as the *hallucinatory insanity of drunkards, or alcoholic mania*. The central feature of the illness, in the beginning, is the occurrence of auditory hallucinations despite an otherwise clear sensorium; i.e., the patients are not confused, disoriented, or obtunded, and they have an intact memory. The hallucinations may take the form of unstructured sounds such as buzzing, ringing, shots, and clicking (the "elementary hallucinations" of Bleuler) or they may have a musical quality, like a low-pitched hum or chant. The most common hallucination, however, is the human voice. When the voices can be identified, they are attributed often to the patient's family, friends, or neighbors,—and rarely to God, radio, or radar. The voices may be addressed directly to the patient, but more frequently they discuss the patient in the third person. In the majority of cases the voices are maligning, reproachful, or threatening in nature and are disturbing to the patient; a significant proportion, however, are not unpleasant and leave the patient undisturbed. The voices are intensely real and vivid, and they tend to be exteriorized; i.e., they come from behind the door, from the corridor, or through the floor. Another quality of these formed auditory hallucinations (and of visual ones) is the appropriateness of the patient's emotional response to them. The patient may call on the police for protection or put up a barricade against invaders; such a patient may even attempt suicide to avoid what the voices threaten. The hallucinations are most prominent during the night, and their du-

ration varies greatly: they may be momentary, or they may recur intermittently for days on end and, in exceptional instances, for weeks or months.

Most patients, while hallucinating, have no appreciation of the unreality of their hallucinations. As improvement occurs, doubt begins to be expressed about their reality, there is a reluctance to talk about them, and the patient may even question whether he or she had been sane during the episode. Full recovery is characterized by the realization that the voices were imaginary and by the ability to recall, sometimes with remarkable clarity, the abnormal thought content of the psychotic episode.

A unique feature of this psychosis is the evolution of a *chronic auditory hallucinosis* in a small proportion of the patients. The chronic disorder begins like the acute one, but after a short period, perhaps a week, the symptomatology begins to change. The patient becomes quiet and resigned, even though the hallucinations remain threatening and derogatory. Ideas of reference and influence and other poorly systematized paranoid delusions become prominent. At this stage the illness may be mistaken for schizophrenia, and indeed has been so identified by Bleuler. There are, however, important differences between the two disorders: the alcoholic illness develops in close relationship to a drinking bout and the past history rarely reveals schizoid personality traits. Alcoholic patients with hallucinosis are not distinguished by a high incidence of schizophrenia within their families (Schuckit and Winokur; Scott). Also, such patients, whom we studied long after their acute attack, did not show an increased incidence of schizophrenia. There is some evidence that repeated attacks of acute auditory hallucinosis render the patient more vulnerable to the chronic state which resembles paranoid schizophrenia.

Withdrawal Seizures ("Rum Fits") In this particular setting (i.e., where relative or absolute abstinence follows a period of chronic inebriation) there is a marked tendency to develop convulsive seizures. Over 90 percent of withdrawal seizures occur during the 7- to 48-h period following the cessation of drinking, with a peak incidence between 13 to 24 h. During the period of seizure activity the electroencephalogram (EEG) may be abnormal, but it reverts to normal in a matter of days, even though the patient may go on to develop delirium tremens. Also during the period of seizure activity the patient is unusually sensitive to stroboscopic stimulation and about half the patients respond with generalized myoclonus (photomyoclonus) or a convulsive seizure (photoconvulsion). In contrast, patients with idiopathic epilepsy show this type of response to photic stimulation infrequently.

Seizures occurring in the abstinence period have a number of other distinctive features. There may be only a single seizure, but in the majority of cases the seizures occur in bursts of two to six, or even more, and an occasional patient develops status epilepticus. The seizures are grand mal in type, i.e., major generalized convulsions with loss of consciousness. A focal seizure or seizures should always suggest the presence of a focal lesion (most often traumatic) in addition to the effects of alcohol. Almost one-third of the patients with generalized seizure activity go on to develop delirium tremens, in which case the seizures invariably precede the delirium. The postictal confusional state may blend imperceptibly with the onset of the delirium, or there may be a clearing of the postictal state over several hours or even a day or two, before the delirium sets in. Seizures of this type occur in patients who have been drinking for many years, and must be distinguished from other forms of epilepsy beginning in adult life.

It is suggested that the term *rum fits*, or *whiskey fits*— i.e., the names used by alcoholics themselves—be reserved for seizures which possess the attributes described above. This would serve to distinguish this form of seizure activity, which occurs only in the immediate abstinence period, from that which occurs in the inter-drinking period long after withdrawal has been accomplished. It is also important to note that the "idiopathic" or posttraumatic forms of epilepsy may be influenced by alcohol. In patients with these latter types of epilepsy, a seizure or seizures may be precipitated by only a short period of drinking (e.g., a weekend, or even one evening of heavy social drinking); interestingly, in these circumstances, the seizures occur not when the patient is intoxicated, but usually the morning after, in the "sobering-up" period.

EEG findings in alcoholic subjects with rum fits do not support the notion that the seizures merely represent latent epilepsy made manifest by alcohol. Instead, the EEG reflects a sequence of changes induced by alcohol itself: a decrease in the frequency of brain waves during the period of chronic intoxication; a rapid return of the EEG to normal immediately after cessation of drinking; the occurrence of a brief period of dysrhythmia (sharp waves and paroxysmal discharges) which coincides with the flurry of convulsive activity; and again,

a rapid return of the EEG to normal. Except for the transient dysrhythmia in the withdrawal period, the incidence of EEG abnormalities in patients who have had rum fits is not greater than in the normal population, in sharp contrast to patients who are indeed subject to seizures (see page 23).

Delirium Tremens This is the most dramatic and grave of all the alcoholic complications. It is characterized by profound confusion, delusions, vivid hallucinations, tremor, agitation, and sleeplessness—as well as by increased activity of the autonomic nervous system, i.e., dilated pupils, fever, tachycardia, and profuse perspiration. The clinical features of delirium have been presented in detail in Chap. 19.

Delirium tremens develops in one of several settings. The patient, an excessive and steady drinker of many years' duration, may have been admitted to the hospital for an unrelated illness, accident, or operation, and 2 to 4 days later becomes delirious. Or, following a prolonged spree the patient may have already experienced several days of tremulousness and hallucinosis, or one or more seizures, and may even be recovering from these symptoms, when delirium tremens suddenly develops.

In the majority of cases delirium tremens is benign and short-lived, ending as abruptly as it begins. Consumed by the relentless activity and wakefulness of several days' duration, the patient falls into a deep sleep and then awakens lucid, quiet, and exhausted, with virtually no memory of the events of the delirious period. Less commonly, the delirious state subsides gradually; more rarely still, there may be one or more relapses, several episodes of delirium of varying severity being separated by intervals of relative or complete lucidity—the entire process lasting for as little as several days or as long as 4 to 5 weeks. When the delirium occurs as a single episode, the duration is 72 h or less in over 80 percent of the cases.

Between 5 and 15 percent of cases of delirium tremens, as defined above, end fatally. In many of these there is an associated infectious illness or injury, but in a few no complicating illness is discernible. Patients frequently die in a state of hyperthermia or peripheral circulatory collapse; in some, death comes so suddenly that the nature of the terminal events cannot be determined. Reports of a negligible mortality in delirium tremens can usually be attributed to a failure to distinguish between delirium tremens and the minor forms of the withdrawal syndrome, which are far more common and almost invariably benign.

Closely related to typical delirium tremens and about as common are the *atypical delirious-hallucina-*

tory or *confusional states,* in which one facet of the delirium tremens complex assumes prominence to the practical exclusion of the other symptoms. One patient may simply exhibit a transient state of quiet confusion, agitation, and peculiar behavior lasting several days or weeks. Another might present a vivid hallucinatory-delusional state and abnormal behavior, consistent with various false beliefs. Unlike typical delirium tremens, the atypical states present as a single circumscribed episode without recurrences, are only rarely preceded by seizures, and do not end fatally. This may be another way of saying that they are a partial or less severe form of the disease.

Pathologic examination is singularly unrevealing in patients with delirium tremens. Edema and brain swelling have been absent in the authors' pathologic material except when shock or hypoxia had occurred terminally. There have been no significant microscopic changes in the brain. Abnormalities of the blood nonprotein nitrogen, carbon dioxide, CSF, serum sodium, chloride, glucose, potassium, and calcium occur unpredictably. The EEG findings have been discussed in relation to withdrawal seizures.

Pathogenesis of the Tremulous-Hallucinatory-Delirious State This has been a matter of considerable controversy. The idea that it simply represents the most severe form of alcohol intoxication is untenable. The symptoms of toxicity—consisting of slurred speech, uninhibited behavior, staggering gait, stupor, and coma—are distinctive and different from the symptom complex of tremor, hallucinations, fits, and delirium. The former symptoms are associated with an elevated blood alcohol level, whereas the latter become evident only when the blood alcohol is reduced. Finally, the toxic symptoms increase in severity as more alcohol is consumed, whereas tremor and hallucinosis and even full-blown delirium tremens may be nullified by the administration of alcohol.

Although much discussed in the past, there is no evidence that endocrine abnormality or nutritional deficiency plays a role in the genesis of delirium tremens and related symptoms. Instead, the illness and its symptoms are of neural origin: the parts of the nervous system that become habituated to alcohol appear to overact when it is withdrawn. The duration of the illness seems to correspond to the time required for neuronal excitability to return to normal. The lesion is a biochemical one, of obscure nature still.

It is evident, from observations in both man and experimental animals, that the most important and the one indispensable factor in the genesis of delirium tremens and related disorders is the withdrawal of alcohol, following a period of chronic intoxication. Further, these observations indicate that the emergence of withdrawal symptoms depends upon a *decline* in the blood alcohol level from a previously higher level and not necessarily upon the complete disappearance of alcohol from the blood. The mechanism(s) by which the withdrawal of alcohol produces symptoms is only beginning to be understood. It has been shown that the early phase of alcohol withdrawal (beginning 7 to 8 h after cessation of drinking) is regularly attended by a drop in serum magnesium levels and a rise in arterial pH values, on the basis of respiratory alkalosis. Possibly the compounded effect of these two factors, both of which are associated with hyperexcitability of the nervous system, are responsible for seizures and for other symptoms which characterize the early phase of withdrawal. The elevation in pH is explained as withdrawal release of the neurons of the "respiratory center," which had been previously rendered insensitive to circulating CO_2. In the "rebound" phase these cells become more sensitive than normal to CO_2, with resultant hyperventilation and respiratory alkalosis. As an explanation of delirium tremens, however, hypomagnesemia is probably not important, since the serum magnesium level has frequently been restored to normal before the onset of the delirium.

Treatment of Delirium Tremens and Minor Withdrawal Symptoms The general aspects of management of the delirious and confused patient have been described on page 283.

More specifically, the treatment of delirium tremens begins with a careful search, followed by appropriate treatment, for associated injuries (particularly head injury with cerebral lacerations or subdural hematoma), infections (pneumonia or meningitis), pancreatitis, and liver disease. Because of the frequency and seriousness of these complications, skull and chest roentgenograms should be obtained and lumbar puncture should be performed routinely. In severe forms of delirium tremens, the temperature, pulse, and blood pressure should be recorded at 30-min intervals in anticipation of peripheral circulatory collapse and hyperthermia, which, added to the effects of injury and infection, are the usual causes of death in this disease. In the case of shock, one must act quickly, utilizing whole-blood transfusions, fluids, and vasopressor drugs. The occurrence of hyperthermia demands the use of a cooling mattress in addition to specific treatment for any infection that may be present.

A very important element in treatment is the correction of fluid and electrolyte imbalance. Severe degrees of agitation and perspiration may require the administration of 6000 to 8000 ml fluid daily, of which 1500 to 2000 ml should be normal saline solution. The specific electrolytes and the amounts in which they are added are governed by the laboratory values for these electrolytes. Occasionally, the withdrawal syndrome is characterized by hypoglycemia, in which case the administration of glucose becomes of prime importance. Rarely, alcoholic patients present with severe ketoacidosis and normal or only slightly elevated blood glucose concentrations; usually such patients recover promptly, without the use of insulin.

A special danger attends the use of glucose solutions in alcoholic patients. Typically these persons have subsisted on a diet disproportionately high in carbohydrate (alcohol is metabolized almost entirely as carbohydrate) and low in thiamine, and their reserves of B vitamins may have been further reduced by gastroenteritis and diarrhea. The administration of intravenous glucose may serve to consume the last available stores of thiamine and precipitate Wernicke's disease. For this reason it is good practice to add B vitamins in all cases requiring parenterally administered glucose, even though the alcoholic disorder under treatment, e.g., delirium tremens, is not primarily due to vitamin deficiency.

In respect to the use of drugs, it is important to distinguish between mild withdrawal symptoms, which are essentially benign and responsive to practically all sedative drugs, and delirium tremens, which has a serious mortality and is relatively unresponsive to drugs. In the case of minor withdrawal symptoms, the purpose of medication is to ensure rest and sleep. In delirium tremens, the object of drug therapy is to blunt the psychomotor overactivity and prevent exhaustion and to facilitate the administration of parenteral fluid and nursing care; one should not attempt to suppress agitation at all costs, since to accomplish this might require an amount of drug that would seriously depress respiration.

A wide variety of drugs is effective in controlling withdrawal symptoms. Some of the more commonly used ones are prochlorperazine (Compazine), chlorpromazine (Thorazine), promazine (Sparine), meprobamate, hydroxyzine (Vistaril), chlordiazepoxide (Librium), and diazepam (Valium). There is little difference in the therapeutic efficacy of these drugs, and it is not certain that any one of them can prevent hallucinosis or delirium tremens, or shorten the duration or alter the mortality rate of the latter disorder. In general, phenothiazine

drugs should be avoided because they reduce the threshold to seizures. At the moment, chlordiazepoxide and diazepam are the most popular drugs for the treatment of withdrawal symptoms, although the advantages of oral administration of these drugs over paraldehyde have not been proved by controlled studies (see review of Gessner). Paraldehyde has the advantage of being extremely safe, provided it is freshly prepared and kept in brown, tightly stoppered bottles to prevent deterioration and the accumulation of acetaldehyde. If the patient can take medication orally, doses of 8 to 12 ml in orange juice should be given. It may also be administered rectally. The intramuscular route should be avoided if possible, since it may damage nerves. It should be given intravenously only with great caution because of the danger of respiratory depression. If parenteral medication is necessary, sodium phenobarbital or sodium amytal in doses of 120 mg, repeated at 3- to 4-h intervals, may be given intramuscularly (provided there is no serious liver disease); or 10 mg diazepam may be given intravenously and repeated once or twice at 20- to 30-min intervals, until the patient is calm but awake. Adrenal corticotropic hormone (ACTH) and cortisone have no place in the treatment of the withdrawal syndrome. These hormones do not significantly modify the course of the abstinence syndrome. In addition, they have many serious disadvantages: the masking of infection, a deleterious effect on tuberculosis and peptic ulcer, and a tendency to produce a negative nitrogen balance and excessive excretion of potassium. All these complications are of more than theoretical interest in the alcoholic patient.

Treatment of "Rum Fits" Most cases do not require the use of anticonvulsant drugs, since there may be only a single seizure or a brief flurry of seizures which have either ceased before the patient is seen by a physician or by the time that certain medicines, such as phenytoin, become effective. The parenteral administration of sodium phenobarbital early in the withdrawal period could conceivably prevent "rum fits" in patients with a previous history of this disorder or in those who might be expected to develop seizures on withdrawal of alcohol. Also, the long-term administration of anticonvulsants is not practical: if such patients remain abstinent, they will be free of seizures; if they resume drinking, they usually abandon their medicines. In rare instances, withdrawal seizures take the form of status epilepticus; such cases should be managed like status or any other type (see page 229). Alcoholics with a history of idiopathic or posttraumatic epilepsy should drink only in moderation or not at all, because of the tendency of even short periods of drinking to precipitate seizures; such patients must be maintained on anticonvulsant drugs.

NUTRITIONAL DISEASES OF THE NERVOUS SYSTEM

These diseases comprise a relatively small but serious group of illnesses in chronic alcoholics. The role of alcohol in their causation is purely secondary, serving mainly to displace food in the diet. These illnesses are discussed in Chap. 38, "Diseases of the Nervous System Due to Nutritional Deficiency."

DISEASES OF UNCERTAIN PATHOGENESIS, ASSOCIATED WITH ALCOHOLISM

Also discussed in Chap. 38 are several disorders (*alcoholic cerebellar degeneration, central pontine myelinolysis, Marchiafava-Bignami disease*) in which a nutritional-metabolic etiology seems likely but has not been firmly established. Certain disorders of skeletal and cardiac muscle associated with alcoholism (*alcoholic myopathy and cardiomyopathy*) are described in Chap. 48, under the acute and subacute myopathic paralyses. There remain to be discussed several diverse disorders that have been associated with alcoholism, but whose causal relationship to alcohol abuse or to nutritional deficiency or to some other factor is not clear.

Alcoholic Deteriorated State (Alcoholic Dementia)   The syndrome designated as alcoholic dementia, or deteriorated state, has never been delineated satisfactorily, either clinically or pathologically. In the *Comprehensive Textbook of Psychiatry* it is defined as "a gradual disintegration of personality structure, with emotional lability, loss of control, and dementia." To other psychiatrists (Strecker et al.) the alcoholic deteriorated state denotes "the common end reaction of all chronic alcoholics who do not recover from their alcoholism or do not die of some accident or intercurrent episode." Purported examples of this state show a remarkably diverse group of symptoms, including jealousy and suspiciousness; blunting of moral fiber and other personality and behavioral disorders; deterioration of work performance, personal care and living habits; disorientation, impaired judgment, and defects of intellectual function, particularly of memory; and even certain physical manifestations, such as dilatation of facial capillaries, a "bloated look," flabby muscles, chronic gastritis, tremors, and recurrent seizures. Some early authors were apparently impressed with similarities between the alcoholic deteriorated state and general paresis, hence the term "alcoholic pseudoparesis." Mercifully the latter term no longer appears in medical writings. Recently, Seltzer and Sherwin have attempted to sharpen the definition of alcoholic dementia. It is their contention that patients with the latter disorder can be distinguished from patients with senile de-

mentia by their stable course and absence of language abnormality, and from patients with Korsakoff's psychosis by their difficulties with constructional tasks and prominent behavioral disturbances in addition to amnesia. In none of their patients designated as alcoholic dementia was the brain examined pathologically.

Courville described a series of cerebral cortical changes which he attributed to the toxic effects of alcohol and which he considered to be the basis of the alcoholic deteriorated state and alcoholic pseudoparesis: progressive atrophy of the cortex of the frontal lobes, associated with opacity and thickening of the overlying meninges and enlargement of the lateral ventricles; swelling, pyknosis, and "pigmentary atrophy" of nerve cells; irregular loss of the smaller pyramidal cells of the superficial and intermediate laminae; and secondary degeneration and loss of nerve fibers. Some of these changes such as neuronal pyknosis are insignificant artifacts, and many of the others are not specific. Opacity of the meninges and moderate dilatation of the lateral ventricles, for example, are observed both in alcoholics and nonalcoholics as well as in persons who had betrayed no neurologic or psychiatric abnormalities during life. Some of the cellular changes noted by Courville may have reflected a state of hepatic failure or terminal anoxia, and others reflect nothing more than the effects of aging or artifacts of tissue fixation and staining. In our experience, the majority of cases that come to autopsy with the label of "alcoholic dementia" or "deteriorated state" prove to have the lesions of the Wernicke-Korsakoff syndrome. Traumatic lesions of varying degrees of severity are commonly added. Other cases show the lesions of anoxic or hepatic encephalopathy, communicating hydrocephalus, Alzheimer's disease, ischemic necrosis or some other disease quite unrelated to alcoholism. Practically always, in our material, the clinical state can be accounted for by one or a combination of these disease processes, and there has been no need to invoke a hypothetical toxic effect of alcohol on the brain.

Alcoholic paranoia and jealousy are outmoded terms that were used in the past to designate what was thought to be a special type of paranoid reaction in chronic alcoholics, in which the patient, usually a male, developed ideas of infidelity on the part of his wife. The delusions of jealousy that might occur acutely in the course of alcoholic intoxication or withdrawal, or chronically, as part of the "alcoholic deteriorated state," were generally not included under this rubric. The notion that pathologic jealousy merits classification as a distinctive complication of alcoholism is not warranted, since the morbid jealousy which develops in alcoholics differs in no essential way from that in nonalcoholics. Nevertheless, among individuals with the syndrome of morbid jealousy, chronic alcoholism may be an important associated factor (11 of 66 cases reported by Langfeldt). Among the alcoholic patients, the delusions of jealousy may at first be evident only in relation to episodes of acute intoxication, but later they evolve, through a stage of constant suspicion and efforts to detect infidelity, into definite morbid beliefs which persist during periods of sobriety as well.

"Cerebral Atrophy" in Chronic Alcoholics   This disorder, like the "alcoholic deteriorated state," does not constitute a clinical-pathological entity. To some authors (e.g., Courville, see above) the concept of "alcoholic cerebral atrophy" is a pathologic one, but usually this diagnosis is made on the basis of radiologic findings. Several pneumoencephalographic studies of chronic alcoholics have shown a symmetrical enlargement of the lateral ventricles in more than half the cases, and a smaller number have also shown a widening of the sulci, mainly of the frontal lobes (Brewer and Perrett, Haug). More recently, similar findings have been reported in chronic alcoholics examined by CT scanning (see review of Carlen et al.).

The clinical correlates of these radiologic findings are quite unclear. In some patients "cerebral atrophy" is associated with an overt complication of alcoholism; we found, for example, that about one-quarter of our autopsied patients with the Wernicke-Korsakoff syndrome showed enlargement of the lateral and third ventricles and convolutional atrophy of the frontal lobes. In other patients there is a history of recurrent seizures, or evidence of liver disease, cerebral trauma, or some other event that might have resulted in ventricular enlargement. In some alcoholic individuals, however, the finding of large ventricles comes as a surprise, no symptoms or signs of neuropsychiatric disease being found in the course of the usual neurologic and mental status testing.

The term "alcoholic cerebral atrophy," implies that chronic ingestion of alcohol causes an irreversible loss of cerebral tissue, a concept to which there is a serious objection. One cannot assume that dilated ventricles and sulci, observed in a single CT scan, represent an irreversible tissue loss. Such CT changes may in fact be reversible, as has been observed in patients with Cush-

ing's syndrome, anorexia nervosa, Lennox-Gastaut syndrome (treated with ACTH), as well as in alcoholic patients (Carlen et al.). This reversibility would suggest that a shift of fluids had occurred in the brain (over many months), rather than loss of tissue. Until this matter has been studied further, it would be preferable to refer to the asymptomatic ventricular enlargement in alcoholics as such, rather than as cerebral atrophy.

Fetal Alcohol Syndrome (FAS)   That parental alcoholism may have an adverse effect on the offspring has been a recurrent theme in medical lore. The documented occurrence of such a relationship was lacking, however, until the turn of the century, when Sullivan reported that the mortality among the children of drunken mothers was almost two and one-half times greater than among children of nondrinking women of "similar stock." The increased mortality was attributed by Sullivan and later by Haggard and Jellinek to postnatal influences such as poor nutrition and chaotic home environment rather than to the intrauterine effects of alcohol. Following Sullivan's studies there appeared isolated clinical reports in which damage to the fetus was ascribed to alcoholism in the mother, but in general this idea was rejected and relegated to the category of superstitions about alcoholism.

In the past decade, the effects of alcohol abuse on the fetus have been rediscovered, so to speak. Lemoine et al., Ulleland, and Jones and Smith have described a distinctive pattern of abnormalities in infants born of severely alcoholic mothers. The affected infants are small in length in comparison to weight, and most of them fall below the third percentile for head circumference. They are distinguished also by the presence of short palpebral fissures (probably a reflection of microphthalmia) and epicanthal folds; maxillary hypoplasia, micrognathia, and cleft palate; dislocations of the hips, flexion deformities of the fingers, and a limited range of motion of other joints; cardiac anomalies (usually spontaneously closing septal defects); anomalous external genitalia; and capillary hemangiomata. The newborn infants suck and sleep poorly, and many of them are irritable, hyperactive, and tremulous; the latter symptoms resemble those of alcohol withdrawal, except that they persist. In one series of 23 infants born to alcoholic mothers there was a neonatal mortality of 17 percent (Jones et al.), and among the infants who survived the neonatal period, almost half failed to achieve normal weight, length, and head circumference or remained backward mentally to a varying degree, even under optimal environmental conditions.

The pathologic changes that underlie the FAS

have been studied in a small number of cases. Clarren et al. found extensive leptomeningeal neuroglial heterotopias and an obstructive hydrocephalus, probably secondary to the dense heterotopias around the brainstem. Neuronal ectopias in the cerebral white matter and agenesis of the corpus callosum were also present. Peiffer et al. described a broader spectrum of malformations, including cerebellar malformations similar to those of the Dandy-Walker syndrome, schizencephaly, agenesis of the corpus callosum, and signs of arrhinencephaly.

Although the relationship of this syndrome to severe maternal alcoholism seems undoubted, the mechanism by which alcohol produces its effects is not fully understood. It is noteworthy that infants born to nonalcoholic mothers who had been subjected to severe dietary deprivation during pregnancy (during World War II) were small and often premature, but these infants did not show the pattern of malformations that characterizes the FAS. Alcohol readily crosses the placenta in humans and animals, and in the mouse, rat, chick, miniature swine, and beagle dogs, alcohol has been shown to have both embryotoxic and teratogenic effects. Thus, the evidence to date favors a toxic effect of alcohol, rather than a nutritional or genetic factor.

The critical degree of maternal alcoholism that is necessary to produce the FAS and the critical stage(s) in gestation during which it occurs are not known. The various teratogenic effects described above were estimated to have occurred between the fourth week and the sixth month of gestation, a reflection perhaps of the varying periods during gestation when the fetus was exposed to particularly high alcohol levels. Cases observed to date have occurred only in infants born to severely alcoholic mothers who continued to drink heavily throughout their pregnancy—an average of 6 oz of absolute alcohol (or 12 oz of 86-proof whiskey) daily, according to Rosett et al. Preliminary data, derived from the collaborative study being sponsored by the National Institutes of Health, indicate that about one-third of the offspring of such women have the FAS. Prospective studies of these problems, and of the effects on the fetus of lesser degrees of maternal alcoholism are in progress. A current account of these studies is contained in the seminar edited by Rosett.

NEUROLOGIC DISORDERS CONSEQUENT UPON ALCOHOLIC CIRRHOSIS AND PORTAL-SYSTEMIC SHUNTS

This category of alcoholic disease is discussed in Chap. 39 in connection with the acquired metabolic disorders of the nervous system.

TREATMENT OF ALCOHOL ADDICTION

Following recovery from the acute medical and neurologic complications of alcoholism, the underlying problem of alcohol dependence remains. To treat only the medical complications and to leave the management of the drinking problem to the patient alone is shortsighted. Almost always, drinking is resumed, with a predictable recurrence of medical illness. For this reason the physician must be prepared to deal with the addiction or at least to initiate treatment.

The problem of excessive drinking is formidable, but not necessarily as hopeless as it is made out to be. A common misconception among physicians is that specialized training in psychiatry and an inordinately large amount of time are required to deal with the addictive drinker. Actually, a successful program of treatment can be initiated by any interested physician, using the standard techniques of history taking, establishing rapport with the patient, and setting up of a schedule of frequent visits, though not necessarily for prolonged periods. Useful points at which to undertake this task are during convalescence from a serious medical or neurologic complication of alcoholism, or in relation to loss of employment, arrest, or threatened divorce. Such a crisis may help convince the patient, more than any argument presented by family or physician, that the drinking problem has reached serious proportions.

The requisite for successful treatment is total abstinence from alcohol; for all practical purposes, this represents the only permanent solution. It is generally agreed that any attempts to curb the drinking habit will fail if the patient continues to drink. There are said to be alcohol addicts who have been able to reduce their intake of alcohol and eventually to drink in moderation, but they represent a very small proportion of the addict population. Also, it is frequently stated that alcoholics must recognize that they are alcoholics—i.e., that their drinking is beyond their control—and must express willingness to be helped. Undoubtedly there is truth in both these statements, but nevertheless these statements should not be interpreted to mean that alcoholic patients must gain this recognition and willingness entirely on their own initiative and that they will be helped only after they do so. The physician can do a great deal to help such patients understand the nature of their problem and thus to motivate them to accept treatment. The help of family, employer, courts, and clergy should be enlisted in an attempt to convince these patients that abstinence is preferable to chronic inebriety. Alcoholic patients must be made fully aware of the medical and social consequences of continued drinking and must also be made to understand that because of some constitutional peculiarity (like that of the diabetic, who cannot handle sugar) they are incapable of drinking in moderation. These facts should be presented in much the same way as one would explain the essential features of any other disease; there is nothing to be gained from adopting a punitive or moralizing attitude. Yet patients should not be given the idea that they are in no way to blame for their illness; there appears to be an advantage in making patients feel that they are responsible for doing something about their drinking.

The prevalent belief that an alcoholic will not stop drinking under duress also requires qualification. In fact, one of the few careful studies of this matter disclosed that relatively few patients would have sought help unless pressure had been exerted by family or employer; furthermore, patients who came to the clinic under duress of this sort did just as well as those who came voluntarily.

If an earnest and sustained effort by the physician fails to convince the patient that alcohol offers a problem, it is usually impossible to modify the alcoholic tendency. The only way to make such individuals discontinue drinking is to commit them to a psychiatric hospital or special institution for the management of alcoholism, in the hope that with forced abstinence and improvement in their physical state they will gain insight and later accept psychiatric or other forms of therapy.

On the other hand, if patients come to realize that their drinking is beyond control and that they need to do something about it, their chances of being helped are raised considerably. Indeed, under these circumstances, many persons stop drinking of their own volition for several months or years. Some of these patients, despite the best of intentions, will relapse. This should not serve as an excuse to abandon treatment; many patients have attained a state of prolonged sobriety after several false starts.

A number of methods have proved valuable in the long-term management of patients. The more important of these are the use of Antabuse, aversion treatment, psychotherapy, and the participation in social organizations for combating alcoholism.

Antabuse (tetraethylthiuram disulfide, disulfiram) interferes with the metabolism of alcohol, so that a patient who takes both alcohol and Antabuse accumulates an inordinate amount of acetaldehyde in the tissues, resulting in nausea, vomiting, and hypotension, sometimes pronounced in degree. It is no longer considered necessary to demonstrate these effects to patients; it is sufficient to warn them of the severe reactions that may result if they drink while they have the drug in their bodies. Treatment with Antabuse is instituted only after the patient has been sober for several days, preferably longer. It should never be given to patients with cardiac or liver disease. The drug is taken each morning, or at another suitable time daily, in a dosage of 0.5 g, preferably under supervision. This form of treatment is of particular value in the spree or periodic drinker, in whom relapse from abstinence usually represents an impulsive rather than a carefully planned or premeditated act. The patient taking Antabuse, aware of the dangers of mixing liquor and the drug, is "protected" against the impulse to drink, and this protection may be renewed every 24 h by the simple expedient of taking a pill. The willingness with which such patients accept this form of treatment also serves as a rough index of their motivation to control the alcoholism. Should the patient drink while taking Antabuse, the ensuing reaction is usually severe enough to require medical attention, and a protracted spree can thus be prevented. Antabuse may cause a polyneuropathy if continued over a period of months or years, but this is a rare complication.

The aversion treatment consists of the simultaneous administration of a drink of alcohol and an injection of emetin. The violent nausea and vomiting which ensue are intended to create in the patient a strong revulsion for alcohol. This form of treatment, as well as other types of conditioned-reflex treatment, has been successfully employed in special clinics but has not gained widespread popularity.

Alcoholics Anonymous (AA), an informal fellowship of former alcoholics, has proved to be the single most effective force in the rehabilitation of alcoholic patients. The philosophy of this organization is embodied in their "twelve steps," a series of propositions about alcohol and alcoholism which guide the patient to recovery. The AA philosophy stresses in particular the practice of making restitution, the necessity to help other alcoholics, trust in God, the group confessional, and the belief that the alcoholic is powerless over alcohol. AA philosophy also embodies the 24-h plan, in which the alcoholic strives for just 24 h of abstinence (a concept inspired by the Sermon on the Mount) as a means of facilitating the maintenance of sobriety. Although accurate statistics are lacking, it is stated that about one-third of the members who express more than a passing interest in the program attain a state of long-sustained or permanent sobriety (Baekeland et al.).

The methods used by AA are not suited to every patient; some prefer the more personalized approach offered by special clinics and centers for the treatment of alcoholism. The physician should, therefore, be fully aware of all the community resources which are available for the management of this problem, and should be prepared to take advantage of them in appropriate cases.

Finally, it should be noted that alcoholism is frequently associated with psychiatric disease of other type, particularly sociopathy (antisocial or psychopathic personality) and manic-depressive disease. In the latter case, the prevailing mood is far more often one of depression than of mania, and is more often encountered in women, who are more apt to drink under these conditions than are men. In these circumstances expert psychiatric help should be sought.

REFERENCES

BAEKELAND F, LUNDWALL LK, KISSIN B: Methods for the treatment of chronic alcoholism: A critical appraisal, in Israel Y (ed): *Research Advances in Alcohol and Drug Problems,* vol 2. New York, Wiley, 1975, pp 247-328.

BLEULER E: Brill AA (trans): *Textbook of Psychiatry,* New York, Macmillan, 1930, pp 163 and 342-345.

BREWER C, PERRETT L: Brain damage due to alcohol consumption: An air-encephalographic, psychometric and electroencephalographic study. *Br J Addict* 66(3): 170, 1971.

CARLEN PL et al: Reversible cerebral atrophy in recently abstinent chronic alcoholics measured by computed tomography scans. *Science* 200:1076, 1978.

CLARREN SK et al: Brain malformations related to prenatal exposure to ethanol. *J Pediat* 92:64, 1978.

COURVILLE CB: *Effects of Alcohol on the Nervous System of Man.* Los Angeles, San Lucas Press, 1955.

EWING JA, ROUSE BA, PELLIZZARI ED: Alcohol sensitivity and ethnic background. *Am J Psychiatry* 131:206, 1974.

GESSNER PK: Drug therapy of the alcohol withdrawal syndrome, in Majchrowicz E, Noble EP (eds): *Biochemistry and Pharmacology of Ethanol,* vol II. New York, Plenum, 1979, pp 375-435.

GOODWIN DW et al: Alcohol problems in adoptees raised apart from alcoholic biologic parents. *Arch Gen Psychiatry* 28:238, 1973.

GORDON GG et al: Effect of alcohol (ethanol) administration on sex-hormone metabolism in normal men. *N Engl J Med* 295:793, 1976.

HAGGARD HW, JELLINEK EM: *Alcohol Explored.* Garden City, NY, Doubleday Doran, 1942.

HAUG JO: Pneumoencephalographic evidence of brain damage in chronic alcoholics. A preliminary report. *Acta Psychiatr Scand Suppl* 203:135, 1968.

ISBELL H et al: An experimental study of the etiology of "rum fits" and delirium tremens. *Q J Stud Alcohol* 16:1, 1955.

JONES KL, SMITH DW: Recognition of the fetal alcohol syndrone in early infancy. *Lancet* 2:999, 1973.

——— et al: Outcome in offspring of chronic alcoholic women. *Lancet* 1:1076, 1974.

LANGFELDT G: The erotic jealousy syndrome. A clinical study. *Acta Psychiatr Neurol Scand* 36(suppl 151):7, 1961.

LEMOINE P et al: Les enfants de parents alcooliques: Anomalies observées à propos de 127 cas. *Ouest-Med* 25:477, 1968.

LINDENBAUM J, LIEBER CS: Hematologic effects of alcohol in man in the absence of nutritional deficiency. *N Engl J Med* 281:333, 1969.

MENDELSON JH, MELLO NK: Medical progress: Biologic concomitants of alcoholism. *N Engl J Med* 301:912, 1979.

MILES WR: The comparative concentrations of alcohol in human blood and urine at intervals after ingestion. *J Pharmacol Exp Ther* 20:265, 1922.

NATIONAL INSTITUTE ON ALCOHOL ABUSE AND ALCOHOLISM: *First Special Report to the U.S. Congress on Alcohol and Health,* US Department Of Health, Education, and Welfare Publication HSM 72-9099. Washington, US Government Printing Office, 1971.

PEIFFER J et al: Alcohol embryo- and fetopathy: Neuropathology of 3 children and 3 fetuses. *J Neurol Sci* 41:125, 1979.

ROEBUCK JB, KESSLER RG: *The Etiology of Alcoholism: Constitutional, Psychological, and Sociological Approaches.* Springfield, Ill, Charles C Thomas, 1972.

ROSETT HL: A clinical perspective of the fetal alcohol syndrome. *Alcoholism Clin Exp Res* 4:119, 1980.

——— et al: A pilot prospective study of the fetal alcohol syndrome at the Boston City Hospital, Part I: Maternal drinking. *Ann NY Acad Sci* 273:118, 1976.

SCHUCKIT MA, HAGLUND RMJ: An overview of the etiological theories on alcoholism, in Estes NJ, Heinemann ME (eds): *Alcoholism: Development, Consequences and Interventions.* St Louis, Mosby, 1977, pp 15-27.

———, WINOKUR G: Alcoholic hallucinosis and schizophrenia: A negative study. *Br J Psychiatry* 119:549, 1971.

SCOTT DF: Alcoholic hallucinosis—an aetiological study. *Br J Addict* 62:113, 1967.

SEEVERS MH: Morphine and ethanol physical dependence: A critique of a hypothesis. *Science* 170:1113, 1970.

SELTZER B, SHERWIN I: Organic brain syndromes: An empirical study and critical review. *Am J Psychiatry* 135:13, 1978.

STRECKER EA, EBAUGH FG, EWALT JR: *Practical Clinical Psychiatry.* New York, McGraw-Hill, 1951, pp 150-170.

SULLIVAN WC: A note on the influence of maternal inebriety on the offspring. *J Mental Sci* 45:489, 1899.

ULLELAND C: The offspring of alcoholic mothers. *Ann NY Acad Sci* 197:167, 1972.

VICTOR M: Treatment of alcoholic intoxication and the withdrawal syndrome. A critical analysis of the use of drugs and other forms of therapy. *Psychosom Med* 28(no 4, pt 2):636, 1966.

———: The pathophysiology of alcoholic epilepsy. *Res Publ Assoc Res Nerv Ment Dis* 46:431, 1968.

———: The alcohol withdrawal syndrome. *Ann NY Acad Med* 215:210, 1973.

———, ADAMS RD: The effect of alcohol on the nervous system. *Res Publ Assoc Res Nerv Ment Dis* 32:526, 1953.

———, HOPE J: The phenomenon of auditory hallucinations in chronic alcoholism. *J Nerv Ment Dis* 126:451, 1958.

WOLFE SM, VICTOR M: The relationship of hypomagnesemia and alkalosis to alcohol withdrawal symptoms. *Ann NY Acad Sci* 162:973, 1969.

——— et al: Respiratory alkalosis and alcohol withdrawal. *Trans Assoc Am Physicians* 82:344, 1969.

CHAPTER 41

DISORDERS OF THE NERVOUS SYSTEM DUE TO DRUGS AND OTHER CHEMICAL AGENTS

Subsumed under this title is a diverse group of disorders of the nervous system which result from the introduction into the body of poisonous or injurious substances. In textbooks of neurology, these disorders are customarily designated as *toxic*, and the offending agents are termed *exogenous* if they are introduced from outside the body, and *endogenous* if they are generated from within—a division which cannot always be sharply drawn, as in the case of toxins of certain bacteria that have invaded the body.

The so-called endogenous bacterial toxins (e.g., those of tetanus and botulism) rank among the most powerful nervous system poisons. While few in number and relatively uncommon, they assume importance because their effects are always serious and frequently fatal. In contrast, exogenous poisons that impair nervous system function are so numerous that it would hardly be possible to mention them all, let alone to describe their actions in detail. Falling into this latter category are the myriad of household products, insecticides, industrial solvents, proprietary medicines, water and air pollutants, and other poisons with which we are surrounded in modern life. The primary effect of most of these agents is on organs and systems other than the nervous system, but practically all of them, in large enough amounts, can give rise to neurologic symptoms such as headache, drowsiness, insomnia, confusion, delirium, seizures, and coma. An important principle derives from this fact—that the occurrence of such neurologic symptoms should always raise the suspicion of poisoning.

A full understanding of neurotoxicology would involve a knowledge of the special biochemical affinities that exist between each of the many neurotoxins and the neurons and interstitial tissue of the brain and spinal cord. These affinities are varied with respect to both their topography within the nervous system and their mechanism. Arsenic, for example, forms bonds with sulfhydryl (SH) radicles which are abundant in the axons of peripheral nerves and the endothelial cells of capillaries in the cerebral white matter. This explains the occurrence of polyneuropathy and hemorrhagic leukoencephalopathy in arsenic poisoning, but the molecular pathobiology is unknown. Diphtheria toxin, which causes a delayed polyneuropathy, proves, on more careful analysis, to be a polypeptide chain composed of two fragments. Pappenheimer finds that so-called fragment B bonds with specific surface receptors on sensitive cell membranes, whereas fragment A crosses the plasma membrane of the cell and inhibits protein synthesis through the inactivation of the eukaryotic translocating enzyme called "elongation factor 2"; a cofactor, nicotinamide adenine dinucleotide, must be present if the toxin is to be active. How impaired protein synthesis damages the medullated sheaths of Schwann cells in the most vascular parts of the peripheral nerve is unknown. In the myocardium the toxin decreases the rate of oxidation of long-chain fatty acids by an interference with the metabolism of carnitine.

These few examples provide a glimpse of the complexity of the mechanisms of interaction of toxins and the cells of the nervous system. The elucidation of the mode of action of the several hundred known neurotoxins promises to yield important information as to the biochemical physiology of neurons. For this reason the study of neurotoxins opens one of the most inviting fields of experimental neuropathology.

It would hardly be possible, in the confines of this chapter, to recount the clinical aspects of the many neurotoxins in any degree of completeness. A number of comprehensive references which identify their symp-

763

toms, signs, and active ingredients are listed at the end of this chapter. An up-to-date handbook of toxicology should be part of the library of every physician.

The scope of this chapter on neurotoxicology will be somewhat limited for other reasons. The toxic effects of ethyl, methyl, amyl, and isopropyl alcohol as well as ethylene glycol are considered in the chapter on alcohol, and the adverse effects of antibiotics on cochlear and vestibular function in Chap. 14. Intoxications with some of the drugs used in the treatment of extrapyramidal motor symptoms (e.g., atropine and related belladonna alkaloids), pain and headache (salicylates), convulsive seizures, sleep disorders, psychiatric illnesses, and so forth are considered in the chapters dealing with these particular disorders. Cyanide and carbon monoxide poisoning are discussed in relation to anoxic encephalopathy (Chap. 39). Other drugs are too rare in the United States and western Europe to justify detailed description. The discussion, instead, will be centered on the more common categories of drugs and chemical agents that affect the nervous system selectively or predominantly, as follows:

1. The addicting drugs: opiates and synthetic analgesics and barbiturates. (Alcohol is considered in Chap. 40.)

2. Other sedative-hypnotic drugs; psychotherapeutic, stimulant, and psychotogenic drugs

3. Bacterial toxins

4. Plant poisons, venoms, bites, and stings

5. Heavy metals

6. Industrial toxins

7. Antineoplastic agents

OPIATES AND OTHER SYNTHETIC ANALGESIC DRUGS

The opiates, strictly speaking, include all the naturally occurring alkaloids in *opium,* which is prepared from the sap of the poppy, *Papaver somniferum.* For clinical purposes, opiates refer only to those alkaloids which have a high degree of analgesic activity, i.e., morphine and codeine (3-methoxymorphine). Thebaine, another opium alkaloid which, like morphine, possesses a phenanthrene nucleus, has few or no analgesic properties and is therefore not ordinarily considered an opiate. The terms *opioid* and *narcotic-analgesic* designate drugs with

actions similar to those of morphine. Compounds that are chemical modifications of morphine include diacetylmorphine or heroin (now the most commonly abused opioid), hydromorphone (Dilaudid), codeine (methylmorphine), Pantopon, dihydrocodeinone (Hycodan), dihydroxycodeinone (Eucodal), morphone (Numorphan) and oxycodone (Percodan). A second class of opioids comprises the purely synthetic analgesics meperidine (Demerol), the meperidine derivatives anileridine and alphaprodine (Nisentil), methadone (Dolophine or Amidone), metopon (6-methyldihydromorphinone), racemorphan (Dromoran), levorphan (*l*-Dromoran), *d*-propoxyphene (Darvon), diphenoxylate (the main component of Lomotil), and phenazocine (Prinadol). These synthetic analgesics are similar to the opiates, both in their pharmacologic effects and in the patterns of abuse, the differences being mainly quantitative. In fact, *d*-propoxyphene has such low addictive liabilities that it is not controlled by the federal narcotic laws. The same statement applies to the synthetic analgesic pentazocine (Talwin), and although its addictive quality is relatively low, prolonged use undoubtedly causes physical dependence. Butorphanol and the related drugs nalbuphine and buprenorphine are recently introduced synthetic analgesics, which, like pentazocine, combine the properties of an opioid and an opioid antagonist. Allegedly butorphanol has a greater analgesic effectiveness and respiratory sparing effect than morphine, but further clinical trials are required before the preliminary impressions can be accepted (Vandam).

The clinical effects of the opioids will be considered from two points of view: (1) acute poisoning and (2) addiction.

OPIOID POISONING

Because of the high incidence of addiction, which leads to irregular and nonmedical usage of opioids, poisoning is a not infrequent accident. This may happen as a result of ingestion with suicidal intent, errors in the calculation of dosage, or unusual sensitivity. Children may exhibit an increased susceptibility to opioids, so that relatively small doses prove toxic. This is true also of adults who have myxedema, Addison's disease, chronic liver disease, or pneumonia. Acute poisoning may also occur in addicts who are unaware of the variations in potency of available opioids and that tolerance for opioids declines quickly after the withdrawal of the drug; upon resuming the habit, a formerly well-tolerated dose can be fatal.

Varying degrees of unresponsiveness, shallow respirations, slow respiratory rate (e.g., two to four per minute) or periodic breathing, pinpoint pupils, bradycardia, and hypothermia are the well-recognized clinical manifestations of acute opioid poisoning. In the most advanced stage the pupils dilate, the skin and mucous membranes become cyanotic, and the circulation fails. The immediate cause of death is usually respiratory depression, with consequent asphyxia. Patients who have a cardiorespiratory arrest are sometimes left with a residuum of anoxic encephalopathy. Others who recover from coma may occasionally reveal a hemiplegia, presumably due to vascular occlusion. The only symptoms of mild intoxication are anorexia, nausea, vomiting, constipation, and loss of sexual interest.

Treatment consists of gastric lavage if the drug was taken orally. This procedure may be efficacious many hours after ingestion, since one of the toxic effects of opioids is severe pylorospasm, which may cause much of the drug to be retained in the stomach. Other measures must be directed toward the maintenance of an adequate airway (a cuffed endotracheal tube should be inserted if the patient is comatose) and oxygenation, as described in the following section on barbiturate intoxication. If the patient does not respond rapidly to these measures, naloxone (Narcan) should be administered. This is a specific antidote to the opiates and also to the synthetic analgesics. It is now preferred to N-allylnormorphine (Nalline) because naloxone has no agonistic properties; hence, naloxone will not depress respiration further if the diagnosis of opiate poisoning is mistaken. For opiate poisoning, the dose of naloxone is 0.7 mg per 70 kg *intravenously*, repeated if necessary once or twice at 5-min intervals for an adequate respiratory response. The improvement in circulation and respiration is usually dramatic. In fact, failure of naloxone to produce such a response should cast doubt on the diagnosis of opioid intoxication. If an adequate respiratory response to naloxone is obtained, the patient should be observed carefully for 24 h and further doses of naloxone (50 percent higher than previously found effective) may be given *intramuscularly* as often as necessary. Naloxone has little direct effect on consciousness, however, and the patient may remain drowsy for many hours. This is not harmful, provided respiration is well maintained.

A new oxymorphone-derived antagonist, *naltrexone,* promises to be even more effective than naloxone. Naltrexone is relatively free of agonistic activity and has the additional advantage of being effective orally. It is about twice as potent as naloxone in precipitating abstinence phenomena in patients dependent upon opiates, and its half-life of antagonistic actions is at least twice as long as that of naloxone.

Once the patient regains consciousness, usually in about 8 h, other complaints such as severe pruritus, sneezing, persistent obstipation, and urinary retention may necessitate symptomatic treatment. Nausea and se-

vere abdominal pain, due presumably to pancreatitis (from spasm of the sphincter of Oddi), are other troublesome symptoms. The antidote must be used with great caution in an addict who has taken an overdose of opioid, because in this circumstance it may precipitate withdrawal phenomena.

In addition to the toxic effects of the opioid itself, the addict is exposed to a variety of neurologic and infectious complications, resulting mainly from the injection of crude adulterants (quinine, lactose, powdered milk, and fruit sugars) and from various infectious agents (injections often administered by unsterile methods). Amblyopia, due probably to the toxic effects of quinine in the heroin mixtures, has been reported, as well as transverse myelopathy and several types of peripheral neuropathy. The spinal cord disorder expresses itself clinically by the abrupt onset of paraplegia with a sensory level on the trunk. Pathologically, there is an acute necrotizing lesion involving both gray and white matter over a considerable vertical extent of the thoracic cord and occasionally the cervical cord. In some cases the myelopathy has followed the first intravenous injection of heroin after a prolonged period of abstinence. Damage to single peripheral nerves at the injection site and from compression are relatively common occurrences. Bilateral compression of the sciatic nerves, caused by sitting for a prolonged period in the lotus position while "stoned," has been observed several times. More difficult to understand is the involvement of individual nerves, particularly of the radial nerve, and painful affection of the brachial plexus, independent of compression and remote from the site of injections.

An acute generalized myonecrosis with myoglobinuria and renal failure has been ascribed to the intravenous injection of adulterated heroin. Brawny edema and fibrosing myopathy (Volkmann's contracture) are the sequelae of venous obliteration resulting from the administration of heroin and its adulterants by the intramuscular and subcutaneous routes. Occasionally there may be an inexplicable swelling of an extremity (sometimes massive) into which heroin had been injected subcutaneously or intramuscularly. Infection and venous thrombosis appear to be involved in its causation.

The diagnosis of drug addiction or the suspicion of this diagnosis should always encourage surveillance for infectious complications, particularly abscesses and cellulitis at injection sites, septic thrombophlebitis, hepatitis, and periarteritis. Tetanus, endocarditis (due mainly to *Staphylococcus aureus*), spinal epidural abscess, meningitis, brain abscess, and tuberculosis are found less frequently.

OPIOID ADDICTION

Just 15 years ago there were about 60,000 persons addicted to narcotic drugs in the United States, not including those who were receiving drugs because of incurable painful diseases. This represented a relatively small public health problem, in comparison with the abuse of barbiturates and alcohol; and opioid addiction was of serious proportions in only a few cities—New York, Chicago, Los Angeles, Washington, and Detroit. In the past 10 years a remarkable increase in opioid (principally heroin) addiction has taken place. The precise number of opioid addicts is not known, but was estimated by the Drug Enforcement Administration, in 1970, to be more than 600,000. The peak incidence of heroin dependence occurred in 1972. The incidence declined between 1972 and 1974, then increased again, and has fluctuated at peak or near peak levels since then.

Etiology and Pathogenesis A number of factors, socioeconomic, psychological, and pharmacologic, contribute to the genesis of opioid addiction. In our culture, the most susceptible subjects are young men or delinquent youths living in the economically depressed areas of large cities, but a significant number are now found in the suburbs and in small cities. The onset of opioid use is usually in adolescence, with a peak at 17 to 18 years. Fully two-thirds of addicts start using the drugs before the age of 21. A disproportionately large number are American Negroes and persons of Puerto Rican or Mexican descent. Almost 90 percent of addicts engage in criminal activity, often necessary to obtain their daily ration of drug, but most of these had had arrests or convictions prior to their addiction. Also many of them show psychiatric disorders, psychoneurosis and sociopathy being the most common. Monroe et al. examined a group of 837 opioid addicts, using the Lexington Personality Inventory and found evidence of antisocial personality in 42 percent, emotional disturbance in 29 percent, and thinking disorder in 22 percent; only 7 percent were asymptomatic. Nevertheless, the precise "personality factor" which renders them vulnerable to addiction has not been defined.

Association with addicts is the chief reason for beginning addiction. One addict recruits another person into addiction, and the new recruit does likewise. In this sense opioid addiction is contagious, and as a result of this pattern of opioid abuse, heroin addiction has attained epidemic proportions. A small, almost insignificant, proportion of addicts are introduced to drugs by physicians in the course of an illness.

Opioid addiction evolves in three successive phases: (1) episodic intoxication, or euphoria, (2) pharmacogenic (physical) dependence, or addiction, and (3) the propensity to *relapse after cure.*

Some of the symptoms of opioid intoxication have already been considered. In persons who are distressed by pain or pain-anticipatory anxiety, the administration of opioids produces a sense of unusual well-being, a state that has traditionally been referred to as *morphine euphoria.* It should be emphasized that only a negligible proportion of such persons continue to use opioids habitually after their pain has subsided. The vast majority of potential addicts are not suffering from painful illnesses at the time they initiate opioid use, and in them the initial effects are not aptly described as euphoric. The latter persons, as indicated above, are mainly teenagers who self-administer opioids under the tutelage of their peers and who learn, after several repetitions, to recognize what they refer to as a "high," despite the recurrence of unpleasant symptoms (nausea, vomiting, faintness). The repeated self-administration of the drug ("reinforcement" in the language of operant psychology) is the most important factor in the genesis of addiction. Regardless of how one characterizes the state of mind that is produced by episodic injection of the drug, the individual quickly discovers the need to increase the dose in order to obtain the original effects. Although the initial effects may not be fully recaptured, the progressively increasing dose of the drug does abate the discomfort that arises as the effects of each injection wear off. In this way a new *pharmacogenically induced need* is developed, and the use of opioids becomes self-perpetuating. At the same time a marked degree of tolerance is produced, so that enormous amounts of drugs, e.g., 5000 mg morphine daily, have been administered without the development of toxic symptoms.

The classic pharmacologic criteria of addiction, as indicated in the preceding chapter on alcoholism, are tolerance and physical dependence. The latter refers to the symptoms and signs that become manifest when the drug is withdrawn, following a period of continued use. These symptoms and signs constitute a specific clinical state, termed the *abstinence syndrome.* The mechanisms that underlie the development of tolerance and physical dependence are not fully understood, although they are the subject of much interest and speculation. A complete discussion of the various theories related to physical dependence can be found in the reviews by Wikler (see references at end of chapter).

This concept of addiction permits a distinction to be made between *addicting drugs* (opiates, alcohol, and barbiturates) and *habit-forming drugs* (bromides, cocaine, and marijuana), since no consistent symptoms of physical dependence follow the discontinuation of the latter group, even after prolonged exposure and the development of varying degrees of tolerance. Stated in another way, all addicting drugs are habit-forming, but the opposite is not true. The place of amphetamines in this scheme is uncertain. Undoubtedly they are habit-forming if used in large dosage. Withdrawal of drug, after chronic oral or intravenous use, is regularly followed by deep sleep (mostly REM sleep), from which the patient awakens with a ravenous appetite. Administration of dextroamphetamine reverses the sleep pattern.

The intensity of the opioid abstinence syndrome depends on the dose of the drug and duration of addiction. In respect to morphine it has been found that the majority of individuals receiving 240 mg daily for 30 days or more will show moderately severe abstinence symptoms following withdrawal, whereas mild signs of opiate abstinence can be precipitated by narcotic antagonists in persons who have taken as little as 15 mg morphine or an equivalent dose of methadone or heroin, three times daily for 3 days.

The abstinence syndrome which occurs in the morphine addict may be taken as the prototype of the opioid group. The first 8 to 16 h of abstinence usually pass asymptomatically. At the end of this period yawning, rhinorrhea, sweating, and lacrimation become manifest. At first mild, these symptoms increase in severity over a period of several hours and then remain constant for several days. The patient may be able to sleep during this early period but is restless, and thereafter insomnia remains a prominent feature. Dilatation of the pupils, recurring waves of gooseflesh, and twitchings of the muscles appear. The patient complains of severe aching in the back, abdomen, and legs and of hot and cold "flashes"; requests for blankets are frequent. By the end of about 36 h the restlessness becomes more severe, and nausea, vomiting, and diarrhea usually develop. Temperature, respiratory rate, and blood pressure are slightly elevated. All these symptoms reach their peak intensity 48 to 72 h after withdrawal, and then gradually decline. The opioid abstinence syndrome is rarely fatal. After 7 to 10 days, all clinical signs of abstinence have disappeared, although the patient may complain of insomnia, nervousness, weakness, and muscle aches for several more weeks, and a small deviation of a number of physiologic variables can be detected with refined techniques for up to 10 months (protracted abstinence).

Two types of abstinence changes are recognized— *nonpurposive* and *purposive*. The former comprise the various autonomic and neuromuscular signs already described and are relatively transient in nature. That these symptoms represent an altered physiologic state and are not psychic in origin has been clearly demonstrated experimentally. Signs of physical dependence on morphine and other opioid drugs can be induced in the lower limbs of dogs whose spinal cords have been transected; the flexor and crossed extensor spinal reflexes that are depressed or abolished by the opioid become remarkably exaggerated when the drug is withdrawn. The purposive changes refer to the patient's craving for the drug and the manipulative activity directed toward obtaining it. These symptoms may persist indefinitely and are important in relation to that characteristic of addiction referred to as *habituation, emotional dependence*, or *psychic dependence*. These terms are used interchangeably and refer to the substitution of drug-seeking activities for all other aims and objects in life.

Habituation, or psychic dependence, is regarded as the most important quality of addiction, since it is this feature which governs the initial use of the drug and relapse following apparent cure of addiction. Relapse to the use of the drug may occur long after the nonpurposive abstinence changes seem to have disappeared. The cause for relapse is imperfectly understood. It has been theorized that fragments of the abstinence syndrome may remain as a conditioned response, and that these abstinence signs may be evoked by the appropriate environmental stimuli. Thus, when a "cured" addict is in a situation where narcotic drugs are readily available, or in circumstances that were responsible for the initial use of drugs, the incompletely extinguished drug-seeking behavior reasserts itself.

The characteristics of addiction and of abstinence are qualitatively similar with all the drugs of the opiate group as well as the related synthetic analgesics. The differences are mainly quantitative and are related to the differences in dosage, potency, and the length of action. Heroin is two to three times more potent than morphine but otherwise the same; nevertheless, the heroin withdrawal syndrome encountered in hospital practice is usually mild in degree because of the low dosage of this drug in the street product. Dilaudid and metopon are more potent than morphine and have a shorter duration of action; hence the addict requires more doses per day, and the abstinence syndrome comes on and subsides more rapidly. The length of action of racemorphan is somewhat longer than that of morphine, but withdrawal phenomena are similar to those of morphine in temporal course and intensity. Abstinence symptoms from codeine, while very definite, are less severe than those from morphine. The addiction liabilities of d-propoxyphene are negligible. Abstinence symptoms from methadone are less intense than those from morphine and do not become evident until 3 or 4 days after withdrawal; furthermore, this drug is qualitatively different from morphine insofar as autonomic signs are less severe in the abstinence period. For these reasons methadone is used in the treatment of morphine addiction. Meperidine addiction is of particular importance because of the high incidence among doctors and nurses and because there is still a widespread belief that this drug is nonaddicting. Tolerance to the toxic effects of this drug is not complete, so that the addict may show tremors, twitching of the muscles, confusion, hallucinations, and at times convulsions. Signs of abstinence appear 3 to 4 h after the last dose and reach their maximum intensity in 8 to 12 h, at which time they may be worse than those of morphine abstinence.

Diagnosis of Addiction Diagnosis is usually made when the patient admits to using and needing drugs. Should the patient decide to conceal this fact, one must rely on collateral evidence such as miosis, needle marks, emaciation, or abscess scars. Meperidine addicts are likely to have dilated pupils and muscles that twitch. A method for testing the urine for opiates is now generally available. The finding of morphine or opiate derivatives (heroin is excreted as morphine) in the urine is confirmatory evidence that the patient has taken or has been given a dose of such drugs within 24 h of the test.

Formerly it was necessary to isolate questionable cases and to observe the patient over a period of at least 2 days for signs of abstinence. Through use of the specific morphine antagonist naloxone (Narcan), a diagnosis of addiction to opiates and related analgesic drugs can be made within an hour. Naloxone should be administered only in the presence of another physician or nurse, with the full understanding and permission of the patient. The drug is given intravenously, slowly, using a syringe containing one ampul (0.4 mg). The injection is stopped when pupillary dilatation, increased respiratory rate, lacrimation, rhinorrhea, sweating, and yawning ap-

pear. If, after 5 to 10 min, no such signs appear, a second injection may be given in the same way. If again the patient shows no abstinence signs, one may assume that there is no physical dependence upon opiates. Naloxone may be injected subcutaneously in the same dosage as intravenously. Again, if the patient has taken more than occasional doses of the drug within a week of the test, the administration of naloxone will precipitate symptoms of abstinence. These become evident within 5 min of the first injection, reach their peak intensity in 20 min, begin to decline in 60 min, and disappear after 3 h. Naloxone does not precipitate abstinence symptoms in meperidine addicts unless the patient has been taking more than 1600 mg daily.

Management and Avoidance of Addiction The ambulatory treatment of addiction never succeeds and should therefore not be undertaken, except in special settings, such as a carefully supervised methadone treatment program (see below). Addicts who are refused opiates may ask for methadone, meperidine, or racemorphine on the ground that these drugs are synthetic and nonaddicting. However, these are addicting drugs and have been legally defined as such. The physician should also be aware that to prescribe narcotics for an addict merely for the purpose of preventing abstinence changes is to break both the letter and the spirit of the regulations. Occasional exceptions may be made in cases of seriously ill addicts who are awaiting treatment in a hospital or methadone program, or of patients who are suffering from incurable, painful disease.

An alternate method, and one that is used now almost exclusively, is to substitute methadone for opioid, in the ratio of 1 mg methadone for 3 mg morphine, 1 mg heroin, or 20 mg meperidine. Since methadone is long-acting and effective orally, it need be given only twice daily by mouth—10 to 20 mg per dose being sufficient to suppress abstinence symptoms. After a stabilization period of 3 to 5 days on this dosage of methadone alone, the dosage may be reduced and the drug withdrawn over a similar period of time. Regardless of the method employed, withdrawal is best carried out in an institution with proper facilities for postwithdrawal rehabilitation in a drug-free environment. Such institutions, private or municipal, are available in most large communities.

The physician must be constantly alert to the dangers of addiction, particularly in susceptible individuals, i.e., in those with psychoneurosis, antisocial personality, or alcoholism. The use of opioids should be limited to patients in whom pain is the chief problem. These drugs should not be used primarily as sedatives, for the relief of asthma, or even in patients with chronic pain until all other measures have been exhausted. It follows that it is most important to make a precise diagnosis of the cause of pain, since in some cases measures other than opioids will suffice, while in others, such as hysteria and depression, narcotics are contraindicated.

If narcotics have to be used for the relief of pain, consideration should be given to the choice of the appropriate drug and to the mode of administration. Morphine is still the drug of choice for most patients requiring relief of severe pain for short periods. Meperidine may be useful in patients who cannot tolerate morphine. Patients with chronic pain should be managed with the least potent and smallest effective dosage; doses should be spaced as far apart as possible and discontinued as soon as the need for pain relief has passed. In general, opioids should be administered orally whenever possible, and the intravenous route should be avoided, since this method produces maximum "euphoria" and, hence, the greatest danger of addiction. The oral administration of codeine and aspirin is a useful way to begin treatment of the patient with chronic pain. If these drugs fail to control the pain, the parenteral administration of codeine should be tried. If the more potent opioids are needed, methadone and levorphan should be used because of their effectiveness by the oral route and the relatively slow development of tolerance. Should long-continued injections of morphine or meperidine become necessary, maximum analgesic effect is obtained with 10 mg morphine rather than with 15 mg, as is often prescribed, and with 60 to 70 mg meperidine rather than with 100 mg. In these cases, use of pentazocine (Talwin) might be considered, administered parenterally in doses of 40 to 60 mg. The respiratory depression produced by pentazocine, like that due to opioids, can be counteracted by naloxone.

Ambulatory Treatment of Opiate Addiction The most significant development in the treatment of opiate (almost exclusively heroin) addiction has been the establishment and growth of ambulatory methadone maintenance clinics. The scope of this activity, like the incidence of addiction, cannot be stated precisely, but can be judged by the fact that at present, about 75,000 former heroin addicts are participating in methadone clinics approved by the Food and Drug Administration.

The method of treatment consists of the oral administration of methadone beginning with 40 mg or less once daily and then increasing the dose to an amount sufficient to suppress the craving for heroin and to abolish the euphoria-producing effects of that drug given intravenously (heroin blockade). The daily dosage of methadone required to achieve these effects varies between 60 and 100 mg; some patients can be maintained on as little as 40 mg/day, and with higher dosage they need take the drug only once in 48 h. Recently, a longer-acting form of methadone—l-acetylmethadol—has become available, which can be taken thrice or even twice weekly. In principle, these effects could be achieved by multiple daily injections of heroin or morphine, but the effectiveness of methadone orally, its prolonged duration of action, and the fact that it precludes the desire and need for taking other opioids make methadone far more practical.

Methadone is no longer dispensed in tablet form; it is given only as a liquid (dissolved in fruit juice) which is taken under supervision. The collection of urine samples is also supervised, and these are analyzed for opiates and other drugs, to monitor the patient's adherence to the program. Once this has been established, the patient is allowed to take home a 1- to 3-day supply. These measures are designed to prevent the diversion of methadone into illicit channels. Various forms of individual psychotherapy, group psychotherapy, social service counseling, and vocational guidance are included in most programs and are of great importance. The use of former heroin addicts (who are themselves on methadone treatment) as counselors is considered to be a particularly important adjunct to methadone treatment.

The results of methadone treatment are difficult to assess and vary considerably from one program to another. Even the best programs suffer an attrition rate of about 25 percent after several years. Of the patients who remain, between 75 and 85 percent achieve a high degree of social rehabilitation; i.e., they are gainfully employed and no longer engage in criminal behavior or prostitution. This has been the very notable achievement of the methadone maintenance programs.

Although the effectiveness of methadone treatment in the social rehabilitation of many addicts cannot be doubted, a number of questions about this method remain. The usual practice of methadone programs is to accept only addicts over the age of 16 years, with a history of heroin addiction for at least one year. This leaves untreated the adolescent addict. Although some individuals have been withdrawn from methadone, this has been accomplished so far in a relatively small number, and their capacity to maintain a drug-free existence remains to be determined. This means that the large majority of addicts now enrolled in methadone programs are committed to an indefinite period of methadone maintenance, and the effects of such a regimen are uncertain.

An alternate method of ambulatory treatment of

the opiate addict involves the use of narcotic antagonists. Cyclazocine is the best-known of these. After withdrawal of the opiate, cyclazocine is administered orally, in increasing amounts over a period of 2 to 6 weeks, until a dosage of 2 mg per 70 kg is taken twice daily. The cyclazocine-stabilized individual is highly refractory to the euphoria-producing and pharmacologic effects of opiates. The idea of treatment is to continue the administration of cyclazocine until all drug-seeking behavior is extinguished, after which it is withdrawn. Good results have been achieved with this drug, but only in small numbers of highly motivated patients. More recently, interest has centered on the opiate antagonist naltrexone which is virtually devoid of agonistic activity and twice as potent as naloxone; it has the added advantages of being effective orally and in much smaller doses than naloxone. The value of this kind of *extinction therapy* has not yet been determined, but the results in some patients have been encouraging. The search for improved methods of using opioid antagonists continues; one such agent, buprenorphine, is said to show promise (Jasinski et al.). Also under restricted investigation is a modification of methadone maintenance, using the drug levomethadyl (LAAM).

BARBITURATES

Despite a reduction in the use of barbiturates during the past decade, the incidence of addiction, suicides, and accidental deaths attributable to the improper use of these drugs is a matter of continuing concern to the medical profession. It is estimated that barbiturates account for 20 percent of acute poisonings admitted to general hospitals and that they are responsible for 6 percent of suicides and 18 percent of accidental deaths—figures exceeded by no other single poison. Despite an estimated mortality rate of only 8 percent of hospitalized cases, barbiturates reportedly cause about 15,000 deaths annually in the United States. In 1975, the Domestic Council Drug Abuse Force estimated that the total number of regular users of barbiturates who were "in trouble" (suicidal and accidental overdoses as well as medical complications of barbiturate abuse) to be 300,000.

About 50 barbiturates have been marketed for clinical use, but only the following are encountered with any frequency: pentobarbital (Nembutal), secobarbital (Seconal), amobarbital (Amytal), aprobarbital (Alurate),

thiopental (Pentothal), barbital (Veronal), and phenobarbital (Luminal). In the United States, pentobarbital, secobarbital, and amobarbital are the most commonly abused barbiturates. All the barbiturates are similar pharmacologically and differ only in their speed of onset and duration of action. The clinical problems posed by the barbiturates are different, however, depending on whether the intoxication is acute or chronic, and these two types will be considered separately.

ACUTE BARBITURATE INTOXICATION

This results from the ingestion of large amounts of the drug either accidentally or with suicidal intent. An uncommon form of accidental poisoning occurs in individuals who are intoxicated with barbiturates or with alcohol and who, being confused, ingest more of the drug than was intended. This type of poisoning has been termed *drug automatism.*

The ingestion of barbiturates with suicidal intent is most frequently the act of a depressed person. The hysteric or sociopath may take an overdose as a suicidal gesture and sometimes become seriously intoxicated because of a miscalculation or ignorance of the toxic dosage. At times, no psychiatric disease is present, the drug being taken impulsively or while the individual is inebriated. The combination of alcohol and barbiturate intoxication is frequent and particularly dangerous, since these drugs have an additive effect.

Site and Mode of Action of Barbiturates Barbiturates decrease the excitability of nerve cells, although the mechanism is not fully understood. Attempts have been made to localize the action of barbiturates to certain anatomic regions, or even to specific nuclei within the nervous system, but it would appear that all parts are to some extent sensitive to the drug. Nevertheless, the reticular formation of the thalamus and midbrain is particularly susceptible. There is little experimental evidence to support the notion that the administration of barbiturates first depresses cerebral cortical activity and then sequentially affects the anatomically lower centers. Reflex and other activity of the nervous system are probably depressed simultaneously, although in some cases the spinal reflexes appear to be accentuated in the early stages of poisoning.

Symptoms and Signs The symptoms and signs of acute barbiturate intoxication vary with the type and the amount of drug, as well as with the length of time that has elapsed since it was ingested. Pentobarbital and secobarbital produce their effects quickly, and recovery is relatively rapid. Phenobarbital induces coma more slowly, and its effects tend to be prolonged. The duration of action of these drugs can be judged from the hypnotic effect of an average oral dose. In the case of the long-acting barbiturates, such as phenobarbital, barbital, and diallylbarbituric acid, it lasts 6 h or more; with the intermediate-acting drugs, amobarbital and aprobarbital, 3 to 6 h; and with the short-acting drugs, secobarbital and pentobarbital, less than 3 h.

In general, much larger doses of long-acting barbiturates are required to produce a depth of unconsciousness comparable with that produced by the short-acting ones. The ingestion by adults of more than 3.0 g secobarbital, pentobarbital, amobarbital, or diallylbarbituric acid at one time may be fatal unless intensive and skilled treatment is applied promptly; it has been estimated that to produce a comparable effect, the following amounts of long-acting barbiturates would have to be ingested: 6.0 to 9.0 g phenobarbital, 5.0 to 20.0 g barbital, and 15.0 g aprobarbital. Because of the serious complications of prolonged coma, the fatalities are greater with the long-acting than with the short-acting drugs.

In regard to prognosis and treatment, it is useful to recognize three grades of severity of acute barbiturate intoxication. Mild intoxication follows the ingestion of approximately 0.6 g pentobarbital or its equivalent. The patient is drowsy or asleep, although readily roused if called or shaken. The symptoms resemble those of alcohol intoxication, except that the face is not flushed and the conjunctivas are not suffused. The patient thinks slowly, and there may be mild disorientation, lability of mood, impairment of judgment, slurred speech, drunken gait, and nystagmus. Reflex activity and vital signs are not affected.

Moderate intoxication follows the ingestion of five to ten times the oral hypnotic dose. Here the state of consciousness is more severely depressed and is usually accompanied by depressed or absent deep reflexes, and slow but not shallow respiration. Corneal reflexes are retained, with occasional exceptions. At times the patient can be roused by vigorous manual stimulation. When awakened, the patient is confused and dysarthric and after a few moments drifts back into stupor. At other times the patient is comatose and cannot be roused by any means. In the latter case the depth of coma and seriousness of respiratory depression may be roughly estimated by the response of respiration to the inhalation of 10% carbon dioxide or to painful stimulation such as the application of firm pressure to the sternum or supraorbital ridge. If these stimuli cause an increase in the depth and rate of respiration, the outlook for recovery is good, and only symptomatic treatment is indicated.

Severe intoxication occurs with the ingestion of 15 to 20 times the oral hypnotic dose. The patient cannot be roused by any of the means indicated. Respiration is slow and shallow or irregular, and pulmonary edema and cyanosis may be present. The deep tendon reflexes are usually but not invariably absent. Most often, the patients show no response to plantar stimulation, but in those who do, the plantar responses are extensor. In the most advanced cases the corneal and gag reflexes may also be abolished. Ordinarily the pupillary light reflex is retained in severe intoxication and is lost only if the patient is asphyxiated. In the early hours of coma, there may be a phase of rigidity of the limbs, hyperactive reflexes, ankle clonus, extensor plantar signs, and decerebrate posturing; persistence of these signs indicates a severe degree of anoxic damage. The temperature may be subnormal, the pulse thready and rapid, and the blood pressure at shock levels.

Diagnosis The diagnosis of barbiturate intoxication is made from the history and physical findings. If a reasonable suspicion of the diagnosis exists, then a careful search for drugs or their containers may be rewarding. One should also examine the mouth and gastric contents for any characteristically colored capsules. Acute barbiturate intoxication which presents as a state of coma must be distinguished from other forms of coma by methods outlined on pages 243 to 246. Actually there are few conditions other than barbiturate intoxication which cause a flaccid coma with reactive pupils, hypothermia, and hypotension. Glutethimide poisoning may produce an identical clinical picture, except that the pupils are fixed (a parasympathomimetic action). Laryngeal spasm and sudden apnea also characterize glutethimide intoxication. In the differential diagnosis, hysteria presents the main problem.

The use of gas chromatography provides a reliable means of identifying the type and amount of barbiturate in the blood. The major virtue of this method is in determining the precise cause of coma when this is in question. The blood level also helps to identify the drug as long- or short-acting, thus giving information as to whether the therapeutic problem will be short or prolonged. A blood barbiturate level of 2 mg per 100 ml in a *comatose* patient is usually due to poisoning with secobarbital or pentobarbital; although the immediate mortality is high in such instances, the comatose state will be short. A level of 11.5 to 12.0 mg per 100 ml is usually due to poisoning with barbital or phenobarbital, and the comatose state will be prolonged. Because of the potentiating effects of alcohol, a patient who has ingested both drugs may be comatose with relatively low blood barbiturate levels. For this reason, and also because of differences in individual tolerance, the correlation between blood barbiturate levels and depth of coma is not entirely dependable.

The *EEG* may also be useful in diagnosis, since characteristic patterns accompany barbiturate intoxication. In mild intoxication, the normal activity is replaced by fast activity, in the range of 20 to 30 cycles per second, and is most prominent in the frontal regions. In more severe intoxication, the fast waves become less regular and interspersed with 3- to 4-per-second slow activity. In still more advanced cases, there are short periods of suppression of all activity, separated by bursts of slow (delta) waves of variable frequency. In extreme overdosage, all electrical activity ceases. This is one instance in which a "flat" EEG cannot be equated with brain death, and the effects are fully reversible unless anoxic damage has supervened.

Management   The management of acute barbiturate intoxication depends on its severity. In mild or moderate intoxication, recovery is the rule, and vigorous treatment is not required. If the type and amount of ingested drug cannot be ascertained, it is important to empty the stomach and analyze its contents. In the responsive patient, gastric lavage with a large tube is difficult, and a simpler procedure is to induce vomiting with syrup of ipecac. Once this has been accomplished, the mildly intoxicated patient should be watched closely for signs of deepening coma.

If the patient is unresponsive, special attention should be given to maintaining respiration and urinary excretion, and to the prevention of infection. It is most important to maintain a patent airway, at first by the insertion of an endotracheal tube; suctioning should be used when necessary, and the patient should be turned frequently. Tracheostomy and bronchoscopic suctioning usually become necessary if atelectasis becomes manifest, or if intubation must be maintained for longer than 48 h. If there is any risk of respiratory depression or underventilation, it is advisable to support respiration by machine, in order to provide adequate oxygenation and minimize the risk of atelectasis. Also, early on, an intravenous fluid line should be established to promote the renal clearance of barbiturate and permit rapid administration of drugs and electrolytes. In the unresponsive, intubated patient gastric lavage may be a useful thera-peutic as well as a diagnostic measure. It must be performed within several hours of ingestion of the drug, since barbiturates are absorbed rapidly and completely.

Cases of severe respiratory depression, with cyanosis and pupillary dilatation, represent a serious medical emergency. A clear airway should be secured immediately and some form of assisted respiration begun with an automatic intermittent positive-pressure respirator. If the patient is in shock, the foot of the bed should be elevated, and norepinephrine and whole blood or plasma administered. Catheterization is required to determine the adequacy of urinary output, to obtain samples for laboratory examination, and to prevent distention of the bladder. Since the amount of barbiturate cleared by the kidney is directly proportional to the amount of urine formed, 8 to 10 liters of 5% glucose in saline solution should be given daily. Forced diuresis is also important because toxic amounts of barbiturate have an antidiuretic effect. Coma of any significant duration requires the administration of other electrolytes as well, the amounts being governed by their serum and urinary values. The occurrence of pulmonary and urinary infections calls for the use of appropriate antibiotic treatment.

Hemodialysis has proved to be an effective form of therapy and should be used in all patients with profound coma who fail to respond to the measures outlined above. It is particularly useful in cases of coma due to long-acting barbiturates and is mandatory if anuria or uremia has developed.

The treatment of severe barbiturate intoxication with analeptic drugs (Metrazol, picrotoxin, Megimide), which enjoyed a brief period of popularity, has been generally abandoned; they do not affect the rate of metabolism or the excretion of barbiturate. Alkalinization of the blood, by the use of large amounts of bicarbonate solution, as a means of mobilizing the barbiturate and increasing its rate of excretion, seems to be a useful measure, particularly when phenobarbital is the responsible agent.

Occasionally, in the case of a barbiturate addict who has taken an overdose of the drug, recovery from coma is followed by the development of abstinence symptoms which have to be managed by the methods outlined below.

CHRONIC BARBITURATE INTOXICATION (BARBITURATE ADDICTION)

Chronic barbiturate intoxication, like other drug addictions, tends to develop on a background of some psychiatric disorder, most commonly depression or psychoneurosis with symptoms of anxiety and insomnia, or so-called character disorder. The drug is usually prescribed for nervousness and insomnia; as the desired effects are lost, the patient increases the dose gradually until taking an amount sufficient to produce symptoms when it is withdrawn. Individuals with character disorders are usually introduced to the drug by associates; since the drug is taken for its intoxicating effect, the dose tends to be increased rapidly. Addiction to alcohol or to opiates may predispose to barbiturate addiction. Alcoholics find that barbiturates effectively relieve their nervousness and tremor; they then may continue to take both alcohol and barbiturate, or the barbiturate may replace the alcohol. Heroin and morphine addicts may turn to barbiturates when they are unable to obtain opiates. As with other addicting drugs, the incidence of barbiturism is particularly high in individuals with ready access to drugs, such as physicians, pharmacists, and nurses.

The symptoms and signs of chronic barbiturate intoxication may be described in relation to (1) the toxic effects of the drug, (2) the development of tolerance, and (3) the effects of sudden withdrawal of the drug after a period of prolonged intoxication.

The toxic manifestations of chronic barbiturism are much the same as those of mild acute barbiturate or alcohol intoxication. The barbiturate addict thinks slowly, shows an increased emotional lability, and becomes untidy in his dress and personal habits. The neurologic signs are quite characteristic and include dysarthria, nystagmus, and cerebellar incoordination. Both the mental and neurologic signs fluctuate greatly, being more severe if the drug is taken in the fasting state and tending to increase during the day as more of the drug is ingested. If the dosage is elevated rapidly, the signs of moderate or severe intoxication become manifest.

A characteristic feature of chronic barbiturate intoxication is the development of tolerance, sometimes striking in degree. The average addict will ingest about 1.5 g of a potent barbiturate daily and will not develop signs of severe intoxication unless this amount is exceeded. Tolerance to barbiturates does not develop as rapidly as to opiates. Daily doses of 2 g have been reached, but this takes many months. Individual variations in the degree of tolerance make it difficult to state precisely the minimal amount of drug which must be ingested before the resulting condition is designated as chronic barbiturate intoxication. Most persons can ingest 0.4 g daily for as long as 3 months without developing major withdrawal signs (seizures or delirium). With a dosage of 0.8 g daily, the efficiency at all tasks is greatly reduced, and after the daily ingestion of this amount for a period of 2 months, abrupt withdrawal will result in

serious symptoms in the majority of patients. Even after 2 weeks at this dosage, some patients will show mild withdrawal symptoms, including paroxysmal EEG changes in response to photic stimulation. Individuals taking 0.4 to 0.7 g daily fall into an intermediate category; practically all show some mental dulling and episodes of forgetfulness, and occasionally severe withdrawal symptoms may occur.

Abstinence or Withdrawal Syndrome The withdrawal of barbiturates, following a period of chronic severe intoxication, precipitates a characteristic clinical syndrome. Immediately following withdrawal the patient seemingly improves over a period of 8 to 12 h, as the symptoms of intoxication diminish. After this short period a new group of symptoms appears, consisting of nervousness, tremor, insomnia, postural hypotension, and weakness. With chronic phenobarbital or barbital intoxication, withdrawal symptoms may not become apparent until 48 to 72 h after the final dose. Generalized seizures with loss of consciousness may occur, usually between the second and fourth days of abstinence, occasionally as long as 6 or 7 days after withdrawal. There may be a single seizure, several seizures, or rarely, status epilepticus. The convulsive phase may be followed directly by a delusional-hallucinatory state or a full-blown delirium, indistinguishable from delirium tremens, or a varying degree of improvement may follow the seizures before the delirium becomes manifest. Death has been reported under these circumstances. The abstinence syndrome may occur in varying degrees of completeness; some patients have seizures and recover without developing delirium and others have a delirium without preceding seizures. The abrupt onset of seizures or an acute psychosis in adult life should always raise the suspicion of addiction to barbiturates or other sedative-hypnotic drugs.

The EEG shows a number of changes during chronic barbiturate intoxication and following withdrawal. During chronic intoxication, the predominant pattern is one of fast activity of moderate voltage, interspersed with some 6- to 8-Hz activity chiefly in the frontal and parietal regions. The EEG findings do not correlate closely with the degree of intoxication, but some subjects do develop "EEG tolerance," i.e., a disappearance of the rapid pattern described above, while receiving moderate doses of barbiturate (400 mg daily for 90 days). On withdrawal of barbiturates the fast activity diminishes. Also in the first few days of abstinence, paroxysmal bursts of mixed spike and slow waves or 4-Hz "spike and dome" paroxysmal discharges occur, and these may or may not be associated with seizures. Characteristically, in the withdrawal period, there is a greatly heightened sensitivity to photic stimulation, to which the patient responds with myoclonus or a seizure, accompanied by paroxysmal changes in the EEG. Most of these abnormalities disappear after 4 or 5 days and the EEG pattern is usually completely normal in 2 weeks.

Treatment of Chronic Barbiturate Intoxication This should always be carried out in the hospital. If the diagnosis of addiction is made before signs of abstinence have appeared, the first step in treatment should be the determination of the "stabilization dosage." This is the amount of short-acting barbiturate required to produce mild symptoms of intoxication (nystagmus, slight ataxia, and dysarthria). Usually 0.2 g pentobarbital given orally every 6 h is sufficient for this purpose. The patient is examined 1 h after each dose. If the signs of intoxication are severe, the next scheduled dose is reduced or omitted. If, instead, tremulousness and postural tachycardia appear, an additional 0.1 g of pentobarbital is given, and the next scheduled dose is increased. This method is preferable to a blind reduction of dosage, since patients frequently underestimate the amount of drug taken. In such patients, establishment of the "stabilization dosage" may have diagnostic as well as therapeutic value. A patient who can take 0.8 g or more of pentobarbital daily, without developing signs of intoxication, is probably physically dependent on drugs of this type. Then a gradual withdrawal of the drug is undertaken, 0.1 g daily, the reduction being stopped for several days if abstinence symptoms appear.

An alternate method of managing barbiturate addiction is to stabilize the patient with phenobarbital rather than pentobarbital. The longer-acting barbiturate is safer than the shorter-acting one and permits a withdrawal that is characterized by fewer fluctuations in blood levels (Wesson and Smith). The initial dosage of phenobarbital is calculated by substituting one sedative dose (30 mg) of phenobarbital for each hypnotic dose (100 mg) of the short-acting barbiturate which the patient had been using.

With either of these methods, a severely addicted person can be withdrawn in 14 to 21 days. Patients undergoing withdrawal treatment require careful observation for symptoms of abstinence, and special precautions have to be taken to prevent the smuggling or concealment of drugs.

The patient presenting with severe withdrawal symptoms, such as seizures, is given 0.3 to 0.5 g phenobarbital intramuscularly and then enough to maintain a state of mild intoxication. Most anticonvulsant medicines have been shown to be ineffective against barbiturate withdrawal convulsions. Withdrawal should then be carried out as indicated above. If the abstinence symptoms are not severe, it is not necessary to reintoxicate the patient, but treatment can proceed along the lines laid down for the delirious and confused patient (pages 283 and 756).

After recovery has taken place, whether from symptoms of acute or chronic intoxication, the psychiatric problem requires evaluation and an appropriate plan of therapy. Many of the considerations in the management of alcoholism are equally applicable to the patient addicted to barbiturate and to nonbarbiturate hypnotic drugs.

BARBITURATE PROVOCATION OF OTHER DISEASES

At times the administration of one of the barbiturates may induce an attack of another disease. The most striking example of this is in hereditary porphyria where a severe and sometimes fatal attack of abdominal pain, psychosis, and polyneuropathy may follow the ingestion of a few capsules of secobarbital. With severe liver disease, detoxification of barbiturates may be impaired.

OTHER SEDATIVE-HYPNOTIC DRUGS; PSYCHOTHERAPEUTIC, STIMULANT, AND PSYCHOTOGENIC DRUGS

SEDATIVE-HYPNOTIC DRUGS

This class of drugs, also referred to as depressants, may be divided into two main groups. The first includes the barbiturates (discussed in the preceding section of this chapter), the bromides, chloral hydrate, and paraldehyde. In the past 15 years these drugs have been largely displaced by a second group of sedative-hypnotic drugs, comprising meprobamate and other glycerol derivatives, and the benzodiazepines, the most important of which are chlordiazepoxide (Librium) and diazepam (Valium). The advantages of the latter sedative-hypnotic drugs are their *relatively* low toxicity and addictive potential and their minimal interactions with other drugs.

Bromides are seldom prescribed by physicians at the present time, but are contained in certain "nerve tonics" and proprietary remedies (Nervine, Neurosine), so that cases of bromide intoxication are still encountered occasionally. Acute poisoning with bromide is rare because large doses of the drug are irritating to the gastric mucosa and vomiting prevents the attainment of significant blood levels. Taken in smaller doses, however, bromide tends to accumulate in the body because of its slow excretion by the kidney, and toxic symptoms may appear in a matter of weeks. These symptoms are caused by the bromide ion itself and are not simply a reflection of displacement of the chloride by the bromide ion.

The symptoms of chronic bromide intoxication range from dizziness, drowsiness, irritability, and emotional lability to a quiet confusional state, with impairment of thinking and memory and, in severe cases, to delirium and stupor and coma. Skin manifestations are associated in many cases, taking the form usually of an acnelike eruption and less frequently of proliferative nodular lesions, resembling those of tertiary syphilis. Headache, mild conjunctivitis, gastric distress, anorexia, and constipation may be associated as well. The blood bromide levels and the severity of toxic symptoms do not necessarily correspond. Levels of 75 mg per 100 ml (9 meq/liter) or more are considered abnormal and diagnostic of bromism, if the clinical picture suggests it. However, higher levels are sometimes well tolerated, and symptoms of bromism may persist for some days even after the blood levels have been reduced to normal or near-normal levels.

Treatment consists of removing the source of the bromide and administering sodium chloride (at least 6 g daily, in divided doses). Ammonium chloride may be substituted if an accumulation of sodium is to be avoided and if there is no danger of an uncompensated acidosis or hepatic failure. Confused or delirious patients require sedation, and anorectic and emaciated patients need careful nursing care and special attention to diet. The administration of a mercurial or thiazide diuretic serves to promote a bromide diuresis. Hemodialysis should be utilized in the most severe cases of intoxication.

Chloral hydrate is the oldest and one of the safest, most effective, and cheapest of the sedative-hypnotic drugs. After oral administration, chloral hydrate is reduced rapidly to trichloroethanol, which is responsible for the depressant effects on the central nervous system. A significant portion of the trichloroethanol is excreted in the urine as the glucuronide, which may give a false-positive test for glucose.

In large doses, chloral hydrate is toxic to the heart, kidneys, and liver, but only in the presence of preexisting disease in these organs. Chloral hydrate is a strong gastric irritant, so that it requires dilution and should not be taken on an empty stomach. Tolerance and addiction to chloral hydrate develop only rarely, and for these reasons it is an appropriate medication for the management of insomnia, particularly the type that is associated with depression. Poisoning with chloral hydrate is a rare occurrence and resembles acute barbiturate intoxication, except for the finding of miosis, which is said to characterize the former. In combination with alcohol—the well-known "Mickey Finn," or "knockout drops"—its effects are additive, leading to a rapid onset of coma. Death from poisoning is due to respiratory depression and hypotension; patients who survive may show signs of liver and kidney disease.

Paraldehyde is also an effective and safe hypnotic, providing that certain precautions are taken in its preparation and administration (see Chap. 40). It has a wide margin of safety when administered orally (or rectally), and even three or four times the usual dose (8 to 10 ml) causes no more than prolonged sleep or mild stupor. It is particularly effective in suppressing the tremulousness, restlessness, and insomnia that characterize the early phase (6 to 60 h) of the alcohol withdrawal period, as indicated in Chap. 40.

As remarked above, the foregoing drugs have been replaced to a large extent by two drugs of the *benzodiazepine* group, chlordiazepoxide (Librium) and diazepam (Valium). Indeed, the benzodiazepines are the most commonly prescribed drugs in the world today. According to Hollister, more than 1.4 billion prescriptions for these psychotherapeutic drugs are filled each year. In 1970, one American in five had used a psychotherapeutic drug by prescription.

The benzodiazepines have been used extensively to control anxiety, and they are probably more effective than the barbiturates in this respect. Also, they have been used to control overactivity and destructive behavior in children and the symptoms of alcohol withdrawal. Diazepam is particularly useful in the treatment of delirious patients who require parenteral medication. The benzodiazepines possess anticonvulsant properties, and the intravenous use of diazepam is an effective means of controlling status epilepticus, as described on page 229. In addition, diazepam has been used with moderate success in the treatment of extrapyramidal movement disorders and dystonic spasms.

Other important benzodiazepine drugs are flurazepam (Dalmane), which is widely used in the treatment of insomnia (see page 265), and clonazepam, in the treatment of seizures.

The benzodiazepine drugs, while comparatively safe in the recommended dosages, are far from ideal. They frequently cause unsteadiness of gait and drowsiness and at times hypotension and syncope, particularly in the elderly. In severely disturbed schizophrenic patients, rage, hostility, uncontrollable excitement, confusion, and depersonalization may develop. Nausea, diminished libido, headache, skin rashes, leukopenia, eosinophilia, agranulocytosis, and enhancement of the effects of alcohol have all been reported but are rare. Additional central nervous effects are slurred speech, dysphagia, ataxia, confusion, and faulty memory.

The *carbonic acid derivatives* are capable of modest depressant action and are appropriate for relieving mild degrees of nervousness, anxiety, and muscle tension. Meprobamate (Equanil, Miltown) is the best-known member of this group. With average doses (400 mg three or four times a day) the patient is able to function quite effectively; larger doses cause ataxia, drowsiness, stupor, coma, and vasomotor collapse. Hypersensitivity reactions in the form of fever, pruritis, and erythematous, maculopapular, and occasionally urticarial or bullous eruptions have been reported. Cutaneous petechiae or ecchymoses may also occur, without thrombocytopenia. Diplopia, syncope, menstrual irregularities, angioneurotic edema, peripheral edema, leucopenia, thrombocytopenia, and pancytopenia are rare complications.

It should be emphasized that addiction to meprobamate does occur, and if four or more times the daily recommended dose is administered over a period of weeks to months, withdrawal symptoms (including convulsions) may appear, resembling those which follow withdrawal of barbiturate in a chronically intoxicated patient.

Several of the other nonbarbiturate sedative-hypnotic drugs have the same intoxicating and addicting effects as barbiturates: glutethimide (Doriden), ethinamate (Valmid), ethchlorvynol (Placidyl), methyprylon (Noludar), chlordiazepoxide (Librium), diazepam (Valium), methaqualone (Quaalude), and perhaps oxazepam (Serax). The toxic effects of these drugs consist of slurred speech, nystagmus, ataxic gait, drowsiness, confusion, and coma. Furthermore, if the daily dose exceeds a minimal safe range, a state of physical dependence develops, so that abstinence symptoms appear upon withdrawal of the drug. These include hallucinations, seizures, and delirium, indistinguishable from those of the barbiturate and alcohol withdrawal syndrome. The seriousness of the abstinence syndrome in these cases is emphasized by reports of death following withdrawal of meprobamate, methyprylon, and diazepam. In view of these observations, physicians must exercise caution in prescribing new sedative drugs which are continually being introduced and which are said to possess no addicting or habit-forming properties.

The treatment of addiction to these sedatives follows the same principles that apply to the treatment of barbiturate addiction. Thus if the drug and its dosage can be determined, it should be withdrawn at the rate of one therapeutic dose per day. Should abstinence symptoms appear, the reduction in dosage is stopped for several days. If the offending drug cannot be identified, a barbiturate such as secobarbital should be administered to the point of mild intoxication and then withdrawn at a rate not to exceed 0.1 g daily. It should be noted that phenytoin and phenothiazine derivatives are not effective against abstinence convulsions.

ANTIPSYCHOTIC DRUGS

Since the mid-1950s, a large new series of pharmacologic agents, loosely referred to as tranquilizers, has come into prominent use—mainly for the control of schizophrenia, psychotic states associated with "organic brain syndromes," and certain instances of manic-depressive disease. The mechanism by which these drugs ameliorate disturbances of thought and affect in these psychotic states is poorly understood, but has been attributed to the ability of the drugs to inhibit or partially block dopamine receptors in the brain; probably their parkinsonian side effects can be attributed to this mechanism also.

There are a large number of antipsychotic drugs on the market, and no attempt will be made here to describe or even list all of them. Some have had only an evanescent popularity, and others have yet to prove their value. Chemically these compounds form a heterogeneous group; six categories are of particular clinical importance: (1) the phenothiazines, (2) the thioxanthines, (3) the butyrophenones, (4) the rauwolfia alkaloids, (5) an indole derivative, molindone (Moban), and (6) a dibenzoxazepine derivative, loxapine (Loxitane). The last two drugs, which have been introduced more recently, are about as effective as the phenothiazines in the management of schizophrenia, and their side effects are also the same. The main use of the newer antipsychotic drugs is in patients who are not responsive to the older ones or who suffer intolerable side effects from them. A new antipsychotic agent, clozapine (dibenzodiazepine derivative), is of current interest since it appears to be uniquely free of extrapyramidal side effects. This drug, as well as metiapine and timozide (a diphenylbutylpiperidine) are presently under investigation in the United States.

Phenothiazines This group comprises some of the most widely used tranquilizers, such as chlorpromazine (Thorazine, Largactil), promazine (Sparine), triflupromazine (Vesprin), prochlorperazine (Compazine), perphenazine (Trilafon), fluphenazine (Permitil, Prolixin), thioridazine (Mellaril), and trifluoperazine (Stelazine). In addition to their psychotherapeutic effects, these drugs have a number of other actions, so that certain members of this group are used as antiemetics (prochlorperazine) and antihistaminics (promethazine).

The phenothiazines have had their widest application in the treatment of the psychoses (schizophrenia and to a lesser extent manic-depressive psychosis). Their use outside of psychiatry should be discouraged. Under the influence of these drugs, many patients who would otherwise be hospitalized are able to live at home and even work productively. In the hospital, the use of these drugs has greatly facilitated the care of hyperactive and combative patients.

Side effects of the phenothiazines are frequent and often serious. All of them may cause a cholestatic type of jaundice, agranulocytosis, convulsive seizures, orthostatic hypotension, skin sensitivity reactions, mental depression, and disorders of the extrapyramidal motor system. Jaundice and blood dyscrasias have occurred less often with prochlorperazine, perphenazine, and fluphenazine than with other members of the group, but the extrapyramidal side effects have been relatively more pronounced. Several types of extrapyramidal symptoms have been noted:

1. A *parkinsonian syndrome*—masked facies, tremor, generalized rigidity, shuffling gait, and slowness of movement. These symptoms appear after several weeks of drug therapy.

2. Muscle spasms and dystonia, taking the form of involuntary movements of facial muscles and protrusion of the tongue (so-called *buccolingual or oral-masticatory syndrome*), dysphagia, torticollis and retrocollis, oculogyric crises, and tonic spasms of a limb (dyskinesias). These complications usually occur early in the course of administration of the drug, sometimes after the initial dose, and often can be improved dramatically by the intravenous administration of diphenhydramine hydrochloride (Benadryl).

3. An inability to sit still and an inner restlessness, such that the patient paces the floor constantly (akathisia).

4. Lingual-facial-buccal dyskinesia as well as choreoathetotic and dystonic movements of the trunk and limbs may occur as a late and persistent complication (*tardive dyskinesia*) of long-term therapy with phenothiazines or haloperidol.

Snyder has postulated that the movements are due to hypersensitivity of dopamine receptors in the basal ganglia, secondary to prolonged blockade of the receptors by antipsychotic medication. It is estimated that 40 percent of patients receiving long-term antipsychotic medication develop tardive dyskinesia (Baldessarini and Tarsy).

These extrapyramidal reactions must be recognized at once and the medication discontinued. The purely parkinsonian syndrome and dystonic spasms will usually improve, but the tardive dyskinesias may persist for weeks or months, and often permanently. Administration of antiparkinsonian drugs of the anticholinergic type (trihexyphenidyl, procyclidine, and benztropine) may hasten the recovery from some of the symptoms. Oral, lingual, and laryngeal dyskinesias are affected relatively little by any antiparkinsonian drugs. Amantadine (Symmetrel) in doses of 50 to 100 mg tid has been useful in some cases of postphenothiazine dyskinesia, and reserpine in others. Several other drugs, including deanol, baclofen, pyridoxine, choline and lecithin, have been used in the treatment of tardive dyskinesia with mixed results. No treatment is uniformly successful. Each of these drugs should be tried, since one sometimes has a better effect than another. The authors have noted a tendency for some of the most obstinate forms of tardive dyskinesia to slowly subside even after several years of unsuccessful therapy.

Butyrophenones These drugs (haloperidol, trifluperidol) have much the same antipsychotic effects as the phenothiazines, as well as the same side effects. Unlike the phenothiazines, they have little or no adrenergic blocking action. The butyrophenones are effective substitutes for the phenothiazines in patients who are intolerant of the latter drugs, particularly of their autonomic effects.

Reserpine This is the prototype of the *rauwolfia alkaloids*. It was in relation to the sedative effects of these drugs that the term *tranquilization* was used for the first time. These drugs, so effective in controlling hypertension and vasospasm, are no longer recommended for the treatment of mental disorders, except perhaps in patients who cannot tolerate phenothiazines. When given in therapeutic doses, the rauwolfia alkaloids often provoke a parkinsonian syndrome or a serious depression of mood, which may prove more troublesome than the disorder for which they were prescribed.

Meprobamate, chlordiazepoxide, and diazepam are often referred to as "minor tranquilizers," the implication being that these drugs share the antipsychotic properties of the phenothiazines. This is not the case. In fact, the minor tranquilizers resemble the barbiturates in their pharmacologic (depressant) effects, including the ability to produce tolerance and physical dependence, and are more appropriately referred to clinically as *antianxiety* drugs.

It hardly needs to be pointed out that the tranquilizing drugs have been much abused. This would be suspected just from the frequency with which they are being prescribed. It is stated that in the decade 1955 to 1965, 50 million patients in the United States received chlorpromazine alone. These powerful medications have specific indications, noted above, and the physician should be certain of the diagnosis before using them. The fact that these drugs can produce tardive dyskinesia in nonpsychotic patients is reason enough not to use them for nervousness, apprehension, anxiety, mild depression, and the many normal psychological reactions to trying environmental circumstances. These drugs are not curative, but only suppress or partially alleviate symptoms, and they should not serve as a substitute for, or divert the physician from, the use of other measures for the relief of the abnormal mental state.

ANTIDEPRESSANT DRUGS

Two classes of drugs—the monoamine oxidase (MAO) inhibitors and dibenzazepine derivatives—are particularly useful in the treatment of depression. The adjective *antidepressant*, to describe these drugs, refers to their therapeutic effect, and is used here in deference to common clinical practice. *Antidepressive* or *antidepression* drugs would be preferable, since the term *depressant* still has a pharmacologic connotation which does not necessarily equate with the therapeutic effect. For example, barbiturates and chloral hydrate are depressants in the pharmacologic sense and mood elevators or antidepressants in the clinical sense. These commonly used terms must not be confused—the one referring to a drug that reduces nervous system excitability and the other to the capacity of the drug to ameliorate the symptoms of mental depression.

Monoamine Oxidase Inhibitors The observation that iproniazid, an inhibitor of monoamine oxidase (MAO), had a mood-elevating effect in tuberculous patients initiated a great deal of interest in compounds of this type, and led quickly to their exploitation in the treatment of depression. Iproniazid (Marsilid) proved exceedingly toxic and was soon taken off the market, as were several subsequently developed MAO inhibitors; but other drugs, much better tolerated, have become available. These include isocarboxizid (Marplan), nialamide (Niamid), phenelzine (Nardil), and tranylcypromine (Parnate), the latter two being the most frequently used. Tranylcypromine, which bears a close chemical resemblance to dextroamphetamine, has proved to be the most potent therapeutically, but it has also produced the most serious toxic effects.

The exact mode of action of the MAO inhibitors has not been determined. They have in common the ability to block the oxidative deamination of naturally occurring amines (norepinephrine, epinephrine, and serotonin), and it has been suggested that the accumulation of these neurohormonal substances is responsible for the antidepressant effect. However, many enzymes other than monoamine oxidases are inhibited by MAO inhibitors, and the latter drugs have numerous actions unrelated to enzyme inhibition. Furthermore, many agents with antidepressant effects like those of the MAO inhibitors do not inhibit monoamine oxidase. At the present time, one cannot assume that the therapeutic effect of these drugs has a direct relation to the property of MAO inhibition.

The MAO inhibitors must be dispensed with great caution and a constant awareness of their potentially serious side effects. They may at times cause excitement, restlessness, agitation, insomnia, and anxiety; occasionally, with the usual dose and more often with an overdose, mania and convulsions may occur (especially in epileptic patients). Other side effects are muscle twitching and involuntary movement of an extremity, urinary retention, skin rashes, tachycardia, hepatic disturbance, jaundice, visual impairment, enhancement of glaucoma, impotence, sweating, muscle spasms, and a variety of paresthesias. Orthostatic hypotension of a serious degree may develop.

Patients taking MAO inhibitors must be warned against the use of dibenzazepine derivatives (see below) and also sympathomimetic amines and tyramine, for the combination of drugs may induce a severe hypertensive episode and cerebral vascular accident, headache, atrial and ventricular arrhythmia, pulmonary edema, and even death. Sympathomimetic amines are contained in some of the commonly used nasal sprays, nose drops, and in so-called coryza tablets and in tyramine-containing cheeses, yogurt, beer, and wine. The phenothiazines and central nervous system stimulants should not be given with the MAO inhibitors, since severe reactions and occasional fatalities have followed their concomitant use. Exaggerated responses to the usual dose of meperidine (Demerol) and other narcotic drugs have also been observed; respiratory function may be depressed to a serious degree, and hyperpyrexia, agitation, and pronounced hypotension may occur as well, sometimes with fatal issue. Unpredictable side effects may also accompany the simultaneous administration of barbiturates and MAO inhibitors.

Dibenzazepine Derivatives (Tricyclic Antidepressants) Soon after the first successes in the treatment of depression with MAO inhibitors, a new class of tricyclic compounds appeared. The first of this group was imipramine (Tofranil), which was soon followed by amitriptyline (Elavil), and then by desipramine (Norpramin) and nortriptyline (Aventyl). The first two members of this group have proved to be the most popular. Another important dibenzazepine derivative is carbamazepine (Tegretol) which is widely used in the treatment of lancinating pains (page 129) and seizures (page 228).

The exact mode of action of these agents is unknown, but there is evidence that they block the reuptake of amine neurotransmitters released into the synaptic cleft. Blocking this amine pump mechanism (which ordinarily terminates synaptic transmission) permits the persistence of neurotransmitter substances in the synaptic cleft; this mechanism provides support for the hypothesis that endogenous depression is due to a deficiency of noradrenergic or serotonergic transmission.

The so-called tricyclic antidepressants are presently the most effective drugs for the treatment of patients with depressive illnesses, particularly those with retarded depressions, associated with hyposomnia, early morning awakening, and decreased appetite and libido. After the drug is stopped, the pharmacologic effects persist for a very short time in comparison with the MAO inhibitors, and their side effects are far less frequent and serious.

The tricyclic or dibenzazepine compounds are potent anticholinergic agents and their most prominent and serious side effects (orthostatic hypotension, urinary bladder weakness) are due to peripheral anticholinergic action. They may also produce central nervous system excitement, leading to insomnia, agitation, and restlessness, but usually these effects are controlled readily by the use of phenothiazines or chlordiazepoxide given concurrently or in the evenings. Occasionally they may cause ataxia and blood dyscrasias. The dibenzazepine drugs should never be given with an MAO inhibitor, as indicated above; serious reactions have allegedly occurred when small doses of imipramine were given to patients who had discontinued the MAO inhibitor one week previously.

STIMULANTS

Drugs which act primarily as stimulants of the central nervous system have a relatively limited therapeutic use but assume clinical importance for other reasons. Some of its members, e.g. the amphetamines, are much abused, and others are not infrequent causes of poisoning.

Amphetamine (Benzedrine) This drug and its *d* isomer, dextroamphetamine, are powerful analeptics and in addition have significant hypertensive, respiratory-stimulant, and appetite-depressant effects. They are useful in the management of narcolepsy, but have been much more widely and indiscriminately used for the control of obesity and the abolition of fatigue. Undoubtedly, they are able to reverse fatigue, postpone the need for sleep, and elevate mood, but these effects are not entirely predictable and certainly not indefinite, and the user must pay for the period of wakefulness with even greater fatigue and often with depression. The intravenous use of a high dose of amphetamine produces an immediate ecstasy, "the flash."

Because of the popularity of the amphetamines and ease with which they can be procured, instances of acute and chronic intoxication are observed frequently. The toxic signs are essentially an exaggeration of the analeptic effects—restlessness, excessive speech and motor activity, tremor, and insomnia. In severe cases, hallucinations, delusions, and changes in affect and thought processes may occur, a state that may be indistinguishable from paranoid schizophrenia. Treatment consists of removal of the amphetamine and the administration of antipsychotic drugs. Nitrites may be useful if the blood pressure is markedly elevated.

Methylphenidate (Ritalin) This drug has much the same type of action as dextroamphetamine and is useful in the treatment of narcolepsy. Paradoxically, like amphetamine, it is useful in the management of overactive children.

Picrotoxin This is a powerful nervous system excitant, the main effects of which are to produce convulsive seizures and to reverse respiratory depression induced by drugs, particularly by barbiturates. It has been shown by Eccles and his colleagues that picrotoxin increases neuronal activity by blocking presynaptic inhibition, i.e., blocking the action of inhibitory fibers that synapse with the presynaptic terminals of excitatory fibers. However, the modern treatment of barbiturate intoxication does not include the use of picrotoxin or other analeptics, because of their epileptogenic properties and because barbiturate intoxication can be managed successfully by other means (see preceding section).

Strychnine The action of this drug is to increase neuronal excitability by interfering with postsynaptic inhibition. The therapeutic value of strychnine is negligible, but in children accidental poisoning may occur from ingestion of A.S.&B. cathartic pills or "rat biscuits." Rarely, strychnine is taken with suicidal intent. After a period of heightened irritability and muscle twitching, tonic seizures occur, characterized by opisthotonus, rigid extension of the legs, facial tetanus, and apnea due to spasm of the muscles of respiration. Death from anoxia may follow several seizures.

The immediate need, in the treatment of strychnine poisoning, is to control the convulsions. This calls for the intravenous administration of a short-acting barbiturate or the use of inhalation anesthesia if the appropriate drug is not immediately available; endotracheal intubation is an important safeguard. The patient must then be observed carefully, and if any signs of irritability recur, more sedative should be given. During this period, supportive care is indicated, as for any comatose patient. Morphine, which is principally a medullary depressant, is contraindicated.

Pentylenetetrazol (Metrazol, Cardiazol) This drug is a potent stimulant of all parts of the nervous system. For a number of years it served as the convulsive agent in "shock treatment" of depression and schizophrenia but was abandoned in favor of less dangerous and more effective forms of convulsive therapy. The use of this drug to activate latent epileptogenic foci or to reproduce convulsions, with the purpose of studying the underlying cerebral mechanisms, has been discontinued.

Bemegride and Nikethamide (Coramine) The actions of these two agents are much like those of pentylenetetrazol. For many years it was common clinical practice to administer nikethamide as a final therapeutic gesture in patients dying of cardiac and respiratory failure, but there is little evidence that it has a significant stimulant effect on either heart or respiration. Poisoning with these drugs, which is usually due to parenteral overdosage, is best treated with barbiturates.

Caffeine The therapeutic value of caffeine and other xanthine derivatives stems from their diuretic effect and their ability to stimulate the heart and nervous system. The major use of these agents is to abolish fatigue and maintain wakefulness, and the usual mode of administration is in coffee, a cup of which contains 100 to 150 mg caffeine. Overdosage leads to insomnia, mild delirium, tinnitus, tachycardia, prominent diuresis, and cardiac arrhythmias. The excitatory effects are easily controlled with barbiturates, and fatalities due to caffeine poisoning are extremely rare.

Camphor (Camphorated Oil) Formerly a popular stimulant, camphor is now rarely used therapeutically; however, occasional cases of poisoning are still seen as a result of ingestion of liniment or moth flakes. The manifestations of poisoning are headache, sensation of warmth, confusion, clonic convulsions, and terminal respiratory depression; the characteristic odor of camphor facilitates the diagnosis. Treatment consists of supportive care and the cautious use of barbiturates to control convulsions.

PSYCHOTOGENIC DRUGS

Included in this category is a heterogeneous group of drugs, the primary effect of which is to alter perception, mood, and thinking out of proportion to other aspects of cognitive function and consciousness. This group of drugs comprises *lysergic acid derivatives*—e.g., lysergic acid diethylamide (LSD), *phenylethylamine derivatives* (mescaline or peyote), *psilocybin*, certain *indolic derivatives, cannabis* (marijuana), *phencyclidine* (PCP) and a number of less important compounds. They are also referred to as psychotomimetic drugs, hallucinogens, illusogins, and psychedelics—but none of these names is entirely suitable.

Tolerance to LSD, mescaline, and psilocybin develops rapidly, even on a once-daily dosage. Furthermore, subjects tolerant to any one of these three drugs are cross-tolerant to the other two. Tolerance is lost rapidly when the drugs are discontinued abruptly, but no abstinence syndromes ensue. In this sense, addiction does not develop, although users may become dependent upon them for emotional support. In the case of marijuana, *reverse tolerance* (i.e., increasing sensitization) may be observed initially, but on continued use, tolerance to the *euphoriant* effects of the drug has been observed in one of the few chronic experimental studies that have been made, and the subjects reported "jitteriness" during the first 24 h after abrupt cessation of marijuana cigarette smoking, although no objective withdrawal signs could be detected.

Mescaline, LSD, and psilocybin produce much the same clinical effects if given in comparable amounts. The perceptual changes are the most dramatic: the user describes vivid visual hallucinations, alterations in the shape and color of objects, unusual dreams, and feelings of depersonalization. An increase in auditory acuity has been described, but auditory hallucinations are rare. Cognitive functions are difficult to assess because of inattention, drowsiness, and inability to cooperate in mental testing. The somatic symptoms consist of dizziness, nausea, paresthesias, and blurring of vision. Sympathomimetic effects—pupillary dilation, piloerection, hyperthermia, and tachycardia—are prominent, and the user may also show hyperreflexia, incoordination of the limbs, and ataxia.

The effects of *marijuana*, when taken by inhaling the smoke from cigarettes, are prompt in onset and evanescent. In low doses the symptoms are like those of mild intoxication with alcohol. With increasing amounts, the effects are similar to those of LSD, mescaline, and psilocybin, and they may be quite disabling for many hours. Very large doses result in severe depression and stupor, but death is unusual.

During the past decade the abuse of phencyclidine (PCP, "angel dust") or its many analogues has become a significant problem, since these drugs are relatively cheap, easily available, and quite powerful. PCP is used legally as an animal immobilizing agent and illicitly as a granular powder, frequently mixed with other drugs, that is smoked or snorted. PCP is usually classified as a hallucinogen, although it also has stimulant and depressant properties. The effects of intoxication are like those of LSD and other hallucinogens and resemble those of an acute schizophrenic episode which may last several days to a week or more. PCP will be present in the blood and urine after ingestion of a large amount (10 mg or more).

The fact that small quantities of these drugs can produce gross mental aberrations has stimulated the search for similar endogenous substances that may be responsible for schizophrenia and other psychoses. The

mechanisms involved in producing and antagonizing the *psychotomimetic* effects are also being studied intensively, in the hope of elucidating the mechanisms of the psychoses and finding improved psychotherapeutic agents. Numerous claims have been made that LSD and related drugs are effective in the treatment of mental disease and a wide variety of social ills and that they have the capacity to increase one's intellectual performance, creativity, and self-understanding. At this time, there are no acceptable studies that validate any of these claims.

LSD is not yet an approved drug, and the use of marijuana is governed by the federal narcotic laws. Nevertheless, these drugs are very widely used. They are taken by narcotic addicts as a temporary substitute for more potent drugs; by "drug heads," i.e., individuals who use practically any agent that alters consciousness; and by many troubled, unhappy college and high school students, often for reasons that they cannot ascertain. The unsupervised use of these drugs is attended by a number of serious adverse reactions taking the form of acute panic attacks; long-lasting psychotic states resembling paranoid schizophrenia; *flashbacks* (spontaneous recurrences of the original LSD experience, often precipitated by smoking marijuana and accompanied by panic attacks); or by serious physical injury, consequent upon impairment of the user's critical faculties. Whether prolonged usage leads to permanent damage to the nervous system is not certain; there are some data suggesting that this may happen. The reports claiming that LSD may cause chromosomal damage remain to be validated. A discussion of the legal implications of the illicit use of these drugs and their social impact is beyond the scope of this chapter, but can be found in the appended references.

DISORDERS DUE TO BACTERIAL TOXINS

The most important diseases in this category are tetanus, botulism, and diphtheria. Each is caused by an extraordinarily powerful bacterial toxin which acts primarily upon the nervous system. Other bacterial toxins, e.g., ammonium and other amines which are produced in the colon by the action of urease-splitting organisms and which are thought to be responsible for hepatic encephalopathy, are more appropriately considered with the metabolic disorders.

TETANUS

The cause of this disease is the anaerobic, spore-forming rod, *Clostridium tetani*. The organisms are found in the feces of some humans and many animals, particularly horses, whence they readily contaminate the soil. The spores may remain dormant for many months or years, but when they are introduced into a wound, especially if a foreign body or suppurative bacteria are present, they are converted into their vegetative forms, which produce the exotoxin *tetanospasmin*. In underdeveloped countries, tetanus is still a common disease, particularly in newborns in whom the spores are introduced via the umbilical cord (tetanus neonatorum). In the United States, injection of contaminated heroin is a significant cause of tetanus. About two-thirds of all injuries leading to tetanus occur in the home and about 20 percent in gardens and on farms. In the United States, the incidence of tetanus is about one case per million per year.

Since 1903, when Morax and Marie proposed their theory of centripetal migration of the tetanus toxin, it has been taught that spread to the nervous system occurs via the peripheral nerves, the toxin ascending in the axis cylinders or the perineural sheaths. Modern studies, utilizing fluorescein-labeled tetanus antitoxin, have disclosed that the toxin is widely disseminated via the blood or lymphatics, a mode of spread that probably accounts for the generalized form of the disease. However, in local tetanus direct neuronal invasion seems probable.

The mode of action of tetanus toxin is not fully understood, but is analogous to that of strychnine, interfering with the function of the reflex arc by suppressing spinal and brainstem inhibitory neurons. In tetanus, the elicitation of the jaw jerk, for example, is not followed by the usual abrupt suppression of motor neuron activity which is manifested in the electromyogram as a "silent period." There appears to be a failure of this normal inhibitory mechanism, with a resulting increase in activation of the neurons which innervate the masseter muscles (*trismus*). Of all neuromuscular systems the masseter innervation seems to be the most sensitive to the toxin. Afferent stimuli not only produce an exaggerated effect but also reciprocal innervation is abolished and both agonists and antagonists contract, giving rise to the characteristic muscular spasm. In addition to its generalized effects on the motor neurons of the spinal cord and brainstem, there is evidence that the toxin acts directly on skeletal muscle at the point of injection or entrance

into the organism, accounting perhaps for the localization of signs of tetanus intoxication. The toxin is also thought to act at the cerebral cortical level and upon the sympathetic nervous system, in the hypothalamus.

The incubation period varies greatly, from a day or two to a month or even longer. Long incubation periods are associated with mild and localized types of tetanus.

Clinical Features There are several clinical types of tetanus, generally designated as local, cephalic, and generalized.

Local tetanus This is the most benign form. The initial symptoms are stiffness, tightness, and pain in the muscles in the neighborhood of a wound, followed by twitchings and brief spasms of the affected muscles. Local tetanus occurs most often in relation to a wound of the hand or forearm, or in the abdominal or paravertebral muscles after an operation. Gradually, some degree of continuous involuntary spasm becomes evident. This is referred to as *rigidity, hypertonic contractions,* or *tetanic spasticity,* terms which denote the tautness of the affected muscles and the resistance to passive movement. Superimposed on this background of more or less continuous motor activity are brief intense spasms, lasting from a few seconds to minutes, and occurring in response to all variety of stimulation or "spontaneously." Early in the course of the illness there may be periods when the affected muscles are palpably soft and appear to be relaxed. A useful diagnostic maneuver at this stage is to have the patient perform some repetitive voluntary movements, such as opening and closing the hand, in response to which there occurs a gradual increase in the tonic contraction and spasms of the affected muscles, followed by spread of the spasms to neighboring muscle groups (*recruitment spasm*). Even with mild localized tetanus there may be a slight trismus, a useful diagnostic sign.

Symptoms may persist in localized form for several weeks or months. Gradually the spasms become less frequent and more difficult to evoke, and they finally disappear without residue. Complete recovery is to be expected, since there are no pathologic changes in muscles, nerves, spinal cord, or brain, even in the most severe generalized forms of tetanus.

So-called *cephalic tetanus* follows wounds of the face and head. The incubation period is short, 1 or 2 days as a rule. This form of tetanus differs from the others in that the affected muscles (most often the ocular and facial) are weak or paralyzed. Nevertheless, during accessions of tetanic spasm, the palsied muscles are seen to contract. Apparently the disturbance in the facial motoneurons is sufficient to prevent voluntary movement but insufficient to prevent the strong reflex impulses of facial spasm. Spasms may involve the tongue and throat, with persistent dysarthria, dysphonia, and dysphagia. In a strict sense these cephalic forms of tetanus are examples of local tetanus that frequently become generalized. Many cases prove fatal.

Generalized tetanus This is the most common form of tetanus. It may begin as local tetanus which after a few days becomes generalized, or it may be diffuse from the beginning. Trismus is frequently the first manifestation. In some cases this is preceded by a feeling of stiffness in the jaw or neck, slight fever, and other general symptoms of infection. The localized muscle stiffness and spasms spread quickly to involve other bulbar musculature, as well as muscles of the neck, trunk, and limbs. A state of unremitting rigidity develops in all the involved muscles: the abdomen is boardlike, the legs are rigidly extended, the lips are pursed or retracted (risus sardonicus), and the eyes are partially closed through contraction of the orbicularis oculi or the eyebrows are elevated by spasm of the frontalis. Superimposed on this persistent state of enhanced muscle activity are paroxysms of tonic contraction or spasm of muscles (tetanic seizures or convulsions), which occur spontaneously or in response to the slightest external stimulus. They are agonizingly painful. Consciousness is not lost during these paroxysms. The tonic contraction of groups of muscles results in opisthotonus or in forward arching of the back, flexion and adduction of the arms, clenching of the fists, and extension of the legs. Spasms of the glottal, laryngeal, or respiratory muscles carry the constant threat of apnea or suffocation. Fever and pneumonia are common complications. Death is usually attributable to asphyxia or to heart failure, the result of constantly recurring spasms, or to circulatory collapse, the result of action of the toxin on the sympathetic nervous system.

The *diagnosis* of tetanus is made from these clinical features and a history of preceding injury. The latter is sometimes disclosed only after careful questioning, the injury having been trivial and forgotten. The organisms may or may not be recovered from the wound by the time the patient is seen by the physician, and other laboratory tests are of little value. Tetany, the seizures of strychnine poisoning (identical to tetanic spasms), trismus due to painful conditions in and around the jaw, the dysphagia of rabies, black widow spider bites, hysterical spasms, and extrapyramidal rigidity and dystonia should not be difficult to distinguish from tetanus, when all aspects of these disorders are considered.

The death rate from tetanus is about 50 percent overall; it is highest in newborns, heroin addicts, and in patients with the cephalic form of the disease. The patient usually recovers if there are no severe convulsions during the course of the illness or if the muscle spasms remain localized.

Treatment This needs to be directed along several lines. At the outset, a single dose of antitoxin (3000 to 6000 units of tetanus-immune human globulin) should be given, and a 10-day course of penicillin (1.2 million units of procaine penicillin daily) or tetracycline (2 g daily) is begun. Both of these drugs are effective against the vegetative forms of *C. tetani.* Immediate surgical treatment of the wound (excision or debridement) is imperative, and the tissue around the wound should be infiltrated with antitoxin.

Tracheostomy is a requisite in all patients with recurrent tonic convulsions, and should not be delayed until apnea or cyanosis has occurred. The patient must be kept as quiet as possible. This requires a darkened, isolated room, the judicious use of sedation, and expert and constant nursing care. Short-acting barbiturates (secobarbital or pentobarbital) in combination with chlorpromazine are the most useful drugs. Paraldehyde is an excellent medication, if it can be taken by mouth. The aim of drug therapy is to suppress muscle spasms and to keep the patient drowsy but rousable. All treatments and manipulations should be kept to a minimum; they should be carefully planned and coordinated, and the patient should be sedated beforehand.

Failure of these measures to control the tetanic paroxysms demands that all muscle activity be abolished by the use of *d*-tubocurarine, given intramuscularly in doses of 15 mg hourly, for as long as necessary, breathing being maintained entirely by a positive-pressure respirator.

From all that has been said, the importance of prevention of tetanus is evident. All persons should be immunized and receive a booster dose of toxoid every 10 years. Injuries that carry a threat of tetanus should be treated by an injection of toxoid if the patient has not received a booster injection in the preceding year, and a second dose of toxoid should be given 6 weeks later. If the injured person has not received a booster injection since the original immunization, he or she should receive an injection of both toxoid and human antitoxin; the same applies to the injured person who has never been immunized. An attack of tetanus does not confer permanent immunity and all persons who recover should be actively immunized.

DIPHTHERIA

Diphtheria, an acute infectious disease caused by the *Corynebacterium diphtheriae,* is now quite rare in the United States and western Europe. The faucial form of the disease, which is the most common clinical type, is characterized by the formation of an inflammatory exudate of the throat and trachea, and from this site the bacteria elaborate an exotoxin, which affects the heart and nervous system in about 20 percent of cases.

The involvement of the nervous system follows a predictable pattern. It begins locally, with *palatal paralysis* (nasal voice, regurgitation, and dysphagia) between the fifth and twelfth days of illness. At this time, or shortly afterward, other cranial nerves (trigeminal, facial, vagus, and hypoglossal) may also be affected. *Ciliary paralysis* with loss of accommodation and blurring of vision appear usually in the second or third week. Very rarely the extraocular muscles are involved. The cranial nerve signs may clear without further involvement of the nervous system, or a sensorimotor polyneuropathy may develop between the fifth and eighth weeks of the disease. The latter varies in severity, from a mild, predominantly distal affection of the limbs to a rapidly evolving, ascending paralysis of the Landry-Guillain-Barré type. The neuropathic symptoms progress for a week or two, and if the patient does not succumb to respiratory paralysis or cardiac failure (cardiomyopathy) they stabilize and then improve slowly and completely.

The early bulbar symptoms, the unique ciliary paralysis, and the subacute evolution of a delayed symmetrical sensorimotor peripheral neuropathy distinguish diphtheritic from all other forms of polyneuropathy. The long latency between the initial infection and the involvement of the nervous system has no clear explanation.

The source of diphtheritic infection may be extrafaucial—a penetrating wound, skin ulcer, or umbilicus. All the systemic and neurologic complications of faucial diphtheria may be observed in the extrafaucial form of the disease, after a similar latent period. It is probable, therefore, that the toxin reaches its neural site via the bloodstream; but in addition some action is exerted locally as evidenced by palatal paralysis in faucial cases and by initial weakness and sensory impairment in the neighborhood of the infected wound.

There is no specific treatment for any of the neurologic complications of diphtheria. It is generally agreed that the administration of antitoxin within 48 h of the earliest symptoms of the primary diphtheritic infection lessens the incidence and severity of complications.

The polyneuropathy of diphtheria is discussed further in Chap. 45.

BOTULISM

Botulism is a rare form of food-borne illness, caused by the exotoxin of *Clostridium botulinum.* Outbreaks of poisoning are more often due to home-preserved than to commercially canned products, and vegetables are incriminated more commonly than any other food product. Until 1950, the death-to-case ratio was consistently above 60 percent, but it has declined since then, due probably to improvements in the intensive care of acute respiratory failure and the effectiveness of *C. botulinum* antitoxins. Although the disease is ubiquitous, five western states (California, Washington, Colorado, New Mexico, and Oregon) account for more than half of all reported outbreaks in the United States.

It is now well established, on the basis of observations both in animals and in man, that the primary site of action of botulinus toxin is at the neuromuscular junction, more specifically on the presynaptic endings. The toxin interferes with the release of acetylcholine quanta, by a mechanism that is not fully understood. The defect is similar to that which characterizes the myasthenic syndrome associated with small-cell bronchogenic carcinoma (Eaton-Lambert syndrome) but different from that of myasthenia gravis.

Symptoms usually appear within 12 to 36 h of ingestion of the tainted food. Anorexia, nausea, and vomiting occur in some patients, not in others. As a rule, blurred vision and diplopia are the initial neural symptoms; their association with ptosis, strabismus, and extraocular muscle palsies may suggest a diagnosis of myasthenia gravis early in the illness. In many cases of botulism, however, the pupils are dilated and unreactive. Other symptoms of bulbar involvement—vertigo, deafness, nasality of the voice and hoarseness, dysarthria, and dysphagia—follow in quick succession, and these in turn are followed by progressive weakness of muscles of the neck, trunk, and limbs. Tendon reflexes are lost in cases of severe weakness. These symptoms and signs evolve rapidly, over 2 to 4 days as a rule, and may be mistaken for those of polyneuritis of the Guillain-Barré type. Sensation remains intact, however, and the spinal fluid shows no abnormalities. Severe constipation is characteristic of botulism, due perhaps to paresis of smooth muscles of the intestine. Consciousness is retained throughout the illness, unless severe degrees of anoxia develop. Almost half the patients succumb, usually as a result of paralysis of the muscles of respiration.

The clinical diagnosis can be confirmed by electrophysiological studies. Improvement, in patients who recover, begins within a few weeks, first in ocular movement, then in other cranial nerve function. Complete recovery of paralyzed limb and trunk musculature may take many months. Outbreaks of a neonatal and infantile form of the disease have been reported recently.

The three types of botulinus toxin, A, B, and E, cannot be distinguished by their clinical effects alone, so that the patient should receive the trivalent antiserum as soon as the clinical diagnosis is made. This antitoxin can be obtained from the National Center for Disease Control, in Atlanta. An initial dose of 10,000 units is given intravenously after intradermal testing for sensitivity to horse serum, followed by daily doses of 50,000 units intramuscularly, until improvement begins.

Guanidine hydrochloride (50 mg/kg) has reportedly been useful in reversing the weakness of limb and extraocular muscles. Actually, antitoxin and guanidine change the course of the illness relatively little: recovery, in the final analysis, depends upon the effectiveness of respiratory care, maintenance of fluid and electrolyte balance, prevention of infection, etc.

POISONING DUE TO PLANTS, VENOMS, BITES, AND STINGS

ERGOTISM

Ergotism is the name applied to poisoning with ergot, a drug derived from the rye fungus, *Claviceps purpurea*. Ergot is used therapeutically to control postpartum hemorrhage due to uterine atony; one of its alkaloids, ergotamine, is the drug of choice in the treatment of migraine. Chronic overdosage of the drug is the usual cause of ergotism; in the past, ingestion of bread made from contaminated flour was a common source of chronic poisoning. Acute overdosage in the postpartum state may cause an alarming rise in blood pressure.

Two types of ergotism are recognized: the *gangrenous*, due to a vasospastic, occlusive process in the small arterioles of the extremities, and *convulsive*, or *neurogenic*. The latter is characterized by fasciculations, myoclonus, and spasms of muscles, followed by seizures. In nonfatal cases, a tabeslike neurologic syndrome may develop, with loss of knee and ankle jerks, ataxia, and loss of deep and superficial sensation. The pathologic changes are said to consist of degeneration of the posterior columns, the dorsal roots, and peripheral nerves, but they are poorly described. The relation of these changes

to ergot poisoning is also not clear, since most of the cases have occurred in areas in which malnutrition was endemic.

LATHYRISM

Lathyrism is a neurologic syndrome characterized by the relatively acute onset of pain, paresthesias, and weakness in the lower extremities, progressing to a permanent spastic paraplegia. The pathologic changes, in keeping with the clinical picture, consist of degeneration of the anterior and lateral columns of the thoracic and lumbar segments of the spinal cord.

Lathyrism is a serious medical problem only in India and in some North African countries, where food is scarce and famine commonplace. The etiologic factors have not been positively identified. Generally the malady has been ascribed to consumption of different varieties of the chickpea, *Lathyrus*; but toxins derived from *Vicia sativa*, the common vetch (which often grows alongside the lathyrus species), and malnutrition may also play a part.

MUSHROOM POISONING

Two species of mushroom—*Amanita muscaria* and particularly *Amanita phalloides*—account for most cases of poisoning. *Amanita muscaria* contains the parasympathomimetic alkaloid muscarine, and the symptoms of poisoning, which appear within minutes or an hour or two, are essentially those of parasympathetic stimulation—miosis, lacrimation, salivation, nausea, vomiting, diarrhea, perspiration, bradycardia, and hypotension. Tremor, seizures, and delirium occur in cases of severe poisoning. Treatment consists of the administration of 1 to 2 mg atropine intramuscularly, repeated every 30 min for as long as necessary.

Poisoning with *A. phalloides* is far more serious. This mushroom contains α-amantin, a cytotoxin that binds rapidly to and destroys the cells of the kidneys, liver, striated muscle, and brain. Symptoms appear 6 to 20 h after ingestion and consist of severe nausea, vomiting, and diarrhea, followed by confusion, seizures, coma, and cardiovascular collapse (fatal in 4 to 8 days in about half the cases). Some cases have responded to early intensive hemoperfusion.

VENOMS, BITES, AND STINGS

These are relatively rare but nonetheless important causes of mortality in the Untied States. The venoms of certain species of snakes, lizards, spiders, and scorpions contain neurotoxins which may cause a fatal depression of respiration and curare-like failure of neuromuscular transmission. Ticks, while engorging, may inject a neurotoxin that has similar effects. The serious effects of *Hymenoptera* stings (bees, wasps, hornets, and fire ants) are due mainly to hypersensitivity and anaphylaxis. These are discussed in detail in *Harrison's Principles of Internal Medicine.*

HEAVY METALS

LEAD

Lead Poisoning in Children The causes and clinical manifestations of lead poisoning are quite different in children and adults.

In the United States, the disease occurs most often in 1- to 5-year-old children who inhabit the slum areas of large cities, where old, deteriorated housing prevails. The chewing of leaded paint, the most common sources of which are window sills and painted plaster walls, and the compulsive ingestion of these nonfood items (pica) are the important factors in the causation of lead poisoning. The development of an acute encephalopathy is the most serious complication, leading to death in 5 to 20 percent of cases and to neurologic and mental disturbances in over 25 percent of survivors.

The *clinical manifestations* of lead poisoning develop over a period of 3 to 6 weeks. The child becomes anorectic, less playful and alert, and more irritable. These symptoms may be misinterpreted as a behavior disorder or mental retardation. Intermittent vomiting, vague abdominal pain, clumsiness, and ataxia may be added. If these early signs of intoxication are not recognized and the child continues to ingest lead, more flagrant signs of acute encephalopathy may develop—most frequently in the summer months, for reasons that are not understood. The latter develop in a period of a week or less. Vomiting becomes more persistent, apathy progresses to drowsiness and stupor, interspersed with periods of hyperirritability, and finally coma and seizures supervene. This syndrome evolves most rapidly in children under 2 years of age; in older children, recurrent and less severe episodes are more likely to occur. This clinical syndrome must be distinguished from tuberculous meningitis, viral meningoencephalitis, and other causes of acute increased intracranial pressure. It follows

that lumbar puncture should be done only if necessary for diagnosis and with the utmost caution. Usually, in lead encephalopathy, there is an increase of lymphocytes and protein in the CSF but glucose values are normal.

The brains of children who die of acute lead encephalopathy show massive swelling and herniation of the temporal lobes and cerebellum, multiple ischemic foci in cerebrum and cerebellum, and deposition of proteinaceous material and mononuclear inflammatory cells around many small blood vessels.

Since the symptoms of plumbism are nonspecific, the diagnosis depends upon an appreciation of the causative factors, a high index of suspicion, and certain laboratory tests. The presence of *lead lines* at the metaphyses of long bones and basophilic stippling of red cells are too inconstant to be relied upon, but basophilic stippling of bone marrow normoblasts is uniformly increased. Impairment of heme synthesis, which is exquisitely sensitive to the toxic effects of lead, results in the increased excretion of urinary coproporphyrin (UCP) and of δ-aminolevulinic acid (ALA). These urinary indexes and the blood lead levels bear only an imperfect relationship to the clinical manifestations. In the test for UCP, which is readily performed in the clinic and emergency room, a few milliliters of urine are acidified with acetic acid and shaken with an equal volume of ether. If coproporphyrin is present, the ether layer will reveal a reddish fluorescence under a Wood's lamp. This test is strongly positive when the whole blood concentration of lead exceeds 80 mg per 100 ml. The diagnosis can be confirmed by promoting the lead excretion with calcium disodium edetate (CaNa$_2$ EDTA) three doses (25 mg/kg) at 8-h intervals. Excretion of over 500 μg in 24 h is indicative of plumbism. At a blood lead level of 80 mg per 100 ml, symptoms may be minimal, but acute encephalopathy may occur abruptly and unpredictably, and the child should be hospitalized for chelation therapy. Some children with a blood lead level of 50 mg per 100 ml may have symptoms of severe encephalopathy, whereas others may be asymptomatic. In the latter case, an attempt should be made to discover and remove the source of lead intoxication and the child should be reexamined at frequent intervals. The seriousness of lead encephalopathy in children is indicated by the fact that of those who become stuporous or comatose most remain mentally retarded despite treatment. The physician's aim, therefore, is to institute treatment before the severe symptoms of encephalopathy have become manifest.

The plan of therapy includes the following:

1. Establishment of urinary flow, following which intravenous fluid therapy is restricted to basal water and electrolyte requirements.

2. Combined chelation therapy with 2,3-dimer-captopropanol (BAL) and CaNa$_2$ EDTA for 5 to 7 days in cases of acute encephalopathy. This is followed by a course of oral penicillamine. It should be emphasized that once the absorption of lead has stopped, chelating agents remove lead only from soft tissues and not from bone, where most of the lead is stored. Any intercurrent illness which causes demineralization can cause a mobilization of lead into the soft tissues and an exacerbation of symptoms of lead intoxication.

3. Repeated doses of mannitol for relief of cerebral edema.

4. Microcytic hypochromic anemia is treated with iron, once the chelating agents have been discontinued.

5. Seizures are best controlled with intravenous diazepam.

The prevention of reintoxication demands that the child be removed from the source of lead. While this is axiomatic, it is very difficult to accomplish, despite the best efforts of local health departments and hospital and city social workers. Nevertheless, an attempt to correct the environmental factor must be made in each case.

Lead Intoxication in Adults   This is much less common than in children. The hazards to adults are exposure to dust of inorganic lead salts and to fumes resulting from the burning of lead or processes that require the remelting of lead. Painting, printing, pottery glazing, lead smelting, and storage battery manufacturing are the industries in which these hazards are likeliest to occur. Intoxication with tetraethyl and tetramethyl lead, used as additives in gasoline, presents a special problem; the hematologic abnormalities of inorganic lead poisoning are not found and chelating agents are of no value in treatment. This form of lead intoxication is fatal in 20 percent of cases.

The usual manifestations of lead poisoning in adults are colic, anemia, and peripheral neuropathy. Encephalopathy is decidedly rare; usually it results from consumption of illicit liquor contaminated by lead solder in the pipes of stills. Lead colic, frequently precipitated by an intercurrent infection or by alcohol intoxication, is characterized by severe, poorly localized abdominal pain, often with rigidity of abdominal muscles. There is no fever or leukocytosis. The pain responds to the intravenous injection of calcium salts, at least temporarily, but very little to morphine. Mild anemia is common. A black line of lead sulfide may develop along the gingival margins. Peripheral neuropathy is a rare manifestation and is discussed in Chap. 45.

The diagnostic tests for plumbism in children are

generally applicable to adults, with the exception of bone films, which are of no value in adults. The CaNa$_2$ EDTA-mobilization test is of value in difficult diagnostic cases. The treatment of adults with chelating agents follows the same principles as in children.

ARSENIC

In the past, medications such as Fowler's solution (potassium arsenite) and the arsphenamines, used in the treatment of syphilis, were frequent causes of intoxication, but now it is most commonly the result of the suicidal or accidental ingestion of insecticides or rodenticides containing copper acetoarsenate (Paris green) or calcium or lead arsenate. In rural areas, arsenic-containing insecticide sprays are a common source of poisoning. Arsenic is used also in the manufacture of paints, enamels, and metals, and as a disinfectant for skins and furs. Occasional cases of poisoning are reported in relation to these occupational hazards.

Arsenic exerts its toxic effects by reacting with the sulfhydryl radicals of certain enzymes necessary for cellular metabolism. The effects on the nervous system are those of an encephalopathy or peripheral neuropathy. The latter may be the product of chronic poisoning, or may become manifest between 1 and 2 weeks after recovery from the acute effects. It is described in Chap. 45.

The symptoms of encephalopathy (headache, drowsiness, mental confusion, delirium, and convulsive seizures) may also occur as part of acute or chronic intoxication. In the latter case, they are accompanied by weakness and muscular aching, hemolysis, chills and fever (in patients exposed to arsine gas), mucosal irritation, a diffuse scaly desquamation, and transverse white (Mees) lines 1 to 2 mm in width, above the lunula of each fingernail. Acute poisoning by the oral route is associated with severe gastrointestinal symptoms, with circulatory collapse and death in a large proportion of patients. The CSF is normal. Examination of the brain in such cases discloses numerous punctate hemorrhages in the white matter. Microscopically the lesions consist of pericapillary zones of degeneration, which in turn are ringed by red cells (*brain purpura* or *encephalorrhagia*, incorrectly referred to as *hemorrhagic encephalitis*). These neuropathologic changes are not specific for arsenical poisoning, but have been observed in such diverse conditions as pneumonia, gram-negative bacillary septicemia from urinary tract infections, sulfonamide and phosgene poisoning, dysentery, and others.

The diagnosis of arsenical poisoning depends upon the demonstration of increased levels of arsenic in the hair and urine. Arsenic is deposited in the hair within two weeks of exposure and may remain fixed there for years. Concentrations of more than 0.1 mg arsenic per 100 mg hair are indicative of poisoning. Arsenic also remains within bones for long periods and is slowly excreted in the urine and feces. Excretion of more than 0.1 mg arsenic per liter of urine is considered abnormal; levels greater than 1 mg/liter may occur soon after acute exposure. The CSF protein level may be raised (50 to 100 mg per 100 ml).

Acute poisoning is treated by gastric lavage, fluid replacement, vasopressor agents, and BAL. Once polyneuropathy has occurred, it is little affected by treatment with BAL, but other manifestations of chronic arsenical poisoning respond favorably. There is gradual recovery from the polyneuropathy.

MANGANESE

Manganese poisoning results from the chronic inhalation and ingestion of manganese particles and occurs in miners of manganese ore and among workers who separate manganese from other ore. Several clinical syndromes have been observed. The initial stages of intoxication may be marked by a prolonged confusional-hallucinatory state. Later, the symptoms are predominantly of extrapyramidal type, resembling those of postencephalitic parkinsonism: impassive facies; drooling; faint, monotonous, dysarthric speech; stiffness and awkwardness of the limbs, often with tremor of the hands; "cogwheel" phenomenon and gross rhythmic movements of the trunk and head; and retropulsive and propulsive gait. Corticospinal and corticobulbar signs may be added. Progressive weakness, fatigability, and sleepiness are other prominent clinical features. Rarely, severe axial rigidity and dystonia, like those of Wilson's disease, are the outstanding manifestations.

Neuronal loss and gliosis, affecting mainly the pallidum and striatum, but also the frontoparietal and cerebellar cortex and hypothalamus, have been described, but the pathologic changes have not been carefully studied.

The neurologic abnormalities have not responded to treatment with chelating agents. In the chronic "dystonic form" of manganese intoxication, dramatic and sustained improvement has been reported with the administration of L-dopa; patients with the more common "parkinsonian type" of manganese intoxication have shown only slight improvement with L-dopa.

MERCURY

Chronic mercury poisoning gives rise to a wide array of serious neurologic symptoms, including tremors of the extremities, tongue, and lips; mental confusion; and a progressive cerebellar syndrome, with ataxia of gait and of the arms, intention tremor, and dysarthria. Choreoathetosis and parkinsonian facies have also been described. Changes in mood and behavior are prominent, consisting at first of weakness and fatigability and later of extreme depression and lethargy alternating with irritability. The pathologic changes are characterized by neuronal loss and gliosis of the calcarine cortex and to a lesser extent of other parts of the cortex and a striking degeneration of the granular layer of the cerebellar cortex, with relative sparing of the Purkinje cells.

This form of poisoning occurs in persons exposed to large amounts of the metal used in the manufacture of thermometers, mirrors, incandescent lights, x-ray machines, and vacuum pumps. Since mercury volatizes at room temperature, it readily contaminates the air and then condenses on the skin and respiratory mucous membranes. Nitrate of mercury, used in the manufacture of felt hats, and phenyl mercury, used in the paper, pulp, and electrochemical industries, are other sources of intoxication. Also, the presence of mercury in industrial waste has contaminated many sources of water supply and fish, which are ingested by humans and cause mercurial poisoning. So-called Minamata disease is a case in point. Between 1953 and 1956, a large number of villagers living near Minamata Bay in Kyushu Island, Japan, were afflicted with a syndrome of chronic mercurialism, probably due to the ingestion of fish that had been contaminated with industrial mercurial pollutants. Cerebellar ataxia and impaired vision were prominent symptoms.

In the treatment of chronic mercury poisoning, N-acetyl-dl-penicillamine is probably the drug of choice, since it can be administered orally and appears to chelate mercury selectively, with less effect on copper, which is essential to many metabolic processes.

PHOSPHORUS

Nervous system function may be deranged as part of acute and usually fatal poisoning with inorganic phosphorous compounds (found in rat poisons, roach powders, and matchheads). More important clinically is poisoning with organophosphorous compounds, the best known of which is triorthocresyl phosphate (TOCP).

Organophosphates are widely used as insecticides. Certain ones, such as tetraethylpyrophosphate, have been the cause of major outbreaks of neurologic disorder, especially in children. These substances have an acute anticholinesterase effect but no delayed action. Chlorophos, which is a 1-hydroxy-2,2,2-trichlorethylphosphonate, has in addition a delayed action, as does TOCP.

The immediate anticholinesterase effect is manifested by headache, vomiting, sweating, miosis, and muscular weakness and twitching. Most of these symptoms can be reversed by atropine. The delayed neurotoxic effects are marked limb weakness and areflexia, progressing to atrophy. Sensory loss is slight. Recovery occurs to a variable degree and then signs of corticospinal damage become detectable. The severity of paralysis and its permanence vary with the dosage of TOCP.

Several striking outbreaks of TOCP poisoning have been reported. During the latter part of the prohibition era and to a lesser extent thereafter, outbreaks of so-called jake paralysis were traced to the drinking of an extract of Jamaica ginger that had been contaminated with TOCP. Another was in Morocco in 1959 when lubricating oil containing TOCP was used deliberately to dilute olive oil. Other outbreaks have been caused by the ingestion of grain and cooking oil that had been stored in inadequately cleansed containers previously used for TOCP.

The experimental studies of Cavenaugh and Patangia in the cat revealed a dying back from the terminal ends of the largest and longest medullated motor nerve fibers, including those from the muscle spindles (annulospiral endings). The long fiber tracts of the spinal cord showed a similar dying-back phenomenon. Abnormal membrane bound vesicles and tubules were found by Prineas to accumulate in axoplasm before degeneration. These effects have been traced to the inhibitory action of TOCP on esterases. Johnson found that one of three enzymes which hydrolyzed phenylphenacetate was always inhibited by TOCP. There is still uncertainty as to the details of these reactions, and no treatment for the prevention or control of the neurotoxic effects has been devised.

THALLIUM

In the late nineteenth century, thallium was used medicinally in the treatment of venereal disease, ringworm, and tuberculosis; poisoning was fairly common. Sporadic instances of poisoning still occur, usually as a result of accidental or suicidal ingestion of thallium-containing rodenticides, rarely from overuse of depilatory agents. Patients who survive the effects of acute poisoning develop a rapidly progressive and painful polyneuropathy, optic atrophy, and occasionally ophthalmoplegia—followed, 15 to 30 days after ingestion, by diffuse alopecia. The latter feature should always suggest the diagnosis of thallium poisoning, which can be confirmed by finding the drug in the urine. The use of potassium chloride by mouth may hasten thallium excretion.

OTHER METALS

Iron, antimony, zinc, barium, bismuth, copper, silver, gold, and lithium may all produce serious degrees of intoxication. The major manifestations in each case are gastrointestinal or renal, but certain neurologic symptoms—notably headache, irritability, confusional psychosis, stupor, coma, and convulsions—may be observed in cases of profound poisoning, often as terminal events. Gold preparations, which are still used occasionally in the treatment of arthritis, may, after several months of treatment, give rise to focal or generalized myokymia and a rapidly progressive, symmetrical polyneuropathy (Katrak et al.). Lithium is employed extensively in the treatment of the manic form of manic-depressive disease (see page 1036) or as a salt substitute in the form of lithium chloride. The symptoms of toxicity, in addition to gastrointestinal ones, are tremor and muscular twitchings, followed by blurring of vision, vertigo, choreoathetosis, and mental confusion. Treatment consists of withdrawal of the offending salt and the administration of fluids and sodium chloride.

CLIOQUINOL

This compound, sold as Entero-Vioform, has been used in many parts of the world to prevent traveller's diarrhea and as a treatment for chronic gastroenteritis. In 1971 clinical observations began to appear in medical journals of a subacute myeloopticoneuropathy (SMON). During the 1960s more than 10,000 cases of this neurotoxic disease were collected in Japan by Tsubaki et al. The usual symptoms are gastrointestinal disturbance followed by ascending numbness and weakness of the legs, paralysis of sphincters, and autonomic disorder. Later, vision is affected. In about two-thirds of the cases the onset is acute, and in the remainder, subacute. The occurrence of these neurological complications was found to be related to the prolonged use of clioquinol, though there is still not full agreement on this point. In Japan the drug was withdrawn from the market, and the incidence of SMON immediately fell, supporting the theory that it was caused by clioquinol.

Recovery is usually incomplete. Two patients seen by the authors several years after onset of the disease had been left with optic atrophy and a spastic-ataxic paraparesis.

INDUSTRIAL TOXINS

Some of these, the heavy metals, have already been considered. In addition, a large number of synthetic organic compounds are widely used in industry and are frequent sources of toxicity, and the list is constantly being expanded. These compounds will only be enumerated here: chlorinated diphenyls (e.g., DDT) or chlorinated polycyclic compounds (Kepone), used as insecticides; diethylene dioxide (Dioxane); carbon disulfide; the halogenated hydrocarbons (methyl chloride, tetrachlorethane, carbon tetrachloride, trichloroethylene, and methyl bromide); naphthalene (used in moth repellants); benzine (gasoline); and benzene and its derivatives [toluene, xylene, nitrobenzene, phenol, and amyl acetate (banana oil)].

The toxic effects of these substances, which are not exerted primarily on the nervous system, are much the same from one compound to another. Neural symptoms are also not specific. They consist of varying combinations of headache, restlessness, drowsiness, confusion, delirium, coma, and convulsions, which, as a rule occur late in the illness or preterminally. Some of these industrial toxins (carbon disulfide, carbon tetrachloride, and tetrachlorethane) may cause polyneuropathy, which becomes evident with recovery from acute toxicity.

ANTINEOPLASTIC AGENTS

The increasing use of potent antineoplastic agents has given rise to a diverse group of neurologic complications, the most important of which are summarized below.

VINCRISTINE

This drug is used in the treatment of acute lymphoblastic leukemia, lymphomas, and some solid tumors. Its most important toxic effect, and the one that limits its use as a chemotherapeutic agent, is exerted on the peripheral nerves. Paresthesias of the feet or hands, or both, may occur within a few weeks of the onset of treatment; with continued use of the drug, a progressive symmetrical motor-sensory and reflex loss occurs. Cranial nerves are affected less frequently; ptosis, lateral rectus and facial palsies, and vocal cord paresis are the usual manifestations. Autonomic nervous system function may also be affected: constipation and impotence are frequent complications; orthostatic hypotension, atonicity of the bladder, and adynamic ileus are less frequent. Inappropriate antidiuretic hormone secretion and seizures have been reported, but are relatively uncommon.

The neural complications of vinblastine are similar to those of vincristine, but are usually avoided because vinblastine first produces a serious degree of bone marrow suppression and the drug is discontinued before the nervous system is affected.

PROCARBAZINE

This drug, originally synthesized as an MAO inhibitor, is now an important oral agent in the treatment of Hodgkin's disease and other lymphomas. Next to bone marrow suppression, neural complications are the most frequent, and usually take the form of somnolence, confusion, agitation, and depression. Diffuse aching pain in proximal muscles of the limbs, and mild symptoms and signs of polyneuropathy are less frequent. A reversible ataxia has also been described. Procarbazine, given in conjunction with phenothiazines, barbiturates, narcotics, and alcohol, may produce serious degrees of oversedation; in conjunction with MAO inhibitors it may cause orthostatic hypotension.

L-ASPARAGINASE

This enzyme is used in the treatment of acute lymphoblastic leukemia in children. It gives rise to a wide range of serious toxic reactions. Drowsiness, confusion, delirium, stupor and coma, and diffuse slowing of the electroencephalogram are the usual neurologic ones. These effects may occur within a day of onset of treatment and clear quickly when the drug is withdrawn, or they may be delayed in onset, in which case they may persist for several weeks. The cerebral abnormalities are attributed to the systemic metabolic derangements induced by L-asparaginase, including liver dysfunction.

5-FLUOROURACIL

This is a pyrimidine analogue and DNA inhibitor, used mainly in treatment of cancer of the breast, ovary, and gastrointestinal tract. A small proportion of patients receiving this drug develops dizziness, ataxia of the trunk and the extremities, dysarthria, and nystagmus. These abnormalities need to be distinguished from metastatic involvement of the cerebellum and so-called carcinomatous cerebellar degeneration. The drug effects are usually mild and subside within 1 to 6 weeks after discontinuation of therapy. The anatomic basis of this cerebellar syndrome is not known.

METHOTREXATE

This drug, a folic acid analogue, is used in the treatment of acute leukemia, choriocarcinoma, certain solid tumors, and polymyositis. Since it does not cross the blood-brain barrier, it does not cause signs of neural toxicity when administered by the oral or intravenous route. Given intrathecally, to treat meningeal leukemia or carcinomatosis, it may have serious neurotoxic effects. Signs of meningeal irritation—headache, nausea and vomiting, stiff neck, fever, and spinal fluid pleocytosis—are common. Other neurologic abnormalities, such as tremor, ataxia, dementia, delayed meningoencephalopathy, and transient and permanent paraplegia, have been attributed to the toxic effects of methotrexate, but are difficult to separate from the effects of the neoplasms or of radiation. Critical neuropathologic studies of such cases by Shapiro and his colleagues have shown necrotizing lesions in the cerebral tissues.

CISPLATIN

A new antineoplastic agent, cisplatin (*cis*-diamminedichloroplatinum) has recently become available for the treatment of certain gonadal and head and neck tumors. The dose-limiting factor in its use is nephrotoxicity and vomiting. In addition, certain neurologic complications have been reported. Approximately one-third of patients receiving this drug experience tinnitus or high-frequency hearing loss (4000 to 8000 Hz) or both. These toxicities are dose-related, cumulative, and only occasionally reversible. Rarely, seizures and retrobulbar neuritis occur. They seem to represent idiosyncratic reactions to the drug and are not dose-related. Peripheral neuropathy manifested primarily by numbness and tingling in fingers and toes is being observed with increasing frequency; this toxic manifestation appears to be related to the cumulative dose administered, and it seems to improve after the drug has been discontinued. It is likely that the neurotoxic potential of this new drug will be more precisely defined as its use increases.

REFERENCES

GENERAL

ARENA JM: *Poisoning: Toxicology-Symptoms-Treatments*, 4th ed. Springfield, Ill, Charles C Thomas, 1979.
BOURNE PG (ed): *Acute Drug Abuse Emergencies: A Treatment Manual.* New York, Academic, 1976.
DREISBACH RH: *Handbook of Poisoning: Diagnosis and Treatment*, 10th ed. Los Altos, Calif, Lange, 1980.
GILMAN AG, GOODMAN LS, GILMAN A (eds): *The Pharmacological Basis of Therapeutics*, 6th ed. New York, Macmillan, 1980.
HAMILTON A, HARDY HL: *Industrial Toxicology*, 3d ed. Acton, Publishing Sciences Group, 1974.

OPIATES AND SYNTHETIC ANALGESICS

BALL JC, CHAMBERS CK (eds): *The Epidemiology of Opiate Addiction in the United States.* Springfield, Ill, Charles C Thomas, 1970.
DOLE VP, NYSWANDER ME: Methadone maintenance and its implication for theories of narcotic addiction. *Res Publ Assoc Res Nerv Ment Dis* 46:359, 1968.
HOLLISTER LE: Effective use of analgesic drugs. *Annu Rev Med* 27:431, 1976.
JASINSKI DR et al: Human pharmacology and abuse potential of the analgesic buprenorphine. *Arch Gen Psychiatry* 35:501, 1978.
MARTIN WR: Realistic goals for antagonist therapy. *Am J Drug Alcohol Abuse* 2:353, 1975.
————, JASINSKI DR, MANSKY PA: Naltrexone, an antagonist for the treatment of heroin dependence: Effects in man. *Arch Gen Psychiatry* 28: 784, 1973.
MONROE JJ, ROSS WF, BERZINS JI: The decline of the addict as "psychopath": Implications for community care. *Int J Addictions* 6:601, 1971.
RICHTER RW et al: Neurological complications of heroin addiction. *Bull NY Acad Med* 49:3, 1972.
VANDAM LD: Butorphanol. *N Engl J Med* 302:381, 1980.
WIKLER A: Theories related to physical dependence, in Mule SJ, Brill H (eds): *The Chemical and Biological Aspects of Drug Dependence.* Cleveland, CRC Press, 1972, pp 359-377.
————: Characteristics of opioid addiction, in Jarvik ME (ed): *Psychopharmacology in the Practice of Medicine.* New York, Appleton-Century-Crofts, 1977, p 417.
————: *Opioid Dependence: Mechanisms and Treatment.* New York, Plenum, 1980.
ZINBERG NE: The crisis in methadone maintenance. *N Engl J Med* 296:1000, 1977.

BARBITURATES AND OTHER SEDATIVE-HYPNOTIC DRUGS

BLOOMER HA, MADDOCK RK JR: An assessment of diuresis and dialysis for treating acute barbiturate poisoning, in Mathew H (ed): *Acute Barbiturate Poisoning.* Amsterdam, Excerpta Medica, 1971, chap 15.

CLEMMESEN C, NILSSON E: Therapeutic trends in the treatment of barbiturate poisoning: The Scandinavian method. *Clin Pharmacol Ther* 2:220, 1961.

ESSIG C: Chronic abuse of sedative-hypnotic drugs, in Zarafonetis CJD (ed): *Drug Abuse.* Philadelphia, Lea & Febiger, 1972, pp 205-215.

HARVEY SC: Hypnotics and sedatives, in Gilman AG, Goodman LS, Gilman A (eds): *The Pharmacological Basis of Therapeutics,* 6th ed. New York, Macmillan, 1980, chap 17.

ISBELL H et al: Chronic barbiturate intoxication: An experimental study. *Arch Neurol Psychiatry* 64:1, 1950.

PLUM F, SWANSON AC: Barbiturate poisoning treated by physiological methods. *J Am Med Assoc* 163:827, 1957.

WESSON DR, SMITH DE: *Barbiturates: Their Use, Misuse, and Abuse.* New York, Human Sciences Press, 1977.

DEPRESSANTS, STIMULANTS, AND PSYCHOTOGENIC DRUGS

BALDESSARINI RJ: Drugs and the treatment of psychiatric disorders, in Gilman AG, Goodman LS, Gilman A (eds): *The Pharmacological Basis of Therapeutics,* 6th ed. New York, Macmillan, 1980, chap 19.

————, Tarsy D: Tardive dyskinesia, in Lipton MA et al (eds): *Psychopharmacology: A Generation of Progress.* New York, Raven, 1978, pp 993-1004.

DiPALMA JR (ed): *Drill's Pharmacology in Medicine.* New York, McGraw-Hill, 1971.

GREENBLATT DJ, SHADER RI: The clinical choice of sedative-hypnotics. *Ann Intern Med* 77:91, 1972.

HOLLISTER LE: *Clinical Pharmacology of Psychotherapeutic Drugs.* New York, Churchill-Livingstone, 1978.

IVERSEN SD, IVERSEN LL: *Behavioral Pharmacology.* New York, Oxford, 1975.

MARKS J: *The Benzodiazepines: Use, Overuse, Misuse, Abuse.* Baltimore, University Park Press, 1978.

PETERSON RC, STILLMAN RC: Phencyclidine: An overview, in Peterson RC, Stillman RC (eds): *Phencyclidine (PCP) Abuse,* Research Monograph Series 21. Washington, National Institute on Drug Abuse, 1978, chap 1.

SNYDER SH: Receptors, neurotransmitters and drug responses. *N Engl J Med* 300:465, 1979.

WIKLER A: Drug dependence, in Baker AB, Baker LH (eds): *Clinical Neurology,* vol 2. New York, Harper & Row, 1975, chap 21.

TETANUS

ABEL JJ, FIROR SM, CHALIAN W: Researches on tetanus: IX. Further evidence to show that tetanus toxin is not carried to central neurons by way of axis cylinders of motor nerves. *Bull Johns Hopkins Hosp* 63:373, 1938.

STRUPPLER A, STRUPPLER E, ADAMS RD: Local tetanus in man. *Arch Neurol* 8:162, 1963.

WEINSTEIN L: Current concepts: Tetanus. *N Engl J Med* 289:1293, 1973.

ZACKS SI, SHEFF MF: Studies on tetanus: V. In vivo localization of purified tetanus neurotoxin in mice with fluorescein-labelled tetanus antitoxin. *J Neuropathol Exp Neurol* 25:422, 1966.

DIPHTHERIA

FISHER CM, ADAMS RD: Diphtheritic polyneuritis: A pathological study. *J Neuropathol Exp Neurol* 15:243, 1956.

McDONALD WI, KOCHEN RS: Diphtheritic neuropathy, in Dyck PJ, Thomas PK, Lambert EH (eds): *Peripheral Neuropathy.* Philadelphia, Saunders, 1975, chap 63, pp 1281-1300.

PAPPENHEIMER AM: Diphtheria toxin. *Annu Rev Biochem* 46:69, 1977.

BOTULISM

CHERINGTON M: Botulism: Ten-year experience. *Arch Neurol* 30:432, 1974.

GANGAROSA EJ: Botulism in the United States, 1899-1967. *J Infect Dis* 119:308, 1969.

KOENIG MG et al: Type B bolulism in man. *Am J Med* 42:208, 1967.

LAMBERT EH: Defects of neuromuscular transmission in syndromes other than myasthenia gravis. *Ann NY Acad Sci* 135:367, 1966.

MAYER RF: The neuromuscular defect in human botulism, in Locke S (ed): *Modern Neurology.* Boston, Little, Brown, 1969, pp 169-186.

PETTY CS: Botulism: The disease and toxin. *Am J Med Sci* 249:345, 1965.

ZACKS SJ, METZGER JF, SMITH CW, BLUMBERG JM: Localization of ferritin-labelled botulinus toxin in the neuromuscular junction of the mouse. *J Neuropathol Exp Neurol* 21:610, 1962.

LEAD

ALBERT JJ et al: Prevention, diagnosis, and treatment of lead poisoning in childhood. *Pediatrics* 44:291, 1969.

CHISHOLM JJ JR: Treatment of lead poisoning. *Mod Treat* 8:593, August 1971.

————: Management of increased lead absorption and lead poisoning in children. *N Engl J Med* 289:1016, 1973.

PERLSTEIN MA, ATTALA R: Neurologic sequelae of plumbism in children. *Clin Pediatr* 5:292, 1966.

ARSENIC

JENKINS RB: Inorganic arsenic and the nervous system. *Brain* 89:479, 1966.

MANGANESE

MENA I, MARIN O, FUENZALIDA S, COTZIAS GC: Chronic manganese poisoning: Clinical picture and manganese turnover. *Neurology* 17:128, 1967.

MERCURY

KARK RAP, POSKANZER DC, BULLOCK JD, BOYLEN G: Mercury poisoning and its treatment with *N*-acetyl-*dl*-penicillamine. *N Engl J Med* 285:10, 1971.
RUSTAM H et al: Evidence for neuromuscular disorder in methyl mercury poisoning. *Arch Environ Health* 30:190, 1975.

ORGANOPHOSPHATES

CAVENAUGH JB, PATANGIA GN: Changes in the central nervous system of the cat as the result of tri-*o*-cresyl phosphate poisoning. *Brain* 88:165, 1965.
JOHNSON MK: A phosphorylation site in brain and the delayed neurotoxic effect of organophosphorus compounds. *Biochem J* 111:487, 1969.

PRINEAS J: The pathogenesis of the dying-back polyneuropathies. *J Neuropathol Exp Neurol* 28:571, 1969.

THALLIUM

BANK WJ et al: Thallium poisoning. *Arch Neurol* 26:456, 1974.

GOLD

KATRAK SM et al: Clinical and morphological features of gold neuropathy. *Brain* 103:671, 1980.

CLIOQUINOL

TSUBAKI T et al: Neurological syndrome associated with clioquinol. *Lancet* 1:696, 1971.

ANTINEOPLASTIC AGENTS

OSTROW S et al: Ophthalmologic toxicity after *cis*-dichlorodiammineplatinum (11) therapy. *Cancer Treat Rep* 62:1591, 1978.
SHAPIRO WR, CHERNIK NL, POSNER JB: Necrotizing encephalopathy following intraventricular instillation of methotrexate. *Arch Neurol* 28:96, 1973.
WEISS HD, WALKER MD, WIERNIK PH: Neurotoxicity of commonly used antineoplastic agents. *N Engl J Med* 291:75, 127, 1974.

CHAPTER 42

DEGENERATIVE DISEASES OF THE NERVOUS SYSTEM

The adjectival term *degenerative* has no great appeal to the modern neurologist. For one thing, it has an unpleasant literary connotation, referring, as it does, to a state of moral degradation or deviant sexual behavior, as the consequence of a psychopathic tendency. Even more important, however, it is not a satisfactory term medically, since it implies an inexplicable decline from a previous level of normalcy to a lower level of function—an ambiguous conceptualization of disease that satisfies neither theoretician nor scientist. Unquestionably some of the diseases included in this category depend on genetic factors, or at least they appear in more than one member of the same family and are, therefore, more properly designated as *heredodegenerative.* An even larger number of diseases, not differing in any fundamental way from the heredofamilial ones, occurs only sporadically i.e., as isolated instances in given families. Gowers in 1902 suggested the term *abiotrophy* for diseases of this type, by which he meant a lack of "vital endurance" of the affected neurons, resulting in their premature death. This concept embodies an untested, unproven hypothesis—that aging and degenerative disease of cells are based on the same process, and contemporary neuropathologists are understandably reluctant to attribute to simple aging the diverse processes of cellular disease that are constantly being revealed by ultrastructural techniques.

There are, within recent memory, numerous examples of disease that formerly were classed as degenerative but now are known to have a metabolic, toxic, or nutritional basis or to be caused by a "slow virus." It seems reasonable to expect that with increasing knowledge, more and more diseases whose cause is now unknown will find their way into these categories. Until such time as the causation of all neurologic diseases is known, there has to be a name and a place for a group of diseases that have no known cause and are united only by the common attribute of gradually progressive disintegration of part or parts of the nervous system. In deference to traditional practice, they are being put together under the rubric of degenerative diseases.

The reader may be perplexed by the inconsistent use of the terms *atrophy* and *degeneration,* both of which are applied to diseases of this category. Spatz has argued that on purely histopathologic grounds they are different. Atrophy specifies a gradual decay and loss of neurons, leaving in their wake no degradative products and only a sparsely cellular, fibrous gliosis. Degeneration refers to a more rapid process of neuronal, myelin, or tissue breakdown, with resulting degradative products that call forth a more vigorous reaction of phagocytosis and cellular gliosis. The difference is both in speed and type of breakdown. It is of some interest that many of the diseases that are characterized by degeneration, in Spatz's sense of the term, are of established metabolic origin, but virtually none of the purely atrophic ones have been shown to have a metabolic basis.

GENERAL CLINICAL CHARACTERISTICS

The diseases included in the degenerative category *begin insidiously, after a long period of normal nervous functioning, and pursue a gradually progressive course which may continue for many years, even a decade or longer.* In this respect they differ from the known metabolic diseases. Frequently it is impossible to assign a date of onset. Sometimes, the patient or the patient's family gives a history of an abrupt appearance of disability, particularly if some injury, infection, or other dramatic event coincided with first symptoms. In such instances a skillfully taken history will elicit the fact that the patient or the family suddenly became aware of a condition which had, in fact, already been present for some time, but had attracted little attention. Whether trauma or other stress can actually evoke or aggravate a degenerative disease is a question that cannot be answered with certainty, but it seems highly improbable that this could happen. Instead, these disease processes by their very nature appear to develop de novo, without relation to known antecedent events, and their symptomatic expressions become possible only when the degree of neuronal loss reaches or exceeds the "safety factor" for that system. In other words, the degree of correspondence between the clinical state and its pathologic basis is only relative.

The familial occurrence of disease is of great importance, but it must be emphasized that such information is often difficult to obtain on first contact with the patient. The family may be small and widely scattered, so that the patient is unaware of the health of other members. Then, too, the patient or the patient's relatives may be ashamed to admit that a neurologic disease has "tainted" the family. Furthermore, it may not be realized that an illness is hereditary if other members of the family have a much more or much less severe form of the disorder than the patient. Sometimes, in the latter case, only the careful examination of other family members will disclose the presence of an hereditary disease. It must be remembered, however, that familial occurrence of a disease does not prove heredity, but may indicate instead that more than one member of a family has been exposed to the same infectious or toxic agent.

In general, the degenerative diseases of the nervous system run a ceaselessly progressive course, uninfluenced by all medical and surgical measures, so that dealing with a patient with this type of illness may be an anguishing experience for all concerned. However, some symptoms can be alleviated by wise and skillful management, and the physician's interest may be of great help even though curative measures cannot be offered.

The bilateral symmetry of the lesions and clinical manifestations is another noteworthy feature of the degenerative diseases, and it alone may distinguish members of this group from many other diseases of the nervous system. This principle requires qualification, however, for in the earliest stages of some degenerative diseases (e.g., paralysis agitans, amyotrophic lateral sclerosis) there may be greater involvement of one limb or one side of the body. Sooner or later, however, despite the asymmetric beginning, the inherently symmetric nature of the process asserts itself.

Many of the degenerative diseases are characterized by the selective involvement of anatomically and physiologically related systems of neurons. This feature is exemplified by amyotrophic lateral sclerosis, in which the pathologic process is limited to motor neurons of the cerebral cortex, brainstem, and spinal cord, and by certain forms of progressive ataxia in which only the Purkinje cells of the cerebellum are affected. Many other examples could be cited (e.g., Friedreich's ataxia) in which certain neuronal systems disintegrate, leaving others unscathed. These degenerative diseases have therefore been called *system diseases* or *neuronal atrophies*, and many of them turn out to be strongly hereditary. It must be realized, however, that selective involvement of systems of neurons is not an exclusive property of the degenerative diseases, since several disease processes of known cause have similarly circumscribed effects on the nervous system. Diphtheria toxin, for instance, selectively affects the myelin of the peripheral nerves near the spinal ganglia, and triorthocresyl phosphate affects both the corticospinal tracts of the spinal cord and the spinal motor neurons. Another example is the special vulnerability of the Purkinje cells to hyperthermia. Conversely, several of the conditions included among degenerative disease (according to the criteria of Spatz) are characterized by pathologic changes that are diffuse and unselective.

As one would expect of any pathologic process that is based on the slow disintegration of neurons, not only do the cell bodies disappear but also their dendrites, axons, and myelin sheaths—unaccompanied by an intense tissue reaction or cellular response. The CSF, therefore, shows little if any change—at most a slight increase in protein content. Moreover, since these diseases invariably result in tissue loss rather than in new tissue formation (as occurs with neoplasms or inflammations), radiologic examination shows either no change or an enlargement of the CSF compartments. The blood-brain barrier tends not to be altered. These negative laboratory findings help distinguish the neuronal atrophies from other large classes of progressive disease of the nervous system, viz., tumors, infections, and other processes of inflammatory type.

CLASSIFICATION

Since grouping of the degenerative diseases in terms of etiology is impossible (save that many are hereditary, or genetic) we resort, for practical reasons, to dividing them according to the presenting clinical syndromes and their pathologic anatomy. Although this simple descriptive approach is the most elementary mode of classification of naturally occurring phenomena, it is a necessary prelude to diagnosis and scientific study, and preferable to a haphazard listing of diseases by the names of the neurologists or neuropathologists who first described them.

I. Syndrome of progressive dementia, other neurologic signs being absent or inconspicuous
   A. Diffuse cerebral atrophy
      1. Alzheimer's disease
      2. Nonspecific types
   B. Circumscribed cerebral atrophy (lobar sclerosis)—Pick's disease
   C. Other types of dementia
      1. Arteriosclerotic
      2. Post-traumatic
      3. Postencephalitic
II. Syndrome of progressive dementia in combination with other neurologic abnormalities
   A. Huntington's chorea
   B. Cortical-striatal-spinal degeneration (Jakob) and the dementia–Parkinson–amyotrophic lateral sclerosis complex (Guamanian and others)
   C. Diffuse cerebral sclerosis
   D. Cerebrocerebellar degeneration (Greenfield)
   E. Familial dementia with spastic paraparesis
   F. Cortical-basal ganglionic degeneration
III. Syndrome of gradual development of abnormalties of posture and movement
   A. Paralysis agitans (Parkinson's disease)
   B. Striatonigral degeneration
   C. Progressive supranuclear palsy (Steele-Richardson-Olszewski)
   D. Dystonia musculorum deformans (torsion spasm)
   E. Hallervorden-Spatz disease
   F. Spasmodic torticollis and other restricted dyskinesias
   G. Familial tremor
IV. Syndrome of progressive ataxia
   A. Predominantly spinal forms of hereditary ataxia
      1. Friedreich's
      2. Strümpell-Lorrain
   B. Predominantly cerebellar forms of hereditary ataxia
      1. Holmes' familial cortical cerebellar atrophy
      2. Late cerebellar cortical atrophy of Marie-Foix-Alajouanine
   C. Cerebellar-brainstem atrophies
      1. Olivopontocerebellar
      2. Dentatorubral
      3. Azorean disease
   D. Carcinomatous and other cerebellar degenerations
V. Syndrome of slowly developing muscular weakness and atrophy (nuclear amyotrophy).

A. Without sensory changes: motor system disease
   1. Amyotrophic lateral sclerosis
   2. Progressive spinal muscular atrophy
   3. Progressive bulbar palsy
   4. Primary lateral sclerosis
   5. Hereditary forms of progressive muscular atrophy and spastic paraplegia
B. With sensory changes (see Chap. 45)
   1. Hereditary sensory neuropathies
   2. Hereditary sensorimotor neuropathies [peroneal muscular atrophy (Charcot-Marie-Tooth); hypertrophic interstitial polyneuropathy (Déjerine-Sottas); heredopathia atactica polyneuritiformis (Refsum); etc.]
VI. Syndrome of progressive blindness
   A. Hereditary optic neuropathy (Leber)
   B. Pigmentary degeneration of retina (retinitis pigmentosa)
   C. Stargardt's disease
VII. Syndromes characterized by neurosensory deafness
   A. Pure neurosensory deafness
   B. Hereditary hearing loss with retinal diseases
   C. Hereditary hearing loss with diseases of the nervous system

DISEASES CHARACTERIZED CHIEFLY BY PROGRESSIVE DEMENTIA

ALZHEIMER'S DISEASE

This is the most common and important of the degenerative diseases of the brain. Some clinical aspects of the intellectual deterioration that characterize this disease have already been described in Chap. 20, under the neurology of dementia, and the relationship of this disease to the aging process has been fully discussed in Chap. 28. There it was pointed out that some degree of shrinkage in size and weight of the brain, i.e., "atrophy," is an inevitable accompaniment of advancing age, but that these changes are rarely of major clinical significance. By contrast, severe degrees of diffuse cerebral atrophy that evolve relatively rapidly are invariably associated with dementia and the underlying pathologic changes in these cases most often prove to be those of Alzheimer's disease (see below). When these changes occur in old age (and the definition of when old age begins is quite arbitrary), it is usual to speak of senile dementia; when a pathologically identical progressive dementia appears *before* the senile period, the term *Alzheimer's disease* is frequently used. This practice of giving Alzheimer's disease and senile dementia the status of separate diseases is probably attributable to the relatively young age (51 years) of the patient originally studied by Alzheimer. The illogicality of such a division is at once apparent, since the two conditions, except for their age of onset, are clinically and pathologically indistinguishable.

Clinical Features Although Alzheimer's disease has been described at every period of adult life, the majority of our patients have been in their late fifties or early sixties or older. It is one of the most frequent mental illnesses, making up some 20 percent of all patients in psychiatric hospitals. It has been estimated by Larsson et al. that the aggregate morbidity risk up to the age of 80 is 5 percent. In England, Kay and his colleagues found that 4.2 percent of elderly people in the general population were suffering from dementia. In the United States, in 17 series comprising 15,000 persons over the age of 60 years, the mean incidence of moderate to severe dementia was calculated to be 4.8 percent (Wang). A number of familial cases have been well documented, but there is not sufficient evidence to indicate that the disorder is truly hereditary. Nearly all our own cases have been sporadic, and males and females have been about equally affected.

The onset of mental changes is usually so insidious that neither the family nor the patient can date the time of its beginning. Occasionally, however, it is brought to attention by an unusual degree of confusion in relation to a febrile illness, an operation, mild head injury, or the taking of medication.

The gradual development of forgetfulness is the major symptom. Small day-to-day happenings are not remembered. Seldom-used names are particularly elusive. Little-used words from an earlier period of life also tend to be lost. Appointments are forgotten and possessions misplaced. Questions are repeated again and again, the patient having forgotten what was just discussed. It is said that remote memories are preserved and recent ones lost (Ribot's law of memory), but this is only relatively true; it is difficult to check the accuracy of ancient memories.

Once the memory disorder has become pronounced, other failures in mentation are increasingly apparent. The patient's speech is halting because of failure to recall the needed word. The same difficulty interrupts writing. Comprehension of spoken words seems at first to be preserved, until it is observed that the patient does not carry out a complicated request, but even then it is uncertain whether the request was not understood or was forgotten. Almost imperceptible at first, all these disturbances of language become more apparent as the disease progresses. Finally, there is a failure to speak in a full sentence; to find words requires a continuous search; and little that is said or written is fully comprehended. Occasionally there is a rather dramatic repeti-

tion of every spoken phrase (echolalia). The deterioration of verbal skills has then progressed to an obvious dysphasia.

Skill in arithmetic calculation suffers a similar deterioration. Faults in balancing the checkbook, mistakes in figuring the price of items and in making the correct change—all these and others progress to a point where the patient can no longer carry out the simplest business affairs. This type of conceptual loss is called *acalculia*, or *dyscalculia*.

Visuospatial orientation begins to fail. The car cannot be parked; the arms do not find the correct sleeves of the dressing gown; the corners of the tablecloth cannot be oriented with the corners of the table; the patient turns in the wrong direction on the way home or becomes lost. The route from one place to another cannot be described nor can given directions be understood. As this state worsens, the simplest of geometric forms and patterns cannot be copied.

The patient also eventually forgets how to use common objects and tools while retaining the necessary motor power and coordination for these activities. The razor is no longer correctly applied to the face; the latch of the door cannot be unfastened; and eating utensils are no longer used properly. Finally, only the most habitual and virtually automatic actions are preserved. Tests of commanded and demonstrated actions cannot be executed or imitated. *Ideomotor apraxia* is the term applied to the advanced forms of this motor incapacity (pages 41 and 42).

As these many deficits declare themselves, the patient at first seems unchanged in overall motility, behavior, temperament, and conduct. Social graces, whatever they were, are retained in the initial phase of the illness, but, gradually, troublesome alterations in these spheres appear. Restlessness and agitation or their opposites—hypokinesia and placidity—become evident. Dressing, shaving, and bathing are neglected. A poorly organized paranoid delusional state, sometimes with hallucinations, may become manifest. The patient may suspect his elderly wife of having an illicit relationship or his children of stealing his possessions. Imprudent business deals may be made. A stable marriage may be disrupted by an infatuation with a younger person. Sexual indiscretions may astonish the community. The affect coarsens; the patient is more egocentric and indifferent to the feelings and reactions of others. A gluttonous appetite sometimes develops, but more often eating is neglected, with gradual weight loss. Later, grasping and sucking reflexes can be readily elicited, sphincteric continence fails, and the patient sinks into a state of relative akinesia and mutism, as described in Chap. 20. Difficulty in locomotion, a kind of unsteadiness with shortened steps but without motor weakness and rigidity, frequently supervenes. Later, elements of cerebellar ataxia, parkinsonian akinesia and rigidity, and tremor can be perceived in the motor disability. Ultimately the patient loses the ability to stand and walk, being forced to lie inert in bed, having to be fed and bathed. The legs may curl into a *paraplegia in flexion*, in this instance of cerebral–basal ganglionic origin (see page 85).

The course of this pathetic illness usually extends over a period of 5 or more years, and, surprisingly, throughout this period the corticospinal functions, corticosensory functions, visual acuity, and visual fields remain relatively intact. If there are hemiplegia, homonymous hemianopia, etc., either the diagnosis of Alzheimer's disease is incorrect or the disease has been complicated by a stroke, tumor, or subdural hematoma. The tendon reflexes are but little altered and the plantar reflexes remain flexor. There is no true sensory or cerebellar ataxia. Convulsions are rare. Occasionally, widespread myoclonic jerks or mild choreoathetotic movements are observed. Eventually, in a bedfast state, an intercurrent infection such as aspiration pneumonia or some other disease mercifully terminates life.

The sequence of neurologic disabilities may not follow this described order, and one or another deficit may take precedence, presumably because the disease process affects one particular part of the brain earlier or later in one patient than in another. This allows for a relatively restricted deficit to become the source of early medical complaint, long before the full syndrome of dementia has declared itself. We have observed five limited deficits of this type, as follows:

1. *Dysnomia.* Forgetting words, especially proper names, which is so often a problem for the older person, may first bring the patient to a neurologist. Later the difficulty involves all common nouns and progresses to the point where fluency of speech is seriously impaired. Every sentence is broken by a pause and search for the wanted word. If not found, a circumlocution is substituted or the sentence is left unfinished. Repetition of the spoken words of others, at first flawless, later brings out a lesser degree of the same difficulty. Other components of language function may be relatively intact, but before

long the patient clearly does not understand all that she or he hears or reads. In contrast, nonverbal memory, judgment, and calculation may be preserved. Usually the EEG is normal or shows only a mild degree of slowing, and the lateral ventricles are either of normal size or slightly enlarged (especially the temporal lobes).

2. *Korsakoff's amnesic state.* The early stages of Alzheimer's disease may be dominated by a disproportionate failure of retentive memory, with integrity of other cognitive abilities. Such a restricted disability constitutes the *senile amnesic state,* or *presbyophrenia.* Retentive memory may become impaired to the point where nothing that is learned is retained for more than a minute or two. Yet the patient, if a business executive, for example, may continue to make acceptable decisions if his or her work utilizes long-established habit patterns. Again the temporal horns tend to be enlarged more than the rest of the ventricular system.

3. *Spatial disorientation.* Parietal lobe function, commonly deranged in the course of Alzheimer's disease, may fail while other functions are preserved. As remarked above, losing one's way in familiar surroundings, inability to interpret a road map or to distinguish right from left or to park or garage a car or a boat, difficulty in arranging a tablecloth or in dressing are all manifestations of a special failure to orient the schema of one's body with that of surrounding space.

4. *Paranoia and other personality changes.* Not uncommonly, the initial event in the development of dementia is the occurrence of paranoia or bizarre behavior. Patients become convinced that relatives are stealing their possessions or that an elderly and even infirm husband or wife is guilty of infidelity. They may hide their belongings, even relatively worthless ones, and go about spying on family members. Hostilities arise, and wills may be altered irrationally. Many of these patients are constantly worried, tense, and agitated.

Of course, paranoid delusions may be part of a depressive psychosis and of many other dementias, but the senile patients in whom paranoia is the presenting problem seem not to be depressed, and their cognitive functions are for a time well preserved. It is tempting to think that a very early senile change has exposed a lifelong trait of suspiciousness, but this is purely hypothetical.

Sometimes other oddities of behavior will announce the oncoming dementia. Social indiscretions, rejection of an old friend, embarking on an imprudent financial venture, or an amorous pursuit that is out of character are examples of these types of behavioral change.

5. *Gait disorder.* While it is true that most patients with Alzheimer's disease walk normally until relatively late in their illness, not infrequently, in the older patients, a short-stepped gait and poor balance may call attention to the disease (see page 85).

It has been our impression that each of these restricted cerebral disorders is only relatively pure. Careful testing of mental function, and this is of diagnostic importance, frequently discloses subtle abnormalities of other functions. Patients with disproportionate affection of some temporal or parietal lobe function usually show impairment on the performance parts of the Wechsler Adult Intelligence Scale. Moreover, within several months to a year or two, the more generalized aspects of mental deterioration become apparent. If one of the foregoing restricted deficits remains uncomplicated over a period of years, one is justified in suspecting some cause other than senile degeneration, such as embolic infarction of one part of the temporal or parietal lobe; or perhaps the initial illness was a herpes simplex encephalitis of the temporal lobes. Also, as stated earlier, a visual field defect, cortical sensory loss, or hemiparesis is seldom if ever due to Alzheimer's disease alone.

Pathology The brain presents a diffusely atrophied appearance. Cerebral convolutions are narrowed and sulci are widened. The third and lateral ventricles are symmetrically enlarged to a varying degree. Usually the atrophic process is most pronounced in the frontal and temporal lobes, but cases vary considerably. Microscopically, there is widespread loss of nerve cells, most marked in the cerebral cortex but often present in the basal ganglia as well. Residual neurons lose dendrites and crowd upon one another due to loss of neuropil. Astrocytic proliferation follows as a compensatory or reparative process. In addition, three microscopic changes give this disease its distinctive character: (1) deposits of amorphous material, scattered throughout the cerebral cortex and most easily seen with silver-staining methods (so-called *senile plaques*), (2) the presence within the nerve cell cytoplasm of thick, fiberlike strands of silver-staining material, often in the form of loops, coils, or tangled masses (*Alzheimer neurofibrillary change*), and (3) granulovacuolar degeneration of neurons, most evident in the pyramidal cell layer of the hippocampus. Electron-microscopic studies have shown the neurofibrillary tangle to be composed of clusters of twisted tubules that are different from the normal microtubules of nerve cells. The senile plaques contain a core of amyloid, surrounded by products of degenerated nerve cells and nerve terminals, mainly dendritic, containing lysosomes, abnormal mitochondria, and often twisted tubules. Also,

amyloid can be found in the walls of some of the small blood vessels near the plaques, the so-called dyshoric, or congophilic, angiopathy. A number of the cases with amyloid angiopathy have been familial (Corsellis).

It is of passing historical interest that Alzheimer was not the first to describe senile plaques, the hallmark of this pathologic state. These miliary lesions ("Herdchen") had been observed in senile brains by Blocq and Marinesco in 1892, and were named "senile plaques" by Simchowicz, in 1910. In 1907, Alzheimer described the case of a 51-year-old woman who died after a 5-year illness characterized by progressive dementia. Throughout the cerebral cortex he found the miliary lesions, but he also noted—thanks to the use of Bielschowsky's silver impregnation method—a clumping and distortion of fibrils in the neuronal cytoplasm, the change which now, appropriately, carries Alzheimer's name.

The *pathogenesis* of the aforementioned changes is unknown. Of interest are the observations of a reduction of choline acetyltransferase, the key enzyme in the synthesis of the neurotransmitter acetylcholine, in the cerebral cortex of patients with senile dementia (Bowen et al., Davies and Maloney). These findings suggest that impairment of cholinergic transmission may play a part in the clinical expression of the disease. The initial report of transmission of Alzheimer's disease in chimpanzees, using brain tissue from two familial cases of the disease, has not been reproduced, and the association between Alzheimer's disease and an infectious agent has not been demonstrated with any certainty (Goudsmit et al.). The role of vascular changes in pathogenesis is controversial. It is definite that Alzheimer's disease is not related to any of the usual types of arteriosclerosis. There are, however, small-vessel changes, accounting for the reduced cerebral blood flow reported by many investigators, recently by Yamaguchi et al. This small-vessel change is probably secondary to the cerebral atrophy since a lesser degree of reduction in blood flow is found in the brains of mentally intact, old individuals.

Associated pathologic states The histologic changes of Alzheimer's disease have a number of rather interesting and unusual associations, which should be added at this point. The Alzheimer changes are far more common in the brains of patients with Parkinson's disease than in the brains of age-matched controls (Hakim and Mathieson). As a corollary, large numbers of Lewy bodies (a characteristic feature of Parkinson's disease) have been found in 10 percent of the brains of 96 patients with Alzheimer's disease (Woodard). These findings undoubtedly explain the high incidence of dementia in patients with Parkinson's disease (see further on, under paralysis agitans). Another association between the two diseases is apparent in the Guamanian Parkinson-dementia complex, which is also discussed below. In this latter entity, the symptoms of dementia and parkinsonism are related to neurofibrillary changes in the cerebral cortex and substantia nigra, respectively; senile plaques and Lewy bodies are unusual findings.

There are instances, such as those reported by Malamud and Lowenberg and by Loken and Cyvin, in which dementia had begun in late childhood, with the finding at postmortem examination of the typical Alzheimer lesions in the cerebral cortex and basal ganglia. The clinical picture in these juvenile and early adult cases has been more varied than in the older ones. In some, paucity of speech, mutism, tremor, stooped posture, grasp and suck reflexes, pyramidal and cerebellar signs leading to inability to stand or walk have appeared at various stages of the disease.

The finding of fibrillary changes, like those of Alzheimer's disease, in boxers ("punch-drunk" syndrome, or "dementia pugilistica") is another interesting ramification of this disease process (page 608). Hydrocephalus is present also, but there is insufficient information as to its nature, whether it is a low-pressure tension hydrocephalus from multiple subarachnoid hemorrhages or a hydrocephalus ex vacuo from cerebral atrophy.

Alzheimer's disease in relation to mongolism, first emphasized by Jervis, is now widely recognized. The characteristic plaques and neurofibrillary tangles appear in the third decade and increase with age, and are present in the majority of patients with Down's syndrome after 30 years of age. Relatively few of these patients, however, manifest a deterioration of behavior from their previously subnormal level (deterioration occurred in only 3 of 20 cases recently described by Ropper and Williams).

Pick's lobar sclerosis has, on occasion, been associated with the histologic alterations of Alzheimer's disease, as was pointed out by Moyano and later by Berlin. The latter refers to this combination as *the double disease*. Other unusual combinations have been reported wherein Alzheimer's disease and Simmond's hypopituitarism or neurosyphilis were conjoined. These isolated combinations are probably a matter of chance and prove nothing. However, where the association is more frequent, as in mongolism and dementia pugilistica, one must consider both endogenous and exogenous factors in causation. From time to time other atypical examples come to light, such as the cases of familial dementia with spastic paraplegia reported by Worster-Drought and by van Bogaert and their associates (see further on in this chapter).

Diagnostic Studies By far the most important is the CT scan. In advanced cases of Alzheimer's disease the lateral and third ventricles are enlarged usually to about twice normal size, and the cerebral sulci are widened. However, early in the disease, the changes do not exceed those found in many mentally intact old persons. For this reason, one cannot rely on the CT scan for the diagnosis of Alzheimer's disease. It is, however, valuable in excluding brain tumor, subdural hematoma, multi-infarct dementia, and obstructive hydrocephalus. Still to be corroborated is the finding in CT scans of cerebral white matter of a diminished "CT number" (Hounsfield unit or delta number)—a number related to the coefficient of attentuation of the brain tissue (see Naeser et al.). The same evidences of cerebral atrophy are revealed by pneumoencephalography. The EEG undergoes a diffuse slowing in the theta and delta range but only late in the course of the illness. The CSF is normal, though occasionally the total protein is slightly elevated.

Differential Diagnosis Formerly, when virtually all forms of presenile and senile dementia were untreatable, there was no advantage to either the patient or the family in ascertaining the cause of the cerebral disease. Such patients were customarily left alone at home or committed to an institution for care of the chronically ill or to a psychiatric institution. Now that a few treatable dementing diseases have been discovered, a great premium attaches to correct diagnosis. The physician is compelled to exercise care in their detection even though they may be relatively infrequent.

The treatable forms of dementia are those due to general paresis; low-pressure hydrocephalus; chronic subdural hematomas; nutritional deficiencies (Wernicke-Korsakoff and Marchiafava-Bignami disease, pellagra, vitamin B_{12} deficiency with subacute degeneration of the spinal cord and brain); chronic drug intoxication (e.g., barbiturates, bromides, and alcohol); certain endocrine-metabolic disorders (myxedema, Cushing's disease, chronic hepatic encephalopathy); certain forms of frontal and temporal lobe tumors; and the pseudodementia of depression. To exclude these several diseases requires admission to a hospital where examinations of blood and CSF, EEGs, and special radiologic studies of the cerebrum can be undertaken (CT scan, scintigraphic cisternography).

The most difficult problem in differential diagnosis, in the authors' experience, has been the distinction between a late-life depression and senile dementia, especially when some degree of both are present. Multi-infarct dementia may be difficult to separate from senile dementia, for patients with the latter illness may have had a single, clinically inevident stroke. Low-pressure hydrocephalus may be confused with senile and multi-infarct dementia. The differential diagnosis of these several conditions is discussed in Chaps. 29, 33, and 53.

Treatment There is no evidence that any of the proposed forms of therapy for the Alzheimer-senile dementia complex—transcerebral vasodilators, stimulants, L-dopa, massive doses of vitamins B, C, and E, or others—has any effect whatsoever. There is no harm in using vitamins, however, for they keep the neurologic problem on a medical plane and provide repeated medical surveillance which proves helpful in counseling the family. The use of chlorpromazine and related drugs may suppress some of the aberrant behavior, where this is a problem, and make life more comfortable for the patient and the family.

The general management of the demented patient should proceed along the lines outlined in Chap. 20.

PICK'S LOBAR ATROPHY

As the name implies, this is a special form of cerebral degeneration in which the atrophy is circumscribed (most often in the frontal and temporal lobes), with involvement of both gray and white matter—hence the term *lobar* rather than cortical. Arnold Pick of Prague first described its gross characteristics but gave no microscopic details; he was interested particularly in disproving a tenet advanced by Wernicke that the manifestations of senile brain atrophy were always diffuse and nonfocal. In a series of publications Pick elaborated upon the aphasic symptoms of this condition. Alzheimer in 1911 presented the first careful study of the microscopic changes. The most complete analyses of the pathologic changes are those of Spatz, van Mansvelt, and Tissot et al., and since the recognition of Pick's disease rests essentially on these pathologic rather than on clinical criteria, they will be described first.

In contrast to Alzheimer's disease, where the atrophy is relatively mild and diffuse, the pathologic change in Pick's disease is a severe wasting of the frontal and temporal lobes. The atrophy may extend to the island of Reil and the amygdaloid-hippocampal structures. The parietal lobes are involved less frequently. The affected gyri become paper-thin; the brain resembles the kernel of a dried walnut. The cut surface reveals not only a markedly thinned cortical ribbon but a grayish appearance and reduced volume of the white matter. The corpus callosum and anterior commissure share in the atrophy. The overlying pia-arachnoid is thickened, and the ventricles are enlarged. The pre- and postcentral, superior temporal, and occipital convolutions resist the onslaught of the disease and stand out in striking contrast to the wasted parts. Pick insisted that the disease involves essentially the association areas of Flechsig. In some instances, atrophy of the caudate nuclei has been pronounced, almost to the degree seen in Huntington's chorea. The thalamus, subthalamic nucleus, substantia nigra, and globus pallidus may also be affected.

The salient histologic feature is a loss of neurons most marked in the three outer cortical layers. Surviving neurons are often swollen and contain argentophilic (Pick) bodies within the cytoplasm. In some cases, however, the alterations in neurons are not demonstrable. There is a loss of medullated fibers in the white matter beneath the atrophic cortex. A heavy astrocytic gliosis is seen in both the cortex and subcortical white matter. Most neuropathologists consider the loss of myelinated fibers to be consequent to neuronal loss; Spatz believed that the site of primary damage was in the axon near the cell body, with swelling of the latter as an "axonal reaction." Senile plaques and Alzheimer neurofibrillary changes are frequently seen in the atrophic zones, and there is granulovacuolar degeneration of neurons in the hippocampus, as in Alzheimer's disease.

Symptomatology Whether the diagnosis is possible during life is doubtful, and our clinical predictions as to the existence of the disease have been erratic. In our opinion, the gradual onset of forgetfulness and confusion with respect to place and time, slowness of comprehension, inability to cope with unaccustomed problems, depreciation of social and work habits, and impairments in personality and behavior do not in any way distinguish Pick's disease from Alzheimer's and other degenerative diseases. Several experienced neurologists have commented that the patient with Pick's disease is likely to be apathetic and indifferent rather than irritable and bad-humored. Focal disturbances are said to be early and prominent in Pick's disease, pointing to a lesion in the frontal, temporal, or parietal lobes. According to Malamud and Lowenberg, memory, orientation, and attention tend to be well preserved in patients whose disease is limited to the temporal lobes, in contrast to Alzheimer's disease. Language disorder has been reported in two-thirds of all cases of Pick's disease. At first the patient speaks less but language is intact; later he or she may forget and misuse words and fail to understand much of what is heard or read. Speech becomes a "medley of disconnected words and phrases" and eventually is reduced to an incomprehensible jargon. Finally, the patient is altogether mute, seemingly without impulse to speak or ability to form words. Verbal perseveration, palilalia, and echolalia have been described. Bulimia and alterations in sexual behavior occur to a distressing degree in some patients (Tissot et al.).

Wilson distinguished two patterns of behavior: in one, the patient is talkative, lighthearted and gay or anxious and uneasy, constantly on the move, occupied with trifles, and attentive to every passing incident; in the other behavior pattern, the patient is taciturn, inert, emotionally dull, and lacking in initiative and impulse.

Exceptionally, cerebellar ataxia or shuffling gait, weakness, rigidity and pseudocontractures of limbs, and marked grasping and sucking dominate the picture, the latter reflecting frontal lobe involvement. Extrapyramidal rigidity and spasticity may also appear. Van Mansvelt remarks upon seven or eight cases in which there was an associated amyotrophic lateral sclerosis, a relationship which we have been unable to corroborate in a pathologic study of several cases of Pick's disease.

The cause of Pick's disease is unknown. Sjögren et al. concluded from a genetic survey of the cases in Stockholm that it was probably transmitted as a dominant trait with polygenic modification. Women seem to be affected more often than men. Van Mansvelt emphasized the possible importance of trauma. No chemical, vascular, or other factor of causal importance has been identified.

The course of the illness is usually 2 to 5 years, occasionally longer, and nothing can be done therapeutically except to postpone the end by careful nursing.

OTHER DEMENTING DISEASES

There are other forms of progressive, diffuse brain atrophy leading to dementia that show none of the pathologic features of either Alzheimer's or Pick's disease, or any of the other hereditary diseases associated with dementia [Wilson's disease, Creutzfeld-Jakob disease, amyotrophic lateral sclerosis (ALS), etc.].

In Sweden, for example, Sjögren has found familial cases of this type, as have Schaumburg and Suzuki in this country, and we have seen occasional sporadic ex-

amples. The clinical picture in these cases has been indistinguishable from that of Alzheimer's disease, and autopsy has disclosed widespread cerebral atrophy, most pronounced in the frontal and temporal lobes. Microscopically these cases were characterized by a diffuse neuronal loss, slight glial proliferation, and secondary demyelination of the white matter, but no other histologic changes of note. Other instances of sporadic and familial presenile dementia have shown subcortical gliosis or nonspecific cellular changes (pyknosis of nerve cells and nuclei, loss of Nissl substance). Some examples of the latter type have in the past been described under the rubric of Kraepelin's disease. The pathologic changes are not sufficiently well described to permit classification; some could be explained on the basis of anoxic damage or a variety of other metabolic illnesses. There are no valid grounds for considering Kraepelin's disease as a clinical-pathological entity. A relatively pure degeneration of thalamic neurons has also been found in relation to a progressive dementia (see Corsellis). The clinical tableau of each of these diseases lacks specificity and therefore will not be described.

In addition to these unclassified forms of dementia, there are other somewhat better characterized dementing diseases, such as the following:

1. *Arteriosclerotic dementia* refers to an impairment of intellectual function due to multiple infarcts, and as would be expected, vascular lesions in special regions such as the medial temporal lobes, the medial frontal lobes, corpus callosum, and the nondominant parietal lobe induce certain special psychic aberrations already described in Chaps. 21 and 33. In all such instances the history of one or more strokes can usually be elicited, and the focal deficit will have had the characteristic temporal profile of such an event. The degree of focal neurologic deficit may be small in comparison to the cognitive impairment, especially if many "silent areas" had been involved. Slow progression of dementia unpunctuated by strokes or only by some minor cerebrovascular incident is usually indicative of the Alzheimer-senile dementia complex, even in the face of hypertension and atherosclerotic occlusion of coronary and other arteries. Multiple lacunae produce a picture of pseudobulbar paresis with its typical labile emotionality, slurred speech, dysphagia, lively facial and mandibular reflexes, etc., but again this rarely happens without at least one incident of stroke. It is now generally agreed that the so-called progressive subcortical encephalitis of Binswanger is a form of arteriosclerosis with multiple infarcts (lacunar and larger infarcts) that tend to be localized to the cerebral white matter and to be associated with dementia.

2. *Severe trauma* may also leave in its wake certain lasting cerebral deficits, usually under circumstances where prolonged coma and stupor have followed the injury. Enduring mental enfeeblement is exceptional, however, except in association with severe neurologic disability of other type (page 604). Surprisingly, McMenemey quotes a number of cases in which a relatively minor cranial injury had initiated a dementia in which the histologic changes of Alzheimer's disease were eventually demonstrated. The authors can only assume that trauma had called attention to an unrelated, ongoing Alzheimer disease.

3. In exceptional instances, *hypoxic encephalopathy and acute inclusion-body (herpes simplex) encephalitis* have left the individual relatively intact, except for impairment of memory and difficulty in learning and assimilating new information. In several such cases, examined pathologically many years later, we have observed destructive lesions limited to the inferomedial portions of both temporal lobes. Unless one knew about the initial event and had accurate information concerning the long-term stability of the intellectual deficit, it would be impossible to differentiate such states clinically from the progressive cerebral degenerative diseases.

DISEASES IN WHICH DEMENTIA IS ASSOCIATED WITH OTHER NEUROLOGIC ABNORMALITIES

HUNTINGTON'S CHOREA

This disease, distinguished by the triad of dominant inheritance, choreoathetosis, and dementia, commemorates the name of George Huntington, a medical practitioner of Pomeroy, Ohio. In 1872, in a paper read before the Meigs and Mason Academy of Medicine and published later that year in the *Medical and Surgical Reporter* of Philadelphia, Huntington gave a succinct and graphic account of the disease, based on observations of patients that his father and grandfather had pointed out to him in the course of their practice in East Hampton, Long Island. Reports of this disease had appeared previously, but lacked the accuracy and completeness of Huntington's description. Vessie, in 1932, was able to show that practically all the patients with this disease in the eastern United States could be traced to about six individuals who had emigrated in 1630 from the tiny East Anglian village of Bures, in Suffolk, England. One remarkable family was traced for 300 years through 12 generations, in each of which the disease had expressed itself.

To quote Huntington, the rule has been that

"When either or both of the parents have shown manifestations of the disease . . . one or more of the offspring invariably suffer of the disease, if they live to adult life. But if by any chance these children go through life without it, the thread is broken and the grandchildren and great-grandchildren of the original shakers may rest assured that they are free from disease." Davenport, in a review of 962 patients with Huntington's chorea, found only five who had descended from unaffected parents. Possibly, in these latter patients, a parent had the trait, but in very mild form. More likely, they represented sporadic instances of Huntington's chorea, i.e., ones in whom a mutation had occurred from the normal gene to the mutant, disease-producing form.

In university hospital centers this is one of the most frequently observed types of hereditary nervous disease. Seldom does a month pass without one coming to our notice. Males are said to be more often affected, but we have been unable to substantiate this point. The usual age of onset is in the fourth and fifth decades, but 5 to 10 percent begin before the twentieth year, and some even in childhood. Once begun, the disease progresses relentlessly, until only a restricted hospital existence is possible, and some other disease mercifully terminates life.

Until the time of manifest symptoms and signs, it has been impossible to foretell which of the children of a patient will be stricken with the disease. Based on the hypothesis that the disease is related to an enhanced sensitivity of striatal neurons to dopamine, the claim has been made that a "challenge" with 3.0 g L-dopa daily (which tends to induce choreoathetosis in parkinsonian patients) for a period of a month will cause chorea in prospective victims. Of 30 subjects (all at 50 percent risk for Huntington's disease) who were treated in this way, 10 developed transient chorea, and 5 of these 10 subjects, within 8 years of the provocative test, have developed Huntington's chorea. Of 20 subjects at risk who had no chorea while receiving L-dopa, one has since been found to have the disease. A longer period of observation of these patients will be required to determine the predictive value of this test (Klawans et al.). Until this information becomes available, L-dopa should not be administered to patients at risk of developing the disease.

Symptomatology The mental disorder assumes several subtle forms long before the deterioration of cognitive function becomes evident. Slight alterations of character are often the source of annoyance to others. Patients begin to find fault and complain about everything and to nag other members of the family; they may be suspicious, irritable, impulsive, eccentric, or excessively religious, or may exhibit a false sense of superiority. Poor self-control may reflect itself in outbursts of temper, alcoholism, or sexual promiscuity. These emotional disturbances and changes in character may reach such proportions as to constitute a virtual psychosis. Disturbances of mood, particularly depression, are common and may constitute the most prominent symptoms early in the disease. Invariably, intellect begins to fail. Memory is among the first faculties to be reduced and also the power to recall the names of common objects. Inattentiveness makes work difficult. The gradual dilapidation of intellect follows the pattern of all types of dementia, with elements of agnosia and apraxia. Often the process is so slow that even though the patient is mentally impaired, some degree of functional capacity is retained for many years.

The abnormality of movement is at first slight and the patient is merely considered to be fidgety or restless and "nervous." Slowly it becomes more pronounced until the entire musculature is involved. Seldom in the advanced stage of the disease is the patient still for more than a few seconds. The disorder of movement has been described fully in Chap. 4.

As Wilson has pointed out, the relation of the choreic to mental symptoms "abides by no general rule." Most often the psychic disorder accompanies the chorea, but it may follow the onset of chorea, sometimes by several years. In some cases the illness develops in the reverse order. Thus, either the chorea or the mental changes may be present for a long time without the other. A recurrent theme in older medical writings, unproven in our opinion, is that Huntington families have an inordinately high incidence of other neuropathic or psychopathic tendencies—mental retardation, constitutional psychopathy, neuroses, and the like. Of undoubted neuropsychiatric importance is the high suicide rate in Huntingtonians. Also there is a high incidence of trauma; nearly half the patients with Huntington's chorea dying at the Massachusetts General Hospital have had chronic subdural hematomas.

Children with Huntington's chorea may exhibit the first signs of the disease before puberty (even under the age of 4) and several small series of such cases have been described. Mental deterioration at this early age is more often accompanied by seizures and rigidity than by

chorea. However, a rigid form of the disease is known also to occur in adults. Earlier onset in successive generations (*anticipation*) has been reported in the past, but has not been confirmed by the more recent study of Chandler et al. The latter authors have shown that the disease is generally more severe in cases of early onset (15 to 40 years) than in those of later onset (55 to 60 years). Furthermore, in the patients with early onset of the disease, the emotional disturbance tends to be initially prominent and precedes the chorea and intellectual loss by many years; with older age of onset, choreiform movements and progressive dementia are more often the initial components and have their onset at nearly the same age.

Pathology Gross wasting of the head of the caudate nucleus and putamen bilaterally is the characteristic abnormality, usually accompanied by a moderate degree of gyral atrophy in the frontal and temporal regions. The caudatal atrophy alters the configuration of the frontal horns of the lateral ventricles; the inferolateral borders do not show the usual bulge created by the head of the caudate nucleus, and in addition the ventricles are diffusely enlarged. In CT scans the bicaudate-cranial index is increased in the majority of patients. This finding corroborates the clinical diagnosis in the moderately advanced case.

The articles of Alzheimer (1911), Ramsay Hunt (1917), and Dunlap (1927) contain the most authoritative descriptions of the microscopic changes. In the striatum the majority of the small cells disappear and are replaced by fibrous astrocytes; the large cells are relatively preserved. The preserved neurons in Huntington's chorea exhibit no special alterations. The anterior parts of the putamen and caudatum are more affected than the posterior parts. With the neuronal loss the myelinated fibers also disappear. In our own cases we have not been impressed with changes in the globus pallidus, subthalamic nucleus, red nucleus, or cerebellum; but slight changes have been seen in the substantia nigra. In the atrophic parts of the cerebral cortex, there is slight neuronal loss in layers 3, 5, and 6, with replacement gliosis. Cases are reported with typical striatal lesions but normal cortices, where only senile chorea had been present during life. Several neuropathologists have observed marked cell loss and gliosis in the subthalamic nuclei in children or young adults with chorea and behavior disorders.

The biochemical defects in Huntington's chorea are only beginning to be understood. Since at least a partial explanation for L-dopa induced involuntary movements is an excess quantity of dopamine (in contrast to Parkinson's disease where there is a decrease), it has been postulated that the abnormal movements of Huntington's chorea represent a heightened sensitivity of striatal receptors to dopamine. The induction of *tardive dyskinesias* by the chronic administration of phenothiazines would support such a concept. Probably there is a disturbance in the metabolism of other putative neurotransmitters as well. Spokes reports noradrenaline to be increased in the striatum and lateral pallidum. Bird and Iversen found that glutamic acid decarboxylase and choline acetyltransferase are reduced in these areas. γ-Aminobutyric acid (GABA) and acetylcholine are also reduced since they are dependent on the activity of these two enzymes. Enna has shown that the GABA-binding sites on striatal neurons are not depleted beyond what would be expected from loss of nerve cells. Therefore one would expect that the strategy of facilitating GABA-nergic transmission would be effective. So far however, the treatment of Huntington's chorea with GABA-mimetic drugs has met with only limited success (Shoulson et al.).

Diagnostic Problems Once the disease has been observed in its fully developed form it requires no great clinical acumen to recognize it. The main difficulty arises in patients who lack a family history but in whom the progressive chorea, emotional disturbance, and dementia beginning in adult life are typical. Sometimes it is learned later that the family history was incomplete or falsified, or that an illness in a parent had been misinterpreted. Chorea that begins in late life, with only mild or questionable intellectual impairment and without a family history of similar disease, is another source of difficulty; referring to it as *senile chorea* does not solve the problem. Indeed, senile chorea may have more than one cause. We have seen it appear with infections and drug therapy, only to disappear after a few weeks. *Recurrent chorea* in early adult life always raises the question of a late form of Sydenham's chorea, an illness in which neither family history nor mental deterioration are seen. Dominant inheritance of other progressive neurologic disorders, beginning in adolescence or adult life (polymyoclonus with or without ataxia, double athetosis) always raises questions of atypical Huntington's chorea; these matters are impossible to resolve clinically. Even the pathologic picture may not settle the matter, for the typical lesions of Huntington's chorea in the striatum are seen in striatonigral degeneration and in other diseases.

Therapy The authors have not been impressed with any of the currently available drugs. Levodopa makes the chorea worse and, in the rigid form of the disease, evokes chorea. Phenothiazines (particularly fluphena-

zine) and butyrophenones (haloperidol), the drugs most favored at the present time, seldom suppress the chorea except early in the illness when the movement disorder is mild. They seem to act by inducing rigidity. They may help alleviate eccentricities of behavior or emotional lability. Drugs which facilitate GABA and acetylcholine synthesis have been unsuccessful. The juvenile form of the disease is probably best treated with antiparkinsonian drugs. The disease pursues a steady progressive course and death occurs, on an average, 15 to 16 years after onset, sometimes much earlier or later.

CORTICOSTRIATOSPINAL DEGENERATION [PARKINSON DEMENTIA (PD) AND AMYOTROPHIC LATERAL SCLEROSIS (ALS) COMPLEX]

In 1921, Jakob, under the title "spastic pseudosclerosis," described a chronic disease of middle to late adult life which was characterized clinically by abnormalities of behavior and intellect; weakness, ataxia, and spasticity of the limbs (chiefly the legs); extrapyramidal symptoms such as rigidity, slowness of movement, tremors, athetotic postures, and hesitant, dysarthric speech; and normal spinal fluid. The lesions were diffuse and consisted mainly of an outfall of neurons in the frontal, temporal, and central motor gyri, the corpus striatum, ventromedial thalamus, bulbar motor nuclei, and spinal cord. In one of Jakob's cases, there were prominent changes in the anterior horns and corticospinal tracts in the spinal cord, like those of amyotrophic lateral sclerosis (ALS). This latter finding probably gave rise to Wilson's concept of the disease as a *corticostriatospinal degeneration*. A degenerative and probably familial disorder that had been described earlier by Creutzfeldt was considered by Spielmeyer to be sufficiently similar to the one of Jakob to warrant the designation Creutzfeldt-Jakob disease.

The disorder described by Creutzfeldt and Jakob has been a source of endless controversy because of its indeterminate character. On the one hand, it has been confused with the subacutely evolving myoclonic dementia (sometimes called Heidenhain's disease, when visual disorder is prominent, or "subacute spongiform encephalopathy") which is now known to be an infection akin to Kuru, due to a transmissible agent. The authors believe that this latter disease, which is described on page 525, bears at best only a superficial resemblance to the one described by Creutzfeldt and Jakob, and that the two disorders should be clearly separated. Unfortunately, the eponym is so entrenched in medical usage that any attempt to remove it stands little chance of success.

On the other side, the disease described by Creutzfeldt and Jakob merges with progressive dementia and spastic paraplegia, with progressive dementia and ALS, with the Parkinson-dementia-ALS complex of Guam, and with the corticopallidospinal degeneration of Davison. One is tempted to conclude that it should not be reckoned with as a disease type, and certainly everyone agrees that the term *pseudosclerosis* (also used for the Westphal-Strümpell form of hepatolenticular degeneration) is worthless. Wilson's arguments for retaining the entity described by Jakob are rational, but the authors doubt that it refers to a disease *sui generis.*

The authors have observed patients in which extreme rigidity, pyramidal signs, and evidences of amyotrophic lateral sclerosis have developed over a period of several years. In the later stages of the disease the patient while alert is totally helpless, unable to speak, swallow, or to move the limbs. Only eye movements are retained. Intellectual functioning is better preserved than movement but is difficult to assess. All other bodily functions are preserved. The course is slowly progressive and ends fatally in 5 to 10 years. There is no family history, and there are no clues as to causation.

DIFFUSE CEREBRAL SCLEROSIS

In the older neurologic literature one finds numerous references to a state of the brain, found sometimes among the insane, in which the tissue is unduly firm. Distinction was drawn customarily between "lobar sclerosis" in which one lobe or parts of lobes were affected (usually consequent to birth injury) and a diffuse or generalized sclerosis.

Advances in neuropathology have negated the value of this ancient concept of disease. It has been found that many diseases both of the poliodystrophic and leukodystrophic type reach an end stage of sclerosis. The reader will find more precise descriptions of these changes on pages 660 and 670 under Schilder's and Tay-Sachs diseases.

CEREBROCEREBELLAR DEGENERATION

See below under cerebellar degenerations.

FAMILIAL DEMENTIA WITH SPASTIC PARAPARESIS

From time to time the authors have encountered families in which several members during middle adult years have developed a spastic paraparesis and a gradual failure of intellect. The mental horizon of the patient narrowed gradually, and the capacity for high-level thinking diminished; in addition the examination showed appropriately exaggerated tendon reflexes, clonus, and Babinski signs. In one such family this illness had occurred in two generations; in another, three brothers in a single generation were afflicted.

Worster-Drought, Greenfield, and McMenemey have reported the pathologic findings in two cases of this type. In addition to senile plaques and neurofibrillary changes, there was demyelination of the subcortical white matter and corpus callosum and a "patchy but gross swelling of the arterioles" which gave the staining reactions for amyloid (Scholz's perivascular plaques). Van Bogaert et al. have published an account of similar cases which showed the characteristic pathologic features of Alzheimer's disease.

Adult forms of metachromatic leukoencephalopathy, as in the families described by Austin, may present with a similar clinical picture. Another interesting association of familial spastic paraplegia is with progressive cerebellar ataxia. Fully a third of the cases we have seen with such a spastic weakness were ataxic and would fall in the category of spinocerebellar degenerations.

CORTICAL-BASAL GANGLIONIC SYNDROMES

Over the years the authors have observed several elderly patients, both men and women, in whom a progressive unilateral extrapyramidal rigidity, resembling that of Parkinson's disease, was associated with a cortical sensory defect. The patients, although able to exert considerable muscle power, could not voluntarily direct their efforts. Attempts to move a limb in one direction to accomplish some purposeful act might result in a totally inappropriate movement, always with great enhancement of the rigidity in the limb and in other affected parts. In other attempts an arm or leg might be elevated persistently, sometimes without the patient being aware of it—a kind of involuntary catalepsy. With progression of the disease the limbs on both sides of the body and the cranial muscles were involved; and a variable combination of apraxia, rigidity, sensory ataxia, and action tremor finally rendered the patient helpless, unable to sit, stand, speak, or take care of basic needs. Mental deterioration of nonspecific type occurred late, but only in some cases. The condition progressed for 5 years or more before some medical complication overtook the patient.

Postmortem examination has disclosed a combination of findings that stamps the disease process as unique. Cortical atrophy (mainly in the parietal lobes) is associated with degeneration of the substantia nigra and, in one instance, of the dentatorubrothalamic fibers. The atrophy is mild (unlike that of Pick's disease), more on one side than the other, with loss of neurons and their medullated fibers in all layers of the cortex. There is moderate gliosis in the cortex and white matter. Many of the residual nerve cells are swollen and chromatolyzed with eccentric nuclei, a state to which Rebeiz and his colleagues have given the name *achromasia*. It resembles the central chromatolysis of axonal reaction. No Alzheimer fibrillary changes, senile plaques, granulovacuolar changes, amyloid deposits, or Lewy bodies are seen.

Marinescu has described a rather different state resembling more a severe form of Alzheimer's disease, but with signs of both pyramidal and extrapyramidal disease (rigidity, tremor, nystagmus, incoordination, confusion, disorientation, and loss of memory). Again there was amyloidosis of blood vessels ("Scholz's perivascular plaques," see above) in the cerebral white matter as well as in the liver and kidney. The disease bears some resemblance to the corticostriatospinal degeneration of Creutzfeldt and Jakob.

DISEASES CHARACTERIZED BY ABNORMALITIES OF POSTURE AND MOVEMENT

PARALYSIS AGITANS (PARKINSON'S DISEASE)

This rather common disease, known since ancient times, was first cogently described by James Parkinson, in 1817. In his words, it is characterized by "involuntary tremulous motion, with lessened muscular power, in parts not in action and even when supported; with a propensity to bend the trunk forward, and to pass from a walking to a running pace, the senses and intellect being uninjured." Strangely, his essay contains no reference to rigidity or to slowness of movement, and, in the authors' opinion, it stressed unduly the reduction in muscular power. The same criticism can be leveled against the term *paralysis agitans*, which appeared for the first time in Marshall Hall's textbook *Diseases and Derangements of the Nervous System*, in 1841.

Certain biometric data are of interest. The degenerative form of the disease begins most frequently between 40 and 70 years of age with the peak age of onset in the sixth decade. It is infrequent before 30 years of age (only 4 in 380 cases in one series) and although some observers comment on a higher incidence in men, we have not been impressed with a sex difference. Trauma, emotional upset, overwork, exposure to cold, etc. have been suggested as predisposing or exciting factors, but there is no convincing evidence to support such claims. The malady is observed in all countries, all ethnic groups, and all socioeconomic classes. Familial cases are on record, but the evidence is rather unsubstantial, especially when one allows the possibility that the cases may be examples of postencephalitic parkinsonism or striatonigral degeneration.

The disease is frequent. In the United States there are approximately a half-million patients; about 1 percent of the population over the age of 50 years is affected. The incidence in all countries where vital statistics are kept is the same. Considering its frequency, coincidence in a family on the basis of chance occurrence might be as high as 5 percent.

Symptomatology The core syndrome of expressionless face, rigidity, poverty and slowness of voluntary movement, "resting" tremor, stooped posture, and festinating gait has been fully described in Chap. 4, and only certain diagnostic problems and variants in the clinical picture will be considered here. The early symptoms may be difficult to perceive and are often overlooked. Advancing years have a way of rendering the spine and limbs less pliable and elastic; and in the senium the gait may become short-stepped and then reduced to a shuffle, and the voice tends to become soft and monotonous. Hence it is all too easy to simply attribute the early symptoms to the effects of age. The patient may for a long time not be conscious of the inroads of the disease; at first the only complaints will be of aching, fatigue, and malaise. A slight stiffness and slowness are ignored until one day it occurs to the physician or to a member of the family that the patient has Parkinson's disease. Infrequency of blinking, as pointed out originally by Pierre Marie, is often a helpful early sign. The usual rate (about 15 to 20 blinks per minute) is reduced in the parkinsonian patient to 5 to 10. And with it there is a slight widening of the palpebral fissures (Stellwag's sign). When seated, the patient makes fewer little shifts and adjustments of position than the normal person, and the fingers straighten and assume a flexed and adducted posture at the metacarpal-phalangeal joints.

The characteristic tremor, which usually involves a hand, is often listed as the initial sign; but in at least half the cases, observant family members will have remarked earlier on the relative immobility and the poverty of movement. Other warning symptoms are aching in the neck, shoulders, back, and hips which may be passed off as osteoarthritis, a surmise which may be correct except that parkinsonian rigidity may have aggravated the pain.

The tremor of the fully developed case takes several forms, as was remarked in Chap. 5. A rather coarse 4-per-second "pill-rolling" tremor of the thumb and fingers is the most frequent, and is typically present when the hand is motionless, i.e., not used in voluntary movement (hence the term *resting tremor*). Complete rest, however, abolishes or reduces the tremor, and a volitional movement usually but not always dampens it momentarily. The rhythmic beat coincides with an alternating burst of activity in agonists and antagonists in the EMG. Arm, jaw, tongue, eyelids, and foot are less often involved. The least degree of tremor is felt during passive movement of a rigid part (cogwheel phenomenon or Negro's sign). The tremor shows surprising fluctuations from moment to moment and is aggravated by excitement.

Lance et al. have called attention to another type of tremor in paralysis agitans—a fine, 7- to 8-per-second, slightly irregular action tremor of the outstretched fingers and hands. Unlike the slower tremor, this one quickly vanishes with relaxation and persists throughout voluntary movement. Electromyographically, it lacks the alternating bursts of action potentials seen in the more typical tremor. The patient may have either type of tremor or both.

The authors have been less impressed with rigidity and hypertonus as important early findings. When present, they tend to appear in the more advanced stages of the disease. Once rigidity develops, it is constantly present, and can be felt by the palpating finger and seen as a salience of muscle groups. When the examiner passively moves the limb, a mild resistance appears from the start (without the short free interval of the spastic limb) and it continues evenly throughout the movement, being altered only by the cogwheel phenomenon.

The basic postural hypertonus predominates in the flexor muscles of trunk and limbs and confers upon the patient the characteristic flexed posture. Particulars of the parkinsonian disorders of muscle tone and of stance and gait are discussed in Chaps. 4 and 6.

As regards the quality of volitional and postural movements, a few additional points may be made. The patient is clearly slow in attempts to deliver a quick hard blow and in a series of successive movements of identical type is increasingly hampered. This is called bradykinesia. Attempts at alternating movements, at first successful, become progressively impeded and finally are blocked completely or adopt the rhythm of the patient's tremor. Originally it was thought that rigidity interferes with facility of movement, but the observation that ap-

propriately placed surgical lesions can abolish rigidity without affecting the disorder of movement refutes this interpretation. Thus the difficulty is not one of rigidity but of brady- or *akinesia*, and this latter factor also underlies the characteristic poverty of movement, shown by infrequency of swallowing, slowness of chewing, disinclination to adjust the position of the body and limbs, lack of small "movements of cooperation" as in arising from a chair without first adjusting the feet, absence of arm swing in walking, etc. As was stated, the patient is able to generate normal or near-normal power, especially in the large muscles, but in the small ones strength is somewhat diminished. According to Hallett and Khoshbin, the parkinsonian patient cannot complete a quick movement by a single burst of agonist-antagonist-agonist sequence of energizing activity, like the normal patient (see also page 34).

As the disorder of movement worsens, all accustomed activities show the effects. Handwriting becomes small (micrographia), tremulous, and cramped, as was first noted by Charcot. The voice softens and the speech seems hurried and monotonous; the voice becomes less audible and finally the patient only whispers. Exceptionally, "mumbling" is an early complaint. The consumption of a meal takes an hour. Each morsel of food must be swallowed before the next bite is taken. Walking becomes reduced to a shuffle; the patient frequently loses balance, and in walking forward or backward must "chase the body's center of gravity" in order to avoid falling (festination). Defense reactions are faulty. Persistent extension or clawing of the toes and other dystonic postures may enter the picture.

These various motor impediments and tremor often begin in one limb and spread to one side (monoplegic and hemiplegic pattern) and later to both sides until the patient is quite helpless. Yet in the excitement of some unusual circumstance (a fire, for example) the patient is capable of brief but remarkably effective movement (*kinesis paradoxica*).

The tendon reflexes vary as they do in normal individuals, from being barely elicitable to brisk. Even when parkinsonian symptoms are confined to one side of the body, it can be shown that the reflexes are equal on the two sides, and the plantar responses are flexor. There is inability to inhibit blinking in response to a tap over the bridge of the nose (Meyerson's sign). Commonly there is an impairment of upward gaze and convergence. Bradykinesia may extend to eye movements, in that the patients may show a delay in the initiation of gaze and slowing of eye movements (decreased maximal saccadic velocity). There are no sensory changes. Drooling is troublesome; an excess flow of saliva has been assumed, but the problem actually is one of inability to swallow the normal amount. Seborrhea and excessive sweating are also secondary, the former to failure to wash the face with the usual frequency, the latter to the effects of the constant motor overactivity. Syncope becomes frequent in some cases, and was found by Rajput and Rozdilsky to be related to cell loss in the sympathetic ganglia.

As indicated earlier in this chapter, dementia is commonly associated with Parkinson's disease. In the series reported by Lieberman et al., 168 of 520 patients (32 percent) with Parkinson's disease had moderate to severe dementia—an incidence that was tenfold higher than that in their age-matched spouses. The demented patients, in addition to being somewhat older, were more severely involved in a shorter time and responded less well to L-dopa than the nondemented ones.

Diagnosis As pointed out on page 521, the epidemic of encephalitis lethargica (von Economo's encephalitis) that spread over western Europe and the United States after the First World War left great numbers of parkinsonian cases in its wake. The interval between the encephalitis and the development of extrapyramidal signs varied from months to years. The earlier age of onset, the more rapid progression of symptoms and signs followed by stabilization, and the presence of a variety of other neurologic disorders (psychopathic behavior, tics, spasms, oculogyric crises and other restricted motor disorders, breathing arrhythmias, hyperphagia, bizarre movements, postures and gaits) distinguished this disease from the one described by Parkinson. Strangely, no instances of this form of encephalitis were recorded before the period 1914-1918, and virtually none have been seen since 1930; hence postencephalitic parkinsonism has nearly disappeared. Rarely, a Parkinson-like syndrome has been described with other forms of encephalitis (Coxsackie B, Japanese B, and St. Louis viral infections).

In England and Europe an "arteriopathic" or "arteriosclerotic" form of Parkinson's disease is much diagnosed, but the authors have never been convinced of its reality. Pseudobulbar (spastic bulbar) palsy from a series of lacunar infarcts (see page 552) can create a clinical picture simulating Parkinson's disease, but unilateral and bilateral corticospinal tract signs, hyperactive facial reflexes, pathologic emotionality, and other characteristic features of spastic bulbar palsy distinguish it from Parkinson's disease. The rigidity (the hallmark of the arteriosclerotic form) is in reality a combination of spasticity and rigidity. Of course, the parkinsonian patient in advancing years is not impervious to cerebrovascular disease, and the two conditions then overlap.

Senile (or essential) tremor is distinguished from that of Parkinson's disease by its fine, quick quality and

tendency to become manifest during volitional movement and to disappear when the limb is in a position of repose, and by the lack of associated slowness of movement, flexed postures, etc. The head is more often involved in senile tremor than in Parkinson's disease. Some senile tremors are familial. Some of the slower forms are indistinguishable from the tremor of Parkinson's disease.

Progressive supranuclear palsy (see further on in this section) is characterized by rigidity and dystonic postures of the neck and shoulders, masklike facies, and a tendency to topple upon attempting to walk—all of which are suggestive of Parkinson's disease. Paralysis of vertical gaze and eventually of lateral gaze with retention of certain reflex eye movements establishes the correct diagnosis.

Paucity of movement, unchanging attitudes and postural sets, and slightly stiff and unbalanced gait may be observed in retarded depression and also in the syndrome of low-pressure hydrocephalus. Since as many as 25 to 30 percent of parkinsonian patients are depressed, the separation of these two conditions may be difficult. The authors have seen patients, called parkinsonian by competent neurologists, whose movements became normal when antidepressant drugs or electroconvulsive therapy were given.

The rapid onset of Parkinson's syndrome, especially in conjunction with other medical diseases, should always raise suspicion of phenothiazine effects; reserpine, tranquilizing and antidepressant medication, chlorpromazine, and haloperidol, all cause a slight masking of the face, stiffness of the trunk and limbs, lack of arm swing, fine tremor of the hands, and mumbling speech. Also they may evoke a curious restlessness, a "muscular impatience," an inability to sit still, much like that which occurs at times in the parkinsonian patient. Bing called this state *akathisia*, adapting a term that Haskovec had earlier applied to the restlessness of certain neurotic individuals. Spasms of neck, facial, and jaw muscles (open mouth, protruded tongue, retrocollis or torticollis, grimacing) may also be provoked by such drugs. A mild, localized rigidity from local tetanus was studied by one of the authors (R.D.A.) in a patient who had been referred as a case of acute parkinsonism.

Early in the course of paralysis agitans, when only a slight asymmetry of stride or an ineptitude of one hand are present, and tremor has yet to appear and impart the unmistakable stamp of the disease, a number of small signs may be helpful in diagnosis. Lack of increased tendon reflexes in the affected limb or of a Babinski sign eliminates a corticospinal lesion, and lack of a grasp reflex excludes a premotor cerebral disorder. Blepharoclonus, Meyerson's sign, digital impedance (tendency to a block in performance of rapid alternating movements or to assume a tremor rhythm), and lack of arm swing are all indicative of early Parkinson's disease.

Pathology   Quite remarkable is the obscurity of the morbid anatomy of paralysis agitans. A lack of familiarity with the detailed anatomic structure of the basal ganglia and midbrain, and a tendency to confuse minor senile changes with those of the disease led to many false postulations in early writings—imputing the primary change to muscles, or to lesions of the striatum, pallidum, and various afferent and efferent systems of basal ganglionic fibers. Even so thorough a student of basal ganglia disease as S. A. K. Wilson did not mention, in his textbook of neurology, the obvious cell loss in the substantia nigra, and Bielschowsky only listed it as one of many structures that are slightly affected.

All modern neuropathologists accept the loss of pigmented cells in the substantia nigra and other pigmented nuclei (locus ceruleus, etc.) as the most constant finding in both paralysis agitans and postencephalitic Parkinson's disease. This structure is visibly pale in gross specimens and is seen to be markedly depleted of cells under the microscope, a combination which enables one to state with confidence that the patient must have suffered from Parkinson's disease. Also, many of the remaining cells of the nigra and locus ceruleus contain eosinophilic cytoplasmic inclusions, called *Lewy bodies*. These are seen in practically all cases of paralysis agitans. They may be present in postencephalitic cases as well, but in the latter neurofibrillary tangles are more usual. Both of these cellular abnormalities appear occasionally in the substantia nigra of aging, nonparkinsonian individuals, however. Possibly these individuals would have developed paralysis agitans if they had lived a few more years. Other depletions of cells are widespread, but they are minor and inconsistent and their significance is less clear. In the sympathetic ganglia there is slight neuronal loss and Lewy bodies, and this is also true of several of the lower brainstem nuclei as well as of the putamen, caudatum, pallidum, and substantia innominata. The lack of a consistent lesion in either the striatum or pallidum is noteworthy, in view of the reciprocal connections between the striatum and nigra and the

depletion of striatal dopamine that characterizes the parkinsonian state.

Treatment   Although there is no known treatment that will halt or reverse the neuronal degeneration that presumably underlies Parkinson's disease, methods are now available which can afford considerable relief from symptoms. Treatment can be medical or surgical, or both. Surgical measures are rarely necessary, and reliance is placed almost exclusively on drugs, particularly on L-dopa and to a lesser extent on anticholinergic and other agents.

At present, L-*dihydroxyphenylalanine* (L-*dopa*) is unquestionably the most effective agent for the treatment of Parkinson's disease, and the therapeutic results, even in those with far-advanced disease, are far better than have ever been obtained with other drugs. The theoretic basis for the use of this compound rests on the observation that striatal dopamine is depleted in patients with Parkinson's disease. Initially, 500 mg of L-dopa should be given daily, in several divided doses. The daily dose should be increased by 500 mg each week until 4.0 to 5.0 g/day are being given. The combination of L-dopa with a decarboxylase inhibitor (Sinemet) prevents its rapid destruction in the blood and permits the control of symptoms more quickly and with a much lower dose (10 to 25 mg inhibitor with 100 to 250 mg L-dopa, three or four times a day).

L-Dopa is not without serious toxic effects, so that it is not universally applicable. Approximately two-thirds of patients tolerate the drug and experience few serious side effects; and one-third of them will show dramatic improvement, especially in hypokinesia. Many patients are at first troubled by nausea, especially if the medication is not taken with meals, and a few have hypotensive episodes. Nausea can be allayed by antiemetic medication, but usually it disappears with continued use of the drug. Psychiatric symptoms may also present problems, and they are to be expected in 15 to 25 percent of patients. With L-dopa therapy, mood may improve and activity increase, with the danger in frail elderly patients of accidental fractures and heart failure or myocardial infarction. Excitement and aggressiveness appear in a few. An increase in or a return of libido may lead to sexual assertiveness. In many parkinsonian patients, however, there is depression, even to the point of suicide; delusional thinking may occur in these circumstances. This combination of disorders is extremely difficult to treat, and one must turn to a medical antidepressant regimen, as described in Chap. 53.

The most common and troublesome effect of L-dopa, and the limiting factor in its use, is the induction of involuntary movements—restlessness, grimacing, lingual-labial dyskinesia, and choreoathetosis and dystonia of the limbs, neck, and trunk. Above a certain daily dose, which varies from patient to patient (usually 3 to 5 g), very few patients escape these effects, forcing a reduction in dosage. Often some degree of dyskinesia must be accepted as the price to be paid for the therapeutic effect.

If involuntary movements are induced by relatively small doses of L-dopa, the therapeutic effect may be enhanced to some extent by the addition of other dopaminergic agents such as amantidine or bromocriptine. *Amantadine,* an antiviral agent, is thought to act by releasing dopamine from striatal neurons; it is given in doses of 50 to 100 mg three times daily. Its benefit appears almost immediately; both hypokinesia and rigidity are reduced and tremor to a lesser degree. The side effects are similar to L-dopa but much milder. Edema of the legs has been troublesome in some of the treated patients. Amantadine is effective in combination with L-dopa and anticholinergic drugs. Given alone or in combination with the latter, it offers an alternative treatment for patients with early Parkinson's disease or those who do not tolerate L-dopa. *Bromocriptine* is an ergot derivative, whose action in Parkinson's disease is explained by its stimulating effect on dopamine receptors. The drug should be introduced cautiously, 10 mg twice daily, and the dosage increased very slowly, up to 100 mg/day. It has a longer action than L-dopa and causes nausea and vomiting less often, but otherwise the action and side effects of the two drugs are much the same. Furthermore, bromocriptine is much more expensive than L-dopa.

Anticholinergic agents related to atropine are now used mainly in conjunction with L-dopa, but occasionally, in patients who cannot tolerate the latter drug, they are used as the mainstay of treatment. Several synthetic preparations are available, including trihexyphenidyl (Artane), cycrimine (Pagitane), procyclidine (Kemadrin), biperiden (Akineton), and benztropine mesylate (Cogentin). Whereas these drugs differ little from one another in their overall effectiveness in large groups of patients, an individual patient may respond better to one of them than to another, and occasionally after one has been given for a prolonged period, change to another may be attended by some additional improvement—perhaps only from the psychological effect of a change in regimen. In order to obtain maximum benefit from the use of these drugs, they should be given in gradually increasing dosage to the point where toxic effects begin to appear: dryness of the mouth (which can be beneficial when drooling of saliva is a problem), blurring of vision

from pupillary mydriasis (for which corrective spectacles may be indicated), constipation, and sometimes urinary retention (especially with prostatism). Unfortunately, mental slowing, confusional states, hallucinations, and impairment of memory—especially in patients with already impaired mental function—are frequent side effects of these drugs and sharply limit their usefulness. The optimum dosage level is the point at which the greatest relief from tremor is achieved within the limits of tolerable side effects. Occasionally further benefit may accrue from the addition of one of the antihistaminic drugs, such as diphenhydramine or phenindamine. In some patients, particularly in those in whom tremor is prominent, ethopropazine (Parsidol) 30 to 60 mg daily in divided doses, is useful. An important note of warning: under no circumstance should a medication program with anticholinergic agents be stopped suddenly. If this is done, the patient is likely to become totally immobilized and incapacitated by an abrupt and severe increase of tremor and rigidity.

Long-term treatment with L-dopa has not prevented the slow advance of the disease. Late complications appear in approximately 80 percent of treated patients, and those who initially benefit the most are liable to the late development of abnormal movements. In some instances the patient becomes so sensitive to L-dopa that as little as an excess of 50 to 100 mg will precipitate violent choreoathetosis, and if the dose is lowered by the same amount, the patient develops disabling rigidity. Frequently and unpredictably, in a matter of minutes or from one hour to the next, the patient may change from a state of relative mobility to one of complete or nearly complete immobility—the so-called *on-off phenomenon.* Some patients function quite well in the morning and much less well in the afternoon, or vice versa. In such cases, one must literally titrate the dose of L-dopa and space the doses during the 24-h day; combining it with anticholinergic medicines and amantadine is helpful. Sometimes temporarily withdrawing L-dopa and at the same time substituting other medications will control the on-off phenomenon and the severe choreoathetosis.

From what has been said, it is clear that the best combination of drugs and their dosages will vary from patient to patient. The patients who can be expected to benefit the most from treatment with anti-Parkinson drugs are those with relatively mild disease in whom relief from the symptoms is sufficient to warrant toleration of some side effects. In those more severely affected, the relief is partial, and eventually a degree of incapacity is reached which is not significantly responsive to the most carefully planned regimen of medications. With the advent of L-dopa therapy the authors have the impression that the disease process is slowed and a much larger proportion of patients can be kept in a stable state for many years. One of the authors has under his care three surgeons and three physicians, and all are maintaining a full schedule of professional work after 5 years of L-dopa therapy. Observing such good therapeutic results, it is only natural to ask whether these benign forms had always existed. It is difficult to answer this question, but there are cases on record in which patients were alive after having the disease for 50 years.

Success with L-dopa has practically obviated the need for surgical therapy. The latter involves the stereotactic placement of lesions in the central nuclei of the brain, either in the globus pallidus or ventrolateral thalamus, contralateral to the side of the body chiefly affected. The best results occur in patients who are relatively young and in good health with sound mentality, in whom unilateral tremor or rigidity, rather than akinesia, are the predominant symptoms.

Finally, in the management of the patient with Parkinson's disease, one must not neglect the maintenance of optimum general health and neuromuscular efficiency by a planned program of exercise, activity, and rest; and expert physical therapy may be of great help in achieving these ends. In addition, the patient often needs much emotional support in meeting the stress of the illness, in comprehending its nature, and in carrying on courageously in spite of it.

STRIATONIGRAL DEGENERATION

Closely related to paralysis agitans clinically but with an entirely different pathologic basis is a state termed by Adams, van Bogaert, and Vander Eecken *striatonigral degeneration*. We found this lesion by chance in four middle-aged patients without family history of similar disease, in three of whom a clinical picture of Parkinson's syndrome had been described. In one of the three, examined by the authors, the typical rigidity, stiffness, and akinesia had begun on one side of the body, then spread to the other, and progressed over a 5-year period. A flexed posture of trunk and limbs, slowness of all movements, poor balance, mumbling speech, and a ten-

dency to faint were other elements in the clinical picture. Mental function was intact, and there were no reflex changes, no release of sucking and grasping reflexes, and no cerebellar signs, tremor, or involuntary movements. The other two patients had been seen by competent neurologists who had made a diagnosis of Parkinson's disease. Some of the symptoms had been partially relieved by anticholinergic drugs.

In each case the postmortem examination disclosed extensive loss of neurons in the zona compacta of the substantia nigra, but there were no Lewy bodies or neurofibrillary tangles in the remaining cells. More striking, however, were the degenerative changes in the putamens and caudate nuclei. These structures were greatly reduced in size and had lost most of their neurons—more of the small than the large ones, and more on the side opposite the first clinical symptoms. The findings were suggestive of the striatal lesion of Huntington's chorea, except that the cell loss was greater in the putamen than caudatum. Secondary pallidal atrophy (mainly a loss of striatopallidal fibers) was present. In the fourth patient there was in addition a widespread olivopontocerebellar degeneration, but the clinical notes on this case were incomplete, and we could not be sure whether a cerebellar ataxia had been present at any time. Since then, however, we have seen several other patients in whom the changes of olivopontocerebellar and striatonigral degeneration were combined, and in whom the symptoms and signs of cerebellar ataxia had been prominent and had preceded the parkinsonian manifestations. These cases provide a link between olivopontocerebellar and striatonigral degeneration.

Many more cases have been reported in recent years, but have not added much to the clinical picture except to make more clear that a prominent orthostatic hypotension may be associated with this illness. In some of these latter cases, a loss of neurons in the intermediolateral cell column of the spinal cord has been demonstrated, but studies of the sympathetic ganglia are incomplete. The nosologic position of this disease and its relationships to other neuronal atrophies are presently unresolved problems.

CT scans should be useful in showing the loss of tissue in the putamens. The treatment involves the same drugs as are used in Parkinson's disease. The syncope should be treated as outlined on page 256.

PROGRESSIVE SUPRANUCLEAR PALSY (PSP)

In 1963 Richardson, Steele, and Olszewski crystallized medical thought about a clinicopathologic entity to which there had been only ambiguous reference in the past. The condition is no longer unusual. In 1972, when Steele reviewed the subject, 73 cases (22 with postmortem examinations) had been described in the medical literature, and several examples are to be found in every large neurologic center. No toxic, encephalitic, racial, or geographic factor has been incriminated as a possible cause.

Clinical Features   Characteristically the disease has its onset in the sixth decade (range 45 to 73 years) with some combination of difficulty in balance, abrupt falls, visual and ocular disturbance, slurred speech, dysphagia, and vague changes in personality, often with an apprehensiveness and fretfulness suggestive of an agitated depression. At first the neurologic and ophthalmologic examinations may be rather unrevealing, and it may take a year or longer for the characteristic syndrome—comprising supranuclear ophthalmoplegia, pseudobulbar palsy, and axial dystonia—to develop fully. Difficulty in voluntary movement of the eyes, usually downward, is a relatively early development, and so is impairment or loss of the fast component of optokinetic and caloric-induced nystagmus. Later all vertical motions of the eyes are lost, and then the lateral ones as well. If the eyes are fixed on a target and the head turned, however, full movements can be obtained, proving the supranuclear, nonparalytic character of the gaze disorder. Bell's phenomenon (reflexive up-turning of eyes on forced closure of eyelids) and ability to converge the eyes are also lost, and the pupils then become small. In the late stages the eyes may be fixed centrally, and all oculocephalic and vestibular reflexes may be lost.

Along with the oculomotor disorder, the neck gradually stiffens and becomes extended (in one of our cases it was sharply flexed), but this is not an invariable finding. The limbs become slightly stiff and rigid, with Babinski signs in a few cases. The signs of pseudobulbar palsy are always prominent. The face becomes "masked" and less expressive, speech is slurred, the mouth hangs open, and swallowing is difficult. The walking difficulty has proved difficult to analyze. Walking becomes more and more awkward with a curious tendency to topple and fall repeatedly, but with only mild ataxia of the limbs. Some patients tend to lean and fall backward. One of our patients, a large man, fell repeatedly, wrecking household furniture as he went down, yet an analysis of his stance and gait provided no clue as to the basic defect. In some ways this "toppling phenomenon" is similar to that seen in lower brainstem lesions such as occurs in lateral medullary infarction. Finally the patient becomes anarthric, immobile, and quite helpless. Dementia of some degree is probably

present in all the cases, but is mild in most of them. The CSF remains normal.

Postmortem examinations have disclosed a bilateral loss of neurons and gliosis in the periaqueductal gray matter, the superior colliculus, subthalamic nucleus of Luys, red nucleus, pallidum, dentate nucleus, pretectal and vestibular nuclei, and to some extent in the oculomotor nucleus. The cerebral and cerebellar cortices are usually spared. Loss of the medullated fiber bundles arising from these nuclear structures has been observed. A remarkable finding has been the neurofibrillary degeneration of many of the residual neurons.

The cause and nature of this disease are quite obscure. Attempts to transmit it to primates by the inoculation of fresh brain tissue from 10 patients have failed. The disease should be suspected whenever an older adult develops extrapyramidal symptoms, particularly dystonia of the neck, ocular palsies, a picture of pseudobulbar palsy, or inexplicable imbalance and falling. Some patients whom we have seen had earlier been thought to have Parkinson's disease or ocular myasthenia (there may be a partial response to tensilon), but the resemblances are superficial. However, there is a small group of parkinsonians with gaze palsies, especially of upward gaze which must be distinguished (see above).

L-Dopa has been slightly beneficial in some of our patients and combinations of L-dopa and anticholinesterase drugs in others. Unfortunately, these medications were of help for only a short period of time.

DYSTONIA MUSCULORUM DEFORMANS (TORSION SPASM)

Dystonia as a symptom has been discussed on page 57. Here we are concerned with a disease of which dystonia is the major manifestation. Schwalbe's account, in 1908, of three siblings of a Jewish family who were afflicted with progressive involuntary movements of trunk and limbs, probably represents the first description of the disease. In 1911, Oppenheim contributed other cases and coined the term *dystonia musculorum deformans*, in the belief that the disorder was primarily one of muscle and always associated with deformity. Flatau and Sterling, in the same year, first suggested that the disease might have a hereditary basis, and gave it the more accurate name *torsion dystonia of childhood*. At first thought to be a manifestation of hysteria, it gradually came to be established as a morbid entity with a curious preference for Russian and Polish Jews. Wider experience has defined a primary form of dystonia that affects non-Jews, and also symptomatic forms of dystonia due to encephalitis lethargica, Wilson's disease, Hallervorden-Spatz disease, and Huntington's chorea, among many other disorders (see classification of Eldridge and Fahn).

The interesting epidemiologic study of Eldridge, who analyzed all reported cases up to 1970, revealed two patterns of inheritance, one an autosomal recessive, the other dominant. The recessive form begins in early childhood, is progressive over a few years and restricted to Jewish patients, often with superior intelligence. The dominant form begins later, usually in late childhood and adolescence, progresses more slowly, and is not limited to any ethnic group.

Symptomatology The first manifestations of the disease may be rather subtle. The patient (usually a child between 6 and 14 years, less often an adolescent), begins intermittently to invert one foot, or to extend one leg and foot in an unnatural way, or to hunch one shoulder, raising the question of a nervous tic. As time passes, however, the motor peculiarity becomes more persistent and interferes increasingly with the patient's activities. Soon the muscles of the spine and shoulder or pelvic girdles become implicated in involuntary spasmodic twisting movements. The spasms are intermittent at first, and in free intervals muscular tone and volitional movements are normal. Indeed, in some instances the muscles are hypotonic. Gradually the spasms become more frequent; finally they are continuous, and the body is grotesquely contorted. For a time recumbency relieves the spasms; but later, position has no influence. The hands are seldom involved, though at times they may be fisted. Cranial muscles do not escape, and in a number of instances a slurring staccato-type speech has even been the opening sign. In two of our patients, severe dysarthria and dysphagia were the first signs of the disease, caused by dystonia of the tongue, pharyngeal, and laryngeal muscles, and in another it was blepharospasm. Other manifestations of the movement disorder include torticollis, tortipelvis, dromedary gait, propulsive gait, action tremor, myoclonic jerks during voluntary movement, and mild choreoathetosis of the limbs. Excitement worsens the condition, and sleep abolishes it; but as the years pass the postural distortion may become fixed to the point where it does not disappear even in sleep. Tendon

reflexes are at all times normal; corticospinal signs are absent; there is no ataxia, sensory abnormality, convulsive disorder, or dementia.

Pathology No agreement has been reached concerning the pathologic substratum of the disease. In several reported cases the ferrocalcinosis of Hallervorden-Spatz disease, the lesions of Wilson's disease or of kernicterus, or the *état marbré* of hypoxia were observed in the lenticular nuclei. Obviously in these cases the dystonia was symptomatic of another disease. However, in the hereditary form, which is the subject of this section, one cannot be certain of any specific lesions that would account for the clinical manifestations. The brain is grossly normal and the ventricular size is not increased. According to Zeman and Dyken, who have reviewed all the reported autopsy studies, neuronal lipofuscinosis and numerical reduction of neurons in the striatum and pallidum is no greater than in age-matched controls. This does not mean that there are no lesions, only that the techniques being used (random sections for light microscopy) are inadequate for their demonstration. Dopamine β-hydroxylase is elevated in the plasma of patients with the autosomal dominant form of the disease. Also the plasma norepinephrine levels are raised (Ziegler et al.).

Treatment Early in the course of the illness the belladonna group of drugs seemingly has a slightly beneficial effect. L-Dopa is of disputed value. The drug has suppressed the symptoms in some cases, but a longer follow-up of such therapy by Barbeau has shown no lasting benefit. The most spectacular results have been obtained by Cooper, using stereotactic techniques (cryo- or chemothalamectomy) to make lesions that are centered in the ventrolateral nuclei of the thalamus. Some frightfully deformed children, unable to sit or stand, have been restored to near normalcy. Approximately 70 percent were moderately to markedly improved by unilateral or bilateral operations. The improvement was usually sustained, according to Cooper's 20-year follow-up. Tegretol in doses up to 1200 mg/day has been beneficial in some cases, according to Geller et al. In some patients who have the dominant type of the disease, the motor disability has been limited, and changed little over the years. In one case seen by the authors, a dystonia of one leg disappeared and did not return in the next 15 years, while that of his sister progressed.

Other degenerative diseases have been described which combine hereditary dystonia with neural deafness and intellectual impairment (Scribanu and Kennedy); with parkinsonism (Allen and Knopp); and with amyotrophy in a paraplegic distribution (Gilman and Romanul).

Another sizable group of dystonic patients are adults without a family history. We have observed the dystonia to be relatively restricted in these patients and to overlap with spasmodic torticollis, as pointed out by Marsden.

HALLERVORDEN-SPATZ DISEASE

See Chap. 37 (page 688).

SPASMODIC TORTICOLLIS AND OTHER RESTRICTED DYSKINESIAS

With advancing age, a large variety of degenerative *movement disorders* come to light. Supposedly there is loss of neurons in certain parts of the motor system. Groups of muscles begin to manifest arrhythmic involuntary spasms. The patient's lack of success in suppressing them and the recognition that they are beyond voluntary control distinguish them from the common tics, habit spasms, and mannerisms described in Chap. 5. If the muscle contraction is frequent and prolonged, it is accompanied by an aching pain that may mistakenly be blamed for the spasm. Worsening under stress and improvement during quiet and relaxation are typical of this group of disorders.

Surely the most frequent and familiar type is *torticollis*, wherein an adult, more often a woman, becomes aware of turning of the head to one side as she walks. Usually it gradually worsens to a point where it may be more or less continuous, but in some patients the condition remains mild for years on end. On the assumption that the illness has a psychogenic basis, many patients receive psychotherapy, but always without benefit. When followed over the years, the condition is observed to remain limited to the same muscles (mainly the scalene, sternocleidomastoid, and upper trapezius). Occasionally torticollis is combined with dystonia of the arm and trunk, or with tremor, facial spasms, or dystonic writer's cramp. There is little if any response to various drugs. Section of the spinal accessory nerves and upper cervical roots (anterior) bilaterally is the only form of treatment that has given satisfactory results in severe cases. In milder ones, sectioning of one sternomastoid muscle or spinal accessory nerve may be helpful. Biofeedback techniques have lately been introduced (replacing "progressive relaxation") and are said to be beneficial. Perhaps this is so in milder forms of the disorder, but we have not been impressed with the results in well-established cases.

Other restricted dyskinesias involve the neck in combination with facial muscles, the orbicularis oculi (*blepharospasm* and *blepharoclonus*), the throat and respiratory muscles ("*spastic dysphonia*," orofacial dyskinesia, and *respiratory and phonatory spasms*). All these conditions, once started, are persistent, unpleasant, and relatively unresponsive to all modes of therapy other than denervative surgical procedures. Dedo reports that section of one recurrent laryngeal nerve and postoperative speech therapy have restored the voice nearly to normal in more than half of 34 patients with spastic dysphonia. Presumably, the abnormality lies in the basal ganglia, but its pathologic substratum has never been divulged. No lesion was found in the one case of spasmodic torticollis examined by Tarlov.

Torticollis, retrocollis, and other restricted forms of dyskinesia are discussed further on pages 75 and 76.

SYNDROME OF PROGRESSIVE ATAXIA

The cerebellum and its major connections are subject to a number of diseases that are more or less confined to these parts of the nervous system. Many of these diseases are so chronic that one would expect close correspondence between symptomatology and anatomic pathology, yet attempts to determine these relationships have been singularly disappointing. Traditionally, the classic examples of cerebellar deficit are subsumed under the chronic system atrophies, but all efforts to give some semblance of order to the anatomy and pathology of the various reported types have been unsuccessful. Wilson remarked in 1940 that "The group of degenerative conditions strung together by the common feature of ataxia is one for which no very suitable classification has yet been devised," a statement which is as appropriate today as when it was written.

The difficulties in nosologic classification and clinical-anatomic correlation stem from several obvious and some inapparent sources. First, many of the clinical and anatomic studies have been incomplete, especially on the anatomic side. Rarely have all parts of the cerebellum been examined in quantitative fashion, and often myelin-stained sections of the spinal cord either were not made or were marred by uninterpretable artifacts; axis cylinder and glial stains were either omitted or inadequate. Equally incomplete in many cases has been the examination of noncerebellar parts of the nervous system. Second, the established and conventional types of disease seem to be infrequent in comparison to aberrant and transitional types. Hence, one is never certain that the patient under study is a typical example. At times it seems to the authors that every new patient deviates from known types in some way. Third, a large part of the neocerebellum has no assigned functions. It plays no recognizable role in motor function, and whatever it contributes to auditory and visual reflexes is obscure. Thus, an undeveloped cerebellar hemisphere may be discovered at postmortem examination in an individual who has had no symptoms of cerebellar deficit during life. Also, cerebellar symptoms from acute lesions have a way of disappearing, a phenomenon attributed to compensation by other parts of the nervous system. Finally, it is well known that lesions of the brainstem, spinal cord, and frontal lobe may cause a cerebellar type of ataxia with no visible abnormality being noted in the cerebellum itself—a situation exemplified by the cases described by Marie as hereditary cerebellar ataxia (see below). This is possible because of the manifold links between cerebrum, brainstem, and spinal cord and the cerebellum.

Greenfield has reviewed the many early clinical and pathologic reports of heredofamilial spinocerebellar diseases. Becker has drawn attention to at least 60 different diseases and syndromes. He points out that in many of the reported conditions it is not possible to decide if one is dealing with a variant of a known genetic entity or a new and separate disease caused by a pathogenic gene. A recent monograph, edited by Kark et al., reviews the subject of the inherited ataxias and considers the role of metabolic, viral, and immunologic factors in their causation. A modification of Greenfield's classification is presented below, but it must be admitted that many of the fresh cases being published today are difficult to place for reasons that have just been given.

I. *Predominantly* spinal forms of hereditary ataxia
   A. Friedreich's ataxia
   B. Non-Friedreich, predominantly spinal ataxias
II. *Predominantly* cerebellar forms of hereditary ataxia
   A. Cortical cerebellar atrophies
      1. Holmes type of cerebello-olivary atrophy
      2. Late cortical cerebellar atrophy of Marie-Foix-Alajouanine
   B. Cerebellar-brainstem atrophies
      1. Olivopontocerebellar atrophy of Déjérine and André-Thomas (cerebellopetal)
      2. Dentatorubral atrophy (Ramsay Hunt; Woods and Schaumburg; and others) (cerebellofugal)

PREDOMINANTLY SPINAL ATAXIAS

Friedreich's Ataxia This is the prototype of all forms of progressive ataxia. Friedreich, a pioneer neurologist in Heidelberg, began in 1861 to report on a form of familial progressive ataxia that he had observed among nearby villagers. Already it was known through the writings of Duchenne in Paris that locomotor ataxia was the prominent feature in syphilis of the spinal cord, i.e., tabes dorsalis, and it was Friedreich who proved that a nonsyphilitic hereditary type also existed. This possibility was greeted with some skepticism, but soon Duchenne himself affirmed the existence of the new disease and other case reports appeared in England, France, and the United States. In 1882, in a thesis on this subject by Brousse of Montpélier, the name of Friedreich was attached to the new entity.

As new cases appeared, it was noted that in about half of them the disease had its onset before the tenth year and sometimes as early as the third or fourth; Mollaret could find no examples with onset after the age of 25 years. Bell and Carmichael identified two inheritance patterns, the common one being autosomal recessive with average age of onset at 11.75 years, and the other dominant with average age of onset at 20.4 years. The disease is invariably and steadily progressive, and within 5 years of the onset walking is no longer possible in many cases. Most of the patients are reduced to a wheelchair existence or are bedridden by the end of the third decade of life. Patients with the recessive type of the disease succumb earlier than those with the dominant type (median ages at death being 26.5 and 39.5 years respectively), but the average duration of the disease has been substantially the same in both types. Males are said to be somewhat more susceptible.

Symptomatology Ataxia of gait is nearly always the initial symptom. Occasionally it begins rather abruptly after a febrile illness, and one leg may become clumsy before the other. A "hemiplegic" pattern, the arm and leg on one side becoming ataxic before the other, has been remarked upon but is exceptional; usually both legs are affected simultaneously. Difficulty in standing steadily and in running are early symptoms, and Wilson has commented on fatigability, leg pains, and postexertional cramps—symptoms which we have seldom elicited. The hands usually become clumsy months or years after the gait disorder, and dysarthric speech appears after the arms are involved (rarely is it an early symptom).

In some patients pes cavus and kyphoscoliosis precede the neurologic symptoms, and in others they follow by several years. The characteristic foot deformity is a high plantar arch with retraction of the toes at the metatarsal-phalangeal joints and flexion at the interphalangeal joints (hammer toes).

In the fully developed state the abnormality of gait is of mixed sensory and cerebellar type, aptly called tabetocerebellar by Charcot. According to Mollaret, the author of an authoritative monograph on this disease, the cerebellar component is said to predominate, but in our small series we have been as much impressed with the sensory (tabetic) aspect. The patient stands with feet wide apart, constantly shifting position to maintain balance. Friedreich referred to the constant teetering and swaying movements as *static ataxia.* In walking, as with all sensory ataxias the movements of the legs tend to be brusque, with sudden lurches, the feet resounding irregularly as they strike the floor. Usually closure of the eyes causes the patient to fall (Romberg sign), and attempts to correct the imbalance may result in abrupt, wild movements. Often there is a rhythmic tremor of the head. The arms become grossly ataxic, and both action and intention tremors are manifest. Speech is slow, slurred, explosive, and finally almost incomprehensible. Breathing, speaking, swallowing, and laughing may be so incoordinate that the patient nearly chokes while speaking. Holmes remarked upon an ataxia of respiration that causes "curious short inspiratory whoops." Facial, buccal, and arm muscles may display tremors and sometimes choreiform movements.

Mentation has been preserved in all of our patients. However, emotional lability has been sufficiently prominent to be commented upon. Horizontal nystagmus may be present in the primary position, and is increased on lateral gaze. Rotatory and vertical nystagmus are rare. Deafness has been recorded along with vertigo, and inexcitability of labyrinths and blindness with optic atrophy have more rarely been conjoined. Ocular movements usually remain full, and pupillary reflexes are normal. The facial muscles may seem slightly weak, and deglutition may become impaired. Amyotrophy occurs late in the illness and is usually slight, but it may be extreme in cases where a neuropathy is conjoined (see below). The tendon reflexes are abolished in nearly every case; rarely they may still be present when the patient is examined early in the illness. Plantar reflexes are extensor, and flexor spasms may occur even with complete absence of tendon reflexes. The abdominal reflexes are usually retained until late in the illness. Loss of vibratory and position sense are invariable from the beginning, and later there may be some diminution of touch, pain, and temperature sensation as well.

Abortive and atypical forms are numerous. Peroneal muscular atrophy is sometimes associated with Friedreich's ataxia, and the same is true of the heredi-

tary areflexic dystasia of Roussy and Levy. These disorders are discussed with the hereditary neuropathies, on pages 910 and 912. Hereditary forms of optic atrophy, retinitis pigmentosa, and deafness are occasionally combined with Friedreich's ataxia as well.

Many of the patients have died as a result of cardiac arrhythmia or congestive failure. Russell has called attention to a cardiopathy in which the muscle fibers degenerate, and presumably the conducting system in the heart is similarly affected. Kyphoscoliosis and restricted respiratory function are important contributary causes of death.

Pathology The spinal cord is small. The posterior columns and the corticospinal and spinocerebellar tracts are all depleted of medullated fibers, and there is a fibrous gliosis that does not replace the bulk of the lost fibers. The nerve cells in Clarke's column and the dorsal root ganglia, especially lumbosacral ones, are reduced in number—but seldom to a degree that would explain the tract degeneration. Betz cells are also diminished in some cases, but the corticospinal tracts are relatively intact down to the medullary-cervical junction. The nuclei of cranial nerves VIII, X, and XII all exhibit a reduction of their nerve cell population. Slight to moderate neuronal loss is seen in the dentate nuclei, and the superior cerebellar peduncles are thin. Depletion of Purkinje cells in the superior vermis and neurons in corresponding parts of the inferior olivary nuclei has been described in some cases.

The myocardial muscle fibers are degenerated, and replaced by myophages and fibroblasts.

Kark and Blass and their colleagues have found reduced levels of pyruvate dehydrogenase and lipoamide dehydrogenase (LAD) in platelets and cultured skin fibroblasts in the majority of their patients with Friedreich's ataxia. Barbeau (1980) has been unable to duplicate these findings, although he consistently finds a decrease in serum LAD activity in patients with Friedreich's ataxia; the latter abnormality is probably not a primary one, however. Some of their patients also had Kearns-Sayre myopathy and retinitis pigmentosa; hence, the clinical classification of the patients with these abnormalities is unclear.

Clinical-pathologic correlations The pes cavus is not greatly different from that seen in diseases that cause mild hypertonus of the long extensors and flexors of the feet, and in diseases (polyneuropathies) that cause amyotrophy of intrinsic feet muscles, occurring at a time when the bones of the feet are malleable. The kyphoscoliosis is probably due to spinal muscular imbalance. The tabetic aspects of the disease are explained by the degeneration of the columns of Goll and Burdach, and the cerebellar ataxia is attributed to a degeneration of the spinocerebellar tracts or the superior vermis or the dentatorubral pathways, or some combination of both. Loss of large neurons in the sensory ganglia causes abolition of tendon reflexes and contributes to the sensory impairment. Corticospinal lesions account for the weakness and Babinski signs.

Diagnosis Friedreich's disease and its variants raise questions of Marie's hereditary ataxia; familial spastic paraparesis with ataxia, or the Strümpell-Lorrain syndrome (see further on in this chapter); and peroneal muscular atrophy and the Lévy-Roussy syndrome which are discussed in Chap. 45.

Rodriguez-Budelli et al. report improvement of the ataxia with parenteral and oral doses of physostigmine (60-mg tablets). Kark and Blass et al. claim that a diet high in fat and low in carbohydrate to counteract the effects of a presumed lipoyl acetyltransferase deficiency has resulted "in growth spurt, weight gain, improvement in fixed neurological signs and increased resistance to neurological deterioration after fevers." These claims require confirmation.

Non-Friedreich, Predominantly Spinal Ataxias In the large literature on cerebellar ataxias, there are a respectable number of cases that resemble Friedreich's ataxia except that the limbs are spastic and the tendon reflexes hyperactive. The unanswered question is whether they represent a variant of Friedreich's ataxia or a different disease. The cases usually cited are those reported by Sanger Brown, and also some of the cases of the Strümpell-Lorrain form of familial spastic paraplegia and of Behr's optic atrophy with spasticity—both the latter groups sometimes have a prominent ataxic component. Cerebellar atrophy has not been a prominent feature, and we would prefer to adopt the position that they are forms of spinocerebellar degeneration which are transitional between Friedreich's ataxia and some of the other heredoataxias with cerebellar atrophy. In the few autopsied cases, the main abnormality has been in the spinal cord and the spinal cerebellopetal (spinocerebellar) tracts.

PREDOMINANTLY CEREBELLAR FORMS OF HEREDITARY ATAXIA

Soon after the publication of Friedreich's descriptions of a spinal type of hereditary ataxia, reports began to appear of other somewhat different diseases in which the ataxia was related to degenerative changes in the cerebellum and brainstem rather than the spinal cord. Claims of their independence from the spinal type were based largely on later age of onset, more definite hereditary transmission, the persistence or hyperactivity of tendon reflexes, and more frequent concurrence of ophthalmoplegia and optic atrophy. Several of these clinical features, particularly briskness of tendon reflexes, are obviously alien to Friedreich's ataxia.

By 1893 Pierre Marie thought it desirable to create a new category of hereditary ataxia that would embrace all of the non-Friedreich cases. He collated the familial cases of progressive ataxia that had been described by Fraser, Nonne, Sanger Brown, and by Klippel and Durante (see Greenfield for references), and proposed that all were examples of an entity to which the name *heredo-ataxie cerebelleuse* should be applied. Marie's proposition was based almost entirely on clinical observations—not his own, but those made by the aforementioned authors. Later, as more members of these families died, postmortem examinations disclosed that Marie's hereditary cerebellar ataxia included not one but several diseases. Indeed, as pointed out by Holmes (1907b) and more recently by Greenfield, in three of the four families the cerebellum showed no significant lesions at all. Yet there was by now no doubt of a separate class of predominantly cerebellar atrophies, some purely cortical and others associated with a variety of noncerebellar lesions. The trouble is, however, that the clinical pictures and underlying pathologic lesions of the subtypes became less rather than more distinct as new cases were found. We can do no more than put all the cases with major cerebellar lesions together and tentatively subdivide them according to the type of lesion and its noncerebellar linkages.

Familial Cortical Cerebellar Atrophy Holmes in 1907 described a family of eight siblings of whom three brothers and one sister were affected by a progressive ataxia, beginning with a reeling gait and followed by clumsiness of the hands, dysarthria, tremor of the head, and a variable nystagmus. The ataxia began insidiously in the fourth decade and progressed slowly over many years.

The late cortical cerebellar atrophy of Marie, Foix, and Alajouanine, reported in 1922, is probably the same disease. In their patients also, the onset was in later life (average age 57 years). The onset was rather abrupt in some, though usually insidious, and the progress was extremely slow (survival 15 to 20 years). Ataxia of gait, instability of trunk, tremor of the hands and head, and slightly slowed, hesitant speech conformed to the usual clinical picture of a progressive cerebellar ataxia. Nystagmus was rare. Intelligence was usually preserved. The patellar reflexes were increased in many cases, the ankle jerks were often absent, and the plantar reflexes were said to be of extensor type in some cases. (It should be noted that this latter finding is always difficult to interpret, for withdrawal responses are often mistaken for extensor reflexes.)

Postmortem examination disclosed a symmetrical atrophy of the cerebellum most obvious on the upper surface (anterior lobe), the vermis being more affected than the hemispheres. The Purkinje cells were absent in the lingula, centralis, pyramis, and reduced in number in the quadrangularis, flocculus, biventral, and pyramidal lobes. The granule cells were affected, but less than the Purkinje cells. The white matter was slightly pale. The roof nuclei and pontine nuclei were normal. There was cell loss in the dorsal and medial parts of the inferior olivary nuclei. A questionable pallor was noted in the corticospinal and spinocerebellar tracts in the spinal cord.

The pathologic findings in Holmes' cases were essentially the same. Both familial and sporadic cases of this type have since been reported. The similarity of the pathology to that of *alcoholic cerebellar degeneration* always raises the question of a nutritional cause of single cases (Chap. 38).

Striatonigral degeneration (described above) may also be combined with a cortical cerebellar atrophy. As in olivopontocerebellar atrophy, cerebellar ataxia is then superseded by a parkinsonian syndrome.

CEREBELLAR ATROPHY WITH PROMINENT BRAINSTEM LESIONS

Menzel in 1891 described a male patient whose illness began at 28 years of age with ataxia of gait and of the limbs, dysarthria and dysphagia, and retained reflexes. When the patient died 18 years later, there was a conspicuous atrophy of the cerebellum involving mainly the middle cerebellar peduncles, pontine and olivary nuclei, and to a lesser extent the dentate nuclei and superior cerebellar peduncles. Some loss of Purkinje cells and thinning of the granule cells was noted, but these changes were less conspicuous than the loss of fibers in the pontine and cerebellar white matter. The dorsal col-

umns and spinocerebellar and corticospinal tracts were also degenerated, along with a slight loss of cells in the anterior horns of the spinal cord and motor nuclei of the brainstem. Greenfield concluded that this was an example of olivopontocerebellar degeneration, but with "additional and anomalous" features. The latter (presumably spinal) features are of considerable interest, since they relate the Menzel type of hereditary ataxia to the Friedreich type.

Many other families with roughly similar lesions have since been reported (see review by Konigsmark and Weiner). Most of them were middle-aged at the time of death; the pattern of inheritance was usually autosomal dominant but occasionally recessive; and a variety of other clinical findings were present in single cases (hemiballismus, athetosis, contractures of legs, fixed pupils, ophthalmoplegia, ptosis, gaze palsy, retinal degeneration, mental retardation and epilepsy, claw foot and scoliosis, incontinence, parkinsonian symptoms and signs, dementia).

Olivopontocerebellar Atrophy A sporadically occurring form of a closely related disorder was described by Déjerine and André-Thomas, who named it *olivopontocerebellar atrophy*. Here the same brainstem lesions were seen, but the spinal cord was not affected. Hence it could hardly be designated as "spinocerebellar," and it differed in this respect from the Menzel form. The onset was in the fifth decade of life and the main manifestations were ataxia—first in the legs, then the arms and hands and bulbar musculature—a symptomatology common to all the cerebellar atrophies. As more and more cases of this type were collected (Rosenhagen collected 45 from the literature and added 11 of his own), a hereditary pattern (dominant) was evident in some, and degeneration of one or more long tracts in the spinal cord was found in several. About half the cases (25 of 45) later developed the symptoms of Parkinson's disease with degeneration of nigral cells and, in a few, of striatal cells. Thus there was overlap with the Menzel type of disease on one side and Parkinson's disease on the other.

Of considerable interest in both the Menzel and Déjerine-André-Thomas types is the extensive degeneration of the middle cerebellar peduncles, the cerebellar white matter, and the pontine, olivary, and arcuate nuclei; loss of Purkinje cells has been variable. Opinion is divided as to whether this is a degeneration of myelin with relative sparing of pontine neurons and their axons, or a terminal "dying-back" of axons of these nuclei with secondary myelin degeneration. Greenfield favors the latter idea, which seems to us the most plausible.

Dentatorubral Degeneration In 1921, Ramsay Hunt published an account of six cases (two in twin brothers) in which myoclonus was combined with progressive cerebellar ataxia. The age of onset in the four nonfamilial cases was 7 to 17 years, but the cerebellar ataxia followed the myoclonus by an interval of 1 to 20 years. Hunt named this disorder *dyssynergia cerebellaris myoclonica*. In the twin brothers there were signs of Friedreich's ataxia, and in an autopsy of one of the latter, the posterior columns and spinocerebellar tracts were degenerated, but not the corticospinal tracts. The only lesion in the cerebellum was a sclerosis and atrophy of the dentate nuclei with degeneration of the superior cerebellar peduncles. Louis-Bar and van Bogaert in 1947 reported a similar case, and they noted, in addition to the above findings, degeneration in the corticospinal tracts and loss of fibers in the posterior roots. Thus the pathology was identical to that of Friedreich's ataxia except for the more severe atrophy of dentate and other roof nuclei.

Earlier (1914), under the name *dyssynergia cerebellaris progressiva*, Hunt had drawn attention to a progressive disease in young adults manifested by what he considered to be a pure cerebellar syndrome. One of the three patients described in this paper died 13 years after the onset of her illness, and necropsy disclosed cavitary lesions in the lenticular nuclei, cerebellum, and pons, associated with Alzheimer (type 2) glia cells diffusely distributed throughout the brain and nodular cirrhosis of the liver—i.e., findings typical of Wilson's progressive lenticular degeneration. Hunt's reports emphasize the hazard of classifying cerebellar ataxias on the basis of clinical findings alone, a point made effectively by Holmes in relation to Marie's hereditary cerebellar ataxia (see above).

Azorean Disease of the Nervous System In recent years a number of hereditary ataxias, aside from Andrade's amyloid polyneuropathy, have been observed in patients of Portuguese descent from the Azores. One of these was described by Woods and Schaumburg in 1972 under the name *nigrospinodentatal degeneration with nuclear ophthalmoplegia*. The disorder was characterized by an autosomal dominant pattern of inheritance and by a slowly progressive ataxia beginning in adolescence or early adult life, in association with hyperreflexia, extrapyramidal (parkinsonian) rigidity, bulbar signs, distal motor weakness, and ophthalmoplegia. The conjunction of Parkinson's syndrome with cerebellar ataxia was reminiscent of the cases of olivopontocerebellar degeneration. Postmortem examination disclosed a degeneration of the dentate nuclei and spinocerebellar tracts, and a loss of anterior horn cells and neurons of the pons, substantia nigra, and oculomotor nuclei. The heredoataxia was unaccompanied by signs of polyneuropathy, unlike the hereditary ataxia in Portuguese emigrants described by Nakano et al. as Machado disease, this being the name of the progenitor of the afflicted family.

A similarly affected Azorean family named Joseph was described by Rosenberg et al. (1976), under the name of *autosomal dominant striatonigral degeneration*, and was considered by these authors to be a new genetic disorder. The disease had its onset in early adult life and was characterized by progressive ataxia of gait, followed by dysarthria, nystagmus, slowness of eye movements, reduced facial mobility, slow lingual movements, fasciculations of face and tongue, dystonic postures, rigidity of the limbs, cerebellar tremor, hyperreflexia, and Babinski signs. A striatonigral degeneration was found in the one autopsied case, but the pictures of the lesions are unconvincing; surely they bear no resemblance to the lesions of striatonigral degeneration reported by Adams et al. The diagnosis of striatonigral degeneration was disputed also by Nielsen and by Romanul who were able to study the brain of the patient reported by Rosenberg et al.

Under the name *Azorean disease of the nervous system*, Romanul et al. described yet another family of Portuguese-Azorean descent, the members of which suffered a progressive ataxia of gait, parkinsonian features, limitation of conjugate gaze, fasciculations, arreflexia, nystagmus, cerebellar tremor, and extensor plantar responses; the pathologic changes closely resembled those described by Woods and Schaumburg. Romanul et al. compared the genetic, clinical, and pathologic features of their cases with those of the three other Portuguese disorders and proposed that all of them represent a single genetic entity with variable expression.

OTHER CHRONIC CEREBELLAR ATAXIAS OF DEGENERATIVE TYPE

To be briefly mentioned here are the hereditary ataxias with optic atrophy of André-van Leeuwen and van Bogaert; an autosomal recessive syndrome of cerebellar ataxia with pigmentary retinal degeneration and congenital deafness of Hallgren; an autosomal dominant hereditary ataxia with muscular atrophy, retinal degeneration and diabetes mellitus; Friedreich's ataxia with juvenile parkinsonism of Biemond and Sinnige; an autosomal recessive ataxia with total albinism of Skre and Berg; and an autosomal recessive ataxia with cataracts, oligophrenia, pyramidal signs, and stunting of growth of Marinesco and Sjögren (see Kark, Rosenberg, and Schut for references). No metabolic abnormalities have been detected in any of these disorders. Familial incidence in itself does not establish a genetic causation for it is now known that a number of slow virus infections, such as subacute spongiform encephalopathy, may begin with cerebellar ataxia. Also an immunologic defect, like the one underlying ataxia-telangiectasia, may cause cerebellar degeneration. The metabolic ataxias are discussed further in Chap. 37 and the slow virus ataxias in Chap. 32.

SYNDROME OF MUSCULAR WEAKNESS AND WASTING WITHOUT SENSORY CHANGES

MOTOR SYSTEM DISEASE

This general term is used to designate a progressive degenerative disorder of motor neurons in the spinal cord, brainstem, and motor cortex, manifested clinically by muscular weakness, atrophy, and corticospinal tract signs in varying combinations. It is a disease of middle life, for the most part, and progresses to death in a matter of 2 to 6 years, or longer in exceptional cases.

Customarily, motor system disease is subdivided into several types, on the basis of the particular grouping of symptoms and signs. The most frequent form, in which amyotrophy and hyperreflexia are combined, is called *amyotrophic lateral sclerosis*. Rather less frequent are cases in which weakness and atrophy occur alone, without evidence of corticospinal tract dysfunction. For these the term *progressive spinal muscular atrophy* is used. Where the weakness and wasting predominantly affect the muscles innervated by the motor nuclei of the lower brainstem i.e., the muscles of the jaw, face, tongue, pharynx, and larynx, it is customary to speak of *progressive bulbar palsy* ("bulb" being the old name for medulla oblongata).Very rarely the clinical state is dominated by spastic weakness, hyperreflexia, and Babinski signs; such cases are classed as *primary lateral sclerosis*. Special types of familial, progressive muscular atrophy also occur in infancy and childhood. The best known form is the Werdnig-Hoffmann type or *infantile muscular atrophy;* but there are other familial cases beginning in later childhood, adolescence, or adult life. In some of these a spastic weakness is the main feature; others are

characterized by a slowly progressive amyotrophy. For the nonfamilial forms there is no reason to believe that the subgroups are anything other than variants of a single pathologic process—a motor cell atrophy. In 5 to 10 percent of patients the disease occurs as an autosomal dominant inherited disorder (Mulder).

History For the original delineation of amyotrophic lateral sclerosis credit is usually given to Charcot. With Joffroy in 1869 and with Gombault in 1871 he studied the pathologic aspects of the disease, and in a series of lectures given from 1872 to 1874 he gave a lucid account of the clinical and pathologic findings. Although called Charcot's disease in France, amyotrophic lateral sclerosis (the term which Charcot recommended) has been preferred in the English-speaking world. Duchenne had earlier (1858) described "labioglossolaryngeal paralysis" which Wachsmuth in 1864 shortened to "progressive bulbar palsy." Charcot called attention to its nuclear origin in 1869 and Déjerine in 1882 established its relationship to amyotrophic lateral sclerosis. Most authors credit Aran and Duchenne with the earliest descriptions of progressive spinal muscular atrophy, which, they believed, was of myogenic origin. This interpretation was of course incorrect, and Cruveilhier, a few years later, noted the slender anterior roots. Soon thereafter the disease was brought into line with amyotrophic lateral sclerosis as a myelopathic or spinal muscular atrophy.

Amyotrophic Lateral Sclerosis (ALS) In its most typical form, uselessness of a hand, awkwardness in tasks requiring fine finger movements, stiffness of the fingers, and slight weakness or wasting of the hand muscles are the first indications of the disease. Cramping beyond what seems natural and twitching of the forearm, upper arm, and shoulder girdle muscles also appear. As the weeks and months pass, the other hand and arm may be similarly affected. Before long, the triad of atrophic weakness of the hands and forearms, slight spasticity of the legs, and generalized hyperreflexia—all in the absence of sensory change—leaves little doubt as to the diagnosis. Loss of power is paralleled by diminution of muscle bulk, yet despite the atrophy, the tendon reflexes are notable for their liveliness. Abductors, adductors and extensors of fingers and thumb tend to become weak before the long flexors, on which the handgrip depends, and the dorsal interosseous spaces are hollowed, giving rise to the "cadaveric" or "skeleton hand." The muscles of the upper arm and shoulder girdles are involved later.

All the while the thigh and leg muscles seem relatively normal, and there may come a time when the patient walks about with useless, dangling arms. Later the atrophic weakness spreads to the neck, tongue, pharyngeal and laryngeal muscles, and eventually those in the trunk and lower extremities yield to the onslaught of the disease.

The affected parts may ache and feel cold, but true paresthesias, except from poor positioning and nerve pressure, do not occur. Sphincteric control is usually well-maintained even after both legs have become weak and spastic, and the abdominal reflexes may be elicitable even when the plantar reflexes are extensor. Extreme spasticity is rarely seen, at least not like that in nonatrophic muscles of other diseases. Coarse fasciculations are usually evident in the weakened muscles, but may not be noticed by the patient until the physician calls attention to them.

Variants We have observed many other patterns of neuromuscular involvement. The leg may be affected before the hand. A foot drop with weakness and wasting of the pretibial muscles may be falsely blamed on a peroneal nerve compression until weakness of the gastrocnemius and other muscles betrays a widespread involvement of lumbosacral neurons. This crural amyotrophy in our experience is nearly as frequent as the brachial-manual type. Another variant is the early involvement of thoracic, abdominal, or posterior neck muscles. The pattern of proximal or shoulder girdle amyotrophy, as in Wohlfart-Kugelberg-Welander disease, is also well known and simulates muscular dystrophy. On several occasions we have observed a pattern of involvement of arm and leg on the same side—sometimes called the *hemiplegic*, or *Mills, variant*. Again the first manifestations may be spasticity and weakness of the legs (*primary lateral sclerosis*) or of an arm, and only after a year or two do the hand and arm muscles weaken, waste, and fasciculate. Exceptionally, cramps or fasciculations of the limb muscles may precede recognizable weakness and wasting by several months. ALS has been observed in conjunction with presenile and senile dementia, and with Parkinson's disease. The complex is similar to that observed among the natives of Guam.

The course of this illness, irrespective of its particular mode of onset and pattern of evolution, is inexorably progressive. Half the patients are dead within 3 years and 90 percent within 6 years (Mulder and Espinosa).

Progressive Muscular Atrophy Usually this consists of symmetrical wasting of intrinsic hand muscles, slowly advancing to the more proximal parts of the arms; less often the legs and thighs are the sites of atrophic weakness while innervation of the upper extremities remains intact. Rarely, the proximal parts of the limbs are affected before the distal parts. These nuclear amyotrophies tend to progress at a slower pace than amyotrophic lateral sclerosis, some patients surviving for 15 years or longer. Some of the most chronic varieties are familial. Otherwise they differ only in that the tendon reflexes are diminished or absent, and signs of corticospinal tract disease cannot be detected. Fascicular twitchings and cramping are variably present.

Progressive Bulbar Palsy Here reference is made to cases in which the first and dominant symptoms relate to weakness of muscles of the jaw, face, tongue, pharynx, and larynx. This weakness gives rise to an early defect in articulation, in which there is difficulty in the pronunciation of lingual (*r, n, l*), labial (*b, m, p, f*), dental (*d, t*), and palatal (*k, g*) consonants. As the condition worsens the syllables lose their clarity and run together until finally speech becomes unintelligible. We have observed other cases in which slurring is due to spasticity of the tongue, pharyngeal, and laryngeal muscles. Defective modulation of the voice with variable degrees of rasping and nasality is another characteristic. The pharyngeal reflex is lost, and the palate and vocal cords move imperfectly or not at all during phonation. Mastication and deglutition are impaired; the bolus of food cannot be manipulated and may lodge between the cheek and teeth; and the pharyngeal muscles do not force it properly into the esophagus. Liquids and small particles of food find their way into the trachea or reflux into the nose. The facial muscles, particularly of the lower face, weaken and sag. Fasciculations and focal loss of tissue of the tongue are usually early manifestations; eventually the tongue becomes shriveled, and lies useless in the floor of the mouth. The chin may also quiver from fascicular twitchings, but the disease should never be diagnosed on the basis of fasciculations alone, i.e., in the absence of weakness or atrophy. Fasciculations may be entirely benign or a part of the syndrome of myokymia or of "continuous muscular activity" (see page 1000).

The jaw jerk may be present at a time when the muscles of mastication are markedly weak. In fact, spasticity of the jaw muscles may be so pronounced that the slightest tap on the chin will evoke clonus, and, rarely, attempts to open the mouth elicit a "bulldog" reflex (jaws snap shut involuntarily). The signs of spastic weakness may at all times surpass those of atrophic weakness, and pathologic laughter and crying may infrequently reach extreme degrees. This is the only common clinical situation in which spastic and atrophic bulbar palsy coexist. Strangely, the ocular muscles always escape, and we have never observed an instance of the sporadic disease with sensory loss. Cases have been reported, but they are so rare that the diagnosis must remain in doubt.

There is little need for laboratory investigation once one is familiar with the clinical picture, but there are a few aids. The electromyogram reveals widespread fibrillations and fasciculations, and motor nerve conduction studies reveal only a slight slowing. The CSF protein is normal or sometimes slightly elevated.

As with other forms of motor system disease, the course of bulbar palsy is inexorably progressive. Eventually the weakness spreads to the respiratory muscles, and deglutition fails entirely; the patient dies of inanition and aspiration pneumonia, usually within 2 to 3 years of onset. About 25 percent of cases of motor system disease begin with bulbar symptoms but rarely, if ever, does the sporadic form of progressive bulbar palsy run its course as an independent syndrome (pure heredofamilial forms of progressive bulbar palsy and progressive ocular palsy in the adult are known, but are rare). Practically always, after a few months, the other manifestations of ALS become evident. The earlier the onset of the bulbar involvement in the course of ALS, the shorter the course of the disease.

Pathology   The principal finding is a loss of nerve cells in the anterior horns of the spinal cord and motor nuclei of the lower brainstem. Many of the surviving nerve cells are small, shrunken, and filled with lipofuscin. Lost cells are replaced by fibrous astrocytes. Large neurons tend to be affected before small ones. The anterior roots are thin, and the muscles show typical denervation atrophy of different ages. In amyotrophic lateral sclerosis, the corticospinal tract degeneration is most evident in the lower parts of the spinal cord, but it can be traced up through the brainstem to the posterior limb of the internal capsule and corona radiata by fat stains which show the macrophages that have accumulated in response to the myelin degeneration. There is loss of Betz cells in the motor cortex. Other fibers in the ventral and lateral funiculi are depleted, imparting a characteristic pallor in myelin stains. McMenemey interprets this as evidence of involvement of nonmotor neurons and, hence, objects to the term *motor system disease.* However, we regard this as due to a loss of the collaterals of motor neurons which contribute to the lamina propria. One observes the same effect in poliomyelitis.

Neuropathologic studies of cases of ALS with dementia are few in number. In addition to the usual affection of motor neurons, these cases have shown an exten-

sive neuronal loss and gliosis involving the premotor area, particularly the superior frontal gyri, and the inferolateral cortex of the temporal lobes. The histologic changes of Alzheimer's or Pick's disease have not been seen; neurofibrillary degeneration has been observed but was inconsequential in comparison to that which characterizes the Guamanian Parkinson-dementia-ALS complex (Finlayson et al.).

Diagnosis   Motor system disease may be simulated by a central spondylotic bar or ruptured cervical disk, but usually with these latter conditions there are pain in the neck and shoulders, limitation of neck movements, and sensory changes, and the lower motor neuron affection is restricted to one or two spinal segments. A mild corticospinal hemiparesis or monoparesis due to multiple sclerosis may for a time be difficult to distinguish from early ALS. Progressive muscular atrophy may be differentiated from peroneal muscular atrophy (Charcot-Marie-Tooth) by the lack of family history and the complete lack of sensory change. The proximal, girdle form of motor system disease may be misdiagnosed as the Erb type of limb-girdle muscular dystrophy. The spastic form of bulbar palsy may suggest the pseudobulbar palsy of lacunar disease. A crural form of progressive muscular atrophy may be confused with diabetic mononeuropathy multiplex or polymyositis. There is also a rare form of subacute poliomyelitis (possibly viral) in patients with lymphoma or carcinoma; it leads to an amyotrophy that progresses to death over a period of several months.

Also, some patients who have recovered from acute poliomyelitis may develop progressive muscular atrophy some 20 to 30 years later; the nature of this relationship is quite obscure, although the concurrence of these events is probably greater than can be explained by chance.

All these caveats notwithstanding, amyotrophic lateral sclerosis or the more discrete forms of motor system disease rarely offer any difficulty in diagnosis.

Treatment   There is no specific treatment for this disease, and only supportive measures can be utilized. It has been our practice to give the patient some idea of the seriousness of the condition, but not to make a devastating statement that it is invariably fatal. Usually it is advisable to give medication of some type "to try to halt the disease," even though none is known to be effective. Lately guanidine hydrochloride and small injections of cobra venom have been said to arrest the process, but no convincing evidence has been forthcoming to support these claims.

Heredofamilial Forms of Progressive Muscular Atrophy and Spastic Paraplegia   *Werdnig-Hoffmann disease (infantile progressive spinal muscular atrophy)*   This is the classic form of a spinal muscular atrophy of hereditary type. It is described fully in Chap. 50, along with the early-life myopathies, since these are the disorders from which it always needs to be distinguished.

Chronic proximal spinal muscular atrophy (PSMA, Wohlfart-Kugelberg-Welander syndrome)   This is a somewhat different form of heredofamilial spinal muscular atrophy which, as the name indicates, involves the proximal muscles of the limbs predominantly, and is only slowly progressive. It was first clearly separated from other forms of motor system disease and from muscular dystrophy by Wohlfart and by Kugelberg and Welander in the mid-1950s. In about a third of the cases, the onset is before 2 years of age and in 50 percent, between 3 and 18 years. Males are preponderantly affected, especially among patients with juvenile and adult onset. The usual form of transmission is by an autosomal recessive gene, but families with dominant and sex-linked inheritance have been described.

The disease begins insidiously, with weakness and atrophy of the pelvic girdle and proximal leg muscles, followed by involvement of the shoulder girdle and upper arm muscles. Unlike the sporadic form of spinal muscular atrophy, the Kugelberg-Welander variety is bilaterally symmetric from the beginning, and fasciculations are observed in only half the cases. Ultimately the distal limb muscles are involved, and tendon reflexes are lost. Bulbar musculature and corticospinal tracts are spared, although Babinski signs and an associated ophthalmoplegia (presumably neural) have been reported in rare instances.

The presence of fasciculations and the EMG and muscle biopsy findings, all of which show the characteristic abnormalities of neural atrophy, permit distinction from muscular dystrophy. Only a few cases have been examined postmortem, and they have shown loss and degeneration of the anterior horn cells.

In addition to the characteristic changes of denervation, muscle biopsies from these cases have disclosed necrosis of single muscle fibers with phagocytosis and attempts at regeneration, changes which may account for elevated creatine phosphokinase levels (Mastaglia and Walton). The nature of these latter changes—whether a primary process in muscle or in some way secondary to denervation—remains to be settled.

The disease progresses very slowly, and some patients survive to old age without serious disability. In general, the earlier the onset, the less favorable the prognosis; however, even the most severely affected patients retain the ability to walk for at least 10 years after the onset. Admittedly, it is difficult to make a sharp distinction between these latter cases of Kugelberg-Welander disease and certain instances of Werdnig-Hoffmann disease with onset in late infancy and early childhood and prolonged survival (Byers and Banker). Some of these cases of "nuclear amyotrophy," as Wilson called them, have been mistaken for Erb's limb-girdle dystrophy (see Chap. 49).

Hereditary spastic paraplegia or diplegia   This disease was described by Seeligmüller in 1874 and later by Strümpell in Germany and Lorrain in France, and has now been identified in nearly every part of the world. The pattern of inheritance is usually dominant, and the onset may be in any age period from childhood to the senium. The clinical picture is that of a gradual development of spastic weakness of the legs with increasing difficulty in walking. The tendon reflexes are hyperactive and the plantar reflexes extensor, and, in the pure form of the disease, sensory and other nervous functions are entirely intact. If the onset is in childhood, the feet are usually arched and shortened and there is a pseudocontracture of calf muscles, forcing the child or adolescent to "toe-walk." Sometimes the knees are slightly flexed, or the legs are fully extended and adducted. Weakness is variable and is difficult to estimate. Sphincteric function is usually retained. The arms are variably involved. In some, the hands are stiff, movements are clumsy, and speech is mildly dysarthric. Conjoined findings such as nystagmus, ocular palsies, optic atrophy, ataxia (both cerebellar and sensory), epilepsy, and dementia have all been described in isolated families.

The few available pathologic studies have shown that, aside from the degeneration of the corticospinal tracts throughout the spinal cord, there is a thinning of the columns of Goll, mainly in the lumbosacral regions, and of the spinocerebellar tracts, even though no sensory abnormalities had been detected during life. These were the pathologic findings described by Strümpell in his original (1880) report of two brothers with spastic paraplegia; one of them in addition had shown a cerebellar syndrome, but again there were no sensory abnormalities. A reduction in number of Betz and anterior horn cells has also been reported.

In the differential diagnosis of this disorder, one must always consider an indolent spinal cord or foramen magnum tumor, familial multiple sclerosis (the clinical diagnosis in Strümpell's original cases), Arnold-Chiari malformation, and the compression of the cord by a variety of congenital bony malformations at the craniocervical junction (see Chap. 35).

Available medications to suppress spasticity have not been successful in the authors' hands.

Other Hereditary Forms of Motor System Disease   Examples of *familial amyotrophic lateral sclerosis (ALS)* in adults have long been recognized. The authors have had several under their care, beginning in the third, fourth, or fifth decades of life and being transmitted from one generation to another. Less well known, however, were the cases of this type that occurred between the infancy-early childhood period (the Werdnig-Hoffmann type) and adulthood—until Emery collected all the familial spinal muscular atrophies of northern England and Scotland and found types that begin at every age. Moreover, a number of forms have been combined with familial spastic paraplegia. Families with later age of onset have tended to have more definite signs of corticospinal tract disease.

A remarkable number of subtypes have been recognized, both of the spinal and brainstem muscular atrophies and of the familial spastic paraplegias. It is not possible to describe all of them, but the following are the major ones, beginning with the lower motor neuron variants.

Progressive bulbar paralysis of childhood (Fazio-Londe syndrome)   Fazio in 1892 and Londe in 1893 described children, adolescents, and young adults who developed progressive bulbar palsy. As subsequent cases were identified, the full picture of facial diplegia, dysarthria, dysphagia, and dysphonia was observed and noted to become increasingly pronounced until the time of death some years after onset. In some there was a late development of corticospinal signs. Also jaw and oculomotor weakness appeared in some instances of the disease, and in one there was progressive deafness. Pathologic verification has been obtained in a few such patients, with loss of motor neurons in the hypoglossal, ambiguus, facial, and trigeminal motor nuclei. In a few, the nerve cells in the oculomotor nuclei were also diminished. This disease, the few times we have encountered

it, needs to be differentiated from a pontomedullary glioma and brainstem multiple sclerosis.

Ophthalmoplegia with neural disease   Weakness of ocular movement or gaze disorders have been observed in cases in Friedreich's ataxia and spastic paraplegia, and in some of the early cases of hereditary ataxia reported by Sanger Brown. Ferguson and Critchley have described a heredofamilial syndrome comprising gaze palsies, spastic paraparesis, cerebellar ataxia, and optic atrophy. Drachman has discussed these and other cases of presumably neural origin under the term *ophthalmoplegia plus*. His chapter and that of Rowland in the *Handbook of Clinical Neurology* summarize the extensive literature on the heredodegenerative ocular palsies.

Variants of familial spastic paraplegia   The literature contains a number of reports of familial spastic paraplegia combined with other neurologic abnormalities. Some of the syndromes had developed early in life and in conjunction with moderate degrees of mental retardation. Nevertheless the rest of the neurologic picture appeared many years after birth and was progressive. Because of limitations of space, each entity cannot be described in detail. The following list includes the best-known entities.

1. *Hereditary spastic paraplegia with spinocerebellar and ocular symptoms (Ferguson-Critchley syndrome)*. This condition, featured by a disorder of gaze, was remarked upon above. Far more impressive has been a spinocerebellar ataxia beginning during the fourth and fifth decades of life accompanied by weakness of legs, alterations of mood, pathologic laughter and crying, dysarthria and diplopia, dysesthesias of limbs, and poor bladder control. The tendon reflexes are lively, with bilateral Babinski signs. Sensation is diminished distally in the limbs. The whole picture resembles multiple sclerosis. In other cases, running through several generations of a family, the extrapyramidal features were more striking; such cases overlap with the following syndromes.

2. *Hereditary spastic paraplegia with extrapyramidal symptoms*. Action and static tremors, parkinsonian rigidity, dystonic tongue movement, and athetosis of the limbs have all been found in combination with spastic paraplegia. Gilman and Romanul (1975) have re-

viewed the literature on this subject. The picture of parkinsonism with spastic weakness and corticospinal signs has been the most frequent combination, in the authors' experience.

3. *Hereditary spastic paraplegia with optic atrophy.* Known as Behr's syndrome, this will be described below in connection with Leber's hereditary optic atrophy. Some of the members of the large family reported by Bruyn and Went also had athetosis. The onset was in childhood.

4. *Hereditary spastic paraplegia with retinal degeneration (Kjellin and Barnard-Scholz syndromes).* Spastic paraplegia with amyotrophy, oligophrenia, and central retinal degeneration constitutes the syndrome described in 1959 by Kjellin. While the mental retardation is stationary, the spastic weakness and retinal changes are of late onset and progressive. When ophthalmoplegia is added, it is called the Barnard-Scholz syndrome.

5. *Hereditary spastic paraplegia with mental retardation or dementia.* Many of the children with progressive spastic paraplegia were noted either to have been mentally retarded since early life or to have regressed mentally as other neurologic symptoms developed. Examples of this syndrome and its variants are too numerous to be considered here, but are contained in the review of Gilman and Romanul. The recessive syndrome of Sjögren-Larsson, with onset in infancy of spastic weakness of the legs in association with mental retardation, stands somewhat apart because of the associated ichthyosis.

If the term *hereditary spastic paraplegia* is to have any neurologic significance, it should only be applied to the relatively rare, pure form of the progressive syndrome. The more common "atypical" cases with amyotrophy, cerebellar ataxia, tremors, dystonia, athetosis, optic atrophy, retinal degeneration, amentia, and dementia should be put in separate categories and their identity retained for nosologic purposes until such time as some biochemical data related to pathogenesis are forthcoming. Separable also are all the congenital nonprogressive types of spastic diplegia and athetosis.

SYNDROME OF PROGRESSIVE BLINDNESS

There are two main classes of progressive blindness in children, adolescents, and adults—progressive optic neuropathy and retinal (pigmentary or tapeto-) degeneration. Of course there are many congenital anomalies and retinal diseases beginning in infancy that result in blindness and microphthalmia. Some of them of neurologic interest were described briefly in Chap. 12.

LEBER'S HEREDITARY OPTIC NEUROPATHY

While familial amaurosis was known in the early eighteenth century, it was Leber who in 1871 gave the definitive description of this disease and traced it through many genealogies. The pattern of inheritance cannot be explained by conventional Mendelian principles. Male preference is revealed in most families, but this cannot be adequately explained on the basis of an X-linked transmission, since females are affected and transmit the carrier state to their daughters more frequently than would be expected. In most patients the onset of visual loss is between 18 and 25 years, but the range of age of onset is much greater. A few of the affected women had their first symptom at the menarche. In some families the disease has been followed for five and six generations (Carroll and Mastaglia).

The visual loss usually has an insidious onset and a subacute or slow evolution, but it may begin so abruptly as to suggest a diagnosis of retrobulbar neuritis. In the latter instance aching in the eye or brow may accompany the visual loss. Subjective visual phenomena are reported by some. Usually both eyes are affected simultaneously—though in some one eye is affected first, followed by the other after an interval of several weeks or months. In practically all cases, the second eye is affected within a year of the first, but rarely after a longer period. In the unimpaired eye, abnormalities of pattern-reversal visual evoked potentials may be found before impaired visual acuity is recognized (Carroll and Mastaglia).

Once started, the visual impairment progresses over a period of weeks to months. Usually central vision is impaired before peripheral, and there is a stage in which bilateral central scotomata are readily demonstrated. Disturbances of color vision are said to be characteristic; blue-yellow deficiency is present, while red and green perception is relatively preserved. In the more advanced stages, however, the patients are totally colorblind. Constriction of the fields may be added later. Usually there is no nystagmus. At first the disks may have blurred margins, but soon they become atrophic. Peripapillary telangiectasia and tortuosity of the more peripheral vessels have also been noted in the early stages of the disease (Smith et al.). Improvement of vision and recovery have been reported, but one must then question the accuracy of the diagnosis. Of some importance is the fact that the visual impairment is seldom complete; and although patients are declared legally blind because of the large central scotomata, they still can do certain types of work.

The optic nerve lesion has been examined on a number of occasions. The central parts of the nerves are degenerated from papillae to the lateral geniculate bodies, the papillomacular bundles being particularly affected. Presumably axis cylinders and myelin degenerate together, as would be expected from the loss of nerve cells in the superficial layer of the retina. Both astrocytic glial and endoneurial connective tissue are increased.

As so often happens in heredofamilial diseases, Leber's optic atrophy may be combined with degeneration in many other parts of the nervous system. Behr in 1909 reported six cases in which corticospinal and cerebellar signs came on with optic atrophy in early life. In others, tremor and mental retardation have been associated, and epilepsy and imbecility were found in some members of the family studied by Ferguson and Critchley; spastic ataxia was seen in another.

Important in differential diagnosis is the recognition of congenital optic atrophy (of which recessive and dominant forms are known) and of retrobulbar neuritis of multiple sclerosis.

RETINITIS PIGMENTOSA

This remarkable retinal abiotrophy, known since Helmholtz first invented the ophthalmoscope in 1851, usually begins in childhood and adolescence. Unlike Leber's disease, which affects only the third neurons of the visual system, it involves all layers, both the neuroepithelium and pigment epithelium. For this combination Leber proposed the term *tapetoretinal degeneration*, thinking it preferable to retinitis pigmentosa, since there is no evidence of inflammation. The incidence of this disorder is two or three times greater in boys than in girls. The inheritance is more often recessive than dominant; in the former, consanguinity, which increases the likelihood of disease by approximately 20 times, plays an important part. Sex-linked types are also known.

The first symptom is usually a failure of twilight vision (nyctalopia). Under dim light the visual fields tend to constrict, but slowly, as the disease progresses, there is permanent visual impairment in all degrees of illumination. The perimacular zones tend to be the first and most severely involved, giving rise to partial or complete ring scotomata. Peripheral loss sets in later. Usually both eyes are affected simultaneously, but rare cases are on record where one eye was affected first and more severely. Color vision is lost relatively late. The electrical activity of the eye (measured by the electroretinogram,

which depends on the activity of all the components of the retina) is extinguished, in contrast to Leber's hereditary optic atrophy, where it is retained.

Ophthalmoscopic examination shows the characteristic triad of pigmentary deposits that assume the appearance of bone corpuscles, attenuated vessels, and pallor of the optic disks. The pigment is due to clumping of epithelial cells that migrate from the pigment layer to the degenerating, superficial parts of the retina. The pigmentary degeneration spares only the fovea, so that eventually the world is perceived as though the patient were looking through narrow tubes.

Diseases to which retinitis pigmentosa may be linked are oligophrenia, obesity, syndactyly and hypogonadism (Bardet-Biedl syndrome); hypogenitalism, obesity and mental deficiency (Laurence-Moon syndrome); Friedreich's and other types of spinocerebellar and cerebellar ataxia; spastic paraplegia and quadriplegia with Laurence-Moon syndrome; neurogenic amyotrophy, progressive external ophthalmoplegia with or without heart block (Kiloh-Nevin and Kearns-Sayre syndromes); deaf mutism; Leber's optic neuropathy; myopia and color blindness; and polyneuropathy and deafness (Refsum's syndrome).

Differential diagnosis includes Batten's form of cerebromacular degeneration, Pelizaeus-Merzbacher disease and Gaucher's disease, and retinal infections such as syphilis, toxoplasmosis, and cytomegalic inclusion disease.

Virtual blindness is the outcome in many cases, but in others the visual failure stops short of that. It is doubtful if any of many proposed medical therapies (sympathectomy, steroids, vitamins A and E) have any effect in halting the progress of the disease.

STARGARDT'S DISEASE

This is a bilaterally symmetric, slowly progressive macular degeneration, differentiated from retinitis pigmentosa by Stargardt in 1909. In essence it is a hereditary (usually recessive) tapetoretinal degeneration or dystrophy (the latter term preferred by Waardenburg), with onset between 6 and 20 years, rarely later, and leading to a loss of central vision. The region of the macula becomes gray, yellowish, or brown with pigmentary spots, and the visual fields show central scotomata. Later the periphery of the retina may become dystrophic. The lesion is well visualized with fluorescein angiography. Activity in the electroretinogram is diminished or abolished.

This disease is clearly different from retinitis pigmentosa. According to Cohan et al. it may be associated with epilepsy, Refsum's syndrome, Kearns-Sayre syndrome, Bassen-Kornzweig syndrome, Sjögren-Larsson syndrome, with spinocerebellar and other forms of cerebellar degeneration, familial paraplegia, and the syndrome of *hyperkinesia with statokinetic trembling* of Vancea and Tudor.

SYNDROME OF PROGRESSIVE DEAFNESS

There is an impressive group of hereditary, progressive cochleovestibular atrophies that are linked to atrophies and degenerations of the nervous system. These are the subject of an informative review by Konigsmark. Such neuro-otologic syndromes must be put alongside a group of five diseases that affect exclusively the auditory and vestibular nerves (dominant, progressive nerve deafness; dominant, low-frequency hearing loss; dominant midfrequency hearing loss; sex-linked, early-onset neural deafness; and hereditary episodic vertigo and hearing loss). The latter ones are of interest to neurologists because they disturb both balance and hearing.

HEREDITARY HEARING LOSS WITH RETINAL DISEASES

Konigsmark separates three syndromes: those with typical retinitis pigmentosa, those with Leber's optic atrophy, and those with other retinal changes.

With respect to retinitis pigmentosa, four syndromes are recognized. Retinitis pigmentosa in combination with congenital hearing loss is referred to as Usher's syndrome. Retinitis pigmentosa and hereditary hearing loss may also be combined with polyneuropathy (Refsum's syndrome); with hypogonadism and obesity (Alstrom's syndrome); and with dwarfism, mental retardation, premature senility, and photosensitive dermatitis (Cockayne's syndrome).

Hereditary hearing loss with optic atrophy forms the core of four syndromes: dominant optic atrophy, ataxia, muscle wasting, and progressive hearing loss (Sylvester's disease); recessive optic atrophy, polyneuropathy, and neural hearing loss (Rosenberg-Chutorian syndrome); optic atrophy, hearing loss, and juvenile diabetes mellitus (Tunbridge-Paley syndrome); opticocochleodentate degeneration with optic atrophy, hearing loss,

quadriparesis, and mental retardation (Nyssen-van Bogaert's syndrome).

Hearing loss has also been observed with other retinal changes, two of which might be mentioned. *Norrie's disease* with retinal malformation, hearing loss, and mental retardation (oculoacousticocerebral degeneration); *Small's disease* with recessive hearing loss, mental retardation, narrowing of retinal vessels, and muscle atrophy. In the former, the infant is born blind, with a white vascularized retinal mass behind a clear lens; later the lens and cornea become opaque. The eyes are small, and the iris is atrophied. In the latter the optic fundi show tortuosity of vessels, telangiectases, and retinal detachment. The nature of the progressive generalized muscular weakness in Small's family (three children in one sibship) has not been ascertained.

HEREDITARY HEARING LOSS WITH DISEASES OF THE NERVOUS SYSTEM

Several conditions are known in which hereditary deafness accompanies degenerative disease of the peripheral or central nervous system.

1. *Hereditary hearing loss with epilepsy.* The seizure disorder is mainly one of myoclonus. In one dominantly inherited form (Hermann's disease) photomyoclonus is associated with mental deterioration, hearing loss, and nephropathy. In May-White disease, also dominant, myoclonus and ataxia accompany hearing loss. Congenital deafness and mild chronic epilepsy of recessive type have also been observed (Latham-Munro disease).

2. *Hereditary hearing loss and ataxia.* Here Konigsmark was able to delineate five syndromes, the first two of which show a dominant pattern of heredity, the last three a recessive pattern: piebaldism, ataxia, and neural hearing loss (Telfer syndrome); hearing loss, hyperuricemia, and ataxia (Rosenberg-Bergstrom syndrome); ataxia and progressive hearing loss (Lichtenstein-Knorr syndrome); ataxia, hypogonadism, mental deficiency, and hearing loss (Richards-Rundles syndrome); ataxia, mental retardation, hearing loss, and pigmentary changes in skin (Jeune-Tommasi syndrome).

3. *Hereditary hearing loss and other neurologic syndromes.* These include dominant sensory radicular neuropathy (Denny-Brown); progressive polyneuropathy, kyphoscoliosis, skin atrophy, eye defects (myopia, cataracts, atypical retinitis pigmentosa), bone cysts and osteoporosis (Flynn-Aird syndrome); chronic polyneuropathy and nephritis (Lemieux-Neemeh syndrome);

congenital pain asymbolia and auditory imperception (Osuntokun's syndrome); and bulbopontine paralysis (facial weakness, dysarthria, dysphagia, and atrophy of the tongue with fasciculations) with progressive neural hearing loss. The onset of the latter syndrome occurs at 10 to 35 years of age; the pattern of inheritance is recessive. The disease progresses to death. It resembles the progressive hereditary bulbar paralysis of Fazio-Londe, except for the progressive deafness and loss of vestibular responses.

References which describe the details of these many syndromes are contained in Konigsmark's review, listed below. The syndromes are summarized here in order to increase awareness of the large number of hereditary neurologic diseases for which the clue is provided by the detection of impaired hearing and labyrinthine functions.

REFERENCES

ADAMS RD, VAN BOGAERT L, VANDER EECKEN H: Striatonigral degeneration. *J Neuropathol Exp Neurol* 23:584, 1964.

ALLEN N, KNOPP W: Hereditary parkinsonism-dystonia with sustained control by L-dopa and anticholinergic medication, in Eldridge R, Fahn S (eds): *Advances in Neurology*, vol 14: *Dystonia*. New York, Raven Press, 1976, pp 201-215.

ALZHEIMER A: Uber eine eigenartige Erkankung der Hirnrinde. *Allg Z Psychiatr* 64:146, 1907.

———: Über eigenartige Krankheitsfälle des späteren Alters. *Z Gesamte Neurol Psychiatr* 4:356, 1911.

AUSTIN JG et al: Metachromatic leukodystrophy. *Arch Neurol* 18:225, 1968.

BARBEAU A: Biochemistry of Huntington's chorea, in Barbeau A, Chase TN, Paulson GW (eds): *Advances in Neurology*, vol 1. New York, Raven Press, 1973, pp 473-516.

———: Biochemistry of Friedreich's ataxia, in *Spinocerebellar Degenerations*. Tokyo, University of Tokyo Press, 1980, pp 303-311.

BECKER PE: Genetic approaches to the nosology of nervous system defects, in Bergsma D: *Birth Defects: Original Article Series*, vol 7: *Nervous System*, pt VI. New York, Alan R Less, 1971, pp 10-22.

BEHR C: Die komplizierte, hereditär-familiäre Optikusatrophie des Kindesalters. Ein bisher nicht beschriebener Symptomkomplex. *Klin Mbl Augenheilk* 47 (Part 2):138, 1909.

BELL J: On hereditary ataxia and spastic paraplegia, in Fisher RA (ed): *Treasury of Human Inheritance*, vol IV: *Nervous Diseases and Muscular Dystrophies*, pt III. London, Cambridge University Press, 1939, pp 141-281.

BERLIN L: Presenile sclerosis (Alzheimer's disease) with features resembling Pick's disease. *Arch Neurol Psychiatry* 61:369, 1949.

BIRD ED, IVERSEN LL: Huntington's chorea: Postmortem measurement of glutamic acid decarboxylase, choline acetyltransferase and dopamine in basal ganglia. *Brain* 97:457, 1974.

BLASS JP, KARK RAP, MENON NK: Low activities of the pyruvate and oxoglutarate dehydrogenase complexes in five patients with Friedreich's ataxia. *N Engl J Med* 295:62, 1976.

BOWEN DA et al: Neurotransmitter-related enzymes and indices of hypoxia in senile dementia and other abiotrophies. *Brain* 99:459, 1976.

BRUYN GW, WENT LN: A sex-linked heredodegenerative neurological disorder associated with Leber's optic atrophy: I. Clinical studies. *J Neurol Sci* 159, 1964.

BYERS RK, BANKER BQ: Infantile muscular atrophy. *Arch Neurol* 5:140, 1961.

CARROLL WM, MASTAGLIA FL: Leber's optic neuropathy. *Brain* 102:559, 1979.

CHANDLER JH, REED TE, DeJONG RN: Huntington's chorea in Michigan: III. Clinical observations. *Neurology* 10:148, 1960.

COHAN SL, KATTAH JC, LIMAYE SR: Familial tapetoretinal degeneration and epilepsy. *Arch Neurol* 36:544, 1979.

COOPER IS: 20-year followup study of the neurosurgical treatment of dystonia musculorum deformans, in Eldridge R, Fahn S (eds): *Advances in Neurology*, vol 14. New York, Raven Press, 1976, pp 423-453.

CORSELLIS JAN: Aging in the dementias, in Blackwood W, Corsellis JAN (eds): *Greenfield's Neuropathology*. Chicago, Year Book, 1976, chap 18, pp 796-848.

———, BRIERLY JB: An unusual type of presenile dementia. *Brain* 77:571, 1954.

CREUTZFELDT HG: Über eine eigenartige herdförmige Erkrankung des Zentralnervensystems. *Z Gesamte Neurol Psychiatr* 57:1, 1920.

DAVENPORT CB: Huntington's chorea in relation to heredity and eugenics. *Proc Nat Acad Sci* 1:283, 1915.

DAVIES P, MALONEY AJF: Selective loss of central cholinergic neurons in Alzheimer's disease. *Lancet* 2:1403, 1976.

DAVISON C: Spastic pseudosclerosis (cortico-pallido-spinal degeneration). *Brain* 55:247, 1932.

DEDO HH: Recurrent laryngeal nerve section for spastic dysphonia. *Ann Otol Rhinol Laryngol* 85:451, 1976.

DRACHMAN DA: Ophthalmoplegia plus: A classification of the disorders associated with progressive external ophthalmoplegia, in Vinken PJ, Bruyn GW (eds): *Handbook of Clinical Neurology*, vol 22. Amsterdam, North-Holland, 1975, chap 9, pp 203-216.

DUNLAP CB: Pathologic changes in Huntington's chorea, with special reference to corpus striatum. *Arch Neurol Psychiatry* 18:867, 1927.

ELDRIDGE R: The torsion dystonias: Literature review and genetic and clinical studies. *Neurology* 20:1, 1970.

———, FAHN S (eds): *Advances in Neurology*, vol 14: *Dystonia*. New York, Raven Press, 1976.

EMERY AEH: Review of the nosology of progressive muscular atrophy. *J Med Genet* 8:481, 1971.

ENNA SJ: Huntington's chorea: Changes in neurotransmitter receptors in the brain. *N Engl J Med* 294:1305, 1976.

FERGUSON F, CRITCHLEY M: A clinical study of an heredofamilial disease resembling disseminated sclerosis. *Brain* 52:203, 1929.

FINLAYSON MH, GUBERMAN A, MARTIN JB: Cerebral lesions in familial amyotrophic lateral sclerosis and dementia. *Acta Neuropathol* 26:237, 1973.

FLATAU E, STERLING W: Progressive Torsionsspasmus bei Kindern. *Z Gesamte Neurol Psychiatr* 7:586, 1911.

GELLER M, KAPLAN P, CHRISTOFF N: Treatment of dystonic symptoms with carbamazepine, in Eldridge R, Fahn S (eds): *Advances in Neurology*, vol 14: *Dystonia*. New York, Raven Press, 1976, pp 403–411.

GILMAN S, ROMANUL FCA: Hereditary dystonic paraplegia with amyotrophy and mental deficiency: Clinical and neuropathological characteristics, in Vinken PJ, Bruyn GW (eds): *Handbook of Clinical Neurology*, vol 22. Amsterdam, North-Holland, 1975, chap 19, pp 445–465.

GOUDSMIT J et al: Evidence for and against the transmissibility of Alzheimer's disease. *Neurology* 30:945, 1980.

GREENFIELD JG: *The Spino-Cerebellar Degenerations*. Springfield, Ill, Charles C Thomas, 1954.

HAKIM AM MATHIESON G: Basis of dementia in Parkinson's disease. *Lancet* 2:729, 1978.

HALLETT M, KHOSHBIN S: A physiological mechanism of bradykinesia. *Brain* 103:301, 1980.

HIRANO A, KURLAND LT, KROOTH RS, LESSELL S: Parkinsonism-dementia complex, an endemic disease on the Island of Guam: I. Clinical features. *Brain* 84:642, 1961.

———, MALAMUD M, KURLAND LT: Parkinsonism-dementia complex on the Island of Guam. II: Pathological features. *Brain* 84:662, 1961.

HOLMES GM: A form of familial degeneration of the cerebellum. *Brain* 30:466, 1907a.

———: An attempt to classify cerebellar disease with a note on Marie's hereditary cerebellar ataxia. *Brain* 30:545, 1907b.

HUNT JR: Dyssynergia cerebellaris progressiva—a chronic progressive form of cerebellar tremor. *Brain* 37:247, 1914.

———: Progressive atrophy of the globus pallidus. *Brain* 40:58, 1917.

———: Dyssynergia cerebellaris myoclonica—primary atrophy of the dentate system: A contribution to the pathology and symptomatology of the cerebellum. *Brain* 44:490, 1921.

———: The striocerebellar tremor. *Arch Neurol Psychiatry* 8:664, 1922.

HUNTINGTON G: On chorea. *Med Surg Reporter* 26:317, 1872.

JAKOB A: Über eigenartige Erkrankungen des Zentralnervensystems mit bemerkenswertem anatomischen Befunde (spastische Pseudo-sclerose-encephalomyelopathie mit disseminierten Degenerationsherden). *Z Gesamte Neurol Psychiatr* 64:147, 1921.

———: Über eine der multiplen Sklerose klinischnahestehende Erkrankung des Centralnervensystems (spastische Pseudosklerose) mit bemerkenswertem anatomischen Befunde. *Med Klin* 17:372, 1921.

JERVIS GA: Early senile dementia in mongoloid idiocy. *Am J Psychiatry* 105:102, 1948.

KANTER W, WOOTEN F, ELDRIDGE R: Dopamine-beta-hydroxylase and the torsion dystonias, in Eldridge R, Fahn S (eds): *Advances in Neurology*, vol 14: *Dystonia*. New York, Raven Press, 1976, pp 303–307.

KARK RAP, ROSENBERG RN, SCHUT LJ (eds): *Advances in Neurology*, vol 21: *The Inherited Ataxias*. New York, Raven Press, 1978.

KAY DWK, BEAMISH P, ROTH M: Old age mental disorder in Newcastle-upon-Tyne: 1. A study of prevalence. *Br J Psychiatry* 110:146, 1964.

KJELLIN KG: Hereditary spastic paraplegia and retinal degeneration (Kjellin syndrome and Barnard-Scholz syndrome), in Vinken PJ, Bruyn GW (eds): *Handbook of Clinical Neurology*, vol 22. Amsterdam, North-Holland, 1975, chap 20, pp 467–473.

KLAWANS HL et al: Levodopa and presymptomatic detection of Huntington's disease—eight year follow up. *N Engl J Med* 302:1090, 1980.

KONIGSMARK BW: Hereditary diseases of the nervous system with hearing loss, in Vinken PJ, Bruyn GW (eds): *Handbook of Clinical Neurology*, vol 22. Amsterdam, North-Holland, 1975, chap 23, pp 499–526.

———, WEINER LP: The olivopontocerebellar atrophies: A review. *Medicine* 49:227, 1970.

KUGELBERG E: Chronic proximal (pseudomyopathic) spinal muscular atrophy: Kugelberg-Welander syndrome, in Vinken PJ, Bruyn GW (eds): *Handbook of Clinical Neurology*, vol 22. Amsterdam, North-Holland, 1975, chap 3, pp 67–80.

LANCE JW, SCHWAB RS, PETERSON EA: Action tremor and the cogwheel phenomenon in Parkinson's disease. *Brain* 86:95, 1963.

LARSSON T, SJÖGREN T, JACOBSEN G: Senile dementia. *Acta Psychiatr Scan Suppl* 39:167 1963.

LEBER T: Ueber Hereditäre and congenital angelegte Schnervenleiden. v. *Graefes Arch Ophthal* 17:249, 1871.

LIEBERMAN A et al: Dementia in Parkinson disease. *Ann Neurol* 6:355, 1979.

LOKEN H, CYVIN K: Case of clinical juvenile amaurotic idiocy with histological picture of Alzheimer's disease. *J Neurol Neurosurg Psychiatry* 17:211, 1954.

LOUIS-BAR D, VAN BOGAERT L: Sur la dyssynergie cérébelleuse myoclonique (Hunt). *Mschr. Psychiatr Neurol* 113:215, 1947.

MALAMUD W, LOWENBERG K: Alzheimer's disease: Contribution to its etiology and classification. *Arch Neurol Psychiatry* 21:805, 1929.

MARIE P: Sur l'hérédo-ataxie cérébelleuse. *Sem Med* 13:444, 1893.

————, Foix C, Alajouanine T: De l'atrophie cérébelleuse tardive a prédominance corticale. *Rev Neurol* 38:849, 1082, 1922.

Marinescu G: Sur une affection particulière simulant, au point de vue clinique, la sclérose en plaques et ayant pour substratum des plaques du type senile spécial. *Arch Roum Pathol Exp Microbiol* 4:41, March 1931 (*Rev Neurol* 2:453, October 1931).

Marsden CD: The problems of adult onset idiopathic torsion dystonia and other isolated dyskinesias of adult life, in Eldrige R, Fahn S (eds): *Advances in Neurology*, vol 14: *Dystonia*. New York, Raven Press, 1976, pp 259-277.

Mastaglia FL, Walton JN: Histologic and histochemical changes in skeletal muscles from cases of chronic juvenile and early adult spinal muscular atrophy (the Kugelberg-Welander syndrome). *J Neurol Sci* 12:15, 1971.

McMenemey WH: The dementias and progressive diseases of the basal ganglia, in Blackwood W et al (eds): *Greenfield's Neuropathology*, 2d ed. London, Arnold, 1963, chap 9, pp 520-580.

Mollaret P: La Maladie de Friedreich. Paris, Legrand, 1929.

Moyano BA: Coloracion de la neuroglia por el metodo de Holzer. *Sem Med* 2:1919, 1930.

Mulder DW (ed): *The Diagnosis and Treatment of Amyotrophic Lateral Sclerosis*. Boston, Houghton-Mifflin, 1980, p 41.

————, Espinosa RE: Amyotrophic lateral sclerosis: Comparison of the clinical syndrome in Guam and the United States, in Norris FH, Kurland LT (eds): *Motor Neuron Diseases*. New York, Grune & Stratton, 1969, pp 12-19.

Naeser MA, Gebhardt C, Levine HL: Decreased computerized tomography numbers in patients with presenile dementia. *Arch Neurol* 37:401, 1980.

Nakano, KK, Dawson DM, Spence A: Machado disease. A hereditary ataxia in Portuguese emigrants to Massachusetts. *Neurology* 22:49, 1972.

Nielsen SL: Striatonigral degeneration disputed in familial disorder. *Neurology* 27:306, 1977.

Pick A: Über die Beziehungen der senilen hirnatrophie zur Aphasie. *Prager Med Wochenschr* 17:165, 1892.

Rajput AH, Rozdilsky B: Dysautonomia in Parkinsonism: A clinicopathologic study. *J Neurol Neurosurg Psychiatry* 39:1092, 1976.

Rebeiz JJ, Kolodny EH, Richardson EP: Corticodentatonigral degeneration with neuronal achromasia. *Arch Neurol* 18:20, 1968.

Richardson JC, Steele J, Olszewski J: Supranuclear ophthalmoplegia, pseudobulbar palsy, nuchal dystonia and dementia. *Trans Am Neurol Assoc* 88:25, 1963.

Rodriguez-Budelli M, Kark RAP, Blass JP: Action of physostigmine on inherited ataxias, in Kark RAP, Rosenberg RN, Schut LJ (eds): *Advances in Neurology*, vol 21: *The Inherited Ataxias*. New York, Raven Press, 1978, pp 195-203.

Romanul FCA: Azorean disease of the nervous system. *N Engl J Med* 297:729, 1977.

———— et al: Azorean disease of the nervous system. *N Engl J Med* 296:1505, 1977.

Ropper AH, Williams RS: Relationship between plaques, tangles and dementia in Down syndrome. *Neurology* 30:639, 1980.

Rosenberg RN et al: Autosomal dominant striatonigral degeneration: A clinical, pathologic and biochemical study of a new genetic disorder. *Neurology* 26.703, 1976.

Rosenhagen H: Die primäre Atrophie des Brächenfusses und der unteren Oliven. *Arch Psychiat* 116:163, 1943.

Rowland LP: Progressive external ophthalmoplegia, in Vinken PJ, Bruyn GW (eds): *Handbook of Clinical Neurology*, vol 22. Amsterdam, North-Holland, 1975, chap 8, pp 177-202.

Russell DS: Myocarditis in Friedreich's ataxia. *J Path Bacteriol* 58:739, 1946.

Schaumburg HH, Suzuki K: Non-specific familial presenile dementia. *J Neurol Neurosurg Psychiatry* 31:479, 1968.

Schwalbe W: Eine eigentümliche tonische Krampffor mit hysterischen Symptomen. Berlin, G Schade, 1908.

Scribanu N, Kennedy C: Familial syndrome with dystonia neural deafness and possible intellectual impairment: Clinical course and pathologic features, in Eldridge R, Fahn S (eds): *Advances in Neurology*, vol 14: *Dystonia*. New York, Raven Press, 1976, pp 235-245.

Shoulson I et al: Huntington's disease: Treatment with muscimol, a GABA-mimetic drug. *Ann Neurol* 1:506, 1977.

Sjögren T, Sjögren H, Lindgren AGH: Morbus Alzheimer and Morbus Pick: A genetic, clinical and pathoanatomical study. *Acta Psychiat Neurol Scand*, suppl 82, 1952.

Smith JL, Hoyt WF, Susac JO: Ocular fundus in acute Leber optic neuropathy. *Arch Ophthalmol* 90:349, 1973.

Spatz H: Die Systematischen Atrophien. *Arch Psychiat* 108:1, 1938.

————: Pick's Disease, in *Proceedings of the 1st International Congress on Neuropathology*. London, Arnold, 1952, vol 2, p 375.

Spielmeyer W: *Histopathologie des Nervensystems*. Berlin, Springer-Verlag, 1922, pp 223-229.

Spokes EGS: Neurochemical alterations in Huntington's chorea. A study of post-mortem brain tissue. *Brain* 103:179, 1980.

Stargardt K: Über familiäre, progressive Degeneration in der Maculagegend. v. *Graefes Arch Ophthal* 71:534, 1909.

Steele JC: Progressive supranuclear palsy. *Brain* 95:693, 1972.

Tissot R, Constantinidis J, Richard J: *La Maladie de Pick*. Paris, Masson et Cie, 1975.

Van Bogaert L, Van Maere M, De Smedt E: Sur les formes familiales précoces de la maladie d'Alzheimer. *Monatsschr Psychiatr Neurol* 102:249, 1940.

Van Mansvelt J: Pick's disease: A syndrome of lobar cerebral atrophy. Clinicoanatomical and histopathological types, Thesis, Utrecht, 1954.

VESSIE PR: On the transmission of Huntington chorea for 300 years—the Bures family group. *J Nerv Ment Dis* 76:553, 1932.

VICTOR M, ADAMS RD, MANCALL EL: A restricted form of cerebellar degeneration occurring in alcoholic patients. *Arch Neurol* 1:577, 1959.

WAARDENBURG PJ: Über familiär-erbliche Fälle von seniler Maculadegeneration. *Genetica* 18:38, 1936.

WANG HS: Dementia in old age, in Smith LW, Kinsbourne M (eds): *Aging and Dementia*. New York, Spectrum, 1977, pp 1–4.

WELLS C, DUNCAN GW: Danger of over-reliance on computerized cranial tomography. *Am J Psychiatry* 34:811, 1977.

WILSON SAK: *Neurology*. Baltimore, Williams & Wilkins, 1940.

WOHLFART G, FEX J, ELIASSON S: Hereditary proximal spinal muscular atrophy: A clinical entity simulating progressive muscular dystrophy. *Acta Psychiatr Neurol Scand* 30:395, 1955.

WOODARD JC: Concentric hyaline inclusion body formation in mental disease: Analysis of 27 cases. *J Neuropathol Exp Neurol* 21:442, 1962.

WOODS BT, SCHAUMBURG HH: Nigrospinodentatal degeneration with nuclear ophthalmoplegia, in Vinken PJ, Bruyn GW (eds): *Handbook of Clinical Neurology*, vol 22. Amsterdam, North-Holland, 1975, chap 7, pp 157–176.

WORSTER-DROUGHT C, GREENFIELD JG, McMENEMEY WH: A form of familial progressive dementia with spastic paralysis. *Brain* 67:38, 1944.

YAMAGUCHI F et al : Noninvasive regional cerebral blood flow measurements in dementia. *Arch Neurol* 37:410, 1980.

ZEMAN W: Pathology of the torsion dystonias (dystonia musculorum deformans). *Neurology* 20 (pt 2):79, 1970.

———, DYKEN P: Dystonia musculorum deformans. Clinical, genetic and pathoanatomical studies. *Psychiatr Neurol Neurochir* 70:77, 1967.

ZIEGLER MG et al: Plasma norepinephrine and dopamine-β-hydroxylase in dystonia, in Eldridge R, Fahn S (eds): *Advances in Neurology*, vol 14: *Dystonia*. New York, Raven Press, 1976, pp 307–318.

CHAPTER 43

DEVELOPMENTAL DISEASES OF THE NERVOUS SYSTEM

Under this broad heading are subsumed a diversity of developmental malformations and diseases acquired during the intrauterine period of life. Taxonomically they include many unrelated pathologic processes of different origins: some stem from germ plasm abnormalities; others are associated with triplication, deletion, and translocations of chromosomes; and still others are due to the effects of a variety of noxious agents acting at different times on the nervous system, i.e., during the embryonal, fetal, and paranatal periods of life.

It would be intellectually satisfying if all the morbid states that originate in the intrauterine period could be separated into genetic (hereditary) or nongenetic (congenital) forms, but in many instances the biologic information and the pathologic changes in brain at this early age have not been characteristic of one group or another and do not allow such a division. For example, in the large group of diseases in which the neural tube fails to close (rachischisis), more than one member of a family may be affected, but it cannot be stated whether a genetic factor is operative or an exogenous factor has acted upon several members. Even what appears to be an outright malformation of the brain may be no more than a reflection of the timing of a pathologic process that has affected the nervous system and other organs early in the embryonal period, derailing later processes of development. Teratology, the scientific study of neurosomatic malformations, is replete with such examples.

The authors do not wish to imply that medical and biologic ideas about these conditions are completely unsettled, for there are diseases that are transmitted from one generation to another, affecting both of identical (monovular) twins and only one of fraternal (biovu-lar) twins. In these, a genetic determinant cannot be questioned, for the unaffected fraternal twin shares the same intrauterine environment as the twin sibling. Then, too, a few diseases destroy parts of the brain in utero in specific ways; others affect it in nonspecific ways but leave little doubt as to the action of an exogenous pathogen.

A perusal of the following pages makes it evident that there is a great variety of structural defects of the nervous system; in fact, every part of the brain, spinal cord, nerves, and musculature may be affected. However, certain principles are applicable to the entire group. *First*, the abnormality of the nervous system is frequently accompanied by an abnormality of some other structure or organ (eye, nose, cranium, spine, ear, and heart), which implicates a certain period of embryogenesis. This principle is far from absolute, however, for in certain maldevelopments of the brain that must have originated in the embryonal period, all other organs are normal. One can only assume that the brain is more vulnerable than any other organ to prenatal as well as natal influences. *Second*, a maldevelopment of whatever cause should be present at birth and remain stable thereafter, i.e., be nonprogressive; but again there are exceptions: the abnormality may have affected parts of the brain that are not functional at birth so that an interval of time must elapse postnatally before the symptoms of a defect can appear. *Third*, the birth should have been nontraumatic. However, the occurrence of a traumatic birth is not proof of a causative relationship between the injury (or infection) and the abnormality, because a defective nervous system may interfere with the birth process or may be excessively vulnerable to an intoxication or infection. *Fourth*, if the birth abnormality has occurred in other members of the family of the same or previous generations, it is usually genetic—although, as noted above, this does not exclude the possible adverse effects of exogenous agents.

A textbook on principles of neurology is not the place to present a detailed account of all the hereditary and congenital developmental abnormalities that might affect the nervous system. Instead we shall only outline the major groups and discuss a few of the more common disease entities. In the classification in Table 43-1 we adhere to a division in accordance with the main presenting abnormality or abnormalities. Represented are all the common problems that cause families to seek consultation with the pediatric neurologist: (1) structural defects of the cranium, spine, and limbs, and of eyes, nose, ears, jaws, and skin; (2) disturbed motor function—retardation in development or abnormal movements; (3) mental retardation; and (4) epilepsy. The following discussion will be focused on each of these clinical states.

NEUROLOGIC DISORDERS ASSOCIATED WITH CRANIOSPINAL DEFORMITIES

One has only to walk through an institution for the mentally retarded to appreciate the remarkable number of physical disfigurements that attend abnormalities of the nervous system: heads small and large, encephaloceles with absence of cranium, dwarfed bodies, and odd physiognomies—some of them appallingly grotesque. Indeed, a normal-appearing individual stands out in such a crowd, and will be found frequently to have an inherited metabolic defect or birth injury.

The intimate relationship between the cranium and the growth and development of the brain deserves comment. In embryonic life the most rapidly growing parts of the neural tube induce special changes in and at the same time are influenced by the overlying mesoderm (a process known as induction); hence abnormalities in the formation of skull, orbits, nose, and spine are regularly associated with anomalies of brain and spinal cord. During early fetal life the cranial bones and vertebral arches enclose and protect the developing brain and spinal cord; throughout the period of rapid brain growth, as pressure is exerted on the inner table of the skull, the latter accommodates to the increasing size of the brain. This adaptation is facilitated by the membranous fontanels, which remain open until maximal brain growth has been attained; only then do they ossify (close).

Table 43-1
Classification of congenital neurologic disorders

I. Neurologic disorders associated with craniospinal deformities
  A. Enlarged head
    1. Hydrocephalus
    2. Hydranencephaly
    3. Macrocephaly
  B. Craniostenoses
    1. Turricephaly
    2. Scaphocephaly
    3. Brachycephaly
  C. Microcephaly
    1. Primary (vera)
    2. Secondary to cerebral disease
  D. Combinations of cerebral, cranial, and other anomalies
    1. Syndactylic craniocerebral anomalies
    2. Other craniofacial anomalies
    3. Oculoencephalic defects
    4. Oculoauriculocephalic anomalies
    5. Dwarfism
    6. Dermatocephalic anomalies
  E. Rachischisis
    1. Anencephaly, cephalic and spinal meningocele, meningoencephalocele, Dandy-Walker syndrome, meningomyelocele
    2. Arnold-Chiari malformation
    3. Platybasia and cervical-spinal anomalies (Chap. 35)
  F. Chromosomal abnormalities
II. The phakomatoses
  A. Tuberous sclerosis
  B. Neurofibromatosis
  C. Cutaneous angiomatosis with CNS abnormalities
III. Restricted developmental abnormalities of the nervous system
  A. Möbius' syndrome
  B. Congenital apraxia of gaze
  C. Other restricted congenital abnormalities (Horner's syndrome, unilateral ptosis, anisocoria, etc.)
IV. Congenital abnormalities of motor function (*cerebral palsy*)
  A. Cerebral spastic diplegia
  B. Infantile hemiplegia, double hemiplegia, and quadriplegia
  C. Congenital extrapyramidal disorders (double athetosis; erythroblastosis fetalis and kernicterus)
  D. Congenital and acquired ataxias
  E. The flaccid paralyses
V. Prenatal and paranatal infections
  A. Rubella
  B. Cytomegalic inclusion disease
  C. Congenital neurosyphilis
  D. Toxoplasmosis
  E. Other viral and bacterial infections
VI. Epilepsies of infancy and childhood
VII. Mental retardation

In addition, statural growth is controlled by the nervous system, as shown by the fact that the majority of mental retardates are dwarfed in varying degree. Thus disorders of craniovertebral development assume importance not merely because of their unsightly appearance but also because they may reflect an abnormality of the underlying brain and spinal cord, i.e., they become diagnostic signs.

CRANIAL MALFORMATIONS AT BIRTH

Certain alterations in the size and shape of the head observed in the infant, child, or even adult always signify a pathologic process that affected the brain before birth or in infancy. The size of the cranium reflects the size of the brain, and the tape measure is the most useful tool in pediatric neurology. No examination is complete without a measurement of the circumference of the head. A newborn whose head circumference is below the third percentile for age and sex, and whose fontanels are closed, may be judged to have a developmental abnormality of the brain. A head that is normal in size at birth but fails to keep pace with body length reflects a later failure of growth and maturation of the cerebral hemispheres (microcephaly or microencephaly).

ENLARGEMENT OF THE HEAD

This can be due to hydrocephalus, hydranencephalus, or excessive brain growth (macrocephaly or macroencephaly). The *hydrocephalic head* is distinguished by several features—frontal bossing, a tendency for the eyes to turn down so that the sclera are visible between the upper lids and irides (sunset sign), prominence of scalp veins due to blockage of blood flow into the dural sinuses, separation of the cranial sutures, thinning of the scalp, and a "cracked-pot" sound on percussion of the skull.

The *hydranencephalic* head (hydrocephalus and destruction or failure of development of parts of the cerebrum) is often associated with enlargement of the skull. When it is transilluminated with a strong flashlight in a darkened room it glows like a jack-o'-lantern. Hydranencephaly is not a well-defined entity. It can be caused by intrauterine vascular occlusion or diseases such as toxoplasmosis and cytomegalic virus disease, in which parts of each cerebral hemisphere are destroyed. Destruction of the cerebral mantle in the embryonal period may lead to the formation of huge porencephalic defects with subsequent failure of development (evagination) of brain. In the marginal parts of the porencephaly the cortex is malformed, but this indicates only that the lesion preceded neuronal migration. The lack of resistance of defective brain to ventricular pressure enlarges the head. In still other cases, there appears to be a pri-

mary failure of development, more specifically varying degrees of failure of evagination. Yakovlev and Wadsworth speak of these as *schizencephalies*.

The *macrocephalic head* (a large head with normal or only slightly enlarged ventricles) may be indicative of the syndrome of macrocephalic idiocy; but it also is suggestive of an advancing metabolic disease that enlarges the brain, as in the later phases of *Tay-Sachs disease, Alexander's disease,* and *spongy degeneration of infancy. Subdural hematomas* may also enlarge the head and cause bulging of fontanelles and separation of sutures. Usually the infant is irritable, listless, and takes nourishment poorly. CT scans disclose the subdural blood or fluid (hygroma) and small ventricles.

CRANIOSTENOSES

Some of the most arresting cranial deformities are caused by an obscure malady in which the cranial sutures (membranous junctions between bones of the skull) close prematurely. When the lambdoid and coronal sutures are both affected, the thrust of the growing brain enlarges the head in a vertical direction (*tower skull, or oxycephaly,* also referred to as *turricephaly* and *acrocephaly*). The orbits are shallow, the eyes bulge, and skull films show islands of bone-thinning (Lückenschädel); and often there is a marked degree of syndactyly and a variable degree of mental retardation. When only the sagittal suture is involved, the head is long and narrow (*scaphocephalic*), and the closed suture projects, keel-like, in the midline. With premature closure of the coronal suture, the head is excessively wide and short (*brachycephalic*). The nervous system is usually normal in these restricted craniostenoses. If recognized in early infancy, the surgeon can make artificial sutures that may permit the shape of the head to become more normal. Once brain growth has been completed, nothing can be done. When several sutures are closed so as to diminish the cranial capacity, intracranial pressure may increase, impairing cerebral function and later causing papilledema. Obviously an operation is then needed to enlarge the skull. When for any reason an infant lies with the head turned constantly to one side, the occiput on that side becomes flattened, as does the opposite frontal bone. The other occiput and frontal bone bulge, so that the maximum length of the skull is not in the midline, but on a diagonal. This condition is called *plagiocephaly,* or *wry head.* Craniostenosis of one-half of a coronal suture may also distort the skull in this way.

MICROCEPHALY

There is a form of hereditary microcephaly called *microcephaly vera* in which the head is extremely small (circumference less than 45 cm in adult life). In contrast, the face is of normal size, the forehead is narrow and recedes sharply, and the occiput is flat. The stature is only moderately reduced. Such individuals can be recognized at birth by their primitive anthropoid appearance and later by their lumbering gait, extremely low intelligence and lack of communicative speech. Vision, hearing, and cutaneous sensation are spared. Tendon reflexes in the legs are brisk, and the plantar reflexes may be extensor. Skull films show that the cranial sutures are present, and there are convolutional markings. There are two types of inheritance of microcephaly vera, autosomal recessive and sex-linked. The brain often weighs less than 300 g (normal 1350 to 1400 g), and shows only a few primary and secondary sulci. The cerebral cortex is thin and unlaminated and grossly deficient in neurons. In a few reported cases there has been an associated cerebellar hypoplasia or an infantile muscular atrophy.

COMBINED CEREBRAL, CRANIAL AND SOMATIC ABNORMALITIES

Many of the diseases that interfere with cerebral development also deform the cranial and facial bones, the eyes, the nose, and the ears. Such somatic stigmata therefore assume significance as indicators of altered cerebral structure and function. Moreover, they constitute irrefutable evidence that the associated neural abnormality is in the nature of a maldevelopment, either hereditary or the result of a disease acquired during the embryonic period.

There are so many of these cerebrosomatic anomalies that one can hardly retain visual images of them, much less recall all the physicians' names by which they are known. Of necessity one turns to atlases, one of the best of which has been composed by our colleagues Holmes, Moser et al., and is based on clinical material drawn from the Massachusetts General Hospital, the Fernald School, and Shriver Institute. The interested reader should turn to this book or to the one by Gorlin et al. for specific information. Ford's monograph *Diseases of the Nervous System in Infancy, Childhood, and Adolescence,* and *The Practice of Pediatric Neurology,* by Swaiman and Wright, are other valuable references.

There is some advantage in grouping these anomalies according to whether the hands and extremities, the face, the eyes, the ears, and the skin are associated with a cerebral defect. For the convenience of the reader and for the purpose of conveying some notion of the number and variety of these anomalies, many of them are summarized below. Unfortunately, no very useful leads as to their origin have been forthcoming.

The Syndactylic Craniocerebral Anomalies Commonly, fusion of two fingers or two toes or the presence of a tab of skin representing an extra digit is present from birth in an otherwise normal individual. However, when syndactylism of variable degree is accompanied by premature closure of cranial sutures, the nervous system usually proves to be abnormal as well. The following are summaries of some of the better-known syndromes.

1. *Acrocephalosyndactyly types I and II (typical and atypical Apert's syndrome).* Type I: turribrachycephalic skull, flat occiput, complete syndactyly of hands and feet ("mitten hands," "sock feet"), protuberant and widely spaced eyes, flat and underdeveloped maxilla and nasal bridge but well-developed chin (relative prognathism), moderate to severe mental retardation, dilated cerebral ventricles. Type II, or atypical form: less-severe extent of syndactyly, probably a phenotypic variant of type I.

2. *Acrocephalosyndactyly III (Saethre-Chotzen syndrome).* Transmission as an autosomal dominant trait, various types of craniostenosis, low frontal hairline, beaked nose with deviated nasal septum, hypertelorism, ptosis, prognathism, cryptorchidism, sometimes low-set ears, proximally fused and shortened digits, moderate degree of mental retardation.

3. *Acrocephalosyndactyly IV (Pfeiffer's syndrome).* Autosomal dominant heredity, turribrachycephaly, protruding, widely spaced eyes and divergent strabismus, antimongoloid obliquity of palpebral fissures, low-set ears, irregularly aligned teeth, broad enlarged thumbs and great toes, partially flexed elbows (radiohumeral or radioulnar synostoses), mental retardation mild and variable.

4. *Acrocephalopolysyndactyly (Carpenter's syndrome).* Autosomal recessive heredity, premature fusion of all cranial sutures with acrocephaly, flat bridge of nose, medial canthi displaced laterally, epicanthal folds and micrognathia, microcorneas and corneal opacities, hypogenitalism in males, excess digits and syndactyly, obesity, cardiac abnormality in some, subnormal intelligence.

5. *Acrocephalosyndactyly with absent digits.* High, bitemporally flattened head, widely spaced, prominent eyes, small posteriorly rotated ears, flexed arms, high-arched palate, defect in parietal bones, absent toes and syndactylic fingers, moderate mental retardation.

6. *Acrocephaly with cleft lip and palate, radial aplasia and absent digits.* Microbrachycephaly due to craniostenosis, hypertelorism, misshapen ears, curved mandible, cleft lip and palate, absent radial bones, severe mental retardation.

7. *Dyschondroplasia, facial anomalies, and polysyndactyly.* Probably inherited as an autosomal recessive trait with keel-shaped skull and ridge running up through center of forehead (metopic suture), macrostomia, micrognathia, upward slant of eyes, high palate, thick alveolar ridges, short neck, short arms and legs, postaxial polydactyly and short digits, genu recurvatum, redundancy of skin, rib anomalies and short sternum, overfolding of helices of ears, moderate mental retardation.

In all the foregoing types of syndactylism and cranial abnormality, which may be regarded as variants of a common syndrome, the diagnosis can be made at a glance, because of the deformed head, protuberant eyes, and abnormal hands and feet. The mental retardation proves to be variable, usually moderate to severe, but occasionally intelligence is normal or nearly so. The brain has been examined in only a few instances and then not in a fashion to display fully a developmental abnormality.

Other Craniocephalic-Skeletal Anomalies In the following group of anomalies, the cranium, face, and other parts have special peculiarities, but craniostenosis is not a consistent feature.

1. *Craniofacial dysostosis (Crouzon's syndrome).* This malformation is inherited as an autosomal dominant trait and consists of variable types and degrees of craniosynostosis, broad forehead with prominence in the anterior fontanel region, shallow orbits with proptosis, midline facial hypoplasia and short upper lip, malformed auditory canals and ears, high narrow palate, crowded, malaligned upper teeth, moderate mental retardation.

2. *Median cleft facial syndrome (frontonasal dysplasia; hypertelorism of Greig).* Autosomal dominant type of heredity in some cases, widely spaced eyes, broad nasal root, cleft nose and premaxilla, V-shaped frontal hairline, sometimes median frontal lipomas, dermoids and teratomas, heterotypic anterior frontal fontanel

(midline cranial defect), strabismus and epibulbar dermoids, sometimes absence of entire prolabium and premaxilla and midline cleft in upper lip, mild to severe mental retardation. Surgical repair possible.

3. *Chondrodystrophia calcificans congenita (chondrodysplasia punctata, Conradi-Hünerman syndrome).* Autosomal recessive or dominant transmission with prominent forehead; flat nose; widely separated eyes; cataracts (in 18 percent); short neck and trunk with kyphoscoliosis; dry, scaly, atrophic skin; cicatricial alopecia; punctate calcifications of epiphyses of long bones and vertebral column with irregularly deformed vertebral bodies; mental retardation infrequent. Severe shortening of limbs in some cases.

4. *Orofaciodigital syndrome.* All the patients are female. It has been suggested that this condition is inherited as a dominant trait which is lethal in males. There are pseudoclefts involving the mandible, tongue, maxilla, and palate; lateral displacement of medial canthi; broad root of nose; hypertrophied buccal frenuli; hamartomas of tongue; sparse scalp hair; subnormal intelligence in one-third to one-half of cases.

5. *Pyknodysostosis.* Autosomal recessively inherited condition with large head and frontal-occipital bossing, underdeveloped facial bones, micrognathia, unerupted and deformed teeth, dense and defective long bones with shortened limbs, short and broad terminal digits of fingers and toes, kyphosis and scoliosis in some cases, mental retardation in 25 percent.

6. *Craniotubular bone dysplasias and hyperostoses.* Included under this title are several different genetic disorders of bone, characterized by modeling errors of tubular and cranial bones. Some are inherited as an autosomal recessive trait, and others as a dominant trait. Frontal and occipital hyperostosis, overgrowth of facial bones, and widening of long bones occur in various combinations. Hypertelorism, broad nasal root, nasal obstruction, seizures, visual failure, deafness, prognathism, and retardation of growth are the major signs. The serum alkaline phosphatase may be elevated.

Oculoencephalic Defects In this category of anomalies there is simultaneous failure or imperfect development of eye and brain. One member of this group, the oculocerebrorenal syndrome of Lowe has already been mentioned on page 675, and of course a number of the mucopolysaccharidoses cause corneal opacities, skeletal changes, and psychomotor regression. Also congenital syphilis, rubella, toxoplasmosis, and cytomegalic inclusion disease may affect retina and brain; hypoxia at birth requiring treatment with oxygen may injure the brain and lead to *retrolental fibrodysplasia*.

1. *Anophthalmia with mental retardation*. A sex-linked recessive disease, in which the child is born without eyes; the orbits and maxillae remain underdeveloped, but adnexal tissues of eyes (lids) are intact; occasional kyphoscoliosis and equinovarus deformities of feet; subnormal intelligence.

2. *Norrie's disease*. Also inherited as a sex-linked recessive trait; eyes are present at birth and some sight may be present; retrolental opacities; later eyes become shrunken and recessed (phthisis bulbi); some patients have short digits; outbursts of anger; hallucinations; regression of psychomotor function (?).

3. *Oculocerebral syndrome with hypopigmentation*. Autosomal recessive type of heredity with absence of pigment of hair and skin; small, cloudy, vascularized corneas and small globes (microphthalmia); marked mental retardation; athetotic movements of limbs; flexion contractures of elbows; spasticity of legs; persistent grasp and sucking reflexes.

4. *Microphthalmia with corneal opacities, spasticity, and mental retardation*. Microcephaly, broad flat nose, small eyes, corneal opacities, eccentric pupils, stiff extended spastic legs, severe mental retardation.

Oculoauriculocephalic Anomalies   These are less important from the neurologic standpoint.

1. *Mandibulofacial dysostosis (Treacher Collins syndrome, Franceschetti-Zwahlen-Klein syndrome)*. Autosomal dominant heredity with abnormalities of external ears, atresia of external auditory canals, middle and inner ear anomalies, downward palpebral slant, colobomas of lower eyelids, malar, mandibular, and zygomal hypoplasia, microphthalmia and colobomas of iris in a few, mental retardation rare.

2. *Oculoauriculovertebral dysplasia (Goldenhar's syndrome)*. Autosomal dominant or recessive type of heredity with preauricular appendages, auricular deformities, epibulbar dermoids (lipodermoids), small receding chin, hypoplasia of the soft and bony tissues of the mandible and face (hemifacial microsomia) and vertebral anomalies (hemivertebrae, cervical spine anomalies, spina bifida). Congenital ophthalmoplegia and mild mental retardation are present in some patients.

3. *Oculomandibulodyscephaly with hypotrichosis (Hallermann-Streiff syndrome)*. Brow and parietal bones prominent, fontanels do not close, long, tapering, beaked nose, mandibular hypoplasia, congenital cataracts and microphthalmia, teeth may be present at birth (others missing), skin thin and tense, hair thin and sparse, short stature (25 percent of cases), slight mental retardation.

Dwarfism   Midgets are abnormally small but perfectly formed people of normal intelligence; they differ from dwarfs in whom not only statural growth but bodily proportions are markedly abnormal. The majority of oligophrenic patients fall below average for height and weight, but there is a small group whose height is well below 135 cm ($4\frac{1}{2}$ ft), and who stand apart by this quality alone.

1. *Nanocephalic dwarfism (Seckel's bird-headed dwarfism)*. The uncomplimentary term *bird head* has been applied to individuals with a small head, large-appearing eyeballs, beaked nose, and underdeveloped chin. Such a physiognomy is not unique to any disease, but when combined with dwarfism it includes a few more or less specific syndromes. Up to 1976 approximately 25 cases had been reported, some with other skeletal and urogenital abnormalities such as medial curvature of middle digits; occasional syndactyly of toes; dislocations of elbow, hip, knee; premature closure of cranial sutures; and clubfoot deformity. They are short at birth and remain so, living until adolescence or adult years. Retardation is severe. A recessive autosomal type of inheritance is probable. At autopsy the brain is found to have a simplified convolutional pattern, and one of our patients had a type of myelin degeneration similar to that of Pelizaeus-Merzbacher disease.

2. *Russell-Silver syndrome*. Possibly an autosomal dominant pattern of inheritance with short stature of prenatal onset, craniofacial dysostosis, short arms, *congenital hemihypertrophy* (arm and leg on one side larger and longer), pseudohydrocephalic head, (normal-sized cranium with small facial bones), abnormalities of genital development in one-third of cases, delay in closure of fontanels and in epiphyseal maturation, elevation of urinary gonadotropins.

3. *Smith-Lemli-Opitz syndrome*. Autosomal recessive inheritance with monocephaly (one cerebral ventricle), broad nasal tip and anteverted nares, wide-set eyes, epicanthal folds, ptosis, small chin, low-set ears, enlarged alveolar maxillary ridge, cutaneous syndactyly, hypospadius in boys, short stature, subnormal neonatal activity, normal amino acids and serum immunoglobulins.

4. *Rubinstein-Taybi syndrome*. Microcephaly but no craniostenosis, downward palpebral slant, heavy eyebrows, beaked nose with nasal septum extending below alae nasi, mild retrognathia, "grimacing smile," strabismus, cataracts, obstruction of nasolacrimal canals, broad thumbs and toes, clinodactyly, overlapping digits, excessive hair growth, hypotonia, lax ligaments, stiff gait, seizures, hyperactive tendon reflexes, absence of corpus callosum, and mental retardation.

5. *Pierre Robin syndrome*. Possible autosomal recessive pattern of inheritance with microcephaly but no craniostenosis, small and symmetrically receded chin ("Andy Gump" appearance), glossoptosis (tongue falls back into pharynx), cleft palate, flat bridge of nose, ears low-set, mental deficiency and congenital heart disease in half the cases.

6. *DeLange syndrome*. The phenotype shows some degree of variability, but the essential diagnostic features are intrauterine growth retardation and stature falling below the third percentile at all ages, microbrachycephaly, generalized hirsutism and eyebrows that meet across the midline (synophrys), anteverted nostrils, long upper lip, and skeletal abnormalities (flexion of elbows, webbing of second and third toes, clinodactyly of fifth fingers, transverse palmar crease). All are severely retarded in mental development which with craniofacial abnormalities is diagnostic. There are no chromosomal abnormalities. A polygenic inheritance has been postulated, but most cases are sporadic.

Neurocutaneous Anomalies with Mental Retardation It comes as no surprise that skin and nervous system should share in pathologic states that impair development, since both have a common ectodermal derivation. Nevertheless, it is difficult to find a common theme to the diseases that affect both organs. In some instances it is clear that ectoderm has been malformed from early intrauterine life; in others a number of acquired diseases of skin must be considered. For reasons to be elaborated later, neurofibromatosis, tuberous sclerosis, and Sturge-Weber encephalofacial angiomatosis need to be set apart as a different category of disease.

Hemangiomas of the skin are without doubt the most frequent cutaneous abnormalities that are present at birth, and usually they are entirely innocent. Many recede in the first months of life. On the other hand, an extensive vascular nevus, located in the territory of the trigeminal nerve and sometimes in other parts as well, causes permanent disfigurement and usually portends a cerebral lesion.

Other neurocutaneous diseases are summarized below. A more complete review of these diseases will be found in the article by Adams, listed in the references. The importance of recognizing the cutaneous abnormalities relates to the fact that the nervous system is usually abnormal, and often the skin lesion appears before the neurologic symptoms are detectable. Thus the skin lesion becomes a prognosticator of potential neurologic involvement.

1. *Basal-cell nevus syndrome*. This condition is transmitted as an autosomal dominant trait, and is characterized by superficial pits in the palms and soles; multiple solid or cystic tumors over the head, face, and neck appearing in infancy or early childhood; mental retardation in some cases; frontoparietal bossing; hypertelorism and kyphoscoliosis.

2. *Congenital ichthyosis, hypogonadism, and mental retardation*. This disorder is inherited as a sex-linked recessive trait. Aside from the characteristic triad of anomalies, there are no special features.

3. *Xeroderma pigmentosum*. An autosomal recessive pattern of inheritance. Skin lesions appear in infancy, taking the form of erythema, blistering, scaling, scarring, and pigmentation on exposure to sunlight; old lesions are parchmentlike, covered with fine scales and telangiectasia; skin cancer later; loss of eyelashes, symblepharon, dry bulbar conjunctivae; microcephaly, hypogonadism, and mental retardation (50 percent of cases).

4. *Sjögren-Larsson syndrome*. An autosomal recessive disease with congenital ichthyosiform erythroderma; normal or thin scalp hair; sometimes defective dental enamel; and pigmentary degeneration of retinae, spastic legs, and mental retardation.

5. *Poikiloderma congenitale* (*Rothmund-Thompson syndrome*). Autosomal recessive heredity; diffuse, pink coloration of cheeks spreading to ears and buttocks, later replaced by macular and reticular pattern of skin atrophy mixed with striae, telangiectasia, and pigmentation; skin changes appear from the third to sixth month of life; sparse hair in half of cases; cataracts; small genitalia; abnormal hands and feet; short stature and mental retardation.

6. *Linear sebaceous nevus syndrome*. Genetics uncertain, linear organoid nevus of one side of face and trunk, lipodermoids on bulbar conjunctivae, vascularization of corneas, mental retardation, focal seizures, and spike and slow waves in EEG.

7. *Incontinentia pigmenti* (*Bloch-Sulzberger syndrome*). Only females affected, dermal lesions appear in first weeks of life and consist of vesicles and bullae followed by hyperkeratoses and streaks of pigmentation, scarring of scalp, and alopecia; abnormalities of dentition; hemiparesis; quadriparesis; seizures; mental retardation; up to 50 percent eosinophiles in blood. Status of this disease is uncertain.

8. *Focal dermal hypoplasia*. Also a disease limited to females, areas of dermal hypoplasia with protrusions of subcutaneous fat, hypo- and hyperpigmentation, scoliosis, syndactyly in a few, short stature, thinness, intelligence occasionally subnormal.

CEREBRAL ABNORMALITY IN MULTIPLE CONGENITAL ANOMALY SYNDROMES

Actually there is little information about the state of the cerebral tissues in the aforementioned neural-somatic syndromes, and in many of them the nervous system has never been examined. In some instances the brain is small with virtually no sulcation, a state known as lissencephaly (smooth brain). In others only a few sulci are present, resulting in an admixture of microgyria and macrogyria (pachygyria). In all these major malformations, the cerebral cortex is thickened, and the architecture is abnormal in that the inner cortical layers (layers 4, 5, and 6) are superficial to a band of medullated fibers beneath which there is a layer of neurons that have failed to migrate to their normal superficial position. This type of cortex has been referred to as undifferentiated. Other types of cortical dysgenesis, such as the one described by Morel as poikilotypic, or the one described by one of the authors as the "driftwood cortex," are special examples of disturbances in cellular migration.

RACHISCHISIS (DYSRAPHISM)

Included under this heading are the disorders of fusion of dorsal midline structures of the primitive neural tube, a process that takes place during the first 3 weeks of postconceptual life. The entire cranium may be missing at birth and the undeveloped brain lies in the base of the skull, a small vascular mass without recognizable nervous tissue. Such a state, called *anencephaly*, is the most frequent of the rachischises and has many associations with other conditions in which the vertebral laminae fail to fuse. Its incidence is 0.1 to 0.7 per thousand births and

females predominate 3 to 7:1. The concordance rate is low, being the same in identical and fraternal twins, but the incidence of the malformation is several times the expected rate if one child in the sibship has already been afflicted. Anencephaly is more frequent in certain geographic areas, e.g., Ireland. Most such fetuses are stillborn or live only a few hours. On the other hand, the cranial defect may be small or hidden, presenting as a polypoid lesion of the forehead or of the nasal cavity, or as a *meningoencephalocele* connected with the brain through a small opening in the skull. Another favorite site is the occipital region, where parts of one or both occipital lobes or the cerebellum, or both, form a protruding mass sometimes as large as the head itself. The small nasal encephaloceles may cause no neurologic signs, and if they are innocently snipped off, CSF rhinorrhea may result. The larger occipital ones are associated with blindness, ataxia, and mental retardation.

A failure of development of the midline structure of the cerebellum forms the basis of the *Dandy-Walker syndrome* (Fig. 43-1). A cystlike structure, representing the greatly dilated fourth ventricle, expands in the midline, causing the occipital bone to bulge posteriorly and

Figure 43-1

Dandy-Walker syndrome. CT scan of a 14-year-old, mildly retarded girl. A large midline cyst, representing the greatly dilated fourth ventricle, occupies the posterior fossa.

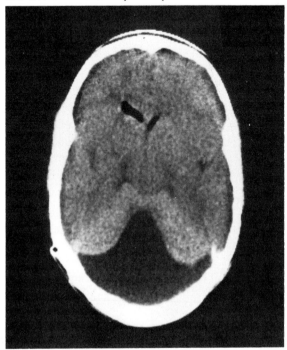

displacing the tentorium and torcula upward. In addition the corpus callosum may be deficient or absent, and there is dilatation of the aqueduct, third, and lateral ventricles.

Somewhat less frequent are abnormalities of closure of the vertebral arches. These are *spina bifida occulta, meningocele* and *meningomyelocele* of the lumbosacral or other regions.

In *spina bifida occulta* the cord remains inside the canal, and there is no external sac, although a dimple or wisp of hair in the overlying skin may mark the site of the lesion. In *meningocele* there is a protrusion of dura and arachnoid through the defect in the vertebral laminae, forming a cystic swelling; the cord remains in the canal, however. In *meningomyelocele*, the cord is extruded also and is closely applied to the fundus of the cystic swelling. Like anencephaly, the incidence of spinal rachischisis (myeloschisis) varies widely from one country to another, and the disorder is more likely to affect a second child (6 to 7 percent) if one child has already had it. Exogenous factors (e.g., potato blight), have been suspected in the genesis of both this and anencephaly. Unfortunately, meningocele is only one-tenth as frequent as meningomyelocele.

Typically the child is born with a large lumbosacral meningomyelocele covered by delicate, weeping skin. It may have ruptured in utero or during birth, but more often the covering is intact. Stroking the sac may elicit involuntary movements of the legs. As a rule the legs are motionless; urine dribbles, keeping the patient constantly wet; there is no response to pinprick over the lumbosacral zones; and the tendon reflexes are absent. In contrast, craniocervical structures are normal unless an Arnold-Chiari malformation is associated. The neurologic abnormalities of the legs prove that the sac contains elements of spinal cord or cauda equina. Differences are noted in the neurologic picture depending on the level of the lesion. If entirely sacral, bladder and bowel sphincters are affected, but legs escape; if lower lumbar and sacral, the buttocks, legs, and feet are more impaired than hip flexors and quadriceps; if upper lumbar, the feet and legs are sometimes spared and ankle reflexes retained, and there may be Babinski signs.

Pathology and Treatment The dreaded complications of these severe spinal defects are ascending meningitis and progressive hydrocephalus from an Arnold-Chiari malformation, which is often associated (see below). Transverse sections through the meningomyelocele show spinal roots and meninges matted together with connective tissue and incompletely covered by skin. The spinal cord is often included, and may appear incomplete with a defect in the posterior half, a widened central canal,

and duplication of the central canal and parts of the central gray matter. The leg muscles are extremely small owing to lack of innervation.

Opinions as to the proper management are in a state of flux. Excision of the meningomyelocele in the first few days of life is advised if the objective is to prevent a fatal meningitis. Later (after a few weeks or months), as hydrocephalus reveals its presence by rapid increase in head size and enlargement of the ventricles in the CT scan, a ventriculoatrial or ventriculoperitoneal shunt is required if the hydrocephalus is to be controlled. In some centers this mode of therapy has been routine for several years, but the long-term results have not been encouraging. Lorber and others report that 80 to 90 percent of their surviving patients are mentally retarded to some degree and are paraplegic—thus totally dependent on others for their care. The decision to undertake these rather formidable surgical procedures is being questioned more and more frequently, especially if the initial assessment indicates severe neurologic deficits (particularly cerebral ones). In mothers suspected of having an affected child, the diagnosis can often be confirmed by the presence of α-fetoprotein in the blood and amniotic fluid and checked by ultrasound or plain films of the fetus. Some parents on receiving this information demand abortion.

Delayed Effects of Failure of Midline Fusion Meningomyelocele and its complications are so strictly pediatric and surgical that the neurologist seldom becomes involved except in the initial evaluation of the status of the nervous system, the treatment of meningeal infection, or shunt failure with decompensation of hydrocephalus. Of greater interest to the neurologist are a series of closely related abnormalities which begin to produce symptoms for the first time in the adolescent or adult. These include sinus tracts with meningeal infections, myeloschisis with low tethering of spinal cord and a delayed radicular or spinal syndrome, diastematomyelia, cysts or tumors with spina bifida and a progressive myeloradiculopathy, and an adolescent or adult Arnold-Chiari malformation and syringomyelia.

Sinus tracts in the lumbosacral or occipital regions are of importance, for they may lead to bacterial meningitis at any age. They are often indicated by a small dimple in the skin or by a tuft of hair along the posterior surface of the body in the midline. (The pilonidal sinus, in the opinion of the authors, should not be included in this group.) They may be associated with dermoid cysts in the central part of the tract. Evidence of such tracts should be sought in every instance of meningitis, especially when the infection has recurred.

There are, in addition, other *congenital cysts* and *tumors*, particularly lipoma and dermoid, which may produce progressive symptoms and signs by compressing the spinal cord or by implicating nerve roots.

Diastematomyelia is another unusual abnormality of the spinal cord often associated with spina bifida. Here a bony spicule or fibrous band protrudes into the spinal canal from the body of one of the thoracic or upper lumbar vertebras, splitting the spinal cord in two, each half being surrounded by a dural sac. This longitudinal fissuring and apparent doubleness of cord is spoken of as diplomyelia. With growth, this leads to a *traction myelopathy*.

Several clinical *syndromes of delayed progressive disease* (in adolescence or adult) have been delineated:

1. Progressive spastic weakness in some of the weak muscles of the legs in a patient known to have had a meningocele or myelomeningocele. Presumably the spinal cord, which is securely attached to the lumbar vertebras, is stretched during the period of rapid lengthening of the vertebral column.

2. An acute cauda equina syndrome following some unusual activity or accident (e.g., rowing or a fall in a sitting position), in patients who have had an asymptomatic or symptomatic spina bifida or meningocele. The implicated sensory and motor roots are believed to be injured by sudden or repeated stretching. Weakness of bladder control, impotence (in the male), and numbness of the feet and legs or foot drop comprise the clinical syndrome.

3. Progressive cauda equina syndrome in the lumbosacral region.

4. Syringomyelia (page 642).

Also there are a variety of neurologic problems associated with spinal abnormalities, particularly in the cervical region [fusion of atlas and occiput or of cervical vertebras (Klippel-Feil syndrome), congenital dislocation of the odontoid process and atlas, platybasia and basilar impression]. These spinal abnormalities are reviewed in Chap. 35, with diseases of the spinal cord.

Arnold-Chiari Malformation (ACM)   Encompassed by this term are a number of congenital anomalies at the base of the brain, the most consistent of which are (1) an extension of a tongue of cerebellar tissue, posterior to the medulla and spinal cord, into the cervical canal and (2) a displacement of the medulla into the cervical canal, along with the inferior part of the fourth ventricle. These and associated anomalies were first clearly described by Chiari (1891, 1896), who divided them into four types. Arnold's contribution to our understanding of these malformations was relatively insignificant, but the double eponym is so widely accepted that a dispute over priorities at this late date will probably not alter its usage. In recent years the term Arnold-Chiari malformation (ACM) has come to be restricted to Chiari's types I and II—i.e., to the cerebellomedullary malformation without and with a meningomyelocele, respectively. Type III is no more than an occipital meningoencephalocele, and the status of type IV remains uncertain (mainly it consists of cerebellar hypoplasia).

Several other morphologic features are characteristic. The medulla and pons are elongated, and the aqueduct is narrowed. The displaced tissue (medulla and cerebellum) occludes the foramen magnum; and the remainder of the cerebellum, which is small, is also displaced so as to obliterate the cisterna magna. The foramens of Luschka and Magendie open into the cervical canal, and the arachnoidal tissue around the herniated brainstem and cerebellum is fibrotic. All these factors are probably operative in the production of hydrocephalus, which is always associated. Just below the herniated tail of cerebellar tissue there is a kink or spur in the spinal cord, pushed posteriorly by the lower end of the fourth ventricle. In this type of malformation, a meningomyelocele is nearly always found; a hydromyelia of the cervical cord is also common.

Developmental abnormalities of the cerebrum (particularly polymicrogyria) may coexist, and the lower end of the spinal cord (i.e., filum terminale) may extend as low as the sacrum. There are usually bony abnormalities as well. The posterior fossa is small; the foramen magnum is enlarged and grooved posteriorly. Often the base of the skull is flattened or infolded by the cervical spine (basilar impression).

Clinical manifestations   In type II ACM (with meningomyelocele) the problem is essentially one of progressive hydrocephalus. Cerebellar signs cannot be discerned in the first few months of life. However, lower cranial nerve abnormalities—laryngeal stridor, fasciculations of the tongue, sternomastoid paralysis (head lag), facial weakness, deafness, bilateral abducens palsies—may be present in varying combinations. If the patient survives to later childhood or adolescence, one of the syndromes that occurs with type I ACM may become manifest.

In type I ACM (without meningocele or other signs of dysraphism), neurologic symptoms may not develop until adolescence or adult life. The symptoms may be those of (1) increased intracranial pressure, (2) progressive cerebellar ataxia, or (3) syringomyelia; or the patient may show a combination of disorders of cranial nerves, cerebellum, medulla and spinal cord, usually in conjunction with headache. Often the disease is mistaken for multiple sclerosis, foramen magnum or high cervical cord tumor, etc. The physical habitus of such patients may be normal, but about 25 percent have signs of an arrested hydrocephalus or a short "bull neck." When basilar impression and ACM coexist, it is impossible to decide which of the two is responsible for the clinical findings.

Diagnosis and Treatment Pantopaque or metrizamide myelography, performed with the patient supine, provides the most consistent means of corroborating the clinical diagnosis. The tongue of cerebellar tissue and the kinked cervical cord obstruct the upward flow of Pantopaque and give a highly characteristic radiologic profile. The latter may be visible in a CT scan. Vertebral angiography may also be helpful, disclosing the displacement of the posterior inferior cerebellar arteries. CSF is usually normal, but may show an elevated pressure and protein level in some cases.

The treatment of basilar impression and ACM is far from satisfactory. If clinical progression is slight or uncertain, it is probably best to do nothing. If progression is certain and disability is increasing, upper cervical laminectomy and enlargement of the foramen magnum are indicated. Often this procedure halts the progress of the illness or results in improvement. The surgical procedure must be done cautiously. Opening of the dura and extensive manipulation of the malformation or excision of tissue may aggravate the symptoms or even cause death.

CHROMOSOMAL ABNORMALITIES (CHROMOSOMAL DYSGENESES)

A mid-twentieth century discovery of outstanding significance was the recognition of a group of developmental anomalies of the brain and other organs associated with a demonstrable abnormality of an autosomal or sex chromosome. Lejeune was the first to note a triplication of the twenty-first chromosome in Down's syndrome, and there followed the discovery of a number of other trisomies as well as deletions or translocations of certain of the autosomal chromosomes, and a lack or an excess of one of the sex chromosomes. Such an event must take place sometime after the formation of the oocyte during the long period it lies fallow in the aging ovary, or during the process of conception or germination and first cell divisions. All the cells in the embryo may be affected or only part of them, the latter condition being called *mosaicism*.

The manner in which triplication or some imperfection of a chromosome is able to derail the pathways of ontogenesis is a mystery. One can imagine that the sequential release of genes and their transcription of nuclear and messenger RNA to form certain basic proteins might affect the development of organs—especially the development of the brain, whose embryogenesis, growth, and maturation are the most complex and protracted of any.

Certain of the chromosomal abnormalities are incompatible with life, and it has been found that the cells of many unexplained abortuses and stillborns show abnormal karyotypes. On the other hand, the organism may survive and exhibit any one of the following syndromes: (1) mongolism (Down's syndrome, trisomy 21); (2) one type of arrhinencephaly (trisomy 13, Patau's syndrome); (3) trisomy 18 (Edwards' syndrome); (4) cri-du-chat syndrome (deletion of short arm of chromosome 5); (5) monosomy 21 (antimongolism); (6) ring chromosomes; (7) Klinefelter's syndrome (XXY); (8) Turner's syndrome (XO); (9) others (XXXX, XXX, XYY, YY, XXYY). An account of these less-frequent chromosomal aberrations can be found in the article by Lemieux.

Mongolism or Down's Syndrome Described first in 1866, by Langdon Down, this is the best known of the chromosomal dysgeneses. The frequency is 1 in 700 births. Familiarity with the condition permits its recognition at birth, but it becomes more obvious with advancing age. The round head, open mouth, stubby hands, slanting palpebral fissures, and short stature create an unforgettable clinical picture. The ears are low-set and oval with small lobules. The palpebral fissures slant slightly upward and outward owing to the presence of medial epicanthal folds which partly cover the inner canthi. The bridge of the nose is poorly developed. The mouth tends to hang open and the tongue is usually enlarged, heavily fissured, and protruding. Gray-white specks of depigmentation are seen in the irides (Brushfield's spots). The little fingers are often short (hypoplastic middle phalanx) and incurved (clinodactyly). The hands are broad with a single transverse (simian) palmar crease and other characteristic dermal markings. Lenticular opacities and congenital heart lesions (septal defects) are not infrequent. At birth the mongoloid infant is of average size, but at later periods of life the child is characteristically small. The stature of the average adult mongoloid seldom exceeds that of a 10-year-old child. Most mongoloid children do not walk until 3 to 4 years of age; their acquisition of speech is delayed, but over 90 percent talk by 5 years. The intelligence quotient (IQ) is variable, and that of a large group follows a gaussian curve; the median IQ is 40 to 50, and the range is 20 to 70.

One cannot distinguish mongolism associated with a triplication of chromosome 21 from that with a translocation. There is a strong correlation between the type with trisomy 21 and age of the mother, whereas the less-frequent translocation is found equally in the off-spring of young and old mothers. Mosaics have atypical forms of the syndrome, and some are of normal intelligence. Laboratory tests are not helpful in clarifying the mechanism of the disorder; abnormalities include decreased serotonin, increased alkaline phosphatase in the white cells, increased glucose diphosphate in red cells, and a 50 percent increase in superoxide dismutase. The latter enzyme derives from a gene located on the long arm of chromosome 21 and is a convenient marker of the trisomy, but is not believed to be responsible for the dysmorphism or mental retardation.

The pathologic findings have been difficult to define. The brain is approximately 10 percent lighter than average. The convolutional pattern is rather simple. The frontal lobes are small, and the superior temporal gyri are thin. There are claims of delayed myelination of cerebral white matter, and also of immature and poorly differentiated cortical neurons. Surprisingly, Alzheimer's neurofibrillary changes and senile plaques are practically always found in mongoloids beyond 30 years of age, but only in a small proportion of these cases are the changes associated with a presenile dementia. There is a high incidence of leukemia, and the cardiac lesion may lead to heart failure.

Now it is possible to make the diagnosis by demonstrating the chromosomal abnormalities in cells of the amniotic fluid. One could eliminate a considerable proportion of the population of mongoloids by doing amniocentesis on all pregnant women over 35 years of age and aborting those with positive tests.

The other chromosomal dysgeneses will only be synopsized.

1. *Trisomy 13 (Patau's syndrome).* Frequency 1:2000 live births, more female than male, average maternal age 30.8 years, microcephaly and sloping forehead, microphthalmus, coloboma of iris, corneal opacities, low-set ears, cleft lip and palate, capillary hemangiomata, polydactyly, flexed fingers, posterior prominence of heels, dextrocardia, umbilical hernia, impaired hearing, hypertonia, severe mental retardation, death in early childhood.

2. *Trisomy 18.* Frequency 1:4000, more female than male, maternal age 34.4 years, growth slow, occasional seizures, mental retardation severe, hypertonia, ptosis and lid abnormalities, low-set ears, small mouth, mottled skin, clenched fist with index finger over third, syndactyly, rocker-bottom feet, shortened big toe, ventricular septal defect, umbilical and inguinal hernias, short sternum, small pelvis, small mandible, death in early infancy.

3. *Cri-du-chat syndrome.* Abnormal cry like a kitten, severe mental retardation, hypertelorism, epicanthal folds, brachycephaly, moon face, antimongoloid slant of palpebral fissures, micrognathia, hypotonia, strabismus.

4. *Ring chromosomes.* Mental retardation with variable physical abnormalities.

5. *Klinefelter's syndrome.* Only males. Eunuchoid appearance; wide arm-span, sparse facial and body hair; high-pitched voice; gynecomastia; small testicles; usually mentally retarded; high incidence of psychosis, asthma, and diabetes.

6. *Turner's syndrome.* Only females. Triangular face, small chin, occasionally hypertelorism and epicanthal folds, widely spaced nipples, clinodactyly, cubitus valgus, hypoplastic nails, short stature, webbed neck, delayed sexual development, mild mental retardation.

Several generalizations can be made about these chromosomal dysgeneses. First, the autosomal ones are often lethal, and they almost always have a devastating effect on cerebral growth and development, whether the infant survives or not. Somatic, nonnervous anomalies are regularly present, an association so constant that one may safely predict that a normally formed infant will not have a detectable chromosomal defect. The physiognomy and bodily configuration of only the mongoloid and trisomy 13 (and possibly trisomy 18) are of predictive value, however. Surprisingly, some of the most grotesque disfigurements, like anencephaly and multiple congenital anomalies, are rarely related to a morphologic abnormality in chromosomes. In contrast, an insufficiency of sex chromosomes exerts only the most subtle effects on brain, intellect, and personality, and to some extent this is true of supernumerary sex chromosomes (XYY, for example).

The abnormality of the brain underlying the mental retardation in these several chromosomal dysgeneses has not been ascertained. The cerebra are slightly small, but only minor changes are seen in the convolutional pattern and cortical architecture. These brain anomalies are under active study.

THE PHAKOMATOSES (CONGENITAL ECTODERMOSES)

As was stated, there are two broad categories of neurocutaneous diseases, one in which the infant is born with a special variety of skin disease or develops it in the first weeks of life; the other in which particular forms of cutaneous abnormality, though often present in minor degree at birth, later evolve as quasineoplastic disorders. The latter, to which van der Hoeve (1920) applied the term *phakomatoses* (from the Greek *phakos*, meaning "mother spot," "mole," or "freckle") includes tuberous sclerosis, neurofibromatosis, and cutaneous angiomatosis with CNS abnormalities. These diseases have been shown to possess many common features such as hereditary transmission, selective involvement of organs of ectodermal derivation (nervous system, eyeball, retina and skin), slow evolution of lesions in childhood and adolescence, tendency to form benign tumors ("hamartomas"), and disposition to fatal malignant transformation. These disorders are discussed below.

TUBEROUS SCLEROSIS (BOURNEVILLE'S DISEASE, EPILOIA)

Tuberous sclerosis is a congenital disease of hereditary type in which a variety of lesions arise in the skin, nervous system, heart, kidney, and other organs due to a limited hyperplasia of ectodermal and mesodermal cells. It is characterized clinically by the triad of adenoma sebaceum, epilepsy, and mental retardation.

It is stated that Virchow had recognized scleromas of the cerebrum in the 1860s and that von Recklinghausen had reported a similar lesion combined with multiple myomata of the heart in 1862, but Bourneville's articles, appearing between 1880 and 1900, presented the first systematic account of the disease and related the cerebral lesions to those of the skin of the face. Vogt (1890) fully appreciated the significance of the neurocutaneous relationship and formally delineated the triad of adenoma sebaceum, epilepsy, and mental retardation. Epiloia, a term introduced by Sherlock in 1911, has never

gained general acceptance. These and other historical aspects are reviewed in a recent monograph on tuberous sclerosis, edited by Gomez.

Epidemiology The incidence of the disease is estimated to be from 5 to 7 per 100,000. It has been described in all parts of the world, and is equally frequent in all races and in both sexes. Heredity is evident in approximately one-third of reported cases (a dominant autosomal gene of variable penetrance). The remaining cases are attributed to a gene mutation, the frequency of which is calculated to be 1 in 20,000 to 1 in 50,000. The disease involves many organs aside from skin and brain and may assume a diversity of forms, the least severe of which, i.e., the *forme fruste*, is difficult to diagnose; hence, one cannot be certain of the true incidence of the disease. Among the feebleminded in institutions the frequency ranges from 0.1 to 0.7 percent. Increasing numbers of reports of patients whose mentality is preserved and who have never had convulsions are to be found in the recent medical literature. It is likely that data drawn from surveys of mental hospital populations have tended to exaggerate the overall frequency of mental retardation in this disorder (Gomez).

Etiology and Pathogenesis Tuberous sclerosis is a genetic disease but its pathogenesis remains unknown. The chromosomes are morphologically unchanged. As was said earlier, the lesions involve cells derived from ectoderm as well as mesoderm. The cellular elements within the lesions are abnormal both in number and size. The tumorlike growths in different organs may include cells of more than one type (e.g., fibroblast and angioblast or glioblast and neuroblast), and their number is locally excessive. Something has gone awry with the proliferative process in embryologic development, yet it is usually kept under control, and only rarely does the growth undergo malignant transformation and metastasize. Highly specialized cells within the lesions may attain giant size; neurons three to four times normal size may be observed in the cerebral scleroses. These facts emphasize the blastomatous character of the process and suggest that some inhibitory growth factor is lacking at crucial moments in embryonic life and later, accounting for both the hyperplasia and hypertrophy of well-differentiated cells. How the trait underlying this disease is transmitted remains a mystery. The focal character of the pathologic process would seem to exclude a systemic metabolic abnormality.

Clinical Manifestations The disease may be present at the time of birth (the diagnosis has been made by CT scan in neonates), but more often the infant is judged at first to be normal. As a rule, attention is initially drawn to the disease by the occurrence of focal or generalized seizures or by retarded psychomotor development. As with any condition that leads to mental retardation, the first suspicion is raised by delay in reaching the milestones of natural maturation. Whatever the initial symptom, the convulsive disorder and mental retardation become more prominent within 2 to 3 years. The facial cutaneous abnormality, the so-called adenoma sebaceum, appears later in childhood, usually between the fourth and tenth years, and is progressive thereafter.

As the years pass, the seizures, which may at first have been focal, change pattern. In the first one to two years they take the form of salaam spasms or flexion myoclonus with hypsarhythmia (irregular dysrhythmic bursts of high-voltage spikes and slow waves in the EEG); later the seizures change to more typical generalized motor and psychomotor attacks or atypical petit mal; any one of the seizure types may be brief, especially if the patient is receiving anticonvulsant medication. Seizures are always the most reliable index of the cerebral lesions, and focal neurologic abnormalities, which one might expect to occur from the number and size of the cerebral lesions, are distinctly uncommon.

Mental function continues to deteriorate slowly. Exceptionally there may be a spastic weakness or mild choreoathetosis of the limbs; in a few cases there is obstructive hydrocephalus. As in any state of imbecility or idiocy, a variety of nonspecific motor peculiarities such as constant crying, muttering, rocking and swaying movements, and digital mannerisms may be observed. Behavioral, moral, and affective derangements may also be added to intellectual deficiency, resulting in what may be loosely classified as a primary type of psychosis.

The lack of parallelism among the epilepsy, mental deficit, and cutaneous abnormalities has been noted by all experienced clinicians. Some patients are subject to recurrent seizures while retaining relatively normal mental function; in others only the relatively trivial skin lesions or a retinal phakoma may suggest the diagnosis. In such cases, recognition may elude competent neurologists and dermatologists.

Limitation of space does not allow more than a catalog of other visceral abnormalities. In about half the cases, gray or yellow plaques (in reality gliomatous tumors) may be found in the retina in or near the optic disk or at a distance from it. It is from this lesion, called phakoma, that van der Hoeve derived the term that is applied to all neurocutaneous diseases of this class. About half of all benign rhabdomyomas of the heart are associated with tuberous sclerosis, and other benign tumors of mixed cell type have been found in the kidneys, liver, lungs, thyroid, testes, and gastrointestinal tract. Cysts of pleura or lungs, bone cysts in digits, and zones of marbling or densification in bones are some of the less-common associated abnormalities.

The well-developed facial lesions, pathognomonic of tuberous sclerosis, are present in 90 percent of patients over 4 years of age. Typically they are red to pink nodules with a smooth, glistening surface, which tend to be limited to the nasolabial folds, cheeks, chin, and sometimes the forehead and scalp. Although called "adenoma sebaceum," these nodules are actually angiofibromas; the sebaceous glands are only passively involved. The earliest manifestation of facial angiofibromatosis may be a mild erythema over the cheeks and forehead, intensified by crying. The occurrence of large plaques of connective tissue on the forehead are usually expressive of a severe form of the disease.

On the trunk the diagnostic lesion is the "shagreen patch" (in reality a plaque of subepidermal fibrosis) found most often in the lumbosacral region. It appears as a flat, slightly elevated, flesh-colored area of skin 1 to 10 cm in diameter, with a "pigskin," "elephant hide," or "orange peel" appearance. Another common site of fibromatous involvement is the nail bed. Subungual fibromas usually appear at puberty and continue to develop with age. Other common skin changes, not in themselves diagnostic, include fibroepithelial tags (soft fibromas), café au lait spots, and port-wine hemangiomas.

In approximately 85 percent of patients with tuberous sclerosis, congenital hypomelanotic macules (formerly called "partial albinism" or "vitiligo") appear before any of the other skin lesions (Fitzpatrick et al.). They are arranged in linear fashion over the trunk or limbs and range in size from a few millimeters to several centimeters; their configuration is oval, with one end round and the other pointed, in the shape of an ash leaf. A Wood's lamp which transmits only ultraviolet rays, facilitates the demonstration of these lesions. These hypopigmented spots have been recognized for many years, but only recently have Gold and Freeman and Fitzpatrick et al. emphasized their frequency and their value in the diagnosis of tuberous sclerosis during infancy, before the other cutaneous lesions appear.

Pathology The brain exhibits a number of anomalies that are at once diagnostic. Broadening, unnatural whiteness, and firmness of parts of some of the cerebral convolutions are simulated by no other disease. These are the *tubers* after which the disease is named. On the surface of the brain, they range in width from 5 mm to 2 or 3 cm. Their cut surface reveals a lack of demarcation of cortex from white matter and the presence of white flecks of calcium; the latter, which are readily seen in CT scans, are called *brain stones*. The floors of the lateral ventricles may be encrusted with white or pink-white masses resembling the gutterings of a candle. When calcified, they appear in radiographs as curvilinear opacities which follow the outline of the ventricle. Rarely, nodules of abnormal tissue are observed in the basal ganglia, thalamus, cerebellum, brainstem, and spinal cord.

Under the microscope the tubers are seen to be composed of interlacing rows of plump fibrous astrocytes (much like an astrocytoma). Elsewhere in the cerebral cortex, derangements of architecture result from the presence of abnormal-appearing glial cells. Monstrous neurons and glial cells, often difficult to distinguish, and displaced normal-sized neurons contribute to the chaotic histologic appearance of cerebral cortex and ganglionic structures. Gliomatous deposits may block the aqueduct or floor of the fourth ventricle, causing an obstructive hydrocephalus. Neoplastic transformation of abnormal glial cells, a not infrequent occurrence, usually takes the form of a large-cell astrocytoma, less often of a glioblastoma; sometimes meningiomas are added.

The phakomas of the retina are composed mainly of neuronal and glial components, but occasionally there is an admixture of fibrous tissue.

Diagnosis When the full combination of mental, convulsive, and dermal abnormalities are conjoined, the diagnosis is self-evident. It is the early stage of the disease and the *forme fruste* that give trouble, and here the experienced dermatologist can be of great help. Epilepsy, i.e., flexion spasms in infancy, and delay in psychomotor development are by no means diagnostic of tuberous sclerosis, since they occur in many diseases. It is in these cases and also in every sizable population of the epileptic or mentally retarded, especially when the family history is unrevealing, that a search for the dermal equivalents of the disease—the hypomelanotic nevus, adenoma sebaceum, collagenous patch, phakoma of retina, or subungual or gingival fibroma—is so rewarding. The finding of any one of these lesions provides confirmation of the partial and atypical case. Adenoma sebaceum may occasionally occur alone and is easily confused with acne vulgaris in the adolescent. The history of epilepsy

and/or the demonstration of a dull mentality is helpful but not necessary for the diagnosis of tuberous sclerosis (Gomez). Useful laboratory measures for corroborating the disease are EEG, CT scans, searching for multiple calcific densities within the brain, and plain films of the skull to show localized patches of hyperostosis on the inner surface of cranial bones. CT scans also reveal ventricular deformity and tumor deposits along the striatal and thalamic borders.

Treatment Nothing can be offered in the way of prevention other than to counsel affected individuals against childbearing. The slow march of the disease, once it has begun, cannot be halted. Anticonvulsant therapy of the standard type suppresses the convulsive tendency more or less effectively and should be applied assiduously. It is rather pointless to attempt to excise tumors, especially in individuals who are severely affected. However, there are patients who are not mentally impaired and who can benefit from dermabrasion of their facial lesions, with the knowledge that they will slowly regrow; and neurosurgeons have partially excised brain tumors that were causing recalcitrant epilepsy or increased intracranial pressure.

Course and Prognosis In general, the disease advances so slowly that years must elapse before one is sure of the progression. Of the severe cases, approximately 30 percent die before the fifth year, and 50 to 75 percent before attaining adult age. Worsening is mainly in the mental sphere. Status epilepticus accounted for many deaths in the past, but improved anticonvulsant therapy has reduced this hazard. Neoplasias take their toll, and the authors have had several such patients who died of malignant gliomas arising in striatothalamic zones (see Gomez).

NEUROFIBROMATOSIS OF VON RECKLINGHAUSEN

Neurofibromatosis is a comparatively uncommon hereditary disease in which the skin, nervous system, bones, endocrine glands, and sometimes other organs are the sites of a variety of congenital abnormalities, often taking the form of benign tumors. The typical clinical picture, usually identifiable at a glance, consists of multiple circumscript areas of increased skin pigmentation accompanied by dermal and neural tumors of various types.

History The condition known as multiple idiopathic neuromas was the subject of a monograph by R. W. Smith in 1849, and even at that time he referred to examples recorded by other writers. It was von Recklinghausen, however, in 1882, who gave the definitive account of its clinical and pathologic features. The articles of Yakovlev and Guthrie (1931) and of Lichtenstein (1949) and the monograph of Crowe et al. (1956) provide a complete analysis of the clinical, pathologic, and genetic data and include extensive bibliographies.

Incidence and Epidemiology Crowe and his associates, at the Institute of Human Biology of the University of Michigan, calculate the frequency of the disease to be 30 to 40 per 100,000 and expect one case of it in every 2500 to 3300 births. Approximately half their cases have affected relatives, and in all instances the distribution of cases within a family is consistent with an autosomal dominant mode of inheritance. They provide evidence that the remaining sporadic cases are due to a mutation of the dominant gene. The disease has been observed in all races in different parts of the world, and males and females are about equally affected.

Cause and Pathogenesis The genetic nature of neurofibromatosis is established. The location of the abnormal gene in the human karyotype of chromosomes remains unknown. Chromosome counts and morphologic features do not deviate from normal. The pathogenesis also remains obscure. Cellular elements derived from the neural crest (i.e., Schwann cells, melanocytes, and possibly endoneurial fibroblasts, the natural components of skin and nerves) multiply excessively in multiple foci, and the melanocytes function abnormally; but the time when this proliferative process begins and the mechanism by which it is accomplished are as unclear as in tuberous sclerosis.

Clinical Manifestations In the majority of patients, spots of hyperpigmentation and cutaneous and subcutaneous tumors are the basis of clinical diagnosis. These appear in increasing number during late childhood and adolescence. Exceptionally, a neurofibroma of a spinal or cranial nerve root, disclosed during neurosurgical intervention, may be the initial manifestation of the disease. In the study of a large series of patients with neurofibromatosis, approximately one-third were discovered to have the cutaneous manifestations while being examined for symptoms of some other disease; that is to say, the neurofibromatosis was asymptomatic and incidental.

Usually these are the cases with the slightest degree of cutaneous abnormality. Of the remainder, many consulted a physician because of the disfigurement produced by the tumors or because some of the neurofibromas were producing symptoms.

Canale et al. (1964) noted that neurologic symptoms had led to hospital admission in one-third of their series of 92 cases. Typical syndromes were traced most often to unilateral or bilateral tumors of the eighth cranial nerve (nerve deafness, dizziness, headache, and staggering), trigeminal neuromas (facial pain and numbness), optic nerve gliomas (progressive monocular blindness, optic atrophy, nystagmus, enlargement of optic foramen, abnormal contour of sella turcica, and failure to thrive, if the hypothalamus is invaded), other cranial nerve involvement, spinal-root tumors with or without compression of the spinal cord, and multiple cranial or spinal meningiomas. Seldom are the more peripheral tumors of nerve or skin painful or distressing.

Patches of cutaneous pigmentation, appearing shortly after birth and occurring any place on the body, constitute the most striking clinical expression of the disease. They vary in size from a millimeter or two to many centimeters, and in color from a light to dark brown (café au lait), and are rarely associated with any other pathologic state. In a survey of pigmented spots in the skin, Crowe and associates found that 10 percent of the normal population had one or more lesions of this type, but any patient with more than six spots, some exceeding 1.5 cm in diameter, nearly always proved to have von Recklinghausen's disease. Of their 223 patients with neurofibromatosis, 95 percent had at least one spot, and 78 percent had more than six large ones. Frecklelike or diffuse pigmentation of the axillae and small, round whitish spots are characteristic and almost pathognomonic of the syndrome (Crowe, 1964).

Multiple cutaneous and subcutaneous tumors appearing in late childhood or early adolescence are the other principal features of the disease. The cutaneous tumors are situated in the dermis and form discrete, soft or firm papules varying in size from a few millimeters to a centimeter or more (*molluscum fibrosum*). In shape they assume many forms—flattened, sessile, pedunculated, conical, lobulate, etc. They tend to be flesh-colored or violaceous and often are topped with a comedo. When pressed, the soft tumors tend to invaginate through a small opening in the skin, giving the feeling of a seedless raisin or a scrotum without a testicle. Crowe et al. (1956) speak of this phenomenon as "button-holeing," and find it useful in distinguishing the lesions of this disease from other tumors, e.g., multiple lipomas. Any given patient may have from a few of these dermal tumors to thousands.

The subcutaneous tumors, which are also multiple, take two forms: (1) firm, discrete nodules attached to a nerve or (2) an overgrowth of subcutaneous tissue, sometimes reaching enormous size. These latter, which are called *plexiform neuromas* (also pachydermatocele, elephantiasis neuromatosis, *le tumeur royale*), occur most often in the face, scalp, neck, and chest and may cause hideous disfigurement. When palpated, these growths feel like a bag of worms or strings; the bone underlying the tumor may enlarge.

Other abnormalities associated with neurofibromatosis include bone cysts, pathologic fractures, cranial bone defects with pulsating exophthalmos, bone hypertrophy, precocious puberty, pheochromocytoma, scoliosis, syringomyelia, nodules of abnormal glial cells in brain and spinal cord, and obstructive hydrocephalus due to overgrowth of glial tissue around the sylvian aqueduct and fourth ventricle. Mental deficiency occurs in approximately 10 percent of patients with this disorder and usually is not profound; Rosman and Pearce have ascribed it to congenital malformation of the cerebral cortex (cortical dysgenesis). The incidence of seizures is about 20 times higher than that in the general population.

Pathology The cutaneous tumors are characterized by a rather thin epidermis whose basal layer may or may not be pigmented. The collagen and elastin of the dermis is replaced by a loose arrangement of elongated connective tissue cells. It lacks the compactness of the normal dermal collagen, which accounts for the palpable opening in the skin.

The pigmented (café au lait) lesions contain only the normal numbers of melanocytes and the dark color of the skin is due instead to an excess of melanosomes in the malpighian cells; abnormally large melanosomes, measuring up to several microns in diameter, appear in some of the basal cells of the epidermis.

The nerve tumors are composed of a mixture of fibroblasts and Schwann cells, except the optic nerve tumors, which contain a combination of astrocytes and fibroblasts. Occasionally, along spinal roots or sympathetic chains, one may find a tumor made up of partially or completely differentiated nerve cells (a typical ganglioneuroma). Clusters of abnormal glial cells may be found in the brain and spinal cord, and, according to Bielschowsky, they form a link with tuberous sclerosis. Clinically, however, the two diseases are quite independent.

Malignant degeneration of the tumors is found in 2 to 5 percent of cases; peripherally they become sarcomas and centrally, astrocytomas or glioblastomas.

Diagnosis If skin tumors and café au lait spots are numerous, the identification of the disease offers no diffi-

culty. A history of the illness in antecedent and collateral family members makes recognition even more certain. Uncertainty arises most frequently in cases of acoustic or other cranial or spinal neurofibromas or schwannomas with no skin lesions or only a few random ones. This tendency for the central forms of neurofibromatosis to be accompanied by a paucity of skin lesions is well recognized. Plexiform neuromas with muscle weakness, due to nerve involvement, and abnormalities of underlying bone may be confused with other tumors, especially in young children who tend to have few café au lait spots and few cutaneous tumors. Enormous hypertrophy of a limb, which may also occur, requires differentiation from other developmental anomalies.

Crowe and his associates believe that 80 percent of patients with von Recklinghausen's disease can be diagnosed by the presence of more than six café au lait spots. Of the remaining 20 percent, those over 21 years of age will be found to have multiple cutaneous tumors, axillary freckling, and a few pigmented spots; in those under 21, with no dermal tumors and only a few café au lait patches, a positive family history and radiographic demonstration of bone cysts will be helpful in some instances. The finding of a few café au lait spots and typical cutaneous tumors may help the neurologist diagnose a progressive spinal syndrome, a cerebellopontine angle syndrome, bilateral deafness, progressive blindness, an occasional case of precocious puberty, hydrocephalus, or mental retardation.

Treatment The skin tumors should not be excised unless they are cosmetically objectionable or show an increase in size, suggesting malignant change. The effects of radiotherapy are so insignificant that they do not justify the risk of heavy exposure. Plexiform neuromas about the face offer difficult problems. Here one must resort to plastic surgery, but the results are not always satisfactory because the growths may involve cranial nerves superficially (with risk of greater paralysis after surgical excision) or alter the underlying bone, the latter being either eroded from pressure or hypertrophied from increased blood supply. Cranial and spinal neurofibromas are amenable to excision, and the gliomas and meningiomas usually demand surgical measures. Peripheral nerve tumors that have undergone malignant (sarcomatous) degeneration pose special surgical problems. Affected individuals should be advised not to have children—a precaution that may not be necessary, because fertility, especially in males, seems to be reduced by the disease.

CUTANEOUS ANGIOMATOSIS WITH ABNORMALITIES OF THE CENTRAL NERVOUS SYSTEM

There are six diseases in which a cutaneous vascular anomaly is associated with an abnormality of the nervous system: (1) encephalofacial (encephalotrigeminal) angiomatosis with cerebral calcification (Sturge-Weber syndrome); (2) dermatomal hemangiomas and spinal vascular malformations (sometimes with limb hypertrophy as in Klippel-Trenauney-Weber syndrome); (3) familial telangiectasia (Osler-Rendu-Weber disease); (4) hemangioblastoma of cerebellum and retina (Lindau and von Hippel disease); (5) ataxia-telangiectasia (Louis-Bar disease); and (6) angiokeratosis corporis diffusum (Fabry's disease). The latter three disorders are considered elsewhere: ataxia-telangiectasia and Fabry's disease on pages 680 and 698, respectively, and von Hippel-Lindau disease on pages 459 and 633.

Meningofacial (Encephalofacial) Angiomatosis with Cerebral Calcification (Sturge-Weber Syndrome) In this condition an extensive vascular nevus is observed at birth to cover a large part of the face and cranium on one side (in the territory of the ophthalmic division of the trigeminal nerve). The lesion varies in extent, the most limited being an involvement of only the upper eyelid, and the most extensive being the entire head and even other parts of the body. The nevus is deep red (*port-wine nevus*), and its margins may be raised or flat; soft or firm papules, evidently composed of vessels, cause surface elevations and irregularities. The orbital tissue, especially the upper eyelid, is almost invariably involved, and congenital glaucoma (buphthalmos) may develop later in the eye on that side, causing blindness. The increased cutaneous vascularity may result in overgrowth of connective tissue and underlying bone, giving rise to a deformity like that of the Klippel-Trenauney-Weber syndrome (see below). Indications of cerebral affection appear later in childhood; the most frequent clinical manifestations are unilateral seizures followed by increasing degrees of spastic hemiparesis with smallness of arm and leg, hemisensory defect, and homonymous hemianopia, all on the side contralateral to the trigeminal nevus. Skull films (usually negative after birth) taken at the end of the second year reveal a characteristic *tramline calcification* which outlines the convolutions of the parietooccipital cortex. CT scans at an earlier age show hyperdensity of the involved cortex.

This condition is generally referred to as the Sturge-Weber syndrome, since it was W. Allen Sturge, in 1879, who first described a child with sensorimotor seizures contralateral to a facial "port-wine mark," and Parkes Weber (1922, 1929) who first demonstrated radiographically the atrophy and calcification of the cerebral hemisphere homolateral to the skin lesion. This eponym overlooks the important intervening contributions of Kalischer (1897, 1901), who first described the meningeal angioma in conjunction with the facial one; of Volland (1913), who demonstrated the intracortical calcific deposits; and of Dimitri (1923), who described the characteristic double-contoured radiographic shadows. Krabbe (1932, 1934) showed conclusively that the calcification lay not in the blood vessels (as Dimitri and many others had concluded) but in the second and third layers of the cortex (see Wohlwill and Yakovlev for historical review and bibliography).

It must not be thought that all cranial hemangiomas affect the cerebrum; facial nevi, especially the flat midline ones and the elevated strawberry nevi, are of no neurologic significance. Rarely, a cerebral meningeal angiomatosis may be present without skin lesions. The involvement of the upper eyelid is of greatest importance and nearly 100 percent of such cases are associated with cerebral lesions. There seems to be a close correlation between the maldevelopment of the embryonic vasculature of eyelid and forehead and that of the occipitoparietal parts of the brain. When the nevus lies entirely below the ophthalmic division, i.e., below the upper eyelid and nose, a cerebral lesion is usually absent, although in a few instances such an angioma has been associated with a vascular malformation of the meninges overlying the brainstem and cerebellum. In angiograms the abnormal meningeal vessels, which are largely veins, are not well seen; thus they can be distinguished from the arteriovenous malformations described in Chap. 33. They are rarely the source of subarachnoid or cerebral hemorrhage, and they do not enlarge to form a "mass lesion." The cortical lesion is of destructive type; lost neurons are replaced by glial tissue which calcifies. Possibly diversion of blood to the meninges during seizures causes an ischemia of the cerebral cortex. Barlow believes the seizures to be responsible for the progressive neurologic deficits and suggests that they be prevented by carefully regulated medical therapy or possibly surgical excision of the discharging foci. However, the magnitude of the cerebral lesion usually contraindicates a neurosurgical approach. Radiotherapy offers no hope of reducing the skin blemish, and sensitive individuals usually try to hide it with cosmetics.

While of congenital origin, the cause and pathogenesis of the encephalotrigeminal syndrome are unknown. Familial coincidence has been observed but is exceptional. The chromosomes appear to be normal.

Dermatomal Hemangiomas with Spinal Vascular Malformations Hemangiomas of the spinal cord may rarely be accompanied by vascular nevi in the corresponding dermatome of skin, as was first pointed out by Cobb. These lesions differ in no important way from the encephalofacial nevi and, like them, tend to conform to a dermatomal pattern. They are nearly always unilateral and are most frequent in the arm and trunk. When the cutaneous lesion involves an arm or leg, there may be enlargement of the entire limb or fingers in combination with underdevelopment of certain parts (Klippel-Trenauney-Weber syndrome). Some of these angiomatous syndromes, as well as the ones described by Wyburn-Mason, combine a spinal or retinodiencephalic arteriovenous malformation (AVM) with a trunkal or facial nevus. Such cases provide a link to the common AVMs described in Chap. 33.

Familial Telangiectasia (Osler-Rendu-Weber Disease) This, a vascular anomaly transmitted as an autosomal dominant trait, affects the skin, the mucous membranes, the gastrointestinal and genitourinary tracts, and occasionally the nervous system. The basic lesion is probably a defect in the vessel wall and bleeding is thought to be due to the mechanical fragility of the vessel. The lesions range from the size of a pinhead to 3 mm or more; they are bright red or violaceous and blanch under pressure. Located sparsely in the skin of any part of the body, they first appear during childhood, enlarge during adolescence, and may assume spidery forms, resembling the cutaneous telangiectases of cirrhosis, in late adult life. The lesions cause trouble only because of their hemorrhagic tendency. During adult years they may give rise to severe and repeated epistaxis or gastric or intestinal or urinary tract hemorrhages. Chronic blood loss may result in an iron-deficiency anemia.

The angiomas of this disease may form in either the spinal cord or brain where they can produce apoplectic syndromes; or an intermittently progressive focal cerebral syndrome may result from enlargement of the vascular lesions or from a succession of small hemorrhages. An unexplained gastrointestinal, genitourinary, intracranial, or intraspinal hemorrhage warrants a search for these small cutaneous lesions, which are easily overlooked. Pulmonary fistulae constitute another important feature of the generalized vascular dysplasia; patients with such lesions are peculiarly subject to brain abscesses. While cautery eradicates a bleeding lesion, satellite ones tend to form. The treatment may require

the application of oxidized cellulose (Oxycel or Gelfoam).

RESTRICTED DEVELOPMENTAL ABNORMALITIES OF THE NERVOUS SYSTEM

In the course of clinical practice one encounters a remarkable number of limited disorders of the nervous system, many of which are transmitted from generation to generation as a mendelian dominant trait. Only a few of the more striking examples will be described here. The reader may turn to books on genetics for an account of such oddities as unilateral ptosis, hereditary Horner's syndrome, pupillary inequalities, jaw winking, absence of a particular muscle, etc.

BIFACIAL AND ABDUCENS PALSIES (MÖBIUS' SYNDROME)

The syndrome of congenital facial diplegia with convergent strabismus is generally referred to as Möbius' syndrome, although it had been described earlier by von Graefe. Its presence at birth is manifested by the lack of facial movements and full eye closure. The most complete review of the subject in the English literature is that of Henderson. In his analysis of 61 cases of the congenital facial diplegia syndrome, there were 45 instances of abducens palsy, 15 of external ophthalmoplegia, 18 of lingual palsy, 17 of clubfeet, 13 of brachial disorders, 6 of mental defect, and 8 of pectoral muscle defect. Thus the overlap with other neuromuscular and CNS abnormalities is evident. In early life there is difficulty in sucking, everted lower lip, and open mouth. Usually it can be distinguished from the facial palsy of forceps or birth injury by its bilaterality and other associated weaknesses. Occasionally more than one family member is affected. The cause of this peculiar condition is not known. The few adequate pathologic studies have shown a lack of nerve cells in the motor nuclei of the brainstem. This syndrome is also referred to on pages 944 and 978.

Partial paralysis of facial muscles, which dates from birth and cannot be attributed to obstetric trauma, is not infrequent. In a common type, the lower lip on the involved side remains immobile when the child smiles or cries; the lip on the unaffected side is drawn downward and outward, resulting in a prominent asymmetry of the lower face. Often it is not appreciated that the side that droops during crying is the normal side (Hoefnagel and Penry).

CONGENITAL LACK OF LATERAL GAZE (OCULOMOTOR APRAXIA OF COGAN)

Children with this congenital defect are unable to turn their eyes to either side on command. Attempting to look to the right, the child turns the head to the right (there is no associated apraxia of head turning, as in the acquired condition), but the eyes lag and turn to the left. As a result, the patient has to overshoot the mark with the head in order to attain fixation straight ahead. Once the eyes fixate, the head returns to the primary position. To compensate for the deficiency of eye movements the patient develops jerky thrusts of the head, which characterize all attempts at voluntary gaze. Caloric stimulation of the labyrinth causes tonic movement (cold to the side of stimulus, warm to the opposite side) but not nystagmus, as in the normal person. Also, optokinetic nystagmus cannot be induced. Vertical movements are normal, however. These children are slow to walk, and Ford has observed one such child whose sibling had an absence of the vermis of the cerebellum. A similar ocular condition may occur in conjunction with ataxia-telangiectasia. The anatomic basis of the condition is unknown.

CONGENITAL ABNORMALITIES OF MOTOR FUNCTION

In this group of congenital disorders, a major disturbance of motor function, usually nonprogressive, has been present since infancy or early childhood. The popular term for these conditions is *cerebral palsy*. The name is not altogether appropriate, nor is it useful from the viewpoint of the physician, collocating, as it does, diseases of widely differing etiologic and anatomic types; the hereditary and acquired, the intrauterine, natal, and postnatal diseases lose their identity. Nevertheless, the term has been adopted as a slogan for fund-raising societies and for a major rehabilitation movement throughout the United States, and it will not soon disappear from medical terminology.

Motor abnormalities which have had their onset early in life are numerous and diverse in their clinical manifestations. To ascertain the etiologic and pathogenic factor(s), it is helpful to categorize a given case according to the extent and nature of the motor abnormality. A careful history of possible prenatal, perinatal, or postnatal insults to the developing nervous system must always be sought; certain correlations of these factors with the resulting pattern of neurologic deficit are outlined below. Most patients with these motor abnormalities of infancy and childhood reach adult years.

CEREBRAL SPASTIC DIPLEGIA (LITTLE'S DISEASE)

Little's original contribution, in 1862, was entitled "On the influence of abnormal parturition, difficult labours, premature birth, and asphyxia neonatorum, on the mental and physical condition of the child, especially in relation to deformities." He emphasized the prenatal or natal origin, the "spastic rigidity of the limbs" (legs more than arms), and the nonprogressive course. Little was of the opinion that asphyxia caused the cerebral damage.

Two main groups can be identified: (1)The first is associated with *prematurity*, and is characterized predominantly by spastic paraparesis (motor disturbances in the upper extremities are mild) and a relatively slight diminution of head size and intelligence. Approximately 20 percent of patients in cerebral palsy clinics in the United States have a spastic diparesis or diplegia and of these 75 to 80 percent are premature babies. Ten to 20 percent of babies who weigh less than 1500 g at birth will develop spastic diplegia and the frequency of diplegia is closely related to the degree of prematurity. The neuropathology is unsettled. Mental function is usually preserved; 5 percent have hearing defects. The incidence of this form of cerebral spastic diplegia has declined significantly since the introduction of neonatal intensive care, and there is reason to believe that it can virtually be eliminated by expert management of premature infants. (2) The second group is associated with *term birth and difficult parturition*, in which the major insult is intrapartum asphyxia and attendant fetal distress. Such infants require resuscitation and have low Apgar scores, which in this circumstance have important predictive value. Most of such infants will develop severe spastic quadriplegia and show mental retardation. The pathologic lesions of the brain in this second group consist of hypoxic-ischemic infarction in distal fields of arterial flow, primarily in the cortex and white matter of parietal and posterior frontal lobes.

The pattern of paralysis is actually more variable than the term spastic diplegia implies; several types may be distinguished; the paraplegic, diplegic, pseudobulbar, and generalized. Pure paraplegic and pseudobulbar types are relatively rare. Usually all four extremities are involved, but the legs are much more affected than the arms, which is the real meaning of diplegia. As a rule, damage to the nervous system is suspected at birth or soon thereafter because of some abnormality of breathing, sucking and swallowing, or responsiveness. If the motor system is affected (corticospinal, extrapyramidal, or cerebellar), hypotonia with retained tendon reflexes and hypoactivity are the rule. Only after the first few months will spasticity appear, first in the adductors of the legs. The plantar reflexes are often ambiguous, but definite extensor responses are pathologic at any age. Also, stiff, awkward movements of the legs, which are maintained in an extended, adducted posture when the infant is lifted by the axillae, do not usually attract attention until several weeks or months have passed. Seizures occur in approximately a third of the cases, and it is not uncommon to observe a delay in all developmental sequences, especially those which depend on the motor system. Once walking is attempted, usually at a much later date than in the normal child, the characteristic stance and gait become manifest. The legs are advanced stiffly in short steps, each describing part of an arc of a circle; adduction of the thighs is often so strong as to lead to actual crossing (scissors gait); the lower legs are slightly splayed, and the feet are flexed and turned in with the heels not touching the ground. In the adolescent and adult, the legs tend to be short and small, but the muscles are not markedly atrophic, as in spinal muscular atrophy and in dystrophy. Passive manipulation of the limbs reveals spasticity in the extensors and adductors and also slight shortening of the calf muscles. The hands and arms may be affected only slightly, if at all; there may be awkwardness and stiffness of the fingers, and, in a few, pronounced weakness and spasticity. In reaching for an object the hand may overpronate. Speech may be well articulated or noticeably slurred, and in some instances the face is set in a spastic smile. The deep tendon reflexes are exaggerated, those in the legs more than in the arms; and the plantar reflexes are extensor in the majority of cases. Usually there is no disturbance of sphincteric function, though delay in acquiring voluntary control is usual. Athetotic postures and movements of the face, tongue, and hands are present in some patients and may actually conceal the spastic weakness; ataxic and hypotonic forms also exist (see further on). The mentality in the pure form of diplegia is relatively normal.

Surprisingly, there is little exact information concerning the cause, mechanism, and morbid anatomy of this syndrome. As was said, a higher incidence of spastic diplegia is known to be associated with prematurity. Physical injury at birth as the responsible factor must be extremely rare, and the existence of an antenatal lesion in some cases, as suggested originally by Freud, can no longer be doubted. Clinical study is handicapped by the fact that anoxic damage to the cerebral cortex and white matter may occur in utero when the fetus cannot be tested; and the possibility of silent injuries to the nonfunctioning cerebrum at any age can never be excluded.

These prenatal and parturitional types of spastic diplegia must be distinguished from the familial types of spastic paraparesis, which have already been discussed in Chap. 42.

INFANTILE HEMIPLEGIA, DOUBLE HEMIPLEGIA, AND QUADRIPLEGIA

Hemiplegia is a common condition of infancy and early childhood. The functional difference between the two sides may be noticed soon after birth or not until after the first 4 to 6 months of life. In other cases, the child is in excellent health for a year or several years before the abrupt onset of hemiplegia. In hemiplegia that dates from earliest infancy, the parents may be the first to notice that movements of prehension and exploration are carried out with only one arm. A manifest hand preference at an early age should always raise the suspicion of a unilateral motor defect. The affection of the leg is usually recognized later, i.e., during the first attempts to stand and walk. Mental defect may be associated with infantile hemiplegia but is less common than with cerebral diplegia and much less common than with bilateral hemiplegia. There may also be a speech delay, regardless of the side of the lesion, but when present, one should look for bilaterality of the motor abnormality and mental retardation. Convulsions occur in 35 to 50 percent of children with congenital hemiplegia, and these may persist throughout life. If hemiplegia occurs during early childhood, seizures often accompany the onset. They may be generalized, but are frequently unilateral and limited to the hemiplegic side. Often, after a series of seizures, the weakness on the affected side will be increased for several hours or longer (Todd's paralysis). Gastaut has described a hemiconvulsive-hemiplegic syndrome in which the progressive paralysis and cerebral atrophy are attributed to the convulsions. In our experience, however, the destruction of tissue, as shown by CT scan, suggests that a vascular or encephalitic lesion has occurred and has resulted in both destruction of brain tissue and seizures.

Double hemiplegia is a much less frequent condition. The bilateral weakness of the face, arms, and legs arises under conditions of severe acquired cerebral disease and at any age. The arms are severely affected, in contrast to their minimal involvement in cerebral diplegia.

Encephaloclastic (destructive) disorders underlie most of the cases of infantile hemiplegia and of bilateral hemiplegias. The pathologic change is essentially that of ischemic necrosis. In many cases, the lesions must have been incurred in utero. The lesions reflect not only the effects of anoxia but also those of circulatory insufficiency (ischemia), the result of hypotension or circulatory failure. The ischemia of circulatory failure tends to affect the tissues lying in arterial border zones, and there may also be venous stasis with congestion and hemorrhage (occurring particularly in the deep central structures such as the basal ganglia and periventricular matrix zones). Myers has reproduced such lesions in the neonatal monkey brain by reducing the maternal circulation over a period of several hours. As the lesions heal, there develop the same ulegyric sclerotic changes in the cortex and white matter of the cerebrum and the "marbling" (*état marbré*) that characterize the brains of patients with spastic diplegia and with double athetosis (see below).

The quadriplegic state differs from bilateral hemiplegias in that the bulbar musculature is not involved in the former. The condition is relatively rare but may result from a bilateral cerebral lesion. However, one should also be alert to the possibility of a high cervical cord lesion. In the infant, this is usually the result of a fracture dislocation of the cervical spine, incurred during a difficult breech delivery. Similarly, in *paraplegia*, with weakness or paralysis limited to the legs, the lesion may be either a cerebral or a spinal one. Sphincteric disturbances and a loss of somatic sensation below a certain level on the trunk always point to a spinal localization. Congenital cysts, tumors, and diastematomyelia are more frequently causes of paraplegia than of quadriplegia. A recently recognized type of infantile paraplegia is spinal cord infarction from thrombotic complications of umbilical artery catheterization.

CONGENITAL EXTRAPYRAMIDAL SYNDROMES

The spastic and rigid cerebral diplegias discussed above shade almost imperceptibly into the congenital extrapyramidal syndromes. Patients with these syndromes are found in every cerebral palsy clinic, and ultimately they reach adult neurology clinics as well. Corticospinal tract signs may be completely absent, and the student, familiar only with the syndrome of pure spastic diplegia, is always puzzled as to their classification. Some cases of

this extrapyramidal type are undoubtedly attributable to severe perinatal hypoxia and others to diseases such as erythroblastosis fetalis with kernicterus. In order to state the probable pathologic basis and future course of these illnesses, it is desirable to separate the extrapyramidal syndromes due to prenatal and natal diseases, which usually become manifest during the first year of life, from the acquired or hereditary postnatal syndromes such as familial athetosis, dystonia musculorum deformans, and hereditary cerebellar ataxia, which become manifest later. The latter have been discussed in Chaps. 37 and 42.

Congenital Choreoathetosis (Double Athetosis) Double athetosis is probably the most frequent of the congenital extrapyramidal disorders. Like the spastic states, it may not be recognized at birth, but only after several months or a year have elapsed. Chorea and athetosis dominate the clinical picture, but various combinations of these involuntary movements with hemiballismus, dystonia, and even myoclonus and ataxic tremor may be found in a single case. Furthermore, in all instances there is in addition a primary defect in voluntary movement.

Choreoathetosis in infants and children varies greatly in severity. In some the abnormal movements are so mild as to be misinterpreted as restlessness or "the fidgets"; in others, every attempted voluntary act precipitates violent involuntary movements, leaving the patient nearly helpless. The clinical appearance of the choreoathetosis and of other involuntary movements has been discussed in Chap. 4.

An initial hypotonia, followed by retardation of motor development, is the rule in these cases. Erect posture and walking may be delayed until the age of 3 to 5 years, and may never be attained in some patients. Tonic neck reflexes or fragments thereof are commonly noted. The plantar reflexes are characteristically flexor, though they may be difficult to interpret because of the continuous flexion and extension of the toes. Sensory abnormalities are not elicited. Because of the motor and speech impairment, patients are often erroneously classified as mentally defective. In some this conclusion is doubtless correct, but in others intellectual function is adequate, and a few can be educated to a high level.

With growth and development, new postures and motor capacities are acquired. The less severely affected patients can even make successful occupational adjustments. The more severely affected ones, even with all the help that can be provided by rehabilitation clinics, rarely achieve a degree of motor control that permits them to lead an independent life. One sees some of these unfortunate persons bobbing and twisting along in public places.

The most frequent pathologic finding in the brain

has been a whitish, marblelike appearance of the putamen, thalamus, and the border zones of the cerebral cortex. These whitish strands represent foci of nerve cell loss and gliosis with peculiar condensations of myelinated fibers and even myelination of astroglial fibers (hypermyelination)—the so-called *status marmoratus* (*état marbré*). This lesion does not develop after infancy, i.e., after the myelination glia have completed their developmental cycle.

Kernicterus   Kernicterus is another important cause of extrapyramidal motor disorder in children and adults. Such cases raise the broader question of the neurologic sequelae of erythroblastosis fetalis secondary to Rh and ABO incompatibilities.

The symptoms of kernicterus appear in the jaundiced neonate on the second or third postnatal day. The infant becomes listless, sucks poorly, develops respiratory difficulties, and becomes stuporous as jaundice intensifies. The serum bilirubin is over 25 mg per 100 ml. In acidotic and hypoxic infants (e.g., those with prematurity and hyaline membrane disease) the kernicteric lesions develop with much lower levels of serum bilirubin (see below).

The majority of infants with this disease die within the first week or two of life. Many of those who survive are mentally retarded, deaf, totally unable to sit, stand, or walk, and spend their lives in homes for the feebleminded. There are exceptional patients, however, obviously less damaged, who are mentally normal or at most only slightly backward. These are the ones who develop a variety of persistent neurologic sequelae—choreoathetosis, dystonia, and rigidity of the limbs—a picture not too different from that of cerebral spastic diplegia with involuntary movements. Kernicterus should always be suspected if an extrapyramidal syndrome is accompanied by bilateral deafness and palsy of upward gaze.

Neonates who die in the acute stage of kernicterus show a characteristic yellow staining of nuclear masses in the basal ganglia, brainstem, and cerebellum—a finding from which the disease takes its name. In surviving patients the pathologic changes consist of symmetrically distributed nerve cell loss and gliosis in the subthalamic nucleus of Luys, the globus pallidus, thalamus, and oculomotor and cochlear nuclei; these lesions are the result of the hyperbilirubinemia. In the newborn, unconjugated bilirubin can pass through the poorly developed blood-brain barrier into these central and brainstem nuclei, where it is directly toxic. Acidosis and hypoxia exacerbate the effect. Also, in the newborn, the development of hyperbilirubinemia is enhanced by the transient deficiency of the enzyme glucuronyl transferase, essential for the conjugation of bilirubin. *Hereditary hyperbi-lirubinemia*, due to lack of this enzyme (*Crigler-Najjar syndrome*), may have the same effect on the nervous system as hyperbilirubinemia due to the excessive hemolysis of Rh incompatibility.

Phototherapy and exchange transfusions with female blood, designed to prevent high levels of unconjugated serum bilirubin, have been shown to protect the nervous system. If the blood bilirubin level can be held to less than 20 mg per 100 ml (10 mg per 100 ml in prematures), the nervous system may escape damage. The effective use of these measures has greatly reduced the incidence of kernicterus.

CONGENITAL AND ACQUIRED ATAXIAS

The combination of cerebral diplegia with cerebellar ataxia has already been mentioned. In these patients difficulty in standing and walking cannot be attributed to spasticity or paralysis. Again, hypotonia is the initial motor abnormality, and the cerebellar defect becomes manifest at a later time, when the patient begins to sit, stand, and walk. These defects may be of such severity that the individual is never able to sit or stand. Yet the muscles are of normal size, and voluntary movements, though weak, are possible in all the limbs. In less-severe cases, sitting, standing, and walking are merely delayed, and with maturation of the corticospinal systems of fibers cerebellar ataxia and tremor become manifest. Relative improvement may occur in later years. The tendon reflexes are present, and the plantar reflexes are either flexor or extensor. Many of these patients suffer a degree of retardation of speech and mental development that results in their placement in homes for the feebleminded. In only a few cases have the pathologic changes been studied. Aplasia or hypoplasia of the cerebellum has been observed but sclerotic lesions of the cerebellum are more common. Since the introduction of the CT scan, the diagnosis can be verified while the patient is alive.

As to causes of this condition, radiation of the abdomen during the first trimester of pregnancy is said to have resulted in cerebellar hypoplasia. A cerebral and cerebellar lesion may coexist in patients with congenital ataxia, which is the reason for the term *cerebrocerebellar diplegia*.

Aside from the congenital ataxias (of which some are cerebellar and others probably cerebral in type), there are other forms of childhood ataxia which have an acute onset and which persist during adolescence and adult life. A few of these are familial. The progressive hereditary ataxias are also likely to begin at a later age than the congenital ones; some are intermittent or episodic, and others are persistent and progressive. They are discussed in Chap. 37.

THE FLACCID PARALYSES

The cerebral form, first described by Foerster and called *cerebral atonic diplegia*, has already been mentioned. It can usually be distinguished from spinal and peripheral nerve paralysis and muscular dystrophy by the retention of postural reflexes (flexion of the legs at the knees and hips when the patient is lifted by the axillae), the preservation of tendon reflexes, and the coincident failure of mental development.

The syndrome of infantile spinal muscular atrophy (Werdnig-Hoffmann disease) is the leading example of flaccid paralysis of lower motor neuron type. Perceptive mothers may be aware of a paucity of fetal movements in utero, and in most cases the motor defect becomes evident soon after birth. Several other types of familial progressive muscular atrophy have been described in which the onset is in late childhood, adolescence, or early adult life. Weakness, atrophy, and reflex loss without sensory change are the main features and are discussed in further detail in Chaps. 42 and 50. A few patients suspected of having infantile or childhood muscular atrophy prove, with the passage of time, to be merely rather inactive, "slack" children, whose motor development has proceeded at a slower rate. A few may remain weak throughout life, with thin musculature. These and several other myopathologic entities, e.g., *central core disease, rod-body myopathy, pleoconial, megaconial, and myotubular myopathies,* are described in Chap. 50. Rarely polymyositis and acute idiopathic polyneuritis may manifest themselves as a syndrome of congenital hypotonia.

Infantile muscular dystrophy and lipid and glycogen storage diseases may also produce a clinical picture of progressive atrophy and weakness of muscles. The diagnosis of *glycogen storage* disease (usually the Pompe form) should be suspected when progressive muscular atrophy is associated with enlargement of the tongue, heart, liver, or spleen. The motor disturbance in this condition may be related in some way to the abnormal deposits of glycogen in skeletal muscles, though it is more likely due to degeneration of anterior horn cells which are distended with glycogen and other substances.

Brachial plexus palsies, well-known complications of dystocia, usually result from forcible extraction of the fetus by traction on the shoulder in a breech presentation, or from traction and tipping of the head in a shoulder presentation. The effects of such injuries are sometimes lifelong. In adults, their early onset is betrayed by the small size and inadequate osseous development of the affected limb. Either the upper brachial plexus and the fifth and sixth cervical roots or the lower brachial plexus and the seventh and eighth cervical and first thoracic roots suffer the brunt of the injury. Upper plexus injuries (*Erb's*) are about 20 times more frequent than lower ones (*Klumpke's*). Sometimes the entire plexus is involved (see page 918).

Facial paralysis, due to forceps injury to the facial nerve immediately distal to its exit from the stylomastoid foramen, is another common peripheral nerve affection in the newborn. The failure of one eye to close and the difficulty in sucking make this condition easy to recognize. It must be distinguished from the congenital facial diplegia that is often associated with abducens palsy i.e., Möbius' syndrome (see above). In most cases of facial paralysis due to physical injury, function is recovered after a few weeks; in some, the paralysis is permanent and may account for an asymmetry observed in later life.

INTRAUTERINE AND NEONATAL INFECTIONS

Throughout the intrauterine period the embryo and fetus are subject to particular types of infection. Since the infective agent must reach the fetus through the placenta, it is evident that the permeability of the latter at different stages of gestation and the immune status of the maternal organism are determinative.

Until the third to fourth month of gestation the large microbial organisms such as bacteria, spirochetes, protozoa, and fungi cannot invade the embryo, even though the mother harbors the infection. Viruses may do so, however—specifically rubella, cytomegalic inclusion disease, herpes simplex viruses, and possibly others. The rubella virus enters embryonal tissues during the first trimester, *Treponema pallidum* in the fourth to fifth postconceptional month, and toxoplasma after that period. Bacterial meningitis (except for that due to *Listeria monocytogenes*, described below) is essentially a paranatal infection contracted during parturition. Neonatal herpes simplex encephalitis, due to the type 2 (genital) virus, is also usually acquired during passage through an infected birth canal.

Embryonal and fetal infections are difficult to diagnose, for the mother may be entirely asymptomatic. Isolation of the organism from fetal and neonatal tissues is possible, but the demonstration of antibodies and other immune responses may be impossible because of the early stage of the infection or imperfections of the infant's immunity.

RUBELLA

Gregg, in 1941, first reported the association of maternal rubella and congenital cataracts in the neonate. His observations were quickly verified, and soon it became widely known that cataracts, deafness, congenital heart disease, and mental retardation constituted a kind of tetrad, diagnostic of this disease. That a virus could affect all these tissues, causing in essence a noninflammatory developmental disorder of multiple organs, was a novel concept, and it raised the exciting prospect that other viruses might have similar effects. Surprisingly, however, only the cytomegalovirus and possibly herpes simplex viruses (most often type 2) have been incriminated in embryonal neuropathology. A large number of other viruses (e.g., influenza, hepatitis) have been implicated in human teratogenesis, but in none is the relationship beyond doubt.

It is now well established that most instances of congenital rubella infection occur in the first 10 weeks of gestation, and that the earlier the occurrence of infection, the greater the risk to the fetus. However, there is considerable risk even beyond the first trimester (Hardy, 1973).

Following the massive rubella epidemic of 1964 and 1965, the congenital rubella syndrome has been expanded to include a wider range of defects: low birth weight; bilateral deafness of neurocochlear type; microphthalmia, pigmentary degeneration of the retina, salt and pepper chorioretinitis, cloudy cornea, glaucoma and cataracts of special type; hepatosplenomegaly, jaundice and thrombocytopenic purpura; patent ductus arteriosus or interventricular septal defect. One, a few, or varying combinations of these abnormalities may occur. The mental retardation is severe and may be accompanied by seizures and motor defects such as hemiplegia or spastic diplegia.

Infection of the fetus after the first trimester results in a less impressive neonatal syndrome. The infant may seem lethargic and fail to thrive. The cranium is abnormally small. Only a cardiac abnormality, deafness, or chorioretinitis may provide clues to diagnosis. The CSF is abnormal with mononuclear pleocytosis and elevated protein. The infection may persist for a year or two.

The maternal infection may be inapparent but even when evident the fetus may be spared in 30 percent of cases. Diagnosis can be verified in the neonate by the demonstration of IgM antibodies to the virus or by the isolation of the virus from the throat, urine, stool, or CSF. Recently the virus has been obtained from cells in the amniotic fluid.

The *neuropathology* is of considerable interest. In the nervous system of abortuses (the procedure performed because of proven maternal rubella in the first trimester) one of the authors (R.D.A.) found no visible lesions by light microscopy even though the virus had been isolated from the brain by Enders. At this period of development there is no possibility of an inflammatory reaction because of an absence of polymorphonuclear leukocytes, lymphocytes, and mononuclear cells in the fetus. At birth the brain is usually of normal size, and there may be no discernible lesions. In a few, a mild meningeal infiltration of lymphocytes, a few zones of necrosis, and calcification of vessels are seen. Smallness of the brain and delay in myelination have been observed in children dying at 1 to 2 years of age. None of the brains in our series have been malformed. Rubella virus continues to be recovered from the CSF for at least 18 months after birth. Recently a delayed progressive rubella encephalitis in childhood has been reported (page 524).

The obvious approach to the problem of congenital rubella infection is to make sure that every woman has been vaccinated against rubella or has had the infection prior to pregnancy. The widespread use of rubella vaccine has reduced the chance of major epidemics, but sporadic infections continue to occur, and an outbreak of epidemic proportions is still possible because of laxity of vaccination programs. There is no effective treatment for the established infection.

CYTOMEGALIC INCLUSION DISEASE (CID)

For many years it was known that in the tissues of some infants who died in the first weeks and months of life there were swollen cells containing intranuclear and cytoplasmic inclusions. This cytologic change seemed related to the fatalities. In 1956 and 1957, three different laboratories isolated what have come to be called the human cytomegaloviruses (see Weller, 1970).

Infection of the fetus occurs in the first trimester of pregnancy, or later, by way of an inapparent maternal viremia and active infection of the placenta. Only a small proportion of women known to harbor the cytomegalovirus give birth to infants with active infection. Early infection of the fetus may result in a malformation of the cerebrum; later, there is only inflammatory necrosis in parts of the normally formed brain. In the premature or in the full-term infant, the clinical picture is one of jaundice, petechiae, hematemesis, melena, hepato-splenomegaly, microcephaly, mental defect, and convulsions. Cells in the urine may show cytomegalic changes. The clinical picture resembles that of severe rubella infection. There are disseminated inflammatory foci in the cerebrum, brainstem, and retinas. In the centers of aggregates of lymphocytes, mononuclear cells, and plasma cells are microglial cells containing inclusion bodies; some astrocytes are similarly affected. The granulomas later calcify. Often there is hydrocephalus.

Several studies indicate that about 1 percent of infants born in the United States excrete virus in their urine and may continue to do so for as long as 4 years postnatally. Of the infected infants, about 17 percent have some degree of nervous system damage (Hanshaw, 1971). The latter may be limited to simple mental retardation or sensorineural deafness. Why one infected fetus develops normally and another develops CNS disease is not understood.

Congenital cytomegalovirus infections pose a much greater problem than rubella. There is no way of identifying the infected fetus prior to birth or to prevent inapparent infections in the pregnant woman. Also, recent evidence suggests that some infected infants (with viruria) may appear normal at birth but develop neural deafness and mental retardation several years later (Reynolds et al.).

There is no known treatment. The difficulties in prenatal diagnosis of maternal infection preclude abortion.

CONGENITAL NEUROSYPHILIS

The clinical syndromes and pathologic reactions of congenital neurosyphilis are similar to those of the adult. Such differences as exist are determined principally by the immaturity of the nervous system at the time of spirochetal invasion.

The syphilitic infection may be transmitted to the fetus at any time from the fourth to the seventh months. The fetus may die, with resulting miscarriage or stillbirth, or may survive only to be born with florid manifestations of secondary syphilis. The dissemination of the spirochetes throughout the body, the time of appearance of the secondary manifestations, and the time of formation of syphilitic reagin in the blood are all governed by the same biologic laws that are operative in adult syphilis.

At birth the spirochetemia may not have had time to cause syphilitic reagin to appear; hence a negative VDRL reaction in umbilical cord blood does not exclude syphilis. In unselected groups of syphilitic mothers, 25 to 80 percent of fetuses are infected, and in 20 to 40 percent of those infected the CNS is invaded, as judged by the finding of abnormal CSF. In general, the incidence of congenital neurosyphilis is approximately the same as adult neurosyphilis, and the types (asymptomatic and symptomatic meningitis, meningovascular disease, hydrocephalus, general paresis, and tabes dorsalis) are also the same except for the rarity of tabes dorsalis. The Hutchinson triad (dental deformities, interstitial keratitis, and bilateral deafness) is infrequently observed in complete form; deafness is rare. The sequence of neurologic syndromes is the same as for the adult, all stemming basically from a chronic spirochetal meningitis. The latter may become symptomatic in the first weeks and months of postnatal life, meningovascular lesions and hydrocephalus reaching maximal frequency during the 9-month to 6-year period. Congenital paresis usually appears between the ninth to fifteenth years and juvenile tabes during adolescence. The pathologic basis of each neurosyphilitic syndrome is, respectively, meningoarteritis (vascular syphilis), meningoencephalitis (general paresis), and meningoradiculitis (tabes dorsalis).

The authors have observed fewer and fewer cases of congenital neurosyphilis as the years pass. If all syphilitic mothers are treated before the fourth month of pregnancy, the fetus will not be infected. If the infant is normal at birth and has had no signs of meningeal invasion, or only an asymptomatic meningitis that is actively treated until the CSF is normal, vascular lesions of brain and spinal cord, hydrocephalus, general paresis, and tabes dorsalis will not develop. If cases of meningovascular syphilis, general paresis, and tabes dorsalis are treated for 3 to 4 weeks with penicillin until the CSF is rendered acellular and the protein reduced to normal, the neurologic disorder will be arrested, and often there is a functional improvement.

The various neurosyphilitic syndromes are described fully in Chap. 31. Only those features pertinent to the congenital forms are mentioned below.

1. *Meningovascular syphilis* declares itself by a stroke with involvement of cerebrum, brainstem, or spinal cord in the first months or years of life. It enters the differential diagnosis of *infantile hemiplegia*. Other neurologic deficits may occur as well. Many infarctive lesions may leave the patient mentally backward, and any one of them may become epileptogenic.

2. *Early hydrocephalus* and *retarded psychomotor development* should always raise the possibility of congenital syphilis though less than 1 percent of cases

have a syphilitic basis. Such children may be permanently retarded.

3. *Congenital paretic neurosyphilis.* Approximately half the patients who decline mentally because of neurosyphilis during late childhood will have been defective physically and mentally since infancy. The other half will have developed normally. In 23 personally observed patients the initial symptom was either mental or physical. If already feebleminded, the patient becomes more deficient; or, if intelligence had been normal, behavior becomes eccentric and school performance declines. Silliness, forgetfulness, irascibility, and inattentiveness are noteworthy behavioral abnormalities. There may be outbursts of agitation and depression. Approximately half the cases have seizures. Peculiar choreiform movements, twitches, and action tremors are frequent. The tendon reflexes are hyperactive, and plantar reflexes extensor. The pupils are fixed to light and sometimes to accommodation, and tend to be dilated rather than miotic. Optic atrophy and chorioretinitis may be conjoined.

4. *Congenital tabetic neurosyphilis.* Failing vision and urinary incontinence are the usual early symptoms. Sensory ataxia and lightning pains are rare. The legs are areflexic but not weak, and the bladder hypotonic and dilated. The pupils are more frequently dilated than miotic, and optic atrophy and strabismus are often present.

Congenital syphilis must be considered a potential albeit an increasingly rare cause of epilepsy and amentia. Once the syphilitic infection has been treated in early life and rendered inactive (acellular CSF, normal protein), the occurrence of a congenital luetic infection can only be substantiated by an accurate history, the finding of the syphilitic stigmata in the eyes, teeth, and ears, or a positive serologic reaction in the CSF.

TOXOPLASMOSIS

This tiny protozoan, occurring freely or in pseudocyst form, was established by Cowan and his associates as a frequent cause of meningoencephalitis in utero or in the perinatal period of life. The disease exists in all parts of the United States, but is more frequent in western European countries. The mother is most often infected by handling uncooked infected mutton or other animal foods, but she is nearly always asymptomatic.

The precise times of placental and fetal invasion are not known, but presumably they are late in the gestational period. The clinical syndrome usually becomes manifest in the first days and weeks of life when seizures, spastic paralysis of the extremities, progressive hydrocephalus, and chorioretinitis appear. The retinal lesions

consist of large pale areas surrounded by deposits of pigment. If severe, the maculae are destroyed, and optic atrophy and microphthalmus follow. In older infants, we have several times observed hemiplegias, first on one side then on the other, followed by hydrocephalus. The latter is present in about one-third of the cases. The CSF contains a moderate number of white blood cells, mostly lymphocytes and mononuclear cells, and increased protein in the range of 100 to 400 mg per 100 ml. The glucose values are normal. Less than 10 percent of infected children recover. In these latter cases the infection must have been mild and soon burned itself out.

Granulomatous masses and zones of inflammatory necrosis abut on the ependyma or meninges. The organisms, 6 to 7 μm in length and 2 to 4 μm in width, are visible in and near the lesions. Microcysts may be found also, lying free in the tissues without inflammatory reaction. The necrotic lesions calcify rapidly and after several weeks or months are readily visible in plain films of the skull. These appear as periventricular and multiple nodular densities.

We have observed the disease coming on later in life—in childhood, adolescence, and even late adult years. Then it gives rise to a rapidly evolving meningitis and multifocal encephalitis in conjunction with myocarditis, hepatitis, and polymyositis. The latter syndrome is described on page 503 as are the diagnostic tests and treatment. Infections such as rubella, syphilis, CID, and herpes simplex must be considered in the differential diagnosis.

OTHER VIRAL AND BACTERIAL INFECTIONS

Several other infections of late fetal life or the neonatal period will only be mentioned here, for to describe them all would be tedious and would elucidate no new neurologic principles. Meningitis due to a small gram-positive rod, *Listeria monocytogenes,* may be acquired in the usual way, at the time of passage through an infected birth canal, or in utero, as a complication of maternal and fetal septicemia due to this organism. In the latter case, it causes abortion or premature delivery. *Neonatal meningitis* is a particularly devastating and often fatal type of bacterial infection, not easily diagnosed unless the pediatrician is alert to the possibility of a silent meningitis in every neonatal infection (page 479).

Herpes simplex encephalitis may destroy large parts of the brain, particularly of the temporal lobes, and is frequently fatal. Coxsackie B, polioviruses, and arboviruses (Western equine) seem to be able to cross the placental barrier late in pregnancy and cause encephalitis or encephalomyelitis in the fetus at term which is indistinguishable from the disease in the very young infant.

EPILEPSIES OF INFANCY AND CHILDHOOD

In Chap. 15 the major types of seizures were discussed in some detail. In bringing up this subject here, attention is drawn to the fact that epilepsy is mainly a disease of infancy and childhood. The largest number of epileptics fall into these age periods, and some of the most interesting and unique types of seizure are peculiar to these epochs of life.

One principle that emerges is that the form which the seizures take in early life are in part age-linked. Neonatal seizures are focal; infantile seizures take the form of myoclonic flexor (sometimes extensor) spasms; and petit mal is essentially a disease of childhood (4 to 13 years). Further, certain epileptic states tend to occur during certain epochs of life—febrile seizures from 6 months to 6 years and generalized or temporal spike-wave activity with benign motor and complex partial seizures from 6 to 16 years. In general, idiopathic epilepsy, so-called because the cause cannot be determined, is predominantly a pediatric neurologic problem. This is not to say that seizures of unknown cause do not occur in adult life, but rather that the proportion of such seizures is much greater in childhood and steadily diminishes once adulthood is reached.

The characteristics of certain forms of infantile and childhood seizures not observed in adult life will be commented upon in the following paragraphs.

NEONATAL SEIZURES

One might question whether a fully organized convulsion, like grand mal, is within the capabilities of the neonatal brain. Most convulsive phenomena at this age are fragmentary, confined to muscles in a particular part of the body—one side of the face, turning of the eyes, arrest of respirations, clonic movements of an arm or leg or one side of the body. Nonetheless, a more widespread, patterned fit may occur on occasion. Neonatal seizures due to metabolic diseases, birth injury, and encephalitis

all have the same appearance but a somewhat different course.

INFANTILE SPASMS (SALAAM SEIZURES)

These seizures, which have been described briefly in Chap. 15, begin in the first weeks of life and continue for several years, ceasing by the age of 1 to 5 years. Flexion of the trunk and of the arms and legs is the usual pattern; less often there is extension of the neck and trunk. Their frequency varies from 1 to 2 per day to as many as 50 to 100. They do not recur at any other period in later life. There is a core syndrome, of obscure (probably metabolic) origin, that presents this way and is accompanied by mental deterioration. The EEG shows giant slow waves (hypsarrhythmia). This disorder has no established neuropathologic basis. The spasms respond to ACTH for reasons not known, but the mental regression is usually uninfluenced by treatment with this hormone. In a variety of other diseases, seizures begin in early infancy with fragmentary motor seizures and progress to infantile spasms (tuberous sclerosis, phenylketonuria, Sturge-Weber disease, etc.).

FEBRILE SEIZURES

These are organized, generalized motor seizures which appear usually on the ascending limb or at the peak of a febrile episode. They affect infants and children between the ages of 6 months and 6 years, after which they cease, and the patient goes through the remainder of life without convulsions. There is a family predisposition to this type of seizure. Imprecision of diagnosis allows other forms of epilepsy, unrelated to fever per se, to contaminate the group; hence some of the patients are said to develop severe psychomotor seizures, atypical petit mal, and the Lennox-Gastaut syndrome (see Chap. 15).

PETIT MAL

Typical petit mal (*absence*) usually begins about 4 to 5 years of age; spells are frequent throughout childhood and tend to disappear during adolescence and adult life. If seizures continue beyond childhood they tend to take other forms, such as grand mal, psychomotor epilepsy, or partial tonic or clonic motor seizures. Exceptions occur, with petit mal persisting well into adult life. Petit mal usually signifies idiopathic epilepsy, and is seldom seen with cerebral tumors, trauma, etc. Atypical forms of petit mal, in distinction to the typical absence, have grave implications. These are discussed in Chap. 15.

Each of these many special forms of epilepsy of

infancy and childhood has its temporal position in the life cycle and is more age-related than disease-related. It is not unusual for an epileptic child to exhibit each type during the span of years from birth to adult life. Neonatal seizures respond best to small doses of phenobarbital (15 mg tid). Treatment and management of other types are discussed in Chap. 15.

MENTAL RETARDATION

In concluding this chapter, it is important to remind oneself that only a small proportion of cases of mental retardation (about 10 percent) can be traced to the congenital anomalies of development and related disorders that have been reviewed in the preceding pages. When this group is studied clinically, a reasonably accurate diagnosis of the brain disease can be made in approximately 50 percent of cases. When examined by conventional histopathologic methods, gross lesions are found in approximately 90 percent of cases and in fully three-quarters of them an etiologic diagnosis is possible. Interestingly, the destructive vascular and hypoxic-ischemic lesions and other diseases (chromosomal, metabolic, and genetic) that are found in this group, are much the same as would be found if the group had been selected on the basis of cerebral palsy rather than severe mental retardation (see Table 43-3). Noteworthy is the fact that the cerebra in the remaining 10 percent of the "pathologically retarded" are grossly and microscopically normal. It is a remarkable fact that current technology does not enable the neuropathologist to visualize a lesion which has caused a lifelong idiocy, and if one includes cases which had less severe degrees of mental retardation, the number of morphologically normal cases increases.

Here it is important to repeat a point made in Chap. 27, that the larger proportion of the mentally deficient do not have recognizable cerebral lesions, but are the segment of the normal population that is the opposite of genius. On the gaussian curve of human intelligence (see Fig. 27-4) they represent the lowest 3 percent, the group that lies between the second and third standard deviations from the mean. Lewis was one of the first to call attention to this large group of simple mental retardates, and he referred to them as *subcultural*. In many of the families other members of the same and previous generations are feebleminded or have other mental disorders so that the term *familial* has been applied to the group. There are several types of hereditary mental retardation, but they have not been well-defined clinically or pathologically. Some of them are characterized by maldevelopment of the cerebral cortex. Males, in general, tend to be affected more frequently than females and there has arisen a recent interest in the "fragile X chromosome" which some geneticists hold accountable for at least part of this sex difference. Some of the translocations and deletions of parts of chromosomes are also found in this group of familial retardates. Nevertheless, it appears that factors other than purely genetic ones are operative in this group. The majority come from families in the lowest social and economic strata. A high incidence of prematurity and complicated births, exposure to toxic substances such as lead, and undernutrition also characterize this group. Of course, these factors may affect only a single child in a family.

The factor of malnutrition as a worldwide cause of mental retardation has received considerable attention in recent years. Animal experiments (Winick) demonstrate that severe undernutrition during critical periods in early life will lead to biochemical, morphological, and behavioral changes in the brain, and these may be permanent (see Chap. 38). However, the data proving that human mental retardation is widely caused by malnutrition is far from convincing. Although there seems to be little doubt that severe protein-calorie deficiency in the first 8 months of life may retard mental development, the authors are more impressed with the fact that the nervous system tends to resist nutritional deficiency more than any other organ. Examples abound of infantile cachexia, as in cystic fibrosis, where, after a lag in development, dietary supplementation has resulted in rapid improvement in nervous functioning—"catching up" to normal levels—and a spurt of brain and head growth, even with temporary separation of sutures. In most of the groups of malnourished children who remain feebleminded it has not been possible to eliminate the effects of polygenic inheritance, impoverished environment, and infectious disease.

The action of exogenous toxins during parturition is another factor to which importance has recently been attached. A low-grade lead intoxication in utero or during infancy, insufficient to cause flagrant lead encephalopathy, is believed to be associated with a lowering of IQ, but so far much of the clinical evidence is statistical. Severe maternal alcoholism has been linked to a dysgenetic syndrome (see Chap. 40, under fetal alcohol syndrome). Surprisingly, maternal addiction to opiates, while causing withdrawal symptoms in the infant for weeks or even months (Wilson et al.), has not resulted in permanent injury to the nervous system. However the follow-up period was not of sufficient duration to be sure of this. Trimethadione, when taken as an anticonvulsant during pregnancy, is said to cause a slight increase in the incidence of mental retardation; phenytoin is reported to have no effect on mental development but does result in a slight (two-to-threefold) incidence of cleft-lip and palate and other selected congenital malformations (Monson et al.).

In all the aforementioned conditions the neuropathology is essentially unknown. For the most part the cases would fall in the category of mental retardation without morphologic changes, akin to the 10 percent of the severely retarded with normal brains and to practically all of the less severely retarded. There is now an active interest in devising new cytopathologic methods for exposing the defect which must surely have a structural component. The nerve cell is being visualized more completely by the Golgi method in order to study its dendritic branchings and synaptic surfaces. Abnormalities of this type have been reported by Huttenlocher and by Purpura, but this work is just beginning. Still to come is the quantitative analysis of neuronal populations of the thalamic nuclei and cortex and the density of neuropil.

As an aid to the pediatrician and neurologist who must assume responsibility for the diagnosis and management of backward children, the following descriptions may be of some value. The differentiation of the various classes of mental backwardness by clinical criteria is facilitated if they are subdivided into the dysmorphic, the neurologic, the systemic, and the simple, or uncomplicated (see Table 43-2 for a framework of reference).

Table 43-2
Types of mental retardation

I. Mental defect with associated developmental abnormalities in nonnervous structures
  A. Those affecting cranioskeletal structures
    1. Microcephaly
    2. Macrocephaly
    3. Hydrocephalus (including myelomeningocele with Arnold-Chiari malformation and associated cerebral anomalies)
    4. Down's syndrome (mongolism)
    5. Cretinism (congenital hypothyroidism)
    6. Mucopolysaccharidoses (Hurler, Hunter, and Sanfilippo types)
    7. Acrocephalosyndactyly (craniostenosis)
    8. Arthrogryposis multiplex congenita (some cases)
    9. Rare specific syndromes: De Lange
    10. Dwarfism, short stature: Russell-Silver dwarf, Seckel's bird-headed dwarf, Rubinstein-Taybi dwarf, Cockayne-Neel dwarf, etc.
    11. Hypertelorism, median cleft face syndromes, agenesis of corpus callosum
  B. Those affecting nonskeletal structures
    1. Neurocutaneous syndromes: tuberous sclerosis, Sturge-Weber, neurofibromatosis (uncommon)
    2. Congenital rubella syndrome (deafness, blindness, congenital heart disease, small stature)
    3. Chromosomal disorders: Down's syndrome, some cases of Klinefelter's syndrome (XXY), XYY, Turner's (XO) syndrome (occasionally), and others.
    4. Laurence-Moon-Biedl syndrome (retinitis pigmentosa, obesity, polydactyly)
    5. Eye disorders: toxoplasmosis (chorioretinitis), galactosemia (cataract), congenital rubella
    6. Prader-Willi syndrome (obesity, hypogenitalism)
II. Mental defect without developmental anomalies in nonnervous structures, but with focal cerebral and other neurologic abnormalities
  A. Cerebral spastic diplegia
  B. Cerebral hemiplegia, unilateral or bilateral
  C. Congenital choreoathetosis or ataxia
    1. Kernicterus
    2. Status marmoratus
  D. Congenital ataxia
  E. Congenital atonic diplegia
  F. Syndromes resulting from hypoglycemia, trauma, meningitis, and encephalitis
  G. Associated with other neuromuscular abnormalities (muscular dystrophy, Friedreich's ataxia, etc.)
  H. Cerebral degenerative diseases (lipidoses)
  I. Lesch-Nyhan syndrome
III. Mental defect without signs of other developmental abnormality or neurologic disorder (epilepsy may or may not be present)
  A. Simple mental retardation, familial mental retardation, subcultural mental retardation
  B. Some cases of encephaloclastic disease (hypoxia, hypoglycemia)
  C. Infantile autism
  D. Associated with inborn errors of metabolism (phenylketonuria, other aminoacidurias, organic acidurias)
  E. Congenital infections (some cases of congenital syphilis, cytomegalic inclusion disease)

Some of the clinical aspects of mental retardation, particularly of the "subcultural" type, have been discussed in Chap. 27. There it was pointed out that mental retardation manifests itself most obviously in the spheres of motor, language, social, and intellectual development. The severely retarded infant with an IQ of less than 20 (idiot level in the older classifications) often does not sit up, walk, or stand; and if any one of these motor activities is acquired, it appears late and is imperfectly performed. Language never develops; at most a few words are understood and uttered, or the patient vocalizes in a meaningless way. Such a patient is continuously idle and interacts little with people and objects in his or her surroundings. There is no effort to make known bodily needs for water, food, excretion, etc. Only primitive emotional reactions are exhibited. Physical growth is usually retarded, nutrition may be poor, and susceptibility to respiratory infections is increased. Sphincteric control may never be accomplished. A variety of physical deformities, particularly microcephaly, is common in this group; affections of the nervous system which have their onset later in life are usually not attended by bodily disfigurement.

If the mental defect is less pronounced [IQ of 20 to 45 (i.e., imbecile), or 45 to 70 (i.e., moron)], and if specific motor defects do not coexist, then sitting, walking, and speech are acquired, but only after a delay in many cases. The existence of a cerebral defect may be noted for the first time when the child fails to speak normally during the second and third years of life, and seems not to be able to learn the usual household and play activities as well as other children. However, delay in speech development must not by itself be taken as a mark of mental retardation, for some children who can obviously comprehend what is said to them and communicate by gesture are slow in talking. Also the deaf child may be singled out by an indifference to noise and reduced vocalization—but otherwise normal development. Toilet training also may be difficult to accomplish in the retarded child; but, again, it may be delayed in an otherwise normal child.

Within the spectrum of mental retardation, even within a group of persons of similar IQs, there are vast differences in overall behavioral functioning. Some retardates are pleasant and amiable, and achieve a rather satisfactory social adjustment; this is especially true of the subcultural group. At the opposite extreme is the ill-understood syndrome of autism, associated with varying degrees of retardation, in which the child or older person fails to manifest any kind of interpersonal, social contact—including communicative language—and demon-strates a limited interest in inanimate objects (see page 412). It is impossible to list all variations of mental retardation here, but the point should be made that all aspects of intellectual life and personality are affected in differing degrees. Many retarded individuals are dull, apathetic, and underactive. Others display an incessant hyperactivity, characterized by a very short attention span, a restless inquisitive searching of the environment, and low frustration tolerance; they may be destructive or recklessly fearless, and may seem strangely impervious to injury. Some display a peculiar *anhedonia* and are indifferent to either punishment or reward. Strangely, as with the mentally normal but hyperactive, inattentive child, improvement in these children can often be achieved by using amphetamines and related drugs. Other aberrant types of behavior, such as violent aggressiveness and even self-mutilation, are not uncommon. Rhythmic rocking, rolling, head-banging, and bouncing movements are features of the motor activities of retarded persons, and may be performed hour after hour without fatigue, often to the accompaniment of bleating sounds, squeals, and other ejaculations. Here the abnormality is not the appearance of rhythmic movements of

Table 43-3

Causes of severe and mild mental retardation in 1372 patients at the W. E. Fernald State School

Disease category	Number of patients IQ<50	Number of patients IQ>50	Percent of all patients
Acquired destructive lesions	278	79	26.0
Chromosomal abnormalities	247	10	18.7
Multiple congenital anomalies	64	16	5.8
Developmental abnormality of brain	49	16	4.7
Metabolic and endocrine diseases	38	5	3.1
Progessive degenerative disease	5	7	0.9
Neurocutaneous diseases	4	0	0.3
Psychosis	7	6	1.0
Mentally retarded (cause unknown)	385	156	39.5

the body—which are to be observed at one period in the development of many normal children—but their persistence. Music may encourage rhythmic movement, and it gives pleasure to many retarded children and adults.

It is apparent that the clinical and behavioral characteristics of retarded individuals cannot be adequately described by a single parameter, the IQ; many other factors determine the social success of the retarded child and should give direction to the education and training of such a child. These include recognition of specific sensory or motor handicaps, such as blindness and deafness as well as athetosis or hemiplegia; specific language or speech deficits; behavioral disturbances, such as lack of socialization and hyperactivity; and the presence of seizures. Measures can be taken which help the handicapped person to compensate for these deficiencies. This becomes a primary consideration in functional diagnosis and in guiding the parents or guardians.

The least severely retarded individual (IQ of 45 to 70) grows and develops in many ways not different from normal ones, and can be taught useful occupational skills. A few of these persons can work under careful supervision. All scholastic pursuits are relatively unsuccessful, and vocational training is of more value than other types of education.

CONCLUSIONS

Viewed in their entirety these many genetic and acquired anomalies of development pose a formidable problem to medicine and science. In the United States, significant fetal abnormalities occur at a rate of about 3 percent of live births and a large but imprecisely determined number of individuals are lost to spontaneous abortion or stillbirth.

As regards the disease processes themselves, once they have acted to prevent development or to destroy the immature brain, little or nothing can be done medically. The lesion is completed. If the pathologic process is encountered in a stage of evolution, effective therapy may prevent further damage. An objective of more fundamental importance is the identification of pathogenic factors and the control or elimination of them as ways of preventing cerebral maldevelopment or injury before they occur.

A number of maternal health factors have been recognized within recent years as having injurious effects on the fetal brain. Rubella is now being controlled by vaccination of all young women or girls before the child-bearing age. Congenital syphilis has been eliminated by widespread serologic testing and by treatment of all syphilitic women in the first half of pregnancy. Kernicterus has been greatly reduced by preventing high levels of bilirubinemia. Although more than 50 medications are suspect as fetal pathogens, only thalidomide, folic acid antagonists, steroid hormones, and alcohol are convincingly dangerous. Evidence of others being harmful may be forthcoming, but until such time it seems advisable for the pregnant woman to take only those drugs that are absolutely essential to her health. The same must be said of street drugs, which may possess teratogenic effects, and of maternal alcoholism, which undoubtedly can cause deficiency of growth, microcephaly, mental retardation, and other anomalies. Smoking diminishes the birth weight of neonates by more than 150 g, but whether this predisposes to cerebral damage is uncertain. Nutritional deficiency is surely associated with an increase of associated disease and subnormal mentality and should be corrected at all costs.

In mothers of advanced age or with diseases that place the fetus at risk, amniocentesis before the twentieth week of fetal life is advisable. The information which it yields at least warns of the possibility of disease in the neonate and offers the option of abortion. This is but a glimpse of future prospects. Increasing knowledge of the specific defects that underlie the congenital and hereditary diseases and newer methods (e.g., fetoscopy) for the direct measurement of these defects promise to control and eliminate many congenital diseases.

REFERENCES

ADAMS RD: Neurocutaneous diseases, in Fitzpatrick TB et al (eds): *Dermatology in General Medicine*, 2d ed. New York, McGraw-Hill, 1979, chap 23, pp 1206-1246.

BARLOW CF: *Mental Retardation and Related Disorders.* Philadelphia, Davis, 1978.

BIELSCHOWSKY M: Über tuberose Sklerose und ihre Beziehungen zur Recklinghausenschen Krankheit. *Z Gesamte Neurol Psychiatr* 26:133, 1914.

CANALE D, BEBIN J, KNIGHTON RS: Neurologic manifestations of von Recklinghausen's disease of the nervous system. *Confin Neurol* 24:359, 1964.

COBB S: Haemangioma of the spinal cord associated with skin naevi of the same metamere. *Ann Surg* 62:641, 1915.

COGAN DC: A type of congenital ocular motor apraxia presenting jerky head movements. *Trans Am Acad Ophthalmol* 56:853, 1952.

COWAN D, WOLF A, PAIGE BH: Toxoplasmic encephalomyelitis: VI. Clinical diagnosis of infantile or congenital toxoplasmosis; survival beyond infancy. *Arch Neurol Psychiatry* 48:689, 1942.

CROWE FW: Axillary freckling as a diagnostic aid in neurofibromatosis. *Ann Intern Med* 61:1142, 1964.

————, SCHULL WJ, NEEL JV: *A Clinical, Pathological and Genetic Study of Multiple Neurofibromatosis.* Springfield, Ill, Charles C Thomas, 1956.

FITZPATRICK TB et al: White leaf-shaped macules, earliest visible sign of tuberous sclerosis. *Arch Dermatol* 98:1, 1968.

FORD FR: *Diseases of the Nervous System in Infancy, Childhood and Adolescence,* 6th ed. Springfield, Ill, Charles C Thomas, 1973.

GASTAUT H et al: H.H.E. syndrome: Hemiconvulsion, hemiplegia, epilepsy. *Epilepsia* 1:418, 1960.

GOLD AP, FREEMAN JM: Depigmented nevi, the earliest sign of tuberous sclerosis. *Pediatrics* 35:1003, 1965.

GOMEZ MR: *Tuberous Sclerosis.* New York, Raven Press, 1979.

GORLIN RS, PINDBORG JJ, COHEN MM JR: *Syndromes of the Head and Neck.* New York, McGraw-Hill, 1976.

GREGG NM: Congenital cataract following German measles in the mother. *Trans Ophthalmol Soc Australia* 3:35, 1941.

HANSHAW JB: Congenital cytomegalovirus infection. A fifteen year perspective. *J Infect Dis* 123:555, 1971.

HARDY JB: Clinical and developmental aspects of congenital rubella. *Arch Otolaryngol* 98:230, 1973.

HENDERSON JL: The congenital facial diplegia syndrome: Clinical features, pathology and etiology. *Brain* 62:381, 1939.

HOEFNAGEL D, PENRY JK: Partial facial paralysis in young children. *N Engl J Med* 262:1126, 1960.

HOLMES LB et al: *Mental Retardation: An Atlas of Diseases with Associated Physical Abnormalities.* New York, Macmillan, 1972.

HUTTENLOCHER PR: Synaptic and dendritic development and mental defect, in Buchwald NA, Brazier MA (eds): *Brain Mechanisms in Mental Retardation.* New York, Academic, 1975, pp 123–138.

JOHNSON KP: Viral infections of the developing nervous system, in Thompson RA, Green JR (eds): *Advances in Neurology,* vol 6. New York, Raven Press, 1974, pp 53–67.

LEMIEUX BG: Chromosomal aberrations, in Swaiman KF, Wright FS (eds): *The Practice of Pediatric Neurology.* St Louis, Mosby, 1975, unit I, chap 26, pp 277–302.

LEWIS EO: Types of mental deficiency and their social significance. *J Ment Sci* 79:298, 1933.

LICHTENSTEIN BW: Neurofibromatosis (Von Recklinghausen's disease of the nervous system). *Arch Neurol Psychiatry* 62:822, 1949.

LORBER J: Spina bifida cystica. Results of treatment of 270 cases with criteria for selection in the future. *Arch Dis Child* 47:854, 1972.

MONSON RR et al: Diphenylhydantoin and selected congenital malformations. *N Engl J Med* 289:1049, 1973.

MYERS RE: Experimental models of perinatal brain damage: Relevance to human pathology, in Glueck L (ed): *Intrauterine Asphyxia and the Developing Fetal Brain.* Bethesda, Md, Year Book, 1977.

PENROSE LS: *The Biology of Mental Defect.* New York, Grune & Stratton, 1949.

PURPURA DP: Normal and aberrant neuronal development in the cerebral cortex of human fetus and young infant, in Buchwald NA, Brazier MA (eds): *Brain Mechanisms in Mental Retardation.* New York, Academic, 1975, pp 141–171.

REYNOLDS DW et al: Inapparent congenital cytomegalovirus infection with elevated cord IgM levels. Causal relation with auditory and mental deficiency. *N Engl J Med* 290:291, 1974.

ROSMAN NP, PEARCE J: The brain in neurofibromatosis. *Brain* 90:829, 1967.

SPILLANE JD: Developmental abnormalities in the region of the foramen magnum, in Bowman PW, Manter HV (eds): *Mental Retardation.* New York, Grune & Stratton, 1960, p 182.

SRABSTEIN JC et al: Is there a congenital varicella syndrome? *J Pediatr* 84:239, 1974.

SWAIMAN KF, WRIGHT FS: *The Practice of Pediatric Neurology.* St Louis, Mosby, 1975.

VAN DER HOEVE J: Eye symptoms of tuberous sclerosis of the brain. *Trans Ophthalmol Soc UK* 40:329, 1920.

WEBER F PARKES: Association of extensive haemangiomatous naevus of skin with cerebral (meningeal) haemangioma, especially cases of facial vascular naevus with contralateral hemiplegia. *Proc R Soc Med* 22:25, 1929.

WELLER TH: Cytomegaloviruses: The difficult years. *J Infect Dis* 122:532, 1970.

————: The cytomegaloviruses: Ubiquitous agents with protean clinical manifestations. *N Engl J Med* 285:267, 1971.

WILSON GS, DESMOND MM, VERNIAND W: Early development of infants of heroin-addicted mothers. *Am J Dis Child* 126:457, 1973.

WINICK M: *Malnutrition and Brain Development.* New York, Oxford, 1976.

WOHLWILL FJ, YAKOVLEV PI: Histopathology of meningofacial angiomatosis (Sturge-Weber's disease). *J Neuropathol Exp Neurol* 16:341, 1957.

YAKOVLEV PI, GUTHRIE RH: Congenital ectodermoses (neurocutaneous syndromes) in epileptic patients. *Arch Neurol Psychiatry* 26:1145, 1931.

————, WADSWORTH RC: Schizencephalies. A study of the congenital clefts in the cerebral mantle. *J Neuropathol Exp Neurol* 5:116, 169, 1946.

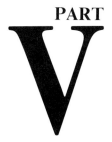
DISEASES OF PERIPHERAL NERVE AND MUSCLE

CHAPTER 44

LABORATORY AIDS IN THE DIAGNOSIS OF NEUROMUSCULAR DISEASE

The clinical suspicion of neuromuscular disease, evinced by the recognition of any one of the symptoms or syndromes that will be discussed in the succeeding chapters, now finds ready confirmation in the laboratory. The intelligent use of the laboratory requires some knowledge of the biochemistry and physiology of muscle fiber contraction, nerve action potentials, and neuromuscular conduction. These subjects will therefore be reviewed briefly, as an introduction to the descriptions of the laboratory methods and findings.

BIOCHEMISTRY AND PHYSIOLOGY OF NEUROMUSCULAR DISEASE

Biochemical tests in common use include the measurement of serum electrolytes and enzymes and the detection of myoglobin in the urine. Also, in certain circumstances, measurements of urinary creatine and creatinine may be useful. The quantitative measurement of certain essential constituents of muscle (carnitine, carnitine palmityl transferase, phosphorylase, acid maltase, phosphofructokinase) is now possible by application of microchemical methods to small pieces of muscle taken at biopsy. Abnormalities of these constituents have proved to be specific for certain myopathies, and will be mentioned in the sections that deal with these particular diseases.

ELECTROLYTES AND NEUROMUSCULAR ACTIVITY

This is not the place to review all the biochemical and biophysical data that explain nerve impulse formation and conduction. Since the early studies of Hodgkin (1951) and of Hodgkin and Huxley (1952), tomes have been written on these subjects. Suffice it to say that the nerve and muscle fibers, like other bodily cells, maintain a fluid internal environment that is distinctly different from the external or interstitial medium. The main intracellular constituents are potassium (K), magnesium (Mg), and phosphorus (P), whereas those outside the cell are sodium (Na), calcium (Ca), and chloride (Cl). In both nerve and muscle the intracellular concentrations of these ions are held within a narrow range by electrical and chemical forces, which maintain the membranes in electrochemical equilibrium (*"resting membrane potential"*). These forces are the result of selective permeability of the membranes to various ions and the continuous expulsion of Na by a kind of pump mechanism ("the sodium pump"). The function of the pump mechanism is dependent on the enzyme ATPase, which is localized in the membranes. The resulting electrochemical equilibrium is such that the inside of the cell is kept negative in respect to the outside by a potential difference of 70 to 90 mV.

This resting membrane potential shows an interesting dependence on the concentrations of K and Na. The interior of the cell is some 30 times richer in K than the extracellular fluid, and the concentration of Na is 10 to 12 times greater in the extracellular fluid. In the resting state the chemical forces that promote diffusion of K ions out of the cell (down their concentration gradient) are counterbalanced by electrical forces (the external positivity opposes further diffusion of K to the outside). At the resting potential, the situation of Na ions is the opposite; they tend to diffuse into the cell, both because of their concentration gradient and because of the relative negativity inside the cell. Because the membrane is less permeable to Na than to K, the amount of K leaving the cell exceeds the amount of Na entering the cell, thus creating the difference in charge across the membrane (the outside of the cell is positive relative to the inside).

The permeability of the cell membrane to Na is

controlled by the electrical potential of the membrane. As the latter is depolarized by slight electrical or chemical change, there is an increased permeability to Na. The subsequent movement of K outward repolarizes the membrane and thereby reduces its permeability to Na. These slight fluxes of ions in the resting state are known as *passive decay*. If a greater degree of depolarization occurs, a situation arises in which the outward movement of K is unable to stabilize the membrane. It then becomes even more depolarized and progressively more permeable to Na, and an "explosive" regenerative Na current develops; Na rushes down its chemical and electrical gradients into the cell. Eventually an equilibrium potential is reached where the interior of the cell becomes about 40 mV positive. This is the *action potential* that lasts only a millisecond or less, before the membrane loses its permeability to Na and becomes much more permeable to K. The resulting efflux of K repolarizes the membrane to a resting level. During this time the nerve and muscle fibers are refractory, at first absolutely then relatively, to another depolarizing stimulus. If the process of recovery is delayed, this *depolarization inactivation* prevents the development of further action potentials until the membrane regains its resting potential.

Action currents in the axon and muscle cell occur when one region of the membrane becomes depolarized. As the action currents flow into the depolarized zone, the contiguous membrane becomes depolarized; the de-

polarization may reach the threshold for development of an action potential, and a new zone of increased Na permeability then spreads in this way, in a kind of all-or-none fashion, down the length of the nerve or muscle membrane. This is the *conducted action potential*.

As the motor nerve impulse passes centrifugally from parent axon into its branches, transmission "breaks down" especially if the repetition rate is excessive and impulses arrive too frequently at branch points. Impulses may then fail to invade certain terminal branches. This happens in myasthenia gravis and other neuromuscular diseases and may result in an EMG picture indistinguishable from that of a myopathy (see further on).

These events, the hallmarks of all excitable tissues, are clearly influenced by the concentration of K ions in the extracellular fluids.

THE NEUROMUSCULAR JUNCTION (MOTOR END PLATE)

This interface between the finely branched nerve fiber and the muscle fiber, where nervous activity is translated into muscle action, has special properties (Figs. 44-1 and 44-2). The nerve fiber, as it indents the muscle cell membrane, always leaves a *synaptic cleft* between the axolemma and sarcolemma (Fig. 44-2). Quanta of relatively fixed size of acetylcholine (ACh) in the nerve terminals, liberated by the arrival of action potentials, diffuse into and attach to the receptor sites on the sarcolemma. Calcium ions facilitate this release, whereas botulinus toxin and a high concentration of Mg ions interfere with it. The ACh is the chemical transmitter and acts on the postsynaptic part of the motor end plate by causing a

Figure 44-1

Motor end plate showing relationship between various structures in nerve and muscle. Last segment of myelin, with Schwann nucleus (S), terminates abruptly, leaving axis cylinder covered by sheaths of Schwann and Henle. End-plate nuclei (EP) of muscle fiber lie embedded in sarcoplasm and have same staining reactions as sarcolemmal nuclei (M). Ramifications of

axis clinder (telodendria) lie in grooves or pouches in granular sarcoplasm, each lined by spiny "subneural apparatus" of Couteaux, which is continuous with membranous sarcolemma and also Schwann membrane. Nucleus (S) of sheath of Schwann commonly lies near point of branching of axon. Sheath of Henle has small nuclei (H) and fuses with endomysial sheath of muscle fiber. (Courtesy of D Denny-Brown.)

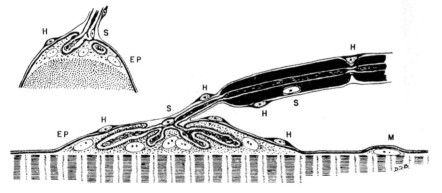

local increase in the conductance of Na and K and other small ions. It produces a depolarization known as the *end-plate potential*. Small end-plate potentials are continuously formed and regenerated as the membranes repolarize, similar to the process of passive decay described above. If the ACh release exceeds a certain threshold (if hundreds of quanta of ACh are released), an independent all-or-nothing action potential invades the muscle cell membrane and spreads up and down its surface much like the nerve action potential. The sarco-

lemma, once depolarized, is refractory to another action potential until repolarized. Molecules of ACh combine briefly with cholinesterase at receptor sites and are hydrolyzed.

THE CHEMISTRY OF MUSCLE CONTRACTION

The plasmalemma (the plasma membrane of the sarcolemma), the transverse tubules, and the sarcoplasmic reticulum each play a role in the control of the activity of muscle fibers. The structural components involved in excitation contraction and relaxation of muscle are illustrated in Fig. 44-3. Following nerve stimulation, an ac-

Figure 44-2

Normal human end plate. The nerve terminal with its synaptic vesicles is seen in upper part of picture. The adjacent nucleus is that of a Schwann cell. Below the nerve terminal the postsynaptic region is composed of folds and clefts. The synaptic space contains homogeneous material. The line indicates 1 μm. × 30,000. (From Engel et al.)

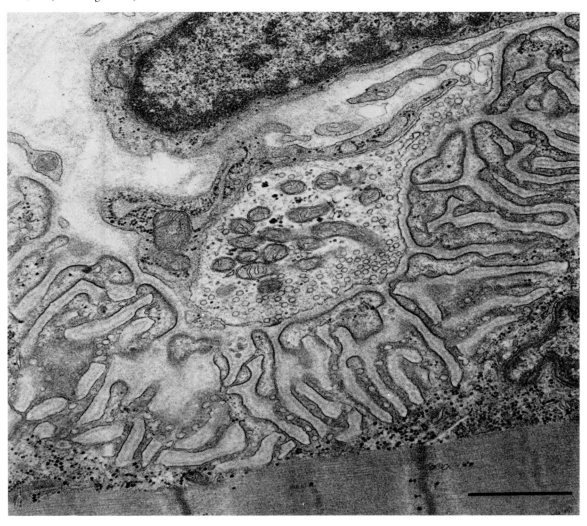

tion potential is transmitted by the plasmalemma from the motor end-plate region to both ends of the muscle fiber. Depolarization spreads quickly to the interior of the fiber along the walls of the transverse tubules, probably by a conducted action potential. The transverse tubules and the terminal cisternae of the sarcoplasmic reticulum come into close proximity at points referred to as *triads.* Here, by a mechanism that is not understood, depolarization of the transverse tubules is transmitted to the sarcoplasmic reticulum, which releases Ca stored in its interior. The main events which follow the release of Ca are fairly well established. Calcium binds to the regulatory protein, *troponin,* thereby removing the inhibition exerted by the troponin-tropomyosin system upon the contractile protein, *actin.* This allows an interaction to take place between the cross bridges of the myosin molecules in the thick filaments and the actin molecules of the thin filaments and enables myosin adenosine triphos-

phatase (ATPase) to split adenosine triphosphate (ATP) at a rapid rate, thereby providing the energy for contraction. This chemical change produces a force which causes the filaments to slide past each other. Relaxation occurs as a result of active (energy-dependent) Ca reuptake by the sarcoplasmic reticulum.

The pyrophosphate bonds of ATP, which supply the energy for muscle contraction, must be replenished constantly by a reaction that involves interchanges with the muscle phosphagen, creatine diphosphate, where high-energy phosphate bonds are stored. These interactions in both contraction and relaxation require the action of creatine phosphokinase (CPK). Myoglobin, another important muscle protein, functions in the transfer of oxygen, and a series of oxidative enzymes are involved in this exchange. The intracellular Ca which, as noted above, is released by the muscle action potential, must be reaccumulated within the cisternae before actin and myosin filaments can slide back past one another in relaxation. The reuptake of Ca requires the expenditure of considerable energy. When ATP is lacking, the muscle remains shortened, as in the *contracture* of phospho-

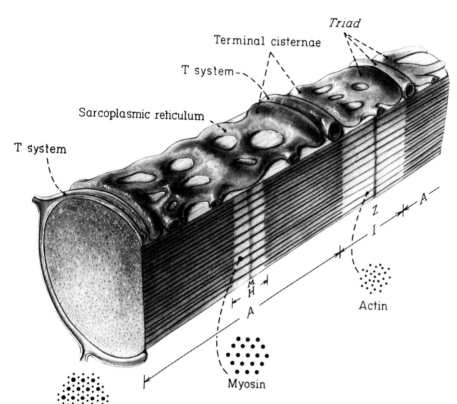

Figure 44-3
Schematic illustration of the major subcellular components of a myofibril. The transverse (T) system, which is an invagination of the plasma membrane of the cell, surrounds the myofibril midway between the Z lines and the center of the A bands; the T system is approximated to, but apparently not continuous with, dilated elements (terminal cisternae) of the sarcoplasmic reticulum on either side. Thus, each sarcomere (the repeating Z-line-to-Z-line unit) contains two "triads," each composed of a pair of terminal cisternae on each side of the T tubule. (From Peter.)

rylase deficiency (McArdle's disease) or phosphofructose kinase deficiency. The same sort of shortening occurs under normal conditions in some of the "catch muscles" of certain mollusks and is the basis of rigor mortis in mammals.

Many glycolytic and other enzymes (transaminases, aldolase, CPK) are also implicated in the metabolic activity of muscle, particularly under relatively anaerobic conditions. Muscle fibers differ in their relative content of oxidative and glycolytic enzymes; the latter determine the capacity of the muscle fiber to sustain anaerobic metabolism during periods of contraction with inadequate blood flow. Muscle cells rich in oxidative enzymes contain more mitochondria and larger amounts of myoglobin (appear red), have slower rates of contraction and relaxation, fire more tonically, and are less fatigable than muscle fibers poor in oxidative enzymes. The latter fire in bursts and are utilized in quick phasic rather than sustained postural reactions. The amount of myosin ATPase activity, which governs the speed of contraction, is low in oxidative-rich fibers and high in glycolytic-rich fibers. The Ca-activated myosin ATPase stain at pH 9.4 has been used to classify these two types of fibers in microscopic sections. Type I (oxidative-rich) fibers have a low content of myosin ATPase, and type II (phosphorylative-rich) fibers have a high content of this enzyme. Other less well-differentiated histochemical types have also been identified. All the fibers within one motor unit are of the same type.

The mechanical events of muscle contraction (twitch) last much longer than the action potential and depend upon the following factors: (1) an end-plate potential of sufficient magnitude to produce muscle contraction, (2) the availability and rate of release of Ca ions from the sarcoplasmic reticulum, (3) the rate of hydrolysis of ATP, (4) the rate of sarcomere shortening, (5) the elasticity of the muscle fiber and surrounding connective tissues, and (6) the rate of reuptake of Ca ions by the sarcoplasmic reticulum. Factors (2) and (3) affect the latency of onset of the twitch (i.e., the interval between the action potential and beginning of contraction); (4) and (5) determine the velocity of rise to peak tension at a given length; and (6) determines the duration of the twitch (viz., the period of full tetanic tension attained during the twitch). The total twitch time is the sum of all the above plus the time required for the twitch to be transmitted to the tendon.

If a second action potential arrives after the refractory phase of the previous action potential but before the muscle has relaxed, the contraction will be prolonged. Thus, at frequencies of anterior horn cell firing of 10 to 20 per s, the twitches fuse into a sustained contraction or *tetanus*. In this fashion the mechanical phenomena are smoothed into a continuous process, even though the electrical potentials present as a series of depolarizations, separated by intervals during which the muscle membrane resumes its resting polarized state.

At the motor end plate, repolarization is possible only if ACh is inactivated by acetylcholinesterase. The latter is located at the receptor site on the muscle fiber. If this chemical reaction does not occur, the end plate remains depolarized and therefore is unable to respond to further nerve impulses. Anticholinesterase drugs, such as neostigmine (Prostigmine), pyridostigmine (Mestinon), edrophonium (Tensilon), physostigmine (Eserine), succinylcholine, decamethonium, diisopropyl fluorophosphate (DFP), tetraethylpyrophosphate (TEPP), and several of the so-called nerve gases and pyrophosphate insecticides, act in this way to paralyze muscle. These substances are called *depolarizing blocking agents* because they maintain the end-plate region in a depolarized state, refractory to activation by the arrival of further action potentials (and quanta of ACh). The quaternary ammonium ions (such as curare), the so-called *competitive blocking agents*, paralyze muscles by occupying the receptor sites on the muscle fiber so that acetylcholine cannot reach them. Antibodies to the end-plate receptor protein (in myasthenia gravis) act in the same way.

Biochemical changes underlie not only an impairment of neuromuscular activity (paresis, paralysis) but also excessive irritability, tetany, spasm, and cramp. In the latter, spontaneous discharges may occur, or a single nerve impulse may initiate a train of action potentials in nerve and muscle, as in the tetany of hypocalcemia and in idiopathic facial spasm. In tetany, ischemic paresthesias also arise on the basis of irritability of the neurilemma. The common cramps of calf and foot muscles (painful, sustained, involuntary contractions with motor unit discharges at frequencies of up to 200 per second) may in part be due to increased excitability of the motor axons. Quinine, procaine amide, diphenhydramine (Benadryl), and warmth reduce the irritability of nerve and muscle fiber membranes.

To summarize, the muscle fiber which is wholly dependent on the nerve for its stimulus to contract may be physiologically paralyzed in a number of ways. The nerve may fail to conduct impulses; the neuromuscular junction may not release acetylcholine, or once released, it may not be inactivated by cholinesterase; the receptor zone on the muscle cell may be blocked by a competing substance; the sarcolemma may not distribute the nerve impulse to all parts of the muscle fiber; and finally, the metabolic or contractile elements of the muscle may not react, or, once contracted, may not relax. Similarly, the mechanisms involved in fasciculations, cramps, and muscle spasms may be traced to a number of different points in the neuromuscular apparatus. There may be an unstable polarization of the nerve fibers as in dehydration with salt depletion and in tetany, or unexplained hyperirritability of the motor neuron, as in amyotrophic lateral sclerosis. The threshold of mechanical activation or electrical reactivation of the sarcolemmal membrane may be reduced, as in myotonia; or, impairment of an energy mechanism within the fiber may slow the contractile process, as in hypothyroidism; or a deficiency of ATP under anaerobic conditions may prevent relaxation, as in the contracture of McArdle's disease. By a mechanism not understood, lesions of the most peripheral branches of nerves (shown electromyographically by prolongation of the terminal latencies of nerve conduction) may give rise to continuous activities of motor units. This is expressed clinically as a rippling appearance known as myokymia or neuromyotonia.

EFFECTS OF ABNORMALITIES OF SERUM ELECTROLYTES

Diffuse muscle weakness or the occurrence of muscle twitchings, spasms, and cramps, should always raise the question of a disorder of serum electrolytes. The latter reflect the ionic concentrations in extracellular fluids. The ECG and EMG may reveal alterations of their intracellular levels in the heart and skeletal muscle. If the plasma level of *potassium falls below 2.5 meq/liter or rises above 7 meq/liter,* weakness of extremity and trunk muscles results. Below a level of 2 meq/liter or above 9 meq/liter, there is almost always flaccid paralysis of these muscles and later of the respiratory ones as well, only the extraocular and other muscles of the cranium being spared. In addition, the tendon reflexes are diminished or absent. The reaction of muscle to percussion is also reduced or abolished, suggesting impairment of transmission along the sarcolemmal membranes themselves. *Hypocalcemia* of 7 mg per 100 ml or less (as in rickets or hypoparathyroidism) or relative reduction in the proportion of ionized calcium (as in hyperventilation) causes increased irritability and spontaneous discharge of sensory and motor nerve fibers, i.e., tetany, and sometimes convulsions from similar effects upon ce-

rebral neurons; frequent repetitive and finally prolonged spontaneous discharges appear in the EMG, and convulsive effects are reflected in the EEG. *Hypercalcemia* above 12 mg per 100 ml (as in vitamin D intoxication, hyperparathyroidism, and carcinomatosis) causes weakness and lethargy, perhaps on a central basis. *Reduction in the plasma concentration of magnesium* also results in tremor, tetanic muscle spasms, and convulsions; a considerable *increase in magnesium levels* leads to muscle weakness and depression of central nervous function (confusion). The weakness of muscle may be due, in part at least, to reduced release of acetylcholine at the motor end plate.

CHANGES IN SERUM LEVELS OF ENZYMES ORIGINATING IN MUSCLE CELLS

In all diseases which cause extensive damage to striated muscle fibers, intracellular enzymes leak out of the fiber and enter the blood. Those which are now being measured in most hospital laboratories are the transaminases, lactic acid dehydrogenase, aldolase, and creatine phosphokinase (CPK). Of these, the level of CPK in serum has proved to be the most sensitive measure of muscle damage. Since high concentrations of this enzyme are found in heart muscle and brain, raised serum values may be due to myocardial or cerebral infarction as well as to the necrotizing diseases of striated muscle (polymyositis, muscle trauma, muscle infarction, Meyer-Betz paroxysmal myoglobinuria, and the more rapidly advancing muscular dystrophies). For serum CPK levels to be interpretable, one has to be certain that heart or brain are undamaged. This problem has been overcome to a large extent by the recent development of techniques for the quantitation of serum isoenzymes of CPK. These isoenzymes are referred to as MB, MM, and BB, and their measurement provides a highly sensitive and tissue-specific means for the detection of damage to myocardium, skeletal muscle, and nervous tissue, respectively.

The MM form of CPK is found in highest concentration in striated muscle. If the normal level is 0 to 65 IU per liter of serum, it may exceed 1000 IU in patients with destructive lesions of striated muscle. Even more interesting is its rise in some children with progressive muscular dystrophy before there is enough destruction of fibers for the disease to be clinically manifest, at least as judged by crude tests of muscle strength. Moreover, the unaffected female carriers of the Duchenne pseudohypertrophic form may often be identified because many of them show slightly elevated serum levels of CPK. Alterations of serum enzyme levels are nonspecific for dystrophy since they occur in all types of disease which destroy the muscle fiber. Moreover, in the more slowly evolving types of dystrophy, such as that of Landouzy-Dejerine, the serum levels of CPK may be normal. It would be expected that the values would always be normal in denervation paralysis with muscular atrophy, but unfortunately they may be slightly elevated in some patients with progressive spinal muscular atrophy and amyotrophic lateral sclerosis. Also, vigorous exercise may elevate CPK in normal persons, and sometimes CPK may be persistently elevated without evidence of muscle or other diseases.

ENDOCRINOPATHIES

In a number of disorders of endocrine glands, muscle weakness may be a prominent feature, and occasionally it may even become a chief complaint. While these diseases are discussed in detail elsewhere (Chap. 49), it should be noted that such weakness, local or generalized, acute or chronic, may occur in the absence of changes in serum electrolytes or enzymes. Specific hormone assays are then necessary for diagnosis. This is particularly true of thyrotoxicosis, where severe muscle paresis may appear without the classic signs of Graves' disease.

MYOGLOBINURIA

The red pigment, myoglobin, responsible for much of the color of muscle, is an iron-protein compound present in the sarcoplasm of striated skeletal and cardiac fibers. Of the total body hematin compounds, about 25 percent is in muscle, the remainder in red blood corpuscles and other cells. Destruction of striated muscle, regardless of the process, liberates myoglobin, and because of its relatively small size, the molecule filters through the glomeruli and appears in the urine, imparting to it a burgundy red color. Because of the low renal threshold, the excretion of myoglobin is so rapid that the serum remains uncolored. In contrast, because of the high renal threshold, the hemoglobin released by destruction of red blood corpuscles colors both the serum and urine. Myoglobinuria should thus be suspected when the urine is deep red and the serum normal in color. As in hemoglobinuria, the guaiac and benzidine tests are positive. The urine does not fluoresce, as it does in porphyria. The most sensitive method for measuring myoglobin in the urine and serum is by radioimmunoassay techniques (Rosano and Kenny). The final demonstration depends on spectroscopic analysis, which shows an absorption band at 581 nm. The conditions giving rise to myoglobinuria are listed on page 957.

CREATINURIA

Creatine, an amino acid, is a prominent constituent of striated muscle tissue. It may be ingested (exogenous creatine), but it is also synthesized in the liver from glycine, arginine, and methionine and then delivered to the skeletal muscles, which contain more of this compound than any other organ (150 mg per 100 g fresh-weight muscle tissue). Creatinine, the anhydride of creatine, is a degradation product which is excreted in the urine. The creatinine content of muscles is low (about 5 mg per 100 ml), since it diffuses readily through the sarcolemma. The serum level of creatine in normal males varies from 0.2 to 0.6 mg per 100 ml; in females from 0.4 to 0.9 mg per 100 ml. Creatinine serum levels range from 0.8 to 1.4 per 100 ml and are increased only in serious renal disease. Adult 24-h urine excretion of creatine averages from 60 to 150 mg in normal men and 100 to 300 mg in women. Creatinine excretion is remarkably constant at 1.0 to 1.6 g per day. In diseases such as progressive muscular dystrophy, the creatine content of the muscle fiber is diminished, and there is a decrease in creatinine excretion, increase in creatine excretion, and hypercreatinemia. The same alterations occur with reduction in muscle mass in neurogenic atrophy, polymyositis, hyperthyroidism, Addison's disease, and male eunuchoidism. Ingestion of 1 to 3 g creatine will not significantly raise its level in blood or urine in a normal person, for the muscles are not saturated, but in an individual with a reduced muscle mass, creatinemia and creatinuria result. This type of creatine tolerance test thus merely indicates reduction in functional muscle mass.

ELECTRODIAGNOSIS OF NEUROMUSCULAR DISEASE

Long ago it was discovered that muscle would contract when a pulse of electric current was applied to the skin, near the point of entrance of the muscular nerve (*motor point*). The effective electrical pulse is brief, less than a millisecond, as induced by a rapidly alternating (faradic) current. After denervation, an electrical pulse of longer duration (several milliseconds) is required to produce the same response; the brief, faradic stimulus becomes ineffective and only a constant (galvanic) stimulation succeeds. This change, in which the galvanic stimulus remains effective after the faradic one has failed, was the basis of *Erb's reaction of degeneration*, and varying degrees of this change were plotted in the form of *strength-duration curves*. For decades, this was the standard electrical method for evaluating denervation of muscle.

ELECTROMYOGRAPHY AND THE NORMAL ELECTROMYOGRAM (EMG)

The foregoing method of evaluating denervation, though still valid, is outmoded. Now, reliance is placed on the demonstration of fibrillations and characteristic changes in motor unit potentials by the insertion into muscle of coaxial needles. This type of study is based on the concept of the "motor unit" introduced by Sherrington and presented on page 33.

Skeletal muscles must be tested laboriously, one at a time, because of the varying topography of muscle and peripheral nerve diseases, which may involve some muscles and not others, or only parts of muscles. Normal findings in one or a few muscles do not exclude the possibility of pathologic phenomena elsewhere. External plate or surface electrodes, such as those used in electrocardiography or electroencephalography, can be used to record motor unit potentials, but they are unable to record potentials from single motor units. The latter requires the use of concentric needle electrodes, 0.3 to 0.8 mm in diameter, which are inserted into the muscle to be studied. The tip of the wire in the lumen of the needle will be in proximity to several muscle fibers, belonging to one or two motor units; this is the recording electrode. The shaft of the needle, in contact over most of its length with intercellular fluid and many other muscle fibers, is the indifferent reference electrode.

The following is a summary of the electrical events that occur in relation to the recording electrode. When the nerve impulse travels along the surface of the muscle, current begins to flow through the normally polarized region under the recording electrode to the depolarized zone. As shown in Fig. 44-4, the recording electrode becomes positive relative to the reference electrode, and the beam of the cathode ray oscilloscope (CRO) is deflected (by convention) downward (at A). When the depolarized zone moves under the recording electrode, the latter rapidly becomes negative and the beam is deflected upward (at B). As the depolarized zone continues to move along the sarcolemma, away from the recording electrode, the membrane under the latter slowly becomes repolarized. Current once again begins to flow outward through the membrane toward the dis-

tant depolarized region, and the electrode becomes relatively positive once again (at C). It then returns to its resting isopotential position. The net result is a triphasic action potential recorded on the CRO, as in Fig. 44-4. This configuration is typical of fibrillations that are recorded at a distance from the end-plate zone and are seen only when single muscle fibers are separated from their nerve supply. Fibrillation potentials are so brief (<5 ms) that the inertia-free CRO must be used to record them; ink-writing apparatus does not have the necessary frequency response.

As indicated above, single fibers do not act alone in normally innervated muscle but are merged in motor unit activity, which involves the almost simultaneous activity of a hundred or more muscle fibers extending for a distance of several millimeters. The potential recorded from a motor unit necessarily has a greater duration and amplitude than a fibrillation potential. The typical configuration of a motor unit potential is also triphasic, as indicated in Fig. 44-8. Up to 10 percent of normal motor unit potentials consist of four or more phases (*polyphasic potentials*).

Normally, resting muscle is electrically silent; the small tension spoken of as muscle tone has no EMG

Figure 44-4

The shaded area represents the zone of the action potential which is negative to all other points on the fiber surface. It is shown at three points in its course (from left to right) along the fiber. At each point, the correspondingly lettered portion of the triphasic muscle-action potential displayed on the cathode ray oscilloscope (CRO) reflects the potential difference between the active (vertical arrow) and reference (Ref.) electrodes. Polarity in this and subsequent figures is negative upward as depicted. The time calibration is on the CRO screen.

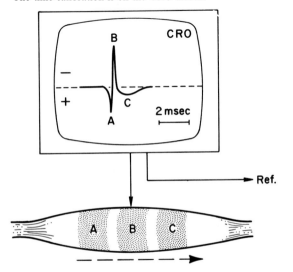

equivalent. Insertion of the coaxial needle into the muscle injures and mechanically stimulates many fibers, causing a burst of potentials of short duration (<300 ms, according to Goodgold and Eberstein). This is referred to as normal insertional activity. When muscle is voluntarily contracted, the action potentials of motor units begin to appear on the CRO. One can observe the way force is built up by watching the recruitment of motor units firing initially at rates of 4 to 5 per second and then at incrementally higher rates as force is increased. As more and more units are recruited, a great crowd of them appears on the CRO screen, firing at rates of 20 to 30 per second (Fig. 44-5A). Since individual motor unit potentials can no longer be distinguished, this is referred to as a complete *interference pattern*. The largest units are up to 5 mV in amplitude. As muscles relax, more and more units drop out, and the rate of firing decreases. If a muscle is weakened by denervation or if voluntary contraction is inadequate for other reasons, there will obviously be fewer motor unit potentials.

If the recording needle electrode is placed near the motor end plate, potentials can be recorded from the normal resting muscle ("end-plate noise"), consisting mainly of miniature end-plate potentials (MEPPs). These small potentials need to be distinguished from fibrillation potentials.

THE ABNORMAL ELECTROMYOGRAM

Clinically important deviations from the normal EMG include (1) increased insertional activity, (2) the occurrence of "spontaneous" activity during relaxation (fibrillations, positive sharp waves, and fasciculations), (3) abnormalities in the amplitude, duration, and shape of single motor unit potentials, (4) a decrease in the number of motor unit potentials, (5) variation in amplitude of motor unit potentials on weak voluntary contraction of muscle, and (6) the demonstration of special phenomena, such as myotonia, coupling (tetany), bizarre high-frequency potentials, or electrical silence during obvious shortening of the muscle (contracture).

Insertional Activity At the moment the needle is inserted into muscle, there is usually a brief burst of action potentials which cease once the needle is stable, providing it is not in a position to irritate an intramuscular nerve fiber. Increased insertional activity is seen in all forms of denervation as well as in polymyositis and disorders that dispose to muscle cramps. In cases of advanced denervation or myopathy, where muscle fibers have been largely replaced by connective tissue and fat, insertional activity may be decreased.

"Spontaneous" Activity Spontaneous activity of single muscle fibers and of motor units, known respectively as *fibrillation* and *fasciculation*, is abnormal. The two phenomena are often confused. Fibrillation is the contraction of *single muscle fibers* and appears when the muscle fiber has lost its nerve supply. Fasciculation consists of synchronous contraction of *groups of muscle fibers* integrated by a single axon into a motor unit. (Both are discussed below.)

Fibrillation When a motor neuron is destroyed by disease, or when its axon is interrupted, the distal part of the axon degenerates, a process which takes several days. The muscle fibers formerly innervated by the branches of the dead axon, viz., the motor unit, are dis-

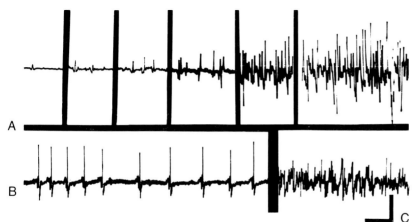

Figure 44-5
Patterns of motor unit recruitment. A. Normal. With each increment of voluntary effort, more and larger units are brought into play until, with full effort at the extreme right, a complete "interference pattern" is seen in which single units are no longer recognizable. B. After denervation, only a single motor unit is recorded despite maximal effort. It is seen to fire repetitively. C. With myopathic diseases, a normal number of units is recruited, though the amplitude of the pattern is reduced. Calibrations: 50 ms (horizontal) and 1 mV in A and B; 200 μV in C (vertical).

connected from the nervous system. For reasons which are still obscure, the chemosensitive region of the sarcolemma at the motor end plate "spreads" after denervation to involve the entire surface of the muscle fiber. Then, 10 to 25 days after death of the axon, the denervated fibers develop spontaneous activity; i.e., even while no effort is being made by the patient to contract the muscle, each fiber contracts at its own rate and without relation to the activity of neighboring fibers. There results a totally random conglomeration of brief, di- or triphasic fibrillation potentials (Fig. 44-6A), having a duration of 1 to 5 ms and rarely exceeding 300 μV in amplitude. When brief, spontaneous potentials of this sort are observed at two or three different locations outside the end-plate zone of a resting muscle, one may conclude that some of the fibers are denervated. Fibrillation potentials may be seen, in considerable numbers, in certain primary diseases of muscle, such as polymyositis, or occasionally in dystrophy; nevertheless, if numerous, they can be taken as a mark of denervation hypersensitivity. Diseases such as poliomyelitis, which damage spinal motor neurons, or injuries of peripheral nerves or anterior spinal roots, frequently produce only partial denervation of the involved muscles. In such muscles, one electrode placement may record fibrillation potentials at

rest from denervated fibers and normal potentials during voluntary contraction from nearby healthy fibers. Fibrillation continues until the muscle fiber is reinnervated by the outgrowth of new axons from nearby healthy nerve fibers, or until the muscle fiber degenerates and is replaced by connective tissue, a process which may take many years. In addition, one often observes *positive sharp waves*, i.e., spontaneous diphasic potentials, as their name suggests, of longer duration and slightly greater amplitude than fibrillations (Fig. 44-6A). These positive sharp waves probably arise from fibers which have been damaged by the recording needle electrode.

Fasciculation Fasciculation is the spontaneous or involuntary contraction of a motor unit or a small group of motor units. Such contractions may cause a visible dimpling or twitching of the skin, though ordinarily they are of insufficient force to move a joint. The form of the accompanying EMG potential, like that of an ordinary motor unit, is relatively constant for any one fasciculating unit. Commonly, it will have three to five phases, a duration of 5 to 15 ms (somewhat less in the facial muscles), and an amplitude of several millivolts (Fig. 44-6B). Fasciculations usually fire irregularly. They are evidence of motor unit irritation, and not necessarily of denervation. Occasional fasciculations, particularly in the calves and hands, occur in many normal persons and constantly in some of them, and need not be taken as evidence of disease at all. Shivering induced by low temperature and twitchings associated with low serum calcium levels are also forms of fasciculatory activity. Whether or not fasciculations are due to denervation in any particular case cannot be decided on the basis of their configuration, firing rate, or rhythm, but only by the presence or absence of associated fibrillations and certain changes in motor unit potentials (see below).

Fasciculation occurs in chronic, slowly advancing, destructive diseases of the anterior horn cells, such as amyotrophic lateral sclerosis and progressive spinal muscular atrophy. In these diseases, fasciculation potentials are numerous and may exceed 15 ms in duration. They are seen often in the early stages of poliomyelitis but only occasionally in the chronic phase of the disease, perhaps because the affected cells die rapidly. They are also seen with compressive anterior root lesions, such as those caused by herniation of the nucleus pulposus (ruptured disk); large numbers of axons may be affected, with the result that the fasciculations (or even cramps) may be more prominent than with disease of anterior horn cells. Fasciculations have also been observed early in the course of acute idiopathic polyneuritis and other peripheral nerve lesions, giving way to fibrillation upon death of the axon. In all these cases, the damaged neu-

Figure 44-6

A. *Fibrillations and positive sharp waves. This spontaneous activity was recorded from a totally denervated muscle—no motor unit potentials were produced by attempts at voluntary contraction. The fibrillations (above arrow) are 1 to 2 ms in duration, 100 to 300 μV in amplitude, and largely negative (upward) in polarity following an initial positive deflection. A typical positive sharp wave is seen above the star. B. Fasciculation. This spontaneous motor unit potential was recorded from a patient with amyotrophic lateral sclerosis. It has a serrated configuration and it fired once every second or two. Calibrations: 5 ms (horizontal) and 200 μV in A; 1 mV in B (vertical).*

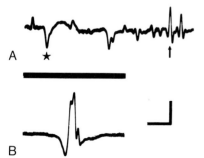

ron seems to be "irritated" by the disease process, fires repetitively, and, in doing so, produces activity in all the muscle fibers that it innervates.

Abnormalities in Amplitude, Duration, and Shape of Motor Unit Potentials   *Motor unit potentials in denervation* Figure 44-7 depicts, schematically, ways in which disease processes affect the motor unit and the appearance, in each case, of the motor unit potential in the EMG. Early in the course of denervation, many motor units with functional connections to the spinal cord are unaffected, and though the number of motor unit potentials appearing during contraction is reduced, the configurations of the remaining ones are quite normal. In time, the remaining motor unit potentials often increase in amplitude, perhaps two to three times normal, and become longer in duration and *polyphasic* (more than four phases). Such large and sometimes *giant potentials* (Fig.

44-8*C*) are believed to arise from motor units containing more than the usual number of muscle fibers and are spread out over a greatly enlarged territory within the muscle (Fig. 44-7*C*). Presumably, new nerve twigs have sprouted from undamaged axons and have reinnervated previously denervated fibers, thus adding them to their own motor units. Some of these units may become extremely polyphasic and prolonged, a finding pathognomonic of reinnervation (Fig. 44-8*B*). These units are to be differentiated (1) from polyphasic potentials of normal duration, which make up as much as 10 percent of the total number of motor unit potentials in normal muscle, and (2) from polyphasic motor unit potentials of short duration and low amplitude, which are characteristic of myopathies and myasthenia gravis of long standing.

The motor unit potential in myopathy Diseases such as polymyositis, the muscular dystrophies, and other myopathies that destroy scattered fibers within a motor unit or render them nonfunctional obviously reduce the population of fibers per motor unit, as in Fig. 44-7*B*. Therefore, when such a unit is activated, its potential is of lower voltage and shorter duration than normal (Fig. 44-8*D*), and it may also appear polyphasic, as the compound motor unit potential becomes fragmented into its constituent single fiber potentials. When most of the muscle fibers are affected, the motor unit potentials are very small and of short duration. Both these types of voluntary motor unit potentials, with their characteristic high-pitched crackling sound from the audio monitor, occur in all forms of progressive mus-

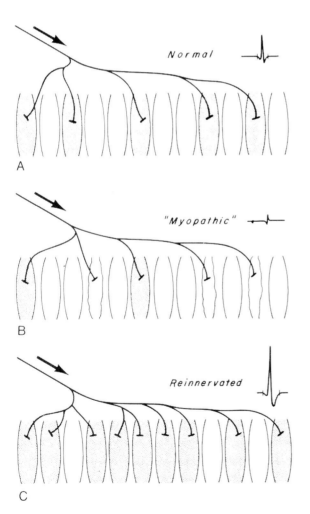

Figure 44-7

The shaded muscle fibers are functional members of one motor unit, whose axon enters from the upper left and branches terminally to innervate the appropriate muscle fibers. The action potential produced by each motor unit is seen in the upper right: its duration is measured between the two vertical lines. The normal-appearing but unshaded fibers belong to other motor units. A. Hypothetical situation, with five muscle fibers in the active unit. B. In this myopathic unit, only two fibers remain active, the other three (shrunken) have been affected by one of the primary muscle diseases. C. Four fibers which belonged to other motor units and had been denervated have now been reinnervated by terminal sprouting from an undamaged axon. Both the motor unit and its action potential are now larger than normal. Note that only under these abnormal circumstances do fibers in the same unit lie next to one another.

cular dystrophy and, unfortunately, are indistinguishable from those of polymyositis, dermatomyositis, and other chronic myopathies. Fibrillation potentials are often seen in the myositides and occasionally in the progressive muscular dystrophies, perhaps because of the destruction of terminal nerve twigs by the inflammatory process. In myasthenia gravis, where transmission of impulse fails at the neuromuscular junction, a single motor unit potential may vary in amplitude during sustained weak contraction; and with fatigue, isolated muscle fibers (as shown in single muscle fiber recordings) do not contract synchronously with all the other fibers of their unit. This phenomenon is called "jitter."

Abnormalities of the interference pattern Diseases which reduce the population of functional motor neurons or axons within the peripheral nerve obviously decrease the number of motor units which can be recruited in the affected muscles. The number of motor units available for activation no longer can produce a complete interference pattern but only a *single unit pattern* (Fig. 44-5*B*) or an *incomplete interference pattern*.

If muscle power is reduced in diseases such as polymyositis or muscular dystrophy, where individual muscle fibers are affected, there will be little or no reduction in the number of motor units available for recruit-

ment, though each unit will consist of fewer muscle fibers than normal. A maximal voluntary effort will then be associated with a normally complete interference pattern despite marked weakness. Because fewer muscle fibers are firing, the amplitude of the pattern will be reduced from normal. A highly complex interference pattern of less than usual amplitude, in the face of dramatic weakness, is the hallmark of the so-called myopathic EMG (Fig. 44-5*C*).

Special Abnormalities in the EMG The phenomenon of myotonia (see pages 943 and 1002) is characterized by high-frequency repetitive discharges which wax and wane in amplitude and frequency, producing a "divebomber" sound on the audio monitor. It is elicited mechanically by percussion or movement of the needle electrode. This electrical picture is also seen following voluntary contraction or electrical stimulation of the muscle via its motor nerve. The motor unit potentials appear normal during voluntary contraction, but they are not followed by the silence which normally occurs on relaxation; instead there is a burst of potentials which may take as long as several minutes to subside (Fig. 44-10*A*). These EMG findings correspond to the clinical failure of voluntary relaxation of muscle following a forceful contraction. Some of the potentials of this prolonged discharge have the duration, amplitude, and form of single fiber activity, while others appear to have

Figure 44-8
Single voluntary motor unit potentials. A. Normal. B. Prolonged polyphasic potential seen with reinnervation. C. "Giant unit"—normally shaped but of much greater amplitude than normal. D. Brief, low-amplitude "myopathic" units. Calibrations: 5 ms (horizontal) and 1 mV in A and B; 5 mV in C; 100 μV in D (vertical).

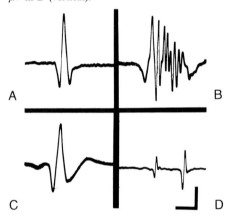

Figure 44-9
Compound action potentials evoked in hypothenar muscles by electrical stimulation of the ulnar nerve at the wrist. A. Patient with myasthenia gravis—typical pattern of decrement in first four responses followed by slight increment. At this rate of stimulation (4 per second) the decrement in response does not continue to zero. B. Patient with Eaton-Lambert syndrome and oat-cell carcinoma—typical marked increase toward normal amplitude with rapid repetitive stimulation (20 per second). Horizontal calibration: 250 ms.

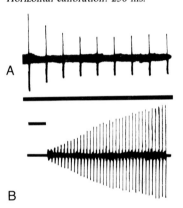

the characteristics of motor unit potentials. If the muscle is activated repeatedly at short intervals, the late discharge becomes briefer and briefer and eventually disappears (Fig. 44-10*B*), as the patient becomes able to relax the exercised muscle at will.

Pseudomyotonia, or bizarre high-frequency discharges without waxing and waning, is seen in some myopathies and in certain types of denervation and reinnervation. High-frequency *coupling* of action potentials into doublets, triplets, or higher multiples of single units, indicating instability in repolarization of the nerve fiber, occurs in tetany.

The *contracture of* McArdle's disease has no consistent electrical counterpart (the EMG is relatively silent). This feature is important in the definition of this syndrome.

ELECTRONEUROGRAPHY

Disease of peripheral nerves may produce the electromyographic evidences of denervation discussed above, but more quantitative observations of neural function can be made by studies of the electrical activity of nerves themselves. Hagbarth and colleagues have, by means of

Figure 44-10

A. Myotonia congenita (Thomsen's disease). The five lines are a continuous record of activity in the biceps brachii following a tap on the tendon. The initial response is within normal limits, but it is followed by a prolonged burst of rapid activity, gradually subsiding over a period of many seconds or minutes. B. Same electrode placement as in A. Response to the fifth of a series of tendon taps. "Warm-up" has occurred, and the characteristic prolonged myotonic activity is no longer evident.

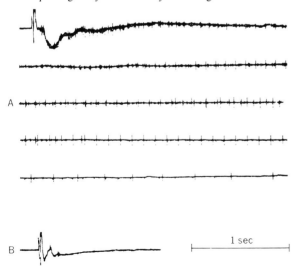

fine-needle electrodes within peripheral nerves in situ, recorded single fiber activity from muscle afferents and from autonomic and other subgroups of fibers within peripheral nerves. This methodology promises to be of critical importance in understanding many aspects of the physiology of peripheral nerves. It has yet to be used widely as a clinical diagnostic tool.

CONDUCTION STUDIES OF NERVE

Techniques are now available for percutaneous stimulation of peripheral nerve fibers and the recording of the muscle action potentials, from stimulation of motor nerves, and nerve action potentials, from stimulation of sensory nerves. The results of these *motor and sensory nerve conduction studies*, expressed as amplitudes, conduction velocities, and distal latencies, are more objective than the results of electromyography and yield certain information unavailable from EMG studies.

Hodes et al. in 1948 were the first to measure nerve conduction velocities in patients. An accessible nerve is stimulated through the skin by surface electrodes, and the resulting compound action potential is recorded by electrodes on the skin (1) over the nerve more proximally in the case of orthodromic activity in large sensory fibers stimulated in the digital nerves or (2) over the muscle more distally in the case of motor fibers in a mixed nerve (Fig. 44-11). The conduction time from the most distal stimulating electrode, measured in milliseconds from the stimulus artifact to the onset of the response, is termed the *distal or peripheral latency*. If a second stimulus can be applied to a mixed nerve more proximally (or if recording electrodes can be placed more proximally in the case of activity in sensory fibers), a new and longer conduction time can be measured. When the distance (in millimeters) between the two sites of stimulation of motor fibers or recording of sensory fibers is divided by the difference in conduction times (in milliseconds), a *maximal conduction velocity* (in meters per second) is obtained which describes the velocity of propagation of the action potentials in the largest and fastest nerve fibers. These velocities in normal subjects vary from a minimum of 40 or 45 m/s, to a maximum of 75 to 80 m/s, depending upon which nerve is studied. Values are lower in infants, reaching the adult range by the age of 2 to 4 years. Normal values have also been established for distal latencies from the distalmost site on various mixed nerves to the appropriate muscles; when one stimulates the median nerve at the wrist, for example (Fig. 44-11*A*), the latency for conduction through the carpal tunnel to the abductor pollicis brevis muscle in the thenar eminence is always less than 4.5 ms in normal adults. Similar tables of normal values have been compiled for orthodromic sensory conduction velocities and sensory distal latencies.

When motor fibers in a mixed nerve are stimulated, the compound action potential of many hundreds of microvolts can easily be recorded from electrodes on the skin over the muscle. However, when one attempts to measure sensory potentials, activity must be recorded from nerve fibers themselves; one then lacks the "ampli-

Figure 44-11

The median nerve is stimulated percutaneously (1) at the wrist and (2) in the antecubital fossa with the resultant compound muscle action potential recorded as the potential difference between a surface electrode over the thenar eminence (arrow) and a reference electrode (Ref.) more distally. Sweep 1′ on the CRO depicts the stimulus artifact followed by the compound muscle action potential. The distal latency, A′, is the time from the stimulus artifact to the take-off phase of the compound muscle action potential and corresponds to conduction over distance A. The same is true for sweep 2′, where stimulation is at 2 and the time from the artifact to the response is A′ + B′. The maximum motor conduction velocity over segment B is calculated by dividing distance B by the time B′.

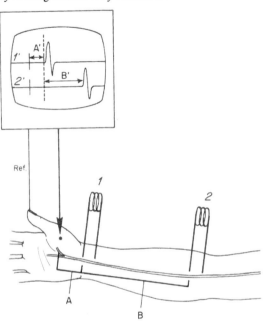

fication" provided by all the muscle fibers in one motor unit, as noted above, and much greater electronic amplification is required. Abnormal sensory potentials are sometimes very small or absent even when powerful computer-averaging techniques are used, and sensory conduction measurements are often difficult or impossible to record. In contrast, it is always possible to obtain a reliable motor conduction velocity as long as some functional nerve fibers remain. These conduction velocities reflect the status of surviving fibers and, if the latter are unaffected by the disease process, may be normal despite widespread axonal degeneration or segmental demyelination. Thus, following incomplete transection of a nerve, the maximal motor conduction velocity may be normal in the few remaining fibers, although the muscle involved is almost paralyzed and its action potential very low.

Disease processes which preferentially affect larger fibers in peripheral nerves should reduce the maximal conduction velocity slightly because the remaining fibers with smaller diameters conduct more slowly. Such a reduction in velocity can be determined by comparing values recorded from the patient with those from a control group of the same age and sex.

In most neuropathies, only a part of the axons are affected (either by the "dying-back" phenomenon or wallerian degeneration), and nerve conduction velocities are then relatively uninformative. This is true for typical alcoholic, nutritional, carcinomatous, uremic, other metabolic, and most diabetic neuropathies, in which conduction velocities range from low in the normal range to 35 or 40 m/s. On the other hand, diseases such as acute idiopathic polyneuritis, diphtheria, infantile metachromatic leukodystrophy, Krabbe's disease, and Charcot-Marie-Tooth disease (as it is seen in most kinships) affect Schwann cells primarily and produce segmental demyelination, with conduction velocities as low as 10 to 15 m/s.

Focal compression of nerve, as in entrapment syndromes, also produces localized slowing or blocks in conduction, perhaps because of segmental demyelination at the site of compression. The demonstration of such localized changes of conduction affords ready confirmation of nerve entrapment; for example, if the distal latency of the median nerve (Fig. 44-11*A*) exceeds 5.0 ms while that of the ulnar nerve remains normal, compression of the median nerve in the carpal tunnel is likely. Similar focal slowing of conduction may be recorded from the ulnar nerve at the elbow or peroneal nerve at the fibular head when they are compressed (see pages 921 and 925).

In addition to the study of distal latency and conduction velocity, the amplitude of the recorded muscle action potential (from stimulation of motor fibers) and the amplitude of the nerve action potential (from stimulation of sensory fibers) can yield valuable information about peripheral nerve function. These amplitudes can be used as an index of the number of nerve fibers responding to a given stimulus. In diseases characterized by axonal loss, the amplitudes of the responses will be low, reflecting the degree of axonal loss, even though the conduction velocities and latencies may be normal. In addition to a lower amplitude, segmental demyelination or loss of the larger and faster conducting fibers can cause a dispersal of the response. Complete or partial blocks in conduction which occur as a result of segmental demyelination can be localized by comparing amplitudes of the response after stimulation of the nerve proximal and distal to the lesion. The use of amplitudes requires scrupulously consistent technique and the establishment of normal values by individual laboratories.

Repetitive Stimulation Studies Skeletal muscle may be stimulated by the application of brief electrical pulses to the skin overlying a motor nerve, and by adjusting the strength of the stimulus, one maximal muscle response may be obtained for each stimulus; the form of the response will depend on the number of motor units activated and the number sampled by the recording apparatus. If repeated stimuli are given, each response will have the same form and amplitude until fatigue supervenes. A normal response will follow each stimulus even with rates of stimulation up to 25 per second for periods of 60 s or more, before a decrement of action potential appears. The latter is due to the failure of some muscle fibers to respond, presumably because of failure of the nerve impulse to be transmitted through certain branching points of the terminal axon.

In certain disorders, notably myasthenia gravis, the initial motor unit potentials produced by voluntary contraction or electrical stimulation are normal. After a few stimuli at rates of 1 to 10 per second (optimal rate 3 per second) the amplitude of the potentials decreases, though not to zero, and then, after four or five stimuli, may increase somewhat (Fig. 44-9A). This partial block of neuromuscular transmission in myasthenics is similar to the one produced by curare and can be partially corrected with neostigmine. Similar decremental response of the action potentials to repetitive stimulation may occur in poliomyelitis and certain other diseases of the motor unit, but the pattern described for myasthenia is not present.

The myasthenic syndrome of Eaton-Lambert, often associated with oat-cell carcinoma of the lung, is characterized by a different type of defect of neuromuscular transmission. Following rapid (up to 50 per second) repetitive stimulation of nerve, the muscle action potentials, which are small or practically absent with the first stimulus, increase in voltage with each successive one until a more nearly normal amplitude is attained (Fig. 44-9B). Neostigmine has no effect on this phenomenon, but it may be reversible with guanidine (20 to 35 mg/kg per day in divided doses) which stimulates the release of ACh. The effects of the myasthenic syndrome are similar to those produced by botulinus toxin or by neomycin and other antibiotics (pages 784 and 993).

ELECTRODIAGNOSTIC STUDIES OF SPINAL REFLEXES

Information about the conduction of impulses through the proximal segments of a nerve, not obtainable by routine nerve conduction techniques, may be provided by the study of the H reflex and the F wave. In 1918, Hoffman, after whom the H reflex was later named, showed that submaximal stimulation of mixed motor-sensory nerves, insufficient to produce a direct motor response, produces a muscle contraction (H wave) after a latency that is much longer than that of the direct motor response (M wave). This reflex is based on activation of fusimotor afferent fibers, and the long delay in muscular response reflects the time required for the sensory impulses to reach the spinal cord, make a single synapse with an anterior horn cell, and then be transmitted along motor fibers to the muscle (Fig. 3-1). With more intense stimulation of the nerve, the response is blocked by antidromic conduction along motor fibers. Stimuli of increasing frequency, but low intensity, cause a progressive depression and finally obliteration of H waves. The latter phenomenon has been used to study spasticity, rigidity, and cerebellar ataxia in which there are differences in the frequency-depression curves of H waves.

The F response, first described by Magladery and McDougal in 1950, is evoked by a stimulus of a motor-sensory nerve *greater* than that required for the short-latency motor potential and H wave; and it persists after supramaximal stimulation. Again, after a longer latency than occurs in the direct motor response, there is a muscle contraction (F wave). It is induced by the antidromic discharge of a group of motor neurons which then induce muscle contraction an interval of time after the direct centrifugal (orthodromic) muscle response.

When conduction studies of the distal segments of peripheral nerves are normal, prolonged latencies of the

H and F waves can be taken as evidence of disease in their most proximal segments.

BIOPSY MYOPATHOLOGY

Muscle biopsy can be of great diagnostic value, but both surgical and microscopic techniques must be exacting. The muscle chosen for study should be accessible; there should be evidence that it has been affected but not totally destroyed by the disease in question, and it should not have been the site of a recent injection or electromyographic study, since the trauma of the needles produces focal necrotizing and inflammatory lesions. Muscle biopsy is helpful in distinguishing several basic disorders in patients with neuromuscular disease.

1. *Denervation atrophy.* Reduction in size of fibers in motor units, with enlargement of intact units (due to collateral regeneration of nerves) and delayed degenerative changes in some fibers. This change typifies all peripheral nerve and spinal cord diseases and is particularly well shown in histochemical stains for ATPase, phosphorylase, and oxidases, where the pattern of fiber types is altered (i.e., muscle fibers of similar histochemical types form large groups).

2. *Segmental necrosis of muscle fibers with myophagia and various manifestations of regeneration.* These are the typical changes in idiopathic polymyositis (in combination with infiltrates of inflammatory cells), infective polymyositis (in the presence of trichina, toxoplasma, etc., as well as inflammation), and paroxysmal myoglobinuria, and may be observed also in Duchenne and other rapidly progressive muscular dystrophies.

3. *Unusual changes of muscle fibers.* Sarcoplasmic masses and ringbinden in myotonic dystrophy, glycogen masses in glycogen storage diseases, rod (nemaline), central core, aggregates of lipid bodies, and other cytoplasmic changes (such as aggregation and other abnormalities of mitochondria) in certain congenital myopathies. Here, histochemical stains for fiber typing and electron microscopy are important diagnostic techniques.

4. *Alterations in number and size of fibers as a reflection of abnormalities of growth, maturation, and aging.* Many states of dwarfism and congenital myopathies of myotubular type present principally with numerical or volumetric changes, which must be distinguished from denervation, disuse effects, cachexia, and work hypertrophy.

5. *Disorders of the conduction apparatus (neuromuscular junctions) in which nerve fibers and muscle fibers appear to be intact.* Here the abnormality can be revealed only by performing motor point biopsy (to include the motor end plate) and using electron microscopy and special staining techniques for nerve terminals, acetylcholinesterase, and the outlining of acetylcholine receptors. Myasthenia gravis, botulism, Eaton-Lambert syndrome, and myasthenic syndrome with motor end-plate acetylcholinesterase deficiency fall into this category.

Further details of pathology will be presented with the descriptions of specific muscle diseases.

As a rule, the biopsy procedure requires no more than a cleanly excised block of muscle 1.0 to 2.0 cm which is prevented from contracting by a clamp or by tying at full length to a stick, and is then fixed in 10% neutral formalin, embedded in paraffin, sectioned in a cross and longitudinal fashion, and stained by hematoxylin and eosin or Gomori trichrome methods. Special techniques should be applied if it is desirable to visualize particular qualities of a disease. Various histochemical stains for enzyme content of muscle fibers are required to establish the diagnosis of many of the unusual myopathies. The latter require rapid freezing rather than formalin fixation. Electron microscopy, performed on carefully selected blocks of muscle and nerve fixed in glutaraldehyde, is useful in confirming abnormalities detected by histochemical staining and provides a refined means of studying other myopathies. Sural nerve biopsies, processed by the fixation, staining, and embedding techniques of electron microscopy, can provide very useful histopathologic data, even when examined by ordinary microscopy. These biopsies can also be studied physiologically in vitro where fibers of all sizes can be stimulated and their activity recorded—in contrast to routine nerve conduction studies where only the largest fibers can be sampled. All these special techniques are of interest to research workers and are available in centers where nerve and muscle diseases are under investigation.

USE OF LABORATORY TESTS IN THE STUDY OF MUSCLE DISEASE

None of the results of the diagnostic laboratory procedures described above may be taken as an infallible index of a specific disease of muscle. Each procedure is subject to technical error and the findings to misinterpretation. A biopsy specimen may be excised from an unaffected muscle or portion of a muscle and, because of this sampling error, be negative in the face of clinical evidence of obvious disease; rough excision and improper fixation and staining may produce artifacts which may be misinterpreted as marks of disease when, in fact, the muscle is microscopically normal. Similarly, EMG study may fail to record fibrillations in obviously denervated muscle, or a few fibrillations may be seen in an otherwise typical dystrophic process. As in the study of all disease, laboratory data have significance only if evaluated in the light of the clinical findings.

REFERENCES

ADAMS RD: *Diseases of Muscle: A Study in Pathology,* 3d ed. New York, Harper & Row, 1975.

BUCHTAL F, ROSENFALCK A: Evoked action potentials and conduction velocity in human sensory nerves. *Brain Res* 3:1, 1966.

ELMQUIST D, LAMBERT EH: Detailed analysis of neuromuscular transmission in a patient with the myasthenic syndrome associated with bronchogenic carcinoma. *Mayo Clin Proc* 43:689, 1968.

ENGEL AG, JERUSALEM M, TSUJIHATA M, GOMEZ MR: The neuromuscular junction in myopathies. A quantitative ultrastructural study, in Bradley WG, Gardner-Medwin D, Walton JN (eds): *Recent Advances in Myology.* New York, Elsevier, 1975, pp 132-143.

FRANZINI-ARMSTRONG C: Membrane particles and transmission at the triad. *Fed Proc* 34:1382, 1975.

GOODGOLD J, EBERSTEIN A: *Electrodiagnosis of Neuromuscular Diseases,* 2d ed. Baltimore, Williams & Wilkins, 1978.

HAGBARTH KE: Exteroceptive, proprioceptive, and sympathetic activity recorded with multielectrodes from human peripheral nerves. *Mayo Clinic Proceedings* 54:353, 1979.

HODES R, LARRABEE MG, GERMAN W: The human electromyogram in response to nerve stimulation and conduction velocity of motor axons: Studies on normal and on injured peripheral nerves. *Arch Neurol Psychiatry* 60:340, 1948.

HODGKIN AL: Ionic basis of electrical activity in nerve and muscle. *Biol Rev* 26:339, 1951.

————, HUXLEY AF: Currents carried by sodium and potassium ions through the membranes of the giant axon of *Loligo. J Physiol* 116:449, 1952.

HUXLEY HE: Molecular basis of contraction in cross-striated muscles, in Bourne GH (ed): *The Structure and Function of Muscle,* 2d ed, vol 1: *Structure.* New York, Academic, 1972, pt 1, chap 7, pp 301-387.

KATZ B: *Nerve, Muscle and Synapse.* New York, McGraw-Hill, 1966.

MAGLADERY JW, McDOUGAL DB: Electrophysiological studies of nerve and reflex activity in normal man. *Johns Hopkins Med J* 86:265, 1950.

PETER JB: Skeletal muscle: Diversity and mutability of its histochemical, electron-microscopic, biochemical and physiologic properties, in Pearson CM, Mostofi FK (eds): *The Striated Muscle,* Baltimore, Williams & Wilkins, 1973, chap 1, pp 1-18.

ROSANO TG, KENNY MD: A radioimmunoassay for human serum myoglobin. Method development and normal values. *Clin Chem* 23:69, 1977.

SUMNER AJ (ed): *The Physiology of Peripheral Nerve Disease.* Philadelphia, Saunders, 1980.

CHAPTER 45

DISEASES OF THE PERIPHERAL NERVES

Disease of the peripheral nervous system stands as one of the most difficult subjects in neurology. Since the structure and function of this system are relatively simple, one might suppose that our knowledge of its diseases would be complete. Such is not the case. At present an etiologic diagnosis cannot be made in about 40 percent of patients who enter a general hospital with a peripheral nerve disease (usually of chronic progressive type), and the pathologic changes have not been fully determined in any one of them. Moreover, the physiologic basis of many of the neural symptoms continues to elude experts in the field.

In recent years there has been a surge of interest in disease of the peripheral nervous system which promises to change this rather discouraging state of affairs. Electron-microscopic studies, new quantitative histometric methods, and refined physiologic techniques are rapidly expanding our knowledge of the structure and function of peripheral nerves under conditions of disease. These methods permit more precise correlations between structural and functional changes than has been possible until now, and biochemical advances hold promise of providing a better understanding of disease processes as well.

GENERAL CONSIDERATIONS

It is important to have a clear concept of the extent of the peripheral nervous system and of the possible mechanisms whereby it can be affected by disease.

The peripheral nervous system (PNS) includes all nervous structures lying outside the pial membrane of the spinal cord and brainstem. The optic nerves and olfactory bulbs are not included, for they are special extensions of the brain. The parts of the PNS within the spinal canal and cranial cavity and attached to the ventral and dorsal surfaces of the cord and ventrolateral surfaces of the brainstem are called the *spinal* and *cranial nerve roots*, respectively. The dorsal (afferent or sensory) roots consist of central axonal processes of the dorsal root and cranial ganglion cells; on reaching the spinal cord and brainstem they extend for a variable distance into the posterior columns (funiculi) and spinal trigeminal and other tracts in the medulla and pons. The peripheral axons of the dorsal root ganglion cells are the sensory nerve fibers. They terminate as freely branching endings or in specialized corpuscular endings in skin, joints, and other tissues. The ventral (efferent, or motor) roots are composed of the emerging axons of anterior and lateral horn cells; they terminate on muscle fibers, or in sympathetic or parasympathetic ganglia. Traversing, as they do, the subarachnoid space, and lacking epineural and perineural sheaths (Fig. 45-1), the cranial and spinal roots (both sensory and motor) are bathed by cerebrospinal fluid (CSF), the lumbosacral roots having the longest exposure.

The vast extent of the peripheral ramifications of cranial and spinal nerves is noteworthy, as are their thick protective and supporting sheaths of perineurium and epineurium, and their unique vascular supply through longitudinal arrays of richly anastomosing nutrient arterial branches that run in the epineurium and perineurium (see Fig. 45-4). The nerves traverse narrow foramens (intervertebral and cranial) and a number pass through tight channels peripherally (e.g., median nerve between the carpal ligament and tendon sheaths of flexor forearm muscles). These anatomic features explain the susceptibility of certain nerves to compression and entrapment.

Sympathetic and parasympathetic motor fibers from the spinal cord end in ganglia whose cells in turn send axons (unmedullated) to peripheral nerves and thence to blood vessels, sweat glands, and viscera. The medullated nerves are coated with short segments of myelin of variable length (250 to 1000 μm), each of which is enveloped by a Schwann cell plasma membrane. This latter characteristic is noteworthy because some anatomists define the PNS as that part of the nervous system which is invested by Schwann cells. Each myelin segment has an intimate symbiotic relation to the axon but is always morphologically independent.

These anatomic features enable one to conceptualize the possible mechanisms by which disease may affect the peripheral nerves. Pathologic processes may be directed at any one of several groups of nerve cells, e.g.,

those of the anterior or lateral horns of the spinal cord, the dorsal root ganglia, or sympathetic ganglia. Each cell type exhibits specific vulnerabilities to disease processes, and if destroyed—as are the motor nerve cells in poliomyelitis—there results secondarily a degeneration of the axons and myelin sheaths of the peripheral fibers of these cells. On the other hand, the function and structure of the peripheral nerves might be affected by disease processes that involve the ventral and dorsal columns (funiculi) of the spinal cord, which contain the fibers of

Figure 45-1

Diagram showing the relationships of the peripheral nerve sheaths to the meningeal coverings of the spinal cord. The epineurium (EP) is in direct continuity with the dura mater (DM). The endoneurium (EN) remains unchanged from the peripheral nerve and spinal root to the junction with the spinal cord. At the subarachnoid angle (SA) the greater portion of the perineurium (P) passes outward between the dura mater and the arach- *noid (A), but a few layers appear to continue over the nerve root as part of the root sheath (RS). At the subarachnoid angle, the arachnoid is reflected over the roots and becomes continuous with the outer layers of the root sheath. At the junction with the spinal cord, the outer layers of the root sheath become continuous with the pia mater (PM). (From FR Haller, FM Low, Am J Anat 131:1, 1971.)*

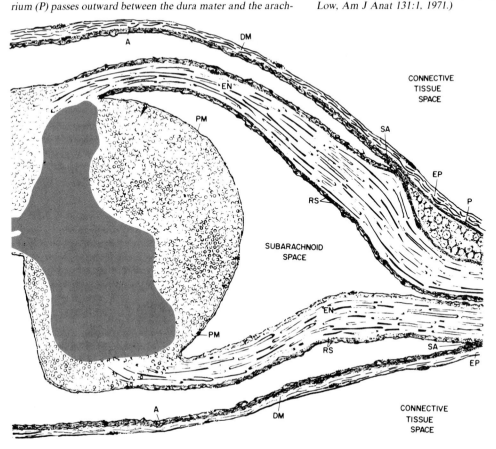

exit and entry of anterior horn and dorsal root ganglion cells, respectively. The myelin here is constituted differently than in peripheral nerves, being enveloped by oligodendrocytes rather than Schwann cells, and the fibers are supported by fibrous astrocytes rather than fibroblasts. Because of the intimate relation of the roots to the CSF and to specialized arachnoidal cells (villi), a pathologic process in the CSF or leptomeninges may damage the exposed spinal roots. Disease of the connective tissues may affect the peripheral nerves which lie within their sheaths. Diffuse or localized arterial diseases may injure nerves by narrowing or obliterating their nutrient arteries. Noxious agents which selectively damage the Schwann cells or their membranes which compose the myelin sheaths cause demyelination of peripheral nerves, leaving axons intact. Finally, one might suppose that axons of the motor or sensory nerve, or sympathetic fibers of varying size and length, or the end organs to which they are attached might each have its particular liability to disease.

Much of this is theoretical and somewhat speculative. At present we can cite examples of diseases that are based on only a few of these potential disease pathways, e.g., diphtheria, in which the bacterial toxin acts directly on the membranes of the Schwann cells near the dorsal root ganglia and adjacent nerves (the most vascular parts of the peripheral nerve); polyarteritis nodosa, which causes widespread occlusion of vasa nervorum; tabes dorsalis, in which there is a treponemal meningoradiculitis that centers on the posterior roots (mainly of the lumbosacral segments) that lie next to the arachnoidal villi (for resorption of CSF); and poisoning with arsenic, which combines with the axoplasm of the largest nerves, via sulfhydryl bonds. However, analogous anatomic pathways are probably implicated in other diseases whose mechanisms remain to be divulged.

Pathologically, several distinct processes are recognized, although they are not disease-specific and may be present in varying combinations in any given patient. The major ones are wallerian degeneration, segmental demyelination, and axonal degeneration (diagrammatically illustrated in Fig. 45-2). The myelin sheaths are the most susceptible element of the nerve fiber, for they may break down as part of a primary process involving the Schwann cells (or some component thereof) or secondarily, consequent to disease affecting their axons. Focal degeneration of the myelin sheath with sparing of the axon is called *segmental demyelination*. Degeneration of myelin secondary to axonal disease has been called medullary-axonic and may occur either distal to the most proximal site of axonal interruption (wallerian degeneration) or as a "dying-back" phenomenon in more generalized, metabolically determined polyneuropathies (axonal degeneration). Wallerian degeneration of axons causes a breakdown of the myelin into blocks or ovoids in which lie fragments of axons (digestion chambers of Cajal). Degeneration of myelin secondary to neuronal disease has been called neuronolytic (Adams and Richardson) and here also the myelin breaks up into fragments. When the myelin sheath degenerates (the axon being left intact), the highly structured lipoprotein disintegrates into fine particles which are then converted, through the action of macrophages, into neutral fats and cholesterol esters, and carried by these cells to the bloodstream.

In segmental demyelination, recovery of function may be rapid because the intact but denuded axon needs only to become remyelinated. In contrast, with wallerian or axonal degeneration, recovery is slower, often requiring months to a year or more, because the axon must first regenerate and reconnect to muscle, sensory organ, blood vessel, etc., before function returns. When a nerve is severed and continuity is not reestablished, regenerating axonic filaments and connective tissue at the end of the central portion of the interrupted nerve form a pseudoneuroma. When nerve cells are destroyed, no recovery of their function is possible except by collateral regeneration from axons of intact nerve cells.

These few pathologic reactions cannot in themselves differentiate the 40 or more diseases of the peripheral nerves, but when considered in relation to the selective effects of pathologic processes on various types and sizes of fibers, to the topography of the lesions, and to the time course of the process, a set of criteria is provided whereby many diseases can be differentiated. Then, too, there are special pathologic changes that characterize certain diseases of the peripheral nervous system. In acute idiopathic polyneuritis and infectious mononucleosis there are infiltrations of lymphocytes, plasma cells, and other mononuclear cells in roots, sensory and sympathetic ganglia and nerves; frequently the destruction of myelin has a perivenous distribution. In polyarteritis nodosa, a characteristic *necrotizing panarteritis* with occlusion of vessels and focal infarction of peripheral nerves and, less often, with rupture of vessels and hemorrhage into nerves (mononeuropathy multiplex) are the dominant findings. Deposition of amyloid in endoneurial connective tissue and the walls of vessels affecting the nerve fibers secondarily either by compression or ischemia are the distinctive features of amyloid polyneuropathy. Diphtheritic polyneuropathy is typified by the predominantly demyelinative character of the nerve fiber change, the location of this change in and around the roots and sensory ganglia, the subacute course, and the lack of inflammatory reaction. Other polyneuropathies (carcinomatous, nutritional, porphyric, arsenical, and uremic) are topographically symmetric but are not presently distinguishable from one another by histopathologic means. The least is known about the familial types of polyneuropathy; although genetic factors are clearly involved, their biochemical mechanisms and pathology are just beginning to be recognized.

Concerning the pathogenesis of the mononeuropathies, our knowledge is also incomplete. Compression producing local or segmental ischemia, violent stretch, and laceration of nerves are understandable, and the pathologic changes they cause have been reproduced in animals. Of infections localized to single nerves, only leprosy, sarcoid, and zoster represent identifiable disease states. For the larger number of acute mononeuropa-

thies the pathologic changes have yet to be defined, since they are usually benign, reversible states which provide no opportunity for complete pathologic examination.

SYMPTOMATOLOGY

There are a number of motor, sensory, reflex, autonomic, and trophic symptoms and signs that are more or less typical of peripheral nerve disease and provide the criteria for diagnosis.

IMPAIRMENT OF MOTOR FUNCTION

Whereas anesthetic agents, nerve toxins, cooling, and ischemia may temporarily cause weakness or paralysis, persistent impairment of motor function over days, weeks, or months always signifies segmental demyelination, axonal interruption, or destruction of motor neurons. The degree of weakness is proportional to the number of alpha motor neurons affected, although kinesthetic loss adds to the motor deficit.

Figure 45-2

Diagram of the basic pathologic processes affecting peripheral nerves. In wallerian degeneration, there is degeneration of the axis cylinder and myelin distal to the site of axonal interruption (arrow), and central chromatolysis. In segmental demyelination the axon is spared. In axonal degeneration there is a distal degeneration of myelin and axis cylinder as a result of neuronal disease. Both wallerian and axonal degeneration cause muscle atrophy. Further details in text. (Courtesy of A Asbury.)

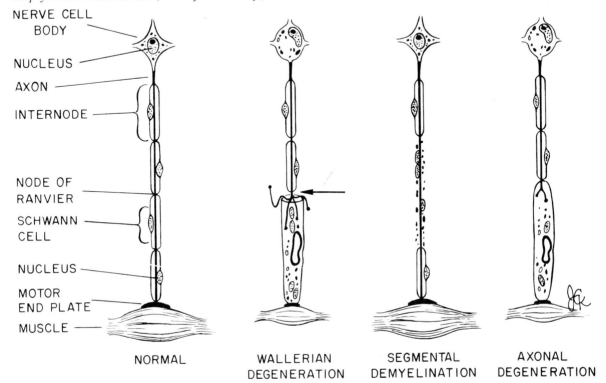

NERVE CELL BODY
NUCLEUS
AXON
INTERNODE
NODE OF RANVIER
SCHWANN CELL
NUCLEUS
MOTOR END PLATE
MUSCLE

NORMAL   WALLERIAN DEGENERATION   SEGMENTAL DEMYELINATION   AXONAL DEGENERATION

A feature of most polyneuropathies is a characteristic distribution of the paralysis. Most often the muscles of the feet and legs are affected first and most severely, and later and usually less severely, those of the hands and forearms. In milder form, only the lower legs are involved. Most of the nutritional, metabolic, and toxic neuropathies take this form. The pathologic changes in such cases begin in the distal parts of the largest and longest nerves and advance along the affected fibers toward their nerve cell bodies ("dying-back" neuropathy," "distal axonopathy"). One explanation for this process is that the primary damage is to the neuronal perikaryon, which fails in its function to synthesize proteins and to deliver them to the distal parts of the axon. A somewhat different theory has been proposed recently by Spencer et al. They postulate that neurotoxic compounds inhibit nerve fiber enzymes required for energy synthesis and that the neuronal soma fails to meet the increased demand for enzyme replacement in the axon, causing the concentration of enzymes to drop and the axon to degenerate in the distal regions. Still another plausible hypothesis would be that functional impairment is in proportion to the number of affected Schwann cells and myelin segments, there being more in long nerves.

Another pattern of paralysis is involvement of all the muscles of the limbs as well as of the trunk and neck, leading often to respiratory paralysis. The vast majority of neuropathies requiring respiratory care are the acute idiopathic variety (Landry-Guillain-Barré syndrome). This disease may at times seem to affect proximal limb muscles more than distal ones. Porphyric, diphtheritic, and certain toxic polyneuropathies are less frequently manifested by such a pattern, but fatalities, when they do occur, are usually due to respiratory paralysis.

Bibrachial paralyses are rare but may occur in porphyria, amyloid polyneuropathy, and Tangier disease; occasionally Guillain-Barré disease begins in the cranial nerves and upper extremities. Bifacial and other cranial nerve paralyses are most likely to occur with acute idiopathic polyneuritis and less frequently with polyarteritic and some of the rare metabolic neuropathic diseases (Refsum's, Bassen-Kornzweig, Tangier, and Riley-Day).

Atrophy of affected muscles proceeds slowly over several months and its degree is proportional to the number of damaged nerve fibers. The atrophy is a product of disuse, especially in demyelinative neuropathies, and of disuse and denervation in diseases which interrupt the axons or destroy motor neurons. Atrophy, therefore, does not coincide with or correspond to acute paralysis and is least prominent in the demyelinative neuropathies such as diphtheritic and some cases of acute idiopathic polyneuritis. In chronic neuropathies, the paralysis and atrophy parallel one another. Finally there is a loss of the denervated muscle fibers which begins in 6 to 12 months; the majority of them have degenerated in 3 to 4 years. If reinnervation takes place within a year, motor function and muscle volume may be completely restored.

TENDON REFLEXES

The rule is that diminution or loss of tendon reflexes is an invariable sign of peripheral nerve disease and that reflexes can be diminished out of proportion to weakness because of involvement of annulospiral afferents from the muscle spindles. Another hypothesis is that slowing of conduction velocities in sensory and motor fibers may prevent the reflex by dispersing the volley of impulses initiated by the tendon tap. Early in an acute polyneuropathy the reflexes may be diminished, but not absent, and may be perceptibly more reduced from day to day. In the newly recognized class of small fiber neuropathies, however, tendon reflexes may occasionally be retained, even with marked loss of perception of painful and thermal stimuli and loss of autonomic function.

FASCICULATIONS AND CRAMPS

In most polyneuropathies fasciculation and cramp are not important findings. However, occasionally one observes a state of mild motor polyneuropathy which upon recovery leaves the muscles in a state which Schultze and Kny called *myokymia* and Isaacs, *continuous muscular activity*. Others refer to it as *neuromyotonia* (see Chap. 52). All the affected muscles ripple and quiver and occasionally cramp. Use of the muscles increases this activity, and there is a reduction in their efficiency which the patient senses as a stiffness and heaviness. Stimulation of a motor nerve, instead of causing a brief burst of action potentials in the muscle, results in a prolonged or dispersed series of potentials lasting several hundred milliseconds. Also the distal latencies are slowed. Evidently, branched axons involved in collateral innervation have an unstable polarization which may last for years.

SENSORY LOSS

Sensation, like motor function, tends to be affected in the distal segments of the limbs, and more in the legs than the arms. In most polyneuropathies, all sensory modalities (sense of touch-pressure, pain and temperature, vibratory, and joint-position) are impaired or lost, although one modality may seemingly be disturbed out of proportion to the others; or superficial sensation may be disturbed more than deep sensation. Vibratory sense is often affected more than position and touch senses. Gilliat and Willison suggest that this is due to slowing of conduction of afferent volleys of high-frequency impulses. As the disease worsens, there is spread of sensory loss to more proximal parts of the limbs.

Another pattern of sensory loss in peripheral nerve diseases has been recognized—that of primary loss of pain and temperature with either sparing or lesser impairment of touch-pressure, vibratory, and position senses. This is reminiscent of the dissociated sensory disturbances of syringomyelia except that it is predominantly lumbosacral. Originally known as lumbosacral syringomyelia, Thévenard was the first to question its anatomical basis, and now it is generally agreed that most such examples are due to hereditary sensory neuropathy. This pseudosyringomyelic dissociation of sensation may extend over arms, trunk, and even the cranial surfaces in certain familial neuropathies such as those associated with primary amyloidosis, congenital absence of pain, the Riley-Day syndrome, and Tangier disease. Exceptionally all forms of sensation may be lost over the entire body, and, as in one of the families studied by Adams et al., motor power and autonomic functions are preserved.

PARESTHESIAS AND DYSESTHESIAS

These abnormalities of sensation have been described in Chap. 8. They are among the most troublesome of all neuropathic symptoms. They tend to be especially marked in the hands and feet. Tingling, electric, novocainelike sensations are the most frequent types of paresthesias. Some sensory neuropathies are attended only by these paresthesias and numbness; others are extremely painful. The pains may be described as aching, sharp-cutting, or crushing, or may resemble the lightning pains of tabes dorsalis. Perversion of sensation is commonplace, e.g., tingling or burning pain induced by tactile stimuli. Under these conditions a given stimulus induces not only an aberrant sensation but one which radiates unnaturally (local sign is lost) and persists after the stimulus is withdrawn.

As remarked on page 712 the patient's reaction may seem to indicate a hypersensitivity ("hyperesthesia"), but more often the sensory threshold is actually raised and only the sensory experience or response is exaggerated (hyperpathia).

These paresthesias and dysesthesias are particu-

larly common in one type of alcoholic beriberi ("burning feet"), in the aged, and in diabetic polyneuropathy. They occur in the feet and hands or all through the limbs in the polyneuropathy of Fabry's disease, and, in limited regions, they occur in herpes zoster, in some cases of diabetic and other types of vascular neuropathy, and in other sensory neuropathies of obscure nature. A particularly intense form of burning pain is that which typifies the causalgia of Weir Mitchell; usually this is due to a partial lesion (traumatic, inflammatory, or neoplastic) of the ulnar, median, posterior tibial, or peroneal nerve (see page 922).

The mechanism of the thermal and painful dysesthesias is not understood. It has been theorized that loss of large touch-pressure fibers disinhibit the pain-receiving nerve cells in the posterior horns and spinal cord (see page 94). An argument against this explanation is that there is no pain in Friedreich's ataxia where these larger neurons degenerate and in certain of the purely sensory polyneuropathies in which perception of tactile stimuli is lost. Pain seems to be a prominent though not invariable feature when a peripheral nerve disease affects the unmyelinated and small myelinated nerve fibers.

SENSORY ATAXIA AND TREMOR

Proprioceptive deafferentation with retention of a reasonable degree of motor function is the basis of ataxia of gait and of limb movement, as discussed in Chap. 8. Action tremor of fast-frequency type may also appear during certain phases of a polyneuropathy. We have the impression that it is due to either a loss of input or slowed nerve conduction from muscle-spindle afferents. Corticosteroid therapy greatly enhances the tremor. During action the tremor may resemble the intention tremor of cerebellar disease.

Ataxia without weakness is, of course, characteristic of tabes dorsalis, but it can be nearly duplicated by diabetic polyneuropathy which also affects posterior roots (diabetic pseudotabes). Several other chronic sensory neuropathies have prominent ataxic features and the movements, though strong, are thereby rendered grossly ineffective. Characteristic of this sensory (tabetic) ataxia are the brusque, flinging, slapping movements of the legs.

DEFORMITY AND TROPHIC CHANGES

In a number of chronic polyneuropathies, the feet, hands, and spine become deformed. This is most apt to occur when the disease begins during childhood. Austin has pointed out that foot deformity is found in 30 percent of patients with hereditary hypertrophic polyneuropathy, and spine curvature in 20 percent. The feet are pulled into a position of talipes equinus because of the weakening of the pretibial and peroneal muscles and unopposed action of the calf muscles. The atrophic paralysis of the intrinsic foot muscles allows the long extensors of the toes to dorsiflex the proximal phalanges and the long flexors to heighten the arch, shorten the foot, and pull the distal phalanges into flexion. The result is the *claw foot—le pied en griffe* of the French. The *claw hand* has a similar basis. In early childhood unequal weakening of the symmetric paravertebral muscles leads to kyphoscoliosis.

Denervation atrophy of muscle is the main trophic disturbance resulting from interruption of the motor nerves. Analgesia of distal parts makes them susceptible to burns, pressure sores, and other forms of injury which are easily infected and heal poorly. Possibly, reflex hyperemia is not regulated properly, deterring the normal tissue responses in infection; paralyzed limbs, even in hysterical paralysis, if left dependent, are often cold, swollen, and pale or blue. These are probably secondary disuse effects. In an anesthetic limb the skin becomes tight and shiny, the nails curved and ridged, and subcutaneous tissues thickened. If the autonomic fibers are interrupted, it is warm and pink. Chronic subcutaneous and osteomyelitic infections may result in loss of digits, and in some sensory neuropathies fingers and toes may be lost without pain. This is a prominent feature of the recessive form of hereditary sensory neuropathy, and we have observed it in dominant forms as well. In diabetic polyneuropathy there may also be ischemia and gangrene from vascular disease. In certain of the familial polyneuropathies, analgesic joints, when traumatized, may develop a Charcot arthropathy, like that of tabes dorsalis and syringomyelia.

AUTONOMIC DISORDERS

Anhidrosis and orthostatic hypotension, the two most frequent manifestations of autonomic paralysis, may be major features of certain types of polyneuropathy. They occur most frequently in amyloid and certain other hereditary *small fiber* polyneuropathies, in diabetic polyneuropathies, and in certain of the congenital types. In addition we have observed them in pure autonomic polyneuropathies and in the so-called Shy-Drager syndrome (see page 375).

Other manifestations of autonomic paralysis are small or medium-sized unreactive pupils that are unusually sensitive to certain drugs (page 374), lack of tears and saliva, sexual impotence, weak bladder and bowel sphincters and overflow incontinence, and weakness and dilatation of esophagus and colon. Some of these abnormalities are found in diabetic and amyloid polyneuropathy. In general these autonomic disturbances correlate with degeneration of unmyelinated Remak fibers in the peripheral nerves.

APPROACH TO THE PATIENT WITH PERIPHERAL NEUROPATHY

The clinician is faced with two problems: (1) establishing the existence of disease of the peripheral nervous system and (2) ascertaining its nature and the possibilities of treatment. The former is not difficult when one becomes familiar with the classic symptomatology of peripheral nerve diseases described above. At times, however, the typical manifestations are lacking or are difficult to ascertain. In these circumstances it is necessary to resort to a number of laboratory procedures, such as (1) biochemical tests to identify those metabolic, nutritional, or toxic states which will produce neuropathy, (2) nerve conduction studies (velocities, amplitudes of evoked potentials, distal latencies), (3) needle examination of muscles, which helps to distinguish primary disorders of muscle (myopathies) from those which are secondary to denervation and neuromuscular block, (4) CSF examination (increase in protein and sometimes in cells with radicular and meningeal involvement), and (5) nerve (sural) and muscle biopsy.

Having established that the patient has a disease of the peripheral nerves, one must attempt to determine its nature. This is accomplished most readily by allocating the case in question to one of the categories in Table 45-1, in which the peripheral nerve diseases are classified according to their mode of evolution and clinical presentation. Stated another way, whenever one of the categories or syndromes of neuropathic disease can be identified, the physician is justified in considering any one of the several diseases comprising that category.

Diseases of the peripheral nerves are considered in the most comprehensive fashion in three publications: the two-volume monograph *Peripheral Neuropathy*, edited by Dyck, Thomas, and Lambert; the two volumes (7 and 8) on diseases of the nerves in the *Handbook of Clinical Neurology*, edited by Vinken and Bruyn; and

Table 45-1
Principal neuropathic syndromes

I. Syndrome of acute ascending motor paralysis with variable disturbance of sensory function
   A. Acute idiopathic polyneuritis (inflammatory polyradiculoneuropathy), Landry-Guillain-Barré (LGB) syndrome, acute immune-mediated polyneuritis (AIMP)
   B. Infectious mononucleosis and polyneuritis
   C. Hepatitis and polyneuritis
   D. Diphtheritic polyneuropathy
   E. Porphyric polyneuropathy
   F. Certain toxic polyneuropathies (triorthocresyl phosphate, thallium)
   G. Rarely, paraneoplastic polyneuropathy
   H. Rarely, vaccinogenic (typhoid-paratyphoid, smallpox, rabies) or serogenic polyneuritis

II. Syndrome of subacute sensorimotor paralysis
   A. Symmetric polyneuropathies
      1. Deficiency states: alcoholism (beriberi), pellagra, vitamin B_{12} deficiency, chronic gastrointestinal disease
      2. Poisoning with heavy metals and industrial solvents: arsenic, lead, mercury, thallium, methyl *n*-butyl ketone, *n*-hexane, methyl bromide, organophosphates (TOCP, etc.), acrylamide
      3. Drug intoxications: isoniazid, ethionamide, hydralazine, nitrofurantoin and related nitrofurazones, disulfiram, carbon disulfide, vincristine, chloramphenicol, phenytoin, amitriptyline, dapsone, stilbamidine, trichlorethylene, thalidomide, Clioquinol, etc.
      4. Uremic polyneuropathy
   B. Asymmetric polyneuropathies
      1. Diabetes
      2. Polyarteritis nodosa (including Wegener's granulomatosis)
      3. Subacute idiopathic polyneuritis
      4. Sarcoidosis
      5. Ischemic neuropathy with peripheral vascular disease

III. Syndrome of chronic sensorimotor polyneuropathy
   A. Acquired
      1. Carcinoma, myeloma, and other malignancies
      2. Paraproteinemias
      3. Uremia (occasionally subacute)
      4. Beriberi (usually subacute)
      5. Diabetes
      6. Hypothyroidism
      7. Connective tissue diseases
      8. Amyloidosis
      9. Leprosy

IV. Genetically determined neuropathies
   A. Inherited polyneuropathies of predominantly sensory type

1. Dominant mutilating sensory neuropathy in adults
2. Recessive mutilating sensory neuropathy of childhood
3. Congenital insensitivity to pain
4. Other inherited sensory neuropathies [including those associated with spinocerebellar degenerations and Riley-Day syndrome and the universal anesthesia syndrome (Adams et al.)]
   B. Inherited polyneuropathies of mixed sensorimotor-autonomic types
      1. Idiopathic group
         a. Dominant peroneal muscular atrophy (Charcot-Marie-Tooth)
         b. Dominant hypertrophic polyneuropathy of Déjerine-Sottas, adult and childhood forms
         c. Roussy-Lévy polyneuropathy
         d. Polyneuropathy with optic atrophy, with spastic paraplegia, with spinocerebellar degeneration, with mental retardation, and with dementia
      2. Inherited polyneuropathies with a recognized metabolic disorder (see also Chap. 37)
         a. Refsum's disease
         b. Metachromatic leukodystrophy
         c. Globoid-body leukodystrophy (Krabbe's disease, see Chap. 37)
         d. Adrenoleukodystrophy (Chap. 37)
         e. Amyloid polyneuropathy of Andrade
         f. Porphyric polyneuropathy
         g. Anderson-Fabry disease
         h. Abetalipoproteinemia and Tangier disease

V. Syndrome of chronic relapsing polyneuropathy
   A. Idiopathic polyneuritis
   B. Porphyria
   C. Beriberi or intoxications
   D. Refsum's disease

VI. Syndrome of mononeuropathy or multiple neuropathies
   A. Pressure palsies
   B. Traumatic neuropathies (including irradiation and electrical injuries)
   C. Idiopathic brachial and sciatic neuropathy
   D. Serum and vaccinogenic (typhoid-paratyphoid, smallpox, rabies) neuropathy
   E. Zoster
   F. Neoplastic infiltration of roots and nerves
   G. Leprosy
   H. Diphtheritic wound infections with local neuropathy
   I. Migrant sensory neuropathy

the monograph on peripheral nerve disease by Asbury and Johnson. The interested reader is referred to these sources for bibliographic details and amplification of some of the clinical points that are made in this chapter.

SYNDROME OF ACUTE ASCENDING MOTOR PARALYSIS WITH VARIABLE DISTURBANCE OF SENSORY FUNCTION

Only minor semiologic differences separate the polyneuropathies of (1) acute idiopathic type (Landry-Guillain-Barré), (2) acute infectious mononucleosis, (3) viral hepatitis, (4) diphtheria, (5) porphyria, (6) certain intoxications. The first of these is by far the most common.

ACUTE IDIOPATHIC POLYNEURITIS [LANDRY-GUILLAIN-BARRE (LGB) DISEASE, ACUTE INFLAMMATORY POLYRADICULONEUROPATHY, ACUTE IMMUNE-MEDIATED POLYNEURITIS (AIMP)]

This inflammatory disease occurs in all parts of the world and in all seasons; it affects children and adults of all ages and both sexes. Its cause is unknown. A mild respiratory or gastrointestinal infection precedes the neuritic symptoms by 1 to 3 weeks in approximately half the patients. Other preceding events include surgical procedures, viral exanthems and other viral illnesses, antirabies and A/New Jersey (swine) influenza vaccination, and lymphomatous disease (particularly Hodgkin's disease).

Historical It has been difficult to find the earliest description of this disease. The important landmarks are Landry's report of an acute, ascending, predominantly motor paralysis with respiratory failure and death; Osler's febrile polyneuritis; the account by Guillain, Barré, and Strohl of a benign childhood polyneuritis with albuminocytologic dissociation in the CSF (increase in protein without cells); elaboration of the clinical picture by many British and American investigators; the negative virologic studies by Sabin and Aring (for details of the historical and other aspects of this disease see reference to Asbury, Arnason, and Adams).

Incidence Our experience with this disease at the Massachusetts General and Cleveland Metropolitan General Hospitals has shown it to be nonseasonal and nonepidemic. Year after year about 10 to 15 patients have been admitted to each institution. The frequency in the Boston area has ranged from 2 to 8 per 100,000. Males and females are equally susceptible. The age range of 160 patients in the period 1963-1979 was 8 months to 81 years, with attack rates highest in persons 50 to 74 years of age.

Symptomatology The major clinical manifestation is weakness, which evolves, more or less symmetrically, over a period of several days. Proximal as well as distal muscles of the limbs are involved, usually the lower extremities before the upper; the trunk, intercostal and neck muscles are affected later, and the cranial muscles the last. The weakness can progress to total motor paralysis with death from respiratory failure within a few days. Pain occurs in about a third of the cases. Paresthesias (tingling and numbness) are frequent but tend to be evanescent; occasionally they are absent throughout the illness. Objective sensory loss occurs to a variable degree and in a few is barely detectable; when present, deep sensibility tends to be more affected than superficial.

The weakness develops so rapidly that muscle atrophy does not occur. Hypotonia and reduced and then absent reflexes are consistent findings. There is in some cases tenderness on deep pressure of muscles. At an early stage the arm muscles may be less weak than the leg muscles or are spared entirely. Facial diplegia, occurring in about half of all cases, and other cranial palsies usually come later, after the arms are affected. Disturbances of autonomic function (sinus tachycardia, and less often bradycardia and facial flushing, fluctuating hypertension and hypotension, loss of sweating or episodic profuse diaphoresis) are common, but rarely do these abnormalities persist for more than a week or two. Retention of urine occurs rarely, and catheterization is seldom required for more than a few days.

Variants of this clinical picture are frequent. Whereas in most patients the paralysis ascends from legs to trunk, arm, and cranial muscles (Landry's ascending paralysis) and reaches a peak of severity within 10 to 14 days (90 percent of our cases), occasionally cranial and arm muscles are affected first, or simultaneously with those of the legs. Again, in the milder cases, the legs may be affected and the arms little if at all. A syndrome comprising complete ophthalmoplegia with ataxia and areflexia, and thought to represent a variety of acute idiopathic polyneuritis, has been described by Fisher. Cases with steady or stepwise progression over weeks or months, some of which show asymmetries of involvement, with recovery in some parts and worsening in others, are other variants. A relapsing form is also known and was noted in approximately 10 percent of our cases.

The body temperature is usually normal, and lymphadenopathy and splenomegaly do not occur. T-wave and other electrocardiographic changes of minor degree have been reported frequently but are evanescent. The CSF is under normal pressure and is acellular in all but 10 percent of patients; in the latter a pleocytosis of 10 to 50 cells per cubic millimeter (rarely as high as 200 cells per cubic millimeter), predominantly lymphocytes and mononuclear cells, is found. Several days after the onset of symptoms the protein level begins to rise, reaching a peak in 4 to 6 weeks. The increase in CSF protein is probably a reflection of the widespread inflammatory disease of the nerve roots. In the peripheral blood, there is a moderate leukocytosis and shift to immature forms early in the illness, but the blood picture soon returns to normal. Nerve conduction velocities are slowed soon after the paralysis develops while denervation potentials (fibrillations), if they are to appear at all, come later. Transient diabetes insipidus, hyponatremia, and glomerulonephritis are rare complications.

Pathologic Findings These have had a consistent pattern and form. Even when the disease is fatal within a few days, perivascular lymphocytic infiltrates have been found. Later the characteristic inflammatory cell infiltrates and perivenous demyelination are combined with segmental demyelination and a variable degree of wallerian degeneration. Infiltrates are scattered throughout the cranial nerves, ventral and dorsal roots, dorsal root ganglia, and along the entire length of the peripheral nerves. Infiltrates of inflammatory cells (lymphocytes and mononuclear cell) are also found in lymph nodes, liver, spleen, heart, and other organs, and reflect the systemic nature of the disease.

Pathogenesis and Etiology Most of the evidence suggests that the clinical manifestations of this disorder are the result of a cell-mediated immunologic reaction directed at peripheral nerve. Waksman and Adams demonstrated that a peripheral nerve disease, clinically and pathologically indistinguishable from acute idiopathic polyneuritis, develops in animals about 2 weeks after immunization with peripheral nerve homogenate (experimental allergic neuritis or EAN). Recent investigations have indicated that the antigen in this reaction is a basic protein found only in peripheral nerve myelin (Abramsky et al.). The steps in this proposed reaction are diagramatically illustrated in Fig. 45-3. All attempts to isolate a virus or microbial agent have failed, but the occurrence of a similar polyneuritis with the Epstein-Barr and cytomegalus viruses opens again the possibility of a viral etiology.

Differenital Diagnosis Acute idiopathic polyneuritis (LGB syndrome) is not only one of the most frequent forms of polyneuropathy seen in a general hospital but also the most rapidly evolving and potentially fatal form. Any polyneuropathy which brings the patient to the brink of death within a few days will usually be of this type. The predominantly motor paralysis is its other major characteristic. Because of the latter feature, one must include poliomyelitis (distinguished by epidemic occurrence, meningeal symptoms, fever, purely motor and usually asymmetric areflexic paralysis) and acute myelitis (marked by sensorimotor paralysis below a given spinal level and sphincteric paralysis) in the differential diagnosis. Other forms of acute polyneuropathy described below must also be differentiated from this syndrome.

Treatment The essence of therapy is respiratory assistance and careful nursing, for the disease remits naturally in the majority of cases and recovery is nearly always complete. Not every patient needs respiratory assistance, but since the patient's condition may rapidly deteriorate, he or she should be in a hospital where such aid is available. A therapeutic trial of prednisone (45 to 60 mg/day) with a low-salt diet and precautions against peptic ulceration is sometimes warranted in the acute stage of the disease, in an attempt to stave off tracheostomy, but should be discontinued in a few days if a definite response is not observed. Respiratory assistance should be instituted at the first sign of dyspnea (vital capacity below 800 ml) or decrease in oxygen saturation of the blood. Tracheostomy may become necessary at this time, especially if the patient has difficulty in clearing secretions from the pharynx and tracheobronchial tree, but may be postponed and an endotracheal tube used for a few days if the physician is uncertain. Once tracheostomy is performed, careful tracheal toilet is required and control of infections by the use of an appropriate antibiotic. Support of the blood pressure in the face of hypotension by vasopressor agents is another essential part of the therapeutic regimen. The best results are obtained by placing the patient in an efficient respiratory care unit, skilled in maintaining adequacy of ventilation and circulation before respiratory failure occurs. Under these conditions the mortality from the disease can be reduced to less than 2 percent. Without competent respiratory assistance approximately 25 percent of patients succumb. Death nowadays in properly equipped hospitals is due to complications (usually bacterial) of prolonged tracheostomy, machine failure, uremia, or suicide. Pulmonary embolism is rare in our material. Occasionally, in the acute stages of the disease, death occurs suddenly, without adequate explanation.

The question of corticosteroid therapy is unsettled. When a group treated in this way was compared with a control group, there was no difference in duration of the illness and outcome. Nevertheless we have observed dramatic improvement in some cases.

In several hospital centers, plasmapheresis is being used to treat both the acute and relapsing forms of the LGB syndrome. Again, dramatic improvement has been reported in some patients but not in others. Until a controlled trial of plasmapheresis has been carried out, anecdotal reports of the efficacy of this method should be interpreted with caution. Such a trial is now under way (Asbury et al., 1980).

Physiotherapy (passive movement and positioning

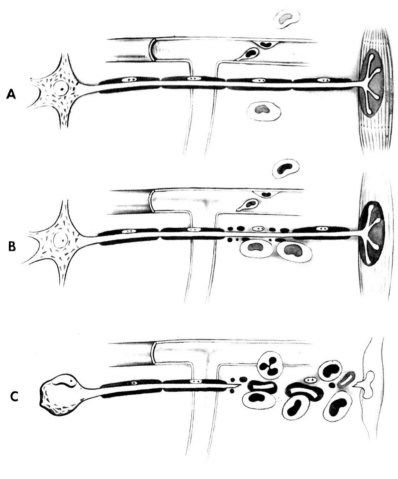

Figure 45-3

Diagram of probable cellular events in idiopathic polyneuritis. A. Lymphocytes attach to the walls of endoneurial vessels, migrate through the vessel wall, enlarging and transforming as they do so. At this stage no nerve damage has occurred. B. More lymphocytes have migrated into the surrounding tissue. The first effect upon the nerve is breakdown of myelin, the axon being spared (segmental demyelination). This change appears to be mediated by the mononuclear exudate, but the mechanism is uncertain. C. The lesion is more intense, polymorphonuclear leukocytes being present as well as lymphocytes. The axon is interrupted in addition to myelin sheath damage; as a result, the muscle undergoes denervation atrophy and the nerve cell body shows central chromatolysis. If the axonal damage is distal, the nerve cell body will survive, and regeneration and clinical recovery is likely. If, as in D, axonal interruption has occurred proximally because of a particularly intense root or proximal nerve lesion, the nerve cell body may die and undergo dissolution. In this situation, there is no regeneration, only the possibility of collateral reinnervation of muscle from surviving motor fibers. (From Asbury et al, 1969.)

of limbs to prevent pressure palsies and, later, mild resistance exercises) should begin once the condition of the patient has stabilized. The decision to discontinue respiratory aid and to close the tracheostomy are based on the degree of recovery of the patient's respiratory function.

Prognosis More than 95 percent of surviving patients are restored to completely normal function and the remaining ones are left with only mild motor or reflex deficits in the feet and legs. Speed of recovery varies. Often it occurs within a few weeks or months; but if nerves have degenerated, their regeneration may require 6 to 18 months.

If there is respiratory failure, the average period of machine-assisted respiration has been 50 days and the period of hospitalization, 108 days.

A small number of patients suffer one or more relapses of acute polyneuropathy, and in the latter cases the nerves may gradually become palpably enlarged. Also, as indicated above, an illness that begins as an acute inflammatory polyradiculoneuropathy may fail to stabilize and continues to progress steadily; or, there may be an incomplete remission followed by a chronic, slowly progressive neuropathy. The chronic forms are described in a later section of this chapter.

INFECTIOUS MONONUCLEOSIS WITH POLYNEURITIS

Three neurologic syndromes have been described with infectious mononucleosis: (1) an acute or subacute ascending sensorimotor paralysis, identical to that of the LGB syndrome described above, (2) aseptic meningitis, and (3) meningoencephalitis. All three appear during the midphase of the infection. The polyneuritis varies in severity and has rarely been fatal. The few autopsied cases have shown heavy infiltrations of lymphocytes, monocytes, and sometimes plasma cells in the nerves, roots, and meninges. The CSF may contain only a few or as many as several hundred mononuclear cells, and the protein level is raised. The diagnosis is suggested by the other typical physical and laboratory findings in this disease.

VIRAL HEPATITIS WITH ACUTE POLYNEURITIS

An acute polyneuritis, indistinguishable clinically and pathologically from the LGB type, may complicate viral hepatitis. The polyneuritis usually follows the jaundice by several days or weeks and probably has the same relation to it as to preceding respiratory or intestinal infections. Usually the type of hepatitis has remained unclear. Recovery from the hepatitis and polyneuropathy has been the rule, but is not invariable.

It should be pointed out that neuropathy is associated with liver disease under two other conditions: (1) A mild and usually asymptomatic (nutritional?) polyneuropathy has been described with chronic liver disease of diverse types. (2) A mild sensory neuropathy, due to xanthomatous involvement of the connective tissue sheaths of cutaneous nerves, is occasionally encountered in patients with biliary cirrhosis (Thomas and Walker).

These *hepatic polyneuropathies*, in which the nerve lesions appear to be a consequence of the liver disease, should not be confused with conditions in which the polyneuropathy and liver disease are both complications of a systemic disease such as alcoholism and malnutrition, infectious mononucleosis, polyarteritis nodosa, amyloidosis, and certain intoxications.

DIPHTHERITIC POLYNEUROPATHY

Some of the neurotoxic effects of *C. diphtheriae* and mode of action of the exotoxin elaborated by the bacillus are described in Chap. 41. Local action of the exotoxin may paralyze pharyngeal and laryngeal muscles within 1 or 2 weeks after the onset of the infection, and shortly thereafter may also cause blurring of vision due to loss of accommodation, but these and other cranial nerve symptoms may be overlooked. The first signs of polyneuropathy, coming 5 to 8 weeks later, take the form of an acute to subacute limb weakness with paresthesias and distal loss of vibratory and position sense. The weakness characteristically involves all four extremities at the same time or may descend from arms to legs. After a few days to a week or more, the patient may be unable to stand or walk, and occasionally the paralysis is so severe and extensive as to impair respiration. The CSF protein level is usually elevated (50 to 200 mg per 100 ml). After the pharyngeal infection is controlled, death in diphtheria is due usually to cardiomyopathy or to polyneuropathy with respiratory paralysis.

Pathologic Findings Postmortem examination discloses a demyelination without inflammatory reaction of spinal roots, sensory ganglia, and adjacent spinal nerves. Axons, anterior horn cells, peripheral nerves distally, and muscle fibers remain normal.

Differential Diagnosis The disease should be considered in all cases of acute polyneuropathy. Throat cultures may demonstrate *Corynebacterium diphtheriae* many weeks after the throat infection has subsided. Usually the history of nasal voice, dysphagia, blurred vision, numb lips, and a throat infection several weeks before the onset of the neuropathy provide the clues to the diagnosis. The ECG may be abnormal at the time of onset of the polyneuropathy. Occasionally a similar clinical picture or a localized mononeuropathy has followed a wound infection with *C. diphtheriae*, as indicated in Chap. 41.

Treatment Antitoxin is of no value once the polyneuropathy begins. Treatment is purely symptomatic, along the lines indicated for acute idiopathic polyneuritis. The prognosis for full recovery is excellent, once respiratory paralysis is circumvented.

PORPHYRIC POLYNEUROPATHY

A severe, rapidly advancing, more or less symmetric polyneuropathy, often with abdominal pain, psychosis (delirium or confusion), and convulsions mark the disease known as *intermittent acute porphyria* (pyrroloporphyria, or Swedish type). This type of porphyria is inherited as an autosomal dominant trait and is not associated with cutaneous sensitivity to sunlight. The metabolic defect is in the liver and is marked by increased production and urinary excretion of porphobilinogen and of the porphyrin precursor, δ-aminolevulinic acid. The peripheral and central nervous systems may also be affected in *variegate (South African) porphyria*. In this latter type, the skin is markedly sensitive to light and trauma, and porphyrins are at all times found in the stools. Both of these *hepatic* forms of porphyria are to be distinguished from the rare *erythropoietic (congenital photosensitive)* porphyria, in which the nervous system is never affected.

The most extensive study of intermittent acute porphyria was reported by Waldenstrom in 1937. The initial and often the most prominent symptom is moderate to severe colicky pain. It may be generalized or localized and is unattended by rigidity of the abdominal wall or tenderness. Radiographs show intestinal distention and spasm. Constipation is frequent. Attacks last for days to weeks and repeated vomiting may lead to inanition. In latent forms, the patient may be asymptomatic or complain only of slight dyspepsia.

The neurologic manifestations vary considerably. Usually the initial manifestation is a polyneuropathy involving principally the motor nerves, less often both sensory and motor nerves, and sometimes autonomic nerves. It may begin in the feet and legs and ascend, or more characteristically, it begins in the hands and arms (sometimes asymmetrically) and spreads in a few days to the trunk and legs. Occasionally it is predominantly proximal in distribution. Sensory loss, often involving the trunk, is present in half the cases. Facial paralysis, dysphagia, and ocular palsies are features of the most severe affections, simulating acute polyneuritis of the LGB type. The CSF protein level is usually normal.

The course of the polyneuropathy is variable. In mild cases the symptoms may regress in a few weeks. If severe, it may progress to a fatal respiratory or cardiac paralysis in a few days, the advance occurring without warning; or it may progress in a saltatory fashion over a period of weeks, finally resulting in a severe sensorimotor paralysis that requires months to regress. A disturbance of cerebral function (confusion, delirium, visual field defects, and convulsions) is more likely to precede the severe than the mild forms of polyneuropathy, but it may not appear at all. The cerebral manifestations usually subside in a few days to weeks though one of our patients was left with a homonymous hemianopia.

Tachycardia and hypertension are frequent in the acute phase of the disease, and fever and leukocytosis also may occur; these are said to be indexes of the activity of the pathologic process. The disease is characterized by recurrent attacks, often precipitated by drugs such as sulfonamides, griseofulvin, estrogens, barbiturates, phenytoin, and the succinimide anticonvulsants. The possibility of sensitivity to the latter drugs must always be kept in mind when treating convulsions in the porphyric patient. The first attack rarely occurs before puberty, and the disease is most likely to threaten life during adolescence and early adulthood. Death may result from respiratory paralysis or cardiac arrest and sometimes from uremia and cachexia.

In sum, the most characteristic clinical features are acute onset, initial psychotic symptoms, predominantly motor disorder, often an early bibrachial distribution of weakness, trunkal sensory loss, abdominal pain, and tachycardia.

Pathologic Findings The changes in the peripheral nervous system vary according to the stage of the illness at which death occurs. If the patient dies in the first few days, the myelinated fibers may appear entirely normal, despite an almost complete paralysis. If symptoms had been present for weeks, degeneration of both axons and myelin sheaths will be found in most of the peripheral nerves. No inflammatory reaction, vascular lesion, or other change distinguishes this form of polyneuropathy. The relation between the abnormality of porphyrin biosynthesis in the liver and nervous dysfunction has never been satisfactorily explained.

Diagnosis is confirmed by the demonstration of large amounts of porphobilinogen and δ-aminolevulinic acid in the urine. The urine turns dark when standing due to the formation of porphobilin, an oxidation product of porphobilinogen.

In general the *prognosis* for ultimate recovery is excellent, though relapse of the porphyria may result in further involvement of the peripheral nervous system (see *relapsing polyneuropathy*, further on).

Treatment consists of respiratory support, use of beta blockers (propranolol) if tachycardia and hypertension are severe, intravenous glucose to suppress the heme biosynthetic pathway, pyridoxine (100 mg twice a day) on the supposition that vitamin B_6 depletion has occurred. Goldberg recommends intravenous levulose (see Ridley). Positioning of limbs to prevent pressure neuropathies is important.

CERTAIN TOXIC POLYNEUROPATHIES

Triorthocresylphosphate (TOCP) and thallium poisoning are examples of acute polyneuropathies that may take life in a few days (see Chap. 41). The former causes severe and permanent motor paralysis that ultimately proves to be due to involvement of both upper and lower motor neurons. *Thallium salts,* when taken in sufficient amount may also produce a clinicial picture that resembles that of the LGB syndrome. If taken orally there is first abdominal pain, vomiting, and diarrhea followed within a few days by pain and tingling in the toes and fingertips and then rapid weakening of muscles of the legs, hands, and arms. Initially the weakness is always distal. As it progresses, the tendon reflexes diminish. Pain sensation is reduced more than touch, vibratory, and position sense. All cranial nerves except the first and eighth may be affected. Facial palsies, ophthalmoplegia, nystagmus, optic neuritis with visual impairment, and vocal cord palsies are the most prominent cranial nerve abnormalities. The CSF protein rises to over 100 mg. Death may occur in the first 10 days, due to cardiac arrest. The early onset of painful paresthesias, pain localized to joints, back, and chest, and rapid loss of hair (within a week or two) help differentiate this neuropathy from LGB, porphyria and other neuropathies. Relative preservation of reflexes is also noteworthy. From lesser degrees of intoxication there may be recovery. Thallium salts act like potassium and a high intake of KCl hastens the excretion of thallium; chelating agents are of unproven value.

Occasionally, the *polyneuropathy associated with polyarteritis nodosa* develops as rapidly as acute idio-

pathic polyneuritis, and muscle biopsy may be needed to distinguish these disorders. However, most cases of neuropathy due to polyarteritis evolve more slowly and the syndrome assumes a symmetric or asymmetric distribution. For this reason it will be described in the next section.

We have observed a few patients with occult carcinoma and Hodgkin's disease who developed an acute polyneuropathy, as rapid in its evolution as the LGB syndrome, and acute episodes of this type have also been described in patients with Refsum's disease. Rarely, vaccination or protective inoculations against typhoid, rabies, and smallpox or injections of antitoxin in foreign serum have produced a generalized and sometimes painful sensorimotor polyneuritis. The usual picture, however, is a brachial plexitis and these conditions are more appropriately discussed with the brachial plexus neuropathies (see further on in this chapter.)

SYNDROME OF SUBACUTE SENSORIMOTOR PARALYSIS

SUBACUTE SYMMETRIC POLYNEUROPATHIES

The neuropathic conditions in this category develop over a period of a few weeks, reach their peak of severity at the end of this time, and last for a variable period. Pain, dysesthesias and paresthesias, "hyperesthesia," and tenderness of muscles are often prominent features, in addition to weakness and atrophy of muscles, and loss of sensation and tendon reflexes. A symmetric syndrome of this type usually proves to be due to alcoholism and nutritional deficiency (beriberi), to poisoning with arsenic, lead, nitrofurantoin, hydralazine, antabuse, or isoniazid. Occasionally an illness that begins as an acute idiopathic polyneuritis evolves at this slower pace.

Deficiency States In the Western world, nutritional polyneuropathy is usually associated with alcoholism. As pointed out in Chap. 38, all data point to the identity of so-called alcoholic neuropathy and beriberi. A common nutritional factor is responsible for both, though in any given case it often remains unclear whether the deficiency is one of thiamine, pyridoxine, pantothenic acid, or a combination of the B vitamins. We have not been able to define a form of polyneuropathy due to the direct toxic effect of alcohol alone. Neuropathic beriberi and other forms of deficiency neuropathy (Strachan's syndrome, pellagra, vitamin B_{12} deficiency, and malabsorption syndromes) are described fully in Chap. 38.

Arsenical Polyneuropathy Of the neuropathies caused by metallic poisoning, that due to arsenic is particularly well known. In cases of chronic poisoning, the symptoms develop rather slowly, over a period of weeks, and have the same sensory and motor distribution as the nutritional polyneuropathies. Gastrointestinal symptoms may result from the oral ingestion of arsenic and may precede the polyneuropathy which is nearly always coupled with anemia, jaundice, brownish cutaneous pigmentation, hyperkeratosis of palms and soles, white transverse banding of the nails (Mees' lines), and an excess of arsenic in the urine and hair.

The ingestion of a single large dose of arsenic may be followed in 14 to 21 days by a more rapidly advancing polyneuropathy. The condition may be preceded by severe gastrointestinal symptoms and mental disturbances, convulsions, confusion, and coma, i.e., arsenical encephalopathy (brain purpura).

Diagnosis and treatment of arsenical poisoning are discussed further in Chap. 41.

Lead Neuropathy Lead neuropathy is an uncommon disorder. It occurs following chronic exposure to lead, and its most characteristic feature is the predominantly motor affection involving mainly the upper extremities. The radial nerves are most frequently involved, producing wrist and finger drop with few or no sensory manifestations. Less commonly, weakness of the proximal muscles of the arm and shoulder girdle occurs, and foot drop in the lower extremities. As pointed out in Chap. 41, lead neuropathy is a disease of adults; it seldom occurs in children, in whom lead poisoning usually results in an encephalopathy.

The diagnosis of lead neuropathy is established by the history of lead exposure, the characteristic motor involvement, associated medical findings (anemia, basophilic stippling of red cell precursors in the bone marrow, lead line along the gingival margins, colicky abdominal pain, and constipation), and urinary excretion of lead and coproporphyrins. Blood lead levels of more than 80 μg per 100 ml are always abnormal. In patients with lower levels, the doubling of the 24-h urinary lead excretion following an infusion of $CaNa_2$ EDTA indicates a significant degree of lead intoxication. Coproporphyrin in the urine is abnormal in any amount, but is found in porphyria, alcoholism, iron defi-

ciency, and other disorders, as well as in lead intoxication. Treatment consists of terminating the exposure to lead and eliminating lead from the bloodstream and the bones by the measures described in Chap. 41. For this purpose, penicillamine is preferable to BAL or edetate, because it can be administered orally and is relatively safe.

Other Metals and Industrial Solvents Poisoning with mercury, thallium (more chronic form of intoxication), and sometimes gold may produce a sensorimotor polyneuropathy similar to arsenical polyneuropathy; these intoxications are discussed in Chap. 41. Exposure to manganese, bismuth, antimony, zinc, and copper may give rise to systemic signs of poisoning; some of them affect the central nervous system, but one cannot be certain that any of them specifically involves the peripheral nerves. A distal, symmetrical, sensorimotor (predominantly sensory) neuropathy may follow exposure to certain hexacarbon industrial solvents, such as *n-hexane* (found in contact cements) and *methyl n-butyl ketone* (used in the production of plastic-coated and color-printed fabrics), to dimethylaminopropionitrile (or DMAPN, used in the manufacture of polyurethane foam), and to the fumigant *methyl bromide*. TOCP and acrylamide, another agent that has been incriminated in the causation of polyneuropathy, have been used to study the biology of neuropathy in experimental animals. Both of these agents cause axonal degeneration in the distal ends of the motor nerves.

Detailed accounts of the clinical and experimental neurotoxicology of these neuropathic agents can be found in the recent monograph edited by Spencer and Schaumburg.

Isonicotinic Acid Hydrazide (Isoniazid, INH) Neuropathy Isoniazid-induced polyneuropathy was a common occurrence in the early 1950s, when this drug was first used for the treatment of tuberculosis. Symptoms of neuropathy appeared in about 10 percent of patients receiving therapeutic doses of the drug (10 mg/kg daily), between 3 and 35 weeks after treatment was begun.

The initial symptoms of the neuropathy are a symmetrical numbness and tingling of the toes and feet, spreading, if the drug is continued, to the knees, and occasionally the hands. Aching and burning pain in these parts then become prominent. In addition to sensory loss, examination discloses a loss of tendon reflexes and weakness in the distal parts of the limbs, almost exclusively of the legs. Severe degrees of weakness and loss of deep sensation are observed only rarely.

INH produces its effects on peripheral nerve by interfering with pyridoxine metabolism, perhaps by inhibiting the phosphorylation of pyridoxine (the collective name for the B_6 group of vitamins), and decreasing the tissue levels of its active form, pyridoxal phosphate. The administration of 150 to 450 mg of pyridoxine daily, in conjunction with isoniazid, completely prevents the neuropathic disorder. The same mechanism is probably operative in the neuropathies that occasionally complicate the administration of the INH-related substances *ethionamide*, used in the treatment of tuberculosis, and the antihypertensive agent *hydralazine*.

Nitrofurantoin Neuropathy   The introduction in 1952 of nitrofurantoin for the treatment of bladder infections was soon followed by reports of neurotoxicity attributable to this drug. The earliest symptoms are pain and tingling paresthesias of the toes and feet, followed shortly by similar sensations in the fingers. If the drug is not discontinued, this disorder may progress to a severe, symmetric, sensorimotor polyneuropathy. Neuropathic symptoms appear after the drug has been administered in high dosage for several weeks or months, but a few patients have experienced paresthesias after briefer periods. Patients with chronic renal failure and azotemia are particularly prone to neurotoxicity from nitrofurantoin, presumably because the diminished excretion in the urine results in high tissue levels of the drug. To make matters more difficult, the uremic state itself may be responsible for a clinically similar polyneuropathy, so that the distinction between uremic and nitrofurantoin neuropathy in the presence of chronic renal failure may be impossible. The neuropathologic studies of Lhermitte et al. reveal an axonal degeneration in peripheral nerves and sensory roots.

Other nitrofurantoin compounds, *furaltadone* and *nitrofurazone*, are also used as chemotherapeutic agents. Neurotoxicity has been reported, but it is of little clinical importance, since it is a rare complication and the drugs are not in common use.

Other Drug-Induced Neuropathies   The development of a sensorimotor neuropathy, similar to that produced by isoniazid, is occasionally associated with the chronic use of *disulfiram* (Antabuse). Its neurotoxic effects have been attributed to the action of *carbon disulfide*, which is produced during the metabolism of disulfiram and is known to produce polyneuropathy, many cases having occurred in workers in the viscose rayon industry who were exposed to carbon disulfide in high concentration.

Peripheral neuropathy commonly complicates the use of *vincristine*, an antineoplastic agent widely used in treatment of the reticuloses and leukemia (see page 790). Loss of ankle jerks is an early manifestation of vincristine neuropathy, along with paresthesias, mild sensory loss, and weakness of the fingers and toes, in that order. Weakness is observed first in the extensor muscles of the fingers and wrists, later in the dorsiflexors of the toes and feet, and if the dosage of vincristine is not reduced, weakness may spread rapidly to involve the proximal muscles of the limbs. Neuropathy is the main limiting factor in the use of this drug. Reduction in dosage is followed by rapid improvement of neuropathic symptoms, and many patients are then able to continue the use of vincristine in low dosage, such as 1 mg every 2 weeks, for many months.

A relatively mild sensory neuropathy associated with optic neuropathy occasionally complicates *chloramphenicol* therapy. Patients who have taken *phenytoin* for many years may show absence of ankle and patellar reflexes, a mild, distal symmetrical impairment of sensation, and a reduced conduction velocity in the peripheral nerves of the legs. The chronic administration of *metronidazole* (used in the treatment of Crohn's disease) and of *amitriptyline* may occasionally have the same effect. A predominantly motor neuropathy may be induced by the chronic administration of *dapsone*, a sulfone used to treat leprosy. *Stilbamidine*, used in the treatment of kala azar, may produce a purely sensory neuropathy, predominantly in the distribution of the trigeminal nerves. The anesthetic agent *trichlorethylene* also has a predilection for cranial nerves, particularly the fifth. Neurotoxicity is apparently due to dichloroacetylene, formed in the course of decomposition of trichlorethylene.

Clioquinol (discussed in Chap. 41) and *thalidomide*, each of which can produce severe polyneuropathy, have been withdrawn from the market, but patients are still seen with the residual neurotoxic effects of these drugs. Several industrial solvents and organophosphorous compounds are important causes of neuropathy and are also discussed in Chap. 41.

SUBACUTE ASYMMETRIC POLYNEUROPATHIES

The most notable examples of this syndrome are certain forms of neuropathy that accompany diabetes, polyarteritis nodosa and other vasculitides, and a more or less obscure form of idiopathic polyneuritis. Rarely, sarcoidosis presents in this fashion.

Diabetic Neuropathy   Only about 15 percent of patients with diabetes mellitus have both symptoms and signs of neuropathy, but nearly 50 percent either complain of neuropathic symptoms or display slowing of nerve conduction velocity. Neuropathy is most common in diabetics over 50 years of age, is uncommon in those under 30 years of age, and is rare in childhood.

A number of clinical syndromes have been delineated:(1) diabetic ophthalmoplegia, (2) acute mononeuropathy, (3) a rapidly evolving, painful, asymmetric, predominantly motor, multiple neuropathy (so-called *mononeuropathy multiplex),* which usually undergoes remission, (4) a symmetric, proximal motor weakness and wasting without pain and with variable sensory loss, which pursues a subacute or chronic course, (5) a distal, symmetric, primarily sensory polyneuropathy affecting feet and legs more than hands in a chronic, slowly progressive manner, and (6) an autonomic neuropathy involving bowel, bladder, and circulatory reflexes. These forms of neuropathy often coexist, particularly the autonomic and the distal symmetric types.

Diabetic ophthalmoplegia is usually due to an isolated third nerve lesion; much less commonly the sixth nerve is involved. This disorder is described on page 183. Isolated affection of practically all the major peripheral nerves has been described in diabetes, but the ones most commonly involved are the femoral and sciatic. The acute mononeuropathies, cranial and peripheral, are presumably due to ischemic infarction of the nerve. The outlook for recovery is good.

Painful, asymmetric multiple neuropathy tends to occur in older patients with mild or unrecognized diabetes. Occasionally it may complicate long-standing diabetes. Pain often begins in the low back or hip and spreads to the thigh and knee on one side. It usually has a deep, burning character with superimposed lancinating jabs, and there is a propensity for the discomfort to be most severe at night. Muscle weakness and atrophy are most evident in the pelvic girdle and thigh, although the distal muscles may also be affected. The upper extremities are usually spared. Deep and superficial sensation may be intact or mildly impaired, conforming to either a multiple nerve or root distribution, or to both. The vesical and anal sphincters may be involved, and the knee jerk is often lost on the affected side. Recovery from this type of neuropathy is the rule, although months and even years may elapse before it is complete. There is a tendency for the same syndrome to recur after a lapse of months or years in the opposite lower extremity. This form of neuropathy is often referred to as *diabetic amyotrophy,* a term which draws attention to one facet of the syndrome but is otherwise uninformative.

There is a second type of proximal diabetic neuropathy, characterized by a symmetric weakness and wasting of insidious onset and gradual evolution over several months. The proximal muscles of the upper limbs and scapulae, especially the deltoid and triceps, and of the lower limbs, particularly the iliopsoas, quadriceps, and hamstrings, are involved in varying degrees. Pain is not a consistent feature as it is in the acute asymmetric type, and sensory changes, if present, are distal, symmetric, and usually mild in degree.

The *distal, symmetric, primarily sensory form* is the most common type of diabetic neuropathy. Persistent and often distressing numbness and tingling, usually confined to the feet and lower legs and becoming worse at night, are the main symptoms. The ankle jerks are rarely preserved. Trophic changes in the form of deep ulcerations and neuropathic joints are occasionally encountered, presumably due to severe sensory denervation of skin and joints. Muscle weakness is usually mild, but in some patients a distal sensory neuropathy is combined with a subacute proximal weakness and wasting of the types described above.

The clinical picture may be dominated by deep sensory loss, ataxia, and atony of the bladder, with only slight weakness of the limbs, in which case it resembles tabes dorsalis (hence the term *diabetic pseudotabes).* The similarity is even closer if lancinating pains in the legs, unreactive pupils and neuropathic arthropathy are present. Loss of nerve fibers is a prominent pathologic finding in the distal symmetric form of neuropathy. In addition, evidence of segmental demyelination and remyelination of remaining axons is apparent in teased nerve fiber preparations. Since myelin is formed from the cell membranes of Schwann cells, one may infer that the Schwann cell is a primary target of the pathologic process in this type of diabetic neuropathy. The nerve fiber loss could hardly be explained by this same process, however. The blood vessels in these nerves do not appear abnormal by light microscopy, but there is an ultrastructural alteration of their basement membranes.

Symptoms of autonomic involvement include impairment of sweating and of vascular reflexes, nocturnal diarrhea, atonic bladder, sexual impotence, and occasionally postural hypotension. The basis of this type of involvement is not well understood.

In all these forms of diabetic neuropathy, the CSF protein may be elevated, 50 to 200 mg per 100 ml, and rarely, even higher. The usual explanation for this phenomenon is involvement of spinal roots and ganglia.

Thomas and Lascelles have reviewed the neuropathology. They confirm the loss of axons in peripheral nerves and the segmental demyelination. The latter finding is believed to be secondary to changes in the axon.

Unmyelinated fibers are also reduced in number in some specimens. Similar lesions are found in the posterior roots and posterior columns of the spinal cord, and in the rami communicantes and sympathetic ganglia. Obliterative vascular lesions were well illustrated by Raff et al. Under the electron microscope the basal membranes of intraneural capillaries are seen to be thickened and duplicated.

Many uncertainties persist about the pathogenesis of the diabetic neuropathies. Both the cranial (diabetic ophthalmoplegia) and peripheral mononeuropathies, as well as the painful, asymmetric, predominantly proximal neuropathy of sudden onset are thought to be ischemic in origin, secondary to disease of the vasa nervorum (Fig. 45-4). In the other forms of diabetic neuropathy the available data favor a metabolic basis, as yet undefined. The several biochemical findings and their interpretations are reviewed by Thomas and Eliasson. One can only conclude after reading their article that a convincing biochemical pathogenesis has yet to be educed.

The only known treatment is regulation of the diabetes and the maintenance of the blood glucose level in a relatively normal range, since the prevailing view is that there is some relationship between peripheral nerve damage and inadequate diabetic control. Vitamin supplements may have some merit. Prognosis in the distal, symmetrical, sensory neuropathy is uncertain, but in the other types improvement and eventual recovery may be expected over a period of months. During that time the management of the painful forms of neuropathy may be trying, because analgesic medication is required and one is faced with the possibility of drug addiction.

Neuropathies with Other Forms of Ischemic Disease One-half to two-thirds of patients with artherosclerotic ischemic disease of the legs will be found to have localized sensory changes or impairment of reflexes. Usually the effects of ischemia on skin and muscle are so prominent that the neurologic changes are overlooked. The literature on this subject is to be found in the articles of Hutchinson and of Asbury, listed in the references.

Angiopathic Neuropathies A number of mononeuropathies and polyneuropathies are known to be caused by small vessel arteritis. These include polyarteritis nodosa, rheumatoid arthritis, lupus erythematosus, systemic sclerosis, cranial arteritis and Wegener's granulomatosis (see review by Conn and Dyck).

Polyarteritis nodosa with polyneuropathy Perhaps 75 percent of cases of polyarteritis nodosa show involvement of the nutrient arteries of peripheral nerves (autopsy figures), but a symptomatic form of neuropathy develops in only about half this number. Yet involvement of the peripheral nerves may be the principal clue to the diagnosis of the underlying disease when, up to that time, the main components of the clinical picture— abdominal pain, hematuria, fever, eosinophilia, hypertension, vague limb pains, and possibly asthma—have not fully declared themselves or have been misinterpreted.

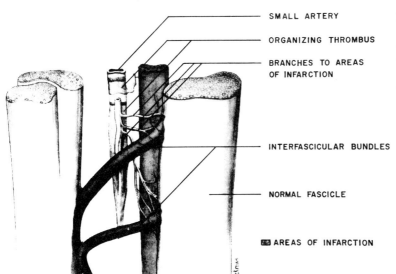

SMALL ARTERY

ORGANIZING THROMBUS

BRANCHES TO AREAS OF INFARCTION

INTERFASCICULAR BUNDLES

NORMAL FASCICLE

▨ AREAS OF INFARCTION

Figure 45-4
Three-dimensional drawing reconstructed from serial cross sections of left obturator nerve, taken from an elderly diabetic with mononeuropathy multiplex. Note organized thrombus in the interfascicular artery. Arteriolar branches from occluded segments supply three infarcted fascicles. The tendency for infarcts to occur in bridging interfascicular bundles is shown. (From Raff et al.)

The polyneuropathy associated with polyarteritis nodosa may be diffuse and more or less symmetric in distribution, but more often it takes the form of a *mononeuropathy multiplex*, i.e., a random affection of two or more individual nerves. The onset in this latter form is usually abrupt, with symptoms of pain or numbness in the distribution of an affected nerve, followed in hours or days by motor or sensory loss in the distribution of that nerve, and then by involvement, in a saltatory fashion, of other peripheral nerves. Both spinal and cranial nerves may be affected. No two cases are identical. The CSF protein level is usually normal. Muscle biopsy, taken near the motor point so as to include nerve twigs, is useful in corroborating the clinical impression in the majority of cases.

Mononeuropathy multiplex due to polyarteritis calls for treatment with corticosteroids. Spontaneous remission and therapeutic arrest are known, but most cases have a fatal outcome.

Rheumatoid arthritis One to five percent of patients with rheumatoid arthritis will have involvement of one or more nerves at some time in the course of their disease. Apart from pressure neuropathies, there is a form of rheumatoid arteritis that may result in acute ischemic necrosis and demyelination of single or multiple nerves. The arteritis is of fibrinoid type and immune globulins are demonstrable in the wall of the vessel. Most of the affected patients have had arthritis for more than 10 years, and the disease is severe. They often have, in addition to the neuropathy, rheumatoid nodules, skin vasculitis, weight loss, fever, a high titer of rheumatoid factor and low serum complement.

Most polyneuropathies that complicate rheumatoid arthritis are chronic in nature and are described further on, under the chronic polyneuropathies associated with the connective tissue diseases.

Lupus erythematosus Approximately 10 percent of patients with this disease will exhibit symptoms and signs of peripheral nerve involvement. It usually appears in the established and more advanced stages of the disease but rarely has been the initial presentation. In several of our cases the polyneuropathy has taken the form of a symmetric, progressive sensorimotor paralysis, beginning in the feet and legs and extending to the arms. In some, the weakness and areflexia were more prominent than the sensory loss; the latter involved mainly vibratory and position senses. Mononeuropathy has also been seen. The elevation of CSF protein in some cases suggests root involvement. The neuropathy is due to occlusion of the nutrient arteries.

Wegener's granulomatosis (necrotizing granulomatous vasculitis of upper and lower respiratory tract, glomerulonephritis, and systemic vasculitis) This disorder has given rise to two neurologic syndromes—one a symmetric or asymmetric polyneuropathy indistinguishable from the other angiopathic neuropathies described above, the other a direct involvement of lower cranial nerves as they issue from the skull and pass through the retropharyngeal tissues. The latter needs to be differentiated from carcinoma, chordoma, sarcoidosis, and zoster.

Subacute Asymmetric Idiopathic Polyneuritis As has been stated, a few patients with an illness which at first glance has all the appearance of acute idiopathic polyneuritis will continue to become worse over a period of weeks or months, either gradually or in a stepwise manner. In a number of these patients, as the months pass, some symptoms improve as others appear, resulting in a markedly asymmetric neuropathy. The nerves may be palpably enlarged, and the level of protein in the CSF extremely high (600 to 1500 mg per 100 ml), with a virtual Froin syndrome (xanthochromia and spontaneous clotting). The high concentration of protein may induce headache, papilledema, and high CSF pressure (without hydrocephalus), possibly because of an increased CSF volume resulting from the osmotic effect of the protein. The pathology of this particular form of neuropathy has not been defined; and its relation to the acute variety of idiopathic polyneuritis has also not been settled.

Ultimately most patients recover to some extent, though late fatality is known to occur. Corticosteroids in full doses have proved to be beneficial in the majority of cases but may have to be continued over a period of months.

A special variety of possibly the same disease, hypertrophic mononeuropathy, presents as an enlargement and tenderness of two or three nerves (back of neck and head or supraclavicular region) and raises suspicion of a nerve tumor (neurofibroma). A biopsy reveals the *onion bulb* type of enlargement of hypertrophic polyneuritis. There may be inflammatory cells in the interstitial tissue. Several patients whom we have followed responded well to corticosteroids only to relapse sometime later, after the treatment was terminated.

Sarcoidosis Sarcoidosis is a rare cause of subacute or chronic polyneuropathy of asymmetric type. It may be associated with lesions in muscles (polymyositis), or with signs of CNS involvement (stalk of the pituitary with diabetes insipidus, and cerebellum with ataxia).

An isolated facial palsy is the most frequent manifestation of single peripheral nerve involvement; in other cases, multiple cranial nerves are affected successively (see later section in this chapter). Weakness and reflex and sensory loss in the distribution of one or more spinal nerves or roots may be added. The occurrence of large, irregular zones of sensory loss over the trunk is said to distinguish the neuropathy of sarcoidosis from other forms of mononeuropathy multiplex.

SYNDROME OF CHRONIC SENSORIMOTOR POLYNEUROPATHY

In this syndrome, impairment of sensation, weakness, and muscular atrophy progress over a period of months or years. The time of onset is often uncertain. In infants the condition may be mistaken for muscular dystrophy or infantile muscular atrophy until sensory testing becomes possible. In the developing child whose musculature naturally increases in power and volume, it may be difficult to decide whether the disease is progressive. Ataxia of limbs may be pronounced at a stage when sensory loss exceeds paresis. The atrophy of muscle and trophic changes in the skin are more marked than in the acute and subacute forms of polyneuropathy, which is why the syndrome must be differentiated from the other forms of severe muscular atrophy, i.e., motor system disease, distal type of muscular dystrophy, and syringomyelia. The feet and hands may be extremely wasted, deformed (talipes equinus, claw hand), and subject to painless injuries, loss of tissue, and Charcot's joints, while proximal structures are sound. Symmetry of distribution is the rule (tuberculoid leprosy is an exception), and in some of the familial sensory neuropathies only the nerves of the legs may be involved. The CSF protein level may remain elevated over a period of years.

There are two main categories of chronic polyneuropathy, one acquired and the other familial. These will be discussed separately.

ACQUIRED FORMS OF CHRONIC POLYNEUROPATHY

Carcinomatous and Myelomatous Polyneuropathy A slowly developing (over a period of months), predominantly distal, symmetric sensory or sensorimotor polyneuropathy may occur as a remote effect of carcinoma or multiple myeloma, and less frequently, lymphoma. Severe weakness and atrophy, ataxia, and sensory loss of the limbs may advance to the point where the patient is confined to a wheelchair or bed; the CSF protein level is often moderately elevated. All these symptoms may oc-

cur months or even a year or more before a small malignant tumor is found.

A mixed sensorimotor polyneuropathy is five times more frequent than a purely sensory one. It may spread slowly from lower to upper extremities, reaching its peak in a few months. Usually the condition remains unchanged until death, but on occasion improvement has been obtained with steroids, and partial remission has occurred in some cases after excision or radiation of the tumor. The sensory polyneuropathy described by Denny-Brown is characterized by severe ataxia with retention of strength. All modalities of sensation are impaired over the limbs and even the face, and the reflexes disappear. Occasionally the evolution of the sensorimotor variety is subacute (weeks) and in a few instances the development seems to have been as rapid as that of the Landry-Guillain-Barré syndrome.

These forms of polyneuropathy are manifest clinically in 2 to 5 percent of all patients with malignant disease. Carcinoma of the lung accounts for about 50 percent of the cases of sensorimotor polyneuropathy and 75 percent of the cases of pure sensory neuropathy (Croft and Wilkinson). Actually, however, these neuropathies have been joined to tumors of every type. They may also accompany a solitary plasmacytoma of bone or multiple myeloma. Thus polyneuropathy must be added to polymyositis or dermatomyositis, with which it is frequently conjoined, as a neurologic complication of malignant tumors. Also the other remote neurologic effects of neoplasia may coexist: a peculiar type of myasthenia (Eaton-Lambert syndrome; Chap. 51), spinocerebellar degeneration, limbic encephalits, and multifocal leukoencephalopathy (Chap. 30).

The *pathology* of the neuropathy has not been completely defined. In the purely sensory type, there is a loss of nerve cells in the dorsal root ganglia, with secondary degeneration of the dorsal nerve roots and posterior columns of the spinal cord. In the sensorimotor type the pathologic picture is usually indistinguishable from that of a nutritional or metabolic disease of nerves. The degeneration is greater in the distal than in the proximal segments of the peripheral nerves, but extends into the roots in advanced cases. Dorsal root ganglion cells may be lost in small numbers. If the histologic examination is performed early in the course of the neuropathy, there are sparse infiltrates of lymphocytes distributed in foci around blood vessels. Their relation to both segmental demyelination and axonal degeneration of myelinated fibers is unclear. Unlike carcinomatous and lymphomatous mononeuropathy multiplex, where tumor cells infiltrate nerves, no tumor cells are seen in the nerves or spinal ganglia. Degeneration of the dorsal columns and chromatolysis of anterior horn cells are probably secondary to changes in the peripheral nerves and roots.

The *prognosis* is poor. Even though the polyneuropathy may stabilize and not progress or even remit with therapy, most of the patients succumb to the tumor within a year.

The *cause* of the polyneuropathy is not known. The presence of infiltrates of inflammatory cells in the sensory ganglia, nerves, spinal roots, and spinal cord and the occasional association with multifocal leukoencephalopathy suggest a viral infection. Croft et al. found circulating antibodies to nerve in four cases of sensory neuropathy but not in the more common sensorimotor neuropathy. This raised the question of an immunologic mechanism. A vitamin deficiency has also been proposed, but the administration of vitamins has been of no value.

Therapy consists of removing or controlling the tumor growth, which has resulted at times in improvement of neuropathic signs. Corticosteroid therapy has helped some patients. In cases of myelomatous polyneuropathy, particularly if the myeloma is "solitary," radiotherapy may result in prolonged remission of both the myeloma and neuropathy.

Neuropathies Associated with Paraproteinemias and Dysproteinemias Occasionally, we have observed patients with relatively mild chronic sensorimotor neuropathies, in whom no associated metabolic disturbance other than an abnormality of the immunoglobulins is found. In general, three such disorders have been recognized (exclusive of multiple myeloma): (1) isolated macroglobulinemia (increase in IgM), (2) cryoglobulinemia (IgG or IgM, or a mixture of both fractions), and (3) ataxia-telangiectasia (specific disorder of IgA).

Macroglobulinemia is the term applied by Waldenstrom to a systemic condition occurring mainly in elderly persons and characterized by fatigue, weakness, and a bleeding diathesis. A significant proportion of cases with hyperproteinemia are complicated by a diffuse slowing of retinal and cerebral circulation (Bing-Neel syndrome), giving rise to episodic confusion, coma, and sometimes to strokes, as well as by a peripheral neuropathy. The latter may be subacute but is more often chronic in nature, sometimes markedly so, and either asymmetric, in a multiple nerve trunk pattern (particu-

larly at the onset of the neuropathy), or symmetric and distal in distribution. In several of our cases the polyneuropathy was symmetrical and sensorimotor in type, and limited to the feet and legs, with mild ataxia and loss of knee and ankle jerks. The CSF protein is usually elevated and the globulin fraction increased.

Cryoglobulinemia is characterized by a serum protein that precipitates on cooling, and may occur without any apparent associated condition (essential cryoglobulinemia) or, more frequently, with a wide variety of disorders such as myeloma, lymphoma, connective tissue disease, and chronic infection. Peripheral neuropathy occurs in a small proportion of both types of cases. It develops insidiously, on a background of Raynaud's phenomenon and purpuric eruptions of the skin. Originally, the neuropathic symptoms consist only of pain and paresthesias which are often precipitated by exposure to cold. Later, weakness and wasting gradually develop, often asymmetrically, more in the legs than in the arms and more or less in the distribution of the vascular changes.

The pathology of the neuropathies associated with macroglobulinemia and cryoglobulinemia have been incompletely studied, and the mechanisms by which these disorders cause neuropathy is quite obscure. In one of our most completely autopsied cases there was widespread distal axonal degeneration of nondescript type without amyloid deposition or inflammatory cells, yet in other reported cases amyloid has been found.

The use of prednisone or the alkylating agent chlorambucil have at times led to improvement in the general and neuropathic symptoms, although recovery has been incomplete.

In *ataxia-telangiectasia*, in which there is a diminution in gamma globulin, a peripheral nerve dysfunction is manifested at first by hyporeflexia and decreased nerve conduction velocities, and then by the slow evolution of a symmetric and predominantly distal atrophic paralysis and sensory loss, the legs being affected more than the arms (see page 680).

Uremic Polyneuropathy Polyneuropathy is probably the most common complication of chronic renal failure. It has been stated by Robson to be present in some degree in two-thirds of all patients about to begin dialysis therapy. Bolton's figures are very much the same; 70 percent of patients being dialyzed regularly had uremic polyneuropathy, and in 30 percent the neuropathy was of moderate or severe degree. Usually the neuropathy takes the form of a painless, progressive, symmetrical sensorimotor paralysis of the legs and then of the arms. In some patients, the neuropathy begins with burning dysesthesias of the feet or with sensations of creeping, crawling, and itching of the legs and thighs which tend to be worse at night and are relieved by movement (restless legs syndrome of Ekbom; see page 264).

The combination of muscle weakness and atrophy, areflexia, sensory loss, and the graded distribution of the neurologic deficit in the limbs leave little doubt about the peripheral nerve character of the disorder. Usually the neuropathy evolves slowly over many months, at times in subacute fashion. Rare instances of acute noninflammatory sensorimotor polyneuropathy have also been reported (Asbury et al.). The neuropathy has been observed with all types of chronic kidney disease. More important to the development of neuropathy than the nature of the renal lesion is the duration and severity of the renal failure and symptomatic uremia (not merely azotemia).

With long-term hemodialysis, the symptoms and signs of polyneuropathy stabilize, but they improve in relatively few patients. In fact, rapid hemodialysis may occasionally worsen the polyneuropathy temporarily. Peritoneal dialysis has been more successful than hemodialysis in improving the neuropathy. Complete recovery, occurring over a period of 6 to 12 months, usually follows successful renal transplantation for the reason given below.

The pathologic findings are those of a nonspecific axonal degeneration with secondary segmental demyelination. The changes are most intense in the distal segments of the nerves, with the expected chromatolysis of their cell bodies. Amyloid deposits in the nerves have not been found; there is no evidence of vitamin deficiency or of diabetes during life, although the latter diagnosis may be difficult to establish in the uremic patient. There are no signs of polyarteritis nodosa at autopsy.

The cause of uremic polyneuropathy is unknown. The "middle molecule" theory is currently the most plausible. The end stage of renal failure is associated with the accumulation of toxic substances in the 300- to 2000-molecular-weight range. Furthermore, the degree of elevation of these substances, which include methylguanidine and myoinositol, has been shown to correlate with the degree of neurotoxicity (Funck-Brentano et al.). These toxins (and the clinical signs of neuropathy) are not greatly reduced by chronic hemodialysis. On the other hand, the transplanted kidney deals effectively with substances of wide ranging molecular weights, which would account for the invariable improvement of neuropathy after transplantation.

Alcoholic and Diabetic Neuropathy In all cases of alcoholic (nutritional) polyneuropathy in which treatment is delayed or for some reason not obtained, the weakness and atrophy of the legs, and to a lesser extent the arms,

may reach an extreme degree. Thus this disease, though subacute in its evolution, becomes a frequent cause of chronic polyneuropathy. Certain cases of diabetic neuropathy behave similarly.

Chronic Polyneuropathy with Connective Tissue Diseases In clinics devoted to patients with connective tissue diseases, occasional examples of either subacute or chronic polyneuropathy or mononeuropathy are observed. The latter are usually related to rheumatoid arthritis, and are difficult to distinguish from pressure palsies. A small proportion of patients with rheumatoid arthritis develop a symmetric, predominantly sensory, and variably painful polyneuropathy. Some of the most painful polyneuropathies we have seen, extending over long periods of time, have had only minimal sensory loss, weakness, or reflex changes in the limbs, and the diagnosis has been difficult. An unexpected rise in the CSF protein level or electromyographic evidence of denervation may sometimes be an important lead.

Pallis and Scott have made an extensive study of the patterns of nerve involvement with rheumatoid arthritis. They divide the neuropathies into five groups, according to whether the upper extremity or lower extremity is involved and whether the involvement takes the form of multiple pressure palsies or a distal sensory loss in the digits. They, too, allude to a rare symmetric sensorimotor polyneuropathy. All these complications occur late, after the rheumatoid arthritis has been present for years. Of course, the carpal tunnel syndrome is frequent with rheumatoid arthritis.

Little is known of the mechanism or pathology of the neuropathies associated with rheumatoid arthritis. Several types of arterial lesions have been described in the nerves of these patients, particularly in a rare, subacutely evolving mononeuropathy multiplex which occurs in the setting of long-standing, severe, destructive joint changes and a high titer of rheumatoid factor (Dyck et al.). This angiopathic neuropathy of rheumatoid arthritis and that of lupus erythematosus and polyarteritis have been discussed in a preceding section of this chapter.

Perhaps more of the obscure polyneuropathies fall into this group of connective tissue diseases than is presently realized.

Amyloid Neuropathy Amyloid, defined as an amorphous extracellular substance with specific functional properties and fine fibrillar ultrastructure, has wide medical ramifications. Small amounts of it are often found in routine autopsies of older individuals, hence it must be regarded as an aging phenomenon. More importantly, it is a consequence of many chronic infections and is often associated with multiple myeloma, medullary carcinoma of the thyroid and other malignancies. Then there are hereditary forms, in which no antecedent or associated disease can be discerned. Finally there are sporadic instances in which a peripheral neuropathy is associated with amyloid deposition in the heart, kidneys, and gastrointestinal tract (primary systemic amyloidosis). The peripheral nervous system is regularly affected in the familial and primary systemic forms but not in those secondary to infection.

The following forms of amyloid neuropathy have been identified: (1) chronic familial polyneuropathy, (2) familial amyloidosis with carpal tunnel syndrome, (3) polyneuropathy or carpal tunnel syndrome associated with multiple myeloma, and (4) peripheral neuropathy in primary systemic amyloidosis.

Insofar as the sporadic form of amyloid neuropathy does not differ clinically or pathologically from the familial form, they will be discussed together, under the genetically determined neuropathies (see further on).

Leprous Polyneuritis This is the classic example of an infectious neuritis, being due to the direct invasion of nerves by the acid-fast *Mycobacterium leprae*, and is probably the most common disease of peripheral nerves in the world today. The disease is particularly frequent in India and Central Africa, but there are many lesser endemic foci, including the parts of Florida, Texas, and Louisiana that border on the Gulf of Mexico.

The initial lesion in leprosy is an innocuous-appearing macule or papule, which is often hypopigmented and lacking in sensation and which results from the invasion of cutaneous nerves by *M. leprae*. The disease may progress no further than this stage, which is spoken of as *indeterminate leprosy,* or it may evolve in several ways depending mainly upon the resistance of the host. The bacilli may be locally invasive, producing a circumscribed epithelioid granuloma that implicates cutaneous and subcutaneous nerves and results in a characteristic patch of superficial sensory loss (*tuberculoid leprosy*). The subcutaneous sensory nerves may be palpably enlarged. If a larger nerve in the vicinity of the granuloma is invaded (the ulnar, median, peroneal, and facial nerves are most frequently affected in this way), a senso-

rimotor deficit in the distribution of that nerve is added to the patch of cutaneous anesthesia.

Unchecked proliferation and hematogenous spread of bacilli results in diffuse infiltration of skin, ciliary bodies, testes, lymph nodes, and nerves (*lepromatous leprosy*). Widespread invasion of the cutaneous nerves produces a symmetric pattern of pain and temperature loss, involving the pinnae of the ears, dorsal surfaces of hands, forearms and feet, and anterolateral aspects of the legs—a distribution that is apparently determined by the relative coolness of these parts of the skin. Eventually the anesthesia spreads to involve most of the cutaneous surface. Extensive sensory loss is followed by loss of motor function owing to invasion of muscular nerves where they lie closest to the skin (ulnar nerve is most vulnerable). There is a loss of sweating in areas of sensory loss, but otherwise the autonomic nervous system is unaffected. In distinction to other polyneuropathies, tendon reflexes are usually preserved in leprosy, despite widespread sensory loss. Probably this depends upon sparing of the muscular nerves. Because of widespread anesthesia, injuries may be unrecognized, with resultant infections, trophic changes, and loss of tissue. Variations in host immunity result in patterns of disease having both tuberculoid and lepromatous characteristics (*dimorphous leprosy*).

All forms of leprosy require long-term treatment with sulfones, dapsone (DDS) being the most commonly used.

Polyneuropathy with Hypothyroidism While characteristic disturbances of skeletal muscle are known to complicate hypothyroidism (see Chap. 48), the demonstration of a polyneuropathy has been infrequent. However, a number of elderly myxedematous patients complain of weakness and numbness of feet, legs, and, to a lesser extent, the hands for which no other explanation can be found. Loss of reflexes, diminution in vibratory, joint-position, and touch-pressure sensations, and weakness in the distal parts of the limbs are the usual findings. The neuropathic manifestations are seldom severe. Nerve conduction velocities are significantly diminished, and the protein content of the CSF is usually increased, to more than 100 mg per 100 ml in some patients; probably this is a reflection of the increased protein content of the serum. Convincing evidence of the etiology is the subjective improvement and complete or near-complete reversibility of neuropathic signs following treatment with thyroid hormones. In biopsies of nerve, an edematous protein infiltration of the endoneurium and perineurium, a kind of metachromatic mucoid material, has been seen. Dyck and Lambert noted segmental demyelination in teased fiber preparations, and in electron-microscopic sections, a slight increase in glycogen, acid mucopolysaccharides, and aggregates of glycogen and cytoplasmic laminar bodies in Schwann cells.

GENETICALLY DETERMINED NEUROPATHIES

There has been much difficulty in classifying the chronic familial polyneuropathies. Dyck has proposed a scheme which divides them according to their main clinical features. Three large groups are thus separated: (1) a *pure motor type*, which includes all the progressive spinal muscular atrophies, hitherto called myelopathic motor neuron diseases, (2) a *predominantly sensory type*, often with mutilating trophic lesions, and (3) *mixed sensorimotor and autonomic* abnormalities. The second and third types each include four or five subgroups. All diseases of this general type, which he designates as *system atrophies*, are notable for their hereditary nature, chronicity, fiber loss with few or no products of degeneration, progressivity, and symmetry of involvement.

We are reluctant to group motor system diseases with the neuropathies but would accept the other two categories, the predominantly sensory and sensorimotor groups. We would agree also that the distinction drawn between system atrophies and degenerations in the hereditary neuropathies probably has no validity. Special neuropathologic features such as pseudohypertrophy of nerves are also not acceptable as the basis of classification. Far better in our view is a division of hereditary polyneuropathies into those with an established gene-controlled biochemical mechanism and those in which the biochemical mechanism is unknown. These considerations have influenced us to propose the classification given in Table 45-1. It is evident from that classification that the major proportion of the familial polyneuropathies is of "degenerative" type. Some are associated with certain abnormalities of the CNS, whereas others are relatively pure. For convenience of exposition several of the hereditary metabolic polyneuropathies have already been discussed in Chap. 37, with the metabolic diseases of the nervous system. Here we will consider the other inherited neuropathies.

INHERITED POLYNEUROPATHIES OF PREDOMINANTLY SENSORY TYPE

Common to the several diseases comprising this group are lancinating pains, ulcers of the feet and hands, osteomyelitis of bones of the feet and hands leading to osteolysis, stress fractures, recurrent episodes of cellulitis and lymphangitis, and insensitivity to pain. Since similar symptoms and signs occur in syringomyelia, leprosy, and tabes dorsalis there has been uncertainty in many writings, especially those cited for historical interest, as to whether the reported clinical cases were examples of one or another of these diseases.

According to Dyck and Ohta, Leplat in 1846 described plantar ulcers (*mal perforant du pied*) as did Nélaton in 1852. Morvan in 1883 reported his observations with adult patients who had developed suppuration of the pulps of insensitive fingers (whitlows). It is now generally agreed that Morvan's cases were examples of syringomyelia whereas the family described by Nélaton was probably an example of a recessive form of childhood sensory polyneuropathy, since familial syringomyelia in children is a rarity. Other examples of foot ulceration were later ascribed to lumbar syringomyelia or dysraphism, again an interpretation which has not been supported by postmortem studies. We would agree with Dyck and Ohta that most such cases are examples of sensory polyneuropathy.

Dominant Mutilating Sensory Polyneuropathy in Adults
The characteristics of this group of polyneuropathies include autosomal dominant mode of inheritance; onset in early or middle adult life; normal life expectancy; involvement mainly of feet with calluses of soles and later episodes of blistering, ulceration, and lymphangitis, followed by osteomyelitis and osteolysis; analgesia or shooting pains; distal sensory loss with greater affection of pain and thermal sensation than of touch and pressure; loss of sweating; diminution or absence of tendon reflexes; and only slight loss of muscular strength.

The plantar ulcer under the head of a metatarsal bone is the most dreaded complication and may develop into an osteomyelitis. Infection of the pulp of the fingers and paronychias are uncommon. Some patients have a mild pes cavus and weakness of peroneal and pretibial muscles with foot drop and steppage gait. Lancinating pains may occur in the legs, thighs, and shoulders, and, exceptionally, the pain may last for days and be as disabling as in tabes dorsalis; however, in the majority of patients there is no pain whatsoever. Neural deafness was present in one of Denny-Brown's patients. In the latter case, which was studied postmortem, there was a loss of small nerve cells in the lumbosacral dorsal root ganglia. The spinal roots were thin, and the fibers in the posterior columns of the spinal cord and peripheral nerves were diminished in number. Myelinated fibers and unmyelinated ones were both affected. Both axonal atrophy and segmental demyelination have been demonstrated in teased nerve preparations by Dyck. Sensory nerve conduction is abolished.

Recessive Mutilating Sensory Polyneuropathy of Childhood   Several sibships have been reported with multiple cases of a sensory neuropathy manifested by an apparent insensitivity to pain. Walking is delayed; there is pes cavus deformity and the first movements are ataxic. Ulcerations of tips of toes and fingers and repeated infections of acral parts result in the formation of paronychias and whitlows. The tendon reflexes are absent, but muscular power is well-preserved. Light-touch, pain, thermal, vibratory, and position senses are all impaired in the distal parts of the extremities and trunk. The lesions and electrical findings are similar to those in the dominantly inherited sensory neuropathy.

In both types of sensory neuropathy measures must be taken to prevent stress fractures, acral mutilation, and infection. This is more difficult in the small child who does not fully understand the problem.

Congenital Insensitivity to Pain   In *congenital indifference* to pain, a syndrome in which the patient throughout life seems totally unreactive to the pain of injury, there is no loss of the ability to distinguish pinprick and other painful stimuli from nonpainful ones. Furthermore, the nervous system of such individuals seems to be normal. There is, however, another variety characterized by universal analgesia. In 1963 Swanson et al. described two brothers and about the same time Biemond reported two siblings in whom, in addition to complete *insensitivity* to pain, there was anhidrosis and mild mental retardation. During childhood, Swanson's patients had high fever when the environmental temperature was raised, and one possibly had orthostatic hypotension. One of the patients died in his twelfth year and was found to have an absence of small neurons in the dorsal root ganglia, an absence of Lissauer's tracts, and a decrease in the size of the descending spinal tracts of the trigeminal nerves. Sweat glands were present in the skin but were not innervated. Biemond observed similar neuropathologic changes in an autopsied case. Nothing was said about the anatomic basis of low IQ (70) or the autonomic disorder.

Other Forms of Inherited Sensory Neuropathy   Included here are the neuropathy of Friedreich's ataxia, which has been discussed in Chap. 42, and the Riley-Day syndrome, which is discussed further on in this

chapter, with the neuropathies that have recognized metabolic abnormalities. However, we have seen other unclassifiable examples of an almost pure sensory or sensorimotor type. Some years ago a young man and woman with universal anesthesia affecting head, neck, trunk, and limbs came to our attention (Adams et al.). All forms of sensation were affected. The patients were areflexic but retained full motor power; the movements were ataxic. Autonomic functions were impaired but not abolished. In a sural nerve biopsy nearly all fibers—large and small, myelinated and unmyelinated—had disappeared. Surprisingly there were no trophic changes, ulcers, osteomyelitis, etc. Another of our families with ulcers and loss of digits had a symmetric sensory and motor polyneuropathy of the extremities with areflexia. The inheritance was of dominant type, with onset in adolescence.

We continue to observe unclassifiable cases such as these every year. In general the mutilating effects are the result of injury to analgesic parts of the body.

INHERITED POLYNEUROPATHIES OF MIXED
SENSORIMOTOR-AUTONOMIC TYPES (IDIOPATHIC)

Peroneal Muscular Atrophy (Charcot-Marie-Tooth Disease)   This disease is inherited as an autosomal dominant (occasionally recessive) trait, with onset during late childhood or adolescence. Described in 1886 almost simultaneously by Tooth in England and by Charcot and Marie in France, all their names were attached to it, even though similar cases had been recorded earlier by Eulenberg (1856), Friedreich (1873), Ormerod (1884), and Osler (1880). Because of changes in the spinal cord and its occasional overlap with Friedreich's ataxia, the early observers considered it to be an hereditary myelopathy and did not class it with the neuropathies; but the evidence that supports this latter nosologic grouping is now unassailable.

Essentially this is a chronic degeneration of peripheral nerves and roots, resulting in distal muscle atrophy, beginning in the feet and legs and later involving the hands. The extensor hallucis and digitorum longus, the peronei, and the intrinsic muscles of the feet are affected early and produce an equinovarus deformity and *pied en griffe* (see page 892). Later, all muscles of the legs and sometimes the lower third of the thigh become weak and atrophic. The thin legs have been likened to those of a stork or, if the lower thigh muscles are affected, to an "inverted champagne bottle." Eventually the nerves to the calf muscles degenerate and power of flexion of the feet diminishes. After a period of years, atrophy of hand and forearm muscles develops. The hands become clawed (*main en griffe*). The wasting seldom extends above the elbows or above the middle third of the thighs. Paresthesias and cramps are invariably present to some degree and there is always some impairment of deep and superficial sensation in the feet and hands, shading off proximally, but it may be rather slight in degree. Rarely, the sensory loss is severe, and perforating ulcers may be associated. The tendon reflexes are absent in the involved limbs. The illness progresses very slowly, and it seems to stabilize for long periods.

The walking difficulty, which is the main disability, is due to a combination of sensory ataxia and weakness. Foot drop and instability of the ankles are additional handicaps. The feet and legs may ache after use and cramps may be troublesome, but otherwise pain is exceptional; the feet are often cold, swollen, and blue, secondary to inactivity of the muscles of the feet and legs and their dependent position. There is usually no disturbance of autonomic function. Fixed pupils, optic atrophy, congenital nystagmus and endocrinopathies, epilepsy, and spina bifida, which have been reported occasionally in association with peroneal muscular atrophy, probably represent coincidental hereditary disorders.

The age of onset varies, but we have not seen cases beginning in early childhood. An onset in middle adult life is not unknown, especially in mild forms. When combined with tremor, it may be difficult to draw a line between this disease and the Roussy-Lévy syndrome. One of our patients had a long family history of benign action tremor and peroneal muscular atrophy; but we discovered, in analyzing this genealogy, that some family members had tremor, some had peroneal muscular atrophy, and some had both. Restricted forms are known to affect only the peroneal and pectoral or scapular muscles (scapuloperoneal form of Dawidenkow). Other variants are (1) a rare type which begins in the proximal muscles of the arms (Hanel) and (2) the *"familial claw foot with absent tendon jerks"* of Symonds and Shaw.

Laboratory data are of little help. The CSF is usually normal. Nerve conduction velocities are diminished, and giant polyphasic units are seen in the EMG, with few fibrillation potentials.

Pathologic findings Degenerative changes in the nerves result in depletion of the population of large sensory and motor fibers leaving only the condensed endoneurial connective tissue. As best as one can tell, axons and myelin sheaths are both affected, the distal parts of the nerve more than the proximal. Anterior horn cells are slightly diminished in number and some are chromatolyzed. Dorsal root ganglion cells suffer a similar fate.

The disease involves sensory posterior root fibers with degeneration of the posterior columns of Goll more than of Burdach. The autonomic nervous system remains intact. The muscles contain large fields of atrophic fibers (group atrophy). Some of the larger fibers have a target appearance and may show degenerative changes, a finding which has led some workers to postulate a myopathic effect. We believe such an idea to be untenable because similar changes may follow poliomyelitis, a disease exclusively of motor neurons. Claims of a coincidental myelopathy and degeneration of spinocerebellar and corticospinal tracts probably indicate that the associated disease was really Friedreich's ataxia.

Treatment No treatment is known. Stabilizing the ankles by arthrodeses is indicated if foot drop is severe and the disease has reached the point where it is not progressing. Fitting the legs with light braces and the shoes with springs, to overcome foot drop, can be helpful.

Differential diagnosis and nosologic differentiation involve distal dystrophies (Chap. 49), late forms of familial motor system disease, Friedreich's ataxia, Roussy-Lévy syndrome (Chap. 42), and other familial polyneuropathies.

Progressive Hypertrophic Neuropathy (Déjerine-Sottas Disease) This type of neuropathy is inherited usually as a recessive and occasionally as a dominant trait. It begins in childhood or in infancy, earlier than peroneal muscular atrophy, and is slowly progressive. Pain and paresthesias in the feet are early symptoms, followed by development of symmetric weakness and wasting of the distal portion of the limbs. Talipes equinovarus postures with claw feet as well as claw hands are common. Sensation is impaired in a distal distribution, and the tendon reflexes are absent. Miotic, unreactive pupils, nystagmus, and kyphoscoliosis have been observed in some cases. There are no important changes in autonomic functions. Trunk and cranial parts of the body are spared. The ulnar, median, radial, posterior neck, and peroneal nerves stand out like tendons and are easily followed with the gently roving finger. The enlarged nerves are nontender. Patients are usually much more disabled than with peroneal muscular atrophy and are confined to a wheelchair at an early age.

It is important to emphasize that the occurrence of hypertrophic neuropathy is not confined to the particular inherited disease described above. If one groups all patients in whom the nerves are diffusely enlarged (incorrectly called "hypertrophic"), several different diseases, both genetic and acquired, are included. Enlarged nerves have been described in some cases of recurrent idiopathic polyneuritis, familial amyloidosis, Refsum's disease, peroneal muscular atrophy, and other diseases. Basically any pathologic process that causes recurrent segmental demyelination and subsequent repair and remyelination may have this effect. In some patients with a history of early childhood hereditary polyneuropathy, the nerves are not palpably enlarged, yet the diagnosis can be established by biopsy of a cutaneous nerve. In Déjerine-Sottas disease the CSF protein is persistently elevated for the reason that the spinal roots are affected. Indeed they may enlarge to the point of blocking the subarachnoid space and compressing the spinal cord. Nerve conduction velocities are markedly reduced in this disease even when there is little or no functional impairment. The treatment is purely symptomatic.

Under the microscope the enlargement of nerves is seen to be due to a great increase in connective tissue (perineurial more than epineurial) and the fields of collagen often appear impregnated with an amorphous eosinophilic protein precipitate resembling mucus. However the identifying lesion is the "onion bulb" which consists of a whorl of overlapping, intertwined, attenuated, Schwann cell processes which encircle naked or finely medullated axons. Onion bulbs are seen in recurrent polyneuritis, Refsum's disease (see below), certain instances of peroneal muscular atrophy, and other remitting and relapsing polyneuropathies in either diffuse or localized forms.

Hereditary Areflexic Dystasia (Roussy-Lévy Syndrome)
In 1926 Roussy and Lévy reported seven cases of a familial malady of singular symptomatology that had not previously been described. Its close relation to Friedreich's ataxia and the amyotrophy of Charcot-Marie was recognized. For many years thereafter—in fact until the present day—the existence of this entity was, by reason of these latter relationships, disputed; and the original authors felt called upon to defend their thesis twice more in the medical literature.

The condition in question is a sensory ataxia (dystasia) with pes cavus and areflexia, affecting mainly the lower legs and later progressing to involve the hands. Some degree of sensory loss, mainly of vibratory and position sense, has been described in all cases. Atrophy of the muscles of the legs, with the electrical reactions of

denervation, are prominent. None of the patients has had evidence of cerebellar ataxia. Kyphoscoliosis is described in several. The abdominal reflexes are preserved, but in some an uncertain extensor plantar reflex has been obtained on one or the other side. Although the feet may be cold or slightly discolored, no autonomic effects are documented. The nerves are not palpably enlarged. Electrocardiographic abnormalities similar to those of Friedreich's ataxia have been noted in one family. Action tremor is variable.

The onset of many cases is during infancy, possibly dating from birth; the course is benign. Lapresle was able to find and reexamine four of the original seven cases of Lévy and Roussy 30 years later, and found that the condition had changed little if at all in its general format. There are no complete postmortem studies.

The authors have been faced repeatedly with the question of diagnosis of this syndrome when a patient has presented with either an ataxic gait or pes cavus and leg atrophy but without the usual signs of Friedreich's ataxia or of peroneal muscular atrophy. The pattern of inheritance, slow course, lack of cerebellar, brainstem, and corticospinal tract signs, and prominence of atrophy serve to exclude Friedreich's ataxia. The very early onset, prominence of a "tabetic" picture with sensory ataxia yet definite atrophy, and the kyphoscoliosis, differentiate it from peroneal muscular atrophy. Our position is that it represents another type of chronic familial neural atrophy of different onset and course than peroneal muscular atrophy, but until a specific biochemical defect of one or the other disease has been discovered, final differentiation is impossible. We are not impressed with the recorded evidence of a myelopathy with pyramidal involvement in either peroneal muscular atrophy or the dystasia of Roussy-Lévy, based as it is on the interpretation of a wavering plantar reflex in a deformed foot with contracture of long extensor muscles of the great toes.

INHERITED POLYNEUROPATHIES WITH A RECOGNIZED METABOLIC DISORDER

Heredopathia Atactica Polyneuritiformis (Refsum's Disease) This is a rare disorder which is inherited as an autosomal recessive trait and has its onset in late childhood, adolescence, or early adult life. Diagnosis is based on a combination of clinical manifestations—retinitis pigmentosa, cerebellar ataxia, and chronic polyneuropathy, coupled with an increase in blood phytanic acid. Cardiomyopathy and neurogenic deafness are present in most patients and pupillary abnormalities, cataracts, and ichthyotic skin changes are present in some. Also, anosmia and night blindness with constriction of the visual fields may precede the neuropathy by many years. Usually the latter develops gradually, sometimes rapidly. The polyneuropathy is sensorimotor, distal, and symmetric in distribution, affecting the legs more than arms. All forms of sensation are reduced and tendon reflexes are lost. The CSF protein is moderately increased.

Although the nerves may not be palpably enlarged, "hypertrophic" changes with onion bulb formation are invariable pathologic features. A metabolic defect in the utilization of dietary phytol—the increase of which was discovered by Klenk and Kahlke—has been corroborated by Steinberg et al. and by others; a failure of oxidation of phytanic acid, a tetramethylated 16-carbon fatty acid, allows its accumulation. The relation between this increase in phytanic acid and the polyneuropathy is uncertain. Clinical diagnosis is confirmed by the finding of increased phytanic acid in the blood; the normal level is less than 0.3 mg per 100 ml, but in patients with this disease it constitutes 5 to 30 percent of the total fatty acids of the serum lipids. Diets low in phytol may be beneficial, but this is difficult to judge, for after an acute attack there may be a natural remission. In other patients there is a very slow and gradual progression of the disease, and in still others a more rapid progression with death from cardiac complications.

Abetalipoproteinemia (Bassen-Kornzweig Syndrome, Acanthocytosis) This rare, autosomal recessive disorder is characterized by (1) near-absence of β-lipoprotein and a low level of cholesterol in the serum, (2) retinal (macular) degeneration, (3) acanthocytosis (a thorny or spiky appearance of the red cells, best seen in wet preparations of fresh blood), and (4) a chronic, progressive neurologic deficit, usually beginning in childhood.

Patients with this disorder first come to medical attention as infants because of steatorrhea and retarded growth. The brunt of the neurologic disorder falls upon the cerebellum and peripheral nervous system. The first neurologic finding is diminution or absence of tendon reflexes detected as early as the second year of life. Later, when the patient is able to cooperate in sensory testing, a loss of vibratory and position sense is found in the legs. Cerebellar signs (ataxia of gait, trunk and extremities, titubation of the head and dysarthria), muscle weakness, ophthalmoparesis, Babinski signs, and loss of pain and temperature sense are the other neurologic abnormalities, in more or less this order of frequency. Mental backwardness occurs in some patients. There are no signs of autonomic disorder. Irregular progression occurs over a few years and many patients are no longer able to stand and walk by the time they reach adolescence.

Skeletal abnormalities include pes cavus and kyphoscoliosis, which are secondary to the neuropathy. Constriction of the visual fields and ring scotomata are manifestations of the macular degeneration and retinitis pigmentosa. Cardiac enlargement and failure are serious and late complications.

Neuropathologic findings consist of *demyelination of peripheral nerves* and degeneration of nerve cells in the spinal gray matter and cerebellar cortex. Diagnosis is confirmed by the finding of acanthocytes, low serum cholesterol, and β (low-density)-lipoproteins. What is known about the pathogenesis and treatment is discussed in Chap. 37 (page 686).

A closely related disease, also with familial hypobetalipoproteinemia, has been described by van Buchem et al. It is associated with a malabsorption syndrome, an ill-defined weakness, ataxia and dysesthesia of the legs, and Babinksi signs, but no sensory loss.

Tangier Disease This is an exceedingly rare familial disorder which also is inherited as a recessive trait. It is marked by a deficiency of α-lipoprotein, low cholesterol, diminution of phospholipids, and high triglyceride levels in the serum. The presence of enlarged, yellow-orange (cholesterol-laden) tonsils is said to be a constant manifestation. About half of the reported cases have had neuropathic symptoms, taking the form of an asymmetric sensorimotor neuropathy, which fluctuates in severity. The polyneuropathy may come in attacks, viz., is recurrent, as in the two sisters reported by Engel et al.; onset of symptoms was in childhood and in infancy, respectively. The sensory loss is predominantly for pain and temperature and extends over the entire body and at times the face. Tactile and proprioceptive sensory modalities tend to be preserved.

The muscular weakness affects either the lower or upper extremities, or both, and particularly the hand muscles, which may undergo atrophy and show denervation potentials by EMG. Nerve conduction is slowed. Tendon reflexes are lost or diminished. Facial muscles may be involved. Transient ptosis and diplopia have been reported.

Fat-laden macrophages are present in the bone marrow and elsewhere. No complete pathologic studies are available. There is no known treatment.

Anderson-Fabry Disease (Fabry's Disease) The genetic and metabolic aspects of this inherited disorder have already been considered (page 698). Here, some additional remarks will be made about the painful neuropathic component.

The pain, which is usually the initial symptom in childhood and adolescence, often has a burning quality or occurs in brief lancinating jabs, mostly in the fingers and toes, and may be accompanied by paresthesias of the palms and soles. Changes in environmental temperature and extreme exertion may induce pain. These abnormalities are due to the accumulation of glycolipid (ceramide trihexoside) in peripheral nerves, both perineurally and intraneurally, as well as in the cells of the spinal ganglia and the anterior and intermediolateral horns of the spinal cord. Ohnishi and Dyck have demonstrated a preferential loss of small myelinated and unmyelinated fibers and small cell bodies of dorsal root ganglia. Involvement of these latter cells and the associated degenerative changes in the afferent fibers are thought to be the likely cause of the painful sensory phenomena (Kahn).

Later in the illness there occur progressive impairment of renal function (usually mild in degree) and cerebral and myocardial infarction, but the most characteristic feature is an eruption of dark red macules and papules, up to 2 mm in diameter, over the trunk and limbs, most closely clustered over the thighs and lower trunk (*angiokeratoma corporis diffusum*).

Phenytoin or carbamazepine (Tegretol) may be helpful in alleviating the pain and dysesthesias, but there is no specific therapy for the disease.

Metachromatic Leukodystrophy (see also Chap. 37) Massive sulfatide accumulation throughout the central and peripheral nervous systems, and to a lesser extent in other organs, occurs in this disorder, apparently because of congenital absence of the degradative enzyme, sulfatase. The abnormality is transmitted as an autosomal recessive trait. Progressive cerebral deterioration is the most obvious clinical aspect, but hyporeflexia, muscular atrophy, and diminished nerve conduction velocity are expressive of a neuropathy. Early in the course of the illness, the weakness, hypotonia, and areflexia may suggest Werdnig-Hoffmann disease; in older children there may be a complaint of paresthesias and demonstrable sensory loss. Bifacial weakness has been reported. Sensory and motor conduction velocities are slowed. Metachromatically staining granules accumulate in the cytoplasm of Schwann cells in all peripheral nerves, as well as in the central white matter. Sural biopsy may be used

to establish the diagnosis, even early in the course of the illness.

Familial Dysautonomia (Riley-Day Disease) This is a recessively inherited disorder which affects Jewish children predominantly. The condition is manifest at birth (poor sucking, failure to thrive, unexplained fever, episodes of pneumonia). Hyporeflexia and impairment or loss of pain and temperature sensation with relative preservation of pressure and touch modalities are the main neuropathic manifestations. Motor fibers are probably involved as well, but only to a slight degree, shown less by weakness than reduced conduction velocity in peripheral nerves. The neuropathy at a later age continues to be overshadowed by the other manifestations of the disease which include repeated infections and abnormalities of the autonomic nervous system (lack of flow of tears and corneal ulceration, blotchiness of skin, defective temperature control, cold hands and feet, excessive sweating, lability of blood pressure, hypertension and postural hypotension, difficulty in swallowing, esophageal and intestinal dilatation, emotional instability, recurrent vomiting, and stunted growth). The tongue shows an absence of fungiform papillae.

Nerve biopsy reveals a diminution in small myelinated and unmyelinated fibers, which explains the impairment of pain and temperature sensation. In autopsy material, sympathetic and parasympathetic ganglion cells and, to a lesser extent, nerve cells in the sensory ganglia are diminished in number. Patients excrete increased amounts of homovanillic acid and decreased amounts of vanillylmandelic acid and methoxyhydroxyphenylglycol. Weinshilboum and Axelrod have shown a significant decrease in serum dopamine β-hydroxylase, the enzyme that converts dopamine to norepinephrine. There is no treatment for the disease.

Other examples of congenital polyneuropathy with absence of autonomic function, probably different from the above diseases and the Riley-Day dysautonomia, have been reported. A congenital failure of development of neural elements derived from the neural crests is postulated.

The Amyloid Neuropathies *Familial amyloid polyneuropathy* Andrade, in 1937, discovered that a chronic familial illness, known as "foot disease" among the inhabitants of Oporto, Portugal, was actually a special type of amyloid polyneuropathy. He was not the first to have seen amyloid in degenerating nerve but deserves credit for identifying the disease as one of the heredofamilial polyneuropathies. By 1969 he had studied 148 sibships including 623 individuals among whom there were

249 with polyneuropathy. Descendants of this family have been traced to Africa, France, and Brazil. Soon other foci of the disease were reported in Japan (Araki et al.), in the United States (by Kantarjian and DeJong), in Germany (Delank et al.) and in Poland, Greece, and Sweden. As far as one can tell these are separate unrelated probands in different ethnic groups. The pattern of inheritance in all instances is autosomal dominant; males and females are affected with about equal frequency.

Cohen and Benson, whose review contains the important references to this subject, are impressed with the degree to which the lower extremities are affected and they distinguish this group from two others—one in which the hands (rarely arms) are involved and another which affects first the legs and later the arms, as occurs in the large group of cases in the United States recorded by Van Allen et al. The authors question the validity of this division, for in all of our patients the lower extremities were affected first and more severely and the disease extended to the hands and arms much later. Thus, the patients would fall at first into one category and then into another. We suggest that these two apparent categories are but different phases of one disorder. The type affecting the hands alone, the carpal tunnel syndrome, is a special problem.

The age of onset of familial amyloid polyneuropathy is between 25 and 35 years. The disease progresses slowly and terminates fatally in 10 to 15 or more years. The initial symptoms are usually numbness, paresthesias, and sometimes pain in the feet and lower legs. Weakness is minimal, and the tendon reflexes, while diminished, may not be lost early in the course of the illness. Unlike most other polyneuropathies, pain and temperature sensation are reduced more than touch, vibration, and position (pseudosyringomyelia). Autonomic involvement stands as another characteristic—loss of pupillary light reflexes and miosis, anhidrosis, vasomotor paralysis with orthostatic hypotension, alternating diarrhea and constipation, and impotence. These autonomic changes tend to be more extensive than the sensory ones. Difficulty in walking also develops, and has its basis in a combination of faulty position sense and mild muscle weakness. Later, tendon reflexes are abolished and the legs become thin. The nerves are not enlarged.

Cases vary somewhat. Irregularities in cardiac rhythm due to bundle branch or AV block and cardiac enlargement occur early in some and late in others. Weight loss may be pronounced, owing to anorexia and disordered bowel function and the later development of a malabsorption syndrome, and the liver may become enlarged. Vitreous opacities (veils, specks, and strands) may progress to blindness, but this has been rare, and in a few there has been an impairment of hearing. Albuminuria, the nephrotic syndrome, and uremia terminate life in a few of the patients. The CSF may be normal or have an elevated protein content (50 to 200 mg per 100 ml); the blood is normal except for anemia in cases of amyloidosis of the bone marrow.

The neuropathic picture in patients with *primary systemic amyloidosis* is much the same as that of hereditary amyloid polyneuropathy. The former type is more frequent in men (27 of 31 cases reported by Kelly et al.) and, as a rule, has a considerably later age of onset (mean age 63 years) than the familial type. About one-half of the sporadic cases present with neuropathic symptoms and signs and the other half with renal, cardiac, hematologic, or gastrointestinal complications, which are usually responsible for the patient's death.

Familial amyloidosis with carpal tunnel syndrome Falls et al. in 1955 and later Rukavina et al have described a large group of patients of Swiss stock living in Indiana who developed, in the fourth and fifth decades, a characteristic syndrome of acroparesthesias due to deposition of amyloid in the connective tissues in and beneath the carpal ligaments. There was sensory loss and atrophic muscle weakness in the distribution of the median nerves, which were compressed. Section of the carpal ligaments relieved the symptoms. Some of the patients were said to have later developed an involvement of other nerves of the upper extremities. Vitreous deposits were frequent in this form of the disease.

Multiple myeloma with amyloid neuropathy Although multiple myeloma is frequently associated with amyloidosis or with a symmetric sensorimotor polyneuropathy that is not due to infiltration with myeloma cells, amyloid neuropathy as a complication of myeloma has proved to be extremely rare. In the few such cases that have been seen, the clinical and pathologic manifestations did not differ from amyloid neuropathy of other type. Bilateral median nerve compression due to amyloid deposition in the carpal ligaments is a relatively frequent complication of myeloma, however.

Other unclassifiable syndromes We have observed two cases of amyloid neuropathy in elderly persons with diabetes mellitus. Severe, chronic, sensorimotor, areflexive polyneuropathy with slightly enlarged nerves and elevated CSF protein were the identifying features. The diabetes was moderately severe and difficult to control and ended fatally, due presumably to Kimmelstiel-Wilson lesions in the kidney.

In the syndrome of urticaria, deafness and amyloid nephropathy (described by Muckle and Wells), in the syndrome of progressive amyloid cardiopathy, and in that of amyloid nephropathy, the peripheral nerves may also be affected, but only late in the course of the disease. Localized trigeminal neuropathy due to amyloid deposition in the gasserian ganglion has been reported (Daly et al.).

Pathologic findings In familial amyloid polyneuropathy amyloid deposits are demonstrable in the blood vessels and interstitial (endoneurial) tissues of the peripheral somatic and autonomic nerves, and in the spinal and autonomic ganglia and roots. There is loss of nerve fibers, the unmyelinated and small myelinated ones being more depleted than the large myelinated ones. The anterior horn and sympathetic ganglion cells are swollen and chromatolysed due to involvement of axons, and the posterior columns of the spinal cord degenerate.

The pathogenesis of the fiber loss is not fully understood. On the basis of their findings in a sporadic case of amyloid polyneuropathy, Kernohan and Woltman suggested that amyloid deposits in the walls of the small arteries and arterioles interfered with the circulation in the nerves and that amyloid neuropathy was essentially an ischemic neuropathy. In other cases, however, the vascular changes are relatively slight and the degeneration of the nerve fibers appears to be related to their compression and distortion by the endoneurial deposits of amyloid. Amyloid is also seen in the tongue, gums, heart, gastrointestinal tract, kidneys, and many other organs.

In all the amyloid polyneuropathies, the only specific diagnostic test is skin, muscle, gingival or rectal mucosa biopsy, in which amyloid can be demonstrated by appropriate stains and electron microscopy. The serum proteins are not altered (except in multiple myeloma and the paraproteinemias), nor are there other changes in the blood. An extra chromosome with a subterminal centromere was seen in 10 percent of the dividing marrow cells in the German cases of lower limb amyloid polyneuropathy.

In personally observed cases we have been impressed with the prominence of autonomic effects, the

pseudosyringomyelia, and the relative sparing of motor nerves and retention of reflexes, at least early in the disease. The constellation of these clinical features should always raise suspicion of the disease. Diagnosis is affirmed by the demonstration of amyloid in the vitreous, by the abnormal ECG, renal abnormalities, and biopsy.

Unfortunately, there is no specific therapy. Life is prolonged by medical measures to maintain renal and cardiac function, the use of fludrocortisone acetate (Florinef) to prevent orthostatic syncope, and nutritional supplements to counteract weight loss.

SYNDROME OF CHRONIC RELAPSING POLYNEUROPATHY

Two diseases most regularly take this form: idiopathic polyneuritis and porphyria, in which the attacks recur spontaneously or because of the administration of barbiturates. Other rare examples are Refsum's disease and Tangier disease. Idiopathic polyneuritis has no proved cause; enlargement of nerves may occur with repeated attacks, and it is probable that some patients classed originally as Déjerine-Sottas disease fall into this category. Also it is obvious that patients who have recovered from an episode of alcoholic-nutritional or toxic polyneuropathy may develop a recurrence of their disease if subjected again to intoxication or nutritional deficiency.

DIFFERENTIAL DIAGNOSIS OF THE CHRONIC POLYNEUROPATHIES

This is the group that has given the authors the most difficulty. We would agree with Prineas, who analyzed all the cases of polyneuropathy in two general hospitals in Newcastle-upon-Tyne over a period of 10 years, that the cause of most of the acute and many of the subacute and relapsing forms can usually be established by the clinical and laboratory methods presently available in teaching centers. It is the chronic ones which may continue to baffle the neurologist despite the respectable advances that have been made in this field of medicine.

Of course, many of the chronic polyneuropathies are heredofamilial, the recessive types tending to begin in early childhood, the dominant ones in late childhood, adolescence, and early adult life. With the genealogic data, the diagnosis of the hypertrophic polyneuropathy of Déjerine-Sottas and the peroneal muscular atrophy of Charcot-Marie-Tooth, the two major types, can usually be made on clinical grounds alone. Sporadic cases become more difficult but can be categorized usually on the basis of biometric and clinical data, aided by electromyography, nerve conduction studies, CSF examination, and nerve and muscle biopsy.

The several new but rare chronic hereditary diseases of nerve express themselves mainly by three syndromes: (1) progressive pseudosyringomyelic syndrome with autonomic paralysis, (2) progressive sensorimotor paralysis, and (3) chronic sensory polyneuropathy with ataxia.

One should always suspect familial amyloidosis and Riley-Day dysautonomia when there is a prominent impairment of autonomic function and of pain and thermal sensation, out of proportion to other sensory and motor symptoms. Each of these diseases can be affirmed by proper laboratory tests. Occasionally, however, we have seen a patient with this syndrome when tests for amyloid and disordered catecholamine metabolism were normal. Bassen-Kornzweig, Tangier, and Refsum's diseases are being entertained as diagnostic possibilities now that the methods for confirming the diagnosis have become more widely available. They are so rare, however, that such a search is seldom rewarding.

The syndrome of chronic sensorimotor paralysis involving legs more than arms and distal parts more than proximal parts should in an adult always lead to a search for occult neoplasia (carcinoma, multiple myeloma, or plasmacytoma) or macroglobulinemia. In exceptional cases, the tumor remains hidden for 2 or 3 years after the onset of neuropathy. In our experience a toxic, endocrine, or nutritional cause is seldom found. Unusual causes of nutritional deficiency, such as celiac disease and other malabsorption syndromes (Whipple's disease, chronic hepatic disease), have usually been obvious enough when present, so that the experienced clinician rarely overlooks them. The most difficult type of case is the older person with a mild nonprogressive sensorimotor polyneuropathy who has mild hypothyroidism, marginally low vitamin B_{12} levels in the blood, a somewhat unbalanced diet, and an abnormal glucose tolerance curve. It is easy to imagine any one of these abnormalities to be relevant, but hard to prove that any one of them is.

In the chronic sensory polyneuropathies—some painful, some not, some very ataxic—the sensory form of occult carcinoma is the primary consideration. Milder degrees may be seen with biliary cirrhosis (xanthomatous polyneuropathy of Thomas and Walker). When confined to the feet and legs, a sporadic example of hereditary sensory neuropathy must be considered. However, there are a few patients that the authors are seeing from year to year in whom the cause is not disclosed by any of the available tests. We have helplessly watched

some of these patients become reduced to a bed and wheelchair existence and others suffer from pain until they become addicted to opiates in spite of our admonitions.

Other peripheral nerve syndromes, whose anatomical bases are not well established, include (1) pure panautonomic polyneuritis (Chap. 26) and (2) possibly myokymia and continuous muscular activity (Chap. 52). Of course, tetany is essentially a peripheral nerve phenomenon, an unstable polarization of the axolemma due to diminished ionized serum calcium.

SYNDROME OF MONONEUROPATHY OR MULTIPLE NEUROPATHY

The distinguishing feature of this group of neuropathies is that one or several individual peripheral nerves is involved by the disease process. The diagnosis rests on the finding of motor, reflex, or sensory changes confined to the territory of a single nerve, and the presence of other data pointing to its causation. A plexus of nerves or part of a plexus may be involved. Certain neuropathies of this group, in which several individual nerves are affected in a random manner (mononeuritis or mononeuropathy multiplex), are due to leprosy, sarcoid, diabetes, and polyarteritis nodosa, and have already been discussed.

COMMON BRACHIAL NEUROPATHIES

Brachial plexus neuropathies comprise an interesting group of neurologic disorders. Some may develop without apparent cause and manifest themselves by sensorimotor derangements ascribable to cords of the plexus. Others result from trauma in which the arm is hyperabducted or the shoulder violently separated from the neck. Difficult births are an important source of traction injuries. Rarely, the brachial plexus or other peripheral nerves may be damaged at the time of electrical injury, either from lightning or from household or industrial sources. Direct compression of parts of the plexus by adjacent skeletal anomalies, fascial bands, or tumors represents another category of plexus injury. Partial plexus derangement may result from a parenteral injection of foreign serum or vaccine. *Neuralgic amyotrophy* of obscure origin, also called paralytic brachial neuritis, stands as a special clinical entity, often difficult to distinguish from other types of brachial pain. Some of these latter are, surprisingly, familial; others occur in epidemic form. There are plexus lesions of presumed toxic nature, as in those which follow heroin injection. Finally, there may be impairment of function of the brachial plexus or portions thereof many months or up to 5 to 10 years after x-ray irradiation.

These introductory remarks are intended to convey the idea that most brachial plexus disorders are due to trauma, tumors, compression, injections of serum, vaccine, or drugs, obscure (viral?) infections, and the delayed effects of radiotherapy.

For the anatomic plan of the brachial plexus and its relation to blood vessels and bony structures one of the more detailed monographs on the peripheral nerves should be consulted. The one by Haymaker and Woodhall is recommended (see references). For quick orientation it is enough to remember that the brachial plexus is formed from the anterior and posterior divisions of cervical roots 5, 6, 7, and 8, and the first thoracic nerve roots (see Fig. 45-5). The fifth and sixth cervical roots merge into the upper trunk, the seventh root forms the middle trunk, and the eighth cervical and first thoracic roots form the lower trunk. Each trunk divides into an anterior and posterior division. The posterior divisions of each trunk unite to form the posterior cord of the plexus. The anterior divisions of the upper and middle trunks unite to form the lateral cord. The anterior division of the lower trunk forms the medial cord. Two important nerves emerge from the upper trunk (dorsal scapular nerve to the rhomboid and levator scapulae muscles, and long thoracic nerve to the anterior serratus). The posterior cord gives rise mainly to the radial nerve. The medial cord gives rise to the ulnar nerve, medial cutaneous nerve to the forearm, and medial cutaneous nerve to the upper arm. This cord lies in close relation to the subclavian artery and apex of the lung and is the part of the plexus most susceptible to traction injuries and to compression by tumors that invade the costoclavicular space. The median nerve is formed by the union of parts of the medial and lateral cords.

Lesions of the Whole Plexus The entire arm is paralyzed and hangs uselessly at the side; the sensory loss is complete below a line extending from the shoulder diagonally downward and medially to the middle third of the upper arm. Biceps, triceps, and finger jerks are abolished. The usual cause is vehicular trauma.

Upper Brachial Plexus Paralysis This is due to injury to the fifth and sixth cervical nerves and roots, caused most commonly by forceful separation of the head and shoulder during difficult delivery, by pressure in the supraclavicular region during anesthesia, by injections of foreign serum or vaccines, and by idiopathic neuralgic amyotrophy. The muscles affected are the biceps, deltoid, brachialis anticus, supinator longus, supraspinatus and infraspinatus, and rhomboids. The arm hangs at the side, internally rotated and extended at the elbow. Hand motion is unaffected. The prognosis for spontaneous recovery is generally good though it may be incomplete; injuries of the upper brachial plexus and spinal roots

Figure 45-5

Diagram of the brachial plexus: the components of the plexus have been separated and drawn out of scale. Note that peripheral nerves arise from various components of the plexus: roots [indicated by (C) 5, 6, 7, 8, and (T) 1]; trunks (upper, middle, lower); divisions (anterior and posterior); and cords (lateral, posterior, and medial). The median nerve arises from the heads of the lateral and medial cords. (From Haymaker and Woodhall.)

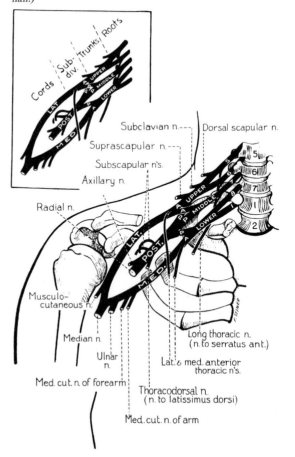

which are incurred at birth (Erb-Duchenne palsy) may persist throughout life.

Lower Brachial Plexus Paralysis   This is usually the result of traction on the abducted arm in falls or during operations on the axilla, or of infiltration or compression by tumors arising from the apex of the lung (superior sulcus or Pancoast's syndrome). Injury may occur during birth, particularly with breech deliveries (Déjerine-Klumpke paralysis). There is weakness and wasting of the small muscles of the hand and a characteristic claw-hand deformity. Sensory loss is limited to the ulnar border of the hand and the inner forearm; and if the first thoracic motor root is involved, there may be an associated paralysis of the cervical sympathetic nerves with a Horner's syndrome.

Lesions of the Cords of the Brachial Plexus (see Fig. 45-5)   A lesion of the *lateral cord* causes weakness of the muscles supplied by the musculocutaneous nerve and the lateral root of the median nerve; it manifests itself mainly as a weakness of flexion and pronation of the forearm. The intrinsic muscles of the hand innervated by the medial root of the median nerve are spared.

A lesion of the *medial cord* causes weakness of muscles supplied by the medial root of the median nerve and the ulnar nerve. The effect is that of a combined median and ulnar nerve palsy. A lesion of the *posterior cord* results in weakness of the deltoid muscle, extensors of the elbow, wrist, and fingers, and sensory loss on the outer surface of the upper arm.

The most frequent causes of injury to the cords are dislocation of the head of the humerus, direct axillary trauma (stab wounds), pressure of a cervical rib, and supraclavicular compression during anesthesia. All cords of the plexus may be injured, or they may be injured in various combinations.

Costoclavicular Syndrome   This is discussed in Chap. 10 (pages 149 to 151).

Brachial Plexus Neuropathy (Neuralgic Amyotrophy, Brachial Neuritis)   This illness, of obscure nature, may develop abruptly in an otherwise healthy individual, or it may complicate an infection, or an injection of serum, vaccine, antibiotic, etc. Magee and DeJong in 1960, and Tsairis et al., in 1972 have reported large series of cases and amplified a well-known clinical picture that the authors have observed repeatedly. Our patients have nearly all been adults ranging from 25 to 65 years of age. Males are slightly more susceptible (2.4:1.0). Beginning as an ache in and around the shoulder, at the root of the neck or base of the skull, and suspected at first of being only a "wry neck," the pain may become severe; it is followed after a period of 3 to 10 days by the rapid development of muscular weakness, sensory changes, and reflex impairment. The pain is made worse by movements which involve the muscles in the region. In a few cases, the neurologic disorder occurs without antecedent pain. Unlike radicular lesions, which almost never cause complete paralysis of a muscle, here a muscle such as the serratus anterior, deltoid, biceps, or triceps may be totally or almost totally paralyzed. Rarely all the muscles of the arm are involved (4 of 99 of Tsairis' cases). Motor nerve conduction becomes slowed in 7 to 10 days. In a small proportion of cases both shoulders and arms are affected. Most of the neurologic deficits in our cases have been localized around the shoulder and upper arm; sometimes the hand has been affected. Either the biceps or triceps reflex may be abolished. The term "neuralgic amyotrophy" was given to this symptom complex by Parsonage and Turner.

Such patients usually have no fever, leukocytosis, or increased sedimentation rate. Occasionally the CSF shows a mild pleocytosis (10 to 50 white blood cells per cubic millimeter) and slightly increased protein, but more often it is entirely normal. Duchowny et al. have described a patient in whom a typical brachial neuritis occurred as part of a febrile illness that proved to be due to cytomegalus virus infection. A few outbreaks have been recorded and have prompted the suggestion that the Coxsackie virus is the cause. No data concerning pathology is available.

The pain usually subsides with the onset of weakness, but in some cases it lasts for weeks. Recovery of paralysis and restoration of sensation are usually complete in a matter of 6 to 12 weeks, but sometimes not for a year or longer. One must differentiate this disorder from the following conditions: spondylosis or ruptured disk with root involvement, brachialgia from bursitis or "cuff syndrome," polymyalgia rheumatica, and serogenic and vaccinogenic plexitis.

Brachial Neuropathy Following Radiotherapy   This is usually a complication of irradiation of the axilla for carcinoma of the breast. Stoll and Andrews studied a group of 117 such patients who were treated with high-voltage, small-field therapy, using either 6300 or 5775 rads in divided doses. Of those receiving the larger dose, 73 percent developed weakness and sensory loss in the hand and fingers between 4 and 30 months after treatment, most of them after 12 months. In one autopsied case, the brachial plexus was ensheathed in dense fibrous tissue; below this zone, both myelin and axons had degenerated (wallerian degeneration), presumably as a result of *entrapment* of nerves in fibrous tissue; possibly a vascular factor was also operative.

Herpes Zoster Plexitis, Neuritis, and Ganglionitis   See Chap. 32.

Serum- and Vaccine-Induced Brachial Neuropathy   Formerly, when animal antisera were in common use, this entity was rather frequent, but now it is a rarity. Three to 10 days after the administration of horse tetanus antitoxin there is the acute onset of severe pain in one or both shoulders and upper arms, coinciding with the development of other systemic manifestations or serum sickness. Several days after the onset of pain, as with brachial neuritis of other types, weakness about the shoulder is noted, usually in the distribution of the upper (lateral) trunk of the brachial plexus. Or there may be only an isolated mononeuropathy (most often of the axillary, suprascapular, musculocutaneous, or long thoracic nerve). The most common isolated palsy is that of the serratus anterior.

Plexitis following vaccines is similar. It has been seen after injection of tetanus toxoid, typhoid-paratyphoid vaccine, triple vaccine (pertussis, diphtheria, and tetanus), and rarely after vaccination for smallpox.

No pathologic data are available. The disease has not been reproduced in the experimental animal Therapy is purely symptomatic. Recovery may occur within a few weeks or may take up to 2 years, or even longer. In 10 to 20 percent of cases there is residual weakness and wasting of the affected muscles.

Heredofamilial Brachial Plexus Neuropathy   This term designates the acute brachial neuropathy that occurs in families. Some of the affected individuals have had multiple attacks with recovery in between. Lower cranial nerve involvement and mononeuropathies in other limbs were conjoined in some instances (see Taylor). Again the clinical course is benign.

Madrid and Bradley have examined the sural nerves from two patients with familial recurrent brachial neuropathy. In teased, single nerve fibers they found sausagelike areas of thickened myelin and redundant loops of myelin with secondary constriction of the axon. In addition, nerve fibers showed a considerable degree of segmental demyelination and remyelination. To this ab-

erration of myelin formation they applied the term "tomaculous neuropathy" (from the Latin *tomaculum*, "sausage"). These changes were not observed in the sural nerve of a sporadic case of recurrent acute brachial plexus neuropathy.

The genetic vulnerability to brachial neuropathy is comparable to the familial occurrence of multiple pressure palsies reported by Earl et al. Indeed, sausage-like swellings of the myelin sheaths have also been found in the nerves of patients with hereditary pressure-sensitive neuropathy (Behse et al.). This would suggest that the nerves of patients with familial brachial plexus neuropathy may also be unduly sensitive to pressure or ischemia. Why the sensitivity should be largely restricted to the brachial plexus is not clear, however.

Brachial Mononeuropathies   *Long thoracic nerve (of Bell)*   This nerve is derived from the fifth, sixth, and seventh cervical nerves and supplies the serratus anterior muscle. Paralysis of this muscle results in winging of the medial border of the scapula when the outstretched arm is pushed forward against resistance, and inability to raise the arm over the head. It is injured most commonly by carrying heavy weights on the shoulder or by strapping the shoulder on the operating table. It is also involved at times in diabetes, serum neuritis, neuralgic amyotrophy (brachial neuritis), or following systemic illnesses. Occasionally it arises de novo.

Suprascapular nerve   This nerve is derived from the fifth (mainly) and sixth cervical nerves and supplies the supraspinatus and infraspinatus muscles. Lesions may be recognized by the presence of atrophy of these muscles and weakness of abduction of the arm (supraspinatus) and of external rotation of the arm at the shoulder joint (infraspinatus). The latter is tested by having the patient flex the forearm and then, pinning the elbow to the side, attempt to move the forearm backward against resistance. This nerve is often involved together with other nerves of the plexus in cases of brachial neuritis. Lesions of this nerve have also been reported in gymnasts and during infectious illnesses.

Axillary nerve   This nerve arises from the posterior cord of the brachial plexus (mainly from C5 root with a smaller contribution from C6) and supplies the teres minor and deltoid muscles. It may be involved in dislocations of the shoulder joint, fractures of the neck of the humerus, serum- and vaccine-induced neuropathies, brachial neuritis, or no cause may be apparent. The anatomic diagnosis depends on recognition of paralysis of abduction of the arm (in testing this function the angle between the side of the chest and the arm must be greater than 15° and less than 90°), wasting of the deltoid muscle, and slight impairment of sensation over the outer aspect of the shoulder.

Musculocutaneous nerve   This nerve is derived from the fifth and sixth cervical roots and is a branch of the lateral cord of the brachial plexus. It innervates the biceps brachii, brachialis, and coracobrachialis muscles. Lesions of the nerve result in wasting of these muscles and weakness of flexion of the supinated forearm. Sensation may be impaired along the radial and volar aspects of the forearm (lateral cutaneous nerve). Isolated lesions of this nerve are usually the result of fracture of the humerus.

Radial nerve   This nerve is derived from the sixth to eighth (mainly the seventh) cervical roots and, as was stated, is the termination of the posterior cord of the brachial plexus. It innervates the triceps, brachioradialis, and supinator muscles; the extensor muscles of the wrist and fingers; and the abductor of the thumb. A complete radial nerve lesion results in paralysis of extension of the elbow, flexion of the elbow when this movement is attempted with the forearm midway between pronation and supination (due to paralysis of the brachioradialis muscle), supination of the forearm, extension of the wrist and fingers, and extension and abduction of the thumb. Sensation is impaired over the posterior aspects of the forearm and a small area over the radial aspect of the dorsum of the hand. The nerve may be injured in the axilla, for example in "crutch" palsy, but is more frequently compressed at a lower point where the nerve winds around the humerus. Common types of injury at this latter site are pressure palsies incurred during sleep and fractures. It is susceptible to lead intoxication and is frequently involved as part of a neuralgic amyotrophy.

Median nerve   This nerve is derived from the fifth cervical to the first thoracic roots, but mainly from the sixth cervical root, and is formed by the union of the medial and lateral cords of the brachial plexus. It innervates the pronators of the forearm, long finger flexors, and abductor and opponens muscles of the thumb, and it is a sensory nerve to the palmar aspect of the hand. Complete interruption of the median nerve results in inability to pronate the forearm or flex the hand in a radial direction, in paralysis of flexion of the index finger and terminal phalanx of the thumb, in weakness of flexion of the remaining fingers, in weakness of abduction and opposition of the thumb, and in sensory impairment over the radial two-thirds of the palmar aspect of the hand and over the dorsum of the distal phalanges of the index

and third fingers. The nerve may be injured in the axilla by dislocation of the shoulder and in any part of its course by stab, gunshot, or other types of wounds. The wrist is the most common site of external injury. Compression of the nerve at the wrist (carpal tunnel syndrome) may be the result of occupational exposure to repeated trauma; of infiltration of the transverse carpal ligament with amyloid (as occurs in multiple myeloma); or of thickening of connective tissue in cases of rheumatoid arthritis, acromegaly, and hypothyroidism. Frequently, the cause of the carpal tunnel syndrome is not apparent. Incomplete lesions of the median nerve between the axilla and wrist may result in causalgia (see below).

Ulnar nerve   This nerve is derived from the eighth cervical and first thoracic roots. It innervates the ulnar flexor of the wrist, the ulnar half of the deep finger flexors, the adductors and abductors of the fingers, the adductor of the thumb, the third and fourth lumbricals, and muscles of the hypothenar eminence. Complete ulnar paralysis is manifested by a characteristic claw-hand deformity, the result of wasting of the small hand muscles and hyperextension of the fingers at the metacarpophalangeal joints and flexion at the interphalangeal joints. The flexion deformity is most pronounced in the fourth and fifth fingers, since the lumbrical muscles of the second and third fingers, supplied by the median nerve, counteract the deformity. Sensory loss occurs over the fifth finger, the ulnar aspect of the fourth finger, and the ulnar border of the palm.

The ulnar nerve is most commonly injured at the elbow, by fracture or dislocation involving the joint. *Delayed ulnar palsy* may occur many years after an injury to the elbow which has resulted in a cubitus valgus deformity of the joint. Because of the deformity, the nerve is stretched in its groove over the ulnar condyle, and its more superficial location renders it vulnerable to compression. A shallow ulnar groove, quite apart from abnormalities of the elbow joint, may expose the nerve to compressive injury. Anterior transposition of the ulnar nerve is a simple and effective form of treatment for these types of ulnar palsy. Yet another site of compression is just distal to the medial epicondyle, where the ulnar nerve runs beneath the aponeurosis of the flexor carpi ulnaris (cubital tunnel). Flexion at the elbow causes a narrowing of the tunnel and constriction of the nerve. This type of ulnar palsy is treated by incising the aponeurotic arch between the olecranon and medial epicondyle. Prolonged pressure on the ulnar part of the palm may result in damage to the deep palmar branch of the ulnar nerve, causing weakness of small hand muscles but no sensory loss. The site of the lesion is localizable by nerve conduction studies.

Causalgia is the name applied by Weir Mitchell to a rare (except in time of war) type of peripheral neuralgia consequent upon partial injury to the median or ulnar nerve, and occasionally the sciatic nerve. It is characterized by intense burning pain in the hand or foot, most pronounced in the digits, palm of the hand, or sole. These parts are exquisitely sensitive to contactual stimuli, so the patient cannot bear the contact of clothing or drafts of air; even ambient heat or cold or noise intensify the causalgic symptoms. The affected extremity is kept protected and immobile, often wrapped in a cloth moistened with cool water. Sudomotor and vasomotor abnormalities are the rule. The skin of the affected part is moist and warm or cool and soon becomes shiny and smooth, at times scaly and discolored. The most plausible explanation of causalgic pain is that it is due to a short-circuiting of impulses, the result of an artificial connection between efferent sympathetic and sensory somatic fibers at the point of the nerve injury. This theory would explain not only the vasomotor and sudomotor abnormalities, but the exacerbations of pain with all types of emotional stimuli. "True causalgia" of this type can be counted upon to respond favorably to procaine block of the appropriate sympathetic ganglia and, over the long run, to regional sympathectomy.

The term *causalgia* should be applied only to the painful burning syndrome that follows injury to a major nerve in the extremity and not to the less clear-cut variations of this disorder that follow less specific forms of trauma. The latter, which are characterized by varying degrees of cyanosis, edema, excessive sweating, and trophic changes in the painful extremity, have been described under a plethora of titles—Sudeck's atrophy, minor causalgia syndrome, shoulder-hand syndrome, reflex dystrophy, and sympathetic dystrophy, to mention the more common ones. In some of these cases, as in "true" causalgia, complete relief from pain and modification of the physical abnormalities can be obtained with sympathetic block; but in others, this response is lacking.

Under the title of *migrant sensory neuropathy*, Wartenberg described an ascending neuritis beginning in the foot or hand and involving sensory nerves. It can be extremely painful, even causalgic. The findings are predominantly sensory. The pathology and cause are unknown. After months, the condition remits, presumably with regeneration.

LUMBOSACRAL PLEXUS AND CRURAL NEUROPATHIES

The twelfth thoracic, first to fifth lumbar, and first, second, and third sacral spinal nerve roots compose the lumbosacral plexuses and innervate the muscles of the lower extremities (see Fig. 45-6). The following are the common plexus and crural nerve palsies.

Lumbosacral Plexus Lesions Extending as it does from the upper lumbar area to the lower sacrum and passing near several lower abdominal and pelvic organs, this plexus is exposed to a number of injuries and diseases, most of them secondary. The cause of involvement may be difficult to ascertain, because the primary disease is not within reach of the palpating fingers, either from the anterior abdominal side or through anus and vagina; even refined radiologic techniques may not reveal it. Differential diagnosis involves exclusion of spinal root (cauda equina) lesions by examination of CSF and myelography. The clinical findings help to focus studies on the appropriate part of the lumbosacral plexus. Valuable diagnostic aids include the presence of autonomic disturbances (present with nerve but not with root lesions), roentgenograms of spine, bone scans, aortic arteriography, intravenous pyelography, barium enema, and electromyography.

Characteristically, plexus lesions produce unilateral muscle weakness and sensory and reflex changes that are not confined to the territory of a single root or nerve. If pain is present, it may occasionally be accentuated by straight leg raising (Lasègue's sign) or movement of the hip, but raising the intraspinal pressure by coughing, sneezing, and jugular compression has no effect on it. The main effects of upper plexus lesions are a weakness of flexion and adduction of the thigh, and of extension of the leg, with sensory loss over the anterior thigh and leg; these effects must be distinguished from the symptoms of femoral neuropathy (see below). Lower plexus lesions weaken the posterior thigh, leg, and foot muscles and abolish sensation over the first and second sacral segments (sometimes the lower sacral segments also). Lesions of the entire plexus, which occur infrequently, cause a weakness or paralysis of all leg muscles, with atrophy, areflexia, anesthesia from toes to perianal region, and autonomic loss with warm, dry skin. Usually there is edema of the leg as well.

The types of lesions that involve the lumbosacral plexus are rather different than those affecting the cervical plexus. Trauma is a rarity except with massive pelvic, spine, and abdominal injuries, because the plexus is so well protected. Occasionally a pelvic fracture will damage the sciatic nerve as it issues from the plexus. In contrast, some part of the plexus may be damaged during surgical procedures on abdominal and pelvic organs, for reasons that may not be entirely clear. For example, hysterectomy has on a number of occasions led to neurologic consultation in our hospitals because of numbness and weakness of the anterior thigh. Either the cords of the upper part of the plexus were compressed by retraction against the psoas muscle or, in vaginal hysterectomy (when thighs are flexed, abducted, and externally rotated), the femoral nerve was compressed against the inguinal ligament. A similar type of injury may be associated with childbirth. Lumbar sympathectomy has also been associated with upper plexus lesions; the most disabling sequelae are burning pain and hypersensitivity of the anterior thigh. Appendectomy, pelvic explorations, and hernial repair may injure branches of the upper plexus (ilioinguinal, iliohypogastric, and genitofemoral nerves), with severe pain and slight sensory loss in the

distribution of one of these nerves. The pain may last for months or a year or more.

The lumbar plexus may be compressed by an aortic, atherosclerotic aneurysm. Usually there is pain which radiates to the hip, anterior thigh, and occasionally to the flank. Slight weakness in hip flexion and altered sensation over the anterior thigh are the findings on examination. Plexus involvement with tumors is commonplace and at times presents special difficulties in diagnosis. Carcinoma of both the cervix and the prostate may seed itself along the perineurial lymphatics and cause much pain in the groin, thigh, knee, or back without much in the way of sensory, motor, or reflex loss. The pain may be bilateral. The CSF and spinal canal (by myelography) are normal. Testicular, uterine, and colonic tumors, or retroperitoneal lymphomas, by extending along the paravertebral gutter, implicate various parts of the lumbosacral plexus. The neurologic symptoms are projected at a distance in the leg, and may or may not be confined to the territory of any one nerve. Pelvic and rectal examinations may be negative and intravenous pyelography and visualization of the lym-

Figure 45-6

Diagram of the lumbar plexus (left) *and the sacral plexus* (right). *The lumbosacral trunk is the liaison between the lumbar and the sacral plexuses. The three divisions of the sciatic nerve are indicated. (From Haymaker and Woodhall.)*

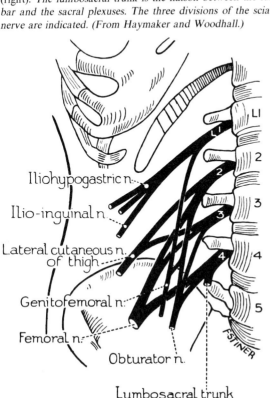 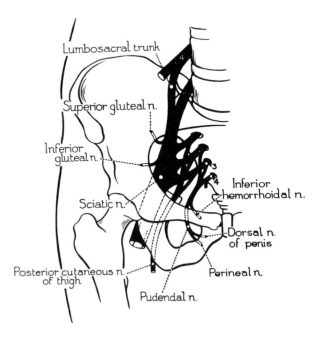

phatic system may be the only means of showing such lesions. If all these examinations are negative, exploratory laparotomy may be necessary.

Reference has already been made to femoral nerve injury during parturition, but other puerperal complications are also observed. Back pain in the latter part of pregnancy is common, but there are rare instances in which the patient complains of severe pain in the back of one or both thighs during labor, and after delivery has numbness and weakness of the leg muscles, with diminished ankle jerks. The attribution of these symptoms to pressure of the fetal head on the sacral portion of the plexus(es) is conjectural. Protrusion of an intervertebral disk may also occur during delivery.

A *neuralgic amyotrophy* or *lumbosacral plexitis,* analogous to the brachial variety, is also observed from time to time. After causing widespread unilateral or bilateral sensory, motor, and reflex changes, lumbosacral plexitis may leave the patient with dysesthesias which are as troublesome as those following herpes zoster (which may also occur at this level). Some patients have had an exploration of the cauda equina (for ruptured disk) even though loss of sweating and warmth of feet should have indicated interruption of autonomic fibers by lesions in peripheral nerves. *Diabetic amyotrophy,* due to involvement of the lumbar plexus(es), has a vascular origin, but probably there are also nondiabetic vascular lesions, which give rise to algesic paresis of proximal muscles. The plexus lesions of polyarteritis nodosa, unilateral or bilateral, may also be manifest as a mononeuropathy multiplex. The incidence of mononeuropathy multiplex in diabetes rises if there is associated occlusive vascular disease of the lower extremities (80 to 90 percent according to Hutchinson and Liversedge). Diabetic mononeuropathy multiplex is discussed in an earlier part of this chapter and protruded intervertebral disk syndromes are described in Chap. 10.

Lateral Cutaneous Nerve of the Thigh   This nerve is derived from the second and third lumbar roots. It is a sensory nerve supplying the anterolateral aspect of the thigh, from the level of the inguinal ligament almost to the knee. The nerve penetrates the psoas muscle, crosses the iliacus and passes into the thigh by coursing between the two prongs of the attachment of the lateral part of the inguinal ligament to the anterior superior iliac spine. Compression (entrapment) may occur at the point where it passes between the two prongs of attachment of the inguinal ligament.

Compression of the nerve results in uncomfortable paresthesias and sensory impairment in its cutaneous distribution, a condition known as *meralgia paresthetica* (meros-thigh). Usually numbness and mild sensitivity of the skin to clothing are the only symptoms, but occasionally there is a persistent, distressing burning pain. Touch and pinprick are reduced in the territory of the nerve; there is no weakness of the quadriceps or diminution of knee jerk. The symptoms are characteristically worsened in certain positions, usually with prolonged standing or walking. Occasionally, in an obese person, sitting is the most uncomfortable position. Obesity, pregnancy, and diabetes mellitus are contributory factors. Usually the neuropathy is unilateral; Ecker and Woltman found only 20 percent of their cases to be bilateral.

Most of our patients with meralgia paresthetica have requested no treatment once they learned of its benign character. A few with the most painful symptoms have demanded a neurectomy, but it is always wise to perform a xylocaine block first so that the patient can decide whether the persistent numbness is preferable. In one specimen of nerve obtained at operation we found a discrete traumatic neuroma. Hydrocortisone injections at the point of entrapment have helped in a few cases.

Obturator Nerve   This nerve arises from the third and fourth and to a lesser extent from the second lumbar roots. It supplies the adductors and to some extent the internal and external rotators of the thigh. The adductors have the added function of flexion at the hip. The nerve may be injured by the fetal head or forceps during the course of a difficult labor or compressed by an obturator hernia. Rarely, it is affected in diabetes, polyarteritis nodosa, and osteitis pubis; and rarely also by retroperitoneal spread of carcinoma of the cervix, uterus, and other tumors.

Femoral Nerve   This nerve is formed from the second, third, and fourth lumbar roots. Within the pelvis it passes along the lateral border of the psoas muscle and enters the thigh beneath Poupart's ligament, lateral to the femoral artery. Branches arising within the pelvis supply the iliacus and psoas muscles. Just below Poupart's ligament the nerve divides into anterior and posterior divisions. The former supplies the pectineus and sartorius muscles and carries sensation from the anteromedial surface of the thigh; the posterior division provides the motor innervation to the quadriceps and the cutaneous innervation to the medial side of the leg from knee to internal malleolus.

Following injury to the femoral nerve, there is weakness of extension of the leg and wasting of the quadriceps muscle; if the nerve is injured proximal to the origin of the branches to the iliacus and psoas muscles, there is weakness of hip flexion. The knee jerk is abolished.

The commonest cause of femoral neuropathy is diabetes. The nerve may be injured during pelvic operations (see above), and may be involved by pelvic tumors. Bleeding into the iliac muscle, observed in patients receiving anticoagulants and in hemophiliacs, is a relatively common cause of isolated femoral neuropathy (Goodfellow et al.). The presenting symptom of iliacus hematoma is pain in the groin, spreading to the lumbar region or thigh, in response to which the patient assumes a characteristic posture of flexion and lateral rotation of the hip. A palpable mass in the iliac fossa and the signs of femoral nerve compression follow in a day or two. Infarction of the nerve may occur in the course of diabetes mellitus and polyarteritis nodosa. Not infrequently the nerve suffers acute damage of indeterminate cause. Biemond states this to be true of 60 percent of his cases; Calverley and Mulder find fewer occult cases, which is more in keeping with the authors' experience.

Sciatic Nerve This nerve is derived from the fourth and fifth lumbar and first and second sacral roots. It supplies motor innervation to the hamstring muscles and all the muscles below the knee; it carries sensory impulses from the posterior aspect of the thigh, the posterior and lateral aspects of the leg, and the entire sole. In complete sciatic paralysis, the knee cannot be flexed and all muscles below the knee are paralyzed. Weakness of gluteal muscles and pain in the buttock and posterior thigh point to nerve involvement in the pelvis. Lesions beyond the sciatic notch spare the gluteal muscles but not the hamstrings.

The sciatic nerve is commonly injured by fractures of the pelvis or femur, by gunshot wounds of the buttock and thigh, and by the injection of toxic substances such as paraldehyde into the lower gluteal region. Tumors of the pelvis (sarcomas, lipomas) or gluteal region may compress the nerve. Sitting for a long period with legs flexed and abducted (lotus position) under the influence of narcotics or lying flat on a hard surface in coma may severely injure one or both sciatic nerves. The nerve may be involved by neurofibromas, by infections, and by ischemic necrosis in diabetes mellitus and polyarteritis nodosa. Cryptogenic forms also occur and are actually more frequent than those of identifiable cause. A ruptured lumbar disk often simulates sciatic neuropathy. Partial lesions of the sciatic nerve occasionally result in causalgia.

Common Peroneal Nerve Just above the popliteal fossa the sciatic nerve divides into the *tibial nerve (medial, or internal, popliteal nerve)* and *the common peroneal nerve (lateral, or external, popliteal nerve)*. The latter swings around the head of the fibula to the anterior aspect of the leg, giving off the musculocutaneous branch (to the peroneal muscles) and continuing as the *anterior tibial, or deep peroneal, nerve.* Branches of the latter supply the dorsiflexors of the foot and toes, and carry sensory fibers from the dorsum of the foot and lateral aspect of the lower half of the leg. Pressure or sleep palsy, or tight plaster casts, obstetrical stirrups, habitual and prolonged leg crossing while seated, and tight knee boots are the most frequent causes of injury to the common peroneal nerve, the compression being to that part of the nerve which passes over the head of the fibula. It may also be affected in diabetic neuropathy and injured by fractures of the upper end of the fibula.

Tibial Nerve This, the other of the two divisions of the sciatic nerve in the popliteal fossa, gives branches to all of the calf muscles, i.e., the plantar flexors of the foot and toes, after which it continues as the posterior tibial nerve. This nerve passes through the tarsal tunnel, an osseofibrous channel along the medial aspect of the calcaneus which is roofed by the flexor retinaculum. The canal also contains the tendons of the tibialis posterior, flexor digitorum longus, and flexor hallucis longus muscles and the vessels to the foot. The posterior tibial nerve terminates under the flexor retinaculum by dividing into medial and lateral plantar nerves (supplying the small muscles of the foot).

Complete interruption of the tibial nerve results in a calcaneovalgus deformity of the foot, which no longer can be plantar-flexed and inverted. There is loss of sensation over the plantar aspect of the foot.

The posterior tibial nerve may be compressed in the tarsal tunnel (entrapment syndrome) by thickening of the tendon sheaths or the adjacent connective tissues or osteoarthritis. Tingling pain and burning over the sole of the foot develop after standing or walking for a long time. Usually there is no motor deficit. Relief is obtained by severing the flexor retinaculum.

ENTRAPMENT NEUROPATHIES

Reference has been made in several places in the preceding pages to entrapment neuropathies. A nerve, passing through a tight canal, is trapped and subjected to constant movement or pressure, forces not applicable to nerves elsewhere. The epineurium and perineurium become greatly thickened, strangling the nerve, with the additional possibility of demyelination. Function is

Table 45-2
Entrapment neuropathies

Nerve	Site of entrapment
Median nerve	Carpal tunnel
Ulnar nerve	
Elbow	Bicipital groove, cubital tunnel
Wrist	Palmar fascia–pisiform bone
Anterior interosseous (pronator syndrome)	Between heads of pronator muscle
Lateral femoral cutaneous (meralgia paresthetica)	Inguinal ligament
Obturator nerve	Obturator canal
Posterior tibial	Tarsal tunnel, medial malleolus–flexor retinaculum
Plantar (Morton's metatarsalgia)	Plantar fascia: heads of third and fourth metatarsals

gradually impaired, sensory more than motor, and the symptoms fluctuate with activity and rest.

Listed in Table 45-2 are the more common entrapment neuropathies.

REFERENCES

ABRAMSKY O, TEITELBAUM D, ARNON R: Experimental allergic neuritis induced by a basic neuritogenic protein (P₁L) of human peripheral nerve origin. *Eur J Immunol* 7:213, 1977.

ADAMS RD, RICHARDSON EP JR: The demyelinative diseases of the human nervous system: A classification; a review of salient neuropathological findings; comments on recent biochemical studies, in Folch-Pi J (ed): *Chemical Pathology of the Nervous System*. New York, Pergamon, 1961, pp 162–195.

——, SHAHANI BT, YOUNG RR: A severe pansensory familial neuropathy. *Trans Am Neurol Assoc* 98:67, 1973.

ASBURY AK: Ischemic disorders of peripheral nerves, in Vinken PJ, Bruyn GW (eds): *Handbook of Clinical Neurology*, vol 8. Amsterdam, North-Holland, 1970, chap 11, pp 154–164.

——, ARNASON BG, ADAMS RD: The inflammatory lesion in acute idiopathic polyneuritis. *Medicine* 48:173, 1969.

——, JOHNSON PC: *Pathology of Peripheral Nerve*. Philadelphia, Saunders, 1978.

——, VICTOR M, ADAMS RD: Uremic polyneuropathy. *Arch Neurol* 8:113, 1963.

—— et al: Guillain-Barré syndrome: Is there a place for plasmapheresis? *Neurology* 30:1112, 1980.

AUSTIN JH: Observations on the syndrome of hypertrophic neuritis (the hypertrophic interstitial radiculoneuropathies). *Medicine* 35:187, 1956.

BEHSE F et al: Hereditary neuropathy with liability to pressure palsies—electrophysiological and histopathological aspects. *Brain* 95:777, 1972.

BIEMOND A: Femoral neuropathy, in Vinken PJ, Bruyn GW (eds): *Handbook of Clinical Neurology*, vol 8. Amsterdam, North-Holland, 1970, chap 18, pp 303–310.

BOLTON CF: Peripheral neuropathies associated with chronic renal failure. *Can J Neurol Sci* 7(2):89, 1980.

CALVERLEY JR, MULDER DW: Femoral neuropathy. *Neurology* 10:963, 1960.

COHEN AS, BENSON MD: Amyloid neuropathy, in Dyck PJ, Thomas PK, Lambert EH (eds): *Peripheral Neuropathy*. Philadelphia, Saunders, 1975, chap 53, pp 1067–1091.

CONN DL, DYCK PJ: Angiopathic neuropathy in connective tissue diseases, in Dyck PJ, Thomas PK, Lambert EH (eds): *Peripheral Neuropathy*. Philadelphia, Saunders, 1975, chap 57, pp 1149–1165.

CROFT PB, WILKINSON M: The incidence of carcinomatous neuromyopathy in patients with various types of carcinoma. *Brain* 88:427, 1965.

—— et al: Sensory neuropathy with bronchial carcinoma: A study of four cases showing serological abnormalities. *Brain* 88:501, 1965.

DALY DD, LOVE JG, DOCKERTY MB: Amyloid tumor of the Gasserian ganglion: Report of a case. *J Neurosurg* 14:347, 1957.

DENNY-BROWN D: Hereditary sensory radicular neuropathy. *J Neurol Neurosurg Psychiatry* 14:237, 1951.

DUCHOWNY M, CAPLAN L, SIBER G: Cytomegalus virus infection of the adult nervous system. *Ann Neurol* 5:458, 1979.

DYCK PJ: Inherited neuronal degeneration and atrophy affecting peripheral motor, sensory and autonomic neurons, in Dyck PJ, Thomas PK, Lambert EH (eds): *Peripheral Neuropathy*. Philadelphia, Saunders, 1975, chap 41, pp 825–867.

——, LAMBERT EH: Polyneuropathy associated with hypothyroidism. *J Neuropathol Exp Neurol* 29:631, 1970.

——, OHTA M: Neuronal atrophy and degeneration predominantly affecting peripheral sensory neurons, in Dyck PJ, Thomas PK, Lambert EH (eds): *Peripheral Neuropathy*. Philadelphia, Saunders, 1975, chap 40, pp 791–824.

——, THOMAS PK, LAMBERT EH (eds): *Peripheral Neuropathy*. Philadelphia, Saunders, 1975.

EARL CJ, FULLERTON PM, WAKEFIELD GS, SCHUTTA HS: Hereditary neuropathy with liability to pressure palsies. *Q J Med* 33:481, 1964.

ECKER AD, WOLTMAN HW: Meralgia paresthetica: A report of one hundred and fifty cases. *J Am Med Assoc* 110:1650, 1938.

EKBOM KA: Restless legs syndrome. *Neurology* 10:858, 1960.

ENGEL WK, DORMAN JD, LEVY RI, FREDRICKSON DS: Neuropathy in Tangier disease. *Arch Neurol* 17:1, 1967.

ENGLAND AC, DENNY-BROWN D: Severe sensory changes and trophic disorders in peroneal muscular atrophy (Charcot-Marie-Tooth type). *Arch Neurol Psychiatry* 67:1, 1952.

FALLS HF et al: Ocular manifestations of hereditary primary systemic amyloidosis. *Arch Ophthalmol* 54:660, 1955.

FISHER CM: An unusual variant of acute idiopathic polyneuritis (syndrome of ophthalmoplegia, ataxia and areflexia). *N Eng J Med* 255:57, 1956.

———, WILLIAMS HW, WING ES: Combined encephalopathy and neuropathy with carcinoma. *J Neuropathol Exp Neurol* 20:535, 1961.

FUNCK-BRENTANO JL, CUEILLE GF, MAN NK: A defense of the middle molecule hypothesis, *Kidney Int* 13(suppl 8):S31, 1978.

GILLIAT RW, WILLISON RG: Peripheral nerve conduction in diabetic neuropathies. *J Neurol Neurosurg Psychiatry* 25:11, 1962.

GOODFELLOW J, FEARN CB, MATTHEWS JM: Iliacus haematoma: A common complication of haemophilia, *J Bone Joint Surg* 49B:748, 1967.

HAYMAKER W, WOODHALL B: *Peripheral Nerve Injuries,* 2d ed. Philadelphia, Saunders, 1953.

HUTCHINSON EC: Ischaemic neuropathy and peripheral vascular disease, in Vinken PJ, Bruyn GW (eds): *Handbook of Clinical Neurology,* vol 8. Amsterdam, North-Holland. 1970, chap 10.

KAHN P: Anderson-Fabry disease: A histopathological study of three cases with observations on the mechanism of production of pain. *J Neurol Neurosurg Psychiatry* 36:1053, 1973.

KELLY JJ et al: The natural history of peripheral neuropathy in primary systemic amyloidosis. *Ann Neurol* 6:1, 1979.

KERNOHAN JW, WOLTMAN HW: Amyloid neuritis. *Arch Neurol Psychiatry* 47:132, 1942.

KOPELL HP, THOMPSON WAL: *Peripheral Entrapment Neuropathies.* Baltimore, Williams & Wilkins, 1963.

LAPRESLE J, SALISACHS P: Roussy-Lévy syndrome, in Vinken PJ, Bruyn GW (eds): *Handbook of Clinical Neurology,* vol 21. Amsterdam, North-Holland, 1975, chap 9, pp 171–179.

LHERMITTE F, et al: Polynévrites au cours de traitements par la nitrofurantoine. *Presse Med* 71:767, 1963.

MADRID R, BRADLEY WG: The pathology of neuropathies with focal thickening of the myelin sheath (tomaculous neuropathy). *J Neurol Sci* 25:415, 1975.

MAGEE KR, DEJONG RN: Paralytic brachial neuritis. *J Am Med Assoc* 174:1258, 1960.

MEDICAL RESEARCH COUNCIL: *Aids to the Examination of the Peripheral Nervous System,* Memorandum no 45 (superseding war memorandum no 7). London, HM Stationery Office, 1976.

OHNISHI A, DYCK PJ: Loss of small peripheral sensory neurons in Fabry disease. *Arch Neurol* 31:120, 1974.

PALLIS CA, SCOTT JT: Peripheral neuropathy in rheumatoid arthritis. *Br Med J* 1:1141, 1965.

PARSONAGE MJ, TURNER JWA: Neuralgic amyotrophy. The shoulder girdle syndrome. *Lancet* 1:973, 1948.

PRINEAS J: Polyneuropathies of undetermined cause. *Acta Neurol Scand* 46(suppl 46): 1970.

RAFF MC, SANGALANG V, ASBURY AK: Ischemic mononeuropathy multiplex associated with diabetes mellitus. *Arch Neurol* 18:487, 1968.

REFSUM S: Heredopathia atactica polyneuritiformis: Phytanic acid storage disease (Refsum's disease), in *Spinocerebellar Degenerations,* Japan Medical Research Foundation Publication no. 10. Tokyo, University of Tokyo Press, 1980, pp 313–338.

RIDLEY A: Porphyric neuropathy, in Dyck PJ, Thomas PK, Lambert EH (eds): *Peripheral Neuropathy.* Philadelphia, Saunders, 1975, chap 46, pp 942–955.

RILEY CM, MOORE RH: Familial dysautonomia differentiated from related disorders: Case report and discussions of current concepts. *Pediatrics* 37:435, 1966.

ROBSON JS: Uraemic neuropathy, in Robertson RF (ed): *Some Aspects of Neurology.* Edinburgh, Royal College of Physicians, 1968, pp 74–84.

RUKAVINA JG et al: Primary systemic amyloidosis: A review and an experimental genetic and clinical study of 29 cases with particular emphasis on the familial form. *Medicine* 35:239, 1956.

SELBY G: Diseases of the fifth cranial nerve, in Dyck PJ, Thomas PK, Lambert EH (eds): *Peripheral Neuropathy.* Philadelphia, Saunders, 1975, chap 26, pp 553–569.

SPENCER PS, SCHAUMBURG HH (eds): *Experimental and Clinical Neurotoxicology.* Baltimore, Williams & Wilkins, 1980.

——— et al: Does a defect of energy metabolism in the nerve fiber underlie axonal degeneration in polyneuropathies? *Ann Neurol* 5:501, 1979.

STOLL BA, ANDREWS JT: Radiation induced peripheral neuropathy. *Br Med J* 1:834, 1966.

SWANSON AG, BUCHAN GC, ALVORD EC JR: Anatomic changes in congenital insensitivity to pain: Absence of small primary sensory neurons in ganglia, roots and Lissauer's tract. *Arch Neurol* 12:12, 1965.

TAYLOR RA: Heredofamilial mononeuritis multiplex with brachial predilection. *Brain* 83:113, 1960.

THÉVENARD A: L'Acropathie ulcero-mutilante familiale. *Rev Neurol* 74:193, 1942.

THOMAS PK, ELIASSON SG: Diabetic neuropathy, in Dyck PJ, Thomas PK, Lambert EH (eds): *Peripheral Neuropathy.* Philadelphia, Saunders, 1975, chap 48, pp 958–981.

———, LASCELLES RG: The pathology of diabetic neuropathy. *Q J Med* 35:489, 1966.

———, WALKER JG: Xanthomatous neuropathy in primary biliary cirrhosis. *Brain* 88:1079, 1965.

TSAIRIS P, DYCK PJ, MULDER DW: Natural history of brachial plexus neuropathy: Report on 99 cases. *Arch Neurol* 27:109, 1972.

VAN BUCHEM FSP, POL G, DE GIER J, BOTTCHER CJF, PRIES C: Congenital β-lipoprotein deficiency. *Am J Med* 40:794, 1966.

VINKEN PJ, BRUYN GW (eds): *Handbook of Clinical Neurol-*

ogy, vols 7 and 8: *Diseases of Nerves*. Amsterdam, North-Holland, 1970.

WAKSMAN BH, ADAMS RD: Allergic neuritis: An experimental disease of rabbits induced by the injection of peripheral nervous tissue and adjuvants. *J Exp Med* 102:213, 1955.

WALDENSTROM J: Studien über Porphyrie. *Acta Med Scand Suppl* 82: 1937.

————: The porphyrias as inborn errors of metabolism. *Am J Med* 22:758, 1957.

WARTENBERG R: *Neuritis, Sensory Neuritis, and Neuralgia*. New York, Oxford, 1959.

WEINSHILBOUM RM, AXELROD J: Reduced plasma dopamine-β-hydroxylase activity in familial dysautonomia. *N Eng J Med* 285:938, 1971.

WILLIAMS IR, MAYER RF: Subacute proximal diabetic neuropathy. *Neurology* 26:108, 1976.

CHAPTER 46

DISEASES OF THE CRANIAL NERVES

The cranial nerves are susceptible to many disorders that rarely if ever affect the spinal peripheral nerves; for this reason alone they deserve to be considered separately. Some of the cranial nerve disorders have already been discussed: viz., disorders of olfaction, in Chap. 11; vision and extraocular muscles, in Chaps. 12 and 13; cochlear and vestibular function, in Chap. 14; craniofacial pain, referable to the trigeminal and glossopharyngeal nerves, in Chap. 9. There remain to be discussed the disorders of the seventh (facial) nerve and of the lower cranial nerves (IX to XII), as well as certain aspects of disordered trigeminal nerve function; these are considered below.

THE FIFTH, OR TRIGEMINAL, NERVE
(See Fig. 46-1)

This is a mixed sensory and motor nerve. It conducts sensory impulses from the greater part of the face and head, from the mucous membranes of the nose and mouth, and from the cornea and conjunctiva. The cell bodies of the sensory part of the nerve lie in the gasserian, or semilunar, ganglion. The proximal axons of these cells form the sensory root. On entering the pons, they divide into short ascending and long descending branches. The former are concerned mainly with touch and deep sensation and terminate in the principal and mesencephalic nuclei, respectively. The long descending branches form the spinal trigeminal tract and are concerned mainly with pain and temperature sensation (facial pain has been relieved after medullary trigeminal tractotomy). The spinal trigeminal tract, together with its nucleus, extends from the junction of the pons and medulla to the uppermost segments of the spinal cord. From the nucleus, second-order fibers cross to the oppo-

site side and ascend to the thalamus in the most medial part of the spinothalamic tract.

The peripheral branches of the gasserian ganglion form the three sensory divisions of the nerve. The first (ophthalmic) division passes through the superior orbital fissure; the second (maxillary) division leaves the middle fossa through the foramen rotundum; and the third (mandibular), through the foramen ovale.

The motor portion of the fifth nerve, which supplies the masseter and pterygoid muscles, has its origin in the midpons; the fibers pass underneath the gasserian ganglion and become incorporated into the mandibular nerve.

Because of their wide anatomic distribution, complete interruption of both the motor and sensory fibers of the trigeminal nerve is rarely observed. On the other hand, partial affection of the trigeminal nerve, particularly of the sensory part, is common. The various brainstem and cranial nerve syndromes in which the fifth nerve is involved are listed in Tables 46-1 and 46-2.

The most striking disorder of the trigeminal nerve is *tic douloureux*, which has been described on page 129. Herpes zoster involving the gasserian ganglion is discussed fully in Chap. 32. Attention has also been drawn to the occasional occurrence of schwannoma of the fifth nerve or its involvement by a meningioma (page 463).

Anesthesia and analgesia of the face may be induced by stilbamidine, which formerly was used in the treatment of kala azar and multiple myeloma, and by inhalation of the fumes of trichloracetic acid; pain and itching may occur during recovery. An idiopathic form of bitrigeminal anesthesia has also been observed. These nerves may be involved in leprosy. Tonic spasm of the masticatory muscles, known as *trismus*, is symptomatic of tetanus (see also Chap. 41), although it may occur in patients treated with phenothiazine drugs; lesser degrees

may be associated with disease in and around the jaws
and teeth.

A restricted form of acute and chronic benign trigeminal neuropathy has been the subject of a number of
reports. In some instances, Horner's syndrome was also
present. In some, it has been associated with lupus erythematosus or "progressive systemic sclerosis" and Sjögren's syndrome. In the majority of patients, however,
the cause was undetermined, and in these, recovery is
the rule over a period of several weeks to months. A few
of the recovered cases have later developed tic douloureux and multiple sclerosis (see Selby for references).

THE SEVENTH, OR FACIAL, NERVE

The seventh cranial nerve is mainly a motor nerve supplying all the muscles concerned with facial expression
on one side. The sensory component is small (the nervus
intermedius of Wrisberg); it conveys taste sensation
from the anterior two-thirds of the tongue and probably
cutaneous sensation from the anterior wall of the external auditory canal. The taste fibers at first traverse the
lingual nerve (a branch of the mandibular), and then
join the chorda tympani. Secretomotor fibers innervate
the lacrimal gland through the greater superficial petrosal nerve, and the sublingual and submaxillary glands
through the chorda tympani (Fig. 46-2).

Several other anatomic facts are worth remembering. The motor nucleus of the seventh nerve lies anterior

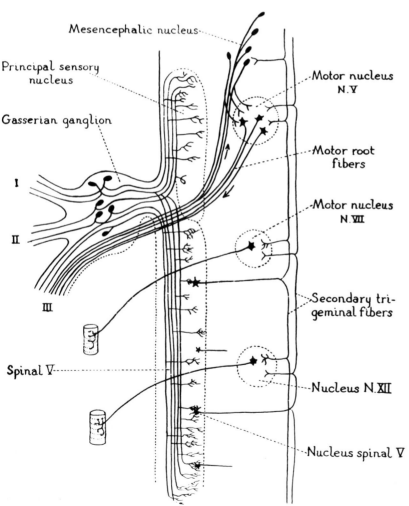

Figure 46-1
*Scheme of the trigeminal nuclei and
some of the trigeminal reflex arcs. I,
ophthalmic division; II, maxillary division; III, mandibular division. (From
MB Carpenter, Human Neuroanatomy, 7th ed. Baltimore, Williams &
Wilkins, 1976.)*

and lateral to the abducens nucleus, and the intrapontine fibers of the facial nerve hook around the abducens nucleus before emerging from the pons, just lateral to the corticospinal tract. The facial nerve enters the internal auditory meatus with the acoustic nerve and then bends sharply forward and downward around the anterior boundary of the vestibule of the inner ear. At this angle *(genu)* lies the sensory ganglion (named *geniculate* because of its proximity to the genu). The nerve continues its course in its own bony channel, the facial canal, and makes its exit from the skull at the stylomastoid foramen. It then passes through the parotid gland and subdivides into five branches to supply the facial muscles, the stylomastoid muscle, and the posterior belly of the digastric muscle. Within the facial canal, just distal to the geniculate ganglion, it gives off the branch to the sphenopalatine ganglion, i.e., the greater superficial

petrosal nerve; somewhat more distally, it gives off a small branch to the stapedius and is joined by the chorda tympani.

A complete interruption of the facial nerve at the stylomastoid foramen paralyzes all muscles of facial expression. The corner of the mouth droops, the creases and skin folds are effaced, the forehead is unfurrowed, the palpebral fissure is widened, and the eyelids will not close. Upon attempted closure of the lids, the eye on the paralyzed side is seen to roll upward (Bell's phenomenon). The lower lid sags also, and the punctum falls away from the conjunctiva, permitting tears to spill over the cheek. Food collects between the teeth and lips and

Figure 46-2

Scheme of the seventh cranial (facial) nerve. The motor fibers are represented by the heavy black line. Parasympathetic fibers are represented by regular dashes; special visceral afferent (taste) fibers are represented by long dashes and dots. A, B, and C denote lesions of the facial nerve at the stylomastoid fora-

men, distal to the geniculate ganglion, and proximal to the geniculate ganglion. Disturbances resulting from lesions at each of these sites are described in the text. (From MB Carpenter, Human Neuroanatomy, 7th ed, Baltimore, Williams & Wilkins, 1976.)

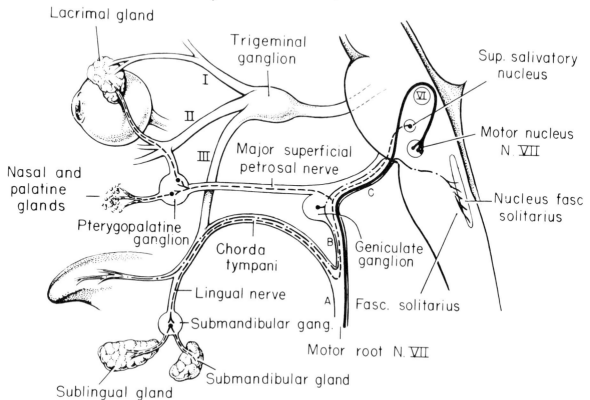

saliva may dribble from the corner of the mouth. The patient complains of a heaviness or numbness in the face, but sensory loss can usually not be demonstrated. Taste is intact.

If the lesion is in the facial canal above the junction with the chorda tympani but below the geniculate ganglion, all the above symptoms occur; in addition, taste is lost over the anterior two-thirds of the tongue on the same side. If the nerve to the stapedius is paralyzed, there is hyperacusis (painful sensitivity to loud sounds), and the sound produced by moving the jaw and facial muscles is no longer present in the ear on the affected side. If the geniculate ganglion or the motor root proximal to it is involved, lacrimation may be reduced. Lesions at this point may also affect the adjacent eighth nerve, causing deafness, tinnitus, or dizziness. Intrapontine lesions that paralyze the face often affect the abducens nucleus and the corticospinal and sensory tracts.

If the peripheral facial paralysis has existed for some time and return of motor function has begun but is incomplete, a kind of contracture (in reality a continuous diffuse muscle contraction) may appear. The palpebral fissure becomes narrowed and the nasolabial fold deepens. Attempts to move one group of facial muscles result in contraction of all of them (associated movements, or synkinesis). Spasms of facial muscles develop and persist indefinitely, being initiated by every facial movement; this condition, called *hemifacial spasm,* occurs not frequently in adults who have never had a facial palsy. Anomalous regeneration of the seventh nerve fibers may result in other curious disorders. If fibers originally connected with the orbicularis oculi become connected with the orbicularis oris, closure of the lids may cause a retraction of the corner of the mouth; or if visceromotor fibers originally innervating the salivary glands later come to innervate the lacrimal gland, anomalous tearing (crocodile tears) may occur whenever the patient salivates. With the passage of time, the corner of the mouth and even the tip of the nose become pulled to the unaffected side.

BELL'S PALSY

The most common disease of the facial nerve is *Bell's palsy,* presumably due to an inflammatory reaction in or around the nerve near the stylomastoid foramen. This disorder affects men and women more or less equally and occurs at all ages. The incidence is not dispropor-

tionately high in diabetics and in pregnant women, contrary to popular belief. The onset is acute; about one-half of the cases attain maximum paralysis in 48 h and practically all cases within 5 days. Pain behind the ear may precede the paralysis by a day or two. In a small proportion of patients a hypesthesia in one or more branches of the trigeminal nerve can be demonstrated. The explanation of this finding is not clear. Impairment of taste is present to some degree in almost all patients, but rarely persists beyond the second week of paralysis. In some cases there is mild pleocytosis in the CSF.

Fully 80 percent of patients recover within a few weeks or in a month or two. Recovery of taste precedes recovery of motor function, and if the former occurs in the first week, it is a good prognostic sign. Incomplete paralysis in the first 5 to 7 days is the most favorable prognostic sign. Electromyography may be of value in distinguishing temporary conduction defects from a pathologic interruption of nerve fibers; evidence of denervation after 10 days indicates a long delay in recovery, until regeneration occurs, and sometimes it is incomplete.

Protection of the eye during sleep, massage of the weakened muscles, and a splint to prevent drooping of the lower part of the face are the measures generally employed in the management of such cases. There is no evidence that surgical decompression of the facial nerve is effective, and it may be harmful. The administration of prednisone during the first week after onset may be beneficial.

OTHER CAUSES OF FACIAL PALSY

Tumors which invade the temporal bone (carotid body, cholesteatoma, and dermoid) may produce a facial palsy, but the onset is insidious and the course progressive. Fracture of the temporal bone (usually with damage to the middle or internal ear), otitis media, and middle ear surgery are relatively uncommon causes of facial palsy. Ramsay Hunt syndrome, due presumably to herpes zoster of the geniculate ganglion, consists of severe facial palsy associated with a vesicular eruption in the external auditory canal and other parts of the cranial integument; often the eighth cranial nerve is affected as well (see Chap. 32). Acoustic neuromas and aneurysmal dilatations of the basilar artery frequently involve the facial nerve. Vascular lesions or tumors are the common forms of pontine disease which may cause facial palsy. Bilateral facial paralysis (facial diplegia) occurs in acute idiopathic polyneuritis and in a variety of sarcoidosis known as *uveoparotid fever (Heerfordt's syndrome)*. *Melkersson-Rosenthal syndrome* comprises a triad of recurrent facial paralysis, facial (particularly labial) edema, and less constantly, plication of the tongue. The syndrome begins in childhood or adolescence and is quite rare; the cause is unknown. The facial nerve is frequently involved in leprosy.

All these forms of nuclear or peripheral facial palsy must be distinguished from the supranuclear type. In the latter the frontalis and orbicularis oculi muscles are involved less than those of the lower part of the face, since the upper facial muscles receive upper motor neuron innervation from both hemispheres, and the lower facial muscles, from the opposite hemisphere alone. In supranuclear lesions there may be a dissociation of emotional and voluntary facial movements, and often some degree of paralysis of the arm and leg or an aphasia (in dominant hemisphere lesions) is conjoined.

A curious disorder is the *facial hemiatrophy of Romberg*. It occurs mainly in females and is characterized by a disappearance of fat in the dermal and subcutaneous tissues on one side of the face. It usually begins in adolescence or early adult years and is slowly progressive. In its advanced form the affected side of the face is gaunt and the skin is thin, wrinkled, and rather dark; the hair may turn white and fall out, and the sebaceous glands become atrophic; the muscles and bones are as a rule not involved. The condition is a form of *lipodystrophy*, and the localization within a dermatome indicates the operation of some neural factor of unknown nature.

The facial muscles on one side may be involved in irregular clonic contractions of varying degree (*hemifacial spasm*). This condition may be due to an irritative lesion of the facial nerve [e.g., an acoustic neuroma, an aberrant artery pressing on the nerve (relieved by surgery), or basilar artery aneurysm], or may represent a transient or permanent sequela of a Bell's palsy, as stated above. A fine fibrillary activity of facial muscles may be caused by a plaque of multiple sclerosis in the region of the facial nucleus and its fibers of exit. A clonic or tonic contraction of one side of the face may be the sole manifestation of a cerebral cortical seizure. An involuntary recurrent spasm of both eyelids (*blepharospasm*) occurs in elderly persons as an isolated phenomenon, and there may be varying degrees of spasm of the other facial muscles (see also page 76). Relaxant and tranquilizing drugs are of little help in this disorder, although in many cases it may subside spontaneously. In very severe and persistent instances, the only effective treatment has been crushing of the nerves to the orbicularis oculi muscles or surgical relief of pressure on the nerve root by an aberrant blood vessel.

Hypersensitivity of the facial nerve occurs in tetany (Chvostek test of spasm of facial muscles on tapping in front of the ear).

THE NINTH, OR GLOSSOPHARYNGEAL, NERVE

This nerve arises from the lateral surface of the medulla by a series of small roots which lie just rostral to those of the vagus nerve. The glossopharyngeal, vagus, and accessory nerves leave the skull together through the jugular foramen and are then distributed peripherally. The ninth nerve has a sensory component with cell bodies in the inferior (petrosal) ganglion (the central processes of which end in the nucleus solitarius) and the small superior ganglion (the central fibers of which enter the spinal trigeminal tract and nucleus). It also receives the nerve of Hering from the carotid body. The somatic efferent fibers of the ninth nerve are derived from the nucleus ambiguus, and the visceral efferent (secretory) fibers, from the inferior salivatory nucleus. These fibers contribute to the motor innervation of the striated musculature of the pharynx (mainly of the stylopharyngeus, which elevates the pharynx) and the glands in the pharyngeal mucosa.

The sensory functions of the ninth nerve are not entirely clear. It is commonly stated that this nerve mediates sensory impulses from the faucial tonsils, the posterior wall of the pharynx, and part of the soft palate, and taste sensation from the posterior third of the tongue. However, an isolated lesion of the ninth cranial nerve is a rarity, and the effects are not fully known. In one personally observed case of bilateral surgical interruption of the ninth nerves, verified at autopsy, there had been no demonstrable loss of taste or other sensory or motor impairment. This suggests that the tenth nerve may be responsible for these functions, at least in some individuals. There is some evidence that the ninth nerve, through its innervation of the carotid sinus, plays a part in the reflex control of circulation.

One may occasionally observe a glossopharyngeal palsy in conjunction with vagus and accessory nerve involvement due to a tumor in the posterior fossa or an aneurysm of the vertebral artery. The nerves are compressed as they pass through the jugular foramen. Hoarseness due to vocal cord paralysis, some difficulty in swallowing, deviation of the soft palate to the sound side, anesthesia of the posterior wall of the pharynx, and weakness of the upper trapezius and sternomastoid muscles comprise the clinical picture (see Table 46-1, jugular foramen syndrome).

Glossopharyngeal neuralgia is a syndrome which in many respects resembles trigeminal neuralgia. It is described on page 130. Rarely, herpes zoster may involve the glossopharyngeal nerve.

THE TENTH, OR VAGUS, NERVE

This nerve has an extensive sensory and motor distribution. It has two ganglia: the jugular, which contains the cell bodies of the somatic sensory nerves (which inner-

vate the skin in the concha of the ear); and the nodose, which contains the cell bodies of the afferent fibers from the pharynx, larynx, trachea, esophagus, and the thoracic and abdominal viscera. The central processes of these ganglia terminate in relation to the nucleus of the spinal trigeminal tract and the tractus solitarius, respectively. The motor fibers of the vagus are derived from two nuclei in the medulla, the nucleus ambiguus and the dorsal motor nucleus. The former supplies somatic motor fibers to the striated muscles of the larynx, pharynx, and the palate; the latter supplies visceral motor fibers to the heart and other thoracic and abdominal organs. The distribution of vagal fibers is illustrated in Fig. 46-3.

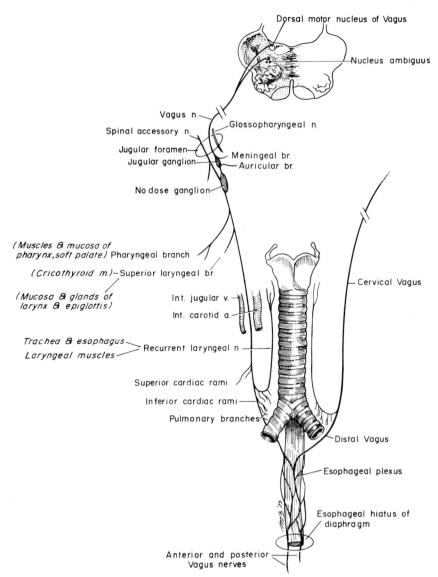

Figure 46-3

Anatomical features of the vagus nerve. Note the relationship to the spinal-accessory and glossopharyngeal nerves at the jugular foramen and the long course of the left recurrent laryngeal nerve.

Complete interruption of the intracranial portion of one vagus nerve results in a characteristic paralysis. The soft palate droops on the ipsilateral side and does not rise in phonation. Deviation of the uvula to the normal side on phonation is an inconstant sign. There is loss of the gag reflex on the affected side and of the *curtain movement* of the lateral wall of the pharynx, whereby the faucial pillars move medially as the palate rises in saying "ah." The voice is hoarse, often nasal, and the vocal cord lies immobile in a "cadaveric" position, i.e., midway between abduction and adduction. With partial lesions, movements of abduction are affected more than those of adduction (Semon's law). There may also be a loss of sensation at the external auditory meatus and back of the pinna. Usually no change in visceral function can be demonstrated.

Complete bilateral paralysis is said to be incompatible with life, and this is probably true if the nuclei are involved in the medulla by poliomyelitis or some other disease. However, in the cervical region both vagi have been blocked with procaine (Novocain) for the treatment of intractable asthma, without mishap. The pharyngeal branches of both vagi may be affected, as in diphtheria; the voice has a nasal quality, and regurgitation of liquids through the nose occurs during the act of swallowing.

The vagus nerve may be implicated at the meningeal level by tumors and infectious processes and within the medulla by vascular lesions, e.g., the lateral medullary syndrome of Wallenberg, by motor system disease and occasionally by tumors. Dysphagia is then invariably present. Herpes zoster may attack this nerve. Polymyositis and dermatomyositis, which cause hoarseness and dysphagia owing to direct involvement of laryngeal and pharyngeal muscles, may be confused with disease of the vagus nerves.

The recurrent laryngeal nerves, especially the left (which has a longer course than the right), are damaged most often as a result of thoracic disease. There is no dysphagia with lesions at this level, since the branches to the pharynx have already separated from the nerve. Aneurysm of the aortic arch, an enlarged left atrium, tu-

Table 46-1
Cranial nerve syndromes

Site	Cranial nerves involved	Eponymic syndrome	Usual cause
Sphenoidal fissure	III, IV, ophthalmic V, VI	Foix	Invasive tumors of sphenoid bone, aneurysms
Lateral wall of cavernous sinus	III, IV, ophthalmic (occasionally maxillary) V, VI	Tolosa-Hunt Foix	Aneurysms or thrombosis of cavernous sinus, invasive tumors from sinuses and sella turcica; sometimes recurrent, benign granulomatous reactions, responsive to steroids
Retrosphenoidal space	II, III, IV, V, VI	Jacod	Large tumors of middle cranial fossa
Apex of petrous bone	V, VI	Gradenigo	Petrositis, tumors of petrous bone
Internal auditory meatus	VII, VIII		Tumors of petrous bone (dermoids, etc.), acoustic neuroma
Pontocerebellar angle	V, VII, VIII, and sometimes IX		Acoustic neuromas, meningiomas
Jugular foramen	IX, X, XI	Vernet	Tumors and aneurysms
Posterior laterocondylar space	IX, X, XI, XII	Collet-Sicard	Tumors of parotid gland, carotid body, secondary and lymph node tumors, tuberculous adenitis
Posterior retroparotid space	IX, X, XI, XII, and Bernard-Horner syndrome	Villaret MacKenzie	Same as above, and granulomatous lesions (sarcoid, fungi)
Posterior retroparotid space	X and XII, with or without XI	Tapia	Parotid and other tumors of, or injuries to, the high neck

mors of the mediastinum and bronchi are much more frequent causes of an isolated vocal cord palsy than are intracranial diseases.

When confronted with a case of vocal cord palsy, the physician must attempt to determine the site of the lesion. If it is intramedullary, there are usually ipsilateral cerebellar signs, loss of pain and temperature sensation over the ipsilateral face and contralateral arm and leg, and an ipsilateral Bernard-Horner syndrome. If the lesion is extramedullary but intracranial, the glossopharyngeal and spinal accessory are frequently involved (jugular foramen syndrome, Table 46-1). If it is extracranial in the posterior laterocondylar or retroparotid space, there may be a combination of ninth, tenth, eleventh, and twelfth cranial nerve palsies and a Bernard-Horner syndrome. Combinations of these lower cranial nerve palsies, which have a variety of eponymic designations (see Table 46-1), are caused by tumors of various types or chronic inflammations of lymph nodes. If there is no sensory loss in the palate and pharynx and no palatal weakness, the lesion is below the origin of the pharyngeal branches, which leave the vagus nerve high in the cervical region. The usual site of disease is then the mediastinum.

THE ELEVENTH, OR ACCESSORY, NERVE

This is a purely motor nerve. Its fibers arise from the anterior horn cells of the upper five cervical cord segments and enter the skull through the foramen magnum. Intracranially, the accessory nerve travels for a short distance with that part of the tenth nerve which is derived from the most caudal cells of the nucleus ambiguus (together, the two roots are referred to as the *vagal-accessory nerve* or the *cranial root of the accessory nerve*). The two roots leave the skull through the jugular foramen. The aberrant vagus fibers then rejoin the main trunk of the vagus, and the fibers derived from the cervical segments of the spinal cord form the external ramus and innervate the sternocleidomastoid and trapezius muscles. Only the latter fibers constitute the accessory nerve in the strict sense.

A complete lesion of the accessory nerve results in weakness of the sternocleidomastoid muscle and upper part of the trapezius (the lower part of the trapezius is innervated by the third and fourth cervical roots through the cervical plexus). This can be demonstrated by asking the patient to shrug the shoulders; the affected trapezius

will be found to be weaker, and there will often be evident atrophy of its upper part. With the arms at the sides, the shoulder on the affected side droops and the scapula is slightly winged; the latter defect is accentuated with lateral movement of the arm (with serratus anterior weakness, winging of the scapula occurs on forward elevation of the arm). When the patient turns the head forcibly against the examiner's hand, the sternomastoid of the opposite side does not contract firmly beneath the fingers. This muscle can be further tested by having the patient press the head forward against resistance or lift the head from the pillow.

Motor system disease, poliomyelitis, syringomyelia, and spinal cord tumors may involve the cells of origin of the spinal accessory nerve. In its intracranial portion, the nerve is usually affected along with the ninth and tenth cranial nerves by lesions of the jugular foramen (glomus tumors, neurofibromas, metastatic carcinoma). In the posterior triangle of the neck, the eleventh nerve can be damaged during surgical operations and by external compression or injury. A benign disorder of the eleventh nerve, akin to Bell's palsy, has been described by Eisen and Bertrand; it begins with pain which subsides in a few days, and is followed by weakness and atrophy in the distribution of the nerve. About one-quarter to one-third of eleventh nerve lesions are of this idiopathic type, and the majority of patients recover. Double sternomastoid and trapezius palsy, which occurs with primary disease of muscles, e.g., polymyositis and muscular dystrophy, may be difficult to distinguish from a lesion of both accessory nerves.

HYPOGLOSSAL NERVE

This also is a purely motor nerve, which supplies the somatic musculature of the tongue. It arises as a series of rootlets which issue from the medulla between the pyramid and inferior olivary complex. The nerve leaves the skull through the hypoglossal foramen and innervates the genioglossus muscle, which acts to protrude the tongue; the styloglossus, which retracts and elevates its root; and the hypoglossus, which causes the upper surface to become convex. Complete interruption of the nerve results in paralysis of one side of the tongue. The tongue curves slightly to the healthy side as it lies in the mouth, but on protrusion it deviates to the affected side owing to the unopposed push of the healthy genioglossus muscle. In the mouth the tongue cannot be moved with natural facility. The denervated side becomes wrinkled and atrophied, and fasciculations and fibrillations can be seen.

Lesions of the hypoglossal nerve roots are rare.

Occasionally an intramedullary lesion damages the emergent fibers of the hypoglossal nerve, the corticospinal tract, and medial lemniscus. The result is paralysis and atrophy of one side of the tongue, together with spastic paralysis and loss of vibration and position sense in the opposite arm and leg. Poliomyelitis and motor system disease may destroy the hypoglossal nuclei. Lesions of the basal meninges and the occipital bones (platybasia, Paget's disease) may involve the nerve in its extramedullary course, and it is sometimes damaged in operations on the neck.

SYNDROME OF BULBAR PALSY

This syndrome is the result of weakness or paralysis of those muscles which are supplied by the motor nuclei of the lower brainstem, i.e., the motor nuclei of the fifth, seventh, and ninth to twelfth cranial nerves. (Strictly speaking, the motor nuclei of the fifth and seventh lie outside the "bulb," which is the old name for the medulla oblongata.) Involved are the muscles of the jaw and face, the sternomastoid and upper part of the trapezius, and the muscles of the tongue, pharynx, and larynx. If weakness develops rapidly, as may happen in diphtheria or poliomyelitis, there is no time for muscle atrophy. The more chronic diseases, e.g., progressive bulbar palsy (a form of motor system disease), result in marked wasting and fasciculation of the facial, tongue, sternomastoid, and trapezius muscles. These disorders need to be differentiated from pseudobulbar palsy (see pages 41 and 355).

MULTIPLE CRANIAL NERVE PALSIES

As will be readily understood, several cranial nerves may be affected by a single disease process. One of the clinical problems that arises is whether the lesion lies within or outside the brainstem. Lesions lying on the surface of the brainstem are featured by involvement of adjacent cranial nerves (often occurring in succession) and late and rather slight involvement of the long sensory and motor pathways and segmental structures lying within the brainstem. The opposite is true of intramedullary, intrapontine, and intramesencephalic lesions. The extramedullary lesion is more likely to cause bone erosion or enlargement of the foramens of exit of the cranial nerves (seen radiographically). The intramedullary lesion involving cranial nerves often produces a crossed sensory or motor paralysis (cranial nerve signs on one side of the body and tract signs on the opposite side). In this way, a number of distinctive syndromes, to which eponyms have been attached, are produced. These are listed in Table 46-2.

Involvement of multiple cranial nerves outside the brainstem is frequently the result of trauma (sudden onset), localized infections such as zoster (acute onset), granulomatous disease (subacute onset), or compression by tumors and saccular aneurysms (chronic development). Of the tumors, neurofibromas, schwannomas, meningiomas, cholesteatomas, carcinomas, and sarcomas have all been observed. Nasopharyngeal tumors may implicate several lower cranial nerves in succession, as do also platybasia and adult Arnold-Chiari malformation. A purely motor disorder without atrophy raises the question always of myasthenia gravis (see Chap. 51). Owing to their anatomic relationships, the multiple cranial nerve palsies form a number of distinctive syndromes, listed in Table 46-1 and in the chapter on intracranial neoplasms (Table 30-3).

From time to time one observes a benign form of multiple cranial nerve involvement on one or both sides of the face. The disease may recur over a period of years with variable degrees of recovery between attacks. Th condition is called *polyneuritis cranialis multiplex*. Sarcoidosis is found to be the cause of some. Others have been associated with tuberculosis. The syndrome of recurrent pain behind one eye, ipsilateral ocular palsies, and sensory loss in the distribution of the ophthalmic division of the fifth nerve has been attributed, on uncertain grounds, to nonspecific granulomatous infiltration of the cavernous sinus; it responds well to the administration of steroids. The question of *viral infections of cranial nerves* is always raised by acute palsies of the facial, trigeminal, and auditory nerves, especially when the affection is bilateral, involves several nerves in combination, or is associated with pleocytosis of CSF. Actually, the only proved virus etiology in this group of cases is that of herpes zoster, and in every instance when we have searched for this virus in cases of Bell's palsy or vestibular neuronitis the results have been negative. Since perceptive deafness, vertigo, and other cranial nerve palsies have been observed in conjunction with the parainfectious encephalomyelitides of varicella, measles, rubella, mumps, and scarlet fever and also with Landry-Guillain-Barré syndrome, an immune-mediated mechanism must be considered. Nothing is known of the pathology of the cranial nerve lesion, nor has a virus been isolated in these latter diseases. Treatment is purely symptomatic; fortunately the prognosis for complete recovery is excellent.

Table 46-2
Brainstem syndromes which involve cranial nerves

Eponym	Site	Cranial nerves involved	Tracts and nuclei involved	Signs	Usual cause
Weber's syndrome	Base of midbrain	III	Corticospinal tract	Oculomotor palsy with crossed hemiplegia	Vascular occlusion; tumor; aneurysm
Claude's syndrome	Tegmentum of midbrain	III	Red nucleus and brachium conjunctivum	Oculomotor palsy with contralateral cerebellar ataxia and tremor	Vascular occlusion; tumor; aneurysm
Benedikt's syndrome	Tegmentum of midbrain	III	Red nucleus, corticospinal tract, and brachium conjunctivum	Oculomotor palsy with contralateral cerebellar ataxia, tremor and corticospinal signs	Softening; hemorrhage; tuberculoma; tumor
Nothnagel's syndrome	Tectum of midbrain	Unilateral or bilateral III	Superior cerebellar peduncles	Ocular palsies, paralysis of gaze, and cerebellar ataxia	Tumor
Parinaud's syndrome	Tectum of midbrain	Supranuclear mechanism for upward gaze	Superior colliculi	Paralysis of upward, and sometimes downward gaze; fixed pupils; divergence of eyes	Pinealoma, hydrocephalus
Millard-Gubler syndrome and Raymond-Foville syndrome	Base of pons	VII and often VI	Corticospinal tract	Facial and abducens palsy and contralateral hemiplegia; sometimes gaze palsy to side of lesion	Softening or tumor
Avellis' syndrome	Tegmentum of medulla	X	Spinothalamic tract. Sometimes descending pupillary fibers, with Bernard-Horner syndrome	Paralysis of soft palate and vocal cord and contralateral hemianesthesia	Softening or tumor
Jackson's syndrome	Tegmentum of medulla	X, XII	Corticospinal tract	Avellis' syndrome plus ipsilateral tongue paralysis	Softening or tumor
Wallenberg's syndrome	Tegmentum of medulla	Spinal V, IX, X, XI	Lateral spinothalamic tract. Descending pupillodilator fibers. Spinocerebellar and olivocerebellar tracts	Ipsilateral V, IX, X, XI palsy, Bernard-Horner syndrome, and cerebellar ataxia. Contralateral loss of pain and temperature sense	Occlusion of vertebral or posterior-inferior cerebellar artery

REFERENCES

BRODAL A: *The Cranial Nerves.* Springfield, Ill, Charles C Thomas, 1959.

EISEN A, BERTRAND G: Isolated accessory nerve palsy of spontaneous origin. A clinical and electromyographic study. *Arch Neurol* 27:496, 1972.

GROVES J: Bell's (idiopathic) facial palsy, in Hinchcliffe R, Harrison D (eds): *Scientific Foundations of Otolaryngology.* London, Heinemann, 1976, pp 446-459.

MAYO CLINIC AND MAYO FOUNDATION: *Clinical Examinations in Neurology,* 4th ed. Philadephia, Saunders, 1976.

SELBY G: Diseases of the fifth cranial nerve, in Dyck PJ, Thomas PK, Lambert EH (eds): *Peripheral Neuropathy.* Philadelphia, Saunders, 1975, chap 26, pp 533-569.

CHAPTER 47

PRINCIPLES OF CLINICAL MYOLOGY: DIAGNOSIS AND CLASSIFICATION OF MUSCLE DISEASES

GENERAL CONSIDERATIONS

The striated muscle tissue constitutes the principal organ of locomotion as well as a vast metabolic reservoir. Disposed in more than 600 separate muscles, this tissue comprises as much as 40 percent of the weight of adult human beings. Intricacy of structure undoubtedly accounts for its diverse susceptibilities to disease, and for this reason reference to the following anatomic characteristics provides an appropriate introduction to this chapter.

A single muscle is composed of thousands of muscle fibers which course for variable distances along its longitudinal axis. Some fibers extend the entire length of the muscle; others are joined end to end by connective tissue. Each fiber is a relatively large and complex multinucleated cell varying in length from a few millimeters to several centimeters (34 cm in the human sartorius muscle) and in diameter from 10 to 100 μm. Although the muscle fiber represents an indivisible anatomic and physiologic unit, disease may affect only one part of it, leaving the remainder to atrophy, degenerate, or regenerate, depending on the nature and severity of the disease. The nuclei of each cell, which are oriented parallel to the longitudinal axis of the fiber and may number into the thousands, lie beneath the cytoplasmic membrane (true sarcolemma) and hence are called "sarcolemmal nuclei." The cytoplasm (sarcoplasm) of the cell is abundant and contains myofibrils, various organelles such as mitochondria and ribosomes, and endoplasmic (sarcoplasmic) reticulum. The myofibrils in turn are composed of longitudinally oriented interdigitating filaments (myofilaments) of contractile proteins (actin and myosin). Droplets of stored fat, glycogen, various proteins, many enzymes, and myoglobin, the latter imparting the red color to muscle, have been identified within the sarcoplasm or its organelles.

The individual muscle fibers are enveloped by delicate strands of connective tissue (endomysium) which provide their support and permit unity of action. Blood vessels, of which there may be several for each fiber, and nerve fibers lie within the endomysium. Muscle fibers are bound into groups or fascicles by similar reticular tissue and sheets of collagen (perimysium), which also bind together groups of fascicles and surround the entire muscle (epimysium). These latter connective tissue tunics are also richly and variably vascularized, different types of muscle having different arrangements of arteries and veins; and fat cells (lipocytes) are embedded within the interstices. The muscle fibers are attached by their ends to tendon fibers, which in turn connect with the skeleton. By this means contraction maintains posture and effects movement.

Other notable characteristics of muscle are its natural mode of contraction, i.e., through innervation, and the necessity of intact innervation for the maintenance of its natural trophic state. Each muscle fiber receives a nerve twig from a motor nerve cell in the anterior horn of the spinal cord or nucleus of a cranial nerve, which joins the muscle fiber at a point called the *neuromuscular junction* or *motor end plate*. As was pointed out on page 33, groups of muscle fibers with a common innervation from one anterior horn cell constitute the *motor unit*, which is the basic physiologic unit in all reflex, postural, and voluntary activity.

Acetylcholine (ACh), ACh receptors, and acetylcholinesterase (AChE), which play a special role in neuromuscular transmission, are concentrated at the neuromuscular junction. ACh is synthesized in the motor nerve terminal and stored in vesicles, i.e., "quanta," each containing about 10,000 molecules. Quanta of ACh are released at the nerve ending, cross the narrow synaptic cleft, and combine with specialized receptors on the muscle cell. Single quanta of ACh are released spontaneously and produce miniature end-plate potentials (MEPPs) of about 1 μV. A nerve impulse triggers the release of many ACh quanta, producing a much larger end-plate potential (EPP), which excites the muscle membrane and leads to muscle contraction. The process is terminated by the action of the enzyme AChE, which breaks down ACh.

In addition to the motor nerves, there are two types of sensory receptors (proprioceptors), the muscle spindles and Golgi tendon organs, which participate in reflex activity (see page 34), and finally there are free nerve endings which subserve the sensation of pain and autonomic endings on blood vessels and possibly on muscle fibers. All muscles are not equally susceptible to disease despite the apparent similarity of their structure. In fact, practically no disease affects all muscles in the body, and each disease has as one of its features a characteristic topography within the musculature. These topographic differences between diseases provide incontrovertible evidence of unspecifiable, but unique, structural qualities not presently disclosed by the light or electron microscope. The factors responsible for the selective vulnerability of certain muscles are not known. One factor may relate simply to fiber size; consider, for example, the large diameter and length of the fibers of the glutei and paravertebral muscles in comparison with the smallness of the ocular muscle fibers. The number of fibers composing a motor unit may be of significance; in the ocular muscles, a motor unit contains only 6 to 10 muscle fibers, but in the gastrocnemius, there are as many as 1800 fibers. The eye muscles have a much higher metabolic rate than the large trunk muscles. Differences in patterns of vascular supply may permit some muscles to withstand the effects of hypoxia or vascular occlusion better than others. Subtle metabolic differences between fibers within any one muscle have been revealed by enzyme studies, certain fibers being richer in glycolytic and poorer in oxidative enzymes than others. Doubtless other differences will be discovered.

These anatomic and biochemical qualities suggest some of the ways in which muscle can be affected by disease. Thus, one may envisage causative agents which affect each of the different components of sarcoplasm, namely, an enzyme, an essential substrate, the filamentous proteins, the endoplasmic reticulum, or the sarcolemma itself. Again, the endomysial connective tissue could be the primary pathway in disease, since it so closely invests the muscle fiber. Inadequacy of blood supply in relation to the requirement of oxygen by active

muscle, or frank ischemia from vascular occlusion, could be another mechanism of disease. Finally, the nerve or its cell of origin in the spinal cord is known to bear the brunt of certain pathologic processes, paralyzing all the muscle fibers which it innervates and depriving them of the unique trophic influences which they normally receive from the nerve.

Normal muscle possesses a limited capacity to regenerate, a point often forgotten. Acute destructive processes of the muscle fiber, e.g., inflammatory or metabolic, are usually followed by fairly complete restoration of the muscle cells, providing some part of each fiber has survived and the endomysial sheaths of connective tissue have not been disturbed. Unfortunately, many pathologic processes of muscle are chronic and unrelenting and destroy the muscle fibers completely. Under such conditions any regenerative activity fails to keep pace with the disease, and the loss of muscle fibers is permanent.

APPROACH TO THE PATIENT WITH MUSCLE DISEASE

The number and diversity of diseases of striated muscle greatly exceed the number of symptoms and signs by which they express themselves clinically; thus, different diseases share certain common symptoms and even syndromes. To avoid excessive repetition in the description of individual diseases, we shall discuss in one place all their clinical manifestations, a subject which we call *clinical myology*.

The physician is put on the track of a myopathic disease by eliciting complaints of muscle weakness, pain, stiffness, spasm, and masses in muscles, or a change in muscle volume. Of these, the symptom of weakness is by far the most frequent and, at the same time, the most elusive. As was remarked in Chap. 23, when speaking of weakness the patient often means excessive fatigability. Although fatigability is a feature of a few muscle diseases, such as myasthenia gravis, it is far more frequently a complaint of patients with anxiety, depression, and chronic systemic disease. To distinguish between fatigability and weakness, inquiry should be made into the patient's capacity to perform certain common activities such as walking, running, climbing stairs, arising from a sitting, kneeling, squatting, or reclining position. Also difficulty in working with the arms above shoulder level usually reflects muscle weakness and not a fatigue state. Particular complaints may reveal a localized muscle weakness; e.g., drooping of the eyelids, diplopia and strabismus, change in facial expression and voice, and difficulty in swallowing indicate a paresis of the levator palpebrae, extraocular, facial, pharyngeal, and laryngeal muscles. Of course, the impairment of muscle function may be due to a neuropathic or a central nervous system disturbance rather than to a myopathic one, but usually these conditions can be separated by the methods indicated further on in this chapter and in Chaps. 3 and 23.

EVALUATION OF MUSCLE WEAKNESS AND PARALYSIS

Reduced strength of muscle contraction, manifested in diminished power of single contractions (peak power), resistance to opposition, and endurance, and in the impaired performance of demanded movements (i.e., work potential), is the indubitable sign of muscle disease. In such testing the physician may encounter difficulty in enlisting the patient's cooperation. The tentative, hesitant performance of the hysteric or malingerer poses difficulties which can be surmounted by resort to the techniques described in Chap. 3. In infants and small children, who cannot follow commands, one assesses muscle power by their resistance to passive manipulation or observing their performance while they are engaged in certain activities. The patient may be reluctant to fully contract muscles in a painful limb, and indeed pain itself may reflexly diminish the power of contraction (algesic paresis). Estimating the strength of isometric contractions that do not require the painful part to be moved is a way around this difficulty. Sometimes the weakness of a group of muscles is not evident when the patient is at rest but only becomes manifest after a period of activity; e.g., the feet and legs may "drag" only after walking a long distance. The physician, upon being told this by the patient, conducts the examination under circumstances that duplicate the complaint(s).

Weakness of muscle contraction acquires added significance when associated with other abnormalities, such as tenderness of muscle, change in tendon reflexes, alteration of muscle volume, twitching, and spasm. Also severe weakness of certain muscle groups may result in abnormalities of posture and gait. A waddling gait indicates affection of the medial glutei (or dysplasia of hip joints); excessive lumbar lordosis and protuberance of the abdomen indicate weakness of the iliopsoas and abdominal muscles; kyphoscoliosis points to an asymmetric weakness of the paravertebral muscles; and flaring of shoulder blades is a sign of weakness of lower trapezii, serratus magnus, and rhomboid muscles. Equinovarus deformities of the feet may be the result of pseudocontracture of the calf muscles.

Ascertaining the extent and severity of muscle weakness requires a systematic examination of all the main groups of muscles from forehead to feet. The patient is asked to contract each group quickly with as much force as possible, while the examiner opposes the movement and offers a graded resistance in accordance with the degree of residual power. Alternatively, the patient is asked to produce a maximal contraction, and the examiner estimates power by the force needed to "break" or overcome it. If the weakness is unilateral, one has the advantage of being able to compare it with the strength of muscles on the normal side. If it is bilateral, the physician must refer to a concept of what constitutes normalcy, based on experience in muscle testing. Ocular, facial, lingual, pharyngeal, laryngeal, cervical, shoulder, upper arm, lower arm and hand, truncal, pelvic, thigh, and lower leg and foot muscles are examined sequentially. A practiced examiner can survey these muscle groups in 2 to 3 min. A word of caution: in using one's hands to oppose the patient's attempts to contract the large and powerful trunk and girdle muscles, one may fail to detect slight to moderate degrees of weakness. These muscle groups are best tested by asking the patient to squat and kneel and then to assume the erect posture; to walk on the toes and heels; and to lift a heavy object (textbook of medicine) over the head.

In order to quantitate the degree of weakness, which indicates the severity of affection, and to compare one examination with another, which is necessary to determine the course of the disease and the effects of therapy, a rating scale should be used. Most widely used is the one proposed by the Medical Research Council of Great Britain which recognizes five grades of muscle strength, as follows: 0, complete paralysis; 1, minimal contraction, with gravity eliminated; 2, weak contraction, against gravity; 3, moderate weakness; 4, minimal detectable weakness; and 5, normal strength. Some physiatrists add further gradations, specified as 4+ for barely detectable weakness and 4− for easily detected weakness, etc. With practice, one can distinguish true weakness from unwillingness to cooperate, feigned weakness, and inhibition of movement by pain.

QUALITATIVE CHANGES IN THE CONTRACTILE PROCESS

In the *myasthenic states* there is a rapid failure of contraction in the most affected muscles during sustained contraction. For instance, in looking at the ceiling for a few minutes the eyelids progressively droop; and after closing the eyes and resting the levator palpebrae muscles, the power returns and the ptosis lessens or disappears. Similarly, holding the eyes in a lateral position will induce diplopia and strabismus. This reaction, in combination with restoration of power by the administration of neostigmine or edrophonium (Tensilon), are the most valid criteria for the diagnosis of myasthenia gravis (see page 990).

In addition to myasthenic weakness, there are other abnormalities that may be discovered by observing, during one or a series of maximal actions of a group of muscles, the speed and efficiency of contraction and relaxation. In myxedema, for example, slow waves of contraction in a muscle such as the quadriceps may be seen on change in posture (*contraction myoedema*); often it is associated with percussion myoedema and prolonged duration of the tendon reflexes. Slowness in relaxation is another indication of hypothyroidism, accounting for the complaints of uncomfortable tightness and firmness of proximal limb muscles.

A prolonged failure of relaxation with afterdischarge is characteristic of the myotonic phenomenon, which characterizes certain diseases—congenital myotonia (of Thomsen), myotonic dystrophy (of Steinert), and the paramyotonia of von Eulenberg. True myotonia, with its prolonged discharges of action potentials, requires strong contraction for its elicitation, is more evident after a period of relaxation, and tends to disappear with repeated contractions (see page 1002). This persistence of contraction is demonstrable also upon tapping a muscle (*percussion myotonia*), a phenomenon easily distinguished from the electrically silent local bulge (*myoedema*) induced by a sharp tap of a muscle in the myxedematous or cachetic patient.

Increase in power in a series of several voluntary contractions in the absence of myotonia is a feature of the inverse myasthenic syndrome, which is associated in about 50 percent of reported cases with small-cell carcinoma of the lung. It, too, has its electromyographic equivalent—a rapid increase in the voltage of a series of action potentials (see page 883).

The effect of cold on muscle contraction may also prove informative; either paresis or myotonia, lasting for a few minutes, may be evoked or enhanced by cold, as in the paramyotonia of von Eulenberg.

Myotonia and myoedema must be distinguished from the recruitment and spread of involuntary spasm induced by strong and repeated contractions of limb muscles in patients with *mild or localized tetanus*. This is not a primary phenomenon of muscle but is due to an abolition of inhibitory spinal mechanisms.

The repeated contraction of forearm or leg muscles, after the application of a tourniquet (exceeding arterial pressure) to the proximal part of a limb, will often elicit latent tetany. The special mode of development of tetany, as well as its duration, its enhancement by hyperventilation, and the presence of accompanying tingling, prickling paresthesias, separate tetany from ordinary cramp and also from true contracture.

In *true contracture* a group of muscles, after a series of strong contractions, may remain shortened for many minutes, unable to relax because of failure of the metabolic mechanism necessary for relaxation; and the muscle in this shortened state remains silent in the electromyogram, in contrast to the high-voltage, rapid discharges observed with cramp, tetanus, and tetany. Such contracture occurs in McArdle's disease (phosphorylase deficiency), where it is aggravated by arterial occlusion, but it has been seen in phosphofructokinase deficiency and possibly in another disease, as yet undefined, where the tourniquet has no effect and phosphorylase seems to be present in adequate amounts, at least as judged by histochemical stains (see page 1001). True contracture is to be distinguished from paradoxical myotonia, in which the myotonia is absent after the first strong contraction but then appears and gradually increases with each successive contraction.

Pseudocontracture (*myostatic contracture*), which inevitably follows all conditions which occasion prolonged fixation and complete inactivity of the normally innervated muscle, is another common disorder, but here the shortened state of the muscle, which may persist for days or weeks, has no established anatomic, physiologic, or chemical basis. It is distinguished from *ankylosis* by the springy nature of the resistance, coincident with increased tautness of muscle and tendon during passive motion, and from *Volkmann's contracture*, where there is evident fibrosis of muscle and surrounding tissues due to ischemic injury, usually after a fracture of the forearm.

TOPOGRAPHY OR PATTERNS OF PARALYSIS

As was stated above, in almost all the diseases under consideration, some of the muscles are affected and others are spared. Each disease exhibits its own pattern. Moreover, the topography or distribution of involvement tends to follow a similar pattern in all patients with the same disease. Thus, topography of involvement becomes another valid diagnostic attribute of muscular disease, ranking next in importance after altered quantity and quality of contraction.

The following patterns of muscle involvement constitute a core of essential clinical knowledge in this field:

1. *Ocular palsies presenting more or less exclusively as diplopia, ptosis, or strabismus,* sometimes in association with exophthalmos, enophthalmos, and pupillary change. As a rule, primary diseases of muscle do not involve the pupil, and in most instances their effects are bilateral. In lesions of the third, fourth, or sixth cranial nerves, the neural origin is revealed by the pattern of ocular muscle palsies or abnormalities of the pupil, or both. When weakness of the orbicularis oculi (muscle of eye closure) is added to ocular palsies and ptosis, it nearly always signifies myopathic disease

Myasthenia gravis, progressive external ophthalmoplegia (ocular myopathy), oculopharyngeal dystrophy, exophthalmic ophthalmoplegia of thyroid disease, ocular myositis, curare-sensitive nonmyasthenic ophthalmoplegia, myotonic dystrophy of Steinert, Kearns-Sayre syndrome (external ophthalmoplegia with retinitis pigmentosa, heart block, short stature, and elevated CSF protein), congenital myotubular myopathy, nuclear ophthalmoplegia (e.g., Moebius' syndrome), and botulism are the principal conditions to be considered. When ptosis or weakness of eye closure or both occur in combination with weakness of other skeletal muscles, one should think of myotonic, facioscapulohumeral, limb-girdle, or oculopharyngeal dystrophy, and the nemaline and myotubular forms of congenital myopathy.

2. *Bifacial palsy presenting as an inability to smile and expose teeth and to close eyes.* Varying degrees of bifacial weakness are observed in myasthenia gravis, and ptosis and ocular palsies are conjoined in about 90 percent of cases. The same is true of myotonic dystrophy. More severe or complete facial palsy occurs in facioscapulohumeral and related dystrophies, in congenital myopathies (centronuclear, nemaline, carnitine) in the Guillain-Barré syndrome (nearly always with other signs of neuropathy), in polymyositis (rare) and in combination with abducens palsies in Moebius' syndrome. Very rarely, Bell's palsy is bilateral. Sometimes bilateral facial paralysis occurs as a manifestation of sarcoid or as part of a cranial polyneuritis of unknown cause (see page 937).

3. *Bulbar palsy presenting as dysphonia, dysarthria, and dysphagia with or without weakness of jaw or facial muscles.* Myasthenia gravis is the most frequent cause of this syndrome and must also be considered whenever there is the solitary finding of a hanging jaw or fatigue of the jaw while eating or talking, but usually ptosis and ocular palsies are conjoined (>90 percent of cases). These combinations of palsies are also observed in myotonic dystrophy and botulism. Progressive bulbar palsy of lower motor neuron type may be the basis of this syndrome, and the diagnosis is most obvious when the tongue is withered and twitching. Platybasia and the Arnold-Chiari malformation may reproduce some of the findings of bulbar palsy by involving the lower cranial nerves; diphtheria and bulbar poliomyelitis are now rare diseases that may present in this way. Pure dysphonia and dysphagia may be the first manifestations of polymyositis.

The neurologic condition known as spastic bulbar paralysis, or pseudobulbar palsy, is readily distinguished by the lack of atrophy of muscle, the mode of onset (usually sudden), and the associated clinical findings (see pages 41 and 355). Athetosis and dystonic spasms of masseter, facial, and bulbar muscles, as in the faciocervical dyskinesias of phenothiazine intoxication are also readily recognizable by the occurrence of spasms without increase in stretch reflexes.

4. *Cervical palsy presenting with inability to hold the head erect or to lift the head from the pillow.* The patient may be unable to hold up the head owing to weakness of the posterior neck muscles, or to lift it from a pillow because of weakness of the sternocleidomastoids and other anterior neck muscles. In advanced forms of this syndrome, the head may hang with chin on chest, unless it is held up by the patient's hands.

The hanging head with weakness of posterior neck muscles occurs most often in idiopathic polymyositis, often combined with slight dysphagia, dysphonia, and weakness of girdle muscles. The major types of progressive muscular dystrophy, when advanced, usually affect the anterior neck muscles disproportionately, so that the head cannot be lifted from the pillow. Rarely, syringomyelia, syphilitic meningoradiculitis, loss of anterior horn cells in conjunction with carcinomatosis, and motor system disease may differentially paralyze various neck muscles.

5. *Bibrachial palsy presenting sometimes as the dangling-arm syndrome.* Weakness, atrophy, and fasciculations of hands, arms, and shoulders characterize the common form of motor system disease, namely, amyotrophic lateral sclerosis. Primary diseases of muscle hardly ever weaken these parts disproportionately. Rarely, a diffuse weakness of both arms may occur in the early stages of acute idiopathic polyneuritis and por-

phyric and other polyneuropathies, but it soon becomes part of a more generalized paralysis.

6. *Bicrural palsy presenting as lower leg weakness with inability to walk on the heels and toes, or as paralysis of all leg and thigh muscles.* Symmetrical weakness of the lower legs is usually due to polyneuropathy although peroneal and anterior tibial muscles are often weakened in dystrophy. Diabetic polyneuropathy may weaken thigh and pelvic muscles asymmetrically with little sensory change. In total leg and thigh weakness, one first thinks of a disease of the spinal cord, in which case there is often loss of control of the bladder and bowel sphincters, as well as loss of sensory function below a certain level. Motor system disease may begin in the legs, asymmetrically as a rule, and affect them out of proportion to other parts. Thus the differential diagnosis of leg weakness involves more diseases than do the restricted paralyses of other parts of the body.

7. *Limb-girdle palsies presenting as inability to raise the arms or to arise from a squatting, kneeling, or sitting position.* Two groups of diseases most often manifest themselves in this fashion—polymyositis and dermatomyositis, and the progressive muscular dystrophies. The Duchenne and Leyden-Moebius types of dystrophy tend first to affect the muscles of the pelvic girdle, gluteal region, and thighs, resulting in a lumbar lordosis and protuberant abdomen, a waddling gait, and difficulty in arising from the floor and climbing stairs without the assistance of the arms. The Landouzy-Déjerine type affects muscles of face and shoulder girdles foremost, and is manifested by incomplete eye closure, inability to whistle and to raise the arms above the head, winging of the scapulae, and thinness of the upper arms ("Popeye" appearance).

In the milder forms of polymyositis, weakness may be limited to either the neck muscles or those of the shoulder or pelvic girdles. Similarly, the early or mild forms of dystrophy may selectively involve only the peroneal and scapular muscles (scapuloperoneal dystrophy). A metabolic myopathy, such as the adult form of acid maltase deficiency and the familial (hypokalemic) type of periodic paralysis may affect only the pelvic and thigh muscles. Proximal muscles are occasionally implicated in progressive spinal muscular atrophy, as in the syndrome first described by Wohlfart et al. and by Kugelberg and Welander, which unfortunately adds to confusion in diagnosis. In a number of the congenital polymyopathies, cataloged by Bethlem, a relatively nonprogressive weakness affects girdle muscles more than distal ones.

8. *Distal limb palsies presenting usually as foot drop with steppage gait (and pes cavus), weakness of all* lower leg muscles, and later wrist drop and weakness of hands (claw hand). The principal cause of this neuromuscular syndrome is a familial polyneuropathy, such as the peroneal muscular atrophy of Charcot-Marie-Tooth, hypertrophic polyneuropathy of Déjerine and Sottas, and the hereditary polyneuropathy of Refsum. Rarely chronic nonfamilial polyneuropathies may also present such a picture, but once more, there are exceptions, such as some forms of familial progressive muscular atrophy and distal types of progressive muscular dystrophy (Gowers, Welander). Steinert's myotonic dystrophy also weakens peroneal and posterior tibial muscles as well as those of the forearm, sternomastoid, face, and eyes. Despite these exceptions, the generalization that girdle weakness means myopathy and distal weakness neuropathy is clinically useful.

9. *Generalized or universal paralysis: limb and cranial muscles, involved either in attacks or as part of a persistent, progressive deterioration.* When acute in onset and episodic, this syndrome is usually a manifestation of familial hypokalemic or hyperkalemic periodic paralysis. One variety of the former type is associated with hyperthyroidism, another with aldosteronism. Generalized paresis (rather than paralysis) that has an acute onset and lasts many weeks is a feature of a peculiar group of diseases called paroxysmal myoglobinuria of Meyer-Betz, and at times of a severe form of idiopathic or parasitic (trichinosis) polymyositis. Idiopathic polymyositis may involve all limb and trunk muscles but usually spares the facial and ocular muscles, whereas the weakness in trichinosis is mainly in the ocular and lingual muscles. In infants and young children, a chronic and persistent generalized weakness of all muscles except those of the eyes always raises the question of Werdnig-Hoffman spinal muscular atrophy or, if mild in degree and relatively nonprogressive, of congenital myopathy or polyneuropathy. In these diseases of infancy, paucity of movement, hypotonia, and retardation of motor development may be more obvious than weakness.

Universal ascending paralysis, developing over a few days, with involvement of cranial (including ocular) muscles, is usually due to acute idiopathic polyneuritis. Insidious onset and slow (months to years) progression of paralysis, atrophy, and fasciculation of limb and trunk muscles, without sensory loss, characterizes motor system disease. Here the eye muscles are nearly always spared. Mild degrees of generalized weakness are features of a number of metabolic myopathies, such as thyrotoxic myopathy, glycogen storage diseases, vitamin D deficiency, and rickets.

10. *Paralysis of single muscles or a group of muscles.* This is almost always neuropathic, rarely spinal. Muscle disease does not need to be considered except possibly in certain atypical forms of familial periodic paralysis (see page 994).

From this exposition of the topographic aspects of weakness one can appreciate that each neuromuscular disease exhibits a predilection for particular groups of muscles. As a corollary, a given pattern of weakness should always suggest certain possibilities of disease and exclude others.

Diagnosis also depends on features of the paralysis other than its topography, such as mode of onset and tempo of progression, the coexistence of medical disorders, and certain laboratory findings (serum enzymes, electromyogram, and biopsy findings). Other differentiating features, such as the natural course of the disease, age of onset, and its genetic determinants figure prominently in the delineation of muscle diseases.

CHANGES IN MUSCLE MASS

Alteration of muscle bulk stands as another feature of disease which can be observed in all except the most obese patients. There are, of course, innate differences in muscle development, a greater salience of muscle in the male than in the female, and differences due to use and disuse. Greatly increased size and strength of muscles (hypertrophia musculorum vera) may be observed in *congenital myotonia* (circus freaks with phenomenal muscular development often have this disease), in rare instances of a pathologic cramp syndrome, in the Bruck-deLange syndrome of congenital hypertrophy of muscle, athetosis and feeblemindedness, and in some patients destined to develop muscular dystrophy. Far more often, muscle enlargement in progressive muscular dystrophy takes the form of *pseudohypertrophy,* where increase in size is accompanied by weakness. Here large and small fibers are mixed with fat cells which have replaced many of the degenerated muscle fibers. Other muscles in the same patient are atrophied. Other diseases may also cause pseudohypertrophy. We have seen it in amyloidosis, sarcoidosis, eosinophilic monomyositis, and rarely in certain of the congenital myopathies. When pain is present, it may impair the power of contraction more than actual loss of muscle fibers. Hypothyroidism is often accompanied by an increase in volume of certain muscles,

simulating hypertrophia musculorum vera and congenital myotonia (see page 1002).

Cachexia, malnutrition, and lipodystrophy tend to reduce muscle bulk without reducing the power of contraction proportionately (pseudoatrophy). Denervation due to lesions of the peripheral nerve or spinal cord, which if complete leads to a loss of bulk up to 85 percent of the original volume within 3 months, is invariably attended by paralysis. The most severe degrees of atrophy usually signify denervation or dystrophy.

TWITCHES, SPASMS, AND CRAMPS

Fascicular twitches during rest, if pronounced and combined with muscular weakness and atrophy, usually signify motor neuron disease (amyotrophic lateral sclerosis, progressive muscular atrophy, or progressive bulbar palsy); but they may be seen in lesser degree in other diseases of gray matter of the spinal cord (e.g., syringomyelia or tumor), in lesions of anterior roots (e.g., protruded intervertebral disk), and in peripheral neuropathies. Widespread fasciculations may occur with severe dehydration, after an overdose of neostigmine, or with organophosphate poisoning. Slow and persistent fasciculations, spreading in a wavelike pattern along the entire length of a muscle and associated with slight reduction in speed of contraction and relaxation, are part of the syndrome of continuous muscular activity (page 1000). The same sequence, evolving at a slightly slower pace, may occur in small fiber neuropathies. Fasciculations that occur during muscular contraction, in contrast to those at rest, indicate a state of heightened irritability of muscle, often for reasons that are not known, or a condition which leaves muscle with some paralyzed motor units, so that during contraction small and increasingly larger units are not enlisted smoothly. One may observe this latter phenomenon years after poliomyelitis has left a muscle weakened. *Benign fasciculations,* a common finding in otherwise normal individuals, can usually be distinguished by the lack of muscular weakness and atrophy; and *myokymia* is a less common condition in which repeated twitchings impart a rippling appearance to the muscle. The recurrent twitches of the eyelid or muscles of the thumb which are experienced by most normal persons are often referred to as myokymia but are probably more closely related to benign fasciculations.

Cramps at rest or with movement (action cramps) are frequently reported in motor system disease, tetany, dehydration after excessive sweating and salt loss and other metabolic diseases (uremia, hypocalcemia, and hypomagnesemia) and in certain muscle diseases (e.g., some of the myoglobinurias, rare cases of Becker's muscular dystrophy and congenital myopathies). However, there is a benign form (*idiopathic cramp syndrome*), in which no other neuromuscular disturbance can be found. One form of it is known as *myokymia with persistent spasm*. A particularly malignant and progressive form of painful spasm is known as the *stiff-man syndrome;* this appears to be a disease of the central nervous system, of unknown nature. Continuous spasm, intensified by the action of muscles, with no demonstrable disorder at a neuromuscular level, is a common manifestation of tetanus and also follows the bite of the black widow spider. All these conditions must be distinguished from sensations of cramp without muscle spasm. The latter is a dysesthetic phenomenon.

All the aforementioned phenomena are discussed in Chap. 52.

PALPABLE ABNORMALITIES OF MUSCLE

Altered structure and function of muscle are not accurately revealed by palpation. Of course, the difference between the firm hypertrophied muscle of a well-conditioned athlete and the slack muscle of a sedentary person is as apparent to the palpating fingers as to the eye, and the persistent contraction in tetanus, cramp, contracture, etc., is easily felt. The muscles in dystrophy are said to have a "doughy" or "elastic" feel, but we find this difficult to judge. In the Pompe type of glycogen storage disease, attention may be attracted to the musculature by an unnatural firmness and increase in bulk. The swollen, edematous, weak muscles in acute paroxysmal myoglobinuria or severe polymyositis may feel taut and firm but are usually not tender. Areas of tenderness in muscles which otherwise function normally, a state called *myogelosis,* has been attributed to fibrositis or fibromyositis, but their nature has not been divulged by biopsy.

A mass may develop in part of a muscle, or throughout a muscle, and poses a series of special clinical problems, which will be discussed on pages 1005 and 1006.

TENDON (STRETCH) REFLEXES

The tendon reflexes are impaired in the majority of neuromuscular diseases, but particularly in those which involve peripheral nerves. In muscular dystrophy and polymyositis they tend to be reduced in proportion to the reduction in muscular power. In the myopathy of hypothyroidism, in which contraction and relaxation of muscle is slowed, there is a characteristic prolongation of the tendon reflex; the opposite condition of quickening and brevity of the tendon reflex is less reliably demonstrated in hyperthyroidism.

MUSCLE PAIN

Severe pain localized to a group of muscles occurs in wryneck, fibrositis and fibromyositis, acute brachial neuritis, radiculitis, and Bornholm's disease or pleurodynia, but little is known of its cause in any of these diseases. Cramping can also cause pain, and the latter is a prominent complaint in most of the muscle spasm and cramp syndromes mentioned above. Tenderness of muscle is a variable state normally. It tends to be more definite in polyneuritis, poliomyelitis, and polyarteritis nodosa than in polymyositis, the various forms of dystrophy, and other myopathies, in which there is usually no increase in the sensitivity of muscle tissue. In polymyositis, if pain is present, it usually indicates coincident involvement of connective tissues and joint structures. The myalgic states are considered further on pages 1004 and 1005.

DIAGNOSIS OF MUSCLE DISEASE

The clinical recognition of myopathic diseases is facilitated, as a rule, by a prior knowledge of a few syndromes. The ones listed in Table 47-1 occur with regularity. A description of these syndromes and the diseases which comprise each of them forms the content of the chapters that follow. Diagnostic accuracy will be aided by an intelligent use of laboratory examinations, such as chemical analyses of serum and urine, electromyography, nerve conduction studies, and muscle biopsy. These methods and the principles underlying them are discussed in Chap. 44.

Table 47-1
Syndromic classification of muscle diseases

I. Acute (evolving in days) or subacute (weeks) paretic or paralytic disorders of muscle*
    A. Rarely fulminant myasthenia gravis or myasthenic syndrome from a "mycin" antibiotic or hypokalemia
    B. Idiopathic polymyositis and dermatomyositis
    C. Viral polymyositis
    D. Acute paroxysmal myoglobinuria
    E. "Alcoholic" polymyopathy
    F. Familial (malignant) hyperpyrexia precipitated by anesthetic agents

---

*The acute and subacute primary disorders of muscle need to be differentiated from acute spinal cord or peripheral nerve diseases, in which paralysis is often severe and widespread and atrophy may or may not be present (poliomyelitis, acute idiopathic polyneuritis, or other forms of polyneuropathy; see Chap. 45).

Table 47-1 (*continued*)
Syndromic classification of muscle diseases

    G. First attack of episodic weakness may enter into differential diagnosis (see below)

    H. Botulism

    I. Organophosphate poisoning

II. Chronic (i.e., months to years) weakness or paralysis of muscle usually with severe atrophy

    A. Progressive muscular dystrophy

        1. Duchenne type

        2. Facioscapulohumeral type (Landouzy-Déjerine)

        3. Limb-girdle types

        4. Distal type (Gowers, Welander)

        5. Myotonic dystrophy (Steinert's disease)

        6. Progressive ophthalmoplegic, oculopharyngeal, and Kearns-Sayre types

    B. Chronic idiopathic polymyositis (may be subacute)

    C. Chronic thyrotoxic and other endocrine myopathies

    D. Chronic, slowly progressive, or relatively stationary polymyopathies†

        1. Central core, multicore, and minicore diseases

        2. Rod-body and related polymyopathies

        3. Mitochondrial and centronuclear polymyopathies

        4. Other congenital myopathies (reducing-body, fingerprint, zebra body, fiber-type atrophies and disproportions, focal lysis of myofibrils)

        5. Glycogen storage disease

        6. Lipid myopathies (carnitine deficiency myopathy, undefined lipid myopathies)

III. Episodic weakness of muscle

    A. Familial (hypokalemic) periodic paralysis

    B. Normokalemic or hyperkalemic familial periodic paralysis (adynamia episodica hereditaria of Gamstorp)

    C. Paramyotonia congenita (von Eulenberg)

    D. Nonfamilial hyper- and hypokalemic periodic paralyis (including primary hyperaldosteronism)

    E. Acute thyrotoxic myopathy (also thyrotoxic periodic paralysis)

    F. Conditions in which weakness fluctuates

        1. Myasthenia gravis, immunologic type

        2. Myasthenia associated with:

            a. Lupus erythematosus disseminatus

            b. Polymyositis

            c. Rheumatoid arthritis

            d. Nonthymic carcinoma

        3. Familial and sporadic nonimmunologic types of myasthenia

        4. Eaton-Lambert syndrome

---

†The chronic myopathies need to be distinguished from the progressive muscular atrophies and other forms of motor system disease (amyotrophic lateral sclerosis, progressive bulbar palsy) and infantile spinal muscular atrophy (Werdnig-Hoffmann disease), as well as chronic neural muscular atrophies such as peroneal muscular atrophy (Charcot-Marie-Tooth), hypertrophic polyneuritis (Déjerine-Sottas), amyloid polyneuropathy, chronic nutritional, arsenical, leprous, and other polyneuropathies (see Chaps. 45 and 50).

Table 47-1 (*continued*)
Syndromic classification of muscle diseases

IV. Disorders of muscle presenting with myotonia, stiffness, spasm, and cramp

    A. Congenital myotonia (Thomsen's disease), paramyotonia congenita, myotonic dystrophy, and Schwartz-Jampel syndrome

    B. Hypothyroidism with pseudomyotonia (Debré-Semelaigne and Hoffmann syndromes)

    C. Tetany

    D. Tetanus

    E. Black widow spider bite

    F. Myopathy resulting from myophosphorylase deficiency (McArdle's syndrome), phosphofructokinase deficiency, and other forms of contracture

    G. Contracture with Addison's disease

    H. Idiopathic cramp syndromes

    I. Myokymia and syndromes of continuous muscle activity

V. Myalgic states‡

    A. Connective tissue diseases (rheumatoid arthritis, mixed connective tissue disease, Sjögren's syndrome, lupus erythematosus, polyarteritis nodosa, scleroderma, polymyositis)

    B. Localized fibrositis or fibromyositis

    C. Trichinosis

    D. Myopathy of myoglobinuria and McArdle's syndrome

    E. Myopathy with hypoglycemia

    F. Bornholm's disease and other forms of viral polymyositis

    G. Anterior tibial syndrome

    H. Other

        1. Hypophosphatemia

        2. Hypothyroidism

        3. Psychiatric illness (hysteria, depression)

VI. Localized muscle mass(es)

    A. Rupture of a muscle

    B. Muscle hemorrhage

    C. Muscle tumor

        1. Rhabdomyosarcoma

        2. Desmoid

        3. Angioma

        4. Metastatic nodules

    D. Monomyositis multiplex

        1. Eosinophilic type

        2. Other

    E. Localized and generalized myositis ossificans

    F. Fibrositis (myogelosis)

    G. Granulomatous infections

        1. Sarcoidosis

        2. Tuberculosis

        3. Wegener's granulomatosis

    H. Pyogenic abscess

    I. Infarction of muscle in the diabetic

---

‡Pain and tenderness of muscle are characteristic also of many forms of polyneuropathy (see Chap. 45).

REFERENCES

ADAMS RD: Thayer lectures: I. Principles of myopathology. II. Principles of clinical myology. *Johns Hopkins Med J* 131:24, 1972.

————: *Pathology of Muscle Disease.* New York, Hoeber, 1975.

BETHLEM J: *Myopathies.* Philadelphia, Lippincott, 1977.

BROOKE MH: *A Clinician's View of Neuromuscular Diseases.* Baltimore, Williams & Wilkins, 1977.

DUBOWITZ V: *Muscle Disorders in Childhood.* Philadelphia, Saunders, 1978.

WALTON JN (ed): *Disorders of Voluntary Muscle,* 4th ed. Edinburgh, Churchill Livingstone, 1981.

CHAPTER 48

POLYMYOSITIS AND OTHER ACUTE AND SUBACUTE MYOPATHIC PARALYSES

Of importance from a diagnostic standpoint is the principle that primary diseases of muscle seldom if ever are the cause of acute, widespread paralysis. Diffuse paralytic states of rapid evolution, i.e., over the period of a few days, are usually due to idiopathic polyneuritis (Guillain-Barré syndrome) and infrequently to poliomyelitis and other neuritides; one must also consider certain spinal cord diseases (Chaps. 35 and 45). Nevertheless, there are exceptions to this clinical rule, the most notable being disorders of neuromuscular transmission. For example, botulinus toxin can paralyze muscles within a few hours by blocking acetylcholine (ACh) release. Rarely, myasthenia gravis or a myasthenic syndrome related to aminoglycide antibiotic therapy may develop over several days, or a week or two. In a thyroid "storm" there may be a widespread weakness of muscles, the defect evidently being within the contractile mechanism of the muscle fibers. Hypokalemic paralysis as in hyperaldosteronism and the initial attack of familial periodic paralysis due to either hypo- or hyperkalemia may come on within a few hours. Finally, in patients with a paroxysm of myoglobinuria, due to an infection or a metabolic myopathy, especially if there is unusually strenuous exertion, may be followed within hours by a rapidly developing paresis of limb muscles, usually in association with pain in the muscles.

Thus the occurrence of sudden and acute paralysis always raises the consideration of neurologic as well as myologic disease. In the relatively rare instances of the latter, diagnostic suspicions are affirmed by measurements of electrolytes, muscle enzymes [creatine phosphokinase (CPK) and aldolase], and thyroid hormones in the serum, by nerve conduction studies and electromyography, and by urinary analysis for myoglobin.

Paralyses of widespread distribution of subacute evolution (over the period of a few weeks) are attributable to a wider spectrum of diseases, some clearly myologic such as infective and idiopathic polymyositis and dermatomyositis and several of the metabolic polymyopathies. These will be the subject material of this chapter.

THE INFECTIVE (AND PRESUMABLY INFECTIVE) FORMS OF POLYMYOSITIS

TRICHINOSIS

The main features of this infection have been discussed in Chap. 31 (page 504). With respect to the myopathic aspect of the illness, the authors have been most impressed with the ocular muscle weakness which results in strabismus and diplopia and with weakness of the tongue which results in dysarthria. The involved muscles are slightly swollen and tender in the acute stage of the disease, and there is conjunctival and orbital edema. As the trichinae become encysted, over a period of a few weeks, the symptoms subside, and recovery is complete. Many, perhaps the majority, of the infected patients are asymptomatic throughout the invasive period and as much as 1 to 3 percent of the population in certain regions of the country will be found at autopsy to have calcified cysts in the muscles, with no history of parasitic illness.

The diagnosis is always suggested by an eosinophilia (>700 per cubic millimeter), and there are many eosinophils in the muscle infiltrates. A skin test using trichina antigen is also available, and it turns positive in the third week of the disease. Precipitin, complement fixation, and bentonite flocculation tests are available. Biopsy of almost any muscle (usually the deltoid or gastrocnemius), regardless of whether they are painful or tender, is the most reliable method of diagnosis.

No treatment is required in most cases. If the infestation is severe, thiabendazole 25 mg/kg daily for 5 to 7 days and prednisone 40 to 60 mg/day, are recommended.

TOXOPLASMOSIS

An acute to subacute systemic illness due to the encephalitozoan toxoplasma, with some indication of retinal, myocardial, liver, and brain involvement, has occasionally been encountered in adults. In one such case we detected toxoplasmic pseudocysts in skeletal muscle. Wherever the pseudocysts had ruptured, there was focal inflammation. Some muscle fibers had undergone segmental necrosis, but this was not prominent, accounting for the relative paucity of muscle symptoms. In fact, most infections with toxoplasma are asymptomatic (10 to 30 percent of the population). The immunocompromised patient is particularly susceptible. Sulfadiazine and trisulfapyramadine are effective therapeutic agents (cf. *Harrison's Principles of Internal Medicine*). See Chap. 31 for further discussion.

OTHER PROTOZOAN AND FUNGAL INFECTIONS

Sarcosporoidosis, echinococcosis, cysticercosis, trypanosomiasis (Chagas disease) actinomycosis, tuberculosis, and syphilis are all known to affect skeletal muscle on occasion, but the major symptoms relate more to involvement of other organs. Hence they will not be discussed further. The reader who seeks more details may refer to the monograph on the pathology of muscle diseases by Adams (see references).

VIRAL INFECTIONS

Most patients with pleurodynia (epidemic myalgia, Bornholm's disease) have had negative muscle biopsies, and there is no clear explanation of the pain. However, group B Coxsackie virus has been isolated from striated muscle of patients with epidemic myalgia. In recent years a number of patients with viral influenza were found to have a necrotizing myositis, and virus was seen under the electron microscope in infected muscle fibers; malaise, myalgia, slight weakness and stiffness were the reported clinical manifestations. From the descriptions it seems difficult to decide how much of the weakness was only apparent, because of the myalgia. Recovery was complete within a few weeks. In one patient with generalized myalgia and myoglobinuria, the influenza virus was isolated from muscle (Gamboa et al.).

Viral myositis is an established entity in comparative myopathology, but its existence in humans has been in doubt. These new observations suggest that the intense muscle pain in certain viral illnesses might be due to a direct viral infection of muscle. However, there are many cases of influenzal myalgia, mainly of the calves and thighs, such as those reported by Lundberg and more recently by Antony et al., where it was not possible to establish a cause of the muscular disorder.

SARCOIDOSIS

Patients with established sarcoidosis may develop a polyneuritis or mononeuritis multiplex (see Chap. 45). As pointed out in Chaps. 31 and 35, a granulomatous meningoencephalitis or -myelitis are also established entities. The response to corticosteroid therapy is at times quite dramatic. Much more puzzling to the authors, however, have been patients with an illness whose clinical features are virtually indistinguishable from those of idiopathic polymyositis, described further on; muscle biopsy reveals inflammation with Langhan's giant cells or a noncaseating granulomatous lesion. Several of the reported cases have been middle-aged or elderly adults with no signs of sarcoidosis of the nervous system, lungs, bone, skin, or lymph nodes.

The question which must be asked is whether the finding of a few giant cells in myositic muscle is a sufficient basis for the diagnosis of sarcoidosis. We doubt that it is, but the matter cannot be settled until we have better laboratory tests than are now available. More acceptable are the rare cases with sarcoid lesions of both nerve and muscle—a neuromyositis—of subacute evolution and unassociated with neoplasia.

IDIOPATHIC POLYMYOSITIS AND DERMATOMYOSITIS

DEFINITION

These are relatively common diseases which affect primarily the striated muscle and skin, and sometimes connective tissues as well. The term used varies according to the distribution of the pathologic process. If restricted clinically to the striated muscles, the disease is called polymyositis; if the skin is involved, it is designated as dermatomyositis; and if connective tissues also are implicated, the term of choice is polymyositis or dermatomyositis with rheumatoid arthritis, rheumatic fever, lupus erythematosus, diffuse sclerosis, or scleroderma.

HISTORY

Polymyositis has been known since the original descriptions by Wagner in 1863, and the dermatomyositic form was first reported by Unverricht in 1887. A survey of the literature since that time and a detailed statement of present knowledge are found in the monograph of Adams and the review of Currie (see references).

ETIOLOGY

The cause of idiopathic polymyositis and dermatomyositis, as the term indicates, is unknown. All attempts to isolate an infective agent have been unsuccessful. Several electron microscopists have observed virus particles of two types in muscle fibers, but their causative role has not been proved. Rising titers of antibodies have not been demonstrated, nor has a polymyositic illness been induced in animals by injections of infected muscle. A disease which resembles polymyositis has been provoked in laboratory animals by injections of sterile muscle extracts with Freund's adjuvants, suggesting an autoimmune mechanism. Its close association with diseases of connective tissue favors the notion of common etiology or pathogenesis, and also is in keeping with an autoallergic inflammation. It must be conceded, however, that the category of disease called polymyositis is not precise and probably has been used to include diseases of viral origin and others of noninflammatory type, namely, metabolic myopathies.

CLINICAL MANIFESTATIONS

Polymyositis and dermatomyositis tend to assume several clinical forms, as follows:

Polymyositis *A subacute symmetric weakness of proximal limb and trunk muscles without dermatitis or with minimal skin lesions.* The onset is usually insidious and the course progressive over a period of several weeks or months. The disease may develop at almost any age and in either sex. However the majority of patients range from 30 to 60 years of age, and females outnumber males two to one. A febrile illness or benign infection may precede the muscle weakness, but in most patients the first symptoms develop in the absence of these or other apparent initiating events.

The patient first becomes aware of a painless weakness of the proximal limb muscles, especially of the hips and thighs and certain actions such as arising from a deep chair or from a squatting or kneeling position, climbing or descending stairs, walking, putting an object on a high shelf, or combing the hair become increasingly difficult. In restricted forms of the disease only the neck muscles or quadriceps may be involved. Pain of an aching variety in the buttocks, calves, or joints is experienced by only a small proportion of patients (15 percent) and often indicates a combination of polymyositis and arthritis or other connective tissue disease.

When the patient is first seen, all the muscles of the trunk, shoulders, hips, upper arms, and thighs are usually involved. The facial, posterior and anterior neck muscles (the head may loll), the pharyngeal and laryngeal muscles (dysphagia and dysphonia) are usually involved as well. Ocular muscles are never affected except in rare combinations of polymyositis and myasthenia gravis; and the forearm, hand, leg, and foot muscles are spared in all but about 25 percent of cases. The muscles are usually not tender, and atrophy and reduction in tendon reflexes, though present, are not so pronounced as in cases of chronic denervation atrophy. When reflexes are disproportionately reduced, one must think of carcinomatosis with polymyositis and neuritis or other more obscure forms of neuromyositis. The skin and mucous membranes and joints are unchanged.

In our cases of polymyositis and dermatomyositis a surprising number of cardiac abnormalities have been observed. Most of these were relatively minor ECG changes, but several patients have had arrhythmias of significance. Among the fatal cases about half showed clinical evidence of severe cardiac disease and had necrosis of myocardial fibers at autopsy, usually with only modest inflammatory changes. As a rule, evidence of systemic infection is absent. Exceptionally there is a low-grade fever, especially if joint pain coexists, and a patch or a few patches of dermatitis may be present at one stage of the illness.

Dermatomyositis The skin changes may precede, accompany, or follow the muscle syndrome and take the form of a localized or diffuse erythema, maculopapular eruption, scaling eczematoid dermatitis, or even an exfoliative dermatitis. Particularly characteristic is the occurrence of a lilac-colored (heliotrope) change in the skin over the bridge of the nose, cheeks, forehead, and around the fingernails. Itching may be troublesome in some cases. Periorbital and perioral edema are common findings particularly in more fulminating episodes. The skin lesions are frequently observed over the joints, particularly in childhood. The skin changes are quite transient in some cases, and in others they consist of only a patch or more of dermatitis. These evanescent and restricted manifestations are emphasized because they are frequently overlooked, and may provide the clues to diagnosis in otherwise difficult cases.

In the healing stage, the skin lesions become whitened and atrophic, with a flat, scaly base. Periarticular and subcutaneous calcification may occur but is not common. Signs of other connective tissue diseases are more frequent than in examples of pure polymyositis. The limb weakness is usually proximal but may be diffuse, i.e., distal and proximal, just as in polymyositis. Raynaud's phenomenon is reported in nearly a third of the patients. Others will develop a mild form of scleroderma. Esophageal weakness may be demonstrated by fluoroscopy in approximately 30 percent of all patients. The superior constrictors are involved almost universally, but careful analysis by cinefluorography may be required to demonstrate the abnormality.

Connective Tissue Diseases with Polymyositis or Dermatomyositis One-third to one-half of our cases of polymyositis or dermatomyositis have occurred in patients who have or have had symptoms of rheumatic fever, rheumatoid arthritis, scleroderma, lupus erythematosus or mixtures of the aforementioned diseases (mixed connective tissue disease). Sjögren's syndrome (keratoconjunctivitis sicca, pharyngitis sicca, diminished secretion of salivary glands, and rheumatoid arthritis) may also be associated with polymyositis. In such cases, there is greater muscular weakness and atrophy than can be accounted for by the original disease. Inasmuch as arthritis may limit motion because of pain, result in disuse atrophy, and cause mono- or polyneuritis, the interpretation of diminished strength in this disease is not easy. Sometimes one must depend on muscle biopsy, EMG findings, and measurements of creatine and creatinine excreted in the urine and of muscle enzymes in the serum. Malaise, aches, and pains may be the only symptoms in the early stages of the disease.

Carcinoma with Polymyositis or Dermatomyositis This syndrome is placed in a separate category, although the muscle and skin changes are indistinguishable from those described above. Approximately 15 percent of all adults who have polymyositis or dermatomyositis are found to have a carcinoma or some other tumor, and if polymyositis-dermatomyositis appears after the age of 50 years, the proportion of patients with carcinoma is much higher. The incidence of this neoplastic syndrome is slightly higher in men than in women. Over 1000 examples have been reported in the literature, being linked most often with bronchogenic carcinoma. Some cases of thymoma are accompanied by polymyositis. The tumors, however, have arisen in nearly every organ of the body. The muscle and skin tissues show no evidence of tumor cells. In about half the cases, the polymyositis antedates the clinical manifestations of the malignancy, sometimes by 1 or 2 years. The relationship is not understood, but it has been theorized that a tumor catabolite may provoke cross-sensitization to a component of muscle or combine with one to form a complex allergen (Waksman).

Dermatomyositis of Childhood Idiopathic polymyositis occurs in children, but much less frequently than in adults. Some of the myositic illnesses in children are relatively benign and do not differ from those in adults. Skin lesions are often conjoined. However, far more common in children is a distinctive syndrome, which is generally designated as dermatomyositis, but which differs in many respects from the adult form of the disease. This childhood form of dermatomyositis is equally distributed between the sexes. It begins as a rule with rather typical skin changes, accompanied by anorexia and fatigue. Erythematous discoloration of the upper eyelids, frequently with edema, is a particularly characteristic initial sign. The erythema spreads to involve the periorbital regions, nose, malar areas, and upper lip, as well as the skin over the knuckles, elbows, and knees. Symptoms of weakness, stiffness, and pain in the muscles usually follow but may precede the skin manifestations. The muscular weakness is generalized, but always more severe in the muscles of the shoulders and hips and proximal portions of the limbs. A tiptoe gait, the result of flexion contractures at the ankles, is a common abnormality. Tendon reflexes are depressed or abolished, commensurate with the degree of muscle weakness. Intermittent low-grade fever, substernal and abdominal pain (like that of peptic ulcer), melena, and hematemesis are common symptoms.

The mode of progression of dermatomyositis of childhood, like that of the adult form, is variable. In some cases, the weakness advances rapidly, involving all the muscles—including those of chewing, swallowing, talking, and breathing—and leading to total incapacitation. Perforation of the gastrointestinal tract (with or without the contributing effects of steroids or gastric intubation) is usually the immediate cause of death. In other patients there is slow progression or arrest of the disease process, and in a small number there may be a remission of muscle weakness. Flexion contractures at the elbows, hips, knees, and ankles, and subcutaneous calcification and ulceration of the overlying skin, with extrusion of calcific debris, are common manifestations in chronic cases.

LABORATORY FINDINGS

In all forms of polymyositis, regardless of the clinical associations, the creatine excretion in the urine is usually elevated to a moderate degree, and creatinine excretion is low. The serum levels of the several types of transaminase and other tissue enzymes such as CPK and aldolase are elevated in the majority of cases. Serum alpha$_2$ and gamma globulin values may be raised. Tests for circulating rheumatoid factor (latex fixation and sensitized sheep cell procedure) and antinuclear antibody reactions are positive in less than half the cases. Myoglobin is occasionally found in the urine, when the muscle affection is acute and severe. The sedimentation rate may be normal or elevated. Lupus erythematosus preparations of blood smears are negative in 90 to 95 percent of cases. The electromyogram reveals a typical "myopathic pattern," i.e., many abnormally brief action potentials of low voltage and, in addition, numerous fibrillation potentials and salvos of pseudomyotonic activity (see Chap. 44). As stated, the electrocardiogram has been abnormal in many of our cases. The muscle biopsy, if taken from an affected muscle, usually demonstrates the typical pathologic changes of the disease. Poor sampling results in a negative biopsy in 15 to 25 percent of cases.

PATHOLOGIC CHANGES

The principal changes in idiopathic polymyositis consist of widespread destruction of segments of muscle fibers, with the expected cellular reaction thereto—phagocytosis (myophages) and infiltration with inflammatory cells (lymphocytes, mononuclear leukocytes, plasma cells, and rare neutrophilic leukocytes). Evidence of regenerative activity in the form of proliferating sarcolemmal nuclei, basophilic (ribonucleic acid–rich) sarcoplasm, and new myofibrils is almost invariable. Many of the residual muscle fibers are small, with increased numbers of sarcolemmal nuclei. Either the degeneration of muscle fibers or the infiltrations of inflammatory cells may predominate in any given biopsy specimen, though at autopsy both types of change are in evidence. There are also inflammatory changes in the skin and other organs.

Probably because of sampling error, only part of the complex of pathologic changes may be divulged in any one biopsy specimen. There may be necrosis and phagocytosis of individual muscle fibers without infiltrates of inflammatory cells, or the reverse may be observed. Repeated attacks of a necrotizing myositis appear to exhaust the regenerative potential of the muscles so that fiber loss, fibrosis, and residual thin and large fibers in haphazard arrangement may eventually impart a dystrophic aspect to the lesions. For all these reasons the pathologic picture can be correctly interpreted only in relation to the clinical and other laboratory data.

Among adult patients with polymyositis, we have observed no important differences in the muscle lesions in those with connective tissue diseases, those with and without skin lesions, and those with the paraneoplastic form.

The muscle lesions in dermatomyositis of childhood differ from those of the adult form, in that the fundamental changes are in the small intramuscular blood vessels. Vasculitis, endothelial alterations (electron-microscopically, tubular aggregates in the endothelial cytoplasm are particularly characteristic), and occlusion of vessels by fibrin thrombi are the main abnormalities. Occlusion of small vessels also involves the intrafascicular nerves, so that the affected muscle shows both zones of infarction and denervation atrophy. The same vascular changes underlie the lesions in the connective tissue of skin, subcutaneous tissue, and gastrointestinal tract.

DIFFERENTIAL DIAGNOSIS

This is secure if there is rapidly evolving proximal weakness with dysphagia and dysphonia with or without dermatitis, typical changes in a muscle biopsy, EMG abnormality of myopathic type with fibrillations, and elevated serum levels of CPK. All these criteria are satisfied in only 25 to 30 percent of our cases, even in those responsive to steroids. One must often accept the diagnosis, therefore, when only part of the criteria are met.

The following problems arise repeatedly in connection with the diagnosis of polymyositis:

1. *The patient with proximal muscle weakness incorrectly diagnosed as progressive muscular dystrophy.* Points in favor of polymyositis are (*a*) lack of family history, (*b*) older age at onset, (*c*) more rapid evolution of weakness, (*d*) evidence, past or present, of other connective tissue diseases, (*e*) high serum CPK and aldolase values, (*f*) many fibrillation potentials in EMG, (*g*) marked degeneration and regeneration in muscle biopsy and finally, if there is still doubt, (*h*) unmistakable improvement with corticosteroid therapy.

2. *The patient with a connective tissue disease (rheumatoid arthritis, scleroderma, lupus erythemato-*

sus) *suspected of having polymyositis in addition.* Pain in rheumatoid arthritis prevents strong exertion (algesic pseudoparesis). Points against the coexistence of polymyositis are (*a*) lack of weakness out of proportion to muscle atrophy, (*b*) normal EMG, (*c*) normal serum CPK and aldolase, and (*d*) normal muscle biopsy, except possibly for infiltrations of chronic inflammatory cells in the endomysial and perimysial connective tissue (interstitial nodular myositis). Also, polymyalgia rheumatica must be differentiated. This syndrome is characterized by pain, stiffness, and tenderness in the muscles of the neck and shoulders and arms, and sometimes of the hips and thighs. Biopsy of the temporal artery frequently discloses a giant-cell arteritis (see page 583).

3. *The patient with restricted muscle weakness.* Posterior neck muscle weakness or paralysis, with inability to hold up the head, restricted bilateral quadriceps weakness, and the limited pelvicrural palsies are examples. The head-hanging or lolling syndrome most often proves to be due to polymyositis, and the other syndromes to restricted forms of dystrophy and neural atrophy. Muscle enzymes in the serum may be relatively normal. EMG and biopsy are helpful in diagnosis.

4. *The patient with diffuse myalgia and fatigability.* Points which exclude a polymyositis are (*a*) lack of reduced peak power of contraction and (*b*) normal EMG, serum enzymes and muscle biopsy. Hypothyroidism, McArdle's disease, hyperparathyroidism, steroid myopathy, adrenal insufficiency, hyperinsulinemia, and early rheumatoid arthritis must be ruled out by appropriate studies (see Chap. 49). Most of our patients with diffuse myalgia and fatigability have proved to be neurasthenic or depressed.

5. *The patient with a clinical picture of polymyositis,* in whom the muscle biopsy discloses a noncaseating granulomatous reaction consistent with sarcoid. More than 25 such cases have been reported.

TREATMENT

Our most gratifying results have been obtained by a program which consists of the following:

1. *Prednisone,* 60 mg in three or four divided doses per day. Once recovery begins, as judged by careful tests of strength and serum enzyme levels, the dosage is reduced gradually, in steps of 5 mg; when the dosage has been reduced to 20 mg daily, it is best to give double this amount (i.e., 40 mg) on alternate days. After cautious reduction of prednisone over a period of 6 months or longer, the patient can usually be maintained on doses of 7.5 to 20 mg daily. Corticosteroids should not

be discontinued too soon, for the relapse which may follow is often more difficult to treat than the original symptoms.

2. *Acetylsalicylic acid,* 0.6 g every 4 h except during the night (blood levels of 20 to 30 mg per 100 ml).

3. *Physiotherapy:* gentle massage, passive movement, and then "resistance exercises" as strength returns and the evidences of activity (elevated sedimentation rate and high serum enzyme values) subside.

All patients receiving corticosteroids and aspirin need to be protected by the liberal administration of potassium and antacids. Elderly patients in particular should be reexamined periodically for signs of malignancy.

Very few measures, other than the aforementioned, are of value in the treatment of polymyositis. Some patients who are refractory to prednisone may respond favorably to weekly intravenous infusions of methotrexate or to oral azothiaprine in doses of 150 to 300 mg/day, keeping the WBC level above 3000 per cubic millimeter. Preferably the methotrexate or azothiaprine should be given together with small daily doses (15 to 25 mg) of prednisone. Cyclophosphamide has also been used in such recalcitrant cases. Vitamin E, or alpha tocopherol, which was used extensively in the past, is of no proven benefit.

PROGNOSIS

Only a small proportion of patients with polymyositis succumb to the disease, and then usually from a pulmonary or cardiac complication. The majority improve with corticosteroid therapy. The period of activity of disease is usually around 2 years in both the childhood and adult groups, but most are left with varying degrees of weakness of the shoulders and hips. Approximately 10 percent of our patients have recovered completely, and long-term remission has been achieved in about an equal number. The extent of recovery is roughly proportional to the acuteness and severity of the disease and the duration of symptoms prior to institution of therapy. Patients with acute or subacute polymyositis, in whom treatment is begun soon after the onset of symptoms, may recover almost completely. In more chronic cases, a more modest degree of recovery is to be expected. Even in patients with a coexistent malignancy, muscle weakness may lessen and serum enzyme levels decline in response to corticosteroid therapy, but weakness returns after a few months, and may then be resistant to further treatment.

OTHER ACUTE AND SUBACUTE MYOPATHIES

EOSINOPHILIC MYOSITIS

This term has been applied to three separable but possibly overlapping clinical entities: (1) eosinophilic fasciitis, (2) eosinophilic monomyositis (sometimes multiplex), and (3) eosinophilic polymyositis.

Eosinophilic fasciitis is a rare entity in which an otherwise healthy individual develops a tenosynovitis manifested by local pain, stiffness, and eventual limitation of movement. One muscle after another is affected in a particular region of the body, such as the forearm and hand. Biopsy of the tendon sheath and fascia of the muscle reveals an intense inflammatory reaction with eosinophilic leukocytes predominating in the infiltrates. The muscle per se is not involved; the EMG is negative. In the two cases we have seen there was no eosinophilia in the blood or evidence of involvement of other organs. No parasite or other microbe has been identified. The response to corticosteroids and salicylates seemed to be quite satisfactory.

Painful swelling of a calf muscle, or less frequently some other muscle, has been the chief characteristic of an *eosinophilic monomyositis*. A painful mass forms within the muscle. Biopsy reveals inflammatory necrosis and edema of the interstitial tissues; the infiltrates contain variable numbers of eosinophils. Our most recent case was that of a young woman who developed such an inflammatory mass first in one calf and, three months later, in the other. The response to prednisone in this patient was dramatic; the swelling and pain subsided in 2 to 3 weeks, and power of contraction was then found to be normal. When the connective tissue and muscle are both damaged, a chaotic regeneration of fibroblasts and myoblasts may occur, forming a pseudotumor which persists indefinitely.

Layzer and his associates have described a third form of this disorder which they classify as a true subacute *polymyositis*. Their patients were adults, in whom a predominantly proximal weakness of muscles had evolved over a period of several weeks. In each case the muscle disorder was part of a severe and widespread systemic illness, which included cardiac involvement

(conduction disturbances and congestive failure), vascular disorder (Raynaud's phenomenon, subungual hemorrhages), pulmonary infiltrates, strokes, anemia, neuropathy, and hypergammaglobulinemia. The muscles were swollen and painful. The eosinophil counts in the blood were increased in some patients, but not in others. There was a favorable response to corticosteroids in two patients, but in a third patient the outcome was fatal within 9 months. Layzer et al. tried to relate the syndrome to Loeffler's eosinophilic pulmonary disease. They felt that a lack of necrotizing arteritis distinguished it from polyarteritis nodosa. No infective agent could be isolated. An allergic mechanism seems a likely cause of the lesions, and in the authors' view one cannot exclude an angiitis as a cause of all of the lesions.

The last two of these syndromes have overlapping features as shown by the cases of Stark where a monomyositis was accompanied by several of the systemic features described by Layzer et al.

NECROTIZING POLYMYOPATHY (RHABDOMYOLYSIS) WITH MYOGLOBINURIA

In any disease that results in rapid destruction of striated muscle fibers, myoglobin and other muscle proteins may enter the bloodstream and appear in the urine. The latter is dark red, burgundy-colored, or brownish, much like the urine in hemoglobinuria. However, in hemoglobinuria the serum is initially pink because hemoglobin (but not myoglobin) is bound to haptoglobin, and this complex is not excreted in the urine as readily as myoglobin. Also, the hemoglobin molecule is three times larger than the myoglobin molecule. The hemoglobin-haptoglobin complex is removed from the blood plasma over a period of hours, and if hemolysis continues, the haptoglobin may be depleted so that hemoglobinuria is present without grossly evident hemoglobinemia. Differentiation of the two pigments in urine is difficult. Both are guaiac-positive. Very small differences are seen on spectroscopic examination, which is the most direct and simple method of detection. Electrophoresis on starch gel or cellulose is preferred by many laboratories and immunologic methods are being used to an increasing degree.

Porphyrins are the other substances that color the urine. They change color on exposure to sunlight and are guaiac-negative. Moreover, the associated clinical findings are those of a neuropathy and not a myopathy.

Regardless of the cause of the rhabdomyolysis, the affected muscles become painful and tender within a few hours. Power of contraction is diminished. Sometimes the skin and subcutaneous tissues overlying the affected muscles (nearly always of the limbs and sometimes of the trunk) are swollen and congested. There may be a low-grade fever. Apart from the discoloration of the urine, albumin excretion rises, and there is a leukocytosis. If myoglobinuria is mild, recovery occurs within a few days, and there is only a residual albuminuria. When myoglobinuria is severe, renal damage may ensue and lead to anuria. The mechanism of the renal damage is not clear; probably it is not simply a mechanical obstruction of tubules by precipitated myoglobin, although it is more likely to occur with massive rhabdomyolysis and very high CPK levels in the serum. Alkalinization of the urine by ingestion of sodium bicarbonate is said to protect the kidneys by preventing myoglobin casts, but in severe cases it is of doubtful value, and the sodium may actually be harmful if anuria has already developed. Therapy is the same as in the anuria which follows surgical shock (see *Harrison's Principles of Internal Medicine*).

The following conditions may give rise to rhabdomyolysis and myoglobinuria:

1. Crush injury.

2. Strain or excessive use of muscles, especially those which are confined in the tight pretibial compartment (pretibial syndrome).

3. Extensive infarction of muscle, as in occlusion of the main artery of a limb or a subcutaneous infusion into the lower leg (with resultant swelling and probably ischemia).

4. Idiopathic polymyositis and viral polymyositis, when necrosis is exceptionally severe.

5. Protoplasmic toxins resulting from the bite of a Malayan Sea Snake or the eating of fish or eels poisoned by toxic resins [Haff disease, so-called because it was first reported in patients residing in the bay (*Haff*) area of Konigsberg, Germany].

6. Alcoholic polymyopathy (see below).

7. McArdle's disease and phosphofructokinase deficiency.

8. Familial recurrent, or paroxysmal, myoglobinuria (Meyer-Betz and related diseases) which occurs in families with or without a diffuse chronic myopathy or dystrophy (see below).

9. Malignant hyperthermia, especially with convulsions, following the use of succinyl choline, halothane, and other anesthetic agents (see below).

PAROXYSMAL MYOGLOBINURIA

Recurrent paroxysmal myoglobinuria surely comprises a number of different diseases. Two clinical syndromes

have been described. In the first an infection may have been a precipitating factor, but usually together with physical exertion, and in the second, a period of excessive muscular activity, possibly during a period of fasting or a diet deficient in glucose or fatty acids. The first example was reported in 1911 by Meyer-Betz, and his name has often been attached to all types of paroxysmal myoglobinuria, even though at that time there was no way of identifying myoglobin.

In recent times myoglobinuria has been observed in conjunction with three hereditary metabolic diseases of muscle: myophosphorylase deficiency (McArdle's disease), phosphofructokinase deficiency (Tarui's disease), and carnitine palmityl transferase deficiency. In each of these diseases, which will be described in the following chapter, a period of intense physical activity is followed by aching stiffness of muscle and extremely high levels of CPK. Only exceptionally do episodes of myoglobinuria result in nephrosis and anuria. Usually, the exact conditions of exercise which cause rhabdomyolysis cannot be defined; intensity and duration of muscle contraction are not the complete explanation. Practically none of the patients seen by the authors has had myophosphorylase or phosphofructokinase deficiency. How many are examples of carnitine palmityl transferase deficiency or some other unrecognized disease(s) is not known. With the availability of dialysis none of our patients has died of myoglobinuria, and by limiting their level of physical activity they have been able to lead relatively normal lives. The possibility of warding off an attack of McArdle's disease by frequent ingestion of fructose or glucose and carnitine palmityl transferase deficiency by ingestion of medium-chain fatty acids has not been sufficiently explored.

LIPID STORAGE POLYMYOPATHY

Although it has long been known that lipids are an important source of energy in muscle metabolism (along with glucose) it was not until 1970 that W. K. Engel et al. described the storage of lipid in muscle fibers of twin girls whose complaints were intermittent muscular discomfort and myoglobinuria. It was suggested that there must be a defect in the utilization of long-chain fatty acids. Bressler, in commenting on this observation, predicted three possible biochemical defects: (1) in carnitine, (2) in carnitine palmityl transferase I, or (3) in carnitine palmityl transferase II. His prediction was borne out by the discovery of two separate conditions, one in which the synthesis of carnitine by the liver appeared to be faulty, the other in which there was an enzymatic defect in muscle of carnitine palmityl transferase.

Defect in Carnitine Palmityl Transferase This disorder was mentioned above as one of the causes of paroxysmal myoglobinuria. It occurs in children and young adults and is a systemic disease, inherited as an autosomal or a sex-linked trait. Between attacks of myoglobinuria the function of muscles is normal. Utilization of palmitate by muscle mitochondria is more impaired than utilization of palmityl carnitine. Serum triglycerides are elevated, and there is fat intolerance with reduced clearance of chylomicrons. The exercise that produces the myoglobinuria must be prolonged. There is then a rapid rise in CPK. The liver is probably affected. Histologically the muscle has been normal in some cases and has been found to contain stored lipid in others.

Carnitine Deficiency A. G. Engel et al. observed a woman with progressive muscular weakness of proximal distribution and lipid myopathy. The carnitine levels in muscle were reduced by 80 percent and that of plasma was normal; this suggested a normal synthesis of carnitine and defective transport into muscle. In another patient, however, both liver and muscle levels were reduced, suggesting defective synthesis by the liver. In the latter patient, the administration of carnitine orally restored blood levels and improved strength of muscular contraction. This condition should be considered in adult patients with progressive weakness of proximal limb and trunk muscles. Notable also has been the development of an acute myopathy with severe weakness and myalgia after pregnancy or an infection. In the cases of Angelini et al. the myopathy developed rapidly in the postpartum period. There was ptosis and such severe weakness of girdle muscles as to render the patient bedfast. The CPK was elevated. The EMG showed fibrillation potentials. There was gradual recovery after the patients were given 2 g of carnitine per day.

These cases bring to light the essential role of carnitine as part of a transport mechanism for fatty acids in muscle and other cells.

MALIGNANT HYPERTHERMIA

This may also be a cause of myoglobinuria, but its clinical presentation usually takes a different pattern, that of a hyperthermic anesthesia accident. As larger experience

has been gained with this entity, since the original report by Denborough and Lovell in 1960, it has proved to be a metabolic polymyopathy occurring as a dominant trait which renders the individual vulnerable to certain anesthetic agents, particularly halothane and succinylcholine and ether to a lesser extent.

The clinical picture is unforgettable. As halothane anesthesia is induced and suxamethonium is given for muscular relaxation, the jaw muscles unexpectedly become tense rather than relaxed, and soon the rigidity extends to all of the muscles. Thereafter the temperature rises to 42 or 43°C with coincidental tachypnea and tachycardia. The final clinical picture is one of failure of brainstem reflexes, circulatory collapse, and death or of survival with gradual recovery. In some cases there is the same sequence without muscular spasm. The CPK rises to high levels.

The pathogenesis of this reaction has been the subject of a number of investigations. Muscle from affected individuals is abnormally sensitive to caffeine, which induces contracture. It has been postulated that the halothane acts in a manner similar to caffeine, i.e., to reduce calcium from and prevent its reaccumulation in the sarcoplasmic reticulum, thus interfering with relaxation of the muscle. A breed of pigs (Landrace) has been found in which muscle spasm (true contracture) and hyperthermia follow the administration of these same anesthetic agents. The latter are found to increase O_2 consumption by 50 to 60 percent and to deplete the ATP of muscle fibers. A primary defect of phosphodiesterase, the enzyme involved in the degradation of cyclic AMP, has been suggested as another factor. The cause of the fever is not known; it is probably due mainly to the muscle spasm, but an effect of the anesthetic on heat regulating centers cannot be excluded.

Clues as to which patients are at risk for this condition come from several sources. Other members of the family may have collapsed or died during anesthesia. Some of the susceptible individuals exhibit certain myopathic and musculoskeletal abnormalities. As to the former, progressive congenital myopathy, high CPK values, or hypertrophic muscular dystrophy going on to atrophic weakness has been noted in some families. As to the latter, short stature, ptosis, strabismus, highly arched palate, dislocated patellae and kyphoscoliosis are the most frequently observed abnormalities.

The treatment consists of discontinuation of anesthesia at the first hint of masseter spasm or rise of temperature. The intravenous administration of dantrolene or procainamide, which inhibit Ca release from the sarcoplasmic reticulum, may be lifesaving. Halothane inhalation anesthesia and succinylcholine should be avoided in such individuals, as well as any unnecessary surgical procedures done under local anesthesia (see Isaacs and Barlow for review of literature).

ALCOHOLIC MYOPATHY

Several forms of muscle weakness have been ascribed to alcoholism. In one type, a painless and predominantly proximal weakness develops over a period of several days or weeks in the course of a prolonged drinking bout, and is associated with severe degrees of *hypokalemia* (serum levels <2 meq/liter). The urinary excretion of potassium is not significantly increased; depletion is probably the result of vomiting and diarrhea which usually precede the onset of muscular weakness. In addition, serum levels of liver and muscle enzymes are markedly elevated. Biopsies from severely weakened muscles show single-fiber necrosis and vacuolation. Treatment consists of the administration of potassium chloride intravenously (about 120 meq daily for several days), after which oral administration suffices. Strength returns gradually in 7 to 14 days, and enzyme levels return to normal concomitantly.

Another type of myopathic syndrome, occurring acutely in the course of a drinking bout, is manifested by severe pain, tenderness, and edema of the muscles of the limbs and trunk, accompanied in the majority of cases by renal damage and hyperpotassemia (Hed et al.). The muscle affection is generalized in some patients and remarkably focal in others. A swollen, painful, and tender limb or part of a limb may give the appearance of a deep phlebothrombosis or lymphatic obstruction. Myonecrosis is reflected by high serum levels of CPK and aldolase and the appearance of myoglobin in the urine, leading in some cases to fatal myoglobinuric nephrosis. In fact, in a general hospital, alcoholism is by far the commonest cause of rhabdomyolysis and myoglobinuria. Some patients recover within a few weeks, but others require several months, and relapse during another drinking spree is commonplace. Restoration of motor power is attendant upon regeneration, but may be complicated by polyneuropathy and other syndromes of neuromuscular disability associated with alcoholism. Recently, Haller and Drachman have produced the main abnormalities of alcoholic rhabdomyolysis (myonecrosis, elevated CPK, and myoglobinuria) in rats by subjecting the animals to a brief fast following a 2- to 4-week exposure to alcohol; these observations suggest that fasting may precipitate myonecrosis during a drinking bout in humans.

Perkoff and his associates have described yet another muscular disorder in alcoholics, characterized by severe muscular cramps and diffuse weakness, occurring in the course of a sustained drinking bout. They noted a number of biochemical abnormalities in these patients,

as well as in asymptomatic alcoholics who were admitted to the hospital immediately after a protracted period of drinking. These abnormalities consisted of elevated serum levels of CPK, evidence of myoglobin in the urine, and a diminished rise in blood lactic acid in response to ischemic exercise, as occurs in McArdle's disease. In distinction to the latter, however, myophosphorylase levels were not consistently reduced in the alcoholic patients. How these biochemical abnormalities are related to muscle cramps and weakness is a matter of speculation.

From time to time one observes in alcoholics the subacute or chronic evolution of painless weakness and atrophy of the proximal muscles of the limbs, especially of the legs, with only minimal signs of neuropathy in the distal segments of the legs and feet. Cases such as these have been referred to as chronic alcoholic myopathy, but the data are insufficient to warrant this designation. Some of these cases have shown necrosis of muscle fibers with myoglobinuria and most cases, in the authors' experience, have proved to be neuropathic in nature. Treatment follows along the lines indicated for alcoholic neuropathy (page 713), and complete recovery can be expected if the patient abstains from alcohol and commences a regimen of good nutrition.

REFERENCES

ADAMS RD: *Diseases of Muscle: A Study in Pathology,* 3d ed. New York, Harper & Row, 1975.

ANGELINI G et al: Carnitine deficiency: Acute postpartum crisis. *Ann Neurol* 4:558, 1978.

ANTONY JH, PROCOPIS PG, OUVRIER RA: Benign acute childhood myositis. *Neurology* 29:1068, 1979.

BANKER BQ: Dermatomyositis of childhood. Ultrastructural alterations of muscle and intramuscular blood vessels. *J Neuropathol Exp Neurol* 34:46, 1975.

——, VICTOR M: Dermatomyositis (systemic angiopathy) of childhood. *Medicine* 45:261, 1966.

BRESSLER R: Carnitine and the twins. *N Engl J Med* 282:745, 1970.

CURRIE S: Polymyositis and related disorders, in Walton JN (ed): *Disorders of Voluntary Muscle,* 4th ed. Edinburgh, Churchill Livingstone, 1981.

DEMOS MA, GITLIN EL, KAGAN LG: Exercise myoglobinuria and acute exertional rhabdomyolysis. *Arch Intern Med* 134:669, 1974.

DENBOROUGH MA, LOVELL RRH: Anaesthetic deaths in a family. *Lancet* 2:45, 1960.

DiMAURO S et al: Debrancher deficiency. Neuromuscular disorder in 5 adults. *Ann Neurol* 5:422, 1979.

ENGEL AG, ANGELINI C, NELSON RA: Identification of carnitine deficiency as a cause of human lipid storage myopathy, in Milhorat AT (ed): *Exploratory Concepts in Muscular Dystrophy*, vol 2. Amsterdam, Excerpta Medica, 1974, pp 601–618.

ENGEL WK, VICK NA, GLUECK CJ: A skeletal muscle disorder associated with intermittent symptoms and a possible defect in lipid metabolism. *N Engl J Med* 282:697, 1970.

GAMBOA ET et al: Isolation of influenza virus from muscle in myoglobinuric polymyositis. *Neurology* 29:556, 1979.

HALLER RG, DRACHMAN DB: Alcoholic rhabdomyolysis: An experimental model in the rat. *Science* 208:412, 1980.

HED R et al: Acute muscular syndrome in chronic alcoholism. *Acta Med Scand* 171:585, 1962.

ISAACS H, BARLOW MB: Malignant hyperpyrexia. *J Neurol Neurosurg Psychiatry* 36:228, 1973.

KOREIN J, CODDEN DR, MOWREY PH: The clinical syndrome of paroxysmal paralytic myoglobinuria. *Neurology* 9:767, 1959.

LAYZER RB, SHEARN MA, SATYA-MURTI S: Eosinophilic polymyositis. *Ann Neurol* 1:65, 1977.

LUNDBERG A: Myalgia crisis epidemica. *Acta Paediatr Scand* 46:18, 1957.

MEYER-BETZ F: Beobachtungen auf einem eigen-artigen mit muskellähmungen verbundenen Fall von Hämoglobinurie. *Dtsch Arch Klin Med* 85:127, 1911.

PEARSON CM, BECK WS, BLAHD WH: Idiopathic paroxysmal myoglobinuria. *Arch Intern Med* 99:376, 1957.

PERKOFF GR, HARDY P, VELEZ-GARCIA E: Reversible acute muscular syndrome in chronic alcoholism. *N Engl J Med* 274:1277, 1966.

ROWLAND LP, PENN AS: Myoglobinuria. *Med Clin North Am* 56:1233, 1972.

STARK RJ: Eosinophilic polymyositis. *Arch Neurol* 36:721, 1979.

CHAPTER 49

THE MUSCULAR DYSTROPHIES AND OTHER CHRONIC POLYMYOPATHIES

As indicated in the classification of the muscle disorders (Chap. 47), progressive muscular weakness and atrophy of chronic course may occur with four major groups of diseases, the *chronic polyneuropathies,* the various forms of *motor system disease* (also called progressive muscular atrophies), the *progressive muscular dystrophies* and certain *metabolic polymyopathies.* All are or may be of genetic origin.

As a rough clinical indicator, the pattern of muscle involvement is helpful in separating these four categories of disease. In most polyneuropathies, the distal limb muscles are the ones predominantly involved; in the dystrophies and polymyopathies, the affection is mainly of the girdle, proximal limb, or ocular muscles; and in the pure muscular atrophies there is a variable, symmetrical or asymmetrical pattern of involvement. Concurrent sensory loss, reflex impairment out of proportion to weakness, slowed nerve conduction velocities, characteristic EMG changes, elevated CSF protein, and group atrophy in muscle biopsies usually establish the existence of a disease of peripheral nerves. The various types are presented in Chap. 45. Variable patterns of weakness, fasciculations at rest in weak muscles, relatively normal nerve conduction velocities, the presence of fibrillation potentials in the EMG, and typical features of neural atrophy in the muscle biopsy serve to demarcate the progressive muscular atrophies. The latter, usually adjudged a degenerative disease of the anterior horn cells, are more appropriately grouped with degenerative diseases of the nervous system (see Chap. 42). Only the progressive muscular dystrophies and the chronic metabolic polymyopathies will be considered in the following pages.

THE MUSCULAR DYSTROPHIES

The muscular dystrophies are progressive, hereditary degenerative diseases of skeletal muscles. The innervation of the affected muscles, in contrast to that of the neuropathic and spinal atrophies, is sound. Indeed, final proof that the origin of these disorders is in muscle itself comes from the demonstration of intact spinal motor neurons, muscular nerves, and nerve endings, in the presence of severe degenerative changes in the muscle fibers. The characteristic features of more or less symmetrical distribution of muscular weakness and atrophy, intact sensibility, preservation of cutaneous reflexes, and the liability to heredofamilial incidence serve to set this group of diseases apart on clinical grounds alone.

Though some clinicians and researchers have suggested that the term *muscular dystrophy* be applied to other degenerative diseases of muscle, such as those in animals due to vitamin E deficiency and the Coxsackie viruses, and certain inherited metabolic diseases in humans, we would discourage this practice, as one leading to terminologic confusion. The intensity of the cellular response and vigor of the regenerative changes distinguishes the histology of these latter diseases and also implies a fundamental difference in pathogenesis. We therefore reserve the term *dystrophy* for the purely degenerative muscular disease of hereditary type and refer to the others as polymyopathies or myopathies. The more benign and relatively nonprogressive myopathies such as "central core," "nemaline," mitochondrial, and centronuclear diseases, present a greater difficulty in classification. Like the dystrophies, they are primarily diseases of muscle and are heredofamilial in nature, but again we prefer to place them in a separate category because of their nonprogressive or slowly progressive course and the special qualities of their morphology.

HISTORY

The differentiation of dystrophic diseases from those secondary to neuronal degeneration was an achievement of neurologists of the second half of the nineteenth century. As pointed out by Gowers, isolated cases of muscular dystrophy had been described earlier but no distinction was made between neurogenic and myopathic disease. Meryon in 1852 gave the first clear description of progressive weakness and atrophy of muscle in young boys, who at autopsy had intact spinal cord and nerves, a fact which led him to postulate an "idiopathic disease of muscles, dependent perhaps on defective nutrition." The French neurologist Duchenne, who had long devoted himself to the clinical analysis of muscle function, described in 1855 the progressive muscular atrophy of childhood which now bears his name. However, it was not until the second edition of his famous monograph in 1861 that the "hypertrophic paraplegia of infancy" was recognized as a distinct syndrome of unknown pathology, but with speculations about the nature of hypertrophy of muscles. Erb, in 1891, was the first to crystallize the clinical and histologic conception of a group of diseases due to primary degeneration of muscle, which he called muscular dystrophies. The first descriptions of a special facioscapulohumeral dystrophy were published by Landouzy and Déjerine in 1894; progressive ocular myopathy, by Fuchs in 1890; myotonic dystrophy, by Hoffmann in 1896 and by Steinert in 1909; distal dystrophy, by Gowers in 1888, by Milhorat and Wolff in 1943, and by Welander in 1951; and oculopharyngeal dystrophy, by the authors with Hayes in 1962. References to these and other writings of historical importance can be found in the monographs of Adams and of Walton (see references).

CLASSIFICATION OR CLINICAL PRESENTATION

The following classification of the muscular dystrophies is largely based on these clinical studies. Certain forms, namely myotonic dystrophy, and the ocular, oculopharyngeal, and distal dystrophies, are sufficiently distinctive to make their separation relatively easy. There is still uncertainty about the classification of the childhood forms of proximal dystrophy with and without pseudohypertrophy and with and without facial involvement.

Erb, in his comprehensive monograph, divided the dystrophies into those beginning in childhood and those beginning in adult life. The adult forms were again divided into two groups, those with and those without facial involvement; and the childhood forms into two subtypes, those with pseudohypertrophy and those with atrophy. A more strictly genetic approach was taken by Walton and Nattrass, who put in one group the sex-linked childhood pseudohypertrophic form of Duchenne; in a second group, the autosomal dominant facioscapulohumeral form of Landouzy and Déjerine; and in a third group of variable type of inheritance, the limb-girdle cases of Leyden-Moebius and of Erb. The latter group has more recently been found to include cases of spinal muscular atrophy of familial type, as reported by Wohlfart et al. and by Kugelberg and Welander, and some of the facioscapulohumeral cases have proved to be examples of polymyositis and mitochondrial polymyopathy.

The authors, while impressed with the relative purity of the first two of these hereditary syndromes, continue to find many examples which do not run true to form. Also difficult to accept is the conclusion of Erb that all the dystrophies are basically the same when viewed histologically, the cycle of changes in the muscle fiber beginning with enlargement, then going on to atrophy, disappearance of the fiber, and fibrosis. This seems premature when as yet we cannot denominate the primary abnormality in any one of the muscular dystrophies.

For purposes of exposition, we shall consider nine subtypes of progressive, hereditary diseases of muscle in which the pathologic changes consist of degeneration and loss of muscle fibers in a particular topographic pattern.

Severe Generalized Muscular Dystrophy of Childhood (Erb's Childhood Type, Duchenne's Hypertrophic Form) This type of dystrophy usually begins in early childhood and runs a relatively rapid progressive course. The incidence is estimated at 3 per 100,000. The disease has a strong familial liability, occurs predominantly in males, with or without pseudohypertrophy. Approximately 40 percent of patients have a negative family history and are said to represent mutations. However, careful examinations of their mothers will show slight involvement in many of them, as pointed out by Roses et al. The most frequent and best known form is Duchenne's pseudohypertrophic muscular dystrophy, the name being taken from the unnatural enlargement of the calves and other muscles. The disease usually begins in the third year of life and nearly always before the sixth year. In nearly half of the patients there is evidence of disease before the infants begin to walk. Many of the infants are backward in other ways (psychomotor retardation), and the muscle weakness is overlooked. An elevated CPK may be the first clue. In another group of young children the earliest symptoms are an indisposition to walk or run when they should do so; or, having achieved these motor milestones, they appear to be less sprightly than usual, and are prone to fall. Increasing difficulty in running and climbing stairs, swayback, and waddling gait become ever-more obvious as time passes. The iliopsoas, quadriceps, and gluteal muscles are the first to be affected. Later the pretibial muscles weaken (foot drop and toe walking). In the upper limbs the serrati, lower parts of pectorals, latissimus dorsi, biceps, and brachioradialis are affected, more or less in this order.

The enlargement of calves and certain other muscles is progressive in the early stages of the disease, but most of the muscles, even the ones which are originally enlarged, eventually decrease in size; only the gastrocnemii, and to a lesser extent the quadriceps and deltoids, are consistently large and that quality may be evident before weakness is noted. The enlarged muscles have a firm, resilient (rubbery) feel and as a rule are slightly less strong and more hypotonic than healthy ones of the same size. Rarely, all muscles are at first large and exceptionally strong, even the facial muscles, as in one of Duchenne's cases (a "Farnese Hercules"); this is a true hypertrophy.

Muscles of the pelvic girdle, lumbosacral spine, and shoulders become wasted from the onset, and weakness of these groups of muscles accounts for certain clinical peculiarities. Weakness of abdominal and paravertebral muscles accounts for the lordotic posture and protuberant abdomen when standing and the rounded back when sitting. Unequal weakening of the paravertebral muscles may result in scoliosis, but usually the posture is symmetrical in the early stages. Bilateral weakness of the extensors of the knees and hips interferes with equilibrium and with activities such as climbing stairs or rising from a chair or from a stooped posture. In standing and walking patients place their feet wide apart in order to increase their base of support. To rise from a sitting position patients first flex their trunk at the hips, put their hands on their knees, and push their trunk upward by working the hands up the thighs (Gowers' sign). In getting up from a recumbent position patients turn their head and trunk and push themselves sideways to a sitting position. S. A. K. Wilson used an alliterative phrase to describe the characteristic abnormalities of stance and gait—the patient "straddles as he stands and waddles as he walks." According to Duchenne, the waddle is due to bilateral weakness of the gluteus medius (see page 84). Weakening of the muscles which fix the scapulae to the thorax (serratus anterior, lower trapezi-

us, rhomboids) causes a winging of the scapulae, and the scapular angles can sometimes be seen when facing the patient.

Later, weakness and atrophy spread to the muscles of the legs and forearms. The muscles that are selectively affected include the neck flexors, wrist extensors, brachioradialis, the costal part of the pectoralis major, latissimus dorsi, biceps, triceps, anterior tibial, and peroneal muscles. The ocular, facial, bulbar, and hand muscles are usually spared although weakness of the facial and sternomastoid muscles and of the diaphragm have been reported as late events in the disease. As the trunk muscles atrophy the bones stand out like those of a skeleton. The space between lower ribs and iliac crests diminishes with affection of the abdominal muscles.

The limbs are usually flaccid and loose. Shortening and contracture appear late, except for a mild equinus posture of the feet. The tendon reflexes are lost as the muscle tissue disappears. The bones are thin and demineralized and the appearance of ossification centers is delayed. Smooth muscles are spared, but the heart may be hypertrophied, and various types of arrhythmia may appear. The most typical ECG shows prominent R waves in right precordial leads and deep Q waves in the left precordial and limb leads. Death is usually the result of respiratory weakness and pulmonary infections, but in some cases cardiac decompensation may ultimately terminate life. Mild degrees of mental retardation, nonprogressive, are observed in many cases. Death usually occurs during adolescence, and survival beyond the twenty-fifth year is rare.

Becker Type Muscular Dystrophy This is another well characterized dystrophy, closely related to the Duchenne type. Its frequency is difficult to ascertain, perhaps 3 to 6 per 100,000 male births. Like the Duchenne form it is an X-linked disorder, affecting only males and transmitted by females. It causes weakness and hypertrophy in the same muscles as the Duchenne dystrophy, but the onset is much later (mean age, 11 years; range, 5 to 45 years). The course is more benign; the average age at which the patient becomes unable to walk is 25 to 30 years; death occurs usually in the fifth decade, but some patients live to an advanced age. The serum CPK values are 25 to 200 times normal, which with the EMG and muscle biopsy findings, helps to exclude an hereditary spinal muscular atrophy. The EMG shows fibrillations, positive waves, low-amplitude and polyphasic motor unit potentials, and sometimes high-frequency discharges. As in

Duchenne dystrophy the female carrier may occasionally display mild dystrophic weakness.

An *X-linked scapuloperoneal dystrophy* which closely resembles the Duchenne form has also been described. The onset is somewhat later than the Duchenne type and earlier than the Becker type, but the course is benign and muscle hypertrophy is lacking (an autosomal dominant form of scapuloperoneal dystrophy with onset from 10 to 40 years and benign course has also been observed).

Other sex-linked, relatively benign dystrophies of muscle, with or without hypertrophy, have been described. Emery and Dreifuss reported a family in which weakness appeared at the age of 4 to 5 years, and there were "flexion contractures of elbows, mild facial weakness, shortening of Achilles tendons and absence of pseudohypertrophy." Kuhn et al. added another genealogy of muscle dystrophy to the literature that involved early myocardial disease and cramping myalgia.

Considering the similarities between the X-linked muscular dystrophies, one might wonder if their separation is justified. Expert opinion favors the idea of different diseases. Duchenne's and Becker's forms differ in at least one respect, in that color blindness is often associated with Duchenne's dystrophy and not with the Becker form. This suggests a different locus of the abnormal gene on the X chromosome.

Relatively Mild Restricted Muscular Dystrophy (Landouzy-Déjerine Facioscapulohumeral Dystrophy, Erb's Adult Form with Facial Involvement) This is a slowly progressive proximal dystrophy involving primarily the musculature of the shoulders and face, with long remissions and often nearly complete arrest. The pattern of inheritance is usually autosomal dominant. A subvariety is a slowly progressive form without facial weakness.

While less common than the Duchenne type, this form of dystrophy is not rare. The age of onset is usually between 6 and 20 years; cases with onset in early adult life are occasionally encountered. Usually the first manifestations are difficulty in raising the arms above the head and winging of the scapulae, although in some cases facial weakness may have attracted attention, even in early childhood. Weakness and atrophy of muscles are the major physical findings; pseudohypertrophy occurs only rarely and is slight. There is an inability to close the eyes firmly, to purse the lips, and to whistle; the lips have a peculiar looseness and tendency to protrude, likened by some to those of the tapir. The lower parts of the trapezius muscles and the sternal parts of the pectorals are almost invariably affected. In contrast the del-

toids may seem to be unusually large and strong, an appearance that may be mistaken for pseudohypertrophy. The advancing atrophic process also involves the sternomastoid, serratus magnus, rhomboid, erector spinae, latissimus dorsi, and deltoid muscles. The bones of the shoulders become salient; the scapulae are winged and elevated, and the clavicles are prominent. The anterior axillary folds slope down and out as a result of wasting of the pectoral muscles. Usually the biceps waste less than the triceps, but both are affected, as are the brachioradialis muscles, so that the upper arm may be thinner than the forearm (Popeye effect). Pelvic muscles are involved later and to a milder degree, giving rise to a slight lordosis and pelvic instability. At this point the disease may become arrested and cease to progress.

An occasional feature of this group of diseases is the congenital absence of a muscle (one pectoral, brachioradialis, or biceps femoris), or part of a muscle, in patients who later develop the typical affection. The external ocular muscles are known to occasionally become affected late in the illness. Cardiac involvement is rare, but in some of the cases tachycardia, cardiomegaly, and arrhythmias (ventricular and auricular extrasystoles) have occurred. Mental function is normal.

Scapulohumeral (Limb-Girdle) Muscular Dystrophy This term has been used to designate a relatively benign form of dystrophy affecting mainly the shoulder or shoulder and pelvic girdle muscles of males and females. A variant limited to the pelvic muscles is known as the Leyden-Möbius form. The inheritance pattern has varied but most often is autosomal recessive. Wilhelm Erb first described it as a childhood form with atrophy, and Walton and Nattrass gave it a place in their classification.

As new cases were found and studied more completely, it became evident, however, that many of the cases were examples of spinal muscular atrophy of the type described by Wohlfart and by Kugelberg and Welander. Some opinion now favors the view that all such cases be considered as anterior horn cell diseases (see Gardner-Medwin). The proof of this position is uncertain, for few such cases have had a postmorten examination of the spinal cord. The authors adopt an intermediate position, that there is both a dominant and recessive form of limb-girdle dystrophy as well as hereditary forms of spinal muscular atrophy. Furthermore, polymyositis of chronic type may simulate either of these two forms of disease.

Progressive External Ophthalmoplegia (Ocular Myopathy of Von Graefe-Fuchs) This is a slowly progressive myopathy, primarily involving and often limited to the extraocular muscles. Usually the levators of the eyelids are the first to be affected, causing ptosis, followed by progressive ophthalmoparesis. This disorder usually begins in childhood, sometimes in adolescence and rarely in adult life (as late as 50 years). Males and females are equally affected; inheritance is of an autosomal dominant type in some and of recessive or uncertain type in others. Once started, the disease progresses relentlessly until the eyes are motionless. Simultaneous involvement of all eye muscles permits the eyes to remain in a central position so that strabismus and diplopia are uncommon (in rare instances one eye is affected before the other). In an attempt to raise the eyelids and to see under them, the head is thrown back and the frontalis muscle is contracted, wrinkling the forehead (Hutchinsonian facies). The eyelids are abnormally thin because of atrophy of the levator muscles.

The orbicularis oculi muscles are frequently involved, in addition to the extraocular muscles. Thus, in progressive external ophthalmoplegia, as in myasthenia gravis and myotonic dystrophy, there may be a unique combination of weakness in closing *and* opening the eyes. As stated above, this is nearly always myopathic, for it would be unusual for all the oculomotor and facial nerves to be involved bilaterally from lesions of the third, fourth, sixth, and seventh cranial nerves or their nuclei. Other facial muscles, masseters, sternocleidomastoids, deltoids, or peronei are variably weak and wasted in about 25 percent of cases.

The absence of myotonia, cataract, and endocrine disturbances distinguishes progressive external ophthalmoplegia from myotonic dystrophy, with which it might be confused because of the ptosis. The more extensive forms of the disease may resemble mild restricted muscular dystrophy, and indeed Landouzy and Déjerine described ocular palsy in one of their cases. The characteristic feature of progressive external ophthalmoplegia is that ptosis and ocular paralysis precede involvement of other muscles by many years. The relatively early age of onset and absence of dysphagia set it apart from the oculopharyngeal form of dystrophy, and the lack of retinal degeneration and the normality of growth, mentation, and CSF protein distinguish it from the Kearns-Sayre syndrome (see below).

Opinions vary as to whether all cases of progressive external ophthalmoplegia should be assigned a myopathic origin. In chronic diseases such as this, dystrophy and partial denervation are difficult to distinguish on the basis of the appearance of the biopsied eye muscle as pointed out by Ringel et al. The categorization of progressive external ophthalmoplegia is complicated further by its frequent association with a variety of neurologic abnormalities and atypical pigmentary degeneration of the retina. Drachman has lumped all these complicated cases under the title of "ophthalmoplegia plus," in the belief that any further classification has little

value. Nevertheless, the purely myopathic origin of some cases is proven by intactness of neurons in the brainstem nuclei and normality of the cranial nerves. It has been possible to separate at least two distinctive syndromes from this group. One of these is the highly restricted oculopharyngeal dystrophy of late onset, which is described in the following section of this chapter. Another rather uniform syndrome comprises childhood ophthalmoplegia, pigmentary degeneration of the retina, varying degrees of heart block, short stature, and elevated CSF protein (Kearns and Sayre). Because of its special histopathologic features, this latter syndrome will be discussed with the congenital myopathies (page 981). (See review by Berenberg et al. for further discussion of the classification of the progressive ophthalmoplegias.)

Oculopharyngeal Dystrophy This disease is inherited as an autosomal dominant trait and is unique with respect to its late onset (usually after the forty-fifth year) and the restricted muscular weakness, manifested as a bilateral ptosis and dysphagia. E. W. Taylor first described the disease in 1915, and assumed that it was due to a nuclear atrophy (oculomotor-vagal complex); the authors, with Hayes in 1962, showed that the descendants of Taylor's cases had a late-life myopathy (myopathic EMG and biopsy). Later studies by Barbeau traced the original family to an early French-Canadian immigrant who was the progenitor of several hundred descendants with the disease. Since then, other families showing a dominant pattern of inheritance and a number of sporadic cases have been described.

Associated with a slowly progressive ptosis is a difficulty in swallowing and change in voice. Swallowing becomes so difficult that food intake is limited, resulting in cachexia. The latter is prevented at first by cutting the cricopharyngeus muscle, and, failing this measure, by a "feeding gastrostomy" or nasogastric intubation. In some families, the other external muscles of the eyes and shoulder and pelvic muscles become weakened and atrophic to a relatively slight extent. In the only autopsied case, a loss of fibers of modest proportions was widespread in these and many other muscles. The brainstem nuclei and cranial nerves were normal. Like the other mild and restricted polymyopathies the serum CPK and aldolase levels are normal, and the EMG is altered only in the affected muscles.

Dystrophia Myotonica (Myotonic Dystrophy, Steinert's Disease) This form of dystrophy is distinguished by its unique topography, the associated myotonia, and the occurrence of dystrophic changes in nonmuscular tissues (lens of eye, testicle and other endocrine glands, skin, and, in some cases, the cerebrum). The levator palpebrae, facial, masseter, sternomastoid, forearm, hand, and pretibial muscles are consistently involved in the dystrophic process. In this sense, dystrophia myotonica is a distal type of myopathy. It is probable that Gowers' case of an 18-year-old youth with weakened and wasted anterior tibial and forearm muscles and sternomastoids, in conjunction with paresis of orbicularis and frontalis muscles, was an example of this disease, differing from the simple distal muscular dystrophy described by Welander (see below).

Usually the muscular wasting in myotonic dystrophy does not become manifest until the third decade of life, but we have seen a number of infants and young children with the typical facies. Moreover, in recent years a severe, often fatal, neonatal (congenital) form of the disease has been identified (see further on). The small muscles of the hands, along with the extensor muscles of the forearms, are often the first to become atrophied. In other cases, ptosis of eyelids and thinness and slackness of the facial musculature may be the earliest signs, preceding other muscular involvement by many years. Atrophy of the masseters leads to narrowing of the lower half of the face, and the mandible is slender and malpositioned so that the teeth do not occlude properly. This, along with the ptosis, frontal baldness, and wrinkled forehead, imparts a distinctive physiognomy that, once seen, can be recognized at a glance. The sternomastoids are almost invariably implicated and are associated with a general thinness and an exaggerated forward curvature of the neck ("swan neck"). Atrophy of the anterior tibial muscle groups, leading to foot drop, is an early sign in other families.

Pharyngeal and laryngeal weakness results in a weak, monotonous nasal voice. The uterine muscle may be weakened, interfering with normal parturition, and the esophagus is often dilated because of loss of muscle fibers in the striated part. Mild functional changes in the heart are usually due to abnormalities of conduction (bradycardia and lengthened PR interval) and less often to cardiomyopathy. Diaphragmatic weakness and alveolar hypoventilation, resulting in chronic bronchitis and bronchiectasis, is frequent.

The disease progresses slowly, with gradual involvement of the proximal muscles of the limbs and muscles of the trunk. Tendon reflexes are lost or much reduced. Contracture is rarely seen and the thin, flattened hands are consequently soft and pliable. Most pa-

tients are confined to a wheelchair or bed within 15 to 20 years, and death occurs before the normal age from pulmonary infection or heart failure.

The phenomenon of *myotonia* that expresses itself in prolonged contraction of certain muscles following brief percussion or electrical stimulation, and in delay of relaxation after strong voluntary contraction, is the second striking attribute of the disease. Not as widespread as in myotonia congenita (Thomsen's disease), it is, nonetheless, easily elicited in the hands and tongue and sometimes in other muscles. Gentle movements do not evoke it (eye blinks, movements of facial expression, and the like are not impeded), whereas strong closure of the lids and clenching of the fist are followed by a long delay in relaxation.

Myotonia may precede weakness by several years. Indeed, Maas and Paterson have claimed that many cases diagnosed originally as myotonia congenita eventually prove to be examples of myotonia dystrophica. Of interest is the fact that in congenital or infantile cases of myotonic dystrophy, the myotonic phenomenon is not elicited until after the second or third year of life. Moreover, the patient often becomes accustomed to the myotonia and no longer considers it abnormal. The relation of myotonia to the dystrophy is not direct. Certain muscles which show the myotonia best (tongue, flexors of fingers) are seldom weak and atrophic. There may be little or no myotonia in certain families showing cataracts and involvement of muscles in a typical distribution of myotonic dystrophy.

The third characteristic is the association of dystrophic changes in nonmuscular tissues. Feeblemindedness of moderate degree is not infrequent, and the brain weights of several of our cases were 200 g less than normals of the same age. Lenticular opacities, first noted by Greenfield, are best seen with a slit lamp. They consist of small, regular opacities found in the posterior and anterior cortex of the lens just beneath the capsule; they are colored blue, blue-green, and yellow under the slit lamp and are highly refractile. In older patients a stellate cataract slowly forms in the posterior cortex of the lens.

Progressive frontal alopecia, beginning at an early age, is a characteristic feature in both men and women with this disease. Testicular atrophy with androgenic deficiency, reduced libido or impotence, and sterility are frequent manifestations. In some patients gynecomastia and elevated gonadotropin excretion are found. Testicular biopsy may show atrophy and hyalinization of tubular cells and hyperplasia of Leydig cells. Thus all the clinical characteristics of Klinefelter's syndrome may be present. However, the nuclei of skin or bone marrow cells only rarely have shown "sex chromatin mass." The majority of patients have the usual sex chromatin constitution. Ovarian deficiency occasionally develops in the female patient but is seldom severe enough to interfere with menstruation or fertility. The prevalence of clinical or chemical diabetes mellitus is only slightly increased in patients with myotonic dystrophy, but an increased insulin response to a glucose load has proved to be a common abnormality. Numerous surveys of other endocrine functions have yielded rather little of significance.

Congenital Myotonic Dystrophy Brief mention was made above of this unique and potentially lethal form of myotonic dystrophy. That it occurs not infrequently is evident from Harper's account (1975) of 70 patients, personally studied, and 56 others gathered from the medical literature. Profound hypotonia and facial diplegia at birth are the most prominent clinical features; myotonia is notable for its absence. The tented upper lip ("carp mouth") and open jaw impart a characteristic appearance, which allows immediate recognition of the disease in the newborn infant. Difficulty in sucking and swallowing, bronchial aspiration (due to palatal weakness), and respiratory distress (due to diaphragmatic and intercostal weakness and pulmonary immaturity) are present in varying degrees of severity, and the latter disorders are responsible for a previously unrecognized group of neonatal deaths from the disease (24 such deaths among sibs of affected families in Harper's study). In surviving infants, delayed motor and speech development, mild to moderately severe mental retardation, and talipes or generalized arthrogryposis are common. Interestingly, myotonia in the usual childhood form of the disease does not become evident before the second or third year, but is uniformly present after the tenth year.

The affected parent, in the congenital form of this disease, is practically always the mother. Contrariwise, in cases of adult onset, transmission is predominantly paternal. These data suggest that in addition to inheriting the myotonic dystrophy gene, the congenital cases also receive some maternally transmitted factor, the nature of which is presently unknown. The disease in the mother need not be severe, and this feature, coupled with the absence of clinical myotonia in the neonatal period, may lead to the condition being overlooked.

Congenital myotonic dystrophy needs to be differentiated from Möbius' syndrome (page 851), one of the congenital myopathies (Chap. 50), severe spinal muscular atrophy (Chap. 50), and congenital myasthenia gravis (Chap. 51).

Late Distal Muscular Dystrophy (Milhorat, Wolff; Welander) This is a slowly progressive distal myopathy with onset principally in middle adult life. Weakness and wasting of the muscles of the hands, forearms, and

lower legs, especially the extensors, are the main clinical features. Although cases such as these had been reported by Gowers and others, their differentiation from myotonic dystrophy and peroneal muscular atrophy was unclear until relatively recent times.

Milhorat and Wolff, in 1943, presented the findings in 12 individuals of one family affected by "a progressive muscular dystrophy of atrophic distal type." The onset was between 26 and 43 years, and within 5 to 15 years the patients had become disabled. There was one autopsy, confirming the dystrophic nature of the disease. An apparently separate form of distal dystrophy with onset before 2 years of age was described by van der Does de Willebois et al. The inheritance is autosomal dominant. The condition is distinguished from spinal muscular atrophy and polyneuropathy by the high levels of CPK in the serum, EMG, and biopsy.

Welander's account of this disorder, based on the study of 249 Swedish cases, appeared in 1951. In her series the mode of inheritance was autosomal dominant. The changes demonstrated in three autopsies and 22 biopsies were purely dystrophic. Fasciculations, cramps, pain, sensory disturbances, and myotonia were notably absent. Senile cataracts appeared after the age of 70 in three patients and surely can be discounted as having special significance. No endocrine disorders were detected. The central nervous system and peripheral nerves were normal. Progression of the disease was very slow; after 10 years or so some wasting of proximal muscles was seen in a few of the patients.

Other Varieties As remarked earlier, there are many patients with obvious muscular dystrophy who do not conform to any one of the above types, and this calls into question the adequacy of our classification or of any nosologic system that is based on semiology alone. Also, some of these patients, initially called dystrophic, prove on more complete examination to fall into the category of familial, slowly progressive spinal muscular atrophy (Kugelberg and Welander). The differentiation between an anterior horn cell disease (*nuclear amyotrophy* would be a more appropriate term) and muscular dystrophy, on the basis of muscle biopsy alone, may prove difficult because of the late dystrophic features of neural and spinal atrophy. By the intravital staining of nerve terminals with methylene blue, Cöers and Telerman-Toppet have determined a range of "terminal innervation ratios" (number of terminals for each axon). They find that in denervation atrophy the ratio is increased, presumably due to collateral sprouting, while in myopathy the ratio is normal. Of course, there would be no difficulty in separating these two categories of disease if postmortem examinations had been performed.

Since the majority of early-life dystrophies are X-linked, it always comes as a surprise to observe a clinically manifest form of *progressive muscular dystrophy in young girls.* However, this happens occasionally and is the subject of several reports. Explanations easily come to mind: (1) If the female has only one X chromosome as in Turner's XO syndrome, she should have the same muscle affection as the male. (2) Some female carriers also have overt disease, probably through the operation of the Lyon principle of sex heredity. However, neither explanation accounts for several families where only females have been subject to a proven muscular dystrophy, such as the one described by Henson et al. In the latter family, proximal myopathy had its onset at the age of 5 to 20 years and led to severe disability by the age of 30 years. Waddling gait and lumbar lordosis were prominent, and the proximal limb and trunk muscles, especially the deltoids, glutei, hamstrings, and medial parts of the gastrocnemii were the most affected.

A familial hypertrophy of the quadriceps may be the first sign of a dystrophic disease which affects males in their third to fourth decades of life. It spreads slowly to other muscles, mainly of the pelvis and legs. A purely atrophic form of quadriceps dystrophy has also been described. Mild forms of restricted scapuloperoneal dystrophy (see above) probably represent variants of Erb's limb-girdle dystrophy.

A universal dystrophy, with affection of every skeletal muscle in the body, including the eye muscles, and occurring in three members of a family (two males and one female in two successive generations), has come under our observation. The onset was in adult life and progression to a state of severe weakness and atrophy occurred over a period of 10 years; there was no hypertrophy, pseudohypertrophy, cataracts, or myotonia.

We have also seen pure dysphagia with esophageal dilatation (upper striated part) as a probable dystrophic disease. This disorder has its onset in early adult life and is slowly progressive but without other signs of myotonic dystrophy.

From time to time, muscular dystrophy of either the classic or exceptional type occurs in conjunction with one or several more strictly neurologic disorders. Wilson refers to these as "transitional states" implying that the disease process has extended from muscle to nervous tissue. Our view would be that other heredofamilial disorders have a closely related genetic mechanism. Muscular dystrophy, for example, has been noted together with cerebellar ataxia, with an extrapyramidal syndrome, and with spastic weakness of legs. The association of progressive external ophthalmoplegia with mild peripheral neuropathy, cerebellar ataxia, and corticospinal tract disease has already been mentioned. Claims that peroneal muscular atrophy is a combined polyneuropathy and polymyopathy must be examined critically, for there is often a tendency to misinterpret the degenerative muscle changes in the late stages of denervation.

PATHOLOGY

The histologic changes in the several forms of muscular dystrophy are plain to see, but elusive of interpretation. The changes listed in all standard writings on this subject are loss of muscle fibers, residual fibers of larger and smaller size than normal in haphazard arrangement (no grouping), segmental necrosis (degeneration) of muscle fibers with phagocytosis and regenerative activity (abortive?), and increase in lipocytes and fibrosis. The basic problem revolves on the interpretation of these changes: Which are primary and which are secondary? Opinions on this subject are divergent.

The difficulty in resolving this problem can be appreciated if one considers the extreme chronicity of the pathologic process. While the Duchenne form may run its course in a 10- to 15-year period, the span of the disease in the Landouzy-Déjerine and Erb types must be reckoned in decades. The prospect of capturing an image of the fundamental defect at any one instant in a tiny biopsy of one muscle is discouraging. Further, a survey of end-stage pathologic changes at autopsy, when all the fibers in many muscles have disappeared, yields little information concerning the pathogenesis of the fiber loss.

That fibers disappear is undoubted. Undetermined is the manner in which they disappear. Two hypotheses merit consideration: (1) that recurrent segmental necrosis results in destruction of the entire fiber and (2) that progressive atrophy leads eventually to fiber death. Each is difficult to affirm. Segmental necrosis is demonstrated most readily in the Duchenne type of dystrophy. Often several closely approximated fibers are simultaneously affected, which has led to the suggestion, by analogy with the findings in experimental embolism in animal muscle, of a vascular pathogenesis of muscular dystrophy. Physiologic and pathologic studies of the vessels have shown this hypothesis to be fallacious. In the chronic (i.e., benign) forms of dystrophy one often searches in vain for evidence of segmental necrosis.

Whether this is a problem in sampling at the correct moment, there being much less likelihood of showing the necrotic change in a long-drawn-out process, or whether this is due to a different type of involvement, cannot be decided with certainty. One of the authors (R.D.A.) believes that segmental necrosis is a feature of all dystrophic muscle diseases and that its frequent recurrence exhausts the regenerative (restorative) potential of the fiber.

The smallness of residual fibers (atrophy?) is a prominent feature but may have a number of explanations. It could be, as some myopathologists argue, that the underlying disorder is one of gradual failure of metabolism with all sarcoplasmic constituents undergoing volumetric reduction. If studied in three dimensions by serial sections, however, one can see, in the Duchenne type of dystrophy, that regeneration of the muscle fiber, after segmental necrosis, results in the formation of several new, thin fibers. This change raises the question of the regenerative capacity of dystrophic muscle. Walton and Adams and others have found that a single trauma to a relatively sound dystrophic muscle excites the same regenerative changes as trauma to a normal and myositic muscle. Yet the fibers do eventually degenerate and disappear, owing presumably to an exhaustion of regenerative capacity after repeated injuries, or more and more extensive necrosis.

Hypertrophy of muscle is believed by most pathologists to be a work hypertrophy of sound fibers in the face of fiber injury. But there are disturbing examples of true hypertrophy of entire muscles prior to the first sign of weakness. Erb contended that the hypertrophy may be the first expression of the basic abnormality, which then progresses to segmental necrosis (atrophy?). Pseudohypertrophy is due to lipocytic replacement of degenerated muscle fibers, but in its earlier stages the presence of many enlarged fibers contributes to the enlargement of muscle. There is general agreement that increase in lipocytes, fibrosis, and thickening of the walls of blood vessels are secondary changes.

In the earlier stages of Duchenne's pseudohypertrophic dystrophy the most distinctive features are prominent segmental degeneration and phagocytosis of single fibers or groups of fibers and evidence of regenerative activity (basophilia of sarcoplasm, hyperplasia and nucleolation of sarcolemmal nuclei, and the presence of myotubes and myocytes). Vitreous change of sarcoplasm in many fibers scattered throughout the muscle has also been emphasized as an early sign of degeneration and is found more often in Duchenne's dystrophy than in other dystrophies. Mokri and Engel have postulated that degenerative foci in the plasma membrane, which allow calcium to enter the fibers, explain this

change. Also, Schotland, by the use of the freeze-fracture technique, has demonstrated ultrastructural alterations in the intramembranous architecture of the plasmalemma of muscle fibers of dystrophic patients. Thus, in the early and midphases of the disease, plasmalemmal degeneration becomes the initial change leading to fiber necrosis. Nevertheless, the authors remain skeptical of this hypothesis because such vitreous fibers do not progress to a state of necrosis and phagocytosis. Moreover, many of the fibers showing the vitreous change are in a state of contraction (contraction bands); hence it may be no more than a mark of irritability of muscle. Also it occurs as a biopsy artifact in many muscle diseases. In myotonic dystrophy, spiral annulets (ringbinden), sarcoplasmic masses, and rowing of central nuclei are characteristic. No specific pattern of changes demarcates the other dystrophic syndromes.

In the late stages of the dystrophic process only a few scattered muscle fibers remain, almost lost in a sea of fat cells. It is of interest that the late, or burned-out stage of chronic polymyositis resembles muscular dystrophy in that the fiber population is depleted, the residual fibers are of variable size but otherwise normal, and fat cells and endomysial fibrous tissue are increased; lacking only are the hypertrophied fibers of dystrophy. This resemblance informs us that many of the typical changes of muscular dystrophy are nonspecific.

All the dystrophies have been studied electronmicroscopically, but the results have been disappointing insofar as they have provided no information as to the initial or specific lesion. The same is true of histochemical studies.

Finally, it should be restated that in all forms of muscular dystrophy the spinal neurons and their axons in the roots and peripheral nerves are normal.

ETIOLOGY

Known to be a hereditary disease, the central issue in dystrophy is how an abnormal gene induces a degeneration of muscle fibers. Probably it is not overly important whether the degeneration occurs as a consequence of repeated segmental necrosis or of progressive atrophy.

The search for essential data regarding pathogenesis began with a scrutiny of the normal-appearing hypertrophied and atrophied fibers. Under the light and electron microscopes they appear to be normal, although one occasionally observes focal degeneration of myofilaments; smudging and misalignment of Z bands; increased numbers of mitochondria, glycogen and lipofuscin granules, lipid droplets, crystalline inclusions, and filamentous and myelinlike bodies. None of these changes, nor any particular combination of them is specific. Residual fibers show no special histochemical features, and attempts at tissue culture have failed to demonstrate unique properties of the dystrophic fibers.

Biochemical studies have revealed the following abnormalities: decreased glycolytic enzymes and relative normality of mitochondrial oxidative enzymes; increase of cathepsins (lysosomal enzymes); decrease in isoenzyme 5 of lactic dehydrogenase; decreased myoglobin; increased serum CPK, aldolase, LDH, SGOT, and SGPT; decreased protein synthesis; creatinuria and short half-life of labeled creatine; increased serum alpha$_2$ globulin and polysaccharides, and occasionally pentosuria and taurinuria. Most of these abnormalities are the result of degeneration or regeneration of the muscle fiber, and none has been shown to be the basic biochemical defect that leads to necrosis and/or atrophy under conditions of natural activity. (See Pennington's review of the biochemistry of muscular dystrophy.)

As has been indicated above, a number of biochemical and biophysical studies in recent years has implicated an abnormality of the muscle surface membrane in the genesis of muscular dystrophy. Supporting evidence has come also from the study of the membranes of red blood cells. Abnormalities in the phosphorylation of membrane proteins have been reported, as have a variety of morphologic abnormalities (distortion and surface projections: "echinocytes" and "stomatocytes"). Unfortunately, these abnormalities have not been found consistently in patients with muscular dystrophy, nor have they proved to be specific for this disorder. To date, morphological abnormalities of red blood cells (or of lymphocytes or cultured fibroblasts) have failed to provide a reliable diagnostic test for dystrophy.

DIFFERENTIAL DIAGNOSIS

The following are some of the common problems that arise in the diagnosis of muscular dystrophy:

1. *The diagnosis of muscular dystrophy in a child who has not been walking for long, or whose locomotion is delayed.* Tests of peak power on command cannot be used with reliability in small children. The most helpful points are (*a*) unusual difficulty in climbing stairs, or arising from a crouch or from a recumbent position on the floor, showing greater weakness at the hips and knees than at the ankles; (*b*) unusually large, firm calves; (*c*) male sex; (*d*) high serum CPK and aldolase values; (*e*) myopathic EMG; and (*f*) biopsy findings.

2. *The adult patient with diffuse or proximal muscle weakness of several months' duration, raising the question of polymyositis versus dystrophy.* Biopsy may be misleading in showing a few inflammatory foci in an otherwise dystrophic picture. The main points which help to distinguish polymyositis from dystrophy have been indicated in the preceding chapter. As a rule, polymyositis is associated with high CPK and aldolase values (higher than any dystrophy except the Duchenne type, which does not begin in adults), and the EMG shows many fibrillation potentials (rare in adult forms of muscular dystrophy). With these points in mind, there may still be uncertainty, in which instance a trial of prednisone is indicated for a period of 6 months. Unmistakable improvement favors polymyositis; questionable improvement (physician's and patient's judgment not in accord) leaves the diagnosis unsettled.

3. *An adult with a slowly evolving proximal weakness.* Several of the congenital polymyopathies discussed in the next chapter may begin to cause symptoms or to worsen in adult years. These include central core and nemaline myopathy. Examples of a mild form of acid maltase or debrancher enzyme deficiency with glycogenosis, progressive hypokalemic polymyopathy, mitochondrial myopathy, and carnitine polymyopathy have been reported in the adult. Muscle biopsy and histochemical staining of the muscle usually provide the correct diagnosis.

4. *The occurrence of subacute or chronic symmetrical proximal weakness in an adolescent or adult raises the question of spinal muscular atrophy (Kugelberg-Welander type) as well as of polymyositis and muscular dystrophy.* EMG and muscle biopsy usually settle the matter. Some of the same problems arise in an adult with distal dystrophy.

5. *Weakness of a shoulder or one leg of some weeks' standing with increasing atrophy.* Here one must differentiate between a mononeuritis or poliomyelitis and the beginning of motor system disease (progressive spinal muscular atrophy) or a muscle dystrophy. The first two may develop silently, in mild form, and only attract notice when wasting begins (the latter takes 2 to 3 months to reach its peak). Points in favor of these acquired diseases are (*a*) lack of progression of weakness, (*b*) sparing of other muscles, and (*c*) EMG showing denervation effects. Biopsy is seldom performed under such circumstances, for by temporizing the problem eventually settles itself (stabilization or recovery with

poliomyelitis, recovery with mononeuritis). Spinal muscular atrophy declares itself by the presence of fasciculations and relatively rapid progression of weakness and involvement of other muscles.

6. The distinction, in the child or adolescent, between dystrophy and one of the congenital myopathies will be considered in relation to the latter disorders (Chap. 50).

TREATMENT

There is no specific treatment for any of the muscular dystrophies, and the physician is forced to stand by helplessly and witness the unrelenting progression of weakness and wasting. The various preparations recommended in the past, such as vitamin E, inositol, anabolic steroids, amino acid and protein supplements to diet, penicillamine, allopurinol, and digitalis preparations, have all proved to be ineffective.

Quinine has a mild curarelike action at the motor end plate and thus relieves myotonia. Although symptomatic relief of the myotonia is usually achieved, the drug has no effect on the progress of the muscle atrophy or other degenerative aspects of dystrophia myotonica. The usual dose is 0.3 to 0.6 g orally, repeated as needed about every 6 h. Mild toxic symptoms such as tinnitus may develop before enough quinine has been given to obtain satisfactory relief of the myotonia. Some patients find the side effects more distressing than the myotonia and prefer not to take quinine except on occasions when the myotonia is troublesome in a particular activity. Procainamide, phenytoin, ACTH, and corticosteroids are sometimes useful in alleviating myotonia.

Androgens may be administered in cases of myotonic dystrophy and provide symptomatic benefit when deficiency is apparent, but a relation of the hormonal deficiency to the pathogenesis of the muscle disease is not established.

Needless to say, the common complications of muscular dystrophy, notably fractures, pulmonary infections, and cardiac decompensation are treated symptomatically. Surgical management of cataracts, when they are mature, is indicated.

Two factors are of importance in the management of patients with muscular dystrophy: avoiding prolonged bed rest and encouraging the patient to maintain as full and normal a life as possible. These help to prevent the rapid worsening associated with inactivity and to conserve a healthy attitude of mind. Obesity should be avoided; this requires careful attention to diet. Contractures and skeletal deformities in Duchenne's dystrophy can be prevented or delayed by passive and active stretching exercises and the use of light spinal braces. Fasciotomy or tendon-lengthening operations and long leg braces may aid in preserving ambulation for several additional years. Maximum resistance exercises when performed regularly may increase muscle strength slightly. Swimming is another useful exercise. Massage and electrical stimulation are worthless. The education of children with muscular dystrophy should continue with the purpose of preparing them for a sedentary occupation.

Detection of carriers, by measuring CPK, and sex determination of the fetus, by examination of amniotic fluid, are the bases for genetic counseling.

THE CHRONIC METABOLIC POLYMYOPATHIES

The boundaries of this category of disease cannot be sharply drawn at this time. Each year, with advancing knowledge of the chemistry of muscle, a number of diseases, formerly classified as dystrophic, have been added to the list of metabolic myopathies. Limitation of space prevents a detailed description of each entity. Only the most representative forms will be presented on the following pages.

Apropos of the clinical manifestations of this group of diseases, the majority have shown few or no muscular abnormalities prior to a certain age. Then there gradually unfolds a progressive weakness over a period of months or years. The weakness may affect only the lower extremities (hip flexors and extensors and quadriceps) or both the lower and upper extremities. Ocular and facial muscles are affected in some cases. Sometimes the involvement is more diffuse. Clues to its myopathic nature are elevated CPK and aldolase in the serum; brief, low voltage (myopathic) units in the EMG; and a random atrophy or degeneration of fibers in the muscle biopsy. The differential diagnosis includes chronic idiopathic polymyositis and some of the congenital myopathies, described in Chaps. 48 and 50, respectively.

THYROID MYOPATHIES

During the past three decades several myopathic diseases related to alterations in thyroid function have been recognized: (1) chronic thyrotoxic myopathy, (2) exophthalmic ophthalmoplegia (infiltrative ophthalmopathy),

(3) myasthenia gravis associated with toxic diffuse goiter or with hypothyroidism, (4) periodic paralysis associated with toxic goiter, and (5) muscle hypertrophy and slow muscle contraction and relaxation associated with myxedema and cretinism. Although not frequent, several examples of these diseases may be seen in a single year in a large general hospital.

Chronic thyrotoxic myopathy is characterized by progressive weakness and atrophy of skeletal musculature, occurring in conjunction with overt or covert (masked) hyperthyroidism. The thyroid disease is usually chronic, and the goiter is of the nodular rather than the diffuse type. The muscular disorder may reach such an advanced degree as to suggest progressive spinal muscular atrophy (motor system disease). This complication of hyperthyroidism is most frequent in middle age, and men are more susceptible than women. The onset is insidious and the weakness progresses over weeks and months. Exophthalmos need not be present. Muscles of the pelvic girdle and thighs are weakened more than others (Basedow's paraplegia), though all are affected to some extent, even the bulbar and rarely the ocular muscles. However, the shoulder and hand muscles show the most conspicuous atrophy. Tremor and twitching during contraction may occur, but we have not seen fasciculations at rest or fibrillations (in the EMG). The tendon reflexes are normal or lively. Creatine excretion in the urine is increased and tolerance to ingested creatine diminished, but the degree of this impairment has not correlated with the degree of weakness. Serum enzyme levels are not elevated. Electromyograms have disclosed no definite abnormality, and biopsies of muscle, except for slight atrophic changes, have been normal. Administration of neostigmine has no effect. Muscle power and bulk are gradually restored when thyroid activity is reduced to normal levels.

Exophthalmic ophthalmoplegia refers to weakness of the external ocular muscles conjoined with the exophthalmos of Graves' disease (pupillary and ciliary muscles are always spared). The exophthalmos varies in degree, being sometimes absent at an early stage of the disease, and is not in itself responsible for the muscle weakness. Both the exophthalmos and the weakness of the extraocular muscles may precede the signs of hyperthyroidism or follow the effective treatment of it. The extraocular muscle palsies may occasionally be unilateral, especially in the beginning. All external eye muscles may be affected, usually one more than others, accounting for strabismus and diplopia; upward movements are usually limited to the greatest degree. Examination of the eye

muscles from biopsies and autopsy material have shown many degenerated fibers and infiltrations of lymphocytes, mononuclear leukocytes, and lipocytes; hence the term *infiltrative ophthalmopathy*. The condition often runs a self-limited course as does the exophthalmos itself, and therapy is difficult to evaluate. Certainly the maintenance of a euthyroid state is desirable.

In patients with marked periorbital and conjunctival edema, high doses of corticosteroids (about 80 mg prednisone per day) may partially control the ophthalmic disorder, including the extraocular muscle weakness. Because of the hazards of corticosteroid therapy, it should be reserved for patients who would otherwise require surgical intervention. In a number of such cases it has been possible, with corticosteroids, to carry the patient over the crisis and to avoid the trauma of extreme exophthalmos and risks of surgery. If the exophthalmos reaches a degree which threatens injury of the cornea, tarsorrhaphy or decompression by removal of the roof of the bony orbit may save the patient's vision.

Thyrotoxic periodic paralysis resembles familial periodic paralysis (page 993), and consists of attacks of mild to severe weakness of the muscles of the trunk and limbs (usually the cranial muscles are spared), which develops in a few minutes or hours and lasts for part of a day or longer. In some series of periodic paralysis, as many as half the patients have had hyperthyroidism and many of them have been Orientals. Unlike the typical hypokalemic form, thyrotoxic periodic paralysis is not a familial disorder. In most of the thyrotoxic cases, the serum potassium levels have been low during the attacks of weakness and the administration of several grams of KCl has terminated the attack. Treatment of the hyperthyroidism abolishes the symptomatic manifestations of the muscular disorder.

Myasthenia gravis, in its typical neostigmine-responsive and autoimmune form, may accompany hyper- or hypothyroidism. The latter are also believed to be autoimmune diseases. In hyperthyroidism, weakness and atrophy of muscles, characteristic of the aforementioned chronic thyrotoxic myopathy, are added to the myasthenia, without appearing to affect the requirement for or response to neostigmine. In contrast, hypothyroidism, even of mild degree, seems to aggravate the myasthenia gravis, greatly increasing the need for neostigmine and at times inducing a myasthenic crisis. Thyroxine is beneficial and, with respect to myasthenia, restores the patient to the status that existed before the onset of the thyroid insufficiency. However, the myasthenia gravis is independent of the thyroid disease, and each must be treated separately.

Hypothyroidism, whether in the form of myxedema or of cretinism, is often accompanied by a series of changes in skeletal muscle, consisting of increased volume, stiffness, and slowness of contraction and relaxation. These changes probably account for the large tongue and dysarthria that one observes in hypothyroidism. The presence of action myospasm (rare) and percussion myoedema, along with the slowness of tendon reflexes, assists the examiner in making a bedside diagnosis (see page 1001). Cretinism in association with these muscle symptoms is known as *Debré-Semelaigne syndrome*, and myxedema in childhood with a similar muscle picture is called *Hoffmann's syndrome*. These clinical syndromes simulate hypertrophia musculorum vera and myotonia congenita. In neither cretinism nor myxedema, however, is there evidence of true myotonia either by clinical test or EMG, and muscle biopsies have revealed only the presence of large fibers. In the rare instances where myotonia and hypothyroidism coexist, the former appears to be accentuated by the latter.

Patients with the muscle disorder of hypothyroidism show a reduction in creatinine excretion and an increase in creatine tolerance. Transaminase values in the serum are normal, but the CPK level is usually slightly elevated. The administration of thyroxine corrects the abnormality of muscle.

How thyroid secretion affects the muscle fiber in all these myopathies is still a matter of conjecture. Clinical data indicate that this hormone influences the contractile process in some manner, but does not interfere with the transmission of impulses in the peripheral nerves, across the myoneural junctions, or along the sarcolemma. In hyperthyroidism this functional disorder enhances the speed of the contractile process and reduces its duration, the net effect being a weakening, an excess fatigability, and a loss of endurance in muscle action. In hypothyroidism, the speed of the contractile process is reduced and its duration prolonged.

CORTICOSTEROID POLYMYOPATHY

The widespread use of adrenal corticosteroids has created a new muscle disease, probably similar to that which has been produced in rabbits by the administration of cortisone. The proximal limb and girdle musculature becomes extremely weak, to the point where it is difficult to elevate the arms and to arise from a sitting, squatting, or kneeling position, and walking may be hampered. The EMG may show a myopathic pattern of small but abundant action potentials but no fibrillations; biopsies disclose a mild variation in fiber size, with mainly atrophic fibers, but also a few degenerating and regenerating ones, without infiltrates of inflammatory cells. The serum CPK and aldolase levels are raised, and there is a creatinuria.

There is only a poor correlation between total dose of corticosteroid and severity of muscle weakness. Nevertheless, in patients who develop this type of myopathy, the corticosteroid dosage has usually been high and sustained over a period of months or years. All corticosteroids may produce the disorder although fluorinated ones are more culpable than others. Discontinuation or reduction of corticosteroid administration leads to improvement and recovery.

A similar myopathy occurs regularly in patients with Cushing's syndrome but is not always symptomatic. The mechanism of the muscle disease in either type is unknown.

POLYMYOPATHY WITH HYPOKALEMIC PERIODIC PARALYSIS

A rare complication of *familial periodic paralysis* (see page 994) takes the form of a subacute or chronic persistent weakness of thigh and pelvic musculature. Onset may be in the middle adult years, long after a troublesome periodic paralysis during childhood or adolescence has ameliorated or ceased altogether. Biopsy reveals the characteristic vacuolization and hydropia of periodic paralysis, and the degeneration of muscle fibers that may be consequent to it. Slightly elevated levels of muscle enzymes in the serum and a myopathic pattern in the EMG substantiates the diagnosis. The effective control of the acute attacks of paralysis by the administration of potassium appears to slow or halt the progress of the myopathy.

GLYCOGEN STORAGE MYOPATHIES

This relatively rare but interesting group of diseases has gradually enlarged as more has been learned about carbohydrate metabolism of muscle. Following the pioneering work of the Coris (1952) several additional enzymatic steps have been discovered, and deficiencies in each of them has become the basis of the commonly accepted classification, which is presented in the following table. These enzymatic deficiencies alter the metabolism of many cells but most strikingly those of the liver, heart, and skeletal muscle; in about half of the affected individuals a chronically progressive or intermittent myopathic syndrome is the major manifestation of the disease.

The most impressive of these glycogen storage diseases from the standpoint of the clinical myologist are the recessive form of α-1,4-glucosidase (acid maltase) deficiency and of myophosphorylase deficiency. *The acid maltase deficiency* takes two clinical forms. The first is the most malignant. It develops in infancy at the age of 2 to 6 months; dyspnea and cyanosis call attention to enlargement of the heart, and the skeletal muscles are found to be weak and hypotonic. The tongue may be enlarged, giving the infant a cretinoid appearance. Exceptionally, the heart is relatively normal in size, and the CNS and muscles bear the brunt of the disorder. The clinical picture then resembles infantile muscular atrophy (Werdnig-Hoffmann disease). The disease is rapidly progressive and ends fatally in a few months. In the second, or adult, form there is a more benign proximal and truncal myopathy. The weakness is slowly progressive over years, and death is usually the result of paralysis of respiratory muscles. The liver and heart are usually not enlarged. The disease must be differentiated from other chronic adult polymyopathies. Children and adolescents have sometimes suffered an illness that is less severe than the infantile form but more severe than the adult form.

The diagnosis is readily confirmed by muscle biopsy. In routine preparations the sarcoplasm is vacuolated and alcohol fixation permits staining of the stored glycogen. The latter is increased 4 to 5 times above normal and the glycogen particles lie in aggregates, some surrounded by membranes and some free. Electron microscopy shows them to occupy lysosomal vesicles. The myofibrillar content of the fiber is disrupted. Some muscle fibers degenerate. In the more severe infantile form of acid maltase deficiency nerve cells may also accumulate glycogen and degenerate. The difference in severity between infant and adult forms may relate to the completeness of enzyme deficiency, but other factors may be at play.

Table 49-1
Glycogen storage diseases

Type	Name	Clinical and laboratory findings	Enzyme deficiency
I	Von Gierke's disease	Enlarged liver and kidneys, hyperlipidemia, hypoglycemia, ketoacidosis, seizures	Glucose-6-phosphatase
II	Pompe's disease	*Infantile form:* cardiomegaly, hypotonia and weakness, dysphagia, and respiratory difficulty; death in infancy. *Adult form:* proximal weakness, enlarged calves, atonic anal sphincter, respiratory difficulties	α-1,4-Glucosidase (acid maltase)
III	Cori-Forbes disease	Hepatomegaly, hypoglycemia, late onset weakness, slight growth retardation	Amylo-1,6-glucosidase (debrancher)
IV	Anderson's disease	Growth failure, cirrhosis, hepatosplenomegaly, hypotonia with muscle atrophy in lower limbs, slow motor development	α-1,4-Glucan 6-glucosyltransferase
V	McArdle's disease	Episodic spasm and weakness with exercise, sometimes myoglobinuria. Liver, spleen, and heart normal	Myophosphorylase
VI	Hers disease	Growth retardation, hepatosplenomegaly, hypoglycemia and mild ketosis	Hepatic phosphorylase
VII	Tarui's disease	Late onset myopathy with muscle spasms and poor endurance	Muscle phosphofructokinase
VIII		Hepatomegaly, hypoglycemia, increased liver glycogen	Hepatic phosphorylase kinase
Other			Phosphohexoisomerase Phosphoglucomutase Glycogen synthetase deficiencies

There is no effective treatment.

McArdle's myophosphorylase deficiency (type V glycogenosis) expresses itself by the syndrome of recurrent contracture, and the same is true of phosphofructokinase deficiency (type VII). Both will be discussed in Chap. 52.

Of the other forms of glycogenosis only type III (Cori-Forbes disease) may affect muscles and then not consistently. A childhood form, less severe than that of acid maltase deficiency sometimes weakens muscle and diminishes tone, and an adult form with chronic proximal myopathy have been observed. In the series reported by DiMauro and his colleagues several of the patients who developed weakness during adult life complained of rapid fatigue and cramps, and an inability to perform in sports during childhood. Their CPK values were elevated, and the EMG showed fibrillations and fasciculations and paratonic discharges, data which suggest involvement of motor neurons as well as muscle fibers. The enzymatic defect is one of amylo-1,6-glucosidase deficiency.

OTHER METABOLIC MYOPATHIES

Carnitine deficiency and *carnitine palmityl transferase deficiency*, described in Chap. 48, may present in either the child or adult as an acute muscular weakness (following pregnancy or an infection) or a chronic weakness of muscles.

A syndrome of painful muscles and generalized weakness has been reported in hypoglycemia.

In hyperparathyroidism and osteomalacia resulting from renal tubular acidosis (a form of Milkman's syndrome) chronic weakness and atrophy of proximal muscles, fatigability, and discomfort after exercise have been noted. The tendon reflexes are normal or hyperactive. Mild neuropathic changes have been reported (Vicale). In *hypophosphatemic rickets* the skeletal muscles may be markedly weakened; in several reported cases a bone tumor (e.g., an ossifying angioma) was found, and its removal restored muscle power to normal. The oral administration of phosphates to raise the serum phosphorus has been beneficial in nontumorous cases. Some of the latter are accompanied by pain and stiffness.

Generalized weakness is a characteristic of *Addison's disease*, related to the water and electrolyte disturbances and hypotension. Rarely, a contracture of hamstring muscles develops, preventing upright stance. Biopsy has revealed normal muscle tissue; the EMG is normal; and the tendon reflexes are retained.

REFERENCES

ADAMS RD: *Diseases of Muscle: A Study in Pathology,* 3d ed. New York, Harper & Row, 1975.

BARBEAU A: The syndrome of hereditary late onset ptosis and dysphagia in French Canada, in Kuhn EE (ed): *Progressive Muskeldystrophies, Myotonie, Myasthenie.* New York, Springer-Verlag, 1966.

BECKER PE: Two new families of benign sex-linked recessive muscular dystrophy. *Rev Can Biol* 21:551, 1962.

BERENBERG RA et al: Lumping or splitting? "Ophthalmoplegia plus" or Kearns-Sayre syndrome? *Ann Neurol* 1:37, 1977.

CÖERS C, TELERMAN-TOPPET N: Differential diagnosis of limb girdle dystrophy and spinal muscular atrophy. *Neurology* 29:957, 1979.

CORI GT, CORI CF: Glucose-6-phosphatase of the liver in glycogen storage disease. *J Biol Chem* 199:661, 1952.

DIMAURO S: Metabolic myopathies, in Vinken PJ, Bruyn GW, Ringel SP (eds): *Handbook of Clinical Neurology,* vol 41: *Diseases of Muscle II.* Amsterdam, North-Holland, 1979, chap 6, pp 175-234.

DRACHMAN DA: Ophthalmoplegia plus: The neurodegenerative disorders associated with progressive external ophthalmoplegia. *Arch Neurol* 18:654, 1968.

EMERY AEH, DREIFUSS FE: Unusual type of benign X-linked muscular dystrophy. *J Neurol Neurosurg Psychiatry* 29:338, 1966.

GARDNER-MEDWIN D: Clinical features and classification of the muscular dystrophies. *Br Med Bull* 36(2):109, 1980.

GRASSI E et al: Deformed erythrocytes in the muscular dystrophies. *Neurology* 28:842, 1978.

HARPER PS: Congenital myotonic dystrophy in Britain. *Arch Dis Child* 50:505, 514, 1975.

————: *Myotonic Dystrophy.* Philadelphia, Saunders, 1979.

HAZAMA R et al: Muscular dystrophy in six young girls. *Neurology* 29:1486, 1979.

HENSON TE, MULLER J, DEMYER WE: Hereditary myopathy limited to females. *Arch Neurol* 17:238, 1967.

KEARNS TP, SAYRE GP: Retinitis pigmentosa, external ophthalmoplegia and complete heart block. *Arch Ophthalmol* 60:280, 1958.

KUGELBERG E, WELANDER L: Heredofamilial juvenile muscular atrophy simulating muscular dystrophy. *Arch Neurol Psychiatry* 75:500, 1956.

KUHN E et al: Early myocardial disease and cramping myalgia in Becker's type muscular dystrophy: A kindred. *Neurology* 29:1144, 1979.

MAAS O, PATERSON AS: Myotonia congenita, dystrophia myotonica and paramyotonia; Reaffirmation of their identity. *Brain* 73:318, 1950.

MILHORAT AT, WOLFF HG: Studies in diseases of muscle. XIII. Progressive muscular dystrophy of atrophic distal type; report on a family; report of autopsy. *Arch Neurol Psychiatry* 49:655, 1943.

MOKRI B, ENGEL AG: Duchenne dystrophy: Electron microscopic findings pointing to a basic or early abnormality in the plasma membrane of the muscle fiber. *Neurology* 25:1111, 1975.

PENNINGTON RJT: Clinical biochemistry of muscular dystrophy. *Br Med Bull* 36(2):123, 1980.

RINGEL SP, WILSON WB, BARDEN MT: Extraocular muscle biopsy in chronic progressive ophthalmoplegia. *Ann Neurol* 6:326, 1979.

ROSES MS et al: Evaluation and detection of Duchenne's and Becker's muscular dystrophy carriers by manual muscle testing. *Neurology* 27:20, 1977.

SCHOTLAND DL: Duchenne dystrophy—a freeze fracture study,

in Rowland LP (ed): *Pathogenesis of Human Muscular Dystrophies*. Amsterdam, Excerpta Medica, 1977, pp 562–568.

VAN DER DOES DE WILLEBOIS AEM et al: Distal myopathy with onset in early infancy. *Neurology* 18:383, 1968.

VICALE CT: The diagnostic features of a muscular syndrome resulting from hyperparathyroidism, osteomalacia owing to renal tubular acidosis, and perhaps to related disorders of calcium metabolism. *Trans Am Neurol Assoc* 74:143, 1949.

VICTOR M, HAYES R, ADAMS RD: Oculopharyngeal muscular dystrophy. A familial disease of late life characterized by dysphagia and progressive ptosis of the eyelids. *N Engl J Med* 267:1267, 1962.

WALTON JN (ed): *Disorders of Voluntary Muscle*, 4th ed. Edinburgh, Churchill-Livingstone, 1981.

———, Nattrass FS: On the classification, natural history and treatment of myopathies. *Brain* 77:169, 1954.

WELANDER L: Myopathia distalis tarda hereditaria. *Acta Med Scand* 141(suppl 265):1, 1951.

WOHLFART G, FEX J, ELIASSON S: Hereditary proximal spinal muscle atrophy simulating progressive muscular dystrophy. *Acta Psychiatr Neurol* 30:395, 1955.

As skeletal muscle is subjected to increasingly careful study, more and more congenital, developmental, and aging abnormalities are being discovered. All are understandable in relation to the life cycle of the muscle fiber and are therefore presented together in this chapter. Such diseases are of particular importance in pediatric neurology, for most of them attract notice at an early age.

THE DEVELOPMENT AND AGING OF MUSCLE

The commonly accepted view of the embryogenesis of muscle is that muscle fibers form originally by fusion of myoblasts, soon after the latter differentiate from mesenchymal cells. The newly formed fibers are thin, centrally nucleated tubes (appropriately called *myotubes)* in which myofilaments begin to be produced from polyribosomes. As myofilaments become organized into myofibrils, the nuclei of the muscle fiber are displaced peripherally to a subsarcolemmal position.

The mechanisms that determine the number and arrangement of fibers in each muscle are not understood. Presumably the myoblasts themselves possess the genetic information that controls the program of development, but within any given species there are wide familial and individual variations which account for obvious differences in muscle size and power of contractility.

It is stated that the number of fibers which is assigned to each muscle is attained by birth, and growth of muscle thereafter depends mainly on the enlargement of fibers. Although the nervous system and musculature develop independently, muscle fibers continue to grow after birth only when they are active and under the influence of nerve. We are in accord with these principles, although one of the authors (R.D.A.) with DeReuck

found a twofold numerical increase in fibers in several muscles between birth and adult life.

Measurements of muscle fiber diameters from birth throughout life show the growth curve to ascend rapidly in the early postnatal years and less rapidly in adolescence, and to reach a peak during the third decade. After puberty, growth of muscle is less in females than in males, but such differences are greater in the arm, shoulder, thigh, and pelvic muscles than in those of the leg, and ocular muscles are about equal in the two sexes. At all ages, disuse decreases the fiber size by as much as 30 percent (at the expense of myofibrils), and overuse increases the size by about the same amount (work hypertrophy). Type I (oxidative-enzyme-rich) fibers are slightly smaller than type II (phosphorylative-enzyme-rich) fibers.

During late adult life and in the senium, the number of muscle fibers diminishes and variations in size increase. The variations are of two types, *group atrophy* (clusters of 20 to 30 fibers, all reduced in diameter to about the same extent) and *random atrophy*. Enlargement of other fibers is also present. Muscle cells, like others of postmitotic type, are subject to aging (lipofuscin accumulation, autophagic vacuolization, enzyme loss) and to death. Group atrophy, present in 90 percent of gastrocnemii in individuals past 60 years of age, represents denervation effect and corresponds to the 30 percent loss of lumbar motor neurons in old age (Tomlinson et al.).

DERANGEMENTS OF THE LIFE CYCLE OF MUSCLE FIBERS

These have not been fully ascertained, but one can envision the following possibilities: (1) failure of muscle cells to differentiate in a given region (congenital absence of muscle); (2) congenital hypoplasia (local or universal); (3) congenital hyperplasia (local or universal); (4) faulty intrinsic development leading to certain disfigurations of fibers (improper arrangement of nuclei, myofilaments, and other organelles; this conceivably could reduce viability, i.e., cause abiotrophy); and (5) presenile abiotrophy or senescent polymyopathy.

Denervation from spinal or nerve disease at every age has roughly the same effect, viz., atrophy of muscle fibers (first in random distribution then in groups) and later dystrophic degeneration. Segmental necrosis at all ages excites a regenerative response from the intact parts of the fiber. As indicated on page 969, if this occurs repeatedly, the regenerative potential presumably wanes, with ultimate death of the fiber. The latter leads to permanent depopulation of fibers and paralysis.

CONGENITAL ABSENCE OF MUSCLES

It is well known to geneticists that some individuals are born without certain muscles. Not only is this true of certain inconstant ones such as the palmaris longus, which are functionally unimportant, but of more constant and important ones as well. In the most authoritative writings on this subject (LeDouble; Bing), the muscles found to be absent most frequently were the pectoralis, trapezius, serratus anticus, and quadratus femoris, but 27 others were missing in at least one case.

It is of interest that congenital absence of a muscle is usually associated with congenital anomalies of other tissues. It would appear that such a crude anomaly as total failure of mesenchymal cells to differentiate into muscle fibers usually affects the anlage of other nonmuscular tissues. For example, congenital absence of the pectoral muscle is accompanied by aplasia or hypoplasia of the mammary gland as well as syndactyly and microdactyly. Agenesis of the pectoral muscle may also be associated with scoliosis, webbed fingers, and underdevelopment of the ipsilateral arm and hand (Poland's syndrome). An unusual syndrome of congenital deficiency of the abdominal muscles is associated with a defect of ureters, bladder, and genital organs.

There is another group of restricted palsies in which the essential abnormalities appear to lie in the nervous system (nuclear amyotrophies). Congenital ptosis is one of the most frequent and is due to an innervatory defect of the levator palpebrae muscles. Complete paralysis of all muscles supplied by the oculomotor nerve, due apparently to hypoplasia of the third nerve nuclei, has been observed in several members of one family, but has also been seen occasionally in only one member. Congenital Horner's syndrome is another well-known phenomenon and may be familial. Bilateral abducens palsy is often associated with bifacial palsy in the newborn and is known as the Möbius syndrome; this usually nonfamilial anomaly, the cause of which is thought to be a nuclear hypoplasia or aplasia, is discussed with the developmental disorders (page 851). However, a primary muscle defect may also give rise to a bifacial weakness in the Landouzy-Déjerine dystrophy.

In these familial nuclear amyotrophies the muscles develop independently of the nervous system but have no prospect of attaining their natural growth and function because of failure of innervation. It is a kind of congenital denervation hypotrophy.

CONGENITAL CONTRACTURES AND PSEUDOCONTRACTURES OF MUSCLES AND JOINT DEFORMITIES

True *contracture* refers to a state in which shortened muscle is unable to relax because of failure of the metabolic mechanism necessary for relaxation, as in McArdle's disease. *Pseudocontracture*, or *fibrous contracture*, refers to a fixation of limb posture due to destruction of muscles, fibrosis of muscle and periarticular tissues, and shortening of ligaments. If joints are primarily affected so as to impede motion, the condition is *ankylosis* (see page 943).

There are a surprising number of deformities in infants and children that appear to be due to shortening and fibrosis of muscles. Some of the most common are congenital clubfoot (talipes), congenital torticollis, and congenital elevation of the scapula (Sprengel's deformity). In all these conditions the postural distortion is either produced and maintained by a weakened, fibrotic muscle or by a normal one which is contracted and shortened because of the absence of a countervailing antagonist. Trauma to a muscle during intrauterine life or at birth leads to fibrosis and to pseudocontracture in some cases.

In congenital clubfoot the deformity may be one of plantar flexion of foot and ankle (talipes equinus), inversion and adduction (talipes varus), eversion and abduction (talipes valgus), or dorsiflexion of foot and ankle (talipes calcaneus). About 75 percent are equinovarus. Usually both feet are affected. Multiple incidence in one family has been described repeatedly; the inheritance is recessive or sex-linked. Two-thirds of the cases have been males. Several explanations of cause and pathogenesis have been offered: fetal malposition, embryonic abnormality of tarsal and metatarsal bones, a primary defect in nerves or anterior horns of the spinal cord, or a congenital dystrophy of muscle. No one theory applies to all cases; available pathologic data exclude a single cause and pathogenesis (see Adams for pertinent literature on the subject).

Congenital wryneck, or torticollis, begins during the first months of life and is due to shortening of the sternomastoid muscle, which is firm and taut. The head is inclined to one side and the occiput slightly rotated to the side of the affected muscle. This disorder is nonfamilial and is usually ascribed to injury of the sternomastoid at birth. Whether the injury is purely mechanical in nature or ischemic, due to arterial or venous occlusion, is not entirely clear. It gives rise to a sternomastoid tumor (actually a pseudotumor) which appears, on exploration, as a white, spindle-shaped swelling of the muscle belly. The histological findings are similar to those of Volkmann's contracture, i.e., replacement of the muscle fibers by relatively acellular connective tissue, so that an ischemic mechanism appears most likely (see page 943).

Arthrogryposis Multiplex Congenita Multiple congenital contractures, multiple congenital articular rigidities, and amyoplasia congenita are some of the names which have been applied to congenital deformity and rigidity of the extremities. This disorder, now generally referred to as *arthrogryposis* (literal meaning—curved joints), has been shown to have at least two pathologic bases. In the more common *myelopathic* type there is a failure in development of anterior horn cells, resulting in uneven smallness and paresis of limb muscles. Overactivity of normally innervated ones causes the fixed deformities. Often this form is combined with multiple defects in the nervous system and somatic structures, i.e., some degree of mental retardation, webbed fingers, polydactyly, hydrocephalus, malformations of skull, small jaw, absence of sacrum, etc. In the second or *myopathic* form, which is much less common than the first, the nervous system is intact and the muscle disease is that of an infantile muscular dystrophy. In this form of arthrogryposis, there is probably a hereditary factor. It is of interest that in the myopathic variety the limbs are fixed in a position of flexion at the hips and knees and adduction of the legs, in contrast to the variable postures of the myelopathic form. Also, the former type is less frequently conjoined with multiple anomalies than the latter. It cannot be decided, from the available reports, whether there is a neuropathic form of arthrogryposis, in addition to the two well-recognized types.

RELATIVELY NONPROGRESSIVE CONGENITAL POLYMYOPATHIES

Beginning in 1956, with the account by Shy and Magee of a patient whose muscle fibers showed a peculiar central densification of sarcoplasm ("cores"), a series of new diseases of muscle has gradually been delineated. These include the central core, nemaline (rod-body), mitochondrial, centronuclear myopathies, and myopathies with fiber-type disproportion. As the names imply, in each of these diseases there is a basic morphologic abnormality that expresses itself early in life by a retardation of motor development and hypotonia and weakness of limbs. The child may otherwise be normal.

Further study has revealed that the diseases of this group are not confined to infancy. Each of the entities described below has been observed at a later age, even in middle adult life; and if the disease is mild, there is often no way of deciding whether it has been present since birth. Extremely slow progression, in contrast to the more rapid pace of muscular dystrophy, Werdnig-Hoffmann disease, and the other forms of hereditary motor system disease of childhood and adolescence, characterizes most of the congenital myopathies. Yet examples of more rapid progression are known, and prior to muscle biopsy studies the clinical diagnosis was muscular dystrophy in several of the recorded examples. Familial occurrence has also been established, so the clinical line of separation between this group of diseases and the muscular dystrophies remains ambiguous. There is no specific treatment for any of the congenital myopathies.

The lesions in the congenital myopathies are revealed most clearly by the systematic use of histochemical stains and in preparations for phase and electron microscopy. Some of the abnormalities are also revealed by the conventional stains used in light microscopy but are always difficult to distinguish from biopsy and fixation artifacts. Thus as a group, one might say that their discovery is a product of a new histologic technology.

A word of caution must be expressed about the specificity of some of the morphological changes and classifications of the congenital myopathies based on them. It is treacherous to assume that a change in a single organelle or a subtle change in the sarcoplasm of a muscle fiber can be relied upon as the characteristic mark of a pathologic process. Indeed as more careful studies have been made of the following entities, the specificity of the lesions has been questioned. Central cores are found in the same muscle as nemaline bodies, etc., and each of the denotative lesions has been reported in other conditions or lesions, as pointed out by Bethlem and his associates. The following subgroups must be regarded as only tentative.

Central Core Myopathy In the original family of Shy and Magee, five members (four males) in three generations were affected, suggesting a dominant type of inheritance. The youngest was 2 years old; the oldest, 65 years old. In each, there was a general delay in motor development, particularly in walking, until the age of 4 to 5 years, and always the patient had had difficulty in arising from a chair, climbing stairs, and running. The weakness was more in proximal than distal muscles, though the latter did not escape, and shoulder girdle muscles were affected less than those of the pelvic girdle. Facial, bulbar, and ocular muscles were spared. The tendon reflexes were active and symmetrical. Muscle atrophy was not a prominent feature, though poor muscular development was present in one patient and has since been reported in others. There were no fasciculations, cramps, or myotonia. The electrocardiograms were normal.

As additional cases were discovered, milder forms of the disease came to be recognized, with onset of symptoms in adult life. Originally some of these patients were thought to have limb-girdle dystrophy because of the disproportionate involvement of proximal muscles. In other families, such as the one reported by Patterson et al., the onset was in middle adult life with rapid progression of a proximal myopathy. These represent the two extremes of the clinical state. Dislocation of the hips has been found in a few children. In the majority of cases the progress of the disease is extremely slow, with slight worsening over many years, but in an occasional one it has been more rapid. The EMG reveals only short, small action potentials with an adequate interference pattern. Except for an increase in urinary creatine and decrease of urinary creatinine, no chemical abnormalities have been found in the blood or urine.

Pathologically, the majority of the fibers appear of normal size or enlarged, and no focal destruction of fibers can be found. The unique feature of the disease is the presence in the central portions of each muscle fiber of a dense, amorphous, hyaline change in myofibrils. This altered zone characteristically gives a positive periodic acid–Schiff (PAS) reaction and a blue color with Gomori's trichrome stain, contrasting with the normal peripheral fibrils.

In other familial cases, particularly in oculopharyngeal dystrophy but also in other forms of dystrophy, multiple cores or minicores have been seen within muscle fibers. These cores, which represent multiple areas of muscle degeneration, do not run the length of the muscle fiber, thus differing from the cores of central core disease.

Nemaline Myopathy This disorder also expresses itself by hypotonia and impaired motility in infancy and early childhood, but unlike central core disease, the muscles of the trunk and limbs as well as the ocular, facial, lingual, and pharyngeal muscles are strikingly thin and hypoplastic. Tendon reflexes are diminished or absent. The young child with this disease usually suffers from inanition and frequent respiratory infections which may shorten life. Strength slowly improves with growth, the latter process evidently exceeding the advance of the disease. Scoliosis becomes apparent in late childhood and adolescence. The milder cases reach adulthood and then worsen slowly over the years. W. K. Engel and Reznick have observed individuals who showed signs of the disease for the first time in middle age; the weakness was mainly in proximal muscles. The EMG is "myopathic" and serum enzymes are normal or only slightly elevated. The inheritance pattern has been both autosomal dominant and recessive.

By using a Gomori trichrome stain of frozen muscle, the characteristic lesion can be seen under the light microscope. Myriads of bacilli-like rods, singly and in small packets, are seen beneath the sarcolemma. They are composed of material which resembles that of Z bands under the electron microscope. The cause of the disease is unknown but probably the weakness is related to a smallness and reduction in the number of muscle fibers and possibly to focal interruption of their cross striations. In one of the few autopsied cases, the anterior horn cells and their axons were present in normal number but were reduced in size (Robertson et al.). These changes were interpreted as being secondary to the myopathic disorder.

Mitochondrial Myopathies A variety of myopathies have been associated with the presence of overly abundant and large mitochondria (often containing abnormal inclusions and cristae) in many muscle fibers. The terms *mitochondrial* and *lipid storage* have been used interchangeably to designate these myopathies, since the enzymes essential for intramuscular lipid metabolism are contained in the mitochondria, and a defect in the latter results in an abnormal accumulation of lipid bodies in muscle fibers.

One type of benign congenital myopathy has been named *pleoconial* by Shy and his colleagues, because the muscle biopsy disclosed a remarkably large number of enlarged mitochondria. The patient was an 8-year-old boy who had hypotonia and slow motor development since early life. It was reported that he craved salt and that there had been at least three prolonged episodes of flaccid quadriparesis, like periodic paralysis.

A closely related disorder was called *megaconial*,

because of the presence, in the muscle biopsy, of giant mitochondria containing rectangular inclusions. This disorder also was detected in an 8-year-old child who had had hypotonia and weakness of muscles since birth. A sibling had died, probably of the same disease, though it had been called infantile muscular atrophy.

Kearns-Sayre Syndrome This disorder, which was briefly referred to in relation to the adult forms of ocular myopathy (page 965), is characterized by the clinical triad of progressive external ophthalmoplegia, atypical pigmentary degeneration of the retina, and heart block. The syndrome has its onset before the age of 20 years and appears to be sporadic rather than hereditary. Ptosis is usually the first manifestation, followed by ophthalmoplegia; evidence of retinitis and heart block comes later, sometimes by many years. In practically all cases the CSF protein is increased (usually >100 mg per 100 ml), and in the majority the gamma globulin is elevated as well. The defect in cardiac conduction is of varying degrees of severity; many patients have required pacemakers for AV block. The pigmentary degeneration of the retina takes the form of a fine stippling around the optic disks and rarely causes discrete field defects—hence, "atypical." Short stature, delayed sexual maturation, neurosensory hearing loss, signs of impaired cerebellar and vestibular function are usually but not invariably associated. Some patients are retarded mentally. Postmortem examination in a few patients has disclosed a diffuse coarse vacuolation of the cerebral tissue, particularly of the structures concerned with eye movements.

Patients with the Kearns-Sayre syndrome (as well as patients with adult type ocular myopathy) have shown striking mitochondrial abnormalities in skeletal as well as in eye muscles. The type I fibers look ragged and red in a Gomori stain, owing to clusters of mitochondria and lipid inclusions. Electron microscopy discloses large numbers of abnormal mitochondria. In patients with progressive external ophthalmoplegia, accumulations of mitochondria in skeletal muscles have also been associated with excessive glycogen in muscle fibers. Similar accumulations of mitochondria have also been observed in the perinuclear zones of fibers in hypokalemic myopathy, in progressive muscular dystrophy, and in the sarcoplasmic masses of myotonic dystrophy.

It is doubtful that these various myopathies represent a primary defect in mitochondria. It seems more likely that some of them, now grouped with the "mitochondrial" myopathies, will assume a separate status once their basic chemical defects are discovered. A case in point is the identification by A. G. Engel et al. of carnitine deficiency as a cause of lipid storage myopathy. Carnitine deficiency myopathy is discussed in Chap. 48, with other lipid myopathies.

Congenital Myopathy with Fiber-Type Disproportion Brooke first called attention to a congenital polymyopathy with a disparity in size of type I and type II fibers, and since that time there have been several other reports. The infants are weak and floppy, and the condition appears to progress in some cases and improve in others. Histochemical stains (ATPase) reveal a smallness and increased number of type I fibers. Additional clinical features are: normal mental development, ophthalmoplegia, hip dislocations, and "contractures." Disproportion of type II fibers has also been reported, some with fatal outcome. In the report of Eisler and Wilson the onset of the weakness was in midchildhood, and there were no nonmuscular abnormalities. The smallness of type I fibers without evidence of degeneration suggests a trophic defect from one class of anterior horn cells.

Centronuclear Myopathy In this familial disease, hypotonia and weakness become manifest early in life, usually soon after birth. Rarely, in the mildest form of the disease, the diagnosis does not become evident until adult years. Essentially all the striated skeletal muscles are involved to some degree. Ptosis and ocular palsies are combined with weakness of facial, masticatory, lingual, pharyngeal, laryngeal, and cervical muscles in most of the patients. In the limbs, distal weakness keeps pace with proximal weakness. The muscles remain thin and areflexic throughout life. Motor development is necessarily retarded, though improvement with maturation can occur; later, however, motor functions that have been acquired may be lost as the disease slowly advances. Several patients have shown signs of cerebral damage, with seizures and an abnormal EEG, but this may not be part of the disease. Muscle enzyme levels in the serum have not been elevated. EMG shows myopathic potentials and fibrillations. The pattern of inheritance has not been constant. X-linked recessive, autosomal dominant, and autosomal recessive patterns have all been described.

The outstanding pathologic features of the disease are the smallness of muscles and of their constituent fibers, and central nucleation. Surrounding most of the centrally placed nuclei is a clear zone, in which there is a lack of organization of contractile elements. Because of central nucleation, the disease has incorrectly been referred to as *myotubular myopathy*, implying an arrest in development of muscle at the myotubular stage. Actually, the nature of the pathologic process is quite obscure. The small, centrally nucleated fibers do not really resemble typical myotubes. Also, there is evidence, from electron-microscopic studies, of degenerative changes in the central parts of the fibers (in the clear zones surrounding the nuclei), leading in all probability to fiber loss. Such changes argue against a purely developmental abnormality.

INFANTILE MUSCULAR ATROPHY (WERDNIG-HOFFMANN DISEASE)

Of an entirely different type, viz., nonmyopathic, is the infantile malady of progressive spinal muscular atrophy. Pathologic studies show the primary fault to be a progressive degeneration of motor neurons in the spinal cord and brainstem with consequent atrophy of muscle fibers. The disease falls into the category of motor system diseases (page 821) but differs in respect to its early age of onset and heredofamilial nature. It is being considered with the early-life myopathies only because it must always be included in differential diagnosis of the weak and limp ("floppy") infant.

History Werdnig, in 1891 and 1894, and Hoffmann, in 1893, and at the same time Thomsen and Bruce, reported instances of an hereditary progressive muscular atrophy of spinal origin. Soon thereafter, however, it became apparent that this disease was being confused with a nonprogressive form of weakness and hypotonia in childhood which Oppenheim was attempting to delineate under the name of *myatonia congenita* (later this name was changed to *amyotonia congenita;* see below).

Clinical Manifestations In its most frequent form, an infant, usually born normally, is noted from birth to be unnaturally weak and limp. Some mothers report that fetal movement had been less than expected or lacking altogether. The muscle weakness in these children is generalized from the beginning, and death comes early, usually within the first year. Other infants seem to develop normally for several months before the weakness becomes apparent. In these, the trunk, pelvic, and shoulder girdle muscles are at first disproportionately affected, while the fingers and hands, toes and feet, and cranial muscles retain their mobility. Hypotonia attends the

weakness, and since passive displacement of articulated parts is easier to judge than power of contraction at this age, it may be singled out as the dominant clinical characteristic. As a rule the tendon reflexes are unobtainable. Volume of muscle diminishes but is difficult to evaluate because of the coverings of adipose tissue. Fasciculations are seldom visible except in the tongue. Response to skin contact and pinch is undiminished, and sensory perceptions and emotional and social development measure up to age.

As the months pass, the weakness and hypotonia progress gradually and spread to all of the skeletal muscles except the ocular ones. Intercostal paralysis with severe collapse of the chest is the rule. Respiratory movements are paradoxical. The cry becomes feeble, and sucking and swallowing are less efficient. Such infants are unable to sit unless propped, and the head cannot be supported. They cannot roll over or support their weight when placed on their feet. The posture assumed by these infants is characteristic: arms abducted and flexed at the elbow, legs in the "frog position," with external rotation and abduction at hips and flexion at hips and knees. If the effects of gravity are removed all muscles continue to contract; i.e., there is paresis, not paralysis. Until late in the illness these children appear bright-eyed, alert, and responsive.

The disease runs a steadily downhill course. Infants in whom the disease only becomes apparent after several months of life run a less precipitous course than those affected in utero or at birth. Some of the former become able to sit and creep and even to walk with support, and may survive for several years and even into adolescence or early adult life (see below).

The heredity of the disease is consistent with an autosomal recessive pattern.

Laboratory data of confirmatory value are few. Muscle enzymes in the serum are normal. Electromyography reveals fibrillations and/or fasciculations, proving the denervative basis of the weakness. Motor unit potentials are diminished in number and some are larger than normal (giant or polyphasic potentials). Motor nerve conduction velocities fall in the low normal range. Muscle biopsy reveals a typical picture of group atrophy and many of the groups of normal fibers are hypertrophied.

Pathologic Findings Aside from the aforementioned multiple, successive motor unit atrophy of muscle, which is universal except in ocular muscles, the essential abnormalities are in the anterior horn cells in the spinal cord and the motor nuclei in the lower brainstem. Nerve cells are greatly reduced in number, and many of the remaining ones are in varying stages of degeneration; a few are chromatolytic and contain cytoplasmic inclusions. Occasionally neuronophagia has been observed. There is replacement gliosis and secondary degeneration in roots and nerves. Other systems of neurons, including the corticospinal and corticobulbar, remain intact.

Differential Diagnosis Some of the problems in clinical diagnosis relate to the variants of the typical syndrome. As indicated above, many babies with the disease never enjoy a period of normal motor development, being slack and feeble from birth or even before; and this proves to be the most malignant form of the disease. Others manifest their first symptoms later in life, and then the disease pursues a milder course. Byers and Banker noted in these latter patients that the tendon reflexes might be elicited, a rarity in other forms. In the mildest variant, the advance is so slow that the patient may survive to adolescence or even adulthood, severely disabled with muscular atrophy, contractures of the limbs, and spinal deformity. Cranial musculature is spared, however, except for mild atrophy and fasciculation of the tongue. Such cases bridge the gap between the common forms of Werdnig-Hoffmann disease and the hereditary forms of spinal muscular atrophy, most of which begin in adolescence (Wohlfart et al., Kugelberg and Welander).

The major problem in diagnosis is to distinguish Werdnig-Hoffmann disease from an array of other diseases that cause hypotonia and delayed motor development in the neonate and infant. The congenital polymyopathies, as described in the preceding section, frequently present in this way. The preservation of tendon reflexes and relative lack of progression of muscle weakness distinguish these latter disorders. Of course, the muscle biopsy, if studied properly, yields the correct diagnosis.

Certain forms of muscular dystrophy, notably myotonic dystrophy, may become manifest in the neonatal period and interfere with sucking and motor development. As a rule, the weakness is not as severe or diffuse as that in Werdnig-Hoffmann disease. Also, a number of polyneuropathies may cause a serious degree of weakness in early childhood. Unfortunately, in respect to the latter, adequate sensory testing is not possible at this age, but the CSF protein is often elevated; diagnosis is greatly facilitated by measurement of nerve conduction velocities (which are reduced) and nerve-muscle biopsy.

Mental retardation with a flaccid rather than spastic weakness of the limbs is another major category of disease that must be distinguished. This may be difficult. Reliance must be placed on tests of sensory perception and psychosocial development, which are invariably delayed. Also, certain of the leukodystrophies may weaken muscles and abolish tendon reflexes, but usually there is evidence of cerebral involvement. The same may be said of mongolism, cretinism, achondrodysplasia, and certain forms of lipid and glycogen storage diseases. Finally, very sick children with celiac disease, cystic fibrosis, and other chronic diseases may be hypotonic, to the point of simulating neuromuscular disease. Usually the tendon reflexes are not abolished in these purely medical states, and strength returns as the medical problem is corrected.

There remains, after the assiduous study of the "floppy infant," a group of cases of hypotonia and motor underdevelopment that are presently unclassifiable. The term *amyotonia congenita* (Oppenheim), once applied to all this group, is obsolete. Oppenheim provided no information about the clinical course of his patients and no pathologic data, so that the nature of the cases he described can never be settled with finality. Walton has devised the term *benign congenital hypotonia* to designate patients who manifest limp and flabby limbs in infancy and delay in sitting up and walking and who improve gradually, some completely and others incompletely. Some of the cases of fiber-type disproportion and centronuclear myopathy fall into this category (see above). This hardly constitutes a homogeneous category of disease. The nature of the cases with complete recovery is quite obscure. One would suspect that among this group there are examples of congenital myopathy that await differentiation by application of modern histochemical and ultrastructural techniques. Neither amyotonia congenita nor benign congenital hypotonia is a categorization that serves the purpose of precise diagnosis, and should be retained only until other parameters of the pathologic process are discovered.

REFERENCES

ADAMS RD: *Diseases of Muscle: A Study in Pathology*, 3d ed. New York, Harper & Row, 1975.

BANKER BQ, VICTOR M, ADAMS RD: Arthrogryposis multiplex due to congenital muscular dystrophy. *Brain* 80:319, 1957.

BETHLEM J, ARTS WF, DINGEMANS KP: Common origin of rods, cores, miniature cores, and focal loss of cross striations. *Arch Neurol* 35:555, 1978.

BING R: Ueber angeborene Muskeldefecte. *Virchows Arch [Pathol Anat]* 170:175, 1902.

BROOKE MH: Congenital fiber type disproportion, in Kakulas BA (ed): *Clinical Studies in Myology*. New York, American Elsevier, 1973.

BYERS RK, BANKER BQ: Infantile muscular atrophy. *Arch Neurol* 5:140, 1961.

DeREUCK J, ADAMS RD: The Metrics of Muscle, in Kakulas BA (ed): *Basic Research in Myology,* International Congress Series. Excerpta Medica Foundation, 1973, pp 1-11.

EISLER T, WILSON JH: Muscle fiber type disproportion. *Arch Neurol* 35:823, 1978.

ENGEL AG, ANGELINI C, NELSON RA: Identification of carnitine deficiency as a cause of human lipid storage myopathy, in Milhorat AT (ed): *Exploratory Concepts in Muscular Dystrophy,* vol 2. Amsterdam, Excerpta Medica, 1974, pp 601-618.

ENGEL WK, REZNICK JS: Late onset rod-myopathy: A newly recognized, acquired, and progressive disease. *Neurology* 16:308, 1966.

HENDERSON JL: The congenital facial diplegia syndrome; clinical features, pathology and aetiology. *Brain* 62:381, 1939.

KUGELBERG E, WELANDER L: Heredofamilial juvenile muscular atrophy simulating muscular dystrophy. *Arch Neurol Psychiatry* 5:500, 1956.

LeDOUBLE AF: *Traité des variations du système musculaire de l'homme.* Paris, Schliger Frères Editeurs, 1897.

LICHTENSTEIN BW: Congenital absence of the abdominal musculature: Associated changes in the genitourinary tract and the spinal cord. *Am J Dis Child* 58:339, 1939.

OPPENHEIM H: Ueber allgemeine und localisierte Atonie der Muskulatur (Myatonie) in frühen Kindesalter. *Monatsschr Psychiatr Neurol* 8:232, 1900.

PATTERSON VH et al: Central core disease: Clinical and pathological progression within a family. *Brain* 102:581, 1979.

ROBERTSON WC, KAWAMURA Y, DYCK PJ: Morphometric study of motoneurons in congenital nemaline myopathy and Werdnig-Hoffmann disease. *Neurology* 28:1057, 1978.

SHY GM, GONATOS NK, PEREZ M: Two childhood myopathies with abnormal mitochondria. *Brain* 89:133, 1966.

———, MAGEE KR: A new congenital non-progressive myopathy. *Brain* 79:610, 1956.

TOMLINSON BF, WALTON JN, REBEIZ JJ: The effects of aging and cachexia upon skeletal muscle: a histopathologic study. *J Neurol Sci* 8:201, 1969.

WALTON JN: The limp child. *J Neurol Neurosurg Psychiatry* 20:144, 1957.

WOHLFART G, FEX J, ELIASSON S: Hereditary proximal spinal muscular atrophy. A clinical entity simulating progressive muscular dystrophy. *Acta Psychiatry Scand* 30:395, 1955.

CHAPTER 51

MYASTHENIA GRAVIS AND EPISODIC FORMS OF MUSCULAR WEAKNESS

The connecting thread between the various types of muscle disease included in this chapter is the fluctuant or episodic nature of the weakness. Its variability, strictly interpreted, implies important physiological rather than structural changes, located at the neuromuscular junction or in the transmitting mechanism of the sarcolemma, transverse tubules, and endoplasmic reticulum (see Chap. 44). In *myasthenia gravis* and in the *myasthenic syndromes* that occur with lupus erythematosus, rheumatoid arthritis, etc., there is usually some degree of weakness at all times, but it is made worse by activity. In the *periodic paralyses*, weakness occurs only in discrete attacks, associated with a derangement of potassium metabolism. These two categories of muscle disease form the subject matter of this chapter.

MYASTHENIA GRAVIS

This proves to be a group of maladies which exhibit several striking clinical features, the most important of which is a *fluctuant weakness* of certain voluntary muscles, particularly those innervated by motor nuclei of the brainstem, i.e., ocular, masticatory, facial, deglutitional, and lingual. Manifest weakening during continued activity, quick restoration of power with rest, and dramatic improvement in strength following administration of anticholinesterase drugs such as neostigmine, are other notable features.

HISTORY

Several students of medical history affirm that Thomas Willis, in 1685, gave an account of a disease that could be none other than myasthenia gravis. Others give credit to Wilks (1877) for the first description, and for having

noted that the medulla was free of disease, in distinction to other types of bulbar paralysis. The first reasonably complete accounts were those of Erb (1878), who classed the disease as a bulbar palsy without anatomical lesion, and of Goldflam (1893). For many years thereafter the disorder was referred to as the Erb-Goldflam syndrome. Jolly (1895) was the first to use the name myasthenia gravis, to which he added the term *pseudoparalytica*, to indicate the lack of structural changes at autopsy. Also it was Jolly who originally demonstrated that myasthenic weakness of muscle could be reproduced by faradic stimulation of its motor nerve and that the "fatigued" muscle would then respond to galvanic stimulation. Interestingly, he suggested the use of physostigmine as a form of treatment, but there the matter rested until Remen, in 1932, and Walker, in 1934, demonstrated the therapeutic value of the drug.

Campbell and Bramwell (1900) and Oppenheim (1901) each analyzed over 60 cases and crystallized the medical conception of the disease. The relationship between myasthenia gravis and the thymus gland was first noted by Laquer and Weigert in 1901, and in 1949 Castleman and Norris described in detail the pathologic changes in the gland.

In 1905 Buzzard published a detailed clinico-pathologic analysis of the disease, commenting on the relation to thymic abnormalities and the infiltrations of lymphocytes (lymphorrhages) in muscle. He postulated the action of an autotoxic agent causing the paralysis of muscle, the lymphorrhages, and the thymic lesions. He also commented on the close relation of myasthenia gravis to Graves disease and Addison's disease, which are also now considered to have an autoimmune basis. In 1960, Simpson and Nastuk et al. theorized that an autoimmune mechanism must be operative in myasthenia gravis. Finally in 1973 and thereafter Patrick, Lindstrom, Lennon, Lambert, and A. G. Engel created an experimental form of myasthenia gravis and showed that the mechanism of the block in neuromuscular transmission is due to antibodies to receptor substance at the end plate.

These and other references to the early historical features of the disease are to be found in the reviews by Viets and by Adams; A. G. Engel's chapter in the *Handbook of Clinical Neurology* is an excellent modern reference.

CLINICAL MANIFESTATIONS

Myasthenia gravis, as the name implies, is a muscular weakness having a grave prognosis. Repeated or persistent activity of a muscle group exhausts its contractile power, leading to a progressive paresis, and rest restores strength, at least partially. The demonstration of these two attributes, assuming the patient cooperates fully, is enough to establish the diagnosis.

The onset is usually insidious, but there are instances of fairly rapid development, sometimes initiated by an emotional upset or infection (usually respiratory). Symptoms may first appear during pregnancy or the puerperium, or in response to drugs used during anesthesia. Once started, a slow progression follows. Usually the muscles of the eyes, and somewhat less often of the face, jaws, throat, and neck, are the first to be affected and only in exceptional cases is the initial complaint referable to the limbs. However, as the disease advances, it may spread to other muscles.

The special vulnerability of certain muscles to myasthenia accounts for the mode of clinical presentation. In more than 90 percent of cases the levator palpebrae or extraocular muscles are involved. Ocular palsies and ptosis are usually accompanied by weakness of eye closure (orbicularis oculi), a combination observed regularly only in this disease and muscular dystrophy, viz., in purely myopathic states. The muscles of facial expression, mastication, swallowing, and speech are next most frequently affected. The flexors and extensors of the neck, the muscles of the shoulder girdle, and flexors of the hips are less often involved. Of the trunk muscles the erector spinae are the most frequently affected. Nevertheless, in the most advanced cases, all muscles are weakened, including the diaphragm, abdominal, and intercostal muscles, and even the external sphincters of the bladder and bowel. The incidence of involvement of any group of muscles closely parallels the likelihood of their being initially affected by the disease. Clinically, myasthenia gravis is most accurately conceived as a fluctuating oculofaciobulbar palsy. In cases with affection of the trunk and limbs, the clinical rule, that in myopathy the proximal muscles are more vulnerable than distal ones, holds firm.

To rephrase the topographic attributes of the illness in terms of symptoms, drooping of the eyelids and intermittent diplopia are the most common complaints. Facial mobility and expression are altered. The natural smile becomes transformed into a snarl. The jaw may hang so that it must be propped up by the patient's hand. Chewing tough food may be difficult, and the meal may have to be terminated because of inability to masticate and to swallow. It may be more difficult to eat after talking, and the voice fades and becomes nasal after a long conversation. Women may complain of inability to fix their hair because of fatigue of the shoulders, or of difficulty in applying lipstick because of inability to purse and roll the lips.

A peculiarity of myasthenic muscle contraction is a sudden lapse of sustained posture, or interruption of movement by a kind of irregular tremor, similar to that of normal muscle nearing the point of exhaustion. A dynamometer or ergogram demonstrates the rapidly waning power of contraction and repetitive stimulation of a motor nerve at slow rates, while recording muscle action potentials, reflects the same disorder in a more quantitative fashion (see page 883; also, Fig. 44-9).

Weakened muscles in myasthenia gravis undergo atrophy in only a limited number of cases (about 10 percent of females and 20 percent of males); the atrophy is rarely marked in degree. Tendon reflexes are seldom altered. Even repeated tapping of a tendon does not tax muscles to the point where contraction fails. Smooth and cardiac muscles are not involved. Normal pupillary responses to light and accommodation in the face of weakness of extraocular muscles and orbicularis oculi are virtually diagnostic of myasthenia gravis, especially if strength is restored after a period of rest.

Other nervous functions are preserved. The weakened muscles, especially those of the eyes and back of the neck, may ache, but pain is seldom an important complaint. Paresthesias of the face, hands, and thighs are sometimes reported but are not accompanied by demonstrable sensory loss. Anosmia and ageusia have been mentioned as rare findings, but whether or not they are coincidental has not been decided. The tongue may display one central and two lateral longitudinal furrows (trident tongue), as was pointed out by Buzzard.

Some statistical features of the disease are of clinical significance. Its prevalance is variously estimated to be from 1 in 10,000 to 1 in 50,000 of the population. The disease may begin at any age, but onset in the first decade or after the age of 70 is rare; the peak age of onset is between 20 and 30 years. Under the age of 40, females are affected two to three times as often as males, whereas in later life, the incidence in males and females is about equal. Of patients with thymomas, the majority are older (50 to 60 years), and males are more numerous.

The course of the illness is extremely variable. Rapid spread from one muscle group to another occurs in some, but in others the disease remains unchanged for months before progressing. Remissions may take place without explanation, but these happen in less than half the cases and are seldom longer than a month or two. If the disease remits for a year or longer and then recurs, it tends to be progressive. In Simpson's opinion, and this coincides with our observations, the danger of death from myasthenia gravis is greatest in the first year after the onset of the disease. A second period of danger in progressive cases is from 4 to 7 years after onset. After this time the disease tends to stabilize, and the risk of severe relapse diminishes. Fatalities then relate mainly to respiratory complications (infection, aspiration). Restricted ocular myasthenia, observed mainly in adult men, also carries a good prognosis.

Thymic tumors occur in some 10 percent of patients, predominantly in older males. This brings up an interesting suggestion—that the myasthenic process in older men differs in several ways from that in young females: (1) older males with thymomas react somewhat differently to anticholinesterase drugs than young females without thymomas; (2) weakness in young women tends to be more generalized than in older men, in whom the weakness tends to be restricted to ocular, pharyngeal, and respiratory muscles; (3) there are differences in HLA phenotype (early onset in females has a strong association with HLA-B8 and -D/DR3). Another difference that may be significant is the finding of a higher incidence of antibody to receptor substance in the older male patients.

A biologic trait of interest is the coincidence of myasthenia gravis and thyrotoxicosis in about 5 percent of patients. Also, rheumatoid arthritis, lupus erythematosus, and polymyositis are associated more often than could be explained by chance. These diseases, believed to be of autoimmune nature, could conceivably be indicative, along with myasthenia gravis, of a genetically determined defect in immune responsivity.

Familial occurrence is known but rare and usually proves to be a nonimmunologic form of myasthenia (see below). We have seen the disease in father and daughter. There are several reports of myasthenia in only one of identical twins, so that direct inheritance is probably not a factor in the autoimmune form. About 10 to 15 per-

cent of babies born to myasthenic mothers show signs of myasthenia. This is a transitory phenomenon, lasting 1 to 12 weeks, and recovery is complete, without later relapse. Obviously, this *neonatal myasthenia* is due to some factor transmitted from the mother; antireceptor antibodies which have passed through the placenta are found in affected newborns.

PATHOLOGY

Reference has already been made to the involvement of the thymus gland in myasthenia gravis. True neoplasms of the gland are found in about 10 percent of patients (see below), and fully 80 percent of the remaining patients show a striking degree of follicular hyperplasia. The cells in the centers of the follicles are histiocytes and they are surrounded by a cuff of densely packed lymphocytes. The germinal centers are exactly like those observed in any lymph node. The changes in the thymus gland resemble the reaction in the thyroid in Hashimoto's thyroiditis. Since the latter has been reproduced in animals by injecting extracts of thyroid with Freund's adjuvants, it is probable that the so-called thymitis of myasthenia gravis is of similar nature.

Thymic tumors are localized growths, despite the potential malignancy of their cell type. Two forms have been described though it is unclear to the authors how separable they are. One is composed of reticular (histiocytic) cells like those in the center of the follicles; the other is predominantly lymphocytic and specified as lymphosarcomatous. Overlapping of the two types is common in our material. Thymic tumors may be unattended by myasthenia, though in all of our cases myasthenia has eventually developed, sometimes 15 to 20 years after the tumor was first recognized. The relation of thymitis to thymoma is not understood, but one may speculate that the latter is a thymitis in which the removal of some restraining influence has permitted neoplastic transformation of local type, such as may happen in ataxia telangiectasia.

As regards the nervous system, all current studies confirm Erb's original contention that it is a disease without anatomic lesion. The brain and spinal cord are normal unless damaged by hypoxia and hypotension from cardiorespiratory failure. The muscle fibers, except for slight reduction in volume (disuse effect?), are generally intact. In fatal cases with extensive paralysis, isolated fibers of esophagus, diaphragm, and eye muscles may be seen to have undergone segmental necrosis with variable regeneration (Russell). Scattered aggregates of lymphocytes (lymphorrhages) are also observed, as originally noted by Buzzard, but none of these changes in muscle explain the widespread and severe weakness.

A morphologic abnormality of the neuromuscular junction, studied by vital staining with methylene blue, was first reported by Cöers and Woolf. Two types of alteration were described, one in which the end plates are elongated and side branches are lacking, the other in which the end plates are enlarged and associated with profuse ramification of the terminal nerve fibers. The relationship of these changes to the block in neuromuscular transmission was not entirely clear, however, and it seems logical to assume that the subterminal branching

Figure 51-1

End plate from a patient with myasthenia gravis. The terminal axon contains abundant presynaptic vesicles, but the postsynaptic folds are wide, and there are few secondary folds. The loose junctional sarcoplasm is filled with microtubules and ribosomes. The synaptic cleft (asterisk) is widened. The line indicates 1 μm. (From Santa et al.)

of nerve fibers represents a purely secondary (reactive) type of collateral regeneration.

Of major importance was the demonstration by A. G. Engel and his associates of a reduction in area of the nerve terminal, a simplification of the postsynaptic region (sparse, shallow, abnormally wide or absent secondary synaptic clefts), and a widening of the primary synaptic cleft (Fig. 51-1; compare with Fig. 44-2). The observation of regenerating axons near the junction, the many simplified junctions, and the absence of nerve terminals supplying some postsynaptic regions, suggested to these authors that there was an active process of degeneration and repair of the neuromuscular junction in myasthenia gravis. Following these observations, Fambrough and his associates, by means of radioactive α-bungarotoxin binding, demonstrated a decrease in the number of acetylcholine (ACh) receptor sites on the postsynaptic part of the neuromuscular junction.

ETIOLOGY

The establishment of an immunologic mechanism, operative at the neuromuscular junction, is certainly one of the most significant developments in the field of myol-

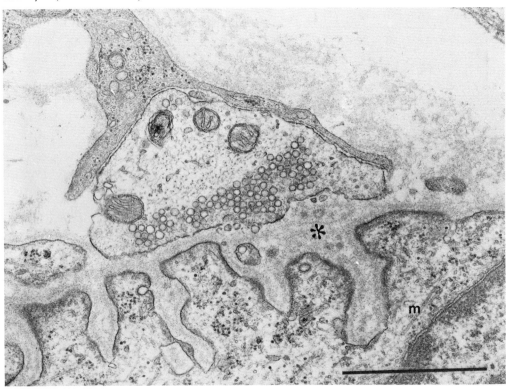

ogy in the last decade. Almost accidentally it was discovered by Patrick and Lindstrom that repeated immunization of rabbits with acetylcholine (ACh) receptor protein, purified from the electric organ of the eel, caused a muscular weakness, which Lennon recognized as being similar to myasthenia gravis. In collaboration with Lambert and A. G. Engel it was also demonstrated that the experimentally induced myasthenia had clinical, pharmacologic, and electrophysiologic properties identical with those of human myasthenia gravis [decreased miniature end-plate potentials (MEPPs) and decremental response on neuromuscular stimulation at 3 Hz] and that labeled antibodies were attached to the receptor site in proportion to the degree of decrease of the MEPPs. It was also shown that humoral antibodies to receptor protein could transfer the myasthenic weakness to normal animals and that the weakness, as well as the physiologic abnormalities, could be reversed by the administration of anticholinesterase drugs. Antibodies to ACh receptor protein were then found to be present in 90 percent of patients with myasthenia gravis, and also in infants with neonatal myasthenia gravis and in animal species known to have a naturally occurring myasthenia. The presence of receptor antibodies in human patients proves to be a sensitive and reliable test of the disease.

How the antibodies act at the receptor surface of the end plate has also been investigated, and the matter is not entirely settled. The nicotinic ACh receptors are located on the crests of the folds in the sarcolemma beneath the nerve fiber terminals, in a density of approximately 30,000 per square micrometer, and are also present in mammalian thymus gland. The receptor substance is a highly specialized glycoprotein, spanning the lipid layer of the postsynaptic membrane, with a molecular weight of 300,000 daltons. Each receptor molecule has multiple binding sites for ACh. Attachment of the latter to the receptor molecule opens an ionic channel in the receptor membrane for the influx of Na and the efflux of K. The neurotoxin α-bungarotoxin, a small polypeptide, has a high affinity for the binding site, and like the receptor antibodies, it blocks the attachment of ACh or destroys in some manner the receptor membrane; C3 complement is also involved in the immunologic blockade. Hypotheses concerning the way in which ACh receptor antibodies might inhibit ACh binding are reviewed by Lennon.

However, the level of receptor antibodies in the bloodstream does not correlate with the severity of the myasthenia, which Lennon explains as a matter of heterogeneity of antigen specificities to ACh receptors. What about the 10 percent of patients who have no antibodies? It is of interest that Lambert and A. G. Engel

and their associates have found two new types of myasthenia which are responsive to anticholinesterase drugs but which have a different mechanism from myasthenia gravis. Such cases may be congenital and of lifelong duration and have a tendency to be familial. There are no receptor antibodies on the postsynaptic membrane. In one of the diseases reported by Engel et al. there is a depletion of ACh at the end plate and a denotative repetitive action potential when the muscle is stimulated. In the other the receptor membrane appears to be abnormal. These new diseases are nonimmunologic forms of myasthenia and fall more in the category of the Eaton-Lambert syndrome.

Thus the evidence that an autoimmune mechanism is responsible for the functional disorder of muscle in most cases of myasthenia gravis appears to be incontrovertible. What is not known is what stimulates the production of these antibodies and where they are formed. Lennon offers an attractive hypothesis. She proposes that the site of the disease is in the thymus, where there are known to be myogenic cells. A virus with a tropism for thymic cells that have ACh nicotine receptors might injure such cells and induce antibody formation. It might at the same time have a potential for oncogenesis, accounting for the 10 percent of myasthenic patients with thymic tumors. The loss of immune tolerance, basic to all autoimmune diseases, is not understood. This failure is postulated to be related to the activity of either suppressor lymphocytes or circulating blocking agents.

DIAGNOSIS

In patients who present with the typical myasthenic facies—unequally drooping eyelids, relatively immobile mouth with down-turned corners, a smile that looks more like a snarl, a hanging jaw supported by the hand—the diagnosis can hardly be overlooked. However, only a minority of patients present in this stage of the disease, and seldom is there a clear recognition—even by the patient—that the muscles tire during activity. Ptosis, diplopia, difficulty in speaking or swallowing, or weakness of limbs are at first mild and inconstant. The finding that sustained activity of small cranial muscles results in weakness (e.g., increasing droop of eyelids while looking at the ceiling for 2 to 3 min) and that contraction improves after a brief rest is virtually diagnostic, however, even in the early stages of the disease. Any other affected group of muscles may be critically tested in similar fashion. If the diagnosis remains in doubt, the EMG and certain pharmacologic tests may be useful.

The rapid reduction in the amplitude of compound muscle action potentials evoked during repetitive stimulation of a peripheral nerve at a rate of 3 per second (*decrementing response*) and reversal of this response by neostigmine or edrophonium, has been a reliable confirmatory finding, and it can be obtained from facial, hand, or proximal limb muscles, which may or may not be clinically weak. Single-fiber electromyography represents an even more sensitive method of detecting the defect in neuromuscular transmission by demonstrating increased variability of the interpotential interval ("jitter") or blocking of successive discharges from single muscle fibers belonging to the same motor unit. During a progressive phase of the disease or during steroid therapy, a *slight incrementing* response may be obtained (Mayer and Williams), not to be confused with the marked incrementing response that characterizes the Eaton-Lambert syndrome (see below). Also characteristic of myasthenic syndrome is the postactivation potentiation of single evoked action potentials, followed by exhaustion (see page 992). Since the eye muscles exert a pull on the globe, which is reflected in intraocular tension, the increase of the latter in response to edrophonium can also be measured. Nerve conduction velocities and terminal latencies are usually normal.

Equally valuable at this point are the edrophonium (Tensilon) test, the neostigmine test, and rarely the curare sensitivity test. These are performed in the following fashion:

Edrophonium (Tensilon) Test After the strength of certain of the cranial muscles has been estimated, 10 mg (1 ml) of the drug is injected intravenously. Initially 2 mg (0.2 ml) is injected, and if this dose is tolerated, the other 8 mg (0.8 ml) is injected after 30 s. The clinical effect is obtained in 30 to 60 s and lasts 4 to 5 min. A positive test consists of visible (objective) improvement in muscle contractility and the report of subjective improvement by the patient. The latter alone is not dependable. There is a danger (rare) of ventricular fibrillation and cardiac arrest.

This test is also of aid in determining whether or not increasing weakness is due to a *cholinergic crisis* (overdose of neostigmine). In this latter condition, there

is no improvement with Tensilon; instead, weakness may actually increase, and there may be fasciculations about the eyes and face. The test is best done about 2 h after the last dose of neostigmine or pyridostigmine. The effect of the Tensilon is gauged by observation of the respiratory and bulbar muscles, since weakness in these muscles may increase while there is no change in the ocular muscles.

Neostigmine Test Neostigmine methylsulfate is injected intramuscularly in a dose of 1.5 mg. Atropine sulfate (0.6 mg) should be available to counteract muscarinic effects (nausea, vomiting, sweating, salivation). The drug may be given intravenously in a dose of 0.5 mg but then should always be preceded by atropine sulfate to obviate the danger of ventricular fibrillation and cardiac arrest. Objective and subjective improvement occurs in 10 to 15 min and reaches its peak at 30 min, lasting 2 or 3 h. Oral prostigmine may also be given as a test dose. The effect is still slower in onset and lasts more than 2 to 3 h.

A negative test does not exclude myasthenia gravis but is a strong point against the diagnosis. A trial of oral prostigmine, 15 mg every 4 h during the day, is sometimes recommended in doubtful cases, but we have been misled more often than helped by it.

Curare Test Only when diagnosis is uncertain after the edrophonium and prostigmine tests should this be considered, and then only in a hospital where respiratory assistance can be given. The curarizing dose in normal persons is 3 mg of *d*-tubocurarine per 18 kg (40 lb). Only 2 percent of this dose is given intravenously to the patient suspected of having myasthenia; if there is no respiratory difficulty in 5 min, then 5 percent of the dose is injected. A definite increase in weakness at this low dosage indicates either myasthenia gravis or the Eaton-Lambert syndrome.

Measurement of Receptor Antibodies in Blood This test is sensitive and useful, but only a few laboratories are prepared to do it. Also, it is awkward and time-consuming to send the serum to one of the centers where the test is being done.

DIFFERENTIAL DIAGNOSIS

We have sometimes been puzzled by the following clinical problems:

1. *The concurrence of myasthenia gravis and thyrotoxicosis.* As indicated on page 972, thyrotoxicosis

may produce its own type of myopathy. There is no certain evidence that thyrotoxicosis aggravates myasthenia gravis, and some have even observed a see-saw relationship which we have not confirmed. The diagnosis of myasthenia must rest on objective clinical findings and be confirmed by the laboratory tests already described. The ophthalmoplegia of thyrotoxicosis can usually be distinguished by the presence of an associated exophthalmos (early in the disease exophthalmos may be absent) and the lack of response to neostigmine. Lupus erythematosus and polymyositis are diagnosed by finding the signs of these diseases in combination with those of myasthenia (see Chap. 48).

2. *The neurasthenic patient who complains of weakness when actually referring to fatigability.* There is no ptosis, strabismus, or dysphagia, though a neurotic individual may complain of diplopia (usually of momentary duration, when drowsy) and also of tightness in the throat (globus hystericus). A number of such patients claim improvement with neostigmine, but objective weakness and reversal thereof can never be ascertained. Conversely, myasthenia may be mistaken for hysteria or other emotional illness, mainly because the physician is unfamiliar with myasthenia (or with hysteria) and has been overly impressed with the precipitation of the illness by an emotional crisis.

3. *Progressive external ophthalmoplegia and other restricted myopathies* may be mistaken for myasthenia gravis. It should be emphasized that the ocular muscles may be permanently damaged by myasthenia and cease to respond to neostigmine. Another possibility is that restricted ocular myasthenia may not respond to anticholinesterase drugs from the beginning and the diagnosis of myasthenia is erroneously excluded. One must then turn to other muscles for clinical and electromyographic confirmation of the diagnosis.

4. *Illnesses with dysarthria and dysphagia, but without ptosis or obvious strabismus;* these may be mistaken for multiple sclerosis or some other neurologic disease.

5. Rarely, one encounters a typical syndrome of *myasthenic polymyopathy with hypersensitivity to neostigmine.* Here there is improvement on minute doses of neostigmine and worsening on the usual dose. The basis of this state has never been ascertained.

TREATMENT

The treatment of this disease involves the careful use of two groups of drugs, the anticholinesterases and corticosteroids, and/or thymectomy.

Anticholinesterase Drugs The two drugs that have given the best results in counteracting myasthenic weakness are neostigmine (prostigmine) and pyridostigmine (Mestinon). The oral dose of neostigmine ranges from 7.5 to 45.0 mg every 2 to 6 h. The dose of pyridostigmine is twice that of neostigmine. Delayed-action forms of both drugs are available. The average maintenance dose of neostigmine is approximately 150 mg (10 tablets) per day. The addition of potassium or ephedrine to fortify the anticholinesterase activity contributes little.

A *cholinergic crisis* is most likely to be encountered in patients receiving high doses of anticholinesterase drugs. The muscarinic effects of neostigmine (nausea, vomiting, pallor, sweating, salivation, colic, diarrhea, miosis, bradycardia), ones which occur in the normal person intoxicated with this drug, are coupled with increasing myasthenic weakness. An impending cholinergic effect is betrayed by constricting pupils; (they should not be allowed to contract to less than 2 mm). If the blood pressure falls, 0.6 mg atropine sulfate should be given slowly by the intravenous route. If the muscarinic effects are not present and weakness from overdose of neostigmine is suspected, the Tensilon test should be done (see above).

Corticosteroids The usual form is prednisone in a dose of 40 to 45 mg/day, preferably given in twice this dose every other day. Since worsening in the first week or 10 days is expected, hospitalization and careful observation for respiratory difficulty is advisable. Improvement occurs in the next few weeks, and, once obtained, the dosage of prednisone can be reduced slowly to the lowest point where it is still effective. Potassium supplements and antacids are prescribed liberally, as with any corticosteroid treatment regime. The anticholinesterase drugs are given simultaneously, and as the patient improves, their dosage may be adjusted downward.

Thymectomy Removal of the thymus gland is indicated in practically all cases of *thymoma.* An exception would be an elderly person enfeebled by age and other diseases; radiation of the tumor could then be substituted. The operative approach is through the anterior thorax, with adequate exposure to remove all tumor tissue. If the removal is incomplete, radiotherapy should be given.

Thymectomy is recommended in practically all patients with uncomplicated myasthenia gravis who, after a period of treatment with anticholinesterase drugs, are responding poorly. In patients with myasthenia restricted to the ocular muscles for a year or two, the prognosis is so good that operation is unnecessary. The remission rate is approximately 40 to 50 percent if the procedure is done in the first year or two after onset of the disease, and progressively lower if operation is postponed beyond this time. In favorably responding cases, levels of circulating receptor antibody are reduced or disappear entirely. A suprasternal approach has been developed and results in less postoperative pain and morbidity, but the transsternal approach is preferable because it assures a more complete removal of thymic tissue. As improvement occurs the dosage of neostigmine can be reduced.

For the moderately severe myasthenic, in whom a remission has not been induced by thymectomy and who is unresponsive to anticholinesterase drugs, a trial of corticosteroids is worthwhile and, if beneficial, may be continued for years. Some physicians use corticosteroids from the beginning, in preference to anticholinesterase drugs. Of course one would hesitate to undertake such a program in children because of the complications of long-term hyperadrenocorticism, and in neonatal myasthenia only neostigmine is required.

Plasmapheresis and Immunosuppression   For the severe myasthenic who does not respond adequately to anticholinesterase drugs, thymectomy, or prednisone, one must resort to other measures. Striking temporary remissions may be obtained by the use of plasmapheresis and this may be lifesaving. Antilymphocyte serum has reportedly been helpful in some cases. Immune suppression with azothiaprine has been accompanied by clinical improvement and reduction in the levels of receptor antibodies (Reuther et al.). Eventually there may be a remission, hence the justification for using every possible measure to support the patient until this happens. Occasionally the administration of paralyzing doses of d-tubocurarine for several weeks, while sustaining respiration mechanically, restores the patient's sensitivity to neostigmine.

THE MYASTHENIC-MYOPATHIC SYNDROME OF
EATON-LAMBERT

This special form of myasthenia, observed often with oat-cell carcinoma of the lung, was first described by Eaton and Lambert, in 1957. Unlike myasthenia gravis,

the muscles of the trunk and the pelvic and shoulder girdles are the ones that most frequently become weak, fatigable, and atrophic. Often the first symptoms are difficulty in arising from a chair, climbing stairs, and walking, and the shoulder muscles are affected later. While ptosis, diplopia, dysarthria, and dysphagia may occur, and may even be the presenting symptoms, this is less frequent. Increasing weakness after exertion stamps the condition as myasthenic, but as Eaton and Lambert originally pointed out, there may be a temporary increase in muscle power during the first few contractions. The tendon reflexes are often suppressed but if abolished should raise the question of an associated carcinomatous polyneuropathy. Fasciculation is not seen. Other complaints are aching pain (suggesting arthritis), dryness of the mouth, and paresthesias. There may be other neurologic manifestations of neoplasia (polyneuropathy, polymyositis or dermatomyositis, multifocal leukoencephalopathy, cerebellar degeneration).

The onset is usually subacute and the course variably progressive. The myasthenia may precede discovery of the tumor by months or years. In addition to lung tumors, this syndrome has been associated with carcinoma of the breast, prostate, stomach, and rectum. In about one-half of patients no tumor is found. In the tumor cases, death usually occurs in a few months to years from the effect of the tumor itself.

Also unlike myasthenia gravis, the response to neostigmine and pyridostigmine is variable. On the other hand, d-tubocurarine, suxamethonium chloride, gallamine, and other relaxing drugs have a deleterious effect and when given during anesthesia may dramatically increase the weakness and even result in fatality.

Electrodiagnostic studies have shown no abnormality in the peripheral nerves. A single stimulus of nerve may yield a low-amplitude muscle action potential (in contrast with myasthenia gravis, where it is normal or nearly so), whereas at fast rates of stimulation (50 per second) there is a marked increase in the amplitude of action potentials (incrementing response). Elmquist and Lambert, from a series of studies of excised muscle, deduced that there is a defect in the release of acetylcholine quanta from the nerve terminals akin to that which occurs in paralysis due to botulinus toxin (see page 784). In contrast to myasthenia gravis the extent of the receptor surface in the myasthenic syndrome is actually increased, and no receptor antibody is present. Some factor(s) elaborated by oat-cell carcinoma appears to interfere with ACh release, according to Lindstrom and Lambert.

Muscle biopsy has shown no specific pathologic changes.

Elicitation   of   the   Eaton-Lambert   syndrome

should lead to a search for occult tumor, especially of the lung. If none is found the search should be repeated at regular intervals. Guanidine hydrochloride, 125 to 250 mg three or more times a day, has been more effective than neostigmine or pyridostigmine in the few cases we have managed; but others report transient benefit from the anticholinesterase drugs.

The only illnesses that might be confused with this myasthenic syndrome are hysterical paralysis, where the patient may do better with encouragement on successive voluntary contractions, and arthritis, where pain hampers the first movements more than successive ones. Then the electrodiagnostic tests are of value.

MYASTHENIC WEAKNESS WITH ANTIBIOTICS AND OTHER DRUGS

Many drugs may cause a worsening of myasthenia gravis, and certain ones such as quinidine, propranolol, and lithium may occasionally unmask a previously unsuspected instance of the disease. However, in some individuals who have had no previous neuromuscular disorder, the administration of drugs may produce a myasthenic syndrome. Argov and Mastaglia list more than 30 drugs in current clinical use (other than anesthetic agents) that may interfere with neuromuscular transmission. Of these, the most important are the antibiotics. According to McQuillen et al. and Pittinger et al., who have reviewed this subject, myasthenic weakness has been reported with 18 different antibiotics but particularly with neomycin, kanamycin, cholistin, streptomycin, polymyxin B, and certain tetracyclines. It has been shown that these drugs impair transmitter release by interfering with calcium-ion fluxes at nerve terminals. Infusion of calcium improves neuromuscular transmission, and there is a slight increase in power with neostigmine. Guanidine chloride has no effect.

The administration of D-penicillamine has also caused a type of myasthenia. The weakness is typical in that rest improves strength as do prostigmine and Tensilon, and the electrophysiologic findings are also typical. In such cases, Vincent et al. found anti-ACh receptor antibodies in the serum; hence, one must assume that this is a form of autoimmune myasthenia gravis. In these respects it differs from the weakness caused by aminoglycosides.

EPISODIC (KALEMIC) PARALYSES

At least four hereditary syndromes of recurrent muscle weakness have now been identified:

1. Familial periodic paralysis (hypokalemic)

2. Hyperthyroidism with periodic paralysis

3. Adynamia episodica hereditaria of Gamstorp (normo- or hyperkalemic)

4. Congenital paramyotonia of von Eulenberg with periodic paralysis (hyperkalemic)

In addition, transitory episodes of weakness are known to be associated with other derangements of potassium metabolism, such as occur with aldosteronism and renal failure (hyperkalemia) and with excess diuretic and laxative medication (hypokalemia).

In each of the periodic paralyses, the patient may, over a few hours, develop a disorder of trunk and limb muscles which varies from a diffuse weakness to total paralysis, and the condition subsides after a few hours or days, leaving the musculature entirely normal. Clinical differences between these several syndromes are small, except in the von Eulenberg form, where evocation of the attacks by cold and a restricted myotonia are added features.

Periodic paralysis can be readily distinguished from cataplexy, which lasts only a few seconds or minutes, and is precipitated by emotion; from episodes of sleep paralysis, which also are very brief; and from syncope, where physical weakness is always combined with pallor and a disorder of consciousness. In textbooks, the differential diagnosis of episodic paralysis also includes "drop attacks" of the aged, myoclonic and akinetic epilepsy with falling attacks, and hydrocephalic attacks with limb weakness, but the resemblances to these states are remote.

FAMILIAL OR HYPOKALEMIC PERIODIC PARALYSIS (PAROXYSMAL MYOPLEGIA)

This is the best-known form of periodic paralysis. The history of the disease is difficult to trace. References to it can be found in writings of the early eighteenth century, but the first clear descriptions were given by Hartwig, in 1874, followed by Westphal (1885) and by Oppenheim (1891). Goldflam (in 1895) was the first to call attention to the remarkable vacuolization of the muscle fibers. In 1937, Aitken and his associates first described the occurrence of hypokalemia during attacks of paralysis and reversal of the paralysis by the administration of potassium, thus setting the stage for subsequent studies of the normo- and hyperkalemic forms of periodic paralysis. For English-speaking readers, Talbott's monograph serves as the best review of the subject and includes the historical references as well as all cases that had been reported prior to 1941; and the more recent articles of Grob et al., and McArdle, bring the subject up to date.

A strong heredofamilial incidence characterizes fully three-quarters of all cases, as the name implies. The usual pattern of inheritance is autosomal dominant. Recessive inheritance is also known to occur. One suspects that in the sporadic cases an intensive exploration of family records might have divulged affected antecedents. Males are more susceptible, in a ratio of 3:1, but a sex-linked hereditary pattern has not been proved. Association with other neurologic or psychiatric conditions, e.g., migraine, is in all probability coincidental. The disease has been observed in all parts of the world.

Clinical Manifestations   The onset of the disease is in late childhood or adolescence. In Talbott's review of 152 cases, there were 40 in which symptoms began before the tenth year of life and 92 before the sixteenth year. The typical attack comes on during sleep, after a day of unusually strenuous exercise; a meal rich in carbohydrates favors its development. Certain prodromata—a sense of well-being before retiring, or of weariness and fatigue—are reported but are difficult to evaluate. Excessive hunger or thirst, dry mouth, palpitation, sweating, diarrhea, and nervousness are also mentioned but do not necessarily precede an attack. Usually the patient awakens to discover a mild or severe weakness of the limbs. However, diurnal attacks also occur, especially after a nap following a large meal. The attack evolves over minutes to several hours, and at its peak may render the patient so helpless as to be unable to call for assistance. Once established, the weakness lasts a few hours, if mild, or several days, if severe.

The distribution of the paralysis varies. Limbs are affected earlier and often more severely than trunk muscles and proximal muscles are possibly more susceptible than distal ones. Legs are often weakened before the arms, but exceptionally the order is reversed. The muscles most likely to escape are those of the eyes, face, tongue, pharynx, larynx, diaphragm, and sphincters, but on occasion even these may be involved. At its peak, tendon reflexes are reduced or abolished and cutaneous reflexes may also disappear. Sensibility is preserved. As the attack subsides, strength generally returns first to the muscles that were last to be affected. Headache, exhaustion, diuresis, and occasionally diarrhea may follow the attack.

Attacks of paralysis tend to occur every few weeks and lessen in frequency with advancing age. Rarely, death may occur from respiratory paralysis or derangements of the conducting system of the heart.

Atypical forms include weakness of one limb or certain groups of muscles, bibrachial palsy (inability to lift arms or comb hair), and transient weakness during accustomed activities. Earlier descriptions of daily brief attacks, some associated with exposure to cold or coupled with muscular hypertrophy or exophthalmic goiter, preceded recognition of the other types of periodic paralysis and cannot be evaluated. A number of patients have developed a slowly progressive proximal myopathy, with vacuolated and degenerated fibers and myopathic action potentials, during middle adult life, long after attacks of periodic paralysis have ceased.

Laboratory Findings   The attacks are accompanied by reduction in serum K levels, as low as 1.8 meq/liter, i.e., levels that would not be associated with paresis in normal subjects or in patients with the hyperthyroid form of the disease. The fall in serum K is not associated with an increase in urinary K excretion; presumably the K enters the muscle fibers. The serum K levels return to normal during recovery. It has been calculated that as much as 100 meq K may move from the extracellular fluid compartment into muscle during an attack. Grob et al. found the intramuscular K to increase after ingestion of carbohydrate, administration of glucose, and injection of insulin and possibly epinephrine. Although these shifts in K are of undoubted importance in the pathogenesis of muscle weakness, the marked sensitivity to small reductions of serum K and to cold suggest that other factors, as yet undefined, are also of importance.

The muscular paralysis is associated with a decrease and eventual loss of muscle action potentials evoked by supramaximal stimulation of peripheral nerve and of voluntary motor unit potentials, recorded by needle examination. Decline in strength precedes loss of motor unit potentials and of propagation of the latter from the neuromuscular junction over the surface of the fiber. The polarization potentials of muscle fibers measured by intracellular recordings are normal, yet the muscle fiber does not propagate the action potential. ECG changes also begin at levels slightly below normal (about 3 meq/liter); they consist of prolonged PR, QRS, and QT intervals and lowering of T waves.

Pathologic Changes   The nervous system is entirely normal. The muscle fibers are relatively large and of similar size. The most striking change is vacuolization of sarcoplasm. The myofibrils are separated by round or oval vacuoles containing clear fluid, presumably water, and a few PAS-positive granules. Isolated muscle fibers may undergo segmental degeneration. Electron-microscopic studies have shown that the vacuoles arise by progressive dilatation of the sarcoplasmic reticulum.

Treatment The daily administration of 5 to 10 g of KCl orally in aqueous solution prevents attacks in many patients, and apparently this program can be maintained indefinitely. When not successful, a low-carbohydrate, low-salt, high-K diet, combined with a slowly released K preparation, may be effective.

For an acute attack, 10 g of KCl should be given, or some other K salt if this is not tolerated. This dose may be insufficient, and if there is no improvement in 1 or 2 h, another 5 g may be required. Under exceptional conditions KCl may have to be given intravenously. Regular exercise (not too strenuous) to keep the patient fit is desirable.

THYROTOXICOSIS WITH PERIODIC PARALYSIS

This, too, is a form of hypokalemic periodic paralysis. It occurs mainly in young adult males, with a special predilection for those of Japanese and Chinese extraction. In Japan, Okinaka et al. found that 8.9 percent of males with thyrotoxicosis had periodic paralysis but only 0.4 percent of females, and for the Chinese, the corresponding figures were 13.0 and 0.17 percent (McFadzean and Yeung). The paralytic disorder is unrelated to the severity of the hyperthyroidism. In the naturally occurring variety of familial periodic paralysis, the induction of hyperthyroidism is said not to increase the frequency or intensity of attacks. Therefore it seems likely that the thyrotoxicosis has unmasked another type of hereditary periodic paralysis, although a familial occurrence in the thyrotoxic cases is exceptional. Clinically, the attacks of paralysis are much the same as those of familial hypokalemic type, except for a greater liability to cardiac irregularity KCl restores power in a paralytic attack, and treatment of the hyperthyroidism prevents their recurrence.

HYPERKALEMIC PERIODIC PARALYSIS (ADYNAMIA EPISODICA HEREDITARIA)

Soon after the recognition of hypokalemia in familial periodic paralysis and its treatment with K replacement, another type of periodic paralysis was found in which the serum K was elevated and an attack would actually be induced by the administration of potassium salts. Tyler et al. (1951) studied such a family and concluded that it was an entity distinct from the usual type of familial periodic paralysis. Five years later, Gamstorp reported two families and named the newly defined state *adynamia episodica hereditaria*. As further examples were reported, it was noted that in many of them there were minor degrees of myotonia, which brought the condition into relationship with paramyotonia congenita described in 1886 by von Eulenberg (see below). Drager et al. insist that the latter disease and that described by Tyler and Gamstorp are identical; Gamstorp does not agree. The dispute cannot be settled until the basic biochemical abnormality of each condition is elucidated.

Clinical Manifestations Onset is usually in infancy and childhood. Characteristically, the attacks of weakness occur when the patient is resting in a chair, about 20 to 30 min after exercise. The paresis begins in the legs, thighs, and lower back and spreads to the hands, forearms, and shoulders. Only in the severest attacks are the neck and ocular muscles involved. Attacks are usually brief, 30 to 60 min, or somewhat longer, and recovery is hastened by exercise. If the patient continues to be active, further attacks may be averted, but then, with rest, they tend to recur. In young, active children the attacks may occur every day; others have them less frequently. During late adolescence and adult years, when the patient becomes more sedentary, the attacks may diminish and cease. In certain muscle groups, particularly ocular, it is difficult to separate the effects of paresis from those of myotonia. Indeed when an attack of paresis is prevented by continuous movement, firm painful lumps may form in the calf muscles. Some patients with repeated attacks may be left with a permanent weakness and wasting of the proximal limb muscles.

PARAMYOTONIA CONGENITA OF VON EULENBERG

In this disease, similar attacks of periodic paralysis are associated with myotonia. The myotonia can be elicited even in a warm environment, but more characteristically, a widespread myotonia, often coupled with weakness, is induced by cold. The weakness may be diffuse, as in adynamia episodica hereditaria, or limited to the part of the body that is cooled. Once started the weakness persists for several hours, even after the body is rewarmed. Percussion myotonia can be evoked in the tongue and thenar eminence. Immersion of the arm and hand in ice water elicits both myotonia and weakness after a period of about 30 min.

Laboratory Findings In these latter two diseases (adynamia and paramyotonia), the serum K is usually above normal range, but paralysis has been observed at levels of 5 meq/liter or even lower. McArdle finds that each patient has a critical level of serum K that if exceeded will be associated with weakness. The administration of KCl, raising serum K to above 7 meq/liter, a level which has no effect on normal individuals, invariably induces an attack in the patient. There is evidence that during the attack intramuscular K falls and Na rises, and that between attacks they are normal. There may also be a hypocalcemia during attacks. The EMG of the weakened muscle shows a dropping out of some motor unit potentials and a reduced voltage and duration of others (as though some muscle fibers in each motor unit are no longer contracting). Other fibers show the typical hyperirritability and afterdischarge of myotonia. The polarization of the resting muscle fiber is reduced between attacks and even more so during the attack. There are no histologic changes in the fibers.

Treatment Many of the attacks are too brief and mild to require treatment. If severe, intravenous calcium gluconate (1 to 2 g) often restores power. If after a few minutes this treatment is unsuccessful, intravenous glucose or glucose and insulin and chlorothiazide should be tried.

The continuous use of diuretics such as chlorothiazide (about 0.5 g daily), keeping the serum K below 5 meq/liter, prevents attacks. Acetozolamide or some longer-acting carbonic anhydrase inhibitors have also proved effective. When the myotonia is more troublesome than weakness, procainamide, and sometimes phenytoin, are useful.

Some patients with paramyotonia, as with other forms of periodic paralysis, slowly develop a mild polymyopathy which causes persistent weakness.

NORMOKALEMIC PERIODIC PARALYSIS

In this condition, described by Poskanzer and Kerr in 1961, the attacks tend to be more severe and prolonged than in the hyperkalemic form, and there is no myotonia or sensitivity to cold. Urinary K does not increase during paralysis. The paralysis is induced and made worse by the administration of K salts. Like other forms of periodic paralysis, the inheritance follows an autosomal dominant pattern. Acetozolamide, 250 mg tid, and appropriate daily doses of 9α-fluorohydrocortisone, prevented attacks in the patients reported by Poskanzer and Kerr, but these measures were unsuccessful in the family reported by Meyers et al. Also, the affected members of

the latter family had shorter attacks that were not provoked by large doses of K.

HYPOKALEMIC WEAKNESS IN PRIMARY ALDOSTERONISM

Hypokalemic weakness due to hypersecretion of the major adrenal mineralocorticoid aldosterone was first described by Conn, in 1955. In *primary aldosteronism,* the cause of the hypersecretion is in the adrenal itself—usually an adrenal cortical adenoma, less often adrenal cortical hyperplasia. The disorder is not common (occurring in about 1 percent of unselected hypertensive patients), but its recognition is essential since it can be treated effectively. Persistent aldosteronism is frequently associated with hypernatremia, polyuria, and alkalosis, which predisposes the patient to attacks of tetany as well as to hypokalemic weakness. Conn et al. (1964), in an analysis of 103 patients with primary aldosteronism, found that persistent muscular weakness was a major complaint in 73 percent; intermittent attacks of paralysis occurred in 21 percent, and tetany in 21 percent. These manifestations were much more frequent in women than in men, in contrast to the preponderance of men among patients with hypokalemic periodic paralysis of familial type. Rarely, the typical syndrome of primary aldosteronism is produced by the chronic ingestion of licorice; this is due to its content of glycyrrhizic acid, a potent mineralocorticoid that causes sodium retention and potassium diuresis.

The muscle fibers of patients with primary aldosteronism show necrosis and vacuolation. Ultrastructurally, the necrotic areas are characterized by a dissolution of myofilaments with degenerative vacuoles; nonnecrotic fibers contain membrane-bound vacuoles and show dilatation of the sarcoplasmic reticulum and abnormalities of the T system, suggesting that a vulnerability of the latter structures may be responsible for the muscle fiber necrosis (Atsumi et al.).

DIFFERENTIAL DIAGNOSIS OF THE PERIODIC PARALYSES

The nocturnal occurrence of severe and prolonged attacks of periodic paralysis, with onset in early life, suggests the hypokalemic type. Infusions of carbohydrate after heavy exercise provokes attacks which can be verified by measurements of serum K and electrodiagnostic testing. Such patients should be checked for hyperthyroidism, but this latter form of periodic paralysis is rare in North America, except in adult Oriental males. In our experience, hyperkalemic patients have all had some degree of sensitivity to cold and restricted myotonia. Moreover their attacks are brief and more frequent in early childhood. In the normokalemic type, the attacks are both severe and prolonged. The paralytic disorders due to renal disease and aldosteronism are not familial, and the serum electrolyte disorders are severe in degree, in distinction to the familial hypokalemic types.

REFERENCES

ADAMS RD: *Diseases of Muscle: A Study in Pathology*, 3d ed. New York, Harper & Row, 1975, chap 12, pp 504–548.

AITKEN RS et al: Observations on a case of familial periodic paralysis. *Clin Sci* 3:47, 1937.

ALMON RR, ANDREW CG, APPEL SH: Serum globulin in myasthenia gravis: Inhibition of α-bungarotoxin binding in acetylcholine receptors. *Science* 186:55, 1974.

ARGOV Z, MASTAGLIA FL: Disorders of neuromuscular transmission caused by drugs. *N Engl J Med* 301:409, 1979.

ATSUMI T et al: Myopathy and primary aldosteronism: Electron microscopic study. *Neurology* 29:1348, 1979.

BUZZARD EF: The clinical history and postmortem examination of 5 cases of myasthenia gravis. *Brain* 28:438, 1905.

CÖERS C, WOOLF AL: *The Innervation of Muscle: A Biopsy Study*. Springfield, Ill, Charles C Thomas, 1959.

CONN JW: Primary aldosteronism: A new clinical syndrome. *J Lab Clin Med* 45:6, 1955.

———, KNOPF RF, NESBIT RM: Clinical characteristics of primary aldosteronism from an analysis of 145 cases. *Am J Surg* 107:159, 1964.

———, ROVNER DR, COHEN EL: Licorice-induced pseudoaldosteronism. Hypertension, hypokalemia, aldosteronopenia and suppressed plasma renin activity. *J Am Med Assoc* 205:492, 1968.

DRACHMAN DB et al: Myasthenic antibodies cross-link acetylcholine receptors to accelerate degradation. *N Engl J Med* 298:136, 186, 1978.

DRAGER GA, HAMMILL JF, SHY GM: Paramyotonia congenita. *Arch Neurol Psychiatry* 30:1, 1958.

EATON LM, LAMBERT EH: Electromyography and electric stimulation of nerves and diseases of motor unit: Observations on myasthenic syndrome associated with malignant tumors. *J Am Med Assoc* 163:1117, 1957.

ELMQUIST D, LAMBERT EH: Detailed analysis of neuromuscular transmission in a patient with the myasthenic syndrome, sometimes associated with bronchial carcinoma. *Mayo Clin Proc* 43:689, 1968.

ENGEL AG: Evolution and content of vacuoles in primary hypokalemic periodic paralysis. *Mayo Clin Proc* 45:774, 1970.

———: Myasthenia gravis, in Vinken PJ, Bruyn GW (eds): *Handbook of Clinical Neurology*, vol 41. Amsterdam, North-Holland, 1980, pp 95–145.

———, LAMBERT EH, SANTA T: Study of long-term anticholinesterase therapy. *Neurology* 23:1273, 1973.

———, TSUJIHATA M, LAMBERT EH, LINDSTROM JM, LENNON VA: Experimental autoimmune myasthenia gravis: A sequential and quantitative study of the neuromuscular junction ultrastructure and electrophysiologic correlations. *J Neuropathol Exp Neurol* 35:569, 1976.

———, ———, LINDSTROM JM, LENNON VA: The motor endplate in myasthenia gravis and in experimental autoimmune myasthenia gravis. *Ann NY Acad Sci* 274:60, 1976.

FAMBROUGH DM, DRACHMAN DB, SATYAMURTI S: Neuromuscular junction in myasthenia gravis: Decreased acetylcholine receptors. *Science* 182:293, 1973.

GAMSTORP 1: Adynamia periodica hereditaria. *Acta Paediatr Scand Suppl* 108:1, 1956.

GROB D, LILJESHAND A, JOHNS RJ: Potassium movement in patients with periodic paralysis. *Am J Med Sci* 23:356:1957.

LAMBERT EH, LINDSTROM JM, LENNON VA: End-plate potentials in experimental autoimmune myasthenia gravis in rats. *Ann NY Acad Med* 274:300, 1976.

LENNON VR: Humoral factors in myasthenia gravis. *Nature* 258:11, 1975.

———: Immunologic mechanisms in myasthenia gravis—a model of a receptor disease, in Franklin E (ed): *Clinical Immunology Update—Reviews for Physicians*. New York, Elsevier/North-Holland, 1979, pp 259-289.

LINDSTROM JM, LAMBERT EH: Content of acetylcholine receptor and antibodies bound to receptor in myasthenia gravis, experimental autoimmune myasthenia gravis, and Eaton-Lambert syndrome. *Neurology* 28:130, 1978.

MAYER RF, WILLIAMS IR: Incrementing responses in myasthenia gravis. *Arch Neurol* 31:24, 1974.

MCARDLE B: Metabolic and endocrine myopathies, in Walton JN (ed): *Disorders of Voluntary Muscle*, 4th ed. Edinburgh, Churchill Livingstone, 1981, chap 19.

MCFADZEAN AJS, YEUNG R: Periodic paralysis complicating thyrotoxicosis in Chinese. *Br Med J* 1:451, 1967.

MCQUILLEN MP, CANTOR HE, O'ROURKE JR: Myasthenic syndrome associated with antibiotics. *Arch Neurol* 18:402, 1968.

MEYERS KR, GILDEN DH, RINALDI CF, HANSEN JL: Periodic muscle weakness, normokalemia and tubular aggregates. *Neurology* 22:269, 1972.

NASTUK WL, PLESCIA OJ, OSSERMAN KE: Changes in serum complement activity in patients with myasthenia gravis. *Proc Soc Exp Biol Med* 105:177, 1960.

OKINAKA S et al: The association of periodic paralysis and hyperthyroidism in Japan. *J Clin Endocrinol* 17:1454, 1957.

PATRICK J, LINDSTROM JP: Autoimmune response to acetylcholine receptor. *Science* 180:871, 1973.

———, ———, CULP B, MCMILLAN J: Studies on purified eel acetylcholine receptor and antiacetylcholine receptor antibody. *Proc Natl Acad Sci USA* 70:3334, 1973.

PITTINGER CB, ERYASE Y, ADAMSON R: Antibiotic induced paralysis. *Anesth Analg* 49:487, 1970.

POSKANZER DC, KERR DNS: A third type of periodic paralysis with normokalemia and favorable response to NaCl. *Am J Med* 31:328, 1961.

REMEN L: Zur Pathogenese und Therapie der Myasthenia gravis pseudoparalytica. *Dtsch Z Nervenheilkd* 128:66, 1932.

REUTHER P, FULPIUS BW, MERTENS HB, HERTEL G: Anti-ace-
tylcholine receptor antibody under long-term azothiaprine
treatment in myasthenia gravis, in Dau PC (ed): *Plasmapheresis and the Immunobiology of Myasthenia Gravis.* Boston,
Houghton-Mifflin, 1979, pp 329-348.

RUSSELL DS: Histological changes in myasthenia gravis. *J Pathol Bacteriol* 65:279, 1953.

SANTA T, ENGEL AG, LAMBERT EH: Histometric study of neuromuscular junction ultrastructure. I. Myasthenia gravis.
Neurology 22:71, 1972.

SIMPSON JA: Myasthenia gravis: A new hypothesis. *Scot Med J*
5:419, 1960.

TALBOTT JH: Periodic paralysis: A clinical syndrome. *Medicine*
20:85, 1941.

TYLER FH, STEPHENS FE, GUNN FD, PERKOFF GT: Studies on
disorders of muscle. VII. Clinical manifestations and inheritance of a type of periodic paralysis without hypopotassemia.
J Clin Invest 30:492, 1951.

VIETS HR: A historical review of myasthenia gravis from 1672
to 1900. *J Am Med Assoc* 153:1273, 1953.

VINCENT A, NEWCOM-DAVIS J, MARTIN V: Antiacetylcholine
receptor antibodies in D-penicillamine associated myasthenia
gravis. *Lancet* 1:1254, 1978.

WALKER MB: Treatment of myasthenia gravis with physostigmine. *Lancet* 1:1200, 1934.

CHAPTER 52

DISORDERS OF MUSCLE CHARACTERIZED BY CRAMP, SPASM, PAIN, AND LOCALIZED MASSES

Quite apart from spasticity and rigidity, which are due to a disinhibition of spinal motor mechanisms (see pages 40 and 55), there are forms of muscular stiffness and spasm that can be traced to abnormalities of the lower motor neuron or the sarcolemma of the muscle fiber and its intrinsic conducting apparatus. Thus, muscles may go into spasm because of an unstable depolarization of their axons, as occurs in myokymia, hypocalcemic tetany, pseudohypoparathyroidism, and motor system disease. The contraction of muscle may be normal but persists despite attempts at relaxation (myotonia); or, after one or a series of contractions the muscle may be slow in decontracting, as occurs in hypothyroidism; or, in the contracture of McArdle's phosphorylase deficiency and phosphofructokinase deficiency, muscle may lack the energy to relax.

Each of these conditions evokes the complaint of cramp or spasm, which is variably painful and interferes with free and effective voluntary activity. Each condition has its own identifying clinical characteristics, registered also in the EMG, and most of them respond favorably to therapy. Premium attaches, therefore, to the clinical differentiation of these phenomena.

MUSCLE CRAMP

As mentioned on page 946, everyone at some time or other has experienced muscle cramps. Usually they occur during the night, after a day of unusually strenuous activity; less often they occur during the day, with exertion. A random restless or stretching movement will induce a hard contraction of a muscle (most frequently of the foot or leg) which cannot be voluntarily relaxed. The muscle is visibly and palpably taut and painful, and the condition is readily distinguished from an illusory cramp, in which the patient experiences only a sensation of cramp but where little or no contraction of muscle occurs, as in intermittent claudication and in certain diseases of peripheral nerve. Massage and vigorous stretch of the cramped muscle will cause the spasm to yield, though for a time the muscle remains excitable and subject to recurrent cramps. Visible fasciculation may precede and follow the cramp, indicating an excessive excitability of the motor neuron supplying the muscle. Sometimes the cramp is so violent that the muscle appears to have been injured. It remains sore to touch and painful upon use for a day or longer. Particularly alarming are cramps of precordial chest muscles or diaphragm. Fear of heart or lung disease may be aroused. In the EMG the cramp is attended by high-frequency action potentials, and the precramp phase by runs of activity in motor units. Why cramps should be painful is not known; probably the demands of the overactive muscle exceed metabolic supply, causing a relative ischemia and accumulation of metabolites. Overwork of muscle with or without impairment of circulation is also painful.

Cramps are known to increase in frequency under certain conditions and with certain diseases. They are frequent during pregnancy for reasons not fully understood. Dehydration and sweating favor cramping, and athletes try to prevent this by ingestion of sodium chloride. Exertional cramps are frequent in motor system disease and less so in chronic polyneuropathies.

Quinine sulfate (300 mg at bedtime and repeated in 4 h if necessary), or 300 mg tid for diurnal cramping, is the most useful medication; diphenhydramine hydrochloride (Benadryl) 50 mg or procainamide 0.5 to 1.0 g may be used if quinine cannot be tolerated.

TETANY AND PATHOLOGIC CRAMP

As pointed out on page 946, a reduction in ionizable calcium and magnesium are associated with involuntary cramplike spasms; in their mildest form they tend to be distal (carpopedal spasm), but they may involve any of the muscles, except those of the eyes. Stimulation of a muscle through its nerve at certain frequencies (15 to 20 times per second) characteristically reproduces the spasms, and hyperventilation and ischemia increase the tendency. Indeed the Trousseau sign—carpal spasms with occlusion of the blood supply to the arm—takes advantage of this phenomenon. That hypocalcemic tetany is attributable to an unstable depolarization of the axonal membrane of the nerve fiber is shown by (1) the sensitivity of nerve to percussion (tapping over the facial nerve near its foramen of exit induces a facial twitch or Chvostek's sign), (2) the appearance of fast-frequency doublets and triplets of motor unit potentials in the EMG, (3) evocation of spasm by application of a tourniquet to proximal parts of a limb (causing ischemia of segments of nerve beneath the tourniquet), (4) the regular association of tingling, prickling paresthesias from excitation of sensory nerve fibers. Hypocalcemia also causes a change of lesser importance in the muscle fibers themselves; hence nerve block does not completely eradicate tetany.

A condition resembling tetany, but without measurable hypocalcemia is the *pathologic cramp syndrome* (*pseudotetany*). Here all skeletal muscles may be continuously or intermittently locked in spasm, and every strong postural or voluntary movement leads to cramp. When this phenomenon is repeated again and again, the overly active muscles begin to hypertrophy. Satoyoshi has described a group of such patients who in addition to the widespread severe cramping of muscle also showed universal alopecia, amenorrhea, intestinal malabsorption, and sometimes epiphyseal destruction and retarded growth. The serum Ca is normal, and the EMG shows only high-frequency discharges. In about half of the authors' cases, stimulation of nerve at 15 per second produced cramp discharges, as in tetany. Muscle biopsy is normal except for a few ringbinden. Calcium and diazepam are of no value, but some patients have responded to phenytoin, quinine, or chlorpromazine. Jusic et al. have described a familial (autosomal dominant) form of cramp of distal limb muscles beginning in childhood and persisting throughout life.

STATES OF CONTINUOUS FASCICULATION, MYOKYMIA, CONTINUOUS MUSCLE ACTIVITY, NEUROMYOTONIA, AND "STIFF MAN" SYNDROME

This is a confusing group of clinical states which are not fully differentiated.

As is well known, a few random fasciculations in the calf muscles are to be seen in most normal individuals. They are of no significance but can be a source of worry to physicians and nurses who have heard or read that fasciculations are an early sign of amyotrophic lateral sclerosis. A simple clinical rule is that fasciculations in relaxed muscle are never indicative of motor system disease unless there is an associated weakness, atrophy, or reflex change.

Frequently a normal individual will experience intermittent twitching of one muscle or even a part of a muscle such as one of the muscles of the thenar eminence or of the orbicularis oculi. It may continue for days. Lay persons refer to it as "live flesh." Electromyographically this twitching, like that of the benign fasciculations described above, tends to be more constant in localization and more rhythmic than the malignant fasciculations of amyotrophic lateral sclerosis, but such distinctions are not entirely reliable.

There is a *state of widespread, continuous fasciculations* that may last for months or even years, and is accompanied by weakness and fatigability. No reflex changes, sensory loss, nerve conduction or EMG abnormality (other than fasciculations), or increase in serum muscle enzymes are found. Low energy and fatigability suggest an endogenous depression, yet the fasciculations are indeed prominent. We suspect that this fasciculatory state reflects a disease of the terminal motor nerves, but the evidence is thin. Eventual recovery can be expected.

Myokymia is a term that refers to a continuous, rippling, more or less tonic contraction of muscles. It may be generalized or limited to one part of the body such as the muscles of the shoulders or of the lower extremities. In some patients cramping is frequently associated, and indeed muscles about to cramp may twitch or show spontaneous rippling contractions; the cramping may be associated with sweating. Other patients with the same condition never have cramps. Obviously myokymia and cramping are two different conditions. Some of the patients complain of a slight weakness and inability to perform motor tasks in a normal fashion. In addition to intermittent discharge of motor units, several of our patients have shown a slowing of distal latencies in nerve conduction tests, and muscle biopsies have revealed a few groups of atrophic fibers. These findings suggest a mild distal motor neuropathy. CPK and aldolase levels are normal. This state is sometimes called *neuromyotonia,* with the implication that a neuropathy has led to a pseudomyotonia. Possibly this represents a phase of nerve regeneration. In several of our cases the response to phenytoin (100 mg tid) has been dramatic. Usually the condition recedes after several years.

The relation of myokymia to a state called *continuous muscular activity* is ambiguous. Isaacs described patients whose muscles began at some point to "work" continuously. Twitching and spasms were evident, as well as generalized muscle stiffness and reduced or abolished reflexes. Slight muscle atrophy is present in some cases. The muscle activity persists throughout sleep. General and spinal anesthesia do not suppress the muscular activity, but curare does; nerve block may have no effect or may reduce it, as in the case of Lütschg et al. The EMG shows continuous motor unit discharges. The reported cases have varied. Some resemble the myokymia described above; others have continuous spasms and cramps which cause the muscles to be hard and unavailable for voluntary movements. The stiffness and slowness of movement makes walking laborious ("armadillo syndrome"), and in some cases all voluntary movement is blocked. Again phenytoin has reduced or abolished the continuous muscle activity and the spasm, permitting normal or nearly normal function.

The condition in which the spasms are continuous, forcing the patient to lie helplessly in bed, the feet in equinus position, the legs extended, conforms to the one originally described by Moersch and Woltman in 1956 as *"stiff man" syndrome.* Since then more than 40 isolated examples have been observed all over the world. The onset is usually in middle life, and men are affected more often than women. At first there is intermittent and then more or less continuous stiffness and spasms of limb and trunk muscles. Muscles of respiration, swallowing, and of the face may be involved in the more advanced cases, but trismus, a common feature of tetanus, does not occur. Any noise or attempted passive or voluntary movement precipitates severely painful spasms of all the involved musculature. Once started, the condition continues for many years with little or no change. Unlike the syndrome of continuous muscular activity, spinal anesthesia and *d-*tubocurarine abolish the spasms. This would suggest a disinhibition of alpha motor neurons, akin to that which occurs in tetanus. In other instances, however, the spasms have ceased during sleep, unlike established tetanus. Again these physiologic and pharmacologic differences are difficult to understand. They suggest different levels of disorder in the central nervous system. Sometimes in reading reports of such cases one wonders how certain extrapyramidal motor

abnormalities (dystonia, phenothiazine dyskinesias) can be excluded. The most effective treatment has been diazepam (Valium) in doses up to 40 to 50 mg/day.

CONTRACTURE (PSEUDOMYOTONIA)

McArdle's phosphorylase deficiency and phosphofructokinase deficiency provide examples of an entirely different type of painful shortening and hardness of muscle. In both these diseases an otherwise normal child, adolescent, or adult begins to complain of weakness and stiffness and sometimes pain on using the limbs. Muscle contraction and relaxation are normal when the patient is at rest, but strenuous activity, especially under conditions of ischemia, causes the muscles to shorten, unable to relax. The primary abnormality in McArdle's disease is a defect in myophosphorylase (hereditary?), which prevents the conversion of glycogen to glucose-6-phosphate. Phosphofructokinase deficiency interferes with the conversion of glucose-6-phosphate to glucose-1-phosphate; the defect is also present in red blood cells (Layzer et al.).

Unlike muscles in cramp and other involuntary spasms, the contracted muscles no longer use energy, and they are more or less electrically silent; moreover they do not produce lactic acid. This condition is spoken of as *pharmacologic contracture.* Ischemia contributes to this condition by denying glucose to the muscle, which cannot function adequately on fatty acids and nonglucose substrates. The diagnosis of either disease is confirmed by the failure of blood lactate to rise in the cubital vein after a 3-min period of ischemic exercise. Histochemical stains of biopsied muscle reveal an absence of phosphorylase activity (in McArdle's disease) or of phosphofructokinase activity. The only known treatment is a planned reduction in activity. Fructose taken orally is said to be helpful in some cases.

A kind of pseudomyotonia also accompanies *hypothyroidism,* where the muscle fibers contract and relax slowly. This response is readily demonstrated in eliciting tendon reflexes, particularly the Achilles reflex. The muscles are large, are subject to myoedema, and when used may show waves of slow contraction. The basis of this disorder appears to be a slowness in the reaccumulation of calcium ions in the endoplasmic reticulum and in the disengagement of thin actin and thick myosin filaments. The EMG does not reflect the abnormality.

TETANUS

In *tetanus*, the skeletal muscles are persistently contracted, owing to the effect of the tetanus toxin on spinal neurons whose natural function is to inhibit the motor neurons (see also page 782). As the condition develops, activities that normally excite the neurons, i.e., voluntary contraction, startle, visual and auditory stimulation, all evoke involuntary spasms. Sleep tends to quiet them, and they are suppressed by spinal anesthesia and curare. The EMG shows the expected interference pattern of action potentials. Once the muscle is involved in persistent contraction, it is said that the shortened state is not abolished by procaine block or severance of nerve (in animals), but this so-called *myostatic contracture* has not been demonstrated in humans.

The black widow spider (*Latrodectus* species) produces a toxin which, within a few minutes of the bite, leads to cramps and spasms, and then a painful rigidity of abdominal, trunk, and leg muscles. If death does not occur in 24 to 48 h, recovery is complete. Little is known of the nature or site of action of this toxin. Presumably it causes a hyperexcitability of alpha motor neurons.

Other conditions that give rise to involuntary spasm of muscle are myotonia, which is discussed below, under Thomsen's disease, and phenothiazine and other extrapyramidal dyskinesias, discussed on page 75.

CONGENITAL MYOTONIA
(Thomsen's Disease)

This is an uncommon hereditary disease of skeletal muscle which begins in early life and is characterized by myotonia and muscular hypertrophy.

HISTORY

This disease was first brought to the attention of the medical profession in 1876, by Julius Thomsen, a Danish physician who himself suffered from the disease as did 20 other members of his family over four generations. His designation *ataxia muscularis* was not apt, but he left no doubt as to the nature of the condition which featured "tonic cramps in voluntary muscles associated with an inherited psychical indisposition." The latter association was not borne out by subsequent studies and is now believed to be fortuitous.

Strümpell in 1881 assigned the name *myotonia*

congenita to the disease, and Westphal in 1883 referred to it as *Thomsen's disease*. Erb provided the first description of its pathology and called attention to two additional unique features, muscular hyperexcitability and hypertrophy. In 1923, Thomsen's great-nephew, K. Nissen, extended the original genealogy to 35 cases in seven generations. In 1948, Thomasen updated the subject in a monograph that is still a useful reference.

ETIOLOGY

The cause of the disease is genetic. From the careful studies of Becker, two forms are now recognized. In one, the type described by Thomsen, the myotonia is inherited as an autosomal dominant trait. The myotonia has its onset early, usually by the time the child begins to walk. In about half the patients in this group, the myotonia is worsened by exposure to cold, but episodes of paralysis do not occur. Hypertrophy of muscles is absent or slight. In the second type the inheritance is autosomal recessive, but males predominate in a ratio of 3:1. Here the myotonia begins later in childhood, and even as late as adult life, and tends to be more severe than in the dominant type. It spreads from the leg muscles, where it begins, to those of the trunk, arms, and face. Hypertrophy is invariably present. There may be an associated mild distal weakness and atrophy.

The assertion that all cases of myotonia congenita eventually convert to myotonic dystrophy, long a point of dispute, has not been confirmed by DeJong, who found, in a study of 100 cases, that the two diseases can be distinguished at all ages. Personal observations accord with this finding. It is for this reason that we have not classified myotonia congenita with the dystrophies.

CLINICAL FEATURES

Tonic spasm of muscle after forceful voluntary contraction stands as the cardinal feature of the disease and is most pronounced after a period of inactivity. Repeated contractions "wear it out," so to speak, and later movements in a series become more swift and effective. Rarely the converse is observed—where the first movements of a series are less likely to induce myotonia than are later ones (*myotonia paradoxica*). The spasm is painless, unlike cramp. Close observation reveals a softness of the muscles during rest, and the initial contraction appears not to be significantly slowed unless there is preexistent myotonia.

The congenital nature of the dominant form of the disease may be evident even in the crib, where the infant's eyes are noted to open slowly after crying or sneezing, and the legs are conspicuously stiff as the first steps are attempted. In the recessive form, myotonia may not become evident until adult years, which probably explains some cases of so-called *myotonia acquisita* or *tarda* (other cases are probably examples of myotonia evoked by hypothyroidism or of myotonic dystrophy).

When severe, the myotonia tends to affect all skeletal muscles, being especially prominent in the lower limbs. Attempts to walk and run are sometimes impeded to the extent that the patient stumbles and falls. Other limb and trunk muscles are also thrown into spasm as are those of the face and upper limbs. Small, gentle movements such as blinking or elicitation of a tendon reflex do not initiate myotonia, whereas strong closure of the eyes, as in a sneeze, sets up a spasm that may prevent complete opening for many seconds. Spasms of extraocular muscles occur in some instances, leading to strabismus. Loosening of one set of muscles after a succession of contractions does not prevent the appearance of myotonia in another set, nor in the same ones if used in another pattern of movement. Smooth and cardiac muscles are never affected.

Myotonia can be induced in most cases by tapping a muscle belly with a percussion hammer. Unlike the lump or ridge produced in hypothyroid or cachectic muscle (myoedema), the myotonic contraction involves an entire fasciculus or a muscle and persists for several seconds. The tongue, if tapped, shows a similar phenomenon. The effect of an electrical (faradic) stimulus delivered to the motor point in a muscle also induces a prolonged contraction (Erb's myotonic reaction).

In severe cases of the recessive type, muscular hypertrophy may reach herculean proportions, and such adolescents and young adults may gain occupation as "strong men" in circuses. The hypertrophy affects particularly the muscles of the thighs, forearms, and shoulders. When relaxed, the large muscles have a natural consistency, but if the myotonia is severe and persistent, they feel firm and tense all the time. The power of large muscles may seem to be reduced, but this is related to difficulty in initiating movements, possibly owing to an inability to relax antagonists.

PATHOLOGIC FINDINGS

Biopsy reveals no abnormality other than enlargement of muscle fibers, and this change occurs only in hypertrophied muscles. As often happens in fibers of increased volume, central nucleation is somewhat more frequent. However, central rowing of nuclei, so prominent in myotonic dystrophy, is not seen, nor are the sarcoplasmic masses and peripheral disorganization of myofibrils that occur in the latter disease. The large fibers contain increased numbers of normally structured myofibrils. Peripheral ringbinden or spiral annulets are visible in some fibers. In well-fixed biopsy material, examined under the electron microscope, Schroeder and Adams were unable to discern any morphologic changes in sarcolemma, transverse or longitudinal endoplasmic reticulum, myofilaments, or other organelles. There are no changes in the peripheral or central nervous system.

PATHOGENESIS

In view of the absence of morphologic changes and the prominence of the myotonic phenomenon in individual muscle fibers, one must assume the existence of a physiologic change in the sarcolemma or some other part of the conducting apparatus of the muscle fibers. The EMG shows that the tension in contracting muscle fibers is slow to diminish, due to persistence of very fine electrical potentials. Some of the latter are of the same size as fibrillation potentials, but others are larger (normal motor unit potentials). The small potentials indicate independent, incoordinate activity of single fibers. Their activity continues after the volley of nerve impulses that initiated the contraction has ceased. Denny-Brown and Foley, stimulating single muscle fibers directly, obtained this myotonic afterdischarge only by a volley of stimuli, never by a single stimulus, and the series of myotonic fibrillation potentials progressively diminished in size, as they do in natural myotonia. Percussion elicits myotonia because it, too, provides a brief but relatively intense repetitive excitation. Thus myotonia can be distinguished electrophysiologically from contracture of other types (e. g., that produced by perfusion of muscle with veratrum alkaloids). Myotonia probably has a biochemical basis. Denny-Brown considers it to be a by-product of the preceding contraction. In addition Denny-Brown and Nevin noted that strong myotonia in one group of muscles may evoke reflex afterspasm in antagonist and synergist muscles, a reaction which depends on the operation of spinal mechanisms.

Substances such as the cholesterol-lowering agent diazacholesterol are capable of inducing myotonia in normal muscle (and cataracts), presumably by altering the membrane resistance of the fibers and decreasing chloride conductance. This suggests that myotonia depends on some basic alteration of the sarcolemma itself. Quinine, procainamide, and calcium lessen the duration of myotonic bursts; these substances are known also to act on the sarcolemma and endoplasmic reticulum.

DIAGNOSIS

In patients with very large muscles one must consider not only myotonia congenita but also familial hyperdevelopment, hypothyroid polymyopathy, hypertrophic polymyopathy (hypertrophia musculorum vera), and the Bruck-DeLange syndrome (congenital hypertrophy of muscles, mental retardation, and extrapyramidal movement disorder). The demonstration of myotonia by percussion and EMG study usually resolves the problem, although it should be noted that in exceptional cases of Thomsen's disease the persistence of contraction may be difficult to demonstrate. In hypothyroidism, the EMG may show pseudomyotonic discharges (page 881). However, true myotonia does not occur, myoedema is prominent, the contraction and relaxation of tendon reflexes is slowed, and there are other signs of thyroid deficiency.

In patients who complain of spasms, cramping, and stiffness, myotonia must be distinguished from myokymia, "the syndrome of persistent muscle activity" (Isaacs), the Schwartz-Jampel syndrome (see below), the pathologic cramp syndrome, the "stiff man" syndrome, and the contracture of phosphorylase or phosphofructose kinase deficiency. The distinguishing features of each of these states have been described in the preceding sections of this chapter. In none of them is there myotonia by percussion or by EMG. The only exception is the Schwartz-Jampel syndrome of hereditary stiffness combined with short stature and muscle hypertrophy. This is probably a form of myotonia and should be set apart from myokymia and the syndrome of continuous muscle activity (Isaacs).

Diagnostic uncertainty may arise in those patients who later prove to have myotonic dystrophy when only myotonia is noted in early life. The myotonia in these latter cases is usually mild and in several families which we have followed, some degree of weakness and a typical facies could be perceived even in early childhood. Also in paramyotonia congenita there is myotonia of early onset, but again it tends to be mild, involving mainly the orbicularis oculi, levator palpebrae, and tongue, and the diagnosis is seldom in doubt because of the cold-induced episodes of periodic paralysis.

TREATMENT

Quinine sulfate, 0.3 to 0.6 g, and procainamide, 250 to 500 mg tid, are clearly beneficial in myotonia congenita.

Phenytoin, 100 mg tid, has also been useful in some cases. It is reported that corticosteroids in moderate doses are capable of reducing myotonia, but the authors have had no experience with this treatment. The adverse effects of prolonged treatment with corticosteroids would probably outweigh their benefits.

SCHWARTZ-JAMPEL SYNDROME

Blepharospasm, dwarfism, pinched face with low-set ears, blepharophimosis, diffuse metaphyseal and epiphyseal bone dysplasia with flattened vertebrae, and a generalized myotonic muscular disorder were crystallized as a syndrome by Schwartz and Jampel in 1962. The syndrome has also been reported under the name of *myotonic chondrodystrophy.* The EMG displays typical myotonic discharges. Fariello et al., who have reviewed the 12 reported instances of this syndrome, do not believe that the reported cases constitute a homogeneous group. The only constant feature is the disturbed muscle function. The stiff muscles disturb gait. Pathologic studies of muscle have yielded inconsistent findings: group atrophy, dilated T system, Z-band streaming, and dilatation of mitochondria. The three latter changes are nonspecific and often artefactual. Treatment with procainamide, phenytoin, diazepam, or barbiturates is ineffective. Presently this should be regarded as the fourth myotonic syndrome, the other three being myotonia congenita, myotonic dystrophy, and the paramyotonia of von Eulenberg.

MYALGIC STATES

Diffuse muscle pain, which merges with malaise, is a frequent expression of a large variety of systemic infections, e.g., influenza, brucellosis, dengue, Colorado tick fever, glanders, measles, malaria, relapsing fever, rheumatic fever (cf. "growing pains"), salmonellosis, toxoplasmosis, trichinosis, tularemia, and Weil's disease. When the pain is intense, and especially if it is localized to the lower chest and abdomen, the most likely diagnostic possibility is epidemic myalgia (also designated as pleurodynia, "devil's grip," and Bornholm's disease). As indicated in Chap. 48, group B Coxsackie virus has been isolated from the striated muscles of patients with pleurodynia, and muscle biopsies of patients with viral influenza have been found to show both necrotizing myositis and virus particles. Poliomyelitis also may be accompanied by intense pain at the onset of neurologic involvement, and later the paralyzed muscles may ache. Nothing is known about the pathologic basis of the muscular pains of this disease. Herpes zoster is another well-known cause of segmental pain, and is related to inflammation in spinal nerves and dorsal root ganglia, which may precede the vesicular skin eruption by as long as 72 to 96 h.

Fibromyositis and *myogelosis* would appear by definition to represent an inflammation of the fibrous tissues of the muscles, fascia, aponeuroses, and probably nerves as well. Unfortunately, the pathologic changes remain obscure. Only some clinical facts are at hand. A muscle or group of muscles becomes painful and tender after exposure to cold, dampness, or minor trauma, or for no reason that can be discerned. The neck and shoulders are the most common sites. Firm, tender zones, sometimes several centimeters in diameter, can be palpated within the muscles, and active contraction or passive stretching of the involved muscles increases the pain—points of diagnostic value. In Europe, the term *myogelosis* has been applied to this condition, but it has never gained popularity in the United States. Usually the condition clears up in a few days, and local heat and massage are found to give comfort while symptoms are present. The condition is a "favorite" with physiotherapists and osteopaths, who believe their physical measures and adjustments to be helpful, as they may be. Rarely a similar syndrome is the forerunner of what proves, after some days, with the onset of neurologic signs, to be a radiculitis, brachial neuritis, or an outbreak of herpes zoster.

Diffuse muscular soreness and aching may at times be the initial symptoms in rheumatoid arthritis, preceding the signs of joint involvement by a period of weeks or months. The muscles are tender, but since this may be found in otherwise normal individuals, particularly women, it is difficult to interpret. Often the patient observes that aching pain occurs not at the time of activity but some hours or even a day or two later, resembling the discomfort following the excessive use of unconditioned muscles. However, a program of conditioning exercises does not alleviate the pain. An increased sedimentation rate, a positive latex-fixation test, or other laboratory aids may clarify the diagnosis. Muscle biopsy may reveal a nonspecific interstitial nodular myositis. Occasionally a localized weakness of muscle, a slightly reduced tendon reflex, or a zone of impaired cutaneous sensation within the territory of a nerve will indicate the existence of a disease of the peripheral nervous system—an interstitial mononeuritis or mononeuritis multiplex (see page 901)—which can sometimes be confirmed by the finding of infiltrates of lymphocytes, mononuclear leukocytes, and plasma cells in a nerve or muscle biopsy.

In thin, asthenic adults who exhibit this rather vague symptomatology without other abnormalities, the authors have found it difficut to exclude hysteria or other neurosis and depression. Before calling for a psychiatric consultant, it is important in every such individual to search for evidence of a rheumatic state, brucellosis, as well as the myopathy which may accompany hypothyroidism, hyperparathyroidism and renal tubular acidosis, hypophosphatemia, hypoglycemia, the intrinsic phosphorylase defect (McArdle's disease), phosphofructokinase defect, and paroxysmal myoglobinuria. Patients with these latter diseases often complain of soreness, stiffness, and lameness after any strenuous muscular effort. Nevertheless, the majority of the diffuse myalgic states sent to the authors with a question of polymyositis have turned out to be examples of an overlooked endogenous depression.

LOCALIZED MUSCLE MASSES

Masses may be found in one or many muscles in a variety of clinical settings, and the clinical findings in each one have a different significance.

Muscle rupture is usually caused by a violent strain attended by an audible snap and then a bulge which appears when the muscle contracts. A weakening in contractile power and mild discomfort are usually noted by the patient. The biceps muscle is the one most often affected. Treatment is immediate surgical repair; if delayed, little can be done for the condition.

Hemorrhage into muscle may occur as a consequence of trauma, as a complication of the use of anticoagulants, in hematologic diseases, or after a minor trauma in a patient with Zenker's degeneration who is convalescing from typhoid fever or other infection.

Tumors include *desmoid tumor* (a benign massive growth of fibrous tissue in parturient women and after surgery), *rhabdomyosarcoma* (a highly malignant tumor with strong liability to local recurrence and metastasis), and *angioma*.

Thrombosis of arteries or, more often, of *veins* causes congestion and infarction of muscle. A special type of muscle infarction occasionally involves the anterior thigh in patients with diabetes mellitus (Banker and Chester). The major symptoms are the sudden onset of pain and swelling of the thigh, with the formation of a tender, palpable mass. Recurrent infarction of the same or opposite thigh is characteristic. The stereotypical clinical picture obviates the need for diagnostic muscle biopsy. The extensive infarction of muscle is due to the occlusion of many medium-sized muscular arteries and arterioles, most likely the result of embolization of atheromatous material from eroded aortic plaques.

Recognition of this complication and immobilization of the limb are of prime practical importance, since muscle biopsy and early ambulation may cause serious hemorrhage into the infarcted tissue.

MYOSITIS OSSIFICANS

This refers to the deposit of bone within the substance of a muscle. Two types are recognized. One is a localized form which appears in a single muscle or group of muscles after trauma, and the other is a progressive, widespread ossifying process in many muscles of the body, entirely unrelated to trauma.

Localized (Traumatic) Myositis Ossificans After a muscle tear or a single blow to the muscle, or after repeated minor trauma, a painful area develops in the muscle. It is gradually replaced by a mass of cartilaginous consistency, and within 4 to 7 weeks' time, a solid mass of bone can be felt and seen in roentgenograms. As would be expected, this most frequently happens in vigorous adult men, and the thigh muscles and to a lesser extent the pectoralis major and biceps brachii are the usual sites of the abnormality. The mass tends to subside after several months if the patient desists from the activity which produced the trauma.

Generalized Myositis Ossificans This disease, also referred to as *myositis ossificans progressiva*, is rare, although Lutwak, in 1964, was able to collect 264 cases from the literature. The cause is unknown, but it is probably inherited as an autosomal dominant trait. It consists of widespread bone deposition along the fascial planes of muscles, and has its onset in infancy and childhood in 90 percent of cases.

Pathology The first stage is believed to be an interstitial myositis or fibrositis. Biopsies of early indurated swellings have revealed extensive proliferation of interstitial connective tissue in which little inflammatory cell reaction is found. Within a few weeks the connective tissue becomes less cellular and retracts, compressing the adjacent muscle fibers. Osteoid and cartilage formation occur at a later stage, developing in the connective tissue and enclosing relatively intact muscle fibers.

Clinical manifestations Nearly 75 percent of all reported cases have had congenital anomalies, the most frequent of which is a failure of development of the great toes or thumbs and less often other digits. The first symptom is often a firm swelling and mild tenderness in a vertebral or cervical muscle. There is, in addition, a mild discomfort during muscle contraction, and the overlying skin may be reddened and slightly swollen. A trauma may be recalled as the initiating factor, but as the months pass, other muscles not injured in any recognizable way become similarly involved. At first radiographs reveal no important changes, but within 6 to 12 months calcium deposits are observed and one can feel stony-hard masses within the muscles. As the disease advances, limitation of movement and deformities become increasingly evident. Calcified bridges between adjacent muscles and across joints lead to scoliosis; rigidity of spine, jaw, and limbs; and limited expansion of the thorax. Ultimately, the patient is virtually converted into "stone."

Diagnosis The principal problem in diagnosis is to differentiate this condition from *calcinosis universalis,* which usually occurs in relationship to scleroderma or polymyositis. In calcinosis universalis there is said to be calcinosis (calcium deposits) in the skin, subcutaneous tissues, and connective tissue sheaths around the muscles, whereas in myositis ossificans there is actual bone formation within the muscles. The pathologic data are too meager to justify this sharp distinction. The prolonged ingestion of large doses of vitamin D may also produce widespread deposition of masses of calcium around muscles, joints, and subcutaneous tissue. Calcific deposits, perhaps true ossification, may occur in the soft tissues around the hips and knees of paraplegics, and rarely following a hemiplegia ("paralytic myositis ossificans").

Prognosis The disease may undergo spontaneous remissions and may halt for many years at a stage where the patient is capable of adequate function. In other cases, progression leads to marked debilitation and respiratory embarrassment, the final illness often being a terminal pneumonia or other infection.

Treatment The administration of diphosphonate (10 to 20 mg/kg orally), a compound that inhibits the deposition of calcium phosphate, has been said to cause regression of new swellings and to prevent calcification (Russell et al.). Some of the calcium deposits in calcinosis universalis have receded in response to prednisone, and because of the unclear relationship of this disease to generalized myositis ossificans, it is probably advisable to try this form of therapy as well. Excision of bony deposits may be undertaken if it is certain that they are the cause of particular disabilities.

REFERENCES

ADAMS RD: *Diseases of Muscle: A Study in Pathology*, 3d ed. New York, Harper & Row, 1975.

BANKER BQ, CHESTER CS: Infarction of thigh muscle in the diabetic patient. *Neurology* 23:667, 1973.

BECKER PE: Genetic approaches to the nosology of muscle disease: Myotonias and similar diseases, pt 7: Muscle, in Bergsma D (ed): *The Clinical Delineation of Birth Defects*. Baltimore, Williams & Wilkins, 1971.

DEJONG JG: *Dystrophia Myotonica, Paramyotonica, and Myotonia Congenita*. Assen, Netherlands, Van Gorcum, 1955.

DENNY-BROWN D, FOLEY JM: Evidence of a chemical mediator in myotonia. *Trans Assoc Am Physicians* 62:187, 1949.

———, NEVIN S: The phenomenon of myotonia. *Brain* 64:1, 1941.

ERB W: *Die Thomsen'sche Krankheit (Myotonia Congenita)*. Leipsig, Vogen, 1886.

FARIELLO R et al: A case of Schwartz-Jampel syndrome with unusual muscle biopsy findings. *Ann Neurol* 3:93, 1978.

HARPER PS: *Myotonic Dystrophy*. Philadelphia, Saunders, 1979.

ISAACS H: Continuous muscle fibre activity in an Indian male with additional evidence of terminal motor fibre abnormality. *J. Neurol Neurosurg Psychiatry* 30:126, 1967.

JUSIC A, DOGAN S, STOJANOVIC V: Hereditary persistent distal cramps. *J. Neurol Neurosurg Psychiatry* 35:379, 1972.

LAYZER RB: Motor unit hyperactivity states, in Vinken PJ, Bruyn GW (eds): *Handbook of Clinical Neurology*, vol 41: *Diseases of Muscle II*. Amsterdam, North-Holland, 1979, chap 10, pp 295-316.

———, ROWLAND LP: Cramps. *N Engl J Med* 285:31, 1971.

———, ———, RANNEY HM: Muscle phosphofructokinase deficiency. *Arch Neurol* 17:512, 1967.

LÜTSCHG J et al: The syndrome of "continuous muscle fiber activity." *Arch Neurol* 35:198, 1978.

LUTWAK L: Myositis ossificans progressiva: Mineral, metabolic and radioactive calcium studies of the effects of hormones. *Am J Med* 37:269, 1964.

MOERSCH FP, WOLTMAN HW: Progressive fluctuating muscular rigidity ("stiff-man syndrome"): Report of a case and some observations in 13 other cases. *Mayo Clin Proc* 31:421, 1956.

NISSEN K: Beiträge zur Kenntnis der Thomsen' Schen Krankheit (Myotonia congenita), mit besonderer berücksichtigung des hereditären Momentes und seinen Beziehungen zu den mendelschen Vererbungsregeln. *Z Klin Med* 97:58, 1923.

RUSSELL RGG et al: Treatment of myositis ossificans progressiva with a diphosphonate. *Lancet* 1:10, 1972.

SATOYOSHI E: A syndrome of progressive muscle spasm, alopecia and diarrhea. *Neurology* 28:458, 1978.

SCHROEDER JM, ADAMS RD: The ultrastructural morphology of the muscle fiber in myotonic dystrophy. *Acta Neuropathol* 10:218, 1968.

STRÜMPELL A: Tonische Krämpfe in willkürlich bewegten Muskeln (myotonia congenita). *Klin Wochenschr* 18:119, 1881.

THOMASEN E: *Myotonia, Thomsen's Disease, Paramyotonia, Dystrophia Myotonica*. Aarhus, Denmark, Universitetsforlaget i Aarhus, 1948.

THOMSEN J: Tonische Krämpfe in willkürlich beweglichen Muskeln in Folge von erebterpsychischer Disposition (ataxia muscularis?). *Arch Psychiatr Nervenkr* 6:706, 1876.

PSYCHIATRIC DISORDERS

To understand mental disorders one must know something of how the brain functions, know something of human psychology, and at the same time be sensitive and responsive to other human beings. The first two of these require special study; the third is more an innate quality, found in all good physicians.

Mental disorders pose a number of special problems not met in other fields of medicine. In the first place there are such wide variations in personality and behavior that the point where the normal ends and abnormal begins is often difficult to ascertain. Secondly, the methods of study of mental illness are quite subjective, depending mainly on the physician's almost intuitive perceptions of the "vital secrets" and occult purposes of the patient and on the powers of description and narration of patients in revealing their symptoms, and these latter capacities vary with intelligence, education, and status of cerebral function. Thirdly, the clinical entities that will be presented in the following pages are wholly unverifiable. Neither by laboratory test nor postmortem examination can one corroborate the clinical impression.

There is another, more abstruse and essentially theoretic problem of which one must be aware in attempting to study mental disorder. Physicians find that there are two different and seemingly antithetical approaches to disordered nervous function—one proceeding along strictly medical or neurologic lines, the other psychological. They must learn to utilize two types of data, one drawn from their own observations of the patient's behavior, the other from the introspections of the patient. It must be emphasized that the terms *neurologic* and *psychological* in this context do not necessarily refer to the activities of neurologists and psychiatrists. They are merely convenient terms for two distinct modes of approach to mental disorders; both may be and frequently are used by the neurologist and the psychiatrist, as will be made clear.

The neurologic approach begins with the premise that all the clinical manifestations of a nervous disorder are expressions of a pathologic process (disease) within the nervous system. This latter may be obvious (such as a tumor or cerebral infarct), or it may be impossible to detect with the light or even the electron microscope (such as the encephalopathy of delirium tremens). In all instances the pathologic process is traceable to some genetic, chemical, or physical factor acting on normal tissue and the visible lesion represents only the most advanced and irreversible stage of a dynamic morbid process. The particular clinical effect, qua symptom or sign, whether it be paralysis, sensory loss, visual or auditory perceptual failure, ataxia, aphasia, tremor, confusion, coma, convulsion or hallucination, depends on the nature of the lesion and its locus within the nervous system. The clinical manifestations, therefore, are interpretable in terms of neurophysiology and neuroanatomy.

The symptoms and signs of the disease, i.e., the expressions of the pathologically altered nervous system, take two forms, either of overactivity or excitation (positive effects) or of loss of function (negative effects)—or first one, then the other. An example of an excitatory lesion would be a convulsive seizure. A destructive lesion abolishes the function of a certain part of the nervous system (negative effects), but at the same time there may be a disinhibition of other intact parts, resulting in their overactivity. As pointed out in Chaps. 3 and 4, grasp and suck reflexes are explained in this way. No doubt, in the delirious patient, as in the paralyzed one, something has also been lost in the course of disease and something new in behavior has emerged, presumably because of the uninhibited activity of the undamaged parts of the nervous system. There are, however, many cerebral disorders where such distinctions between negative and positive effects are uncertain; we lack knowledge of the basic pathophysiology of such processes as perceiving, thinking, remembering, symbolization, etc., and are unable to reduce them to this simple formulation.

This brings us face to face with other problems posed by the more complex diseases of the cerebrum. Quite apart from differences in symptoms related to anatomic localization and nature of the pathologic process, the status of the nervous system at the time of onset of the disease makes a difference. Level of intelligence, degree of education, facility with language(s), peculiarities of personality and character, stability of emotional control are all reflected in symptoms. Thus in a syndrome like dementia or a partial aphasia, while the deficit symptoms may be much the same from patient to patient, the unbalanced behavior may differ widely even with the same disease in the same parts of the cerebrum. Only with some knowledge of the patients' natural endowment, education, premorbid personality, etc., can such differences be understood.

In assaying the symptoms of cerebral diseases the examiner must depend on two separate types of information—one subjective, the other objective. Subjective information is provided through the patients' awareness of their own deficits and their capacity to report and describe them; objective information has to do with changes in behavior that can be recognized by others. For example, information about hallucinations comes mainly from the patients' descriptions of their abnormal sensory experience, and the objective side may not be evident or is uncertain. Interestingly, in cerebral diseases causing complex disorders of perception, speech, and thinking, there is usually an impairment of introspective ability (lack of insight) as well as a change in behavior. This dual loss provides the most certain proof that activities of the mind and behavior depend on the same physiologic processes in the brain. It leads inevitably to a psychophysical monism, the position on the mind-body problem most acceptable to thoughtful neurologists. One of the ideas most difficult to grasp and appreciate, though it follows clearly from the neurologic concept of disordered nervous function, is that there is no essential difference between diseases called *physical* or *organic* and others called *functional*. Every functional disorder must have a structural basis.

The methodology used in the neurologic analysis, already described in Chap. 1, is merely a series of techniques for eliciting in a systematic fashion the altered activities of the nervous system. The standard procedure of history taking and physical examination requires supplementation by additional tests of biochemical, physiologic, and psychological type. Pathologic examination provides the final confirmation of diagnosis. The goals of the neurologic methodology and of neuropathology (the scientific study of nervous diseases) are to determine if a disease exists in the patient and, if so, to ascertain its cause and mechanism and the possibilities of prevention and therapy. A complete theory of a disease must incorporate all its essential elements—genetic, biochemical, physiologic, psychological as well as pathologic.

A second mode of approach to disordered nervous function, which one may term the psycho-logical approach, makes many of the same assumptions as the neurologic one. For example it assumes that in many patients the psychological disorder is an expression of structural changes in the brain at the molecular, chemical, or tissue level. Again, the latter may be determined by a genetic abnormality, a developmental defect, or an acquired lesion of many types. The main premise, however, is that there is an additional category of nervous disorders, which, within broad limits, is understandable solely in terms of a reaction to previous or present life experiences. Certain abnormalities of personality, degree of emotional maturity, and the capacity to adjust to social situations are thought to stem from an inadequate development of personality and/or hurtful experiences in early life. Some of these experiences are easily remembered (i.e., "conscious"), others are forgotten (i.e., "unconscious") and recalled with difficulty or through the free association method of psychoanalysis. In either case the principal approach is to reconstruct a kind of autobiography of the individual and to search it for the roots of the present difficulty. Particular emphasis is placed on three lines of data, traced from early life to the present: key events in the patient's life, their temporal association with medical illnesses, and psychiatric symptoms. The purpose of this approach is not only to determine causality but to understand the patient's current reactions in the light of past experiences and to use this understanding to effect change. By frank discussion the physician endeavors to demonstrate the relationship of the patient's symptoms to abnormal behavior patterns and reactions, and thereby to assist in bringing about an understanding of the problems.

Psychiatrists have formulated a number of psychological mechanisms whereby symptoms are produced, and they speak of them in a language rather unfamiliar to most physicians—e.g., conflict, repression, projection, displacement of affect, conditioning, and arrest of libido. Some of the more narrowly trained psychoanalysts believe that all theories of mental disorder must be cast in pyschological terms and that anatomic, biochemical, and pathologic terms have no place in such a formulation. Needless to say, most contemporary psychiatrists do not accept this restrictive psychological concept of nervous disorders.

A HOLISTIC AND ECLECTIC POSITION

It seems to the authors that both the neurologic and the psychological concept and approach have their place in medicine. But the two methods operate at different levels and are of principal use in different types of nervous aberrations.

In the *diagnosis* of a disease of the nervous system one begins always with a careful recording of the symptoms and signs and their temporal aspects, obtained through a detailed history and physical and ancillary examinations. The interpretation of such data leads to diagnosis. Here the psychological method is of little value, and the neurologic method stands as the only valid system of thought. It permits one to approach the problem of nervous disease as one does any other medical problem.

In *theorizing* about disease and in investigating its causes, this broad neurologic or medical approach is essential, for it accepts data from all the medical sciences and is able to incorporate all biologic as well as psychological facts. Here the psychological method has limited application, and although yielding useful data concerning the evolution of particular symptoms and their form and content, will never provide a complete explanation of disease.

However, in the *diagnosis* and *management of social maladjustments,* which constitute such a large and important part of psychiatry, the psychological approach takes precedence. Worry over loss of a job, domestic difficulty, the illness of a child, the death of a loved one, with all their potential physiologic disturbances, would be acceptable to every thoughtful person as derangements consequent upon the social problem. Indeed, only when the connection between the social event and its physical effects are not perceived do the effects become medical problems. These are suitably looked upon as reactions to life's difficulties and dealt with entirely at a psychological level. In the *management of all diseases,* knowledge of the patient's personality and general reactions is quite indispensable. This is a province of medicine where the psychological approach is of practical value, and the physician who knows the patient and how to deal with him or her as a troubled individual functions with great effectiveness.

This brings us to one of the crucial problems in neurology and psychiatry—that of defining a disease of the nervous system and in distinguishing it from a social or psychological maladjustment. Failure to do this has resulted in much confusion as to the legitimate spheres of medical activity and has been an obstacle to research. The authors propose as a *definition of nervous disease any condition in which there is a visible lesion in the nervous system or in which there is reasonable evidence of its existence on the basis of stereotypy of clinical expression and of genetic and collateral laboratory data. An abnormal psychological reaction is defined as a disorder of psychic function and behavior caused by a maladjustment in social relations not based directly on a known disease process or lesion.*

Simple as this division might seem, it is not easily applied to every abnormal nervous state. How does one interpret disturbances of impulse control, hyperactivity, inability to learn at the accustomed pace, failure to read or master arithmetic, criminality, and inadequacy in adjustment to school, work, marriage, and society? Some of these disturbances, as pointed out in Chap. 27, are surely due to specific retardations in development; others may be due to lack of proper training and education, unstable home environment, etc. Obviously in such a complex situation it may at times be quite impossible to separate cause and effect. An individual whose nervous system is affected by disease and who is unable to learn or to form stable social relationships may create an abnormal environment. Or a serious environmental stress may decompensate a patient with an obvious nervous disease.

Certain mental abnormalities have an uncertain status vis-à-vis this division and are currently subject to double interpretations, depending on one's premises. A persistent anxiety state without obvious cause in a previously healthy adult would be viewed by many psychiatrists as a neurosis—a psychophysical reaction of fear to some unconscious threat. Many neurologists would consider it a genetic disease closely allied to endogenous depression, in which some biochemical disturbance, as mysterious as was hyperthyroidism a century ago, has developed de novo. Since the nature of the condition is unsettled, it is understandably treated by physicians using both psychological methods and drugs. Anyone who proposes to investigate it, we would argue, should do so with a completely open mind and be prepared to review critically any reasonable hypothesis as to its cause.

There is also disagreement about depression, mania, paranoia, and schizophrenia—the major mental disorders in psychiatry. Most psychiatrists and all neurologists regard them as genetically determined diseases of the nervous system, the mechanism, anatomy, and biochemistry of which are still obscure. Environmental stress at times seems important in their evocation and exacerbation. Only a few psychiatrists insist, still, that such states represent deviate ways of living or abnormal psychological reactions. It seems reasonable to assume that the more comprehensive methodology of neurology and the medical sciences will eventually lead to their solution.

PSYCHOSOMATIC MEDICINE

In the recent past there has been great interest in a large category of disease called *psychosomatic.* Included here were peptic ulcer, mucous and ulcerative colitis, hay fever, bronchial asthma, urticaria, angioneurotic edema, essential hypertension, hyperthyroidism, rheumatoid arthritis, amenorrhea, and migraine—diseases in which a stressful life situation or emotional upset appeared to have been associated with their development, exacerbation, or prolongation. Three lines of evidence were adduced that purportedly set these diseases apart from others: (1) observations showed the function of the offending organ to be excited and possibly deranged by strong emotions; (2) analyses of the biographies and personalities of patients with these diseases allegedly disclosed an inordinately high incidence of resentment, hostility, dependence, aggressiveness, suppressed emotionality, inability to communicate matters of emotional concern or to differentiate reality and subjective falsification—attributes which are difficult or impossible to define and quantitate; (3) longitudinal histories drawn from the memories of the patients were said to reveal a relationship between personal crises and outbreaks (relapses) of the chronic disease. Medical therapy failed, it was argued, when these psychological phenomena were disregarded.

Some 45 years have passed since these ideas were first proclaimed, and an enormous literature followed, with the establishment of pathetically few unassailable facts. It became clear that these "psychosomatic" diseases are not neuroses in that (1) they have different symptoms and (2) the psychosomatic diseases have in most instances a known and easily demonstrable pathologic basis. No complete proof of psychic causation of the psychosomatic diseases has been adduced. Treatment has been concerned mainly with the relief of symptoms and has been directed for the most part by nonpsychiatric specialists. There is no evidence that the therapeutic results obtained by a purely psychiatric methodology are better than those of a competent internist.

With the growth of the field of psychosomatic medicine, there was, on the part of many physicians, an overemphasis of the psychological aspects of disease, out of all proportion to the somatic. As pointed out by Wolff in his scholarly exposition of the "mind-body" relationship, the logical fallacy of "psychogenic" or "psychosomatic" concepts is that they imply a mind acting in opposition to the body. Nevertheless, interest in the psychosomatic diseases contributed to the growing awareness of the diseased patient and not merely of the disease in isolation. First suggested by Claude Bernard and ably espoused and elaborated by Walter Cannon and Adolph Meyer is the view that a person must always be regarded as a complex psychobiological unit functioning in relationship to the immediate physical and social environment. Disease represents a faulty or inadequate adaptation of the organism to the environment. Sometimes the maladaptation can be traced to a single agent in the environment, such as a tubercle bacillus, without which the disease could not develop. Seldom, however, even in such a straightforward disease as tuberculosis, or, to take another example, the withdrawal syndrome of delirium tremens, can the problem be reduced to a single physical or psychic factor. Hence a rigid, narrowly physical or psychological approach always proves to be inadequate and must be supplanted by a broader psychobiological one which attempts to weigh each of many factors in the equation of disease. At present this is difficult, especially with the so-called psychosomatic diseases, since not all the factors are known. Until such time as new facts are obtained, the physician must cope with a huge population of patients with inadequate methods of diagnosis and treatment. Fortunately most of these patients suffer from relatively minor ailments which time and reassurance alleviate, or from neuroses that are not disabling.

PLAN OF PSYCHIATRY SECTION

In the chapters that follow there will be a consideration of the affective disorders, the neuroses, the schizophrenias, paranoid states, and sociopathies. The magnitude of these disorders and their clinical and social importance can hardly be overestimated. All physicians should know something about these categories of psychiatric disease. Neurologists in particular need to be familiar with them, if only for the purpose of differentiating them from other neurologic diseases and initiating intelligent management.

Emphasis throughout these chapters will be on the biologic characteristics and the diagnosis of each state. This is in keeping with a significant trend in psychiatry, stimulated by the development of rigorous diagnostic criteria (the Feighner Research Diagnostic Criteria; see also the monograph edited by Rakoff et al. and the monograph by Goodwin and Guze). The prevention of suicide, the choice of appropriate therapy, communication with the patient's family and physician, predictions about the course of the illness (prognosis)—all begin with accurate diagnosis. Finally, strict diagnostic criteria are important in psychiatric research.

In adhering to the bias of neurologic medicine we do not wish to depreciate the importance of psychological medicine. Our position on this matter has been fully stated in the preceding pages and needs no further belaboring. Theoretic aspects of personality and psychopathology and psychoanalytic concepts of symptom formation will be given little space, largely because the authors find themselves relatively unfamiliar with and unable to evaluate many of the tenets of these aspects of psychiatry. The reader interested in these aspects of the subject will find them well presented in the references at the end of each chapter.

REFERENCES

COBB S: *Emotions and Clinical Medicine.* New York, Norton, 1950.

FEIGHNER JP et al: Diagnostic criteria for use in psychiatric research. *Arch Gen Psychiatry* 26:57, 1972.

GOODWIN DW, GUZE SB: *Psychiatric Diagnosis,* 2d ed. New York, Oxford University Press, 1979.

RAKOFF V et al (eds): *Psychiatric Diagnosis.* New York, Brunner-Mazel, 1977.

WOLF S, WOLFF HG: *Human Gastric Function: An Experimental Study of Man and His Stomach.* New York, Oxford, 1947.

WOLFF HG: The mind-body relationship, in Bryson L (ed): *An Outline of Man's Knowledge of the Modern World.* New York, McGraw-Hill, 1960.

CHAPTER 53

THE NEUROSES

Though numbered as the most frequent types of mental illness, the neuroses are among the least understood. They were established as clinical entities in the late nineteenth century, but there are still major, unresolved issues with respect to their nature, classification, and etiology. When Freud made his original observations on hysteria and obsessional neurosis, he chose to designate them as psychoneuroses, implying a psychogenesis; but even Freud was uncertain of the etiology and speculated that the underlying cause of anxiety neurosis would probably be traced to a biologic factor. We have, therefore, retained the term *neurosis*, thinking it perferable to *psychoneurosis*, but of course this does not settle one of the great uncertainties about the neuroses—whether they actually have a physical basis or are merely expressions of social maladjustments, i.e., natural reactions to undue stress.

Neuroses express themselves by certain symptoms, altered patterns of behavior, and sometimes physical signs. They bear no obvious relationship to the patient's immediate situation, and hence are not readily explicable as reactions to environmental stress. In this respect they differ from the natural emotional states to which everyone is subject. Patients who are told that their trouble is a question of "nerves" or "emotional problems," for which no reason is evident to them, become perplexed, worried, and ashamed. There is implied in such an explanation a loss of self-control and weakness of will. One can imagine the patient's relief when an understanding physician explains the condition as a recognized medical problem and offers a positive therapeutic program.

DEFINITIONS

Descriptively the neuroses include the following clinical syndromes: (1) anxiety neurosis, (2) neurasthenia, (3) phobic neurosis, (4) obsessive-compulsive neurosis [(3) and (4) are also called *psychasthenia*], (5) hysteria, (6) hypochondriasis, and (7) neurotic depression. The International Classification of Diseases recognizes one additional type called "depersonalization neurosis," with which we have had little experience. Most such cases we would probably classify under (5). Although each of these syndromes is identifiable and separable when occurring in pure form, experience shows that many patients exhibit symptoms of more than one type, and therefore are considered to have "mixed neurosis."

It is difficult to furnish a definition which satisfactorily covers the essential attributes of these seven (or eight) neuroses. Such varied syndromes, as different as neurasthenia and panic, do not lend themselves to a unitary explanation. Common to all neurotic states is a degree of psychological functioning that allows the individual to function reasonably well as a student, member of a family unit, or worker. He is not totally disabled like a psychotic patient; the neurotic disorder is seen as a "part reaction" and is relatively benign. This distinction between neurosis and psychosis is ephemeral, for mild endogenous depressions occur in individuals with previously normal mental function and disable the patient little if at all. Episodes of worsening or outbreak of neurotic symptoms are viewed by many psychiatrists as psychological decompensations of a neurotic personality under stress. In psychiatric writings, the central issue is *anxiety*, which runs as a leitmotif through all the neuroses. Even in hysterical neurosis, in which patients seem indifferent to their physical disabilities, there is a strong undercurrent of anxiety. In psychoanalytic theory, anxiety is looked upon as the individual's response to a danger that threatens from within, in the form of a forbidden instinctual drive that is about to escape from the individual's control. The intensity of the anxiety is thought to be proportional to the intensity of the disguised threat, i.e., one of which the patient is unaware but which must be suppressed. The anxiety is seen as a signal to which the mind reacts by erecting psychological defenses. Thus each neurotic syndrome is perceived as a particular defense mechanism for dealing with anxiety. These and other psychodynamic theories of the neuroses are discussed in detail by Nemiah in the *Comprehensive Handbook of Psychiatry* (see References at end of chapter).

INCIDENCE

There are few reliable data as to the frequency of neuroses in a general population or the relative incidence of the various types of neurosis. An analysis of 1045 consecutive psychiatric consultations at the New England Center Hospital, during the years 1955 and 1956, disclosed that the dominant syndrome in about 20 percent was an anxiety state. In addition, symptoms of anxiety were present in some cases of depression, hysteria, and schizophrenia. In contrast to the high incidence of anxiety neurosis, frank hysteria was diagnosed in only 6 percent of cases, and all the other neuroses together with schizophrenia, alcoholic psychoses, sociopathic states, and the dementias comprised only 10 percent. As indicated on page 1026, depression in one form or another was the most common psychiatric illness (50 percent); psychiatric disease was either absent or could not be diagnosed in the remaining 13 percent of this series.

Such information as is available suggests that the incidence of the neuroses is much the same in an urban population (midtown New York) and a rural one (Stirling County, Nova Scotia), which would indicate that socioeconomic, racial, and cultural factors are of relatively little importance. Further, in times of calamity, such as the bombing of London, the incidence of neurotic symptoms was said not to have increased. Thus one tends to dismiss as an oversimplification the notion that neuroses are merely a by-product of life in civilized society. Neurosis of all types occurs in both sexes, except for hysteria which, with the qualifications to be indicated, is a disease of females. The onset is in late childhood, adolescence, and early adult life. Admittedly, neurotic symptoms may be recognized for the first time after this age, but a good clinical rule is to suspect any mental illness that appears for the first time after the age of 40 years to be a depressive psychosis or degenerative disease of the brain.

ANXIETY NEUROSIS
(Neurocirculatory Asthenia)

The term *anxiety neurosis* was introduced by Freud, in 1894, to describe a syndrome consisting of general irritability, anxious expectation, anxiety attacks, somatic equivalents of anxiety, and nightmares. In anxiety neurosis this symptom complex occurs in pure form, i.e., it constitutes the entire illness. However, as indicated on pages 347 and 1033, it may also occur in a number of other psychiatric diseases—manic-depressive psychosis, schizophrenia, hysteria, and phobic neurosis. Its closest link is with depression which it resembles in another respect, viz., a strong hereditary factor. *Anxiety reaction* is the term proposed by the American Psychiatric Association, and has largely replaced *anxiety state*. *Anxiety neurosis* is the term preferred by the authors.

CLINICAL PRESENTATION

Anxiety neurosis is a chronic disease, punctuated by recurrent attacks of acute anxiety or panic. The acute attacks are the hallmark of the disease, and many psychiatrists are reluctant to make a diagnosis of anxiety neurosis in their absence. Fully developed, they are nearly as dramatic as a seizure. They begin with a distressing presentiment of imminent dissolution. Patients are assailed by a feeling of strangeness, as though their body had changed or the surroundings were unreal. They are frightened, most often by the prospect of imminent death (angor animi), of losing their mind or self-control, or of smothering. "I am dying," "This is the end," "Oh, my God, I'm going," or "I can't breathe" are the characteristic expressions of alarm and panic. The heart races, breathing comes in rapid gasps, pupils are dilated, and the patient sweats and trembles. Hyperventilation induces paresthesias of fingers, tongue, and lips and, rarely, carpopedal spasms. The palpitation and breathing difficulties are so prominent that a cardiologist is often called. The symptoms abate spontaneously after 15 to 30 min, leaving the patient shaken, tense, perplexed, and often embarrassed.

Such attacks may occur several times a day, or at infrequent intervals. They may occur in situations where there are no easily recognizable sources of fear, in a public place, or when the patient is sitting quietly at home; or the attacks may awaken the patient from sleep. Except in minor details all the attacks are alike in any one individual.

Between attacks patients may feel relatively well or may experience the symptoms of the panic attack in lesser but persistent fashion. Most patients complain of chronic fatigue, palpitation, difficulty breathing, chest pain, dizziness, faintness, headache, and apprehension—an uneasy concern about the possibility of further attacks.

Anxiety neurosis may begin with an acute panic attack, but more frequently the onset is insidious—feelings of tenseness, nervousness, fatigue, weakness, and giddiness having been present for weeks or months before the first panic attack. From the history alone, two patterns of chronic anxiety neurosis are discernible. In one, there is a nearly lifelong history of poor exercise tolerance, little stamina, inability to do heavy physical work or participate in vigorous sports (running and swimming), tenseness, nervousness, and intolerance of crowds. In the other, the patient is vigorous and symptom-free until a chronic nervous state begins. Most patients with chronic symptoms first consult a physician complaining of cardiorespiratory symptoms, but in a significant number gastrointestinal symptoms (dyspepsia, loss of appetite, or "irritable colon") are the initial symptoms. The former often come to light at the time of induction into the armed services and have been designated, since shortly after the American Civil War, as *neurocirculatory asthenia*, "irritable heart," or "soldier's heart."

The physical examination between acute attacks yields relatively little of diagnostic value. The thorough study of Cohen et al. disclosed slight tachycardia, sighing respirations, yawning, flushed face and neck, tremor of outstretched hands, and brisk tendon jerks.

The onset of both acute and chronic anxiety neurosis is rare before the age of 18 and seldom begins after 35 to 40 years (average age of onset, 25 years). It is twice as frequent in women as men. There is a high familial incidence of this illness. In one study (Wheeler et al.) there was a prevalence of 40 percent among the grown children of patients with anxiety neurosis, compared to a prevalence of about 5 percent in the general population. An exact pattern of inheritance has not been established, but most closely approximates that of mendelian autosomal dominance.

The course of anxiety neurosis is variable. The symptoms fluctuate in severity, without apparent relation to environmental stress. A 20-year follow-up study by Wheeler and his associates showed that symptoms of anxiety neurosis were still present in 88 percent, but were moderately or severely disabling in only 15 percent. Most of the patients were able to work and to enjoy a normal family and social life; their only liability to further psychiatric illness was to recurrent anxiety neurosis or anxious depressions. So-called psychosomatic illnesses and other psychiatric illnesses do not occur more frequently than in the general population. The life span of patients with anxiety neurosis is not shortened. They rarely commit suicide, but we have observed exceptions to this rule.

ETIOLOGY

Anxiety neurosis has been attributed to constitutional weakness of the nervous system, to social and psychological factors, some of which have already been discussed, and more recently, to certain physiologic and biochemical derangements. None of these factors provides a satisfactory explanation of the primary disorder, however.

The symptoms of fear resemble those of an anxiety attack in many ways, though nearly always the symptoms of the latter are longer in duration and less distinct. The most important distinction, however, is that with fear the cause is known and with anxiety it is not.

On the physiologic and biochemical side it has been observed that anger provokes an excessive secretion of norepinephrine, whereas fear is accompanied by increased secretion of epinephrine. Actually fear activates the whole autonomic nervous system, but the increase in epinephrine is more than counterbalanced by a parasympathetic discharge. The responsiveness of the autonomic nervous system remains heightened in chronic anxiety. Easton and Sherman report that in six patients who had been having anxiety attacks infusion of isoproteronol reproduced their attacks whereas it had no such effect in controls. This suggests a hyperresponsivity of beta-adrenergic receptors. Others (Bourne et al.) dispute this theory pointing out that some normal individuals will have the same reaction. Another interesting observation is that the blood lactic acid levels are abnormally high, especially after mild exercise, and injections of lactic acid are said to trigger anxiety symptoms. The presence of these physiologic derangements does not mean that they are causal; more likely they are secondary to the inactivity and apprehension associated with the syndrome.

DIFFERENTIAL DIAGNOSIS

Shorn of the psychological components of apprehension and fear, the anxiety attack consists essentially of an autonomic discharge. Some of the autonomic symptoms are duplicated by chromaffin tumors, hyperthyroidism, and the menopause. The prominence of chest pain and respiratory distress during an acute anxiety attack may cause it to be mistaken for myocardial ischemia. Strict criteria for the clinical diagnosis of these latter disease states readily permit their differentiation from anxiety neurosis.

Of greater importance is the distinction between anxiety neurosis and depression. Symptoms of depression are frequently added to those of anxiety neurosis, and the majority of patients with depression have symptoms of anxiety. Indeed, there are many psychiatrists who believe that anxiety neurosis is only a variant of depression. As has been mentioned, an anxiety state appearing for the first time after the fortieth year usually proves to be a depression. The uncovering of paranoid symptoms in a patient with an anxiety state should always raise the question of depression, as should the presence of symptoms such as self-depreciation and feelings of hopelessness.

Schizophrenia may begin with prominent anxiety symptoms. Here the differentiation rests on the finding of the characteristic thought disorder of schizophrenia, which may emerge only after several interviews. Hysteria also includes anxiety symptoms, as do phobic and obsessive-compulsive neurosis, but each has other distinguishing attributes.

TREATMENT

Rather little information is available as to the efficacy of different methods of treatment. There is no evidence that sophisticated psychotherapy is of more value than an explanation of the nature of the illness and reassurance that the symptoms have no ominous significance. A cardiac consultation and some simple tests (ECG, chest films) may be needed to reinforce the diagnosis of the primary physician and to alleviate fear of heart disease. Brief admission to a hospital for this purpose is often justified. Propranolol (Inderal), 10 to 20 mg tid, blocks many of the autonomic accompaniments, and diazepam (Valium), 5 mg tid, or chlordiazepoxide (Librium), 10 mg tid, may also suppress symptoms to some extent. If depressive symptoms are in evidence, amitriptyline 150 mg/day in divided doses should be given. As with all neuroses, the physician must develop and maintain a psychotherapeutic program involving discussion, reassurance, and explanation as to the nature of the illness.

The remission rate with simple medical measures is about 50 percent within 3 months, and the rate is not much higher with the most intense psychotherapy (58 percent in one series). Patients whose anxiety state persists should always be suspected of having an endogenous depression.

NEURASTHENIA

Literally the word means "nervous weakness," and the closest equivalent as a medical symptom is chronic fatigability. The latter was discussed in Chap. 23, as one of the cardinal manifestations of disease. Once considered an important neurosis, the diagnosis of neurasthenia is now obsolete. The careful study of patients with the complaint of chronic fatigue usually reveals that they are suffering from anxiety neurosis or depression. When lifelong, it may resemble more a character disorder than a neurosis (the asthenic psychopathy of Kahn; see Table 55-1). In the authors' experience, most patients designated as chronic neurasthenics are depressed and will recover under the influence of antidepressive therapy.

PHOBIC NEUROSIS

In this state patients are overwhelmed by an intense and irrational fear of some object, situation, or disease. Though acknowledging that there are no rational grounds for this fear (hence it is not a delusion), they are nonetheless powerless to suppress it.

Mild phobias of darkness, solitude, animals, and high places are commonplace in childhood; some persist into adult life and may be culturally acceptable, such as fear of snakes or mice. In phobic neurosis, however, the patient is chronically fearful of a particular object or situation and may be panic-stricken or incapacitated by the phobia. For example, it may be impossible for the patient to leave the house or neighborhood except when attended by a relative or friend, or to mingle in a crowd (ochlophobia). The patient may be unable to eat certain foods, ride in cars or planes, have sexual intercourse, eat in public, urinate in the presence of others, etc. Feelings of helplessness, pessimism, and despondency may result. Often there are obsessive-compulsive tendencies as well, and some patients are hypochondriacal. The authors have observed a number of patients whose phobic (or obsessive-compulsive) neurosis decompensated as an endogenous depression developed. Recovery from the depression returned them to their earlier and milder phobic state.

OBSESSIVE-COMPULSIVE NEUROSIS

Like the pure phobic states, a neurosis dominated by obsessions and compulsions is rare, occurring in not more than 1 to 2 percent of patients seeking help in a psychiatric outpatient clinic. On the other hand, minor compulsions (not stepping on cracks in the sidewalk, etc.), like minor phobias, are common in children, cause little or no distress, and disappear in later life. Certain irrational habits and rigid obsessional ways of thinking are frequent and persistent but excite little attention medically until they interfere with some diagnostic procedure or the therapy of some disease.

Obsessive-compulsive or *obsessional neurosis,* as it is usually designated, begins, as do the other neuroses, in adolescence or early adult years. The two sexes are equally affected. Onset is usually gradual and cannot be accurately dated, but in some cases it is precipitated by some event in the life of the patient, such as death of a relative, sexual conflict, etc.

Obsessions may be defined as imperative and distressing thoughts and impulses which persist in the patient's mind despite a desire to be rid of them. Obsessions are of various forms. The most common are the *intellectual obsessions,* in which phrases, rhymes, ideas, or vivid images (these are often absurd, blasphemous, obscene, and some may be frightening) constantly intrude into consciousness; *impulsive obsessions,* in which the mind is dominated by an impulse to kill oneself, to stab one's children, or to perform some other objectionable act; *inhibiting obsessions,* in which every act must be ruminated upon and analyzed before it is carried out—a state aptly called *doubting mania.* Every effort of will or deliberate attempt at distraction fails to rid the patient of the obsessive thought. It engulfs the mind, rendering the person miserable and inefficient. Probably the most disturbing of these obsessions are the impulsive ones, in which patients constantly struggle with the fear that they will put some terrible thought into execution. Even as they tell of the obsession they seek reassurance that they will not yield to it. Fortunately, such patients rarely obey their pathologic impulses. Phobias are essentially *obsessive fears* and should probably be included in this category of neurosis. The most common phobias are those of open places, closed places, high places, dogs, dirt, sprays and other contaminants, traveling, syphilis, cancer, insanity, and death.

Compulsions are acts that result from obsessions. These are single acts or a series of acts (rituals) which the patient feels must be carried out in order to put the mind at ease or relieve nervousness. Examples are repeatedly checking the gas jets or the locks on doors, adjusting articles of clothing, repeated hand washing, wiping with a clean handkerchief objects which have been touched, tasting foods in specific ways, touching objects in a particular sequence, etc.

Certain motor disturbances, namely habit spasms or tics, are (in a sense) motor compulsions. They consist of repetitive movements of the shoulders, arms, hands, and certain of the facial muscles (see Chap. 5). Their outstanding feature, which separates them from involuntary movements of extrapyramidal type, is that they are accomplished with an accompanying awareness that they must be done to relieve tension (see page 77). Unlike compulsions, however, tics are not based on obsessive thoughts.

In all these obsessions and compulsions, and in the phobias, patients recognize the irrationality of their ideas and behavior, yet are powerless to control them, much as they desire to do so. It is this insight into the obsessional experience and the struggle against it that distinguish obsessions from delusions.

The majority of these patients are tense, irritable, and apprehensive. They suffer a curious feeling of insufficiency or incompetency in being unable to expel their troublesome thoughts. The most distraught emotional state, as indicated above, is related to the fear that an idea may eventuate in reality. These patients may complain of typical anxiety attacks, and after the condition has persisted for a time they may become depressed. Fatigue, anorexia, and general lack of interest, which are often present, are probably related to the anxiety and depression.

MECHANISMS OF PHOBIC AND OBSESSIVE NEUROSES

Janet believed that individuals with phobias and obsessions differ from normal in that they have less power of mental inhibition and that the processes of attention do not function normally, which is why distracting and irrelevant thoughts cannot be eliminated. Indecisiveness was thought to be another common manifestation of this state. For all these defects Janet suggested the term *psychasthenia;* by this he vaguely implied a genetic origin but offered no evidence on this point.

The psychoanalysts theorize that psychasthenic behavior is the result of the imperfect repression of some disagreeable wish. They conceive of this wish as having both an ideational and an emotional or affective content. If the disagreeable wish is completely repressed, the psychic energy may be converted into a physical symptom such as paralysis or anesthesia (conversion hysteria). If repression is imperfect or incomplete, so that only the ideational content is repressed, the psychic energy may be converted into fear (phobia), or into another idea which then becomes an obsession. They attribute the persistence of the phobia or obsession to the emotional energy derived from another idea, which cannot be recalled except by the aid of free association.

To the neurologist, both Janet's and Freud's theories appear to be only partial explanations. One expects that some more basic defect, as yet unexplained, must allow these irrational ideas or fears to dominate the mind.

DIAGNOSIS

Since the prevailing emotional state in patients with phobias and obsessions is one of anxiety and depression, it is necessary to distinguish between phobic and obsessional neuroses, anxiety neurosis, and depressive psychosis. In phobic and obsessive neuroses the depression tends to be inconstant and closely related to a sense of weariness and helplessness in overcoming the irrational fears and obsessive thinking. As the latter improve the depression lightens. In uncomplicated anxiety states, although baseless fears are not uncommon, they are never so persistent or so disabling as in psychasthenia; also the indecisiveness and compulsive tendencies are lacking. Schizophrenia must be considered when an adolescent or young adult begins to harbor peculiar ideas, but then the mental status almost invariably reveals the other disturbances in affectivity, thought, and attention, which are described on pages 1050 and 1051.

TREATMENT OF PHOBIC AND OBSESSIONAL NEUROSES

This is best left to psychiatrists, or at least there should be a trial of psychotherapy in most cases. In the case of phobic neurosis, the aim of treatment is to reduce the patient's fear to the extent that exposure to the phobic situation can be tolerated. The most popular form of therapy in recent years has been so-called *systematic desensitization* (Wolpe), which consists of graded exposure of the patient to the object or the situation which arouses fear.

Those cases of obsessional neurosis which are cyclic in nature, with exacerbations and remissions and with no apparent relationship to environmental factors, have the best prognosis. Some psychiatrists treat this cyclic form like cyclic depressions, with electroconvulsive therapy (ECT) and antidepressant drugs. It is not certain that these measures accomplish more than can be attributed to the spontaneous changes in the disease. More often the course of obsessional neurosis is steady and

severely disabling, and in these patients the outlook for recovery is poor. ECT has helped some patients, in whom there has been a strong element of depression. Tranquilizing drugs are being used, but their efficacy is uncertain.

Cingulotomy has reportedly produced symptomatic improvement in both phobic and obsessional neuroses. This measure, if it is to be used at all, should be considered only as a last resort in exceptionally severe cases, in which the patient has failed to respond to all other methods of treatment and is totally disabled.

HYSTERIA (Hysterical Neurosis, Dissociative State, Conversion Reaction)

Although hysteria has been known since ancient times, it was the French physician Briquet who in 1859 first described the syndrome as we know it today. Later, Charcot elaborated on certain manifestations of the disease, and interested Freud and Janet in it. Charcot believed that the symptoms could be produced and relieved by hypnosis (mesmerism). Janet postulated a dissociative state of mind to account for certain features such as trance and fugue states. Freud and his students conceived of hysterical symptoms as a product of "ego defense mechanisms," in which psychic energy, the product of unconscious psychic conflicts, is converted into physical symptoms. This latter explanation has been widely accepted, so that the term *conversion* has been incorporated into the nomenclature of the neurosis and the terms *conversion symptoms* and *conversion reaction* have come to be equated with the disease hysteria. In the authors' opinion, the term *conversion symptoms*, if it is used at all, should refer only to certain unexplained symptoms, such as amnesia, paralysis, blindness, aphonia, etc., which mimic neurologic disease. *Hysteria* should be viewed as a disease practically confined to women and characterized further by a distinctive age of onset, natural history, and many somatic symptoms and signs, which typically include "conversion symptoms" and dissociative reactions.

The term *hysteria* has a number of other connotations, most of them pejorative. Lay people refer to individuals showing tantrums or losing self-control in the face of an emotional crisis as "hysterical." Some psychiatrists dub any dramatic, histrionic, manipulative, or "seductive" behavior as hysterical (referring to the *hysterical personality*), or equate hysteria with hypersuggestibility and susceptibility to hypnosis. These are traditional ideas based on the incorrect belief that these qualities are typical of hysteria.

In clinical neurology one encounters two types of patients with hysteria: (1) young women with a chronic illness marked by multiple and often dramatically presented symptoms and somatic abnormalities for which no cause is evident; (2) men and women who develop physical symptoms or remain inexplicably disabled for the purpose of obtaining compensation, avoiding military duty, imprisonment, etc. This latter state is called *compensation neurosis* or *compensation hysteria*.

CLASSIC, OR FEMALE, HYSTERIA (BRIQUET'S DISEASE)

This neurosis usually has its onset in the teens or early twenties. A few cases may begin before puberty. Once established, hysteria is a life-long illness and symptoms continue to recur intermittently, though with lessening frequency, throughout adult years, even to an advanced age. There are, no doubt, cases of lesser severity which exhibit symptoms only a few times or perhaps only once, just as there are mild forms of all diseases. The patient may be seen for the first time during the middle period of life or later, and the earlier history may not at first be obtained. Careful probing, however, will almost invariably reveal that the earliest manifestations of this illness had appeared before the age of 25 years.

Other important data are also brought to light by a careful past history. During late childhood and adolescence, the normal activities of the patient, including education, have usually been interrupted by periods of illness. Rheumatic fever, tuberculosis, or some obscure disease may have been suspected. Later in life, problems in work adjustment and marriage are frequent. There is a notably high incidence of marital incompatibility, separation, and divorce. The patient's life history is punctuated by symptoms which do not conform to recognizable patterns of medical and surgical disease. For these, many forms of therapy, including surgical operations, will have been performed. Rarely has adult life been reached without at least one abdominal operation, usually done because of pain, persistent nausea and vomiting, or some vague gynecologic complaint. The indications for the surgical procedures have usually been unclear, and, further, the same symptoms or others have recurred to complicate the convalescence. The biographies of these patients are also replete with disorders which center about menstrual, sexual, and procreative functions. Menstrual periods may be painfully prostrating, irregular, or excessive. Sexual intercourse may be painful, unpleasant, or unsatisfactory. Pregnancies may be difficult; the usual vomiting of the first trimester may persist all through the gestational period, with weight loss and prostration; labor may be severe and prolonged,

and all manner of unpredictable complications are said to have occurred during and after parturition.

Hysteria is, then, a polysymptomatic disorder, involving almost every organ system. The most frequent symptoms, all statistically significant, which were elicited during a study of 50 unmistakable cases of female hysteria as compared with a control group of 50 healthy women, included the following: headache, blurred vision, lump in the throat, loss of voice, dyspnea, palpitation, anxiety attacks, anorexia, nausea and vomiting, abdominal pain, food dyscrasia, severe menstrual pain, sexual indifference, painful intercourse, paresthesias, dizzy spells, nervousness, and easy crying (Purtell et al.).

The examination of the female hysteric demonstrates a number of useful findings, mostly in the sphere of mental status. The patient's response to questions regarding the chief complaint usually elicits a vague reply or the narration of a series of incidents or problems, many of which prove to have little or no relevance to the question. However, unlike the situation in a psychotic illness, the patient's ideas about most aspects of her life are sensible, and there is no evidence of hallucinations, delusions, disturbance in logical thinking, or loss of appreciation of the reality of the situation. The manner of the patient is often amiable and even ingratiating. The description of symptoms tends to be dramatic and exaggerated and does not accord with the facts as elicited from other members of the family; yet at the same time a rather casual demeanor is manifested. The patient may insist that everything in her life is quite normal and controlled, when, in fact, her medical record is checkered with instances of dramatic behavior and unexplained illness. This calm attitude toward a turbulent illness and seemingly disabling physical signs is so common that it has been singled out as an important characteristic of hysteria, *la belle indifférence*. Other patients, however, are obviously tense and anxious, and frank anxiety attacks are reported by many of them; or the patient may be effusive in her enthusiasms, fickle and flighty, always putting on an act, and demanding constant attention. Her emotional reactions are superficial and she creates scenes that are disturbing to others but are quickly forgotten. If physical disorders are present, attempts by the physician to disprove the somatic nature of the complaints usually meet with anxiety and vehement protest. Memory defects (amnesic gaps) are usually demonstrated while the history is being taken; the patient appears to have forgotten important segments of the his-

PART VI / PSYCHIATRIC DISORDERS

tory, some of which she had clearly described in the past and are part of the medical record.

There are no characteristic physical findings. Although many writers have commented on the rather youthful, girlish appearance and coquettish manner of the patients, this by no means characterizes all of them. The so-called stigmas of hysteria, i.e., corneal anesthesia, absence of gag reflex, spots of pain and tenderness over the scalp, sternum, breasts, lower ribs, and ovaries, are often suggested by the examiner and are too inconsistent to be of much help in the diagnosis. The only limit to the variation and pleomorphism of the physical signs is the patient's ability to produce them by an effort of will. Accordingly, symptoms and signs which are beyond volitional control cannot be accepted as manifestations of hysteria.

SPECIAL HYSTERICAL SYNDROMES

A few hysterical syndromes recur with great regularity, and every physician may expect to encounter them. They may constitute some of the most puzzling diagnostic problems in medicine.

Hysterical Pain　This may involve any part of the body; generalized or localized headache, "atypical facial neuralgia," vague abdominal pain, back pain with camptocormia are the most frequent and most troublesome to the clinician. In many of these patients the response to analgesic drugs has been unusual, and some of them are addicted. They may respond to a placebo as though it were a potent drug, but it should be pointed out that this is a notoriously unreliable means of distinguishing hysterical pain from that of other diseases. The greatest error is to mistake the pain of osteomyelitis, metastatic carcinoma, or brain tumor, before other symptoms have developed, for a manifestation of hysteria. The most helpful diagnostic features of hysterical pain are the inability of the patient to give a clear, concise description of the type of pain, its location, and other features; the dramatic elaborations of its intensity and effects; its persistence, either continuous or intermittent, for long periods of time; the lack of conformation to known pain syndromes; the absence of other diseases which could account for pain; the assumption of bizarre attitudes and postures; and, most important, the coexistence of other symptoms of hysteria.

Hysterical Vomiting　This is often combined with pain and tenderness in the lower abdomen and results in unnecessary appendectomies and removal of pelvic organs in adolescent girls and young women. The vomiting is somewhat unusual, in that it often occurs after a meal, leaving the patient hungry and ready to eat again; it may be induced by unpleasant circumstances. Some of these patients can vomit at will, regurgitating food from the stomach like a ruminant animal. Vomiting may persist for weeks with no cause being found. Weight loss may occur but seldom to the degree anticipated. The usual first-trimester vomiting of pregnancy may continue throughout the entire 9 months, and occasionally pregnancy will be interrupted because of it. Anorexia may be another prominent symptom.

Hysterical Seizures, Trances, and Fugues　These conditions seem to be less frequent than in the days of Charcot, when *la grande attaque d'hystérie* was often exhibited before medical audiences. Nevertheless they do occur and must be distinguished from convulsive seizures and catalepsy. To witness an attack is of great assistance in diagnosis. The lack of aura, initiating cry, hurtful fall, and incontinence; the presence of peculiar movements such as grimacing, squirming, biting, striking at or resisting those who offer assistance; the retention of consciousness during a motor seizure which involves both sides of the body; the long duration of the seizure and abrupt termination by strong sensory stimulation, are all typical of the hysterical attack. Sometimes hyperventilation will initiate an attack and is therefore a useful diagnostic maneuver. Both epilepsy and hysteria may be combined in the same patient, in which instance the resulting illness invariably causes difficulty in diagnosis. Hysterical trances or fugues, in which the patient wanders about for hours or days and carries out complex acts, may also simulate temporal lobe epilepsy or any of the conditions which lead to confusional psychosis or stupor. Here the most reliable point of differentiation comes from observation of the patient, who, if hysterical, is likely to indicate a degree of alertness and promptness of response not seen in confusional states. Following the episode, an interview with the patient, under the influence of hypnosis, strong suggestion, or amobarbital, will often bring to light memories of what happened during the episode; this will exclude the possibility of an epileptic fugue.

Hysterical Paralyses and Tremors　Hysterical palsies usually involve an arm, a leg, one side of the body, or both legs. If the affected limb can be moved at all, muscle action is weak, and often the strength of voluntary

1022

movement is in proportion to the resistance offered. Movements are characteristically slow, tentative, and poorly sustained. One can feel agonist and antagonist muscles contracting simultaneously. When the resistance is suddenly withdrawn, there is no follow-through or rebound, as is normally the case. The muscular tone in the affected limbs is usually normal, but rigidity may sometimes be found. Walking may be impossible, there may be a veritable astasia-abasia, or the gait may be bizarre (see page 85). This discrepancy between the inability to walk and to move the legs is, of course, not unique to hysteria; it also occurs in so-called frontal lobe apraxia and in ataxia from midline cerebellar lesions. If the limb has been held in a rigid posture for a long time, contractures may set in. The features of hysterical tremor, described on page 72, need not be repeated here. The tendon reflexes are always normal, but with hysterical anesthesia of one-half the body, the abdominal and plantar reflexes may be suppressed on the affected side. Anesthesia or hypesthesia is almost always inadvertently induced by the examining physician. Seldom is sensory loss a spontaneous complaint of the patient, although symptoms of "numbness" and paresthesias are not uncommon. The sensory loss may involve one or more limbs below a sharp line (stocking and glove distribution) or may involve one-half the body. Touch, pain, taste, smell, vision, and hearing may all be affected on that side, which is an anatomic impossibility from a single lesion.

Hysterical Amnesia Patients brought to a hospital in a state of amnesia, not knowing their own identity, are usually hysterical or psychopathic males involved in a crime. Usually after a few hours or days, with encouragement, they divulge their life history. Epileptic patients or victims of a concussion or acute confusional psychosis do not come to a hospital asking for help in establishing their identity. Moreover, the complete loss of memory for all previous life experiences by a patient who is otherwise able to comport himself normally is not observed in any other conditions.

In *Ganser's syndrome* (amnesia, disturbance of consciousness, and hallucinations), patients pretend to have lost their minds or to have become insane. They act in an absurd manner, in the way they believe an insane or feebleminded person should act, and give senseless answers to every question asked of them.

Unexplained Hyperpyrexia Among the sporadic cases of unexplained fever which turn up in every diagnostic clinic, there are always a few hysterics. One cannot help but be impressed with the number of student nurses,

nurses, and nurses' aides among this group of patients. Some of them will be found to have no fever if the nurse or doctor checks the temperature. Others have oral temperatures of 37 to 38°C (99 to 100°F), which must be regarded as normal for some individuals. Finally, there are a few well-documented cases of verified hyperpyrexia, said to be of psychogenic origin. In these the possibility of some obscure hypothalamic disorder cannot be excluded. Diagnosis is assisted by a longitudinal history and the elicitation of the other symptoms of hysteria.

Dermatitis Factitia (Hysterical Dermatoneurosis) This condition is seen more often in the psychopathic than in the hysterical patient. The skin eruptions induced by the patient are characterized by erythema, ulcerations, gangrene, and variable degrees of dermatitis. Usually a caustic or irritant chemical or a sharp instrument such as a nail file has been used. The lesions are most commonly observed on parts of the body accessible to the right hand, i.e., right side of the face, neck, anterior trunk, anterior surface of left arm. They are multiple, sharply outlined, appear at variable intervals of time, and do not conform to any of the standard dermatologic diseases. They resist all treatment until protected from the persistent manipulations of the patient, and then they heal promptly.

HYSTERIA IN MEN (COMPENSATION NEUROSIS IN MEN AND WOMEN)

As stated before, hysterical symptoms do occur in men, most often in those trying to avoid serious legal difficulties or military service, or trying to obtain disability payments, veteran's pensions, or compensation following injury. Male sociopaths may also present with this type of illness. Therefore the diagnosis of hysteria in the male should be made with great caution unless some obvious compensation factor is present. In compensation neurosis, as in the classical form of hysteria described above, multiple symptoms are noted in the majority of cases. Furthermore, many of the symptoms are the same as those listed under female hysteria. Descriptions of symptoms tend to be lengthy and circumstantial, and the patient fails to give details which are necessary in diagnosis. A tangible gain from the illness may be discovered by simple questioning. This is usually in the form of monetary compensation, which surprisingly, is often less than the patient could earn if he returned to work. Another interesting feature is the frequency with which the patient expresses extreme dissatisfaction with the medical care given him; he is often hostile toward the physicians and nurses. Many of these patients have already been subjected to an excessive number of hospitalizations when first seen, and rather dramatic mishaps have allegedly occurred in carrying out diagnostic and therapeutic procedures. The majority of these patients have been suspected and many have been accused of malingering in the past, which may be responsible for the aggressive behavior and uncooperative attitude of some of them.

Women who suffer injury at work or are involved in auto accidents may exhibit these same symptoms and signs. Both men and women with hysterical personalities may also be excessively disposed to accidents. This is one of the causes of the *accident-prone syndrome.*

DIAGNOSIS

The method of diagnosis subject to the least error is that employed in medicine generally, i.e., obtaining an informative history (from the patient as well as from sources other than the patient) and performing a physical and mental status examination. The characteristic time of onset, the longitudinal history of recurrent multiple complaints, as outlined above, the manner and attitude of the patient, and the absence of symptoms and signs of other medical and surgical disease will permit an accurate diagnosis in the majority of cases.

So-called projective tests (Rorschach and Thematic Apperception Tests), which for a time were popular with dynamic psychiatrists, are not useful in diagnosis and are now used very little. Evidence of extreme suggestibility and the tendency to dramatize symptoms cannot be taken as absolute criteria of the disease, for they appear under certain conditions in nonhysterical individuals.

TREATMENT

The treatment of hysteria may be considered from two aspects—the correction of the long-standing basic personality defect, and the removal of the recently acquired physical symptoms. Little or nothing can be done about the former. Psychoanalysts have attempted to modify it by long-term reeducation, but their results are unavail-

able, and there are no control studies for the few reports of therapeutic success. One has the impression that in most cases the underlying illness is so pervasive that nothing can be accomplished except to grant that the patient is inadequate in certain respects and requires medical support. Many psychiatrists, for this reason, are inclined to regard the female hysteric with a lifelong history of ill health as having a severe personality disorder (see Chap. 55). In other less-severe cases and especially in those in whom the hysterical symptoms have appeared under the pressure of a major crisis, psychotherapy appears to be helpful, and the patients have been able thereafter to resume their places in society.

The acute symptoms can usually be controlled by persuasion. Here the best tactic is to treat the patient as though she has had an illness and is now in the process of recovering. The earlier this is done after the development of symptoms, the more likely they are to be relieved. In chronically bedridden patients, strong pressure to get out of bed and resume function must be applied. Compensation neuroses are quite difficult to treat, and a settlement of the patient's claim is often necessary before the symptoms subside.

The following therapeutic principles should be observed in the classical cases of female hysteria:

1. Hysteria must be treated as a tangible, definite illness. The patient should not be told, "There is nothing wrong with you," or "It's just your imagination." This at once alienates her, and she almost invariably terminates her relations with the physician. The patient should not be dismissed as a malingerer or a faker of illness.

2. Simple understandable language should be employed in interviews with these patients; abstruse psychological terms should be avoided. It is unnecessary to employ the term *hysteria* in discussions with these patients or their families, since it has a derogatory connotation which the physician should not imply.

3. The care of the patient should be entrusted to one physician.

4. All indicated examinations and laboratory procedures for the investigation of the chief complaints should be conducted before actual treatment is begun. Once treatment is started, one should avoid, if possible, checking or repeating physical or laboratory examinations.

5. Persuasion and suggestion, both direct and indirect, should be employed in the treatment of patients. Illustratively, the patients should be encouraged, told that they are improving, urged to resume work or house-

hold duties and to continue participation in routine activities. Medication should be withheld.

6. There should be several personal interviews in which the patient is permitted to direct the discussion. She should be assured of the privacy of the interview, of the impersonal, "morally neutral" position of the physician, and of the advantages of "thinking things out more thoroughly." Any questions which the patient asks should be answered truthfully in accordance with the physician's knowledge, in simple, direct terms.

7. Every illness in such patients should be evaluated as a possible manifestation of hysteria, but the possibility of other diseases must not be overlooked. Surgical procedures should be used only if strict criteria of surgery-requiring disease are satisfied.

How successful this program will be over a long period of time is not known. The eradication of some recently acquired hysterical symptom is relatively easy. The real test of therapy, however, is whether it enables the patient to adjust satisfactorily to family and society and to perform daily activities effectively, whether it prevents addiction, unnecessary medical treatments, and operations, and whether it makes possible the prompt diagnosis of any medical or surgical disease, which may strike a hysterical patient just as it does any other person.

HYPOCHONDRIACAL NEUROSIS AND NEUROTIC DEPRESSION

Hypochondriasis, the morbid preoccupation with bodily functions or physical symptoms, is a common expression of emotional disease. Typically, hypochondriacal symptoms occur in association with other neurotic, psychiatric, and organic syndromes, and many psychiatrists have questioned its status as a nosologic entity. It is no longer included as a diagnostic category in the *Diagnostic and Statistical Manual* of the American Psychiatric Association. Some psychiatrists still speak of the *hypochondriacal personality,* in which concern for health and relationships with physicians are involved in chronic patterns of maladaptation, and of *hypochondriacal neurosis,* which is a decompensation from a healthier, more mature level of adjustment. Unlike hysterical neurosis and psychophysiologic disorders, in which there also may be morbid preoccupations with physical processes, this neurosis entails no disorder of bodily function. These and other features of hypochondriasis are discussed in the following chapter.

Also, there is dispute about the existence of *neurotic depression* as a diagnostic entity. That disagreement about this category of illness should exist is not surprising, considering the number of private meanings that are attached to it (see also Chap. 54). A review of some of the writings on this subject discloses that neurotic depression has been distinguished from endogenous depression on the basis of the following criteria: (1) patients with endogenous depressions recover spontaneously, or in response to electroshock or antidepressive drug treatment, in contrast to those with neurotic depressions; (2) patients with endogenous depressions suffer guilt and remorse, whereas the neurotics tend to blame others for their distress; (3) absence of diurnal variation of mood in neurotic depressions, and of insight in endogenous depression; (4) certain differences in heredity, body build, and premorbid personality; and (5) absence of psychotic symptoms (delusions, hallucinations, etc.).

Certainly not all psychiatrists agree that a valid distinction exists between the psychotic and neurotic forms of depression. Aubrey Lewis, on the basis of a detailed study of 61 hospitalized depressed patients, denied that any of the foregoing criteria had any differentiating significance.

REFERENCES

BOURNE HR, THOMSON PD, MELMON KL: Diagnosis and treatment of β-adrenergic receptor hyperresponsiveness: A critical appraisal. *Arch Intern Med* 125:1063, 1970.

COHEN ME et al: Neurocirculatory asthenia, anxiety neurosis or the effort syndrome. *Arch Intern Med* 81:260, 1948.

EASTON JD, SHERMAN DG: Somatic anxiety attacks and propranolol. *Arch Neurol* 33:689, 1976.

GOODWIN, DW, GUZE SB: *Psychiatric Diagnosis,* 2d ed. New York, Oxford University Press, 1979.

LEWIS A: Melancholia: A clinical survey of depressive states. *J Ment Sci* 80:277, 1934.

NEMIAH JC: Neurotic disorders, in Kaplan HI et al (eds): *Comprehensive Textbook of Psychiatry,* 3d ed. Baltimore, Williams & Wilkins, 1980, chap 21, pp 1483–1517.

PURTELL JJ et al: Observations on clinical aspects of hysteria. *J Am Med Assoc* 146:902, 1951.

ROBINS E et al: Hysteria in men. *N Engl J Med* 246:677, 1952.

WHEELER EO et al: Neurocirculatory asthenia (anxiety neurosis, effort syndrome, neurasthenia): A twenty year follow-up study of one hundred and seventy-three patients. *J Am Med Assoc* 142:878, 1950.

WOLPE J: *Psychotherapy by Reciprocal Inhibition.* Stanford, Calif; Stanford, 1958.

CHAPTER 54

GRIEF, REACTIVE DEPRESSION, ENDOGENOUS DEPRESSION, MANIC-DEPRESSIVE DISEASE, AND HYPOCHONDRIASIS

Depression is the cause of more human misery than any other single disease to which mankind is subject. This statement is taken from an article by Kline, an authority on the subject, and is shared by everyone in the field of mental health. Although it has been known for over 2000 years (melancholia is described in the writings of Hippocrates), there is still disagreement as to its medical status. Is depression a disease state (Kraepelinian concept), or a type of psychological reaction (Meyerian concept)? In other words, is it basically a response to stress and conflict with which a person cannot cope, or a biologic derangement?

Before elaborating on this problem, a few words are necessary to explain the grouping of entities listed in the title of this chapter. Depression, of course, is the symptom that relates all of them to one another, but the setting in which the depression occurs, differences in other clinical attributes, and the fact that each requires somewhat different management permit the recognition of a number of distinctive clinical states. Taken together, they are the most frequent of all psychiatric illnesses. At the New England Center Hospital, for example, as indicated on page 1016, they accounted for an estimated 50 percent of psychiatric and 12 percent of all medical admissions. Grief reactions are ubiquitous but only exceptionally do they demand hospitalization.

Some illnesses in this group, also spoken of as the *affective disorders,* take the form of a relatively pure, uncomplicated depression. Others are mixed with anxiety and agitation and because of their tendency to appear for the first time in middle and late adulthood, have been loosely referred to as *involutional.* Admittedly this term takes license with the concept of involution, for such diseases may occur at any time in late adult life and have no relationship to the climacteric. Some depressions are clearly reactions to real and imaginary life situations. If in proximate relation to the loss of a family member, the condition is called *grief*; if in relation to a life-threatening or disabling medical or neurologic disorder, it is referred to as a *reactive depression. Mania,* which is less frequent than depression, may develop as a relatively pure clinical state or alternate with depression in manic-depressive disease. Lastly there are depressions which present as *hypochondriasis.* Although this latter psychiatric syndrome may rarely occur as a protracted and obstinate neurosis, the presence of an underlying depression must always be considered when assessing a hypochondriacal patient.

The authors have the impression that depressive states are so often associated with obscure physical symptoms that they are more likely to come to the attention of general physicians and internists than are other psychiatric entities. They are frequently misdiagnosed, the symptoms being falsely attributed to anemia, low blood pressure, hypothyroidism, migraine, tension headaches, chronic pain syndrome, chronic infection, "nerves," and "emotional problems." Another reason why physicians should be knowledgeable about this group of illnesses is the danger of suicide, which may be attempted and successfully executed before the depression is recognized. Prompt diagnosis may prevent such a tragedy—a tragedy that is all the more regrettable since depressions can be successfully treated. In the following pages the *"masked depression"* as a diagnostic puzzle will be emphasized.

As remarked in Chap. 24, the term *depression* embraces more than a feeling of sadness and unhappiness. It is a complex of disturbed feelings (affect), particularly of hopelessness and loss of self-esteem, associated with abnormalities of thinking and behavior and prominent physical complaints, the most important of which are insomnia, anorexia, and decreased energy and libido. At one extreme are depressions of psychotic proportions, such as manic-depressive disease, which create chaos in the life of the patient and anyone close to the patient. At the other extreme are the normal reactions to the disappointments of everyday life, such as a loss of a relative or one's job or a failure to gain recognition. Since feelings of sadness, discouragement, and resentment are a natural part of life, the precise point at which they become pathologic may be difficult to specify. There are, however, diagnostic guidelines which should enable the physician to distinguish the endogenous from the reactive forms of depression.

CLASSIFICATION

There are four main types of depression with which the physician should be acquainted:

1. Grief reactions

2. Reactive depression

3. Depression in relation to neurosis

4. Endogenous depression (with or without agitation and anxiety) and manic-depressive disease

Since grief, in one of the forms to be described below, is the most common form of depression that the physician is likely to encounter, an important contemporary view of depression takes the grief reaction as a prototype. However, some psychiatrists question whether depression and grief are the same process. There are two schools of thought. Adolf Meyer and his followers regard depression as a continuum, with sadness and disappointment at one end and psychotic depressions at the other. In the Kraepelinian view, depression is a disease process quite independent of social and psychological forces, and the cause of the illness is "innate." Most writers on depression assume that there are two basic forms of depression: *exogenous* and *endogenous.* Exogenous, or reactive depressions, have an overt external cause, such as a loss of a loved one, loss of one's fortune or position, or a life-threatening illness. In this framework, the grief reaction would exemplify a typical reactive or exogenous depression. In contrast, the endogenous depressions have no apparent external cause; they seem to occur in susceptible individuals as a response to some unknown biologic stimulus. Endogenous depression and manic-depressive psychosis are typical forms of hereditary depression. To date the genetic data cited below support the Kraepelinian theory more than the other.

Another semantic problem relates to the differences between grief reaction, reactive depression, and psychoneurotic depression. All three are, in a sense, exogenous or reactive. In the nomenclature of the American Psychiatric Association reactive and psychoneurotic depressions are the same, both reactive. The authors distinguish between grief as a normal reaction, reactive depression as a prolonged and abnormal grief reaction, and psychoneurotic depression as a depressive state in a person with a psychoneurotic, lifelong social maladjustment. These distinctions are of therapeutic importance.

GRIEF REACTIONS

Grieving is a response to a loss, which may be real (as in the death of a spouse) or, in the opinion of some psychiatrists, symbolized. Psychological analysis of the typical grief reaction discloses the following characteristics (Lindemann):

1. An intense subjective sensation of mental pain accompanied by a feeling of exhaustion.

2. Preoccupation with the image of the deceased.

3. A sense of guilt concerning the relationship to the deceased.

4. Sometimes an inexplicable and unwarranted hostility toward friends and relatives.

5. A loss of the usual pattern of conduct. Bereaved persons are unable either to initiate or to organize their daily affairs and tend to perform routine tasks in an automatic and uninterested fashion.

The authors cannot vouch for the validity of each of these characteristics, but accept them as a reasonable formulation. There is no doubt, however, that a sense of exhaustion and disorganization of daily activities are invariable accompaniments.

The grief reaction lasts as a rule for a period of 4 to 12 weeks, by which time it begins to abate, with gradual resumption of normal activities that come to occupy the mind more and more of the time and expel thoughts of the deceased. Grieving is to be regarded as a natural human reaction to personal tragedy, and its absence in circumstances where it should be called forth is believed by psychiatrists to be abnormal. However, the overt expressions of grief are highly individual, depending on personality and cultural and other factors.

Distortions of the normal reaction to distress or personal loss are not infrequent; they are referred to as *pathologic grief.*

1. The most frequent distortion is *prolongation of the reaction*, i.e., there is no sign of resolution by the end of a 3-month period. Mothers who have lost a child tend to suffer for an unduly long period of time, and the elderly who have lost a spouse may never recover completely. Patients with a history of previous depressive episodes may also remain in mourning for longer periods. In general when a bereaved person has shown no improvement within 3 to 4 months of the loss, one should suspect a pathologic grief reaction and call for psychiatric consultation. Prolonged grief is a not unusual setting for suicide.

2. Another variation of the grief reaction is *delayed* or *postponed grief*. Often in an attempt to sustain the morale of others or to avoid the unpleasant spectacle of mourning, the patient may show little or no reaction to the loss. This "stiff-upper-lip" attitude is frequently admired and consequently reinforced, especially in Anglo-Saxon and Scandinavian cultures. According to some psychiatrists, the potential danger of this suppressed reaction is that the grief may find expression months or even years later in a delayed depression. (We find this interpretation of a depressive reaction rather speculative and would prefer to believe that the patient later develops an endogenous depression, in which past worries and sources of unhappiness are reinstated.)

3. In an effort to overcome sadness the bereaved person may become hyperactive and even euphoric. The elation is interpreted as a defense against depression. It may give way to a sudden reversal of mood, whereupon the individual is plummeted into a depression. In another variation of unacknowledged grief, bereaved persons embark on a series of social and economic adventures that may end in disaster. They may invest or gamble recklessly, turn away from old friends, or take up high-risk sports such as auto racing or skydiving. Rarely do they recognize the self-punitive nature of their activity or the guilt that is believed to lie behind it. Sometimes simply pointing this out helps such patients.

4. Occasionally patients will acquire the same symptoms as the deceased and may be convinced that they have the same disease. This may be the origin of some of the hypochondriacal ideas that accompany depressive reactions. The identification of this variant of grieving requires only that the examiner, after excluding the presence of disease in the patient for want of clinical evidence, inquire about the illness that took the life of the deceased.

Management of the usual grief reaction consists of expressing sympathy and helping the bereaved person to acknowledge the loss and to face the changes required as a result of it. The sooner the patient comes to a realistic acceptance of the loss and the need to restructure his or her life, the more swiftly the process will reach closure. Stoicism should not be encouraged or reinforced. To express sadness through tears, anguish, and even hostility is helpful for many individuals. The practice of treating grief-stricken patients with antidepressants is seldom effective, for it attempts to suppress what is a natural and necessary human reaction. Early on, undue restlessness and anxiety can be relieved by minor tranquilizers, and the insomnia by carefully prescribed hypnotics. Diazepam (Valium), 5 mg tid, or the equivalent dose of chlordiazepoxide (Librium) or oxazepam (Serax) is suitable for daytime sedation and can be used at bedtime for sleep by doubling the dose. Each of these drugs has a wide margin of safety, which decreases the danger of its use as a means of committing suicide. The possibility of suicide must be entertained in managing all depressed patients, including mourners, and care must be taken not to supply them with large doses of hypnotics.

In treating patients with pathologic grief reactions, the practitioner should enlist the help of a psychiatric colleague to see if the plan of treatment is sound; often these patients require specialized psychiatric help.

REACTIVE DEPRESSION

Depressed patients seldom, if ever, express feelings of sadness or despair without mentioning physical concomitants, such as the ease with which they tire, their loss of appetite, reduced interest in life and love, and trouble in falling asleep or premature awakening; it follows that whenever these symptoms become manifest in the course of medical disease they should arouse suspicion of a depressive reaction.

Chronic pain is a particularly frequent somatic manifestation of depression. The pain may be vague in nature and recalcitrant to most straightforward medical and surgical approaches, or in the beginning, it may have been caused by an arthritic hip, ruptured disk, or injury. One should question such individuals about recent losses or changes in status, disappointments, or dissatisfactions. All patients with chronic pain syndromes should be evaluated psychiatrically, as pointed out in Chap. 7.

In a number of major medical illnesses depressive symptoms occur with such frequency as to constitute important diagnostic and therapeutic problems; and in certain chronic, occult diseases, symptoms such as lassitude and fatigue resemble those of a depressive reaction. Hypothyroidism, infectious mononucleosis, infectious hepatitis, carcinoma of the head of the pancreas, metastatic carcinoma of the liver, malnutrition, and frontal lobe tumors may simulate depression for several weeks or months before the diagnosis becomes evident. Drugs such as reserpine, or any of the *Rauwolfia* derivatives, and the phenothiazines may evoke a depressive reaction; and the steroids can induce a peculiar psychiatric state in which confusion, insomnia, and depression or elevation of mood are combined. Depression may emerge during the tapering-off period of steroid medication.

Of even more significance are the depressions which occur on learning of medical and neurologic diseases. Often such an emotional reaction, which the physician has tended to ignore, may be the dominant manifestation of a devastating disease that threatens the life pattern and independence of the patient. Recognition of the presence of medical catastrophies such as myocardial infarction, cancer, multiple sclerosis, Parkinson's disease, and stroke is almost always followed by some degree of reactive depression.

An example is the depression that follows myocardial infarction. It begins usually toward the end of the patient's stay in the acute-care ward and continues through the rest of the hospitalization. Usually, too, it is a covert or silent depression and attracts little attention, the clinical manifestations being at first obscured by bed rest and hypnotic-sedative medication. Discouragement and a gloomy attitude toward the future are the principal indications of the state. The patient may not mention these concerns to the physician, assuming them to be trivial or likely to be misinterpreted as signs of fear or weakness of character. Once the patient is home, the depression becomes much more apparent both to him and his family. Fatigability which approaches exhaustion is the primary complaint and interferes with accustomed activities; it may be described as weakness and falsely attributed to a failing heart. Symptoms of irritability, anxiety, and despondency are next in order of frequency, followed by insomnia and feelings of aimlessness and boredom. When the time comes to return to work, fearful anticipation mounts and often results in long, unwarranted delays in ending the convalescent period. These are more apt to intrude themselves when the patient's occupation is physically or mentally stressful.

Though it is true that most of these patients ultimately recover without medical assistance (the disorder is, in this sense, self-limited), the toll that depression exacts in terms of suffering and anguish is enormous. Depression is probably the main cause of extended convalescence and retarded rehabilitation following myocardial infarction. Much of it could be prevented by proper intervention.

The first step in management is recognition of the depressive state. This can be greatly simplified if one assumes that all patients after coronary thrombosis are liable to depression and if a plan to deal with this is started during the acute stage of the illness. Such a program carries no risk for those unusual individuals who may not be depressed, and offers considerable benefit to those who are. One begins by assuring the patient that a sense of sadness and discouragement is normal and to be expected. Next, the patient should be advised that regular activities may not need to be curtailed as much as anticipated. This can be supplemented by giving examples of public figures, such as former Presidents Eisenhower and Johnson, who returned to active life following severe heart attacks. The patient is then given a program of graduated activity consistent with his or her cardiac condition. Physical conditioning is the best antidote for depression in the coronary patient; it raises self-esteem and reinstates a feeling of independence even when bed rest is still required. Once established, this schedule of activity should be carried through convalescence and maintained long after the patient has returned to work.

It is also important, in treating postcoronary depression, to instruct the patient about the disease. Patients have their own ideas about illness, which often do not conform to the facts. Misconceptions must be actively uncovered and corrected. The most prevalent misbeliefs surrounding myocardial infarctions include the following: exertion, even when mild, can kill you; sexual intercourse should never again be attempted; myocardial infarctions tend to recur at orgasm; recurrence is apt to take place on the anniversary of the first infarction; one is likely to die at the same age as did a parent from heart disease; recurrent infarctions are more likely to take place in sleep. After these and other misunderstandings have been corrected, the patient should be told which activities to continue and which to forgo. The spouse and children should be included in the discussions. Warning the patient what to expect almost always reduces the actual stress of an event and spares much torment. If the physician warns that it is normal to feel weak on returning home from the hospital and that this is not a sign of a failing heart, the patient is less apt to be alarmed when a sense of weakness does occur. The family should not be overprotective.

Sodium amytal, 100 mg tid, in combination with dextroamphetamine, 5.0 mg morning and noon, has been one of the most successful treatments of depressions of this type. The tricyclic antidepressants and monoamine oxidase (MAO) inhibitors are generally considered unsafe for use with coronary patients. Electric-shock therapy has been successfully and safely employed in postmyocardial infarction patients but should be used only if there is an endogenous depression severe enough to warrant it.

An analogous depressive reaction occurs in patients with strokes, and should be managed along the lines indicated above. Other neurologic diseases, such as paralysis agitans (Parkinson's disease), are complicated by a depressive reaction in one-quarter to one-half the cases. In this latter disorder, weakness and fatigability, the principal psychological manifestations, are added to the akinesia, and the resulting therapeutic problem becomes formidable. Another hazard in this disease is the tendency for L-dopa itself to provoke a depression, sometimes with suicidal tendencies, and other mental symptoms, such as paranoid ideation and psychotic episodes. The treatment of depression with MAO inhibitors is contraindicated in patients receiving L-dopa.

Cancer is another illness which is almost invariably attended by a depressive reaction. Aside from the prognosis, an important determinant of the severity of this depressive response is the attitude of the physician. In the nineteenth century, physicians tended to be quite open with their patients and gave an honest diagnosis and a straightforward prognosis. A mid-twentieth century survey of physicians' attitudes toward the truthful disclosure of these vital factors in patients with cancer revealed a disinclination toward candor. There seemed to be a direct relationship between the seriousness of the prognosis and the degree to which truth was rejected. Thus, over 90 percent of dermatologists but less than 20 percent of gynecologists chose to be frank, a disparity which relates to the control each of these specialists can exert over the malignancy. Basal-cell carcinoma can usually be removed entirely and survival ensured; the outlook in carcinoma of the cervix is far less hopeful. Thus the type of tumor, rather than the patient's personality, appeared to determine what was said. It was assumed that the patient, upon hearing that intervention offered uncertain success, would fall into a hopeless depression and that it would therefore be wiser to withhold information that could serve no useful purpose.

In the last two decades there has been a gratifying change in the psychological management of the cancer patient. It is now generally agreed that the patient should learn the truth in most instances and that withholding or distorting information seriously undermines the doctor-patient relationship. Furthermore, the facts of the illness, if presented with a ray of hope, can be coped with more readily than a tangle of half-truths, hollow reassurances, and furtive falsifications. The notion that patients can be kept blissfully unaware of their jeopardy while their closest relatives are fully informed is not sensible. This approach, which has aptly been called "the conspiracy of silence," not only fails to accomplish its purpose but isolates the patient at a time when all available human support is needed. In being truthful, physicians need not thrust all the harsh realities on each patient the moment the biopsy report returns, but they should make available whatever information is requested and maintain open communications with the patient throughout the course of the illness. Though some individuals cannot bear to hear the truth and ask not to be told, most patients want to know and should be told. It is important to remember that the cancer patient often phrases crucial questions indirectly, especially when fearful of the answer. Such persons might talk of buying a new house in an effort to get the doctor's opinion as to whether they will be around long enough to justify the expense. Such questions ought not to pass unnoticed. The physician should ask the patient what he or she means or to rephrase the question to bring out the hidden meaning.

A worry common to patients with cancer, yet seldom mentioned openly, is that the doctor will give up on them. This is particularly so in this era of the specialist, in which often no one physician is in overall charge. A firm, supportive doctor-patient relationship with mutual trust and respect is the best insurance against the fear of abandonment. Once this has been established, patients are usually able to cope with their depression without specific help from the physician. However, the latter should be ready to supply minor tranquilizers such as diazepam, 2 to 10 mg qid, if necessary. The dose may be doubled or tripled for use as a hypnotic at bedtime. If depression persists, it is justifiable to try a tricyclic antidepressant or a MAO inhibitor.

NEUROTIC DEPRESSION

This term has little precision. One view is to regard it simply as a condition of depression that occurs in an individual who exhibits or who has in the past exhibited the symptoms of anxiety neurosis or one of the other neurotic syndromes (hysteria, or phobic or obsessive-compulsive neurosis). Theoretically there is no illogic in assuming that a person harboring neurotic traits should on occasion (one chance in 20) be subject to an hereditary depression. Of course, a depression in response to a serious illness or a grief reaction, in other words a reactive depression, is as likely to occur in a neurotic individual as in a normal one.

The separation of this state from endogenous depression and reactive depression has not received universal acceptance. Some psychiatrists such as Mapother find no basis for separating neurotic from endogenous depression; others stress that there are differences in terms of heredity, prominence of vegetative signs, and delusional thinking, all being more positive in endogenous depression. Still others use the term *neurotic depression* synonymously with reactive depression. To further confuse the issue, some psychiatrists simply use the term *neurotic* to distinguish a relatively mild depression from a more severe or psychotic depression, and others use the term even more loosely, to designate depressions in persons with chronic character disorders or maladaptive personality patterns.

Our position on this controversy is to regard depressive symptoms as probably endogenous whenever there is not an obvious life circumstance to explain them, but if the patient has been neurotic throughout life, we give more attention to possible psychogenic mechanisms and to be more cautious in recommending electroconvulsive therapy (see page 1025 for further discussion).

ENDOGENOUS DEPRESSION AND MANIC-DEPRESSIVE PSYCHOSIS

DEFINITIONS AND EPIDEMIOLOGY

Manic-depressive disease or psychosis is a disorder of affect (mood) which consists of episodes of depression or mania, or both. Although it has been regarded traditionally as a periodic or cyclic condition in which one major mood swing is followed by an equal but opposite excursion, this is seldom the case. Depression is far more prevalent than mania, and the mixed variety, containing both extremes, is relatively uncommon. As a consequence, manic-depressive psychosis has been divided into two subtypes: a *unipolar group*, in which only an endogenous depressive illness occurs, and a *bipolar group*, in which mania occurs, with or without depression (contrary to one's initial impression of the term—that bipolar patients have *both* mania and depression).

The disease was given its name by Kraepelin in 1896, and it is with him that our current clinical concept of this disorder originates. He viewed the manic and depressive attacks as opposite poles of the same underlying process, and pointed out that unlike dementia praecox (his name for schizophrenia), manic-depressive psychosis entails no intellectual deterioration with recurrent episodes.

The incidence of manic-depressive disease cannot be stated with precision, mainly because of differing criteria for diagnosis. Apparently, British psychiatrists make the diagnosis of this disease more frequently than their American colleagues. Studies of large groups of patients from isolated areas of Iceland and the Danish islands of Bornholm and Samsø, indicate that 5 percent of men and 9 percent of women will develop symptoms of depression or mania, or both, sometime during their lives (Goodwin and Guze). The estimate for an American urban community (New Haven, Connecticut) is higher; the lifetime expectancy for an attack of major depression, with sexes combined, is 18 percent (Weissman and Myers). For Western nations in general, if attention is limited to manic-depressive illness, lifetime expectancy is 1 to 2 percent (Klerman).

Manic-depressive psychosis occurs most frequently in middle and later adult years, with a peak age of onset between 55 and 65 for both sexes. However, a small proportion of patients experience the first attack in childhood, adolescence, or early adult life. The disease is two or three times more frequent among women. It was reported, in the 1930s, to be more common in individuals of Jewish and Irish heritage and among those in upper socioeconomic strata, but subsequent studies have not confirmed these findings. The manic form tends to occur at an earlier age than the depressive, but episodes of depression are far more frequent than are episodes of mania at any age. The bipolar variety occurs in about 10 percent of patients with affective disorders.

CLINICAL PRESENTATION

The fully developed form of depression may evolve within a few days (acute onset) or merge gradually with vague prodromal symptoms that had been present for months. The symptoms and signs of depression were described in Chap. 24. It need only be stressed that the patient expresses feelings of sadness, helplessness, discouragement, and despondency, with loss of self-esteem and reduced energy for mental and physical activity. There is heightened irritability, as well as a lack of interest in all activity that was formerly pleasurable. Overwhelmed by feelings of worry and hopelessness, and by indecisiveness, these patients become increasingly dependent and incapable of acting in their own behalf. In despair, they express the desire for death and may become suicidal with very little warning. As pointed out in Chap. 24, any combination of weakness, easy fatigue, pain, anorexia, insomnia, loss of libido, and anxiety may dominate the clinical picture and may therefore simulate several medical diseases. At its worst the illness takes the form of a depressive stupor; patients become mute, indifferent to nutritional needs, and neglectful even of bowel and bladder functions. Their condition at this time resembles catatonia. They must be fed and their other needs attended to until therapy (usually electroconvulsive therapy) brings about an improvement. In some forms, delusional thought disorder and self-accusatory hallucinations (paranoid beliefs; conviction of hopeless disease when it does not exist) are prominent features. These are called psychotic depressions.

The *manic phase* is, in most ways, the mirror opposite of the depressed phase, being characterized by a flight of ideas, hyperactivity, and an increased appetite and sex urge. With a minimum of sleep the patient awakes in the morning filled with enthusiasm and expectation. The manic person appears to possess great drive and confidence, yet lacks the ability to carry out plans. Headstrong, impulsive, socially intrusive behavior is characteristic. Judgment is so poor in this disease that the patient may make reckless investments and spend fortunes in gambling and shopping sprees. Setbacks do not perturb the patient but rather act as goads for new activities. Euphoria and expansiveness sometimes bubble over into delusions of power and grandeur, which in turn may make the patient offensively aggressive. Up to a point, the mirth and good spirits may be contagious, and others may join in on the laughter; however, if thwarted, the warmth and good humor can suddenly change to anger. Irritability rather than elation may be the prevailing mood. The threshold for paranoid thinking is low, which makes the patient sensitive and suspicious. Personal neglect reaches the point of dishevelment and poor personal hygiene. In its most advanced form, a condition described as *delirious mania*, the patient becomes totally incoherent and altogether disorganized in behavior. At this stage visual and auditory hallucinations and paranoid delusions may be rampant; furthermore, as the term implies, the patient may be disoriented, with clouded sensorium. Fortunately, this extreme is rarely encountered.

Hypomania represents a milder degree of the disorder, but this term is also used loosely to depict normal behavior in which the individual is unusually energetic and active. In this latter sense hypomania is a personality trait found in many talented and productive persons, and need not arouse concern unless it is totally out of character for the individual. This is best determined by questioning the family.

First attacks of either depression or mania last an average of 6 months if untreated although the range of duration of attacks varies greatly. Modern therapy can reduce this by more than half. About 90 percent of manic-depressive patients recover from their first attack. For those who do not recover, there is often some pertinent reason in terms of their family or environment which serves to retard improvement. Attacks tend to be longer in older age groups. In a small number, the disease is chronic. About one-half of all depressed patients have one or more recurrences.

THE MONOPOLAR ENDOGENOUS DEPRESSION OF MIDDLE AND LATE LIFE

This type of depressive illness was formerly referred to as *involutional melancholia* and separated from other forms of manic-depressive disease by the less definite family history of depression, later age of onset, frequent conjunction with menopause, and greater prominence of anxiety and agitation. Each of these criteria have been challenged (see Winokur and Cadoret), so that now it is doubtful if involutional melancholia is anything more than endogenous monopolar depression of middle and late life. The authors accept this position and in the following paragraphs would only call attention to some of the more common characteristics of this group of patients. Here multiple physical complaints, some of which may be delusional in nature, generally accompany the symptoms of depression. Typically, there is no history of previous episodes.

There appears to have been a steady increase in the prevalence of this disorder over the last 50 years. Rather than an actual increase, however, this probably reflects a growing awareness of the condition by the lay population and an appreciation that such an entity as "middle-life depression" exists and can be treated. As in manic-depressive psychosis, women are affected more often than men, in a ratio of almost 3:1. There is no known cause for this sex difference, but some have speculated that just as many men are depressed, only they deny it or turn to alcohol.

The onset is most apt to be insidious, characterized by increased irritability, insomnia, psychomotor restlessness, easy fatigue, loss of interest in sexual and gustatory pleasures, and ever-mounting feelings of worthlessness and worry about health. These manifestations develop over one or more years before the clinical picture is complete. As time passes, the life of these individuals narrows to a single-minded concern about their physical deterioration, mental decline, or both. Before long, every conversation comes to balance on the fulcrum of symptoms, no matter how hard the patient may try to avoid that topic. In dialogue the rejoinders of such a person become so stereotyped that the listener can soon predict exactly what is going to be said. There is a poverty of ideation, as well as a notable absence of insight. Consciousness is clear, and though there is usually no evidence of a schizophrenic type of thought disorder, paranoia is not infrequently part of the picture. The suspicions and delusions are generally not as fixed or bizarre as in schizophrenia. If hallucinations are present, the possibility of an associated organic disease or drug intoxication must be considered. Frequently, agitation, rather than physical inactivity and mental slowness, is the principal behavioral abnormality. The source of the agitation is an underlying anxiety state. Pacing the floor, particularly in the early morning hours, is characteristic. Furthermore, the patients tend to be overtalkative and vexed in their manner of expression, so that the examiner is acutely aware of their mental distress. Attempts at reassurance may meet with initial success, only to be unseated in the next rush of doubts. These patients remain inaccessible to reason and logic as these apply to their symptoms, even though they may retain the capacity to exercise these functions in other areas of their life.

The most important concern in patients with late-life depression is the risk of suicide. Since so many of these individuals have reputations for being sound, dependable, and stable, one's prevailing attitude toward them is to reject the possibility of self-destruction. Furthermore, consumed as they often are by hypochondriacal ruminations, they may deny being depressed. Because of the high risk of suicide one should seek the advice of a psychiatrist as soon as the diagnosis is suspected.

DIFFERENTIAL DIAGNOSIS

1. *Mild, nonretarded depressions mistaken for chronic medical disease.* Such patients talk of weakness, tiredness, and exhaustion more than depressed mood. In fact, if one suggests they are depressed, they strongly disavow the possibility on the grounds that they have no reason to be. Any alteration of mood, they aver, is only a consequence of their illness. Correct diagnosis is achieved by searching for and eliciting all the standard symptoms of anxiety and depression and by adhering strictly to the criteria of medical disease. The most difficult situation arises when there is a chronic medical disease such as hypothyroidism, brucellosis, rheumatoid arthritis, chronic hepatitis, or influenza combined with a depression. The only solution to this problem is to eliminate the medical symptoms by treatment, and, if disability continues, to treat the depression.

2. *Depression and drug addiction associated with chronic pain.* Among patients who suffer chronic pain one frequently finds all the symptoms and signs of depression. Dependency on analgesic medicines, which in themselves deplete energy and have other side effects, is added. Such patients are to be found among those disabled after multiple operations for ruptured disk or arthritic hips, or those with atypical facial neuralgias, decompensated migraine, chronic rheumatic diseases, intractable angina pectoris, intercostal and occipital neuralgias, etc. Antidepressant medications have helped only a few of our patients, but daily electroshock treatments, to the point of confusion, have almost miraculously eradicated the pain in many of them. Drug addiction can be overcome at this time. An alternative is a locked psychiatric ward, withdrawal of the addicting drug(s), and use of antidepressant medication.

3. *Intractable headaches or anorexia.* The latter sometimes takes the form of anorexia nervosa in a child, adolescent, or young adult.

4. *Anxiety neurosis.* See Chaps. 24 and 54.

5. *Hypochondriasis.* See final section in this chapter.

ETIOLOGY

The following are some of the theories that have been put forth to explain the origin of depression.

Genetic Theories The capacity to experience sadness and depression is common to all people. There is no question that depression can be caused by adverse circumstances; however, in response to the same degree of loss, some individuals are more liable to depression than others. In general, there seems to be a familial diathesis for most depressive illness, but especially for manic-depressive psychosis and endogenous depression. Much work has been done on the inheritance of depression, most of which has dealt with these two affective psychoses. Undoubtedly the frequency of these illnesses is increased in the relatives of affected patients (prevalence rate of 10 to 25 percent in first-degree relatives). Similarly the morbidity risk among first-degree relatives is increased (15 percent, in comparison to 1 to 2 percent risk in the general population). Although the exact pattern of inheritance has not been defined, it is known that depression is not simply transmitted by either an autosomal dominant or recessive gene. If all twin studies are taken together, there is a concordance rate of 68 percent for monozygotic twins and 23 percent for same-sex dizygotic twins, clearly indicative of a genetic factor. The authors, from their personal experience, suspect that a dominant mode of heredity is likely.

Biochemical Theories The biogenic amines (norepinephrine, serotonin, and dopamine) are the key elements in this theory. Following the observations that antidepressant drugs, such as the tricyclic antidepressants and the MAO inhibitors, exert their effect by increasing one or another of the biogenic amines at the central adrenergic receptor sites (limbic system and hypothalamus) and that drugs which often cause depression (such as reserpine) deplete biogenic amines, the theory followed that naturally occurring depressions might be associated with a deficiency of these latter substances. Indeed measurements of 3-methoxy-4-hydroxyphenylglycol (MHPG), a metabolite of norepinephrine, was found to be subnormal in the CSF of patients with endogenous depression and to be elevated in manic states. Also, 5-hydroxyindoleacetic acid (5-HIAA), a deaminated metabolite of serotonin, was reduced in the CSF of depressed patients. However, the findings were not consistent. Some investigators interpreted this to mean that all depressions are not the same. At least two groups emerged; one with low levels of bioamine metabolites, one with normal levels. Maas, in the study of a small group of depressed patients reported that those who had low levels of MHPG responded better to imipramine therapy and those with normal levels, to amitriptyline therapy.

Another set of observations, summarized by Schlesser et al., suggests a disorder of the hypothalamic-pituitary-adrenal axis. In a series of cases of endogenous monopolar and bipolar depressions, the parenteral administration of 1 to 2 mg of dexamethasone failed to suppress serum cortisol levels while the patient was ill, but did so after recovery. In a comparable series of reactive depressions there was a normal suppression of serum cortisol levels. Dextroamphetamine restored to some extent the normal response in the patients with endogenous depressions. This test is believed to separate the two large groups of depressed patients and to predict the response to drug therapy, for only the endogenous depressives responded to antidepressant tricyclic and MAO inhibitory drugs.

Research on the amphetamines, cocaine, electroconvulsive shock treatment, and lithium salts has also produced data that agree with the biogenic-amine hypothesis. Although this possibility has received much attention and is generally well accepted, it leaves many questions unanswered. How is a genetic abnormality transcribed into a disorder of biogenic amines? Why are the therapeutic results so inconsistent with either the tricyclic antidepressants or the MAO inhibitors, both of which should favorably influence the balance of biogenic amines at the proper receptor sites? How can one explain the observation that steroids play a part in the etiology of affective disorders? Further knowledge of the metabolism and physiology of the transmitter function of the biogenic amines is needed before a complete theory can be developed. For readers who seek more information on this subject, the review by Schildkraut is recommended.

Psychoanalytic Theories Karl Abraham was the first psychoanalyst to study manic-depressive patients. He stressed their tendency to have obsessive-compulsive personalities and unusually strong "oral needs." In his estimation, the mother-child relationship was marked by strong ambivalent feelings, which resulted in the infant's constant sense of unfulfillment. This, in turn, set the stage for the deep depressions in adult life. Abraham viewed depression as a regression to an earlier period of development, "the oral stage of hostile dependency," and the manic phase as an acting out of the infant's unbridled freedom.

Freud used mourning as a model for depression. Both, he hypothesized, were a response to the loss of a "love object," i.e., somebody or something greatly valued by the patient. In the case of melancholia, however, the loss involved intense expressions of ambivalent, hostile feelings associated with the object; these unresolved negative feelings were directed inward, resulting in the characteristic feelings of depression. There are a number of other psychoanalytic explanations of depression, and the theories mentioned above are far more complex than these few remarks indicate, but all are purely speculative.

TREATMENT

Enlisting the Help of a Psychiatrist The untrained physician would be rash to attempt the management of these patients without such assistance.

Hospitalization If there is any doubt about the patient's intention of suicide, hospitalization is better than taking a chance. In manic-depressive illness, successive attacks of depression or elation are remarkably similar in the same individual. Thus one can predict the course and content of the present episode on the basis of the last. If suicide attempts were made then, the probability is that they will be made again.

If the depressed patient is psychotic, i.e., suffering from delusions or hallucinations, one of the antipsychotic medications (haloperidol, thioridazine, chlorpromazine) should be given before the antidepressant (see below).

Antidepressant Medication Two categories of antidepressants, the tricyclic compounds and the MAO inhibitors, are the most useful. Imipramine (Tofranil), amitriptyline (Elavil), and doxepin (Sinequan) represent the former; phenelzine (Nardil) and tranylcypromine (Parnate), the latter. In the treatment of depression, most psychiatrists start with imipramine or amitriptyline, because they are safest. Some psychiatrists favor imipramine or desipramine (Norpramin) for the endogenous depressions and amitryptiline for reactive or anxious depressions with prominent sleep disturbances. The starting dose is 50 to 100 mg/day, which is then raised in stepwise fashion if needed. The therapeutic effect of tricyclic medication is often not evident for 2 or 3 weeks after treatment has been initiated. Common side effects are orthostatic hypotension, dry mouth, constipation, tachycardia, and urinary retention; these compounds should not be given to patients with coronary heart disease. If full doses given for 4 to 6 weeks are ineffective, the tricyclic compounds are discontinued and a MAO inhibitor is prescribed, after an interval of at least one week. Phenelzine (Nardil) is regarded as the least likely of the MAO inhibitors to produce serious side effects. The usual starting dose is 15 mg tid, which is gradually increased as needed to a maximum of 45 mg tid. The most serious side effect of MAO inhibitors is a hypertensive crisis; therefore, they should be dispensed with extreme caution in patients with hypertension or cardiovascular or cerebrovascular disease. Patients taking these drugs should avoid foods with a high tyramine content (aged cheese, pickled herring, chicken liver, beer, wines, yeast extract).

Since patients are responsive either to the tricyclic drugs or MAO inhibitors but not to both, it is important to find out which of these drugs have been more helpful in the past. This will guide one in current management. Interestingly, it has been found that members of the same family are apt to have a similar response to the same antidepressant.

Although some psychiatrists would disapprove, the authors have found some patients with depression to respond to dextroamphetamine (5 to 10 mg bid, given in the early part of the day), and sodium amytal, 60 to 120 mg tid. These medications are useful in patients who are only mildly depressed and are still at work, and they have no serious side effects.

Electroconvulsive Therapy (ECT) This is an effective treatment for "involutional melancholia" and the depressed phase of manic-depressive psychosis and can also be used to interrupt manic episodes. The latter often require only two or three treatments. The technique is quite simple. The patient is premedicated with a muscle relaxant, succinylcholine (Anectine) and then anesthetized by an intravenous injection of the short-acting barbiturate methohexital (Brevital). An electrode is placed over each temple and an alternating current of about 400 mA and 70 to 120 V is passed between them for 0.1 to 0.5 s. The Anectine prevents strong and injurious muscle spasm. The patient is awake within 5 to 10 min and is up and about in 30 min. The mechanism by which convulsive therapy works is not known. In treating depression, ECT is usually given every other day for 6 to 14 treatments. The only absolute contraindication is the presence of increased intracranial pressure, such as may occur with a neoplasm or hematoma. Its major drawback is a transient impairment of recent memory for the period of treatment and the days which follow, the degree of impairment being related to the number of treatments given. Placing both electrodes on the nondominant side (unilateral ECT) produces less memory disturbance but is thought to be less effective against the depression.

Until the advent of the antidepressant drugs, ECT was the treatment of choice for the agitated depression of middle and late life. Of all the conditions for which ECT is used, it is the one that is most predictably benefited. Close to 90 percent of patients recover within less than 2 months following a course of 6 to 14 treatments. Prior to the use of ECT, this type of depression could be expected to last for 2 to 7 years before remission occurred. Although some psychiatrists prefer to use drugs, most still favor ECT for this form of depressive illness. It has the advantage of speed and safety, but carries the tariff of amnesia. Since the tricyclic compounds and the MAO inhibitors cause no memory impairment, most patients should first be given a trial of one and then of the other of these antidepressants on the chance of avoiding the use of ECT. These trials, of course, must be conducted in a setting where the chance of suicide is minimized.

Lithium Carbonate   This may be the drug of choice in treating the manic phase of manic-depressive disease. Hospitalization is usually required to protect the manic patient from impulsive and often aggressive behavior which might cause a loss of good standing in the community or jeopardize a career. Chlorpromazine (Thorazine) or haloperidol (Haldol)—or ECT, if these drugs are ineffective—can be used to control the mania until lithium carbonate becomes effective, usually a matter of 4 or 5 days. The usual dosage of lithium is 1 to 3 g daily in divided oral doses, which produces the desired serum level of 1.2 to 1.5 meq/liter. The serum level of lithium must be followed closely, both to ensure that a therapeutic dose is being given and to guard against toxicity (page 789).

Lithium has proved to be most effective in the *milder* degrees of mania, and can be used in such cases without having to hospitalize the patient initially. There is also evidence that continued administration of lithium, given in half the dosage that is used for manic episodes, may prevent further attacks of mania. Evidence for the usefulness of lithium in the treatment of depressive illnesses is incomplete.

Psychotherapy   In all patients with manic-depressive disease, psychotherapy (explanation, reassurance, encouragement) is of value in helping the patient understand his or her illness and coping with it.

As a general rule, manic-depressive illness is best managed by a physician who is willing to follow the patient over a long period of time and who is known to the family. Although the prognosis for any individual attack is relatively good, it is wise to arrange for a plan of action which is set in operation as soon as the first symptoms of a recurrence become manifest. A family physician who has ready access to a psychiatrist best fulfills this need.

SUICIDE

There are approximately 225,000 suicide attempts in the United States each year, of which 25,000 end fatally. All psychiatrists agree that this is a conservative figure. Suicide is the thirteenth leading cause of death in America, a figure which emphasizes the importance of recognizing those depressions with a high potential for self-destruc-

tion. Every physician should be familiar with the few clues we possess to identify those patients who intend to end their lives.

Manic-depressive psychosis, endogenous depression of middle and late life, depression resulting from a debilitating disease, pathologic grief, and depression in an alcoholic or schizophrenic—all carry the risk of suicide. In manic-depressive disease and endogenous depression, it approaches 5 percent, and the risk of suicide over the lifetime of these patients is about 15 percent (Guze and Robins). Most suicides are not impulsive but planned. Furthermore, the intention of suicide is more often than not communicated to someone significant in the life of the patient. The message may be a direct verbal statement of intent, or indirect, such as giving away a treasured possession or revising a will. It is known that successful suicide is three times more common in men than in women and particularly common among men over 40 years of age. Those with a history of suicide in either mother or father carry a higher risk for self-destruction than those without such a history. A previous attempt at suicide adds to the risk. Most successful suicides give as their motive "a concern about ill health." Chronic illnesses such as alcoholism, cancer, heart disease, and progressive, incurable neurologic conditions all contribute to the risk of suicide. Thus, a portrait of a likely prospect for suicide might be an elderly man in poor health through heavy drinking who has recently lost his wife, who has attempted suicide before, and whose father committed suicide. However, no single trait stands out as highly significant in terms of predicting suicide. As a consequence, we are left with our clinical judgment and index of suspicion as our main guides. The only rule of thumb is that all suicidal threats are to be taken seriously and all patients who threaten to kill themselves should be evaluated by a psychiatrist.

Some physicians are reluctant to question the presence of suicidal thoughts in depressed patients on the grounds that this might upset them. More likely it is the physician who is upset by this questioning, for surely mention of suicide will not alarm persons who are determined to end their lives, nor offend those with no such intention. Rather, a query of this type is apt to be appreciated by the depressed patient because it expresses the physician's concern, and indicates that the patient's behavior is being taken seriously. Should a patient's manner or conversation raise a suspicion of suicidal intent, it should be quickly voiced by the physician. This in itself sometimes brings to awareness unrecognized suicidal urges. If there appears to be an immediate danger of suicide, a bed should be obtained in a general hospital (preferably on the psychiatric ward) and a psychiatrist consulted. The point is to get the patient under cover until a psychiatrist arrives, and since a general hospital is far less threatening than a mental institution the patient is more apt to agree to enter. Once such a person has been admitted to the hospital, suicidal precautions should be initiated, including nurses "around the clock." When the psychiatrist arrives, the need for more or less security can be determined. If the patient refuses hospitalization, the family should be assembled, along with an intimate friend or clergyman, if appropriate, to urge the patient's cooperation. Should all efforts fail, the only recourse is a commitment to a psychiatric ward. Commitment procedures and laws vary from state to state, but all provide for temporary confinement of individuals who are thought to be self-destructive. Although an action of this sort is bound to be stressful for all concerned, prudence and caution are more important than the patient's plea for freedom. Hard feelings over a short period of enforced confinement vanish in time, but those who mourn the loss of a loved one through a preventable suicide are apt to be unforgiving.

Patients who arrive at the hospital having attempted suicide should be under constant surveillance, once consciousness is regained, and a psychiatrist should be consulted. It is unwise to allow the family to keep watch, unless their competence is unquestioned. Among patients who have been hospitalized because of a preoccupation with suicide, a particular danger attends the phase of recovery from depression, when the physician may develop a false sense of security. In either case, the psychiatrist should assume the responsibility for setting up a program of therapy and arrange for transfer to a psychiatric ward, if this is necessary, or for outpatient treatment.

HYPOCHONDRIASIS

A few remarks concerning the status of hypochondriasis as a psychiatric illness are in order. It is a condition which may be defined as the constant preoccupation with matters of health and an exaggerated concern about real or imagined signs and symptoms of illness. A hallmark of hypochondriasis is the failure of reassurance to affect either the symptoms or the patient's conviction of being sick. The most common complaint is pain, often vague and variable, most of which is referable to the head, chest, and lower part of the abdomen. It is a curious fact that over 70 percent of hypochondriacal complaints are related to the left side of the body.

Hypochondriasis is considered to be not a specific psychiatric disorder but rather the somatic equivalent of depression or anxiety. As such, it is found in a number of psychiatric conditions such as depression (as described earlier in this chapter), schizophrenia, and the neuroses. It is not uncommon to encounter hypochon-

driacal reactions in otherwise normal individuals during periods of stress. Medical students, for example, traditionally develop symptoms of a variety of diseases during their first exposure to clinical medicine. When adolescents or young adults present hypochondriacal symptoms that are not related to transient episodes of stress, one should suspect a more serious underlying disorder such as schizophrenia.

Though it is estimated that 85 percent of hypochondriasis is secondary to other mental disorders, chiefly depression, in about 15 percent of cases there appears to be no associated emotional illness (*primary hypochondriasis*). The etiology is unknown. In this latter category are the habitués of medical outpatient clinics, who are passed from specialist to specialist, perplexing and angering doctors along the way because their symptoms defy both satisfactory diagnosis and cure. Often referred to as "crocks," these patients seldom benefit from conventional therapy.

The first principle in the management of hypochondriasis is to determine what should be treated. Is the hypochondriasis part of another psychiatric syndrome such as depression, neurosis, or schizophrenia? As a rule this question can best be answered by a psychiatrist, and it is advisable to have each case evaluated in order to institute a suitable program of management. If depressive symptoms are an important part of the clinical picture, the patient should be given a trial of antidepressant medication as described above. Neurotics and schizophrenics should be treated by a psychiatrist.

The treatment of primary hypochondriasis is difficult, if not impossible, unless the physician keeps in mind the therapeutic goals. Since, for a variety of reasons, these patients need to retain their symptoms, the concept of "curing" is inapplicable. The presence of symptoms is thought by some to provide the context for a relationship with a physician. It is the continuation of this relationship, which is often the only dependable human contact in the patient's life, that motivates some hypochondriacs. In this setting it is understandable why reassurance that vigor and health will be restored seldom moves the patient to improve. Physicians are so oriented toward the relief of suffering and the cure of disease that anger and frustration inevitably occur when they meet patients who coexist with their symptoms in an immutable symbiosis. In this situation it is usually the doctor who is the most discomfited. Such patients are best managed by physicians who realize that these patients do not necessarily want or expect a cure, who are content with small gains and the avoidance of unnecessary surgery, and who have an interest in the way symptoms persist rather than in any improvement. Since this type of physician is difficult to find, some hospitals have found it economical to utilize the time of those staff members who are able to provide such care by establishing special clinics under their leadership where all hypochondriacs are evaluated and their course is followed. This is probably the most effective method for managing these cases from the standpoint of the physician as well as the patient.

ANOREXIA NERVOSA

Loss of appetite and of weight are common manifestations of a retarded depression. As was stated above, this illness not infrequently occurs in children and adolescents. The special syndrome called *anorexia nervosa* has been difficult to classify. If it has any clear connection with a psychiatric disease, and this is not established at the present time, it would be with a psychotic depression.

Anorexia nervosa is a disorder of previously healthy girls and young women, mainly from the upper and middle social classes, who become extremely emaciated as a result of voluntary starvation. It is rare in Orientals and blacks and practically never occurs in males.

As a rule, the syndrome begins shortly after puberty but sometimes later, and rarely it may be delayed to the thirtieth year. Some of the patients have been overweight in childhood and especially in the prepubertal period. Dieting is much talked about and is encouraged, especially by the mothers, as a means of becoming more attractive. Sometimes there appears to be a precipitating event, such as leaving home, a disruption of family life, or other stress. In undertaking a diet, food intake is greatly reduced. What is more important, the patient persists in dieting even when she has become painfully thin, and when counselled to eat normally, she will use every artifice to starve herself. Food is hidden, and vomiting may be provoked to empty the stomach after a meal. No amount of persuasion will induce the patient to take adequate amounts of food. The patient shows no concern about her obvious emaciation and remains active. If left alone, these patients waste away and about 5 percent have succumbed to some intercurrent infection.

On physical examination, one is struck with the degree of emaciation; it exceeds that of most of the wasting diseases. Often as much as 30 percent of the body weight will have been lost by the time the patient's family insists on medical consultation. A fine lanugo type of hair covers the body and limbs. The skin is thin and dry without its normal elasticity and the nails are brittle. Pubic hair and breast tissue are normal, and in this respect anorexia nervosa is unlike Simmond's disease. The extremities are often cold and blue. There are no neurologic signs of nutritional deficiency. The patient is alert and cheerfully indifferent to her condition. Any suggestion that she is unattractively thin or seriously depleted is rejected.

Amenorrhea is usually present and may precede the extreme weight loss. Luteinizing hormone (LH) levels are reduced to a pubertal or prepubertal pattern. Clomiphene citrate fails to stimulate a rise in LH or follicle-stimulating hormone (FSH) as it normally does. Administration of gonadotropic releasing factor raises the LH and FSH levels, suggesting a hypothalamic disorder. The basal metabolic rate is low; T_3 and T_4 are low, while levels of physiologically inactive $3,3',5'$-triiodothyronine (reverse T_3) are normal. Plasma thyrotropin (TSH) and growth hormone levels are normal. Plasma cortisol levels are normal and excretion of 17-hydroxysteroids are slightly reduced. In sum, there is evidence of hypothalamic-pituitary dysfunction, but to what extent it is primary or secondary to starvation is not clear.

As to etiology, there are numerous hypotheses. Mayer-Gross, Slater, and Roth remark on constitutional factors. Earlier signs of hysterical tendencies and of obsessional traits are mentioned as being frequent. Neurosis or psychopathy may be found in other members of the family. However, all psychiatrists seem agreed that at the time of the anorexia, the patient does not have symptoms that conform to any of the major neuroses or psychoses. In some reported series, depression is a major factor in 80 percent of patients, and it is said that a high percentage of first-degree relatives have manic-depressive disease. Certainly loss of appetite, lack of self-esteem and interest in personal appearance, and self-destructive thoughts—which are common features of anorexia nervosa—are also the symptoms of depression. A characteristic personality disorder and family constellation are claimed to have been found by psychoanalytically oriented psychiatrists, such as Bruch.

The fact that anorexia nervosa is practically confined to females must figure in any acceptable explanation of the syndrome. Among psychiatric disorders, only hysteria has this sexual predilection. Yet most psychiatrists do not believe anorexia nervosa to be a manifestation of hysteria. The racial-social relationships of the syndrome are also noteworthy. Probably another point of importance is that anorexia nervosa has its onset in relation to the menarche, at a time when the female exhibits rather large fluctuations in appetite and weight. Obesity before or around puberty is more pronounced in girls than boys, as though the appetite-satiety mechanism of the hypothalamus is unstable. Whether the majority of these patients are tipped into this condition by an endogenous depression is debatable. They do not look despondent or admit to being dejected. Moreover endogenous depressions affect both sexes.

The most effective treatment consists of immediate hospitalization, preferably on a psychiatric ward, supportive psychotherapy, assignment of one nurse to sit with the patient as each meal is eaten, a gradual increase of a balanced diet, and the use of imipramine, 150 mg/day. If the patient refuses to eat, tube feeding is the only alternative, and she must understand that it is simply a question of eating voluntarily or being tube-fed. As weight is gained over several weeks the patient becomes more normal in her attitude and will usually continue to recover on this regimen at home. Boyar points out that the menses will not return until the body fat reaccumulates and exceeds 25 percent. Our colleagues report an 80 percent success with such a regime. The long-term results are less clear. In several reports there has been a significant relapse rate, and many of the survivors are said to lapse into a chronic neurotic state.

All the adolescent boys that we have seen with this syndrome have recovered on antidepressant medication.

REFERENCES

BECK AT: *Depression: Clinical, Experimental and Theoretical Aspects.* New York, Harper & Row, 1967.

BOYAR RM: Anorexia nervosa, in Isselbacher KJ et al (eds): *Harrison's Principles of Internal Medicine,* 9th ed. New York, McGraw-Hill, 1980, chap 77, pp 416-418.

BRUCH H: *Eating Disorders: Obesity, Anorexia Nervosa and the Person Within.* New York, Basic Books, 1973.

CASSIDY WL et al: Clinical observations in manic-depressive disease. *J Am Med Assoc* 164:1535, 1957.

FREUD S: Mourning and melancholia, in *The Complete Psychological Works of Sigmund Freud.* London, Hogarth, 1957.

GOODWIN DW, GUZE SB: *Psychiatric Diagnosis,* 2d ed. New York, Oxford University Press, 1979.

GUZE SB, ROBINS E: Suicide and primary affective disorders. *Br J Psychiatry* 117:437, 1970.

KALINOWSKY LB, HIPPUS H: *Pharmacological, Convulsive and Other Somatic Treatments in Psychiatry.* New York, Grune & Stratton, 1969.

KENYON FE: Hypochondriasis: A clinical study. *Br J Psychiatry* 110:478, 1964.

KLERMAN GL: Affective disorders, in Nicholi AM Jr (ed): *The Harvard Guide to Modern Psychiatry.* Cambridge, Mass, Harvard, 1978, pp 253-281.

KLINE N: Practical management of depression. *J Am Med Assoc* 190:732, 1964.

LEWIS A: Melancholia: A historical review, in *The State of Psychiatry: Essays and Addresses.* New York, Science House, 1967.

LINDEMANN E: Symptomatology and management of acute grief. *Am J Psychiatry* 101:141, 1944.

MAAS JW: The clinical and biochemical heterogeneity of the depressive disorders. *Ann Intern Med* 88:556, 1978.

MAPOTHER E: Discussion on manic-depressive psychosis. *Br Med J* 2:872, 1926.

ROBINS E et al: Some clinical considerations in the prevention of suicide based on a study of 134 successful suicides. *Am J Public Health* 49:888, 1959.

SCHILDKRAUT JJ: The biochemistry of affective disorders: A brief summary, in Nicholi AM Jr (ed): *Harvard Guide to Modern Psychiatry.* Cambridge, Mass, Harvard, 1978, pp 81-91.

SCHLESSER MA, WINOKUR G, SHERMAN BM: Hypothalamic-pituitary-adrenal axis activity in depressive illness. *Arch Gen Psychiatry* 37:737, 1980.

SLATER E, ROTH M: *Mayer-Gross, Slater and Roth Clinical Psychiatry,* 3d ed. Baltimore, Williams & Wilkins, 1969.

WEISSMAN NM, MYERS JK: Affective disorders in a U.S. urban community. *Arch Gen Psychiatry* 35:1304, 1978.

WINOKUR G, CADORET R: The irrelevance of the menopause to depressive disease, in Sachar EJ (ed): *Topics in Psychoendocrinology.* New York, Grune & Stratton, 1975, pp 59-66.

—— et al: *Manic-Depressive Illness.* St Louis, Mosby, 1969.

CHAPTER 55

PERSONALITY DISORDERS: ANTISOCIAL PERSONALITY (SOCIOPATHY)

Personality is a descriptive term for the totality of a person's observable behavior and reportable subjective experience. In other words, it designates the whole of the neuropsychic organization and thus includes elements of the individual's character, intelligence, instincts, sentiments, motor control, habits, and memories—in short, all forces from within the organism that govern behavior as well as the prevailing influences of the environment. Personalities are as individualistic as fingerprints. They are a product of genetic, social, and cultural influences, all these elements in some manner normally becoming integrated. The steps by which this is achieved were briefly outlined in Chap. 27.

As might be expected, there are individuals in whom certain portions of the personality do not develop properly or at times do not function in a normal manner. This is most clearly reflected in the techniques individuals use for getting along with people, i.e., in their way of "establishing and maintaining a stable reciprocal relationship with human and nonhuman environment" (Hartman). According to psychoanalytic theory, the nature of the individual's personality is a reflection of his psychological defense mechanisms ("ego defenses"), which automatically come into play in the maintenance of psychic stability. These defensive techniques are seen by the psychoanalysts as a product of certain trends in psychosexual development. Further discussion of these theories is not suitable for a textbook of neurology. The interested reader will find a full review of this subject in the chapter by Vaillant and Perry in the *Comprehensive Textbook of Psychiatry* (see references).

In general, deviant personality types are thought to represent immaturity or inadequacy of development, the effect of which is lifelong. They are not regressions or decompensations after a period of healthy adjustment, and "intrapsychic conflict" is believed not to be involved in their genesis. Disturbances of personality do not have an identifiable onset, as do the symptoms of other mental disorders, but are part of the "warp and woof" of the individual's life history and personal identity. For these reasons, personality disorders are separable from neuroses. This distinction may at times be difficult, for personality disorders may be associated with neurotic symptoms and with specific types of deviant behavior, such as sexual perversions, but biographical data should settle the matter.

The term *personality pattern* or *character disturbance* is currently being used to designate the condition of those individuals whose life style and manners are sources of difficulty. They are aggressive or docile, rigid or pliant, oversensitive or callous, and because of these traits their actions repeatedly defeat their own ends. Yet many such individuals remain rational in most of their conduct and are not classifiable as neurotic or psychotic in the strict sense of the word; they are usually capable of being educated, forming a family, and working, though always with more difficulties than well-balanced individuals.

In Table 55-1 is a list of the types of personality disorders accepted by the American Psychiatric Association, along with their characteristic features and their relative frequency.

It need hardly be stressed that many of these definitions lack precision (how does one measure passivity or aggressivity?) and that they are used indiscriminately by physicians and laity alike. Nevertheless, an understanding of these personality disorders and the traits and peculiarities of patients whose personalities are not necessarily abnormal, may be of great help to the physician. Such knowledge makes it possible to distinguish disorders of personality from the neuroses and other mental disorders; to understand a patient's reactions during a medical illness and to anticipate reactions during future medical illnesses; to prevent the patient from interfering with diagnostic and therapeutic procedures and particularly to make certain predictions about the form that psychiatric illness will assume, should it develop.

In general, there are two groups of personality disorders: one comprising the paranoid, schizoid, cyclothymic, and obsessive-compulsive types, in which there is a relation to particular types of psychiatric illness, and another in which such a relationship is not evident. Thus, among patients who develop paranoid schizophrenia, a

considerable number will have had the attributes described under paranoid personality. Similarly, among patients who develop schizophrenia of other type, the history will frequently disclose a preexistent schizoid personality. In fact, it may be difficult to judge where the personality disorder left off and the schizophrenic illness began. It seems clear from several family studies (re-

Table 55-1
Personality disorders

Type*	Characteristics	Type*	Characteristics
Paranoid (16)	Chronic wariness, suspiciousness, litigiousness; hypersensitivity, jealousy, envy; lack of insight or humor; tendency to blame others; sense of self-importance and entitlement	Asthenic (1)	Chronic weakness, easy fatigability, sense of vulnerability, oversensitive to physically and emotionally taxing situations, little ambition or aggression; low energy level; anhedonia
Cyclothymic (3)	Recurring periods of depression (low energy, pessimism, hopelessness, despair) and elation (high energy, ambition, enthusiasm, optimism) not readily explained by circumstances	Passive-aggressive (78)	Obstructive behavior, stubbornness, intentional errors or omissions; intolerance of authority with struggles over control often creating difficulties in medical settings; externalization of conflicts and blaming others for untoward events
Schizoid (30)	Isolation, seclusiveness, secretiveness; discomfort in relationships; often eccentric and lacking in energy; few friends; detachment; inability to express ideas and feelings, especially anger	Inadequate (17)	Chronic inability to meet ordinary life demands in the absence of mental retardation; severe dependency on others; tendency to become institutionalized or to become dependent on institutions
Explosive (4)	Outbursts of rage and aggression not in keeping with usual personality, often in response to minor provocation; sense of loss of control followed by regret	Antisocial (32)	Unsocialized or antisocial behavior in conflict with society; selfishness, callousness, impulsiveness, lack of loyalty, and little guilt; frustration tolerance is low; tendency to blame others and have a long history of interpersonal and social difficulties and arrests
Obsessive-compulsive (anankastic) (21)	Chronic worries about standards; excessive concern about self-image; tension in relationships, leading to isolation; inability to relax and excessive inhibitions; overly meticulous, conscientious, and perfectionist; predisposition to depression and obsessive-compulsive neurosis	Passive-dependent (30)	Lack of self-confidence, indecisiveness, tendency to cling to and seek support from others
Hysterical (103)	Immaturity, histrionic behavior, excitability, emotional instability, sexualization of relationships, low frustration tolerance, and shallow interpersonal ties; dependency	Immature (12)	Ineffectual responses to social, psychological, and physical demands; lack of stamina; adapts poorly to ordinary situations; a "loser"
		Unspecified (14)	

*Figures in parentheses represent the number of diagnoses of each personality disorder out of a total of 361 patients with the diagnosis of personality disorder at the Psychiatric Service of the University of Iowa (Winokur and Crowe).

viewed by Winokur et al.) that the cyclothymic personality is related to manic-depressive disease. Obsessive-compulsive personality is closely related to obsessive-compulsive neurosis, as one might expect, but it also appears to be related to depressive disease. In particular, it has been stated that patients who develop involutional melancholia do so on a background of an obsessive-compulsive personality.

As has been pointed out in Chap. 54, care must be taken to distinguish between "hysterical personality" and the disease *hysteria*; there are no data to support the idea that a hysterical personality is a determinant in the development of the full-blown hysterical neurosis. Also, there is no evidence that the asthenic, inadequate, and passive-aggressive or -dependent personalities are related to any major psychiatric illnesses or neuroses. In this sense they are "pure" personality disorders, which in themselves may be lifelong sources of distress and difficulties in functioning, but which do not lead to the development of any specific psychiatric illness.

Personality disorders are little influenced by the general physician or the psychiatrist, although often the contacts between physician and such an individual over many years may in themselves serve as a stabilizing force, and, of course, one should never underestimate the powers of further maturation to stabilize the individual, as will be evident in the discussion of the sociopathies. The use of sedatives and tranquilizers should be avoided unless there is evidence that what has been called a personality disorder is really an early stage of schizophrenia.

ANTISOCIAL PERSONALITY (Sociopathy)

Of all the abnormal personality types listed in Table 55-1, the antisocial is the best defined and the one most likely to cause trouble in the community. Formerly the sociopathic state was referred to as psychopathic personality, constitutional psychopathy, and chronic psychopathic inferiority. In the *Diagnostic and Statistical Manual* of the American Psychiatric Association, it is defined as a state in which the individual "is always in trouble, profiting not from experience or punishment, unable to maintain loyalties to any person, group or code. He is frequently callous and hedonistic, showing marked emotional immaturity with lack of sense of responsibility, lack of judgment, and an ability to rationalize his behavior so that it appears warranted, reasonable and justi-

fied." Also included under this heading are sexual deviation and addiction.

Since Prichard first described this condition under the term *moral insanity* in the mid-nineteenth century, there have been many attempts to give it a more precise definition and to avoid using it as a psychiatric wastebasket. At the turn of the century, Koch introduced the term *psychopathic inferiority*, implying that deviations in personality were constitutionally determined. Later the term *psychopathic personality* came into common use. Some authors used this last term indiscriminately to embrace all forms of deviant personalities; others used it in a more restricted sense to define a subgroup of antisocial or aggressive psychopaths. To reduce confusion, the American Psychiatric Association has adopted the term *antisocial personality* to refer to the aggressive or antisocial psychopath. Aubrey Lewis has given a lucid account of the history of the concept of sociopathy.

By far the best modern study of sociopathy is that of L. N. Robins, based on a 30-year follow-up study of 524 cases from a child guidance clinic and 100 controls. Other investigations of note are those of Ehrlich and Keough, who studied 50 patients with sociopathy in a mental hospital, and of Guze et al. who studied psychiatric illness in large numbers of felons and their first-degree relatives. The clinical descriptions which follow are derived largely from these writings.

CLINICAL STATE

This condition, unlike most psychiatric disorders, is manifest by the age of 12 to 15 years, frequently earlier. It consists essentially of deviant behavior in which individuals seem driven to make trouble in everything they do. Every code imposed by family, school, church, and society is broken. Seemingly the sociopath acts on impulse, but after committing the unsocial act, shows no remorse. The most frequent antisocial activities are theft, incorrigibility, truancy, running away overnight, associating with undesirable characters, staying out late, indiscriminate sexual relations, physical aggression or assault, recklessness and impulsivity, lying without cause, vandalism, abuse of drugs and alcohol and later, inability to work steadily or keep a job. In children or adolescents who exhibited 10 or more of these antisocial symptoms, 43 percent were classed as sociopaths in adulthood; if only 8 or 9 of these traits were present, 29 percent were so classed; if 6 to 7, 25 percent; and 3 to 5, only 15 percent. Conversely, not a single adult sociopath was observed who did not manifest antisocial symptoms in earlier life. Interestingly, a number of other problems of childhood and adolescence, such as enuresis, dirty appearance, sleep walking, irritability, nail biting, oversensitivity, poor eating habits, nervousness, being withdrawn or seclusive, unhappiness, tics, and fears were not predictive of adult sociopathy. None of Robins' patients was mentally defective.

As noted above, more than half the deviant children in Robins' study (even those with 10 or more antisocial manifestations) had lost most of their sociopathic traits by adulthood. This does not mean that they remained psychiatrically well, however. Of those who did not continue to be sociopaths, the large majority developed other adult psychiatric illnesses, particularly addiction to alcohol. Only in the group of children with less than three antisocial symptoms did a reasonable number (one-third) remain well in adult life. Thus Robins' observations indicate that the presence of moderate to severe antisocial behavior in childhood carries an exceedingly high risk of development of sociopathy, alcoholism, or other psychiatric disease in adult life.

The criteria used in making the diagnosis of adult sociopathy were persistent disturbances in at least five of the following so-called life areas—poor work record, marital difficulties, financial dependency, multiple arrests, excessive use of alcohol, impulsive actions, sexual promiscuity, vagrancy, leading a "wild life," belligerency, social isolation, disciplinary problems in the Armed Forces, lack of guilt, more than nine somatic complaints or a complaint of medical disability, use of aliases, pathologic lying, and suicide attempts. These findings in the adult were the same, whether the patients were drawn from the community at large (only 12 percent of Robins' adult sociopaths were in prison at the time of their follow-up examination), from a mental hospital, or from a group of prisoners (or parolees or probationers). Furthermore, in each of these groups of adult sociopaths, the manifestations of antisocial behavior in childhood were much the same.

Also of interest are Robins' findings that sociopaths show an unusually high incidence of anxiety, depressive, and particularly "conversion" symptoms, and that the neurotic symptoms are in proportion to the sociopathy, i.e., the larger the number of antisocial manifestations, the larger the number of neurotic symptoms or the greater the disability from them. These latter symptoms and many other somatic complaints frequently bring the sociopath to the attention of the physician.

These manifestations of deviant behavior in childhood and adult sociopathy are five to ten times more frequent in the male than the female. A search for evidence of encephalitis, often postulated as the basis of sociopathy, was not revealing; Robins could elicit no proof of other brain damage. It has been shown that EEG abnormalities, which usually take the form of mild to moderate bilateral slowing, are more frequent in criminals and sociopaths than in the normal population. Furthermore the biologic parents also show a higher frequency of such EEG abnormalities than the general population. These and other findings suggest that there may be a genetic predisposition to antisocial personality. The presence of a chromosomal abnormality, e.g., XYY, which has been found in a small number of sex deviants, has not been studied in a controlled manner in sociopaths.

Surveys of the families of sociopaths have disclosed a high incidence of antisocial behavior, broken homes, alcoholism, and poverty. The two factors which seem to be most closely related to the development of sociopathy are a lack of parental discipline and having an antisocial or alcoholic father. However, as Robins' study has shown, if any of these factors are causal, then they must be mediated through the occurrence of deviant behavior in childhood. In the absence of the latter, broken homes, slum neighborhoods, etc., do not lead to adult sociopathy.

DIAGNOSIS

The following characteristics are most helpful in making a diagnosis of sociopathy and distinguishing this disorder from other psychiatric states:

1. The deviant behavior begins at an early age, always before age 15 and sometimes at age 7 or 8.

2. The clinical picture is one of chronic and repetitive antisocial behavior directed equally toward parents, teachers, and strangers and involving multiple areas of social functioning, e.g., legal and marital difficulties, financial dependency, poor work and poor military records.

3. Certain psychological traits, such as callousness, egocentricity, lack of deep human attachments and loyalties, are prominent.

PROGNOSIS

This is of interest for several reasons. The relation between deviant behavior in childhood and adolescence and the development of sociopathy and other psychiatric illnesses in adult life has already been discussed. In addition it should be noted that in adult sociopaths, improvement of gross antisocial behavior is possible, occurring in somewhat more than a third of such individuals. Improvement occurs most frequently between the ages of 30 and 40 years (median age 35). This bears out the Gluecks' contention that repetitive criminality diminishes with age. Improvement of sociopathic behavior does not necessarily mean that these individuals have become well-adjusted, but that they have married and are maintaining a home and working. Probably maturation, marriage, assumption of family responsibilities, and fear of imprisonment are the main stabilizing forces; at least these are the ones proffered by patients to explain their improvement.

There is no information as to the best methods of *treatment.* Most psychiatrists have been discouraged by the results of psychotherapy, but whether behavioral therapy, psychoanalysis, or drugs have more to offer cannot be determined from available data.

MALINGERING

This problem arises frequently in connection with both hysteria and psychopathic personality, and the physician should know how to deal with it. It is not a medical diagnosis, except under the rare circumstances in which a patient is caught in the act of producing a sign of disease or confesses to have done so. The term *malingering means consciously and deliberately to feign an illness or disability in order to attain a desired goal.* It does not occur as an isolated phenomenon, and its occurrence must be interpreted as a sign of a serious personality disturbance, often one which prevents effective work or military combat, though noteworthy exceptions to this statement can be found.

Certainly there is a close similarity between hysteria and malingering, but the nature of the relationship is nebulous, and there may be great difficulty in establishing a clinical differentiation. Jones and Llewellyn have observed:

> Nothing . . . resembles malingering more than hysteria; nothing, hysteria more than malingering. In both alike we are confronted with the same discrepancy between fact and statement, objective sign and subjective symptom—the outward aspect of health seemingly giving the lie to all the alleged functional disabilities. We may examine the hysterical person and the malingerer, using the same tests, and get precisely the same results in one case as the other.

The following are the main points of difference between the two conditions that are cited by most authors:

1. The conscious or unconscious quality of the motivation, which always seems more unconscious in the hysteric and more conscious in the malingerer.

2. The influence of persuasion, which is usually effective in hysteria and not in the malingerer.

3. The attitude of the patient. The hysteric appears more genuinely ill and invites examination; the malingerer seems less ill and evades examination.

The tendency of the psychopath to malinger has already been mentioned. Most of the more obvious cases of malingering seen by the authors have been psychopaths, and for this reason comment on this phenomenon is made in relationship to this disease.

In the malingerer one observes pain, hyperesthesia, anesthesia, limping gait, tremor, contracture, paralysis, amaurosis, deafness, stuttering, mutism, amnesia, epileptiform seizures and fugues, unexplained gastrointestinal bleeding, pains, and unexplained skin lesions, in short, the same array of symptoms and signs as in the patient with compensation hysteria. A particular form of sociopathy or malingering, which consists essentially of deceiving the medical profession, has been described under the title of *Munchausen's syndrome.* The name, not altogether apt, has been taken from a character in English fiction who invented incredible tales of adventure and daring. Ireland et al., who analyzed 59 well-documented cases (45 men, 14 women), list the following characteristic features, which will be recognized at once by all neurologists with extensive hospital experience: feigned severe illness of a dramatic and emergency nature; factitious evidence of disease, surreptitiously produced by interference with diagnostic procedures or by self-mutilation; a history of many hospitalizations (sometimes more than a hundred), extensive travel, or visits to innumerable physicians; evidence of laparotomy scars and cranial burr holes; pathological lying; aggressive, unruly, evasive behavior; and, finally, departure from the hospital against medical advice. Unlike the usual forms of compensation hysteria, an ulterior motive is not readily discernible. The psychopathology of this syndrome is quite obscure. It has been regarded as a form of sociopathy, malingering, and compensation hysteria, but the distinctions between them are too ambiguous to be of clinical value. Probably the medical profession has placed too great a reliance on degree of conscious awareness of deception. In such "weakminded," unstable, and morally defective individuals, the terms *conscious, unconscious,* and *deception* are too vague and subjective to serve as useful guides in practical work.

HOMOSEXUALITY

The homosexual is one who is motivated in adult life by a preferential erotic attraction to members of the same sex. He or she may or may not engage in overt sexual relations with them. Most psychiatrists exclude from the definition of homosexuality those patterns of behavior which are not motivated by specific preferential desire, such as incidental homosexuality of adolescents and the situational homosexuality of prisoners and sailors.

Figures on incidence are difficult to secure. According to the Kinsey reports, approximately 4 percent of American males are exclusively homosexual and up to 10 percent have been "more or less exclusively homosexual for at least three years sometime between the ages of 16 and 65." He reports that at least 37 percent of the male population has had overt homosexual experiences sometime between puberty and old age. For females the incidence is lower, perhaps half that for males, and approximately 28 percent have had at some time in their life a homosexual experience. It has been estimated, on the basis of the examination of large numbers of men during World War II, that 1 to 2 percent of male adults are exclusively or predominantly homosexual—a figure more in accord with the experience of psychiatrists who deal with this problem.

Two main types of male homosexual are recognized. One is exclusively homosexual, functioning in a homosexual ("gay") society and forming strong emotional and social relationships only with other homosexuals. A second type lives in the heterosexual world and may be married and have children; his homosexual activities are intermittent and carried on in secrecy. The first type may be effeminate, with delicate gestures and suggestive gait, special modes of dress, etc., but many in this group do not conform to an effeminate stereotype. The second type may be overtly masculine in his ways and manners; few, if any, may be recognizable as homosexuals.

The origins of homosexuality are obscure. One hypothesis suggests a genetic patterning of the nervous system (hypothalamus) during early life. Another (Freudian) theory postulates a regression to the earliest ("narcissistic" or "autoerotic") phase in the sexual development of the child. Others postulate that homosexuality is determined by adverse parental attitudes and home experiences. All are unsubstantiated, and attempts to show an endocrine basis for homosexuality have also failed. The most widely held current view is that homosexuality is not a mental or a personality disturbance, though it may at times lead to secondary reactive neurotic or psychotic states (Ross and Talikka).

From the medical point of view it is important to know the types of problem faced by the homosexual. The male homosexual may have few stable relationships, even with other homosexuals, and may spend a great deal of time seeking sexual satisfaction ("cruising"), becoming involved in chance situations which may expose him to robbery, injuries of various sorts, venereal disease, and blackmail. The female homosexual is less likely to attract notice and tends usually to form a stable relationship with another woman. Female and particularly male homosexuals exhibit a high incidence of neurotic symptoms, especially those of anxiety and depression and benefit from supportive psychotherapy and the drugs commonly used to allay these symptoms. Endocrine therapy and psychotropic drugs are not recommended for homosexuality. Other methods of treatment are discouraging, although Bieber has claimed a modicum of success, using psychoanalysis.

Other forms of sexual deviation—pedophilia, exhibitionism, incest, sadism, masochism, voyeurism, fetishism—represent special problems rarely encountered by the neurologist. They will not be included here for that reason.

ALCOHOL AND DRUG ADDICTION

These are unquestionably associated with sociopathy, as indicated in the above pages, but they also represent special problems of immense proportions and have therefore been discussed in Chaps. 40 and 41.

REFERENCES

Bieber I et al: *Homosexuality: A Psychoanalytic Study.* New York, Basic Books, 1962.

Diagnostic and Statistical Manual of Mental Disorders (DSM III). Washington, American Psychiatric Association, 1980.

Ehrlich SK, Keough RP: The psychopath in a mental institution. *Arch Neurol Psychiatry* 76:286, 1956.

Glueck S, Glueck E: *Criminal Careers in Retrospect.* New York, Commonwealth Fund, 1943.

Guze SB, Goodwin DW, Crane JB: Criminal recidivism and psychiatric illness. *Am J Psychiatry* 127:832, 1970.

Hartman H: *Ego Psychology and the Problem of Adaptation.* New York, International Universities Press, 1958.

IRELAND P, SAPIRA JD, TEMPLETON B: Munchausen's Syndrome. *Am J Med* 43:579, 1967.

JONES AB, LLEWELLYN LJ: *Malingering*. Philadelphia, Lippincott, 1918.

KINSEY A et al: *Sexual Behavior in the Human Female*. Philadelphia, Saunders, 1948.

—— et al: *Sexual Behavior in the Human Male*. Philadelphia, Saunders, 1948.

LEWIS A: Psychopathic personality: A most elusive category. *Psychol Med* 4:133, 1974.

ROBINS LN: *Deviant Children Grown Up: A Sociological and Psychiatric Study of Sociopathic Personality*. Huntington, NY, Krieger, 1974.

ROSS MW, TALIKKA A: Homosexual labelling and cultural control: The role of psychiatry. *Psychiatr Opinion* 16:31, 1979.

VAILLANT GE, PERRY JC: Personality disorders, in Kaplan HI et al (eds): *Comprehensive Textbook of Psychiatry*, 3d ed. Baltimore, Williams & Wilkins, 1980, chap 22, pp 1562–1590.

WINOKUR G, CLAYTON PJ, REICH T: *Manic Depressive Illness*. St. Louis, Mosby, 1969.

——, Crowe RR: Personality disorders, in Freedman AM et al (eds): *Comprehensive Textbook of Psychiatry*, 2d ed. Baltimore, Williams & Wilkins, 1975, chap 22-1, pp 1279–1297.

CHAPTER 56

THE SCHIZOPHRENIAS AND PARANOID STATES

Schizophrenia is the most serious unsolved disease in world society, according to *Medical Research: A Midcentury Survey,* sponsored by the American Foundation (see References at end of chapter). Because of its prevalence (it occurs in about 1 percent of the population) and particularly because of its early onset, chronicity, and associated disability, the same conclusion is probably justified today.

SCHIZOPHRENIA

DEFINITIONS

Though an official classification of all the major psychoses acceptable to both neurologists and psychiatrists has not been agreed upon, one major subdivision has been established—that of the "functional psychoses." This category includes (1) schizophrenia, (2) endogenous manic-depressive disease and "involutional" depression, and (3) the paranoid states. It hardly need be repeated that the adjective *functional* has little appeal to neurologists, for reasons given in the introduction to the mental disorders (page 1011).

Neurologists and psychiatrists currently accept the idea that schizophrenia comprises a group of closely related disorders characterized by a special type of disorder of thinking, affect, and behavior. The syndromes by which they most commonly manifest themselves differ from those of delirium, confusional states, dementia, and depression in ways that will become clear in the following exposition. Unfortunately diagnosis depends on the recognition of specific psychological symptoms unsupported by physical findings and laboratory data. This inevitably results in a certain imprecision. In other words, any group of patients classified as schizophrenic will to some extent be "contaminated" by others with diseases that resemble schizophrenia, and variant cases of schizophrenia will probably be rejected. Moreover, there is not full agreement as to whether all the conditions called schizophrenic are the expression of a single disease process. In America, *paranoid schizophrenia* is usually considered to be a type of the common syndrome, whereas in Europe it is believed to be a separate disease.

Even the concept of disease with reference to schizophrenia has been criticized. Extreme opinions have claimed that schizophrenia is a product of the imagination of rigid European psychiatrists, or that it is but a social maladjustment, idiosyncratic behavior, or "creative adaptation to an insane world," but these are seldom taken seriously in medical circles.

HISTORICAL BACKGROUND

Present views of the disease we now call schizophrenia originated with Emil Kraepelin, a Munich neuropsychiatrist, who first clearly separated it from manic-depressive psychosis. He called it *dementia praecox,* adopting the term introduced earlier by Morel. At first, Kraepelin believed that "catatonia" and "hebephrenia," which had previously been described by Kahlbaum and by Hecker, respectively, as well as the paranoid form of schizophrenia, were separate diseases, but later, in 1898, he proposed that they were manifestations of a single disease. Onset in adolescence and early adult life and the chronic course, often ending in marked deterioration of the personality, were emphasized as the denominative attributes of all.

Early in the twentieth century, the Swiss psychiatrist, Eugen Bleuler, substituted the term *schizophrenia* for *dementia praecox.* While an improvement, in that the term *dementia* was already being used to specify the clinical effects of another category of disease, it unfortunately implied a "split personality" or "split mind," a feature thought by Morton Prince to be typical of a neurosis. Nonetheless schizophrenia became and still is the accepted name for the disease. By the "splitting" of psychic functions Bleuler meant the lack of correspondence between ideas and emotions—the inappropriateness of thinking and behavior in relation to the patient's mood and affect (in distinction to manic-depressive disease, in which the patient's morbid thoughts accurately reflect his mood). He introduced the terms *autism* ("divorce from reality") and *ambivalence* to describe particular aspects of schizophrenia. He also called attention to a fourth syndrome, that of *simple schizophrenia*.

Bleuler believed all the schizophrenic syndromes to be composed of primary or basic symptoms, easily remembered as the "four A's" (loose *associations*, flat *affect*, *ambivalence*, and *autism*), and of secondary or "partial phenomena" such as delusions, hallucinations, negativism, stupor, etc. However interesting this concept proved to be, the psychological abnormalities are so poorly understood and so difficult to define precisely that this arbitrary division does not seem justified.

Other theories were those of Adolph Meyer and Sigmund Freud. Meyer, who introduced the "psychobiologic approach" to American psychiatry, sought the origins of schizophrenia, as well as other psychiatric syndromes, in the personal and medical history of patients and their habitual reactions to life events. His term for schizophrenia, *parergasia*, never gained wide acceptance. Freud viewed schizophrenia as a manifestation of a "weak ego" and an inability to use the ego defenses to handle anxiety and instinctual forces. As a result, the patient regressed to infantile levels of psychosexual function and a fixation at the narcissistic stage. Berze in 1914 singled out the "insufficiency and lowering of all psychic activity" as being the fundamental defect in schizophrenia and attributed it to organic damage of unknown nature. None of these theories has been corroborated.

In 1937, Langfeldt proposed his concept that in schizophrenia we are dealing with two principally different types of psychosis, viz., (1) cases which correspond to the disease considered briefly above, i.e., Kraepelin's dementia praecox and Bleuler's schizophrenia (these cases are characterized, among other things, by a poor prognosis) and (2) cases which occur acutely, on a background of a stable premorbid personality, often with clouding of consciousness and demonstrable precipitating factors. For the latter cases, which could be a manifestation of several diseases, Langfeldt proposed the term *schizophreniform psychoses*. The latter cases have a favorable prognosis.

EPIDEMIOLOGY

Schizophrenia has been found in every racial and social group so far studied. Incidence rates are difficult to evaluate because psychiatrists around the world have not used the same criteria for diagnosis. Prevalence rates worldwide range from 100 to 500 per 100,000 (probably 150 is nearest the correct value), and expectancy rates are estimated to be as high as 1000 per 100,000, i.e., one chance in 100 that a person will manifest the condition during his or her lifetime. Presumably there are always some undiagnosed cases in every population which would require the figure to be corrected upward. Most of the statistical data come from North America, Europe, and Japan, and one cannot be certain that the incidence is the same in other parts of the world, but estimates of a worldwide prevalence of 10 to 20 million and of 4 to 5 million new cases per year seem realistic.

Schizophrenics occupy about half the beds in mental hospitals—more hospital beds than patients with any other single disease. They constitute 20 to 30 percent of all new admissions to psychiatric hospitals (100,000 to 200,000 new cases per year in the United States); at any one time about 300,000 schizophrenics are in hospitals and 1.5 million are living outside. The age of admission is between 20 and 40, with a peak at 28 to 34 years.

The incidence of schizophrenia has remained more or less the same over the past several decades. Males and females are affected with equal frequency. For unknown reasons the incidence is higher in social classes showing high mobility and disorganization. It has been suggested that the disease causes a "downward drift" to the lowest socioeconomic stratum, where one finds poverty, crowding, limited education, and associated handicaps, but the same data have been used to support the idea that such social factors cause schizophrenia. The fertility of schizophrenics, formerly lowered by institutionalization, is now approaching that of the general population, which will probably result in an increase in their number.

CAUSE AND MECHANISM

Although there is no universal agreement as to the cause of the disease, an increasing weight of evidence favors a genetic factor. Biologic and psychosocial factors are also considered important. The evidence for each will be presented.

Genetic Factors The early studies of Kallmann showed that the expectancy rate for schizophrenia in 5000 siblings of schizophrenic patients was increased from 0.7 to 0.9 percent (the expected rate for the general population) to 11 percent. In 90 sets of fraternal twins, one of whom had schizophrenia, the incidence of disease in the other twin was also 11 percent, the same as in nontwin siblings. In monozygotic twins (62 sets) the incidence in the second twin was 68 percent. In other words, the closer the relatedness of a family member to a schizophrenic, the greater the risk of schizophrenia. Thus, the prospect of the child of one schizophrenic parent having schizophrenia is the same as for the siblings of schizophrenic patients (about 11 percent, see above); if both parents are schizophrenic, the chances are greater than 50 percent that the child will have the disease. Subsequent family studies have repeatedly confirmed these findings (see Goodwin and Guze for complete tabulation).

There has been much discussion in the literature concerning nature versus nurture, i.e., the relative importance of genetic and environmental factors, in the genesis of the disease. The available studies lend little support to environmental factors. In the study of Rosenthal, Kety, and their associates, a group of children of schizophrenics who had been removed at an early age from their natural parents and placed in adoptive homes were compared with a group of adopted children whose natural parents had no known psychiatric disease. Thus the child of the schizophrenic shared only the genetic background of his parents but not their environment. The incidence of schizophrenia in the first group of children was about twice that of the second. In similar studies both Karlsson and Heston showed that children separated early in life and reared apart from schizophrenic parents had the same disposition to schizophrenia (11 percent) as children of schizophrenics raised in the homes of their biologic parents. Fischer has approached the problem differently. Monozygotic twins, only one of whom was schizophrenic, were identified, and their children were studied; the incidence of schizophrenia in the children of the nonschizophrenic member of the twin pair was the same as in the children of the schizophrenic member.

Although the importance of genetic factors in the etiology of schizophrenia is undeniable, the precise mode of inheritance has not been determined; the best evidence to date favors a single gene of intermediate (partial or incomplete) dominance (Morton et al.; Böök et al.).

Other Biological Factors Body habitus was singled out by Kretschmer as being linked in some way to schizophrenia. He thought slender (leptosomic) individuals tended to develop schizophrenia, if they were to become psychotic, and those with pyknic (stocky) body build became manic-depressive. More careful studies by Sheldon and others have not fully supported this hypothesis.

A great variety of physiologic and endocrine differences between schizophrenic and normal subjects has been claimed. When the observations were controlled, however, the abnormality in question was always found to relate to physical inactivity, neglect, or undernourishment, especially in chronically hospitalized patients, rather than to the disease per se.

There have been many attempts to isolate from the blood of schizophrenic patients some metabolic or toxic substance that could reproduce the clinical state when injected into nonschizophrenic subjects. Such positive results as were claimed have been unverifiable. This is true of the psychotropic copper-containing globulin called *taraxein*, histamine, serotonin or catecholamine metabolites, amino acids, altered macroglobulins, and an erythrocyte-lysing factor. From time to time an aminoaciduria, a folate or vitamin B_{12} deficiency, or some such condition has been discovered in a psychotic patient who is said to have schizophrenia, but isolated findings of this sort, in patients in whom the diagnosis can be questioned, have little meaning.

When certain hallucinogens, such as mescaline and lysergic acid diethylamide (LSD), were first observed to induce hallucinations and abnormalities of thinking, it was hoped that these drugs might provide models of experimental schizophrenia. It was even postulated that in schizophrenia a faulty metabolism of biogenic amines might produce such an endogenous psychotogen. This has never been substantiated. When methionine, a potent source of methyl groups, was observed to exacerbate the symptoms of some schizophrenics, it was thought that evidence of a primary metabolic fault had been discovered. The presence of increased quantities of dimethoxyphenethylamine and N-methylated indoleamines lent support to this idea. However, none of these observations has been unequivocally corroborated.

Since the antipsychotic neuroleptics display an affinity for dopamine receptors, it has been widely concluded that these drugs act by reducing dopaminergic transmission. Other hypotheses have implicated neurotransmitters which interact or maintain a balance with dopamine (norepinephrine, acetylcholine, serotonin, γ-aminobutyric acid). These hypotheses are under active study (for further details see reviews by Kety).

Since psychoses may complicate corticosteroid administration and certain endocrine diseases (Cushing's disease, thyrotoxicosis), there have been many attempts to uncover such abnormalities in the schizophrenic patient. All have failed.

Psychosocial Factors Freud's theory of schizophrenia has already been mentioned. He assumed that the essential disturbance occurred early in life, during the formative period of infantile sexual development. He believed that the schizophrenic process represents a fixation at or possibly a regression to that period of life when the organism thinks illogically and is absorbed in itself, i.e., when it is narcissistic. Though such a proposition is interesting, there is no way of either affirming or refuting it.

A somewhat more physiologically based hypothesis postulates a defect in the attention process by which sensations, thoughts, and feelings are "filtered." This results in altered experiences, and the delusions and hallucinations are said to be attempts to deal with them.

Intrafamily relationships are thought by some to be responsible for engendering schizophrenic traits. The picture is painted of the cold, rejecting, but overprotective mother who induces conflicting reaction patterns in her child. The latter is said to be threatened by the intermittent expression of affection, possibility of separation, coercion to conform to family standards, lack of mutual support, etc. Behind all these suggestions is the notion that disturbed interpersonal relations in the family in some way interfere with the normal maturation of personality. Proof is totally lacking that such an environment is unique to the development of schizophrenia. Furthermore, the extent to which these aberrations of family relationship are primary or secondary cannot be ascertained. Unquestionably such explorations have elucidated hitherto unknown aspects of family life, but just how they relate to schizophrenia is anyone's guess.

CLINICAL MANIFESTATIONS

It is probably fair to say that the most serious students of psychiatry are still uncertain as to what constitutes the

essential clinical abnormality in schizophrenia. Many suggestions have been offered, but no independent means exists of determining their validity. All the many criteria for clinical diagnosis, including those of Bleuler, depend upon (1) the identification of a constellation of clinical symptoms and (2) the natural course of the disease, i.e., chronicity with periodic exacerbations.

From the neurologic point of view the central issue of schizophrenia appears to be a disturbance in thinking and in the perception of self and environment, unlike the conditions seen in deliria, confusional states, dementia, and depression. Some patients with chronic schizophrenia, when in remission, show little evidence of their disease by all tests usually employed in assessing the mental status. If symptomatic but testable, schizophrenics, although oriented and seemingly able to form memories, are vague, preoccupied, and unable to think in the abstract, to understand figurative statements such as proverbs, and to separate relevant from irrelevant data. There is a circumstantiality and tangentiality about their remarks. They fail to communicate their ideas clearly. Their thinking no longer shows respect for the logical limits of time and space. Parts are confused with the whole or are clustered together or condensed in an illogical way; opposites may be considered as identical, and conceptual relationships are distorted. In the analysis of a stimulus situation there is a tendency to be overinclusive rather than underinclusive (in underinclusive analysis, as happens in amentia, dementia, and delirium, the main features are missed). In conversation and in writing, the trend of an argument or thought sequence is often interrupted abruptly.

Such schizophrenic aberrations of thinking are displayed in speech, writing, and even art. In every mode of expression one perceives curious combinations of excessive concreteness, florid symbolism, esoteric interpretations, and the abandonment of accepted rules of logic. Speech is stereotyped, repetitious, and lacking in communicative content.

In more severely affected schizophrenics, thinking is even more disintegrated, and they can do no more than utter a series of meaningless phrases or neologisms, or speech may be reduced to a "word salad." They are unable to attend to the task at hand or to concentrate, with the result that performance becomes variable and unpredictable. At times these patients are talkative and exhibit odd behavior; at other times they are quiet, preoccupied with their own thoughts and concerned about their family or others around them or with imagined diseases. Young patients are often quite hypochondriacal, which brings them to the attention of a physician. At the other extreme, they are mute and idle. With recovery, they may have only fragmentary memories of events during the exacerbation of their illness.

A number of unusual ideas, concerning the relationship of these patients to themselves and to their environment, may appear in their comments. Frequently they express the thought that their body is somehow separated from their mind, that they do not feel like themselves, that their body belongs to someone else, or that they are not sure of their own identity or even sex. This is called *depersonalization*. Closely related is a sense of being under the control of other persons, of hearing their own thoughts or being made to speak them, or to act in ways that are dictated by others, often through the medium of radar, x-ray, etc. (*passivity feelings*). There are frequently *ideas of reference*—that the remarks or actions of others are subtly directed to them. Finally patients may feel that the world about them is changed or unnatural, not in a brief episode like the *jamais vu* of a temporal lobe seizure, but continuously.

Auditory hallucinations are frequent; often the voices are accusatory or threatening, or in control of the patient's actions. The voices may or may not be recognized. Sometimes the voices come from outside the patient, but more often the patient feels that such voices come somehow from within and cannot distinguish them from his or her own feelings and thoughts. Visual, olfactory, and other types of hallucinations also occur. The patient believes in the reality of these hallucinations, and they may be part of a delusional system.

The behavior of the individual experiencing these bizarre ideas and feelings is correspondingly altered. Early in the course of the illness, normal activities may be interrupted. No longer does the patient function properly in school or at work. Associates and relatives are likely to find the patient's ceaseless complaints, fears, and bizarre ideas disturbing. The patient may be idle for long periods, preoccupied with inner ruminations, and may withdraw socially. The emotional response to threatening hallucinations may at first be one of fear, but later the patient comes to tolerate them with a show of indifference and may not let anyone know about them. A panic or frenzy of excitement may lead to a visit to an emergency ward (a high degree of anxiety developing for the first time in a young person should always alert one to the possibility of a developing schizophrenia), or the patient may become mute and immobile, i.e., *catatonic*. However, attacks of catatonia are infrequent, and lack of will, drive, assertiveness, etc., are the more characteristic features of the disease.

Much has been made of the change in affect. Usually the patient's manner is bland or apathetic; he or she may casually express ideas that would be disturbing to a normal person, even smiling or laughing over a morbid idea. To the authors this has not been an impressive feature of the illness. Often one observes agitation and appropriate emotionality in response to a threatening hallucination or delusion, although later there appears increasing indifference and preoccupation, with flat affect, as though the patient had become inured to the abnormal thoughts and feelings.

Other behavioral and delusional features are discussed in relation to the special types of schizophrenia.

SUBTYPES OF SCHIZOPHRENIA

Traditionally, psychiatrists have distinguished a number of syndromes, but in the United States the one recognized most often is the "undifferentiated" type.

Undifferentiated, or Simple, Schizophrenia In this condition the patient typically exhibits thought disorder, bland affect, social withdrawal, and impaired work performance, but not hallucinations and delusions. These abnormalities develop insidiously over months and finally present in an acute schizophrenic episode during which all the aforementioned symptoms worsen. In the acute phase the patient usually needs to be hospitalized and given medication. As a rule, a remission follows, during which the patient is able to function at a level below that which is expected on the basis of previous abilities and intelligence. In the chronic phase the patient resumes a quiet life and can work with supervision but lacks normal drive, initiative, and enterprise. These patients attract notice only because they behave in an odd manner, tending to remain by themselves ("loners"), making no effort to adjust to a social group at school, find work, "have dates," or establish or maintain a family unit. If the parents do not provide support and protection, such persons drift from one odd job to another, always shy, withdrawn, and relatively indifferent to their surroundings. Psychotic manifestations are infrequent. Such individuals are often found among "hobos" and others on the fringes of society.

In this form of schizophrenia, none of the florid characteristics of catatonia or hebephrenia are observed. Since it may easily be confused with other psychiatric illnesses, the precision of diagnosis is variable (see below, under "Differential Diagnosis").

Hebephrenic Schizophrenia This was believed by Kraepelin to be a particularly malignant form. It tends to occur at an earlier age than the other varieties. The thought disorder is pronounced—there is a striking incoherence of ideas, and the frequent occurrence of hallucinations, delusions, and marked emotional disturbances (periods of excitement alternating with periods of tearfulness and depression) leaves little doubt that the patient is psychotic. The visual and auditory illusions and hallucinations are usually more in the nature of symbolic interpretations than abnormal perceptions. Kraepelin remarked on the changeable, fantastic, and bizarre character of the delusions. Motor symptoms, in the form of stereotyped behavior, tics, and mannerisms, are particularly prominent in this form of schizophrenia. Others have been impressed with the fact that hebephrenic patients since their early days have shown an unstable emotional condition; a history of tantrums throughout childhood and of being too pious, shy, fearful, solitary, conscientious, and idealistic may have marked them as odd or "queer." This latter state is sometimes called *schizoid*, but it could as well represent the early phase of the disease (see Chap. 55).

Catatonic Schizophrenia   This is the most readily differentiated type. It was originally described by Kahlbaum and accepted as a variety of mental disturbance *sui generis*, until Kraepelin recognized that it was another form of schizophrenia. There is in this disorder a curious combination of excitement with catatonic stupor. In 60 percent of cases, the onset is relatively acute. After a prodrome of slackening interest, apathy, lack of concentration, and dreamy preoccupation, a state of dull stupor supervenes, with mutism, inactivity, refusal of food, and a tendency to maintain one position, "like a mummy." The facial expression is vacant, the lips pursed; the patient lies supine without motion, or sits for hours with hands on knees and head bowed (*catalepsy*). If a limb is lifted by the examiner it will sometimes be held in that position for hours (flexibilitas cerea). Urine and feces are retained, or there is incontinence. The patients must be tube-fed (or will eat mechanically) and have to be dressed and undressed. Pinprick or pinch induces no reaction. Extreme negativism, every command being resisted, characterizes some cases. Echolalia and echopraxia are occasionally exhibited. Yet all the time these patients know everything that is said to them or is happening around them and will reproduce much of this information during recovery or a temporary remission induced by intravenous sodium amytal. After weeks or months in this state, the patient begins to talk and act

normally, and there is then rapid recovery. In certain phases of catatonia there may be a period of excitement and impulsivity, during which the patient may be suicidal or homicidal.

For reasons that are unclear, this form of schizophrenia is now seen infrequently. A similar catatonic state may occur in the manic phase of manic-depressive psychosis.

Acute Schizophrenia   This term is applied to acute undifferentiated or catatonic forms. This diagnosis is well accepted in the United States, but many psychiatrists are skeptical that such an entity exists, especially when there is no family history of similar disease or of early schizoid behavior. The majority of such episodes turn out to be manic attacks; endocrine psychoses may also simulate schizophrenia (the schizophreniform psychosis of Langfeldt). Yet there is no doubt that schizophrenia may begin acutely or that acute episodes may be an exacerbation of a chronic, progressive form of illness.

Paranoid Schizophrenia   This is one of the most frequent subtypes. The mean age of onset is 42 years (Winokur), somewhat later than the preceding types. Multiple, unsystematized, changeable delusions are expressed, some quite fantastic and accompanied by hallucinations. More often than not they are persecutory, but also they may be religious, depressive, and grandiose in nature. Many such patients settle into a chronic hallucinatory psychosis with disorders of thinking, featured by mistrust and suspiciousness. They appear cold, aloof, and indifferent, and many are hypochondriacal.

European psychiatrists, impressed with the lack of schizoid traits in the premorbid period and in the family history, have insisted that paranoid schizophrenia is a different disease. The studies of Rosenthal and his colleagues in this country tend to bear them out. Also, the clinical and family studies of Winokur indicate that hebephrenic and paranoid schizophrenia are separate illnesses.

There are of course other psychiatric illnesses in which paranoid delusions appear, such as manic-depressive psychosis, dementia, and delirium. Alcoholic auditory hallucinosis stands as a separate illness (see page 753). There is, in addition, a special form of *delusional disorder* (*paranoia*) in which the individual is consumed by a single persecutory, grandiose, or amorous delusional system, without other thought disorders. An exotic form is known as *folie à deux*, in which two closely related persons share a delusional system. These several types of paranoia are discussed further in the latter part of the chapter.

Residual Schizophrenia This term is applied to the condition in which, after one or several acute episodes of schizophrenia, patients become nonpsychotic and function reasonably well, though subnormally. In reality they have schizophrenia in remission.

Childhood Schizophrenia This term designates the disorder of children who have a wide variety of developmental and adjustment problems and become at some time psychotically disturbed; i.e., they become excited, depressed, or hallucinatory and express bizarre ideas. The relation of such illnesses to adult schizophrenia remains unsettled. There is no evidence that such children go on to have schizophrenia later in life. Often organic factors, such as metabolic errors, mental retardation, and infantile autism (Kanner's syndrome), are demonstrable.

Robins and Guze have attempted to simplify the confusing nomenclature of these schizophrenic disorders by dividing them into two major categories, one with relatively poor and the other with relatively good prognosis. *Schizophreniform, schizoaffective, acute, reactive,* and *remitting schizophrenia* are other terms that have been applied to cases with a relatively good prognosis. They suggest that the term *schizophrenia* be reserved for the types of illness that carry a poor prognosis, which are also generally referred to as *process,* or *nuclear, schizophrenia.*

CLINICAL COURSE AND LIFE PROFILE OF SCHIZOPHRENIA

Not infrequently an acute florid illness, with the main attributes of schizophrenia, appears unheralded in an otherwise intact individual. The patient makes a full recovery and remains well thereafter. Such an episodic illness is particularly frequent in college students and soldiers. The most experienced clinicians are uncertain as to whether this type of illness is truly schizophrenia or a psychotic reaction resembling this disease, i.e., a manic attack, toxic confusional state, or an endocrine psychosis. Most of the monophasic illnesses with complete remissions are, in fact, cases of this type. Strong arguments against acute or "good prognosis" schizophrenia being true schizophrenia are the preponderance of manic-depressive disease over schizophrenia in family members of the former group and the response of these patients to drugs that are effective in manic-depressive disease. In contrast, most "real" schizophrenic decompensations follow a long period of emotional and behavioral maladjustment. Some of these cases had been diagnosed as "adolescent turmoil." As stated above, psychosis in childhood is hardly ever recorded in the histories of schizophrenic patients (which is why psychiatrists are hesitant to make a diagnosis of schizophrenia during childhood). Instead, the personality of the patient destined to develop schizophrenia is cold, difficult, withdrawn, eccentric, and easily disorganized by the common problems of life. Another pattern is the unstable, "stormy personality," with periods of alternating aggressiveness and submissiveness, and defiance of authority; envy, disdain, "touchiness," insecurity, and unreasonable fears are other features.

Many schizophrenic patients exhibit neurotic traits before and during their disease. Hypochondriasis, with vague feelings of being unwell, are especially frequent. Fear and anxiety may also be present, along with insomnia, tension, rapid heart action, and headaches. Some of these arise in relation to a disappointment, separation from family, the breaking of an unstable heterosexual relationship, or a physical illness. These symptoms may continue for years before the schizophrenic disorder of thinking is recognized or a frank schizophrenic break occurs.

In a 30- to 40-year follow-up study of schizophrenic and manic-depressive patients, Winokur and Tsuang found that in each group the same proportion (about 10 percent) of patients who were deceased had committed suicide. The risk of suicide in schizophrenia is often not appreciated. Suicide occurs most often among young schizophrenics living apart from their families, frightened and discouraged by their symptoms and the difficulties of independent existence. Sometimes the suicide is in response to terrifying and commanding vocal hallucinations. Homicide also may occur, usually in acting out a delusional system in which the patient becomes convinced that he or she has been harmed by the victim.

Once schizophrenia is clearly recognized, usually after an insidious onset, the chronic pattern establishes itself. The earlier turmoil occasioned by fear, anger, resentment, and delusional thinking subsides. The later phases are characterized by marked poverty of ideation, weakness of impulse, inability to cope with school, the workaday world, and the community. The persistent defect is not so much in intelligence and memory (which may test at a near-normal level or be reduced) as in personality. These patients seem incapable of sustained, goal-directed activity and efficient performance. When other cerebral functions are examined, certain abnormalities have been found. Alertness is not impaired, but attention is difficult to judge. Often patients seem oblivious to what happens around them. Except where muteness is a feature, speech is fluent and no measured alteration of language function or calculation has been reported. In tests of verbal and visual pattern learning and memorizing, Cutting found a surprising degree of impairment in both the acute and chronic schizophrenic (and in retarded depression) which was not attributable to electroconvulsant therapy, seizures, drugs, or other diseases. Interestingly in the acute schizophrenic he found verbal memory more affected than visual pattern memory, in agreement with the findings of Flor-Henry that the left-hemispheric functions are more reduced than the right. In the chronic schizophrenic there was evidence of bihemispheral derangement.

Periodically schizophrenic patients are subject to exacerbations of their illness, sometimes at regular intervals, as though determined by a metabolic disorder, e.g., Gjessing's cases, in which attacks of periodic catatonia were associated with shifts in nitrogen balance (see Lehman). Functional remissions are more frequent and lasting when medication is given and long institutionalization is avoided. Modern therapeutic programs have reduced the number of patients in mental hospitals by 1 to 2 percent per year. However, readmission rates also have risen (revolving-door phenomenon), and the total number of very young and very old patients in hospitals has even increased slightly. The life span of schizophrenics is somewhat reduced, probably because of the malnutrition, neglect, and exposure to infections that occur in public institutions.

NEUROPATHOLOGY

Throughout the modern era of cellular neuropathology, there has been disagreement concerning the status of schizophrenia. Alzheimer and his pupils, who had access to the clinical material of Kraepelin, made a study of 55 cases, including 18 uncomplicated and 6 acute. They reportedly noted hypertrophy (ameboid change) of the astrocytes, to which importance was attached because it was not found in cases of manic-depressive psychosis. Further, in the cerebra of deteriorated patients with chronic schizophrenia, an outfall of neurons in the second and third laminae of the frontal cortex was described, along with nuclear swelling, shrinkage of cell body, and deposits of lipofuscin. Similar findings were subsequently described by Sioli, Orton, and others.

Dunlap, in 1928, in a highly critical analysis, repudiated all earlier interpretations of these alterations. He pointed out that many changes, such as the dark "sclerotic" nerve cells, were artifacts and that lipofuscin was a nonspecific age change. He asserted also that the neuronal loss described by Alzheimer was based on impression and could not be corroborated by quantitative methods. Similarly, the claim of Oscar Vogt of neuronal loss in the cortex was rejected by his contemporaries, W. Spielmeyer and W. Scholz, who were unable to find any consistent cellular abnormality in schizophrenia (see Dunlap for early references).

Unfortunately the matter is not settled even today, for no cases (except those of Vogt) have been rigorously studied by whole-brain serial sections, and no quantitative studies have been made of septal and other little known central nuclei. Golgi and ultrastructural methods, using reliable techniques, have not been undertaken. Of course, the absence of a cellular pathologic change does not rule out a disease process, for in delirium tremens, toxic psychosis, and many metabolic diseases of the brain, the lesion is probably subcellular, i.e., molecular.

Other laboratory investigations have been equally uninformative. The EEG reveals little of interest except minor, uninterpretable changes. The CSF, blood, and urine are normal. Recently a degree of "brain atrophy" (enlargement of ventricles and widening of cerebral sulci) has been reported in the CT scans of a number of chronic schizophrenics. It is said that this has been checked against age-matched controls (Rieder et al.).

DIFFERENTIAL DIAGNOSIS

From the neurological standpoint the concept of Langfeldt has particular appeal. As indicated in the historical remarks, he distinguished the schizophreniform reactions or psychoses from the disease schizophrenia. The authors would equate the schizophreniform psychosis with a delusional-hallucinatory syndrome in which there is little if any disturbance of consciousness. We would agree with Schneider that the syndrome consists of six closely related symptoms that as a group are pathognomonic: (1) auditorization of thought (the patient hears his or her own thoughts), (2) auditory hallucinations which take the form of voices giving a "running commentary" on the patient's current thoughts and actions (e.g., there may be a conversation between two voices which comment on the patient as a third person), (3) thought withdrawal or broadcasting, wherein the patient's thoughts are heard by others, (4) somatic hallucinations in which the patient's movements and deeds are no longer subject to will but are under the control of outside agencies, (5) delusions, some of which are conditioned by things seen or heard, and (6) feelings, impulses, and willed actions that the patient feels are determined by others (passivity feelings). Reduced to the simplest terms these reflect disturbances of thought (equivalent to Bleuler's looseness of associations), hallucinations, and delusions.

Although this syndrome is characteristic of schizophrenia, it may occur in the manic phase of manic-depressive disease, alcoholic auditory hallucinosis, temporal lobe epilepsy, chronic amphetamine intoxication, and rarely in certain endocrine and metabolic disorders where consciousness is not impaired. Whenever this syndrome is recognized, therefore, these several causes need to be differentiated. At the McLean Hospital, only one out of five of the acute schizophreniform psychoses proves to be due to the disease schizophrenia.

The diagnosis of the disease called schizophrenia involves a different constellation of data. The presence of the delusional-hallucinatory syndrome always raises the possibility of schizophrenia, but it must be remembered that in chronic schizophrenia or in the remittent form of the disease, the components of this syndrome may be either absent or too subtle to detect. Other data are required for diagnosis. Feighner, Robins, and Guze, who have drawn up a set of diagnostic criteria for research in all the major psychiatric syndromes, state that the diagnosis of schizophrenia is tenable only if there are (1) a chronic illness of at least 6 months' duration and a failure (after an acute episode) to return to the premorbid level of psychosocial adjustment, (2) delusions or hallucinations without significant perplexity or disorientation (i.e., without clouding of consciousness), (3) verbal productions that are so illogical and confusing as to make communication difficult (if patient is mute, diagnosis should be deferred), and (4) at least three of the following manifestations: (*a*) an adult who is single, (*b*) poor premorbid social adjustment or work history, (*c*) family history of schizophrenia, or (*d*) onset of illness prior to age of 40 years. Important negatives include absence of a family history of manic-depressive disease, absence of an earlier illness with depressive or manic symptoms, and absence of alcoholism or drug abuse within a year of onset of the psychosis.

While these criteria are so strict as to exclude certain patients with a schizophrenic illness, those that are included will be found to constitute a fairly homogeneous group. Morrison et al., who used these criteria, noted that after a 10-year follow-up there was practically no change in diagnosis; they had quite reliably separated schizophrenia, the schizophreniform psychoses (where only the acute delusional-hallucinatory syndrome was present), and manic-depressive psychosis.

The typical chronic cases offer little difficulty in diagnosis, especially if one adheres to the essential criteria of a special disorder of thinking, the presence of hallucinations and delusions, an eccentric behavior pattern and bland affect, a chronic, relapsing course, the presence of a family history, and onset of the disease in adolescence and early adulthood. As a rule, depressed mood, anxiety and agitation, feelings of hopelessness, and psychomotor retardation mark the cyclical and involutional depressions, and restless, overactive, pressured, intrusive, and easily frustrated (irritable) behavior denotes the manic states. Schizophrenics with prominent depressive symptoms who have made repeated suicidal attempts pose an exceptionally difficult problem in diagnosis. Sometimes referred to as *schizothymic*, to this day it is not certain whether they have schizophrenia or manic-depressive disease, or both. When in remission, patients with affective disorders are usually normal, whereas schizophrenic and many schizoaffective psychotics are not. Abrupt onset at any period in life, disorientation, confusion, insomnia, and vivid exteriorized hallucinations set apart the delirious-confusional psychoses. Seldom does schizophrenia appear for the first time after the fortieth year; in older patients who develop mental illness for the first time, the illness usually proves to be a depression, presenile dementia, or some other organic psychosis.

Over the years the authors have encountered the greatest difficulties in the diagnosis of schizophrenia in the following clinical situations:

1. *A schizophrenia-like illness in a patient whose family members are not affected and whose premorbid personality has been normal.* The presence of disturbed thinking, anxiety, depression or euphoria, catatonia, catalepsy, and odd mannerisms may seem compatible with schizophrenia, but such illnesses often terminate, leaving the patient completely normal. Experienced psychiatrists prefer to make no diagnosis or refer to the condition as *schizophrenic reaction*, or *schizophreniform psychosis*, as distinguished from *process schizophrenia*.

2. A similar case of *a patient with an acute illness* having many of the typical features of schizophrenia but *associated with confusion, forgetfulness, and/or clouding of consciousness.* Mood change may be prominent. Thus the illness combines the features of an affective disorder, schizophrenia, and a confusional state. This syndrome is characteristic of corticosteroid psychosis (drug-induced or Cushing's disease), thyrotoxic psycho-

sis, puerperal psychosis, and the so-called exhaustion psychoses of war years. Usually recovery is complete, and "process schizophrenia" is excluded by the fact that the patient remains well.

3. *Adolescents and young adults whose social relationships are disorganized and who are unusually sensitive, resentful, rebellious, fearful, discouraged, in trouble with school authorities and the law, using drugs, etc.* The latter may have caused seizures, hallucinations, and withdrawal symptoms, or may have resulted in addiction. Such patients are usually classified as having "character disorders" that appear to go back to the early years of life; or if they are incorrigible, unable to profit by experience, amoral, and in trouble with social agencies, they are called *psychopaths* or *sociopaths*. Since the diagnosis of schizophrenia depends on the elicitation of a complex of manifestations described above, this type of social maladjustment usually turns out not to be schizophrenia. In other words, if the syndrome does not contain all the cardinal elements of schizophrenia and if the course of the illness is not known or has not been traced back to late childhood and adolescence, one should hesitate to make the diagnosis of schizophrenia.

4. There is the opposite type of diagnostic problem, arising in *an individual who has been only marginally competent because of personality problems and many vague neurotic symptoms* often requiring prolonged psychotherapy. Many such individuals will be found to have the "pseudoneurotic" or simple form of schizophrenia. Errors in diagnosis usually result from a failure to assess mental status carefully, to search for the typical signs of schizophrenia, and to ascertain the life profile of the disorder.

5. *Acute auditory hallucinosis in a chronically alcoholic patient.* This is usually a dramatic illness, at first characterized by threatening, exteriorized auditory hallucinations to which the patient's emotional reaction is appropriate. Mental clarity is another feature. Only later do a few of these patients drift into a quiet hallucinatory, mildly paranoid state, with rather bland affect. The so-called schizoid personality cannot be detected, and there is usually no family history of schizophrenia. Cases of this type that we have studied had their onset between 45 and 50 years of age, i.e., much later than the age of onset of schizophrenia. In European medical circles, this schizophrenia-like illness is now considered different

from the "core" or "process" type of schizophrenia, an opinion which concurs with that of the authors.

6. *A patient who is confused or stuporous and seemingly negativistic, refusing or unable to speak, execute commands, or be activated in any way.* By inference one is tempted, if signs of focal cerebral or brainstem disease are absent, to diagnose catatonic schizophrenia, not realizing that catatonia as a phenomenon can be a manifestation of widespread disease of the associational cortex, of mania, of deliria or confusional states, and of hysteria. The error can be avoided if one makes diagnoses on the basis of positive findings, not on the absence of data. The authors have seen cases of hypoxic encephalopathy, Schilder's disease, and Creutzfeldt-Jakob disease mistaken for schizophrenia because of failure to adhere to this principle.

7. *A patient with a typical delusional-hallucinatory syndrome* who has taken large quantities of dextroamphetamine for weeks or months.

8. *A patient with temporal lobe epilepsy* who, apart from psychomotor seizures, has long periods (weeks or months) of hallucinations, delusions, bizarre behavior, and disorganization of thinking. This has been observed only with temporal lobe seizures, some of which have been demonstrated by depth electrodes as originating in the amygdaloid area. Other types of psychopathology are also associated with temporal lobe epilepsy, such as behavioral disturbances and sexual deviations. In the series reported by Jensen and Larsen, 55 out of 74 patients exhibited mental disturbances (see also Chap. 25).

At the root of all these diagnostic difficulties is the lack of any confirmatory laboratory test or of specific physical or pathologic findings in schizophrenia. Consequently, diagnosis lacks accuracy, allowing cases to be included which only resemble the core type of schizophrenia, and probably others to be overlooked because the symptoms are incomplete or variant. Only by repeated examinations, which over the years reveal the course of the disease, does diagnosis become more secure. Even then there may be the error of arbitrarily excluding cases or syndromes that do not conform to a preconceived idea of the disease.

TREATMENT

It is often possible, once the diagnosis of schizophrenia is established, for an internist or neurologist to assume responsibility for treatment. He soon becomes accustomed to the particular pattern of the patient's behavior and can help support the patient and his or her family during difficult periods. Relapse with psychotic decompensation demands drug therapy, and if there is a hazard of injury or suicide, or difficulty in family management, hospitalization becomes necessary. Most general hospitals now have facilities for the management of such cases, and many of the state hospitals are able to provide short-term treatment. Instead of mere custodial care with restraints, locked doors, and little nursing help, they now have flexible programs of planned activities, physiotherapy, vocational and milieu therapy, etc., which quickly involve the patient as a contributing member of the clinical unit during the active phases of the disease. The aim of hospitalization is to protect the patient, relieve the family of the labor of constant vigilance and supervision, and to assure the administration of drugs until the exacerbation spends itself. The patient can then return to the family and community.

Modern treatment consists essentially of antipsychotic medication. The original drugs were *Rauwolfia* alkaloids and the phenothiazines, particularly chlorpromazine. Several modifications of chlorpromazine have become available, including the piperazine derivatives. The latter [e.g., fluphenazine (Prolixin), trifluoperazine (Stelazine), and perphenazine (Trilafon)] are higher in milligram potency than chlorpromazine. There are also new molecular types such as the thioxanthenes, e.g., chlorprothixine (Taractan); a butyrophenone, *l*-haloperidol (Haldol); an indole, molindone (Moban); and a tricyclic piperazine, *l*-loxapine (Loxitane). Often these drugs are called *tranquilizers*, with the implication that they reduce anxiety. However, the antipsychotic drugs should not be used for this purpose, since they are both less effective and more toxic than the barbiturates and benzodiazepines (Librium, Valium). The antipsychotic drugs not only suppress the psychiatric abnormalities but also have other rather specific ("neuroleptic") effects, probably due to their action as dopamine antagonists in the basal ganglia. Parkinsonian rigidity, motor restlessness (akathisia), dystonia, and several other facial-cervical dyskinesias are common side effects, which once started, may persist long after the drug is discontinued (tardive dyskinesia; see page 777). Many of these extrapyramidal disorders can be controlled by the simultaneous parenteral administration of antihistaminic drugs [e.g., diphenhydramine (Benadryl), 25 mg tid] and the anticholinergic drugs used in the treatment of Parkinson's disease [e.g., benztropine mesylate (Cogentin), 0.2 mg tid]. However, the latter drugs must be given cautiously, for they may hamper the antipsychotic action and, if given in large doses, may themselves induce a toxic psychosis. If it becomes necessary to treat the extrapyramidal side effects, it is usually possible to eliminate the anticholinergic drugs after 2 to 3 months without return of symptoms. In chronically medicated patients, in whom tardive dyskinesias are frequent, an increased dose of the antipsychotic drug may suppress the dyskinesia temporarily. Whenever possible, drug therapy should not be prolonged; the use of the lowest possible dose and drug holidays a few times a year are advised. During periods of remission no drug therapy is needed. However, some psychiatrists believe that continuous antipsychotic medication is useful in preventing hospitalization.

Tolerance and addiction to the antipsychotic drugs do not develop. Turnover rates are low, so that a single dose in 24 h suffices (usually given at bedtime to help with the insomnia). Barbiturates and tranquilizers are reserved for sedation of acutely combative and emotionally disturbed patients.

The dosages of these antipsychotic drugs need to be individualized. The usual daily dose of chlorpromazine is 300 to 500 mg, but up to 1000 mg or more can be given; the dose of other antipsychotic drugs is equivalent. Since most schizophrenic patients have no insight into their illness and the side effects of the medication are unpleasant, the major difficulty is in getting them to take it, in which case a depot form of fluphenazine can be given once every 1 to 3 weeks.

Electroconvulsive therapy (ECT) is now seldom used except in patients who are stuporous or agitated or who have major affective symptoms, or in exceptional instances where there is no response to medication. Insulin therapy has been abandoned, as has leukotomy. One form of the latter (cingulotomy) is still being tried in patients who have failed to respond to all other types of therapy.

Massive doses of vitamin C or B (megavitamins) are of no proven value.

Supportive psychotherapy (explanation, reassurance, encouragement) is of course necessary, as in any prolonged illness, and the family needs the same type of help. The physician should be understanding and sympathetic, but also firm and professional. The general purpose of psychotherapy is to assist the patient to obtain a grasp on reality and to strengthen self-esteem and psychological defenses. Psychoanalytic therapy has been tried with few claims of benefit. Most practicing psychiatrists believe it to have little to offer as a primary mode of treatment.

PARANOIA AND PARANOID STATES

The term *paranoid* designates patients who show

> . . . fixed suspicions, persecutory delusions, dominant ideas or grandiose trends logically elaborated and with due regard for reality once the false interpretation or premise has been accepted. Further characteristics are formally correct conduct, adequate emotional reactions, and coherence of the train of thought. (Rosanoff)

In other words, in pure paranoia there is supposed to be no mental defect other than the delusional system—no dementia, hallucinations, or emotional disturbance. Time was when a large group of the mentally ill were classified as paranoid. But with advancing knowledge of mental illness, fewer and fewer have been left in this category.

The trouble that psychiatrists have taken to couch this definition in negatives implies that paranoia is frequently a feature of other forms of mental illness, notably schizophrenia; manic-depressive, toxic, or alcoholic psychosis; general paresis, etc. This fact about paranoia was known from the beginning, when Heinroth originally described it in 1818 and classified it as a limited disorder of the intellect. Krafft-Ebing, in his monograph on the subject, took pains to distinguish two syndromes: (1) "original paranoia," developing about the time of puberty and attributable to heredity (surely schizophrenia by present-day criteria), and (2) acquired paranoia, developing in late life, particularly in the involutional period (the condition under discussion). Kraepelin remarked that approximately 40 percent of his cases of paranoia developed this symptom early in life and went on to have schizophrenia. The others were true paranoia or a closely related condition which he called *paraphrenia*, a term no longer used.

Figures on the frequency of true paranoia are probably not reliable because they are of necessity based on hospital records. Doubtless there are many individuals with mild forms of the disorder who have never crossed the threshold of a mental hospital. They are relatively harmless, and in their communities are judged to be mildly "cracked," or monomaniacs. Male preponderance is agreed upon (male/female = 2:1), thus differing from schizophrenia, in which males and females are equally affected.

CLINICAL MANIFESTATIONS

It would be inappropriate in a neurology text to give a detailed account of all the many ways in which paranoiacs behave. A simple paradigm will suffice—that of a middle-aged man of uneasy, brooding, asocial, eccentric nature who gradually develops a dominating idea or belief of his own importance, of having in his possession special powers that make him the envy of others who become bent on persecuting him. As the delusion grows he becomes more preoccupied, less efficient, and increasingly suspicious of others, with a tendency to interpret every one of their words, gestures, or actions as having some reference to himself. Only when his behavior becomes noticeably bizarre or when he does something to annoy others does his condition come to medical attention. On examining such a person one is impressed with his capacity for careful reasoning, which betrays good intelligence. Whatever the false belief—delusions of reference, jealousy, and persecution being the most common—the patient's arguments are logical and buttressed cogently by evidence. Also, the views of such patients about other matters are sensible.

As was said, the illness usually does not lead to hospitalization, and if admitted to hospital the patient does not stay long. The querulous paranoiacs are the most annoying. They usually remain in the community, flooding the mails with mimeographed documents accusing people falsely, expressing their worthless opinions about anything and everything.

As the years pass, the patient changes little, though a few such patients may later break down and begin to hallucinate and finally end in a deteriorated state much like schizophrenia. This trend supports Bleuler's opinion, that the illness is often a variant of schizophrenia.

As to causation, there are several interesting ideas. The Freudian school has laid particular emphasis on repressed homosexuality as a major factor. Meyer invoked the long-standing personality disorder, the paranoid constitution. This refers to persons who always have a tendency to biased views, to wonder what others think of them, and to attribute deliberate intentions to indifferent actions. Their behavior seems but an exaggeration of a mild suspiciousness that is part of the personality make-up of most individuals. Finally a break occurs, perhaps preceded by excessive and exhausting work, emotion, an accident or a depressive reaction, after which these individuals can no longer adapt their own ideas to the actual facts of their daily lives. All insight is lost. Cameron has presented a detailed discussion of the psychological mechanisms of paranoia.

The authors' experience with paranoid states in a general hospital has been rather limited. One sees deluded patients, to be sure, but usually their abnormal ideas have referred to health and bodily functions, infidelity of spouse, the theft of possessions, etc.; and the abnormal ideas tend to be unsystematized and part of a confusional psychosis, delirium, or dementia. Rarely, a patient comes to the hospital in some other medical context, and it is found that he or she has been living quietly in the community with a bizarre delusional state and without appearing either depressed or schizophrenic. Of course, paranoid schizophrenics or alcoholics with chronic auditory hallucinosis may also develop some medical problem that brings them to a general hospital. Certainly the neurologist sees delusions most often in depressed patients who decompensate as their depression develops. Among the inmates of a psychiatric hospital for the chronically ill, true paranoia is rare (0.1 percent of admissions, according to Winokur).

MANAGEMENT

The methods and objectives of psychotherapy are discussed fully by Cameron (see References at end of chapter). We have no way of deciding whether psychotherapy has influenced this state. In a general hospital, where nearly all our patients have been depressed or maniacal, we have several times been gratified by the effects of antidepressive medication. In the treatment of patients with pathologic jealousy, Mooney has found phenothiazine drugs to be useful.

From what has been said, the clinical analysis of patients with delusions requires a careful study of mood and intelligence to rule out manic-depressive psychosis and dementia. If either of these two states exists, the treatment proceeds along the lines discussed in Chaps. 54 and 20. A matter of practical importance is for the physician to evaluate carefully the nature of the delusional ideas and try to judge whether the patient is homicidal or suicidal. Occasionally, physicians and others have been killed or maimed by paranoiacs who thought they were being mistreated.

PUERPERAL (POSTPARTUM) PSYCHOSES

The parturitional event, including as it does many biologic factors such as the effects of pain, drugs, eclampsia, hemorrhage, infection, and an abrupt hormonal adjustment, is frequently associated with a disturbance of mood. Obstetricians have repeatedly observed that the woman may feel extraordinarily well immediately postpartum, only to lapse in the next days into a weepy, depressed state in which she is distressed by lack of feeling for her newborn infant. Usually this lasts for only a few days, being quelled by the return home, responsibility for the infant, nursing, etc.

The period after childbirth is one in which there is a strong disposition to psychosis. Opinion varies as to whether there is a special *puerperal psychosis*. Most psychiatrists believe that the psychotic break which may occur at this time is of either schizophrenic or depressive type, and that these illnesses do not differ from those which occur at other times in life.

As neurologic consultants to the Boston Lying-in Hospital, the authors were impressed with an unusual type of psychosis that they saw on an average of two or three times each year. Usually this psychosis has its onset between 48 and 72 h after a delivery that may have been complicated by excessive bleeding or infection. The patient alternates between periods of noisy hyperactivity and of mutism and inactivity. She is disoriented and incapable of thinking clearly. The baby is rejected as not belonging to her (instances of infanticide are not unknown). Although the illness has some features of delirium, its persistence for months is incompatible with that diagnosis, nor does it correspond to either a depressive psychosis or schizophrenia. In some instances this postpartum psychosis was terminated by electroconvulsive therapy and did not recur, but there has been no long-term follow-up study of such cases.

Also, in some patients, a depression has followed each of several pregnancies, disabling the patient for months. Some women with manic-depressive disease have had their early depressive attacks only after delivery. In the few instances where we witnessed an acute postpartum schizophrenic episode in a patient without family history or prepsychotic schizoid personality, the prognosis for full and lasting recovery seemed better than one usually expects in schizophrenia. These are only impressions, however.

In the diagnosis of postpartum psychosis, one must also keep in mind the possibility of eclampsia, and the consequences of pituitary infarction (the latter due to circulatory collapse), and hypotensive-hypoxic cerebral injury.

THE ENDOCRINE PSYCHOSES

One of the most provocative observations in contemporary psychiatry is that apparently normal individuals may become psychotic when they develop hyper- or hypothyroidism, Cushing's disease, or adrenal insufficiency, or when they receive therapeutic doses of ACTH or cortisone. If these conditions were no more than examples of drug-induced psychosis, they would be interesting enough. The fact is, however, that they differ considerably from the usual toxic deliria or confusional states. The syndrome, reminiscent of puerperal psychosis and some cases of "combat exhaustion" seen during World War II, comprises features that are suggestive of manic-depressive psychosis or schizophrenia on the one hand and of the confusional psychoses on the other. These endocrine psychoses have far-reaching medical significance, for they provide experimental models of psychoses that can be created by the manipulation of metabolic factors.

ACTH AND CORTISONE PSYCHOSIS

These syndromes are now occurring far less frequently than when ACTH and cortisone were first introduced into medicine. Presumably these hormones are now more purified, and there are more reliable data as to safe dosage. The psychosis usually develops over a period of a few days after the patient has received the hormone for one or more weeks. The features are extremely variable. Some of the patients become elated, agitated, excited, and talkative, as though under pressure to speak, while others are mute; or the prevailing emotional response may be one of anxiety and panic. Thinking may be confused, illogical, tangential, and incoherent. Hallucinations and sensory misinterpretations may appear. Clouding of the sensorium, disorientation, and confusion, the hallmarks of deliria and the confusional psychoses, have not been prominent in the ACTH and cortisone psychoses. However, the state of awareness is not altogether normal, and at times the patient is frankly bewildered. In the motor sphere there may be incessant activity or immobility, resistiveness, and even negativism verging on catatonia. If the hormone is stopped as soon as the diagnosis is established, the psychosis subsides gradually over several days to weeks, with complete recovery.

The mechanism of this psychosis is not known. From the few available studies it has been learned that the occurrence of the psychosis is not related to the premorbid personality. Although the dosage of ACTH or cortisone has usually been high, there has been no exact correlation between dose level and the occurrence, sever-

ity, and duration of the psychosis. Nor does the mental disturbance appear to be related to the rapidity and intensity of the therapeutic response to ACTH and cortisone. Lithium is often effective in controlling the symptoms, allowing continuation of the corticosteroid therapy. The dose is the same as for manic states (see page 1036).

THYROID PSYCHOSIS

A great deal has been said and written about the pervasive effects of abnormal thyroid function on all organs, including the neuromuscular apparatus and central nervous system. These effects are discussed in Chap. 39, under metabolic diseases of the nervous system (pages 742 and 743).

The hyperthyroid patient often shows minor changes in emotions and mentation. Restlessness, irritability, apprehension, emotional lability, and at times even agitation may occur. Either of two trends may be observed in the relatively rare psychotic thyroid patient. There may be mania with its characteristic increase in psychomotor activity, overtalkativeness, and flight of ideas, or there may be depression with its somber mood, weeping, and anxiety. Visual and auditory hallucinations are present in both groups of cases. The clinical picture is seldom clear. Usually the psychiatrist finds something more than simple mania or agitated depression, i.e., some clouding of the sensorium with perplexity and confusion suggestive of delirium. The condition is said to be related to the premorbid personality, some personality types being more vulnerable, but this point is disputed. The condition is not directly related to the severity of the thyrotoxicosis. Careful studies of cerebral blood flow and metabolism during and after the psychosis have not been done. Treatment of the hyperthyroidism does not result in prompt arrest of the psychic disorder, but usually recovery takes place over a period of months. One must distinguish this illness from other types of recurrent psychosis which happen to be coincidental with or precipitated by hyperthyroidism.

With *myxedema* there is a characteristic slowness and thickness of speech, drowsiness, hypothermia, mental dullness, listlessness and apathy, irritability, and sometimes suspiciousness. The patient may sleep most of the time, having to be awakened for meals. A disturbance of memory, and the lack of genuine symptoms of depression, such as feelings of hopelessness and loss of self-esteem, help to distinguish the mental disorder of myxedema from manic-depressive disease. Nevertheless, unless one thinks of myxedema in all cases of psychomotor retardation, the diagnosis will be missed. Reduced cerebral blood flow and metabolism have been found in myxedema, and with specific therapy these functions are restored to normal.

OTHER ENDOCRINE PSYCHOSES

Mental aberrations much like those in ACTH and cortisone psychoses have been observed in *Cushing's disease.* Mental changes in *Addison's disease* are frequent but varied. Irritability, confusion, disorientation, and convulsions, with or without hypoglycemia, are the main features. Some of the mental abnormalities may be related to the disturbances of electrolyte balance, but the mechanisms are not well understood.

REFERENCES

AMERICAN FOUNDATION: *Medical Research: A Mid-century Survey.* Boston, Little, Brown, 1956.

BLEULER E: *Dementia Praecox or the Group of Schizophrenias,* Zinkin J (trans). New York, International Universities Press, 1950.

BÖÖK JA, WETTERBERG L, MODRZEWSKA K: Schizophrenia in a north Swedish geographical isolate 1900–1977. *Clin Genet* 14:373, 1978.

CAMERON NA: Paranoid conditions and paranoia, in Arieti S, Brody EB (eds): *American Handbook of Psychiatry,* 2d ed. New York, Basic Books, 1974, vol III, chap 29, pp 676–693.

CLARK L et al: Preliminary observations on mental disturbances occurring in patients under therapy with cortisone and ACTH. *N Engl J Med* 246:205, 1952.

CUTTING J: Memory in functional psychoses. *J Neurol Neurosurg Psychiatry* 42:1031, 1979.

DUNLAP CB: The pathology of the brain in schizophrenia. *Res Publ Assoc Nerv Ment Dis* 5:371, 1928.

FEIGHNER JP et al: Diagnostic criteria for use in psychiatric research. *Arch Gen Psychiatry* 26:57, 1972.

FISCHER M: Psychoses in the offspring of schizophrenic twins and their normal co-twins. *Br J Psychiatry,* 118:43, 1971.

FLOR-HENRY P: Lateralized temporo-limbic dysfunction and psychopathology. *Ann NY Acad Sci* 280:777, 1976.

GOODWIN DW, GUZE SB: *Psychiatric Diagnosis.* New York, Oxford University Press, 1979.

GOTTLIEB S, HOPE JM: Prognostic value of intravenous administration of sodium amytal in cases of schizophrenia. *Arch Neurol Psychiatry* 46:87, 1941.

HESTON L: Psychiatric disorders in foster home–reared children of schizophrenic mothers. *Br J Psychiatry* 112:819, 1966.

JENSEN I, LARSEN JK: Mental aspects of temporal lobe epilepsy. *J Neurol Neurosurg Psychiatry* 42:256, 1979.

KALLMANN FJ: The genetic theory of schizophrenia: An analysis of 691 twin index families. *Am J Psychiatry* 103:309, 1946.

KARLSSON JL: *The Biologic Basis of Schizophrenia.* Springfield, Ill, Charles C Thomas, 1966.

KARNOSH LJ, HOPE JM: Puerperal psychosis and their sequelae. *Am J Psychiatry* 94:537, 1937.

KETY SS: Genetic and biochemical aspects of schizophrenia, in Nicholi AM Jr (ed): *The Harvard Guide to Modern Psychiatry.* Cambridge, Mass, Harvard, 1978, chap 6, pp 93–102.

———: The syndrome of schizophrenia: Unresolved questions and opportunities for research. *Br J Psychiatry* 136:421, 1980.

KRAEPELIN E: *Dementia Praecox and Paraphrenia,* Barclay RM (trans), Robertson GM (ed). Edinburgh, E & S Livingstone, 1919.

LANGFELDT G: The prognosis in schizophrenia and the factors influencing the course of the disease. *Acta Psychiatr Neurol Scand Suppl* 13, 1937.

———: The prognosis in schizophrenia. *Acta Psychiatr Neurol Scand Suppl* 110, 1956.

LEHMAN HE: Schizophrenia: Clinical features, in Kaplan HI et al (eds): *Comprehensive Textbook of Psychiatry,* 3d ed. Baltimore, Williams & Wilkins, 1980, chap 15.5, pp 1153–1192.

MALAMUD W, RENDER N: Prognosis in schizophrenia. *Am J Psychiatry* 95:1039, 1939.

MOONEY H: Pathologic jealousy and psychochemotherapy. *Br J Psychiatry* 111:1023, 1975

MORRISON J et al: The Iowa 500: The first follow-up. *Arch Gen Psychiatry* 29:677, 1973.

MORTON LA et al: Recurrence risks in schizophrenia: Are they model dependent? *Behavior Genetics* 9:389, 1979.

RIEDER RO et al: Sulcal prominence in young chronic schizophrenic patients: CT scan findings associated with impairment on neuropsychological tests. *Psychiatry Res.* 1:1, 1979.

ROBINS E, GUZE SB: Establishment of diagnostic validity in psychiatric illness: Its application to schizophrenia. *Am J Psychiatry* 126:983, 1970.

ROSANOFF AJ: *Manual of Psychiatry.* New York, Wiley, 1920.

ROSENTHAL D, KETY SS (eds): *The Transmission of Schizophrenia.* New York, Pergamon, 1968.

——— et al: The adopted-away offspring of schizophrenics. *Am J Psychiatry* 128:307, 1971.

SCHNEIDER K: *Clinical Psychopathology,* Hamilton MW (trans). New York, Grune & Stratton, 1959.

SHELDON WM, STEVENS SS, TUCKER WB: *The Varieties of Human Physique: An Introduction to Constitutional Psychology.* New York, Hafner, 1963.

WINOKUR G: Delusional disorder (paranoia). *Compr Psychiatry* 18:511, 1977.

———, TSUANG M: The Iowa 500: Suicide in mania, depression and schizophrenia. *Am J Psychiatry* 132:650, 1975.

INDEX